RUTHERFORD'S
Vascular Surgery

RUTHERFORD'S
Vascular Surgery

SEVENTH EDITION

Jack L. Cronenwett, MD
Professor of Surgery
Dartmouth-Hitchcock Medical Center
Lebanon, New Hampshire

K. Wayne Johnston, MD, FRCSC
R. Fraser Elliott Chair in Vascular Surgery
Professor of Surgery
University of Toronto
Toronto General Hospital
Toronto, Ontario
Canada

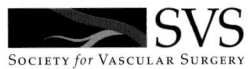

SOCIETY *for* VASCULAR SURGERY

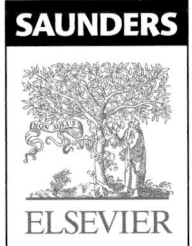

SAUNDERS

ELSEVIER

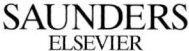

SAUNDERS
ELSEVIER

1600 John F. Kennedy Blvd.
Ste 1800
Philadelphia, PA 19103-2899

BOOK TITLE   RUTHERFORD'S VASCULAR SURGERY   ISBN: 978-1-4160-5223-4
Copyright © 2010, 2005, 2000, 1995, 1989, 1976 by Saunders, an imprint of Elsevier Inc.

Library of Congress Cataloging-in-Publication Data

Rutherford's vascular surgery / [edited by] Jack L. Cronenwett, K. Wayne Johnston; associate editors,
Richard Cambria ... [et al.].—7th ed.
    p. ; cm.
  Rev. ed. of: Vascular surgery / [edited by] Robert B. Rutherford. 6th ed. ©2005.
  Includes bibliographical references and index.
  ISBN 978-1-4160-5223-4
  1. Blood-vessels—Surgery. I. Cronenwett, Jack L. II. Johnston, K. Wayne. III. Rutherford,
Robert B. IV. Vascular surgery. V. Title: Vascular surgery.
  [DNLM: 1. Vascular Surgical Procedures. WG 170 R975 2010]
  RD598.5.V37 2010
  617.4'13—dc22

                                                                              2009001286

Publishing Director: Judith Fletcher
Developmental Editor: Joanie Milnes
Publishing Services Manager: Tina Rebane
Project Manager: Amy Norwitz
Design Direction: Ellen Zanolle

Printed in China

Last digit is the print number: 9 8 7 6 5 4 3 2

This Edition is dedicated to our good friend Robert B. Rutherford, the founder of this textbook, in recognition of his numerous contributions to the field of vascular surgery.

And to the memory of James M. Seeger, an Associate Editor, good friend, and important contributor to vascular surgery education, whose untimely death leaves a void in our hearts.

And to our wives, Debra Cronenwett and Jean Johnston, for their strong support of our academic endeavors.

Richard P. Cambria, MD
Professor of Surgery
Harvard Medical School
Chief of Division of Vascular and Endovascular Surgery
Massachusetts General Hospital
Boston, Massachusetts

Peter Gloviczki, MD
Joe M. and Ruth Roberts Professor of Surgery
Mayo Clinic College of Medicine
Chair of Division of Vascular and Endovascular Surgery
Director of Gonda Vascular Center
Mayo Clinic
Rochester, Minnesota

Louis M. Messina, MD
Professor of Surgery
Vice Chair for Research
Department of Surgery
University of Massachusetts Medical School
Chief of Division of Vascular and Endovascular Surgery
University of Massachusetts Memorial Health Care
Worcester, Massachusetts

Joseph L. Mills, Sr., MD
Professor of Surgery and Chief of Division of Vascular
   and Endovascular Surgery
University of Arizona College of Medicine
Co-Director of Southern Arizona Limb Salvage Alliance
University of Arizona Health Sciences Center
Tucson, Arizona

Bruce A. Perler, MD, MBA
Julius H. Jacobson II Professor of Surgery
Johns Hopkins University School of Medicine
Chief of Division of Vascular Surgery and Endovascular
   Therapy
Director of Vascular Noninvasive Laboratory
Johns Hopkins Hospital
Baltimore, Maryland

James Seeger, MD*
Professor and Chief
Division of Vascular Surgery and Endovascular Therapy
University of Florida College of Medicine
Chief of Vascular Surgery
Shands Hospital at University of Florida
Gainesville, Florida

Anton N. Sidawy, MD, MPH
Professor of Surgery
Georgetown University School of Medicine
George Washington University School of Medicine and
   Health Sciences
Chief of Surgical Services
Veterans Affairs Medical Center
Washington, DC

Fred A. Weaver, MD
Professor of Surgery
Keck School of Medicine of University of Southern
   California, Los Angeles
Chief of Division of Vascular Surgery and Endovascular
   Therapy
University of Southern California University Hospital
Los Angeles, California

*Deceased

Contributors

Ahmed M. Abou-Zamzam, Jr., MD
Associate Professor of Surgery and Chief of Division of Vascular Surgery, Department of Cardiovascular and Thoracic Surgery, Loma Linda University School of Medicine, Loma Linda, California
Lower Extremity Amputation: General Considerations

Christopher J. Abularrage, MD
Vascular and Endovascular Surgery Fellow, Massachusetts General Hospital, Boston, Massachusetts
Takayasu's Disease

Ali F. AbuRahma, MD
Professor of Surgery and Chief of Vascular and Endovascular Surgery, Robert C. Byrd Health Sciences Center, West Virginia University; Medical Director of Noninvasive Vascular Laboratory and Co-Director of Vascular Center of Excellence, Charleston Area Medical Center, Charleston, West Virginia
Complex Regional Pain Syndrome

Stefan Acosta, MD, PhD
Associate Professor and Specialist in Vascular Surgery, Vascular Center, Malmo University Hospital, Malmö, Sweden
Mesenteric Vascular Disease: Venous Thrombosis

Harold P. Adams, Jr., MD
Professor of Neurology and Director of Division of Cerebrovascular Diseases, Carver College of Medicine, University of Iowa; Director of University of Iowa Stroke Center, University of Iowa Hospitals and Clinics, Iowa City, Iowa
Cerebrovascular Disease: Decision Making and Medical Treatment

Gilbert Aidinian, MD
Vascular Surgeon, William Beaumont Army Medical Center, El Paso, Texas
Venography

A. Ruchan Akar, MD, FRCS (CTh)
Associate Professor, Department of Cardiovascular Surgery, Heart Center, Ankara University School of Medicine; Consultant Cardiovascular Surgeon, Ankara University Biotechnology Institute, Dikimevi, Ankara, Turkey
Thromboangiitis Obliterans

Yves S. Alimi, MD, PhD
Professor of Vascular Surgery, Université de la Mediterranee; Chief of Department of Vascular Surgery, University Hospital North, Marseilles, France
Iliocaval Venous Obstruction: Surgical Treatment

George Andros, MD
Medical Director, Diabetic Foot Center, Valley Presbyterian Hospital, Van Nuys, California
Diabetic Foot Ulcers

Juan I. Arcelus, MD, PhD
Professor of Surgery, University of Granada Medical School; Attending Surgeon, Hospital Virgen de las Nieves, Granada, Spain
Acute Deep Venous Thrombosis: Prevention and Medical Treatment

David G. Armstrong, DPM, PhD
Professor of Surgery and Director of Southern Arizona Limb Salvage Alliance (SALSA), University of Arizona College of Medicine, Tucson, Arizona
Podiatry Care

Paul A. Armstrong, DO, FACS
Assistant Professor of Surgery, University of South Florida College of Medicine; Chief of Vascular Surgery, James A. Haley Veterans Affairs Hospital, Tampa, Florida
Vascular Laboratory: Arterial Duplex Scanning

Subodh Arora, MD
Associate Professor of Surgery, George Washington University School of Medicine; Chief of Vascular Surgery George Washington University Medical Center, Washington, DC
Takayasu's Disease

Zachary M. Arthurs, MD
Fellow, Cleveland Clinic, Cleveland, Ohio
Vascular Trauma: Head and Neck

Enrico Ascher, MD, FACS
Professor of Surgery, Mount Sinai School of Medicine; Director of Vascular and Endovascular Surgery, Maimonides Medical Center, New York, New York
Superficial Thrombophlebitis

Marvin D. Atkins, MD
Assistant Professor of Surgery, Texas A&M Health Science Center; Attending Surgeon, Division of Vascular Surgery, Scott and White Hospital and Clinic, Temple, Texas
Carotid Artery Disease: Aneurysms

Robert G. Atnip, MD
Professor of Surgery, Penn State Heart and Vascular Institute, Penn State Milton S. Hershey Medical Center, Hershey, Pennsylvania
Local Complications: Nerve Injury

Faisal Aziz, MD
Vascular Surgery Fellow, Jobst Vascular Center, Toledo Hospital, Toledo, Ohio
Acute Deep Venous Thrombosis: Surgical and Interventional Treatment

Martin R. Back, MD
Associate Professor of Surgery, University of South Florida College of Medicine, Division of Vascular and Endovascular Surgery, Tampa, Florida
Local Complications: Graft Infection

Jeffrey L. Ballard, MD
Clinical Professor of Surgery, University of California, Irvine School of Medicine; Staff Vascular Surgeon, St. Joseph Hospital, Orange, California
Spinal Operative Exposure

Dennis F. Bandyk, MD
Professor of Surgery and Director of Division of Vascular and Endovascular Surgery, University of South Florida College of Medicine, Tampa, Florida
Vascular Laboratory: Arterial Duplex Scanning

John R. Bartholomew, MD
Department of Cardiovascular Medicine, Cleveland Clinic Foundation, Cleveland, Ohio
Atheromatous Embolization

Ruediger G. H. Baumeister, MD
Professor of Surgery and Head of Division of Plastic, Hand, and Microsurgery, Campus Grosshadern, Ludwig-Maximilians-University of Munich, Munich, Germany
Lymphedema: Surgical Treatment

Joseph E. Bavaria, MD
Professor of Surgery, University of Pennsylvania School of Medicine; Vice Chief of Division of Cardiothoracic Surgery and Cardiovascular Surgeon, Hospital of the University of Pennsylvania, Philadelphia, Philadelphia
Vascular Trauma: Thoracic

Carlos F. Bechara, MD
Assistant Professor of Surgery, Division of Vascular Surgery and Endovascular Therapy, Michael E. DeBakey Department of Surgery, Baylor College of Medicine, Houston, Texas
Superior Vena Cava Obstruction: Endovascular Treatment

Michael Belkin, MD
Associate Professor, Harvard Medical School; Chief of Division of Vascular and Endovascular Surgery, Brigham and Women's Hospital, Boston, Massachusetts
Aortoiliac Disease: Direct Reconstruction

Scott A. Berceli, MD, PhD
Associate Professor of Surgery, University of Florida College of Medicine; Chief of Vascular Surgery, Malcom Randall Veterans Affairs Medical Center, Gainesville, Florida
Autogenous Vein Grafts

Michael J. Bernas, MS
Associate Scientific Investigator, University of Arizona College of Medicine, Tucson, Arizona
Lymphatic Pathophysiology

Martin Björck, MD
Professor in Vascular Surgery, Department of Surgery, Uppsala University, Uppsala, Sweden
Mesenteric Vascular Disease: Venous Thrombosis

James H. Black, III, MD
Assistant Professor of Surgery, Johns Hopkins University School of Medicine; Attending Vascular and Endovascular Surgeon, Johns Hopkins Hospital, Baltimore, Maryland
Aneurysms Caused by Connective Tissue Abnormalities

Jan D. Blankensteijn, MD, PhD
Associate Professor of Vascular Surgery, VU University Medical Center, Amsterdam, The Netherlands
Computed Tomography

Thomas C. Bower, MD
Professor of Surgery and Program Director of Vascular Surgery Fellowship, Mayo Clinic College of Medicine, Rochester, Minnesota
Venous Tumors

William T. Brinkman, MD
Assistant Professor of Surgery, Institute of Biomedical Studies, Baylor University, Waco, Texas; Cardiovascular Surgeon, Medical City Dallas, Dallas, Texas
Vascular Trauma: Thoracic

Kathleen E. Brummel-Ziedins, PhD
Associate Professor of Biochemistry, University of Vermont College of Medicine, Colchester, Vermont
Normal Coagulation

Ruth L. Bush, MD, MPH
Associate Professor, Texas A&M University College of Medicine; Vascular Surgeon, Division of Vascular Surgery, Scott and White Hospital and Clinic, Temple, Texas
Carotid Artery Disease: Aneurysms

Keith D. Calligaro, MD
Clinical Professor of Surgery, University of Pennsylvania School of Medicine, Chief, Section of Vascular Surgery and Endovascular Therapy, Pennsylvania Hospital, Philadelphia, Pennsylvania
Renovascular Disease: Aneurysms and Arteriovenous Fistulae

Richard P. Cambria, MD
Professor of Surgery, Harvard Medical School; Chief of Division of Vascular and Endovascular Surgery, Massachusetts General Hospital, Boston, Massachusetts
Aortic Dissection

Piergiorgio Cao, MD, FRCS
Professor of Vascular Surgery, University of Perugia, School of Medicine; Chief of Vascular Surgery, Vascular and Endovascular Surgery Unit, S. Maria Della Misericordia Hospital, Perugia, Italy
Carotid Artery Disease: Stenting

Joseph A. Caprini, MD, FACS, RVT
Clinical Professor of Surgery and Louis W. Biegler Chair of Surgery, University of Chicago Pritzker School of Medicine, Chicago, Illinois; North Shore University Health System, Evanston, Illinois
Acute Deep Venous Thrombosis: Prevention and Medical Treatment

Gregory D. Carlson, MD
Assistant Clinical Professor of Surgery, Department of Orthopedic Surgery, University of California, Irvine School of Medicine; Staff Orthopedic Surgeon, St. Joseph Hospital, Orange, California
Spinal Operative Exposure

T. Johelen Carleton, MD
Vascular Surgery Fellow, University of Rochester School of Medicine and Dentistry, Rochester, New York; Attending Surgeon, Veterans Affairs Medical Center, Phoenix, Arizona
Carotid Artery Disease: Dissection and Other Disorders

Jeffrey P. Carpenter, MD
Professor and Chief of Department of Surgery, University of Medicine and Dentistry of New Jersey/Robert Wood Johnson Medical School; Chief of Surgery, Cooper Health System, Camden, New Jersey
Magentic Resonance Imaging

Elliot L. Chaikof, MD, PhD
John E. Skandalakis Professor of Surgery and Chief of Vascular Surgery and Endovascular Therapy, Emory University School of Medicine, Atlanta, Georgia
Prosthetic Grafts

Kristofer M. Charlton-Ouw, MD
University of Texas, Department of Cardiothoracic and Vascular Surgery, Houston, Texas
Imaging: Evolving Techniques

Stephen W. K. Cheng, MS, FRCS
Professor of Surgery, University of Hong Kong; Chief of Division of Vascular Surgery, Queen Mary Hospital, Hong Kong
Radiation Safety

Jae Sung Cho, MD
Associate Professor of Surgery, University of Pittsburgh School of Medicine, Pittsburgh, Pennsylvania
Thoracic and Thoracoabdominal Aneurysms: Endovascular Treatment

Timothy A. M. Chuter, DM
Professor of Surgery in Residence, University of California, San Francisco; Chief of Endovascular Surgery, University of California, San Francisco Medical Center, San Francisco, California
Abdominal Aortic Aneurysms: Endovascular Treatment

Claudio S. Cinà, MD, Spec Chir It, FRCSC, MSc
Professor of Surgery, University of Toronto, School of Medicine; Professor, Department of Health Policy, Management and Evaluation, University of Toronto; Associate, Department of Biostatistics and Epidemiology, McMaster University; Vascular and Endovascular Surgeon, St. Michael's Hospital, Toronto, Ontario, Canada
Postoperative Management

Daniel G. Clair, MD
Professor of Surgery, Cleveland Clinic Lerner College of Medicine of Case Western Reserve University; Chairman and Program Director of Vascular Surgery, Cleveland Clinic, Cleveland, Ohio
Brachiocephalic Artery Disease: Endovascular Treatment

W. Darrin Clouse, MD
Associate Professor of Surgery, Uniformed Services University of the Health Sciences, Bethesda, Maryland and University of California, Davis, School of Medicine; Chief of Vascular and Endovascular Surgery, David Grant United States Air Force Medical Center, Sacramento California
Upper Extremity Arterial Disease: Amputation

Marc Coggia, MD
Professor of Vascular Surgery, Faculty of Medicine, Versailles Saint Quentin en Yvelines University, Guyancourt; Vascular Surgeon, Ambroise Pare University Hospital, Boulogne-Billancourt, France
Aortoiliac Disease: Laparoscopic Reconstruction

Raul Coimbra, MD, PhD
The Monroe E. Trout Professor of Surgery, University of California, San Diego, School of Medicine; Chief of Division of Trauma, Surgical Critical Care, and Burns, University of California, San Deigo, Medical Center, San Diego, California
Vascular Trauma: Epidemiology and Natural History

Anthony J. Comerota, MD
Adjunct Professor of Surgery, University of Michigan Medical School, Ann Arbor, Michigan; Director of Jobst Vascular Center, Toledo Hospital, Toledo, Ohio
Acute Deep Venous Thrombosis: Surgical and Interventional Treatment

Mark F. Conrad, MD, MMSc
Instructor, Harvard Medical School; Assistant in Surgery, Massachusetts General Hospital, Boston, Massachusetts
Aortic Dissection

Leslie T. Cooper, Jr., MD
Professor of Medicine, Mayo Clinic School of Medicine, Rochester, Minnesota
Vasculitis and Other Arteriopathies

Michael S. Conte, MD
Professor of Surgery and Chief of Division of Vascular and Endovascular Surgery, University of California, San Francisco, School of Medicine, San Francisco, California
Atherosclerosis

Matthew A. Corriere, MD
Assistant Professor of Surgery, Division of Vascular Surgery, Emory University School of Medicine, Atlanta, Georgia
Renovascular Disease: Endovascular Treatment

Robert S. Crawford, MD
Clinical Fellow in Surgery, Harvard Medical School; Clinical Fellow in Vascular Surgery, Massachusetts General Hospital, Boston, Massachusetts
Ischemia-Reperfusion

David L. Cull, MD
Professor of Clinical Surgery, University of South Carolina School of Medicine, Columbia; Vice-Chair of Surgical Research, Academic Department of Surgery, Greenville Hospital System/University Medical Center, Greenville, South Carolina
Hemodialysis Access: Complex

Ronald L. Dalman, MD, FACS, FAHA
Professor and Chief, Stanford University Medical Center, Division of Vascular Surgery, Stanford, California
Arterial Aneurysms

Michael C. Dalsing, MD
E. Dale and Susan E. Habegger Professor of Surgery and Director of Vascular Surgery and Program Director, Indiana University School of Medicine, Indianapolis, Indiana
Chronic Venous Insufficiency: Deep Vein Valve Reconstruction

Alan Dardik, MD, PhD
Assistant Professor of Surgery, Yale University School of Medicine, New Haven; Attending Surgeon, Veterans Affairs Connecticut Healthcare Systems, West Haven, Connecticut
Preoperative Management

R. Clement Darling III, MD
Professor of Surgery, Albany Medical College; Chief of Division of Vascular Surgery, Albany Medical Center Hospital, Albany, New York
Upper Extremity Arterial Disease: Revascularization

Mark G. Davies, MD, PhD, MBA
Professor of Cardiovascular Surgery and Vice Chairman and Program Director, Department of Cardiovascular Surgery, Weill Medical College at Cornell University, Ithaca, New York; Methodist Hospital and Research Institute, Houston, Texas
Intimal Hyperplasia

Stephanie S. DeLoach, MD
Assistant Professor of Medicine, Jefferson Medical College of Thomas Jefferson University, Philadelphia, Pennsylvania
Atherosclerotic Risk Factors: Hypertension

Demetrios Demetriades, MD, PhD
Professor and Vice-Chairman of Surgery, Keck School of Medicine of University of Southern California, Los Angeles; Director, Division of Trauma, Emergency Surgery and Surgical Intensive Care Unit, Los Angeles County and University of Southern California Medical Center, Los Angeles, California
Vascular Trauma: Abdominal

Ralph G. DePalma, MD, FACS
Professor of Surgery, Uniformed Services University of the Healh Sciences, Bethesda, Maryland; National Director of Transplant Services, Department of Veterans Affairs, Washington, DC
Erectile Dysfunction

Paola De Rango, MD
Staff Vascular Surgeon, Vascular and Endovascular Surgery Unit, S. Maria Della Misericordia Hospital, Perugia, Italy
Carotid Artery Disease: Stenting

Hasan H. Dosluoglu, MD, FACS
Associate Professor of Surgery, State University of New York at Buffalo, School of Medicine and Biomedical Sciences, Buffalo, New York; Chief of Surgery and Vascular Surgery, VA Western New York Healthcare System, Buffalo, New York
Hemodialysis Access: Nonthrombotic Complications

Matthew J. Dougherty, MD
Associate Clinical Professor of Surgery, University of Pennsylvania School of Medicine; Section of Vascular Surgery, Pennsylvania Hospital, Philadelphia, Pennsylvania
Renovascular Disease: Aneurysms and Arteriovenous Fistulae

Matt Driskill, MSPT
Teaching Lab Assistant, Program in Physical Therapy, Washington University School of Medicine; Physical Therapist, The Rehabilitation Institute of St. Louis, St. Louis, Missouri
Thoracic Outlet Syndrome: Neurogenic

Audra A. Duncan, MD
Associate Professor of Surgery, Mayo Clinic College of Medicine; Director of Clinical Research Division of Vascular and Endovascular Surgery, Mayo Clinic, Rochester, Minnesota
Local Complications: Lymphatic

Serkan Durdu, MD
Department of Cardiovascular Surgery, Heart Center, Ankara University School of Medicine; Cardiovascular Surgeon, Ankara University Biotechnology Institute, Dikimevi, Ankara, Turkey
Thromboangiitis Obliterans

Jonothan J. Earnshaw, DM, FRCS
Consultant Vascular Surgeon, Gloucestershire Royal Hospital, Gloucester, United Kingdom
Acute Ischemia: Evaluation and Decision Making

Robert T. Eberhardt, MD
Associate Professor of Medicine, Boston University School of Medicine; Co-Director of Noninvasive Vascular Laboratory and Director of Vascular Medical Services, Boston Medical Center, Boston, Massachusetts
Chronic Venous Disorders: General Considerations

James M. Edwards, MD
Professor of Surgery, Divison of Vascular Surgery, Oregon Health and Science University; Chief of Surgery, Portland Veterans Affairs Medical Center, Portland Oregon
Upper Extremity Arterial Disease: General Considerations

Matthew S. Edwards, MD
Associate Professor of Surgery and Public Health Sciences, Department of Vascular and Endovascular Surgery, Wake Forest University Health Sciences Center, Winston-Salem, North Carolina
Renovascular Disease: Endovascular Treatment

John F. Eidt, MD
Professor of Surgery and Radiology and Director of Vascular Surgery Division, University of Arkansas for Medical Sciences, Little Rock, Arkansas
Lower Extremity Amputation: Techniques and Results

Eric Endean, MD
Gordon L. Hyde Professor and Chair in Vascular Surgery, University of Kentucky College of Medicine; Section Head of Vascular Surgery, Albert B. Chandler Medical Center, Lexington, Kentucky
Embryology

Mark K. Eskandari, MD
Associate Professor
Feinberg School of Medicine, Northwestern University; Attending Surgeon, Northwestern Memorial Hospital, Chicago, Illinois
Occupational Vascular Problems

Alik Farber, MD
Associate Professor of Surgery and Radiology, Boston University School of Medicine; Chief of Vascular and Endovascular Surgery and Co-Director of the Noninvasive Vascular Laboratory, Boston Medical Center, Boston, Massachusetts
Biologic Grafts

Peter L. Faries, MD
Professor of Surgery and Professor of Radiology, Mount Sinai School of Medicine; Chief of Vascular Surgery, Mount Sinai Medical Center, New York, New York
Infrainguinal Disease: Endovascular Treatment

Mark F. Fillinger, MD
Professor of Surgery (Vascular), Dartmouth Medical School; Program Director of Vascular Surgery, Dartmouth-Hitchcock Medical Center, Lebanon, New Hampshire
Abdominal Aortic Aneurysms: Evaluation and Decision Making

Steven J. Fishman MD
Associate Professor of Surgery, Harvard Medical School; Children's Hospital Boston, Boston, Massachusetts
Vascular Tumors in Childhood

Tamara N. Fitzgerald, MD PhD
Resident, Yale University School of Medicine, New Haven, Connecticut
Preoperative Management

Thomas L. Forbes, MD, FRCSC, FACS
Professor of Surgery, University of Western Ontario; Chief of Vascular Surgery, London Health Sciences Centre, London, Ontario Canada
Nonatheromatous Popliteal Artery Disease

Charles J. Fox, MD
Assistant Professor of Surgery, Uniformed Services University of the Health Sciences, Bethesda, Maryland; Program Director of Vascular Surgery and Attending Vascular Surgeon, Walter Reed Army Medical Center, Washington, DC
Vascular Trauma: Military

Gail L. Gamble, MD
Assistant Professor of Physical Medicine and Rehabilitation, Feinberg School of Medicine, Northwestern University; Medical Director, Cancer Rehabilitation, Rehabilitation Institute of Chicago, Chicago, Illinois
Lymphedema: Nonoperative Treatment

Robert P. Garvin, MD
Vascular Surgery Faculty, Geisinger Medical Center, Danville, Pennsylvania
Local Complications: Nerve Injury

Randolph L. Geary, MD, FACS
Professor, Department of Vascular and Endovascular Surgery, Wake Forest University School of Medicine, Winston-Salem, North Carolina
Renovascular Disease: General Considerations

David L. Gillespie, MD
Professor of Surgery and Program Director of Vascular Surgery, University of Rochester School of Medicine and Dentistry, Rochester, New York
Venography

Peter Gloviczki, MD
Joe M. and Ruth Roberts Professor of Surgery, Mayo Clinic College of Medicine; Chair of Division of Vascular and Endovascular Surgery; Director of Gonda Vascular Center, Mayo Clinic, Rochester, Minnesota
Superior Vena Cava Obstruction: Surgical Treatment

Christopher J. Godshall, MD
Assistant Professor of Surgery, Department of Vascular and Endovascular Surgery, Wake Forest University School of Medicine, Winston-Salem, North Carolina
Renovascular Disease: Open Surgical Treatment

Olivier Goëau-Brissonnière, PhD
Professor of Vascular Surgery, Faculty of Medicine, Versailles Saint Quentin en Yvelines University, Guyancourt; Chief of Department of Vascular Surgery, Ambroije Pare University Hospital, Boulogne-Billancourt, France
Aortoiliac Disease: Laparoscopic Reconstruction

Heather L. Gornik, MD, MHS
Assistant Professor of Medicine, Cleveland Clinic Lerner College of Medicine of Case Western Reserve University; Staff Physician and Medical Director of Noninvasive Vascular Laboratory, Cleveland Clinic, Cleveland, Ohio
Atherosclerotic Risk Factors: Smoking

Anders Gottsäter, MD, PhD
Associate Professor, Faculty of Medicine, University of Lund, Lund; Senior Registrar in Vascular Medicine, Vascular Centre, Malmo University Hospital, Malmö, Sweden
Renovascular Disease: Fibrodysplasia

Roy K. Greenberg, MD
Associate Professor of Surgery, Cleveland Clinic Lerner College of Medicine of Case Western Reserve Unversity; Staff Physician and Director of Endovascular Research, Cleveland Clinic Foundation, Cleveland, Ohio
Aortic Arch Aneurysms and Dissection

Arin K. Greene, MD, MMSc
Assistant Professor of Surgery, Harvard Medical School, Children's Hospital Boston, Boston, Massachusetts
Vascular Tumors in Childhood

Nathan M. Griffith, PhD
Postdoctoral Neuropsychology Fellow, University of California, Los Angeles, Semel Institute, Los Angeles, California
Acute Deep Venous Thrombosis: Clinical and Diagnostic Evaluation

Geoffrey D. Guttmann, PhD
Associate Professor of Anatomy and Director of Anatomic Studies, Commonwealth Medical College, Scranton, Pennsylvania
Embryology

Raul J. Guzman, MD
Associate Professor of Surgery, Vanderbilt University School of Medicine, Nashville, Tennessee
Local Complications: Anastomotic Aneurysms

Allen Hamdan, MD
Associate Professor of Surgery, Harvard Medical School; Clinical Director of Vascular Surgery, Beth Israel Deaconess Medical Center, Boston, Massachusetts
Lower Extremity Aneurysms

Jaap F. Hamming, MD, PhD
Professor of Surgery and Head of Section of Vascular Surgery; Program-Director Surgical Training, Leiden University Medical Center, Leiden, The Netherlands
Renovascular Disease: Acute Occlusive Events

Kimberley J. Hansen, MD
Professor of Surgery, Department of Vascular and Endovascular Surgery, Wake Forest University School of Medicine, Winston-Salem, North Carolina
Renovascular Disease: Open Surgical Treatment

Linda M. Harris, MD
Associate Professor of Surgery, State University of New York at Buffalo, School of Medicine and Biomedical Sciences; Vice Chair of Department of Surgery; Program Director of Vascular Surgery Fellowship; Interim Division Chief of Division of Vascular Surgery, Kaleida Health, Buffalo, New York
Hemodialysis Access: Nonthrombotic Complications

Olivier Hartung, MD
Vascular Surgeon, Department of Vascular Surgery, Université de la Mediterranee, University Hospital North, Marseilles, France
Iliocaval Venous Obstruction: Surgical Treatment

Peter K. Henke, MD
Associate Professor of Surgery, University of Michigan Medical School; Chief of Ann Arbor Veterans Affairs Hospital, Ann Arbor, Michigan
Venous Pathology

Anil P. Hingorani, MD
Clinical Assistant Professor of Surgery, College of Medicine, State University of New York at Brooklyn; Vascular Surgeon, Maimonides Medical Center, Brooklyn, New York
Superficial Thrombophlebitis

Jamal J. Hoballah, MD, MBA
Professor of Surgery and Chairman, Department of Surgery, American University of Beirut Medical Center, Beirut, Lebanon; Professor of Surgery, Chairman of Division of Vascular Surgery, University of Iowa, Iowa City, Iowa
Technique: Open Surgical

Kim J. Hodgson, MD
Professor and Chairman, Southern Illinois University School of Medicine, Springfield, Illinois
Technique: Endovascular Diagnostic

Douglas B. Hood, MD
Associate Professor of Surgery, Southern Illinois University School of Medicine, Springfield, Illinois
Technique: Endovascular Diagnostic

Wm. James Howard, MD
Professor of Medicine, George Washington University School of Medicine and Health Sciences; Director of Lipid Clinic and Lipid Consultation Service, Washington Hospital Center, Washington, DC
Atherosclerotic Risk Factors: Hyperlipidemia

David B. Hoyt, MD, FACS
Professor and Chairman, Department of Surgery; Executive Vice Dean, University of California, Irvine School of Medicine, Orange, California
Vascular Trauma: Epidemiology and Natural History

Christina Huang, BS
Research Assistant, Yale University School of Medicine, New Haven, Connecticut
Arterial Wall Biology

Thomas S. Huber, MD, PhD
Professor of Surgery, University of Florida College of Medicine; Attending Surgeon, Shands Hospital at University of Florida, Gainesville, Florida
Mesenteric Vascular Disease: Chronic Ischemia

Glenn C. Hunter, MD
Professor of Clinical Surgery, University of Arizona College of Medicine; Chief of Vascular Surgery, Southern Arizona Veterans Affairs Healthcare Service, Tucson, Arizona
Acquired Arteriovenous Fistulae

Mark D. Iafrati, MD
Assistant Professor and Vascular Surgery Fellowship Director, Tufts University School of Medicine; Chief of Vascular Surgery and Director of Vascular Medicine Center, Tufts Medical Center, Boston, Massachusetts
Varicose Veins: Surgical Treatment

Karl A. Illig, MD
Professor of Surgery and Neurosurgery, University of Rochester School of Medicine and Dentistry; Chief of Division of Vascular Surgery, University of Rochester Medical Center, Rochester, New York
Carotid Artery Disease: Dissection and Other Disorders

Kenji Inaba, MSc, FRCSC, FACS
Assistant Professor of Surgery, Keck School of Medicine at University of Southern California, Los Angeles, School of Medicine; Medical Director Surgical Intensive Care Unit, University of Southern California Medical Center, Los Angeles, California
Vascular Trauma: Abdominal

Glenn R. Jacobowitz, MD
Associate Professor of Surgery, New York University School of Medicine; Vice Chief of Division of Vascular Surgery, New York University Langone Medical Center, New York, New York
Congenital Vascular Malformations: Endovascular and Surgical Treatment

Michael J. Jacobs, MD, PhD
Professor of Surgery, University of Maastrizht; Chief of Department of Surgery, Maastrizht University Medical Center, Maastrizht, The Netherlands
Thoracic and Thoracoabdominal Aneurysms: Open Surgical Treatment

Juan Carlos Jimenez, MD
Assistant Professor, Division of Vascular Surgery, David Geffen School of Medicine at University of California, Los Angeles; Attending Surgeon, Division of Vascular Surgery, Ronald Reagan University of California, Los Angeles, Medical Center, Los Angeles, California
Mesenteric Vascular Disease: General Considerations

William D. Jordan, Jr., MD
Professor of Surgery, University of Alabama School of Medicine at Birmingham; Attending Surgeon, University of Alabama Hospital, Birmingham, Alabama
Nonaortic Stents and Stent-Grafts

Lowell S. Kabnick, MD, FACS, FACPh
Associate Professor of Surgery, New York University School of Medicine; Director of New York University Vein Center, New York University Langone Medical Center; Attending Surgeon, Morristown Memorial Hospital, Morristown, New Jersey
Varicose Veins: Endovenous Treatment

Venkat R. Kalapatapu, MD, FRCS
Assistant Professor and Vascular Surgeon, University of Arkansas for Medical Sciences, Little Rock, Arkansas
Lower Extremity Amputation: Techniques and Results

Manju Kalra, MD
Associate Professor of Surgery, Mayo Clinic College of Medicine; Consultant in Division of Vascular and Endovascular Surgery, Mayo Clinic, Rochester, Minnesota
Superior Vena Cava Obstruction: Surgical Treatment

Vikram S. Kashyap, MD, FACS
Associate Professor, Cleveland Clinic Lerner College of Medicine of Case Western Reserve University; Staff, Department of Vascular Surgery, Cleveland Clinic, Cleveland, Ohio
Local Complications: Aortoenteric Fistulae

Karthikeshwar Kasirajan, MD
Assistant Professor of Surgery, Emory University School of Medicine, Atlanta Veterans Affairs Medical Center, Atlanta, Georgia
Acute Ischemia: Treatment

Paulo Kauffman, MD
Assistant Professor of Vascular and Endovascular Surgery, São Paulo University School of Medicine, São Paulo, Brazil
Thoracic Sympathectomy

Lois A. Killewich, MD, PhD
Leonard and Marie Louise Aronsfeld Rosoff Professor of Surgery and Assistant Dean for Continuing Education, University of Texas Medical Branch, Galveston, Texas
Venous Physiology

Esther S. H. Kim, MD, MPH
Associate Staff, Cleveland Clinic, Cleveland, Ohio
Atherosclerotic Risk Factors: Smoking

Ted R. Kohler, MD
Professor of Surgery, Washington University School of Medicine; Chief of Vascular Surgery, Veteran Affairs Puget Sound Healthcare System, Seattle, Washington
Vascular Laboratory: Arterial Physiologic Assessment

Timothy F. Kresowik, MD
Professor of Surgery, University of Iowa Carver College of Medicine; Attending Surgeon, University of Iowa Hospitals and Clinics, Iowa City, Iowa
Cerebrovascular Disease: Decision Making and Medical Treatment

Nicos Labropoulos, PhD, DIC, RVT
Professor of Surgery and Radiology, Stony Brook University School of Medicine; Director of Vascular Laboratory, Stony Brook University Medical Center, Stony Brook, New York
Vascular Laboratory: Venous Duplex Scanning

Brajesh K. Lal, MD
Associate Professor, Vascular Surgery and Bioengineering, University of Maryland School of Medicine, Baltimore, Maryland
Vascular Laboratory: Venous Physiologic Assessment

Gregory J. Landry, MD
Associate Professor of Surgery, Division of Vascular Surgery, Oregon Health and Science University, Portland, Oregon
Raynaud's Syndrome

David L. Lau, MD
Vascular Surgeon, Southern California Permanente Medical Group, Kaiser Downey Medical Center, Bell Flower, California
Brachiocephalic Artery Disease: Surgical Treatment

Lawrence A. Lavery, DPM, MPH
Professor of Surgery, Texas A&M College of Medicine, Scott and White Hospital, Temple, Texas
Diabetic Foot Ulcers

Peter F. Lawrence, MD
Chief of Division of Vascular Surgery, University of California, Los Angeles, Medical Center, Los Angeles, California
Arterial Aneurysms: General Considerations

Jeffrey H. Lawson, MD, PhD
Associate Professor of Surgery and Assistant Professor of Pathology, Duke University School of Medicine; Director of Vascular Surgery Research Laboratory and Director of Clinical Trials for Vascular Surgery, Duke University Medical Center, Durham, North Carolina
Coagulopathy and Hemorrhage

Byung-Boong Lee, MD, PhD
Professor of Surgery, Georgetown University School of Medicine; Clinical Professor of Surgery and Attending Surgeon, Division of Vascular Surgery, Georgetown University Hospital, Washington, DC
Congenital Vascular Malformations: General Considerations

W. Anthony Lee, MD
Associate Professor of Surgery, University of Florida College of Medicine; Attending Surgeon, Shands Hospital at University of Florida, Gainesville, Florida
Mesenteric Vascular Disease: Chronic Ischemia

Luis R. León, Jr., MD, RVI, FACS
Associate Professor of Surgery and Staff Surgeon, University of Arizona College of Medicine; Attending Vascular Surgeon, Tucson Medical Center, Vascular and Endovascular Section, University of Arizona Health Science Center, Tucson, Arizona
Vascular Laboratory: Venous Duplex Scanning

Wesley K. Lew, MD
Research Fellow in Vascular Surgery, Department of Surgery, Keck School of Medicine of University of Southern California, Los Angeles, California
Thrombolytic Agents

Christos Liapis, MD, FACS, FRCS
Professor of Vascular Surgery, University of Athens Medical School; Chairman of Department of Vascular Surgery, Attikon Hospital, Athens, Greece
Atherosclerotic Risk Factors: General Considerations

Howard A. Liebman, MD
Professor of Medicine and Pathology, Keck School of Medicine of University of Southern California; Chief of Division of Hematology, Kenneth Norris Comprehensive Cancer Center, Los Angeles, California
Hypercoagulable States

Michael P. Lilly, MD
Associate Professor, University of Maryland School of Medicine; Director of Maryland Vascular Center and Chief of Department of Surgery, Maryland General Hospital, Baltimore, Maryland
Intraoperative Management

Peter H. Lin, MD
Professor of Surgery and Chief of Vascular Surgery, Division of Vascular and Endovascular Surgery, Michael E. DeBakey Department of Surgery, Baylor College of Medicine, Houston, Texas
Superior Vena Cava Obstruction: Endovascular Treatment

Bengt Lindblad, MD, PhD
Associate Professor, Faculty of Vascular Surgery, University of Lund, Lund; Senior Lecturer in Vascular Surgery, Vascular Center, Malmo University Hospital, Malmö, Sweden
Renovascular Disease: Fibrodysplasia

Thomas F. Lindsay, MD, CM
Professor of Surgery and Chair of Division of Vascular Surgery, University of Toronto Faculty of Medicine; Staff Surgeon, University Health Network, Toronto, Ontario, Canada
Abdominal Aortic Aneurysms: Ruptured

Pamela A. Lipsett, MD
Professor of Surgery, Anesthesiology, Critical Care, and Nursing; Program Director of General Surgery Residency Program; Johns Hopkins University Schools of Medicine and Nursing; Co-Director, Surgical Intensive Care Units, Johns Hopkins Medical Institutions, Baltimore, Maryland
Systemic Complications: Respiratory

Harold Litt, MD
Associate Professor of Radiology, University of Pennsylvania School of Medicine; Chief of Cardiovascular Imaging, Hospital of the University of Pennsylvania, Philadelphia, Pennsylvania
Magnetic Resonance Imaging

Jayme E. Locke, MD, MPH
Chief Resident in Surgery, Johns Hopkins University School of Medicine, Baltimore, Maryland
Systemic Complications: Respiratory

Joann Lohr, MD, FACS, RVT
Director of John J. Cranley Vascular Laboratory and Associate Program Director of Vascular Surgery Residency, Good Samaritan Hospital, Cincinnati, Ohio
Acute Deep Venous Thrombosis: Clinical and Diagnostic Evaluation

G. Matthew Longo, MD
Assistant Professor of Vascular Surgery, University of Nebraska Medical Center, Omaha, Nebraska
Patient Clinical Evaluation

Alan B. Lumsden, MD
Professor of Cardiovascular Surgery, Methodist Hospital; Chairman of Department of Cardiovascular Surgery, Houston, Texas
Imaging: Evolving Techniques

Fedor Lurie, MD, PhD
Clinical Assistant Professor, John A. Burns School of Medicine, University of Hawaii; Vascular Surgeon, Kistner Vein Clinic, Honolulu, Hawaii
Chronic Venous Insufficiency: Treatment of Perforator Vein Incompetence

Thomas G. Lynch, MD
Professor of Surgery, University of Nebraska Medical Center; Chief of Surgical Service, Veterans Affairs Nebraska/Western Iowa Health Care System, Omaha, Nebraska
Patient Clinical Evaluation

William C. Mackey, MD
Andrews Professor and Chairman, Department of Surgery, Tufts University School of Medicine; Surgeon-in-Chief, Tufts Medical Center, Boston, Massachusetts
Cerebrovascular Disease: General Considerations

Robyn A. Macsata, MD
Chief of Vascular Surgery, Veterans Affairs Medical Center, Washington, DC
Hemodialysis Access: General Considerations

Michel S. Makaroun, MD
Professor and Chief, Division of Vascular Surgery, University of Pittsburgh School of Medicine, Pittsburgh, Pennsylvania
Thoracic and Thoracoabdominal Aneurysms: Endovascular Treatment

Thomas S. Maldonado, MD
Assistant Professor of Surgery, New York University Medical School, New York, New York
Splanchnic Artery Aneurysms

Kenneth G. Mann, PhD
Professor, University of Vermont College of Medicine, Colchester, Vermont
Normal Coagulation

George Markose, MBChB, MRCP(UK), FRCR
Consultant Interventional Radiologist, St. George's Hospital Medical School, London, England, United Kingdom
Cerebrovascular Disease: Diagnostic Evaluation

William A. Marston, MD
Professor of Surgery, University of North Carolina School of Medicine, Chapel Hill, North Carolina
Wound Care

Carlo O. Martinez, MD
Postdoctoral Research Fellow, University of Texas Health Science Center, San Antonio, Texas
Arteriogenesis

Jon S. Matsumura, MD
Professor of Surgery, University of Wisconsin School of Medicine and Public Health; Chief of Division of Vascular Surgery, University of Wisconsin Hospital and Clinics, Madison, Wisconsin
Aortic Stents and Stent-Grafts

James F. McKinsey, MD, FACS
Associate Professor of Surgery, Weill Medical College at Cornell University, Ithaca, New York; Site Chief, New York-Presbyterian Medical Center, New York, New York
Local Complications: Endovascular

Robert B. McLafferty, MD
Professor of Surgery, Division of Vascular Surgery, Southern Illinois University School of Medicine, Springfield, Illinois
Arteriography

George H. Meier, MD
Professor and Chief of Vascular Surgery, University of Cincinnati College of Medicine; Medical Director of Vascular Laboratory, University Hospital, Cincinnati, Ohio
Hemodialysis Access: Failing and Thrombosed

Matthew T. Menard, MD
Instructor in Surgery, Harvard Medical School; Associate Surgeon, Brigham and Women's Hospital, Boston, Massachusetts
Aortoiliac Disease: Direct Reconstruction

Louis M. Messina, MD
Professor of Surgery, Division of Vascular and Endovascular Surgery, University of Massachusetts Medical School; Chief of Division of Vascular and Endovascular Surgery and Vice Chair for Research, Department of Surgery, University of Massachusetts Memorial Health Care, Worcester, Massachusetts
Thoracic Outlet Syndrome: Venous

Joseph L. Mills, Sr., MD
Professor of Surgery and Chief of Division of Vascular and Endovascular Surgery, University of Arizona College of Medicine; Co-Director of Southern Arizona Limb Salvage Alliance, University of Arizona Health Sciences Center, Tucson, Arizona
Infrainguinal Disease: Surgical Treatment

J. Gregory Modrall, MD
Associate Professor of Surgery, Division of Vascular and Endvascular Surgery, University of Texas Southwestern Medical School; Chief of Section of Vascular and Endovascular Surgery, Dallas Veterans Affairs Medical Center; Attending Surgeon, University of Texas Southwetern Medical Center, Dallas Texas
Compartment Syndrome

Emile Mohler III, MD
Associate Professor of Medicine, University of Pennsylvania School of Medicine; Director of Vascular Medicine, University of Pennsylvania Health System, Philadelphia, Pennsylvania
Atherosclerotic Risk Factors: Hypertension

Gregory L. Moneta, MD
Professor and Chief of Vascular Surgery, Oregon Health and Science University, Portland, Oregon
Chronic Venous Disorders: Nonoperative Treatment

Mark D. Morasch, MD
Associate Professor of Vascular Surgery and Interventional Radiology, Feinberg School of Medicine, Northwestern University; Attending Surgeon, Northwestern Memorial Hospital, Chicago, Illinois
Vertebral Artery Disease

Stuart I. Myers, MD, FACS
Director of Bryan LGH Medical Center Vascular Institute, Lincoln, Nebraska
Systemic Complications: Renal

A. Ross Naylor, MD, FRCS
Professor of Vascular Surgery, Leicester Royal Infirmary, Leicester, England, United Kingdom
Cerebrovascular Disease: Diagnostic Evaluation

Peter Neglén, MD, PhD
Vascular Surgeon, River Oaks Hospital, Flowood, Missouri
Iliocaval Venous Obstruction: Endovascular Treatment

Louis L. Nguyen, MD, MBA, MPH
Assistant Professor of Surgery, Harvard Medical School; Vascular Surgeon, Brigham and Women's Hospital, Boston, Massachusetts
Epidemiology and Clinical Analysis

Thomas F. O'Donnell, Jr., MD
Emeritus Professor of Surgery, Tufts University School of Medicine; Director of Vein Center, Tufts Medical Center, Boston, Massachusetts
Varicose Veins: Surgical Treatment

Patrick J. O'Hara, MD, FACS
Professor of Surgery, Cleveland Clinic Lerner College of Medicine at Case Western Reserve University; Staff Vascular Surgeon, Cleveland Clinic Foundation, Cleveland, Ohio
Local Complications: Aortoenteric Fistulae

Takao Ohki, MD, PhD
Professor of Surgery and Chairman, Division of Vascular Surgery, Department of Surgery, Jikei University School of Medicine, Tokyo, Japan
Technique: Endovascular Therapeutic

W. Andrew Oldenburg, MD
Associate Professor of Surgery, College of Medicine, Mayo Graduate School of Medicine, Rochester, Minnesota; Head, Section of Vascular Surgery, Mayo Clinic Florida, Jacksonville, Florida
Arterial Tumors

Jeffrey W. Olin, MD
Zena and Michael A. Wiener Cardiovascular Institute and Marie-Josée and Henry R. Kravis Center for Cardiovascular Health, Mount Sinai School of Medicine, New York, New York
Atheromatous Embolization

Christopher D. Owens, MD, MSc
Assistant Professor of Surgery, Division of Vascular and Endovascular Surgery, University of California, San Francisco, California
Atherosclerosis

Giuseppe Papia, MD, MSc, FRCSC
Assistant Professor of Surgery, University of Toronto School of Medicine; Physician Lead in Cardiovascular Instensive Care Unit, Vascular and Endovascular Surgery, Critical Care Medicine, Sunnybrook Health Sciences Centre, Toronto, Ontario, Canada
Postoperative Management

Hugo Partsch, MD
Professor of Dermatology, Medical University, Vienna, Austria
Chronic Venous Disorders: Nonoperative Treatment

Marc A. Passman, MD
Associate Professor of Surgery, University of Alabama School of Medicine at Birmingham, Birmingham, Alabama
Vena Cava Interruption

Himanshu J. Patel, MD
Assistant Professor of Surgery, University of Michigan Medical School, Ann Arbor, Michigan
Thoracic and Thoracoabdominal Aneurysms: Evaluation and Decision Making

Kaushal R. Patel, MD
Kaiser Permanente Medical Center, Los Angeles, California
Vascular Trauma: Extremity

Benjamin Pearce, MD
Assistant Professor, Department of Surgery, Division of Vascular Surgery, University of Texas Health Sciences Center at San Antonio; Vascular Surgeon, University Health System, San Antonio, Texas
Nonaortic Stents and Stent-Grafts

Bruce A. Perler, MD, MBA
Julius H. Jacobson II Professor of Surgery, Johns Hopkins University School of Medicine; Chief of Division of Vascular Surgery and Endovascular Therapy and Director of Vascular Noninvasive Laboratory, Johns Hopkins Hospital, Baltimore, Maryland
Carotid Artery Disease: Endarterectomy

Don Poldermans, MD, PhD
Professor of Medicine, Department of Vascular Surgery, Erasmus Medical Center, Rotterdam, The Netherlands
Systemic Complications: Cardiac

Frank B. Pomposelli, MD
Associate Professor of Surgery, Harvard Medical School; Chief of Vascular and Endovascular Surgery and Chief of Cardiovascular Surgery, Cardiovascular Institute, Beth Israel Deaconess Medical Center, Boston, Massachusetts
Lower Extremity Aneurysms

Lori L. Pounds, MD
Vascular Surgeon, Peripheral Vascular Associates, San Antonio, Texas
Venous Physiology

Richard J. Powell, MD
Professor of Surgery and of Radiology, Section of Vascular and of Radiology, Dartmouth Medical School; Attending Surgeon, Mary Hitchcock Memorial Hospital and Veterans Affairs Hospital, Hanover, New Hampshire
Aortoiliac Disease: Endovascular Treatment

Alessandra Puggioni, MD
Assistant Professor, Mount Sinai School of Medicine, New York, New York; Attending, Department of Vascular Surgery, Maimonides Medical Center, Brooklyn, New York
Chronic Venous Insufficiency: Treatment of Perforator Vein Incompetence

Zheng Qu, BS
Research Associate, Georgia Institute of Technology, Atlanta, Georgia
Prosthetic Grafts

Brendon M. Quinn, MD
Attending Vascular Surgeon, The Heart Institute, Bowling Green, Kentucky
Hemodialysis Access: Complex

William J. Quinones-Baldrich, MD
Professor of Surgery, David Geffen School of Medicine at University at California, Los Angeles; Director of Endovascular Surgery, Ronald Reagan University of California, Los Angeles, Medical Center, Los Angeles, California
Mesenteric Vascular Disease: General Considerations

Joseph D. Raffetto, MD
Assistant Professor of Surgery, Harvard Medical School, Boston, Massachusetts; Chief of Vascular Surgery and Chief of Vascular Laboratory, Veterans Affairs Boston Healthcare System, West Roxbury, Massachusetts; Visiting Research Scientist. Brigham and Women's Hospital, Boston, Massachusetts
Chronic Venous Disorders: General Considerations

Seshadri Raju, MD
Emeritus Professor and Honorary Surgeon, University of Mississippi Medical Center, Jackson, Mississippi; River Oaks Hospital, Flowood Mississippi
Iliocaval Venous Obstruction: Endovascular Treatment

Nabeel R. Rana, MD
Vascular Surgery Fellow, Division of Vascular Surgery, Department of Surgery Southern Illinois University School of Medicine, Springfield, Illinois
Arteriography

Todd E. Rasmussen, MD
Associate Professor of Surgery, Uniformed Services University of the Health Sciences, Bethesda, Maryland; Chief of Division of Surgery and Attending Vascular Surgeon, Wilford Hall United States Air Force Medical Center, Lackland Air Force Base, Texas
Vascular Trauma: Military

Daniel J. Reddy, MD
Professor of Surgery, Wayne State University School of Medicine; Vascular Surgeon, John D. Dingell Veterans Affairs Medical Center, Detroit Michigan
Infected Aneurysms

David Rigberg, MD
Associate Professor of Surgery, David Geffen School of Medicine at University of California, Los Angeles, Los Angeles, California
Arterial Aneurysms: General Considerations

Caron B. Rockman, MD
Associate Professor of Surgery, New York University Medical School, New York, New York
Splanchnic Artery Aneurysms

Stanley G. Rockson, MD
Allan and Tina Neil Professor of Lymphatic Research and Medicine, Stanford University School of Medicine; Chief of Consultative Cardiology and Director of Stanford Center for Lymphatic and Venous Disorders, Stanford University, Stanford, California
Lymphedema: Evaluation and Decision Making

Sean P. Roddy, MD
Associate Professor of Surgery, Albany Medical College; Attending Vascular Surgeon, Albany Medcal Center Hospital, Albany, New York
Upper Extremity Arterial Disease: Revascularization

Lee C. Rogers, DPM
Associate Medical Director, Amputation Prevention Center at Valley Presbyterian Hospital, Los Angeles, California
Podiatry Care

Glen S. Roseborough, MD
Assistant Professor of Surgery, Johns Hopkins University School of Medicine; Attending Vascular Surgeon, Johns Hopkins Hospital, Baltimore, Maryland
Carotid Artery Disease: Endarterectomy

Vincent L. Rowe, MD
Assistant Professor of Surgery, Keck School of Medicine of University of Southern California, Los Angeles, Los Angeles, California
Vascular Trauma: Extremity

Brian G. Rubin, MD
Professor of Surgery, Washington University School of Medicine, Washington University in St. Louis; Attending Surgeon, Barnes-Jewish Hospital, St. Louis Missouri
Abdominal Aortic Aneurysms: Open Surgical Treatment

Eva M. Rzucidlo, MD
Associate Professor of Surgery and Vascular Surgery, Dartmouth Medical School, Hanover, New Hampshire; Associate Professor, Cheshire Medical Center, White River Junction, Vermont; Staff Surgeon, Mary Hitchcock Memorial Hospital, Lebanon New Hampshire; Vascular Surgeon, Dartmouth-Hitchcock Clinic, Lebanon, New Hampshire; Associate Professor, Veterans Administration Hospital, Lebanon, New Hampshire
Aortoiliac Disease: Endovascular Treatment

Mikel Sadek, MD
Instructor, New York University School of Medicine, New York, New York
Infrainguinal Disease: Endovascular Treatment

Hazim J. Safi, MD
Professor and Chairman, Department of Cardiothoracic and Vascular Surgery, University of Texas Medical School, Houston; Chief of Cardiothoracic and Vascular Surgery, Memorial Hermann Hospital, Houston, Texas
Brachiocephalic Artery Disease: Surgical Treatment

Elliot B. Sambol, MD
Fellow in Vascular Surgery, New York-Presbyterian Hospital, New York, New York
Local Complications: Endovascular

Richard J. Sanders, MD
Clinical Professor of Surgery, University of Colorado Health Science Center, Aurora, Colorado
Thoracic Outlet Syndrome: General Considerations

Andres Schanzer, MD
Assistant Professor of Surgery, Division of Vascular and Endovascular Surgery, University of Massachusetts Medical School, Worcester, Massachusetts
Thoracic Outlet Syndrome: Venous

Darren Schneider, MD
Associate Professor of Surgery in Residence, David Geffen School of Medicine at University of California, San Francisco, Surgeon, University of California,, San Francisco Medical Center, San Francisco California
Abdominal Aortic Aneurysms: Endovascular Treatment

Joseph R. Schneider, MD, PhD
Professor of Surgery, Feinberg School of Medicine, Northwestern University, Chicago, Illinois; Vascular Surgeon, Vascular and Interventional Program, Central DuPage Hospital, Winfield, Illinois
Aortoiliac Disease: Extra-anatomic Bypass

Peter A. Schneider, MD
Department of Surgery, University of Hawaii, John A. Burns School of Medicine; Chief of Division of Vascular Therapy, Hawaii Permanente Medical Group, Honolulu, Hawaii
Carotid Artery Disease: Fibromuscular Dysplasia

Olaf Schouten, MD
Department of Vascular Surgery, Erasmus University Medical Center, Rotterdam, The Netherlands
Systemic Complications: Cardiac

Torben V. Schroeder, MD, DMSc
Professor of Vascular Surgery, Faculty of Health Sciences, University of Copenhagen; Consultant Vascular Surgeon, Rigshospitalet, Copenhagen, Denmark
Intravascular Ultrasound

Leo J. Schultze Kool, MD, PhD
Professor of Interventional Radiology, Radbound University Medical Centre, Nijmegen, The Netherlands
Computed Tomography

Paul M. Schumacher, MD, MPH
Fellow in Vascular Surgery, Vanderbilt University Medical Center, Nashville, Tennessee; Attending Surgeon, Sacred Heart Medical Center at Riverbend, Springfield, Oregon
Local Complications: Anastomotic Aneurysms

Geert Willem Schurink, MD, PhD
Professor of Vascular Surgery, University of Maastrizht; Chief of Vascular Surgery, Maastrizht University Medical Center, Maastrizht, The Netherlands
Thoracic and Thoracoabdominal Aneurysms: Open Surgical Treatment

Peter Sheehan, MD
Senior Faculty, Mount Sinai School of Medicine; Director of Diabetes Center of Excellence, Mount Sinai Hospital, New York, New York
Atherosclerotic Risk Factors: Diabetes

Paula K. Shireman, MD
Associate Professor, University of Texas Health Science Center, San Antonio, Texas; Staff Surgeon, South Texas Veterans Health Care System, San Antonio Texas
Arteriogenesis

Gregorio A. Sicard, MD
Professor of Surgery; Chief of Section of Vascular Surgery; and Vice-Chairman, Department of Surgery, Washington University School of Medicine, Washington University in St. Louis; Attending Surgeon, Barnes-Jewish Hospital, St. Louis, Missouri
Abdominal Aortic Aneurysms: Open Surgical Treatment

Anton N. Sidawy, MD, MPH
Professor of Surgery, Georgetown University School of Medicine and George Washington School of Medicine and Health Sciences; Chief of Surgical Services, Veterans Affairs Medical Center, Washington, DC
Hemodialysis Access: General Considerations

Bantayehu Sileshi, MD
Surgical Resident, Duke University School of Medicine, Duke University Medical Center, Durham, North Carolina
Coagulopathy and Hemorrhage

Niten N. Singh, MD
Chief of Endovascular Surgery, Division of Vascular and Endovascular Surgery, Madigan Army Medical Center, Fort Lewis, Washington
Upper Extremity Arterial Disease: Amputation

Stephen T. Smith, MD
Assistant Professor of Surgery, Division of Vascular Surgery, University of Texas Southwestern Medical School; Attending Surgeon, Parkland Memorial Hospital, University Hospital, Dallas Veterans Affairs Medical Center, Dallas, Texas
Thoracic Outlet Syndrome: Arterial

Benjamin W. Starnes, MD, FACS
Associate Professor and Chief, Division of Vascular Surgery, University of Washington School of Medicine, Harborview Medical Center, Seattle, Washington
Vascular Trauma: Head and Neck

W. Charles Sternbergh III, MD
Section Head of Vascular and Endovascular Surgery, Ochsner Clinic, New Orleans, Louisiana
Technique: Endovascular Aneurysm Repair

David H. Stone, MD
Assistant Professor of Surgery, Section of Vascular Surgery, Dartmouth Medical School, Dartmouth-Hitchcock Medical Center, Lebanon, New Hampshire
Graft Thrombosis

Makoto Sumi, MD, PhD
Assistant Professor, Division of Vascular Surgery, Department of Surgery, Jikei University School of Medicine, Tokyo, Japan
Technique: Endovascular Therapeutic

David S. Sumner, MD
Distinguished Professor of Surgery, Emeritus, Southern Illinois University School of Medicine, Springfield, Illinois
Arterial Physiology
Vascular Laboratory: Arterial Physiologic Assessment

Bauer Sumpio, MD, PhD, FACS
Professor of Surgery and Radiology, Yale University School of Medicine; Chief of Vascular Surgery and Program Director of Vascular Surgery, Yale-New Haven Medical Center, New Haven, Connecticut
Arterial Wall Biology

Lars G. Svensson, MD, PhD
Professor of Surgery, Thoracic and Cardiovascular Surgery, Cleveland Clinic Lerner College of Medicine of Case Western Reserve University; Director of Aorta Center, Marfan and CTD Clinic; Director of Quality and Process Improvement; Cleveland Clinic, Cleveland, Ohio
Aortic Arch Aneurysms and Dissection

Spence M. Taylor, MD
Professor and Chairman of Department of Surgery, University of South Carolina School of Medicine; Chairman of Surgery, Greenville Hospital System; Senior Assistant Dean of Academic Affairs, Greenville Hospital System, Greenville, South Carolina
Lower Extremity Arterial Disease: Decision Making and Medical Treatment

Maureen M. Tedesco, MD
Surgical Resident Stanford University Medical Center, Stanford, California
Arterial Aneurysms

Bryan W. Tillman, MD, PhD
Assistant Professor, Division of Vascular Surgery, University of Pittsburgh School of Medicine, Pittsburgh, Pennsylvania
Renovascular Disease: General Considerations

Robert W. Thompson, MD
Professor of Surgery (Vascular Surgery), Radiology and Cell Biology and Physiology, Washington University School of Medicine; Attending Surgeon and Director, Center for Thoracic Outlet Syndrome, Barnes-Jewish Hospital, St. Louis, Missouri
Thoracic Outlet Syndrome: Neurogenic

Carlos H. Timaran, MD
Associate Professor of Surgery, Division of Vascular and Endovascular Surgery, University of Texas Southwestern Medical School; Chief of Endovascular Surgery, North Texas Veterans Affairs Healthcare System, Dallas, Texas
Upper Extremity Aneurysms

Gilbert R. Upchurch, Jr., MD
Professor of Surgery, Leland and Ira Doan Research Professor of Surgery, and Associate Chair of Clinical Affairs, University of Michigan Medical School, Ann Arbor, Michigan
Thoracic and Thoracoabdominal Aneurysms: Evaluation and Decision Making

R. James Valentine, MD
Professor and Vice Chairman, Alvin Baldwin, Jr. Chair in Surgery, University of Texas Southwestern Medical School; Attending Surgeon, Parkland Memorial Hospital, University Hospitals, Dallas Veterans Affairs Medical Center, Dallas, Texas
Thoracic Outlet Syndrome: Arterial

J. Hajo van Bockel, MD, PhD
Professor and Chairman, Department of Surgery, Leiden University Medical Center, Leiden, The Netherlands
Renovascular Disease: Acute Occlusive Events

Frank C. Vandy, MD
Resident in Vascular Surgery, University of Michigan Medical School, Ann Arbor, Michigan
Acute Deep Venous Thrombosis: Pathophysiology and Natural History

Leonel Villavicencio, MD
Distinguished Professor of Surgery, Uniformed Services University School of Medicine, Department of Surgery, Bethesda, Maryland; Senior Consultant and Staff, Department of Surgery, Vascular Surgery, Walter Reed Army Medical Center, Washington, DC
Congenital Vascular Malformations: General Considerations

Katja C. Vogt, MD, DMSc
Consultant Vascular Surgeon, Rigshospitalet, Copenhagen, Denmark
Intravascular Ultrasound

Thomas W. Wakefield, MD
S. Martin Lindenauer Professor of Surgery and Section Head of Vascular Surgery, University of Michgan Medical School; Staff Surgeon, University of Michigan Medical Center, Ann Arbor, Michigan
Acute Deep Venous Thrombosis: Pathophysiology and Natural History

Roger Walcott, MD
Vascular Surgery Fellow, Washington Hospital Center, Georgetown University Hospital, Veterans Administration Hospital, Washington, DC
Atherosclerotic Risk Factors: Hyperlipidemia

Daniel B. Walsh, MD
Professor of Surgery, Dartmouth Medical School, Hanover, New Hampshire; Staff Physician, Dartmouth-Hitchcock Medical Center, Lebanon, New Hampshire
Graft Thrombosis

Kenneth J. Warrington, MD
Assistant Professor of Medicine, Mayo Clinic College of Medicine, Rochester, Minnesota
Vasculitis and Other Arteriopathies

Michael T. Watkins, MD
Associate Professor of Surgery, Harvard Medical School; Director of Vascular Surgery Research Laboratory, Associate Visiting Surgeon, Massachusetts General Hospital, Boston, Massachusetts
Ischemia-Reperfusion

Fred A. Weaver, MD
Professor of Surgery, Keck School of Medicine of University of Southern California, Los Angeles; Chief of Division of Vascular Surgery and Endovascular Therapy, University of Southern California University Hospital, Los Angeles, California
Thrombolytic Agents

Mitchell R. Weaver, MD
Assistant Professor of Surgery, Wayne State University School of Medicine; Senior Staff Vascular Surgeon, Henry Ford Hospital, Detroit Michigan
Infected Aneurysms

Ilene C. Weitz, MD
Assistant Professor of Clinical Medicine, Keck School of Medicine of University of Southern California, Los Angeles; Kenneth Norris Comprehensive Cancer Center, Los Angeles, California
Hypercoagulable States

John V. White, MD
Clinical Professor of Surgery, University of Illinois College of Medicine, Chicago, Illinois; Attending Vascular Surgeon and Chair of Department of Surgery, Advocate Lutheran General Hospital, Park Ridge, Illinois
Lower Extremity Arterial Disease: General Considerations

Jeffrey I. Wietz, MD, FRCPC, FACP, FCCP
Professor of Medicine and Biochemistry and Biomedical Sciences, McMaster University; Director of Henderson Research Centre, Hamilton, Ontario, Canada
Antithrombotic Agents

Marlys H. Witte, MD
Professor of Surgery, University of Arizona College of Medicine; Attending Physician in Surgery (Lymphology), University Medical Center, Tucson, Arizona
Lymphatic Pathophysiology

Nelson Wolosker, MD, PhD
Associate Professor, Department of Vascular and Endovascular Surgery, São Paulo University School of Medicine, São Paulo, Brazil
Thoracic Sympathectomy

Mark C. Wyers, MD
Visiting Assistant Professor, Harvard Medical School; Vascular Surgeon, Beth Israel Deaconess Medical Center, Boston, Massachusetts
Mesenteric Vascular Disease: Acute Ischemia

John W. York, MD
Associate Professor of Surgery, Medical University of South Carolina; Medical Director of Greenville Hospital System Wound Care Center, Greenville, South Carolina
Lower Extremity Arterial Disease: Decision Making and Medical Treatment

Wayne W. Zhang, MD
Assistant Professor of Surgery, Division of Vascular Surgery, Department of Cardiovascular Thoracic Surgery, Loma Linda University School of Medicine, Loma Linda, California
Lower Extremity Amputation: General Considerations

R. Eugene Zierler, MD
Professor of Surgery, University of Washington School of Medicine; Medical Director of D. E. Strandness, Jr. Vascular Laboratory, University of Washington Medical Center, Seattle Washington
Arterial Physiology

Foreword

This seventh edition of *Vascular Surgery* is different, and I think better, than the sixth edition, thanks to some new approaches introduced by my colleagues, Jack Cronenwett and Wayne Johnston, who have drawn from their experiences as associate editors of earlier editions of this textbook and editorship of the *Journal of Vascular Surgery*.

Before my work on the first edition in 1977, the only editorial experience I had was as a co-editor of the *Management of Trauma* during my career as a trauma surgeon and director of the Emergency Department at Johns Hopkins. Shortly after I opted to pursue a career in vascular surgery, Robert Rowan, then head of WB Saunders, commented, "Your chosen specialty is rapidly growing but does not yet have a textbook." He then asked me if I would consider being the editor of one. My initial response was that such a book needed a "name editor" and I was still a nobody in the field.

Bob Rowan persisted with this request after I moved to Colorado, and by then it occurred to me that a vascular surgery textbook edited by a group of "young lions" in the field might not be such a bad idea. Not long afterward I gathered with a group of associates—Victor Bernhard, Wesley Moore, Malcolm Perry, and David Sumner—and the angiographer who worked with Victor, Frank Maddison, to plan the first edition. Realizing that none of us was widely recognized yet, and fearing that the leaders of vascular surgery of the time might consider a textbook by us as somewhat presumptuous, I suggested dedicating the book to them, as our mentors. They might well have done the book themselves had they not been so busy leading our specialty through its early challenges, but their response was gratifying and the book was better received than we might have expected.

Nearly every five years since then, another edition of *Vascular Surgery* has been published, and I continued the strategy of gathering together the most knowledgeable of my colleagues and asking them to serve as assistant or associate editors of one or more sections of the book. Each edition grew and became more comprehensive, growing quickly to two volumes and ultimately to the 2502-page 6th edition. The intent was to provide complete coverage of current vascular surgery practice and to produce a book not to be read from cover to cover, but one that could serve as the ultimate reference. Thanks to Wayne Johnston, the last edition included an online version, with periodic updates. It was marketed as a separate entity but is more integral in this edition.

During the ensuing years, the hard work of many colleagues has not only justified my choice of collaborators and rewarded my own efforts but made me look good. My policy of changing chapter authorship after two editions may have seemed inappropriate to those contributing good chapters, but including them as coauthors of the revised chapters guaranteed a smooth transition, allowing retention of elements that were still current. This was not "change for change's sake," but awareness of the difficulty of improving on a chapter that one has written twice. As the result of this turnover and of the expanding scope and practice of vascular surgery, a majority of chapters in new editions reflected either new first authors or new chapter titles, and sometimes both. Yet, as I look over the table of contents of the 6th edition it is surprising how many colleagues have continued to contribute and stay involved over the years; more than twice the number of contributors remain as those missing. I thank them for their willingness to contribute in one way or another to what has become our specialty's main textbook.

Looking over past editions and seeing the names Charles Anderson, Gene Bernstein, John Cranley, Stanley Crawford, Bob Hobson, George Johnson, Allastair Karmody, Dick Kempczinski, Bill Krupski, John Porter, Ed Saltzman, Gene Strandness, and Charles Witte on those pages reminds us of the tragic toll of illness or injury among my colleagues. I remember them with fondness. In addition, I owe a special thanks to former section editors John Bergan, Victor Bernhard, Tony Comerota, Richard Dean, Julie Freischlag, Kaj Johansen, Dave Kumpe, Tom Riles, Wesley Moore, Malcolm Perry, Lloyd Taylor, David Sumner, and John Wolfe, who toiled with me in earlier editions (and some of whom still contribute chapters) as well as those with me through the 6th edition: Hugh Beebe, Kim Hansen, Peter Gloviczki, Ken Ouriel, Greg Moneta, Bruce Perler, John Ricotta, Russell Samson, Jim Seeger, Tony Sidawy, Jim Valentine, Tom Wakefield, and Fred Weaver.

I am particularly pleased to have this textbook in good hands as I pass the baton to long-time friends and co-editors Jack Cronenwett and Wayne Johnston, especially with the prospects of continued support from the Society for Vascular Surgery as vascular surgery goes forward. In spite of all the hard work, I am quick to admit that this textbook has been good for me and my career, and so it is without regret, and with considerable enthusiasm, that I look forward to its continuing to serve as a valuable renewable resource for present and future vascular surgeons.

Robert B. Rutherford, MD, FACS, FRCS (Glasg.)

Preface

"This book was conceived as a comprehensive treatise on the surgical management of vascular diseases. … Our efforts will have been rewarded if the book proves helpful to any physician who has committed himself or herself to treating patients with vascular disease."

This quotation from the Preface to the first edition of *Vascular Surgery*, published in 1976, exemplifies the vision, purpose, and commitment demonstrated by Robert B. Rutherford as he guided this textbook through six editions over the next 30 years. Known simply as "*Rutherford*," this textbook has become the definitive reference not only for vascular surgeons but also for all physicians who treat vascular disease. Vascular specialists and their patients owe a great debt of gratitude to Dr. Rutherford for his stewardship of this invaluable resource.

When Bob Rutherford decided to pass along the editorship of *Vascular Surgery*, he worked with the publisher, Elsevier, and the Society for Vascular Surgery, which agreed to sponsor the book and appoint future editors.

We were honored to be selected as the first new editors of this textbook, which is now officially and appropriately titled *Rutherfords's Vascular Surgery* in honor of its founding editor. Never has it been truer that we stand on the shoulders of a giant. In fact, our joint work on this project over the past two years has reinforced our admiration for our good friend Bob Rutherford, who single-handedly and tirelessly edited the first six editions. It took two of us to do his work, and we can only hope to live up to his standard.

Never has the discipline of vascular surgery been so exciting! Traditional open surgery remains a rewarding component of practice, but it has been joined by ever-expanding endovascular options as well as better medical therapies. These expanded therapeutic options increase the complexity of decision making and hence increased the challenge of preparing a comprehensive textbook on the treatment of vascular disease. While it is tempting to continually increase the page content of such a comprehensive book, we decided that addition length (and weight!) could not be handled by most readers. Accordingly, we have worked diligently with authors and Associate Editors to minimize repetition. Also, we eliminated the many print pages of references, which are now available online only (where they are Web-linked with the full PubMed citation and abstract for easy research) and substituted a short annotated reference list for the reader seeking additional general reading on each topic.

In keeping with the inclusionary policy of the SVS, we invited many new and younger authors to participate in this edition and expanded the number of authors from countries outside the United States and Canada. Many new chapters have been added to reflect progress and changes in the treatment of vascular disease. We completely revised the structure and order of chapters, so that the two volumes contain chapters with related content, and the two volumes are easily identified by different colored and illustrated covers. Following current publishing guidelines, we have included many subheadings to allow expeditious location of content; also, full-color illustrations are now distributed throughout the book. Numerous new figures have been created for this edition, and all previous figures have been colorized and updated.

Readers increasingly use Web-based resources, and we are pleased that the current textbook is bundled as a print and Web version. The Web version contains all references, as noted above, and will be updated monthly with new relevant references selected from the Journal of Vascular Surgery and the European Journal of Vascular and Endovascular Surgery. It also contains video presentations.

All of this work would not have been possible without the assistance of many others. Bob Rutherford provided substantial guidance and insights as we undertook this project. We were greatly assisted by our hard-working, thorough, and meticulous Associate Editors: Rich Cambria, Peter Gloviczki, Lou Messina, Joe Mills, Bruce Perler, Jim Seeger, Tony Sidawy, and Fred Weaver. Each of them participated in the selection of authors, development and revision of the proposed chapter outlines, and editing of many chapters. Of course, the ultimate value of any multiauthored textbook is determined by the diligence of the authors who prepared the chapters. Realizing the demands of this task, we selected recognized experts and limited their contribution to a single chapter each, so that they could focus on this endeavor. We were rewarded by excellent contributions. We especially appreciate the authors' patience with our admittedly rigorous editorial process. In that regard, we treated these chapters more like journal articles, undoubtedly influenced by our tenure as editors of the *Journal of Vascular Surgery*.

Finally, we appreciate the assistance of many individuals at Elsevier who tolerated our demands for excellence and then exceeded them. Judy Fletcher served as the Publishing Director, Joanie Milnes as the Developmental Editor, and Amy Norwitz as the Senior Project Manager. It was the combined effort of these and many other copy editors, artists, and printers that assembled this final product.

In closing, we echo the hope of Bob Rutherford in his first edition, that this edition will prove helpful to physicians involved in vascular health care. It has been an honor for us to serve as the first SVS editors for the new *"Rutherford."*

Jack L. Cronenwett
K. Wayne Johnston

Contents

Technique | *Section* 12

Fred A. Weaver

CHAPTER 83

Technique: Open Surgical

Jamal J. Hoballah

Based in part on chapters in the previous edition by John J. Ricotta, MD, FACS; Robert B. Rutherford, MD, FACS, FRCS (Glasg.); Frank J. Veith, MD; Evan C. Lipsitz, MD; Nicholas J. Gargiulo, MD; Jacob Cynamon, MD; William C. Krupski, MD; Louis M. Messina, MD; and Ronald J. Stoney, MD.

The management of vascular disease has undergone a major evolution. A decade ago, whenever vascular intervention was deemed necessary, open vascular surgery was the norm. However, with advances in catheter-based technology, endovascular therapy is now the first option in most clinical situations. Endovascular intervention is less invasive, and patient recovery is rapid. The limitations of endovascular therapy are related to specific anatomic considerations and questions of durability.

Open vascular surgery traditionally offered the "gold standard" with respect to durability and efficacy. However, it was associated with the typical morbidity and mortality of all open surgical procedures. These drawbacks included complications of general anesthesia (when used), the physiologic changes of clamping and unclamping major vessels, the significant intraoperative blood loss and fluid shifts in vascular procedures, and the impact of various types of skin, abdominal, and thoracic incisions.

With the goal of decreasing the morbidity of vascular interventions, the shift toward endovascular procedures is well justified. When an endovascular intervention is not anatomically possible, open vascular surgery can be used in a hybrid fashion to modify the anatomy so that endovascular intervention is possible. For example, a bypass to the common iliac artery or aorta may be constructed to allow the safe passage of a large stent-graft for endovascular thoracic aortic aneurysm repair in a patient with a small or occluded iliac artery. Similarly, debranching procedures such as iliorenal and iliomesenteric bypasses in patients with suprarenal aortic aneurysms or carotid-subclavian and carotid-carotid bypasses in patients with thoracic aortic aneurysms can provide a landing zone during the endovascular treatment of a thoracoabdominal or thoracic aortic aneurysm.

Despite advances in endovascular technology and the increase in the number of endovascular interventions, open vascular reconstructions will continue to play a significant role in the management of patients with vascular disease for the foreseeable future.

■ BASIC PRINCIPLES

The key elements of a successful open vascular reconstruction are choosing the right procedure and vascular exposure and then executing the selected procedure correctly. This requires the appropriate instruments and graft and suture materials. In addition, open vascular procedures should be performed under excellent lighting and are often aided by magnifying loupes. For the operating surgeon, maintaining good ergonomic position during the reconstruction is essential to prevent significant work-related discomfort in the neck, shoulders, or back.

Vascular Instruments and Retractors

A vascular instrument tray typically includes vascular clamps, needle holders, forceps, scissors, and various retractors. Depending on the size of the vessel and the location of the surgical reconstruction, the instruments used will vary.

Clamps

Vascular clamps typically have jaws with rows of fine interdigitating serrations that allow clamping of the vessel without slippage or significant crush injury. Although vascular clamps are considered atraumatic, a vascular clamp applied inappropriately can cause significant intimal damage or may tear the artery if placed over a plaque in an inappropriate manner. Even in a soft, minimally diseased artery, a clamp applied with excessive force can damage the arterial wall and intima.

In general, clamps can be divided into those used for large, medium, or small vessels. They vary in shape and angulation to fit into specific anatomic locations, and they can be used as fully or partially occluding clamps. Clamps with special soft plastic inserts (e.g., Fogarty soft jaw) are also available to allow the clamping of prosthetic grafts without damaging the graft material. Types of vascular clamps and their suggested uses are outlined in Table 83-1. For smaller vessels and branches, various sizes of bulldog clamps or intracranial aneurysm clips, such as the Yasargil or Heifitz clips, are available. (See Figs. 83-1 to 83-12 on the Expert Consult Web site.)

Needle Holders, Forceps, and Scissors

Needle holders of various lengths and shapes are available. The choice of needle holder is often dictated by the size of the needle used. A Mayo-Hegar needle holder is typically used with large needles, and Castroviejo needle holders are typically used with small, fine vascular needles. (See Fig. 83-13 on the Expert Consult Web site.)

Table 83-1 Vascular Clamps and Target Vessels

Clamp Type	Vessel
Totally Occluding	
DeBakey aortic aneurysm clamp (side-to-side apposition of aortic wall)	Supraceliac, infrarenal aorta
DeBakey-Bahnson aortic aneurysm clamp	Infrarenal aorta
Howard-DeBakey aortic aneurysm clamp with reverse curve shafts (side-to-side apposition of aortic wall)	Infrarenal aorta
Fogarty aortic clamp (side-to-side apposition of aortic wall)	Infrarenal aorta; aortic grafts, calcified aorta
DeBakey aortic aneurysm clamp (apposition of anterior and posterior walls together)	Infrarenal aorta
Lambert-Kay aortic clamp (apposition of anterior and posterior walls together)	Infrarenal aorta
Wylie hypogastric clamp	Iliac arteries, especially hypogastric arteries
DeBakey peripheral vascular clamp (angled handle)	Iliac arteries
DeBakey peripheral vascular clamp (angled jaw, 45 degrees)	Iliac and common carotid arteries
Henly subclavian clamp	Subclavian and common femoral arteries
Partially Occluding (Side-Biting)	
Lemole-Strong aortic clamp	Aorta; aortic grafts
Satinsky clamp	Aorta, vena cava
Cooley anastomosis clamp	Aorta; aortic grafts
Cooley-Derra clamp	Graft limbs
Cooley pediatric clamp	Common femoral artery, saphenofemoral junction
Self-Compressing (No Applicator Required)	
Gregory carotid "soft" bulldog	Small vessels
Potts bulldog—straight and angled jaw	Small vessels
DeBakey bulldog	Small vessels
Dietrich bulldog	Small vessels
Self-Compressing (Applicator Required)	
Yasargil aneurysm clip	Small vessels and branches
Heifitz clip	Small vessels and branches
Kleinert-Kutz clip—straight, angled, curved	Microvascular anastomoses
Louisville microvessel approximator	Microvascular anastomoses

Adapted from Hoballah JJ. *Vascular Reconstructions: Anatomy, Exposures, and Techniques.* New York: Springer-Verlag; 2000.

The forceps used during vascular procedures typically have very fine, noncrushing jaws, exemplified by the DeBakey forceps. However, similar to vascular clamps, vascular forceps can crush a vessel wall if they are not used appropriately and delicately. Fine-tip ring forceps are very useful during the construction of vein bypasses to infrapopliteal vessels. Metzenbaum and Church scissors are used for the dissection of blood vessels. Stevens tenotomy scissors with sharp tips are used for dissecting tibial vessels. Special Potts scissors with various angulations are used to enlarge and shape arteriotomies and venotomies. Right-angle clamps with various tip sizes are used to encircle blood vessels and branches. (See Figs. 83-14 to 83-19 on the Expert Consult Web site.)

Retractor Systems

Retractors can be self-retaining or hand-held. Self-retaining retractors should be used whenever possible. The Omni-Flex vascular retractor (Omni-Tract Surgical, St. Paul, MN) is frequently used for open aortic surgery, whether transabdominal or retroperitoneal. (See Fig. 83-20 on the Expert Consult Web site.) This retractor system consists of a wishbone that attaches to a post mounted on the operating room table rail, and it typically offers a selection of blades with different depths, widths, and shapes that can be clamped to the wishbone. Shallow, wide blades are typically used to retract the abdominal walls, whereas deeper splanchnic blades may be used to retract the splenic flexure and other parts of the colon. A wide, fence-shaped blade is typically used to retract the small bowel during aortic dissection, and a narrow, deep blade may be used to retract the left renal vein cephalad. This retractor system is useful during thoracoabdominal aortic aneurysm repair. Modifications of this retractor have also been designed for inguinal, carotid, and spine exposures.

Another self-retaining abdominal retractor is the Bookwalter retractor (Codman Johnson & Johnson, Raynham, MA). (See Fig. 83-21 on the Expert Consult Web site.) This retractor is often used when conducting abdominal aortic replacement through mini-laparotomy incisions. The retracting blades in the Bookwalter retractor attach to an oval metal ring placed around the abdominal incision instead of a wishbone.

Several single-instrument self-retaining retractors are available for neck and extremity procedures. (See Figs. 83-22 to 83-24 on the Expert Consult Web site.) The Weitlaner retractor is commonly used for inguinal and popliteal incisions. In obese patients with significant inguinal pannus, a Miskimon retractor can be especially useful owing to its deeper and wider blades, which provide a larger retracting area. Spring retractors are extremely useful when conducting infrageniculate vessel exposure because they tend to occupy

Table 83-2 Suggested Needle Sizes

Vessel Size*	Needle Brand and Size			
	Ethicon	*USSC*	*Davis and Geck*	*Gore-Tex*
Small (calcified tibial)	CC	DV-1	CV-311/DTE-10	PT-9
Small (tibial, internal carotid)	BV-1	CV-1	CV-310/TE-10, 11	TT-9
Small (tibial)	BV	CV	CV-309/TE-9	TT-12
Medium (common carotid, femoral, popliteal)	C-1	CV-11	CV-301/TE-1	TT-13
Large (common iliac)	RB-1	CV-23	CV-331/T31	TH-18
Large (aorta)	V7	V-20	DV-305/T-5	TH-26
Large (posterior wall of aorta)	MH	V26	CV-C00/T-10	TH-35

*For arterial anastomoses, the following suture and needle sizes are recommended: 2-0, 3-0, aorta; 4-0, iliac arteries; 5-0, axillary, common carotid, common femoral, and superficial femoral arteries; 5-0, 6-0, internal carotid, popliteal, and brachial arteries; 7-0, 8-0, tibial and inframalleolar arteries.
Adapted from Hoballah JJ. *Vascular Reconstructions: Anatomy, Exposures, and Techniques*. New York: Springer-Verlag; 2000.

little space. The Gelpi retractor is typically helpful when conducting a first rib resection through a transaxillary approach for thoracic outlet obstruction.

Vascular Sutures and Grafts

Sutures

Nonabsorbable sutures are used for vascular anastomoses and repairs. These sutures typically provide the tensile strength necessary to juxtapose and secure the vessels together until healing is completed. When prosthetic conduits are used in vascular reconstruction, the tensile strength provided by the sutures is needed indefinitely to maintain vascular integrity. Currently, monofilament sutures are most commonly used for vascular reconstructions, although some surgeons still prefer braided polyester multifilament sutures. Vascular sutures are usually double-armed with a needle on each end to allow continuous suturing in both directions from the initial knot.

Commonly used monofilament sutures include polypropylene, polybutester, and polytetrafluoroethylene (PTFE). Polypropylene sutures (Prolene, Surgipro, Surgilene) are made of a monofilament strand of synthetic linear polyolefin. These sutures tend to maintain their tensile strength over time. They have little friction and excellent handling characteristics. They are widely popular and are probably the most commonly used suture material in vascular reconstructions. Polybutester is another type of monofilament suture made of a co-polymer of polyglycol terephthalate and polytrimethylene terephthalate coated with polytribolate to reduce drag and improve tissue passage. PTFE sutures were developed to minimize the needle hole bleeding that is often seen when polypropylene sutures are used with PTFE grafts or patches. They are designed so that there is minimal difference in the diameters of the needle and the suture. They have excellent handling characteristics, with a low tissue friction and low drag coefficient. The needle and suture sizes vary, depending on the vessel. Suggestions are provided in Table 83-2.

Grafts

Selection of a graft type is an integral part of any vascular reconstruction. Polyester grafts of different shapes and structures are available to replace the thoracic aorta. Polyester and PTFE grafts are available as conduits for the abdominal aorta and infrainguinal vessels. Autogenous vein grafts are favored in many small arterial reconstructions. These grafts are discussed in detail in Chapters 87 (Autogenous Vein Grafts), 88 (Prosthetic Grafts), and 89 (Biologic Grafts).

■ BASIC VASCULAR TECHNIQUES

Open vascular surgery is conducted using the general principles of blood vessel exposure and control, along with the basic techniques of vascular reconstruction. These basic vascular techniques include thromboembolectomy, endarterectomy, creation and closure of an arteriotomy, and construction of bypasses or in-line graft replacement using end-to-side or end-to-end anastomoses.

Vascular Exposure and Dissection

An exhaustive discussion of specific vascular exposures is beyond the scope of this chapter; these are addressed in greater detail in procedure-specific chapters. Several excellent resources are also available that describe the vascular anatomy and the variety of exposures available to the vascular surgeon.[1-4]

Initial Vessel Exposure

The basic concept of vascular exposure and dissection is to approach and expose the vessels by the most direct and shortest route possible. Selection of the surgical approach and incision should take into consideration the possibility that the operation may become more complex than originally anticipated and that surgical control and reconstruction may occur at a more proximal or distal location. Anatomic landmarks, location of the pulse, or a combination of the two is typically used to guide placement of the initial skin incision.

Following incision, proper handling of the skin and soft tissue overlying the vessels is essential to prevent significant wound complications. Lymphatics are typically ligated and divided to avoid lymphorrhea and lymphocoele. Use of electrocautery through lymph nodes should be avoided to prevent significant lymph leak or the need to excise lymph nodes, leaving dead space in the wound.

Once the vascular sheath is identified and incised, the adventitia is held and retracted in one direction, and dissection is carried out in the tissue adjacent to the edge of the blood vessel wall. By staying close to the adventitia, the dissection can be maintained in the correct areolar anatomic plane, and the vessel can be circumferentially dissected and encircled with a Silastic loop or umbilical tape. The basic surgical technique of traction with countertraction is essential in vascular exposure. Traction on a vessel loop is often used to retract a vessel during dissection or mobilization. Gentle tension on the vessel loop is recommended to prevent injury to the intima.

"Redo" Vessel Exposure

"Redo" vascular exposure poses a unique challenge, given the fibrous obliteration of the normal anatomic vascular planes. When the surgeon is faced with a "redo" operation, sharp dissection with a No. 15 knife blade may allow better management of the scar tissue than scissors dissection, and it may allow the surgeon to stay in the appropriate dissection plane. An inadvertent arteriotomy caused by a small blade may be easier to repair than arterial disruption caused by dissecting scissors. The most common vessel that requires "redo" exposure is the common femoral artery, and the approach to this vessel is illustrative of "redo" vessel exposure in general.

The principle of dissecting from known to unknown can be useful in preventing branch vessel injury during re-exposure. A significant concern with a "redo" femoral artery exposure is injuring the profunda femoris artery. Consequently, the superficial femoral artery is exposed in the most distal part of the incision, where minimal scarring exists. The dissection is then carried along the medial aspect of the superficial femoral artery and progresses proximally. Typically the common femoral vein is identified during the process, revealing a safe dissection plane. Once the inguinal ligament is reached, the common femoral artery is encircled with a loop. The direction of the dissection is then reversed and continued back distally toward the superficial femoral artery. The area of size transition between the common and superficial femoral arteries exposes the location of the profunda femoris artery. At that level, dissection from the medial and posterior aspect of the common femoral artery identifies a plane that has not been violated and allows dissection of the profunda femoris artery from underneath the common femoral artery. The profunda femoris artery is controlled at its origin by passing a vessel loop underneath the superficial femoral artery and then retrieving it just proximal to the common femoral bifurcation. In cases of extensive scarring, the profunda femoral branch can be controlled with a balloon occlusion catheter after common femoral arteriotomy, to avoid potential injury during profunda dissection.

Anticoagulation

Before interrupting blood flow, the patient must be adequately anticoagulated. Unfractionated heparin at 75 to 100 units/kg is typically administered intravenously approximately 5 minutes before blood flow interruption. The patient's anticoagulation is monitored by measuring the activated clotting time (ACT), aiming at a value greater than 250 seconds.

Distal limb ischemia following aortic reconstruction or other types of vascular procedures is a dreaded complication and is often attributed to distal embolization. However, an important factor in this complication is unrecognized suboptimal anticoagulation. Hence, it is important to maintain adequate anticoagulation throughout the period of blood flow interruption by re-dosing with heparin when necessary, using the ACT for guidance. In patients with known heparin-induced thrombocytopenia, anticoagulation may be achieved with intravenous thrombin inhibitors such as argatroban (see Chapter 34: Antithrombotic Agents).

Blood Vessel Control

Blood vessel control can be achieved using vascular clamping, balloon occlusion, vessel loops, pneumatic tourniquet, Rumel tourniquet, or internal occluders.

Vascular Clamping

Ideally, vascular clamps should be applied to a disease-free segment of the artery. Palpating the artery against a right-angle clamp can help determine the presence and extent of atherosclerotic plaque, which is often in a posterior location and not appreciated by palpating the anterior surface only. In the presence of significant plaque, the artery should be dissected more proximally to identify a less diseased site for clamping. This situation is often encountered when clamping the common femoral artery, where plaque often extends to the level of the inguinal ligament. Further dissection proximal to the external iliac circumflex and inferior epigastric branches, however, usually reveals an external iliac artery that is soft and free of disease. If clamping is necessary across an area of diseased artery, the clamp should be applied in a manner that opposes the soft part of the artery against the plaque without causing plaque fracture or vessel tear.

Occasionally, the plaque burden and calcification are so extensive that the only option is to identify a more proximal location for safe clamp placement. One example is supraceliac aortic control through the lesser sac, when clamping in the infrarenal or suprarenal location is not possible owing to extensive calcification or scarring from previous surgery or an inflammatory process.

Balloon Occlusion

If the plaque is circumferential or occupies more than 50% of the circumference, vascular clamps can fracture the plaque or tear the wall and may not provide vascular control. This can be managed by occluding the artery from within using a balloon occlusion catheter such as the Fogarty balloon catheter. Balloon occlusion can be used to control the external iliac artery in the presence of extensive calcification that

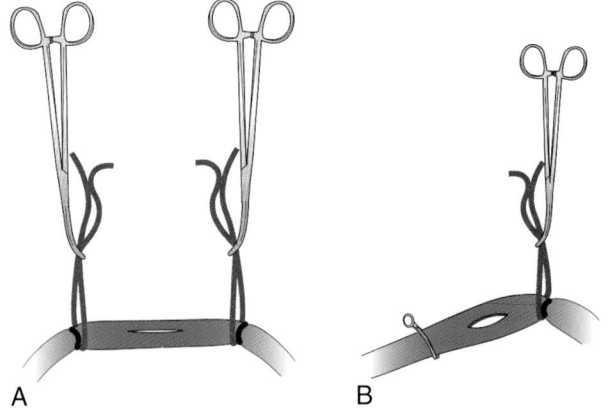

Figure 83-25 A vessel loop on the proximal side of the artery and a small Yasargil aneurysm clamp or bulldog clamp on the distal side of the artery can minimize tension on the anastomosis. **A,** Pulling on both loops can result in tension on the arteriotomy. **B,** Tension on the anastomosis is minimized when one loop is pulled and the other replaced with a bulldog clamp.

extends beyond the most proximal part of the exposure. It is also useful for controlling the right common iliac artery during a left retroperitoneal abdominal aortic aneurysm repair, the profunda femoris artery during repair of a pseudoaneurysm of a femoral anastomosis, or the renal or visceral vessels during a thoracoabdominal aortic aneurysm repair.

Vessel Loops

Vessel loops are ideal for controlling small to medium-sized vessels such as the profunda femoris or popliteal arteries and arterial branches. Silastic vessel loops can be traumatic, however, if excessive tension is applied on them. Further, excessive tension on Silastic vessel loops for simultaneous proximal and distal control of a vessel may make an anastomosis or repair more difficult to construct. One way to avoid excessive tension on the artery in two opposing directions is to apply a vessel loop on the proximal side of the artery and a small Yasargil aneurysm clamp or bulldog clamp on the distal end of the artery (Fig. 83-25).

Pneumatic Tourniquet

A pneumatic tourniquet can be used for vascular control in the extremities and is ideal for infrapopliteal reconstructions. It allows for minimal exposure, dissection, and handling of the arteries and may decrease the risk of spasm or injury caused by clamping of the tibial vessels. The tourniquet can be placed around the thigh or below the knee; usually a soft roll is applied first, followed by the tourniquet. The leg is elevated, and an Esmarch compression wrap is used to expel the venous blood from the leg. The tourniquet is then inflated to a pressure of about 250 mm Hg, or 100 mm Hg above systolic pressure. It is essential to make sure the graft is well aligned and to mark the graft orientation before inflating the tourniquet. Bleeding occasionally occurs despite the tourniquet, and this can sometimes be controlled by increasing the pressure in the tourniquet. An additional clamp on the pro-

funda femoris artery can also help control persistent bleeding. Sometimes calcified and incompressible arteries at the tourniquet site prevent this technique from completely controlling bleeding at the distal arteriotomy.

Other Techniques

Rumel tourniquets can be used for vascular control, but they can cause arterial wall damage in the presence of significant plaque. The Rumel tourniquet may be most useful during an endovascular aortic aneurysm procedure when there is a large sheath in an artery and persistent bleeding from the arteriotomy around the sheath. Cinching the sheath with a Rumel tourniquet at that level can control the bleeding.

When dealing with tibial vessels, direct clamping of the arteries should be avoided to prevent intimal injury or spasm. The use of internal coronary artery occluders in this setting can be useful to achieve vessel control. Florester internal vessel plastic tip occluders (Biovascular, St. Paul, MN) are available in various sizes. However, the surgeon must be comfortable using such occluders, and oversizing should be avoided to prevent intimal damage during insertion.

■ THROMBECTOMY AND THROMBOEMBOLECTOMY

Basic Considerations

Thrombectomy and thromboembolectomy must be mastered by every vascular surgeon because the need to perform these procedures is inevitable. Even the most successfully performed open or endovascular procedure can be complicated by a distal embolic or a thrombotic event. Although numerous techniques are available to achieve pharmacologic or mechanical thrombectomy, the need for balloon thrombectomy cannot be avoided. Balloon thrombectomy allows the removal, inspection, and pathologic examination of the occlusive clot and restores blood flow expeditiously.

A vessel may become acutely occluded owing to a thrombotic or embolic process. Thrombosis frequently occurs proximal and distal to the embolus owing to the stagnant flow—hence the term *thromboembolectomy:* balloon embolectomy is often paired with thrombectomy to remove the thrombus. Several issues need to be addressed during the performance of a thromboembolectomy procedure, including the location and shape of the arteriotomy used to extract the thrombus, selection of the thrombectomy catheter, and performance of the procedure with minimal blood loss and injury to the arterial system. In addition, steering the catheter into the appropriate location and extracting all the offending thrombi are essential to the success of the procedure.

Thromboembolectomy Catheters

A wide variety of thromboembolectomy catheters are available (see Figs. 83-26 and 83-27 on the Expert Consult Web site). The standard ones are balloon catheters that vary in size, length, and maximal balloon inflation. These catheters are typically available in sizes from 2 to 7 Fr. Saline solution is used to inflate the balloon, except for the 2 Fr balloon, which requires air insufflation for easy deflation. The diameter of the fully inflated balloon is 4 mm for the 2 Fr catheter, 5 mm for the 3 Fr, 9 mm for the 4 Fr, 11 mm for the 5 Fr, 13 mm for the 6 Fr, and 14 mm for the 7 Fr.

Size 2 Fr catheters are typically used for very small pedal or hand vessels. The most commonly used catheters are 3 to 5 Fr catheters. A 3 Fr Fogarty catheter is typically used for tibial vessels. A 4 Fr Fogarty catheter is used for vessels the size of the superficial femoral and popliteal arteries; it can also be used for external iliac arteries. A 5 Fr Fogarty catheter is typically used for external iliac or common iliac arteries. Size 6 and size 7 Fr catheters can be used for thrombectomy of an aortic femoral graft or a saddle aortic embolus. A venous thrombectomy catheter with a large, lower pressure balloon is also available.

Standard balloons are made of latex; however, latex-free embolectomy catheters are available for patients with latex allergy. In addition, balloon catheters that can be introduced over guide wires for fluoroscopically assisted thromboembolectomy are also available in sizes 3, 4, 5.5, 6, and 7 Fr.

Special catheters have been devised for adherent clots. The fogarty adherent clot catheter (Edwards Life Sciences, Irvine, CA) features a spiral-shaped, latex-covered stainless steel cable that assumes a corkscrew shape when retracted, thus expanding the surface area to entrap fibrous material. It is marketed for adherent clots resistant to removal by standard elastomeric balloons in both native arteries and synthetic grafts. The fogarty graft thrombectomy catheter (also from Edwards Life Sciences) is designed to remove tough thrombus from synthetic grafts; it has a flexible wire coil at the distal end and expands when retracted to form a double-helix ring that acts as stripper, forming a plane between the graft and the adherent material. This catheter is not intended for native vessels and is marketed for use in PTFE dialysis grafts and aortobifemoral grafts. (See Fig. 83-28 on the Expert Consult Web site.)

Technique

Arteriotomy Location and Shape

The balloon embolectomy catheter is designed to extract thrombi from a site remote from the clot's location. The arteriotomy for clot extraction can be performed in a location proximal or distal to the embolic or thrombotic process. Site selection depends on the ease of exposure, anticipated location of the thrombus, and ease of arteriotomy closure. In patients with acute lower extremity ischemia, the common femoral artery is an ideal site for clot extraction. A patient with an aortic saddle embolus or a popliteal embolus can be managed by thromboembolectomy through the common femoral artery. The common femoral artery and its bifurcation are easy to expose, and closure of the arteriotomy is easily

accomplished in this relatively large artery. Further, the procedure can be performed under local anesthesia. If thromboembolectomy proves to be inadequate, a site closer to the location of the thrombus may be required. Before performing the thrombectomy, it is important to ensure that the patient is adequately anticoagulated.

The selection of a transverse versus longitudinal arteriotomy for catheter access is influenced by the size of the vessel, the cause of the embolus or thrombus, and the presence of plaque in the vessel. A transverse arteriotomy is usually simpler to close and may be preferred when dealing with an embolic process. When the occlusive pathology is due to an atherosclerotic and thrombotic process, or when significant arterial plaque is present, a longitudinal arteriotomy should be used. In such a situation it is not uncommon for an emergency bypass to become necessary, and the longitudinal arteriotomy can be incorporated into one of the anastomoses. If a bypass is deemed unnecessary, a patch is usually needed to close the longitudinal arteriotomy without significant narrowing of the vessel lumen.

Minimizing Blood Loss

During the process of establishing inflow, a balloon catheter is passed proximally for an estimated distance, inflated, and withdrawn through the arteriotomy (Fig. 83-29). As the balloon exits the arteriotomy, the surgeon typically allows brief but unrestricted bleeding to flush any debris or thrombi that may still be present in the proximal part of the vessel. This step can be repeated once or twice to ensure there are no remnants of clot in the artery. A significant amount of blood can be lost in this process. This can be decreased by

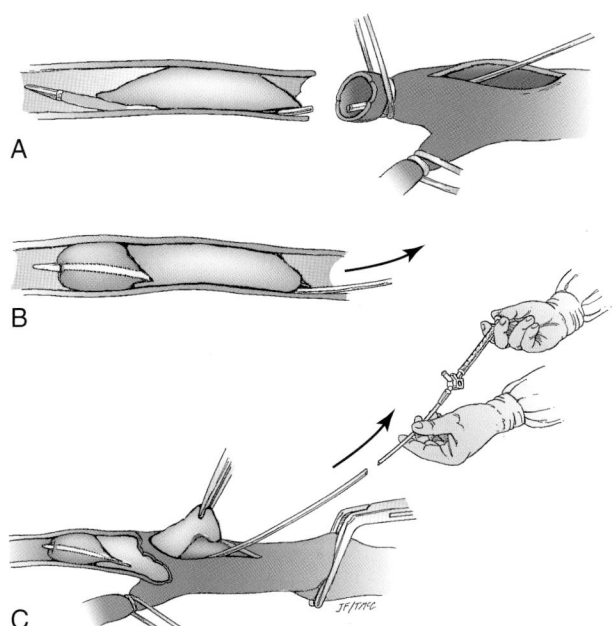

Figure 83-29 Balloon thromboembolectomy catheter is passed proximally for an estimated distance (**A**), inflated (**B**), and withdrawn through the arteriotomy, with bleeding controlled by double-looped Silastic tape (**C**).

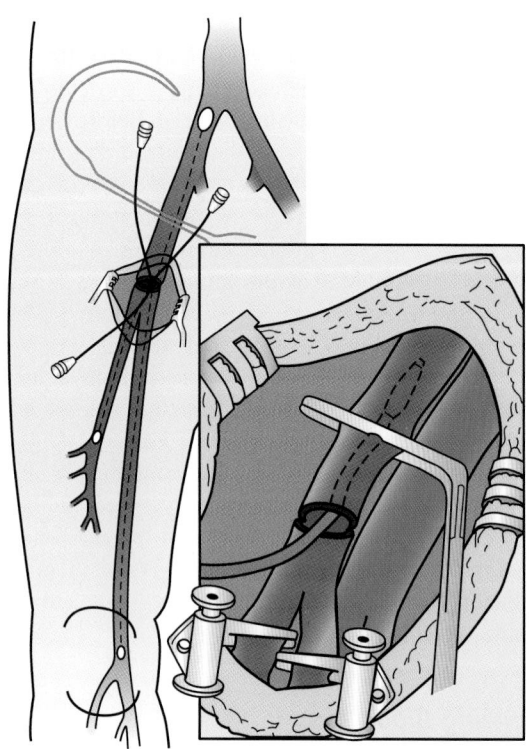

Figure 83-30 The Fogarty soft-jaw clamp may be able to appose the blood vessel walls just enough to prevent bleeding and still allow manipulation of the thromboembolectomy catheter.

applying Silastic double-looped vessel tape around the artery and pulling on the loop while the catheter is being advanced proximally or distally.

When performing thromboembolectomy of a prosthetic bypass or the limb of an aortobifemoral bypass, vessel loops are not adequate to control bleeding. The surgeon can often control bleeding manually by squeezing the arterial wall between the index finger and thumb with one hand and withdrawing the inflated catheter with the other hand. Depending on the anatomy and the presence of scarring, bleeding may be excessive if finger control is used while passing the Fogarty catheter through the proximal artery. In such situations, use of a Fogarty soft-jaw clamp is recommended (Fig. 83-30). The soft jaws are intended to appose the blood vessel walls just enough to prevent bleeding and still allow the thromboembolectomy catheter to be advanced or withdrawn. The jaws are then opened as the inflated thromboembolectomy catheter is being withdrawn. The clamp is reapplied once the balloon catheter is pulled out of the vessel and vigorous blood flushing has occurred.

Minimizing Vascular Injury

Significant vascular injury can occur from thromboembolectomy and inappropriate manipulation of the balloon catheter. Vascular injury can occur from inadvertent placement of the balloon tip or from excessive inflation of the balloon itself. Injury can also occur during insertion, advancement, or withdrawal of the thromboembolectomy catheter. During inser-

tion, it is important to ensure that the catheter is being advanced intraluminally. It can inadvertently pass in a subintimal plane, and inflation and withdrawal of the catheter in that situation can cause arterial dissection or disruption. Injury is also possible because the procedure is commonly performed blindly or without fluoroscopic control. Hence, it is very important to perform the procedure gently and be cognizant of any resistance during passage of the catheter. If the catheter does not advance freely, it may be passing into a side branch or abutting a curve in the artery. Further forceful advancement can result in either perforation or penetration into the subintimal plane.

Another cause of injury is overinflation of the balloon catheter and its withdrawal; this can result in significant shearing of the intima, with intimal disruption and damage. This technique has long been used to experimentally induce intimal damage or to harvest endothelial cells in animal models. Balloon overinflation can also result in rupture of the vessel or pseudoaneurysm formation.

To minimize vascular injury during balloon thromboembolectomy, several steps are necessary. Selection of an appropriately sized thromboembolectomy catheter is a must. Before inserting a thromboembolectomy catheter, it is important to test the balloon, visualize its size, and get a feel for its inflation. It is a good practice to limit the fluid used in the syringe to inflate the balloon to the minimum amount needed for full inflation. This protects against overinflation of the balloon when it is in the vessel. Another helpful maneuver is to externally measure the distance from the arteriotomy to the location of the thrombus. This helps determine whether the catheter has reached its desired destination. In addition, it may help limit unnecessary pushing of the catheter beyond the thrombus.

Once the catheter has reached its maximal advancement or the desired location, the balloon is gently inflated while the catheter is slowly withdrawn until tactile friction is sensed by the surgeon. At that point, the balloon should not be further inflated. The catheter is then retrieved, maintaining the same amount of friction and tension. The balloon may have to be further inflated as the catheter is being pulled into a more proximal location, where the artery's caliber may increase. The inflation, deflation, and withdrawal of the balloon should be a dynamic and variable process to accommodate changes in vessel caliber.

Fluoroscopy-Guided Thromboembolectomy

To achieve successful thromboembolectomy, the catheter should be advanced to the desired location distal to the occluding thrombus and then used to retrieve the thrombus. Once no more thrombus can be retrieved, the arteriotomy can be closed, especially if distal vessel backbleeding is present. However, the presence of adequate backbleeding does not ensure complete thromboembolectomy. A significant intraluminal thrombus burden may still exist despite multiple balloon passes and the presence of generous backbleeding. This is especially true when performing thromboembolectomy of the infrapopliteal vessels. The catheter may repeatedly pass into the peroneal artery while significant thrombus remains in the anterior and posterior tibial arteries.

To avoid leaving behind clinically significant thrombus, the reperfused limb or organ is carefully examined following arteriotomy closure. An angiogram may be obtained if the reperfusion does not appear satisfactory. It may also be obtained before closing the arteriotomy to assess the completeness of the thromboembolectomy. Another option is to perform the thromboembolectomy procedure under fluoroscopic guidance.[5] Fluoroscopy can be used from the start of the procedure, or it can be used selectively to retrieve thrombi that cannot be extracted with non–image-guided thromboembolectomy.

Thromboembolectomy under fluoroscopic guidance can be educational even for a seasoned vascular surgeon. The balloon is first tested under fluoroscopy to appreciate its shape when inflated and deflated, and an angiogram through the arteriotomy can be performed before passing the Fogarty catheter. This may allow a better understanding of the anatomy and the location of the thrombus. Visualizing the catheter as it travels down the leg provides significant information about its location and course. When the balloon is inflated under fluoroscopy, the surgeon can appreciate the degree of inflation required. To best image the balloon, it should be inflated using contrast material diluted to 25%. Overinflation can be avoided, and inadvertent positioning of the catheter into a side branch before balloon inflation can be detected and corrected. Further, if the catheter passes through an area of stenosis, a change in the shape of the inflated catheter indicates the location of the stenosis.

When performing an infrapopliteal thromboembolectomy, the catheter can be directed into the desired tibial vessel by bending its tip and rotating it into the desired location. One approach is to use two balloon catheters; one is inflated at the origin of the tibioperoneal trunk, forcing the second one toward the anterior tibial artery (Fig. 83-31). Another technique is to use a 7 or 8 Fr multipurpose guiding catheter and park the catheter tip at the level of the popliteal trifurcation. The balloon catheter is introduced through the guiding catheter, and using the curve of the guiding catheter, the balloon catheter is directed into the desired location. The balloon is inflated and withdrawn together with the guiding catheter.

Another approach is to use over-the-wire balloon embolectomy catheters. Standard endovascular techniques are used to introduce a wire into the desired vessel, followed by advancement of the thromboembolectomy balloon over the wire. The 5.5 Fr catheter can be advanced over a 0.035-inch wire; the 3 Fr catheter, which is typically the size needed for tibial vessels, is passed over a 0.018-inch wire. The process of withdrawing the catheter over the wire may be frustrating, because often the wire is dislodged and pulled at the same time as the catheter.

The main drawback of thromboembolectomy under fluoroscopic guidance is the inconvenience of using fluoroscopy, especially if skilled radiology technicians are unavailable.

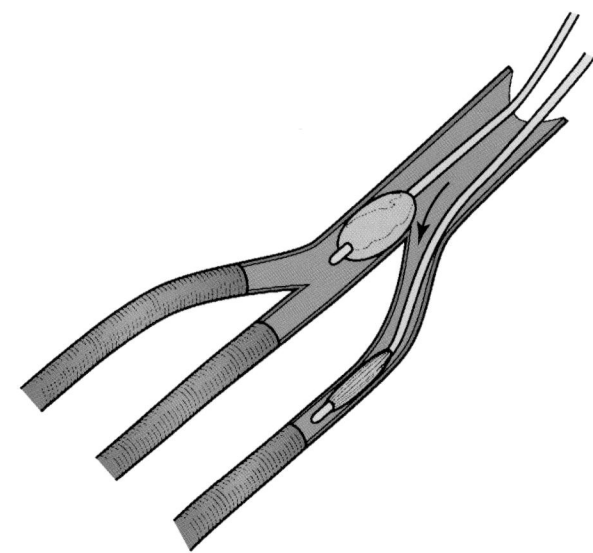

Figure 83-31 One approach to guide the thromboembolectomy catheter into the anterior tibial artery is to use two balloon catheters, inflating one at the origin of the tibioperoneal trunk and thus forcing the second one toward the anterior tibial artery.

However, the advantages of fluoroscopy are significant: it allows the performance of a controlled thromboembolectomy, and it allows the opportunity for endovascular intervention when appropriate, such as balloon angioplasty and stenting of a dialysis graft venous stenosis, distal anastomosis of a femoropopliteal bypass, or occlusive iliac pathology.

Embolectomy in Specific Conditions

The approaches to thromboembolectomy in specific vessels and for specific conditions, such as infrainguinal ischemia, aortic saddle embolus, visceral ischemia, graft occlusion, and iliofemoral venous thrombosis, are available in Appendices 1 and 2 on the Expert Consult Web site.

■ ENDARTERECTOMY

Endarterectomy is a basic vascular procedure that should be mastered by every vascular surgeon.

Basic Considerations

This procedure, which involves the removal of obstructive atherosclerotic plaque from the arterial lumen, can be performed as the sole therapeutic procedure or in combination with bypass. For example, carotid endarterectomy may be the sole intervention for occlusive disease at the carotid bifurcation and is one of the most commonly performed open vascular procedures. Similarly, endarterectomy of the common femoral and profunda femoris arteries may be the sole procedure to treat lower extremity occlusive disease. However, endarterectomy of the common femoral and profunda femoris arteries can also be included in the construction of the femoral anastomosis of an aortobifemoral bypass to ensure a nonobstructed outflow into the profunda femoris artery. It can also be incorporated into the construction of the proximal anastomosis of an infrainguinal bypass. Endarterectomy usually results in removal of the thickened intima and inner media, leaving behind the outer part of the media and the adventitia. It should not be performed in an aneurysmal artery because the remaining adventitial layer is too weak and degenerated to withhold suturing or arterial pressure. Several methods of endarterectomy have been described. These include open, semiclosed, eversion, orificial, and extraction endarterectomy.

Open Endarterectomy

In the open endarterectomy technique, the artery is opened longitudinally at the site of disease. The plaque is then separated from the artery wall in the direction of the arteriotomy and removed (Fig. 83-32). The arteriotomy can be closed primarily or with a patch. Being in the right anatomic vessel wall plane is essential to performing an adequate endarterectomy. This can be accomplished by holding the edge of the adventitia with a forceps and pulling it away from the plaque. A plane is then developed between the plaque and the media or adventitia. Using the Freer elevator or a beaver blade, the outer media or adventitia is typically pushed away from the plaque. The endarterectomy plane is developed on each side of the vessel wall and advanced posteriorly until it becomes

circumferential. When dissecting in the appropriate plane, the dissecting instrument meets little resistance. When a normal part of the wall is reached proximally, the plaque is transected flush with the arterial wall without leaving a significant protruding edge.

Completion of the distal endpoint of the endarterectomy can be challenging. Often the plaque clearly ends as a tongue into a normal soft artery. In this case, the endarterectomy plane is moved to a more superficial level, allowing the plaque to feather out from the wall. This provides a desirable flat distal endpoint, with a very smooth transition from the endarterectomized surface to the nonendarterectomized segment. On other occasions, the plaque may extend farther distally, with no visible end. In that situation, transection of the plaque in the least diseased segment is necessary, which results in a shelf between the endarterectomized and nonendarterectomized segments of the wall. Suture tacking of the intima and plaque to the posterior part of the adventitia is necessary to avoid plaque lifting, dissection, or thrombosis upon vessel reperfusion. To place a tacking suture, one end of the suture is placed 1 mm distal to the endpoint, and the other end is placed at the junction of the endarterectomy and the endarterectomized surface (Fig. 83-33). Multiple sutures are often required to adequately tack the plaque edge to the arterial wall.

Inspection of the completed endarterectomized luminal surface may reveal loose circular fibers in the media and other debris that can be peeled away in a circumferential manner. It is essential to create a debris-free surface area at the endarterectomy site before vessel closure and reperfusion. The endarterectomized surface can be very thrombogenic upon vessel reperfusion. This can be inhibited by the administration of antiplatelet agents before the procedure.

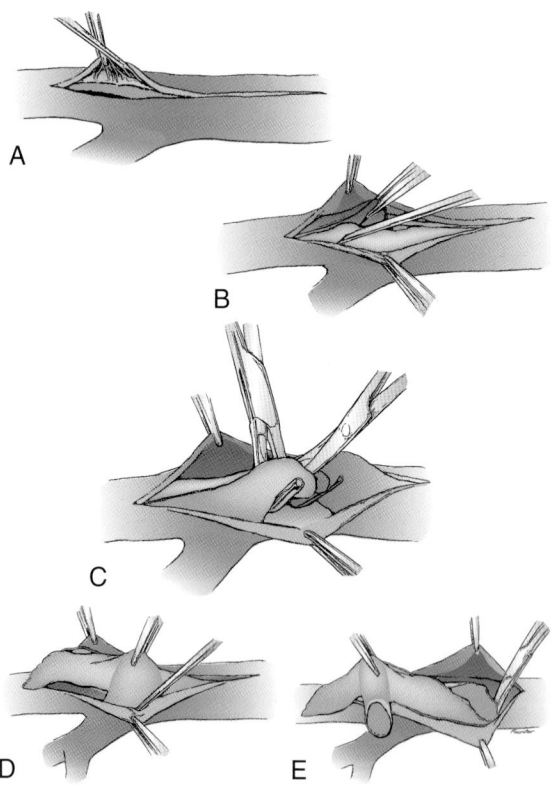

Figure 83-32 A–E, In the open endarterectomy technique, the vessel is opened longitudinally at the site of disease. The plaque is then separated from the vessel wall in the direction of the arteriotomy and removed.

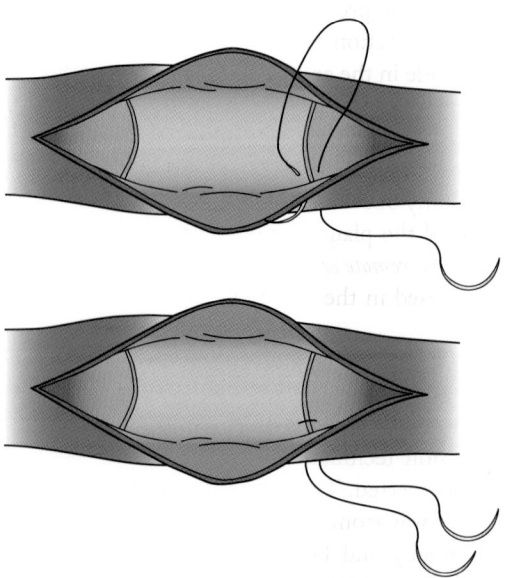

Figure 83-33 Endarterectomy plaque is tacked using multiple interrupted sutures, with one end of the suture placed 1 mm distal to the endpoint and the other end placed at the junction of the endarterectomy and the endarterectomized surface.

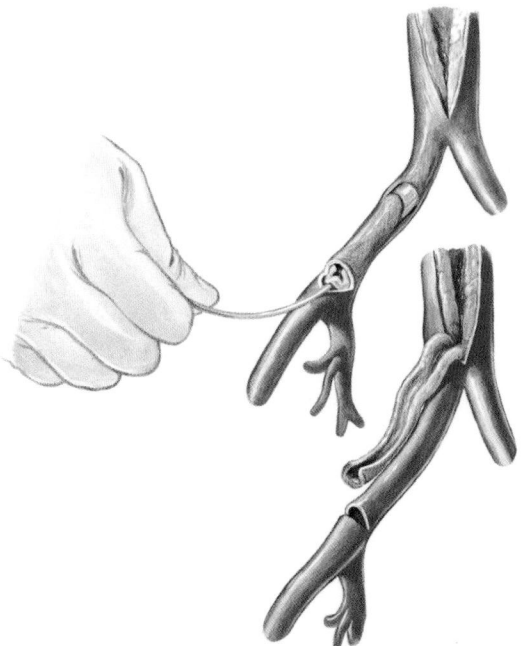

Figure 83-34 Plaque is cored out as a cylinder from the intervening segment, with the help of special ringed intra-arterial strippers.

Semiclosed Endarterectomy

The semiclosed endarterectomy was designed to avoid opening the artery longitudinally for the full extent of disease and thus circumvent a long arteriotomy closure. Typically, the artery is opened in a proximal and a distal location. The plaque is first dissected and transected at the proximal level; then it is cored out as a cylinder from the intervening segment with the help of special ringed intra-arterial strippers, transected again at the level of the distal arteriotomy, and removed (Fig. 83-34). With this technique, closure of what would have been a long arteriotomy is replaced by closure of two small arteriotomies, one proximally and one distally.

In one modification of the semiclosed technique, only one incision is made in the artery. The plaque is crushed manually or with the help of a clamp at the other end, eliminating the need for the second arterial incision, which is usually used to transect the plaque. The disadvantage of this technique is the unpredictability of the endpoint. Moll ring cutters allow sharp transection of the plaque from the remote site (Fig. 83-35), hence the term *remote endarterectomy*. This technique has been successfully used in the external iliac and superficial femoral arteries.

Eversion Endarterectomy

In the eversion technique, the artery is transected and the vessel wall is everted. The adventitia is held with forceps and gently lifted away from the plaque. A plaque core is developed circumferentially and held firmly with the forceps. As the plaque is being extracted from the artery, the adventitia is retracted backward and the artery is pushed forward from within, causing the plaque to protrude and be separated from the outer arterial media and adventitia (Fig. 83-36). It is then

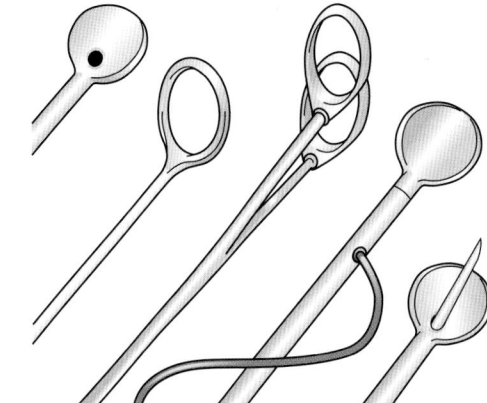

Figure 83-35 Moll ring cutters, spatula, and reentry needle system.

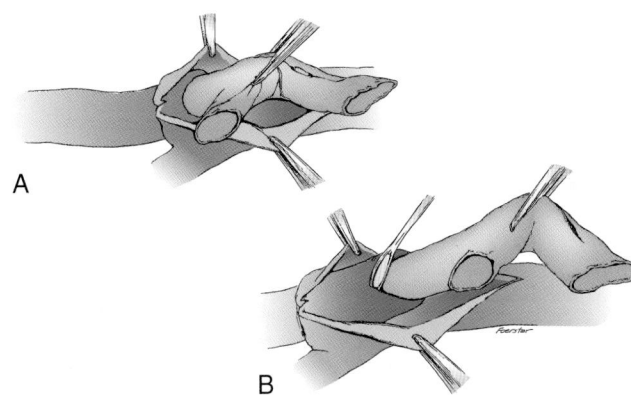

Figure 83-36 A and **B,** As the plaque is being pulled out of the artery, the adventitia is retracted backward and the artery is pushed forward from within, causing the plaque to protrude and allowing it to be extracted from the artery.

transected when an appropriate endpoint is reached. This technique requires mobilization of the proximal artery to allow eversion.

Orificial and Extraction Endarterectomy

Orificial endarterectomy is a modification of the eversion technique used to treat occlusive disease at the orifice of an artery. Typically, the orifice of the artery has been exposed through the lumen of the vessel (Fig. 83-37). The plaque is extruded from the orifice by pushing the artery distal to the plaque toward the orifice in an everting manner.

In extraction endarterectomy, a clamp is introduced into the orifice and used to grab the distal plaque or plaque remnant and extract it from the lumen. Generally, this technique is applicable only if the plaque ends a short distance beyond the orifice. Furthermore, because the endpoint is not under direct vision, it must be carefully assessed intraoperatively to ensure that a distal flap has not been created after restoring blood flow.

Endarterectomy in Specific Conditions

For approaches to endarterectomy in specific vessels and for specific conditions, such as carotid, arch, visceral, aortoiliac,

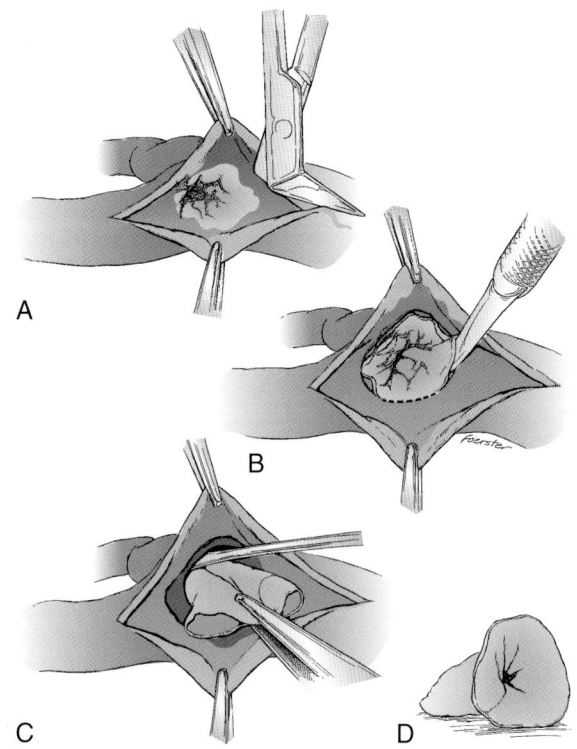

Figure 83-37 A–D, Orificial endarterectomy is a modification of the eversion technique used to treat occlusive disease at the orifice of an artery.

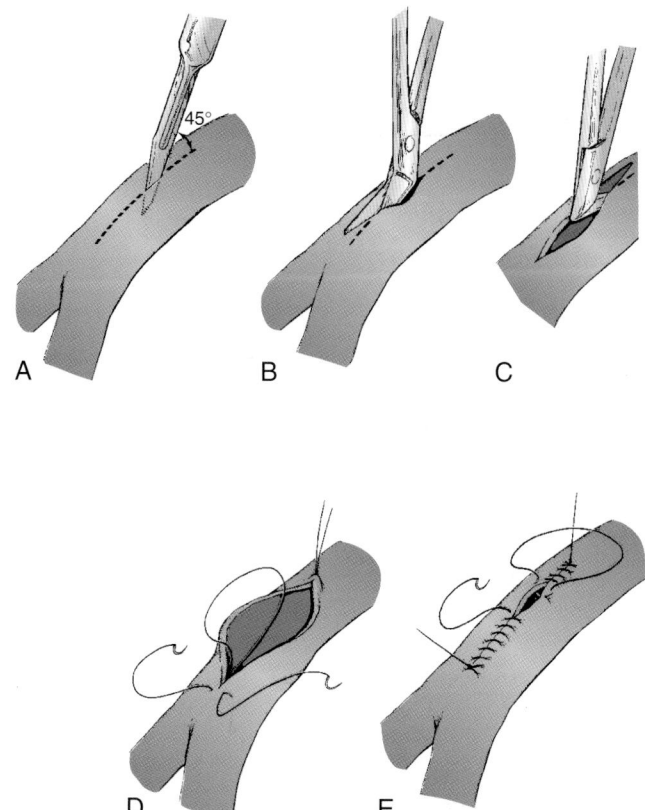

Figure 83-38 A–E, Primary closure is performed most expeditiously using a continuous running suture technique.

and infrainguinal disease, see Appendices 1 and 2 on the Expert Consult Web site.

ARTERIOTOMY CLOSURE

An arteriotomy can be closed either primarily or with a patch. The choice of a closure method depends on various factors, including the size of the artery, the direction and shape of the arteriotomy, and the degree of atherosclerotic involvement of the artery.

Primary Closure

Primary closure of an arteriotomy is a simple method that can be performed expeditiously. Most transverse arteriotomies in nondiseased arteries can be closed primarily. This can even be done in smaller arteries measuring 2 mm in diameter, such as a radial or posterior tibial artery. Similarly, primary closure can be performed in longitudinal incisions if the vessel is not diseased and has a diameter greater than 5 mm. A typical example is closure of a longitudinal arteriotomy in the common carotid artery or common femoral artery. Some narrowing of the lumen can be expected to occur with primary closure. Such narrowing should be minimal when the arteriotomy is transverse, but it can be significant if smaller arteries (<5 mm) are closed longitudinally.

Primary closure is most expeditiously performed using a continuous running suture technique (Fig. 83-38). A basic

concept in the placement of arterial sutures during closure is to include all layers of the vessel wall. Adventitial fibers should be trimmed and not allowed to protrude into the lumen because they can be thrombogenic. The needle is preferentially introduced from the intimal side of the vessel toward the adventitial side, "inside to outside." In the presence of atherosclerotic plaque, a needle introduced from the adventitial side can push the plaque away from the arterial wall and create a site for dissection or thrombus formation.

In the continuous suture technique, the needle is introduced from the adventitial surface of one wall and then from the intimal surface of the opposite wall. For the reasons already cited, it is important that the arterial wall at the incision site and site of closure be free of plaque. Thus, primary closure with a continuous suture is most suitable in disease-free arteries, endarterectomized vessels, prosthetic bypasses, or veins. The bites should be evenly placed throughout the length of the suture line, and the depth and advancement should be carefully monitored. Bites placed too deep can result in focal narrowing of the lumen.

In the presence of atherosclerotic plaque at the arteriotomy site, primary closure may still be possible; however, an interrupted suture technique is preferable. When closing transverse arteriotomies, interrupted sutures can be placed individually and then tied after all are placed, to allow better visualization of each suture placement (Fig. 83-39). This allows placement of all the sutures with the needle being

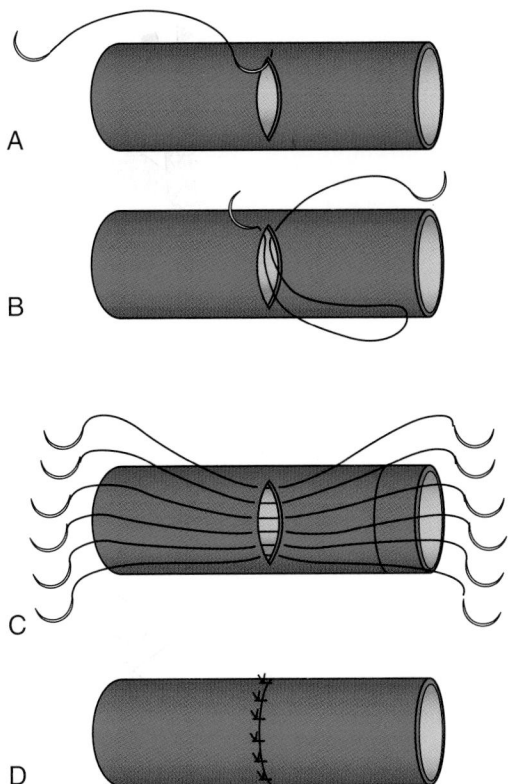

Figure 83-39 A–D, An interrupted suture technique is preferable in the presence of significant plaque.

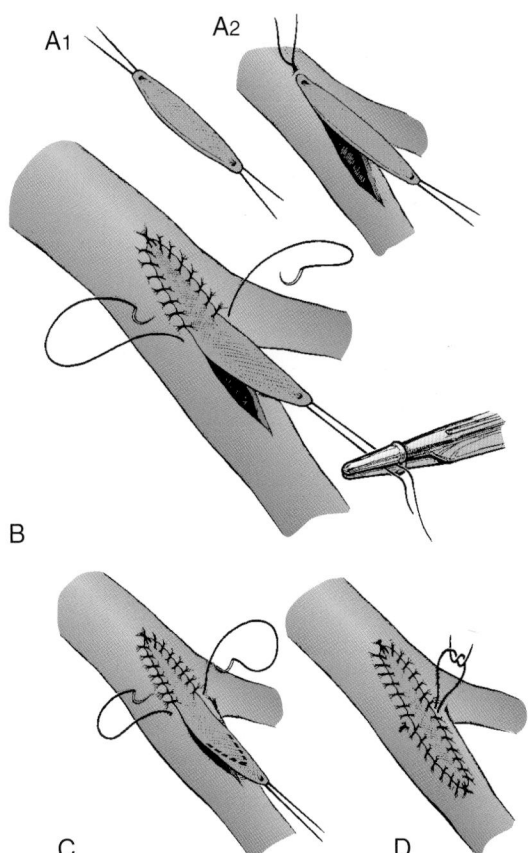

Figure 83-40 A–D, The simplest technique is to place one suture on each apex of the patch and run both sutures on each side of the patch.

introduced from the intimal side and exiting from the adventitial side of the vessel.

Patch Closure

When primary closure is expected to cause significant luminal narrowing of an arteriotomy, patch closure should be performed. Several technical and nontechnical factors may play a role in the decision to perform patch closure. Technical factors include an artery less than 5 mm in diameter, the presence of significant atherosclerotic plaque at an arteriotomy site, a jagged arteriotomy, or a very tortuous artery. Furthermore, if there is loss of area in the vessel wall or an obstructing pathology that cannot be excised, such as neointimal hyperplasia, closure with a patch is indicated. Nontechnical factors include risk factors that predispose to restenosis, such as hyperlipidemia, heavy smoking, female gender, and a history of recurrent stenosis. The advantage of patch closure is that it allows the needle to be introduced constantly from the adventitial aspect of the patch and then from the intimal aspect of the arterial wall. This eliminates the possibility of pushing a plaque fragment into the arterial lumen and precipitating thrombosis or dissection. Patch closure also allows adequate arterial purchase in the patch and in the artery without compromising the lumen. Nevertheless, the bites should be placed carefully, with matching depth and even advancement. Otherwise, undesirable lumen narrowing may occur.

When performing patch closure, the width of the patch should be selected to accommodate the vessel size. An overly wide patch can result in aneurysmal dilatation and excessive redundancy in the arterial patch lumen and act as a nidus for thrombus formation.

Several techniques can be used for closure of a patch. The simplest technique is to place one suture on each apex of the patch and run both sutures on each side of the patch (Fig. 83-40). Alternatively, when suturing in a deep location, the patch can be closed using a parachute technique. In a parachute closure, suturing is started at the apex or a few bites off the apex without tying of the suture (Fig. 83-41). Suturing is continued until approximately three bites are placed on both sides of the center of the apex. The patch is then pulled down while intermittent tension is applied to the suture line.

Closure of a Transected Vessel

The method used to close a transected vessel depends on its size and intraluminal pressure. Small arterial and venous branches are typically controlled by simple ligature with nonabsorbable suture material or the use of metal clips. Vessels with diameters ranging from 3 to 5 mm are usually controlled by suture ligatures, especially if the vessel is short. Larger vessels are typically closed with a running nonabsorbable suture. If the vessel has a low intraluminal pressure, such as

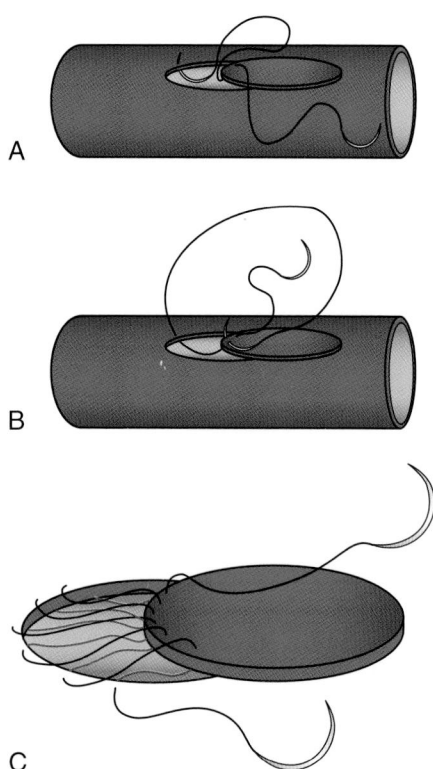

Figure 83-41 A–C, In a parachute closure, the suturing can be started at the apex or a few bites off the apex without tying of the suture.

in a large transected vein or the distal end of a transected artery, an over-and-over continuous running suture is usually sufficient to secure hemostasis. However, if the vessel is the proximal end of a transected artery, a single row of continuous sutures may not be adequate. This is especially true when closing an aortic stump after the removal of an infected aortic prosthesis. In such situations, two rows of sutures are preferred to secure hemostasis. The first row is usually constructed using horizontal mattress sutures, which can be placed using a continuous or an interrupted technique. The second layer is typically a continuous over-and-over running suture. The proximal row is meant to decrease the pressure and tension on the distal suture line (Fig. 83-42).

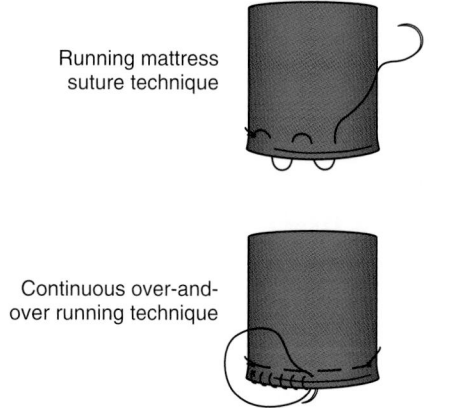

Running mattress
suture technique

Continuous over-and-
over running technique

Figure 83-42 The first row is performed using a running mattress suture technique. The second row is completed using a continuous over-and-over running technique.

REPLACEMENT AND BYPASS PROCEDURES

Vascular replacement or bypass procedures are typically performed to manage occlusive disease or to replace aneurysmal or destroyed vessels. A variety of anastomotic techniques are employed in these procedures. The technique selected depends on the procedure, the vascular pathology, and the anatomic location of the operative field.

Basic Considerations

When creating a bypass to treat lower extremity occlusive disease, the reconstruction should be performed with preservation of the existing circulation. As a result, the proximal and distal anastomoses are typically performed in an end-to-side manner. Such a configuration allows the maintenance of antegrade flow at the level of the proximal anastomosis. Ideally, the distal anastomosis is placed in a disease-free segment of the vessel distal to the occlusive pathology. An end-to-side configuration at the distal anastomosis allows the maintenance of retrograde flow through all patent branches (Fig. 83-43).

Occasionally, atherosclerotic disease in the artery requires the creation of an anastomosis with an end-to-end configuration. When treating aneurysmal disease, the aneurysm is typically replaced by interposing a new conduit using end-to-end anastomoses. Aneurysmal pathology is sometimes treated by an end-to-side bypass proximal and distal to the aneurysm and ligation of the aneurysm, as is done for popliteal artery aneurysms.

End-to-Side Anastomosis

An important step in constructing an end-to-side anastomosis is to align the vessels without a twist or kink. The bypass should be prepared such that the posterior incision in the bypass is parallel to the long axis of the bypass graft; otherwise, a buckle effect may develop at the anastomosis. Anastomotic failure is more likely to be caused by technical imperfections than by the dimensions of the anastomosis.[6] The ideal arteriotomy length is poorly defined and is influenced by the bypass diameter. Some recommend that the length be twice the bypass diameter.[3] Others recommend an arteriotomy greater than 2 cm.[7,8] In coronary artery–vein bypass, a short arteriotomy (4 to 6 mm) is usually recom-

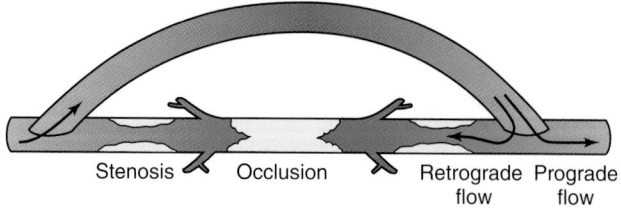

Stenosis   Occlusion   Retrograde   Prograde
                                       flow   flow

Figure 83-43 End-to-side configuration at the distal anastomosis allows the maintenance of retrograde flow through patent branches.

mended.[9] Most often, an arteriotomy measuring 1.2 to 2 times the graft diameter is created. The bypass is transected, and then a slit matching the arteriotomy is made in its posterior aspect. This allows spatulation of the graft end to minimize narrowing at the anastomosis. An arteriotomy shorter than 1.2 times the diameter of the graft results in the bypass's joining the artery at an unfavorably sharp angle. Too long an arteriotomy requires more time for construction, with no proven additional benefits. An end-to-side anastomosis can be performed using an anchor or parachute technique.

Anchor Technique

In the anchor technique, the anastomosis is constructed by first placing a suture at the heel of the bypass and the arteriotomy. The suture is tied, thus stabilizing and anchoring the graft at the heel of the anastomosis. Suturing is continued on one side of the heel to the toe, then halfway down the other side of the anastomosis. The anastomosis is completed by suturing the other end of the heel suture until it meets the previously placed suture (Fig. 83-44). An alternative is to start another suture at the apex and run it in a continuous manner on both sides of the apex toward the heel to complete the anastomosis.

There are numerous other variations of the end-to-side anastomosis. The anchoring sutures placed at the apex or the heel can be either simple or mattress sutures. However, in small vessels, mattress sutures at the apex or the heel may cause narrowing of the lumen. Another option is to place interrupted sutures at the apical part of the anastomosis (instead of a continuous suture line). The theoretical advantages of this variation include allowing the anastomosis to stretch with arterial pulsations and not be limited by the length of the continuous suture line. Further, the needle tip in a running suture can become blunted from repetitive piercing, especially of calcified vessels.

The anchor technique is ideal for superficial vessels and larger arteries. The anchoring sutures facilitate traction and countertraction during the anastomotic procedure.

Parachute Technique

In the parachute variation of the end-to-side anastomosis, the sutures at the heel and the apex are not initially pulled down or tied. Suturing is started a few millimeters from the center of the heel. The bypass is typically held with forceps a few centimeters from the arteriotomy. This allows the placement of sutures in deep areas without the bypass's obscuring the suturing or interfering with suture placement. First, several bites are placed in the bypass and the arteriotomy until the challenging part of the anastomosis is completed. This usually requires a total of three sutures on each side of the center of the heel. Tension is then applied on both ends of the suture, and the bypass is slowly pulled toward the anastomosis, achieving a tight suture line (Fig. 83-45). It is important to avoid excessive, continuous pulling on the suture line during this step because it could result in tearing of the arterial wall.

The parachute technique is especially useful if the vessels are small or in a deep location where visualization of the first few bites at the apex and heel may be suboptimal. Variations in the parachute technique relate to the site where the suture is started: it can be started exactly at the center of the heel or a few bites off-center. The technique of starting a few bites off-center can be challenging to learn. However, with experience, it may become the surgeon's preferred method of performing an end-to-side anastomosis.

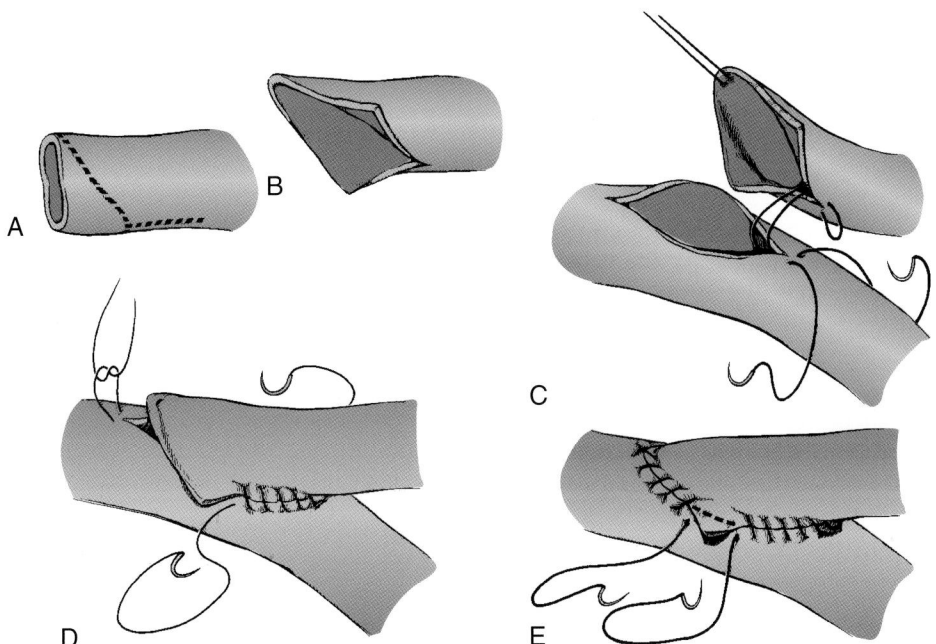

Figure 83-44 A–E, End-to-side anastomosis anchor technique.

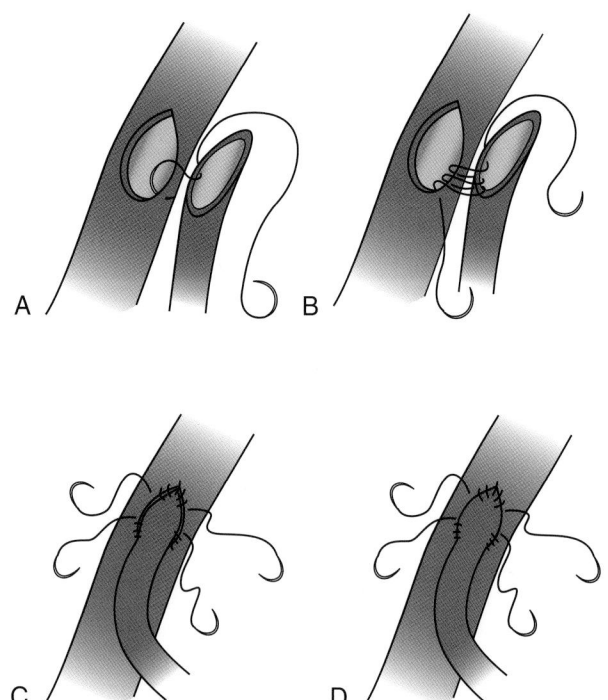

Figure 83-45 A–D, Parachute technique—another variation of the end-to-side anastomosis.

End-to-End Anastomosis

An end-to-end anastomosis is typically performed for replacement of an arterial segment, such as an aneurysmal artery or a vessel that has been destroyed by trauma. An end-to-end anastomosis is also constructed when a composite bypass is needed or when preservation of retrograde or antegrade flow is not essential.

The technique varies, depending on the size of the vessels and their mobility. When constructing an end-to-end anastomosis between two large vessels of comparable diameters, the transection of the vessels and the anastomotic suture line are usually in a plane perpendicular to the long axis of the vessel. If both segments are freely movable, a number of techniques have been developed to simplify suturing in a forward manner, maintaining the most favorable angle for suture placement.

One technique involves placing two diametrically opposed sutures in an anterior and posterior part of the vessel. The sutures are tied, and the anterior part of the anastomosis is constructed first. The vessels are then flipped 180 degrees, placing the posterior wall in an anterior location for completion of the anastomosis (Fig. 83-46). This technique is a modification of the triangulation method first described by Carrell. In the triangulation technique, the anastomosis is divided into three parts rather than anterior and posterior parts (Fig. 83-47).

When the segments are not freely movable, such as when constructing an anastomosis for aortic aneurysmal disease, the back wall is sutured first with a continuous suture using a parachute or an anchor technique, based on the depth of the anastomosis and the surgeon's preference (Fig. 83-48). When

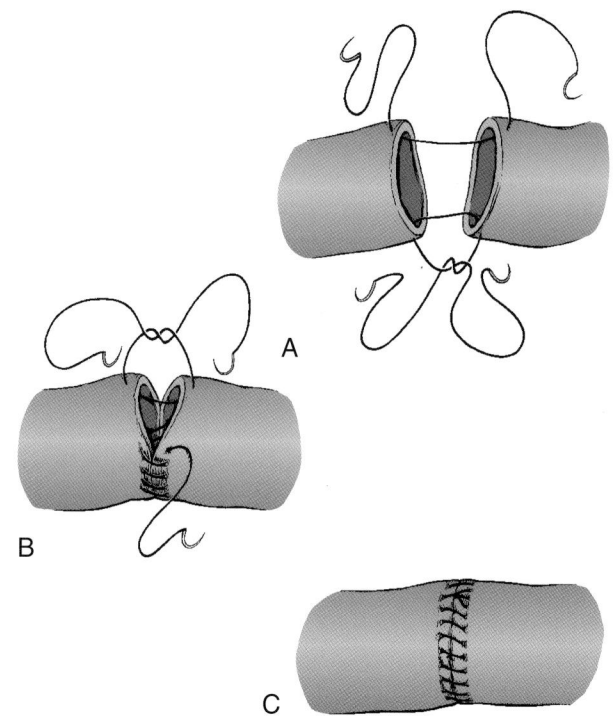

Figure 83-46 A–C, End-to-end anastomosis in large, movable vessels. The vessels are then flipped 180 degrees, placing the posterior wall in an anterior location for completion of the anastomosis.

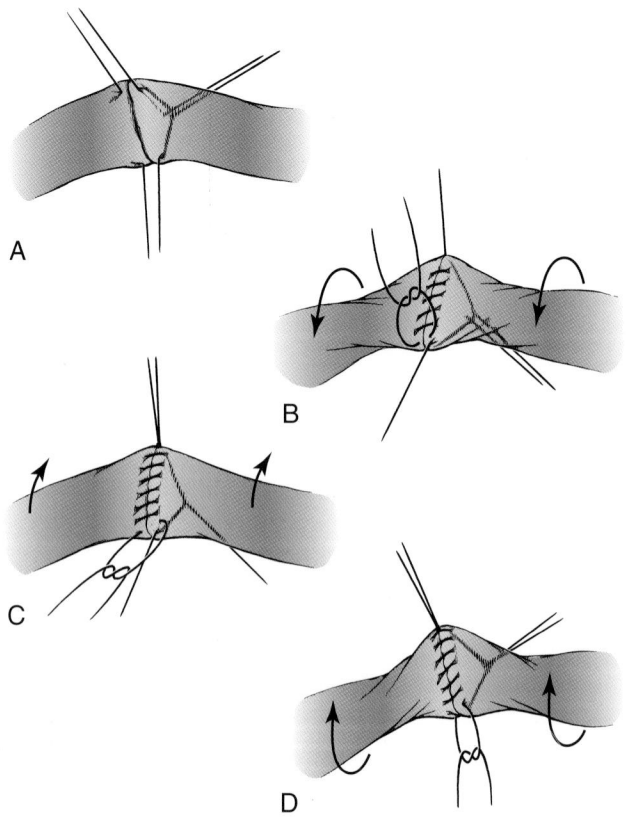

Figure 83-47 A–D, End-to-end anastomosis using the triangulation method.

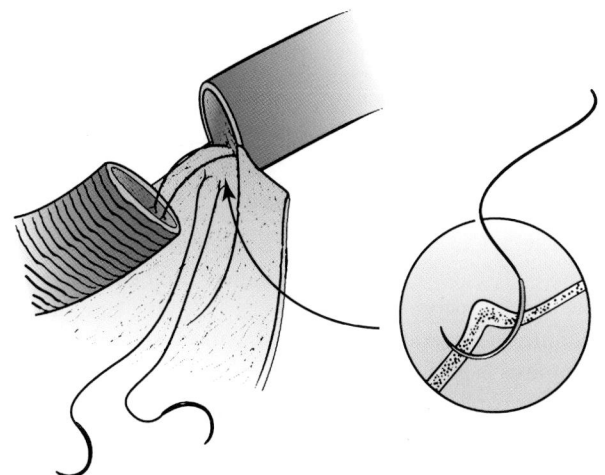

Figure 83-48 When the segments are not freely movable, such as when constructing an anastomosis for aortic aneurysmal disease, the back wall is sutured first with a continuous suture. It is essential to take deep bites because shallow bites may tear.

the back wall is left intact, suturing involves placing a double-layer bite in the posterior wall of the aorta. It is essential to take deep bites; shallow bites may miss the adventitia and do not provide the strength needed to hold the aortic anastomosis.

When constructing an end-to-end anastomosis between two small vessels, it is essential to spatulate the anastomosis to avoid compromising the lumen. Thus, both segments are transected in an oblique manner, and the incision is extended posteriorly. An anchoring suture is started at the center of the heel and continued on each side of it (Fig. 83-49). The suturing may be continued around the apex. Alternatively, another suture is started at the apex and continued on both sides of the apex toward the heel to complete the anastomosis.

Side-to-Side Anastomosis

A side-to-side anastomosis is rarely performed. It can be used, however, to create a side-to-side radiocephalic arteriovenous fistula for chronic hemodialysis or a side-to-side arteriovenous fistula distal to an infrainguinal prosthetic bypass as an adjunctive procedure to improve graft patency by decreasing outflow resistance.[10] A side-to-side configuration can also be used in the construction of a second anastomosis in a sequential bypass for limb revascularization. To perform a side-to-side anastomosis, the vessels need to be dissected and mobilized so they lie adjacent to each other with minimal tension. The anastomosis is created by longitudinal arteriotomy or venotomy where the walls come in direct contact. The posterior wall of the anastomosis is typically constructed first. The anastomosis is usually 6 to 10 mm long.

Adjunctive Techniques for Infrainguinal Bypass Anastomosis

T-Junction

A useful technique to facilitate the construction of an anastomosis in infrainguinal vein bypass is the T-junction technique (Fig. 83-50). In this method, a side branch in the vein is identified. The vein is transected 5 to 10 mm from the branch and then slit along the posterior wall in a fashion to incorporate the side branch in the anastomosis. The shape of that segment of vein looks like a "T." This can be used at the proximal or distal anastomosis and is helpful in minimizing sharp angulation of the bypass and narrowing at the heel of the anastomosis.

Saphenofemoral Junction Vein Cuff

When constructing a greater saphenous vein bypass, the vein can be transected at the saphenofemoral junction with a 1-mm rim of femoral vein (Fig. 83-51). This technique

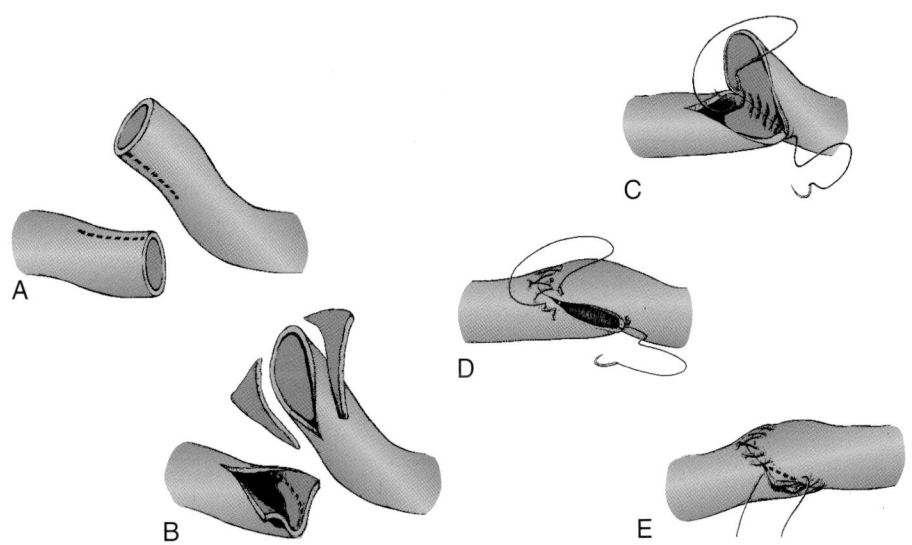

Figure 83-49 A–E, Spatulated end-to-end anastomosis between two small vessels.

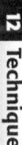

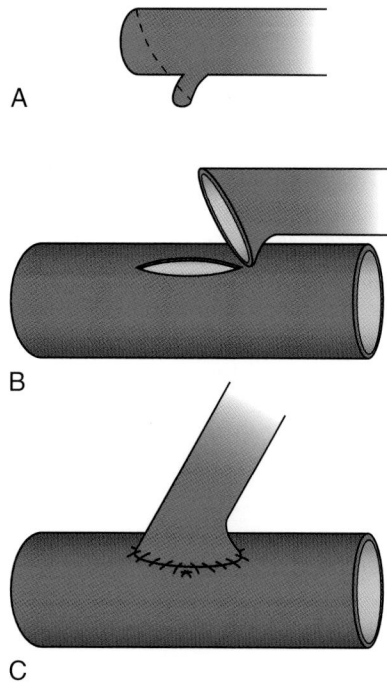

Figure 83-50 A–C, T-junction technique.

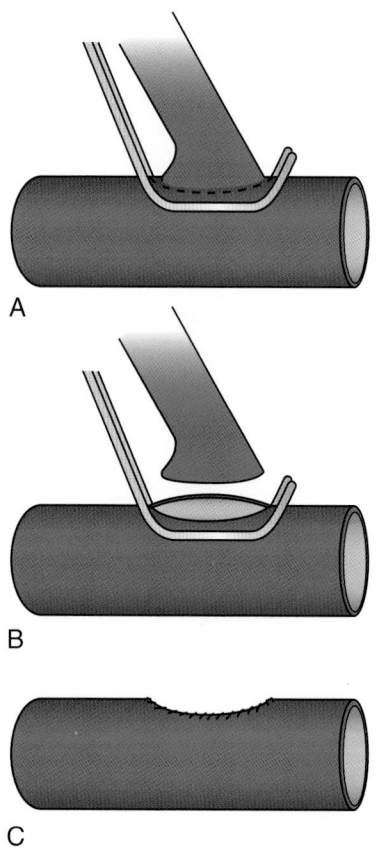

Figure 83-51 A–C, Saphenofemoral junction technique.

provides a large venous hood for construction of the anastomosis, especially if the artery is thickened and the vein is relatively small.

Linton's Patch, Taylor's Patch, and Miller's Cuff Angioplasty

In an attempt to improve the patency of prosthetic bypasses to infrageniculate vessels, a vein segment can be incorporated in the distal anastomosis (Fig. 83-52).[10-13] In the Linton patch technique, the arteriotomy is closed with a vein patch, and the anastomosis is performed between the graft and the patch. In the Taylor patch technique, the graft is sutured to the artery; then a vein patch angioplasty is performed at the apex of the anastomosis.[14] In the Miller cuff technique, a vein segment is interposed as a cuff between the graft and the artery.[15]

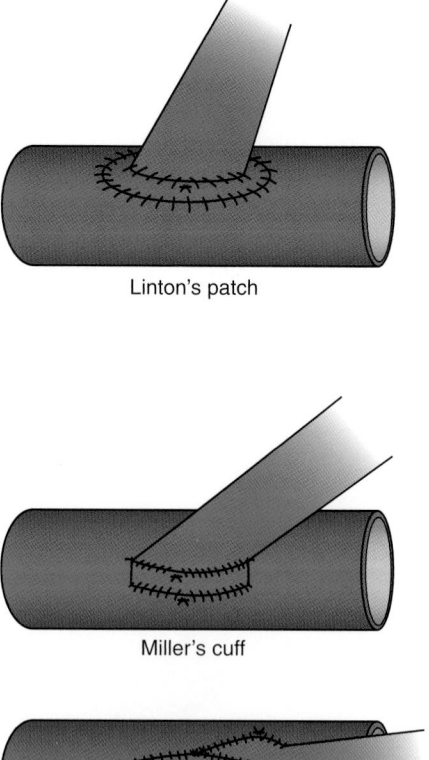

Linton's patch

Miller's cuff

Taylor's patch

Figure 83-52 Venous cuff at the distal anastomosis of prosthetic grafts; Linton's patch, Miller's cuff, and Taylor's patch.

SELECTED KEY REFERENCES

Henry AK. *Extensile Exposure.* 3rd Revised ed. New York: Churchill Livingston, 1995.
This reference (now out of print) provides a wide variety of unusual exposures, some of them of historic in nature, to increase the armamentarium of the vascular surgeon.

Hoballah JJ. *Vascular Reconstructions: Anatomy, Exposures, and Techniques.* New York: Springer-Verlag; 2000.
This atlas provides a short review of vascular anatomy with simple illustrations of vascular exposures, along with detailed, step-by-step illustrations of vascular reconstructions.

Rutherford RB. *Atlas of Vascular Surgery: Basic Techniques and Exposures.* Philadelphia: W B Saunders; 1993.
This atlas, with sections on basic techniques and vascular exposures, provides clear artistic illustrations of common vascular exposures and basic vascular techniques.

Valentine RJ, Wind GG. *Anatomic Exposures in Vascular Surgery.* 2nd ed. Philadelphia: Lippincott Williams & Wilkins; 2003.
This atlas provides a comprehensive, three-dimensional anatomic approach, with clear illustrations of basic and advanced vascular exposures.

REFERENCES

The reference list can be found on the companion Expert Consult Web site at *www.expertconsult.com.*

CHAPTER 84

Technique: Endovascular Diagnostic

Kim J. Hodgson and Douglas B. Hood

This chapter reviews the fundamental concepts related to the performance of diagnostic and therapeutic endovascular procedures. Specific indications, results, and complications are addressed elsewhere in this text. These guidelines concerning the characteristics and attributes of certain catheters, wires, and devices are only generalizations; each clinical situation is unique, with its own nuances. How a given catheter or guide wire (GW) will likely perform in a particular situation must take into account multiple variables, including the extent of tortuosity and angulation present, the working distances involved, and the characteristics of the target vessel or lesion, among many others. Ultimately, the selection of a particular endovascular tool boils down to judgment, which comes only with experience. Once the basics are mastered, however, innovative applications of these techniques are possible, allowing increasingly complex situations to be successfully addressed.

■ ENTRY NEEDLES

There are two basic types of entry needles: single-wall and double-wall puncture types (Fig. 84-1).

Single-Wall Puncture Needles

The single-wall puncture needle is more familiar and more commonly used. It is a beveled, 18-gauge, thin-walled, hollow needle that typically accommodates a 0.035-inch GW. The

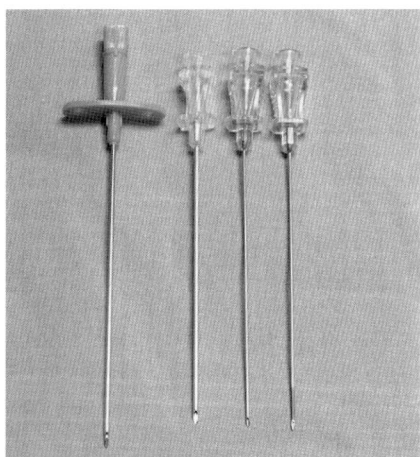

Figure 84-1 A double-wall puncture needle (*left*) and three single-wall puncture needles (*right*).

needle is advanced toward the target vessel until the anterior wall of the vessel is punctured and blood flow returns. A syringe may be attached to the hub of the needle, if desired, but most operators prefer to leave the hub uncapped, with pulsatile blood flow signifying successful entry into the artery. For venous punctures, however, gentle aspiration of an attached syringe may be necessary to get blood on entry into the target vein. Once adequate blood return is ascertained from the target vessel, needle position is stabilized. A soft-tipped GW is then advanced through the needle into the vessel lumen and directed toward the vascular bed of interest. Theoretically, blood return from the hub of the needle may occur while the beveled area is within the wall of the vessel rather than within its center. If the needle tip is partially within the arterial wall, subsequent wire passage may disrupt atherosclerotic plaque in the region and create a dissection plane. Therefore, it is critical to evaluate the quality of blood return through the needle to ascertain that central positioning of the needle tip within the vessel lumen is likely. If blood return is inconsistent or less than expected, gentle manipulation of the needle should be performed in an attempt to improve the quality of the flow before proceeding with guide-wire passage. Fluoroscopic observation of the GW's course is recommended if any resistance to wire advancement is met to ensure that the wire is following the presumed course of the entry vessel. An abnormal course or deflection of the GW tip should prompt reassessment of the situation. The importance of doing this cannot be overemphasized because it minimizes vascular injury not only at the puncture site but also farther along the course of the GW. Similarly, sheaths, catheters, or other devices should never be advanced over the entry GW until radiographic evaluation has confirmed that the wire is properly positioned and follows a straight course.

Smaller, 21-gauge micropuncture needles are now available for a single-wall technique. Use of these smaller needles may reduce the risk of significant injury due to inadvertent puncture of surrounding structures. The smaller needles are typically packaged with a short, 0.018-inch GW and a 4 or 5 French (Fr) introducer with a coaxial dilator. Backbleeding from the smaller entry needle is usually less robust than that obtained after puncture with a standard entry needle. After backbleeding is obtained, the GW is advanced through the needle, and the needle is removed. The introducer and dilator are inserted over the wire, and then the dilator and wire are removed. The remaining introducer is large enough to accommodate a standard 0.035- or 0.038-inch GW, over which a standard working sheath can be inserted. Alternatively, if only a diagnostic catheter is required, a 4 Fr diagnostic catheter can be inserted directly through a 5 Fr introducer. The 21-gauge entry needles are also available with echogenic tips, which make visualization easier during ultrasound-guided vessel puncture.

Double-Wall Puncture Needles

Double-wall puncture needles are two-component systems that combine a blunt-tipped hollow needle with a bevel-tipped stylet that projects slightly from the end of the needle. The double-wall puncture technique involves the intentional passage of the needle-stylet assembly through both walls of the vessel until it contacts the underlying bone. The stylet is then removed, and the remaining outer needle is slowly withdrawn until blood return is noted. The rationale for using a double-wall technique is that blood return from the blunt-tipped needle may indicate a higher likelihood of central lumen positioning, with a lower incidence of GW-induced vessel dissection or injury. However, because a lower incidence of vessel injury has not been well documented, and because it involves the unnecessary puncture of the posterior wall of the vessel, the double-wall technique has not been widely adopted by vascular surgeons. Most prefer the single-wall puncture technique, with its instantaneous feedback from blood return at the time the vessel is punctured.

■ GUIDE WIRES

GWs serve the basic function of facilitating the positioning of diagnostic catheters and therapeutic devices at particular locations. The GW characteristics required to achieve this function depend on the unique anatomic circumstances of a given situation, as well as the nature of the task. To meet these varying requirements, GWs are available in a variety of diameters and lengths and with an assortment of tip shapes, different degrees of tip and shaft stiffness, and antifriction coatings. Additional variables to consider when selecting a wire include radiopacity and the presence of calibration markers along the wire shaft.

Components

Classic GWs have two components: an inner wire called a mandrel and an outer stainless steel coil wrap. The mandrel, or core, which imparts the quality of wire stiffness, usually tapers toward the tip to produce a soft, atraumatic leading edge. The mandrel is typically bonded to the outer coil to prevent separation of these components. Also available are wires in which the inner mandrel is movable, allowing the length of the soft leading edge of the GW to be shortened or lengthened by alternately advancing or retracting its inner core (movable core wires). With infusion wires, the inner mandrel can be completely removed, allowing the channel to be used for the slow infusion of dilute contrast material or therapeutic substances such as thrombolytic drugs.

Tip Shape

To be used successfully, the GW must be manipulated into the desired location without traumatizing the vessel. Tip shape plays a major role in this function. J-tipped configurations are the least traumatic and the least likely to dissect or perforate blood vessels, but these wires may also be the least likely to negotiate a tight stenosis. The most common J-wires have either a 1.5-mm or a 3-mm radius of curvature, resulting in wires that lead with a 3-mm or a 6-mm prow, respectively. GWs are also available with straight or angled tips. In addition, it may be possible to alter the shape of a wire tip by bending it over a thumbnail. Having a shaped tip gives the GW directionality, the ability to steer the leading end of the wire and facilitate its passage into selected branch vessels. Torqueability, which refers to the degree of correlation between the rotation of the ex vivo shaft of the wire by the operator and the corresponding rotation of the in vivo tip of the wire, can also vary among different types of wires. Disposable torque devices designed to grip the wire and facilitate manipulation are frequently used, especially with hydrophilic wires that may be difficult to grip. Regardless of shape, most GW tips are fairly floppy over a distance of 3 to 8 cm, a feature designed to minimize the risk of vessel dissection and perforation. When inserting a GW, one must be certain to lead with the soft tip rather than with the stiffer back end.

Coating

Many GWs in use today have a hydrophilic antifriction coating, often Teflon, to facilitate wire placement and catheter exchanges. It is important to keep all wires clean by wiping them down with a damp gauze pad after each catheter exchange, thereby preventing blood from drying on the wire and hindering catheter passage. It is especially important to keep hydrophilic wires damp because they are slippery when wet, minimizing friction between the wire and catheter; they become sticky when dry, making exchanges difficult. Hydrophilic wires should be wet-wiped before each catheter exchange to reduce the risk of losing wire position during the exchange. It is recommended that hydrophilic wires not be used through entry needles during the initial access procedure owing to the risk of shearing the coating.[1-3]

Stiffness

The ability of a GW to support subsequent catheter passage, particularly around multiple turns, depends largely on the stiffness of the wire shaft. To some extent, stiffness is a function of GW diameter, but within a given size category, there is a range of stiffness. In general, to reduce the risk of vessel injury, it is best to choose the most flexible wire that provides sufficient support to achieve the desired catheter or device position, bearing in mind that larger and stiffer devices, such as stents and endoluminal grafts, may require stiffer wires to reliably negotiate even normal vessel tortuosity. If a GW alone provides insufficient support to achieve the desired catheter position, external support can be provided by an appropriately shaped guiding catheter or guiding sheath.

Length

GWs are generally available in two length ranges. Standard lengths range from 145 to 180 cm. Standard lengths are useful for positioning catheters but may not be long enough to permit catheter exchanges. This maneuver, in which the wire tip is left in its desired position while one catheter is removed from the wire and replaced with another, requires a sufficient length of wire to permit complete withdrawal of the initial catheter without having to relinquish the position of the wire or lose contact with its ex vivo tail. In general, if the target lesion is within 50 to 60 cm of the vascular access site, a standard-length wire is sufficient to allow the exchange of standard catheters and devices. For lesions located farther from the access site, rapid exchange (monorail) devices can be used, or a longer wire can be placed. Exchange-length wires are typically in the 240- to 300-cm range. Some GWs have a "docking" feature that allows a standard-length wire to be transformed into an exchange-length wire by attaching an extension to the back end.

Diameter

GW diameter is specified in fractional inches, ranging from 0.010 to 0.052 inch, with 0.035 inch being the most commonly used size for peripheral vascular work (Table 84-1). With the ongoing trend to reduce device size, however, smaller 0.018- and 0.014-inch systems are increasingly common. GWs are just one component of the instrumentation system being used for a particular task, and one must anticipate several steps ahead during a procedure to select a wire of appropriate diameter that will be compatible with available catheters and devices. Although wires with diameters smaller than the lumen size of a catheter can be used through that catheter, the resultant diminution of support generally renders this an undesirable combination. The most common situation in which a smaller-than-maximum GW is used is when a larger catheter is being exchanged for a smaller catheter that would accommodate only the smaller GW or when pressure gradients are to be measured without losing wire access across the lesion. Occasionally, it may be desirable to inject radiographic contrast material (or another liquid) through a catheter while the GW remains in place. If a smaller-than-maximum GW is used, some of the catheter

lumen remains open to transmit dilute contrast material. However, achievable flow rates are small, and the resultant opacification is sometimes suboptimal. Unfortunately, attempting to compensate for the lower flow channel by infusing full-strength contrast material rarely improves the situation because the increased viscosity inhibits contrast flow through the small lumen.

Small-diameter wires are difficult to visualize under fluoroscopy, a problem that is sometimes addressed by using a highly radiopaque material such as gold or platinum at the tip. Similarly, some wires have radiopaque markers placed at fixed distances that allow calibration for subsequent measurement of vessel diameters.

Selection

Ultimately, GW selection is a function of the task and the given anatomic configuration. Initial diagnostic evaluation is generally performed using a GW that is least likely to cause injury to the vessel wall, such as a J-wire. If lesions are identified that may be amenable to endovascular therapy, it may be useful to switch to a calibrated wire for accurate sizing or to an angled- or straight-tipped wire to traverse the lesions. Working with relatively large or stiff devices or through tortuous vessels may mandate the use of a stiffer wire to get the device to track over the wire without dislodging its tip. In addition to these general guidelines, wire selection is often based on operator familiarity and experience, and the use of multiple wires to address different needs during a given case is not uncommon.

■ DIAGNOSTIC CATHETERS

Diagnostic catheters (DCs) are designed to facilitate the delivery of radiographic contrast material to specific areas of the vascular system, thereby allowing radiographic opacification of the flow channel of the target vessel. Several characteristics of DCs determine how each behaves and for what use it is best suited. Experience with various catheters is necessary to learn which ones work best in various settings (Table 84-2).

Although referred to as diagnostic catheters, these devices are also important for interventional procedures. For diagnostic studies, it is usually necessary only that the catheter tip be

Table 84-1 Endovascular Device Sizing

Device	Measurement Standard	Unit
Entry needle	Outer diameter	Gauge
Guide wire	Outer diameter	Inch
Sheath	Inner diameter	French
Guiding catheter	Outer diameter	French
Diagnostic catheter	Outer diameter	French

Table 84-2 Commonly Used Diagnostic Catheters

Vessel	Catheter Shape	Catheter Name
Contralateral iliac	Self-forming	Cobra 2, IMA, Pigtail, Omni Flush
	Manual-forming	Simmons 1 or 2
Renal, mesenteric	Self-forming	Cobra 2, RDC (renal double curve), SOS Omni
	Manual-forming	Simmons 1 or 2
Axillary, brachial	Self-forming	Kumpe, Cobra 2
Subclavian, carotid	Self-forming	Headhunter H1, Vitek
	Manual-forming	Simmons 1 or 2

engaged in the vessel origin to obtain good images. Interventional work frequently requires GW support well beyond the lesion being treated. Using the shape of the catheter to select a branch vessel allows for passage of a GW into that branch and beyond a lesion, facilitating its subsequent treatment. DCs are also commonly used to perform coil embolization of branch vessels. Similar to GWs, catheters are available with radiopaque markers placed at specified intervals to facilitate the calibration of measuring devices and subsequent measurements of vessel diameter or length.

Structure

Most DCs are made of polyethylene, which has good torqueability (i.e., twisting of the ex vivo portion of the catheter produces a similar degree of rotation of its in vivo tip) and pliability and holds its shape well. Nylon is often used in the construction of high-flow catheters, such as the pigtail, because nylon can withstand higher infusion pressures than polyethylene can. Polyurethane is a softer, more pliable material that yields catheters with poor torqueability but that track GWs well, although the higher coefficient of friction often mandates a friction-reducing coating on either the GW or the lumen of the catheter. To improve the torqueability of polyurethane catheters, a fine wire mesh is often incorporated into the catheter wall.

Characteristics

The primary difference among catheters is the particular shape the tip will assume (or can be made to assume) once it is intravascular and the leading GW has been removed. Other important characteristics include catheter stiffness, tip design, torque response, antifriction properties, and radiopacity. Catheters are typically available in 65- and 100-cm lengths, with the shorter lengths being suitable for placement in the abdominal and the proximal, contralateral lower extremity vessels from a femoral access site. The longer lengths are typically used for arch, brachiocephalic, and distal contralateral lower extremity work. Shorter catheters are available for procedures on hemodialysis access grafts, and longer catheters may be useful for contralateral tibial or cerebrovascular indications.

Diameter

DCs are sized by outer diameter in French units. The inner diameter is generally cited as maximum allowable wire diameter (in fractional inches) and is determined by the thickness of the catheter wall. DC sizes commonly used for peripheral indications range from 4 to 6 Fr and typically have inner diameters of 0.035 or 0.038 inch. Catheters as small as 2 or 3 Fr (microcatheters) can be advanced through the lumen of standard DCs for superselective work. Obviously, the lumen of such a small catheter accommodates a commensurately smaller GW and permits only relatively low contrast infusion rates.

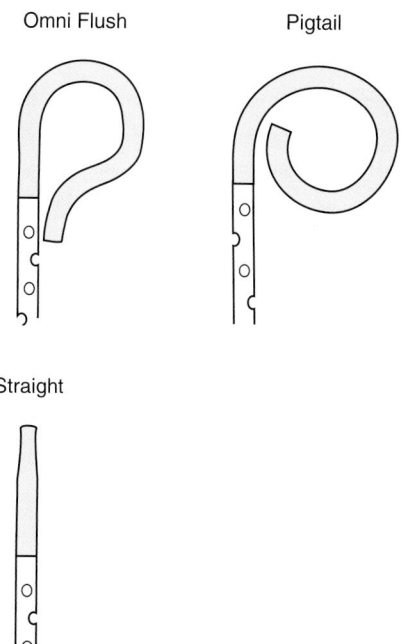

Figure 84-2 Commonly used nonselective diagnostic catheters. *(Courtesy of AngioDynamics, Queensbury, NY.)*

Type

Nonselective Catheters

Nonselective catheters (Fig. 84-2) are intended for contrast infusion in the aorta and vena cava. Generally, optimal visualization occurs when the catheter position is close to the area of interest, thereby maximizing contrast density in this region while minimizing opacification of adjacent, overlapping vessels. Although some nonselective catheters can be used in conjunction with GW support and direction to perform selective catheterization, this is not their primary function.

Nonselective catheters commonly have multiple side holes, allowing the rapid injection of contrast material into larger, high-flow vessels under the high pressure required to achieve adequate opacification. The multiple holes dissipate the stream of contrast, minimizing the potentially injurious "jet effect" of the injectate on the vessel wall if it were to come out of a single end hole. Further, the multiple sites of injection into the flow stream provide more uniform opacification of the target vessel. Virtually all multiple side-hole catheters are self-forming, meaning that they assume their shape spontaneously after removal of the GW when placed into vessels of adequate size.

Selective Catheters

Selective catheters (Fig. 84-3) are designed to engage the orifices of branch vessels and may be advanced farther out the selected vascular tree before contrast infusion. Ancillary uses for selective catheters include pullback pressure measurements, the instillation of pharmacologic agents (e.g., vasodila-

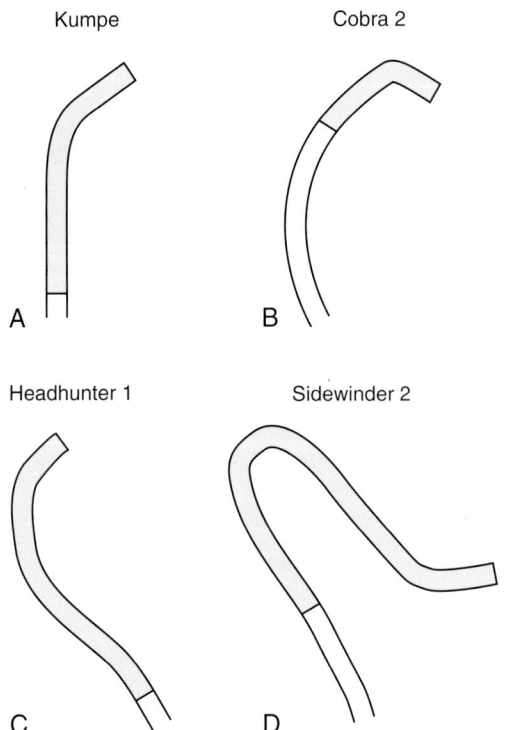

Figure 84-3 Typical selective diagnostic catheters. *(Courtesy of AngioDynamics, Queensbury, NY.)*

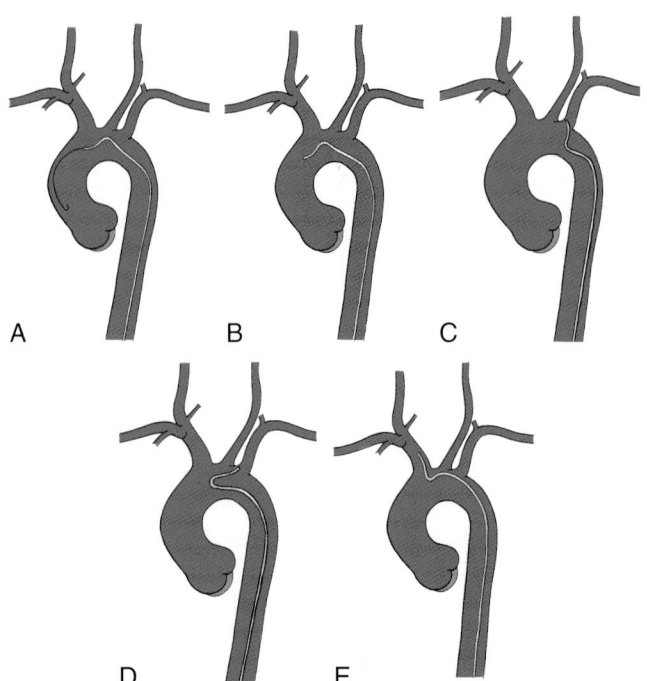

Figure 84-4 Side-branch technique for forming a Simmons catheter. **A,** The straightened catheter is advanced over a guide wire into the aortic arch. **B,** The wire is removed, but the catheter does not spontaneously assume a usable shape because the aortic diameter is too small. **C,** The catheter is rotated and retracted, engaging its tip in the orifice of the left subclavian artery. **D,** The catheter shaft is then advanced with the tip engaged, causing the catheter to fold onto itself and assume its formed shape. **E,** In its formed shape, the Simmons catheter can be used to select a branch vessel without the use of a guide wire. The catheter is advanced under fluoroscopic visualization until its tip is seen deflecting into the branch. The catheter tip is then advanced by retracting the catheter shaft, thereby seating the tip deeper into the branch vessel.

tors, sclerosants), the delivery of embolic material (e.g., coil embolization), and sampling of blood from specific locations (e.g., renal vein renin sampling).

Selective catheters whose curves have an overall radius less than the diameter of the target vessel are generally self-forming and are useful for selecting the origins of a number of branch vessels (see Fig. 84-3A to C). Advancement of the catheter farther into the branch vessel is then performed over a GW. Selection of tip shape is largely dependent on the angulation of the branch of interest.

Selective catheters with a larger radius of curvature do not form spontaneously and need to be manipulated in vivo to assume their designated shape (see Fig. 84-3D). These catheters usually form U-turn configurations. Formation is usually accomplished by engaging the tip in a side branch while advancing the body of the catheter, effectively folding the catheter over on itself (Fig. 84-4). An alternative technique uses wire deflection off the aortic valve (Fig. 84-5). The aortic valve technique is simple to perform and has been well tolerated in our experience; however, one should be aware of the possibility of ectopy if the wire or catheter is advanced into the ventricle. The technique of forming catheters is difficult to explain but critical to master. There is a definite risk of plaque injury and embolization during such catheter manipulation; consequently, forming catheters should be done with extreme care.

Some catheters are shaped to advance deeper into side branches when they are pushed forward, while others are designed so that the tip advances deeper into the branch when the catheter shaft is withdrawn. The operator's challenge is

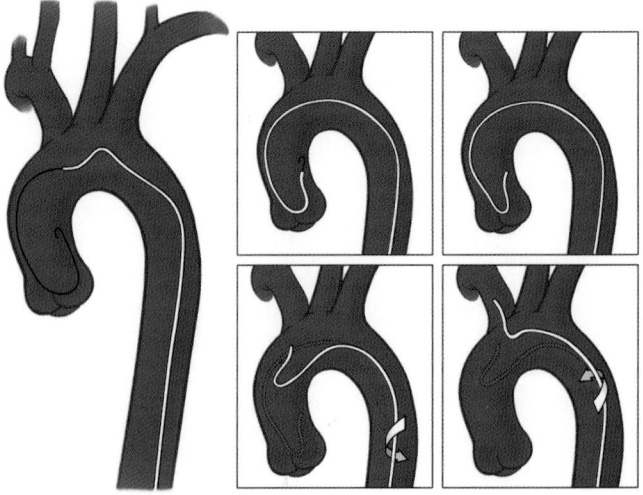

Figure 84-5 Technique of forming a Simmons catheter off the aortic valve.

to carefully analyze the orientation of the aorta and its relevant branches while performing all catheter manipulations under fluoroscopic guidance to reduce the risk of plaque dissection or perforation. One must consider the geometry of all the curves of a particular catheter and envision the shape the catheter will assume when confined by the walls of the vessel into which it is being inserted.

■ SHEATHS AND GUIDING CATHETERS

After vascular access has been achieved using an entry needle and GW, one must consider methods to secure and maintain the access site. If a purely diagnostic procedure is planned and multiple catheter and GW exchanges are unlikely, the size of the puncture wound can be minimized by using a full-length GW as the entry wire and simply advancing the DC directly into the vessel over that wire. This is a reasonable approach when all imaging can be performed through flush aortography (or cavography) without the need for selective catheterizations that require exchanging the pigtail for one or more selective catheters. Each catheter or GW exchange has the potential to traumatize the vessel puncture site by enlarging it, lifting an intimal flap, or both. Further, during each exchange, some blood escapes from the puncture, forming a localized hematoma that may compromise effective compression at the completion of the case. Therefore, unless the desired study can be accomplished with just one catheter and without undue manipulation, we generally recommend that an indwelling sheath be used. Because of the higher profile and irregular surface characteristics of balloon angioplasty catheters and stents, we consider use of a sheath mandatory for interventional procedures to prevent device-related vessel wall injury during exchanges.

Sheaths

Structure and Function

Sheaths are essentially access ports to the vascular system placed at the time of initial vascular access and removed after completion of the diagnostic or interventional procedure. All exchanges of GWs, DCs, and interventional catheters or devices are performed through the lumen of the sheath, which functions to maintain access to the vascular system while minimizing trauma to the vessel wall. Backbleeding from the sheath itself is prevented by a hemostatic valve located in its hub that provides a seal around introduced GWs and catheters (Fig. 84-6). There are limits, however, to the effectiveness of the hemostatic valve, particularly when very small GWs or non-coaxial devices are in place.

A useful feature of sheaths is a side-port connection that allows blood sampling, pressure monitoring, vasodilator administration, or contrast injection during the procedure (see Fig. 84-6). For example, if the entry GW cannot be passed all the way up the iliac at the time of initial vascular access, visualization of the cause of the obstruction can be helpful. Although injecting contrast medium directly through

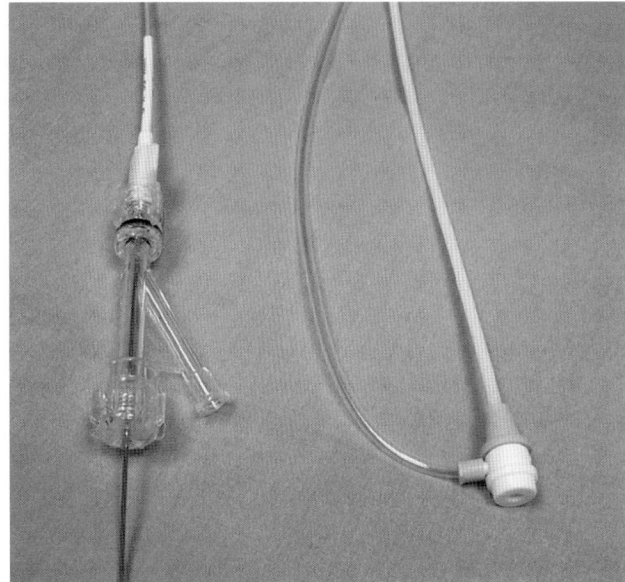

Figure 84-6 Y-adapter on a guiding catheter (*left*) and hemostatic valve of a sheath (*right*).

the entry needle may elucidate the nature of the obstruction, the relevant anatomy is often better visualized by inserting a sheath a limited distance into the vessel and injecting contrast material through the side port. Injection directly through the needle risks dislodgement of the needle, and its small diameter may not permit a sufficient volume of contrast material to be infused rapidly enough for adequate visualization.

Diameter

Sheaths are manufactured in an array of diameters (Fig. 84-7). The diameters most commonly used are 5 to 6 Fr because most diagnostic and balloon catheters are this size. Placement of stents frequently requires sheaths in the 6- to 8-Fr range, whereas iliac and superficial femoral artery (SFA) endografts require approximately 6 to 12 Fr sheaths, and aortic endografts require sheaths as large as 22 to 25 Fr. Nominal sheath size denotes its inner diameter, in contrast to catheters and

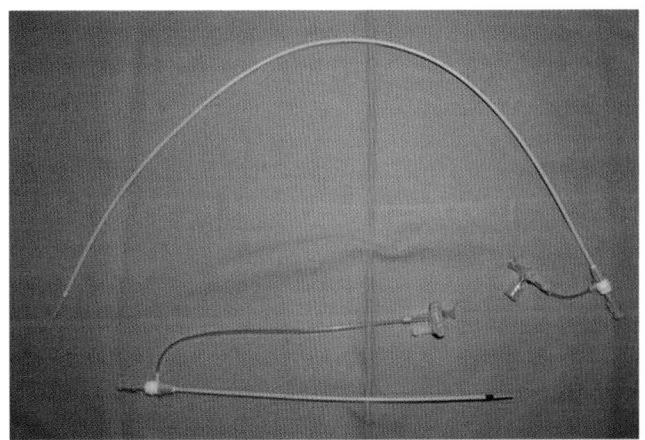

Figure 84-7 Vascular access sheaths.

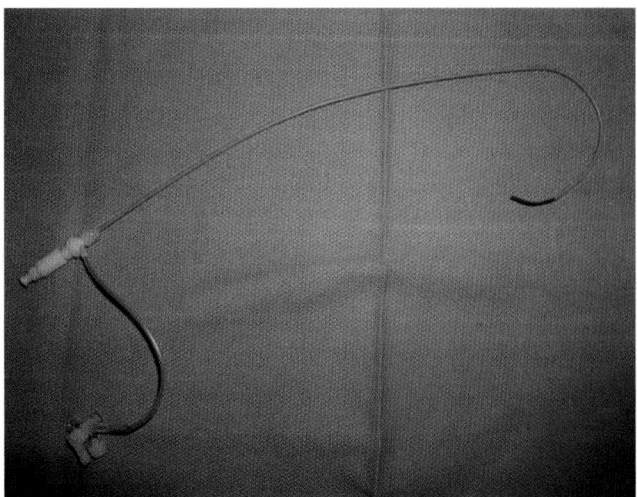

Figure 84-8 Sheath designed for placement across the aortic bifurcation.

other devices that are sized by the outer diameter. Accordingly, a 5 Fr sheath will admit a 5 Fr catheter. A standard 5 Fr sheath has a typical outer diameter of 6 or 7 Fr, which represents a 1 or 2 Fr increase in the size of the vessel puncture wound. In practice, this is not clinically significant, and the benefits of sheaths far outweigh this issue or their relatively modest cost.

Length

There are several basic ranges in sheath length: 3 to 5 cm, 10 to 12 cm, 22 to 25 cm, 30 to 40 cm, and 90 to 100 cm. The 10- to 12-cm length is standard for most peripheral vascular diagnostic and interventional procedures, and the 3- to 5-cm length is used primarily for dialysis access management. Sheaths in the midrange lengths are commonly used for procedures on the contralateral iliac or femoral arteries and the renal arteries. These sheaths may have preshaped tips or kink-resistant internal support to facilitate placement over the aortic bifurcation (Fig. 84-8). Some manufacturers place a radiopaque marker on the end of the sheath that facilitates visualization under fluoroscopic imaging. This is particularly valuable during interventional work when it is critical to know, for example, that the stent is completely outside the sheath before beginning deployment. The longest sheaths are used for interventional procedures on the carotid and contralateral tibial arteries.

Guiding Catheters

Guiding catheters (GCs) are similar to sheaths and perform essentially the same functions during endovascular interventions, but there are important differences. GCs typically do not have hemostatic valves or injection side ports at the ex vivo working end, although these options are available separately. Lengths are typically in the 40- to 100-cm range. GCs are not designed to secure initial vascular access but are intended to be placed through access sheaths and into the target vessel. GCs have preformed tips that aid in the selection of intended vessels. One important distinction is the standard system of sizing, which is different for sheaths and GCs. Like DCs, GCs are sized in French units by the outer diameter, with the inner diameter denoted in fractional inches (e.g., 0.086 inch). Consequently, a 6 Fr sheath accommodates a 6 Fr GC that typically has an inner (working) lumen diameter of 0.060 to 0.070 inch. Depending on the manufacturer's specifications, the inner diameter of a GC may accommodate a 1 or 2 Fr smaller catheter or device (e.g., a 6 Fr GC may accept a 4 or 5 Fr DC). Further, in contrast to sheaths, which come with tapered dilators that create a smooth transition from the GW to the sheath, most GCs have no tapered obturator. Consequently, there is a significant step-off between the wire and the GC (e.g., from the 0.035-inch outer diameter of the GW to the 0.105-inch outer diameter of a typical 8 Fr GC), which can easily snag atheromatous plaque or debris during unprotected passage. Even though most GCs have soft, pliable tips designed to minimize vascular trauma, it is advisable to observe their passage under fluoroscopy. Recently, manufacturers have begun to provide long, tapering obturators with some GCs, analogous to the dilators used within sheaths. Owing to their similarity of purpose, use of an interventional sheath or GC depends on operator selection and is largely a matter of personal preference. The following discussion of clinical applications uses the terms "sheath" and "catheter" interchangeably.

Clinical Applications

One use of sheaths or GCs during endovascular interventions is to provide a mechanism to angiographically evaluate the results of the intervention without losing access to the treated vessel. It is generally advisable that a lesion undergoing treatment remain traversed by a GW or catheter (referred to as "maintaining lesion crossing") at all times until a successful interventional result has been demonstrated. Sheaths allow for contrast injection into the target vessel while the balloon, GW, or both remain in position across the lesion.

Without the use of a sheath, angiographic evaluation of a balloon angioplasty or other endovascular intervention while maintaining lesion crossing is problematic and requires leaving the tip of a catheter just beyond the most distal aspect of the dilated area, removing the GW, and forcefully injecting contrast material through the GW channel of the balloon catheter. In most cases, a sufficient volume of contrast refluxes proximally and allows a general assessment of the adequacy of the intervention. If the result appears satisfactory, the catheter can be withdrawn to a position upstream of the lesion, and formal completion angiography is performed. If a problem is revealed that requires repeat dilatation after the lesion crossing has been surrendered, the lesion must be crossed again, which carries a significant risk of subintimal wire passage and plaque dissection. If lesion recrossing is attempted, it should be performed under fluoroscopic guidance and is most safely accomplished with a J-tipped wire.

An alternative method to assess results in the absence of a sheath and without relinquishing wire traversal is to exchange the standard GW for a smaller, undersized wire. Contrast material can then be injected through the wire lumen of a slightly withdrawn balloon using a Y-adapter at the balloon hub, with lesion crossing maintained by the undersized wire. In general, this maneuver requires use of a wire smaller than necessary to accomplish the other technical requirements of the procedure. Both the contrast-reflux and small-wire angiography techniques may provide adequate imaging in relatively small, low-flow vessels, but obtaining adequate opacification in larger, high-flow vessels can be problematic. Use of an interventional sheath or GC eliminates these difficulties.

A related use of sheaths and GCs is to determine the appropriate position of a balloon catheter or stent before its inflation or deployment. Because contrast injection can be performed while the predeployed device is in place across the lesion, there is an opportunity to make final adjustments in its position before completing the intervention. This is particularly critical when deploying stents at the orifice of branch vessels, such as for renal or subclavian artery lesions, to minimize the risk of excessive stent projection into the aorta. Further, during interventions in which the length of GW that can be positioned beyond the lesion is restricted, such as with renal artery stenosis, there may not be enough of the stiff part of the wire through the lesion for the interventional device to track to its intended site. In this situation, sheaths or GCs can provide substantial external support and guidance to the interventional device. This is particularly valuable when acute vascular angulation is present.

Another advantage of sheaths and GCs is the ability to facilitate the performance of balloon angioplasty of distant contralateral sites or through tortuous arteries by reducing the arterial wall friction effect on the interventional catheter passing through them. In essence, the sheath acts as a reduced friction sleeve through which the interventional catheter is passed. When used over the aortic bifurcation, for example, both crossover sheaths and GCs redirect the force vector of the interventional catheter being passed through them; thus, it is more like the catheter is being introduced from the aorta itself, resulting in improved torqueability and pushability of the interventional catheter. In a similar fashion, sheaths are used to provide a smooth pathway to a lesion when implanting balloon-deployed stents. Without them, there is a risk of either vessel wall trauma or stent dislodgement from the catheter during passage to its intended site of deployment. Last, sheaths are used for the passage of snares and graspers to protect vessel walls along the way to the target lesion.

■ VASCULAR ACCESS

Femoral

Both antegrade and retrograde femoral accesses are used in the contemporary practice of vascular surgery. Access via the common femoral artery (CFA) has the least risk owing to its relatively large size and the fact that it can be effectively compressed against the underlying osseous structures. Selection of an antegrade or retrograde approach is dependent on the envisioned endovascular procedure, the patient's body habitus, and the operator's experience. In general, retrograde puncture of the CFA usually provides the simplest, most reliable entry into the arterial tree and is the most common approach.

Anatomy

A thorough understanding of the anatomic relationship of the CFA and the surrounding bony and ligamentous structures is essential, particularly if the femoral pulse is weak or absent. The risk of puncture site bleeding is significantly increased if the puncture occurs above the inguinal ligament or on the lateral wall of the artery. The latter is usually not a problem if there is a good pulse to guide the way, but an appreciation of the location of the inguinal ligament between the pubic tubercle and the anterior superior iliac spine is critical. Puncture of the external iliac artery cephalic to the inguinal ligament increases the risk of bleeding complications, particularly retroperitoneal bleeding, observed with suprainguinal punctures.[4,5] Punctures overly distal in the SFA or profunda femoral artery (PFA) can also be problematic because of the smaller size of the arteries in this location. The more abundant plaque commonly found in the distal CFA or proximal SFA also results in a greater risk of dissection and thrombosis. Further, the relative abundance of arterial and venous branches and the less adherent perivascular tissues found distal to the femoral bifurcation result in an increased risk of hematoma, false aneurysm, and arteriovenous fistula with low punctures.[6,7]

Femoral Artery Localization

An anatomic landmark that can be used to localize the CFA is the midpoint of the inguinal ligament, with the CFA typically being within 1.5 cm on either side of this point.[8] However, palpation of the superior pubic tubercle and the anterior superior iliac spine may be difficult in obese patients, preventing definitive localization of these structures. Further, both anatomic and radiographic landmarks for the location of the inguinal ligament are poor predictors of its actual location.[9,10]

Fluoroscopic Guidance. Fluoroscopic imaging of the femoral head may be a more reliable method of localizing the CFA (Fig. 84-9). The most medial cortex of the femoral head lies an average of 15 mm (range, 7 to 35 mm) below the inguinal ligament[9] and 33 mm (range, 2 to 66 mm) above the femoral bifurcation.[11] In 77% to 79% of patients, at least part of the CFA lumen is located over the medial third of the femoral head.[10,11] Consequently, puncturing the femoral artery 1 cm lateral to the most medial cortex of the femoral head, as assessed radiographically, appears to be best for both retrograde and antegrade femoral artery catheterizations.

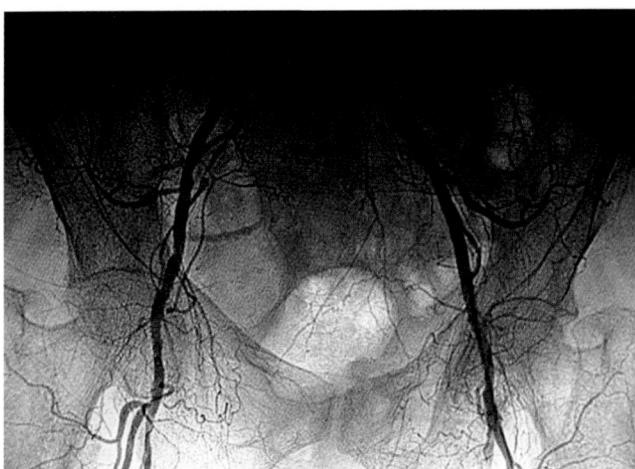

Figure 84-9 Position of the common femoral arteries over the femoral heads.

When using this method, it is important to remember that the femoral head should be centered in the field of view to avoid parallax errors that might otherwise occur. Additionally, any rotation of the patient's pelvis on the angiography table distorts the relationship between the artery and the femoral head. Radiographic visualization of a calcific blood vessel can guide successful puncture in patients with weak or absent femoral pulses.

Ultrasound Guidance. Obese, fully anticoagulated, and pulseless patients are at higher risk for complications at the vascular access site. Under these circumstances, the use of ultrasound guidance for needle entry into the vessel may reduce the incidence of complications.[12,13] The femoral vessels are imaged in a transverse plane using a high-frequency ultrasound probe (5 to 7.5 MHz) in gray-scale mode. The CFA is visualized lateral to the larger common femoral vein; deliberate pressure with the probe should cause the vein to easily collapse. Pulsation can sometimes be seen in the artery. A site free of plaque on the anterior artery wall is chosen for puncture. The tip of the entry needle can be followed through the subcutaneous tissue and directed to the chosen puncture site. Puncture of the arterial wall should be performed as centrally as possible.

Retrograde Femoral Technique

Once the site of intended needle insertion is ascertained, the skin and subcutaneous tissues are anesthetized with 1% lidocaine, and a small skin nick is made with a No. 11 knife blade. The entry needle is then advanced through the skin nick toward the pulse at an angle of 45 to 60 degrees. Keeping the artery between two fingers while advancing the needle with the other hand helps guide the needle and may also stabilize the artery. If the patient feels any discomfort as the needle approaches the artery, more lidocaine can be injected through the entry needle into that region. Shooting pain down the anterior thigh may indicate femoral nerve stimulation from a

laterally positioned needle that should be redirected. Although some interventionists attach a syringe to the needle and apply suction as they advance the needle, we prefer to enter with an open needle; this allows assessment of the puncture quality and needle position by the force with which the stream of blood is expelled. For venous access, however, gentle aspiration is usually required.

Once good blood return is obtained, the J-end of a short entry GW (typically packaged with the sheath) is advanced through the needle. If any resistance is encountered, further advancement under fluoroscopic guidance is mandatory. Once the wire is beyond the tip of the needle and advancing smoothly, it is generally best to image the wire as it passes up the iliac artery. Any areas in which the wire hangs up can be noted for further assessment. It is not uncommon for the wire to curl in the CFA or iliac arteries as it is being advanced. This can frequently be resolved by slight rotation or repositioning of the needle and re-advancement of the GW under fluoroscopic visualization. In some instances, the use of a straight, "floppy-tipped" GW may be more successful. A slight angle can usually be placed on the straight end of the wire by gently bending it over a thumbnail, giving the wire some steerability. If the entry GW becomes kinked or damaged, it should be replaced. Although one can switch to a full-length diagnostic GW (which is often already open and ready to use), it must be a metal-jacketed wire. Wires with hydrophilic coatings should not be passed through an entry needle because of the risk of shearing off the coating by the needle tip if the wire is retracted. Occasionally, significant vessel tortuosity impairs passage of the entry wire. Because significant iliac tortuosity is unilateral in 80% of cases,[14] contralateral cannulation should be considered to minimize the risk of arterial damage if the degree of tortuosity proves problematic or prohibitive for device passage.

Once the wire is successfully positioned in the iliac artery or distal aorta and there is radiographic confirmation that there are no kinks, loops, or significant deviations in the course of the wire, a sheath may be inserted. The needle is withdrawn off the wire, and pressure is held over the puncture site while an assistant threads the sheath and its dilator onto the wire for advancement into the iliac artery. A firm, smooth motion is employed to advance the sheath over the wire. If resistance is met, fluoroscopy can be used to investigate. Any angulation or arching of the wire or sheath creates resistance that may hinder passage. Once the sheath is advanced to the hub, it is important to re-evaluate the situation fluoroscopically before withdrawing the wire because, particularly in obese patients, the sheath may be curled in the subcutaneous tissue rather than within the artery. If the tip of the GW rests against a more proximal stenosis, the wire (and possibly the dilator) may have to be withdrawn while the sheath is advanced to minimize trauma to the lesion. The sheath should never be advanced without a wire and tapering dilator leading the way.

In patients who have undergone multiple femoral catheterizations or previous groin operations, significant resistance to advancement of the sheath may be encountered. In such instances, it is advisable to pass a dilator 1 Fr larger than the intended sheath size over the wire to create a larger track through the scar before attempting to re-advance the sheath. If continued resistance is encountered, one can go 1 Fr larger or re-insert the previous dilator into the vessel and exchange for a stiffer GW that allows the sheath to track better through the scar and into the vessel. Perisheath bleeding from over-dilatation is rarely a problem, and postprocedure hematomas are uncommon because the scar does not allow a place for blood to collect.

Antegrade Femoral Technique

As with retrograde femoral access, the skin is anesthetized over the localized femoral artery before needle insertion. The entry needle is angled at 45 to 60 degrees, with the tip aiming caudad, and access is obtained. However, obtaining antegrade femoral artery access is considerably more difficult than obtaining retrograde access, for three reasons:

1. Body contours tend to interfere with access to the artery.
2. The puncture site is near the origin of the SFA.
3. The position of the proximal anastomosis of an existing lower extremity bypass graft limits available working space between the needle puncture and the first bifurcation.

The last consideration mandates as high a puncture as possible (while still entering the artery below the inguinal ligament), but body habitus often makes this difficult. Antegrade femoral access can be facilitated by placing a roll of towels under the ipsilateral hip for slight hip extension and having an assistant retract the abdomen.

Once needle access is achieved, cannulation of the SFA or a bypass graft at the time of initial sheath placement is desirable. Retraction of a sheath initially placed in the PFA and attempts to manipulate it into the SFA risk inadvertent sheath removal and loss of vascular access (Fig. 84-10). To avoid PFA sheath placement, passage of the entry GW must be carefully observed fluoroscopically, and the wire must be seen following the anticipated course of the SFA or graft before the sheath is advanced over the wire. When in doubt about GW location, one can perform a scout angiogram through the entry needle to identify the origin of the vessel of interest and its course. Alternatively, a small (4 Fr) dilator can be advanced into the artery and an angiogram performed through it. If it turns out to be in the SFA, it can be rewired and the sheath placed in standard fashion. If it is in the PFA and the puncture site is proximal enough on the CFA to allow for GW manipulation, the dilator can be slowly withdrawn while an angled GW is manipulated through the dilator and into the SFA. Any movement of the angiography table or image intensifier between the performance of the scout study and attempted wire passage should be avoided because it will alter the relationship between the anatomic and radiographic landmarks.

Angiographic evaluation sometimes reveals that the puncture has entered the SFA itself. If there is sufficient working room to address the lesion of interest, there is no need to withdraw and repuncture. If, however, it is determined that

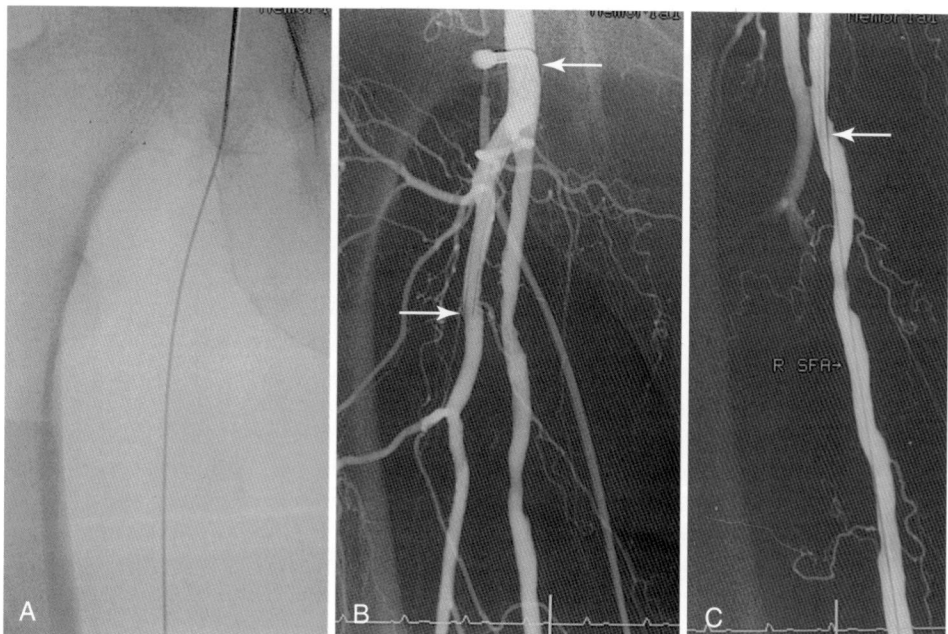

Figure 84-10 A, Initial guide wire placement during antegrade femoral artery puncture demonstrates lateral deviation of the wire, suggesting passage into the profunda femoris artery (PFA). **B,** This was not appreciated, and a sheath was inserted over the wire into the PFA, with subsequent contrast injection confirming its position. The *upper arrow* indicates the puncture site in the common femoral artery, and the *lower arrow* indicates the sheath tip. **C,** Because the puncture site was sufficiently proximal to the femoral bifurcation, the sheath was retracted, and the guide wire was redirected and advanced into the superficial femoral artery (SFA). The *arrow* indicates the sheath tip in the SFA.

the puncture is in the PFA or too distal in the CFA to allow wire manipulation, the needle must be removed, pressure held for 5 to 10 minutes, and the puncture repeated. Alternatively, a closure device can be used and a new access site selected.

On occasion, disease in the SFA prevents the standard entry J-wire from passing into or far enough down the SFA. In such situations, a floppy-tipped straight wire can be used, usually after placing a slight angle on its tip, as described earlier. The remainder of the sheath placement procedure is the same as outlined earlier. One must always check sheath placement radiographically before removing the GW, because subcutaneous curling of the sheath rather than intravascular positioning is not uncommon with antegrade CFA puncture.

Although we do not favor it, some have proposed a technique for converting from a retrograde femoral cannulation to an antegrade approach as a means of gaining antegrade femoral artery access more easily. If one anticipates the need for this technique, the puncture should be relatively high on the CFA with a steep, near-vertical angle to the skin. After retrograde placement of a soft 4 or 5 Fr sheath into the CFA, a curved catheter such as a Simmons, SOS Omni, or Visceral Selective-1 (VS-1) is formed in the abdominal aorta or the ipsilateral iliac artery. The access sheath and catheter are then retracted until the secondary curve of the catheter is at the puncture site, its tip is directed into the ipsilateral SFA or bypass graft, and its position is confirmed angiographically. Wire purchase is then obtained, and the access sheath and DC are exchanged for a sheath inserted in an antegrade direction.

Potential drawbacks of this technique include puncture of the PFA or veins, possible shear injury to the arterial access site, and kinking of the sheath. Higher radiation doses have been documented with the use of this technique, but few significant complications have been reported.[15-18] Proponents of this conversion technique believe that it may have advantages over an antegrade femoral approach, particularly in obese patients.

Popliteal

The technique for retrograde popliteal cannulation is similar to that for standard CFA access, except for the necessary use of ultrasound guidance. Retrograde popliteal access may be useful to avoid difficult and dangerous antegrade femoral punctures in obese patients, in patients with a high CFA bifurcation, in those with extra-anatomic bypass grafts, or in those with local groin issues such as open wounds, infections, or radiation changes. Retrograde access to the popliteal artery also permits the combined treatment of ipsilateral SFA and iliac lesions at the same setting and may facilitate recanalization of the true lumen during subintimal SFA angioplasty.[19,20] However, this technique requires placement of the patient in the prone position, which may not be tolerated in obese patients with obstructive pulmonary disease; in this case, ventilatory support may be required.

The popliteal artery and vein are ultrasonographically imaged in their longitudinal or transverse orientation and punctured under ultrasound guidance. This technique is greatly facilitated by the use of an echogenic-tipped needle. Ultrasound can also demonstrate the healthiest possible site for access, avoiding heavily calcified plaque formations or aneurysmal arteries. The greatest concern with popliteal puncture is the creation of an arteriovenous fistula. Furthermore, if distal embolization were to occur into the runoff arteries, the options for mechanical retrieval or pharmacologic thrombolysis would be limited.

Tibial

Retrograde cannulation of the tibial arteries for limb salvage in the setting of distal lower extremity arterial occlusive disease has been reported.[21,22] This approach may be useful for patients in whom GW advancement across a popliteal or tibial artery lesion has proved unsuccessful from the usual contralateral or antegrade ipsilateral femoral puncture sites. Under roadmapping or using ultrasound guidance, the posterior tibial artery at the medial ankle or the dorsalis pedis artery on the dorsum of the foot is punctured with a radial artery catheterization kit or a micropuncture needle. Once successful puncture is achieved, a small GW (0.014 or 0.018 inch) is advanced into the artery. A 4 Fr dilator, DC, or balloon catheter may be used to support the wire as it crosses the target lesion. After confirming reentry into the true lumen, the traversing wire can be snared from above, brought out through a femoral access site, and used to treat the distal lesion. Alternatively, depending on the condition of the punctured tibial artery, treatment may be accomplished directly from below, with or without placement of a 4 Fr sheath.

Upper Extremity

On occasion, such as in the presence of severe bilateral iliac artery occlusive disease or recently created aortobifemoral or femorofemoral bypass grafts, arterial access must be obtained via an upper extremity approach. This can be achieved through either open or percutaneous subclavian, axillary, brachial, or radial approaches. Vascular surgeons are familiar with the technique for open vascular access, so it is not discussed here, except to say that open exposure is the safest approach; the neural and vascular structures are directly visualized and protected, and the artery can be repaired primarily, minimizing the risk of complications. In surgeons less experienced in percutaneous brachial access, the open technique may be preferred because an increased incidence of complications has been recognized in those who perform percutaneous procedures only occasionally.[23]

A technique for catheterization of the second portion of the subclavian artery or first portion of the axillary artery has been introduced[24]; however, it has not been broadly adopted because it is technically demanding, it has a steep learning curve, and there are concerns about iatrogenic pneumothorax. This technique, when performed by expert surgeons and with the use of supraclavicular and infraclavicular pressure after catheter removal, is associated with high success and low complication rates.

Axillary-Brachial

Of the upper extremity percutaneous access techniques, distal axillary–proximal brachial artery puncture is the most commonly performed and the one that we favor. Unless there is evidence of coexisting subclavian or axillary artery disease, the left side is preferred. It is generally easier to manipulate wires and catheters into the descending aorta from the left than from the right, particularly if the innominate artery originates low on the arch. Further, when approached from the right side, the catheter and wire reside in the flow path to the right vertebral and common carotid arteries, the innominate artery, and the left carotid artery, increasing the risk of neurologic embolic events.

Proper patient positioning is important and is best achieved by having the patient place his or her ipsilateral hand palm-up behind the head. The brachial artery pulse is palpated lateral to the pectoralis major muscle, and the overlying skin is anesthetized. The close proximity of nerve trunks mandates careful, deliberate passage of the needle; direct nerve injury from the needle is uncommon, however, occurring in less than 1% of axillary punctures.[24-26] Patient complaints of shooting pain down the arm should prompt the retraction and redirection of the needle. The mobile axillary-brachial artery often benefits from manual fixation by the surgeon's second hand. Once good arterial blood return is encountered, the GW is advanced into the artery, after which the sheath is advanced over the entry wire as previously outlined.

Having secured arterial access, a full-length angiographic GW (preferably a J-wire) is advanced through the sheath under fluoroscopic guidance and manipulated down the descending aorta, a maneuver best observed in the left anterior oblique projection. A pigtail catheter may be hooked at the origin of the left subclavian artery and used to direct the GW down the descending thoracic aorta. Alternatively, an angled DC can be used to negotiate the GW into the descending aorta. The remainder of the procedure is performed in the usual fashion, typically requiring 100-cm DCs to cannulate the abdominal branches.

In general, it is advisable to use the smallest sheath possible in the upper extremity arteries because their relatively small size increases the risk of vessel thrombosis. Additionally, puncture-related hemorrhage, more common with larger punctures, involves the risk of axillary sheath hematoma with neurologic compromise. Although this complication reportedly occurs in less than 3% of brachial or axillary artery catheterizations,[27-29] it requires immediate recognition and surgical decompression if permanent neurologic dysfunction is to be avoided. The development of peripheral paresthesias warrants close observation, whereas any loss of motor function mandates immediate intervention. Despite attempts to minimize the puncture size, on occasion it is necessary to place a 6 or 8 Fr sheath to allow the passage of interventional devices, and this is usually well tolerated. Brachial artery thrombosis is the most frequent major complication associated with brachial access. We prefer mid to high brachial artery puncture because of its larger size compared with the more distal artery, which has a tendency to spasm when punctured.

Radial

The merits of percutaneous radial artery access for coronary and cerebral angiography have long been recognized.[30] Advantages of this technique include limited patient discomfort, simple and safe postprocedural hemostasis, and early mobilization. However, the small size of the radial artery cannot accommodate the larger sheaths necessary for peripheral arterial interventions. Diagnostic studies of the lower extremities may also be compromised by the unavailability of DCs of sufficient length to reach from the wrist to the leg.

Venous

Knowledge of techniques to access the venous system for diagnostic studies, the performance of vena caval filter placement or renal vein renin sampling, and the treatment of upper or lower extremity deep venous thrombosis is essential for the endovascular surgeon. Venous puncture using ultrasound guidance is increasingly common to avoid the potential morbidity of inadvertent puncture of adjacent arterial structures. Ultrasound is also helpful in localizing superficial veins in the extremities that may be suitable for puncture.

Femoral

The technique of femoral venous puncture parallels that of the femoral artery. The femoral vein is located just medial to the artery, the pulsation of which is typically used as a landmark. If arterial pulsation is absent, the vein can be found approximately 2 cm lateral to the pubic tubercle. As with arterial punctures, it is recommended that the GW be advanced up the iliac vein under fluoroscopic visualization to avoid inadvertent misplacement of the sheath. Although vena caval filters can be inserted via a femoral approach contralateral to a deep venous thrombosis, some prefer a jugular approach.

Jugular

A jugular puncture reduces the risk of instrumentation through thrombus or potential venous injury from the filter delivery system, which may increase the incidence of thrombosis at the access site. Catheterization of the jugular vein for insertion of a vena caval filter is best performed on the right side, which provides a straighter course to the infrarenal vena cava than does a left-sided approach. The jugular vein is punctured just lateral to the carotid artery, either anterior to the sternocleidomastoid muscle or between its sternal and clavicular heads. A sheath is inserted in the typical fashion.

Ultrasound guidance is useful to avoid inadvertent carotid artery puncture.

Subclavian-Axillary

If neither femoral access site can be used owing to proximity of the venous thrombosis and the jugular approach is also unavailable, the subclavian vein is a reasonable alternative. The subclavian vein can be approached through a supraclavicular puncture just lateral to the clavicular head of the sternocleidomastoid muscle, directing the needle toward the contralateral nipple. Alternatively, the axillary vein can be punctured with ultrasound or fluoroscopic guidance. Contrast material injected into a more peripheral vein in the ipsilateral arm can be used to locate the axillary vein and fluoroscopically direct the needle tip, especially when used in conjunction with the roadmapping feature of the imaging equipment.

Extremity

Extremity venography has become more common with the wider acceptance of active clot management in the treatment of deep venous thrombosis. In the upper extremity, access sites include the median antecubital or cephalic vein at the elbow. The basilic vein in the upper arm is also a preferred site owing to its relatively large caliber and direct approach to the axillary and subclavian veins. Because many extremity venous examinations are performed for limb swelling, which makes the superficial veins difficult to visualize, ultrasound-guided puncture is commonly employed. In the lower extremity, access sites include the popliteal vein, approached with the patient in a prone position and using ultrasound. To avoid direct puncture of the popliteal vein, the lesser saphenous vein on the posterior calf may used as an alternative. Access via the posterior tibial veins at the ankle is also common, especially for the management of disease involving the distal popliteal vein.

◼ VASCULAR CLOSURE

Following a diagnostic or therapeutic endovascular procedure, vascular closure is required after sheath removal. For venous access, simple manual pressure for 5 to 10 minutes is sufficient for vascular control. However, arterial access requires more attention, and recently developed technology has provided an alternative to manual compression.

Manual Compression

Manual compression to achieve hemostasis after the removal of arterial access devices is a simple procedure that must be learned and practiced to achieve optimal results. To obtain maximum cooperation, ensure that the patient is comfortable before pulling the device, including draining the bladder if necessary. If the patient is hypertensive, consider antihypertensive medication before sheath removal. If heparin was administered during the procedure, many operators measure the activated clotting time and do not remove the access device until this value has normalized.

The goal of manual compression is to prevent bleeding from the artery while maintaining flow, allowing a platelet plug to seal the puncture site. Pressure should be applied with only as much force as necessary to prevent bleeding. Pressure with one or two fingers is usually sufficient directly at the arteriotomy site. Be aware that the arterial puncture site is usually proximal to the skin entry site for retrograde femoral access and distal to the skin entry for antegrade femoral access. The ipsilateral foot should be exposed while pressure is applied so that its perfusion can be continually assessed. Pressure is usually held for 15 to 20 minutes after the removal of 4 to 6 Fr devices; consider maintaining pressure for up to 30 minutes after the removal of larger devices.

Although manual compression can achieve hemostasis in most cases, there are several drawbacks. A significant time commitment is required—usually 15 to 30 minutes of sustained pressure over the puncture site, followed by 6 to 8 hours of bed rest. This prolonged period of immobilization is often a source of patient discomfort and dissatisfaction, and noncompliance with this regimen is associated with failure of vascular control and bleeding. Access site complications result in increased morbidity and an associated increase in hospital costs. These factors prompted efforts to find an alternative means of achieving hemostasis after percutaneous vascular access and led to the development of arterial closure devices.

Closure Devices

The ideal closure device should provide effective hemostasis, even when used to seal large puncture sites, and should be unaffected by the use of antithrombotic regimens.[31] Deployment should be simple and rapid. The device should be reliable, not cause compromise of the vessel lumen or intra-arterial embolization, and allow for immediate repeat access. The device should enable early postprocedural ambulation and hospital discharge. Patient comfort and acceptance should be high. The rate of hemorrhagic, thrombotic, and infectious complications following use of a closure device should be no greater than that associated with manual compression.

Over the past decade, a number of arterial closure devices have been introduced as an alternative to manual compression. Evaluation of the literature regarding these devices is difficult. New devices are continually being introduced and existing devices modified. Few prospective studies comparing closure devices to manual compression or to other devices have been completed.[32-35] The majority of studies are found in the cardiology literature, with fewer published studies involving patients with peripheral vascular disease.[35-37] However, the use of closure devices appears to offer several advantages. Patients are able to ambulate almost immediately, technician time can be used more efficiently, and patient acceptance is excellent. Sheaths can be removed immediately even in patients receiving anticoagulation.

Types

Arterial closure devices can be separated into two categories. The first type relies on collagen or a procoagulant to augment normal coagulation pathways; examples include Duett (Vascular Solutions, Minneapolis, MN), Angioseal (St. Jude Medical, St. Paul, MN), and Mynx (AccessClosure, Mountain View, CA). Collagen augments normal platelet activation and aggregation and forms a framework onto which clot can deposit. Swelling of the collagen plug also acts as a mechanical seal at the puncture site. In animal studies, the collagen plug is resorbed within 4 weeks. The second type of device relies on suture-mediated or other mechanical means of sealing the puncture site; examples include Perclose and StarClose (Abbott Vascular, Santa Clara, CA), Boomerang (Cardiva Medical, Mountain View, CA), and SuperStitch (Sutura, Fountain Valley, CA). Suture-mediated devices achieve hemostasis by performing a percutaneous, limited surgical closure of the puncture site.

Deployment

A detailed discussion of the deployment technique for each device is beyond the scope of this text, and interested readers are referred to the instructions for use of such devices. There are no clear data recommending any one device over the others. Common to essentially all devices, however, is the advisability of femoral arteriograms in one or more planes to determine the exact site of arterial puncture (e.g., CFA versus SFA) and the extent of underlying atherosclerosis. Although the greatest experience is in patients undergoing cardiac catheterization, these devices can be deployed in patients with peripheral vascular disease if certain guidelines are followed. The mechanical devices should be deployed only in the CFA, which should be at least 5 mm in diameter and free of significant luminal compromise at the puncture site. Vessel calcification should not be considered a contraindication to device usage. Both retrograde and antegrade punctures can be successfully managed with the various devices. Before using a particular device, however, instruction on its proper deployment is mandatory. There is clearly a learning curve before competence is achieved.

■ COMPLICATIONS

Complications from diagnostic arteriography are uncommon.[38] They can be divided into three types: puncture site, catheter related, and systemic. The first two types are addressed here.

Puncture Site

Risk factors for puncture site complications include female gender, small or very large body habitus, diabetes, aggressive anticoagulation, poor access technique (multiple, high, low, or back-wall punctures), large sheath size, small vessel size, poor sterility, and operator inexperience.

The most frequent puncture site complication is hematoma. The incidence of minor hematomas is variable and may be as high as 10%, but major hematomas are unusual. A major hematoma, defined as one requiring transfusion, surgical evacuation, or delay in discharge, occurs in approximately 0.5% of femoral punctures and approximately 1.7% of axillary punctures. An axillary hematoma is less well tolerated than a groin hematoma because of the associated nerve compression. A small hematoma at an axillary puncture site usually requires surgical evacuation to prevent permanent nerve injury earlier than does a similar hematoma in the groin. For femoral access, hematomas are more likely to occur if the puncture site is below or above the femoral head, where compression may be less effective. In general, a stable hematoma that is not associated with nerve compression, compromise of the overlying skin, or hemodynamic instability can be safely observed. Beware of high groin punctures that enter the external iliac artery because of the risk of retroperitoneal hemorrhage, which can cause significant blood loss and hemodynamic instability in the absence of a visible hematoma.

Other puncture site problems, including dissection, thrombosis, pseudoaneurysm, and arteriovenous fistula, are also unusual, occurring in less than 1% of femoral punctures. Clinically significant infection at the puncture site with bacteremia is very rare, and antibiotic prophylaxis is generally not recommended for diagnostic arteriography. When infections do occur, they are most often associated with repeated punctures of the same artery over a short period or with long-term sheath access, as in complex interventional procedures. Infections have also been reported after the use of arterial closure devices. If puncture site infection is encountered, surgical débridement and extra-anatomic bypass grafting may be required.

Catheter Related

Complications due to intravascular catheter manipulation include subintimal passage of the GW or catheter and dissections or emboli caused by catheter movement or contrast injection under pressure. Catheter-related complications reportedly occur in 0.15% to 2.0% of cases, with more recent series reporting a frequency of less than 0.5%. In recent years, these types of complications have decreased in frequency, in part owing to advances in GW and catheter technology. Dissections that are not flow limiting can usually be safely observed. For a severe, flow-limiting dissection, treatment options include stenting to tack up the dissection flap or direct surgical repair.

SELECTED KEY REFERENCES

Dotter CT, Rosch J, Robinson M. Fluoroscopic guidance in femoral artery puncture. *Radiology.* 1978;127:266-267.
   Article delineating the relevant anatomic landmarks for fluoroscopy-guided femoral artery puncture—an essential skill for endovascular procedures, especially in patients with diminished or absent pulses.

Section **12** Technique

Katz SG, Abando A. The use of closure devices. *Surg Clin N Am.* 2004;84:1267-1280.
Excellent review of arterial closure devices, although the development of this technology remains in evolution.

Nice C, Timmons G, Bartholemew P, Uberoi R. Retrograde versus antegrade puncture for infrainguinal angioplasty. *Cardiovasc Intervent Radiol.* 2003;26:370-374.
Technique for converting a retrograde femoral puncture into an antegrade puncture, which may be helpful in obese patients or those with a stoma.

Singh H, Cardella JF, Cole PE, Grassi CJ, McCowan TC, Swan TL, Sacks D, Lewis CA. Society of Interventional Radiology Standards of Practice Committee. Quality improvement guidelines for diagnostic arteriography. *J Vasc Intervent Radiol.* 2003;14:S283-S288.
Guidelines on the appropriate indications for diagnostic arteriography and the assessment of results, including thresholds for the incidence of complications.

Wacker F, Wolf KJ, Fobbe F. Percutaneous vascular access guided by color-duplex sonography. *Eur Radiol.* 1997;7:1501-1504.
Technique of ultrasound-guided femoral artery puncture.

REFERENCES

The reference list can be found on the companion Expert Consult Web site at *www.expertconsult.com.*

CHAPTER 85

Technique: Endovascular Therapeutic

Makoto Sumi and Takao Ohki

Based in part on a chapter in the previous edition by Juan Ayerdi, MD, and Kim J. Hodgson, MD.

Surgical revascularization has been the traditional treatment for a variety of occlusive lesions of the aorta, carotid artery, and lower extremity arterial tree. However, with recent advances in endovascular technology, catheter-based intervention is now a viable option, and percutaneous treatment has replaced open surgical procedures as the first line of treatment for many arterial lesions. The advantages of percutaneous endovascular procedures include the avoidance of general anesthesia and incision-related wound complications, reduced cardiovascular stress, earlier recovery and ambulation, and more easily performed re-intervention when required. However, these advantages apply only in the context of an overall strategy to treat the arterial disease and related symptoms. An important aspect of decision making is the fact that the performance of an endovascular procedure may limit future surgical options. Because no vascular intervention, either endovascular or surgical, is durable forever, there is always the possibility that the patient may require additional interventions in the future. Therefore, endovascular placement of a stent in locations such as the common femoral or popliteal artery, which would complicate or limit the performance of a subsequent bypass, should be avoided if possible.

■ BALLOON ANGIOPLASTY

Dotter and Judkins originally described the mechanism of transluminal angioplasty by the endoluminal passage of progressively larger dilators through an arterial stenosis.[1] Gruntzig developed the concept of balloon angioplasty, whereby stenoses are dilated using polyvinyl chloride balloons.[2] The effect of balloon dilatation is disruption of the obstructing plaque in the arterial media, with stretching of the adventitia and media, thereby increasing luminal arterial diameter. The relatively low risk and ease of re-inflation and re-intervention make balloon dilatation of obstructive lesions an attractive alternative to surgical intervention. Balloon catheters vary in terms of material, size, shape, and compliance. Choosing the correct balloon for the planned procedure entails matching the balloon catheter to the desired procedural result.

Balloon Characteristics

Compliance

Compliance is a measure of the balloon's ability to expand beyond its stated nominal pressure diameter. Very compliant balloons that continue to enlarge even when the nominal diameter has been reached can cause overstretching, injury, and possible rupture of the arterial wall. Compliance is usually measured with the balloon in a 37°C water bath. However, no generally accepted protocol is used by manufacturers to measure and classify balloon compliance. This results in different terminology for the same class of balloon compliance.

With regard to compliance, there are three types of balloons: noncompliant, controlled-compliant, and compliant. Noncompliant balloons have the least expansion of diameter, compliant balloons the most, and controlled-compliant balloons are intermediate (Fig. 85-1A and B).

Noncompliant Balloons. The term *noncompliant* is misleading, because strictly speaking, every balloon exhibits a certain amount of growth if pressure is applied. A more correct expression would be *minimally compliant*. The balloon material polyethylene terephthalate is relatively noncompliant, relatively inexpensive, and easy to handle during the manufacturing process; however, it is not resistant to mechanical irritation, such as from sharp edges of calcified plaques. Most endovascular surgeons prefer noncompliant balloons for postdilatation of stents, which require high pressure because the balloon limits overstretching of both the stent and the vessel wall.

Controlled-Compliant (Semicompliant, Minimally Compliant) Balloons. This intermediate class of compliance is achieved when the balloon is made of nylon. Differently manufactured nylon balloons vary slightly in compliance but are still in the same class. An older term is *semicompliant*, but *controlled-compliant* expresses the fact that the balloon size is predictable. A modern marketing expression is *minimally compliant*, which implies that the compliance is closer to that of a noncompliant balloon. Tables displaying balloon diameter relative to applied pressure (compliance charts) are available.

Compliant Balloons. Polyolefin copolymer and polyethylene balloons are in this class. One potential advantage is the ability to cover a larger range of diameters with a single balloon. This may be advantageous if the treated vessel varies in diameter or if several vessels have to be treated in the same patient.

Profile

Profile is mainly determined by how snugly the balloon wraps around the catheter shaft. A lower profile allows balloon

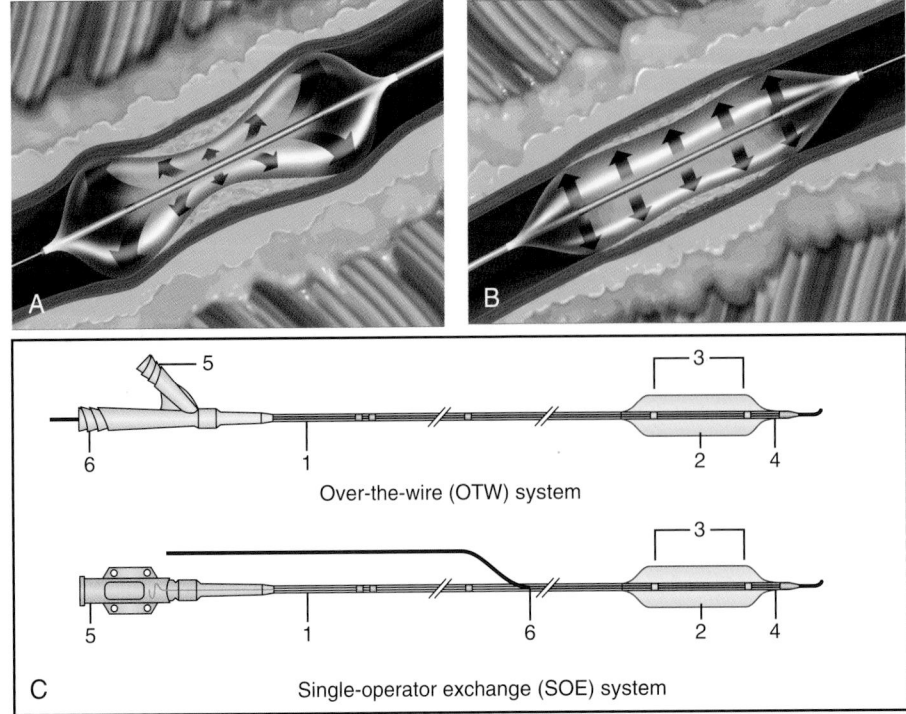

Figure 85-1 A, Compliant balloons (pictured) stretch more than noncompliant or low-compliance balloons. **B,** Noncompliant or low-compliance balloons retain their shape. These balloons are typically applied to fibrous lesions. **C,** Balloon angioplasty catheters. 1, catheter shaft; 2, balloon; 3, marker/balloon size; 4, tapered tip; 5, inflation port; 6, guide-wire exit port.

introduction through smaller catheters and the crossing of tighter lesions and smaller vessels.

Pushability

Pushability is the ability to advance a catheter through the arterial tree. Columnar strength and a low-friction surface contribute to the ease with which a catheter and balloon can be advanced. Hydrophilic coatings on the balloon catheter allow easier passage through the sheath, access vessels, and lesion of interest.

Trackability

Trackability is the catheter's ability to follow the guide wire. Low friction and flexibility allow the negotiation of tortuous vessels.

Wings

Balloons are wrapped around the shaft of the catheter, much like a sail is wrapped around the mast of a ship. After a balloon is inflated, it does not resume its original low profile on deflation. The postdilatation profile is due to the balloon's "memory" of the way it was wrapped around the catheter before inflation. This profile resembles winglike projections.

Burst Pressure

Nominal pressure refers to the inflation pressure required to achieve the inflated balloon diameter specified on the package label and usually ranges from 3 to 10 atmospheres. Burst pressure—usually reported as rated burst pressure (RBP)—is defined as the pressure below which 99.9% of balloons will not rupture. RBP is an important component of product labeling and is monitored by the Food and Drug Administration (FDA), providing the operator with a good idea of the safe range of inflation pressures. RBP commonly ranges from 6 to 16 atmospheres. Mean burst pressure, defined as the pressure at which 50% of balloons will rupture, is higher than RBP and ranges from 10 to 27 atmospheres. Many manufacturers do not routinely disclose data on mean burst pressure.

Balloon Catheter Types
Over-the-Wire Systems

Two techniques of guide wire manipulation when using over-the-wire (OTW) balloons are the "through-wire" and "bare-wire" techniques; they are equally acceptable. The availability of many ultra-low-profile balloons has led most manufacturers to eliminate or markedly curtail the production of balloons that are fixed to a guide wire (Fig. 85-1C).

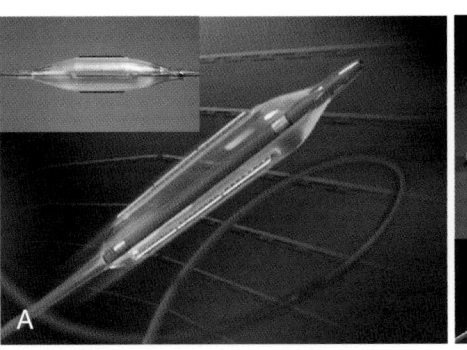 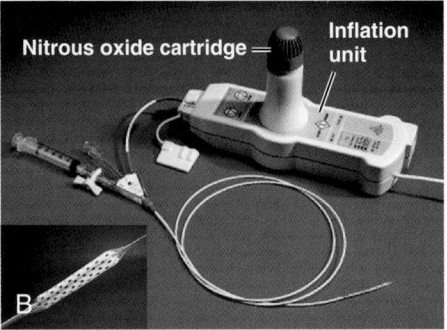

Figure 85-2 A, Peripheral Cutting Balloon device (Boston Scientific Corp., Natick, MA). **B,** PolarCath device (Boston Scientific Corp., Natick, MA). Cryoplasty uses nitrous oxide to inflate the angioplasty balloon.

Through-Wire Technique. In the through-wire technique, the operator advances the guide wire–loaded balloon into the O-ring and through the guiding catheter just proximal to the vessel ostium. The guide wire is then advanced beyond the stenosis, and the balloon is tracked over the wire and through the lesion. If the operator has difficulty with guide wire crossing, the balloon catheter can be advanced into the target vessel for additional support and torque control. If the lesion still cannot be crossed, the balloon catheter can be left in place to function as a transfer catheter, and the operator can fashion a different curve on the guide wire or use a new guide wire if necessary.

Bare-Wire Technique. The bare-wire technique involves advancing the guide wire across the lesion *without* the balloon. This technique may allow better visualization during contrast injections because there is more room within the sheath for contrast material. However, this technique does not permit use of the balloon to enhance support or facilitate wire exchanges.

Single-Operator Exchange Systems

Outside the United States, single-operator exchange (SOE) systems, also commonly referred to as "monorail" or "rapid-exchange" balloons, constitute the overwhelming majority of balloon catheter sales (see Fig. 85-1C). SOE balloons are modified OTW balloons in which only the distal portion of the balloon catheter tracks coaxially over the guide wire; the remaining portion of the catheter shaft does not have a guide wire through-lumen. Compared with OTW balloons, SOE balloons have a lower profile and facilitate single-operator use. Additional advantages include the fact that the guide wire (or an embolic protection device) can be more readily stabilized during balloon catheter exchange, and the procedure time can be shortened owing to faster balloon insertion and exchange. Furthermore, exchange-length guide wires are not necessary with SOE systems requiring only standard-length guide wires. Disadvantages of SOE balloons include less pushability and trackability, the inability to reshape or exchange the guide wire without a transfer catheter, and dif-

ficulty using the balloon catheter for additional guide wire backup support when crossing a difficult lesion.

Cutting Balloon

A cutting balloon is a specialized angioplasty device that consists of a series of cutting blades (or atherotomes) placed longitudinally along the surface of a standard angioplasty balloon (Fig. 85-2A). It was originally introduced for coronary intervention, but given the similar diameters of coronary and infrapopliteal vessels, it has been employed for peripheral arterial interventions. When inflated, these cutting blades score the lesion with incisions to facilitate dilatation of the vessel. Cutting balloons are not widely considered a primary therapy for de novo occlusive lesions because the longest balloon is only 2 cm. They are best suited for lesions such as bypass graft anastomoses, bifurcation stenoses, and no-stent-zone lesions (e.g., common femoral, popliteal, subclavian arteries) in which stenting works poorly. Its ability to dilate the lesion at a much lower pressure (typically 3 to 5 atmospheres) is also considered an advantage. The occurrence of dissection appears to be lower than that seen after percutaneous transluminal angioplasty (PTA). Like standard PTA, cutting balloons have excellent technical success rates (95%), but this advantage is somewhat offset by a relatively restricted range of balloon diameters and lengths that limit the therapy's potential applications.[3] Encouraging results, such as a 1-year limb salvage rate of 86%, were reported by Ansel and colleagues in 73 patients with critical limb ischemia undergoing peripheral interventions using a cutting balloon, with a low adjunctive stenting rate of 20% for severe dissection and inadequate dilatation.[4] However, the long-term efficacy of cutting balloons has yet to be proved superior to that of standard balloon angioplasty.

Cryoplasty

The PolarCath peripheral balloon catheter (Boston Scientific Corp., Natick, MA) is a system that simultaneously dilates and cools the plaque and vessel wall in the area of treatment (Fig. 85-2B).[5,6] When activated, liquid nitrous oxide fills the angioplasty balloon and exposes approximately 500 μm of diseased vessel wall to −10°C of cold therapy, which is intended to induce cell apoptosis and limit the intimal hyperplastic response. In addition, it is believed to reduce the rate of flow-limiting dissections. Although cryoplasty may be applied in a variety of situations, it is commonly used to treat suboptimal PTA or in-stent restenosis. Because cryoplasty is a relatively new therapy, efficacy data are scarce, and 9-month re-intervention rates as high as 15% have been reported in patients with lesions less than 10 cm.[5] The purported advantages of cryoplasty include a reduction in the incidence of neointimal hyperplasia and less trauma to the vessel than standard angioplasty. However, these claims require confirmation by prospective clinical trials.

■ STENTS

It is said that the term *stent* originated from Charles R. Stent, a 19th-century British dentist. He developed an apparatus to make dental molds and called it a stent; it was thereafter used in the context of a mold to maintain an inner cavity. Dotter was the first to apply metallic stents to the human vascular tree. He started the era of intravascular stent placement in 1969 with the introduction of a transluminally placed coil spring endarterial tube graft.[7] Nitinol stents were introduced in 1983 by Dotter[8] and Cragg.[9] Palmaz introduced the balloon-expanding stent in 1985.[10] His stent was the first and, for a long time, the only stent approved by the FDA for vascular use.

The BENESTENT (Belgian Netherlands stent) trial[11] in Europe and the STRESS (Stent Restenosis Study) trial[12] in the United States revealed that Palmaz-Schatz stents offer a major advantage over transluminal balloon angioplasty in maintaining luminal patency. As a result of these positive outcomes, stenting became common in endovascular therapy. Routine stenting is now well accepted for the treatment of aortoiliac, brachiocephalic, and renal artery lesions but is less well accepted at the femoropopliteal level and in the carotid artery.

Stents are differentiated primarily by their method of deployment: balloon-expandable or self-expanding. The prototypical and classic balloon-expandable stent is the Palmaz stent; the self-expanding counterpart is the Wallstent. The metals used for stents include stainless steel, nitinol, tantalum, platinum, and various metal alloys. The construction of stents is variable and includes laser-cut or -etched, woven, knitted, coiled, or welded constructions. Stent properties such as flexibility, radial strength, hoop strength, radiopacity, and foreshortening characteristics can differ. In addition, various stent characteristics such as metal thickness, surface charge, method of cleaning and polishing, source of the metal, corrosion resistance, durability, open area–to–metal surface ratio, "kinkability," and sharpness of the ends may affect the biocompatibility, ease of use, and, ultimately, long-term patency rates. All stents are not alike, and no stent exhibits all the ideal properties (Table 85-1).[13]

Table 85-1 Properties of Balloon-Expandable and Self-Expanding Stents

	Balloon-Expandable Stent	Self-Expanding Stent
Pros	Accuracy in deployment Strong radial force Radiopaque	Flexible Long Crush resistant
Cons	Crushable Rigid Short	Insufficient radial force Insufficient radiopacity Inaccurate deployment
Indications	Orificial lesions Calcified, resistant lesions	Superficial lesions Long lesions Tortuous vessels

Balloon-Expandable Stents

Balloon-expandable stents (Fig. 85-3A) are slotted tubes of malleable metal that are expanded by a coaxial balloon matched to the size of the target vessel. When deployed, the metal tube maintains the inflated balloon diameter, and fixation to the arterial wall is enabled by friction and subsequent endothelialization. The rigid nature of these stents provides resistance against elastic recoil of the vessel, but it also renders them susceptible to irreversible deformation when subjected to an external compressive force.[13] Consequently, these stents are ideal for immobile and well-protected areas of the body such as the renal, mesenteric, iliac, and subclavian arteries and for ostial lesions. Most balloon-expandable stents are made of a stainless steel alloy. Stainless steel is suitable for this purpose because it combines malleability and strength. For this reason, balloon-expandable stents tend to have greater radial and hoop strength than self-expanding stents. They also tend to be more radiopaque. Because of their mode of deployment and the minimal amount of predictable foreshortening, balloon-expandable stents can be placed with a high degree of precision. Its higher radial strength and accurate deployment make the balloon-expandable stent a better choice for ostial lesions, which are often calcified.

The first commercially available balloon-expandable stent was the rigid Palmaz stent, the efficacy of which has been validated in clinical trials.[14-16] Recently, there has been a drive toward manufacturing lower profile, flexible, balloon-expandable stents with complex cell geometry and open or hinged designs. These stents derive their flexibility from the ability of individual cell rings to track independently. However, there are few scientific data comparing the clinical impact of different stent designs and cell configurations. Because most balloon-expandable stents are made of ferromagnetic stainless steel, they cause large susceptibility artifacts (signal loss) on magnetic resonance images.

Self-Expanding Stents

The mode of action of self-expanding stents (Fig. 85-3B) is based on the property of elasticity. These stents self-expand to their nominal diameter when released from a constrained state within the delivery system. Typically, a stent with a nominal diameter greater than that of the target vessel is

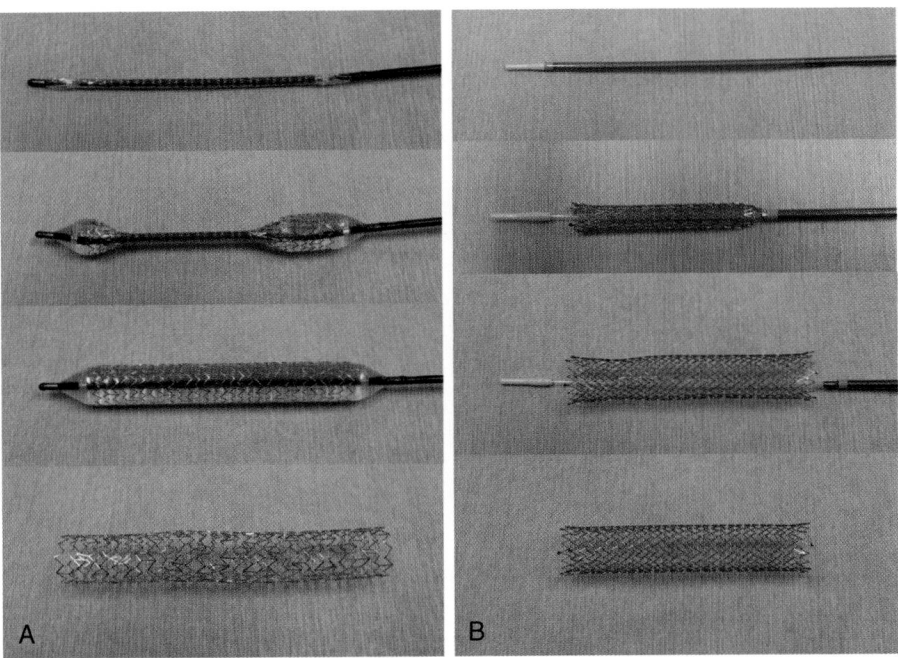

Figure 85-3 A, The balloon-expandable Express LD stent (Boston Scientific Corp., Natick, MA) is crimped onto an angioplasty balloon and deployed by balloon inflation. **B,** The self-expanding SMART stent (Cordis Corp., Bridgewater, NJ) is deployed by passing the delivery catheter over a guide wire and withdrawing a cover sheath.

chosen so that it exerts an outward expansible force, resulting in good vessel wall apposition. The ultimate diameter of the vessel with the stent is the result of equilibrium between the elastic recoil of the vessel and the radial expansion force of the stent.

The elasticity of self-expanding stents is derived from either the design of the stent mesh or the elastic properties of the metal. Nitinol, an alloy of approximately 50% nickel and 50% titanium, provides the most flexibility and memory. In general, self-expanding stents are more flexible than balloon-expandable stents, and they tend to track better when advanced through tortuous anatomy. The self-expanding nature of these stents also provides a certain amount of crush resistance that is not possessed by most balloon-expandable stents. Because most self-expanding stents are made of inert, nonferromagnetic metals, they generally cause less susceptibility artifacts than stainless steel stents on magnetic resonance images. Disadvantages of self-expanding stents include less radiopacity, less accurate deployment, and less radial strength than balloon-expandable stents.

Self-expanding stents can be categorized as having an open-cell or closed-cell design. An open-cell design is defined as a stent that has circumferential sets of strut members, with some but not all curved sections (crowns) connected by a longitudinal connecting link to an adjacent circumferential set of strut members. In comparison, in a closed-cell stent, every curved section of every circumferential set of strut members, except at the distal and proximal ends of the stent, is attached to a longitudinal connecting link. The chief advantage of the open-cell design is greater flexibility before and after stent deployment. Therefore, it is more trackable during insertion

and conforms to the anatomy well after deployment. Poor lesion coverage is one downside of the open-cell design. Poor lesion coverage may lead to distal embolization or plaque protrusion through the stent struts.

Other Stent Types

Other important stent concepts and types are discussed in detail in Chapters 90 (Aortic Stents and Stent-Grafts) and 91 (Nonaortic Stents and Stent-Grafts), including drug-eluting stents and covered stents.

EMBOLIC PROTECTION DEVICES

Percutaneous and surgical interventions in diseased arteries often result in distal embolization of atherosclerotic debris, which is often clinically occult. However, in saphenous vein graft interventions, carotid interventions, and possibly renal artery stenting, distal embolization may result in clinically significant sequelae, including myocardial infarction, stroke, and renal failure. Ohki and coworkers proved that embolic materials are released during angioplasty of carotid artery lesions using an ex vivo human carotid artery model.[17] Accordingly, a number of protection devices have been contrived to prevent distal embolization. Currently, these are most frequently applied to carotid artery stenting (CAS) (see Chapter 96: Carotid Artery Disease: Stenting).

Types of embolic protection devices include distal protection devices (distal occlusion balloons and filters), proximal occlusion balloons, and flow reversal devices (Table 85-2). Filters positioned distal to the area of treatment trap debris

Table 85-2 Embolic Protection Devices

Type of Device	Device (Company)	Advantages	Disadvantages
Distal occlusion balloon	PercuSurge GuardWire (Medtronic CardioVascular, Minneapolis, MN) GuardDOG Guidewire Occlusion System (Possis Medical, Inc., Minneapolis, MN)	Low profile	Crosses lesion without protection Interrupts antegrade flow Does not allow proper visualization
Distal filter device	See Table 85-3	Easy to use Does not interrupt antegrade flow Allows contrast injection during procedure	Crosses lesion without protection Difficult to use in tight lesions, tortuous vessels
Proximal occlusion balloon	Proxis (St. Jude Medical, Inc., St. Paul, MN) MOMA (Invatec, Brescia, Italy)		Antegrade carotid artery flow may be preserved
Proximal occlusion with flow reversal	Gore Neuro Protection System (W. L. Gore, Flagstaff, AZ)	Crosses the lesion under protection	Complex system

and particles during the procedure. They are the easy to use, do not interrupt antegrade flow, and allow for contrast injection during the procedure for lesion and arterial visualization. In contrast, the use of distal occlusion balloons interrupts antegrade flow and may result in intolerance to ischemia during the procedure in some patients. Therefore, appropriate collateral blood flow to the end-organ, as well as its susceptibility to ischemia, should be assessed before deployment. Further, distal occlusion balloons do not allow angiographic visualization of the lesion after balloon occlusion has been applied. Filters and distal occlusion balloons are introduced after sheath placement, and their placement in tortuous vessels may be difficult. Protection is achieved only after the lesion is crossed by the device. Proximal occlusion balloons and flow reversal devices are placed before the lesion is accessed, allowing initial crossing of the stenosis under protection. Similar to distal occlusion balloons, proximal protection devices rely on a good collateral blood flow and may be poorly tolerated by some patients. In general, use of any protection device makes the procedure more complex and difficult; therefore, one needs to consider the risk-benefit ratio of using such a device, especially if one will encounter difficult anatomy. The use and type of device must be assessed on an individual basis, taking into account symptoms, collateral blood flow, anatomy, and the presence of thrombus, tortuosity, or calcification.[18-20]

Distal Protection Devices

Distal Occlusion Balloons

There are two distal occlusion balloons: PercuSurge Guard-Wire and GuardDOG Guidewire Occlusion System. Percu-Surge GuardWire is the more popular type of distal occlusion balloon. The distal occlusion balloon accomplishes distal protection by occluding the vessel, thereby preventing distal emboli. The emboli are then suction-aspirated by a catheter at the end of the procedure and before balloon deflation. Gradual inadvertent deflation of the balloon can occur, resulting in the re-establishment of prograde flow and distal embolization of trapped debris. This can be prevented by continuously monitoring balloon inflation and position with

the fluoroscope and intermittent injection of contrast material to confirm effective balloon occlusion. Balloon overinflation in an effort to minimize embolization increases the risk of vessel spasm or dissection.

Tubler and associates reported on their experience with the PercuSurge GuardWire.[21] They experienced a 5.2% periprocedural neurologic complication rate during CAS, despite the use of the GuardWire. The authors speculated that suction shadow may have been responsible for this phenomenon. Suction shadow occurs when the aspiration catheter fails to aspirate all the emboli either because some emboli are too large for aspiration or because the blood column adjacent to the GuardWire balloon is not effectively aspirated. The advantages of the GuardWire balloon compared with distal filters include increased flexibility and lower profile, both of which may contribute to a higher chance of crossing the lesion.

Distal Filter Devices

The advantage of a filter device over an occlusion balloon is that it can preserve flow during the procedure (Table 85-3). This not only maintains distal blood flow but also permits angiography to be performed during embolic protection.

Table 85-3 Distal Filter Devices

Device (Company)	Pore Size (μm)	Crossing Profile (Fr)	Filter Diameter (mm)
RX Abbott (Abbott Laboratories, Abbott Park, IL)	115	3.5-3.7	4.5, 5.5, 6.5, 7.5
Emboshield (Abbott Laboratories, Abbott Park, IL)	140	3.7-3.9	3, 4, 5, 6
Angioguard XP, RX (Cordis Corp., Bridgewater, NJ)	100	3.2	4, 5, 6, 7, 8
FilterWire EZ (Boston Scientific Corp., Natick, MA)	110	3.2	One size for 3.5-5.5
Spider FX (ev3 Inc., Plymouth, MN)	50-200	3.2	3, 4, 5, 6, 7

However, preservation of flow means the possibility of distal emboli. The filter's ability to capture embolic particles was evaluated in an ex vivo model, and although it captured the vast majority of particles, especially large ones, it did not capture 100%.[22,23] Particles can be released during the initial wire passage phase, and particles smaller than the filter pore can pass through or around the filter. Based on experience with the PercuSurge GuardWire, it is known that 50% of the emboli released during CAS are smaller than 100 μm.[24] Interestingly, all filters currently available have pore sizes larger than 100 μm, which may explain why significantly more particles are captured with the PercuSurge than with filters.[25,26]

Smaller pore size may decrease the chance of microembolization; however, it also results in a higher incidence of filter thrombosis. Filter thrombosis is related to plugging of the filter as a result of capturing too many particles or fibrin deposition.[27] Some manufacturers have made the pore size larger because the thrombosis rate was approaching 20%. Currently, most filters have a pore size of 100 to 150 μm.

In addition to particles flowing through the pore of the filter, some particles may flow around the filter. This is especially true when a filter device is placed in a tortuous vessel in which filter and vessel wall apposition is not complete.

Embolization can also occur during the retrieval phase because filters have a limited volume, and this decreases further when the filter is collapsed during retrieval. Although extremely rare, detachment of the filter from the guide wire has also been reported. Detachment usually occurs when the filter is caught on the stent during retrieval.

All distal protection devices require that either the aspiration catheter or the retrieval catheter be introduced before retrieving the protection device. Both catheters have a large lumen designed to either suction particles (aspiration catheter) or collapse the filter. Introducing these catheters may be problematic if this large opening gets caught on the struts of the stent. With the increasing use of nitinol stents, this has become a more frequent event because nitinol stent struts have a tendency to protrude into the lumen. In some cases, surgical conversion has been required.

Proximal Occlusion Balloons

When analyzing the limitations of distal protection devices, it becomes apparent that there is room for improvement. The advantage of a proximal occlusion balloon is that it is placed before the lesion is manipulated, thereby decreasing the risk of embolization. In addition, the proximal balloon stabilizes the entire system and increases the pushability of the balloon and the stent. Also, unlike the distal occlusion balloon or filter, one can choose a guide wire that increases the chance of lesion crossing.

The occlusion balloon placed proximal to the lesion suspends antegrade flow and preserves downstream vessel collateral flow. The Proxis embolic protection system is designed for proximal protection and aspiration of embolic material during interventional coronary procedures. By providing complete embolic protection, the Proxis system has proved to be effective in reducing the rate of major adverse cardiac events.[28] This device can handle large embolic loads and aspirate embolic particles regardless of size. It also captures vasoactive agents and prevents distal embolization. The MOMA device is another example of a proximal occlusion balloon.[26,29]

Flow Reversal Devices

The limitation of a proximal occlusion balloon relates to the presence of a side branch distal to the balloon that may allow prograde flow and embolization from the target lesion into the target organ (brain). An example is the superior thyroid artery during CAS. However, if the proximal occlusion balloon is coupled with occlusion of the external carotid artery and reversal of flow, this risk is completely eliminated. Reversal of flow is accomplished by connecting the side port of the occlusion balloon catheter to the femoral vein. Because the stump pressure of the internal carotid artery is higher than that of the femoral vein, the blood in the internal carotid artery is drained into the femoral vein. Embolic material is captured by a filter placed within the tubing that connects the proximal occlusion sheath and the femoral vein.

The Gore Neuro Protection System (Parodi antiembolization catheter) uses internal carotid artery flow reversal during CAS.[30,31] This protection device has a guiding sheath with an occlusion balloon attached to the distal end of the sheath. The main lumen has an inner diameter of 7 Fr, which allows the passage of balloons and stents and also maintains some extra room for blood to flow. Once the device is inserted in the common carotid artery, the occlusion balloon attached to the outer surface of the device, as well as the external carotid artery occlusion balloon, is inflated, thereby occluding inflow to the carotid bifurcation while maintaining access to the carotid bifurcation lesion through the main lumen. Once reversal of flow is established, CAS can be safely performed with a guide wire of choice.

This approach has some disadvantages, including interruption of flow during protection, the potential to cause dissection or spasm in the external or common carotid artery, and a larger puncture site for vascular access. In addition, the somewhat bulky sheath (10 Fr outer diameter) may make its introduction into the common carotid artery challenging if the arch anatomy is complex. Although this approach is not perfect, it eliminates many of the issues encountered with distal protection devices.

ATHERECTOMY DEVICES

Atherectomy refers to the physical removal of plaque material from the blood vessel. The presumed benefit of atherectomy is that it debulks or removes obstructing material rather than displacing it, as is done with balloon angioplasty. Atherectomy devices fall into two main categories: excisional (removing and collecting atheromatous material) and ablative (fragmenting the atheroma into small particles).

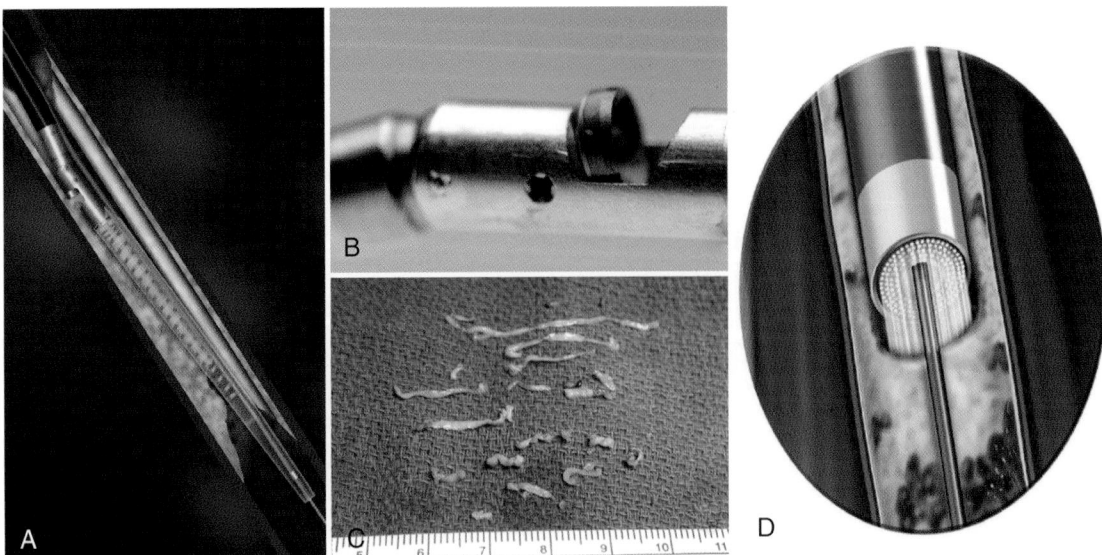

Figure 85-4 A, SilverHawk atherectomy catheter (ev3 Inc., Plymouth, MN). Excised plaque is placed in the nose cone; note the absence of a balloon for cutter apposition. **B,** A carbide cutter spins at 8000 revolutions per minute. **C,** Excised plaque. **D,** Laser atherectomy illustration (Spectranetics Corp., Colorado Springs, CO). The cold-tip laser uses pulsed energy and is characterized by markedly reduced thermal effects.

Excisional: Directional Atherectomy

The Simpson Coronary AtheroCath (Devices for Vascular Intervention, Redwood City, CA) was the original atherectomy device for coronary vessels. In the early 1990s, atherectomy was considered a major advancement in percutaneous coronary intervention. However, concerns were raised regarding high rates of restenosis (both short and long term), with no improved efficacy over balloon angioplasty.[32] The use of this device in the periphery had technical limitations (e.g., limited to vessel diameters >4 mm), and the long-term results were not superior to those of contemporary balloon angioplasty.[33]

The SilverHawk Plaque Excision System (ev3 Inc., Plymouth, MN) was approved in 2003 by the FDA to treat peripheral arterial disease and has become the dominant directional atherectomy device in use (Fig. 85-4A to C). The SilverHawk device debulks without a balloon for apposition. Rather, the device self-apposes the atheroma through a hinge system and contains a carbide cutter with a variable height (depending on the device used) that rotates at speeds up to 8000 revolutions per minute. It shaves atherosclerotic material from the luminal portion of the arterial wall rather than compressing the plaque and is contained within a distal storage chamber. It can be used without balloons or stents, and its palm-sized drive unit, with an on-off thumb switch, allows single-operator use.

Evidence of the benefit of excisional atherectomy with the SilverHawk comes mainly from single-center and multicenter registries. To date, there has been no randomized controlled trial for excisional atherectomy with the SilverHawk in those with critical limb ischemia. The largest of the registries is the TALON Registry, which involves 19 U.S. centers.[34] Midterm (6- and 12-month) outcomes for 601 patients with 1258 symptomatic lesions (mean length, 62.5 mm above the knee

and 33.4 mm below the knee) treated with the SilverHawk device have been reported, with an excellent procedural success rate (98%). Total lesion revascularization at 6 and 12 months was 90% and 80%, respectively. Although these results are encouraging, one needs to be aware of the weakness of data obtained from a registry as opposed to a randomized trial.

Ablative: Excimer Laser

Advances in laser catheter design and refinement of recanalization techniques have resulted in improved results with laser-assisted angioplasty of complex peripheral arterial disease (Fig. 85-4D).[35,36] The 308-nm excimer laser uses flexible fiberoptic catheters to deliver intense bursts of ultraviolet energy in short pulse durations. Tissue is ablated only on contact, with minimal surrounding thermal injury. A unique feature of ultraviolet light is its ability to ablate plaque and thrombus and thus reduce the potential for embolic complications. Excimer laser atherectomy of peripheral arteries has been practiced in Europe since 1994 and has proved to be a useful adjunct for the treatment of long superficial femoral artery (SFA) occlusions.[35] In the Laser Angioplasty for Critical Limb Ischemia trial, 42% of the lesions treated were in the SFA, with the majority of patients having complex occlusive disease.[37] This approach resulted in an excellent limb salvage rate of 93% at 6 months.

▌ THROMBECTOMY DEVICES

Introduction of the Fogarty thromboembolectomy catheter in the early 1960s facilitated the reliable removal of occlusive material through small remote incisions.[38] Totally percutaneous thrombectomy was first implemented in the 1990s, in the

---

Box 85-1 Thrombectomy Devices

ASPIRATION DEVICES
- Export Catheter (Medtronic Vascular, Minneapolis, MN)
- Pronto Extraction Catheter (Vascular Solutions, Inc., Minneapolis, MN)

HYDRODYNAMIC DEVICES
- Angiojet (Possis Medical, Inc., Minneapolis, MN)
- Hydrolyser (Cordis Corp., Bridgewater, NJ)

ROTATIONAL DEVICES
- HELIX Clot Buster Thrombectomy Device (ev3 Inc., Plymouth, MN)

ULTRASONIC DEVICES
- Resolution Ultrasonic Endovascular Ablation System (OmniSonics Medical Technologies, Inc., Wilmington, MA)
- Acolysis (Vascular Solutions, Inc., Minneapolis, MN)

OTHERS
- X-SIZER Catheter (ev3 Inc., Plymouth, MN)
- Trellis Peripheral Infusion System (Bacchus Vascular, Inc., Santa Clara, CA)

---

form of aspiration thrombectomy.[39,40] Since then, many devices have been designed to remove thrombi from the arterial or venous circulation. The main aim of such device development was to obviate the need for major surgical incisions and pharmacologic thrombolysis. However, over time, it has become apparent that mechanical and pharmacologic approaches to the treatment of thrombi are complementary rather than competitive techniques. The following paragraphs discuss the function and technical specifications of the array of devices currently available or under investigation for the treatment of arterial thrombus (Box 85-1). Chapter 158 (Acute Ischemia: Treatment) provides expanded information on the therapeutic use of these devices in the extremity.

Simple Aspiration Catheters

The simplest thrombectomy device is a catheter with a large distal port for the application of suction. Currently there are two aspiration catheters available for use in the coronary and peripheral circulations: Export Catheter and Pronto Extraction Catheter. Both these catheters have a monorail design and are delivered over a 0.014-inch guide wire. The suction lumen is large and extends from the tip of the catheter to the hub, where a syringe is attached for aspiration.

These catheters work most effectively when there is no flow in the artery. In the presence of flow, the catheter aspirates blood instead of thrombus. For maximal efficacy, the catheter is placed in the midst of a thrombus, and suction is applied as the catheter is gradually withdrawn over the monorail. These steps are typically repeated several times. If the catheter becomes clogged, it should be removed and flushed. In small vessels (up to 4 to 5 mm), these catheters seem to work well. When the thrombus burden is large, other mechanical devices are generally required to remove the remaining thrombus. These catheters may be used as a pre-

treatment in some cases, before the use of more bulky devices for thrombectomy (see later), in an effort to minimize distal embolization at the time of the latter's insertion.

Rheolytic Devices

These devices exploit the use of high-speed saline jets to create a Venturi effect at the catheter tip, which results in lysis and aspiration of thrombus. Saline is injected though a narrow injection lumen toward the catheter tip. Using a variety of designs, the jets are then directed backward, toward the proximal portion of the catheter. A low-pressure zone is thus created around these high-speed jets, which has the effect of fragmenting and aspirating the thrombus through the holes in the catheter tip. A large export lumen then carries the aspirated thrombus toward a collection area. Various aspects of fluid delivery, pressure generation, and suction account for the specific advantages and disadvantages of these systems.

These devices are relatively bulky and may cause distal macroembolization during catheter manipulation in thrombus-laden vessels. Although hemodialysis fistulae usually tolerate this downstream embolization into the large-capacitance venous system, this event is typically poorly tolerated in the peripheral arterial circulation.[41] In theory, these devices exert their effect without making contact with the vessel wall. In practice, however, the negative suction effect created at the catheter tip has the potential to draw the vessel wall into the openings in the tip. Angiographically, it is rare to observe evidence of vessel trauma (i.e., frank vessel dissection), but angioscopic and histologic studies commonly demonstrate evidence of endothelial denudation.[42] The asymmetry in the opening of the Hydrolyser device may increase the risk of this complication compared with use of the Angiojet. Reducing the flow rate of the saline solution is likely to reduce the risk of this complication. Hemolysis resulting in anemia may occur during the mechanical disruption of red blood cells in the path of the high-velocity saline jets. Long activation runs of these devices, together with large amounts of applied saline, increase the risk of this complication. One of the effects of hemolysis is the release of adenosine, which may cause significant heart block in some patients. This is commonly seen during coronary artery intervention but has been observed in peripheral arterial and venous interventions as well.

Rotational Devices

These thrombectomy devices mechanically fragment the thrombus and then disperse it. In theory, these devices are more likely to be associated with distal embolization, because there is no attempt to aspirate the thrombus from the vessel. The HELIX Clot Buster Thrombectomy Device (formerly known as the Amplatz Thrombectomy Device) was the first rotational device. It has a 7 Fr outer lumen and is delivered, without the use of a guide wire, to the desired location within the vessel. A compressed gas–driven turbine activates a driveshaft running the length of the catheter. This causes rotation of an encapsulated impeller, housed at the distal end of the device, at approximately 100,000 revolutions per minute. The miniature impeller creates a recirculating vortex that draws thrombus to the catheter tip, where it is macerated into microscopic fragments and dispersed into the bloodstream.

Other Devices

The Trellis catheter is a novel device for the treatment of arterial and venous thrombus. Using a unique design and technology, it allows both localized mechanical lysis and pharmacologic fibrinolysis of thrombus in the arterial circulation. Currently, the FDA has approved the device only for the administration of fibrinolytic agents.

The Trellis device contains a 6 Fr multilumen catheter. Near the distal end of the catheter are two compliant balloons with infusion holes located in between. When inflated, the balloons isolate a treatment zone that effectively maintains the concentration of infused fluid. Depending on the length of thrombus to be treated, catheters with a 10- or 20-cm distance between balloons may be chosen. The device also has a central through-lumen, compatible with a 0.035-inch guide wire, to allow delivery of the device. The mechanical thrombectomy component of the system requires that the guide wire be exchanged for a dispersion wire component, which is a shape-set nitinol cable. Once placed, the shape-set region of the dispersion wire resides between the two balloons of the catheter. The dispersion wire is connected to an integral drive unit that oscillates the wire within the isolated region to further disperse the infused fluid and mechanically lyse the thrombus.

◼ ENDOVASCULAR THERAPEUTIC TECHNIQUES

Percutaneous Transluminal Balloon Angioplasty

Approach to the Lesion

Before PTA, the approach must be planned based on the location of the lesion, its suitability for angioplasty, and the timing of PTA during the procedure. If the location and appearance of the lesion are known as a result of a prior imaging study (e.g., duplex mapping, computed tomographic angiography, magnetic resonance angiography, standard arteriography) and it is deemed suitable for angioplasty, the best puncture site for remote access can be chosen accordingly. When arteriography is performed initially and PTA is added at the same setting, the access site chosen for arteriography can be converted and used for the therapeutic intervention, or a new access site can be selected. The shortest distance that provides adequate working room is usually best. Ideally, the operator should work forehand for best catheter control.

After the lesion has been identified, it is marked with external markers placed on the field, by the observation of body landmarks, by angiographic roadmapping, or by a combination of these techniques. Heparin is usually used; more recently, direct thrombin inhibitors have been employed for periprocedural anticoagulation. When stent placement is anticipated, prophylactic antibiotics may be useful. The lesion should be crossed with an appropriate guide wire and catheter combination before opening an angioplasty catheter. If the guide wire does not pass easily, the operator may decide on a different approach.

A basic principle is to try to pass the wire through the lesion via the true lumen. This is relatively easy in cases of moderate stenosis, but one must be careful when dealing with preocclusive, highly stenotic (>90%) lesions. In this situation, magnified angiographic views, with correct projection of the image intensifier, are needed for precise imaging. The use of a 0.014- or 0.018-inch guide wire as opposed to a 0.035-inch wire and an appropriately shaped guide wire tip is often helpful for crossing severely stenotic lesions. If one manipulates the lesion in a blind fashion or without care, one may convert a stenotic lesion that is readily treatable into an occlusive lesion that not only becomes more complex and difficult to handle but also results in elongation of the treatment area. For example, this may convert a Trans-Atlantic Inter-Society Consensus for the Management of Peripheral Arterial Disease (TASC) type A lesion into a TASC type C or D lesion, with compromised long-term patency (see Chapter 108: Aortoiliac Disease: Endovascular Treatment and Chapter 110: Infrainguinal Disease: Endovascular Treatment). If the lesion is preocclusive, guide wire passage alone may inhibit flow and induce thrombus formation. Therefore, the patient should be adequately anticoagulated, and the operator should proceed directly with PTA.

Arteriography does not require a hemostatic access sheath. When an arteriographic procedure is converted to an angioplasty procedure, a sheath is usually placed to minimize injury to the access vessel. The smallest sheath adequate for the intended balloon catheter is best, because complications increase with increasing sheath French size. Midprocedure sheath changes are cumbersome and inconvenient; therefore, the operator should attempt to place the correct sheath when the decision is made to proceed with PTA. The sheath is selected based on the type and diameter of balloon, catheter size, and need for a stent. To achieve maximal support and allow effective contrast injection, the sheath should be placed as close to the lesion as possible. For example, when treating an internal carotid lesion, the sheath should be placed in the common carotid artery; when treating an SFA lesion from the contralateral femoral puncture, the sheath should be placed in the ipsilateral external or common femoral artery (via the aortic bifurcation). In general, for lower extremity interventions, contralateral femoral access with a sheath up and over the aortic bifurcation is used.

Balloon Catheter Selection

Slight overdilatation at the angioplasty site is generally recommended. Ranges of balloon sizes for specific PTA sites are

Table 85-4 Selection of Balloon Size

Lesion Location	Balloon Diameter (mm)	Balloon Length (cm)
Internal carotid artery	4-6	2
Common carotid artery	6-8	2-4
Vertebral artery	3-5	2
Subclavian artery	6-8	2-4
Axillary artery	5-7	2-4
Aorta	8-18	2-4
Renal artery	5-7	2
Common iliac artery	6-10	2-4
External iliac artery	6-8	2-4
Superficial femoral artery	4-7	2-10
Popliteal artery	3-6	2-4
Infrageniculate artery	2-4	2-4

listed in Table 85-4. The diameter of the normal vessel just distal to the lesion (reference vessel) must be measured to select the appropriate balloon diameter. Digital subtraction technology with software measuring packages or catheters or wires with graduated measurement markers can be used for size comparisons. In general, if there is uncertainty about the final desired diameter, it is best to begin with a smaller diameter balloon and to upsize as needed to avoid overdilatation.

The balloon should be long enough to allow a short distance of overhang into the adjacent healthy vessel. If the lesion is lengthy or is juxtaposed to an area where dilatation is contraindicated, it is best to choose a shorter balloon and to dilate the lesion with several sequential balloon inflations. The length of the catheter shaft must be adequate to cover the distance from the access site to the lesion. For example, if one is treating an iliac lesion from the contralateral femoral access, a standard 80-cm-long shaft is appropriate, whereas treating a more distal popliteal or below-knee lesion from the contralateral femoral artery or a brachial artery requires a 100- to 130-cm-long shaft.

Balloon Catheter Placement

The selected balloon catheter is wiped and the guide wire lumen is flushed with heparinized saline solution. The balloon should be aspirated with 25% to 50% strength contrast solution to exchange the preexisting air inside the balloon shaft with liquid. This maneuver is important to avoid air embolization in case of balloon rupture, better visualize the inflated balloon, and apply precise pressure to the balloon (because air is more compliant than liquid). After placement of the correctly sized sheath, the angioplasty catheter is passed over the guide wire, through the sheath, and into the lesion. The catheter should pass easily through the sheath because the balloon has not yet been inflated. The balloon catheter is tracked along the guide wire and advanced across the lesion using the predetermined markers of the lesion's location.

If the balloon catheter will not track along the guide wire, this may be due to distance, lack of shaft strength, tortuosity, subintimal guide wire positioning, or high-grade stenosis with dense calcification. If this occurs, one should consider a stiffer

guide wire or a longer sheath to maximize pushability and support.

Balloon Inflation

Contrast injection via the sheath is performed to confirm the relative position of the balloon before inflation. The balloon is centered so that its body dilates the portion of the lesion with the most critical stenosis. This is where the force vector contributes substantially to the dilating force. The balloon's appearance at this point is often referred as a "dog bone."

After catheter placement, the balloon is inflated without delay to avoid thrombus formation. The balloon is inflated using a 25% to 50% contrast agent solution so that the outline of the balloon is visible under fluoroscopy. This permits the operator to observe the location and severity of the atherosclerotic waist as it is being dilated. Solution is forced into the balloon using an inflation device, which also measures the pressure required to dilate the lesion.

The balloon is usually inflated for 30 to 60 seconds, deflated, and then re-inflated for another 30 to 60 seconds. A spot film of the inflated balloon is obtained to document its full expansion. After complete deflation of the balloon, but before moving the catheter, fluoroscopy is used to visualize the balloon and ensure that it is fully deflated. Partially flared balloon wings may disrupt fractured atherosclerotic plaque or damage the tip of the access sheath on withdrawal. During removal of the balloon catheter, maintenance of guide wire traversal of the dilated lesion is essential, in case additional treatment is required (Fig. 85-5).

Completion Arteriography

After the balloon catheter is removed, completion arteriography is performed to evaluate the results of PTA. If the lesion was accessed in a prograde manner (e.g., retrograde common femoral access to treat a contralateral lesion, or prograde femoral access to treat an ipsilateral distal lesion), completion angiography should not be performed with an angiographic catheter; placement of an angiographic catheter would require exchange of the guide wire, which would result in loss of guide wire access to the treated lesion. In such situations, completion angiography should be performed via the sheath. Removal of the balloon catheter or stent delivery sheath may be required to obtain room within the sheath for contrast injection. If the lesion was accessed in a retrograde manner (e.g., retrograde femoral access to treat an ipsilateral iliac lesion), the guide wire should be exchanged for an angiographic catheter, which is placed upstream from the lesion. Alternatively, injecting contrast material upstream (against blood flow) via the sheath may be feasible if the tip of the sheath is placed adjacent to the lesion and if the treated lesion is short. If completion arteriography shows a widely patent PTA site without residual stenosis or significant dissection, and vessel contrast evacuation is brisk, the procedure is complete. When residual stenosis or dissection is present, its significance can be evaluated using adjunctive means (Table 85-5). Inadequate

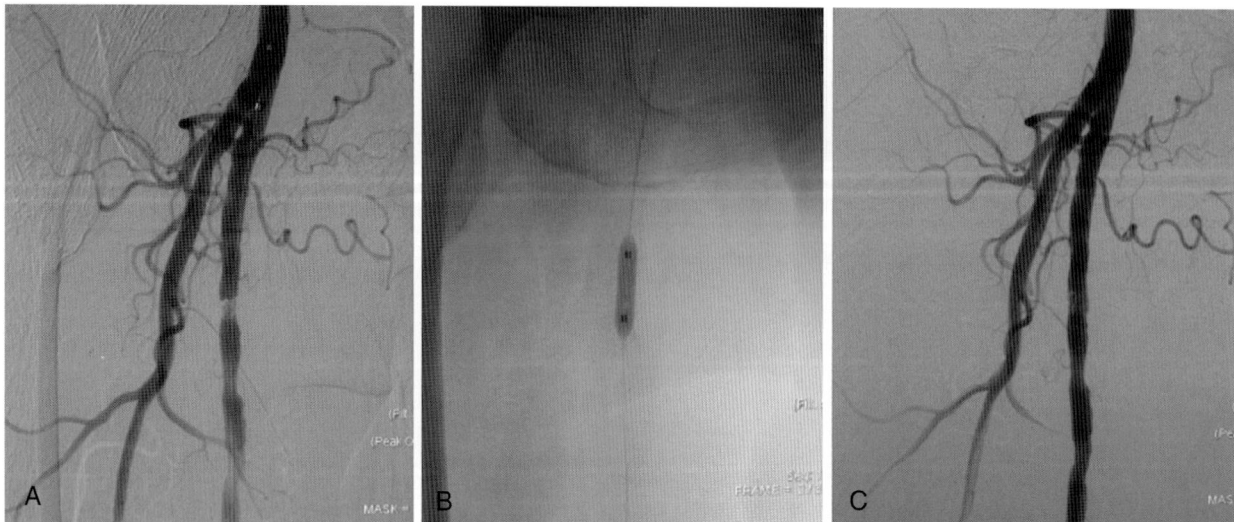

Figure 85-5 Balloon angioplasty. **A,** Preintervention angiography shows a short stenotic lesion of the superficial femoral artery (TASC type A). A guide wire is placed across the lesion. **B,** The balloon diameter is based on the reference vessel diameter. The balloon is inflated using the inflation device, and the fully dilated shape of the balloon is confirmed by fluoroscopy. **C,** Completion angiography.

Table 85-5 Assessment of Percutaneous Transluminal Angioplasty (PTA)

Method	Comments
Completion arteriography	Only method required in most cases; usually performed in same projection used for PTA (anteroposterior)
Oblique views	Useful in assessing posterior wall residual stenosis or postangioplasty dissection
Magnified views	Evaluation for dissection flaps or contrast trapping in arterial wall
Pressure measurement	Only quantitative hemodynamic assessment available; time-consuming; catheter placement across lesion may affect pressure in small-diameter artery
Vasodilator use	Adjunct to pressure measurement when there is no gradient despite appearance of substantial lesion
Intravascular ultrasonography	Expensive; particularly effective in finding and measuring diameter of residual stenosis
Distal pulse examination	Should be done in all cases; no risk; no cost

angioplasty can be treated with stent placement or repeated PTA with more prolonged inflation.

Subintimal Angioplasty

Subintimal angioplasty for the treatment of occluded femoropopliteal arteries was first described by Bolia and associates in 1989.[43] Anatomically favorable lesions are those with a suitable length of relatively normal artery both proximal and distal to the occluded segment, which permits the creation of the subintimal dissection plane and reentry into the native lumen without potentially compromising major branch vessels during the procedure or reducing future bypass options.

Subintimal angioplasty of chronic total occlusions of the femoropopliteal segments can be performed using either an ipsilateral antegrade common femoral artery puncture or a contralateral common femoral artery puncture. An angled hydrophilic guide wire and supporting 4 to 5 Fr rigid catheters with slightly angled tips are used to create a subintimal dissection plane above the level of the occlusion (Fig. 85-6). The wire is then advanced, and a loop naturally forms at the tip of the guide wire. It is important to form a large-loop guide wire configuration. The loop and catheter are then advanced through the subintimal plane until the occlusion is passed. The subintimal dissection plane has a characteristic resistance when entered, traversed, and exited. A loss of resistance is often encountered as the wire reenters the true lumen of the native artery distal to the occlusion. Recanalization is confirmed by advancing the catheter over the guide wire beyond the point of reentry and obtaining an angiogram. In cases in which a contralateral puncture is used, an angioplasty balloon is inflated proximal to the lesion to stabilize the guide wire and allow the necessary force to enter and traverse the subintimal plane. The recanalized segment is then balloon-dilated at 8 to 10 atmospheres using an appropriately sized angioplasty balloon. The technique does not require the use of stents, and these should be placed only in the setting of a flow-limiting dissection or elastic recoil. Patency, adequacy of flow, and preservation of runoff are confirmed by completion angiography. A rapid rate of flow through the recanalized segment, not the presence of a spiral dissection, is believed to be a strong predictor of a successful subintimal angioplasty. If it is difficult to reenter the true lumen after creating the subintimal dissection, reentry devices can be used, as described later and in Chapter 108 (Aortoiliac Disease: Endovascular Treatment) and Chapter 110 (Infrainguinal Disease: Endovascular Treatment).

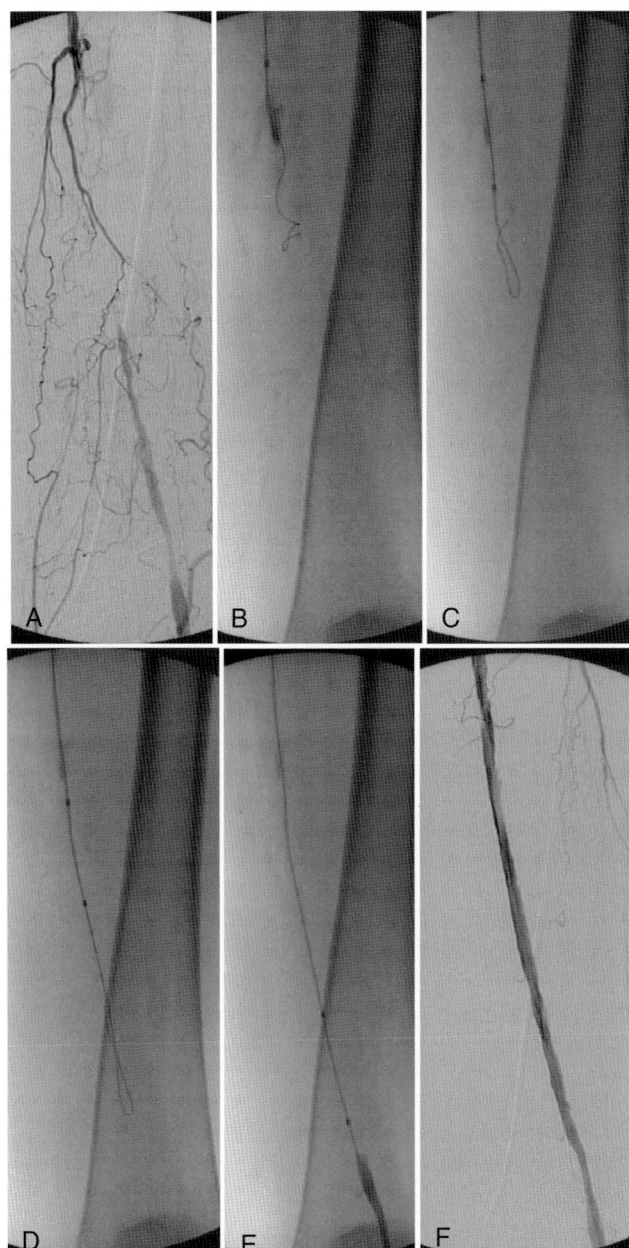

Figure 85-6 A, Preintervention angiogram shows the occluded superficial femoral artery. **B,** A nonlooped hydrophilic guide wire enters the occlusion with a support catheter. **C** and **D,** A small loop (**C**) or large loop (**D**) is used to dissect the superficial femoral artery occlusion. **E,** After the loop has reentered the true lumen, the guide wire is exchanged for a catheter to confirm reentry. **F,** After successful recanalization, the dissection plane is dilated. Completion angiography shows spiral dissection but the presence of rapid flow.

Reentry Devices

OutBack LTD Reentry Catheter

The OutBack LTD reentry catheter (Cordis Corp., Bridgewater, NJ) is either 80 or 120 cm long. It has a single 0.014-inch guide wire lumen and can be delivered through a 6 Fr sheath. The catheter consists of a deployment handle mounted on a rotating hemostasis valve, which is attached to the proximal catheter shaft. At the distal end of the catheter

is a 22-gauge reentry cannula (needle). The device is passed over a 0.014-inch guide wire into the subintimal space adjacent to the desired reentry location. Orienting the catheter under fluoroscopy using the radiopaque markers at the end of the catheter shaft aligns the cannula toward the true lumen. The guide wire is then partially withdrawn before deploying the cannula. By deploying the cannula, the intimal flap is penetrated from the subintimal space. The partially withdrawn guide wire can then be advanced into the true lumen, facilitating recanalization of a chronic total occlusion. Once a guide wire has crossed the lesion, any conventional therapies such as balloon angioplasty or stenting can be performed.

Pioneer Catheter

The Pioneer device (Medtronic, Minneapolis, MN) is 120 cm long, accommodates two 0.014-inch guide wires (one to track the device and one for the reentry needle), and is compatible with a 7 Fr sheath. This device incorporates a distal 25-gauge nitinol reentry needle with an integrated 64-element phased-array intravascular ultrasound transducer to allow directed ultrasound-guided reentry into the true lumen. The device is brought into the subintimal tract over a wire, and color flow is identified in the true lumen under intravascular ultrasound imaging. The catheter is rotated to place the true lumen at the 12 o'clock position, after which the 25-gauge nitinol reentry needle is advanced, and the true lumen is wired. The Pioneer catheter can then be removed, and any conventional intervention can be performed. Difficult reentry may be encountered with highly calcified vessels, a poorly visualized distal true lumen, and a deep subintimal catheter location.

Stenting

Indications

Indications for adjunctive stent placement following PTA include dissection, residual stenosis, presence of a pressure gradient across the PTA site, and acute occlusion.

Dissection. Stent placement should be considered for a significant dissection after angioplasty. Because plaque fracture is the mechanism of angioplasty, some degree of dissection is common. Unfortunately, there is no good method of assessing the severity of dissection or predicting its behavior. As a result, many postangioplasty dissections that would have healed spontaneously are not being given that opportunity and are stented immediately. Stents should be placed for any false channel or for any intimal flaps that impede flow, increase in size during the procedure, or extend into a previously disease-free segment of artery.

Residual Stenosis. After PTA, residual stenosis can usually be resolved with stent placement. The concept of preventing recurrence by eliminating residual stenosis makes empirical sense. A 30% postangioplasty stenosis can be used as a general threshold for continued intervention, although there is no convincing justification for using this particular degree of stenosis.

Pressure Gradient. A resting pressure gradient (>10 mm Hg systolic) after angioplasty usually indicates residual stenosis or dissection that requires treatment. Again, the threshold for treatment is arbitrary.

Occlusion. Balloon angioplasty for chronic total occlusion has poor long-term patency, especially for lesions longer than 2 cm. Stenting improves the durability of endovascular treatment of occlusion.

Recurrence. The use of stents to treat a recurrence after a previous angioplasty is an empirical approach; reasonable results can also be obtained in many patients with PTA alone. Relative indications include an embolizing lesion, significant ulceration, a long lesion, or a highly irregular, calcified plaque. Some proponents favor primary stenting of all iliac angioplasty sites on the basis of improved long-term results. This approach must be balanced against the higher cost of the procedure and the potential for stent-related complications.

The location of the proposed angioplasty site impacts the need for stent placement. For example, aortoiliac angioplasty is fairly durable without stents, so stents can be used selectively with reasonable results. Infrainguinal angioplasty is not very durable, and stent placement offers little improvement. Stent placement clearly improves the results of angioplasty for ostial renal artery lesions, however. Subclavian artery lesions often respond to angioplasty with significant recoil and may require stenting.

Stent Choices and Tips

Stents are either balloon-expandable or self-expandable. These two categories are best exemplified by the stents currently being used for peripheral endovascular work (Table 85-6). Either balloon-expandable or self-expanding stents can be used in the aorta. Short, focal lesions are best treated with balloon-expandable stents. Placement is precise, and a single stent is less expensive. Self-expanding stents are well suited to longer aortoiliac lesions (>2 to 3 cm). Placement of a single self-expanding stent is usually simpler, faster, and less expensive than placement of multiple balloon-expandable stents.

Lesions in the aortic bifurcation are treated by "raising" the aortic flow divider with balloon-expandable stents. Precise "kissing," side-to-side self-expanding stent placement is possible but difficult. Aortic bifurcation plaque usually extends through the common iliac artery orifices. Self-expanding stents are too flexible and lack the hoop strength desirable for orifice lesions.

Nonorificial common and external iliac artery lesions can be treated with either stent type. Focal lesions are treated with balloon-expandable stents, and self-expanding stents are used for longer lesions and those located in tortuous arteries. Self-expanding stents are better for stenting in flexible arteries, such as the SFA and distal subclavian arteries. Lesions in an

Table 85-6 Comparison of Balloon-Expandable and Self-Expanding Stents

	Balloon-Expandable Stent	Self-Expanding Stent
Length change during placement	Shortens by 1%-20%	Shortens by 1%-30% (Wallstent shortens by 30%)
Hoop strength/ radial strength	High	Low
Flexibility	Low	High
Precision of placement	Very precise	Very precise at only one end
Requirement of post-stenting dilatation	Sometimes	Always
Requirement of protective sheath for stent delivery	Always	Sometimes (e.g., entry site in contralateral groin)
Clamping of stented artery	No	Yes

aortic branch orifice, such as the proximal subclavian artery or renal artery, are best treated with balloon-expandable stents.

Technique for Balloon-Expandable Stent

The stent size is selected based on the anticipated diameter of the treated artery. The appropriate sheath and dilator combination are passed through the lesion (Fig. 85-7). The sheath must be of adequate length to pass from the entry site through the lesion. The dilator is removed. A customized cannula is used to temporarily open the hemostatic valve on the sheath. The balloon catheter, with the stent crimped into place, is passed over the guide wire and into the sheath. Using fluoroscopy, the balloon and stent are passed into the appropriate location. The sheath is withdrawn, exposing the balloon and stent. Before deployment, it is important to make sure that the stent is still in the correct place on the balloon. The balloon is then inflated to expand the stent. The stent should be slightly overdilated to embed its metal struts into the plaque. The balloon-expandable stent is passed through a sheath across the lesion to avoid dislodging the stent if it were placed directly across a tight stenosis.

Balloon-expandable stents expand to a "dog bone" shape, with the proximal and distal ends flaring initially and the middle portion of the stent filling out at the completion of balloon inflation. The proximal or distal end of the stent is often only partially dilated into an oval shape, which is not always apparent on completion arteriography. The balloon is deflated after the stent has been fully deployed. The balloon is advanced slightly and re-inflated so that the proximal end of the stent is fully dilated. This maneuver is repeated on the distal end of the stent.

Guide wire control must be maintained across the stent until the reconstruction is complete. If additional stents are required, the dilator is placed back through the sheath, and the dilator and sheath combination is advanced into the appropriate position. If numerous overlapping stents are

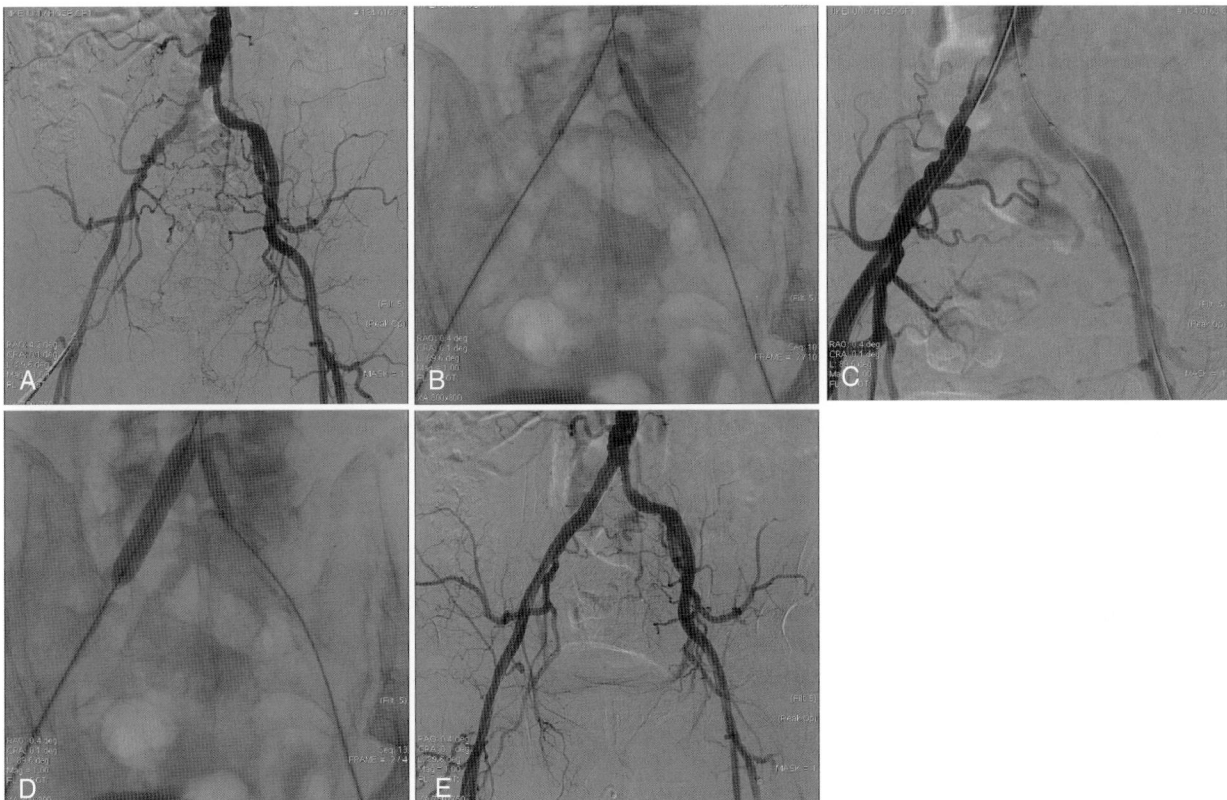

Figure 85-7 Placement technique for balloon-expandable stent. **A,** Preintervention angiography shows a right proximal iliac lesion in the aortic bifurcation. **B,** Bilateral guide wires are placed across the stenosis. The balloons are inflated simultaneously to the same pressure to dilate the lesion ("kissing" balloon). **C,** After dilatation of the lesion, flow-limiting dissection is observed. **D,** The dilator and sheath are advanced through the lesion. The balloon-expandable stent is placed at the desired location within the lesion through the sheath. Another balloon is placed in the left common iliac artery. The balloons are inflated to deploy the stent ("kissing" balloon). **E,** The stenosis is improved.

required, the distal stent is placed first and built proximally to create a "telescope" effect. If dilatation to a larger diameter is required, the deployment balloon is exchanged. Balloon-expandable stents can be dilated to a slightly larger size on one end, if necessary, to match vessel size and taper.

A completion arteriogram is performed in the manner explained previously. These techniques also apply to balloon-expandable covered stents.

Technique for Self-Expanding Stent

Placement of self-expanding stents is performed by withdrawing a covering sheath that encloses the stent on a prepackaged catheter. The selected self-expanding stent should be oversized—at least 2 mm greater than the final desired resting diameter—to provide a constant outward radial force on the endoluminal surface of the artery after the stent has been placed.

The self-expanding stent catheter is removed from its package, flushed, and wiped with a heparin-saline solution. The end stopcock is closed, and the catheter is advanced over the guide wire (Fig. 85-8). Because the apparatus is somewhat flexible, it can be passed over the aortic bifurcation. The stent is marked by radiopaque markers on its proximal and distal

ends, which are observed by fluoroscopy. To deploy the stent, the metal pushing rod is held steady, and the outer sheath is withdrawn. Fluoroscopy visualization is essential to monitor the stent position because the stent often moves forward or "jumps" during deployment. As the pushing rod is held stationary and the outer sheath is withdrawn, the proximal end of the stent begins to expand. The position of the stent is continually assessed. The stent position cannot be moved after the proximal end is deployed.

After the self-expanding stent is deployed, the stent is dilated further, especially in areas of maximal stenosis. It is sometimes difficult to assess whether the stent is fully expanded. If balloon angioplasty is to be used within the stent, the central part of the stent is dilated first. The ends of the stent are not routinely dilated because doing so may result in dissection beyond the area covered by the stent.

Atherectomy
Directional Atherectomy

Stents and angioplasty balloons are known to induce barotrauma and dissection. The SilverHawk atherectomy catheter removes plaque without the use of a balloon, which may reduce the potential for these events. Directional atherectomy

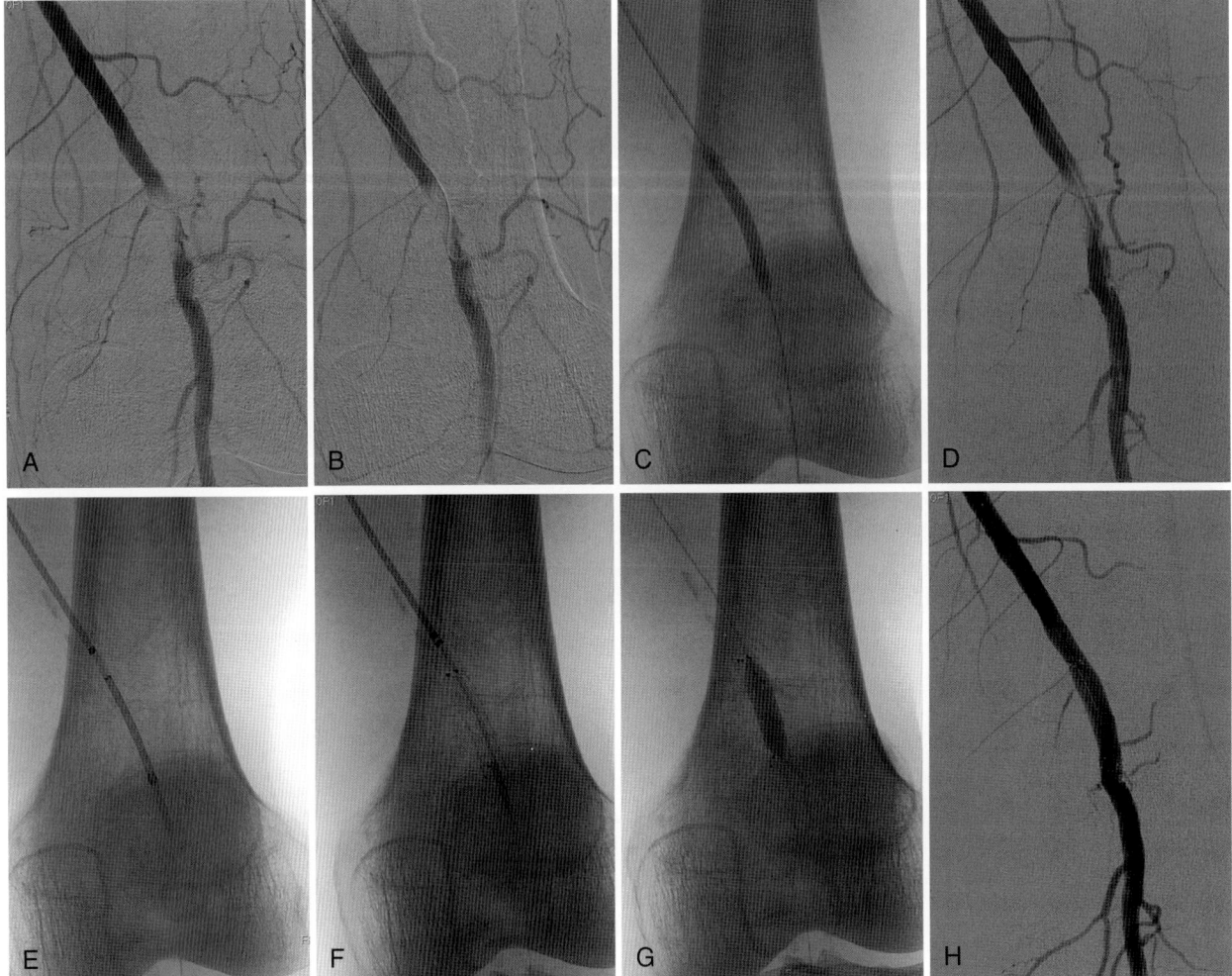

Figure 85-8 Placement technique for self-expanding stent. **A,** Preintervention angiography of the distal superficial femoral artery shows a severely stenotic lesion (TASC type A). **B,** The guide wire is placed across the lesion. **C** and **D,** After dilatation of the lesion, a relevant flow-limiting dissection is observed. **E,** A self-expanding stent of the appropriate diameter and length is placed over the guide wire. **F,** The position of the stent is continuously monitored with fluoroscopy during stent deployment. **G,** Because expansion of the stent is not sufficient, post-stenting dilatation is required. **H,** Completion angiogram shows a satisfactory result.

is best suited for "debulking" noncalcified lesions in the superficial femoral, common femoral, popliteal, and infrapopliteal arteries and for in-stent restenosis. However, the manufacturer recommends that the device not be used for the treatment of in-stent restenosis because of the risk of the cutter's catching on a stent strut.

The atherectomy catheter has a monorail design and an outer diameter of 6 Fr, making it compatible with a 7 Fr sheath. It is advanced over a wire just proximal to the lesion of interest. A mechanism in the handle at the proximal end of the catheter activates the device by opening an articulation between the cylindrical housing and shaft. This brings the cutter in contact with the plaque. The catheter is then advanced distally, removing a thin piece of plaque. Having reached the distal end of the lesion, the device is deactivated, withdrawn proximally, rotated 90 degrees, activated, and then advanced distally to remove more plaque. This process is repeated several times to achieve optimal debulking of the plaque (Fig. 85-9).

Laser Atherectomy

Potential advantages of laser atherectomy include the ability to treat long occlusions and complex disease effectively, thereby providing a better angiographic result and less need for stenting. Contralateral access with subsequent crossover recanalization of the occlusion is the standard approach for recanalizing long SFA occlusions. After the guide wire is placed in the origin of the SFA occlusion, two different laser techniques can be used to cross the lesion. In the OTW approach, the guide wire is navigated through the lesion. The laser catheter is then activated and slowly advanced over the wire to debulk the occlusion. Alternatively, laser ablation can be used in a step-by-step manner: The guide wire is first advanced into the origin of the occlusion; the excimer laser catheter is then advanced beyond the guide wire a few millimeters into the occlusion, without guide wire guidance. For further recanalization of the occluded vessel segment, the activated laser catheter is advanced stepwise for a short distance (<5 mm) without wire guidance, followed by further medium before activating the laser. The laser recanalization procedure is completed by balloon dilatation in a standard fashion with appropriately sized balloon catheters.

Thrombectomy

Aspiration Thrombectomy

With the increasing use of endovascular procedures for the treatment of arterial obstructive lesions, iatrogenic thromboembolic complications due to sheath insertion or balloon angioplasty are becoming more frequent. The first percutaneous technique developed for acute thrombus removal was the catheter aspiration technique. This method, which is still commonly used, involves placing an aspiration catheter adjacent to the thrombus and creating a vacuum with a syringe. Several aspiration catheters are currently available for use in the peripheral vasculature. The advantages of such catheters include ease of use and deliverability to small-caliber distal vasculature. The Export Catheter and Pronto Extraction Catheter (see Box 85-1) have a dual-lumen monorail design that is compatible with a 6 Fr guiding catheter (or a 4 Fr sheath) and a 0.014-inch guide wire. Thrombus is extracted by placing the catheter in the desired site over a guide wire, and manual aspiration is achieved by 30- to 60-mL locking syringes. This technique is most effective for the treatment of small amounts of fresh thrombus.

Rheolytic Thrombectomy

The Angiojet rheolytic thrombectomy system (see Box 85-1) consists of a pump set and drive unit that delivers pressurized saline to the tip of the rheolytic catheter to produce a series of retrograde-directed high-velocity saline jets that entrain thrombus through a Venturi effect. Six Angiojet catheters that can accommodate a wide variety of vessel diameters and clinical applications are currently available. Thrombus is fragmented by the saline jets and aspirated mechanically through the effluent lumen. Advantages of the Angiojet system include the ability to rapidly remove large amounts of thrombus without the need for chemical thrombolysis, which carries the risk of hemorrhagic complications. Disadvantages of the system include the potential for distal embolization, inability to remove chronic or insoluble thrombus, and difficulty delivering the catheter into small vessels such as the tibial or renal arteries. The rheolytic catheter can be used in combination with adjunctive thrombolytic agents (power-pulse technique) for more complete and rapid thrombus removal with less need for high doses of chemical thrombolytics.

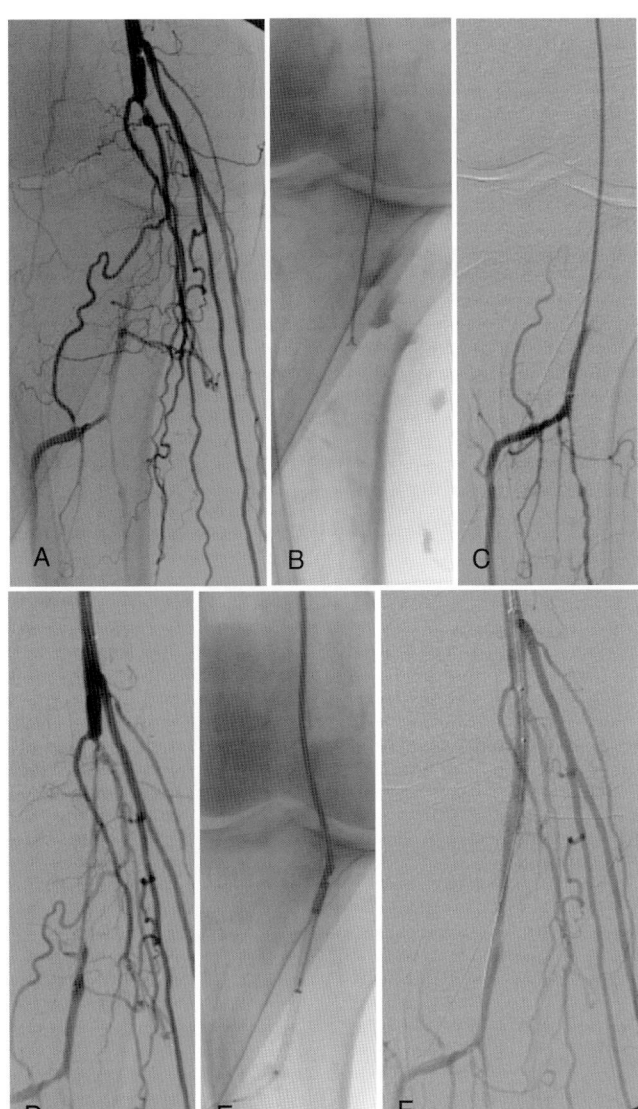

Figure 85-9 A, Preintervention angiography of a popliteal artery occlusion shows below-knee popliteal artery reconstitution. The occlusion length is 7 cm. **B** and **C,** Recanalization of the popliteal artery is performed with the Frontrunner device (Cordis Corp., Bridgewater, NJ) at the desired location. **D,** Angiogram obtained after Frontrunner recanalization. **E,** A SilverHawk atherectomy device is used to recanalize the lesion. **F,** Completion angiography. Note the preservation of all the collateral genicular vessels.

crossing with the guide wire in a step-by-step technique. The last 1 to 2 cm of the occlusion and the patent distal segment of the artery are crossed with the guide wire alone before using the laser, to avoid dissection.

In both techniques, advancement of the activated laser catheter must be performed very slowly, not exceeding 1 mm/sec. Fluoroscopic roadmapping is used throughout the procedure to verify the alignment of guide wires and catheters to the vessel lumen. Because saline more effectively transmits laser light to atherosclerotic tissue, and the absorption of ultraviolet light in contrast medium may induce shock waves that can result in dissection of the vessel wall, it is important to carefully flush the vessel with saline to remove contrast

SELECTED KEY REFERENCES

Dotter CT. Transluminally-placed coilspring endarterial tube grafts. Long-term patency in canine popliteal artery. *Invest Radiol.* 1969; 4:329-332.
   Dotter was the first to apply metallic stents to the human vascular tree.

Dotter CT, Judkins MP. Transluminal treatment of arteriosclerotic obstruction. Description of a new technic and a preliminary report of its application. *Circulation*. 1964;30:654-670.
Dotter and Judkins originally described the mechanism of transluminal angioplasty.

Gruntzig A, Kumpe DA. Technique of percutaneous transluminal angioplasty with the Gruntzig ballon catheter. *AJR Am J Roentgenol*. 1979;132:547-552.
Gruntzig developed the technique of balloon angioplasty whereby stenoses are dilated using polyvinyl chloride balloons.

Krankenberg H, Schluter M, Steinkamp HJ, Burgelin K, Scheinert D, Schulte KL, Minar E, Peeters P, Bosiers M, Tepe G, Reimers B, Mahler F, Tubler T, Zeller T. Nitinol stent implantation versus percutaneous transluminal angioplasty in superficial femoral artery lesions up to 10 cm in length: the femoral artery stenting trial (FAST). *Circulation*. 2007;116:285-292.
The FAST trial randomized patients with SFA lesions to primary stenting or PTA and showed that stenting resulted in improved 1-year patency.

Palmaz JC, Sibbitt RR, Reuter SR, Tio FO, Rice WJ. Expandable intraluminal graft: a preliminary study. Work in progress. *Radiology*. 1985;156:73-77.
Palmaz introduced the balloon-expanding stent in 1985.

Scheinert D, Scheinert S, Sax J, Piorkowski C, Braunlich S, Ulrich M, Biamino G, Schmidt A. Prevalence and clinical impact of stent fractures after femoropopliteal stenting. *J Am Coll Cardiol*. 2005;45: 312-315.
This study showed that SFA stent fracture is more likely in longer lesions and that fracture is associated with an increased risk of in-stent restenosis.

Schillinger M, Sabeti S, Loewe C, Dick P, Amighi J, Mlekusch W, Schlager O, Cejna M, Lammer J, Minar E. Balloon angioplasty versus implantation of nitinol stents in the superficial femoral artery. *N Engl J Med*. 2006;354:1879-1888.
This randomized controlled trial revealed that selective stenting of a short SFA was as good as primary stenting at 1-year follow-up in terms of binary restenosis, target lesion revascularization rate, and severity of symptoms.

REFERENCES

The reference list can be found on the companion Expert Consult Web site at *www.expertconsult.com*.

CHAPTER 86

Technique: Endovascular Aneurysm Repair

W. Charles Sternbergh III

In 1991, Parodi and colleagues published their seminal work on the use of a homemade tube endograft to treat an abdominal aortic aneurysm (AAA).[1] Although prior experimental studies had been published on the topic,[2,3] this first human report was the accelerant that fueled subsequent innovation in the field of endograft technology. Within 5 years, commercially manufactured endografts began to undergo clinical trials in the United States,[4] culminating in the first commercially available devices for endovascular aneurysm repair (EVAR) in September 1999.[5,6] In Europe and Australia, aortic endografts were available earlier because of differences in governmental regulation. Second- and third-generation endografts provided improvements in fixation, sizing versatility, and delivery profile.[7-9] All devices underwent refinements after their initial release, improving both long-term outcome and the applicability of EVAR. Endografts for thoracic endovascular aortic repair (TEVAR) began clinical trials at the turn of the 21st century, culminating in the first commercially available device in the United States in 2005.

In this short span of 10 to 15 years, the treatment paradigms for aortic pathology have undergone a seismic shift. Endovascular repair has become the preferred treatment modality for the majority of abdominal and thoracic aortic aneurysms. Other thoracic pathology, including traumatic transection and type B dissection with malperfusion, is also being treated preferentially with endografts. This is because endovascular repair has demonstrated improved perioperative mortality and major morbidity in both infrarenal[10-12] and thoracic locations[13,14] when compared with traditional open repair. These improvements in perioperative safety and the technique's minimally invasive nature have been the primary drivers of these remarkable changes in practice patterns.

ENDOGRAFT CONFIGURATIONS

Chapter 90: Aortic Stents and Stent-Grafts provides detailed descriptions of specific endograft designs. Bifurcated endografts are currently used in more than 95% of abdominal EVAR cases. These are either modular (AneuRx, Excluder, Talent, Zenith) or unibody (Powerlink). Early designs using a tube endograft (EVT/Ancure) had very limited applicability and poor long-term results, making this design undesirable for fusiform infrarenal aneurysms.[15] Tube endografts are now used only for focal saccular aneurysms or penetrating ulcers that have sufficient normal distal aorta for a dependable seal. Although there are no commercially available devices for this indication, off-label use of "stacked" aortic cuffs or larger iliac

Box 86-1 Relative Indications for Aortouniiliac Endograft Configuration

- Very small (<15 mm) terminal aorta (which would not accommodate a bifurcated device)
- Severe unilateral iliac occlusive disease
- Secondary treatment of migration of a short-body endograft

components is possible for this purpose.[16] Aortouniiliac endografts (ReNu) can be used in conjunction with a contralateral iliac occlusion device and a femorofemoral bypass. The relative indications for this configuration are listed in Box 86-1. Branched and fenestrated endografts (Zenith platform) can be used in juxtarenal or pararenal aneurysms and thoracoabdominal aortic aneurysms when there is inadequate normal aorta to achieve a durable seal adjacent to a critical side branch. These devices are not commercially available in the United States, however.

PREOPERATIVE SIZING AND PLANNING

It is axiomatic that precise sizing and preoperative planning are essential for both initial and long-term success after EVAR. Failure to pay close attention to these critical details predictably increases the risk of a poor outcome. Every patient requires a custom-sized device that conforms to his or her particular anatomy. It is incumbent on the treating physician to master the nuances of precise endograft sizing. These tasks should not be delegated to support staff or device representatives.

Preoperative Imaging

Computed Tomography

Computed tomography (CT) using fine cuts (≤3 mm) is the cornerstone of preoperative imaging for EVAR. Intravenous contrast should be routine unless the patient has severe renal insufficiency. Computed tomographic angiography with three-dimensional reconstruction is useful (Fig. 86-1), particularly when sizing thoracic endografts. The axial, coronal, sagittal, and three-dimensional reconstructions should all be reviewed. Depending on institutional capabilities, these reformatted images may be routinely available. Access to dedicated

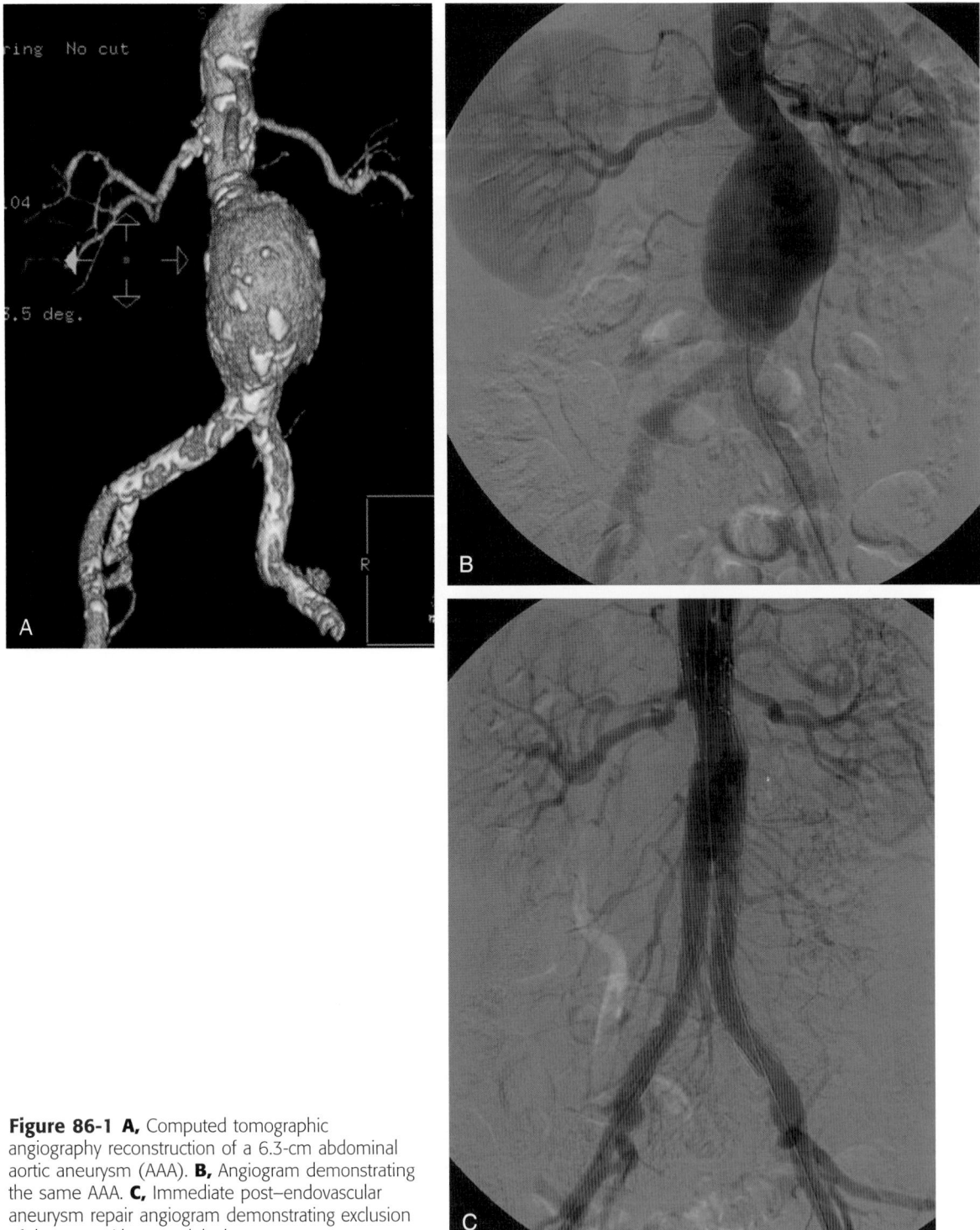

Figure 86-1 A, Computed tomographic angiography reconstruction of a 6.3-cm abdominal aortic aneurysm (AAA). **B,** Angiogram demonstrating the same AAA. **C,** Immediate post–endovascular aneurysm repair angiogram demonstrating exclusion of the AAA without endoleak.

workstations that allow the end user to personally postprocess and manipulate the images is ideal. Alternatively, such image processing can be performed by third parties and provided to the physician electronically. Standard arteriography has little utility in the preoperative evaluation for EVAR and should not be done routinely. With rare exceptions, all anatomic details can be obtained with CT scanning.

Patients with significant renal insufficiency present challenges in terms of preoperative imaging. Frequently, noncontrast CT scanning provides enough anatomic information to proceed with EVAR. Diameter and length measurements can be made from such a study, and if the anatomy appears uncomplicated and there is no clinical suspicion of associated occlusive disease, it may be reasonable to proceed. However, potentially important anatomic information can be missed, including the presence of laminated thrombus in the aortic neck; the patency of important side branches, such as the hypogastrics; and occlusive disease in the common or external iliac arteries. Significant calcification in the iliac arteries, particularly the external iliac arteries, should raise the suspicion of associated occlusive disease. All these anatomic details may negatively impact the performance of EVAR. Finally, if contrast is absolutely necessary, a pigtail catheter can be placed in the perirenal aorta and used to inject diluted contrast material while performing CT scanning. This reduces the amount of contrast material used by about 50% to 75% compared with that required for intravenous administration.

Alternative Imaging

In a patient with severe renal insufficiency who needs better definition of pertinent anatomy before EVAR, other options are available. Intravascular ultrasound can be used to size the aortic and iliac seal zones, evaluate potential eccentric thrombus in the aortic neck, and interrogate the external iliacs for occlusive disease. Direct angiographic imaging can be obtained using carbon dioxide as the contrast agent, with relatively good visualization. Until recently, gadolinium was also an option as a contrast agent. However, gadolinium's association with subsequent renal impairment in patients with significant renal insufficiency has made its use relatively contraindicated.

Endograft Sizing

Aortic Neck Diameter

Aortic neck diameter should be measured at the level of the lowest renal artery and 15 mm caudal. These measurements should be made from the *minor axis* of axial cuts or from reformatted slices that allow a plane perpendicular to the center line. The key here is not to overestimate the diameter based on the tortuosity that is frequently present in the aortic neck. Using electronic calipers, these measurements are made from adventitia to adventitia to size the aortic neck for most devices. Intima-to-intima measurements were used in the pivotal studies of the Excluder endograft (W. L. Gore and Associates, Inc., Newark, DE) and are recommended for this device.

Endografts should be oversized 10% to 20% in comparison to the aortic neck. In practical terms, this usually translates into an endograft that is 3 to 4 mm larger than the aortic neck. Currently, the diameters of EVAR devices range from 20 to 36 mm and can accommodate aortic diameters of 19 to 32 mm. TEVAR devices currently range from 26 to 41 mm, accommodating treatment diameters of 23 to 37 mm. Other sizes, particularly for TEVAR, are in clinical trials and are likely to be available in the near future. These new sizes, both larger and smaller, will allow wider applicability of safe and effective EVAR as well as the treatment of traumatic aortic transection and complicated type B dissection.

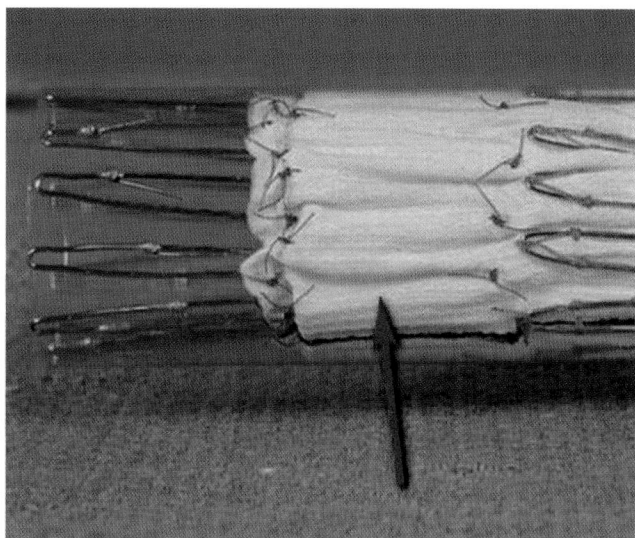

Figure 86-2 Oversizing causes pleating of the fabric (*arrow*). This is a 28-mm Zenith endograft in a 22-mm tube (27% oversize). Such pleating increases the risk of type I endoleak and migration.

Failure to adhere to precise sizing guidelines predictably increases the risk of both immediate and long-term failure. The danger of undersizing is intuitive; if the endograft is not fully apposed to the aortic wall, the risk of type I endoleak is substantial. The risks of oversizing are less obvious. Bench testing has demonstrated that oversizing greater than 20% creates pleats in the fabric (Fig. 86-2). This pleating may contribute to an increased risk of type I endoleak and possibly decreased fixation. The deleterious effects of excessive device size for EVAR are not device specific. In a study of the AneuRx device, oversizing greater than 20% was associated with an increase in late aortic neck dilatation and device migration.[17] In a multicenter study using the Zenith endograft, oversizing greater than 30% was associated with a marked increase in the risk of aneurysm expansion and migration.[18] No effects on late aortic neck dilatation were observed.

Sizing the Conical Aortic Neck

Patients with conical aortic necks—that is, those with a greater than 2- to 3-mm change over the first 15 mm of aortic length—pose an interesting conundrum. In a patient with an aortic neck diameter of 20 mm at the renal arteries that dilates to 24 mm at 15 mm caudal, the larger diameter would suggest the use of a 28-mm endograft. However, that corresponds to a proximal oversizing of 40%. Conversely, if sized according to the smaller diameter (a 24-mm endograft in a 20-mm neck), the size would be inadequate in the caudal area. In such situations, it is prudent to split the difference—minimum 10% oversizing in the larger segment and less than 30% oversizing in the smaller segment. If the degree of size mismatch does not allow such sizing (>3- to 4-mm conical change in the first 15 mm of neck), EVAR is ill-advised.

Length Measurement

Accurate length measurements between proximal and distal landing zones are critical in choosing the correct endograft components. For EVAR cases, counting the axial cuts is very accurate for calculating the distance between the lowest renal artery and the aortic bifurcation in the absence of significant tortuosity or aortic neck angulation. Axial measurements generally *underestimate* the length between the aortic bifurcation and the internal iliac arteries, especially with very tortuous vessels. Conversely, measurements based on centerline calculations frequently *overestimate* the true length needed. In TEVAR cases that include the aortic arch, axial cuts are not nearly as helpful, and even centerline reconstruction measurements can be inaccurate, usually underestimating the true length. If more than one thoracic component is used, a minimum of 5 cm overlap is needed. This component overlap should be even greater if the bridge area is within a large aneurysm without significant laminated thrombus or in an area with significant angulation. Ultimately, knowledge of these imaging limitations allows the experienced operator to use gestalt to choose the appropriate length.

Situations that typically require longer iliac limbs than the measurement suggests include extreme iliac tortuosity, "balleting" of the limbs (AneuRx and Excluder; Fig. 86-3), and the need to extend to the external iliac arteries. It these anatomic circumstances, it is prudent to choose a longer device when in doubt. Modular devices also allow some degree of flexibility at the time of implantation by adjusting the amount of overlap between the components.

Modular devices with variable body lengths (Zenith) provide additional flexibility in sizing. With this device, the contralateral iliac gate is ideally positioned 1 to 2 cm from the aortic bifurcation. Unlike with iliac components, one should choose the shorter length when in doubt about the correct length. Other scenarios that call for a shorter body length include patients with a small (<20 mm) distal aortic neck or those with an eccentric calcific "reef" in the terminal aorta. In these instances, after opening the ipsilateral limb (12 mm diameter), there may be inadequate room for the contralateral gate to open, making cannulation difficult.

Iliac Diameter

Limbs for the iliac arteries should be sized 10% to 20% larger than the minor axis diameter. For nonectatic iliac arteries, this generally translates into an iliac limb diameter 1 to 3 mm larger than the vessel. Particular care should be taken to correctly size the iliac limb if extension to the external iliac is required. Excessive oversizing may increase the risk of limb thrombosis.

Patient Selection

The major anatomic factor in predicting suitability for EVAR is the character of the aortic neck. Length, diameter, angulation, and shape of the aortic neck are important factors. The instructions for use that accompany most current devices suggest a minimum neck length of 15 mm and angulation of less than 45 to 60 degrees. For the Talent device, a minimum neck length of 10 mm is recommended. Taking into account proper sizing and available endograft sizes, aortic diameters up to 32 mm can be accommodated. The shape of the neck is also important for both immediate and long-term success. The ideal is a parallel neck without any eccentric laminated thrombus. Patients with irregularly shaped necks have a greater risk of an inadequate seal. In addition to patients with conical and reverse conical necks, an occasional patient has a localized posterior bulge in the neck ("double bubble") that can compromise the seal zone. Anatomically compromised necks can negatively impact both short- and long-term results of EVAR.

How far can these aortic neck constraints be pushed? Although a patient with a single adverse anatomic variable can often be treated effectively, those whose aortic necks have multiple compromising issues are more problematic. Highly angulated necks are associated with inferior outcomes,[19] but if the neck length is greater than 2 cm and the shape is parallel, the patient may be a reasonable EVAR candidate. Patients with neck lengths of 10 to 15 mm can frequently attain a good outcome in the absence of any other anatomic problems. Note that the ability to safely "push the envelope" anatomically is somewhat device dependent; some devices should never be employed in situations outside the manufacturer's recommendations.[20,21] However, any device will ultimately

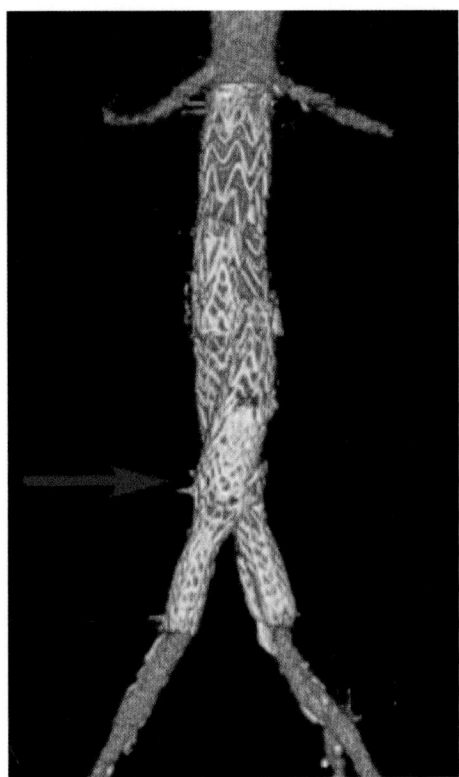

Figure 86-3 "Balleting" of iliac limbs (*arrow*). This technique can facilitate cannulation of the contralateral gate of short-bodied modular endografts. A longer iliac limb is frequently required.

produce unsatisfactory outcomes if the anatomic constraints are profoundly exceeded.[22]

Fenestrated or branched devices may be useful to extend the applicability of EVAR in the case of a compromised aortic neck. Although excellent short-term outcomes have been reported with these customized devices, they are associated with some increased morbidity compared with standard EVAR.[23] In fit patients, open juxtarenal AAA repair has demonstrated excellent outcomes.[24] See Chapter 90: Aortic Stents and Stent-Grafts and Chapter 127: Abdominal Aortic Aneurysms: Evaluation and Decision Making for an expanded discussion of patient selection for endovascular versus open repair.

ANESTHESIA, ACCESS, AND IMAGING

Anesthesia

The choice of anesthetic technique can be tailored to the patient's co-morbidities and body habitus. In all situations it is ideal to be able to control the patient's respirations, either by asking the patient to hold his or her breath or by doing it manually with the respirator. With open vascular access, a regional (spinal) or general anesthetic is favored by most operators. Although local infiltration and intravenous sedation are possible in such scenarios, it may be challenging to keep the patient comfortable, and a substantial amount of intravenous sedation often becomes necessary. The patient's diminished alertness makes effective breath-holding difficult, potentially compromising the precision of proximal endograft placement. A regional anesthetic is the ideal choice in a patient with severe pulmonary disease in whom avoidance of endotracheal intubation is desirable; only light intravenous sedation is used so that the patient can hold his or her breath. In a patient who may need an iliofemoral conduit, general anesthesia is clearly the best choice.

Vascular Access

Access to the femoral vessels can be obtained in an open or percutaneous fashion.

Open Access

With open access, either a vertical or an oblique skin incision can be used. The advantages of a vertical incision include the ease of gaining additional exposure to the femoral artery. If preoperative imaging suggests significant femoral artery occlusive disease that might require endarterectomy and patch angioplasty, this is the preferred incision. If an iliofemoral conduit may be needed, a vertical incision is also preferable. Postoperative wound problems can be minimized by keeping the incision above the femoral crease, which is possible in most patients. The oblique skin exposure is favored by many operators because it may result in fewer wound problems. After the superficial fat is divided in the plane parallel to the oblique skin incision, deeper dissection is vertically oriented. This open exposure may be particularly useful in a morbidly obese patient. If the angle into the femoral vessel is too acute, a small counterincision can be made inferior to the skin incision, just large enough for the needed sheaths.

Percutaneous Access

Percutaneous access is possible for sheath sizes up to 24 Fr. The reported success rates for percutaneous closure with 18 to 20 Fr sheaths is 78% to 91.4%; this increases to 95% to 99% with 12 to 16 Fr sheaths.[25,26] Because 5% to 10% of larger arteriotomies fail to close, the immediate availability of surgical closure is essential. Prudent patient selection and careful study of preoperative imaging of the femoral arteries can maximize the success rate of percutaneous access for EVAR. In particular, preoperative imaging should be closely scrutinized for information about the diameter of the common femoral artery, associated occlusive disease (particularly anterior calcification), and location of the femoral bifurcation relative to the inguinal ligament. Box 86-2 lists relative contraindications for percutaneous access.

This technique involves the off-label use of suture-mediated closure devices in a "preclose" fashion. Ideally, the common femoral artery is accessed 1 to 2 cm proximal to its bifurcation but below the inguinal ligament. Some operators routinely employ a micropuncture set with a 21-gauge needle and 3 Fr introducer rather than a standard 18-gauge needle. Ultrasound guidance has been recommended by some to increase the accuracy of puncture placement.[27] Verification of the wire entry location should be done through a small retrograde arteriogram with the appropriate ipsilateral oblique view to better define the origins of the superior and profunda femoral arteries.

A 0.035-inch guide wire is then advanced into the aorta, and a 7 Fr sheath is placed. The "preclose" technique may be performed with either a single 10 Fr Prostar or two 6 Fr Proglide devices. When using the Proglide devices,[25] the first device is deployed with a 30-degree medial rotation. Maintaining wire access, the second device is deployed with a 30-degree lateral rotation. These devices place a single monofilament suture proximal and distal to the puncture site. These sutures are exteriorized as the delivery device is removed and then tagged for later use. The 7 Fr sheath is then replaced for hemostasis. Alternatively, a single 10 Fr Prostar device can be used.[26] Some operators have suggested the routine use

---

Box 86-2 Relative Contraindications to Percutaneous Access for Endovascular Aneurysm Repair

- Obesity, particularly a large pannus in the groin
- Severely scarred groin
- High femoral bifurcation
- Need for frequent introducer sheath changes
- Significant proximal iliac occlusive disease
- Small iliofemoral arteries
- Anterior calcific femoral disease

of serial Coons dilators to predilate the tract and the arteriotomy after the preclose sutures are placed but before delivery of the sheath for endograft placement. This maneuver may decrease the chance that the "lip" of the dilator-sheath interface will catch on the subcutaneous tissue or the arteriotomy itself.

After EVAR is complete, the delivery sheath is removed while retaining guide-wire access. Hemostasis is maintained with manual compression until the preformed knots (Proglide) are cinched down with a knot pusher. After hemostasis is confirmed, the guide wire is removed and manual compression is reapplied. Reversal of heparin with protamine is suggested at this time. If there is pulsatile bleeding after the two Proglide sutures are tied, a third Proglide device can be placed over the existing wire and deployed. If pulsatile bleeding continues, an open surgical repair should be performed. Replacement of an appropriate size dilator over the existing wire facilitates this exposure by providing a nonhemorrhagic field.

Iliac Occlusive Disease

The iliac vessels should be carefully studied preoperatively with CT so that any potential difficulties in access can be anticipated. Focal iliac occlusive disease can be treated with angioplasty immediately before endograft insertion. Bare metal stents should not be placed initially because the large sheath for the endograft must be placed through them, increasing the possibility of stent migration. If an iliac lesion warrants stent placement and is not covered by the endograft, the stent should be placed after the completion of EVAR. Hydrophilic Coons dilators can be effective in dilating longer segments of occlusive disease and also act as a guide to whether the endograft sheath will pass. These should only be placed over very stiff wires. A word of caution is in order, however. Sometimes a larger sheath can be negotiated into the aorta with significant pressure, only to have catastrophic bleeding from iliac disruption upon removal of the sheath or with repeated placement. This reality should be considered when planning the repair to minimize the need for repeat traversal of the diseased iliac artery.

Iliac Conduit Placement

The ability to surgically place a conduit must be in the "toolbox" of all operators performing EVAR.[28] Although the need for conduits for EVAR is now fairly unusual, the larger French sizes for TEVAR and the higher prevalence of women undergoing the procedure have translated into 10% to 20% usage in most larger series. Patients with diffusely calcified and small external iliac arteries clearly need a conduit in most cases. If the operator is concerned about the access, serious consideration should be given to performing a conduit without trying to access the iliac artery. Visual inspection of the common femoral artery and terminal external iliac artery with open exposure can help in making this decision in equivocal cases. Certainly the worst time to perform a conduit is after

the iliac vessel has been injured, when the potential morbidity and mortality rise considerably.

An iliac conduit is performed through a right or left low retroperitoneal incision. Staying in the retroperitoneal plane, the common iliac artery is readily identified. We favor a standard end-to-side anastomosis with the distal common iliac artery. A 10-mm prosthetic conduit (Dacron or polytetrafluoroethylene) can accommodate the largest sheath needed. The conduit should be tunneled under the inguinal ligament through a femoral counterincision. The distal end of the conduit is then clamped to the drapes and accessed in the usual fashion. After EVAR is completed, most operators elect to anastomose the distal end of the conduit to the common femoral artery in an end-to-side fashion. Alternatively, the conduit can be removed, leaving a small "stump" on the common iliac artery.

Another method of obtaining access is to create an "internal endoconduit" by placing a covered stent in the external iliac artery, which then undergoes aggressive angioplasty to the required diameter of 9 to 12 mm.[29,30] The covered stent is protective of the extensive dissection or free rupture of the native vessel caused by the aggressive angioplasty. Clearly, to be safe, there must be a sufficient proximal and distal seal zone for the covered stent. Such landing zones are not routinely present, however. Prudent patient selection is critical. Although successful outcomes have been reported anecdotally with these techniques,[29,30] larger series are needed to establish the safety of these innovative access procedures before their broader use.

Imaging

Equipment

High-quality fluoroscopy and angiography equipment is essential for successful EVAR. A contemporary fixed-imaging unit with a 15- to 16-inch image intensifier is ideal and is used in many institutions. Portable C-arm fluoroscopy with a modern unit is acceptable but cannot provide the versatility and imaging capabilities of fixed units.

Gantry Positioning

The precision of proximal endograft deployment with EVAR and TEVAR is considerably enhanced by adjusting the gantry of the fluoroscope to be perpendicular to the axis of the aortic neck. A large percentage of infrarenal aortic necks have a modest amount of anterior angulation, which should be adjusted for by adding an appropriate amount of cranial tilt to the fluoroscopy unit; this amount can be estimated based on preoperative imaging. The majority of infrarenal aortic necks have 5 to 15 degrees of cranial angulation, but there may be as much as 30 to 40 degrees. Adjusting the left-right obliquity is also helpful in precisely locating the origin of the lowest renal artery. The left renal artery typically comes off the aorta a bit posterior to the centerline, while the right renal artery most commonly originates somewhat anterior to the centerline. An appropriate amount of left anterior oblique adjustment gives the proper orientation to the renal arteries in most cases. Frequently, this translates to approximately 10 to 20 degrees left anterior obliquity. These adjustments are particularly important in patients with shorter and angulated aortic necks.

Gantry position is also critical in the performance of TEVAR. Significant left anterior obliquity of 30 to 75 degrees is routinely needed to best visualize the aortic arch and the origin of the subclavian, carotid, and innominate vessels. If the distal extent of a thoracic endograft needs to be deployed close to the celiac, a true lateral position (>75-degree obliquity) is required.

■ EVAR DEPLOYMENT

Wire Placement

After bilateral femoral access is achieved (open or percutaneous), a floppy J-wire should be placed in the proximal thoracic aorta and, over a catheter, exchanged for a stiff guide wire (Lunderquist, Amplatz Super Stiff, Meier). These very stiff guide wires should not be routinely advanced in a bare fashion, and never without fluoroscopic visualization. Failure to routinely visualize the location of these stiff wires in the aortic arch increases the risk of inadvertent cannulation of an arch vessel, plaque disruption, and stroke. After the stiff wire is placed, the distal end of the wire should be marked on the operative drape so that a stable position is ensured throughout the procedure. Through the contralateral femoral artery, a pigtail catheter is placed just above the renal arteries, which are usually between L1 and L2. If there is concern about iliac occlusive disease, an angiogram should be taken at the aortic bifurcation, and the occlusive disease treated as detailed earlier. Otherwise, no arteriography should be performed until the undeployed main component is placed in the pararenal area. Particularly in patients with significant iliac or aortic neck tortuosity, placement of the undeployed endograft in the pararenal aorta may alter the relative position of the renal arteries, making the preinsertion arteriography inaccurate.

Delivery of the Main Device

The contralateral gate or limb of the main device should be appropriately oriented by fluoroscopy before insertion (Fig. 86-4A). This orientation should be rechecked as the device is being advanced, and any rotational adjustments can be made while the device is being moved axially. Attempts to rotate the device statically may not translate to the entire device, particularly in tortuous or small iliac arteries. Failure to follow these principles can cause a relative twist in the endograft.

Navigation of the main endograft through extremely tortuous iliac arteries can be challenging. If the endograft is not advancing smoothly, the first step is to change to an extra stiff guide wire such as a Lunderquist. Using this wire and a trackable endograft, it is unusual to be unable to deliver the endo-

graft to the desired location. Rarely, external manipulation of the distal aortoiliac segment may be beneficial. An assistant stabilizes the aorta from the contralateral side of the main device by placing a hand on the lateral edge of the aneurysm, thus helping to reduce any additional tortuosity created by advancement of the endograft.[31] The final step is to reconfirm that unexpected occlusive disease is not contributing to the inability to advance the endograft. If all these maneuvers are unsuccessful, use of a "buddy wire" should be considered. A second extra-stiff wire placed through the iliac artery can help straighten the tortuous segment.

Proximal Endograft Deployment

After the main device is placed in the pararenal aorta and the contralateral gate or limb position is satisfactory, the gantry position of the fluoroscopy unit is adjusted, as detailed earlier. A maximally magnified view should be used, with the lowest renal artery in the center of the screen to minimize parallax errors. Using a contrast injector, a short-burst injection using a high rate–small volume ratio allows good visualization of the renal arteries with a small amount of contrast material. A 30 mL/sec injection rate with a total of 7 to 12 mL of contrast material is usually sufficient, depending on the equipment and body habitus. It is essential that both renal arteries are visualized. If the lowest renal artery is not close to the center of the image, the table or fluoroscopy unit should be adjusted and the image redone.

With devices designed for a slow, stepwise deployment (AneuRx, Zenith), initial deployment should begin 1 to 2 cm above the intended target position and then should be slowly pulled down to immediately below the lowest renal artery. With the initial proximal deployment of these devices, there is an opportunity to further adjust the gantry position to ensure a perfectly perpendicular alignment with the aortic neck. The anterior and posterior aspects of the endograft should be superimposed if the gantry position is parallel to the aortic neck. If they are not, the degree of cranial tilt can be adjusted and the arteriogram repeated. Note that once they are deployed, the AneuRx and Talent endografts cannot be moved craniad; the design of the Zenith generally allows movement in either direction. With the Excluder device, the top of the endograft should be placed at the intended level of delivery and then deployed. Though not mentioned in the instructions for use, a slower, sequential deployment of the Excluder device, partially constrained in the delivery sheath, may facilitate precise delivery in the presence of challenging aortic neck anatomy.[32] The goal is to place the endograft within 2 mm of the caudal edge of the lowest renal artery. The maximum amount of overlap with the aortic neck increases the seal zone and reduces the likelihood of a type IA endoleak. The increased proximal overlap is also important in decreasing the long-term risk of endograft migration, particularly in devices without active fixation.

After the proximal landing zone of the endograft is established, deployment of the endograft continues until the contralateral gate is deployed (Fig. 86-4B). With the AneuRx

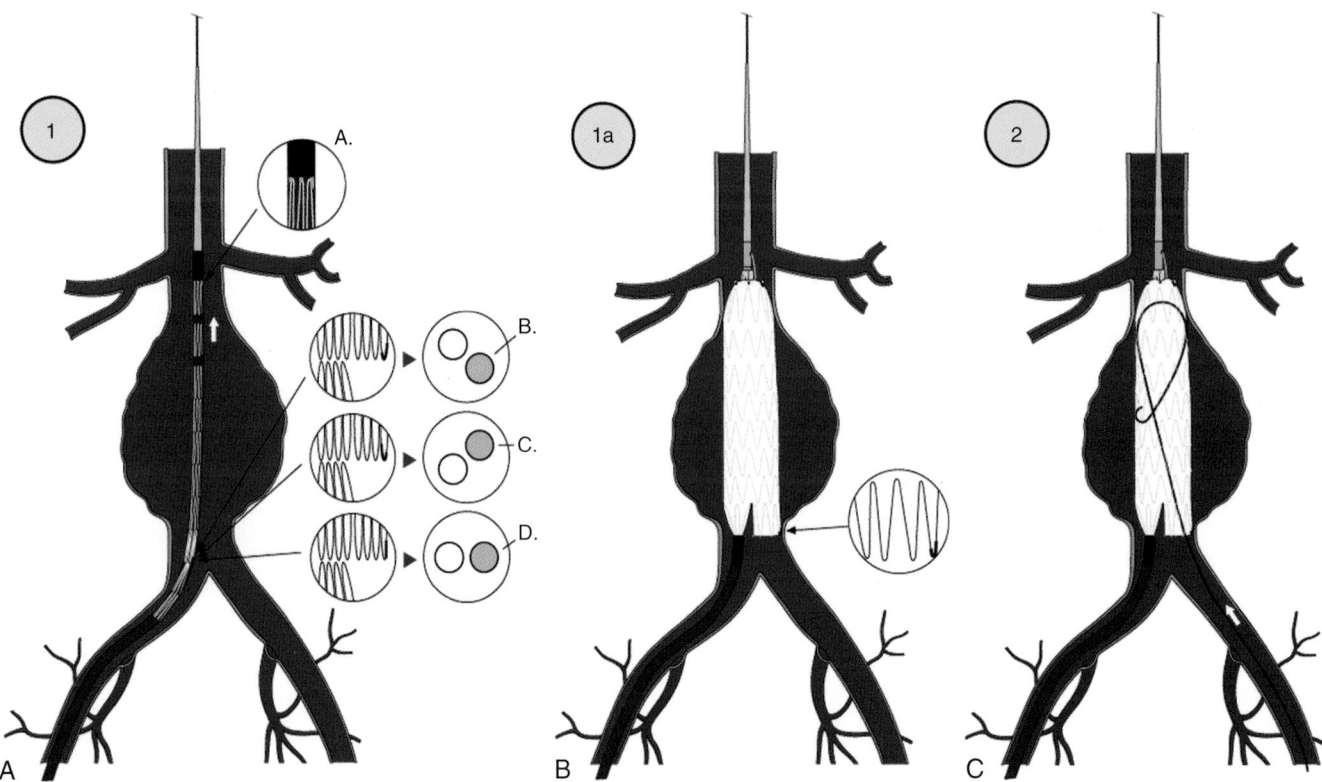

Figure 86-4 A, Placement of the undeployed main body in a position immediately below the lowest renal artery. Note the orientation of the contralateral gate. **B,** Deployment of the main body, stopping after the contralateral gate is opened. **C,** Retrograde cannulation of the contralateral gate.

and Excluder devices, the instructions suggest full initial deployment of the ipsilateral limb. However, some operators may choose to stop after the contralateral gate is deployed to help stabilize the device and minimize intraoperative migration.[32] At this stage in the deployment process, the Zenith device is still attached to the delivery sheath by the proximal and distal trigger wires and cannot have uncontrolled migration. With the Zenith device, some experienced operators deploy the bare suprarenal stent at this stage. This modification to the manufacturer's deployment sequence facilitates precise placement, particularly in very tortuous anatomy. Using this technique with the pigtail still in place, any necessary adjustments can be made before final suprarenal stent deployment.

Accessory Renal Artery Management

Occasionally a patient has a low accessory renal artery, in which case deployment below it would compromise the proximal seal zone. In patients with normal renal function, it is generally safe to cover such an accessory renal artery with the endograft. Embolization of the artery before coverage is generally not required. Patients with significantly impaired renal function present a more difficult situation. Further reduction in a patient's renal function by coverage of an accessory renal artery is far from ideal. However, alternative approaches, including a fenestrated endograft or open repair, have significantly higher morbidity and mortality in a patient with sig-

nificant renal insufficiency. Individualization of the plan is paramount in such situations.

Contralateral Gate Cannulation

For modular devices, the next step is cannulation of the contralateral iliac gate (Fig. 86-4C and D). This step is obviated if a unibody device such as the Powerlink is used. Retrograde cannulation of the gate should be possible in more than 95% of cases. Several "pearls" can facilitate this maneuver. Perhaps the most important step is planning where the gate will be located to facilitate cannulation. Deployment of the gate slightly anterior to the midline is usually complementary to the angle of the iliacs. With short-body devices such as the AneuRx and Excluder, it is sometimes easier put the contralateral gate ipsilateral to the main limb, thus crossing or "balleting" the limbs. This maneuver is particularly helpful if the angle of the proximal common iliac artery is splayed laterally. With a long-body device such as the Zenith, the contralateral gate should be within 1 to 2 cm of the iliac artery; thus, balleting is inadvisable. In cases in which one common iliac artery has significantly more lateral angulation than the other, placing the main device in the *more* tortuous side facilitates contralateral gate cannulation.

Several maneuvers can speed cannulation of the gate:
- After retrieving the pigtail or other angiographic catheter, avoid pulling the wire back into the iliac artery. If there is

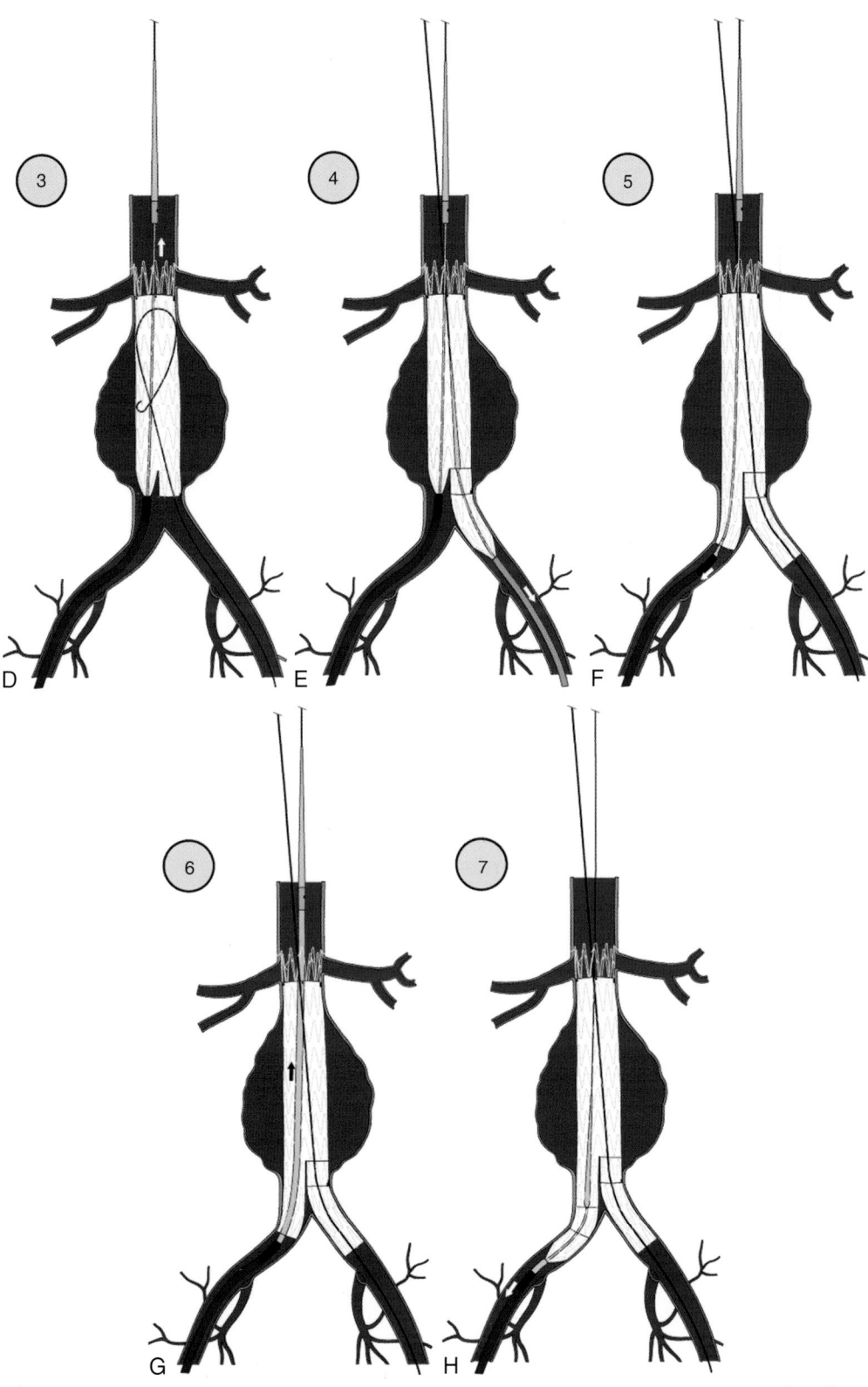

Figure 86-4, cont'd D, Deployment of the suprarenal bare stent. **E,** Deployment of the contralateral iliac limb after a retrograde arteriogram marking the location of the hypogastric artery. **F,** Deployment of the remainder of the main device and retrieval of the cap that housed the suprarenal bare stent. **G,** Placement of the ipsilateral iliac limb. **H,** Deployment of the ipsilateral iliac limb.

severe tortuosity or a narrow distal aortic neck, it can be challenging to regain access to the aneurysm sac.

- Choose a steerable angled wire (e.g., angled glide wire) and an appropriately angled catheter (e.g., DAV, Cook, Inc., Bloomington, IN).
- Use oblique fluoroscopic views to maximally "open" the gate. Using both the catheter and the wire to steer, attempt to place the wire into the gate. If the wire appears to be in the appropriate orientation with the gate but actually is not, the wire must be either anterior or posterior. By changing the obliquity of the fluoroscopic image with the wire in place, it becomes clear whether anterior or posterior deflection is needed. Occasionally, a different-shaped catheter facilitates cannulation.

Confirmation of proper gate cannulation is essential and can be done with angiography or by spinning the pigtail catheter in the area of the aortic neck. The pigtail's inability to freely rotate in this area suggests that the catheter is constrained between the aortic wall and the endograft. Failure to routinely confirm the wire position can result in deployment of the limb outside of the gate. This error should never occur.

Rarely, the contralateral gate cannot be cannulated in a retrograde fashion despite the aforementioned maneuvers. This is usually the result of the gate's failure to open because of a small (<20 mm) distal aortic neck, an eccentric calcific distal aortic "reef" (long-body devices), or extreme tortuosity (short-body devices). In such situations, the gate should be cannulated in an antegrade fashion. This maneuver is most easily accomplished with brachial access. Once a wire is negotiated through the gate in an antegrade fashion from above, it is snared from the iliac artery. Then the wire can be exchanged over a catheter for typical retrograde deployment. An alternative method of antegrade cannulation is to come from the contralateral iliac artery and go "up and over" the flow divider with an appropriately shaped catheter (Simmons 1, Sos). Although this approach seems intuitively attractive, because the access is already established, our experience has been that the anatomic issues that make retrograde cannulation impossible also make this approach problematic and frequently unsuccessful.

If all attempts at gate cannulation are unsuccessful, the final bailout maneuver is to convert the bifurcated device into an aortouniiliac configuration. This maneuver should be needed in less than 1% of cases. With the Zenith device, this is accomplished with a specifically designed converter endograft deployed within the main body, excluding the contralateral gate. A similar configuration can be accomplished with other modular devices either by using stacked aortic or iliac cuffs or by deploying a second main-body device within the existing one, with the contralateral gate oriented 180 degrees opposite the existing contralateral gate. After conversion to such a configuration, an occluder must be placed in the contralateral common iliac artery, and limb perfusion must be re-established with a femorofemoral bypass.

Limb Deployment

Once contralateral gate cannulation is confirmed, the distal landing zone in the iliac artery is established with a retrograde

arteriogram shot through the previously placed iliac sheath (Fig. 86-4E to H). The complementary obliquity should be used to visualize the takeoff of the hypogastric artery (about 20 degrees left anterior obliquity for the right iliac artery and 20 degrees right anterior obliquity for the left iliac artery). If the length of the limb is in question, a marker pigtail can be placed over the wire. More iliac overlap is preferable to less overlap. For the AneuRx device, routine iliac extension to the hypogastric takeoff has been advocated as a means of reducing proximal migration.[33] The absolute minimum overlap into the iliac artery (common or external) is 2 cm in a patient with nontortuous vessels and an AAA less than 6 cm. Patients with larger AAAs or tortuous anatomy should have longer iliac coverage if possible. These patients may have greater conformational changes as the AAA shrinks post EVAR, putting increased axial strain on the components. This scenario can result in craniad migration of the iliac limb and a type IB endoleak.

In patients with extremely tortuous iliac arteries, landing the distal end of the device in the acute bend should be avoided. Any kinks or stenosis in the endograft limbs should undergo aggressive angioplasty, usually with a compliant balloon (Coda, Cook, Inc., Bloomington, IN). If there is significant residual stenosis, consider the placement of a self-expanding bare stent within the endograft.[34] Occasionally, both iliac limbs can be externally compressed by a narrow distal aortic neck. Simultaneous conventional (noncompliant) angioplasty usually resolves this issue. However, if there is significant recoil, the use of bilateral balloon-expandable stents in this location should be considered. Careful review of these potential limb problems can minimize the risk of subsequent limb thrombosis.

A compliant molding balloon (Coda) may be used at the aortic neck, iliac gate, and distal iliac limb to optimize the seal (Fig. 86-5). Use of such a balloon is recommended in the aortic seal zone for the Excluder and Zenith devices. It is important not to overinflate this balloon outside of the endograft, particularly in the iliac artery, because arterial injury can occur.

Completion Arteriography

After the endograft placement is complete, a completion arteriogram is taken through a pigtail catheter placed in the pararenal aorta (see Fig. 86-1C). Use of a power injector with an injection rate of 15 mL/sec and a total amount of 30 mL is recommended. Because the devices' large sheath size often reduces iliac flow, we routinely aspirate these sheaths with 20-mL syringes during the injection. Image acquisition should continue for a minimum of 5 seconds after the contrast material in the iliacs is gone, so late type II endoleaks can be visualized.

The completion arteriogram should be carefully and systematically studied, with the following goals in mind:

- Confirm the patency of the renal and hypogastric arteries.
- Assess the precision of the proximal and distal endograft landing zones. Ideally, the proximal extent of the endograft

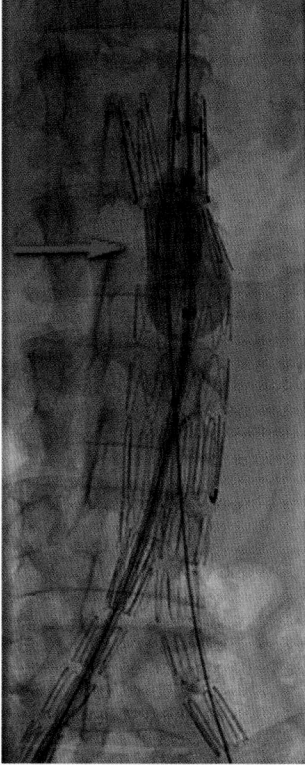

Figure 86-5 Use of a compliant molding balloon (Coda) on the aortic neck to optimize the seal (*arrow*).

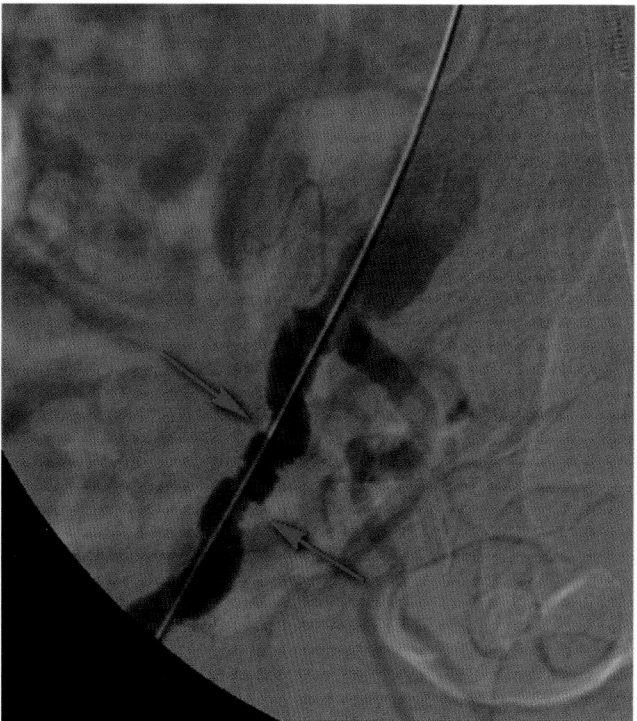

Figure 86-6 "Pseudolesion" of the external iliac artery (*arrows*). This is caused by placement of a super-stiff wire in a tortuous vessel, causing it to "accordion" around the wire. Removal of the stiff wire corrects the stenosis without adjunctive measures.

should be within 2 mm of the lowest renal artery. If this distance is considerably greater and the residual seal zone is less than 10 to 15 mm, placement of an aortic cuff should be considered, even in the absence of a type I endoleak. Likewise, iliac extensions should be placed if there is inadequate overlap with the artery.

- Evaluate for unsuspected external iliac occlusive disease. If significant tortuosity in the iliac vessels exists, the stiff wires in place for endograft deployment should be exchanged for a flexible wire before the final arteriogram. Stiff wires cause the tortuous iliac artery to "accordion," giving the radiographic appearance of severe stenosis (Fig. 86-6). These "pseudolesions" disappear with removal of the stiff wire. True occlusive lesions should be treated.
- Assess for endoleaks. (See Chapter 129: Abdominal Aortic Aneurysms: Endovascular Treatment for definitions of endoleak types.)

EVAR TROUBLESHOOTING

Endoleaks

Every effort should be made to definitively treat any initial type I or III endoleak before leaving the endovascular suite. Type II endoleaks should be observed because the large majority resolve spontaneously without intervention. In general, early endoleaks are almost always type I or III, whereas late-appearing endoleaks are more commonly type II. Frequently, retrograde filling of the lumbar arteries or inferior mesenteric artery can be seen before the contrast material appears in the sac, confirming the type of endoleak.

However, even the late appearance of contrast material in the sac adjacent to the proximal or distal seal zones is worrisome for a type I endoleak and should be aggressively interrogated. Additional magnified views with different obliquity may be helpful in establishing the presumptive type of endoleak.

Aortic Cuffs

Initial type IA endoleak treatment is predicated on the position of the endograft relative to the lowest renal artery. If this distance is less than 3 mm, the seal zone should undergo angioplasty with a compliant molding balloon. If the distance is greater than 5 mm, initial placement of an aortic cuff followed by compliant balloon angioplasty should be performed. As previously stated, it is essential that the proper gantry position be used to accurately assess the distance between the endograft and the renal arteries.

Giant Palmaz Stent Placement

If a type IA endoleak persists despite the aforementioned maneuvers, placement of a giant Palmaz stent may eliminate the endoleak (Fig. 86-7). Placement of this stent provides greater radial strength in the seal zone and eliminates the type I endoleak in most cases. A 4010 or 5010 Palmaz stent is hand-mounted on an appropriately sized valvuloplasty balloon (Braun Z-Med) in a slightly asymmetric fashion, such that more of the proximal extent of the balloon inflates first. The existing main-body delivery sheath, or a sheath of comparable size, is advanced beyond the intended deployment zone. The

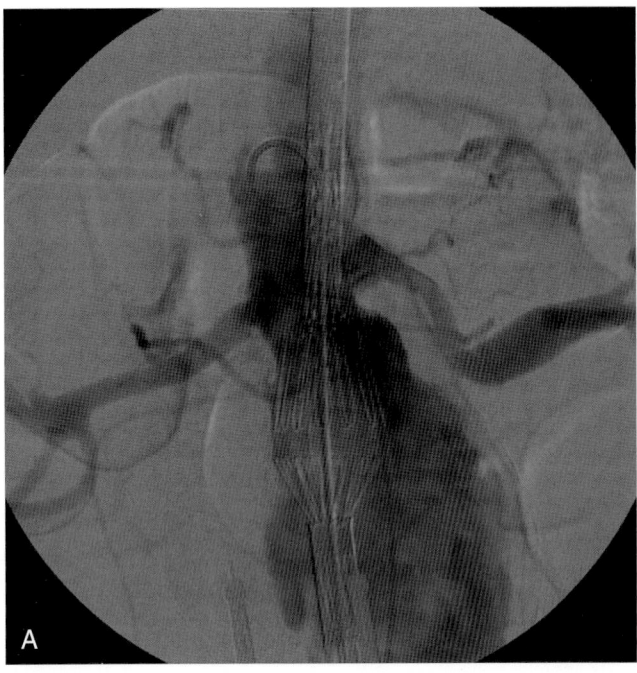

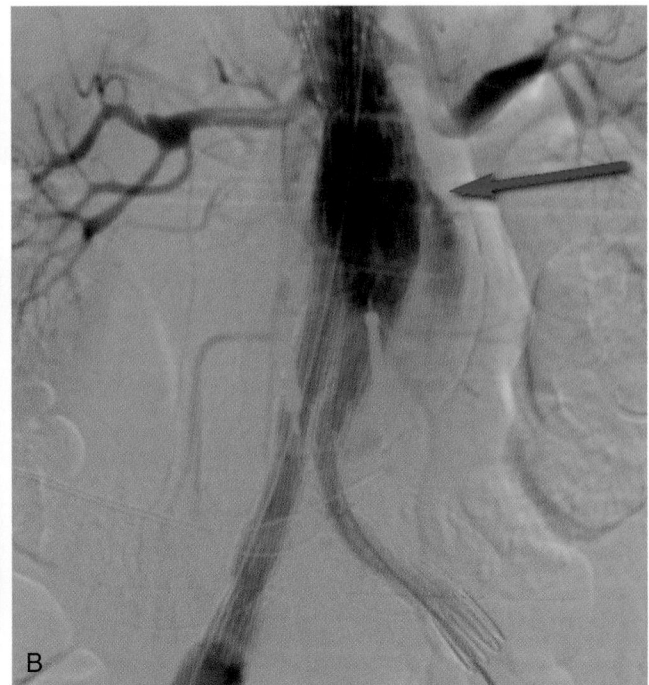

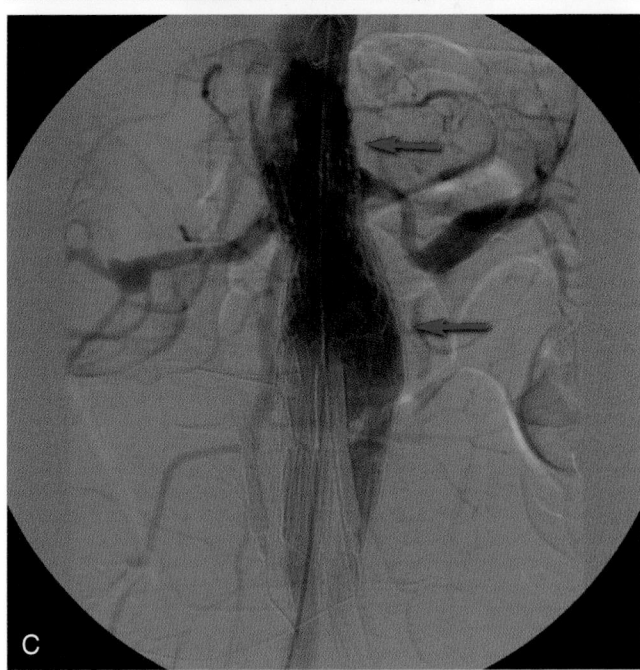

Figure 86-7 A, Short aortic neck immediately before endovascular aneurysm repair. **B,** Type IA endoleak (*arrow*) after initial endograft placement and molding balloon angioplasty. **C,** Resolution of the type IA endoleak after placement of a 5010 "giant" Palmaz stent (*arrows* show proximal and distal extent).

Palmaz stent is then carefully delivered through the sheath with continuous fluoroscopic observation to confirm the position of the stent on the balloon. Keep in mind that the stent will foreshorten significantly as it is expanded: it is 5 cm long at 10 mm of expansion but shortens to approximately 3.8 cm at 28 mm.[35] To prevent the stent from "watermelon-seeding" and to avoid maldeployment during balloon inflation, the distal two thirds of the stent is constrained in the delivery sheath while initial balloon deployment is performed (Fig. 86-8).[35] Because the stent is mounted slightly asymmetrically, no movement should occur. After the proximal portion of the stent is expanded, the sheath is carefully retracted, and the remainder of the stent is deployed.

Type IB endoleaks should be treated initially with repeat angioplasty at the distal seal zone. If this is not successful, extension of the limb with an appropriately sized cuff of limb should be performed. Type III endoleaks almost always resolve with angioplasty, assuming that the correct amount of overlap is present. If the overlap between components is not adequate, place a bridging iliac component.

Renal Artery

Inadvertent partial or complete coverage of a renal artery by the endograft should be a rare occurrence. However, knowledge of bailout strategies can be invaluable. It may be possible

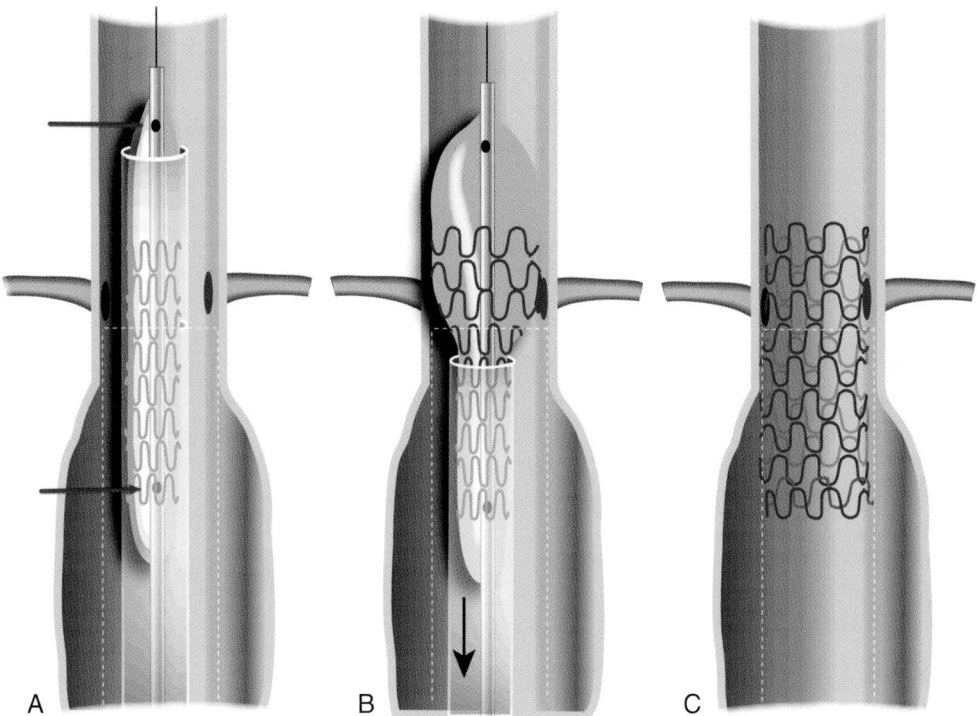

Figure 86-8 Sequence of the modified deployment technique of a "giant" Palmaz stent in the perirenal aorta for repair of a type IA endoleak. The *white dotted lines* represent the previously placed endograft for endovascular aneurysm repair. Details of the endograft have been omitted to enhance the clarity of the giant Palmaz stent device. **A,** The stent (Palmaz 3010, 4010, or 5010) is hand-crimped off-center on a valvuloplasty balloon (*arrows*). The balloon-mounted stent is then positioned at the intended area of deployment through the sheath under fluoroscopic guidance. **B,** The sheath is partially retracted and the balloon is inflated, deploying the proximal (cranial) portion of the stent. The off-center mounting of the stent ensures that it will not "watermelon-seed" craniad; the sheath prevents caudad displacement. **C,** Fully deployed stent. *(Redrawn from Kim JM, Tonnessen BH, Noll ER Jr, Sternbergh WC III. A technique for increased accuracy in the placement of giant Palmaz stents for treatment of type I endoleaks following EVAR. J Vasc Surg. 2008;48:755-777).*

to displace the endograft caudad by pulling on a wire placed over the flow divider and brought out the contralateral femoral artery. Alternatively, a large compliant balloon can be inflated just above the flow divider, and caudad pressure applied. If the body of the device cannot be displaced caudad, placement of a balloon-expandable stent in the renal artery can restore flow in most cases. Depending on the amount of orificial coverage and caudad angulation of the renal artery, a brachial approach can facilitate this maneuver. If none of these endovascular options is successful, extra-anatomic bypass (iliorenal, hepatorenal) is possible. As a last resort, acute open conversion can be considered. In these situations, the risk of the treatment must be carefully considered, because it might be more dangerous than expectant management.

Management of an incidentally discovered renal artery stenosis should follow the same indications as for isolated renal artery disease. The largest question is one of timing. Generally, it is best to treat the renal artery stenosis after EVAR, either at the same setting or staged. The rationale for this approach is the theoretical dislodgement or crushing of the renal stent during manipulation and deployment of the aortic endograft. These concerns are more pronounced when using devices that deploy slightly above the renal arteries and then move caudad (AneuRx, Zenith). An exception to this rule is a

patient with either severe renal insufficiency or hypertension that increases the perioperative risk. In such a case, staged treatment of the renal artery stenosis before EVAR is indicated.

Iliac Aneurysm

External Iliac Extension

Ectatic common iliac arteries up to 2 cm in diameter are suitable landing zones for the iliac limbs of an aortic endograft. However, common iliac arteries greater than 2 cm generally necessitate extension of the endograft to the external iliac artery. When extending to the external iliac artery, one should be particularly mindful of excessive oversizing, which can predispose to limb thrombosis or a type IB endoleak. There is frequently significant iliac tortuosity in these cases, which makes accurate length measurements difficult. When in doubt, a longer limb length should be chosen for external iliac extension.

Internal Iliac Artery

Embolization. When extending to the external iliac artery, the operator must decide how to manage the excluded hypogastric artery. The most common approach is embolization of the proximal hypogastric artery to eliminate the possibility of a type II endoleak. Such embolization can be performed with standard coils or occlusion plugs (Amplazer-II plug). In most circumstances, this is most easily performed antegrade from the contralateral femoral artery. If the takeoff of the internal iliac artery is unusually "splayed" from the external vessel, a retrograde approach can be used. In either case, the key is to provide a stable delivery platform for the coils or plugs. Ideally, the embolization is performed in the proximal internal iliac artery, preserving the distal branches.[36] This approach preserves distal collateral flow and lessens the incidence of buttock claudication. If bilateral internal iliac embolization is planned, a staged approach is strongly recommended.

Coverage of the internal iliac artery without embolization has been described and may be an appropriate choice in many situations.[37,38] The advantages of such a strategy include simplification of the procedure and complete avoidance of compromise to the distal hypogastric branches. Depending on the geometry of the external-internal iliac bifurcation, the endograft extending to the external iliac artery may significantly compromise flow to the internal iliac artery orifice. The theoretical limitation of such a strategy is a persistent type II endoleak that contributes to aneurysm growth. These instances are rare, however.

Preservation. Preservation of flow to the internal iliac artery can be achieved by several different methods. The most intuitive method is the use of a branched endograft designed specifically for this purpose. Though not commercially available in the United States, such devices are undergoing clinical trials and are in use in other parts of the world.[39] Off-label use of main-body devices as an extra modular bifurcation has been described.[40] A second endovascular option is the placement of a covered stent from the internal iliac artery into the ipsilateral external artery. Combined with a contralateral aortouniiliac endograft and a femorofemoral bypass, this provides arterial flow to the internal iliac artery in a retrograde fashion from the external iliac artery.[41] The usually tight angle between the hypogastric and the external iliac artery make this innovative option realistic only in highly selected cases. Finally, a short open bypass or transposition from the external iliac artery to the internal iliac artery may be performed.[42] The anastomosis should be at least 2 cm distal to the takeoff of the external artery to allow sufficient overlap for the endograft.

■ EVAR FOR RUPTURED ABDOMINAL AORTIC ANEURYSM

EVAR for elective repair has demonstrated significant reductions in perioperative mortality and major morbidity when compared with open repair. It is intuitive that such improvements may be magnified in patients with ruptured AAAs and a greatly increased risk of death. Indeed, many but not all reports of EVAR for rupture suggest that endovascular treatment may be the preferred approach for many of these patients.[43-46]

Preoperative Assessment

Effective EVAR for rupture is predicated on the immediate availability of the necessary personnel, endografts, and imaging and an endovascular-equipped operating room. The operator should have significant experience with elective EVAR; perhaps as important, the support personnel need to be comfortable with this procedure. The participation of an "on-call" radiology technologist who has never been involved with EVAR is a recipe for disaster. Some institutions have addressed these concerns by developing specific protocols for the endovascular treatment of ruptured AAAs.[47,48]

With the proliferation of spiral CT scanning in most emergency departments, it is unusual for a patient to be too hemodynamically unstable to obtain this study before transfer to the operating room. The anatomic information obtained is critical in terms of determining a patient's candidacy for EVAR and appropriate sizing. In patients deemed too unstable to obtain a CT scan, on-table angiograms can be used for sizing purposes.

Preoperative resuscitation should mimic that for open ruptured AAA repair, including permissive hypotension to reduce further hemorrhage. The patient needs to be in an operating room with full open capabilities and anesthesia support. Although elective EVAR can be performed in a radiology or cardiology laboratory where surgical backup is available, such a scenario is ill-advised for a patient with a ruptured AAA. Before the initiation of anesthesia, the patient should be prepared for both open and endovascular repair. Induction of general anesthesia can sometimes rapidly decrease vascular tone and cause profound hypotension. Therefore, some operators advocate that vascular access be gained with local anesthesia only. The final choice of anesthetic technique should be tailored to the patient's body habitus and hemodynamic stability and the preferences of the treating anesthesiologist and vascular specialist.

Device Placement
Endograft Selection

An in-hospital stock of endograft components is essential. Such a "rupture kit" should have enough size options to effectively treat most anatomic situations. The device type and configuration (modular, unibody, aortouniiliac) may be less important than the operator's experience with a given device. All available devices can be rapidly implanted by experienced operators. Both the unibody and aortoiliac devices have the advantage of not needing to cannulate the contralateral limb gate. Although this maneuver should not take more than 5 minutes, it can occasionally be more difficult and time-consuming. Such prolonged gate cannulation is problematic in an unstable patient. Conversion of a modular bifurcated device to a uniiliac one can be performed with additional components.

Technique

EVAR for a ruptured AAA should generally mimic the technique for elective repair described earlier. Expedient delivery of the endograft is certainly desirable and is facilitated by experience with the chosen device. Leaving a residual type I endoleak is unacceptable in the setting of a ruptured AAA because there may be continued retroperitoneal bleeding. Some authors believe that sacrifice of a low renal artery to obtain an adequate proximal seal may be reasonable. The operator must individualize such decisions, keeping in mind the patient's preexisting renal function, hemodynamic stability, and ability to withstand an open AAA repair. The significant additional time needed for implantation of a fenestrated endovascular device makes its use problematic in such situations.

Aortic Balloon Occlusion

Balloon occlusion of the visceral aorta can be lifesaving in a patient who is profoundly unstable hemodynamically. A compliant balloon (Coda) should be used. A brachial approach might seem optimal because it allows unfettered access to the femoral arteries for the subsequent EVAR. Unfortunately, the large sheath (12 to 14 Fr) required for this balloon can be problematic in a patient with very small vessels. Open repair of the brachial artery is typically required. In addition, the aortic arch anatomy is usually unknown. With a type III arch, delivery of the balloon to the desired location may be challenging. Many operators advocate a femoral approach for the occlusion balloon because it obviates many limitations of the brachial approach.

Postoperative Issues

Postoperative complications of ruptured AAAs treated by EVAR can parallel those of open repair in some situations. An abdominal compartment syndrome can occur if there is a great deal of retroperitoneal hematoma or bowel edema. Postoperative coagulopathy is also correlated with this serious complication. In patients deemed at risk, serial bladder pressure measurements can be helpful. Poor urine output is also generally associated with this syndrome. Timely decompression of the abdomen is required to reduce the very high mortality in this patient cohort. Colon ischemia is also a potential concern, particularly in a patient with prolonged hypotension or the need for hypogastric artery coverage. Liberal use of sigmoidoscopy can help establish the diagnosis and treatment.

◼ TEVAR

General Considerations

TEVAR in U.S. multicenter trials is associated with significantly reduced perioperative mortality and morbidity.[13,14] This early benefit is sustained through 5 years of follow-up,[13]

making TEVAR the preferred first-line treatment in most anatomically suitable patients.

Device Selection

As with EVAR, careful preoperative sizing and planning for thoracic endograft placement are critical for a successful outcome. A minimum of 2 cm of nonaneurysmal landing zone is required proximally and distally. Oversizing more than 20% in the aortic arch is associated with a greatly elevated risk of subsequent endograft collapse, particularly in patients with a tight arch radius. These patients frequently have poor apposition of the endograft to the inner wall, creating a "bird-beaking" effect. Patients treated for traumatic aortic transection are most susceptible to this complication. These patients are generally younger and have smaller diameter aortas with nonsplayed aortic arches. The smallest available thoracic endograft (26 mm) is too large for many of these patients, necessitating the off-label use of infrarenal aortic cuffs in some instances. Fortunately, smaller diameter devices that conform to the aortic arch are currently being developed and should be commercially available in the near future.

Aortic Arch Landing Zones

The aortic arch is divided into five zones (Fig. 86-9). Zone 0 is proximal to the innominate artery, zone 1 is between the innominate and left carotid arteries, zone 2 is between the left

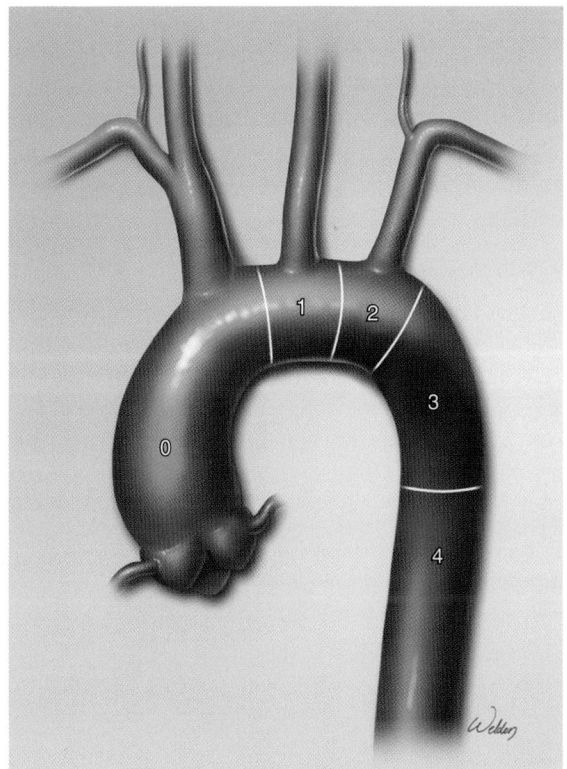

Figure 86-9 Aortic arch proximal landing zones 0 to 4 for thoracic endovascular aortic repair. *(Courtesy of Alan Lumsden.)*

carotid and left subclavian arteries, zone 3 is between the left subclavian artery and 2 cm distal to it, and zone 4 is the thoracic aorta greater than 2 cm from the left subclavian artery. Coverage into zones 0 and 1 always requires adjunctive revascularization of the covered vessels by either debranching or endovascular techniques (see later). Landing in zone 2 with coverage of the left subclavian artery may also require revascularization. The risk of major morbidity, especially stroke, may increase when TEVAR is extended to the more proximal arch zones.

Spinal Cord Drainage

Although the incidence of paralysis or paraparesis has been less with TEVAR than with traditional open repair in most series, it does occur. Spinal cord drainage to a pressure of 10 cm H_2O and avoidance of hypotension are consistently effective in reducing this dreaded complication. Selective—not routine—use of spinal cord drainage is standard with TEVAR in most institutions. Box 86-3 lists patients in whom preoperative spinal cord drainage should be strongly considered. Occasionally, a post-TEVAR patient develops symptoms of spinal cord injury one or more days after the procedure. Prompt placement of a spinal drain and treatment of any relative hypotension can have salutary benefits in this situation.[49]

Left Subclavian Artery Coverage

Coverage of the left subclavian artery is frequently needed to achieve an adequate proximal seal zone. Some patients absolutely require revascularization of the left subclavian artery before TEVAR (Box 86-4). Bypass or transposition of the left subclavian artery to the left common carotid artery is typically

performed either staged or immediately preceding TEVAR (Fig. 86-10). Most reports of TEVAR suggest that in the absence of particular anatomic situations (see Box 86-4), coverage of the left subclavian artery is well tolerated and does not require routine revascularization.[50] The reported incidence of subsequent revascularization for left arm ischemia or vertebral-basilar insufficiency has been less than 10%. However, a recent report from the EuroSTAR registry in a large cohort of patients demonstrated that coverage of the left subclavian artery is significantly associated with an increase in paralysis or paraparesis.[51] Thus, selective revascularization of the left subclavian artery with TEVAR has been reappraised, and some centers now routinely revascularize the vessel.[52]

Technique

Though intuitively simple, TEVAR can be technically challenging and is associated with risks of major morbidity that are rarely experienced with EVAR. Advanced endovascular skills are sometimes required to attain a good outcome (Fig. 86-11). Hence, TEVAR operators should not be endovascular novices.

Vascular Access

The techniques for vascular access discussed for EVAR are applicable to TEVAR as well. However, the need for an iliac conduit is much higher with TEVAR because of the larger sheath requirements (20 to 24 Fr) and the higher relative prevalence of women compared with AAA patients. Thus, the operator should always be concerned that traditional access via the common femoral artery may not be successful and should be prepared to create a conduit if necessary.

Device Positioning and Deployment

After establishing the primary vascular access for endograft delivery, a 4 or 5 Fr sheath is placed in the contralateral femoral or brachial artery in order to position a pigtail catheter proximal to the intended delivery zone. Placement of the pigtail from the brachial approach is especially useful when treating acute type B aortic dissection because it may facilitate true lumen placement of the main delivery guide wire. Through the primary vascular access, a preformed super-stiff wire (Lunderquist) is placed in the proximal ascending aorta through a previously placed catheter. Although use of a single endograft is ideal, variations in proximal and distal landing diameters and length of coverage frequently require the use of two (rarely, three) components. When multiple components are employed, there must be a minimum of 5 cm overlap. Devices with tapering diameters are in development to facilitate the use of fewer components.

When the proximal landing zone is in or adjacent to the arch (zones 0 to 3), a steep left anterior obliquity is needed to maximally "open" the arch. With the use of continuous fluoroscopy, the necessary amount of obliquity can be adjusted

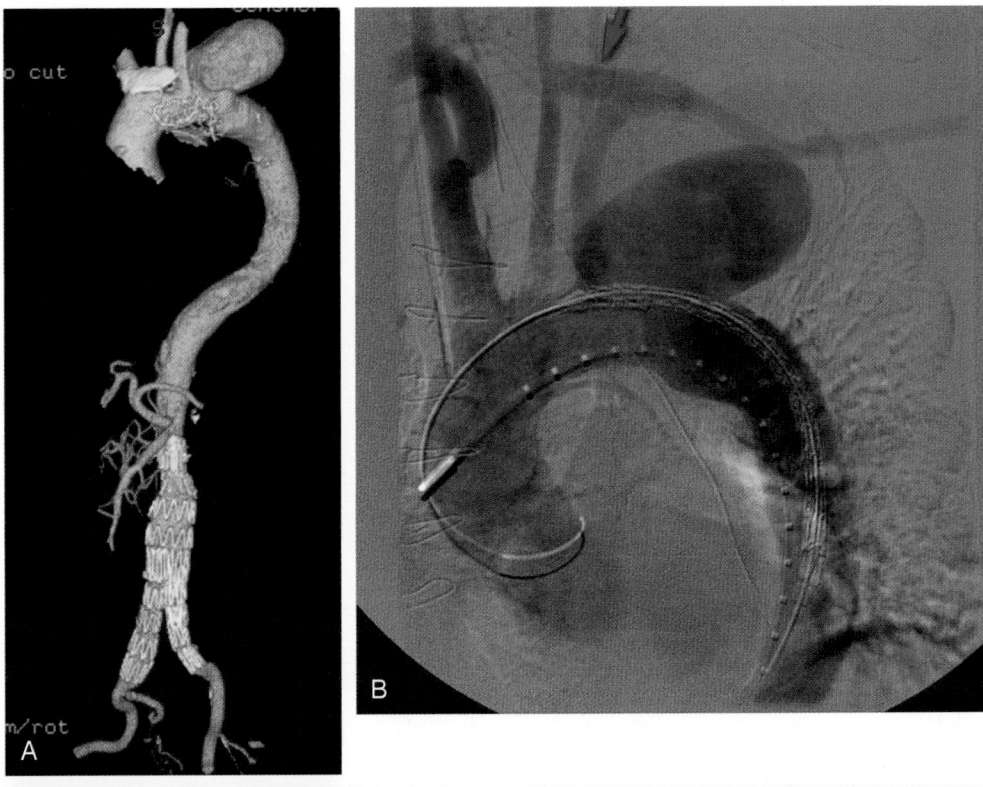

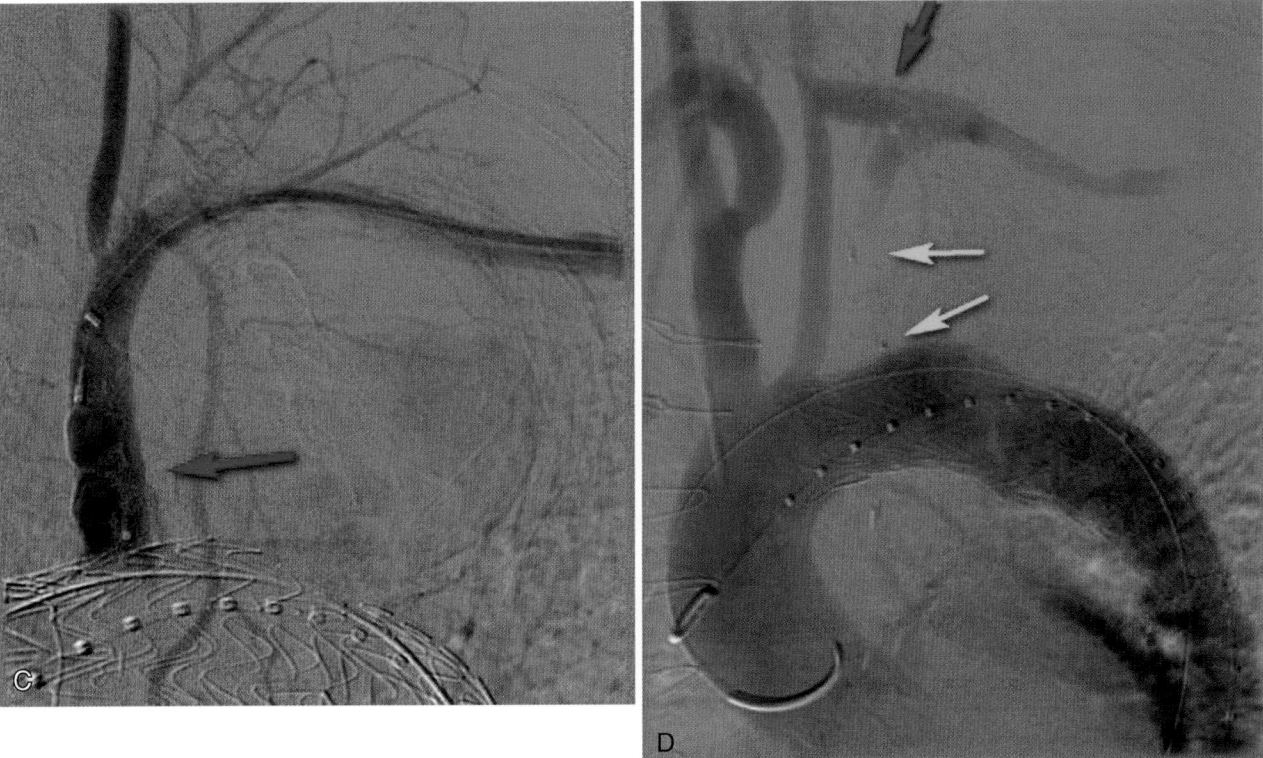

Figure 86-10 A, Three-dimensional computed tomographic angiography reconstruction of a 7.3-cm saccular thoracic arch aneurysm. Note the previous endovascular aneurysm repair. **B,** Angiogram immediately before TEVAR. Note the left carotid–to–subclavian bypass (*arrow*) performed for an existing left internal mammary artery bypass. **C,** Embolization of the proximal left subclavian artery with an Amplazer-II plug using a brachial approach (*arrow*). Note the preservation of the left vertebral artery. **D,** Completion of TEVAR with no endoleak. *Red arrow,* left carotid–to–subclavian bypass; *blue arrows,* proximal and distal extent of Amplazer-II plug.

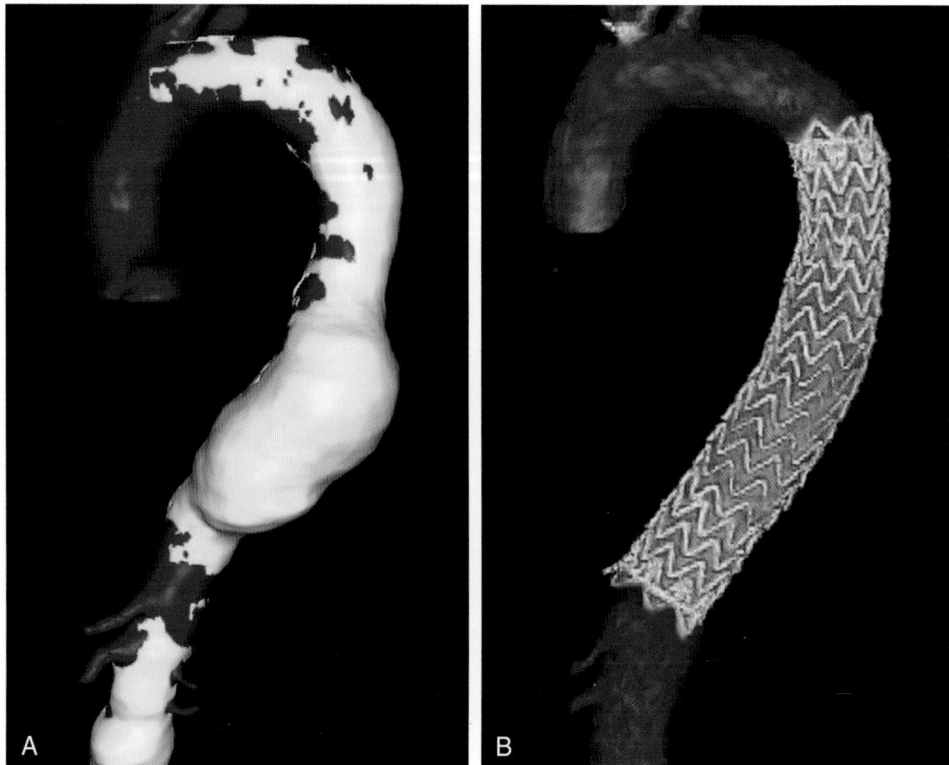

Figure 86-11 A, Three-dimensional computed tomographic angiography reconstruction of a descending thoracic aneurysm. **B,** Post thoracic endovascular aortic repair.

visually by progressively adding more obliquity until the positions of the wire in the ascending aorta and descending aorta are maximally separated. After the desired proximal landing position is demonstrated with an angiogram via the pigtail catheter, the endograft position is adjusted accordingly. The endograft naturally follows the greater curvature of the aortic arch once it is deployed. Thus, it is important to place the device as close to the greater arch curve as possible before deployment. This step is accomplished by applying craniad tension on the delivery wire and endograft delivery sheath. This "tensioning" of the wire should minimize any caudad migration of the device as it is deployed. If two components are used, it is usually helpful to deploy the distal device first, if possible. Deployment of the second, more proximal endograft is thus better supported, providing increased accuracy at the intended landing zone. A compliant molding balloon is usually used at the seal zones, except in cases of aortic dissection. A trilobed compliant balloon has the advantage of some continued aortic flow, and it is less likely to be distally displaced than a standard compliant balloon. However, a standard compliant balloon may provide superior concentric expansion in some situations. If a standard compliant balloon is used in the arch, the operator should consider reducing the blood pressure with a short-acting intravenous medication.

A note of caution is in order regarding the use of compliant balloons in TEVAR. When advancing the molding balloon around the arch through the deployed endograft, it is possible to cause craniad migration of endografts that do not have active fixation. This complication, which can occur owing to friction between the balloon and the outer wall of the endograft, can be avoided by "de-tensioning" the wire off the greater curve of the aorta and a slow, methodical advancement of the balloon.

TEVAR Troubleshooting

Arch Branch Coverage

Inadvertent coverage of an arch branch is one of the most feared intraoperative complications of TEVAR. In such a situation, one should verify the potential problem by repeat arteriography after adjusting the gantry position of the fluoroscope, making it perfectly perpendicular to the leading edge of the endograft. Occasionally, one may find that there is no significant encroachment on the branch vessel. If coverage of a vital branch is confirmed, the first corrective step can be an attempt to move the endograft caudad by traction of a compliant balloon within the device. If this is not successful, retrograde stenting of the branch vessel can be performed (Fig. 86-12).[53] These cases most frequently involve the left carotid artery. Using either an open or a percutaneous approach, a guide wire is passed retrograde from the left common carotid artery into the ascending aorta. A stent is then deployed extending from the edge of the endograft into the proximal common carotid artery. Both self-expanding and balloon-expandable stents have been used in these situations. Alternatively, surgical revascularization with a right-to-left carotid-carotid bypass can be performed.

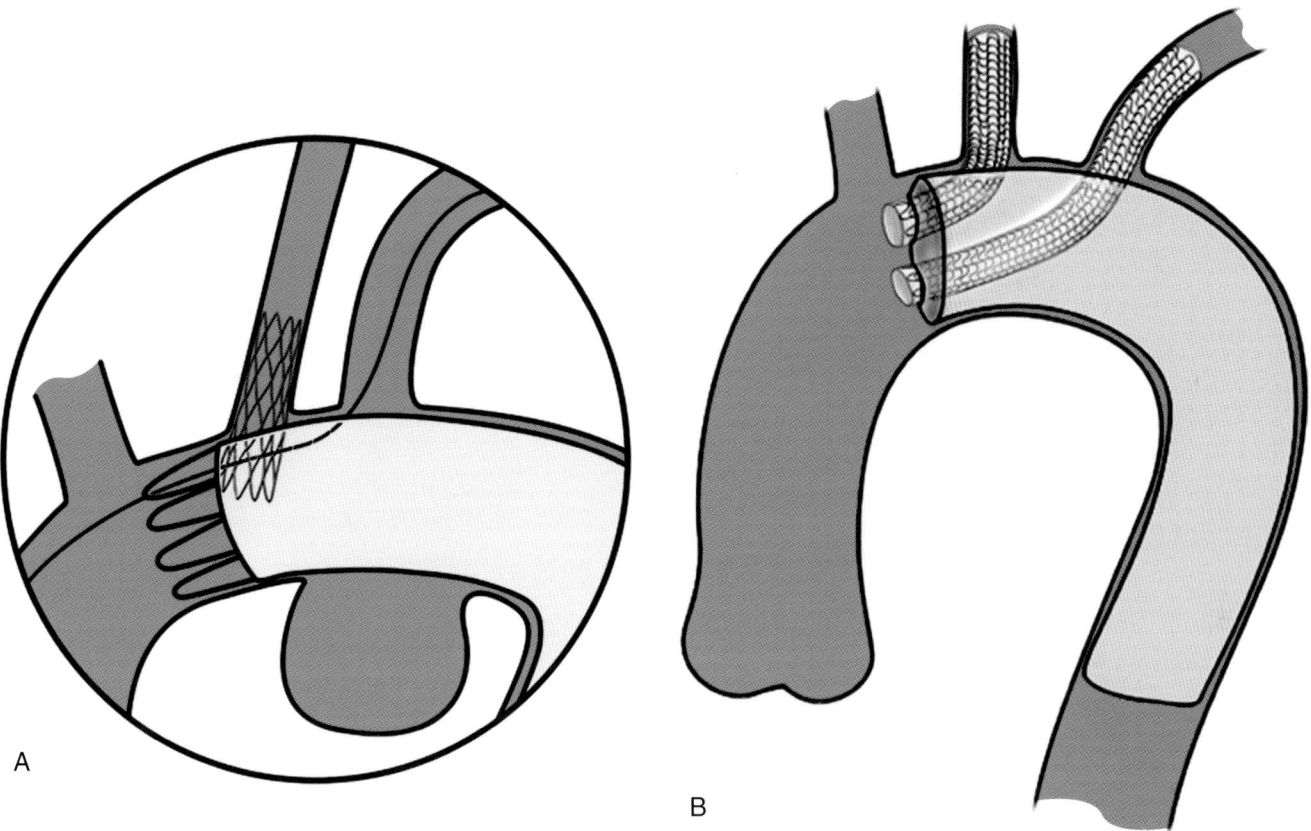

A

B

Figure 86-12 Endovascular debranching with a bare balloon-expandable stent (**A**) or self-expanding covered stents (**B**). *(Redrawn from Criado FJ. A percutaneous technique for preservation of arch branch patency during thoracic endovascular repair [TEVAR]: retrograde catheterization and stenting. J Endovasc Surg. 2007;14:54-55.)*

Endoleak

Management of intraoperative endoleaks is similar to that previously described for EVAR. If re-ballooning is not effective, the seal zone should be extended, if possible. In the case of a proximal endoleak, this may require adjunctive endovascular or surgical debranching of the cervical great vessel. If the seal zone is believed to be adequate, adding radial strength to the endograft–seal zone interface with placement of a balloon-mounted giant Palmaz stent should be considered.

Hybrid TEVAR Techniques

The anatomic limits of TEVAR can be expanded by arch or visceral debranching, providing additional seal zone in patients with extensive aortic aneurysms. The mainstay of arch cervical debranching involves subclavian–left carotid bypass or transposition or carotid-carotid bypass. An innovative endovascular technique is a double-barrel or "endobranching" technique whereby a bare or covered stent is placed in a retrograde fashion from the subclavian or left carotid artery into the arch, followed by overstenting of the thoracic endograft (see Fig. 86-12).[54] The potential downside to this maneuver is compromise of the seal zone and resultant type I endoleak. This technique may be particularly suited for saccular aneurysms on the inner curve of the arch. Although small series

have demonstrated encouraging short-term results, no long-term data are available on the durability of this technique.

Complete arch debranching can be performed by median sternotomy and placement of a branched conduit from the proximal ascending aorta to revascularize all the arch great vessels. Using a side-biting clamp on the medial proximal ascending aorta, a 10- to 14-mm Dacron graft is placed with branches directly to the great vessels or in combination with cervical bypass. An additional limb can be placed through which the thoracic endograft is deployed in an antegrade fashion.

Visceral debranching can be performed with retrograde grafts to both renal arteries, the superior mesenteric artery, and the celiac artery (Fig. 86-13). These grafts usually originate from the iliac artery. A thoracic endograft is then placed across the aneurysmal segment. The considerable morbidity and mortality from these visceral debranching procedures has tempered initial enthusiasm for this approach.[55]

Many clinicians view these hybrid techniques as a bridge to totally endovascular thoracoabdominal aortic aneurysm repair with side branches.[56] Such devices for both the arch and visceral segments are in development and have limited clinical experience. Discussion of this technique is found in Chapters 129 (Abdominal Aortic Aneurysms: Endovascular Treatment), 133 (Thoracic and Thoracoabdominal Aneurysms:

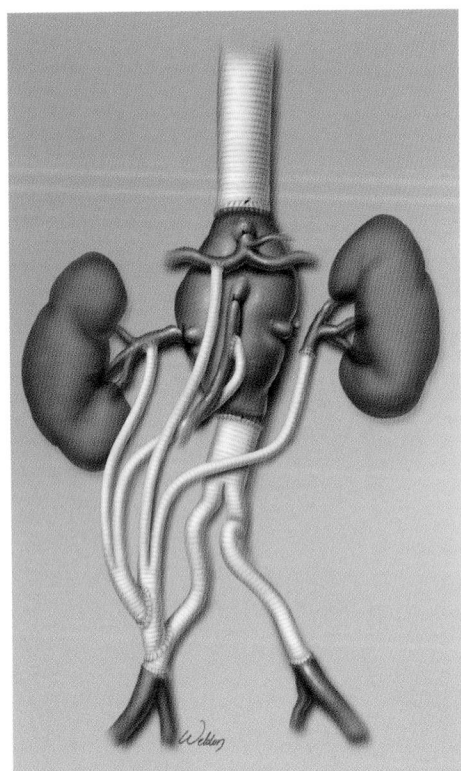

Figure 86-13 Visceral debranching. *(Courtesy of Alan Lumsden.)*

Endovascular Treatment), and 134 (Aortic Arch Aneurysms and Dissection). The initial results with branched endografts have been excellent.[57] Only time will tell whether such technology will be disseminated into widespread clinical practice.

SELECTED KEY REFERENCES

Buth J, Harris PL, Hobo R, van Eps R, Cuypers P, Duijm L, Tielbeek X. Neurologic complications associated with endovascular repair of thoracic aortic pathology: incidence and risk factors. A study from the EUROSTAR registry. *J Vasc Surg.* 2007;46:1103-1110.
Large retrospective analysis of TEVAR suggesting that coverage of the left subclavian artery without revascularization may be associated with a higher risk of spinal cord injury.

Chuter TA, Rapp JH, Hiramoto JS, Scheider DB, Howell B, Reilly LM. Endovascular treatment of thoracoabdominal aortic aneurysms. *J Vasc Surg.* 2008;47:6-16.
Seminal study demonstrating the safety and efficacy of totally endovascular treatment of thoracoabdominal aortic aneurysms in a large group of patients.

Criado FJ. A percutaneous technique for preservation of arch branch patency during thoracic endovascular repair (TEVAR): retrograde catheterization and stenting. *J Endovasc Surg.* 2007;14:54-55.
An innovative method of preserving antegrade flow to brachiocephalic vessels during TEVAR.

Lee WA, Brown MP, Nelson PR, Huber TS. Total percutaneous access for endovascular aortic aneurysm repair ("preclose technique"). *J Vasc Surg.* 2007;45:1095-1101.
Excellent technical overview of percutaneous access for EVAR.

Makaroun MS, Dillavou ED, Wheatley GH, Cambria RP; the Gore Investigators. Five-year results of endovascular treatment with the Gore TAG device compared with open repair of thoracic aortic aneurysms. *J Vasc Surg.* 2008;47:912-918.
Prospective trial demonstrating a sustained benefit of TEVAR relative to open thoracic aneurysm repair.

Schermerhorn ML, O'Malley AJ, Jhaveri A, Cotterill P, Pomposelli F, Landon BE. Endovascular vs open repair of abdominal aortic aneurysm in the Medicare population. *N Engl J Med.* 2008;358:464-474.
Large population-based study confirming the lower morbidity and mortality of EVAR versus open AAA repair.

REFERENCES

The reference list can be found on the companion Expert Consult Web site at *www.expertconsult.com.*

Grafts and Devices | *Section* **13**

Joseph L. Mills, Sr.

CHAPTER 87

Autogenous Vein Grafts

Scott A. Berceli

Based in part on a chapter in the previous edition by Frank B. Pomposelli, Jr., MD, and Frank W. LoGerfo, MD.

Despite ongoing attempts to develop prosthetic or bioengineered materials for bypass grafting in the lower extremities, autologous vein graft remains the conduit of choice for infrainguinal revascularization. Though it was sporadically used for repair of popliteal aneurysms in the early 20th century, the first report of the routine use of autogenous vein for the treatment of occlusive arterial disease was provided in 1944 by Dos Santos, who used segments of vein as patch material after superficial femoral artery endarterectomy.[1] This was followed several years later by the report of Kunlin, who described the use of reversed saphenous vein grafts for the treatment of focal lesions within the superficial femoral artery.[2] Based on these initial reports, expanded use of the saphenous vein for both endarterectomy and grafting was attempted, but creation of the anastomoses with the standard surgical techniques of the day proved difficult. With long-term patency negatively influenced by a high rate of anastomotic stricture and an inability to replicate the promising results of Kunlin, the majority of practitioners in the 1940s and 1950s used arterial homografts or the newly developed prosthetic grafts for infrainguinal arterial reconstruction. Reinvigorating the use of autogenous vein, however, was a small group of surgeons who traveled to Europe to observe Kunlin's vein grafting procedures.[3] Characterized by a spatulated end-to-side anastomosis using a small-caliber running silk suture, these meticulous techniques allowed Linton and Darling, as well as others, to duplicate the reported success with autogenous vein grafting.[4]

In the 1960s, wider interest in the use of autogenous vein was fueled by the observation that acceptable long-term patency of prosthetic bypass grafts could be achieved only with distal anastomoses placed in the above-knee position.[5] Treatment of critical limb ischemia in patients with compromised outflow via femorotibial bypass was a natural extension for autogenous vein grafting, with the first published report by Dale in 1963.[6] Although initial published reports of the use of saphenous vein for tibial bypass grafts suggested it to be notably inferior to femoropopliteal grafts,[7,8] further refinements in the techniques have proved the durability of tibial as well as inframalleolar bypass grafting with autologous vein.[9] Along with these technical improvements in the 1980s came increasing experience with alternative autogenous vein sources (i.e., arm, small saphenous, and femoral

veins),[10] thereby expanding the potential for autogenous tissue reconstruction to 95% of patients undergoing infrainguinal bypass.[11]

HISTOLOGY

Analogous to other vascular structures, veins are composed of three layers—the tunicae intima, media, and adventitia (Fig. 87-1). The intima consists of a continuous monolayer of cuboidal endothelial cells supported by a subendothelial layer of loose connective tissue. In contrast to the arterial endothelium, where cells are tightly packed and highly aligned in the direction of flow, venous endothelial cells are cuboidal with poorly developed interendothelial tight junctions.[12,13] The resulting enhanced permeability to blood solutes, in conjunction with the underlying physiologic differences between arterial and venous endothelium, is thought to be among the

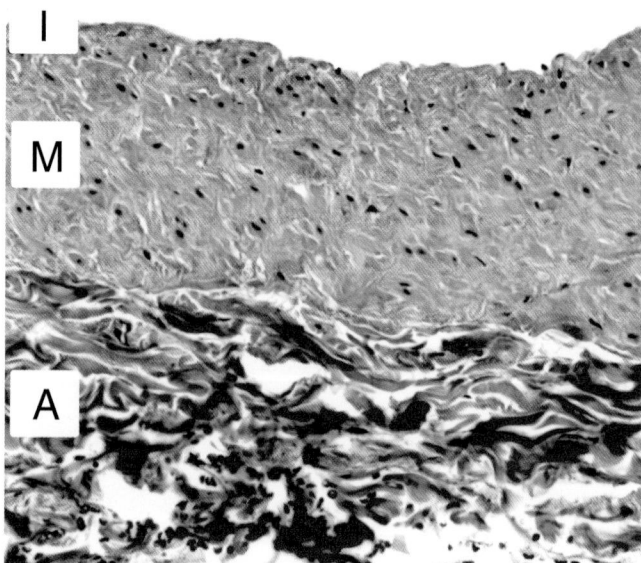

Figure 87-1 Cross-sectional histology of the normal saphenous vein. The intima (I) is composed of a single layer of endothelial cells and a thin basement membrane. The media (M) consists of smooth muscle cells surrounded by a tightly packed extracellular matrix. The adventitia (A) is a loose network of collagen-dominated extracellular matrix with sporadic inflammatory cells and fibroblasts.

underlying mechanisms for the accelerated intimal hyperplasia characteristic of vein grafts.[14]

The intima is separated from the media by a poorly developed internal elastic lamina with large fenestrae that allow diffusion of substances into the wall. The media is composed of vascular smooth muscle cells and extracellular matrix, with type I collagen being the dominant component of this layer. Unlike arteries, which function in a pulsatile pressure environment and correspondingly have high elastin content, veins are exposed to small excursions in pressure and demonstrate only sparse elastin fragments. Transposition of a vein into the arterial circulation induces a marked increase in intraluminal wall tension that greatly exceeds the dynamic range of the elastic elements and therefore leads to a rigid graft with substantial compliance mismatch in comparison to the adjacent artery.[15]

External to a poorly developed external elastic lamina is the adventitia, a loose connection of extracellular matrix with a sparse vasa vasorum. Though traditionally thought to have limited influence on biologic function of the vein, evolving evidence suggests that remodeling of an implanted vein graft is very much dependent on adaptation within the adventitia. Recruitment of myofibroblasts, production of cytokines, and the influx of inflammatory cells into the adventitia are thought to have an important influence on the biology of the early vein graft.

Superficial extremity veins are prone to the development of a range of pathologies such as varicose degeneration, thrombosis with luminal recanalization, and phlebitis with intramural calcification. Limitations in available autogenous conduit not infrequently require these "compromised" vein segments to be included as conduit in a revascularization procedure. Histologic evaluation of harvested vein segments, coupled with long-term clinical follow-up, has demonstrated that grafts with low endothelial cell coverage, stenosis of the lumen, and thick walls are at an increased risk for early graft failure.[16] Grafts with subendothelial spindle-shaped cells, which demonstrate a proliferative smooth muscle phenotype on electron microscopic examination, and calcification within the wall at the time of graft implantation are notably prone to the development of aggressive hyperplastic lesions.[17] Unfortunately, preoperative ultrasound is unable to reliably identify many of these abnormalities.[18]

■ ANATOMY

Lower Extremity Veins

The veins of the lower extremities are classified into three general groups: the deep, superficial, and perforating systems. The deep veins are encompassed by thick fascia and are contained within the muscular compartment of the leg. Superficial veins are bounded deeply by the muscular fascia and superficially by the dermis. Short veins piercing through the fascia and running between the superficial and deep systems are the perforating veins. Increasing interest in accurate description of the venous structures in the leg and confusion

between the clinical and anatomic terminology used in naming them have prompted a review and standardization of the nomenclature. The following descriptions are based on this consensus terminology,[19,20] with reference to the older nomenclature as appropriate.

The *great saphenous vein* (formerly called the greater or long saphenous vein) begins just anterior to the medial malleolus, crosses the tibia, traverses medial to the knee, and ascends in the medial-posterior aspect of the thigh to the groin. Duplicated systems within the great saphenous vein are relatively common and occur at a 25% and 8% incidence in the calf and thigh, respectively.[21] The *accessory great saphenous veins* run parallel to the main trunk within the thigh and leg, in an anterior or posterior location. Although these veins are at times mistaken for the great saphenous vein during surgical exposure, they are usually of inadequate diameter for use in bypass grafting. The saphenous veins, but not their tributaries, are covered by a fibrous sheath termed the *saphenous fascia*. Less well developed than the deep fascia, this fascia, in combination with the deeper muscular fascia, forms a subcompartment that extends along the length of the lower extremity. Recognition of this fascia can be useful in localizing the great saphenous vein during surgical dissection. In the proximal portion of the thigh, the great saphenous vein receives one or two large tributaries from the anterior or posterior accessory great saphenous vein (or both) and enters the fossa ovalis approximately 4 cm inferior and lateral to the pubic tubercle, where it joins with the superficial circumflex iliac, superficial epigastric, and external pudendal veins to create the *confluence of superficial inguinal veins* (formerly called the saphenofemoral junction) on the anterior surface of the *common femoral vein*.

The *small saphenous vein* (formerly called the lesser or short saphenous vein) ascends lateral to the Achilles tendon in the calf. It runs in the subcutaneous adipose tissue in the lower two thirds of the calf, pierces the muscular fascia, and courses between the medial and lateral heads of the gastrocnemius. The small saphenous vein usually joins the popliteal vein in the popliteal fossa about 5 cm proximal to the knee crease. Rarely, the small saphenous vein ends high and empties into the femoral vein or runs superficially up to the posteromedial aspect of the thigh and joins the great saphenous vein directly.

Particularly useful in arterial reconstructions within infected fields, the *femoral vein* (formerly called the superficial femoral vein) has increasingly become a potential source of autogenous conduit. The femoral vein originates from the popliteal vein at the upper margin of the popliteal fossa and courses in the femoral canal. The femoral vein is lateral to the femoral artery in the distal part of the thigh but crosses under and runs medial to the femoral artery in the proximal portion of the leg before joining the *deep femoral (profunda femoris) veins* approximately 9 cm below the inguinal ligament. During harvest of the femoral-popliteal vein segment for use as an autogenous graft, preservation of the junction of the profunda femoris vein with the common femoral vein is critical for maintaining adequate venous outflow from the limb.[22,23]

Upper Extremity Veins

Veins of the upper extremity are also divided into superficial and deep groups, although direction of flow from superficial to deep is not as distinct as in the lower extremity. The *cephalic vein*, which originates on the posterolateral aspect of the wrist, gradually swings across the lateral portion of the forearm, ascends lateral to the biceps muscle into the deltopectoral groove, and passes through the clavipectoral fascia to join the axillary vein. The *basilic vein* swings across the posteromedial side of the forearm, passes lateral to the antecubital fossa, and ascends medially in the arm, where it joins the *brachial veins* to become the *axillary vein*. The *median cubital vein* starts at the apex of the antecubital fossa as a branch of the cephalic vein and ascends medially to enter the basilic vein.

Approximately 10 cm proximal to the antecubital fossa, the basilic vein passes through the deep fascia to reside along the medial side of the brachial artery. Harvest of the basilic vein proximal to this location requires longitudinal division of this fascia and ligation of multiple communicating branches coursing between the basilic and brachial veins. During this portion of the dissection, the medial cutaneous nerve of the forearm is often first identified as it travels anterior to the basilic vein. Injury to this nerve can lead to paresthesias along the medial portion of the forearm.

■ VEIN GRAFT PREPARATION

Preoperative Vein Mapping

As surgeons have increased the complexity of lower extremity reconstruction and become more aggressive with repeat revascularization after graft failure, assessment of available autogenous conduit has evolved into an essential component of preoperative planning. Initial attempts to evaluate available conduit centered around the use of routine preoperative saphenous venography, with information obtained from these studies influencing the operative approach in up to 30% of patients.[24] Though useful in defining the anatomy and dimensions of the greater saphenous system, broad application of this technique was limited by its requirement for percutaneous access, frequent underestimation of conduit diameter, and the small but worrisome risks of nephrotoxicity or chemically induced thrombophlebitis.

With refinements in ultrasound instrumentation and the increasing availability of skilled technologists, investigations into the merits of B-mode imaging for preoperative conduit evaluation were initiated.[25-28] By providing the ability to determine vein size and quality in a physiologic environment and facilitate operative exposure, duplex vein mapping generated significant enthusiasm. Early reports were mixed, however, with concern that duplicate saphenous systems were frequently not identified and diameters measured on B-mode imaging were not representative of in vivo graft geometries.[25] Although the former issue has essentially been solved by increased experience of vascular technologists and an understanding of anatomic variants, difficulties with direct correla-

tion of preoperative mapping and graft size remain. Among the important issues in minimizing this variability is the development of a standard preoperative evaluation protocol.

Warming the examination room, placing warmed blankets on the extremities, and using prewarmed ultrasonic gel minimizes peripheral venous vasoconstriction. Imaging with a high-frequency probe (≥8 MHz) provides maximum resolution with 0.3-mm point-to-point discrimination. Veins are assessed in cross-section to evaluate compressibility, wall thickening, and the presence of intraluminal echoes, and sites of thrombus, intraluminal webs, and sclerotic walls are noted. Vein wall abnormalities have been described in 12% of potential conduits, with preoperative duplex evaluation correctly identifying 62% of these diseased segments.[29] To assess the great saphenous vein, patients are placed in a modified reversed Trendelenburg position and images collected for measurement of lumen diameter at six locations along the length of the limb. Evaluation of the small saphenous vein is performed with the patient in a prone position and the diameter measured at three locations within the calf. If either of the saphenous veins is of good quality but inadequate size, the patient is placed in a standing position and diameter measurements are repeated. Alternatively, a tourniquet may be placed on the proximal part of the thigh to facilitate this reassessment. For segments identified to be of adequate size and quality for bypass grafting, the overlying skin is marked with indelible ink. Routine evaluation of the femoral vein may also be warranted depending on local clinical practice. In addition to lumen diameter, examination should include a thorough assessment for deep venous thrombosis and valvular incompetence. Use of standardized reference zones facilitates the reporting of relevant information, with zones 2, 3, and 4 corresponding to the proximal, middle, and distal portions of the thigh and zones 5, 6, and 7 corresponding to the proximal, middle, and distal portions of the calf, respectively.[30] Evaluation of the upper extremity cephalic and basilic veins should follow a similar protocol. An upper arm tourniquet may be used selectively or routinely to facilitate these measurements. Reference zones have also been established for the upper extremity, where zones 3, 4, and 5 correspond to the proximal, middle, and distal portions of the arm and zones 6, 7, and 8 correspond to the proximal, middle and distal portions of the forearm, respectively.[30] Measurements of upper extremity vein diameter seem even more variable than those of the lower extremity. Although the underlying etiology is open to speculation, this variability should be recognized, and repeat testing of borderline upper extremity veins may prove valuable in preoperative planning.

Despite multiple attempts to define acceptable conduit size, no clear consensus has emerged. Smaller diameter veins have repeatedly been shown to negatively influence long-term patency,[31,32] and a minimum suitable diameter ranging between 2.0 and 3.0 mm has been proposed.[33] Among the confounding issues is the variable effect of the mapping technique on approaching an accurate in vivo graft diameter. These variations are nonlinear and in part dependent on the initial size of the conduit; whereas a 2.5-mm vein increases

27% in diameter when placed in the arterial circulation, a 6-mm vein increases only 8%.[27] In the absence of a universally accepted vein mapping protocol, absolute delineation of a minimum acceptable vein size is problematic, and development of size criteria within an institutional practice is most appropriate.

Vein Handling Considerations

Research over the last decade has uncovered the importance of the endothelium in vascular injury and repair. Previously thought to be a passive monolayer with predominantly barrier functions, endothelial cells have been identified as central mediators in the maintenance of vascular homeostasis. Advanced by the work of Ross and his development of the response-to-injury hypothesis,[34-36] loss of endothelial integrity induces platelet deposition and elaboration of growth factors. Coupled with recruitment of inflammatory mediators, these growth factors stimulate smooth muscle proliferation and matrix deposition, which lead to the formation of an occlusive arterial lesion. Analogous mechanisms are thought to be fundamental in the pathologic remodeling of vein grafts, with early endothelial injury among the initiating events in the development of intimal hyperplasia.[37] Accordingly, maintenance of an intact endothelial monolayer during vein graft harvest is thought to provide improved long-term patency of autogenous vein grafts. Work by LoGerfo[38] and others[39] in a canine model supports this contention by demonstrating that smooth muscle cells are maintained in a contractile (nonproliferative) phenotype and that leukocyte infiltration is reduced when endothelial injury is avoided. Analogous work by Conte's group confirmed that surgical manipulation of human vein segments results in a significant increase in monocyte adhesion.[40] However, direct evidence linking improved endothelial integrity to a reduction in intimal hyperplasia, enhanced outward remodeling, or improved patency is lacking. Nonetheless, significant indirect evidence supports the concept that endothelial preservation minimizes the early biologic perturbations within vein grafts, and therefore harvest techniques aimed at reducing endothelial dysfunction seem reasonable.

Dissection

Precise, atraumatic dissection and minimal direct manipulation of the vein via a "no-touch" technique have been demonstrated to reduce endothelial damage during harvest (Fig. 87-2).[41-44] Though somewhat of a misnomer, the technique involves limited handling of the vein without direct application of forceps or vascular clamps. Major branches are ligated away from the wall to avoid narrowing of the lumen and promote outward remodeling after implantation. Opinions regarding the importance of maintaining continuity of the vein during dissection versus early ligation for intermittent infusion of isotonic fluids are mixed. Despite not being studied in a directed manner, continued continuity of vein has been shown to reduce the formation of small thrombi on the wall, and cannulation and division of the distal vein promote the direct application of antithrombotic and smooth muscle relaxants directly into the lumen. Although limited vein graft handling is universally considered an important component of promoting both short- and long-term graft patency, this concept is challenged by the nearly identical clinical outcomes for reversed, nonreversed, and in situ vein

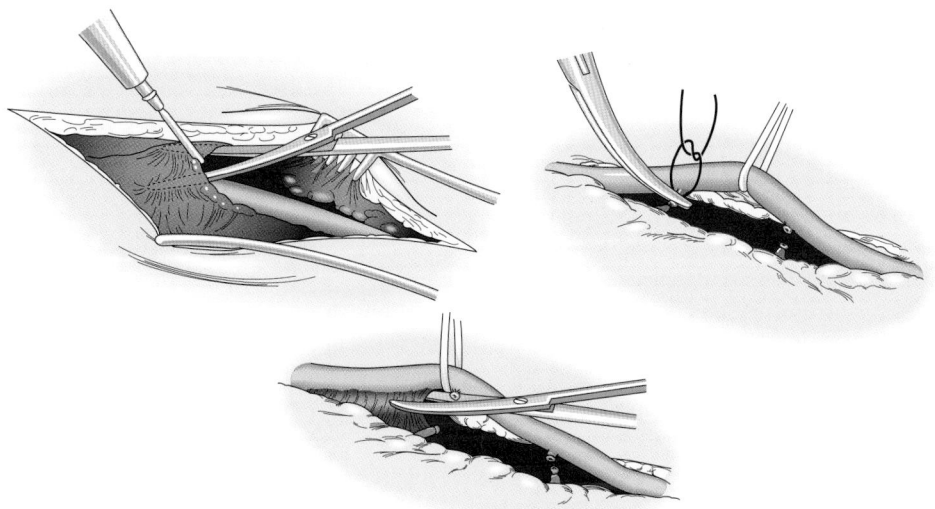

Figure 87-2 "No-touch" technique used in the harvest of autogenous vein. To minimize spasm, papaverine (120 mg/L) is injected into the periadventitial plane before surgical exposure. Side branches are identified and ligated several millimeters away from the wall to prevent luminal narrowing after implantation and outward remodeling of the vein graft. Using a Silastic vessel loop to control the vein without direct manipulation with surgical instruments, the periadventitial tissues are divided and the vein is excised.

grafting techniques.[45,46] If limiting vein manipulation is a dominant factor, one might intuitively expect improved outcomes with in situ grafting, where direct vein manipulation can be essentially eliminated, and compromised outcomes with nonreversed/excised grafts, which require complete mobilization with valvulotomy. The absence of such differences suggests that careful dissection of the vein is prudent, but absent extensive injury, it is of only modest importance to final outcomes.

Though not examined in the setting of peripheral vein grafts, saphenous vein encased by a thick pedicle of surrounding adipose tissue has been used for coronary bypass grafting with promising results. Morphologic and physiologic studies have confirmed reduced endothelial injury and increased expression of endothelial nitric oxide synthase when compared with the standard technique for vein harvest.[47,48] Prospective randomized clinical testing has demonstrated improved short- and long-term patency with use of the pedicle harvest technique, with 90% versus 76% patency rates at 8.5 years for pedicle versus standard grafts.[49,50] Although this technique may not be applicable to the long-segment grafts required for lower extremity revascularization, it is interesting to speculate on the underlying mechanisms for these improved outcomes, which could include decreased endothelial injury, maintenance of an intact vasa vasorum, or the potential delivery of biologic mediators from the surrounding periadventitial tissue.

Distention Pressure

Cannulation of the vein is required before implantation to evaluate the potential diameter of the graft, assess for leaks, and identify adventitial bands compromising the lumen. Use of a standard small-volume syringe can produce intraluminal pressure in excess of 700 mm Hg.[51] A number of investigations have examined the effect of distention pressure on endothelial integrity and almost uniformly have observed that pressure in excess of 100 mm Hg causes patchy endothelial denudation and that pressure in excess of 500 mm Hg leads to disruption of the underlying media.[52-54] The intrinsic biomechanical properties of the graft are negatively impacted, with a resultant decrease in wall compliance secondary to disruption of the elastic elements within the wall.[55] Biologic function is also influenced, with distention injury initiating an increase in c-fos expression, an upstream regulator of platelet-derived growth factor production.[56] Among the few studies to contradict this observation is the work of LoGerfo and colleagues,[54] who observed no significant injury up to a distention pressure of 500 mm Hg and speculated that their aggressive use of papaverine prevented vasospasm and minimized the effect of overdistention. Nevertheless, a variety of pressure-sensing devices have been developed to allow the surgeon to monitor or control distention pressure. Ranging from syringes with intrinsic pressure transducers to reservoir inflation bulbs that generate a fixed pressure, these devices have undergone only sporadic testing and have never been accepted into widespread clinical use.

Irrigating Solution

An array of irrigating solutions ranging from crystalloids to colloids to autogenous blood has been used during vein harvest. Among the first and still the mostly widely used solutions are the isotonic crystalloids normal saline (pH 5.5, 308 mOsm), lactated Ringer's (pH 6.5, 273 mOsm), and Plasma-Lyte (pH 7.4, 292 mOsm). Although the extent of injury and the magnitude of biochemical perturbations with these solutions are variable and depend on confounding variables such as temperature and the use of pharmacologic adjuncts, the bulk of the literature would suggest that simple crystalloid solutions are most damaging to the endothelium.[39,42,51,57] Modified crystalloid solutions such as tissue culture and whole-organ preservation media have also been investigated and have demonstrated modest reductions in endothelial denudation and no improvement in endothelial function when compared with an isotonic saline perfusate.[54,58,59] Without ready access to these solutions in the operating room and because of only modest benefit, these modified crystalloids have not been widely accepted for clinical use. Despite some concern for fibrin deposition, predominantly at higher temperatures, heparinized autologous blood probably provides the best option for use during vein harvest.[39,42,51] Published reports, however, are not unanimous, with several suggesting equivalent results when using standard crystalloid solutions with pharmacologic adjuncts.[58,60]

Temperature

Focusing on maintaining endothelial integrity, LoGerfo and colleagues put forward the concept that warmer perfusate temperatures during active dissection would prevent vasospasm whereas storage of the graft and minimization of metabolic insult would be best accomplished at a much cooler temperature.[54] Supporting this hypothesis, they demonstrated that infusion of 37°C perfusate during active vein harvest and storage of the distended vein at 4°C minimized the extent of endothelial damage. Interestingly, the influence of this dual-temperature approach was most prominent in saline-treated grafts. Subsequent investigations using a single-temperature approach also favored perfusion with a 4°C irrigation solution,[39,54,57] with blood preferred over saline because of the mural edema associated with cold saline infusion.[42]

Although initial studies focused on endothelial morphology as the primary endpoint, further work in the field diversified to examine the effect of solution temperature on biologic activity of the vein graft wall. Nitric oxide–mediated vasodilatation is greatly impaired after storage at 4°C, with room-temperature blood and Plasma-Lyte demonstrating little deterioration when compared with control veins tested immediately after harvest.[61] Analogous studies examining endothelial prostacyclin production and functional thrombomodulin activity support the use of room-temperature perfusates as the best option for preserving metabolic activity.[62,63]

With conflicting experimental evidence, delineation of the most favorable storage temperature is difficult, and reasonable arguments for either cold- or room-temperature treatments can be crafted. Although no definitive recommendation can be proposed, the increased effort required to supply and maintain cold perfusate in the operating suite has prompted most clinicians to favor the use of room-temperature solutions.

Pharmacologic Adjuncts

Unfractionated heparin has universally been included in most vein harvest solutions. Aimed at reducing fibrin deposition and the formation of microthrombi, doses ranging from 4 to 10 U/mL are typically used.[39,57,64]

Prevention of vasospasm is widely identified as being critical in maintaining an intact endothelium, and the use of pharmacologic agents to facilitate this goal may be the most important component of the vein harvest regimen. The most widely studied vasodilator for this purpose is papaverine. Although its exact mechanism of action is unclear, papaverine appears to induce smooth muscle cell relaxation through inhibition of phosphodiesterase and an increase in intracellular cyclic adenosine monophosphate levels. Percutaneous injection of papaverine (120 mg/L) along the outside of the vein before skin incision has been described as an important step to minimize spasm,[64,65] although this can prove challenging in all but the thinnest patients. Application of papaverine along periadventitial tissues and within the lumen perfusate is more easily accomplished and continued throughout vein harvest. Though not rigorously studied as an independent variable, most regimens containing papaverine have shown reduced endothelial injury in comparison to controls.[39,54,57,60]

Other vasodilators have been examined, and a combination of glyceryl trinitrate (8.3 mg/L) and verapamil (16.7 mg/L) appears to be particularly beneficial.[66] In direct comparison to papaverine, glyceryl trinitrate/verapamil demonstrated notable improvement in endothelial coverage.

Even though extensive research has been conducted in this area, no consensus has been reached regarding the optimal techniques for vein graft harvest, with each variable demonstrating unique advantages and shortcomings. Box 87-1 provides a practical summary protocol for the preparation of autogenous vein conduit. The relative importance of these variables is best illustrated by the work of Adcock and coworkers, who examined the combined benefits of papaverine, autologous blood, and limited pressurization in maintaining endothelial integrity.[39] Even though this combined regimen achieved a significant reduction in endothelial loss at the time of implantation, 71% of the endothelial cells exhibited morphologic abnormalities by the second postoperative day (versus 92% for the "standard" regimen). Although the majority of published regimens have sought to optimize variables to maintain an intact endothelial monolayer at the time of implantation, few reports have challenged their techniques to extended exposure in an in vivo environment. Widespread endothelial injury and metabolic perturbation of the harvested vein are probably unavoidable, with only secondary

---

Box 87-1 Recommended Vein Graft Harvest Protocol

HANDLING
- Precise atraumatic technique
- Ligation of tributaries away from the wall
- Lysis of adventitial bands
- Minimization of time from vein excision to implantation

SOLUTION
- Autologous blood (primary)
- Isotonic crystalloid (secondary)

TEMPERATURE
- No definitive recommendation

DISTENTION
- Maximum pressure of 100-150 mm Hg

PHARMACOLOGIC ADJUNCTS
- Heparin (4000-10,000 U/L)
- Papaverine (120 mg/L) *or* Glyceryl trinitrate (8.3 mg/L)/ verapamil (16.7 mg/L)

---

improvements gained by the various methodologies just described.

Minimally Invasive Vein Harvest

Among the significant complications associated with a single continuous incision for lower extremity vein harvest are wound infection and dehiscence, observed in up to 40% of patients.[67] Minimally invasive approaches to saphenous vein harvest have been developed to reduce incisional length and diminish the attendant morbidity. Early investigations of this technique were initiated without specialized instrumentation but used a series of small, sequential incisions overlying the vein. The use of such "skip incisions" significantly improved primary wound healing, with wound complications developing in 28% of patients with a continuous incision as opposed to 9.6% of patients in the "skip incision" group.[68] Over the past 2 decades the concept has evolved with the marriage of endoscopic visualization and specialized instrumentation to facilitate minimally invasive vein harvest. Several different devices have been developed for this purpose, all using three small incisions to access the vein and ligate side branches. Used predominantly for harvesting of vein for coronary bypass surgery, prospective randomized human trials have demonstrated significant reductions in wound morbidity when compared with single-incision saphenectomy.[69-71] Increased manipulation of the vein is inherent with this approach and raises concern about increased endothelial damage and accelerated graft failure. Blinded morphologic examination of harvested human vein specimens[72,73] and clinical outcome studies[71] have demonstrated no significant differences in vein injury or graft patency. Universally noted throughout these reports is the steep learning curve that accompanies endoscopic saphenous vein harvest, with many centers identifying a core group of practitioners who focus on this aspect of the procedure. Although performance of these studies at large-volume medical centers can provide insight into the optimum outcomes with this approach, extrapolation to lower volume centers may not be as promising.

Probably related to the long segments of vein required for lower extremity bypass and the prolonged learning curve inherent in this approach, endoscopic vein harvest for peripheral revascularization has not been uniformly embraced. A small number of centers have championed its use, with mixed results. With no randomized trials comparing single-incision with endoscopic saphenous vein harvest for peripheral bypass, experiences have predominantly been reported through case series with retrospective controls.[74-78] These reports generally support the observations in the cardiac literature and suggest that endoscopic harvest offers reduced wound complications with no notable deterioration in short- and long-term graft patency. Not all reports have been favorable, however, with one investigative team detailing inferior patency rates with little improvement in wound complications after endoscopic vein harvest.[78] Among the important conclusions in this study is the significant learning curve inherent in this technique, with an estimated 40- to 50-patient experience required to become fully competent in harvesting the more difficult below-knee saphenous vein.[79,80] It is noteworthy that the center reporting inferior results performed an average of only one endoscopic harvest per month, probably an insufficient volume to master this technique. Concerns about increased cost of the procedure secondary to additional equipment expenses are relatively unfounded, with these costs more than offset by decreased length of stay during the primary admission and a reduction in the number of readmissions for wound complications.[76]

In an effort to reduce instrument costs while retaining the benefits of a minimally invasive approach, a limited-incision saphenectomy was proposed in which 2-cm-long incisions flanked by 6-cm skin bridges were used to extract the vein with standard surgical instrumentation. When compared with historical controls, this limited-incision approach offered no improvement in wound complications and a notable reduction in long-term patency.[78] The authors speculated that the significant manipulation of the vein required for exposure beneath the skin bridges is the probable cause of the inferior performance of these grafts.

AUTOGENOUS VEIN GRAFT CONFIGURATIONS

In the preoperative planning stage before open lower extremity revascularization, the surgeon is faced with a number of variables concerning the suitability of various inflow and outflow arteries and the length and quality of the available conduit. Invariably, because of some discordance among the available options, assessment of the potential risks and benefits for each choice is required. Preoperative arteriography and duplex vein mapping provide the baseline data through which primary and secondary operative plans are developed. Direct operative assessment of the intended proximal and

Table 87-1 Vein Graft Configurations—Preoperative Planning

Configuration	Advantages	Disadvantages
Reversed	Intraluminal manipulation and valve lysis not required; Option for anatomic or nonanatomic tunnel placement	Potential size mismatch at the anastomoses; Hemodynamic effect of intact valves; Intact valves can complicate graft thrombectomy
Nonreversed	Improved vein-to-artery size match at the anastomoses; Option for anatomic or nonanatomic tunnel placement	Intraluminal manipulation and valve lysis required
In situ	Facilitates the use of limited skin incisions; Reduced manipulation of the vein with the potential benefit of less traumatic injury; Improved vein-to-artery size match at the anastomoses; Subcutaneous position assists in operative graft revision	Not an option when using alternative autogenous conduit (arm vein, small saphenous vein); Intraluminal manipulation and valve lysis required; Subcutaneous position presents an increased risk for graft exposure with wound infection; Construction of the proximal anastomosis may be dictated by length of the proximal saphenous vein

distal anastomotic sites and the quality of the autogenous conduit may initiate re-evaluation and modification of the intended plan during the course of the operation. A summary of the various factors that influence this decision is provided in Table 87-1.

The conduit of choice is the ipsilateral great saphenous vein, with the contralateral saphenous vein being an appropriate secondary option. To preserve the great saphenous vein in the contralateral limb for future revascularization procedures, some surgeons have advocated the use of alternative conduit as a secondary option.[81] Studies examining this issue are in general agreement that in the absence of advanced ischemia (disabling claudication, rest pain, or tissue loss), use of the contralateral saphenous vein is recommended over alternative conduit because of its length, superior performance, and minimal risk to the donor limb.[82-84] Independent risk factors predictive of the need for future vascular intervention in the contralateral limb include age younger than 70 years, diabetes, coronary artery disease, and an ankle-brachial index (ABI) of less than 0.7. In patients demonstrating three out of these four risk factors, the potential for requiring contralateral revascularization within the next 5 years ranges from 25% to 43%, and use of alternative conduit over the contralateral saphenous vein may be a reasonable consideration in this select population.[85]

The approach of using the "best" available autogenous conduit has been advocated[86] and is a practice used routinely by most vascular surgeons. Although vein segments with chronic phlebitis, calcification, or organized intraluminal thrombus are prone to accelerated failure and should be excluded from use,[16,17] other characteristics that define the "best" vein have been an active area of investigation. Even though single-segment saphenous vein has universally been identified as the most durable conduit, an array of single-institution, retrospective studies have attempted to define the effect of such characteristics as vein diameter, graft type, and orientation on long-term patency.[11,31,87-91] Though useful in framing this question, the most comprehensive examination of this issue can be obtained from the prospective, multi-institutional PREVENT III (Prevention of Recurrent Venous Thromboembolism) database.[32,92] Examining conduit diameter and using veins greater than 3.5 mm as the reference standard, this trial found that grafts ranging from 3.0 to 3.5 mm had a 1.5-fold risk and grafts less than 3.0 mm had a 2.4-fold risk for primary failure, with secondary loss of patency in 37% of the grafts smaller than 3.0 mm at 1 year. In terms of graft type, composite veins had a 1.5-fold increase and arm veins a 1.6-fold increase in primary failure when compared with single-segment great saphenous vein. Graft orientation did not influence patency, with reversed and nonreversed configurations demonstrating equivalent patency rates. As these data demonstrate, deviation from using an adequately sized single-segment saphenous vein carries increased risk for failure, and understanding the magnitude of these risks is critical in operative planning and maximizing the potential for a durable outcome.

Reversed Vein Grafts

Excision of the vein plus orientation in a reversed configuration while maintaining antegrade flow with intact valves offers the most straightforward method for vein graft implantation and is suitable for most clinical situations. Difficulty may arise when significant tapering of the saphenous vein in the distal part of the limb creates a size mismatch between the artery and vein graft at both the proximal and distal anastomoses. The proximal vein graft appears to be a common site for luminal narrowing and vein graft failure, and use of small-diameter conduit at this location may accentuate this problem.[93] The size mismatch can be most problematic, however, when performing a tibial or pedal artery anastomosis. A fourfold to fivefold difference in diameters may be encountered, and tailoring the proximal great saphenous vein into a suitable anastomotic configuration can be challenging in these situations.

Examination of normal venous physiology has demonstrated that complete effacement of the valves does not occur during periods of prograde flow. In the low-flow, nonpulsatile hemodynamic environment that characterizes the superficial venous system, the mild to moderate stenosis created by these partially open valves does not translate into significant loss of pressure or impediment to flow. After implantation into the arterial system, the hemodynamic significance of the valves becomes more pronounced. Though not significantly narrowing the lumen during peak systole, a transition to turbulence with localized regions of stasis is noted within the valves.[94]

Lysis of these valves leads to a 15% decrease in hydrodynamic resistance and a 15% to 30% increase in graft flow rates.[95-97] Intact valves have not been proved to adversely influence the long-term patency of reversed vein grafts, but based on these observations, routine valve lysis within these antegrade flow grafts has been proposed.

Less well studied is the biologic effect of the hemodynamic microenvironment within the valve regions, which serve as a nidus for the development of a hyperplastic lesion and focal graft narrowing. Strandness and colleagues prospectively evaluated the long-term remodeling of these valves in reversed saphenous vein grafts.[98,99] Ten percent of the valves were associated with greater than 50% stenosis, but only 2.5% progressed to a critical stenosis requiring operative intervention; these valves accounted for 17% of the total graft revisions within the 18-month follow-up period. Interestingly, valve morphology was dynamic, with 60% of the hemodynamically significant valve lesions showing regression to less than 20% stenosis in a mean period of 3 months.

Nonreversed Vein Grafts

Among the challenges in constructing a reversed-configuration vein graft is significant proximal-to-distal tapering of a vein and the resulting size mismatch at the proximal or distal anastomoses (or both). Although use of an in situ grafting technique can be one solution to this issue, the combination of complete excision of the vein, lysis of the valves, and orientation in a nonreversed configuration offers an alternative technique. Despite the fact that initial attempts with this approach suggested results inferior to the in situ method, these early efforts were probably compromised by the use of an eversion valvulectomy technique and extensive injury to the vein wall.[100] With subsequent refinements in the approach to valve lysis, nonreversed vein grafts have proved as durable as other available techniques.[101-104]

Although nonreversed vein grafts inherently require increased manipulation with the potential for injury during valve lysis, this shortcoming is theoretically offset by the improved hemodynamics offered by this approach. After valve lysis, nonreversed grafts offer a 20% improvement in flow rates over nonlysed, reversed conduits.[96] This hemodynamic effect is most pronounced in smaller diameter vein grafts ranging from 2.0 to 2.5 mm, where the leaflets from intact valves encompass 45% of the luminal cross-sectional area.[95]

In Situ Vein Grafts

The concept of using the great saphenous vein as a graft with mobilization of only the proximal and distal segments while maintaining the interval region within its subcutaneous bed was initially suggested by Rob's group in 1959.[105] Interested in the potential hemodynamic advantages offered by removal of the valves and retrograde perfusion of the conduit, he believed the procedure to be too time-consuming for routine application. Hall, a visiting fellow from Norway, became intrigued by this approach, refined the techniques for routine clinical application, and published the first report of the in situ vein graft technique in 1962.[106] His version of the procedure, requiring valve excision by opening the vein at multiple locations along the graft, was tedious, required significant technical expertise, and failed to gain widespread acceptance. The development of efficient instrumentation for valve lysis provided the opportunity to reduce vein manipulation and maintain an intact vasa vasorum and fueled renewed enthusiasm for the in situ approach. Initial reports of this approach, championed by Leather and colleagues,[107] suggested improved patency over excised vein grafts.[108] These early analyses are compromised by the use of historical controls, however, and contemporary comparisons of in situ versus reversed or nonreversed grafts fail to demonstrate significant differences in long-term outcomes.[46,103,109]

Preparation of the saphenous vein for use in situ as an arterial bypass entails (1) mobilization of the proximal and distal segments for construction of the anastomoses, (2) removal of the valvular obstructions to arterial flow, and (3) interruption of the venous side branches to prevent the formation of arteriovenous fistulae. The objective is to accomplish these tasks in the most expeditious manner while minimizing traumatic injury to the vein.

Proximal and Distal Anastomoses

The common femoral artery serves as the most common source of inflow for infrainguinal revascularization, and the relative position of this artery and the confluence of the superficial inguinal veins dictates construction of the proximal anastomosis. Mobilization of the proximal great saphenous vein is accomplished by secure ligation of the superficial branches, placement of a side-biting vascular clamp across the common femoral vein, transection of the great saphenous vein flush with the wall, and repair of the femoral vein with running nonabsorbable suture. Lysis of the most proximal great saphenous valve can be difficult with standard valvulotomes, but localized eversion of this segment permits excision of the valve under direct vision. Intrinsic atherosclerotic disease in the common femoral artery may dictate more proximal placement of the anastomosis. Additional proximal vein length can be obtained by harvesting a segment of the superficial epigastric vein and extending the venotomy proximally along the posterior surface of this vein to provide an autologous patch for repair of proximal common femoral artery disease. Care should be taken to minimize longitudinal stretching of the graft, which can accelerate the development of intimal hyperplasia.[110] Extensive common femoral or profunda femoris origin disease (or both) may necessitate endarterectomy with patch angioplasty or graft replacement of the common femoral artery. In the absence of significant proximal artery occlusive disease, defined as greater than a 50% reduction in lumen diameter, the superficial femoral, profunda femoris, or popliteal artery can be considered for placement of the proximal anastomosis.[111]

The posterior tibial, peroneal, and dorsalis pedis arteries provide the most straightforward options for placement of the distal anastomosis. Although the below-knee popliteal artery can also be used, fashioning the anastomosis can be problematic because of the nearly 90-degree angle that is formed between the graft and artery. With most hemodynamic analyses detailing an increase in flow separation and activation of proliferative metabolic pathways with right-angle anastomoses, grafts configured to this segment of the popliteal artery may benefit from excision and placement in an anatomic tunnel. Distal anastomoses to the above-knee popliteal artery do not offer the same constraints on their configuration; however, after mobilization of the proximal and distal graft, the segment that remains in situ can be quite short and of limited benefit.

Valve Lysis

Although limited transverse venotomies were used in initial development of the in situ bypass graft, this approach to render the valves incompetent has given way to less invasive techniques. Valvulotomes have undergone a variety of revisions over the last several decades, and the current generation of devices can be classified into three categories—the modified Mills valvulotome, the adjustable valvulotome, and the fixed valvulotome (Fig. 87-3)

The modified Mills valvulotome (see Fig. 87-3A) was initially described in 1976 for application to coronary artery bypass surgery.[112] With limited modification, this device was rapidly adopted for use in peripheral vascular surgery. Introduced into a side branch or the distal end of the vein, the device is advanced through the valve leaflets (Fig. 87-4). The proximal vein graft is distended by arterial inflow or manual infusion to induce valve closure, and the valvulotome is slowly withdrawn until the reverse cutting blade engages the valve leaflet. The tip of the valvulotome is maneuvered toward the center of the lumen and a short burst of inferior traction is applied to transect the valve. The valvulotome is advanced a

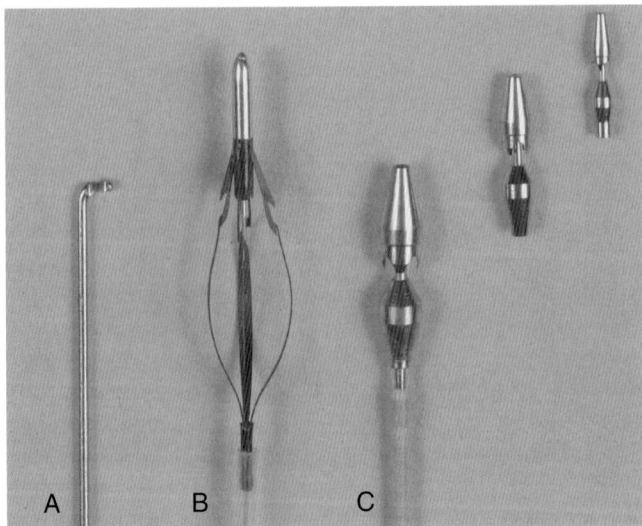

Figure 87-3 Valvulotomes. **A,** Modified Mills. **B,** LeMaitre adjustable. **C,** Uresil fixed with 2-, 3-, and 4-mm cutting heads.

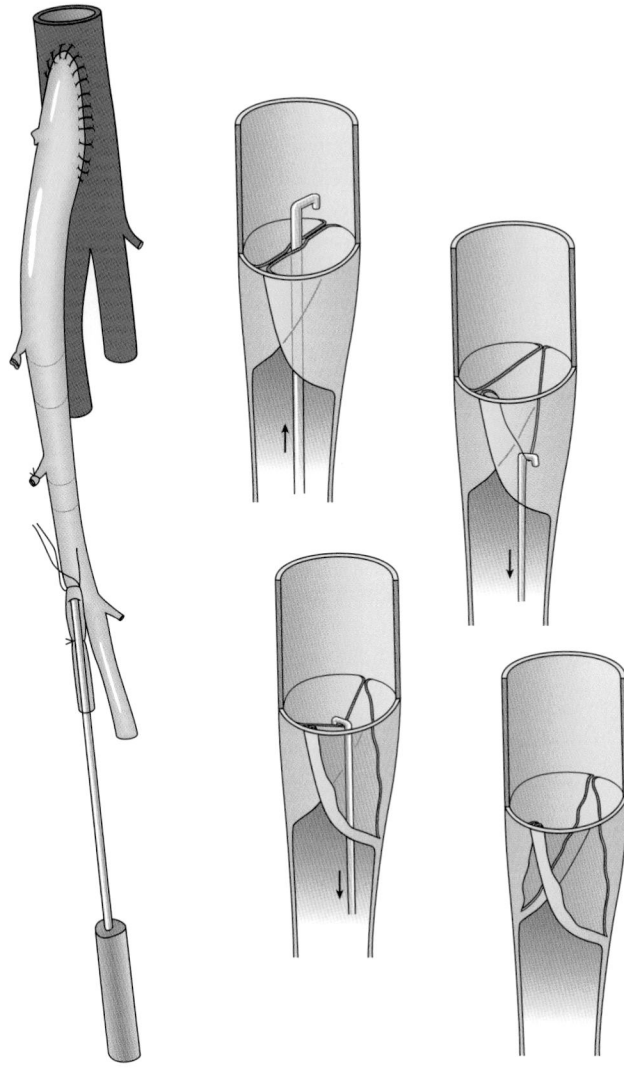

Figure 87-4 Valve lysis using the modified Mills valvulotome. The valvulotome is inserted into a long side branch and advanced into the proximal vein. Competent valves within the graft are maintained in closed position by arterial inflow pressure, and the valvulotome is withdrawn until resistance is encountered. After ensuring that the instrument has not engaged a side branch, a short burst of inferior traction is delivered and the valve leaflet transected. Short advancement and 180-degree rotation of the valvulotome permit division of the opposite valve in analogous fashion.

short distance and rotated 180 degrees, and the steps are repeated for complete division of the opposite valve. With close proximity of a major side branch to most valve sinuses, laceration of the wall can occur as a result of improper positioning, so care must be taken to identify the location of the tip before application of the cutting force.

Popularized by LeMaitre, the expandable valvulotome offers four cutting blades encompassed within a self-centering series of wire hoops (see Fig. 87-3B).[113] The cutting system is mounted on a long flexible shaft to provide a mechanism for remote deployment from the distal end of the graft. With the blades encased in a protective sheath, the device is advanced to the proximal end of the vein graft. The vein is distended,

the cutting system deployed, and the device slowly withdrawn until a valve is engaged. A burst of inferior traction facilitates simultaneous transection of both valve leaflets. Because of the mobility of the wire hoops, the position of the cutting blades is self-adjusting to accommodate vein diameters between 1.8 and 6 mm. Although direct visualization of the vein is not required during valve lysis, the shaft of the device is relatively stiff. Tracking within tortuous segments can be difficult and presents some risk of perforation if the shaft is advanced without regard to the position of the tip.

Fixed-diameter valvulotomes were developed from the original work of Hall, in which a blunt-tipped vein stripper was passed proximally to distally through the graft to avulse the valve leaflets and render them incompetent.[114] The addition of cutting blades and detachable heads of varying size led to the current generation of devices (see Fig. 87-3C).[115] Similar to the expandable valvulotomes, the cutting heads are attached to a long flexible shaft that is introduced distally and passed through the length of the vein. A 2-, 3-, or 4-mm head is secured to the shaft and reintroduced into the lumen of the vein. Similar to with the other devices, the proximal vein is distended and the valves are lysed with a rapid burst of inferior traction. Significant tapering of the vein distally may necessitate advancement of the device and exchange for smaller cutting heads. Direct vision of the head is mandatory to ensure an appropriate size match and avoid laceration of the wall from an oversized head. Such injuries are difficult to repair without narrowing the lumen of the vein and often require this segment of the graft to be discarded.

Visualization studies after the application of valvulotomes report that complete disruption occurs in approximately 70% to 95% of the treated valve leaflets.[116,117] Proximal segments of the vein, where the size mismatch is most pronounced, are most likely to demonstrate only partial valve disruption, and careful attention to this region seems warranted.[116] Limited data providing a direct comparison among the types are available, with one study suggesting incomplete valve lysis to be more common with expandable valvulotomes[117] and another suggesting no differences among the groups.[118] A prospective randomized trial comparing clinical outcomes for fixed and expandable devices failed to show any difference in short-term patency.[118]

Intraoperative angiography, duplex scanning, and angioscopy have been proposed as suitable adjuncts to evaluate the completeness of valve lysis during in situ bypass grafting. Angiography and duplex scanning are relatively insensitive modalities for identifying retained valves and detect only about 20% of such valves; angioscopy is much more sensitive.[119] Used for either direct visualization during valve lysis or graft surveillance, angioscopy is successful, with a sensitivity of identifying retained valve cusps approaching 100%. The clinical implications of identifying these valve abnormalities are uncertain, and several studies suggest no long-term improvement in graft patency with the routine use of angioscopy.[120,121] Potentially the most notable benefit from routine angioscopy may be the identification of significant preexisting venous disease. Veins with preexisting pathology have a high rate of early graft failure, and intraoperative recognition of these compromised vein segments may be the most important role for pre-bypass angioscopy.[68,122] Angioscopy may also be especially important in the evaluation of arm vein conduits because of their documented increased frequency of intrinsic vein abnormalities (see "Arm Vein and Composite Grafts").

Side Branch Ligation

Without the need to mobilize the vein from its subcutaneous bed, multiple options are available for treatment of the venous side branches. The standard approach would be complete exposure of the great saphenous vein with a single continuous incision that extends the length of the leg. Although this open approach simplifies side branch ligation and valve lysis, it has been associated with a wound complication rate in excess of 40% in some reported series.[67,123] These complications are of even more significance because of the superficial location of the in situ bypass. Even though extended rehospitalization and operative débridement may be required, these wounds can usually be managed without loss of graft patency.

Noninvasive identification of the major side branches offers the opportunity for a limited-incision or semi-closed in situ technique. Intraoperative venography and duplex scanning are two readily available options for this task, but these methods can be surprisingly inaccurate and fail to recognize almost 50% of the side branches.[119] Using the angioscope to identify the orifice and transcutaneous illumination to guide the location of the skin incision has proved somewhat more successful, with detection of approximately two thirds of patent side branches.[119,123] Commensurate with the smaller size of the incisions, these approaches offer notable improvement in wound complication rates.[120,123] Graft patency rates are relatively unaffected by the operative approach, but an increased incidence of persistent arteriovenous fistulae has been documented with most semi-closed techniques. Studies examining persistent fistulae have generally recommended their ligation; however, such an aggressive approach has been called into question. Conservative management of these fistulae results in spontaneous closure in a third of cases, eventual revision for reduced distal graft velocity in a third, and a third remaining stable without intervention.[124,125]

Increasing comfort with remote treatment of side branches led to the development of a closed technique in which major side branches are coil-embolized with a coaxial catheter system under angioscopic guidance, and only proximal and distal skin incisions are required for creation of the anastomoses.[126] Although this approach provides a further reduction in wound complications,[127] enthusiasm has waned significantly because of the associated increased expense and operative time required.

Arm Vein and Composite Grafts

The ipsilateral great saphenous vein is clearly the most desired conduit, but reports suggest that it is absent in up to 45% of patients requiring infrainguinal revascularization.[128] Use of single-segment or composite arm grafts provides an important alternative in such challenging patients. The most extensive experience with arm vein bypass is detailed through a series of reports from the Beth Israel Deaconess Hospital.[81,90,129] Preoperative duplex evaluation of the upper extremity veins is critical in the operative planning for patients with inadequate or previously harvested ipsilateral saphenous vein. A summary of the advantages and disadvantages of available arm vein conduits, along with an estimate of their relative frequency of use, is provided in Figure 87-5.[81]

To take advantage of the larger veins in the upper part of the arm, the basilic-cephalic loop graft has been proposed.[130,131] Using the median cubital vein as the connecting segment, the cephalic and basilic veins are harvested in a continuous loop from the antecubital fossa to their termination in the axillary vein. With the larger basilic vein serving as the proximal vein graft, a valvulotome is introduced into a midgraft side branch to facilitate lysis of valves in the basilic and median cubital segments. The cephalic vein segment, which tends to be thin

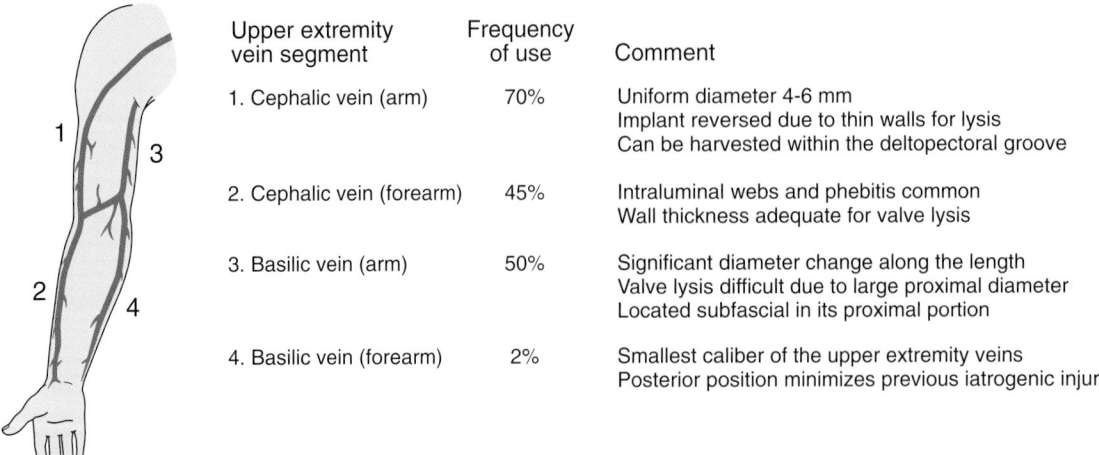

Upper extremity vein segment	Frequency of use	Comment
1. Cephalic vein (arm)	70%	Uniform diameter 4-6 mm Implant reversed due to thin walls for lysis Can be harvested within the deltopectoral groove
2. Cephalic vein (forearm)	45%	Intraluminal webs and phebitis common Wall thickness adequate for valve lysis
3. Basilic vein (arm)	50%	Significant diameter change along the length Valve lysis difficult due to large proximal diameter Located subfascial in its proximal portion
4. Basilic vein (forearm)	2%	Smallest caliber of the upper extremity veins Posterior position minimizes previous iatrogenic injury

Figure 87-5 Superficial upper extremity veins available for use in bypass grafting, including individual considerations and relative frequency of their use.[81]

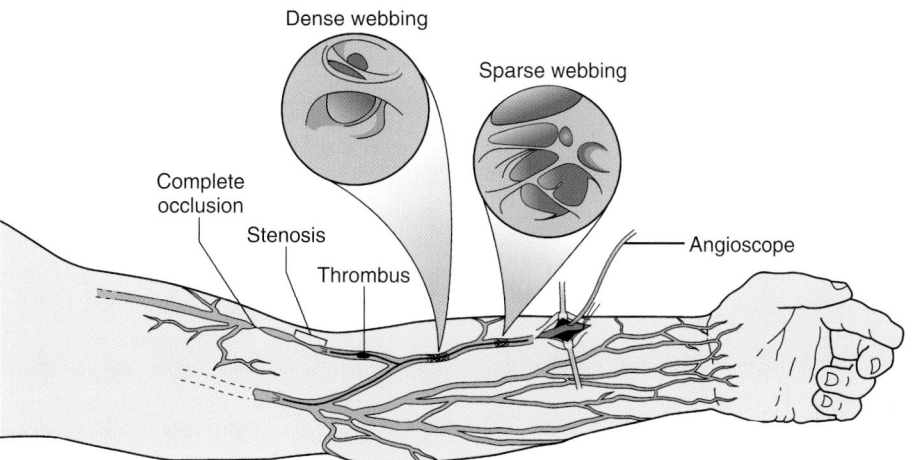

Figure 87-6 Iatrogenic injury to upper extremity veins leading to stenosis or segmental occlusion is common. Although preoperative duplex vein mapping can helpful, intraoperative angioscopy offers the potential for precise localization of these compromised areas.

walled and troublesome for valve lysis, is maintained in a reversed configuration and used for the distal anastomosis.

Similar to the approach when using lower extremity veins, single-segment arm vein is preferable. Through extensive use of the median antecubital vein as a bridge, success can be achieved in up 80% of cases requiring the use of arm vein.[81] Limiting this effort, however, is the inherent iatrogenic injury that occurs from repeated cannulation (Fig. 87-6). Veins that are most superficial and anatomically accessible, such as the forearm cephalic and median antecubital, are most frequently damaged, with 30% to 50% of these veins demonstrating a variety of pathologies.[132] Angioscopic evaluation of the quality of the arm vein and identification of compromised segments are thus fundamental to achieving long-term patency in these grafts. Minor abnormalities such as sparse webbing or an adherent thrombus can be successfully treated by endoluminal repair to restore a widely patent lumen. Other pathologies such as dense webbing or focal stenosis may require local repair with vein patch angioplasty. Marked abnormalities such as sclerosis with long-segment stenosis or occlusion cannot be repaired locally and require resection of the abnormal segment. Using such a treatment strategy, 25% of arm veins required local repair and 16% required resection, with no difference in long-term patency when compared with good-quality arm vein that required no intervention.[81] In the subset of grafts in which a segment of suboptimal-quality vein was used, failure within 6 months of implantation was common.

ETIOLOGY OF VEIN GRAFT FAILURE
Technical Factors

Traditionally, graft occlusions within 30 days of implantation have been thought to be related to technical factors that could potentially have been corrected at the time of graft placement. Although flow-limiting lesions within the bypass graft are a clear component of these failures, estimated at about 20%,[133] the events leading to graft thrombus are clearly more complex. Similar to the etiology of venous thrombosis, Virchow's classic triad is probably at the intersection of early graft failure. Not uncommon is the scenario in which early graft failure prompts re-exploration, which fails to identify any clear underlying cause.[133] Endothelial injury related to manipulation of the graft, hypercoagulability in the early postoperative period, and reduced graft flow because of inflow, outflow, or graft stenosis are factors that contribute to these early failures.

With insufficient time for formation of significant intimal hyperplasia, graft failures within 30 days are thought to be technical if they are associated with one of four categories: inadequate inflow, inadequate outflow, extrinsic lesions, and intrinsic lesions.[134] Inadequate inflow may be secondary to an unrecognized lesion in the proximal arteries or inflow graft. More common is the scenario in which the importance of the proximal lesion is underestimated, only to have its hemodynamic significance unmasked after placement of the distal graft. The resulting increase in flow leads to an accentuated drop in pressure across the lesion and converts a previously innocuous lesion into one that now has important hemodynamic implications. Cardiovascular compromise, such as systemic hypotension or a low cardiac output state (e.g., cardiogenic shock), can also be the cause of inflow-related graft failure.

Inadequate outflow as a result of extensive, preexisting tibial and inframalleolar occlusive disease is an established risk factor for early graft failure; patients demonstrating the most severe disease have a 10-fold increased risk for 30-day graft thrombosis.[135,136] Vasospasm of the target artery is a less well studied but possible contributor to early postoperative outflow compromise. Though difficult to quantify and monitor postoperatively, a subset of patients demonstrate severe luminal narrowing and delayed reperfusion despite minimal atherosclerotic disease in the distal artery (Fig. 87-7).

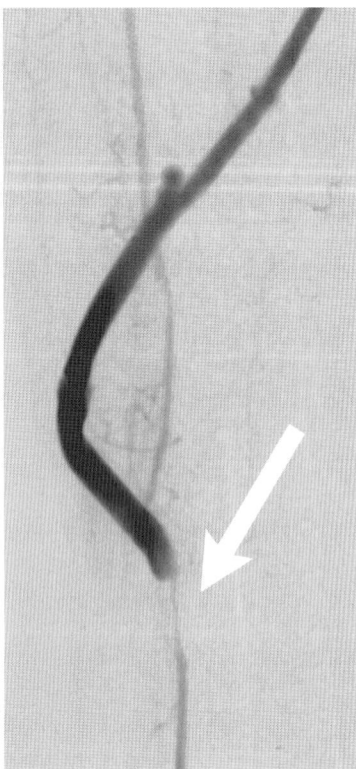

Figure 87-7 Intraoperative digital subtraction arteriogram of a vein bypass graft to the distal anterior tibial artery. Severe distal spasm of the outflow artery (*arrow*) has led to diminished diastolic flow in the graft.

Extrinsic causes of early graft failure include extrinsic compression because of tunneling errors or hematomas that may compromise graft flow. Other extrinsic causes of graft failure, such as hypercoagulability, are systemic. Alterations in the coagulation system are detectable in more than 25% of patients undergoing lower extremity revascularization.[137] Although some studies have suggested that 10% of early graft failures are primarily related to an identified hypercoagulable state,[133] the contribution of transient abnormalities in coagulation is unclear and perhaps underestimated.

Intrinsic vein graft defects include focal, flow-limiting lesions such as a retained valve leaflet, an intimal flap, or inappropriate placement of anastomotic sutures. Limitations in flow can result from the use of an undersized conduit, with vein grafts less than 3.0 mm in diameter being at significant risk for early failure.[136] Independent of luminal narrowing, intrinsic vein graft defects, such as sclerosis and calcification, also contribute to graft thrombosis.[17]

Recent data from the multi-institutional PREVENT III trial have detailed a 5% incidence of thrombosis or re-exploration within 30 days of graft implantation.[92] Whereas endovascular management of these early graft occlusions is of limited value, open surgical revision provides a reasonable opportunity for durable graft salvage, with a 90% 1-year patency rate reported after successful exploration and revision.[138]

Intimal Hyperplasia and Pathologic Remodeling

Surgical manipulation of the vein combined with the acute exposure to elevated shear and tensile forces elicits a complex series of biologic events in the vein wall that begin immediately on implantation. Analogous to the events that occur in generalized wound healing, repair of the damaged vein graft is initiated by the local synthesis of a wide variety of cytokines and growth factors. Chemokines induce the recruitment of neutrophils and mononuclear cells, which further amplifies these pathways. Activated by these chemoattractants and mitogens, smooth muscle cells begin to dedifferentiate from a contractile to a synthetic phenotype and replicate within the media. By tracing the gradient of chemokines, liberated smooth muscle cells migrate from the media to the intima, where continued proliferation and abundant matrix deposition are stimulated. Progressive thickening of the intima leads to narrowing of the lumen, a reduction in graft flow, and intraluminal thrombosis (Fig. 87-8).

Despite the relative uniformity of the surgical trauma and hemodynamic insult, vein graft lesions demonstrate a strong tendency to be focal rather than diffuse.[139] With a peak incidence at 4 to 12 months after implantation, 30% to 45% of autogenous grafts will fail or require revision secondary to significant narrowing of the lumen.[92,140] Stenotic lesions are more likely to be associated with the proximal or distal anastomosis (53% incidence) but occur not infrequently in the midbody of the graft (30% incidence).[93] It has been postulated that these midgraft lesions are associated with valve leaflets; detailed evaluation of this issue demonstrated substantial remodeling within valve sites, but progression to high-grade stenosis was rare and accounted for less than 20% of the

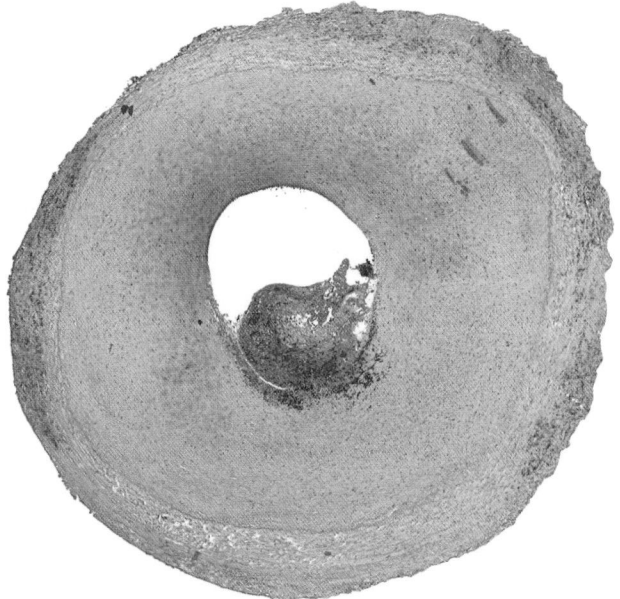

Figure 87-8 Cross-sectional histologic image of an 8-month-old vein graft demonstrating severe intimal hyperplasia. Adherent thrombus is present within the severely compromised lumen.

intrinsic graft lesions requiring repair.[99] Despite such general observations, the underlying biologic mechanisms for development of this segmental pattern of intimal hyperplasia remain poorly understood. Although the local flow environment plays a significant role, physical forces in isolation fail to explain these observations. More likely, critical lesion development occurs at the intersection of localized trauma, ongoing hemodynamic stress, and an altered ability for local repair after injury.

Although much of the emphasis in vein graft pathology has focused on intimal hyperplasia, graft morphology is actually dictated by the balance between outward expansion and wall thickening. As Glagov and coworkers demonstrated, the normal vascular adaptive response is an increase in overall wall circumference to compensate for luminal narrowing in the presence of a developing occlusive lesion.[141] In response to hemodynamic and biochemical stimuli, smooth muscle cells degrade and reorganize the rigid matrix structure of the wall to facilitate these changes. Examination of early vein graft morphology demonstrated a 20% increase in diameter within the first month after implantation; failure of this outward remodeling has been correlated with subsequent graft failure.[142] Inflammatory pathways appear to further modulate this shear-mediated adaptive response, thus providing potential mechanistic insight into the heterogeneity that is observed clinically.[143]

Graft Atherosclerosis

Although the peak incidence of vein graft failure occurs within the first year, delayed progression of intrinsic lesions leads to a 4% annual loss of graft patency in the 2- to 10-year time frame.[9,140] Because studies have focused predominantly on the mechanisms of early graft failure, insight into the pathology of delayed lesion development in peripheral vein grafts is limited. Much of our understanding of late graft failure is derived from coronary bypass grafts examined at the time of autopsy. Replacement of the fibrotic wall with lipid-laden macrophages and intramural calcification is common.[144-146] Degeneration of the vein graft wall with intramural thrombus formation, characteristic of ruptured atherosclerotic plaque, is also frequently observed.[147,148] Supporting these observations is the clinical impact of lipid-lowering therapy on coronary artery graft patency, where reductions in total serum cholesterol significantly enhance vein graft durability.[149-151]

With few relevant animal models, examination of these events in peripheral bypass grafts has been relegated to the analysis of sporadic samples obtained at the time of graft revision. The initial report published by Szilagyi and coauthors in 1973 identified atherosclerotic changes in 8 of 21 grafts ranging in age from 8 to 96 months.[139] These observations are supported by Walton and colleagues, who described apolipoprotein B deposits, ulceration, calcification, and aneurysm formation in the majority of failed grafts that had been implanted for more than 2 years.[152] More recent reports, however, present a more variable picture and predominantly describe a fibrocellular hyperplastic intima with rare athero-

sclerotic degeneration as the cause of late failure.[153] Although investigators have speculated that modulation of early intimal hyperplasia will have an impact on cholesterol-driven atherogenesis and provide an avenue to improve graft patency, this view remains speculative with limited data to support it.[154,155]

◼ PREVENTION OF VEIN GRAFT FAILURE

Intraoperative Evaluation

Despite improvements in surgical technique, 5% of autogenous vein grafts fail within 30 days of implantation.[92] Retained valve leaflets, abnormal twists or kinks, intimal flaps, other unrecognized obstructive lesions, and technical defects at the time of graft placement are estimated to account for between 15% and 25% of early failures.[156,157] The initial technical adequacy of an infrainguinal bypass graft can be judged intraoperatively by the external appearance of the bypass and anastomoses and by the restoration of distal pulses and perfusion. Continuous wave Doppler is a useful intraoperative adjunct that permits evaluation of anastomoses and areas of concern within the body of the graft for localized increases in the audible sound frequency. Though adequate for gross defects, a more detailed assessment to ensure technical success and to optimize short- and intermediate-term graft patency has been advocated. Recent investigations report a 15% intraoperative graft revision rate for abnormalities identified on secondary imaging.[158] Although it is unclear to what extent these irregularities increase the risk for graft failure, the significant morbidity resulting from early reintervention for graft failure supports an aggressive approach to intraoperative repair.[159]

Angiography

Contrast-enhanced angiography remains the diagnostic standard for arterial anatomic imaging and is the most widely used method for intraoperative vein graft assessment. Facilitated by the increasing availability of high-quality intraoperative angiographic equipment, this technique provides the current standard for determination of technical adequacy of a bypass graft. Though particularly useful for identifying a kink or twist in the graft, a patent side branch or branch ligature stenosis, and distal arterial disease requiring sequential bypass,[160] angiography has several notable shortcomings. Limited by a single projection plane and the dense opacification provided by iodinated contrast material, retained valve leaflets and intraluminal webs can be difficult to identify, with one study reporting failure rates approaching 80%.[119] Particularly troublesome is angiographic evaluation of the distal anastomosis and delineation of a structural abnormality versus spasm in the outflow artery (see Fig. 87-7). Significant spasm occurs in approximately 50% of tibial and pedal artery bypasses, but it is of no clinical consequence in the large majority of cases.[161,162] Routine intraluminal injection of papaverine hydrochloride (30 to 60 mg in 1 to 2 mL of 0.9% saline) into the vein graft before performing completion angiography has been advocated to alleviate vasospasm.[163]

With these technical limitations, the use of a standard evaluation algorithm (consisting of visual inspection, palpation, and interrogation with continuous wave Doppler) with selective arteriography has been proposed. Mills and colleagues noted that these simpler techniques failed to identify 80% of the vein graft and outflow abnormalities that were detected by completion angiography and required revision.[164] Focusing on 1-year patency as the primary endpoint, other investigators examining this issue arrived at the opposite conclusion and stated that the additional expense of routine arteriography outweighs its benefit.[165] In the latter retrospective review, where no difference in graft patency was observed in association with routine or selective angiography, patient enrollment was modest and statistical analysis insufficiently powered to allow firm conclusions. Completion angiography provides useful anatomic information, especially with regard to the status of the outflow arteries; its major weakness is that it fails to provide any hemodynamic assessment.

Flow Rate Measurements

Non–imaging-based modalities such as measurement of blood flow rates have been advocated as useful adjuncts in the intraoperative evaluation of vein grafts. Based on the assumption that flow-limiting stenoses could be detected by reductions in flow, investigators identified 80 mL/min as the critical threshold below which there was a high probability of a technical problem within the reconstruction and for which further evaluation with angiography was suggested.[166] Though of interest, this approach has largely been supplanted by duplex imaging. The use of intraoperative flow measurements has also been described as an independent predictor of graft patency. Despite being unreliable in identifying grafts at risk for early (<30 day) failure,[167] an extensive literature confirms the importance of graft flow rates in determining intermediate- and long-term patency.[168-170] Not surprisingly, flow rates demonstrate high correlation with the angiographic runoff score[135] and can serve as a surrogate for this well-established risk factor with limited direct application to intraoperative decision making. More quantitative assessments of graft hemodynamics, such as the resistive index and longitudinal impedance, have also been proposed.[171,172] Similar to flow rate measurements, these parameters have prognostic significance but little utility in therapeutic decision making.

Duplex Scanning

After angiography, duplex scanning has developed into the next most commonly used intraoperative method for evaluation of vein grafts. Duplex uses B-mode imaging and velocity spectrum analysis to detect lesions and grade lesion severity, thus providing both anatomic and hemodynamic assessment. Initially described by Bandyk and coworkers for the assessment of in situ bypass grafts,[173] duplex scanning proved effective in the identification of competent valve leaflets, anastomotic narrowing, arteriovenous fistulae, hemodynamic stenosis caused by small-caliber conduit, and the intraoperative

formation of fibrin-platelet aggregates. With evolving diagnostic criteria, duplex scanning was initially thought to be too sensitive and best suited for use as a screening tool in combination with selective arteriography to better define suspect areas. Subsequent refinements in both instrumentation and interpretation have yielded improved accuracy, with multiple studies supporting the replacement of intraoperative angiography with duplex scanning.[174-176] Although the published literature has been unequivocal regarding the value of intraoperative duplex, application has been limited predominantly to centers of excellence where sufficient skilled vascular technologists are available to support these efforts.

A standardized procedure for intraoperative duplex graft scanning has been proposed by Johnson and colleagues.[158] Before scanning, papaverine (30 to 60 mg) is injected into the distal vein graft segment with a 27-gauge needle. Using a linear-array 7- to 15-MHz transducer (for superficial grafts) or 5-MHz transducer (for tunneled grafts), velocity spectra along the distal anastomosis and outflow artery are recorded while maintaining a 60-degree Doppler angle. The entire length of the graft is then scanned in a distal to proximal direction to evaluate color-flow images and velocity spectra for retained valves and residual arteriovenous fistulae (if applicable). Evaluation is completed with scanning of the proximal anastomosis and inflow artery. Diagnostic criteria for elevated velocities and an appropriate management algorithm are presented in Table 87-2. In one center using this protocol, a normal intraoperative duplex scan has been associated with a reduction in 90-day graft thrombosis to 0.4%.[177]

A significant advantage of this technique is its ability to detect low-flow bypass grafts, defined as an average peak systolic velocity (PSV) of less than 45 cm/sec (see Table 87-2). Subsequent analysis of these low-flow grafts has identified two clinical subgroups based on the presence or absence of diastolic flow. The majority of grafts with high peripheral vascular resistance and absent diastolic flow failed within 6 months of implantation,[178] and surgical revision consisting of either a sequential graft to an alternative target or placement of an arteriovenous fistula has been advocated to salvage these threatened grafts. Low-flow grafts with low peripheral vascular resistance (characterized by antegrade flow throughout the pulse cycle) were at intermediate risk of failure (30% failure rate at 6 months) and may benefit from postoperative anticoagulation.[158]

Angioscopy

Angioscopy provides an alternative image-based modality for intraoperative assessment of vein grafts. Not only does it assist in preparation of the conduit by allowing accurate and complete valvulotomy, detecting unsuspected intraluminal pathology, and assisting in the selection of optimal-quality vein segments for composite grafting, it also provides a tool for assessment of technical errors at completion of the procedure. However, successful application of angioscopy requires an investment in new instrumentation and a commitment to overcome its inherent learning curve. Several groups have

Table 87-2 Intraoperative Duplex Monitoring—Diagnostic Criteria and Management Options

Category	PSV (cm/sec)	V_r	Interpretation and Intraoperative Management
Stenotic Lesion			
Normal/minimal	< 125	1.0-2.0	Normal flow pattern; no further evaluation
Moderate	125-180	2.0-3.0	Residual flow abnormality; rescan after 5 min with papaverine flow augmentation; consider arteriography
Severe	>180, with spectral broadening	2.5-5.0	Significant abnormality, repair defect; if not repaired, perform arteriography to verify normal bypass graft segment
High-grade	>300	>5.0	Critical lesion, typically associated with a pulse pressure deficit and low graft flow
Low-Flow Graft			
Low flow, low PVR	<40	—	Consider systemic anticoagulation / Caveats: large-caliber veins may have low peak systolic flow velocities; reversed veins to pedal outflow arteries may also have low distal graft flow velocities
Low flow, high PVR	<40	—	Consider an adjunctive procedure to increase graft flow (distal arteriovenous fistula, jump/sequential graft to an alternative target)

PSV, peak systolic velocity; PVR, peripheral vascular resistance—low (antegrade flow throughout the pulse cycle) or high (antegrade flow only during systole with minimal diastolic flow); V_r, velocity ratio ($PSV_{at\ lesion}/PSV_{proximal}$).

Adapted from Johnson BL, Bandyk DF, Back MR, et al. Intraoperative duplex monitoring of infrainguinal vein bypass procedures. *J Vasc Surg.* 2000;31:678-690.

examined the potential benefits of completion angioscopy, with a generalized consensus that angioscopy is significantly more sensitive in identifying intraluminal abnormalities than either angiography[179,180] or duplex scanning.[119] The most informative study to date, conducted by Miller and associates, was a 250-patient prospective randomized evaluation of angioscopy versus angiography.[181] Intraluminal abnormalities were identified in a fifth of the enrolled grafts, with 75% of them determined to be of sufficient severity to prompt surgical correction. Intraoperative revisions were fourfold more likely to be performed after angioscopic evaluation and led to a 50% reduction in 30-day graft failure (3% after angioscopy versus 6% after angiography). Although this difference did not reach statistical significance, it suggested that some improvement in early graft patency may be obtained with the use of completion angioscopy and aggressive intraoperative revision of any abnormalities identified. Not examined in this trial were the potential intermediate- and long-term benefits in graft patency afforded by this approach, which may have been even more pronounced than the effects on early patency.

Postoperative Surveillance

Physical Examination and Physiologic Assessment

As initially established by the seminal work of Szilagyi's group[139] and re-enforced by multiple other studies, it is now known that autogenous grafts develop segmental foci of luminal narrowing that lead to reductions in flow and precipitate thrombosis. Attempts to salvage thrombosed grafts outside of the early postoperative period have largely been unsuccessful, with 30% 1-year patency rates after thrombectomy.[182] These observations contributed to the concept of routine graft surveillance, or periodic evaluation to identify grafts with evolving lesions before the development of thrombosis. Resulting from a combination of intimal hyperplasia and pathologic (inward) remodeling, these lesions have a peak incidence within the first 12 months, with 30% becoming hemodynamically significant within this 1-year time frame.[93,183] These observations form the basis for graft surveillance protocols in which frequent evaluations are recommended during the first 12 to 18 months after implantation.

Clinical protocols for graft surveillance focus on physical examination with physiologic assessment of distal perfusion. Patient histories are elicited to detect new onset of claudication or ischemic pain at rest, and physical examination is performed to identify notable changes in the lower extremity pulse. The ABI is used as the quantitative measure of perfusion, with a reduction of greater than 0.15 being considered significant. Changes in any of these parameters should prompt further evaluation to identify the lesion or lesions that have precipitated the hemodynamic deterioration. To improve the sensitivity of physiologic testing, pulse volume recording with a transfer function index protocol has been proposed.[184] Pulse volume recordings are collected from upper extremity (inflow) and ankle (outflow) cuffs and subjected to a Fourier transform algorithm to produce discrete spectra for review. Direct comparison of the frequency response curves provides a numerical value that can be used to identify at-risk grafts. Proof-of-concept testing of this device has suggested accuracy equivalent to that of duplex scanning, but this approach has failed to gain acceptance outside the research arena.

Duplex Scanning

With the recognition that clinical surveillance parameters were insensitive until the lumen was severely compromised,[164,185] duplex scanning was identified as a method for earlier detection of these developing lesions. After an initial focus on reductions in PSV and the absence of diastolic

Table 87-3 Postoperative Duplex Monitoring—Diagnostic Criteria and Management Options

Category	PSV (cm/sec)	V$_r$	Waveform Characteristics	Management
Stenotic Lesion				
Less 20% stenosis (normal)	<150	<1.5	Absent or mild spectral broadening in systole	Rescan in 6 months
20% to 50% stenosis (mild)	>150	1.5-2.0	Spectral broadening throughout systole with no change in waveform	Rescan in 6 months
50% to 75% stenosis (moderate)	>180	>2.5	Severe spectral broadening in systole with reversed-flow components	Rescan in 4-6 weeks; if lesion does not progress during two cycles of testing, increase scan interval to 3 months
Greater than 75% stenosis (severe)	>300	>3.5	Severe lumen reduction with a "flow jet"; damped distal velocity waveform	Recommend repair (urgent if average PSV <45 cm/sec or change in ABI >0.15)
Low-Flow Graft				
Low flow	<40	—		Angiography and repair of a non–flow-limiting stenosis should be considered

ABI, ankle-brachial index; PSV, peak systolic velocity; V$_r$, velocity ratio (PSV$_{at\ lesion}$/PSV$_{proximal}$).

Adapted from Bandyk DF. Infrainguinal vein bypass graft surveillance: How to do it, when to intervene, and is it cost-effective? *J Am Coll Surg*. 2002;194(1 Suppl.): S40-S50.

flow,[186,187] changes in velocity along the length of the graft were recognized as a more useful approach for lesion localization.[188,189] Though not generated through a formal series of receiver operating characteristic curves, a duplex classification has evolved to correlate PSV and the velocity ratio (V$_r$) with the approximate degrees of vein graft stenosis (Table 87-3).[190] Complicating management of vein graft stenosis is the dynamic remodeling that occurs in 12 to 18 months after implantation, during which the appearance and subsequent regression of focal regions of luminal narrowing are frequently observed.[99,191] Retrospective reviews correlating duplex-derived hemodynamic data with lesion morphology suggested a PSV of 300 cm/sec (or a V$_r$ of 4.0) to be the critical threshold above which lesion regression was relatively unlikely (Fig. 87-9).[192,193] Intermediate stenoses (200 cm/sec

< PSV < 300 cm/sec; 2 < V$_r$ < 4) are notably dynamic, with 20% to 30% of these lesions demonstrating significant regression within 2 years. Complicating these retrospective analyses, however, was the preexisting bias that high-grade stenoses mandate intervention, so the natural history of these high-grade lesions has been incompletely defined. Although the number of grafts with high-grade stenoses that did not undergo elective revision is relatively small, the risk of occlusion of these unrepaired grafts appears to be in excess of 75%.[187,193] Predominantly based on these observations, an algorithm for the management of postoperative vein graft stenosis has been proposed,[190] with the key elements of this approach outlined in Table 87-3. Of particular concern are grafts with a PSV of greater than 300 cm/sec and a change in the ABI of greater than 0.15 or significant dampening of the

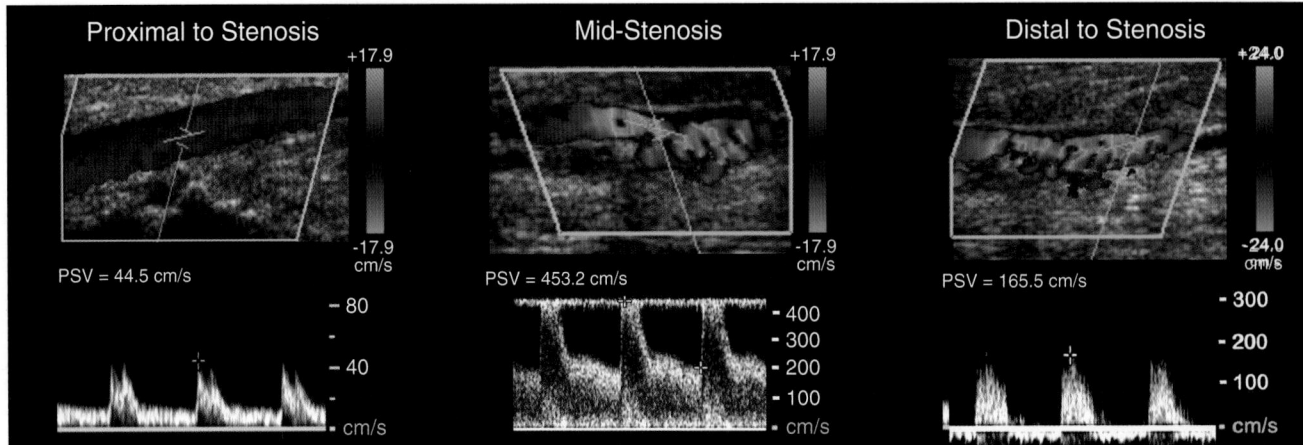

Figure 87-9 Postoperative duplex scan of a vein graft demonstrating markedly elevated peak systolic velocity and spectral broadening within an area of stenosis. Distal to the lesion, disordered flow is evident on color-flow imaging, and a significant reduction in diastolic velocity is observed.

distal waveforms. These findings are generally thought to be preocclusive lesions, and initiation of systemic anticoagulation with prompt repair is indicated.

In parallel with these observational studies, multiple single-institution cohort studies have clarified the role of duplex surveillance in improving patient outcomes. Results from these studies are in general agreement and demonstrate an approximate 15% improvement in graft patency rates with routine duplex evaluation versus clinical follow-up alone.[194-196] Recommendations for the frequency of vein graft surveillance have been proposed and focus on the intermediate period (1 to 18 months), when lesion remodeling is most active. After an intraoperative or early postoperative scan to identify technical problems, outpatient duplex evaluations at 1, 3, 6, 12, and 18 months and annually thereafter are recommended. The development of moderate stenosis or the need for vein graft revision would prompt closer follow-up, with interval scans at approximately 6 weeks until lesion stabilization or regression is confirmed.

The economic benefits of a graft surveillance program have been investigated by a number of investigators, who have focused on major amputation as the dominant outcome variable.[197,198] Duplex scan surveillance was the least expensive ($2823) and resulted in the fewest major amputations (17 per 1000 patients examined) when compared with clinical follow-up alone ($5072 and 77 amputations per 1000 patients).[197] With the recognition that 90% of lesions that will require revision between 1 and 18 months will demonstrate some element of flow abnormality within 4 weeks,[199] investigators have questioned the need for continued aggressive surveillance after normal 1- and 3-month graft scans.[200] Longer-term follow-up has clarified this issue; one study reported that 30% of the flow abnormalities that ultimately required revision were not observed until after 6 months.[201] Annual examination to evaluate for graft atherosclerosis or aneurysmal degeneration and progression of native inflow-outflow arterial disease therefore seems warranted.

Although the large array of cohort studies presents compelling data to support a routine duplex surveillance program, consensus on this issue is not uniform. Three randomized prospective trials were performed to evaluate vein graft surveillance and reached variable conclusions regarding its benefits. The first and smallest of these studies, published by Lundell in 1995, randomized 156 patients after vein bypass grafts to either intense duplex surveillance or intermittent clinical follow-up.[202] Although major amputation was not explored as an endpoint, implementation of an intensive duplex protocol provided a 25% absolute improvement in both primary-assisted and secondary graft patency rates at 3 years. Among the confounding factors in this trial, however, was their use of frequent (every 3 months) follow-up in the duplex group but only annual follow-up in the clinical group. Consequently, a definitive conclusion on the value of duplex scanning versus more frequent clinical follow-up could not be obtained. The second trial randomized 342 patients between duplex and clinical surveillance and demonstrated no difference in graft patency or limb salvage at 1 year.[203] Though

methodologically sound, the duration of follow-up was probably insufficient to realize the full benefit of serial duplex evaluation. The largest trial, in which 594 patients were randomized to a duplex or clinical protocol, demonstrated no difference in major amputation or graft patency at 18 months.[204] Despite the use of a prospective randomized methodology, significant concern has been raised in regard to the validity of these findings.[205,206] Use of nonstandard duplex criteria resulting in an aggressive treatment approach to intermediate stenoses, delay in randomization until 4 to 6 weeks postoperatively (reducing the early benefit of duplex examination), and the short follow-up time were among the major issues that were raised.

Despite these potential methodologic flaws in the randomized trials, the available literature presents two diametrically opposing views on the relative value of a duplex surveillance program. Multiple cohort studies have exhaustively detailed the natural history of vein graft lesions and the perceived benefits of early detection and repair of high-grade lesions, yet all lack an appropriate control group. In contrast, the randomized trials suggest little benefit of duplex surveillance, but such generalization may be limited by notable methodologic flaws. Faced with this dilemma, the 2007 Inter-Society Consensus for the Management of Peripheral Arterial Disease came forth with a grade C recommendation supporting clinical surveillance only, with a focus on history taking for new symptoms, complete vascular examination of the extremity, and resting and postexercise ABI at 6-month intervals for a minimum of 2 years.[207] The consensus statement notes that the previous recommendation for routine duplex scanning after autogenous lower extremity bypass has not yet proved cost-effective. Nevertheless, most surgeons continue a program of vein graft surveillance and remain skeptical of these negative findings.

SELECTED KEY REFERENCES

Adcock OT Jr, Adcock GL, Wheeler JR, Gregory RT, Snyder SO Jr, Gayle RG. Optimal techniques for harvesting and preparation of reversed autogenous vein grafts for use as arterial substitutes: a review. *Surgery.* 1984;96:886-894.
Comprehensive, literature-based review of the techniques available for minimizing endothelial injury during vein graft harvest.

Bandyk DF. Infrainguinal vein bypass graft surveillance: how to do it, when to intervene, and is it cost-effective? *J Am Coll Surg.* 2002; 194(Suppl 1):S40-S50.
Compilation of clinical care algorithms for the use of intraoperative and postoperative duplex scanning to maximize vein graft patency.

Caps MT, Cantwell-Gab K, Bergelin RO, Strandness DE Jr. Vein graft lesions: time of onset and rate of progression. *J Vasc Surg.* 1995; 22:466-474.
Longitudinal evaluation of early and intermediate vein graft lesion development and regression.

Davies AH, Hawdon AJ, Sydes MR, Thompson SG. Is duplex surveillance of value after leg vein bypass grafting? Principal results of the vein graft surveillance randomised trial (VGST). *Circulation.* 2005;112:1985-1991.
Prospective, randomized trial examining the efficacy of routine duplex vein graft surveillance for the prevention of major limb amputation.

Hölzenbein TJ, Pomposelli FB Jr, Miller A, Contreras MA, Gibbons GW, Campbell DR, Freeman DV, LoGerfo FW. Results of a policy with arm veins used as the first alternative to an unavailable ipsilateral greater saphenous vein for infrainguinal bypass. *J Vasc Surg.* 1996;23: 130-140.
Clinical outcomes using a defined treatment algorithm to maximize the use of arm vein for lower extremity bypass.

Marcaccio EJ, Miller A, Tannenbaum GA, Lavin PT, Gibbons GW, Pomposelli FB Jr, Freeman DV, Campbell DR, LoGerfo FW. Angioscopically directed interventions improve arm vein bypass grafts. *J Vasc Surg.* 1993;17:994-1002.
Angioscopic evaluation of the incidence and segmental distribution of intraluminal disease in arm veins used for lower extremity bypass.

Mills JL, Fujitani RM, Taylor SM. The characteristics and anatomic distribution of lesions that cause reversed vein graft failure: a five-year prospective study. *J Vasc Surg.* 1993;17:195-204.
Duplex examination of the incidence, characteristics, and anatomic distribution of lesions that cause graft failure in the intermediate postoperative period.

Schanzer A, Hevelone N, Owens CD, Belkin M, Bandyk DF, Clowes AW, Moneta GL, Conte MS. Technical factors affecting autogenous vein graft failure: observations from a large multicenter trial. *J Vasc Surg.* 2007;46:1180-1190.
Interrogation of the prospective, multicenter PREVENT III trial database to identify technical variables that were significantly associated with early and midterm results of autogenous vein bypass grafting.

REFERENCES

The reference list can be found on the companion Expert Consult Web site at *www.expertconsult.com.*

CHAPTER 88

Prosthetic Grafts

Zheng Qu and Elliot L. Chaikof

Based in part on a chapter in the previous edition by Lian Xue, MD, PhD, and Howard P. Greisler, MD.

Synthetic conduits were introduced to modern arterial reconstructive surgery by Voorhees and Blakemore in 1952 with the development of a vascular graft woven from Vinyon-N fibers, a copolymer of vinyl chloride and acrylonitrile.[1] Despite successful early clinical outcomes, first-generation vascular prostheses lacked long-term durability. Within 5 years, graft dilatation and aneurysmal degeneration were frequent, with an 80% loss in tensile strength.[2,3] A variety of candidate materials for synthetic arterial conduits were examined throughout the 1950s, including solid rigid metals, glass, and silk. Their failure led to the supposition that porosity and resistance to thrombosis were critical features for an arterial substitute. Innovations in polymer science and engineering in the period surrounding World War II led to the synthesis of polytetrafluoroethylene (PTFE; e.g., Teflon) in 1938 and polyethylene terephthalate (PET; e.g., Dacron) in 1941. Both polymers, when engineered as fibers or as a nonwoven fabric, proved to be more durable and biocompatible and have remained commercial standards. In the aortic position, the performance of prosthetic grafts is excellent, with susceptibility to graft infection the remaining major limitation. In the pediatric population, the inability of commercially available prostheses to match the growth of the child is an additional limitation of current synthetic large-caliber conduits.

Prospective randomized clinical studies have confirmed that PET and PTFE differ little in their long-term performance characteristics when used in the infrainguinal position.[4] However, both display significantly lower patency than vein grafts because of greater risk for thrombosis and anastomotic neointimal hyperplasia. The inherent thrombogenicity of available polymeric materials and the presence of a chronic injury site at the anastomosis caused, in part, by a compliance mismatch between the prosthesis and host artery contribute to late graft occlusion. These failure modes exist whether a synthetic conduit is used for lower extremity revascularization or for arteriovenous hemodialysis access, even when the prosthesis has an inner diameter of 6 mm or larger. Currently, coronary and infrageniculate lower extremity revascularization requires the use of conduits smaller than 6 mm in diameter. Despite significant effort by industrial and academic research groups over the past half-century, a durable, synthetic, small-diameter vascular graft does not exist.

Attempts to address these failure mechanisms and the complete absence of a small-diameter conduit have led to collaborative interactions among vascular surgeons, material scientists, biologists, and engineers. Novel materials with improved mechanical responses continue to be synthesized, and new surface engineering schemes along with systemic antithrombotics have been devised to reduce the risk for thrombus formation. As the distinction between "biologic" and "synthetic" continues to be blurred, the design of "living," biologically functional structures may ultimately supplant autologous vein grafts as the ideal small-diameter conduit. Such a development would revolutionize the field.

MATERIALS
Dacron Prosthesis

Dacron is the DuPont trademark for PET, a highly durable polyester thermoplastic polymer that can be processed into synthetic fibers. DeBakey introduced the first knitted Dacron prosthesis in 1957; it was used extensively for arterial reconstruction of the thoracic and abdominal aorta, as well as proximal peripheral vessels.[5] This pioneering work, combined with developmental and clinical studies by Szilagyi, Wesolowski, Sauvage, and Cooley, contributed to the popularization of Dacron grafts.[6]

Historically, weaving and knitting have been the two common techniques for fabrication of Dacron fibers into a tubular conduit. The knit structure involves looping fibers in an interlocking chain, which yields a soft and stretchable fabric. In contrast, a woven structure assembles the yarn in an over-and-under pattern in the lengthwise and circumferential directions (Fig. 88-1).[7-9] Woven grafts are stronger and less porous than knitted grafts but are less compliant and may fray when cut. Typically, highly porous knitted Dacron grafts required "preclotting," a process that involved exposing the graft to an aliquot of the patient's blood before heparinization. Currently, most commercial knitted grafts are impregnated with gelatin,[10] collagen,[11] or albumin.[12] Despite some evidence that coated grafts may induce a greater inflammatory response than preclotted grafts,[13,14] both display similar patency rates.[15,16]

Characteristically, knitted grafts incorporate a velour finish that orients the loops of yarn upward, perpendicular to the fabric surface, thereby increasing the available surface area and enhancing the anchorage of fibrin and cells to promote

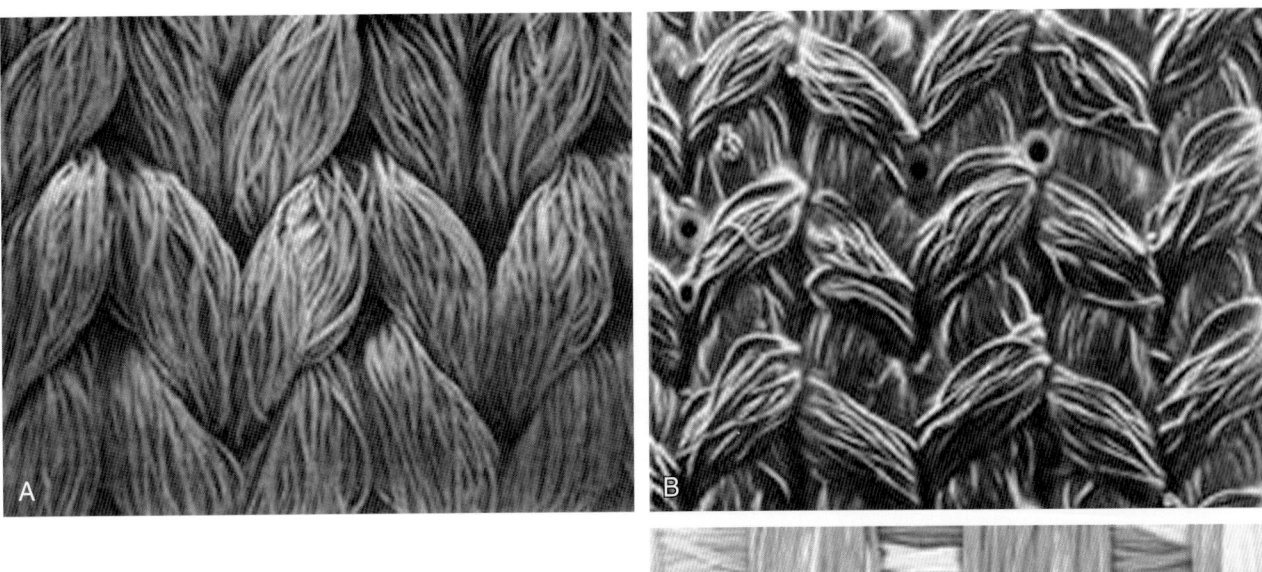

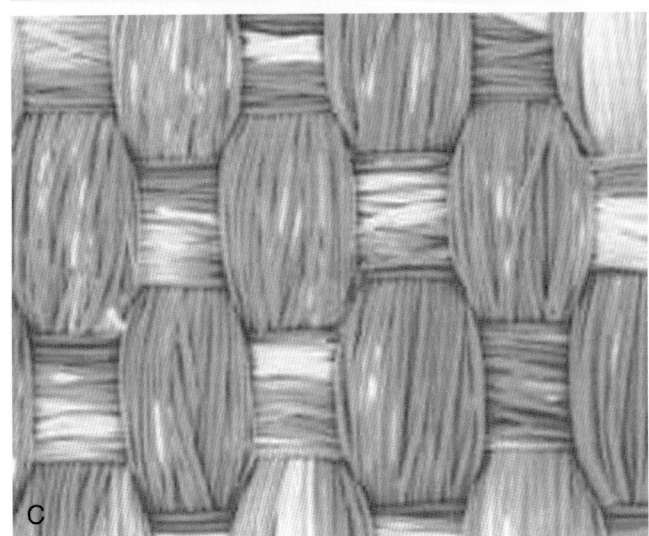

Figure 88-1 Scanning electron microscopy of typical yarn configurations in Dacron grafts. **A,** DeBakey standard-knit Dacron vascular prosthesis (original magnification ×37).[6] **B,** Vascutek Gelsoft Köper knitted prosthesis sealed with gelatin (×40).[7] **C,** Woven Dacron (×50).[8] *(A, from Snyder R, Botzko KM. Woven, knitted, and externally supported Dacron vascular prostheses. In: Stanley JC, ed.* Biologic and Synthetic Vascular Prostheses. *New York: Grune & Stratton; 1982; B, from Hake U, Gabbert H, Iversen S, et al. Evaluation of the healing of precoated vascular Dacron prostheses.* Langenbecks Arch Chir. *1991;376:323; C, from Salzmann DL, Kleinert LB, Berman SS, et al. Inflammation and neovascularization associated with clinically used vascular prosthetic materials.* Cardiovasc Pathol. *1999;8:63.)*

tissue integration. The preference for a velour finish has primarily been motivated by improved handling characteristics with little data demonstrating that internal, external, or double velour grafts exhibit greater patency rates.[17] Dacron grafts are often crimped longitudinally to increase flexibility, elasticity, and kink resistance. However, these properties are lost soon after implantation as a consequence of tissue ingrowth.

Recently, several modifications of Dacron grafts have been approved for clinical use. To reduce surface thrombogenicity, grafts coated with bioactive heparin or passivated with fluoropolymers have been developed.[18] A silver-coated Dacron graft has also been introduced to decrease the occurrence of graft infection. Long-term follow-up studies will be required to determine whether these modifications improve outcomes.

Early versions of knitted grafts were prone to dilatation over time, with a 10% to 20% increase in graft size immediately after implantation,[19] followed by slow expansion.[20] Nonetheless, correlation of graft dilatation and structural failure has not been established.[21] Most Dacron grafts have

been extremely durable. In 1997, the Food and Drug Administration (FDA) disclosed a total of 68 cases of structural failure occurring at an average of 7.4 years after implantation.[22] Given that approximately 60,000 aortic reconstructions are performed annually, the overall rate of graft failure is small.[22] A recent single-center review noted a 0.2% structural failure rate at a mean follow-up of 12 years.[23]

ePTFE Prosthesis

PTFE is a fluoropolymer that was trademarked as Teflon by Dupont in the late 1930s. It is chemically inert, hydrophobic, and mechanically durable. PTFE was initially used as a fiber in textile-based grafts, but today it is predominantly processed into expanded PTFE (ePTFE) tubes by extruding the polymer resin through a die. ePTFE grafts were first implanted in animals in 1972,[24] and Campbell and colleagues reported their initial clinical use in 1976.[25]

Macroscopically, the surface of ePTFE is smoother than Dacron's, and the grafts are soft and pliable. On a microscopic scale, the extrusion process results in a porous morphology

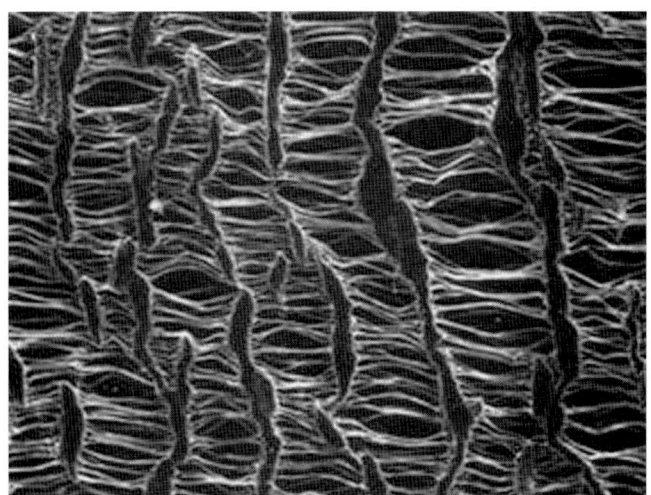

Figure 88-2 Scanning electron microscopy of node-fibril structure in expanded polytetrafluoroethylene grafts (original magnification ×500). *(From Lumsden AB, Chen CY, Coyle KA, et al. Nonporous expanded polytetrafluoroethylene grafts reduces graft neointimal hyperplasia in dog and baboon models.* J Vasc Surg. *1996;24: 825.)*

consisting of solid islands or nodes linked by fibrils (Fig. 88-2). This node-fibril structure occupies about 20% of the total volume of the expanded polymer and results in a higher ratio of pores to material than in Dacron grafts. However, the void space in ePTFE grafts is considerably smaller than the voids in woven or knitted material. Furthermore, the inherent hydrophobic nature of the fluoropolymer establishes a natural barrier to water that prevents permeation of blood. Despite the chemical inertness of ePTFE, plasma proteins and platelets adhere to the surface, and the host response is similar to that with Dacron.[26]

In standard ePTFE grafts, fibril length measures about 30 μm, although there have been experimental variants with a larger fibril length of 60 μm, which in animal models facilitated luminal endothelization.[27] However, these observations have not been replicated in clinical studies. Thin-walled ePTFE has a wall thickness of 200 to 300 μm as compared with a standard wall thickness of 400 to 600 μm. This increases compliance of the graft and improves handling, but with some loss of suture retention strength and an inability to use the prosthesis for repeated dialysis access. Clinical performance of thin- and standard-walled ePTFE is otherwise similar.[28] Stretch ePTFE is a modification of standard ePTFE in which a microcrimping process is applied to compress the fibrils. This property allows the graft to extend longitudinally as the fibrils are stretched to their full length, which provides some improvement in handling characteristics. Kink resistance of ePTFE grafts has been augmented by the application of external plastic rings. A recognized limitation of ePTFE grafts is their relative stiffness, which leads to a compliance mismatch between the prosthesis and host artery that may contribute to anastomotic intimal hyperplasia. In addition, because ePTFE does not display self-sealing characteristics, early access for hemodialysis is precluded by bleeding at the puncture site.

Despite some evidence suggesting that platelet deposition[29-31] and complement activation[32] are lower on ePTFE than on Dacron prostheses, the patency rates of Dacron and ePTFE grafts are similar.[4] Recently, heparin- and carbon-coated ePTFE prostheses have become commercially available, but data confirming increased patency rates over unmodified grafts are limited. It has been suggested that intimal hyperplasia may be related to adverse local hemodynamic effects. This has led to the use of a vein cuff at the distal anastomosis, with reports of improved 3-year patency rates for below-knee femoral-popliteal bypass (45% versus 19%).[33] A recent clinical study has demonstrated that grafts in which a distal PTFE cuff is incorporated have similar patency rates as those with a vein cuff.[34]

Polyurethane Prosthesis

The development of a polyurethane vascular prosthesis was largely motivated by a desire to reduce compliance mismatch. Polyurethane is more elastomeric than Dacron or ePTFE and has been used as a polymeric coating for pacemaker leads, breast implants,[35] and barrier films for dermal wounds.[36] Polyurethane is a copolymer that consists of three different monomer types—a diisocyanate hard domain, a chain extender, and a diol soft domain. At physiologic temperatures, the soft domains provide flexibility whereas the hard domains impart strength. The most common medical-grade polyurethanes are based on soft domains made from polyester, polyether, or polycarbonate. By varying the composition of the monomer repeat units, the mechanical properties of polyurethane prostheses can be tuned.

Polyester-based soft domains were used in the earliest generation of polyurethane vascular grafts. Good biocompatibility was observed in vivo, but the hydrolytic susceptibility of the ester linkage led to chemical deterioration.[37,38] In a small clinical study of below-knee bypass grafts, more than half occluded within 1 year.[39] Biodegradation is also a concern because some degradation products may be carcinogenic. The FDA terminated the use of polyurethane foam in breast implants in 1991 as a result of the release of 2,4-toluene diamine, which caused liver cancer in animals.[40] However, most polyurethanes studied today incorporate a different monomeric diamine subunit.

A more hydrolytically stable polyether-based polyurethane graft was developed later, but the ether linkage remains susceptible to oxidative degradation in vivo.[38] Vectra (Bard, Inc.) is the only commercially available graft based on polyether urethane and is used solely for hemodialysis access.[41] It may be punctured within 24 hours of implantation because of its self-sealing characteristics. A second polyurethane graft known as the Aria graft (Thoratec, Inc.) had been subjected to clinical study but is no longer being produced.[42]

The latest generation of polycarbonate-based polyurethanes is inert to both hydrolysis and oxidation in both in vitro and animal studies.[43-45] The Corvita graft (Corvita Corp.), a composite polyurethane and Dacron prosthesis, did not dilate in dogs after a 1-year implantation period but is no longer in development.[46] The Expedial graft (LeMaitre, Inc.) was a polycarbonate-based polyurethane graft impregnated with heparin. This prosthesis underwent evaluation for hemodialysis application but is no longer under development.[47]

Choice of Prosthetic Graft Based on Indications and Anatomic Location

Although several new vascular grafts have become commercially available in the past decade, little has changed in graft selection. Additional data are available on long-term patency and durability (Table 88-1)[8,18,33,34,49-54]; however, graft selection remains dictated largely by handling characteristics, convenience, surgeon preference, and cost. The following sections evaluate the available arterial substitutes (Table 88-2) and provide general guidelines for their most suitable anatomic application.

Aortic Reconstruction. Synthetic arterial prostheses have performed best as large-diameter replacements for the thoracic or abdominal aorta. Dacron grafts display patency rates of greater than 95% at 5 years.[55] Similar results have been observed for ePTFE grafts, which may be somewhat more resistant to infection.[56,57] Overall, late clinical outcomes appear to be independent of graft type whether used in open surgery or as components of endovascular grafts for the repair of abdominal or thoracic aneurysms.

Infrainguinal Reconstruction. Controversy exists over the preference of a synthetic graft for above-knee revascular-ization. An operative procedure with a synthetic graft is simpler, and some have proposed that the saphenous vein be reserved for future operations[58] because patency rates for secondary revascularization are higher when performed with vein than with prosthetic grafts.[59-61] However, ePTFE grafts have a higher occlusion rate than vein grafts,[62,63] and prosthetic grafts lead to a greater number of secondary operations.[64] Late patency rates are higher with vein than with prosthetic grafts for femoropopliteal bypass (61% to 76% versus 38% to 68%).[64-66] Thus, we agree with the proposition that autologous bypass conduits should be used whenever possible because of their significantly higher long-term durability.[67] Nonetheless, a prosthetic graft may be an appropriate choice in selected patients with disabling claudication and good runoff.

When autologous vein is not available, synthetic grafts are acceptable substitutes. Although ePTFE is currently the most widely used graft material for above-knee femoropopliteal bypass, the patency rates of Dacron and ePTFE prostheses in this position are similar.[4,51,68-70] Heparin-bonded Dacron displayed significantly better patency than did unmodified ePTFE in the above-knee femoropopliteal position at 3 years, but this difference was not apparent at 5 years.[71]

Saphenous vein is preferred for below-knee infrapopliteal bypass because of a patency rate of approximately 70% at 5 years.[65,72,73] Reported patency rates for synthetic grafts in this position range from 18% to 41% at 3 years.[74-77] An adjunctive venous cuff, patch, or boot, as well as an arteriovenous fistula, has been used at the distal anastomosis to improve graft patency (see Chapter 109: Infrainguinal Disease: Surgical Treatment). A prospective, randomized multicenter trial

Table 88-1 Recent Clinical Trials of Modified Prosthetic Vascular Prostheses

Series	Year	Location	Graft Type	Number Studied	Patency Rates	Outcome
Ricco[48]	2006	Aortobifemoral and aortobiiliac	Silver- and collagen-coated Dacron (InterGard Silver)	289	95% at 3 years	No controls
Eiberg et al.[18]	2006	Femorofemoral	Fluoropassivated Dacron (Vascutek, Inc.)	91	94% at 2 years	Patency similar to standard ePTFE
Caldarelli et al.[49]	2004	Femoropopliteal	Heparin-bonded Dacron (InterGard Heparin)	106	46% at 5 years	Patency was not greater than with ePTFE, but the amputation rate was reduced by 50%
Griffiths et al.[33]	2004	Femoropopliteal	ePTFE with distal vein cuff	120	40% at 5 years	Patency improved for BK but not for AK bypass
Panneton et al.[34]	2004	Femoropopliteal	Carbon-coated ePTFE with distal cuff (Distaflo)	44	49% at 2 years	BK only. Patency similar to ePTFE with vein cuff
Bosiers et al.[50]	2006	Femoropopliteal	Heparin-coated ePTFE (Propaten)	99	82% at 1 year	Nonrandomized, no controls
Jensen et al.[51]	2007	Femoropopliteal	Dacron vs. ePTFE	203 vs. 205	70% vs. 57% at 2 years	Patency greater for Dacron than for ePTFE
Scharn et al.[52]	2008	Femoropopliteal	Heparin-bonded Dacron (InterGard Heparin)	59	58% at 5 years	AK only, compared with human umbilical vein grafts
Laurila et al.[53]	2004	Femorotibial	ePTFE with distal vein cuff	59	36% at 2 years	Use of AV fistula with vein cuff did not improve patency rates
Kapfer et al.[54]	2006	Femorotibial	Carbon-coated ePTFE (Carboflo) with distal vein cuff	140	33% at 3 years	Patency similar to standard ePTFE

AK, above knee; AV, arteriovenous; BK, below knee; ePTFE, expanded polytetrafluoroethylene.

Table 88-2 Selected Commercially Available Vascular Grafts in the United States

Material Type	Company	Product	Description
Standard			
ePTFE	Angiotech/Edwards Life Sci	Lifespan	Re-enforced
	Atrium	Advanta VXT	Softwrap technology
		Advanta SST	Trilaminate, allows pulsation
		Advanta VS	60/20-μm through-pore design
		Flixene	Laminated with biomaterial film
	Bard	Impra CenterFlex	Unmodified
	Boston Scientific	Exxcel Soft Vascular Graft	Unmodified
	Braun	VascuGraft	Unmodified
	Vascutek	Maxiflo Ultrathin	Thin wall, external ePTFE wrap
		Maxiflo Wrap	Regular wall, external ePTFE wrap
	WL Gore & Assoc.	Gore-Tex	Unmodified
		Gore-Tex Stretch	Stretch
		Gore Intering	Unibody, intrawall radially supported
Dacron	Braun	Protegraft	Knitted, double velour
	InterVascular	InterGard Ultrathin	Unmodified
	Vascutek	VP1200K	Unmodified
Sealed			
ePTFE	Vascutek	SealPTFE Ultrathin	Gelatin sealed, thin wall
		SealPTFE Wrap	Gelatin sealed, regular wall
		Taperflo	Gelatin sealed, tapered
Dacron	Atrium	Ultramax	Knitted, gelatin sealed, double velour
	Bard	Vasculour II	Knitted, albumin sealed
	Boston Scientific	Hemashield Gold Microvel	Knitted, collagen sealed, double velour
		Hemashield Platinum	Woven, collagen sealed
	Braun	UniGraft	Woven, gelatin sealed, single/double velour
	InterVascular	InterGard Woven	Woven, collagen coated
		InterGard Knitted	Knitted, collagen coated
	Vascutek	Gelseal	Knitted, gelatin sealed
		Gelsoft	Knitted, gelatin sealed
		Gelsoft Plus	Köper knitted, gelatin sealed
Heparin Modified			
ePTFE	WL Gore & Assoc.	Propaten	Carmeda bioactive heparin coating
Dacron	InterVascular	InterGard Heparin	Knitted, collagen coated
Carbon Modified			
ePTFE	Bard	Impra Carboflo	Carbon coated
		Distaflo	Preformed cuff at distal end
		Dynaflo	Preformed cuff at distal end
Silver Modified			
Dacron	Braun	SilverGraft	Antibacterial
	InterVascular	InterGard Silver	Antibacterial
Others			
Collagen based	Artegraft	Artegraft	Cross-linked bovine carotid artery

found that a vein cuff significantly improved the 2-year patency rate of ePTFE grafts (52% versus 29%).[78] Corroborating these results, use of a Miller vein cuff more than doubled the 3-year patency rate of noncuffed grafts (45% versus 19%).[33] Interposition of a Linton patch[79] or Taylor patch[80] has also been found to improve patency. Adopting the geometry of such adjuncts, one study of an ePTFE graft (Fig. 88-3) with an expanded distal cuff (Distaflo, Bard, Inc.) demonstrated 1-year patency comparable to that of grafts that had been modified with a vein cuff.[34]

Extra-anatomic Reconstruction. Axillofemoral, femorofemoral, and axilloaxillary bypasses require a much longer, subcutaneously placed prosthetic graft. This often precludes the use of autologous vessels because of insufficient length. These grafts are often externally supported with a removable continuous spiral coil to reduce kinking and compression. ePTFE and Dacron grafts have similar patency rates in these positions.[81-84] For carotid-subclavian bypass, some reports have indicated better patency rates with either ePTFE or Dacron than with vein grafts.[85-87]

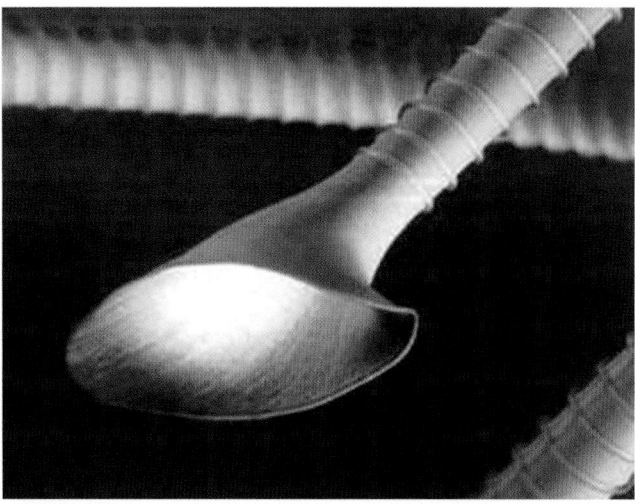

Figure 88-3 Externally supported expanded polytetrafluoroethylene grafts with a modified distal cuff. *(Adapted from Panneton JM, Hollier LH, Hofer JM. Multicenter randomized prospective trial comparing a pre-cuffed polytetrafluoroethylene graft to a vein cuffed polytetrafluoroethylene graft for infragenicular arterial bypass. Ann Vasc Surg. 2004;18:199.)*

Other Locations. Prosthetic grafts display excellent long-term patency for visceral and renal arterial reconstruction as a result of short graft length, high blood flow, and absence of extrinsic mechanical compression. Large-caliber venous reconstruction of the inferior or superior vena cava[49,88-90] and the iliofemoral,[49] jugular,[91] and portal veins,[92] including portosystemic shunts,[93,94] is typically performed with externally supported ePTFE grafts. Adjunctive anticoagulation is generally required, with the exception of patients with portal hypertension.

FAILURE MODES FOR PROSTHETIC VASCULAR GRAFTS

In general, failure of prosthetic vascular conduits can be classified as early, midterm, or late. Technical problems during surgery and the presence of underlying thrombophilia are common causes of early graft failure within the first month after surgery. Graft occlusion occurring between 6 months and 3 years after surgery is usually due to anastomotic intimal hyperplasia. Late graft thrombosis is frequently secondary to progression of distal atherosclerotic disease. Graft infection is relatively uncommon but most often requires removal of the prosthesis. The interaction between blood, host artery, and graft initiates a complex set of biochemical and cellular responses that ultimately limit implant function.

The Blood-Material Interface

The concept of a blood-compatible material has been driven by strategies to minimize activation of prothrombotic responses. Coagulation is a normal defense mechanism that responds almost instantaneously to injury and is a precursor of the inflammatory responses that constitute the healing process. The full cast of this response includes a combination of lipids, proteins, and cells that act in concert to provide localized amplification (Fig. 88-4). A series of negative feedback mechanisms control the propagation and termination of these responses. Because many of these antithrombotic mechanisms are localized to the endothelium, the inability of current prostheses to replicate these complex systems plays a large role in eventual graft failure.

Protein Interactions

One of earliest events that occurs when blood encounters an artificial surface is the adsorption of proteins. The composition of the adsorbed protein layer plays a direct role in the thrombotic response by activating the coagulation and complement cascades. The adsorption process is largely determined by the size, charge, and structure of the protein and related surface physiochemical properties, including topography and chemical composition. Inhibiting the adsorption of thrombogenic proteins in vivo remains a significant challenge.

Protein Adsorption. Transport of proteins to a surface occurs by both convection and diffusion. Convective transport is determined by blood velocity and flow profile. However, very close to the surface, within a region referred to as a boundary layer, protein transport occurs primarily by diffusion.[95,96] Other properties, such as charge, the tendency of a protein to unfold, and hydrophobicity, affect the affinity of bound proteins to the surface. Overall, this dynamic change in surface protein composition over time is referred to as the "Vroman effect." That is, surface composition is initially governed by different rates of diffusion for each molecular species, but at later times specific binding affinities and exchange reactions with other proteins will dictate the equilibrium surface composition of the adsorbed species.[97] Bound protein typically unfolds or denatures to expose domains that trigger events ultimately resulting in thrombosis.

Complement Cascade. Activation of the alternative pathway of the complement system may contribute to surface-induced thrombosis. Binding of C3b or C3 to a foreign surface and subsequent binding of factor B results in the formation of a complement complex that stimulates an inflammatory response. This serves as a prelude to platelet activation, as well as monocyte and neutrophil infiltration, all of which have been implicated in the development of neointimal hyperplasia and may also inhibit endothelialization of the lumen of the graft.[98]

Coagulation Cascade. Although the coagulation system is dealt with in greater detail elsewhere in this text, it bears emphasis that molecular events at both blood- and tissue-material interfaces initiate the coagulation cascade. Binding

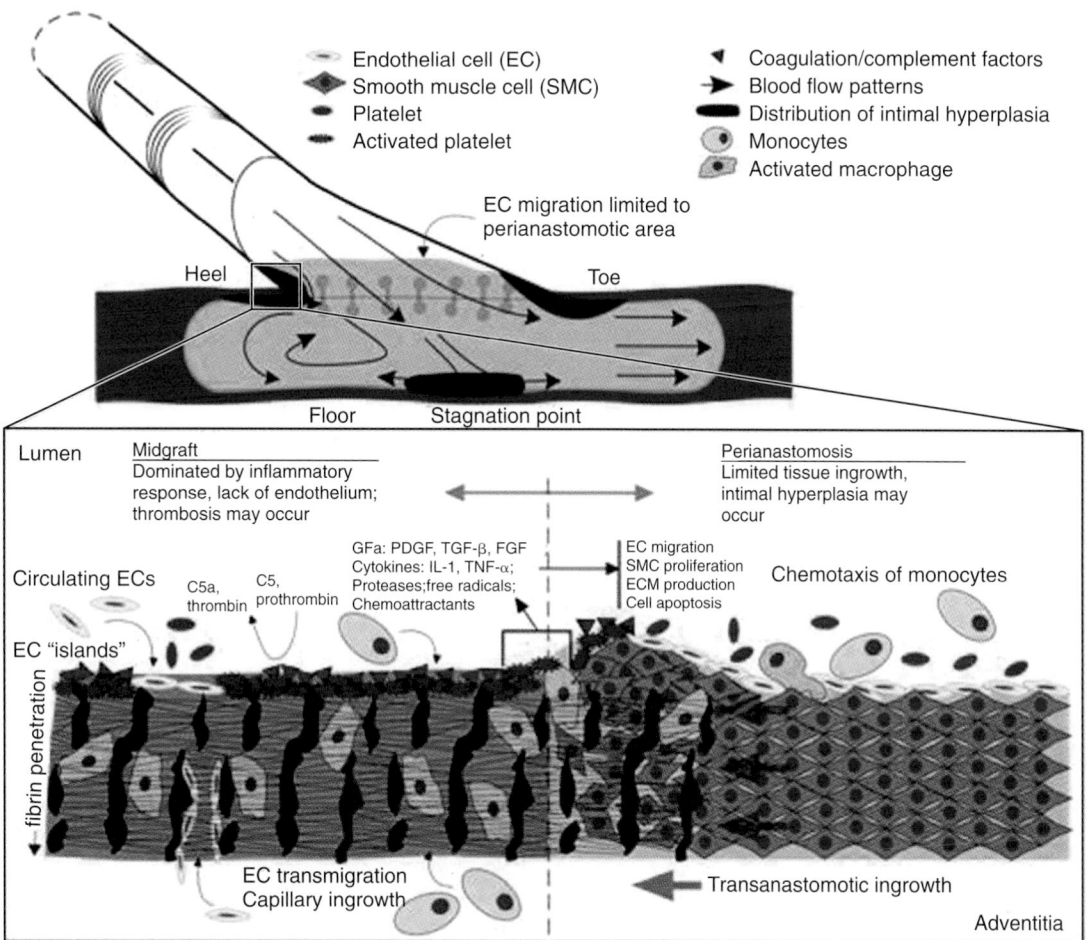

Figure 88-4 Simplified view of biomechanical phenomena at the distal end-to-side anastomosis (graft-artery interface). On a macroscopic scale, fluid dynamics and wall shear stress near the anastomosis encourage intimal hyperplasia. Microscopically, a host of inflammatory and thrombotic responses mediated by cellular and protein components could lead to anastomotic intimal hyperplasia. Incomplete transanastomotic ingrowth results in poor endothelial coverage in the midgraft area, thereby potentiating graft thrombosis. EC, endothelial cell; ECM, extracellular matrix; EGF, epidermal growth factor; FGF, fibroblast growth factor; GFa, growth factors; IL, interleukin; PDGF, platelet-derived growth factor; SMC, smooth muscle cell; TGF, transforming growth factor; TNF, tissue necrosis factor.

of plasma factor XII to a foreign surface results in a conformational change that yields an activated form, XIIa, which catalyzes the activation of factor XI and leads to the production of Xa. Factor Xa converts prothrombin to thrombin, the main effector of this cascade.[99,100] In addition, tissue factor, invariably expressed at sites of injury that occur with the creation of an anastomosis, triggers the formation of factor VIIa, which generates factors IXa and Xa. Both physical and biochemical events serve to enhance or limit propagation of the coagulation cascade. Blood flow modulates this process by controlling the rate at which coagulation proteins and activated factors are delivered to or removed from the graft surface. For example, locally disturbed flow or eddies at an anastomosis may create recirculation regions that localize coagulation factors. Although the negative feedback control of clot propagation is complex, it is important to note that antithrombotic systems include circulating factors that may limit the generation of thrombin, as well as inactivate thrombin after its formation.

Cellular Interactions

Platelets. The platelet is the major cellular component of the thrombotic response[101] and is involved in both complement- and T-cell–mediated immune responses.[102] Adsorption of fibrinogen, fibronectin, or von Willebrand factor onto a graft surface facilitates the deposition and aggregation of platelets. Platelets provide a reactive phospholipid surface for the coagulation cascade to propagate. In turn, thrombin stimulates the release of platelet granule contents, such as serotonin, adenosine diphosphate, and calcium, that support further platelet activation and aggregation. Chemoattractants such as platelet factor 4 and β-thromboglobulin are also released and promote an inflammatory response.

Increased levels of platelet-generated thromboxane and decreased platelet counts continue to be observed 1 year after graft implantation in animals,[103] and clinical studies have revealed persistent platelet deposition on Dacron grafts for at least several months.[104-106] Early studies have shown that antiplatelet agents can reduce platelet deposition onto prosthetic grafts.[107,108] More detailed discussion of adjunctive antiplatelet therapies can be found under "Pharmacologic Adjuncts to Improve Long-term Graft Function."

Neutrophils and Macrophages.

Recruitment of circulating neutrophils to the graft surface is mediated by chemoattractants such as C5a and leukotriene B₄.[109] Neutrophils interact with surface-bound proteins such as fibrinogen, IgG, C3bi, and factor X though cell surface integrins,[110] as well as with glycoproteins on adherent platelets.[111,112] At sites of vascular injury, endothelial cells upregulate adhesion molecules such as intercellular adhesion molecule-1 and vascular cell adhesion molecule-1, which also increase neutrophil and monocyte recruitment.[113,114] Despite their role in the phagocytosis of foreign material and bacteria, neutrophils recruited to a biomaterial surface do not protect against infection.[115]

Although infiltration of neutrophils occurs initially after graft implantation, neutrophils are short lived and are replaced by monocytes, which differentiate into macrophages. Macrophages produce proteases, chemotactic factors, reactive oxygen radicals, complement components, and coagulation factors, and these substances contribute to a chronic inflammatory state that inhibits re-endothelialization. Macrophages form foreign body giant cells in a layer covering the surface of ePTFE grafts.[116,117]

The production of cytokines appears to depend, in part, on the material activating the leukocytes. Monocytes and macrophages produce interleukin-1β, interleukin-6, and tumor necrosis factor-α[118] in greater amounts when in contact with Dacron than when ePTFE is used.[119] In addition, activated macrophages exposed to ePTFE or Dacron express tumor necrosis factor-α, as well as several growth factors that may stimulate smooth muscle cell (SMC) proliferation and contribute to intimal hyperplasia.[120,121]

Endothelial and Smooth Muscle Cells.

Migration of endothelial cells from the perianastomotic area in humans is highly inefficient and results in the formation of a neointima extending no more than a few centimeters from the anastomoses with little coverage of the midportion of the graft. However, scattered islands of endothelial cells have been observed far from the anastomotic regions, which may be due to transmural ingrowth of microvessels from perigraft tissue[27,122-124] or adherence of blood-borne endothelial progenitor cells (EPCs).[125-127] Indeed, Dacron grafts implanted in dogs appear to be rapidly covered with bone marrow–derived hematopoietic stems cells.[128]

Despite efforts to increase endothelial cell coverage, endothelial cells growing onto prosthetic graft surfaces that display a procoagulant phenotype can, in principle, promote rather than retard thrombosis. Furthermore, activated endothelial cells may increase growth factor production and secretion and thereby encourage SMC proliferation. Indeed, subintimal SMC proliferation occurs predominantly in areas that have an overlying endothelium.[129] As an additional example, ePTFE grafts coated with anti-CD34 antibodies and implanted in pigs captured EPCs and increased endothelial

cell coverage. However, at 4 weeks, intimal hyperplasia at the distal anastomosis was significantly greater.[130]

The turnover of SMCs at the anastomotic interface peaks 2 weeks after graft implantation and persists at a level higher than in the native artery. SMCs in the resulting neointima also display increased production of growth factors[131] and secrete higher amounts of collagen.[132,133] Inflammatory cells likewise produce a variety of growth factors that increase proliferation of SMCs and production of extracellular matrix (ECM).[134,135]

Infection

The incidence of graft infection ranges between 1% and 6%,[136,137] and infection is associated with a 50% amputation rate and a 25% to 75% mortality rate.[138] Graft infection is often a result of the assembly of a bacterial biofilm that protects bacteria from antibody and cell-mediated attack[139,140] and reduces antibiotic effectiveness.[141] Attempts to decrease bacterial infection have included binding rifampicin, silver, and other antibacterial compounds onto the luminal surface of grafts. However, the effectiveness of rifampicin-coated[142-144] or silver-coated grafts[48,145] has been difficult to ascertain.

The Tissue-Material Interface

Porosity.

Measurement of porosity depends on the graft material. In textile grafts such as Dacron, porosity is defined by water permeability, whereas the porous nature of ePTFE grafts is defined by the average internodal distance. Optimization of graft porosity was driven by a desire to improve vascular wall healing under the presumption that a transmural angiogenic response would lead to endothelialization of the lumen of the graft.[146] For example, ePTFE grafts with internodal distances of 60 or 90 μm demonstrated enhanced transmural tissue ingrowth and greater luminal coverage of endothelial cells than did grafts with 30-μm pores in a primate model.[27,147,148] Nonetheless, a clinical trial using 90-μm ePTFE grafts failed to show a benefit over standard 30-μm grafts.[149]

Compliance.

Compliance is defined as the percent change in diameter of a cylindrical conduit between diastolic and systolic pressure. Compliance mismatch between a relatively extensible host vessel and stiff graft leads to a region of excessive mechanical stress that may contribute to anastomotic intimal hyperplasia, as well as pseudoaneurysm formation.[150] In addition, native vessels have a dynamic compliance that is inversely proportional to blood pressure. At low physiologic pressure, native vessels may be better able than noncompliant prosthetic grafts to preserve pulsatile energy and optimize flow.[151] When compared with a native artery (compliance of 0.059%/mm Hg) and vein (0.044%/mm Hg), Dacron (0.019%/mm Hg) and ePTFE (0.016%/mm Hg) grafts are relatively noncompliant,[152] whereas polyurethane grafts have a compliance similar to that of the host artery.[152] It also bears noting that the compliance of synthetic grafts may decrease after implantation because of the formation of a surrounding fibrous capsule, which stiffens the graft wall. As a result, the impact of initial compliance on long-term patency may be difficult to assess.[153]

Hemodynamics. Anastomotic intimal hyperplasia is a common cause of prosthetic graft failure, in part because of local flow disturbances and alterations in wall shear stress. Decreased neointimal thickness has been observed with the placement of a distal venous cuff,[154] patch,[155] or arteriovenous fistula[156,157] in animal models, which initially was attributed to increased compliance at the distal anastomosis.[158] However, no difference was noted between grafts with a vein cuff and those in which the vein cuff was wrapped with ePTFE, thus suggesting that modulation of local fluid dynamics plays the dominant role in reducing intimal hyperplasia.[150,159] Indeed, local flow conditions may modulate endothelial cell function.[160] In an end-to-side anastomosis, wall shear stress may drive endothelial cells to an activated, prothrombotic phenotype.[161] Activated endothelium, in turn, promotes SMC proliferation and migration and production of matrix proteins.[162] Thrombus formation may also be potentiated by regions of stasis created by low blood velocity, as well as by high shear rates, which activate platelets locally.[163]

Advances in numerical simulations have yielded valuable data on velocity distributions near the anastomosis, which has led to the rational design of grafts that modulate local blood flow.[163] Indeed, helical grafts have been developed with improved cross-plane mixing, a characteristic that has been reported to improve graft patency in an animal model,[164] as well as in a pilot clinical study.[165]

■ BIOFUNCTIONAL VASCULAR PROSTHESES

Thromboresistant Surface Engineering

The generation of nonfouling surfaces that resist protein adsorption and subsequent platelet deposition and activation has been pursued within a framework in which it is postulated that thermodynamic factors at the blood-material interface drive protein adsorption. Specifically, protein adsorption is favored by electrostatic and hydrophobic interactions between the adsorbed protein and synthetic surface, as well as by the local increase in entropy that occurs upon the displacement of water molecules and counter ions from the first few nanometers of the material surface. Both synthetic and natural materials, including polyethylene oxide (PEO), pyrolytic carbon, albumin, phosphorylcholine, and more recently, elastin-inspired protein polymers, have been investigated for the development of strategies to passivate the prosthetic surface by reducing or eliminating the enthalpic or entropic effects that drive protein and cell adsorption on a molecular level.

Inhibition of Protein and Cell Adsorption

Polyethylene Oxide. In the early 1970s it was observed that PEO passively adsorbed onto glass surfaces prevented the adsorption of viruses, platelets, and thrombin, and subsequent studies have demonstrated that PEO exhibits among the lowest levels of protein or cellular adsorption of any known polymer. This property was attributed to the presence of a hydrophilic ether oxygen in its structural repeat unit, $[CH_2\text{-}CH_2\text{-}O]_n$, which leads to a water-solvated structure that is capable of forming a "liquid-like" surface with highly mobile molecular chains that exhibit no systematic molecular order. Unlike other hydrophilic polymers such as polyhydroxyethylmethacrylate and polyacrylamide, the absence of surface charges and the presence of only small hydrophobic methylene groups in the structural repeat unit were thought to provide few other sites for protein or cellular binding.[166] Surface modification with PEO has been attempted by several methods, including bulk modification, covalent grafting, and physical adsorption. In most cases investigators have been able to demonstrate resistance to protein binding in vitro; however, in vivo results have been inconsistent, and clinical studies of a PEO-modified stent or graft have yet to be performed. For the interested reader, a comprehensive review of the blood compatibility of PEO can be found in a monograph by Lee and colleagues.[167]

Albumin Coating. Albumin as an inert, thromboresistant coating has been pursued since early studies of platelet interactions with various adsorbed proteins on artificial surfaces established that albumin induced significantly less platelet adhesion than did other plasma proteins, including fibrinogen and gamma globulin.[168-171] Some groups have covalently grafted albumin to surfaces,[172-174] whereas others have modified surfaces with long aliphatic chains (C8-C18) or PEO-tethered warfarin to increase selective affinity for endogenous albumin.[175-180] Guidoin and associates developed a glutaraldehyde–cross-linked albumin coating later manufactured by Bard, Inc.[181,182] The Bard albumin-coated Dacron prosthesis was evaluated by Kottke-Marchant and colleagues and found to display reduced platelet and leukocyte adhesion and aggregation in vitro, as well as decreased fibrin production.[183] In a thoracoabdominal bypass model in dogs, however, only small differences were observed between coated and uncoated grafts.[184] In clinical studies, Al Khaffaf and Charlesworth[185] and Kudo and coworkers[186] evaluated this prosthesis in the aortic position and demonstrated performance characteristics similar to those of other noncoated vascular prostheses.

Carbon Coating. Pyrolytic, or graphitic, carbon coating of implantable materials has been investigated for a variety of blood-contacting devices, including vascular grafts, heart valves, and stents.[187-189] In brief, pyrolytic carbon films are produced by chemical vapor deposition, a process in which a hydrocarbon, such as methane, is heated to its decomposition temperature and the graphitic layer allowed to crystallize as a highly ordered layer of carbon atoms. Early animal studies of carbon-coated vascular prostheses demonstrated improved patency rates in comparison to uncoated controls.[190,191] However, surface irregularities on carbon-lined ePTFE grafts have contributed to poor performance in other investigations.[192,193] More recently, 15-month implant studies in sheep documented reduced platelet adhesion and spreading on carbon-coated polyester grafts, but these observations did not affect overall histologic outcomes or patency rates.[194] Furthermore, in a prospective, randomized multicenter study conducted in Germany, 283 patients received either 6-mm carbon-coated (Carboflo, Bard, Inc.) or uncoated ePTFE grafts (Bard, Inc.) for femoral–anterior tibial artery bypass. At 3-year follow-up, no significant differences were observed between the two groups with respect to patency or limb salvage.[54]

Phosphorylcholine Coating.
Planar-supported bilayers of phosphatidylcholine, the predominant glycerophospholipid in animal cell membranes, have been shown to reduce protein and cell adhesion in vitro.[195-199] It has been proposed that this phenomenon is due to the zwitterionic nature of the phosphorylcholine head group, which although carrying both positive and negative charges, is electrically neutral at physiologic pH. Application of supported lipid films as coatings for implantable devices has been limited by the inherent instability of a coating that is formed by individual molecules that "self-assemble" as a monolayer or bilayer film through relatively weak hydrophobic van der Waal interactions.[200] Consequently, methods have been devised to create stable "membrane-mimetic" films through protein anchors,[201,202] heat stabilization,[203] and in situ polymerization of synthetically modified, polymerizable phospholipids.[204-209] In all studies, the protein- and cell-resistant properties of the exposed phosphatidylcholine layer were retained.

Since 1984, a variety of polymethacrylate- and polyurethane-based polymers have been synthesized that incorporate the phosphorylcholine head group within the polymer backbone.[210,211] For example, Yoneyama and colleagues demonstrated excellent in vivo blood compatibility of a segmented polyether urethane/2-methacryloyloxyethyl phosphorylcholine (MPC) polymer blend processed as a coating for Dacron prostheses.[212-214] Chen and associates evaluated 4-mm-diameter ePTFE grafts coated with a copolymer of MPC and laurylmethacrylate in a canine femoral arteriovenous shunt. Significantly reduced platelet deposition was demonstrated, as well as limited neointimal hyperplasia at anastomotic sites.[215,216] Similarly, ultraviolet-polymerizable, acrylate-modified phospholipids assembled on the lumen of an ePTFE graft (d = 4 mm) reduced platelet adhesion in an ex vivo baboon femoral arteriovenous shunt model.[217] Direct chemical grafting of phospholipids on Dacron and ePTFE has been reported to reduce fibrinogen and platelet adhesion in vitro,[218] and polyurethane-based grafts (d = 2 mm) modified with phosphorylcholine prevented thrombus formation after 8 weeks in a rabbit model.[214]

Elastin-Inspired Surfaces.
Elastin is a constituent structural protein in the vascular wall and elicits minimal platelet adhesion and aggregation.[219,220] Because Dacron grafts coated with elastin inhibit SMC migration, it was suggested that elastin may also inhibit neointimal hyperplasia.[221] However,

the intrinsic insolubility of elastin makes purification and processing from tissue difficult. This problem has largely been overcome by the identification of consensus sequences involved in the molecular assembly of elastin, which are used to construct a variety of elastin-mimetic protein polymers.[222-227]

Covalent immobilization of poly(VPGVG) on silicone reduced fibrinogen and immunoglobulin adsorption and inhibited the secretion of proinflammatory cytokines from monocytes in vitro.[228] In a later study, passive adsorption of recombinant elastin peptides onto polyurethane catheters decreased fibrin deposition and increased patency in a rabbit model.[229] Recently, ePTFE grafts (d = 4 mm) coated with a thin film of a recombinant amphiphilic elastin-mimetic protein polymer inhibited platelet deposition in an acute primate ex vivo shunt model.[230]

Inhibition of Thrombin and Fibrin Formation

The endothelial cell presents and releases a number of biologically active constituents that limit thrombotic responses, which can lead to catastrophic graft failure (Fig. 88-5). Consequently, seeding or otherwise reconstituting endothelial cells on a prosthetic surface has been actively pursued as a strategy for generating thromboresistant vascular substitutes. However, this approach poses its own challenges related to cell sourcing, stability, viability, and function.[231-233] Alternatively, promising results have been achieved through biologically inspired or "biomimetic" design in which the antithrombogenic features of the endothelial cell surface are selectively mimicked by introducing bioactive molecules such as heparin, thrombomodulin (TM), or urokinase[234-237] onto the surface of synthetic materials.

Heparin.
The first report of a heparinized surface was published in 1963 by Gott, who demonstrated significantly prolonged in vitro and in vivo clotting times on graphite-coated surfaces ionically bonded with heparin.[188] Since then, heparin-coating technologies have been developed for a number of blood-contacting devices and used most extensively in cardiopulmonary bypass circuits.[238,239] The literature on heparin immobilization is extensive and has been reviewed elsewhere.[240-242] Some of the techniques to immobilize heparin include electrostatic self-assembly via heparin's negatively charged sulfate groups[243,244]; covalent grafting, often via a spacer arm[245-249]; integration into a hydrogel network[250]; and loading into a bulk polymer for controlled release.[251] One technique that has been successfully translated to the clinic is end-point immobilization, in which the reducing end of the linear heparin chain is depolymerized to yield a reactive aldehyde group that can then be conjugated to a primary amine on the graft or stent surface.[252-254]

Several heparin-bonded vascular grafts have recently been assessed in clinical trials. A prospective randomized multicenter study compared InterGard heparin-bonded Dacron grafts with standard ePTFE for femoropopliteal bypass. The patency of heparin-bonded Dacron grafts was superior to that

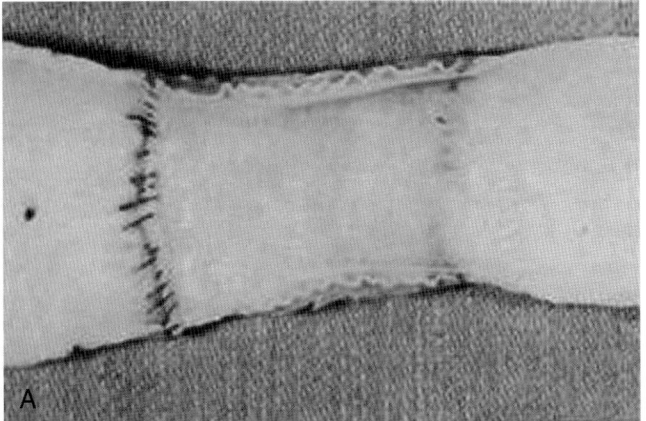
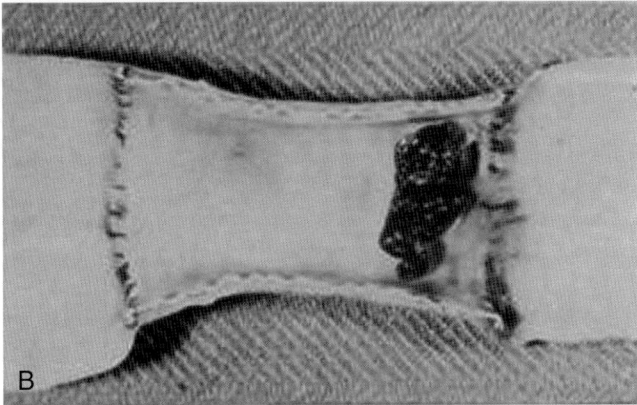
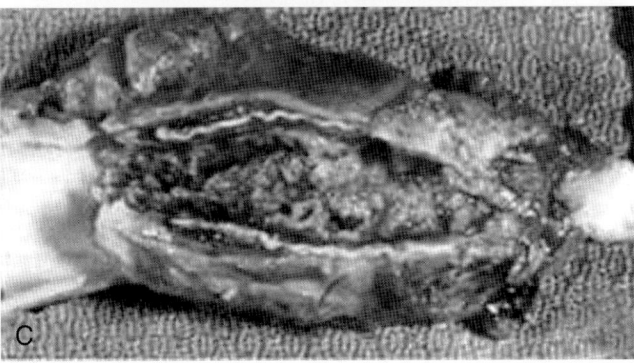

Figure 88-5 Variability of healing in three identical knitted DeBakey Dacron prostheses recovered after 3 months of implantation into three different porcine thoracic aortas. **A,** Excellent healing. **B,** Fibrin deposition on the graft surface. **C,** Progression of fibrin deposition leading to total graft thrombosis. *(From Wesolowski S. Foundations of modern vascular grafts. In: Sawyer PN, Kaplitt MJ, eds.* Vascular Grafts. *New York: Appleton-Century-Crofts; 1978.)*

of ePTFE at 3 years, but a significant difference was not observed at 5 years.[71] Recently, a randomized multicenter prospective study found that heparin-bonded Dacron grafts displayed a 5-year patency rate in the femoropopliteal position comparable to that reported for standard ePTFE and Dacron.[52] A heparin-modified ePTFE graft, marketed as Propaten (W. L. Gore and Associates, Inc.), received FDA approval in 2006. Several nonrandomized clinical trials using Propaten have reported 1- and 2-year patency rates for femoropopliteal bypass that are similar to those previously noted for unmodified grafts.[50,255,256]

Thrombomodulin. Several investigators have immobilized TM onto polymeric surfaces to generate surfaces that actively limit the local generation of thrombin through the production of activated protein C rather than inactivate thrombin after it has already been produced. Specifically, activated protein C inactivates factors Va and VIIIa, thereby limiting Xa and thrombin production. Kishida and colleagues conjugated recombinant human TM to both aminated and carboxylated surfaces, including polyvinyl amine and polyacrylic acid surface-grafted polyethylene and a surface-hydrolyzed polyether urethane urea.[257-259] Similarly, Vasilets and coauthors reported binding TM onto polyacrylic acid surface-grafted PTFE.[260] As an alternative approach, Cutler's group physically adsorbed and cross-linked soluble human TM onto small-caliber ePTFE grafts and reported promising short-term results in vivo.[261] Other investigators such as Sperling and associates[262,263] and Han and coworkers[264] have tethered TM to surfaces via a polyethylene glycol spacer. A disadvantage of all these strategies is the inherent reduction in bioactivity associated with immobilization schemes that involve reactions to any freely available amino or carboxyl functionality on the protein surface, including those near or within the catalytic site of the protein.

Recently, genetically directed synthesis has been used to create a recombinant TM construct that consists of the catalytically active site along with the C-terminal synthetic, non-natural amino acid azido(N_3)-methionine. The azido-functionalized TM construct can be coupled to surfaces directly through the C-terminus by using highly selective reaction schemes with full retention of bioactivity.[265,266] As an additional strategy, TM-containing membrane-mimetic surface assemblies that display prolonged stability and activity in high-shear environments have been produced.[267,268] The ability of surface-bound TM to dramatically reduce tissue factor–induced thrombin production has been characterized in both simulated venous and arterial flow conditions.[267]

Direct Thrombin Inhibitors and Fibrinolytic Agents.

Direct thrombin inhibitors such as recombinant hirudin and argatroban have been used as an additional strategy to produce thromboresistant surfaces. Seifert and colleagues cross-linked hirudin to poly(D,L-lactide-co-glycolide) with glutaralde-hyde,[269] and LoGerfo and coworkers grafted recombinant hirudin to polyurethane and Dacron via a cross-linker–modified albumin base coat.[270-274] Several groups have also reported immobilization of urokinase on surfaces to confer local fibrinolytic activity.[234-237]

Inhibition of Platelet Adsorption

The capacity of aspirin to reduce thrombosis in ePTFE vascular prostheses has been noted in a number of randomized trials.[275] However, prolonged systemic administration of all antiplatelet drugs significantly increases the risk for bleeding and gastrointestinal complications. This has motivated the development of materials that locally inhibit platelet activity by surface immobilization of antiplatelet molecules, such as prostacyclin, or by local delivery of antiplatelet agents, including nitric oxide (NO).

Antiplatelet Drugs. Direct surface immobilization of antiplatelet agents has been studied extensively. Prostacyclin and prostaglandin E_1 have been immobilized on albumin-covered surfaces.[276,277] Likewise, Dacron and ePTFE grafts have been coated with collagen or laminin for covalent conjugation of prostacyclin and prostaglandin E_1.[218] Dipyridamole has also been conjugated to polyurethane vascular grafts, with improved patency rates reported in a sheep model.[278-280] An aspirin-eluting coating for sustained release has been explored by several groups,[281-284] applied to Dacron grafts, and reduced platelet deposition in a canine ex vivo shunt model.[285] Similarly, ePTFE grafts impregnated with alginate containing the prostacyclin analogue iloprost have demonstrated reduced thrombus formation in vitro.[286]

Nitric Oxide. NO inhibits platelet aggregation and prevents SMC proliferation.[287,288] Two types of NO donors, diazeniumdiolates ($[N(O)NO]^-$) and S-nitrosothiols, have been extensively studied as graft modifications for release and generation of NO. Diazeniumdiolate ions are stable solids that readily release NO in physiologic conditions.[289] The earliest studies involved loading the pores of ePTFE grafts with polyethylenimine microspheres that incorporated diazeniumdiolate ions.[290,291] Sustained release over a period of 5 weeks with reduced platelet deposition in comparison to uncoated grafts was observed in a baboon ex vivo shunt model. Diazeniumdiolate has also been conjugated to polyurethane grafts that release NO over a 2-month period.[292,293] A major limitation of diazeniumdiolate polymers is leaching of diamine precursors with the formation of carcinogenic nitrosamines.[294] This has led to the design of leach-resistant lipophilic diazeniumdiolate formulations.[295-297]

S-nitrosothiols are a stable form of NO that is present in circulating blood and may act as an NO donor.[298,299] S-nitrosothiols have been covalently bound to synthetic surfaces with satisfactory in vitro bioactivity.[300] However, S-nitrosothiols may act as an endogenous reservoir of NO that can be activated by copper (II)–based catalysts,[301,302] cysteine-modified polymers,[303,304] and organoditelluride[305] incorporated into polymers.

Outlook

Conclusive evidence is lacking that heparin- or carbon-coated grafts have improved patency over standard grafts. Despite efforts to coat graft surfaces with therapeutic agents, a key limitation is the finite reservoir in these materials, which reduces their efficacy over time. Multifunctional surface modification schemes involving bioactive enzymes, such as TM- or S-nitrosothiol–activating catalysts, are promising areas of current research.

Biohybrid Vascular Grafts

A guiding principle of graft design since the 1950s has been the notion that the presence of an intact, quiescent endothelial lining on the prosthetic graft surface would reduce the risk for thrombosis and neointimal hyperplasia. Both in vitro seeding with endothelial cells and in vivo schemes to induce endothelialization of the graft surface have been investigated.

Endothelial Cell Seeding

In 1978, Herring and coworkers introduced a single-stage technique whereby venous endothelial cells were seeded onto grafts with enhanced patency in a canine model.[306] Though a promising concept, translating these results into clinical practice has been challenging. Zilla and associates noted in an early clinical report the absence of a confluent endothelial cell lining 14 weeks after bypass grafting.[307] A subsequent clinical study revealed that at 30 months the patency of single-stage endothelial cell–seeded ePTFE grafts in the femoropopliteal position was significantly worse than the patency of vein bypass (38% versus 92%).[308] Similarly, endothelial cell–seeded Dacron aortobifurcated grafts did not demonstrate improved late outcome.[309] These disappointing outcomes were attributed to insufficient initial cell density, poor adhesion under flow, and failure to achieve confluence.

Cell density was increased by using a two-stage technique[310,311] and a 3- to 4-week culture period. The two-stage technique has yielded encouraging clinical results, with a randomized study reporting that seeded femoropopliteal grafts had greater patency than nonseeded grafts at 32 months (85% versus 55%).[312] In a follow-up report, the 9-year patency rate was 65% for cell-seeded and 16% for nonseeded grafts.[313] In a subsequent report, similar primary patency rates were observed for 153 seeded ePTFE grafts.[314] A total of 14 patients have received cell-seeded 4-mm ePTFE grafts for coronary bypass, with 91% patency rates noted at 28 months.[315]

Adhesive proteins such as fibronectin, collagen, and fibrin,[316-325] as well as adhesive peptide sequences,[326-328] have been investigated as coatings to increase cell anchorage, but the most appropriate coating for clinical studies is unclear.[329] Other techniques such as electrostatic seeding[330,331] and shear conditioning[332,333] may also increase cell adhesion. Phenotypic modulation of cells through genetic engineering has been pursued in an attempt to increase expression of antithrombotic proteins such as tissue plasminogen activator[334] and NO synthase.[335] EPCs from either bone marrow[336,337] or peripheral blood,[338] as well as the microvasculature in the omentum or subcutaneous fat, have been highlighted as potential sources for endothelial cells.[339-342]

Promoting Endothelialization of Synthetic Grafts In Vivo

ePTFE grafts have been impregnated with fibrin glue containing fibroblast growth factor-1 (FGF-1) and heparin, which in a dog model promoted transmural endothelialization, as well as proliferation of SMCs.[343-345] Polyurethane-based grafts coated with heparin and FGF-2 have accelerated transmural endothelialization.[346] ePTFE grafts coated with an anti-CD34 antibody to capture circulating EPCs increased the rate of endothelialization in pigs.[130]

Outlook

Although endothelial seeding of grafts has met with some clinical success, the requirement for significant infrastructure and associated technical challenges remain significant limitations to its widespread application. The presence of a permanent polymeric scaffold may also induce a chronic inflammatory response and a persistent mechanical mismatch with the native artery.

Tissue-Engineered Constructs

Protein-Based Scaffolds

Two broad approaches have been pursued in the design of a vascular graft that mimics the structural organization of the native artery. Decellularized allogeneic or xenogeneic tubular tissues that contain an intact and structurally organized ECM have received the greatest attention in both animal models and human clinical studies. Since the mid-1980s, a number of schemes have been evaluated in which cells are cultured in vitro as sheets or tubes in a manner that promotes the synthesis of structural ECM proteins.

Decellularization removes most cellular antigenic components in allogeneic and xenogeneic tissue. A combination of physical agitation, chemical surfactant removal, and enzymatic digestion disrupts cells and removes protein, lipids, and nucleotide remnants.[347-350] After decellularization, chemical cross-linking is used to enhance mechanical strength and reduce immunogenicity.[351,352] Glutaraldehyde is the most common cross-linker but may be cytotoxic when released during degradation,[353] so alternative cross-linkers have been explored.[352,354] The addition of external support to provide extra mechanical strength and prevent late dilatation is also common. Clinical studies have not demonstrated a definitive advantage of glutaraldehyde–cross-linked bovine carotid artery[355-357] or human umbilical vein grafts[52] over synthetic grafts.

Efforts to improve the durability and the healing response of decellularized scaffolds have included coating with heparin[358] and FGF,[357] as well as seeding with endothelial cells,[359-361] EPCs,[362] SMCs,[361,363] bone marrow–derived cells,[364] and adipose-derived stem cells.[365] Alternative tubular tissue sources have also been explored, including small intestinal submucosa.[366,367]

Extracellular Matrix Gel Constructs

Collagen is a major ECM component that is responsible for the overall mechanical strength of the vessel wall. The use of exogenous collagen gels as a scaffold for seeding of vascular cells was first reported in 1986 by Weinberg and Bell.[368] Although this report demonstrated enhanced mechanical integrity because of the cellular-driven alignment of collagen, its tensile strength was still insufficient for clinical use even when a Dacron mesh was used as external support. Later reports using collagen scaffolds experienced similar deficiencies in mechanical strength.[369-371]

Additional efforts to improve the mechanical characteristics of collagen-based constructs have included magnetic prealignment of collagen, mechanical conditioning, inhibition of enzymatic degradation, and cross-linking strategies.[372-377] None of these schemes has been able to reproduce the structural organization and density distribution of native matrix proteins.

Resorbable Scaffolds

In 1982, Greisler was the first to show that a woven polyglycolic acid scaffold implanted in rabbit aortas promoted cellular recruitment and tissue regeneration.[378] Subsequent studies revealed that macrophage phagocytosis was responsible for scaffold degradation and that expression of growth factors by macrophages induced proliferation of myofibroblasts in the neoarterial wall.[122,379,380]

Since these initial studies, many groups have seeded resorbable polymer scaffolds with endothelial cells and SMCs. After 8 or more weeks of culture, vessel analogues were produced.[381,382] In 2001, a tissue-engineered vessel produced in this manner was used to reconstruct the pulmonary artery of a 4-year-old child, with no evidence of graft failure at 7 months.[383] Further studies have been conducted with tissue-engineered grafts constructed with autologous bone marrow cells, which were used to repair the pulmonary outflow tract in 42 pediatric patients. All grafts remained patent at a mean follow-up of 16 months.[384]

Cell-Directed Self-Assembly

Cell-directed assembly of endogenously secreted matrix proteins has been explored as an alternative to scaffold-based approaches. Using ascorbic acid to stimulate collagen production by neonatal SMCs and fibroblasts, cellular sheets were generated in vitro that could be layered around a mandrel to form a tubular vessel.[385] Recently, adult dermal fibroblasts were assembled into multilayer vessels (Fig. 88-6) with a burst pressure exceeding 3000 mm Hg.[386] These vessels have been implanted in a small number of human patients for hemodialysis access.[386,387]

Similar to the Sparks mandril approach,[388,389] Silastic tubing has been implanted into the peritoneal cavity of animals to induce the growth of a "living" tube made of granulation tissue that contained mostly fibroblasts and a mesothelial layer lining the lumen.[390] Burst strength greater than 2500 mm Hg was achieved, and 80% of the grafts remained patent after transplantation into the femoral arteries of dogs after 6 months.[391]

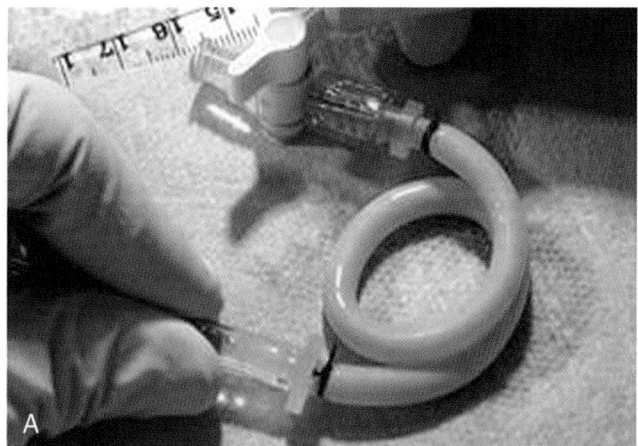

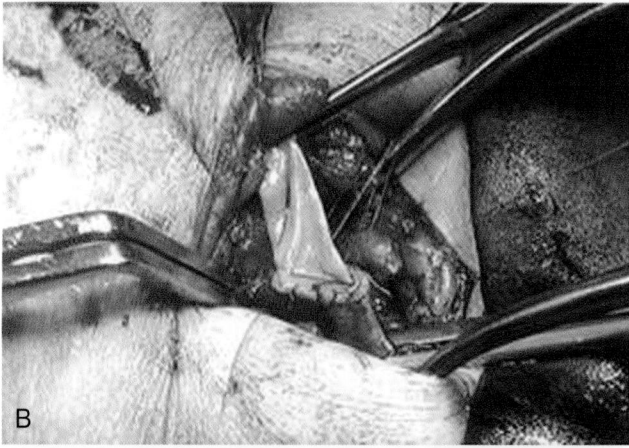

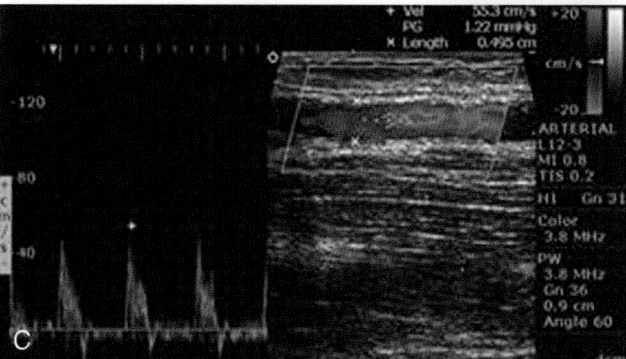

Figure 88-6 The first clinical use of a tissue-engineered blood vessel for high-pressure arterial revascularization (**A**). A completely autologous graft was implanted as an arteriovenous shunt between the humeral artery and the axillary vein (**B**). The tissue-engineered blood vessel resembled native tissue and had normal surgical handling and suturing properties. The vessel synthesized met safety criteria and showed excellent flow under routine Doppler surveillance (**C**). At 6 months, the shunt maintains high flow without signs of restenosis or aneurysm. *(Adapted from L'Heureux N, Dusserre N, Marini A, et al. Technology insight: the evolution of tissue-engineered vascular grafts—from research to clinical practice.* Nat Clin Pract Cardiovasc Med. *2007;4:389.)*

Outlook

Tissue-engineered constructs have been produced with burst pressures that exceed physiologic requirements, and preliminary reports have noted excellent patency for short conduits in high-flow positions. However, several limitations exist, including long culture periods in vitro ranging between 2 and 6 months, as well as reduced proliferative ability of cells isolated from the elderly population. In addition, although SMCs produce adequate amounts of collagen in these schemes, substantial amounts of elastin are not produced, and as a consequence these vessels are relatively noncompliant and may be at risk for late aneurysmal degeneration.

PHARMACOLOGIC ADJUNCTS TO IMPROVE LONG-TERM GRAFT FUNCTION

There is increasing clinical evidence supporting the use of antithrombotic pharmacotherapy to improve long-term prosthetic graft performance in extremity and medium-caliber revascularization. The use of antiplatelet agents such as aspirin and clopidogrel and oral anticoagulants such as the vitamin K antagonists warfarin (Coumadin) and acenocoumarol is discussed.

An early randomized trial in 1983 by Goldman and coworkers found reduced platelet deposition on prosthetic grafts in patients undergoing antiplatelet therapy with aspirin and dipyridamole.[30] Retrospective meta-analyses of clinical studies suggest improvements in graft patency with the use of antiplatelet therapy. In a meta-analysis of 11 randomized controlled studies by the Antiplatelet Trialist's Collaboration in 1994, it was found that in 3000 patients who underwent peripheral artery procedures, antiplatelet therapy with principally aspirin resulted in a 38% reduction in the graft occlusion rate when compared with placebo.[392] This result was corroborated by a later meta-analysis in 1999 showing a 22% reduction in patients receiving antiplatelet therapy versus placebo, but a 44% reduction in comparison to placebo in patients receiving oral anticoagulants and a relative reduction of 62% when anticoagulants were used in conjunction with aspirin versus aspirin alone.[393] This report set the stage for several later prospective trials that investigated the possible benefits of oral anticoagulants.

The Dutch Bypass Oral Anticoagulants or Aspirin study compared the effectiveness of oral anticoagulants with that of aspirin in preventing infrainguinal bypass graft occlusion in a multicenter, open randomized trial involving 2690 patients. The study group concluded at the 21-month follow-up that the use of aspirin at 80 mg/day significantly reduced occlusion in prosthetic grafts when compared with warfarin and was associated with fewer bleeding episodes.[275] The Veteran Affairs Cooperative Trial randomized 665 patients undergoing femoropopliteal bypass to aspirin at 325 mg/day and warfarin with a goal international normalized ratio of 1.4 to 2.8 or to aspirin alone. There was no significant difference in patency rate for the 8-mm bypass subgroup, but there was a significant difference for the 6-mm bypass subgroup (femoropopliteal; 71.4% in the warfarin-plus-aspirin group versus 57.9% in the aspirin-only group; $P = .02$).[394] In both studies, aspirin appeared to provide the most benefit, whereas the addition of warfarin may have increased this benefit. However, the two studies showed that warfarin nearly doubled the risk for major bleeding episodes when compared with aspirin alone.

Based on these results, aspirin is recommended for all patients undergoing prosthetic infrainguinal bypass or clopidogrel for those allergic to aspirin. For patients without unique risk factors for graft occlusion, warfarin is not recommended. However, for those at high risk for occlusion and limb loss, combination therapy with warfarin and aspirin is recommended.[395]

SELECTED KEY REFERENCES

Campbell CD, Brooks DH, Webster MW, Bahnson HT. The use of expanded microporous polytetrafluoroethylene for limb salvage: a preliminary report. *Surgery.* 1976;79:485.
The first clinical application of ePTFE grafts as an arterial substitute.

Clagett GP, Sobel M, Jackson MR, Lip GY, Tangelder M, Verhaeghe R. Antithrombotic therapy in peripheral arterial occlusive disease: the Seventh ACCP Conference on Antithrombotic and Thrombolytic Therapy. *Chest.* 2004;126:609S.
The most recent recommendations on the use of pharmacologic therapy to improve the long-term performance of prosthetic grafts from the American College of Chest Physicians.

DeBakey ME, Cooley DA, Crawford ES, Morris GC Jr. Clinical application of a new flexible knitted Dacron arterial substitute. 1958. *Am Surg.* 2008;74:381.
The first clinical application of Dacron grafts as an arterial substitute.

Herring M, Gardner A, Glover J. Single-staged technique for seeding vascular grafts with autogenous endothelium. *Surgery.* 1978;84:498.
The introduction of autologous endothelial cell seeding of prosthetic grafts.

Heyligers JM, Arts CH, Verhagen HJ, de Groot PG, Moll FL. Improving small-diameter vascular grafts: from the application of an endothelial cell lining to the construction of a tissue-engineered blood vessel. *Ann Vasc Surg.* 2005;19:448.
Reviews current advances in endothelial cell–seeded grafts.

Jordan SW, Chaikof EL. Novel thromboresistant materials. *J Vasc Surg.* 2007;45:A104.
A comprehensive review of current strategies to modify the surface of prosthetic vascular prostheses to reduce thrombogenicity.

L'Heureux N, Dusserre N, Marini A, Garrido S, de la Fuente L, McAllister T. Technology insight: the evolution of tissue-engineered vascular grafts—from research to clinical practice. *Nat Clin Pract Cardiovasc Med.* 2007;4:389.
Brief overview of current progress in tissue-engineered grafts; highlights the clinical, regulatory, and reimbursement hurdles to overcome in the transition from bench to bedside.

Loth F, Fischer PF, Bassiouny HS. Blood flow in end-to-side anastomoses. *Ann Rev Fluid Mech.* 2008;40:367.
Reviews current understanding of mechanical factors and fluid mechanics near the anastomosis in relation to graft failure.

Miller JH, Foreman RK, Ferguson L, Faris I. Interposition vein cuff for anastomosis of prosthesis to small artery. *Aust N Z J Surg.* 1984;54:283.
The first report on the use of a venous interposition cuff to decrease intimal hyperplasia.

Stegmann TH, Haverich A, Borst HG. Clinical experience with a new collagen-coated Dacron double-velour prosthesis. *Thorac Cardiovasc Surg.* 1986;34:54.
Early favorable clinical experience with pre-sealed grafts, which along with other later investigations propelled the widespread adoption of such grafts that continues today.

Tiwari A, Cheng KS, Salacinski H, Hamilton G, Seifalian AM. Improving the patency of vascular bypass grafts: the role of suture materials and surgical techniques on reducing anastomotic compliance mismatch. *Eur J Vasc Endovasc Surg.* 2003;25:287.
Overview of current suture and venous adjunctive techniques to generate the anastomosis.

Tiwari A, Salacinski H, Seifalian AM, Hamilton G. New prostheses for use in bypass graft with special emphasis on polyurethanes. *Cardiovasc Surg.* 2002;10:191.
Summarizes the clinical experience with polyurethane-based vascular grafts.

Voorhees AB, Jaretski AH, Blakemore AH. The use of tubes constructed from Vinyon "N" cloth in bridging arterial defects. *Ann Surg.* 1952;135:332.
The first report of the application of a synthetic vascular substitute to repair the abdominal aorta in dogs.

Weinberg CB, Bell E. A blood-vessel model constructed from collagen and cultured vascular cells. *Science.* 1986;231:397.
The first cell-based vascular graft constructed in vitro that pioneered the field of tissue-engineered grafts.

Zilla P, Bezuidenhout D, Human P. Prosthetic vascular grafts: wrong models, wrong questions and no healing. *Biomaterials.* 2007;28:5009.
Reviews current understanding of prosthetic graft healing and critically evaluates results from research and animal models in comparison to clinical experience.

REFERENCES

The reference list can be found on the companion Expert Consult Web site at *www.expertconsult.com.*

CHAPTER 89

Biologic Grafts

Alik Farber

In the field of vascular surgery the use of surgical bypass is fundamental to the treatment of a wide variety of arterial and venous disorders. In turn, the technical conduct and success of surgical bypass are directly dependent on the conduit used. The ideal conduit should be readily available, easy to handle, resistant to thrombosis and infection, durable, and inexpensive, as well as have characteristics similar to the vessel that it is replacing.

Although the perfect conduit does not exist, autogenous blood vessels are closest to the ideal. Autogenous arterial conduits such as the internal mammary, radial, and gastroepiploic arteries have been used with great success in the coronary circulation.[1-3] The internal iliac and radial arteries have been used in the visceral vascular bed,[4,5] and the superficial temporal artery has been used for extracranial-intracranial bypass.[6] Unfortunately, short conduit length and invasive harvest have limited the use of autogenous arterial grafts to a relatively small number of clinical scenarios.

Autogenous vein has been the preferred conduit for infrainguinal bypass because long lengths of vein can be harvested, removal is inconsequential, and harvest complexity is minimal.[7] Autogenous vein has also been used for the bypass of upper extremity,[8] carotid,[9] coronary,[1] and visceral[10] arterial beds. Finally, it has been preferentially used in the construction of arteriovenous fistulae (AVFs) for hemodialysis.[11]

Although autogenous vascular grafts perform well, there are multiple clinical situations in which these conduits are inadequate, unavailable, or improperly matched to the recipient vascular bed. These unmet demands led to the development of artificial grafts. Although multiple materials have been tried, polyethylene terephthalate (Dacron) and polytetrafluoroethylene (PTFE) have emerged as the standard materials for prosthetic vascular grafts. These grafts have been used with excellent success for the bypass of large vessels such as the aorta[12] and medium-sized vessels such as the subclavian artery.[9] Prosthetic grafts have also been used extensively for dialysis access[11] and with mixed results for infrainguinal revascularization.[13] Dacron and PTFE grafts offer "off-the-shelf" availability and a variety of sizes to permit replacement of even the largest vessels. In general, however, they cannot be used in infected fields and, when compared with autogenous conduits, are at increased risk for infection, structural deterioration, and occlusion. Although patency rates are acceptable for aortic reconstruction because of high flow rates and low outflow resistance, bypass to smaller targets, such as the tibial arteries, is associated with low graft patency.

Limitations of autogenous and prosthetic grafts have fueled exploration for other potential conduits, and this investigative effort has led to the evaluation of biologic grafts for bypass. Biologic grafts, or biografts, are bypass conduits made of nonautogenous biologic vessels modified for use in clinical practice. Allografts or homografts refer to arteries or veins that are transplanted from one individual to another within the same species. Xenografts or heterografts are vessels transplanted from an individual of one species to an individual of another species.

Carrel was first to experiment with fresh allografts and xenografts in dogs during the first decade of the 20th century.[14] The first recorded human use of allografts, obtained from casualties, occurred during World War I.[15] In 1948, Gross and colleagues described the first clinical series of fresh arterial allografts,[16] and less than a decade later, Linton published his series of fresh venous allografts.[17] Various methods of allograft cryopreservation were developed in the 1950s,[17] refined in the 1970s,[18,19] and finally standardized and commercialized in the late 1980s.[20] In parallel, enzymatically treated and tanned bovine carotid artery (BCA) xenografts were evaluated and first described in a clinical setting in 1966.[21] Application of similar techniques to human vessels led to development of the human umbilical vein (HUV) graft by Dardik and Dardik in 1976.[22]

Theoretically, biografts promise to be the optimal vascular conduit. They can potentially offer "off-the-shelf" availability, a wide variety of sizes, excellent handling characteristics, and patency rates similar to those of autogenous vessels. These attractive features prompted scientific investigation and clinical use of these conduits that has spanned the course of almost a century. Although this collective experience with an assortment of biografts in a variety of clinical settings led to specific clinical indications for their use, biologic grafts failed to become the "Holy Grail" of vascular surgery.

GRAFT PROPERTIES

Fresh Vascular Allografts

Fresh arterial and venous allografts have been studied in animal experiments.[14,23,24] In one canine model, fresh venous allografts had a patency rate of 69% at 20 months. Pathologic analysis of explanted veins revealed intimal proliferation, medial inflammation, medial degeneration, and periadventitial fibrosis.[23] In another canine venous allograft experiment, dogs that were immunosuppressed with azathioprine demonstrated slightly better graft patency than did those that were not.[24] Conversely, in a murine model, fresh venous allografts implanted in rats had excellent patency rates and minimal intimal thickening on histologic analysis.[24]

In humans, fresh venous allografts used for infrainguinal bypass had a failure rate of 55% in one series; failed grafts either occluded or became aneurysmal. Patency rates of allografts appeared to be higher in patients whose grafts were harvested from ABO-compatible donors.[25] In another study, fresh arterial allografts placed in the aortic position were noted to be highly immunogenic, with evidence of both a humoral and cellular immune response.[26] These animal and human data suggest that fresh vessel allografts initiate a host immune response. Furthermore, the patency of these grafts appears to vary among species.

Aside from their immunogenicity, the use of fresh vascular allografts in the clinical setting has been hampered by logistic factors. Scarce availability of fresh arteries and veins and a need to successfully store such vessels for future use have led to the development of a number of preservation and modification techniques. These techniques can be divided into those that involve preservation without a planned significant change in graft integrity and those in which the graft is intentionally chemically altered. Cryopreservation is the most common example of the preservation technique, whereas proteolytic enzymatic digestion and dialdehyde starch tanning are examples of the modification technique. In addition to creating a conduit that would be more readily available, there was hope that these techniques would inhibit the host immune response and thereby increase graft patency.[27]

Over the course of the past century, multiple vessel preservation techniques have been tested. Grafts were stored in a number of solutions, including nutrient broths,[16] glycerol,[28] and plasminate.[29] A variety of storage temperatures ranging from room temperature to $-70°C$ were tried.[17,28] Finally, a number of adjunctive sterilization techniques, including ethyl dioxide and irradiation, were attempted.[17] Early techniques focused on preservation without much regard to viability of the vascular tissue. Initial results with preserved vascular grafts were inconsistent, probably because significant cellular and structural damage occurred in many of these vessels and made them nonviable.[25,30]

Cryopreserved Allografts
Methods of Preparation

There is evidence that cryopreservation can result in significant cellular damage unless appropriate precautions are taken.[31] During the cryopreservation process, the extracellular matrix freezes at a higher temperature than cellular cytoplasm. This leads to a vapor pressure gradient between the intracellular and extracellular components. When cooling occurs slowly, this gradient can result in cellular dehydration, whereas rapid cooling can lead to plasma membrane rupture. Work with cell suspensions such as blood and semen has revealed that certain substances, when added during the freezing process, can significantly improve cell viability.[32] These substances, called cryoprotectants, include dimethylsulfoxide and glycerol. Their mechanism of action is to enter cellular cytoplasm and decrease the vapor pressure gradient that exists between the intracellular and extracellular components.[20]

Over the last 20 years, cryopreservation techniques have been optimized and commercialized. Important variables inherent in modern cryopreservation processes include the type and amount of cryoprotectant used, freezing rate, storage temperature, duration of storage, and additives used.[20] The most common cryoprotectant in use today is dimethylsulfoxide at 10% to 20% dilution. The freezing rate varies among protocols, and there is some evidence that rapid freezing at $5°C/sec$ may work best. Storage temperature may vary from $-102°C$ to $-196°C$. The duration of cryopreservation may be important, and longer duration has been shown to have an adverse influence on vessel wall morphology but not on graft patency in one animal model.[33] Finally, there is evidence that the addition of certain additives such as chondroitin sulfate to the storage solution enhances vein viability and function.[34]

Histology and Physiology

Cryopreserved arteries and veins are affected by both cryopreservation and immune rejection; a large body of research has been performed to define and dissect these processes from one another.

Cryopreservation has effects on the mechanical properties, histology, and physiology of the treated vessel. Elasticity and compliance of a vessel are important mechanical characteristics that affect its performance as a conduit. Changes in these properties lead to an increased difference in compliance between the conduit and host vessel, which can adversely affect graft patency. In vitro models comparing the mechanical properties of cryopreserved and freshly harvested arteries and veins reveal that cryopreservation does not significantly affect elasticity, compliance, and the mechanical buffering function of the treated vessel.[19,35,36]

Cryopreservation of blood vessels leads to changes in the intima, media, and adventitia. Although appropriate cryopreservation does not affect the gross morphology of the endothelial layer, histologic changes such as focal microvillous projection, cytoplasmic vacuolization, nuclear prominence, and interruption of tight junctions have been visualized.[33,37] These changes increase with the duration of cryopreservation[33,37] and lead to partial endothelial cell loss.[37-39] Endothelial loss is significant when the cryopreserved graft is exposed to arterial flow. Although autogenous grafts re-establish an endothelial layer, only minimal re-endothelialization is observed in allografts.[20,29] Because of a compromise in intimal integrity, cryopreserved grafts accumulate low-density lipoprotein cholesterol at an accelerated rate as measured in an ex vivo organ perfusion system.[40]

Endothelial vasodilatory function, as measured by response to acetylcholine, thrombin, and calcium ionophore, appears to be retained, albeit somewhat diminished, with cryopreservation.[41,42] With regard to coagulation homeostasis, although cryopreservation of vein grafts is not associated with increased platelet deposition,[42] it does cause decreased thrombomodulin activity.[38] Fibrinolytic activity appears to be similar in both fresh and cryopreserved canine jugular veins, but this activity may be adversely affected by the duration of cryopreservation.[37]

The medial layer of cryopreserved vascular grafts appears to have grossly normal smooth muscle cells, although slight lysis and minimal mitochondrial edema were observed in a rabbit model. In that model, implantation of autologous veins into an arterial circuit led to the preservation of both smooth muscle cells and the elastic lamina. The smooth muscle cells displayed a synthetic rather than a contractile phenotype characterized by dilatation of the endoplasmic reticulum.[33] Despite these findings, collagen synthesis in cryopreserved veins but not fresh veins was diminished in a canine model.[39] Smooth muscle cells in cryopreserved canine saphenous autografts were noted to have a diminished relaxation response to nitric oxide,[42] although contraction induced by norepinephrine, potassium chloride, and serotonin was unaltered.[20]

Immunology

Allogeneic implantation of cryopreserved vessels leads to a different histologic and physiologic picture than that seen with cryopreserved autologous grafts. These observed changes are caused by immune mechanisms. Endothelial loss, encountered when an allograft is exposed to arterial flow, is not appreciably reversed, and exposed subendothelial elements are noted on electron microscopy.[20,29] Smooth muscle cell viability is lost,[23,43] severe medial fibrosis and disruption of elastic fibers occur,[23,29,43] and medial necrosis has been described.[44] Significant lymphocytic infiltration of the media and adventitia has been observed.[29] These alterations in vessel wall biology are not routinely observed with autologous conduits.[44]

Although it is well known that transplanted allograft and xenograft organs elicit an immune response, it was initially believed that the host-mediated immune response of transplanted vessel allografts was minor[45,46] and could be successfully blunted by the cryopreservation process.[27] Recent literature, however, suggests that vascular allografts do trigger a significant immune response.[20,26] Endothelial cells present surface antigens that stimulate a cell-mediated immune response[47] against the donor graft. An IgG-mediated humoral immune response to donor-specific antigens has been described.[26,48] Transplanted canine venous allografts, but not autografts, demonstrated extensive medial fibrosis and lymphocytic infiltration consistent with immunologic rejection.[49] In a human model, analysis of 22 explanted cryopreserved saphenous vein (CSV) allografts revealed moderate to severe intimal, medial, and adventitial inflammatory infiltrates. Immunohistochemical analysis demonstrated an abundance

of activated T lymphocytes containing cytotoxic granules.[50] In another experiment, cryopreservation did not alter antigenic expression and the immunologic response of a murine host to allograft transplantation in a number of studies.[51,52] Chronic immunologic rejection clearly plays a role in allograft biology and appears to be responsible for both diminished patency of cryopreserved vascular grafts and the predilection of these grafts to aneurysmal degeneration.[44]

A number of investigators hypothesized that manipulating the host immune response to vascular allografts may attenuate immune rejection and improve graft patency. Matching of ABO blood groups was suggested by Ochsner and associates, who noted improved patency of allografts transplanted to ABO-matched patients.[25] In animal models, immunosuppression with cyclosporine has been demonstrated to diminish immunologic rejection of aortic[44] and venous allografts.[53,54] Azathioprine has likewise been shown to decrease the effects of rejection in venous allografts.[24]

Based on these findings, attempts were made to improve the results of allograft use in humans by modulating the host immune response. Carpenter and Tomaszewski, in a prospective, randomized trial of 40 CSV allografts implanted in patients treated with low-dose azathioprine, failed to show a significant improvement in graft patency at 1 year.[55] Azathioprine immunosuppression, however, was associated with a decreased presence of T-lymphocyte cytotoxic granules in that study.[50] In another small human trial, a combination of low-dose cyclosporine, azathioprine, prednisone, warfarin, aspirin, and vasodilators was used in patients undergoing CSV bypass. Grafts treated with this immunosuppressive regimen demonstrated increased patency rates. This regimen, however, was associated with an increased incidence of complications and graft aneurysmal degeneration.[56] Finally, in one series, 10 of 30 patients undergoing aortic allograft replacement for prosthetic aortic infection were concomitantly treated with cyclosporine. Although the measured humoral immune response was blunted in patients who received cyclosporine, no differences in graft patency or graft complication rates were appreciated.[26]

Furthermore, an immunologic response evoked by a cryopreserved allograft can induce allosensitization, which may interfere with future organ transplantation. This mostly affects the use of cryopreserved femoral vein (CFV) allografts in hemodialysis access. A case-matched series of 20 patients undergoing creation of hemodialysis access with this graft demonstrated host allosensitization in all patients as measured by the panel-reactive antibody assay.[57] Allosensitization, however, did not occur when the CFV graft was processed to remove cellular elements.[58] Diminution of the immune response by removal of antigenic epitopes has led to multiple attempts to structurally modify biologic grafts.

Structurally Modified Biologic Grafts

In parallel with the development of cryopreservation techniques, further research was conducted to modify blood vessels so that an acceptable vascular substitute could be developed. The goal was to transform a harvested blood vessel into a durable nonimmunogenic graft that could be easily produced and stored. During early experiments in the 1950s, animal arteries were modified by enzymatic digestion of the musculoelastic portion of the vessel wall with ficin, a proteolytic enzyme isolated from figs, to remove immunologically reactive proteins. The resultant collagenous vascular skeleton was strengthened by collagen cross-linking through subsequent tanning with dialdehyde starch.[21,59] This modified graft was then sterilized and stored in a 1% propylene oxide–50% ethanol solution.[21]

In the earliest experiments, modified BCA grafts were implanted as xenografts first in dogs and then in patients with symptomatic lower extremity occlusive disease. Although no graft ruptures had occurred at 3 years of follow-up, early neointimal hyperplasia and diminished patency were observed.[21] An unacceptable late rate of graft infection and aneurysmal degeneration led to a change to glutaraldehyde-based tanning protocols.[59,60]

Bovine mesenteric vein (BMV) has also been modified by a patented process of glutaraldehyde cross-linking and sterilized by gamma radiation.[61] Both BCA and BMV have been used as xenografts in a number of clinical applications.

HUV is a modified biologic conduit that was first evaluated in baboons[22] in the early 1970s and subsequently used in humans[22,62] in 1975. Umbilical vessels are uniform in caliber, valveless, and branchless. The umbilical vein was removed from the umbilical cord by a variety of techniques, including enzymatic digestion and mechanical stripping. After a rinsing process with a cold isotonic solution, this vein was tanned with glutaraldehyde. A polyester fiber mesh was then sutured in place about the length and outside circumference of the graft for added support.[22]

Although thrombosis and aneurysm formation were common in early experiments, tanning and external support modifications significantly reduced these complications. Increased adherence of platelets to the luminal surface of these grafts has been observed in a canine model.[63] Histologic analysis of modified HUV grafts explanted from baboons revealed an early neutrophil and late macrophage response in the vicinity of the surrounding polyester mesh. The inner collagen layer appeared thickened and dense but was free of significant inflammation.[22] The reduced immunogenicity of this graft was hypothesized to be secondary to pretreatment with glutaraldehyde, which was thought to bind to graft histocompatibility antigen sites and thereby shielded them from the host immune response.[64]

Other Grafts

The search for an ideal blood vessel substitute led to the investigation of a number of nonconventional biologic grafts in animal models. Vascular prostheses fashioned from pericardium[65] and small intestinal mucosa[66] have been evaluated. Chemically modified human[67] and bovine[68] ureters have been used as vascular conduits with some success. Modified bovine ureters have been used clinically with acceptable patency rates in one small Australian series.[69]

CLINICAL USE IN PERIPHERAL VASCULAR SURGERY

Indication

Biologic grafts have been used in modern peripheral vascular surgery mostly in three distinct clinical settings: extremity bypass in the absence of suitable autogenous conduit, arteriovenous (AV) access for hemodialysis, and replacement of infected prosthetic grafts.

Extremity Bypass

Acute or chronic ischemia of an extremity is caused by a number of conditions, including atherosclerosis, trauma, embolization, and in situ thrombosis. Treatment of extremity ischemia involves revascularization by endovascular or surgical techniques. When a surgical procedure is indicated and a long arterial segment needs revascularization, surgical bypass is used. This scenario most commonly involves the infrainguinal arteries, and the choice of conduit for such a bypass is crucial to success of the operation. Autogenous great saphenous vein has proved to be the preferred conduit for infrainguinal revascularization.[70,71] When autogenous great saphenous vein is not available, alternative, autogenous conduits such as an arm vein,[72] the small saphenous vein,[73] and composite autogenous vein[74] have been used with good results. The ever-increasing age and complexity of patients with infrainguinal arterial occlusive disease has brought about increasingly frequent clinical scenarios in which autogenous vein is not available and an alternative conduit must be found. Although prosthetic grafts have been used with moderate success above the knee, they have been disappointing when used for infrageniculate bypass.[75,76] Distal modification of prosthetic grafts with a vein cuff or distal AVF may improve patency rates[77-79] but is more cumbersome.

Given the absence of reliable conduit options for infrageniculate bypass when suitable autogenous vein is lacking, the feasibility of biologic grafts has been evaluated. In this setting, CSV allografts,[80] CFA allografts,[43] HUV grafts,[81] BCA xenografts,[59] and BMV xenografts[82] have been used with varying degrees of success.

Arteriovenous Access

End-stage renal disease is a significant public health problem in the United States,[83] its prevalence is increasing steadily, and it is forecast that by the year 2010, more than 500,000 patients will be undergoing hemodialysis.[84] Long-term hemodialysis is best performed through a surgically created AVF that connects the arterial and venous circulations via a conduit. The ideal AV conduit carries high flow for efficient dialysis, is superficial enough for easy access, is sufficiently durable to withstand multiple cannulations, allows rapid sealing of cannulation sites, and is resistant to infection, stenosis, and thrombosis. A mature, native vein AVF comes closest to the ideal, and its use is strongly encouraged.[11] Unfortunately, many individuals lack suitable vein for native AVF construction because of small vein size and previous access procedures or vein harvest for peripheral or coronary bypass. Furthermore, up to 40% of native AVFs fail to mature and therefore cannot be used successfully.[85] Although prosthetic AV grafts are widely used, they have lower patency rates, require more frequent revision, and are at higher risk than vein AVFs for infection.[86] The search for optimal hemodialysis access in patients who are not candidates for a native vein AVF has led to the use of biologic grafts. CFV allografts,[87] BCA xenografts,[88] and BMV xenografts[61] have been used in a variety of settings with variable results.

Replacement of Infected Prosthetic Grafts

Prosthetic graft infection, particularly when the aorta is involved, is one of the most dreaded complications in vascular surgery and is associated with high morbidity and mortality.[89] Treatment of an infected aortic prosthesis includes excision of the infected segment and extra-anatomic prosthetic bypass[89] or reconstruction with an antibiotic-soaked or antibiotic-bonded prosthetic graft,[90] femoral vein,[91] or aortic allograft.[92] Extra-anatomic bypass and aortic ligation are associated with long operative times, risk for remote infection, bypass thrombosis, and aortic stump rupture.[89,93] Antibiotic-soaked prosthetic grafts may work well for infections caused by relatively indolent *Staphylococcus epidermidis* but are much less effective against more virulent organisms.[90] Finally, use of the femoral vein for aortic reconstruction is tedious and associated with harvest-related complications.[91]

Cryopreserved aortic allografts offer "off-the-shelf" availability, good handling properties, and the potential for expeditious in situ repair. Cryopreserved aortic allografts were more resistant than prosthetic grafts to *S. epidermidis* infection in a canine model.[94] Resistance of vascular allografts to infection has led to the wide use of arterial allografts to treat aortoiliac infection,[95] CFV allografts to treat infection involving prosthetic AV grafts,[96] and CSV allografts to replace infected infrainguinal prosthetic bypass grafts.[97]

Biologic Graft Preparation

Cryopreserved Allografts

A number of tissue banks and commercial companies prepare, store, and supply cryopreserved blood vessels. Despite similarities in conduit preparation, many have proprietary cryopreservation protocols.[98] The great saphenous vein, femoral vein, and arterial segments are harvested from multiorgan donors who are screened for an array of viral, bacterial, and fungal infections. Branches are suture ligated and the allografts are sized with calibrated dilators. They are tested for presence of pathogens, rinsed in an antibiotic solution, placed in a proprietary cryoprotectant solution, and stored

in the vapor phase of liquid nitrogen at −110°C to −196°C. Allografts are shipped and stored in a solution of dimethylsulfoxide at −96°C until needed. The vein, but not artery, is usually matched for ABO/Rh compatibility with the recipient to decrease the risk of rejection. At the start of the procedure the allograft is rapidly thawed by submersion in a warm water bath at 37°C to 42°C for 20 minutes. After rinsing in a series of solutions provided by the manufacturer, it is ready for use.

CSV allografts are available in a number of lengths and diameters. Most commonly the vein measures 3 to 5 mm in diameter. These grafts look, feel, and handle like autogenous saphenous vein. During the course of infrainguinal bypass, the allograft is usually reversed and placed in a superficial tunnel for easy access.[80] Postoperative surveillance was not found to be useful in one large series.[80]

CFV allografts are usually less than 25 cm in length and have a diameter between 5 and 7 mm. They have most commonly been used in hemodialysis, particularly in the setting of prosthetic AV graft infection. When used for dialysis access, this allograft is appropriately reversed and tapered to a 5-mm diameter at the arterial anastomosis to decrease the incidence of ischemic steal syndrome.[87] It is allowed to mature for 3 to 4 weeks before it is accessed for hemodialysis. Revision of these grafts is very difficult because of their thin wall and surrounding fibrosis.[96]

Arterial allografts have most frequently been used for aortic replacement in the setting of primary or prosthetic aortic infection. Given this clinical setting and the need to replace a large artery such as the aorta, these allografts have to withstand particularly hostile conditions. To this end, technical modifications for the use of these allografts have been developed, including vigilance in following thawing instructions, use of appropriately long grafts and construction of tension-free anastomoses, taking great care that suture ligation of branches is performed with polypropylene sutures that include the graft wall along with the branches, aggressive excision of infected tissue and wound drainage, circumferential anastomotic reinforcement with allograft strips, use of gentamicin-impregnated fibrin glue, and coverage of the graft with viable tissue such as a pedicled omental or muscle flap.[92,99]

Structurally Modified Allografts

The HUV graft (Fig. 89-1) is shipped and stored in 50% ethanol and provided on a glass mandril. It is irrigated up to 10 times with a low-molecular-weight dextran–containing solution and rinsed with a high-concentration heparin solution (10,000 U/L). This graft does not tolerate traction or the application of standard vascular clamps well. To avoid injury it needs to be passed through a metal or plastic conduit during tunneling and preferably controlled with a tourniquet. To decrease the risk of pseudoaneurysm formation during suturing, both the vein and the Dacron mesh need to be incorporated into the suture line. Finally, infusion of low-molecular-weight dextran was recommended in the early

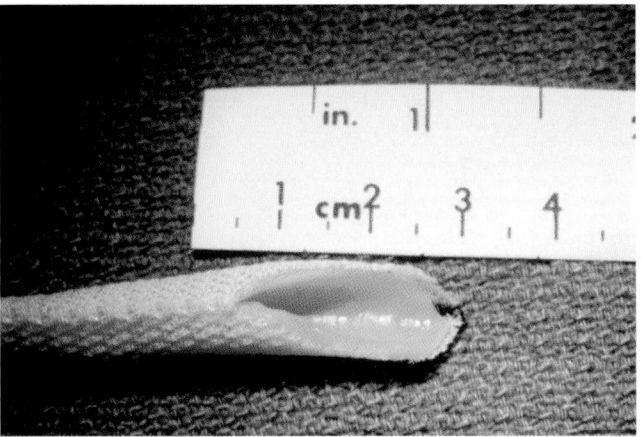

Figure 89-1 Human umbilical vein graft. *(Courtesy of Herbert Dardik.)*

Figure 89-3 Bovine mesenteric vein graft. *(Courtesy of ProCol Vascular Bioprosthesis, Hancock Jaffe Laboratories, Irvine, CA.)*

postoperative period by the manufacturer to decrease the risk for early thrombosis.

Manufacturing of the umbilical vein graft by Synovis Life Technologies, Inc. (St. Paul, MN) stopped in May 2006 in compliance with new U.S. Food and Drug Administration (FDA) guidelines governing combination tissue-medical devices. Currently, a new-generation device that will fulfill FDA regulations is in the process of development.[100]

The BCA graft (Fig. 89-2) is supplied in a specially designed tube containing a proprietary solution of 1% propylene oxide in 40% aqueous ethyl alcohol. It is naturally compliant, soft, and relatively easy to use. It is presently available in 6-, 7-, and 8-mm diameters and 15- to 45-cm lengths (Artegraft; Artegraft, Inc., New Brunswick, NJ). BMV graft (Fig. 89-3) is shipped in a sterile saline solution and is available in 6-mm diameters and 10- to 40-cm lengths (ProCol Vascular Bioprosthesis, Hancock Jaffe Laboratories, Irvine, CA). This graft is compliant and handles much like saphenous vein.[61] Both xenografts require a series of rinsing steps in the operating room before use.

CLINICAL OUTCOMES

Cryopreserved Saphenous Vein Allografts

Numerous reports on the utility of CSV allografts for infrainguinal revascularization have been published (Table 89-1).[55,56,80,101-107] However, this literature suffers from some confounding factors that may affect the interpretation of outcomes. CSV has been distributed by a number of vendors who use similar, but not identical, cryopreservation techniques. There is significant variability pertaining to patients, location of the proximal and distal anastomoses, use of anticoagulation, and use of immunosuppressive agents. The majority of these reports are retrospective, and the two largest studies contain 115[104] and 240[80] grafts. Four prospective studies have been published but include small numbers of patients.[55,56,80,103]

Graft Patency

Although use of CSV allografts has been reported in a number of settings, these grafts are generally used for the treatment of limb-threatening ischemia.[80,104] The primary patency rate of CSV grafts has been noted to be relatively low in most retrospective series (see Table 89-1).[80,101-107] The largest case series reported a 30% primary patency rate at 1 year,[80] similar to the 37% primary patency rate noted in the second largest series.[104] Although Buckley and coauthors published an impressive 87% primary patency rate in their prospective study of 26 patients,[107] Carpenter and Tomaszewski found a dismal 13% primary patency rate in their prospectively monitored patient cohort.[55]

Secondary procedures on failing or failed grafts generally seem to yield little gain. Primary-assisted and secondary patency of CSV grafts was not significantly higher than primary patency in the two largest allograft series.[80,104] Once the graft failed, it was abandoned and secondary grafting was performed when indicated.[80] Other authors, however,

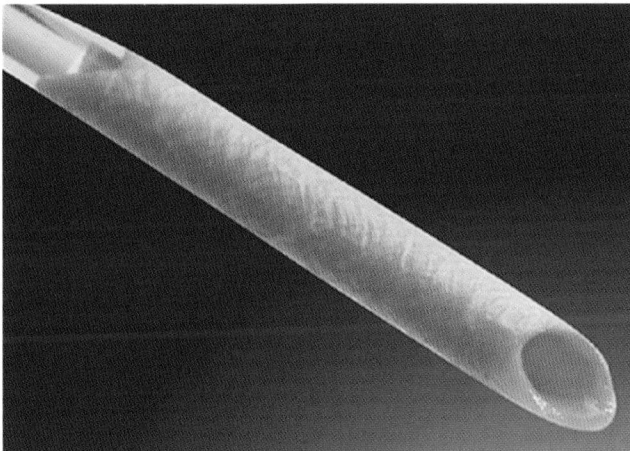

Figure 89-2 Bovine carotid artery graft. *(Courtesy of Artegraft, Inc., North Brunswick, NJ.)*

Table 89-1 Summary of Published Cryopreserved Saphenous Vein Allograft Series Containing More Than 20 Grafts

Series	Number of Grafts	Primary Patency at 1 Year (%)	Secondary Patency at 1 Year (%)	2-Year Limb Salvage (%)
Farber et al.[80]	199	30	NR	71
Harris et al.[101]	80	36.8	NR	62.3*
Harris et al.[102]	25	NR	36	74†
Leseche et al.[103]	25	NR	52	78
Martin et al.[104]	115	37	40	66‡
Shah et al.[105]	43	66	NR	NR
Walker et al.[106]	39	28	46	67‡
Buckley et al.[107]	26	87	NR	80
Carpenter and Tomaszewski[55]	40	13	NR	42†

*At 3 years.
†At 12 months.
‡At last follow-up.
NR, not reported.

almost doubled their secondary patency rates by adopting an aggressive posture toward allograft thrombectomy and revision.[106]

Multiple patient and procedural variables were evaluated for their influence on allograft patency. In the largest published series, multivariate analysis identified that diabetes negatively affected graft patency. Age, gender, hypertension, smoking, renal dysfunction, indication for surgery, history of bypass grafting, and site of distal anastomosis did not have an effect.[80] Other investigators found no significant effect of diabetes on graft patency.[104,106] Shah and associates found that secondary and composite allograft reconstructions adversely affected graft patency.[105]

The Role of Anticoagulation and Immunosuppression

A number of studies have evaluated the effect of anticoagulation on allograft patency. Aspirin and warfarin, alone or in combination, did not improve graft patency in most studies.[55,80,102,104,105] Buckley and colleagues, however, reported an impressive 87% primary patency rate in their prospective cohort of 26 patients who were treated with an intensive anticoagulation protocol consisting of preoperative aspirin, perioperative low-dose heparin and dextran, and postoperative warfarin, aspirin, and dipyridamole.[107] Of note, 42% of grafts in that series underwent distal anastomotic modification with either vein cuffs or AVFs. A limitation of most retrospective studies is that the precise level of therapeutic anticoagulation was not rigorously followed for each individual patient. The true effect of an anticoagulation protocol on allograft patency awaits a prospective randomized study that will closely monitor the adequacy of postoperative oral warfarin therapy.

Immunosuppressive regimens have been evaluated clinically. In a prospective randomized trial of 40 grafts in patients treated with low-dose azathioprine, Carpenter and Tomaszewski failed to show a significant improvement in graft patency at 1 year.[55] Although other immunosuppressive protocols may be effective, potentially serious side effects of

therapy may not justify clinical trials in this patient population.[56]

Limb Salvage

Despite discouraging graft patency, use of CSV allografts has been associated with acceptable limb salvage rates (see Table 89-1). In the largest published series, a 71% 2-year limb salvage rate was achieved.[80] The discrepancy between graft patency and limb salvage can be explained in part by secondary bypass procedures performed after primary graft failure. Others have reported that repetitive bypass grafting significantly extends limb salvage.[108] Another possibility is that the saphenous allografts remained patent long enough to enable healing of lower extremity ulceration in a large proportion of patients. The ulcers may not have recurred despite graft failure.[80,103,104] Unfortunately, this hypothesis can be proven only in a trial in which ulcer healing is prospectively monitored along with limb salvage.

Of the various clinical factors that could potentially influence limb salvage, multivariate analysis found the site of distal anastomosis to be significant.[80] Patients undergoing allograft bypass to the popliteal artery had better limb salvage than did those undergoing tibial bypass. Martin and coworkers found patient age to be inversely related to limb salvage.[104]

Aneurysmal Degeneration

CSV allografts that remain open for a prolonged period are prone to aneurysmal degeneration,[56,80,104] probably related to the immune response mounted by the recipient against the graft. The true incidence of allograft aneurysm formation cannot be accurately determined because the vast majority of these grafts occlude long before a clinically detectable aneurysm can develop. In one series, aneurysmal degeneration developed in 9 grafts, for a 2-year aneurysm incidence of 44%.[80] Martin and coauthors reported a 25% aneurysm formation rate at 2.5 years.[104] The development of aneurysms in allografts necessitates close surveillance of those few patients whose graft remains open for a prolonged period. Because allograft aneurysm rupture has been reported,[56,80] preemptive graft revision is recommended.

Summary and Indications for Use

Although CSV allografts look, feel, and handle like autogenous vein, they are far from being the "Holy Grail" of conduits for infrainguinal reconstruction. Their poor patency rates are worsened by several risk factors, including diabetes, previous bypass, and composite reconstruction. Postoperative anticoagulation has not significantly improved graft patency,[80] although some authors believe that an intensive perioperative and postoperative anticoagulation regimen has merit.[107] Given the immunologic mechanism of graft failure, it is unlikely that anticoagulation alone is sufficient to prevent graft occlusion. Grafts that stay open for extended periods, perhaps as a result of chance matching of important immunologic loci, are prone to aneurysmal degeneration. Finally, CSV allografts are expensive, costing more than $4000 per graft in 2008 dollars.

Given published clinical data, many authors conclude that the use of CSV allografts should be limited.[56,80,101,103,104,109] Nevertheless, these grafts clearly have a place in the armamentarium of the modern vascular surgeon. Because they have been reported to be relatively resistant to graft infection,[97] they have an advantage when revascularization needs to be performed in an infected field. They also have an advantage when distal bypass needs to be extended onto the foot because closure of the wound is considerably easier than if a prosthetic graft is used. Finally, CSV allografts remain patent long enough to allow healing of an ischemic ulcer or minor amputation. The final piece of evidence supporting the continued role of this graft is persistent demand for the product by the vascular surgery community as evidenced by the number of grafts that continue to be sold.

Cryopreserved Femoral Vein Allografts

Femoral vein allografts have been used for hemodialysis access in the setting of prosthetic AV graft infection, multiple graft failures, or compromised venous outflow sites. In one series of 48 allografts, 1-year primary and secondary patency rates of 49% and 75%, respectively, were achieved. No allograft infection or aneurysmal degeneration was noted.[87] In another series of 45 allografts, a cumulative 1-year patency rate of 68% was reported. Although no infection was noted during follow-up, two pseudoaneurysms required repair.[110] Madden and colleagues compared the outcomes of 90 femoral allografts with 100 concurrent PTFE AV grafts and noted similar patency rates. No infections were seen in the allograft group, whereas 10% of the PTFE AV grafts became infected. In 18% of the allografts, however, aneurysmal degeneration developed.[111] Despite these favorable data, others have found the use of CFV for AV access to be associated with a 55% rate of infection, which was particularly common in thigh grafts. Allograft rupture occurred in 46% of infected grafts.[112]

CFV allografts do not have a primary role in hemodialysis access. They may have a secondary role in the setting of infected prosthetic access in a patient with limited reconstructive options. Because of allosensitization they should not be used in patients who are candidates for future kidney transplantation,[57] although decellularized femoral vein allografts appear be safer in that regard.[58] Symptomatic pseudoaneurysms may develop in these allografts and should elicit a low threshold for repair. Finally, CFV placement in the thigh should be avoided.

Cryopreserved Arterial Allografts

Although most experience with arterial allografts has been gained with aortic replacement in the setting of prosthetic graft infection, CFAs have been used for infrainguinal revascularization. Cryopreserved femoropopliteal arterial allografts used for infrageniculate revascularization had a primary patency rate of 51% at 17 months in one series of 17 bypasses.[43] Because of short conduit length, a composite bypass was necessary in 53% of cases. Another series of 35 allografts reported 39% primary patency and 59% secondary patency rates at 18 months. Two grafts required replacement as a result of aneurysmal degeneration.[113] A 5-year primary patency rate of 16% was achieved in a retrospective multicenter trial of 165 fresh and cryopreserved arterial allografts.[114] These results suggest that in lower extremity bypass, cryopreserved arterial allografts have low patency rates, are predisposed to aneurysmal degeneration, do not offer any significant advantage over the use of saphenous vein allografts, and have the additional potential drawback of the need to connect two or more arterial segments together to create a conduit of sufficient length.

Arterial allografts have been used extensively for the management of primary and prosthetic aortic infection. To this end, fresh aortic allografts stored for less than 1 month at 4°C have been used with some success.[92,115-117] An Italian study of 44 patients treated with 13 fresh and 31 cryopreserved aortic allografts did not find a difference in patient outcomes.[116] A French study of 179 patients treated with 111 fresh and 68 cryopreserved grafts, however, did note long-term differences in graft behavior: fresh allografts were associated with allograft rupture and an increased incidence of late graft-related complications.[92]

There are five published studies with more than 40 grafts that provide information about the outcomes of cryopreserved aortic allografts for the treatment of aortic infection (Table 89-2). Most of these represent multi-institutional registries with relatively short follow-up periods.[95,118,119] Although many patients had polymicrobial aortic infection, staphylococcal species were the most common organisms cultured.[95,99,116,119,120] As expected, perioperative mortality rates were high and ranged between 6% and 17%. Factors associated with increased mortality included emergency or urgent surgery and the presence of an aortoenteric fistula.[99,119] Aortic allograft repair in a cohort of patients with aortoenteric fistulae was associated with a mortality rate of 83%.[119]

Table 89-2 Summary of Published Cryopreserved Aortic Allograft Series Containing More Than 40 Grafts

Series	Total Number of Grafts	Number of Aortic Grafts	Follow-up (months)	30-Day Mortality (%)	Number with Perioperative Major Complications (%)	Number of Allograft Ruptures (%)	Amputation Rate (%)	Number of Graft Thromboses (%)	Graft Dilatation (%)
Zhou et al.[95]	42	42	12.5*	7 (17)	21 (50)	0	6 (14)	1 (6)	0
Kieffer et al.[92]	68	68	34†	9 (13)‡	31 (45)	1 (2)	0	2 (3)	NR
Vogt et al.[99]	49	49	27*	3 (6)	10 (20)	5 (10)	NR	NR	NR
Noel et al.[118]	56	56	5.3*	7 (13)	28 (55)	8 (14)	3 (5)	5 (9)	1 (2%)
Verhelst et al.[119]	90	66	36*	16 (17)	40 (44)	12 (13)	1 (1)	8 (9)	7 (8%)

*Mean follow-up.
†Median follow-up.
‡In-hospital mortality.
NR, not reported.

As expected, these patients had very high perioperative complication rates, ranging between 20% and 55%. Allograft rupture was seen in the immediate postoperative period and up to 4 years of follow-up.[99] This devastating complication occurred in 2% to 14% of cases and was associated with high mortality. Allograft aneurysmal dilatation was noted to occur in as many as 8% of patients in one series.[119] Graft stenosis and thrombosis were more often associated with grafts extending to the iliac or femoral arteries.[92] Amputation rates ranged between 1% and 14%. Despite these sobering statistics, 87% and 60% of patients were free of aortic and iliofemoral complications or interventions, respectively, at 7 years in one large single-institution series.[92]

Aortic infection is one of the gravest conditions in peripheral vascular surgery. Therefore, allograft performance needs to be viewed against the results of other treatment options for the management of infected aortic grafts. Graft excision with extra-anatomic bypass was associated with a 30-day mortality of 13% and an amputation rate of 10%.[89,121] Likewise, in situ aortic graft replacement with a rifampicin-bonded prosthetic graft had a perioperative mortality rate of 18%.[90] Although cryopreserved aortic allografts clearly have a place in the management of prosthetic aortic graft infection, their precise role has yet to be defined clearly. They are associated with allograft dilatation and rupture, probably because of previously discussed immunologic mechanisms.[20,23,29,44,43] Graft surveillance protocols have yet to be standardized and validated. Although the use of current immunosuppressive regimens in these very ill patients is not practical, the development of more focused immunosuppressive therapy in the future may better define the role of aortic allografts in the armamentarium of vascular surgeons.

Human Umbilical Vein Grafts

Patency and Limb Salvage

The first large clinical experience with the use of HUV grafts was reported in 1988 by Dardik and coauthors. Nine hundred seven lower limb bypass procedures were performed in 799 limbs of 715 patients. The 5-year primary-assisted patency rate was 57% and 32% for femoropopliteal and femorotibial bypasses, respectively. The 5-year limb salvage rate ranged between 70% and 80%. Fifty-seven percent of the grafts exhibited aneurysmal dilatation at a mean follow-up of 5 years.[81] In 1989, ownership and manufacture of the HUV graft changed hands. In an attempt to address the issue of time-dependent graft degradation, efforts were made to improve the graft manufacturing process. Improved cross-linking with glutaraldehyde and upgraded quality control procedures, including time, temperature, and pressure determinants during manufacture, led to the development of a second-generation graft that was resistant to aneurysmal degeneration.[100] In parallel, Dardik and colleagues attempted to improve the patency of femorotibial HUV grafts by using adjunctive distal AVFs.[79] These investigators published an updated experience with 283 second-generation HUV grafts in 2002. Five-year primary patency rates for this graft were 60% and 50% for below-knee popliteal and tibial bypass, respectively. Five-year limb salvage rates were 80% and 65% for below-knee popliteal and tibial bypass, respectively. No graft aneurysmal degeneration was noted on duplex surveillance of these grafts.[122]

Neufang and associates published their three recent series of patients treated with the HUV graft for popliteal bypass,[123] composite bypass,[124] and composite sequential bypass.[125] Two hundred eleven patients treated by HUV femoropopliteal bypass had 5-year primary and secondary patency rates of 54% and 76%, respectively. Reported complications included early graft thrombosis in 17% and aneurysmal degeneration in 7%. This group did not use adjunctive distal AVFs but did recommend an aggressive anticoagulation protocol with perioperative and postoperative aspirin and clopidogrel, early postoperative heparin, and long-term warfarin to keep the international normalized ratio at 2.5.[123]

Fifty-four patients with critical limb ischemia treated by HUV–autologous vein composite bypass to tibial targets had 4-year primary patency, secondary patency, and limb salvage rates of 53%, 67%, and 88%, respectively. Patients who did not undergo anticoagulation had a significantly higher incidence of early graft thrombosis.[124] HUV–autologous vein

Table 89-3 Life-Table Analyses of Patency and Limb Salvage with Human Umbilical Vein Grafts

Series	Year	Number of Grafts Implanted	Aneurysm Formation (%)	Popliteal Bypass Patency (%)	Crural Bypass Patency (%)
Dardik et al.[81]	1988	907	57	57	33
Batt et al.[126]	1990	105	6	—	29*
Sato et al.[127]	1995	111	NR	—	61
Dardik et al.[122]	2002	283	0	56	43
Sommeling et al.[128]	1990	227	37	55/57 (BK/AK)	19
Johnson et al.[129]	2000	261	1	49	—
Neufang et al.[123]	2007	211	7	54	—

AK, above knee; BK, below knee; NR, not reported.
*At 3 years.

composite sequential femoral-tibial bypasses demonstrated lower long-term patency rates.[125] Patency and limb salvage results in recent studies using HUV grafts are listed in Table 89-3.[81,122,123,126-129]

Comparison of Human Umbilical Vein with Other Grafts

A number of studies compared the utility of HUV grafts with other conduits for infrainguinal revascularization. Cranley and colleagues reported a 3-year cumulative patency rate of 74% for umbilical vein grafts, 41% for PTFE grafts, and 76% for saphenous vein grafts when used for bypass to the popliteal artery in the setting of critical limb ischemia. HUV patency was comparable to PTFE graft patency when tibial targets were evaluated (31% versus 35%, respectively).[130] A small Scandinavian multicenter, prospective randomized trial compared outcomes of HUV grafts with PTFE for below-knee femoropopliteal bypass. The 4-year primary-assisted patency rate was 42% for umbilical vein grafts versus 22% for PTFE.[131] The New England Society for Vascular Surgery Registry revealed HUV to have improved 5-year patency rates in comparison to PTFE grafts for bypass to the below-knee popliteal artery (45% versus 20%, respectively).[132]

Another small, prospective randomized trial evaluated the outcomes of first-generation HUV grafts and PTFE grafts in above-knee femoropopliteal bypass. At 6 years, the primary patency rate of HUV was significantly higher than that of PTFE grafts (71.4% versus 38.7%, respectively). Thirty percent of HUV grafts demonstrated aneurysmal dilatation.[133] The largest randomized trial of HUV grafts was a Veterans Administration–sponsored trial in the United States in which the outcomes of HUV, saphenous vein, and PTFE grafts were evaluated in 752 patients undergoing above-knee femoropopliteal bypass. At 5 years, primary-assisted patency rates were 73%, 53%, and 39% for saphenous, umbilical vein, and PTFE grafts, respectively. Although HUV grafts outperformed PTFE grafts, they were associated with a higher incidence of early graft thrombosis and amputation.[129] This study prompted the manufacturer of this graft to recommend low-molecular-weight dextran in the postoperative period. Some investiga-

Table 89-4 Nonthrombotic Complications of Umbilical Vein Grafts

	First-Generation Grafts (1975-1985)	Second-Generation Grafts (1990-2000)
Total number of grafts	907	283
Failure without thrombosis	49 (5.4%)	2 (0.7%)
Infection	39 (4.3%)	9 (3.2%)
Stenosis	19 (2.1%)	5 (1.8%)
Dissection	1 (0.1%)	1 (0.4%)
Pseudoaneurysm	13 (1.4%)	1 (0.4%)
Aneurysm (surgical repair)	26 (2.9%)	0

Adapted from Dardik H, Wengerter K, Qin F, et al. Comparative decades of experience with glutaraldehyde-tanned human umbilical cord vein graft for lower limb revascularization: An analysis of 1275 cases. *J Vasc Surg.* 2002;35:64.

tors routinely recommend antiplatelet agents, postoperative heparin, and long-term warfarin therapy.[122,123]

Aside from thrombosis, umbilical vein grafts are associated with a number of complications, including infection, stenosis, dissection, and pseudoaneurysm. These complications vary between the first- and second-generation HUV grafts (Table 89-4).[122]

Although HUV grafts have demonstrated adequate outcomes and improved patency rates when compared with PTFE grafts, they have never made it into the mainstream of vascular practice. Many factors, including perceived handling difficulty, complexity of adjunctive distal AVF creation, and industry bias, partially account for this observation. Currently, the HUV graft is no longer commercially available, although a third-generation HUV graft is under development.[100]

Bovine Carotid Artery Xenografts

The BCA xenograft was first used for dialysis access by Chinitz and coworkers, who found that the graft tolerated frequent cannulation and maintained flow sufficient for suc-

Table 89-5 Published Reports Comparing the Cumulative Patency of Bovine Carotid Artery and Expanded Polytetrafluoroethylene Grafts

Series	Year	Grafts (n)	Cumulative Patency (%)		
			6 Mo	12 Mo	24 Mo
Kaplan et al.[139]	1976	BCA (16)	NR	NR	NR
		ePTFE (15)	NR	NR	NR
Butler et al.[138]	1977	BCA (103)	94	83	76
		ePTFE (184)	85	75	74
Tellis et al.[140]	1979	BCA (71)	NR	33*	NR
		ePTFE (66)	NR	62*	NR
Lilly et al.[141]	1980	BCA (113)	NR	73	NR
		ePTFE (83)	NR	84	NR
Anderson et al.[137]	1980	BCA (76)	NR	70*	45*
		ePTFE (100)	NR	87*	73*
Sabanayagam et al.[135]	1980	BCA (402)	57*	21*	NR
		ePTFE (225)	94*	91*	NR
Hurt et al.[142]	1983	BCA (62)	NR	84	72
		ePTFE (78)	NR	65	63
Anderson et al.[136]	2005	BCA (245)	NR	86	NR
		ePTFE (446)	NR	82	NR

Adapted from Scott EC, Glickman MH: Conduits for hemodialysis access. *Semin Vasc Surg.* 2007;20:158.s
BCA, bovine carotid artery; ePTFE, expanded polytetrafluoroethylene; NR, not reported.
*Significant difference between conduits.

cessful hemodialysis.[134] Patency rates of this graft range from 21% to 86% at 1 year and 45% to 76% at 2 years.[135-138] With the advent of PTFE and its use in hemodialysis access in the mid-1970s, multiple studies comparing BCA xenografts with PTFE grafts have been published (Table 89-5).[135-143] A prospective, controlled, randomized trial of 140 BCA and PTFE AV grafts found no significant differences in patency and complication rates.[142] Other trials, however, revealed PTFE grafts to have superior patency rates.[135,137,140] BCA xenografts are associated with higher infection[135,137] and aneurysmal degeneration[135,140] rates than PTFE AV grafts are. A 9% to 20% infection rate[135,137,144] and a 1% to 8% aneurysmal degeneration rate[135,138,140,144] have been observed.

Although BCA xenografts elicit a dense desmoplastic reaction, they are predisposed to aneurysmal degeneration, which is exacerbated by repeated cannulation during hemodialysis. They are prone to infection, and when it occurs, they are very difficult to excise because of intense inflammation and the fragile nature of the graft.[140] Finally, they are more expensive than PTFE grafts. These issues have limited widespread use of this graft for hemodialysis access.[143]

There have been a few published series on the use of different BCA xenografts for infrainguinal revascularization. In one series, 30% of the grafts underwent degeneration within 4 months of insertion.[145] A study of 112 grafts used for femoropopliteal bypass yielded a 1-year primary patency rate of 90%.[146] Another study of 58 grafts used for above-knee femoropopliteal bypass yielded a 56% 5-year primary-assisted patency rate. No graft infections or aneurysmal degeneration was noted.[59] Short available lengths, wide availability of PTFE, and concern about graft degeneration have dampened

enthusiasm for the use of BCA xenografts in lower extremity bypass.

Bovine Mesenteric Vein Xenografts

BMV xenografts have been successfully used for hemodialysis access. In one series of 50 grafts placed in 49 patients who had an average of 3.6 previous AVFs, a primary patency rate of 62% was noted at 30 months. Four infections but no aneurysmal degeneration developed.[147] In one prospective, multicenter registry, 183 patients with previous failed synthetic grafts were treated with a BMV hemodialysis access. Outcomes were compared with a concomitant nonrandomized group of patients who received PTFE grafts. One-year primary and secondary BMV patency rates were 36% and 66%, respectively. Although primary rates were similar to those of PTFE AV grafts, secondary rates were significantly higher for bovine xenografts. Graft infection was less common in the BMV xenograft group, and the pseudoaneurysm formation rate was similar to that seen with PTFE grafts. In six grafts, however, significant dilatation occurred.[61] In another recent series of 62 BMV grafts used for hemodialysis access, 30% primary and 58% secondary patency rates were reported. Thirteen infections occurred and six (10%) grafts required surgical excision. In two patients significant graft dilatation was noted.[148]

BMV xenografts appear to have acceptable patency rates that are similar to those seen with PTFE grafts. Although data are limited, these grafts do not appear to be any more predisposed than PTFE grafts to infection or pseudoaneurysm formation. The significance of the dilatation that occurs in some of these grafts is not yet clear. More research will be required before the role of this graft for hemodialysis access is more precisely defined.

BMV xenografts have been used for infrainguinal revascularization. In one small trial involving six patients, all grafts failed within 4 months.[82] In another trial of 32 patients with critical limb ischemia, a 16% primary patency rate was noted at 1 month. Most of the occlusions occurred within 1 day of the operation.[149] Given these results, this conduit cannot be recommended for infrainguinal bypass.

Future Directions

Biologic grafts differ from one another in composition and method of preparation. They are useful in a number of clinical scenarios and have earned a place in the armamentarium of modern vascular surgeons. They have not, however, delivered on the expectations that many early vascular surgeons had for these conduits. Despite an enormous amount of basic and clinical investigation they failed to become the ideal conduit. In fact, the search for such a conduit is still in progress.

Significant research is currently being conducted in an attempt to create a biologic nonimmunogenic xenograft. New techniques are being used to create cellular arterial scaffolds that may provide an inert backbone for future biologic grafts.[150-152] Re-endothelialization of such grafts may lead to improved performance.[153,154] It is still conceivable that in the future a biologic graft with little or no immunogenicity and characteristics similar to that of a normal artery or vein can be developed.

SELECTED KEY REFERENCES

Dardik H, Wengerter K, Qin F, Pangilinan A, Silvestri F, Wolodiger F, Kahn M, Sussman B, Ibrahim IM. Comparative decades of experience with glutaraldehyde-tanned human umbilical cord vein graft for lower limb revascularization: An analysis of 1275 cases. *J Vasc Surg.* 2002;35:64.
The largest single-center experience with human umbilical vein grafts.

Farber A, Major K, Wagner WH, Cohen JL, Cossman DV, Lauterbach SR, Levin PM. Cryopreserved saphenous vein allografts in infrainguinal revascularization: analysis of 240 grafts. *J Vasc Surg.* 2003; 38:15.
Largest single-center series of cryopreserved saphenous vein allografts for infrainguinal revascularization.

Katzman HE, Glickman MH, Schild AF, Fujitani RM, Lawson JH. Multicenter evaluation of the bovine mesenteric vein bioprosthesis for hemodialysis access in patients with an earlier failed prosthetic graft. *J Am Coll Surg.* 2005;201:223.
Largest multicenter registry of the use of bovine mesenteric vein grafts for dialysis access.

Kieffer E, Gomes D, Chiche L, Fléron MH, Koskas F, Bahnini A. Allograft replacement for infrarenal aortic graft infection: early and late results in 179 patients. *J Vasc Surg.* 2004;39:1009.
One of the largest single-center series of aortic allografts for the treatment of aortic infection.

Madden RL, Lipkowitz GS, Browne BJ, Kurbanov A. Experience with cryopreserved cadaveric femoral vein allografts used for hemodialysis access. *Ann Vasc Surg.* 2004;18:453.
One of the largest single-center series of CFV allografts for hemodialysis access.

Neufang A, Espinola-Klein C, Dorweiler B, Messow CM, Schmiedt W, Vahl CF. Femoropopliteal prosthetic bypass with glutaraldehyde stabilized human umbilical vein (HUV). *J Vasc Surg.* 2007;46:280.
Modern large series of human umbilical vein grafts for femoropopliteal bypass.

REFERENCES

The reference list can be found on the companion Expert Consult Web site at *www.expertconsult.com.*

CHAPTER 90

Aortic Stents and Stent-Grafts

Jon S. Matsumura

This chapter reviews the use of stents and stent-grafts for the endovascular treatment of aortic pathology. A detailed description of stent characteristics and stent-graft construction is presented, with specific attention paid to developments in devices that mitigate the failure modes of older technology. Delivery systems and implantation techniques are addressed in Chapter 86 (Technique: Endovascular Aneurysm Repair), and clinical results are covered in Chapters 129 (Abdominal Aortic Aneurysms: Endovascular Treatment) and 133 (Thoracic and Thoracoabdominal Aneurysms: Endovascular Treatment).

Endovascular aortic aneurysm repair (EVAR) was reported in 1986 by Volodos and colleagues.[1] However, it was Parodi and associates' report in 1991 that developed interest in endovascular treatment with abdominal and thoracic stent-grafts.[2] These early grafts were custom, hand-made devices consisting of graft material placed over balloon-expandable or self-expanding metal stents. The initial designs were single-unit, tubular configurations. Subsequently, groups in Malmö, Montefiore, and elsewhere developed stent-grafts with a distal landing site in the common femoral artery.[3,4] The contralateral iliac artery was occluded, and a femorofemoral bypass graft was constructed to provide arterial inflow for the contralateral leg. The Sydney group, during this same time period, used the concept of modular components, thereby providing adaptability to the varied anatomy of aortoiliac aneurysms.[5]

Commercial interest in EVAR has resulted in rapid acceleration of device innovation to address many major shortcomings of the initial stent-grafts. Current stent-grafts have developed considerably in the past 2 decades, with more durable fixation systems, fatigue resistance, and conformability. These systems have a wide variety of configurations that can treat the majority of infrarenal aortoiliac aneurysms. In the first decade of development, thoracic stent-grafts faced more challenging anatomic and physiologic conditions, and many lessons were learned. Current commercial grafts are at the tubular design stage, with technologies emerging to address branch aortic anatomy.

◼ AORTIC STENTS

Most stents that are used in the aorta are labeled for biliary or tracheobronchial use. Because the market size has been too small to warrant expenditure on a premarket application development path, despite clinical needs that are more diverse than the available endoprostheses, the physician often chooses to use a stent that is not specifically designed for the aortic clinical situation but is the best option available. A specific warning often comes on the package label, "Warning: the safety and effectiveness of this device for use in the vascular system has not been established and can result in serious harm and/or death." Despite these limitations, the endovascular use of aortic stents has become the preferred treatment option for a number of aortic diseases because the overall risks in comparison to the alternatives favor an endovascular approach.

General Categories of Stents

Stents have traditionally been classified as balloon-expandable and self-expanding designs.

Balloon-Expandable Stents

There are many characteristics of balloon-expandable stents that require consideration when deciding what to use for a given patient, including deployment accuracy, crush resistance, length and expandable size, foreshortening, deliverability, tapering, shape, recoil, radiopacity, and corrosion resistance.

Because of the perception that balloon-expandable stents have a higher degree of precision in deployment, they are sometimes selected when treating lesions near critical branch vessels. These stents are often favored in aortic applications because they have sufficient hoop strength or compression resistance to enable them to overcome strong elastic recoil after balloon expansion of stenotic aortic tissue. Hoop strength helps maintain an adequate lumen when treating resilient calcified lesions. Aortic uses require stent sizes larger than most other endoprosthesis applications, and many balloon-expandable stents are dilated to a significantly larger extent than the labeled maximum size, particularly for endovascular repair of aortic aneurysms, where diameters above 25 and even 30 mm are required. At these large diameters, balloon-expandable stents undergo severe foreshortening. A large balloon-expandable stent that is commonly used in the aorta is the Palmaz XL Transhepatic Biliary Stent, P4010 (Cordis Corp., Miami, FL) (Fig. 90-1, right side).

Deliverability of large balloon-expandable stents is a major issue. They often require large sheath access across the lesion and are usually unmounted. The technical art of delivering unmounted stents is rarely practiced in the contemporary era

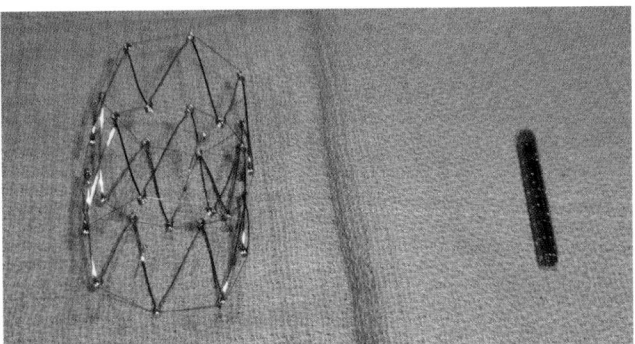

Figure 90-1 Self-expanding (*left*) and balloon-expandable (*right*) stents, frequently used off-label in the aorta.

of premounted stents for most small and medium-sized applications. Unmounted stents must be crimped tightly by the physician onto a large balloon (such as an aortic valvuloplasty balloon), delivered to the target site, and then expanded precisely. These large stents are inflexible and difficult to crimp because of the thickness of the struts, so they can easily slip onto the hub end of the balloon catheter during introduction or migrate off the tip end of the balloon during deployment. Specific techniques that must be used to prevent or recover from these possible catastrophes are discussed in Chapter 129 (Abdominal Aortic Aneurysms: Endovascular Treatment).

Another important characteristic is the ability to taper or mold a stent for treatment of a focal stenosis or coarctation of the aorta. Many physicians prefer to dilate these lesions cautiously to a diameter just large enough to eradicate a significant pressure gradient because full expansion might result in higher risk of aortic rupture. For example, if the focal stenosis and aortic stent are dilated to 10 mm but the adjacent aorta is 18 mm above and below the lesion, tapering the stent into an hourglass shape is favored to minimize later stent migration and avoid leaving bare metal suspended in the aortic lumen. The design pattern of different stents allows them to taper to a variable degree. More recently, specific shaped stents are emerging for niche aortic branch applications.

All balloon-expandable stents demonstrate some degree of recoil after expansion, but it is usually small and clinically negligible. Clinicians should be aware that some newer metals, such as cobalt-chromium alloys, have greater recoil than do their stainless steel predecessors, and balloon sizes and target inflation pressures may be slightly larger to attain the nominal size after recoil. As long as the underlying lesion has similar elastic recoil, rupture or inadequate apposition should not be a clinical issue. Radiopacity is a strong attribute of most balloon-expandable stents, particularly the large sizes used for aortic applications. Finally, clinicians should be aware that the biocompatibility of different metals has not been tested for off-label indications and the potential exists for accelerated corrosion and metal ion leaching, with unknown consequences.

Self-Expanding Stents

Self-expanding stents suitable for off-label aortic use are composed of stainless steel, nitinol, or Elgiloy. Detailed characteristics of each of these metals are presented in Chapter 91 (Nonaortic Stents and Stent-Grafts). Nitinol and Elgiloy self-expanding stents labeled for iliac use are generally available in diameters up to 10 mm and lengths of 6 to 7 cm for that diameter. Nitinol stents have relatively little foreshortening, high radial strength, excellent conformability to eccentric lesions, and good deliverability, and most have radiopaque markers on the ends to improve fluoroscopic visualization.

Elgiloy stents are more radiopaque but less conformable than nitinol. They have the additional advantage of reconstrainable deployment such that up to 80% of the stent can be deployed and then reconstrained and the deployment location readjusted up to three times. This characteristic is useful because of the less predictable foreshortening of Elgiloy stents. There is a more limited selection of stents larger than 10 mm, which are often required for aortic use, and they all require sheaths larger than 6 Fr. The SMART Control (Cordis) nitinol biliary stents come in diameters up to 14 mm and lengths up to 80 mm. The Elgiloy tracheobronchial Wallstent (Boston Scientific, Natick, MA) is available in diameters up to 24 mm and lengths of 90 mm. The Elgiloy and polyester Wallgraft stent-graft comes in sizes up to 14 mm with a length of 70 mm for that diameter. The stainless steel Cook Z-Stent, Gianturco-Rosch Tracheobronchial Design, GTZS-40-5.0 (Cook, Inc., Bloomington, IN) (Fig. 90-1, left side), is available in sizes up to 40-mm diameter. These larger sizes are useful in fashioning custom-made stent-grafts for some aortic applications. These stents also come as a two-stent complex composed of two 2.5-cm-long devices sutured together with nylon suture and have welded barbs for fixation.

◼ CHARACTERISTICS OF STENT-GRAFTS FOR ENDOVASCULAR REPAIR OF ABDOMINAL AORTIC ANEURYSMS AND THORACIC AORTIC PATHOLOGY

Stent-graft diversity has broadened the available characteristics that may be selected for treatment of an individual patient. Various options exist for stent-graft fixation, sealing, patency, sizing, and durable exclusion of aortic aneurysms. Radiopacity, deployment precision, ease of use, and access issues of sheath size and flexibility are additional important attributes. Some of these options are found in most devices, whereas others are unique to specific systems. It is important to note that the clinical value of many of these performance attributes is difficult to quantify, and it is even more difficult to directly compare these attributes among devices.

Because direct randomized trials comparing these devices have not been performed, much of the clinical value of the characteristics discussed in the following text remains in the arguable domains of convinced physicians and manufacturer-sponsored marketing. Indeed, it may be more dependent on the physician's having mastered knowledge of the advantages and disadvantages of a system than on the differences among systems. Hence, education should stress prevention, detection, and treatment of failure modes of devices and not focus on marginal iterative improvements in devices.

Fixation

An essential feature of all stent-grafts is a method of fixation to inhibit migration after deployment. Aortic blood flow delivers constant force that pushes the proximal end of stent-grafts caudad. In tortuous anatomy, vector forces tend to cause separation of components and craniad migration of the distal components. Aortic lengthening forces intercomponent separation. Several mechanisms have been engineered to resist these forces, which may frequently exceed 9 N.[6,7] The magnitude of these forces is graphically illustrated by the rare failures of early EVAR devices (Fig. 90-2).

Positive Fixation, Column Support, and Friction

Positive fixation describes the use of metal hooks, barbs, anchors, or supplemental staples that embed in the aortic wall. In endografts with stents that run the full length of the device, column stiffness helps hold the cranial end of the device in place by "standing" it on the iliac arteries or aortic bifurcation. This concept is supported by finding that long iliac seal zones reduce infrarenal migration.[8] The outward radial force

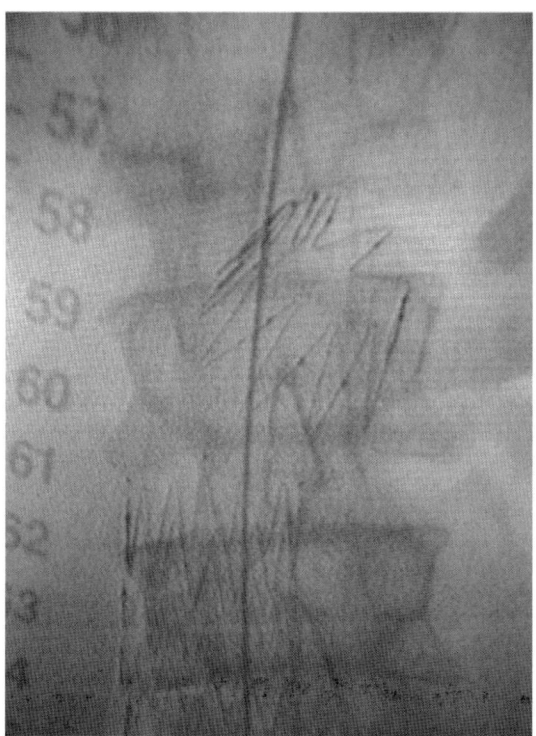

Figure 90-2 Top stent separation of an early endograft design demonstrating forces that promote late migration. *(Courtesy of Geoffrey White, MD.)*

of the stents themselves creates friction that retards migration. Some devices have polyester fuzz or other prosthetic material that induces a fibrotic reaction in the necks that helps hold a device in place. These methods are not exclusive, and several devices include a combination of these characteristics. There is some evidence that positive fixation provides high fixation force, which may lead to low rates of long-term migration.[9]

Infrarenal versus Suprarenal Fixation

Suprarenal fixation is an option in which the fixation component of a bare-metal stent is separated from the sealing component of the infrarenal neck portion of the stent-graft. The suprarenal aortic neck is more resistant to late neck dilatation, and long-term fixation may be improved.[10,11] Concern has been raised about late renal infarction, but data are insufficient to assess the relationship between late renal dysfunction and suprarenal bare stents.[12] If open conversion and complete graft explantation should become necessary, suprarenal fixation may present more difficulties.

Sealing

Almost any endograft will seal in a straight, cylindrical, 15-mm-long neck without thrombus or calcification. However, many patients do not have this type of infrarenal neck, and stent-grafts must therefore be able to address diseased aortic walls and neck anatomy that is angled, conical, eccentric, or reverse taper in shape. Seal zone adjuncts include covered flares that expand beyond the nominal diameter of the main graft, polyester fuzz, and sealing cuffs. Some forms of positive fixation could impair sealing if the protruding elements fail to embed in the aortic wall but instead prevent the sealing elements from coming in contact with the aortic neck, as may happen with a severely calcified area of neck. The basic stent pattern of the seal zone of the device will have a large impact on sealing and conformability; these are critical factors for angulated necks. The stent design also has an impact in that shorter and smaller cell sizes are more likely to seal. Longer cell sizes could possibly lead to channeling and perigraft blood flow. The scallop depth of the cranial border of the graft material of the device will also determine the effective required seal zone of the device.

Limb Patency

The unsupported limbs of early EVAR devices were often plagued by limb occlusion, which prompted frequent off-label use of stents within the limbs. Late fabric erosion with a type III endoleak and aneurysm enlargement or rupture is one complication that illustrates a late pitfall of off-label use without adequate evidence of safety and effectiveness (Fig. 90-3). Although most fully supported endografts provide excellent long-term patency, there is sufficient space between stents or stent rings in some devices that limb kinking, compression, and occlusion may occur uncommonly. Concomi-

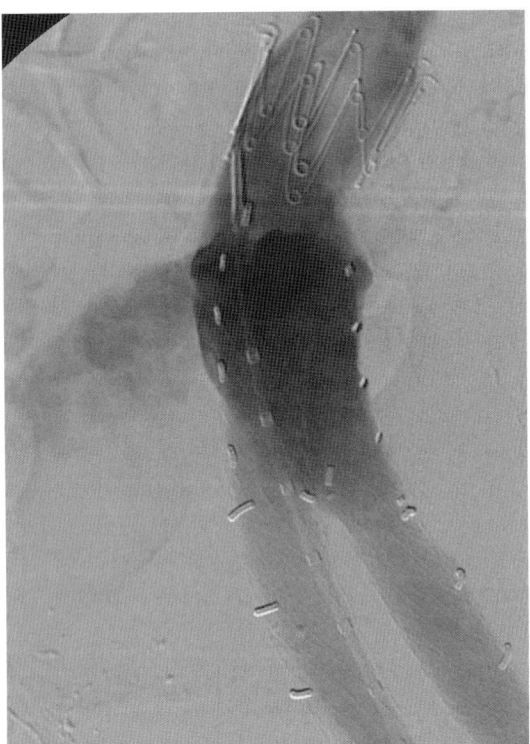

Figure 90-3 Off-label stent use and late type IIIb endoleak. The stents eroded through standard-thickness polyester graft fabric after 6 years. Regulatory trials typically do not extend follow-up beyond 5 years.

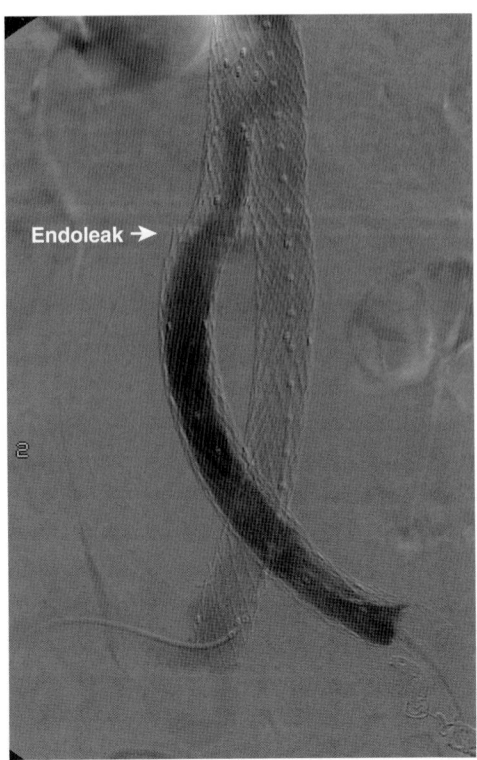

Figure 90-4 Late fabric tear and type IIIb endoleak that led to hemorrhagic rupture of an aneurysm 6 years after implantation. If the greater curve of the device is embedded in aneurysm thrombus, it may be prone to significant fabric degeneration.

tant iliac arterial injury during EVAR, heavy circumferential distal aortic or iliac calcification, an abrupt kink in the limb associated with severe iliac tortuosity, and excessive graft limb oversizing are factors that may lead to limb occlusion.

Sizing

EVAR stent-grafts come in a wide range of aortic diameters, iliac diameters, and graft lengths that are labeled for varying arterial diameters and angulations. Larger-diameter devices allow treatment of more patients with EVAR, although sizing is not directly comparable because of differences in methods of measuring aortic neck diameter and angulation. The complexity of case planning varies with each system because of differences in sizing windows, techniques, tapering zones (if any), and usable seal zones. Some devices have long primary components and may require fewer additional pieces to perform ideal treatment from the lowest renal artery to the hypogastric origins. Some systems have longer main bodies or long component overlap junctions (2 to 3 cm) that provide good long-term intercomponent stability.

Graft Material

The graft material is key to durable exclusion of the aneurysm. The polyester or polytetrafluoroethylene (PTFE) graft material is similar to that used for open surgical repair and is described in Chapter 88 (Prosthetic Grafts). However, the

environment of implantation is the thrombus of the aneurysm, which results in different incorporation than when the graft is placed in the retroperitoneum or an evacuated aneurysm sac. In contrast to open grafts, which become incorporated in fibrous material, stent-grafts are suspended in the thrombus and may develop transudates or holes that do not close.[13-15] The graft material may be abraded by constant wear against metallic stent components or be subject to weave deformation by attachment sutures (Fig. 90-4). Sutures themselves may wear or break, causing subsequent increased movement and abrasion. Furthermore, the materials selected are sometimes thinner to allow compression into smaller delivery catheters, and late deterioration or damage may occur sooner. Some stent-grafts are sutured only at the ends of the stent, whereas others use a composite bonding process without sutures. Many first-generation devices were prone to suture breakage or early graft wear, and graft materials, manufacturing tolerances, and suturing have subsequently been modified to improve durability.

Radiopacity

Stent components are visible with high-quality fluoroscopic equipment, but many EVAR procedures are performed with portable C-arms and thus visualization may be difficult in heavy patients. Delivery systems and stent-grafts have additional radiopaque markers to facilitate rotational orientation, deployment, and gate cannulation. Such markers vary with

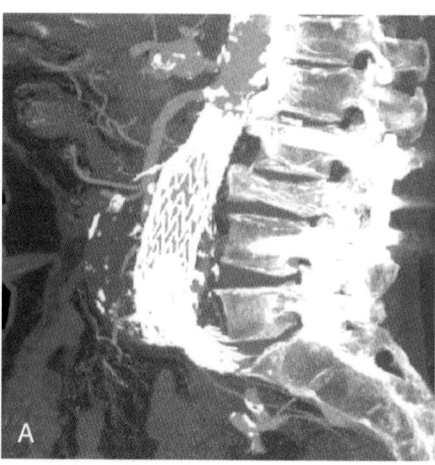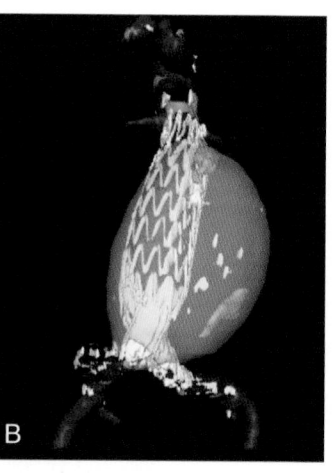

Figure 90-5 Type Ia endoleak (**A**) and caudad migration (**B**).

each graft, and not all are positioned at the very edge of the graft material, which is not itself radiopaque. Some markers are circumferential, whereas others are positioned intermittently around the circumference of the device.

Deployment Precision and Ease of Use

Many methods are used to deliver and deploy the device. Deployment systems are important components of an EVAR system and vary in flexibility, trackability, valve function, outer diameter of the ipsilateral and contralateral sheaths, number of times that a large sheath must be inserted, ability to perform concurrent angiography, and deployment precision. The labeling, torque responsiveness, need for exchange-length wires, difficulty in cannulating a contralateral gate or snaring a contralateral wire, cannulation adjuncts, and other attributes all contribute to the relative complexity of the deployment sequence. Ease of use is only one aspect of deployment system performance. Difficulty delivering and deploying the device may result in potentially fatal iliac artery injury or catastrophic misdeployment and coverage of visceral or renal branches. Procedural techniques are covered in detail in Chapter 86 (Technique: Endovascular Aneurysm Repair).

▪ MECHANISMS OF FAILURE

Several failure modes accompany EVAR.[16,17] The most concerning failure modes are those that are unpredictable and catastrophic (i.e., manifested as hemorrhagic aneurysm rupture).[18-21] Fortunately, most device issues can be prevented by a protocol of radiographic surveillance to monitor, detect, and re-treat problems, when indicated, at an asymptomatic stage. A common issue is endoleaks, which are specifically defined and their management addressed in Chapter 129 (Abdominal Aortic Aneurysms: Endovascular Treatment).[22]

Migration

Migration can be defined as movement of the device greater than 10 mm or any endograft displacement associated with

a new type I endoleak or the need for a secondary procedure (Fig. 90-5). Lower thresholds will detect migration earlier but result in more false positives. Some studies focus only on caudad migration of the proximal end of the main trunk and do not address migration of components or the distal end of the device. Migration in any form can lead to type I and type III endoleaks, and it is a significant risk factor for late rupture. Migration is sometimes associated with severe angulation and aortic neck dilatation when the aorta or iliac arteries dilate above the nominal size of the device.[8,23-27]

Neck Dilatation

Clinically important dilatation occurs in a very small number of patients in the first 5 years after endovascular repair. The cause of late increases in neck diameter may be a continuation of the original aneurysmal process or may be a result of device oversizing, with the continued outward force affecting the structural morphology of the aortic neck. Long-term results are just emerging, and neck enlargement may be a significant long-term disadvantage of an unsutured endovascular attachment system.[11,28,29]

Fracture

Virtually every vascular implant has suffered fatigue fractures, and stent-grafts are no exception; fractures occur in stent struts, anchors, barbs, and hooks, and longitudinal structures are particularly susceptible. Older designs with welded anchors, connecting bars under compression along an inner curve, or longitudinal deployment spines have been abandoned. Poor design predictions, lack of adequate surface polishing, off-label ballooning of devices, and placement in adverse anatomy are additional contributing factors. When fractures do occur, they may lead to further complications such as migration, type I endoleak, or limb occlusion.[30] Pivotal trials of stent-grafts are rarely powered to detect low rates of fracture, even when using diligent central core imaging laboratories, and postmarketing data are important to identify these late events.[31,32]

Limb Occlusion

Obstruction of a limb is usually manifested as an acute onset of claudication, but if the ipsilateral hypogastric artery has been occluded, it may result in a threatened or nonsalvageable extremity.[33] The often-used off-label bell-bottom technique may be preferred when feasible because hypogastric flow is preserved.[34] Most limb occlusions occur with unsupported devices and take place early, but morphologic changes with a shrinking aneurysm sac can lead to kinking of limbs and the necessity for late secondary procedures to reopen and expand the graft limb.[35-38]

Sac Expansion and Graft Material Failure

Aneurysm sac size has been considered a surrogate measure of procedural success, and sac growth has been a cause for concern. Rates of sac enlargement vary with the type of graft placed, and some have been modified as graft material issues have been identified. Ultrafiltration results in sac enlargement without endoleak; it is characterized by a gray, fibrin-rich, gelatinous fluid found in the aneurysm sac after endovascular repair.[13,39,40] Material device failure is manifested later in the follow-up period. It includes fabric tears or disintegration and suture breaks causing separation and dislocation of the structural segments (see Figs. 90-2 to 90-4). Many of the newer designs have tried to address earlier causes of failure. However, the durability of these modified prostheses remains incompletely explored because of short follow-up.[41,42]

Complications Specific to Thoracic Aortic Endovascular Stent-Grafts

Endovascular treatment with thoracic stent-grafts has complications that are unique to thoracic endovascular aortic repair (TEVAR) and some that occur more frequently than with EVAR, such as fatigue, migration, and access issues because of the greater displacement forces and larger devices.

Proximal Aortic Injury

Retrograde dissection by a thoracic stent-graft can be indistinguishable from a spontaneous type A dissection that is forced to reenter in the aorta just above a previously placed TEVAR graft. Nevertheless, these dissections require urgent operative treatment and must be considered potentially device related. There are also reports of aortic perforation and proximal false aneurysm, and these aortic injuries may be more common with uncovered or sharp proximal stents or flares.

Compression/Collapse

Some devices may be subject to graft infolding, compression, or collapse, particularly when used off-label with excessive oversizing (e.g., in the setting of traumatic injury in young

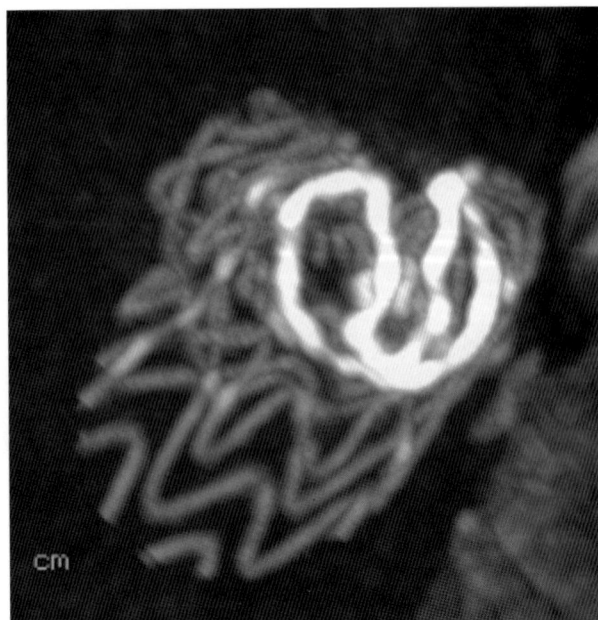

Figure 90-6 A TAG device became compressed after placement in a patient with aortic dissection. This case was successfully re-treated by balloon angioplasty. *(Courtesy of Geoffrey White, MD.)*

patients). High aortic flow, small radius of curvature of the arch, and poorly conformable ends of stent-grafts may also contribute to the compression phenomenon (Fig. 90-6). The compression can be asymptomatic or have catastrophic clinical implications if flow-limiting obstruction is present.[43]

■ CLINICAL APPLICATION: ENDOVASCULAR AORTIC ANEURYSM REPAIR

FDA-Approved Devices

The following sections review devices that have been approved by the U.S. Food and Drug Administration (FDA) as of January 2009. Table 90-1 summarizes some general features of stent-grafts.

Ancure

The Ancure (Boston Scientific, Natick, MA) bifurcated endograft system is a unibody design that is unsupported except at the aortic and iliac attachment sites. The proximal end features polyester fuzz to encourage sealing and ingrowth, as well as positive fixation hooks. The original design had welded hooks that fractured, and thus the device was redesigned with a more durable attachment system. Radiopaque markers run only along the sides of the graft, and the graft material is located at a set level relative to the attachment stents. The largest aortic size is 26 mm, and oversizing is not required. The unsupported limbs require intraoperative adjunctive stenting approximately 30% of the time. The device is complicated to deploy and requires the largest ipsilateral sheath,

Table 90-1 Stent-Graft Features

Feature	Stent-Graft								
	AneuRx	*Zenith*	*Excluder*	*Ancure*	*Talent*	*PowerLink*	*TAG*	*TX2*	*Talent*
Full-length stent support	X	X	X		X	X	X	X	X
Sealing adjuncts			X	X			X		
Modular	X	X	X		X	X	X	X	X
Hook/anchor fixation		X	X	X				X	
Bare proximal or distal attachment		X			X	X		X	X
Maximum main trunk diameter (mm)	28	36	31	26	36	28	40	42	46

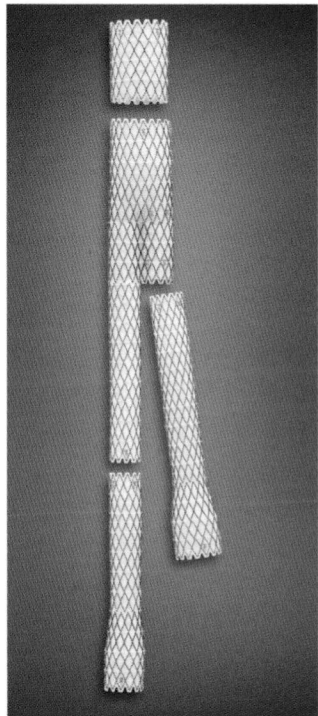

Figure 90-7 AneuRx graft.

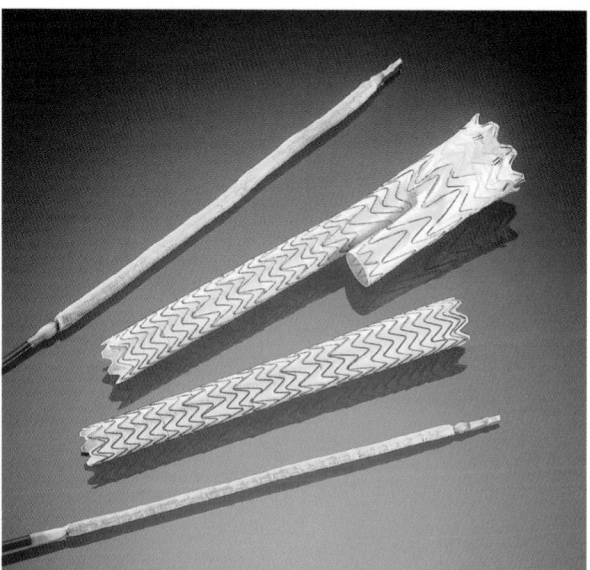

Figure 90-8 Excluder endoprosthesis.

approaching 27 Fr after expansion, and a 12-Fr contralateral sheath. The device is no longer manufactured.

AneuRx

The AneuRx (Medtronic, Santa Rosa, CA) graft is a modular, bifurcated, woven polyester graft supported with a nitinol exoskeleton (Fig. 90-7). The nitinol skeleton expands for friction fixation, and column strength provides some additional support. Radiopaque markers are strategically located near the ends of each component and define the contralateral overlap zone. The device comes in aortic diameters of 20 to 28 mm and iliac diameters of 12 to 24 mm. The ipsilateral sheath is 21 Fr, and the contralateral varies from 16.4 to 19 Fr, but the device can often be inserted bare with the tapered tip and hydrophilic system. When used bare, each device must be reinserted in the iliac artery. Slow deployment and buttressing techniques allow very precise deployment of the proximal end of this device.[44]

Excluder

The Excluder (W. L. Gore & Associates, Flagstaff, AZ) is a modular endoprosthesis composed of PTFE bonded to a nitinol exoskeleton (Fig. 90-8). There are proximal covered flares, positive fixation anchors, and a sealing cuff. Radiopaque markers are positioned at the very end of the graft material peaks, with intermittent shallow valleys. The device comes in aortic diameters of 23 to 31 mm and iliac diameters of 10 to 20 mm. The ipsilateral sheath is 18 to 20 Fr and the contralateral sheath is 12 to 18 Fr. The contralateral gate hole has a gold ring to improve radiopacity. The device is designed for rapid deployment with a simple pull cord, and concurrent arteriography is possible to facilitate distal positioning.

Zenith

The Zenith (Cook, Inc., Bloomington, IN) endograft is a bifurcated, modular, three-component system (Fig. 90-9). It is woven polyester sutured to stainless steel Z-stents and has a suprarenal bare stent component that provides positive fixation at the aortic attachment site. The stainless steel stents themselves provide good radiopacity, and supplemental markers are located near the proximal end of the graft

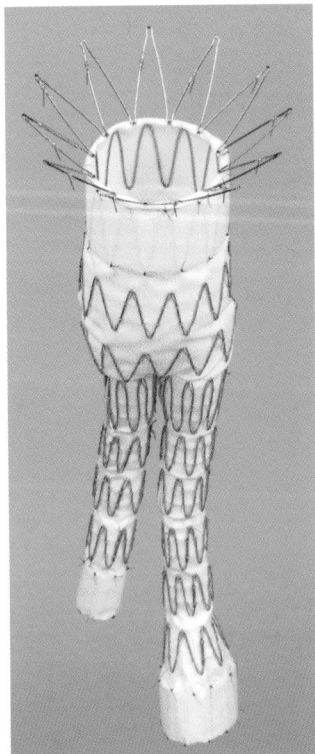

Figure 90-9 Zenith endograft.

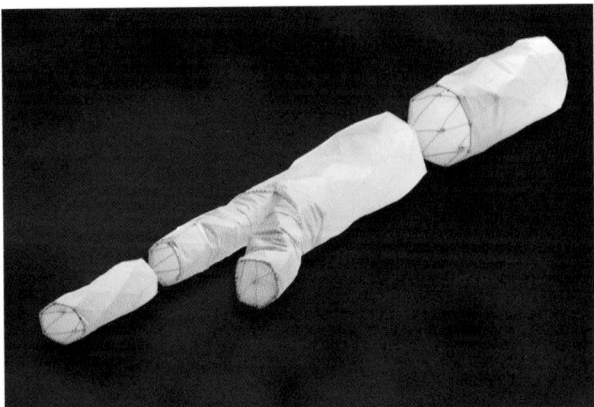

Figure 90-10 PowerLink endograft.

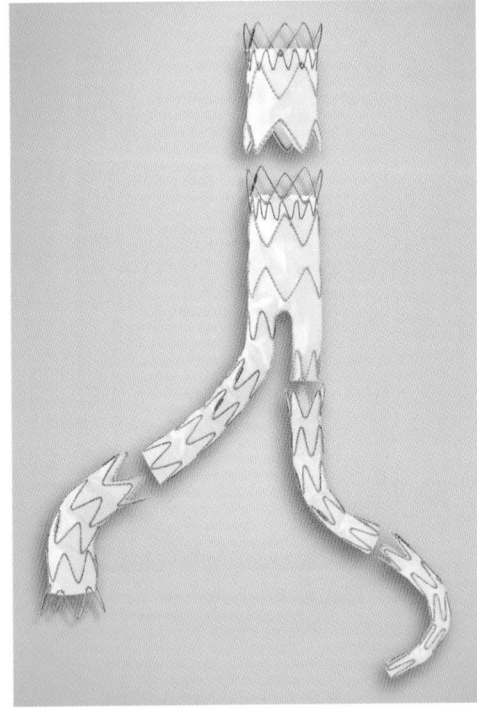

Figure 90-11 Talent system.

material. The device comes in 22- to 36-mm aortic diameters and 8- to 24-mm iliac diameters. The ipsilateral sheath ranges from 18 to 20 Fr and the contralateral sheath from 14 to 16 Fr. The device has a long main body and a staged deployment system, which facilitates cannulation. Because of the staged deployment system, deployment can be very precise.[45] It also permits off-label customized device modification.

PowerLink

The PowerLink (Endologix, Irvine, CA) endograft is a one-piece design that incorporates PTFE graft material with a cobalt-chromium alloy stent (Fig. 90-10). Fixation relies on column strength and placement of the device on the aortic bifurcation. Radiopacity is provided by the cobalt-chromium stents. The device comes in 25- and 28-mm aortic diameters, an iliac diameter of 16 mm, and limb extensions with distal diameters of 16, 20, and 25 mm. Larger aortic extensions with suprarenal fixation are available. The ipsilateral sheath is 21 Fr, the contralateral sheath is 12.5 Fr, and the limb extension sheaths are 17 and 19 Fr, but the device can often be inserted bare. A preloaded hollow 0.035-inch wire facilitates contralateral access. The system usually requires placement of at least one aortic cuff, although the main body is one piece.[46]

Talent

The Talent (Medtronic, Santa Rosa, CA) system is composed of woven polyester graft material sutured to a nitinol lattice (Fig. 90-11). A bare top stent provides suprarenal friction

fixation. For improved conformability and sealing, there is an additional sinusoidal stent at the proximal end that is about 8 mm long from apex to apex, as opposed to the main stents, which are about 16 mm long. It is labeled for a 10-mm or greater proximal neck length and 60 degrees of angulation or less. It is available in 22- to 36-mm diameters and has flared and tapered iliac limbs ranging from 8 to 24 mm in diameter. The ipsilateral sheath ranges from 22 to 24 Fr and the contralateral sheath from 18 to 20 Fr.[47,48]

Emerging Technology

Several devices are under investigation, including modified versions of approved devices. They have the potential to provide options for the management of patients with anatomy that is currently off-label. Such options include prefabricated fenestrations, in vivo fenestrations, branches, larger aortic sizes, conformable designs, staged deployment, articulated deployment, reconstrainable deployment, stapled fixation, and smaller introducers. Several of these options have been introduced into the literature in single-center experiences of the developers of the newer technology. Some of these advances are likely to be considered pioneering work, similar to the original descriptions of Parodi.[2] However, caution is warranted in overly eager acceptance of technologic advances because new features are usually accompanied by discovery of novel failure modes. In fact, many EVAR and TEVAR devices had begun multicenter investigational device exemption trials and later been abandoned after major technical flaws in the implant or delivery system emerged.[31]

Graft Selection (Anatomic) and Primary Device Characteristics

Graft selection is a complex decision in the reality of a competitive commercial marketplace. However, from a clinical perspective, it can be rather simple—use the system that the physician has mastered. For patients with suitable anatomy, physician preference for a familiar device is important. Detailed knowledge of sizing, deployment techniques, failure modes, expected outcomes, and reintervention techniques can result in outcomes superior to those with open repair.[48-52]

There are a few anatomic situations in which one device may be preferred, although even in these situations a surgeon with mastery of one device could probably make that device work for even difficult cases. Larger aortic and iliac diameters can be treated with the Zenith and Talent systems. Disadvantaged iliac access can often be overcome with the Excluder because of the smaller sheath size and flexibility and trackability of the deployment system. Very short lengths from the lowest renal artery to the bifurcation can be treated with the PowerLink graft. Angulated aortic necks are not well treated with any approved system, but more flexible investigational devices and the use of an off-label aortic stent can overcome many challenging necks. Similarly, short necks may be addressed with the Talent system, investigational fenestrated devices, or off-label branch vessel kissing stents.[53]

CLINICAL APPLICATION: THORACIC ENDOVASCULAR AORTIC ANEURYSM REPAIR

FDA-Approved Devices

TAG

The TAG (W. L. Gore & Associates, Flagstaff, AZ) is a modular endoprosthesis composed of PTFE bonded to a nitinol exoskeleton (Fig. 90-12). On both ends of the device are covered flares and a sealing cuff. Radiopaque gold ring markers are positioned near the end of the graft, but flares extend beyond these rings. The device comes in aortic diameters of 26 to 40 mm and lengths of 100 to 200 mm. The

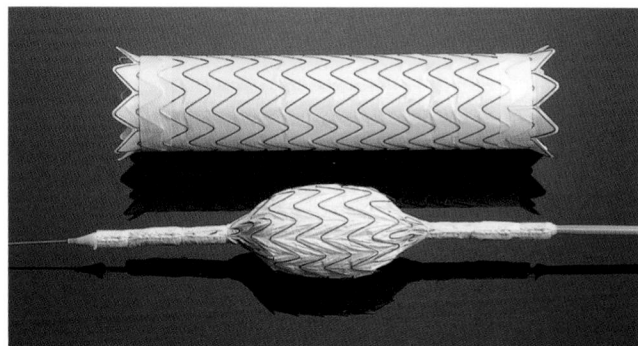

Figure 90-12 TAG endoprosthesis.

sheath ranges from 20 to 24 Fr. At least a 20-mm-long neck is required. The device is intended to be deployed rapidly from the middle section outward by pulling a deployment cord.[54]

Talent

The Talent system (Medtronic, Santa Rosa, CA) is composed of woven polyester graft sutured to a nitinol lattice with a proximal bare stent (see Fig. 90-11). It is available in diameters of 22 to 46 mm. The sheath ranges from 22 to 25 Fr. There is an additional sinusoidal sealing stent at the proximal end that is about 8 mm long. It is labeled for larger-diameter aortic necks that are 20 mm or longer.[55]

TX2

The TX2 endograft (Cook, Inc., Bloomington, IN) is a modular system (Fig. 90-13). Each component is woven polyester sutured to stainless steel Z-stents, with a barbed covered top stent on the proximal components and an uncovered barbed stent at the caudal aortic attachment site of the distal components; these barbed stents provide positive fixation at both ends. The proximal device comes in aortic diameters of 28 to 42 mm, 4-mm tapered devices with top diameters of 32 to 42 mm, and lengths of up to 216 mm. The distal component comes in diameters of 28 to 42 mm and lengths of up to 207 mm, not including the bare distal stent. Sheaths range from 20 to 22 Fr. Because of the staged deployment system, deployment can be very precise, but at least a 30-mm-long neck is required.[56]

Investigational Devices

Many devices have investigational components in larger diameters and lengths, and there are specifically designed devices to address traumatic injury and aortic dissection. A fascinating developmental area is the treatment of thoracoabdominal and arch aneurysms with scalloped or branched endografts.[57,58] These devices are under development worldwide, but none are currently available commercially in the United States. Several other innovative concepts are being explored for branch vessel involvement.[59-61]

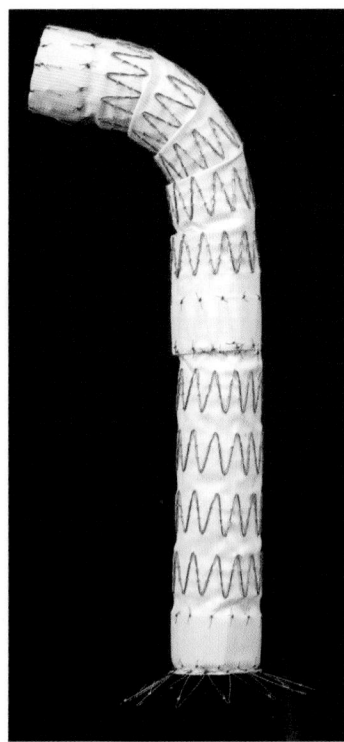

Figure 90-13 TX2 endograft.

Graft Selection (Anatomic) and Primary Device Characteristics

As with EVAR, comprehensive knowledge of sizing, deployment techniques, and failure modes results in excellent outcomes when compared with open repair. However, graft selection for TEVAR is more important than for EVAR. Inappropriate sizing can have catastrophic implications because open thoracic surgical repair is associated with much higher morbidity and mortality. Some patients with focal mid-descending thoracic aneurysms or large ulcers can be treated with any of the approved systems, but many patients may have anatomy that is better suited to a particular system. Such anatomic situations include larger aortic diameters, best treated with the TX2 and Talent systems; tapered short aortas, best treated with the TX2, and poor iliac access, best treated with the TAG and TX2 because of the smaller sheath size and longer devices that require fewer passes through small iliac arteries. The predictability of the staged TX2 deployment system is favored in some situations. Off-label branch vessel kissing stents may be more compatible with the TAG system, with short stent cells allowing sealing in short seal zones.

Innovation has characterized stent-grafts since the very beginning, and clinical research continues to identify the strengths and weaknesses of EVAR and TEVAR. As specific device failure modes are recognized, further engineering will lead to improved performance of these complex devices.

SELECTED KEY REFERENCES

Carpenter JP, for the Endologix Investigators. Midterm results of the multicenter trial of the PowerLink bifurcated system for endovascular aortic aneurysm repair. *J Vasc Surg.* 2004;40:849-859.
Data on the pivotal trial of an EVAR system used to treat smaller aneurysms.

Criado FJ, Fairman RM, Becker GJ. Talent LPS AAA stent graft: results of a pivotal clinical trial. *J Vasc Surg.* 2003;37:709-715.
Data from the pivotal trial of most recently approved endograft system with inclusion of shorter-length infrarenal necks.

Greenberg RK, Chuter TA, Sternbergh WC 3rd, Fearnot NE; Zenith Investigators. Zenith AAA endovascular graft: intermediate-term results of the US multicenter trial. *J Vasc Surg.* 2004;39:1209-1218.
Summary of pivotal trial data with a suprarenal fixation system.

Makaroun MS, Dillavou ED, Wheatley GH, Cambria RP, for the Gore TAG Investigators. Five-year results of endovascular treatment with the Gore TAG device compared with open repair of thoracic aortic aneurysms. *J Vasc Surg.* 2008;47:912-918.
Summary of a multicenter trial with long-term follow-up of both TEVAR and control groups.

Matsumura JS, Cambria RP, Dake MD, Moore RD, Svensson LG, Snyder S, for the TX2 Clinical Trial Investigators. International controlled clinical trial of TEVAR with the TX2: one-year results. *J Vasc Surg.* 2008;47:247-257; discussion 257.
Summary of a recent multicenter trial of TEVAR and open repair.

Peterson BG, Matsumura JS, Brewster DC, Makaroun MS; Excluder Investigators. Five-year report of a multicenter controlled clinical trial of open versus endovascular treatment of abdominal aortic aneurysms. *J Vasc Surg.* 2007;45:885-890.
Summary report of 5-year core laboratory EVAR and control data showing that reintervention does not erase the early postprocedure benefits of EVAR.

Rutherford RB, Krupski WC. Current status of open versus endovascular stent-graft repair of abdominal aortic aneurysm. *J Vasc Surg.* 2004;39:1129-1139.
Classic paper reviewing many of the failure modes of stent-grafts that have been struck by "lightening."

Zarins CK, for the AneuRx Clinical Investigators. The US AneuRx clinical trial: 6-year clinical update 2002. *J Vasc Surg.* 2003;37:904-908.
Update of the AneuRx device, which was one of the first commercially available systems in the United States.

REFERENCES

The reference list can be found on the companion Expert Consult Web site at *www.expertconsult.com.*

CHAPTER 91

Nonaortic Stents and Stent-Grafts

Benjamin Pearce and William D. Jordan, Jr.

Endovascular therapy has rapidly changed the landscape of vascular surgical practice over the past decade. A major thrust into catheter-based therapy was initiated in 1999 with Food and Drug Administration (FDA) approval of endografts for aneurysmorrhaphy. As this important technique became ubiquitous, surgeons began to use stents in other vascular beds both for initial therapy and as secondary treatment after failed vascular grafts. Endovascular therapy with stents is now performed throughout the vascular system, including arteries and veins from the intracranial circulation to the tibial arteries.

As the use of endovascular stents has undergone more critical study, it has become evident that various vascular beds react differently to stent placement.[1-3] Furthermore, angioplasty and stenting alter the biology of the treated vessel, which has implications for both short- and long-term results. The nature of the lesion, as well as the vascular bed to be treated, has specific nuances that should guide the surgeon in choosing an appropriate stent.

This chapter is focused on considerations inherent in stent choice when one is performing endovascular interventions and monitoring patients after treatment. We briefly review the indications for using a stent in conjunction with balloon angioplasty in the nonaortic vascular beds and describe the interaction between vessel and stent. The desired outcome can dictate the optimal stent design for any given lesion. Relevant stent characteristics are described, especially deployment, cell design, precision, treatment length, deliverability, and the use of stent-grafts. Finally, adjunctive techniques and future stent designs that may have an impact on therapy are summarized.

HISTORICAL BACKGROUND

Stenting was initially developed for the treatment of acute technical failure of percutaneous angioplasty. Isolated dilatation of vessels with dilatation catheters was first introduced by Dotter in 1964. The technique was further refined in the 1970s by Gruentzig, who used smaller catheters with balloons attached that could be delivered through the vascular tree from a remote location. Balloon angioplasty became a popular technique in the 1980s but produced results inferior to those of most open surgical procedures because acute occlusion and intermediate restenosis rates were unacceptably high. Acute technical failure occurred as a result of elastic recoil, vasospasm, plaque rupture, or dissection. In addition, balloon

angioplasty can incur recurrent stenosis related to an intense hyperplastic response commonly seen in the first 2 years after the intervention. In initial series of coronary angioplasty, interval restenosis occurred in 30% to 50% of treated lesions.[4-6] Likewise, angiographically detected failure of isolated renal artery angioplasty was noted in 26%,[7,8] failure of iliac primary angioplasty in up to 32%,[1] and failure of femoropopliteal angioplasty in as many as 50%.[9,10] Stenting was introduced to improve results in a number of vascular beds.

Stenting after percutaneous angioplasty improves long-term patency by providing a better technical result. The goals of stenting are to ensure an adequate lumen, maintain flow, and reduce the embolic load. Achieving optimal luminal diameter leads to less impact of in-stent neointimal formation on flow through the stented lesion. Paradoxically, the stent itself has inherent properties that alter the normal vascular resistance to intimal formation and can lead to maladaptive remodeling. Major contributors to negative remodeling include a low-shear environment (<5 dyn/cm^2), direct intimal damage related to the procedure, and interaction between the arterial wall and the stent itself.

STENT-VESSEL INTERACTION

Vessel Injury. The degree of intimal response has been directly linked to the extent of vessel injury. Sullivan and colleagues used an experimental stent with beveled struts to demonstrate this negative remodeling effect in vivo in a swine model.[11] The experimental stent was designed to violate the internal elastic lamina. When compared with Palmaz stents, the experimental stent showed significantly greater neointimal formation in control vessels. Furthermore, the extent of vessel injury demonstrated a linear effect on absolute neointimal formation.

Inflammatory Response. An inflammatory response to stent placement has also been demonstrated histologically. In an early autopsy series after approval of coronary stenting, Farb and associates demonstrated inflammatory cell infiltration in the area of the vessel directly adjacent to the stent struts.[12] The absolute number of inflammatory cells present was significantly increased when the strut violated the internal lamina and penetrated the lipid core of the plaque. Subsequent analysis demonstrated that inflammatory mediators were present more than 6 months after implantation. Other pathologic evaluation has demonstrated that in addition to the effect of the stent itself, bacterial contaminants brought to the vessel with the stent can likewise play a role in neointimal formation.[13]

Fluid Dynamics. Endovascular stents also alter the fluid dynamics of the stented segment. The most widely studied impact of stent placement on flow and negative remodeling is the creation of areas of low (<5 dyn/cm^2) wall shear stress (WSS). Alteration in WSS occurs both from change in luminal diameter and from the presence of the stent itself. In a computational flow model, LaDisa and coworkers demonstrated several characteristics of stent placement that create a low-shear environment.[14,15] The factor that led to the most significant increase in the percentage of vessel wall exposed to a low-shear environment was overdistention of the stented segment. Some degree of stent oversizing is necessary for appropriate apposition of the stent to the vessel wall to take advantage of the structural benefit of the radial force properties of the stent. However, LaDisa and associates demonstrated a 13-fold increase in total native vessel exposed to low WSS with 20% stent oversizing, versus that with 10% oversizing. This low WSS can subsequently lead to greater intimal hyperplasia and recurrent stenosis.

Strut Height. Tolerances for stent construction are very strict, and alteration of strut height by minimal degrees can have a significant impact on shear and neointimal formation. Intuitively, the area of the vessel wall adjacent to the stent struts has the greatest potential for negative remodeling. Eddy currents are created as blood flows over the stent struts and result in low-shear environments. This effect leads to a proportional change in shear with alterations in strut thickness. In addition, the formation of neointima in these areas of low shear has been reproduced in several models, and the thickness of the resultant neointima correlates with strut height. Sprague and colleagues demonstrated how positive remodeling by endothelial cell migration is hampered by low-WSS environments.[16] In normal-shear models, migration of endothelial cells increased 2.5 times in the first week after intervention. However, in low-shear vessels, this migration was delayed up to several months.[17] The clinical effect of these findings was demonstrated in the angiographic restenosis rates of two nearly identical coronary stents that varied only by stent height (50 μm versus 140 μm). A significant difference favored the lower profile design.[18]

Stent Composition. The material composition of the stent itself also plays a role in neointimal formation. The most common bare-metal stent components are stainless steel, nitinol (nickel-titanium alloy), cobalt-chromium alloy, and tantalum. The actual mechanism of vessel injury from stent components is unclear. Corrosive products from alloys have been found within sections of vessel wall, in addition to documented hypersensitivity of some patients to certain metals.[19] Palmaz and coworkers demonstrated that galvanic currents are created within stented arteries and lead to corrosion and subsequent vessel injury.[20]

STENT TYPES AND CHARACTERISTICS

Each stent has intrinsic properties that determine whether it is suitable for any given lesion.[20,21,24-26] Based on the biologic interaction between vessel and stent, an ideal stent will conform to the vessel, be easy to deliver with minimal sheath size, prevent acute failure of the procedure, provide long-term resistance to negative remodeling, be fracture resistant, and be easily visible on radiographs. Generally, stents are divided into two groups based on their construction and mode of deployment—self-expanding (SE) stents and balloon-expandable (BE) stents (Fig. 91-1 and Table 91-1).

Important Characteristics

Between the two groups (SE and BE), the major characteristics that determine suitability are radial force, flexibility, and precision of deployment, including radiopacity. Another

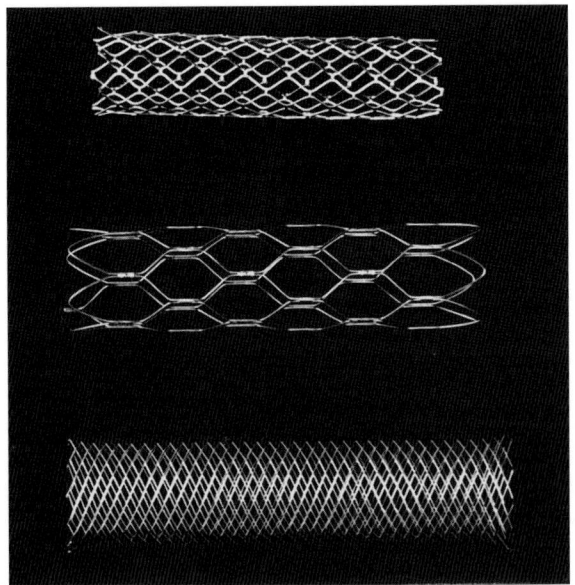

Figure 91-1 Comparison of stents. From top to bottom are the balloon-expandable Palmaz stent, the self-expanding nitinol Symphony stent, and the self-expanding stainless steel Wallstent.

Table 91-1 Comparison of Balloon-Expandable and Self-Expanding Stents in the Treatment of Occlusive Arterial Disease

Stent Characteristic	Types of Stents	
	Balloon-Expandable Stents	**Self-Expanding Stents**
Radial force	High	Low
Flexibility	Low	High
Requires delivery sheath	Yes	No
Radiopacity	High	Variable
Oversizing	No	Yes, 10%
Treats lesions with variable diameter	No	Yes
Resistant to external compression/bending	No	Yes

option, covered stents or stent-grafts of both SE and BE types, have the basic characteristics of the stent and the advantage of a graft.

Radial Force. Radial force is defined as the force required to produce a 50% reduction in luminal diameter of the stent. This outward force provides an improved acute technical result when compared with balloon angioplasty alone. The radial force of the stent maintains its apposition to the vessel wall and tacks down any intimal flaps that might obstruct flow. Radial force also provides the support to resist immediate vessel recoil and acute occlusion. As the stent is incorporated into the vessel, radial force resists deformation and negative remodeling to maintain luminal diameter over time.

Ultimately, radial force is a product of both stent design and composition. The original Palmaz stent is a stainless steel slotted/diamond design. The slotted configuration allows the stent to maintain a low profile for loading onto the balloon. Once expanded, the slots become diamonds that resist further conformational change and provide high radial force. The Wallstent also has a diamond configuration to provide its conformation but is designed to change lengths with its diameter. Therefore, its radial force is related to both its design and the degree of endothelialization within the artery. As the stent becomes more securely anchored, it will resist shortening and actually increase in radial force. Various BE and SE stents can be seen in Figure 91-1.

Conversely, nitinol stents rely on the inherent nature of their metallic composition to provide resistance to deformation. The alloy assumes a predetermined configuration at a desired temperature. At low temperatures the alloy exists in the martensite state (metallurgic property of shape-memory alloys in which the crystalline structure of the alloy is elongated or asymmetric at cooler temperatures), which is flexible and aids in mounting on the catheter shaft and deliverability. At higher temperatures, the crystalline austenite state (metallurgic property of shape-memory alloys in which the crystalline structure is symmetric and face centered) makes the stent rigid to provide more radial force.

Flexibility. Flexibility is determined by the same properties that determine radial force. BE stents require force to change conformation. Thus, these stents will be less able to maneuver around tortuous vessels. Furthermore, force must be applied to the balloon to change from the slotted to the diamond shape. Intuitively and in independent testing, roughly the same external force is required to produce a similar conformational change once deployed, and that new shape will be retained as well. Consequently, BE stents are susceptible to deformation in mobile arteries. In contrast, a nitinol stent in the martensite state can easily be deformed and is more suitable for lesions that require significant maneuverability to reach the target lesion. Interestingly, nitinol will change states not only with a change in temperature but also with external compression. This characteristic provides nitinol stents with improved flexibility in mobile arteries.

Radiopacity. The final consideration for stent suitability is radiopacity. BE stents are generally more visible on radiographic imaging than SE stents, which can be harder to visualize during delivery and deployment. The improved visibility can influence the accuracy of delivery and deployment and must be considered when choosing the appropriate stent (see Fig. 91-4).

Balloon-Expandable Stents

BE stents are optimal in situations that demand high radial force and precise deployment. Unfortunately, the characteristics of the stent that make it ideal also limit its deliverability to lesions. Because it is mounted on a balloon, the stent is at risk for dislodgement during transit to the target or when crossing the lesion. For this reason it is recommended that BE stents be delivered through guiding sheaths already delivered to the site of deployment, preferably over a stiff guide wire. Once delivered to the intended position, the sheath can be retracted and the stent deployed. The balloon is designed to inflate at both ends simultaneously to prevent forward "watermelon seeding" of the stent off the balloon before full deployment.

BE stents will achieve a size corresponding to the degree to which the balloon is expanded. Because the stents are deployed with expansion, vigorous oversizing of the stent with respect to the vessel is not recommended. However, one advantage of BE stents is that they can subsequently be overdistended with a balloon if optimal vessel apposition is not obtained. Such oversizing of the stent with a larger balloon will foreshorten the stent and weaken the struts, a situation that can lead to stent failure.

The innate characteristics of BE stents make them ideal for difficult lesions requiring precise placement. The most common example is an ostial lesion of an aortic branch vessel. BE stents are most widely used for renal artery, "kissing" iliac artery, and subclavian artery stenting. These specific locations are anatomically fixed and thus have little potential for deformation of the stent with movement. Additionally, the plaque at bifurcations tends to be more calcific and prone to dissection. Placement of a stent as the lesion is being dilated will decrease the incidence of propagation of dissection when compared with balloon angioplasty alone.

The construction of the BE stent also accounts for its major limitations. When the segment being treated transitions across branch points from a larger into a smaller artery, BE stents are not appropriate; examples include the iliac and carotid bifurcations. The higher profile needed to deliver both stent and balloon may necessitate predilatation for delivery of the stent to the desired location. Certain situations pose a higher risk for embolization, including end organs such as the renal artery or the carotid arteries, where the kidney and brain are in jeopardy. Predilatation should be done judiciously with small balloons to improve subsequent stent deliverability and to prevent embolism or dissection. Protection devices can also be considered for other territories at risk for embolic complications.

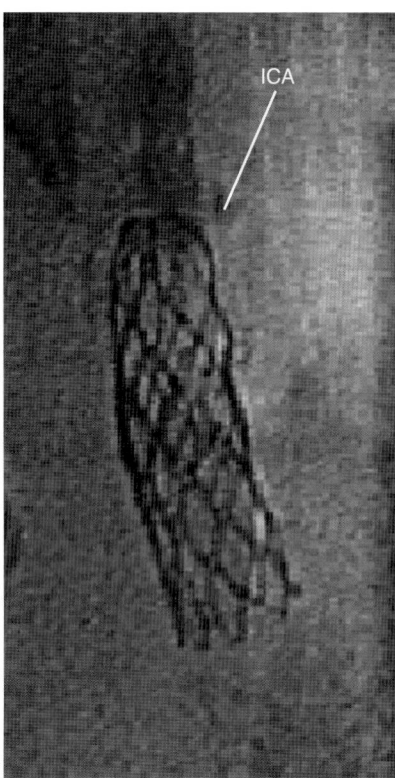

Figure 91-2 This balloon-expandable stent in the cervical portion of the carotid artery is deformed at its distal endpoint, where the carotid artery is mobile and susceptible to external compression. ICA, internal carotid artery.

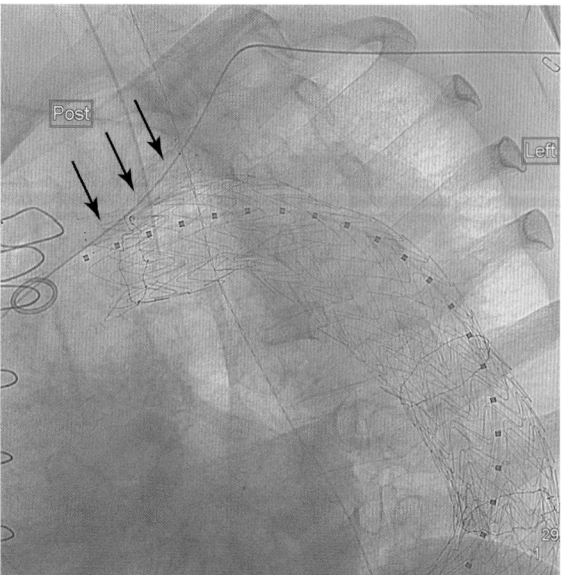

Figure 91-3 A flexible nitinol stent is placed across the subclavian artery origin (*arrows*) to maintain patency when a thoracic endograft has covered the ostium.

In addition, BE stents may retain a new conformation or fracture when stressed by outside forces. This risk of deformation affects the decision to use BE stents across the inguinal ligament or joints. In these positions, the risk of stent compression with fracture and subsequent vessel occlusion is increased (Fig. 91-2). Furthermore, care must be taken when operating in areas with BE stents. Clamping of these stents will also lead to a permanent conformational change or stent fracture that may require redilatation or surgical removal of the stent.

Self-Expanding Stents

SE stents are better suited for tortuous lesions or those traversing vessels of variable diameter. These stents are more flexible than their BE counterparts (Fig. 91-3). Accordingly, they can be delivered through vessels that create more torque within the catheter. To maintain the stent in its constrained form during delivery to the lesion, the stent is covered by an outer sheath on the mounting catheter. When this sheath is withdrawn, the stent is allowed to take its natural shape. As such, SE stents do not require that guiding catheters or sheaths be advanced to the desired lesion. Actual deployment of the stent requires sequential removal of the constraining sheath from the distal end of the catheter (relative to the operator) to the proximal end. It is during this maneuver that the stent can "watermelon seed" in one direction or be

retracted by the operator. This potential "jumping" or "seeding" of the stent can lead to maldeployment of SE stents and must be considered by the operator before the final deployment maneuvers.

Another factor to consider in the use of SE stents is the need for adequate oversizing. As mentioned previously, flow dynamic models demonstrate optimal shear environments at 10% oversizing. However, it is essential to choose a stent that opposes the vessel wall on deployment because SE stents cannot be overdilated. In cases in which an SE stent is undersized for a given vessel, a second stent can be deployed within the first to aid in oversizing. A BE stent is the preferred choice in this circumstance because its increased radial force can overcome the intended size of the SE stent.

Nitinol SE stents have better vessel-matching characteristics because they achieve an optimal diameter based on the ambient temperature. This allows the length of the stent to be controlled dependably, as opposed to stainless steel SE stents. Because SE stents have less radial force and, conversely, improved elasticity, they are ideal for lesions that cross tortuous vessels, joints, or vessel branches. The most common examples are placement within the carotid circulation or in the transition zone from the common to the external iliac artery. SE stents are also used preferentially in more distal branches of the extremities to better accommodate variable vessel diameters when balloon angioplasty produces suboptimal results.

As noted earlier, a final consideration for stent choice is related to *radiopacity*. BE stents are generally more visible on radiographic imaging, whereas SE stents can be harder to visualize during delivery and deployment. The improved visibility can influence the accuracy of delivery and deployment and must be considered when choosing the appropriate stent (Fig. 91-4).

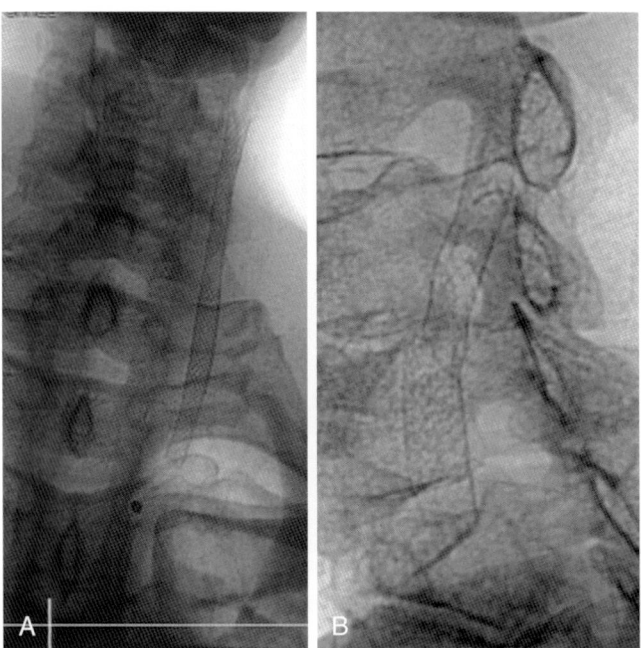

Figure 91-4 Plain radiographs of a stainless steel self-expanding stent (**A**) and nitinol self-expanding stent (**B**) show the better visibility of the stainless steel stent.

Cell Size: Open and Closed Cells

Stent cell size should also be considered when selecting the best stent for clinical use. Cell size refers to the area outlined by connected metallic components of the stent. A large cell size is labeled an "open cell," whereas a small area outlined by the metallic components is considered a "closed-cell" stent. The cell size of the stent and the connection of the wires to each other may influence performance.

A closed-cell stent has consistent interconnection of all stent wires throughout its length. This consistency provides a fixed area of interstices within the stent and uniform coverage of the vessel wall. Such construction decreases the free cell area and, intuitively, may trap fractured plaque at the time of deployment and thus limit subsequent embolic phenomena. However, this configuration makes a stent less flexible and less conformable to vessels. Considering the previously mentioned advantage of the SE stent, a closed-cell stent may have more difficulty matching the tortuosity and change in luminal diameter across a vessel length.

Conversely, open-cell stents are not interconnected throughout the entire stent. Although this feature allows a greater range of movement between the stent components for added flexibility and conformability to lesions, it also results in significantly more vessel wall exposure between the stent struts and greater potential for debris to embolize during deployment or balloon dilatation. Free cell area can vary from 1.08 mm^2 in the smallest closed-cell stent to 11.48 mm^2 in the largest open-cell stent.[21]

The efficacy of cell design in reducing embolic phenomena during stenting has yet to be determined. Cell size relative to a stent has received the most attention in the carotid position, but it may also have implications at other sites. Hart and col-

leagues[22] demonstrated a significant reduction in stroke, transient ischemic attack, and death when closed-cell stents were used versus open-cell stents in a series of 701 carotid stents. The statistical significance was due to a difference in the number of symptomatic lesions. However, a larger evaluation combining patients from 10 European centers demonstrated no significant difference between the two stent designs, even with symptomatic lesions.[23] Because closed-cell stents are less flexible, a bias may exist to use them in straighter, less complicated lesions and thus improve results. Ultimately, the use of open- or closed-cell stents remains the prerogative of the clinician because there is no convincing evidence of the superiority of one over the other. The operator should seek the ideal characteristics for a stent based on the lesion and the location for delivery of the stent.

Covered Stents and Stent-Grafts

Covered stents have expanded the use of endovascular technology beyond their contribution to the treatment of aortic aneurysm. A covered stent may be considered the ultimate closed-cell stent with the inherent applications and limitations of full coverage of the treatment area. Covered stents can be either Dacron (Wallgraft) or polytetrafluoroethylene (Viabahn, iCast, Jostent, Fluency) and can be BE (iCast) or SE (Viabahn, Jostent, Wallgraft). The multiplicity of choices is further complicated by different deployment mechanisms and delivery characteristics that affect clinical utility. Even within the SE category, delivery can vary from distal to proximal (Jostent, Wallgraft) or proximal to distal (Viabahn). This variability allows covered stents to be used in a wide variety of lesions.

Most commonly, covered stents provide the inherent advantage of continuous exclusion of the vessel wall from luminal flow. Historically, this allowed complete exclusion of vessel defects such as aneurysm, arteriovenous fistula, pseudoaneurysm, an embolic source, or perforation. Several case reports have demonstrated the utility of covered stents in acute vascular trauma as well. Depending on the location of the defect, SE or BE stent-grafts can be chosen. In addition, true aneurysms of peripheral arteries are amenable to treatment with covered stents. Popliteal aneurysms can also be treated with covered stents. Isolated iliac aneurysms can be excluded with the iliac limbs of FDA-approved aortic stent-grafts, with possible hypogastric occlusion as indicated for appropriate seal zones. Case series have also reported successful use of covered stents in the subclavian position for aneurysmal degeneration, although special care should be taken to exclude an associated outlet syndrome in these patients, who may require further surgical therapy (rib excision).[27]

In addition, a stent-graft can be used to "trap" debris within the treated lesion. This approach, in theory, lessens the risk of embolization during inflation. The embolic source can be trapped by inflation of a BE covered stent, or an SE covered stent can be deployed, followed by postdeployment molding. Embolization has been shown in both ex vivo and in vivo models of angioplasty in several arterial beds.[28-30] As

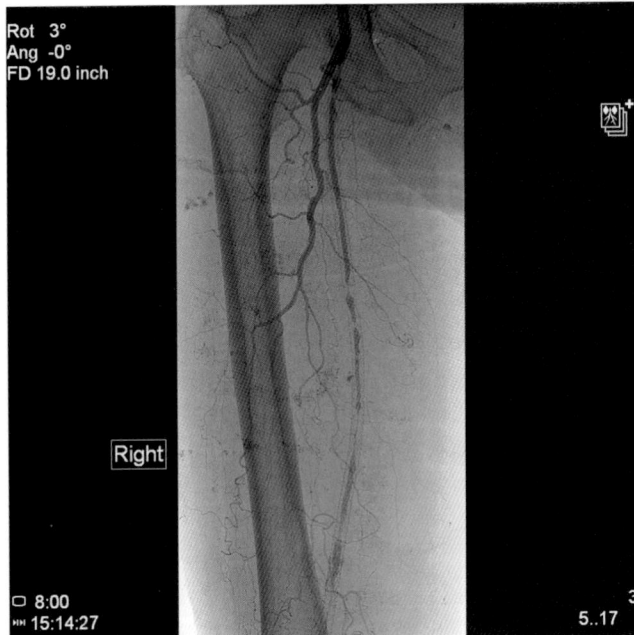

Figure 91-5 Angiographic image of a dense neointimal reaction through the interstices of a stent that was placed in a superficial femoral artery 12 months earlier.

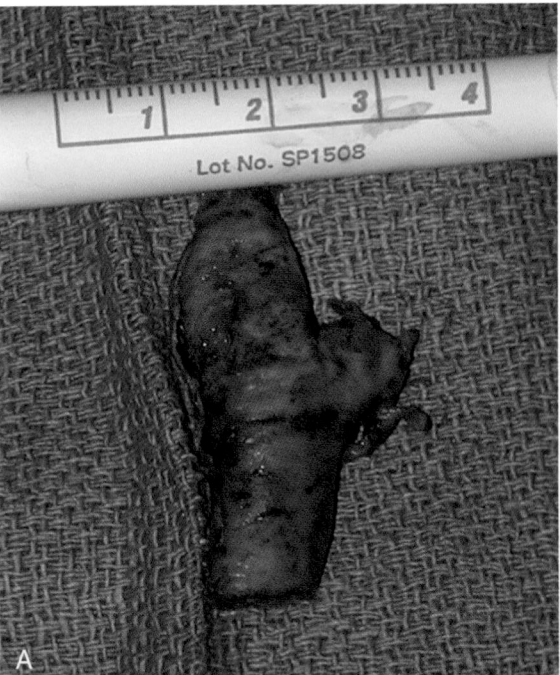

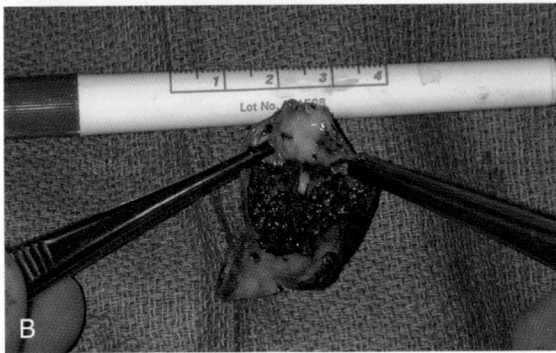

Figure 91-6 A and **B,** Photographs of an endarterectomized carotid plaque that had embolized and caused symptoms. This type of plaque is thought to be at greater risk for periprocedural embolization when an open-cell stent is used to cover the stenosis.

such, use of covered stents may prove to be an effective treatment in the renal, iliac, or subclavian position, where embolization might add significant morbidity. However, covered stents may have limited use in certain locations because they will exclude any branch points or collateral vessels covered by the stent during placement.

Another potential use for covered stents is long-segment treatment of superficial femoral artery (SFA) lesions. In this position, a covered stent provides protection from embolization during deployment. Moreover, the covering theoretically provides a barrier to smooth muscle cell migration and neointimal growth within the body of the treated segment. If the SFA has a large plaque burden, a stent can fail after an aggressive neointimal response by muscular cells in the arterial media (Fig. 91-5). Kedora and associates demonstrated equivalent patency and limb salvage rates between covered stents and prosthetic bypass for the treatment of various lesions in the above-knee position, with comparable runoff.[31] However, no randomized trial has compared percutaneous transluminal angioplasty/covered stent placement versus femoral-to–above-knee popliteal bypass with vein conduit. One must pay diligent attention to collateral flow and anticoagulation when using covered stents in this position. Because a covered stent will exclude all collaterals within the treated segment, stent thrombosis may lead to worse limb ischemia than in the pretreatment limb if these preexisting collaterals are important for protective flow.

■ SELECTION OF STENTS

After consideration of the various stent characteristics, selection of an appropriate stent depends on plaque morphology,

external forces, anatomic location, and branch locations. Foremost, the stent must treat the primary lesion.

Plaque Morphology

If there is concern about microembolization of debris with stent deployment, a covered or closed-cell stent should be used. Procedural and early postprocedural embolization associated with carotid stenting can lead to important clinical sequelae (Fig. 91-6). Additional data on plaque morphology may help predict which lesions are more likely to embolize through the interstices of the stent. Some authors have used ultrasound technology to determine the gray-scale median score to ascertain the embolization potential of a specific carotid plaque.[32] Magnetic resonance imaging or computed tomography may also provide morphologic plaque information about lipid content that can help the clinician choose a stent type (Fig. 91-7).[33]

Additionally, if stenting is indicated in the setting of possible fresh thrombus, one should consider selecting a covered

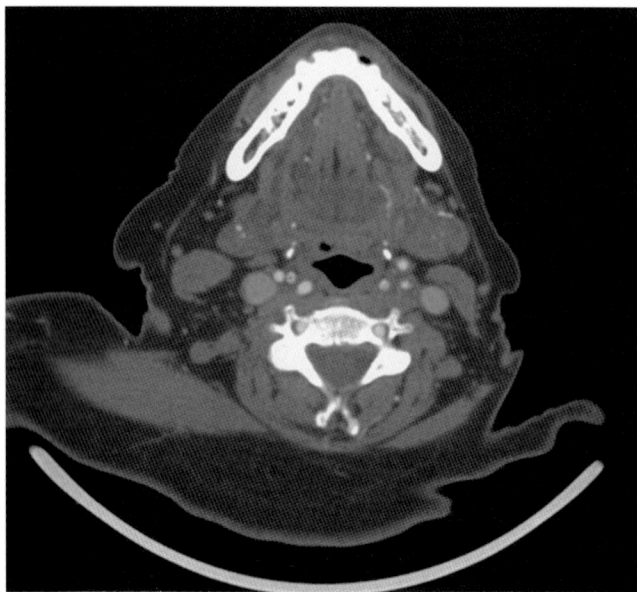

Figure 91-7 Computed tomographic angiogram of a left carotid plaque showing mixed soft and hard atherosclerotic debris that caused an embolic stroke.

stent. Although it may be difficult to differentiate stenotic plaque from organized thrombus, clinical or angiographic evidence of distal embolization in the lower extremity should raise concern about a proximal iliac, femoral, or popliteal lesion that is unstable and prone to repeated embolization during manipulation. If a covered stent cannot be used, one can also consider various embolization protection methods such as filter wires, reversal-of-flow devices, or open arterial exposure to flush debris away from the distal vascular bed.

External Forces

Once the inner surfaces of the artery and the lesion-specific pathology have been considered, the clinician must also review the potential impact of external forces on the stent in the arterial or venous circulation. Extrinsic forces affecting the origin of the supra-aortic trunks are minimal; however, the extra-thoracic carotid and subclavian arteries can be subjected to external compression forces. A narrow thoracic outlet or a cervical rib may compress the subclavian artery and vein. The axillary artery may be compressed by a hypertrophic pectoralis muscle or manipulation in the axilla. A carotid stent can be compressed by neck rotation or vigorous external pressure and become occluded, which may cause an ischemic event (see Fig. 91-2). SE stents are used more often in these mobile areas and are more resistant to external forces.

Anatomic Location

Celiac Artery. The origin of the celiac artery can be compressed by the median arcuate ligament. The radiographic defect can often be corrected by placement of a BE stent, but long-term relief from compression of the arcuate ligament is

rarely maintained. Regardless of stent type, this defect most often requires division of the arcuate ligament (by either open surgical means or laparoscopic methods) before a lasting result is achieved.

Superior Mesenteric Artery and Renal Origins. The superior mesenteric artery and renal origins are typically treated with BE stents because of the extent of disease in the ostia of these vessels, which often includes extensive atherosclerotic plaque from the aortic wall. However, SE stents may prove superior when disease extends farther into the vessel and is associated with dissection. Commonly, more distal lesions of the mesenteric and renal circulations can often be treated with balloon angioplasty because of the high-flow, small-caliber characteristics in these vascular beds.

Left Common Iliac Vein. The left common iliac vein is another anatomic location with reproducible compression from the right common iliac artery. Although most patients are asymptomatic, May-Thurner syndrome is a well-described complication of such venous compression. These patients often appear to have symptoms of venous hypertension of the left leg but may, in fact, have occlusive iliac thrombosis with severe symptoms. After lytic therapy for deep venous thrombosis, the underlying stenosis/compression may become exposed and be an indication for treatment. Because of the external force of the iliac artery, a BE stent would appear to be the first choice for this problem; however, many clinicians have reported success with a large SE stent.

Distal Abdominal Aorta and Iliac Arteries. The distal abdominal aorta and the iliac arteries are prone to extensive plaque formation that can cause ischemic symptoms. Treatment of proximal common iliac stenosis often requires a technique of "kissing balloons" to protect both arterial flow lumina rather than simply "shifting plaque" from one location to another. Stent use in this location also requires this technique to ensure that both stents are deployed simultaneously and that their positions are matched in the distal aorta and proximal iliac arteries. Although both stent types are used in the proximal iliac arteries, the BE type is used more often for short lesions and the SE type for longer lesions that traverse the change in artery caliber past the iliac bifurcation. As one treats more distally in the external iliac artery, consideration is given to the tortuosity of the artery and the transition to smaller diameters, factors favoring SE stents. Occasionally, the more distal segment of the external iliac can be treated better with a precisely placed, short BE stent to avoid excessive material load in this smaller artery. Plaque characteristics that suggest a high risk for embolization would favor treatment with a closed-cell or covered stent in the iliac arteries.

Infrainguinal Arteries. For the infrainguinal arteries, SE stents are used preferentially, with a few exceptions. Stents in the common femoral arteries are generally contraindicated for two reasons. First, the stent could cover the origin of the profunda femoris artery, which may compromise flow into this vital artery. Although arteries often remain patent after they have been "jailed" (e.g., the hypogastric artery and the external carotid), the extent of disease in the common femoral and the potential consequences of occluding the profunda have a more serious effect on long-term salvage of the leg. Second, the common femoral artery remains a major access point for vascular procedures throughout the body, and a stent in this position may adversely affect access into that artery. Ultimately, the common femoral artery is easily accessible surgically with minimal anesthetic risk, and relatively good success is achieved with surgical repair/endarterectomy, which would be difficult to replicate with current stent technology.

Branch Location

Although we have already reviewed the external forces that may affect an artery and the subsequent stent choice, the clinician must also consider the extent of the disease relative to branch points of the artery. When plaque appears radiographically at the origin of a vessel, histologically it will extend into the "parent" artery (Fig. 91-8). For example, ostial renal artery stenosis may appear to be isolated to the renal artery on subtraction angiography when, in fact, the majority of the plaque is in the wall of the aorta (Fig. 91-9). This extensive plaque requires a stent with high radial force and accurate deployment—the BE type. For the same reason, ostial lesions of the great vessels of the aortic arch often require placement of a BE stent to provide the necessary radial force to expand this lesion and the accuracy to deploy the stent with a small portion protruding across the plaque into the aortic flow lumen.

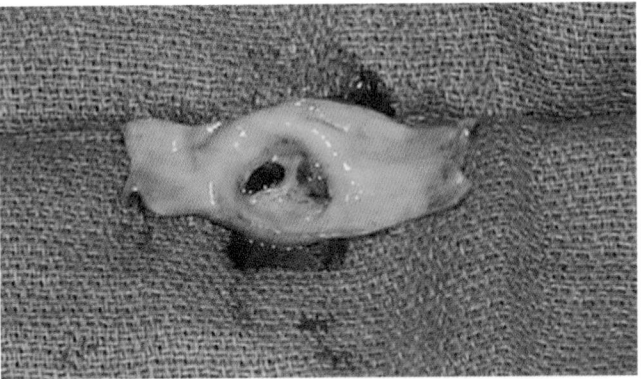

Figure 91-9 This endarterectomized specimen shows the extent of the plaque that originated in the aortic wall but affected flow through the branched vessel.

■ FAILURE MODES

Although stents are designed to maintain patency of the treated vessel, the presence of foreign material in the arterial bed may actually add to long-term failure through neointimal hyperplasia and vessel restenosis/thrombosis. Studies have demonstrated that acute inflammatory changes occur with disruption of the endothelial surface. After the acute phase, the arterial wall continues to react through a remodeling process that includes acute and chronic changes with a smooth muscle response that can be seen as neointimal hyperplasia.[12] This chronic inflammatory change can actually lead to an obstructing lesion and create a more severe recurrent stenosis or in situ thrombosis.

Stents are made of various metallic components that have a long but limited life span under the mechanical stress of the cardiac cycle. Stents are prone to corrosion and subsequent metallic fracture, which can add to the problem of arterial stenosis/occlusion. Stent fracture or failure may be related to metallic corrosion, which may in turn be related to the local vascular environment, external forces, and interaction of other intravascular material.[34-38] When two overlapping stents are placed (a common clinical scenario), the composition of the two stents can be additive in the corrosive process. Figure 91-10 shows surface corrosion of an iliac stent that ultimately failed and was removed during the course of aortobifemoral bypass. The figure shows pitting corrosion that may have contributed to device failure, recurrent stenosis, and eventual iliac artery thrombosis. Figure 91-11 shows two overlapping stents in the coronary circulation that ultimately fractured, probably as a result of galvanic corrosion between the stents. Recurrent stenosis developed at an angulated area of a coronary vein graft.

Stents can also release ions into the local vascular environment that can adversely affect the treated lesion. Both stainless steel and nitinol stents have been shown to release cytotoxic agents that may contribute to smooth muscle necrosis and thereby affect the response of the artery to the stent.[39,40]

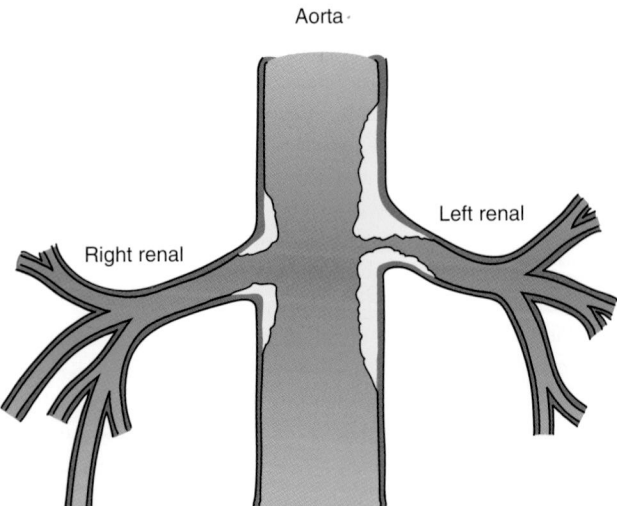

Aorta

Right renal

Left renal

Figure 91-8 The atherosclerotic plaque of a renal artery stenosis originates in the aortic wall, as this drawing depicts. This type of plaque is susceptible to elastic recoil with angioplasty alone and is often better treated with a balloon-expandable stent that protrudes slightly into the aortic lumen to maintain improved luminal flow.

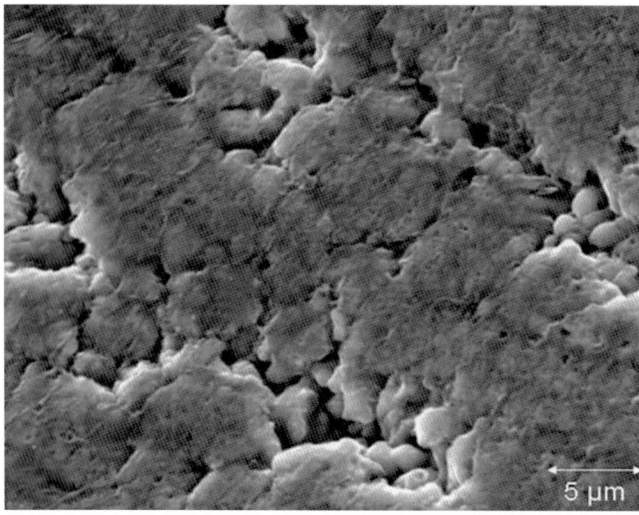

Figure 91-10 Scanning electron microscopy of a nitinol stent that had been deployed in an iliac artery. The stent occluded and the patient ultimately required aortobifemoral bypass. (*Courtesy of Dr. Britta Brott.*)

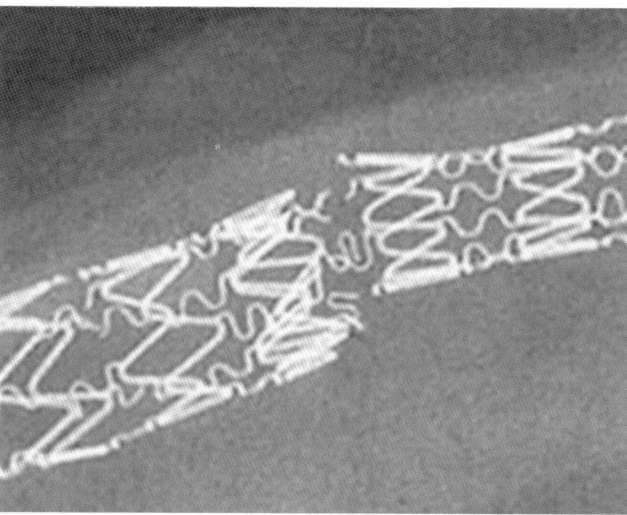

Figure 91-11 Two overlapping coronary stents placed at a tortuous portion in the coronary artery created a stress point that led to stent fracture and recurrent stenosis. (*Courtesy of Dr. Britta Brott.*)

■ NEW DEVELOPMENTS

Drug-Eluting Stents

Many modalities have been investigated to control the hyperplastic response to an arterial implant. Specifically, stents have become a conduit to deliver medication to the local vascular environment in an effort to limit this injury response. Three chemotherapeutic agents have been attached to BE stents for use in the coronary arteries: paclitaxel, sirolimus, and everolimus. These agents have been shown to aggressively inhibit the neointimal response and improve patency rates. Paradoxically, these drug-eluting stents (DESs) have created a new late failure mode of delayed stent thrombosis as a result of the lack of re-endothelialization and minimal incorporation into the associated vessel wall. The raw surface of the stent carries a risk of stent thrombosis as high as 4% after 1 year.[41] When evaluating the use of a DES in the periphery, one must consider that late stent thrombosis (LST) of the femoral artery carries a significantly different risk profile than does LST of a coronary artery.

Approval for DESs in the coronary circulation fueled interest in using these stents in other vascular positions. However, only smaller stents (<3.5 mm) were clinically available, thus limiting their application to small peripheral arteries such as the infrapopliteal, renal, and vertebral arteries. Some clinicians have used these smaller stents in larger arteries by "postdilating" beyond the nominal diameter. However, aggressive postdilatation can cause material fatigue and lead to strut fracture and upregulation of the injury response with resulting hyperplasia and target vessel failure.

Clinical trials of DESs in the SFA have failed to demonstrate improved patency over bare-metal stents. The SIROCCO (Sirolimus-Coated Cordis Self-expandable Stent) trial compared the results of an SE DES with those of a bare-metal SE stent and found after a 2-year interval nearly equivalent restenosis: 22.9% with the DES versus 22.1% with the bare-metal stent.[42] A paclitaxel-coated stent is currently being used in another clinical trial to further investigate the benefit of DESs for lower extremity revascularization.[43]

Absorbable Stents

As discussed, the long-term stent-vessel interaction can result in late failures and, ultimately, occlusion. One method under investigation to counteract this effect is the potential for stents composed of biodegradable material. The long-term benefit of stent implantation is attenuated after approximately 24 months. Bioabsorbable stents could theoretically provide scaffolding for healing of the vessel before the stents are eventually biologically absorbed. Although lower extremity data are not available, absorbable stents in the coronary arteries have shown a 30% reduction in neointimal hyperplasia at 12 months and a 60% reduction at 18 months.[44] Tamai and associates used a poly-L-lactic acid (PLLA) bioabsorbable stent in the coronary arteries of 15 patients and reported a restenosis rate of 10.5% at 6 months.[45] Even at 4 years these investigators found some hyperplasia related to the local stent reaction; however, there were no late stent thromboses in these patients.[46] The biodegradable stents were still evident at 6 months by intravascular ultrasound and coronary angiographic imaging, but the data suggested reduced neointimal hyperplasia in comparison to bare-metal stents.

The clinical effect of this expected degradation may lead to some late events such as embolization with resulting small-vessel ischemia, but this clinical phenomenon has not been well documented. In view of the initial reported success with the PLLA stent, Ormiston and colleagues recently reported success in attaching everolimus to the PLLA stent to obtain the benefit of a medicated stent that reduces the intimal response while potentially removing the nidus for LST.[44]

These investigators found a decreased neointimal response and reduced cardiac events (3.3%) in a series of 30 patients. Even though stent absorption was not complete, no patient suffered LST. Although these investigations are certainly important in the clinical application of vascular stents, the fine balance between modulating the hyperplastic response with medication and promoting the degradation of a vascular foreign body has not been realized.

Considering the success of antiproliferative agents attached to stents, other investigators have delivered these medications to the treatment area with balloon catheters. Tepe and associates reported a restenosis rate of 4.4% (defined as target vessel revascularization) in a clinical trial comparing balloon angioplasty, balloon angioplasty with a paclitaxel-coated balloon, and balloon angioplasty with paclitaxel in the contrast medium.[47] Although there was no difference in amputation rates between these three groups, the angiographic restenosis rate was less in the patients treated with a drug-coated balloon. This mechanism of delivery may enhance the overall vessel response to angioplasty by delivering a high dose of medication without sustained systemic exposure and without long-term inhibition of positive remodeling and subsequent LST.

Avoiding Stents—Debulking the Occlusive Disease

The focus on improving endovascular outcomes has largely been based on stent platforms; however, catheter-based therapy may ultimately prove most effective when no residual foreign material remains in the flow lumen. Treatment options for arterial reconstruction include various methods of atherectomy and modifications of balloon angioplasty.

Various endovascular debulking methods have been used to reduce the burden of atherosclerotic plaque with the intent of reproducing the success of open endarterectomy.[48] Most recent investigations have focused on the SFA because of its high prevalence of atherosclerosis, long-segment disease, resilient downstream target tissue, and resistance to other forms of endovascular treatment. Additionally, because of its superficial location, the SFA can easily be monitored with duplex ultrasound. Two major forms of debulking have been translated into clinical tools for treating the SFA: laser atherectomy and rotational atherectomy.

Laser atherectomy uses a low-energy light source (wavelength of 308 nm) via a fiberoptic catheter to dissolve arterial plaque. Although this technique has the advantage of vaporizing the plaque material, luminal gain is limited to 30% greater than the catheter size, thus limiting it to a maximum lumen diameter of 3.8 mm. Directional catheters can be used to improve that diameter to 6 to 7 mm, but complete clinical efficacy has not yet been established.[49,50]

Rotational atherectomy catheters have been used to "shave" the offending plaque from the intimal surface with a gain in lumen of up to 7 mm in the SFA. These catheters have some potential for distal embolization, which can certainly complicate the revascularization effort by paradoxically causing distal end-organ ischemia.[51] These novel treatments are seeking to miniaturize the endarterectomy process by accomplishing the same task through a catheter that surgeons first advocated as an open endarterectomy procedure in the 1960s. However, catheter-based treatment can only rarely completely remove the intima and the muscular fibers of the media to the external elastic lamina, as surgical endarterectomy accomplishes.

Commonly, after a debulking procedure another catheter treatment is added to avoid a problem with restenosis related to neointimal hyperplasia. One such treatment method includes cryoplasty or a modification of balloon angioplasty that includes hypothermic treatment of the diseased segment. Nitrous oxide is delivered into a balloon catheter at the arterial wall to create a treatment temperature of $-10°$ C to inhibit the proliferative neointimal response.[52] Again, early clinical enthusiasm for this technology has not translated in widespread acceptance or success of this treatment modality.[53]

Progressive miniaturization of revascularization technology remains a persistent goal for clinicians treating vascular disease. One must keep in mind that open surgery has been refined over the last 50 years but the endovascular era is still relatively young. Because simple dilatation of diseased vessels has had limited clinical success, intensive effort has been directed at improving these results with intravascular devices, including stents and antiproliferative medications. Additionally, various techniques to physically remove the disease have shown early promise but limited long-term success. Instead, continued efforts are needed to apply the principles of open revascularization to catheter-based treatment and thus provide improved outcomes with reduced morbidity. Stents have improved some of these catheter-based treatments, but further modifications are necessary to provide more effective therapy for vascular patients.

SELECTED KEY REFERENCES

Dyet JF, Watts WG, Ettles DF, Nicholson AA. Mechanical properties of metallic stents: how do these influence the choice of stent for specific lesions? *Cardiovasc Intervent Radiol.* 2000;23:47-54.
The experiment design of this study is pertinent to all physicians who perform peripheral interventions. The key components of stent choice—flexibility, trackability, radiopacity, and others—are evaluated for several stent types. The results and discussion serve as an excellent guide to optimal stent selection for various lesions.

LaDisa JF Jr, Olson LE, Guler I, Hettrick DA, Audi SH, Kersten JR, Warltier DC, Pagel PS. Stent design properties and deployment ratio influence indexes of wall shear stress: a three-dimensional computational fluid dynamics investigation within a normal artery. *J Appl Physiol.* 2004;97:424-430.
This article provides a mathematical basis for stent selection in avoiding negative shear environments and defines a precise indication for proper stent sizing.

Mauri L, Hsieh W, Massaro JM, Ho KL, D'Agostino R, Cutlip DE. Stent thrombosis in randomized clinical trials of drug-eluting stents. *N Engl J Med.* 2007;356:1020-1029.
Late stent thrombosis continues to be a major limitation to the use of drug-eluting stents. The implications of the need for continued antiplatelet therapy affect both cardiovascular treatments but can have an effect on other patient outcomes such as the need for abdomi-

nal procedures. This article summarizes data on antiplatelet therapy for drug-eluting stents and nuances for proper perioperative management.

Palmaz JC, Bailey S, Marton D, Sprague E. Influence of stent design and material composition on procedure outcome. *J Vasc Surg.* 2002; 36:1031-1039.

Dr. Palmaz's contributions to stent technology are as great as any single individual's. He provides a comprehensive review of several factors that lead to stent failure, including stent topography, metallic composition, corrosion, and contamination.

Sullivan TM, Ainsworth SD, Langan EM, Taylor S, Snyder B, Cull D, Youkey J, Laberge M. Effect of endovascular stent strut geometry on vascular injury, myointimal hyperplasia, and restenosis. *J Vasc Surg.* 2002;36:143-149.

This article demonstrates the potential for vessel injury and negative remodeling that can be caused by the stent itself. It presents a pertinent review of the histologic findings associated with peristent inflammation.

REFERENCES

The reference list can be found on the companion Expert Consult Web site at *www.expertconsult.com.*

Cerebrovascular Disease | *Section* **14**

Bruce A. Perler

CHAPTER 92

Cerebrovascular Disease: General Considerations

William C. Mackey

The primary goal of treatment of cerebrovascular disease is prevention of stroke. Clarification of surgery's role in stroke prevention depended on elucidation of the pathophysiology of stroke, on advances in imaging, on development of surgical and interventional techniques, and on large-scale clinical trials demonstrating the safety and efficacy of such techniques.

BACKGROUND

In 1875, Gowers described the relationship of stroke and extracranial carotid disease in a patient with right hemiplegia, left eye blindness, and left carotid occlusion.[1] In postmortem studies conducted in 1905, Chiari established the association of ulcerated carotid bulb plaque with cerebral embolization.[2] Hunt emphasized the relationship between stroke and extracranial carotid disease in a clinicopathologic study in 1914 in which the clinical history was correlated with postmortem findings.[3] These observations were clinically irrelevant until 1937, when Moniz and colleagues demonstrated the potential for angiography to define carotid pathology before death.[4] Based on images provided by angiographic techniques, neurologists and surgeons began to consider surgical approaches to extracranial carotid disease.

Carrea, a Brazilian surgeon, performed external carotid–to–internal carotid anastomosis for symptomatic common carotid occlusion in 1951, although the paper describing this procedure was not published until 1955.[5] Carrea's ideas may have come from a 1918 report by Lefevre in which he described anastomosis of the external to the internal carotid artery as an alternative to carotid ligation in cases of common carotid trauma.[6] The first report of a procedure in which in-line physiologic flow was restored for the treatment of transient cerebral ischemia was by Eastcott, Pickering, and Rob in 1954.[7] In this procedure, the diseased carotid bifurcation was resected and the internal carotid reanastomosed to the common carotid with good results. The first successful carotid endarterectomy was performed by DeBakey in August 1953 but not reported until 1975.[8] Successful carotid endarterectomies were also reported by Rowe in 1955 and by Cooley and associates in 1956.[9,10] The technique of carotid endarterectomy became more standardized during the 1960s, but its widespread adoption awaited large-scale clinical trials demonstrating safety and efficacy.

The first large-scale clinical trial of carotid surgery, the Joint Study of Extracranial Arterial Occlusion, produced results that for the most part cast doubt on the role of carotid endarterectomy.[11] In this study, surgery was beneficial only for patients with transient ischemic attack (TIA) and unilateral carotid stenosis, whereas it was detrimental for those with stroke and more extensive disease. A large proportion of the subjects in this study had suffered major strokes, and many had stroke with carotid occlusion. This study led to improved patient selection with resultant improvement in surgical results.[11] During the 22 years between publication of the Joint Study of Extracranial Arterial Occlusion and publication of the North American Symptomatic Carotid Endarterectomy Trial (NASCET), imaging modalities, surgical techniques, and patient selection evolved tremendously, but there was no consensus on the role of carotid endarterectomy. Results reported from single centers contrasted with community-based surveys. Representative results from single centers reported perioperative stroke mortality rates of 1% to 3% for asymptomatic patients and 2% to 5% for symptomatic patients, whereas community-based surveys reported stroke mortality rates of 9% to 20%.[12-15] There was substantial doubt about the safety and efficacy of carotid endarterectomy.[16]

Appropriate patient selection for carotid endarterectomy and the current acceptance of carotid endarterectomy as the "gold standard" in stroke prevention for selected patients with symptomatic and asymptomatic extracranial disease are wholly dependent on the modern clinical trials of carotid endarterectomy, most prominently NASCET, the European Carotid Surgery Trial (ECST), the Asymptomatic Carotid Atherosclerosis Study (ACAS), and the Asymptomatic Carotid Surgery Trial (ACST).[17-21] These trials and their role in defining the indications for carotid endarterectomy are discussed in detail later. Similar current trials promise to better define the role of carotid stenting.

EPIDEMIOLOGY AND IMPACT OF STROKE AND CEREBROVASCULAR DISEASE

Incidence and Prevalence

Despite recent declines in incidence and related mortality, stroke remains the third leading cause of death in the United States.[22] About 160,000 Americans die of stroke each year. Around 700,000 strokes occur in the United States each year, approximately 500,000 of which are new strokes and about 200,000 are recurrent strokes.[22] Stroke is especially prevalent in older Americans. In 2005, 2.6% of noninstitutionalized Americans reported having suffered a stroke.[23] Prevalence clearly increases with age: it occurs in 8.1% in those 65 or older and 0.8% in those 18 to 44 years.[23] Men and women report almost equal prevalence, 2.7% and 2.5%, respectively. Stroke is also more prevalent in those with less education, occurring in 4.4% of those with less than 12 years of formal education versus 1.8% of college graduates.[23] Native Americans, African Americans, and those of multiracial lineage are more frequently affected by stroke than whites (prevalence of 6.0%, 4.0%, and 4.6%, respectively, versus 2.3% in whites), whereas Asians and Hispanics (1.6% and 2.6%, respectively) are similar to whites in stroke prevalence. Within the United States there is striking geographic diversity in stroke prevalence, with age-adjusted prevalence ranging from 4.3% in Mississippi to 1.5% in Connecticut.[23]

Current estimates suggest that 87% of strokes are ischemic and 13% are hemorrhagic, with hemorrhagic strokes being approximately equally divided between subarachnoid and intracranial hemorrhage.[23] Ischemic strokes may be subdivided by type: extracranial atherosclerosis, intracranial atherosclerosis, lacunar, cardioembolic, miscellaneous, and cryptogenic.[24] In a recent study of ischemic stroke etiology in New York City, 14.5% were found to be related to atherosclerotic disease (7.3% intracranial and 7.3% extracranial), 19.6% were lacunar, 19.6% were cardioembolic, 1% were of miscellaneous causes, and fully 45% were of cryptogenic or unclear cause.[24] In this study ethnicity and race strongly influenced the relative risks for these various ischemic stroke subtypes, with whites having a higher relative risk than blacks or Hispanics for cardioembolic stroke, and blacks and Hispanics having a higher relative risk than whites for lacunar and atherosclerotic stroke.[24]

The prevalence of cerebrovascular disease depends on the population studied. In one large-scale population-based study of 6727 adults (aged 25 to 84 years), carotid artery stenosis was detected in 3.8% of men and 2.7% of women. Prevalence increased with age, total cholesterol, low-density lipoprotein cholesterol, fibrinogen, systolic blood pressure, and cigarette use.[25] In an even larger population-based screening program for adults aged 45 to 75 years, the prevalence was noted to be 2.5% overall (0.43% in the youngest subjects and 8.1% in the oldest), and the prevalence in males was 1.7 times that of females.[26] In subjects 60 to 79 years of age the prevalence of duplex-detected carotid atherosclerosis has been found to be 10.5% in men and 5.5% in women.[27] In a population-based study of healthy volunteers aged 50 to 79 years, the prevalence of 50% or greater carotid stenosis was noted to be 6.4% and the incidence of 80% stenosis to be 0.4%. This study included clinical follow-up; at 2 years 9.4% of the population had suffered a neurologic event (TIA or stroke), and progression of the carotid lesion occurred in 14%.[28]

Not surprisingly, the prevalence of cerebrovascular disease is much greater in patients with peripheral vascular disease. In one survey of 373 patients evaluated for peripheral arterial disease symptoms, the prevalence of carotid stenosis greater than 30% was 57%. Fully 18% of the patients had symptoms

of cerebral ischemia, and an additional 19% had asymptomatic 60% to 99% stenotic lesions.[29] Similarly, in one vascular surgeon's practice, 21% of patients 65 years or older referred for noncarotid disease were found to have 70% or greater carotid stenosis.[30]

Socioeconomic and Personal Impact of Stroke

Stroke remains the third leading cause of death in the United States, and those who survive the acute event have a markedly shortened life expectancy. Median survival times after a first stroke are 6.8 years for men and 7.4 years for women at age 60 to 69 years, 5.4 years for men and 6.4 years for women at age 70 to 79 years, and 1.8 years for men and 3.1 years for women at 80 years of age.[31]

Still, mortality statistics alone grossly underestimate the full impact of stroke. Only 50% to 70% of stroke survivors regain functional independence, 15% to 30% are permanently disabled, and 20% require institutional care 3 months after the onset of stroke.[31] Among surviving stroke patients, the following disabilities were observed at 6 months[31]:

- 50% had some hemiparesis.
- 30% were unable to walk without some assistance.
- 26% were dependent in performing activities of daily living.
- 19% had aphasia.
- 35% had depressive symptoms.
- 26% were institutionalized in a nursing home.

It has recently been estimated that the mean lifetime health care expenditure for each stroke patient is $140,000 and that in 2007, stroke expenditures nationwide reached $62.7 billion.[31]

Risk Factors

Age, gender, and race are clearly risk factors for stroke, as seen in Figure 92-1.[32] Similarly, the usual cardiovascular risk factors of hypertension, diabetes, smoking, and known cerebrovascular disease seem to have an additive effect on stroke risk, as shown in Figure 92-2.[33] A history of atrial fibrillation adds substantially to stroke risk. Although hypercholesterolemia has been associated with increased risk for coronary disease, myocardial infarction, and other cardiovascular events, its association with stroke has been inconsistent. Recently, low levels of high-density lipoprotein cholesterol have been associated with an increased risk for stroke in elderly men.[34] Despite uncertainty over the relationship between hypercholesterolemia and stroke, there is clear evidence that the use of statin drugs lowers stroke risk. In a very large British study that included 20,536 subjects, simvastatin was found to lower risk for ischemic stroke by 28% when compared with placebo.[35] Use of simvastatin was also associated with a statistically significant lowered incidence of TIA and carotid endarterectomy or stenting. The effect was noted even in those without hypercholesterolemia. Even though the subgroup of patients in this study with preexisting

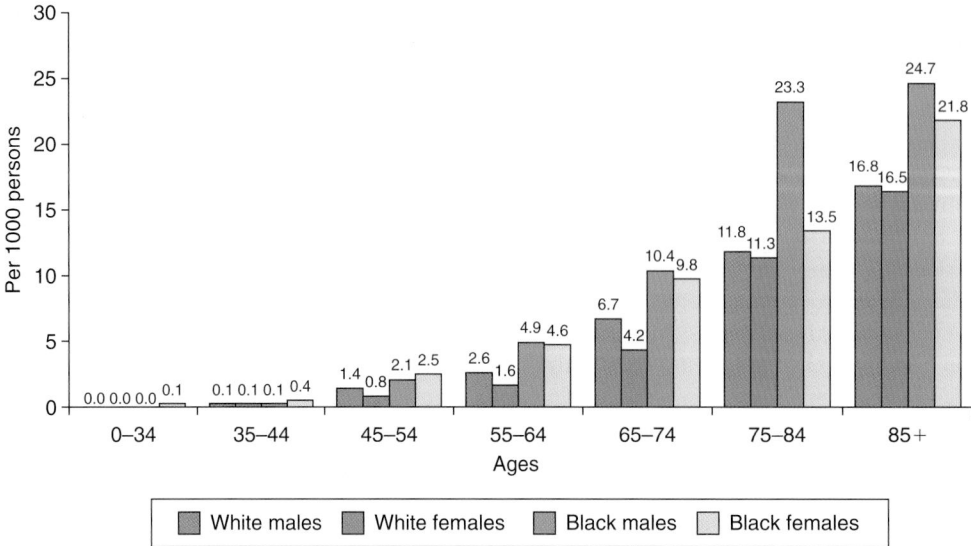

Figure 92-1 Prevalence of stroke by age, gender, and race.

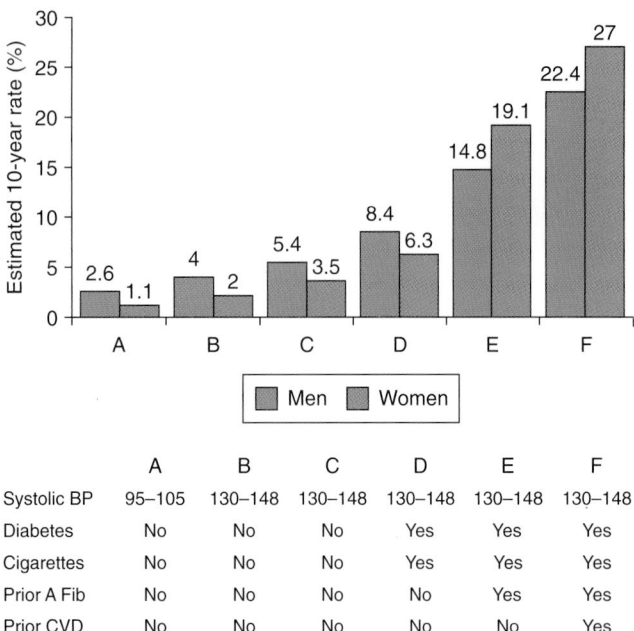

	A	B	C	D	E	F
Systolic BP	95–105	130–148	130–148	130–148	130–148	130–148
Diabetes	No	No	No	Yes	Yes	Yes
Cigarettes	No	No	No	Yes	Yes	Yes
Prior A Fib	No	No	No	No	Yes	Yes
Prior CVD	No	No	No	No	No	Yes

Figure 92-2 Estimated 10-year stroke risk in a 55-year-old adult according to risk factors. A Fib, atrial fibrillation; BP, blood pressure; CVD, cardiovascular disease.

symptomatic cerebrovascular disease did not benefit by a reduction in stroke incidence, they did benefit by a reduction in the incidence of all other major cardiovascular events.[35] Other factors often cited as being associated with increased stroke risk include sedentary lifestyle, excessive alcohol consumption, and obesity.[31]

TIAs represent a major risk factor for stroke. The prevalence of TIAs is 2.7% and 1.6%, respectively, in men and women 65 to 69 years of age and 3.6% and 4.1%, respectively, in men and women 75 to 79 years of age.[31] The 90-day risk for stroke after TIA is 3% to 17.3%, with the greatest risk occurring in the first 30 days.[36-40] In one study of 1707 TIA patients seen in the emergency department associated with a

large medical center, stroke developed in 180 patients (10.5%) within 90 days, and 91 patients (5.3%) suffered a stroke within 48 hours.[41] This high risk for stroke in the immediate aftermath of TIA mandates immediate aggressive evaluation and treatment of all patients with TIA. In addition, TIA confers a poor overall prognosis, with 1-year mortality of up to 25%.[37] The 10-year risk for stroke, myocardial infarction, or vascular death after TIA has been reported to be 43%.[42]

It is clear that asymptomatic carotid stenosis also represents a significant risk factor for stroke. The association of asymptomatic carotid disease and stroke is discussed thoroughly in the section on the natural history of carotid disease.

NATURAL HISTORY OF CEREBROVASCULAR DISEASE

Asymptomatic Carotid Disease

Carotid artery atherosclerosis predisposes patients to TIA and stroke, and the risk for these events is proportional to the severity of the carotid disease. Chambers and Norris monitored 500 patients with cervical bruits and varying degrees of carotid disease graded by Doppler ultrasound.[43] At 1 year, TIA or stroke had occurred in 5 of 239 (2.1%) patients with 0% to 29% stenosis, in 9 of 157 (5.7%) patients with 30% to 74% stenosis, and in 22 of 113 (19.5%) patients with 75% to 100% stenosis. The authors further noted that in this cohort the incidence of cardiac ischemic events was proportional to the severity of carotid stenosis (Fig. 92-3).[43] More recently, Nicolaides and colleagues have demonstrated a linear relationship between the degree of carotid stenosis (calculated by the ECST method) and the neurologic event rate in 1115 patients monitored for 6 to 84 months (mean, 37).[44]

Similarly, O'Holleran and associates showed that the risk for TIA and stroke was related to the degree of carotid

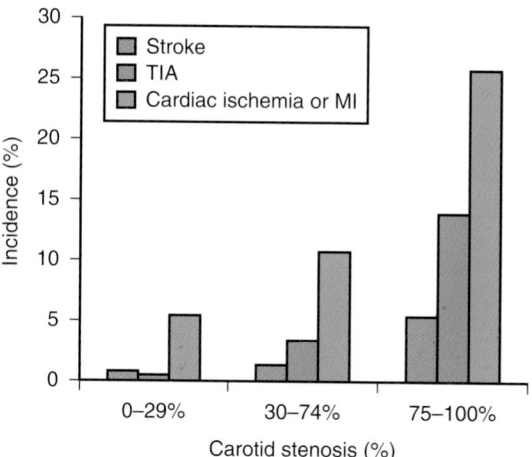

Figure 92-3 Incidence of stroke, transient ischemic attack (TIA), and myocardial ischemia or myocardial infarction (MI) by percentage of carotid stenosis in patients monitored for up to 4 years (mean, 23 months). *(Adapted from Chambers BR. Norris JW. Outcome in patients with asymptomatic neck bruits. N Engl J Med. 1986;315:860-865.)*

stenosis.[45] In their study, 60% of 121 patients with greater than 75% stenosis by B-mode ultrasound but only 12.6% of those 175 patients with less than 75% stenosis had a stroke or TIA during a 5-year follow-up period. These authors further correlated clinical outcome with the echogenicity of the carotid lesions. Calcified plaque was much less likely than soft echolucent plaque to be associated with symptoms.[45] Their findings are summarized in Table 92-1. Nicolaides and colleagues have confirmed these findings in a more recent study. Using the gray-scale median as a measure of plaque echogenicity, they found that dense calcified plaque (gray-scale median >32) was statistically significantly less likely than more echolucent plaque (gray-scale median ≤32) to be associated with computed tomography–detected infarcts.[46] The relationship between plaque echogenicity and risk for neurologic symptoms was confirmed in the Tromsø study, in which the adjusted relative risk for cerebrovascular events in subjects with echolucent plaque was 4.6 (95% confidence interval [CI], 1.1 to 18.9), and there was a significant linear trend (P = .015) for higher risk with increasing plaque echolucency.[47] Current studies are focusing on characterization of plaque morphology by magnetic resonance imaging (MRI) and the relation-

ship of MRI plaque characteristics to natural history. These studies are discussed in detail under "Pathology, Pathogenesis, and Pathophysiology."

From these data it is apparent that both the degree of stenosis and plaque morphology are correlated with clinical outcome in patients with asymptomatic carotid disease.

Plaque progression also correlates with clinical events. Roederer and coworkers found that in asymptomatic patients with initially less than 80% stenosis, progression to greater than 80% was associated with a high incidence of stroke, TIA, or progression to carotid occlusion.[48] Within 6 months of disease progression, these authors noted a 35% risk for ischemic symptoms or carotid occlusion, and within 12 months of disease progression the risk was 46%. Conversely, in only 1.5% of patients whose plaque remained stable did symptoms develop over a 12-month follow-up period.[48]

Further natural history data are available from the medically managed groups in the more recent randomized trials of management of asymptomatic carotid atherosclerosis. These data do not really reflect the natural history of asymptomatic carotid disease, but rather the outcome associated with "best medical management." Optimal medical management is discussed in detail in Chapter 94 (Cerebrovascular Disease: Decision Making and Medical Treatment). In the Veterans Administration Cooperative Trial, medical management of asymptomatic carotid lesions (≥50% stenosis) resulted in a 20.6% incidence of ipsilateral TIA or stroke with 4 years of follow-up.[49] In ACAS, medical management of 60% or greater carotid stenosis was associated with an 11% risk for stroke and a 19.2% risk for TIA, stroke, or death over a 5-year follow-up period.[20] Similarly, in ACST, medical therapy for 70% or greater asymptomatic reduction in carotid diameter was associated with a 5-year risk for stroke of 11% and a 5-year risk for disabling stroke of 5.3%.[21]

Medical therapy can favorably alter the natural history of asymptomatic carotid disease. 3-Hydroxy-3-methylglutaryl coenzyme A reductase inhibitors (statins) may slow the progression of carotid plaque and decrease the incidence of TIA and stroke even in patients with normal cholesterol levels.[35,50] The role of aspirin and other antiplatelet agents in patients with asymptomatic carotid lesions has been established on the basis of several large-scale trials demonstrating benefit in the prevention of several cardiovascular endpoints (cardiac death, stroke death, stroke, and nonfatal myocardial infarction) in

Table 92-1 Risk for Neurologic Events and Carotid Plaque Characteristics in 296 Patients (Mean Follow-up of 46 Months)

Duplex Characteristics	Stenosis (%)	Number of Patients	Number of TIAs (%)	Number of Strokes (%)
Calcified plaque	>75	37	4 (11)	1 (3)
	<75	53	0	0
Dense plaque	>75	42	23 (55)	4 (10)
	<75	76	7 (9)	1 (1)
Soft echolucent plaque	>75	42	32 (76)	9 (21)
	<75	46	10 (22)	4 (9)

TIA, transient ischemic attack.
Modified from O'Holleran LW, Kennelly MM, McClurken M, Johnson JM. Natural history of asymptomatic carotid plaque. *Am J Surg.* 1987;154:659-662.

patients with known atherosclerosis and in patients at risk for atherosclerosis.[51,52]

Symptomatic Carotid Disease

The true natural history of symptomatic carotid disease cannot be absolutely discerned from recent studies, largely because in contemporary practice TIA and stroke have generally been accepted to represent compelling indications for surgical treatment. A randomized study of the management of patients with TIA or stroke that includes a placebo or untreated control group would never be allowed by modern human investigation review committees. The basis for our certainty that TIA or stroke demands treatment lies in several older studies. First, the Canadian Cooperative Study showed that in 139 symptomatic patients, placebo treatment was associated with a 22% risk for stroke or death over a mean follow-up period of 26 months.[53] Similarly, in an American trial of aspirin therapy for patients with symptomatic cerebrovascular disease, Fields and colleagues found a 21% risk for stroke or death at 2 years for placebo-treated patients.[54] Finally, in a French trial, placebo treatment of symptomatic patients was associated with a 3-year risk for stroke or mortality of 19%.[55] In each of these trials medical therapy with aspirin reduced stroke risk. These studies clearly establish that TIA and minor stroke are associated with a high risk for stroke or death (or both) within a few years after the index event. However, these studies included no sophisticated brain or carotid imaging studies, and thus they may have included many strokes and TIAs unrelated to carotid disease.

Because the placebo-controlled trials clearly demonstrated the high risk for subsequent stroke and death associated with untreated TIA or minor stroke events and because aspirin and more recently clopidogrel have been shown to reduce this risk, all modern trials are conducted without placebo control. Current studies compare the "natural" histories of medically and medically plus surgically treated carotid lesions. Future studies will compare outcomes of medical and surgical management with endovascular management.

NASCET has taught us a remarkable amount about the stroke risk associated with symptomatic carotid atherosclerosis.[17] Stroke risk in NASCET-eligible patients randomized to medical therapy was correlated with the presence of risk factors identified at the time of study entry and with the degree of carotid stenosis, as shown in Figure 92-4. For patients with symptomatic severe carotid disease managed medically, the risk for stroke is high and predictable based on well-established risk factors and the severity of carotid stenosis. More recently, the NASCET collaborators have better defined the outcome of moderate and mild carotid disease.[18] Medically managed patients with 50% to 69% and 30% to 50% stenosis had 5-year ipsilateral stroke risks of 22.2% and 18.7%, respectively.[18]

Similar results were noted in ECST, which, like NASCET, compared outcomes in patients with symptomatic carotid artery disease treated by medical management alone versus medical management plus surgery.[19] The results of NASCET

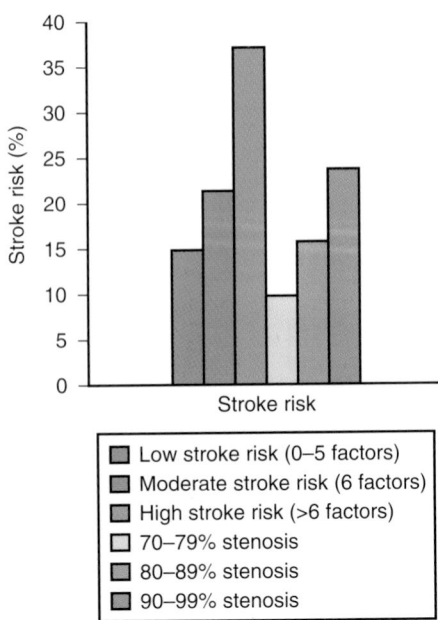

Figure 92-4 Stroke risk at 2 years in medically managed symptomatic patients by number of risk factors and by percent stenosis from NASCET. *(Adapted from North American Symptomatic Carotid Endarterectomy Trial Collaborators. Beneficial effect of carotid endarterectomy in symptomatic patients with high-grade carotid stenosis. N Engl J Med. 1991;325: 445-453.)*

and ECST are not directly comparable because the method of computing the degree of stenosis in the two trials was different, such that 80% and 90% stenosis in ECST was approximately equivalent to 61% and 80% stenosis, respectively, in NASCET. Even with this difference, the outcome in medically managed patients in ECST was similar to those in NASCET. As seen in Figure 92-5, in ECST as in NASCET, stroke risk was high and correlated with the degree of stenosis. In addition, stroke risk was greatest in the first year after initial examination and declined over time. The finding that stroke risk after TIA or minor stroke is highest in the early months after herald events is common to several studies, including the earliest studies of aspirin therapy. In the aspirin trial conducted by Fields and colleagues, the placebo group had a 17.3% risk for cerebral or retinal infarction in the first year after randomization but only a 5% risk in the second year.[11] In NASCET, the ipsilateral stroke risk in the medically managed cohort was approximately 18% in the first year and 8% in the second year.[17]

Our current surgical decision-making process for patients with both symptomatic and asymptomatic carotid disease is based on these randomized controlled trials (NASCET, ECST, ACAS, ACST) and others. These investigations define cohorts of patients in which carotid endarterectomy plus medical management is shown to be superior to medical management alone, as well as other cohorts in which endarterectomy confers no additional benefit when compared with medical management. Current carotid stent trials compare stenting plus medical management against endarterectomy

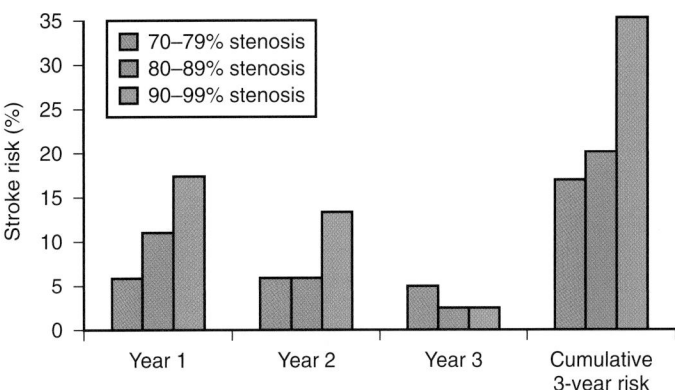

Figure 92-5 Annual and cumulative risk for stroke over a 3-year period by the degree of stenosis in medically managed symptomatic patients in ECST. *(Adapted from European Carotid Surgery Trialists' Collaborative Group. MRC European Carotid Surgery Trial: Interim results for patients with severe (70-99%) or mild (0-29%) carotid stenosis. Lancet. 1991;337:1235-1243.)*

plus medical management but do not include a medical management–alone arm. The results of these trials and their pivotal role in current clinical decision making in the management of carotid atherosclerosis are covered in Chapter 94 (Cerebrovascular Disease: Decision Making and Medical Treatment).

Because there have been no large-scale prospective trials of vertebrobasilar disease, the natural history of this condition is not as nearly well understood. The clinical manifestations of vertebrobasilar disease are discussed later and its management in detail in Chapters 100 (Brachiocephalic Artery Disease: Surgical Treatment), 101 (Brachiocephalic Artery Disease: Endovascular Treatment), and 102 (Vertebral Artery Disease).

■ PATHOLOGY, PATHOGENESIS, AND PATHOPHYSIOLOGY

Atherosclerotic Carotid Plaque

Carotid plaque places asymptomatic patients at risk for TIA and stroke. As shown earlier, the degree of stenosis, plaque density, and plaque progression are correlates of the degree of risk related to carotid artery atherosclerotic lesions. Patients at highest risk for TIA or stroke are those with greater than 80% stenosis secondary to soft, echolucent plaque or those whose plaque progresses from less than 80% to greater than 80% stenosis during follow-up. These clinical findings are consistent with our current understanding of plaque evolution and degeneration.

Benign fatty streaks progress to fibrous plaque. Continued infiltration of lipid into the arterial wall leads to macrophage infiltration, elaboration of growth factors, and chronic inflammation with a slow increase in plaque mass. Macrophage lysis with release of proteolytic enzymes, coupled with further lipid infiltration, results in complex plaque with areas of lipid accumulation, necrotic debris, ongoing chronic inflammation, and calcification.[56] Neovascularity within the arterial wall and overlying plaque results from this cycle of ongoing inflammation and healing. As illustrated in Figure 92-6, areas of intraplaque hemorrhage may "heal" and renew the cycle of macrophage infiltration, calcification, fibrosis, and ongoing plaque evolution. Alternatively, intraplaque hemorrhage can

result in sudden plaque expansion with arterial stenosis or occlusion or in rupture of the fibrous cap with resultant embolization.[56,57] Furthermore, once plaque rupture occurs, the resulting ulcer will act as a nidus for the accumulation of platelet aggregates and other thrombotic debris and thereby put the patient at risk for further episodes of embolization (Fig. 92-7). Figure 92-8 is a color-flow duplex scan showing deeply ulcerated plaque. It is easy to see how this plaque is a potential source of cerebral embolization. Figure 92-9 is a photomicrograph of a typical deeply ulcerated carotid plaque containing loosely adherent thrombotic debris prone to embolization. Given our current understanding of the pathogenesis of cerebrovascular events based on this scenario, it is understandable that low-density plaque (more lipid pool or intraplaque hemorrhage), plaque causing greater stenosis, or plaque showing progression and therefore instability would be associated with a greater risk for cerebrovascular events.

The clinical relevance of this pathologic description of plaque evolution lies in its description of "stable" plaque unlikely to result in TIA or stroke and "unstable plaque" associated with these clinical events. The "Holy Grail" in this field remains imaging findings or biochemical markers that will reliably distinguish between plaque destined to remain stable and that destined to become unstable. The ability to reliably distinguish between stable and unstable plaque will greatly improve patient selection for surgery or stenting, especially in cases of asymptomatic disease. Some current studies using MRI technology suggest that it can reliably measure fibrous cap thickness and integrity and other potentially important features.[58] In a recent prospective study of 154 asymptomatic patients with 50% to 79% stenosis monitored for a mean of 38.2 months, Takaya and colleagues noted 12 cerebrovascular events. MRI findings at study entry of a thin or ruptured fibrous cap (odds ratio [OR], 17.2; $P < .001$), intraplaque hemorrhage (OR, 5.2; $P = .005$), larger area of intraplaque hemorrhage (OR for 10 mm^2, 2.6; $P = .006$), larger lipid-rich or necrotic core (OR for a 10% increase, 1.6; $P = .004$), and greater maximal wall thickness (OR for a 1-mm increase, 1.6; $P = .008$) correlated well with clinical behavior.[58]

The ability to differentiate stable from unstable plaque with imaging studies looms on the horizon, and it is also possible that biochemical markers will provide even earlier pre-

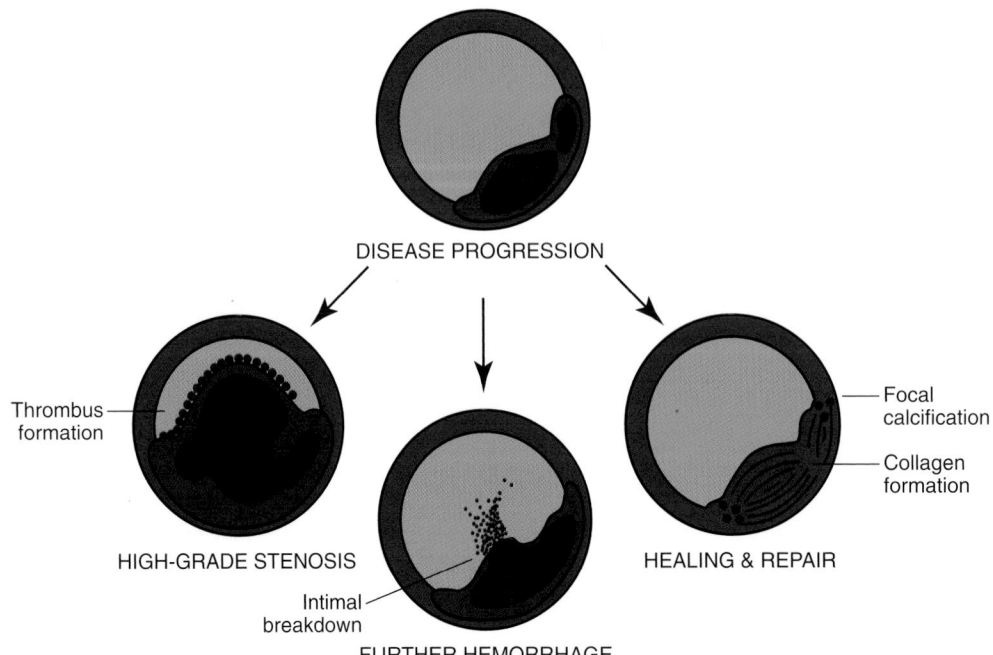

Figure 92-6 Diagram illustrating the possible events after an initial intraplaque hemorrhage. *(Redrawn from Bergan JJ, Yao JST, eds.* Cerebrovascular Insufficiency. *New York, NY: Grune & Stratton; 1983:51.)*

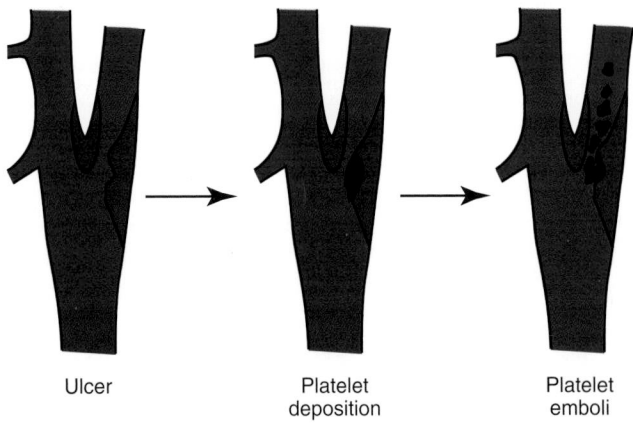

Figure 92-7 After fibrous cap rupture and plaque ulceration, the irregular, thrombogenic surface serves as a nidus for the deposition of platelet aggregates and other thrombotic debris, which can become dislodged and embolize to the brain.

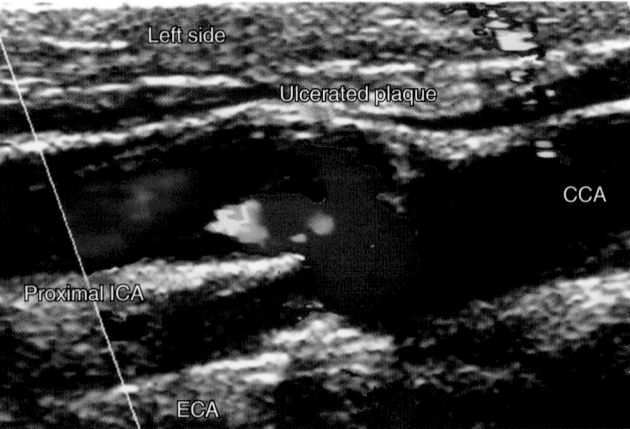

Figure 92-8 Color-flow duplex ultrasonogram of deeply ulcerated carotid plaque in a patient with multiple episodes of transient monocular blindness. CCA, common carotid artery; ECA, external carotid artery; ICA, internal carotid artery.

diction of plaque behavior. Alvarez and coworkers studied matrix metalloproteinase-2 (MMP-2) and MMP-9 and found that serum levels of both were statistically significantly higher in symptomatic than in asymptomatic patients.[59] Furthermore, MMP-9 levels correlated with the presence of unstable plaque as determined by infiltration of plaque by lymphocytes and macrophages.[59] By logistic regression analysis, these investigators determined that the best predictors of unstable plaque were a previous neurologic event and an MMP level of greater than 607 ng/mL (sensitivity, 96%; specificity, 92%; negative predictive value, 94.7%; positive predictive value, 93%).[59]

Similarly, C-reactive protein (CRP) levels have been shown to correlate with the presence of unstable plaque. The same team of investigators that evaluated MMP levels found that mean CRP levels were 27.1 mg/L (258 nmol/L) in patients with unstable plaque but only 4.1 mg/L (39 nmol/L) in those with stable plaque.[60] More recently, another team of investigators has shown that CRP levels correlate with carotid plaque progression.[61] In the study by Arthurs and associates, patients with CRP levels in the highest quartile were statistically significantly more likely to suffer plaque progression as measured by duplex ultrasound than were those with lower CRP levels (OR, 1.8; 95% CI,

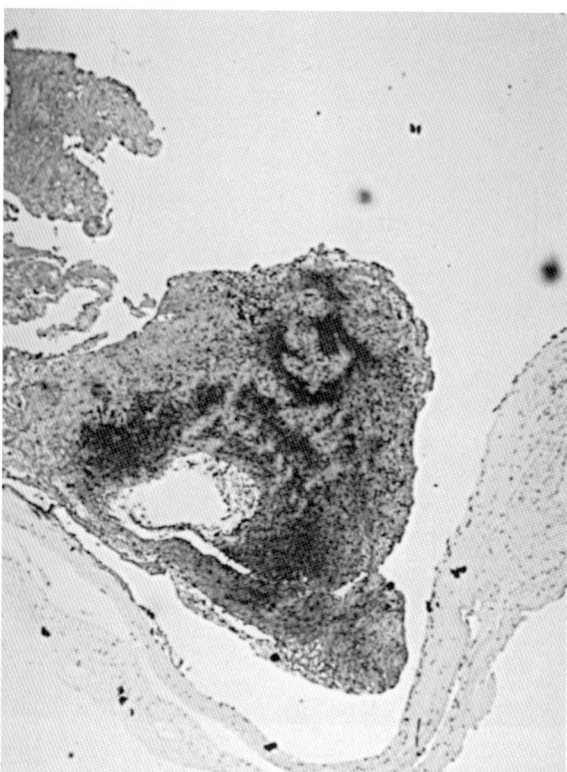

Figure 92-9 Photomicrograph of ulcerated plaque showing organizing thrombus loosely adherent to the wall of the ulcerated plaque. The potential for embolization is apparent.

1.03 to 2.99; $P < .05$).[61] The reliability and clinical applicability of these findings have yet to be determined. If reliable imaging or biochemical markers of plaque instability are determined, asymptomatic patients could be selected for surgery with much greater precision.

Stroke and Transient Ischemic Attack

Carotid plaque causes TIA and stroke through one of two mechanisms, the most common of which is embolization. As mentioned earlier, one potential outcome of plaque degeneration with intraplaque hemorrhage is rupture of the fibrous cap and discharge of plaque contents into the arterial lumen. Evidence for the role of embolization comes from many sources. Hollenhorst used ophthalmoscopy to assess the retinal vessels of patients with transient monocular blindness. He found "bright plaque," which now bears his name, in the retinal arterioles and hypothesized that they represented embolic debris.[62] Fisher noted what he called the "boxcar effect" in the retinal arterioles and suggested that this represented embolic debris, which might explain both transient visual symptoms and transient cerebral ischemia.[63] Our current appreciation of the importance of emboli in the pathogenesis of transient ischemia and stroke comes from multiple studies showing that antiplatelet and anticoagulant therapy decrease the incidence of these events significantly and that removal of the probable source of the emboli during carotid endarterectomy reliably eliminates the symptoms.[17-19,53-55]

Another potential pathogenetic mechanism for TIA and stroke is hypoperfusion. Because cerebrovascular autoregulation maintains cerebral blood flow at nearly constant levels over wide ranges of blood pressure, hypoperfusion or hemodynamic TIA is seen only in patients with severe multivessel disease. In patients with occlusion of one or more of the extracranial vessels and stenosis of the remaining vessels, the autoregulatory mechanism may fail during episodes of hypotension and result in global ischemia (syncope or near syncope) or in more focal events if flow is insufficient focally. Figure 92-10 shows arteriographic images from a patient with multiple spells of near-syncope and bilateral visual loss. Note the right carotid occlusion, the tight left carotid stenosis with carotid kinking just above the carotid stent, the tight left subclavian stenosis with nonvisualization of the left vertebral artery, and the large right vertebral artery.

Vertebrobasilar Insufficiency

Vertebrobasilar spells that occur in association with subclavian steal syndrome represent a common example of hemodynamically based transient cerebral ischemia. In the presence of subclavian occlusion proximal to the vertebral takeoff, exercise of the affected arm may cause flow resistance to drop in the arm because of exercise-induced vasodilatation. This drop in resistance may result in retrograde flow down the ipsilateral vertebral artery with subsequent steal from the vertebrobasilar distribution and posterior circulation symptoms (diplopia, bilateral visual loss, drop attacks, etc). These symptoms subside when the arm is rested.[64] With more severe subclavian disease, steal physiology and symptoms can occur in the absence of ipsilateral arm exercise. Hemodynamic TIAs are more common with vertebrobasilar disease than with carotid disease.

Nonatherosclerotic Disease

Atherosclerosis is the underlying pathology in more than 90% of patients with extracranial cerebrovascular disease, but several other disease states can also cause cerebrovascular symptoms (Box 92-1). These conditions may cause TIA or stroke (or both) via hemodynamic compromise or embolization. The chronic inflammatory arteritides (radiation induced arteritis, giant cell arteritis, and Takayasu's arteritis) generally result in marked and irregular medial thickening with progressive arterial stenosis. Symptoms are often related to hemodynamic compromise from multivessel involvement. Traumatic and spontaneous carotid dissections can result in ischemia from luminal compromise but more commonly result in thromboembolism from dissection-related flaps and pseudoaneurysms. Likewise, fibromuscular dysplasia can cause hemodynamic compromise from luminal narrowing or embolism from the irregular intimal surface. Fibromuscular dysplasia, carotid aneurysms, carotid dissection, arteritides,

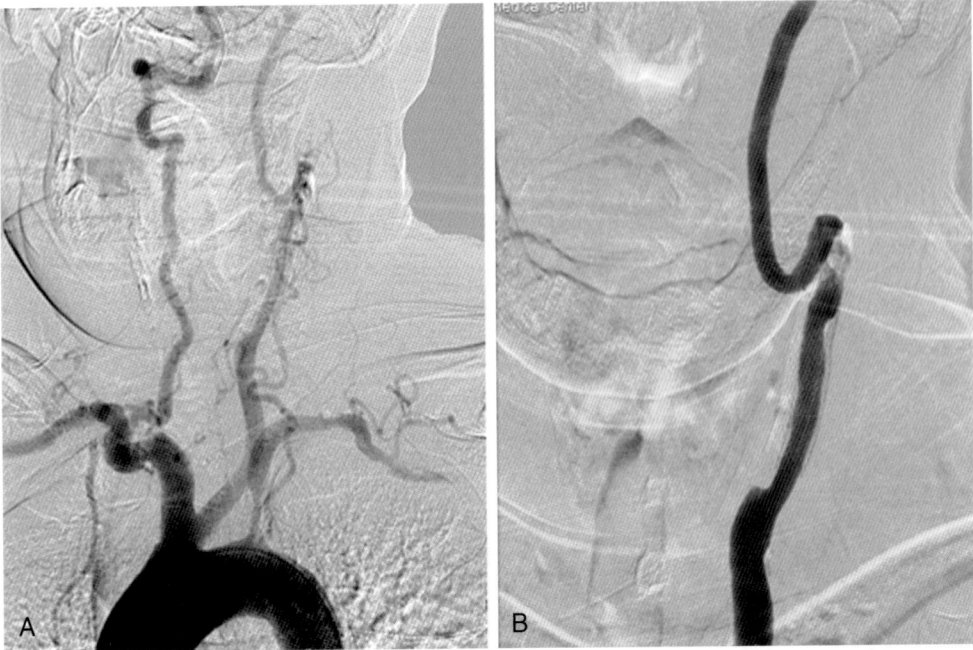

Figure 92-10 Patient with severe multivessel cerebrovascular disease and symptoms of bilateral visual loss and near-syncope. **A,** Note the occluded right carotid, tight stenosis of the left internal carotid, and tight left subclavian artery stenosis. **B,** Close-up detail of left carotid with heavily calcified, stenosing plaque and a kink just distal to the stent.

and Takayasu's arteritis are covered in Chapters 76 (Vasculitis and Other Arteriopathies), 78 (Takayasu's Disease), 97 (Carotid Artery Disease: Fibromuscular Dysplasia), 98 (Carotid Artery Disease: Aneurysms), and 99 (Carotid Artery Disease: Dissection and Other Disorders).

Carotid kinks and coils are encountered in 16% to 34% of the adult population and are only rarely the primary cause of cerebrovascular symptoms.[65] True carotid coils are generally thought to be congenital lesions related to failure of straightening of the normally coiled fetal carotid with descent of the fetal heart.[66] Kinks and redundancies of the carotid, on the other hand, are most often acquired lesions related to gradual arterial lengthening and perhaps cervical spine shortening associated with aging.[67] Even though coils and kinks only rarely cause symptoms by themselves, they may result in areas of turbulence or focal narrowing that may accelerate atherosclerotic degeneration of the involved or adjacent segments. Occasionally, extremely redundant or kinked arteries, or both, may cause cerebrovascular symptoms, which in some cases may be elicited by rotation, flexion, or extension of the neck. More commonly, however, coils and kinks are encountered incidentally on studies carried out on atherosclerotic arteries. It is important that significant kinks and redundancies be eliminated at the time of carotid reconstruction because significant kinking after endarterectomy can lead to carotid thrombosis and stroke.

Management of symptomatic kinks and redundancies in the absence of associated atherosclerotic disease is controversial. Many question whether kinks and redundancies without associated atherosclerotic disease ever cause symptoms.

Box 92-1 Common Nonatherosclerotic Causes of Cerebrovascular Symptoms

- Carotid kinking or coiling
- Carotid aneurysms
- Spontaneous dissection
- Post-traumatic dissection
- Fibromuscular dysplasia
- Radiation-induced arteritis
- Giant cell arteritis
- Takayasu's arteritis
- Cardioarterial embolization

Recently, Ballotta and colleagues randomly assigned 182 symptomatic patients with redundancy or kinking (or both) but without associated atherosclerotic disease to immediate surgery versus initial medical treatment, with surgery being reserved for worsening of symptoms or onset of new symptoms.[68] Patients were monitored for a mean of 6.2 years. Patients in the immediate-surgery group suffered fewer hemispheric or retinal TIAs (10.8% versus 33.3%; $P < .05$), fewer late strokes (0% versus 6.6%; $P = .01$), and fewer carotid occlusions (0% versus 5.5%; $P = .02$).[68] They concluded that symptomatic patients with kinking or coiling from redundancy should undergo carotid reconstruction even in the absence of associated atherosclerotic changes. Surgical management of kinks and redundancies is discussed in detail in Chapter 99 (Carotid Artery Disease: Dissection and Other Disorders).

CLINICAL FINDINGS

Patients with carotid disease may be asymptomatic or have a wide variety of symptoms. Detection of a cervical bruit will often lead to performance of duplex ultrasound, which may reveal severe but asymptomatic disease and prompt referral for surgical evaluation. Furthermore, noninvasive screening of high-risk populations may result in detection of significant asymptomatic lesions.

Transient Ischemic Attack and Stroke: Focal Symptoms

There are many clinical syndromes associated with symptomatic carotid disease. Events related to carotid artery lesions are usually classified as either TIAs or strokes. TIAs are defined as neurologic events that are sudden in onset without a preceding aura, are less than 24 hours in duration, resolve to leave the patient at neurologic baseline, and referable to a definable vascular distribution of the central nervous system. Although by convention the definition of TIA includes events lasting up to 24 hours, most TIAs resolve within a few minutes, and events lasting longer than a few hours and then resolving completely are unusual. TIAs may be related either to hypoperfusion associated with vascular stenosis or occlusion or to embolization. Carotid territory TIAs can involve the eye only (transient monocular blindness or transient monocular field cuts). More insidious chronic monocular visual deterioration can be associated with critical stenosis or occlusion of the ipsilateral internal carotid artery (chronic ocular ischemic syndrome).[69] Patients with chronic ocular ischemic syndrome may suffer from transient visual loss when exposed to bright light (bright light amaurosis), gradual loss of visual acuity, and occasionally, eye pain. Carotid TIAs may also result in speech deficits (dysarthria, dysphasia, or aphasia) if the dominant hemisphere is affected. Motor manifestations range from mild clumsiness of a single limb to hemiplegia opposite the carotid lesion. Sensory manifestations may include numbness or paresthesias on the side opposite the carotid lesion. Headache, mild confusion, and lightheadedness may accompany the aforementioned symptoms, but these nonspecific and nonlocalizing symptoms occurring alone are not usually symptoms of carotid TIA. Common symptoms of carotid territory TIAs are shown in Box 92-2.

Of equal importance with recognition of symptoms likely to be related to carotid disease is recognition of symptoms unlikely to be carotid related. Common symptoms not likely to be related to carotid territory TIA or stroke are shown in Box 92-3.[70] Most of the symptoms listed in Box 92-3 are more likely to be manifestations of cardiac arrhythmias, seizures, migraine, or other conditions unrelated to extracranial cerebrovascular disease.

Reversible ischemic neurologic deficit (RIND) is a term used to describe a focal neurologic event lasting longer than 24 hours but resolving completely within 1 week. The duration of symptoms in patients with RIND suggests that some degree of structural damage to the brain must have occurred,

---

Box 92-2 Common Symptoms of Carotid Territory Transient Ischemic Attack

EMBOLIC SYMPTOMS
- Transient monocular blindness
- Transient monocular field cuts
- Dysarthria
- Dysphasia
- Aphasia
- Monoparesis
- Hemiparesis
- Hemisensory deficit

HYPOPERFUSION SYMPTOMS
- Bright light amaurosis
- Lightheadedness or presyncope associated with any of the above focal deficits

---

Box 92-3 Signs and Symptoms Unlikely to Be Related to Carotid Disease

- Unconsciousness (including syncope)
- Tonic/clonic activity
- March of sensory deficit
- Dizziness alone
- Vertigo alone
- Dysphagia alone
- Dysarthria alone
- Bowel or bladder incontinence
- Visual loss with alteration of consciousness
- Focal symptoms with migraine
- Scintillating scotomas
- Confusion alone
- Amnesia alone

From Toole JF, Dibert SW, Harpold GJ. Transient ischemic attacks and stroke in the distribution of the carotid artery: Clinical manifestations. In: Moore WS, ed. *Surgery for Cerebrovascular Disease*. 2nd ed. Philadelphia, PA: WB Saunders, 1996:73.

---

although it may be very limited and undetectable by clinical imaging studies. The definitions of TIA and RIND are based on clinical events. Correlation of these events with findings on brain imaging studies is imprecise. Approximately 24% of patients with clinical events consistent with TIA will be found on brain imaging studies to have infarction in an anatomic distribution consistent with the transient neurologic event.[71]

Strokes are infarctions of central nervous system tissue related to hypoperfusion, embolization, or intracranial hemorrhage. The stroke deficits related to carotid disease are similar to the temporary deficits seen with TIA. Permanent monocular blindness secondary to retinal infarction, aphasia, monoparesis or hemiparesis/hemiplegia, and hemisensory deficits are the most common manifestations of stroke related to carotid disease. The severity of stroke is graded by using one of a number of stroke severity scales. A commonly used stroke scale is that formulated by the National Institute of Neurologic Diseases and Stroke (NINDS) of the National Institutes of Health (NIH). The NIH stroke scale (Table

92-2) yields a numeric score of 0 (no deficits) to 34 (most severe deficits in all areas). The NIH stroke severity scale can be determined at initial evaluation and at specific intervals throughout the clinical course. A score of 5 or lower is generally considered to represent mild stroke; a score of 6 to 20, moderate stroke; and a score higher than 20, severe stroke. NIH stroke scores at initial examination have been shown to predict outcomes and eventual disposition in patients undergoing thrombolytic therapy and other acute interventions for stroke.[72] The use of scales such as the NIH stroke scale permits comparative assessment of treatment effects in clinical trials by providing a standard measure of stroke severity initially and throughout the clinical course.

Global Ischemia

On occasion, carotid disease can cause symptoms consistent with more global cerebral hypoperfusion. Patients with critical stenosis or occlusion of several extracranial vessels can have decreased mental acuity, orthostatic presyncope, or even vertebrobasilar-like symptoms. In the setting of severe hemodynamic compromise related to multiple vascular lesions, these global symptoms may be properly attributed to carotid disease. With more localized vascular disease or with emboligenic lesions, these symptoms are not usually carotid related. Examples of symptoms related to global hypoperfusion include orthostatic syncope or presyncope, binocular visual loss, ataxia, dizziness, or vertigo. Usually, symptoms related to global hypoperfusion are associated with sudden standing from a seated position or other events likely to cause a fall in cerebral perfusion pressure.

Lacunar Infarcts

There is significant current interest and controversy surrounding a potential role for carotid atherosclerosis in the pathogenesis of lacunar infarctions. Traditionally, these small infarcts, often located in the internal capsule or basal ganglia, which are supplied by the lenticulostriate vessels (small proximal branches of the intracranial carotid), have been thought to be associated with small-vessel disease, lipohyalinosis related primarily to hypertension. Challenging this traditional view of lacunar infarction is a recent study by Tejada and associates in which carotid stenosis was found to be more common on the side of lacunar infarction than on the unaffected side (OR, 5.5; 95% CI, 1.2 to 23; $P < .03$).[73] Furthermore, these investigators found that by multivariate analysis, the only statistically significant independent predictors of multiple lacunar infarctions on one side of the brain were left ventricular hypertrophy (OR, 9.1; 95% CI, 2.5 to 33.6) and ipsilateral carotid stenosis greater than 75% (OR, 14.4; 95% CI, 2.0 to 99.6).[73] Similarly, Roquer and colleagues demonstrated that lacunar infarcts were associated with large-vessel disease in 73 of 217 patients (33.6%) and with small-vessel disease in 144 of 217 (66.4%).[74] Together, these studies suggest that embolization to the lenticulostriate vessels from extracranial carotid disease may be one cause of lacunar

Table 92-2 The National Institutes of Health Stroke Scale

Task	Score	Description
Item 1a: Level of consciousness	0	Normal
	1	Not alert but arousable
	2	Not alert, arousable with difficulty
	3	Unresponsive
Item 1b: Questions (month and patient age)	0	Both answered correctly
	1	One answered correctly
	2	Neither answered correctly
Item 1c: Commands (open/close eyes, grip/release)	0	Both done correctly
	1	One done correctly
	2	Neither done correctly
Item 2: Best gaze	0	Normal
	1	Partial gaze palsy
	2	Forced gaze deviation
Item 3: Visual	0	No visual loss
	1	Partial hemianopia
	2	Complete hemianopia
	3	Bilateral hemianopia (blind)
Item 4: Facial palsy	0	Normal
	1	Minor weakness
	2	Total or near paralysis of the lower face
	3	Complete facial paralysis
Item 5: Motor arm	0	No drift
	1	Drift
	2	Some effort against gravity
	3	No effort against gravity
	4	No movement
	UN:	Amputation or joint fusion
Item 6: Motor leg	0	No drift
	1	Drift
	2	Some effort against gravity
	3	No effort against gravity
	4	No movement
	UN:	Amputation or joint fusion
Item 7: Limb ataxia	0	Absent
	1	Present in one limb
	2	Present in two limbs
	UN:	Amputation or joint fusion
Item 8: Sensory	0	Normal
	1	Mild to moderate sensory loss
	2	Severe to total sensory loss
Item 9: Best language	0	Normal
	1	Mild to moderate aphasia
	2	Severe aphasia
	3	Mute, global aphasia
Item 10: Dysarthria	0	Normal
	1	Mild to moderate (slurring)
	2	Severe (unintelligible)
	UN:	Intubated or other barrier
Item 11: Extinction and inattention	0	Normal
	1	Visual, tactile, spatial, personal inattention
	2	Profound hemi-inattention or extinction
Total score:		

UN, unavailable.

A score of 5 or lower is generally considered to represent mild stroke; a score of 6 to 20, moderate stroke; and a score higher than 20, severe stroke.

infarcts and that patients with lacunar infarction should undergo thorough evaluation of the extracranial carotids.

Cognitive Decline

The role of carotid disease in cognitive decline is another area of significant interest. There is no doubt that dementia may be caused by multiple cerebral infarcts. Multiple lacunar infarctions with arteriosclerotic periventricular white matter lesions characterize Binswanger's disease, one form of multi-infarct or vascular dementia. Cerebral autosomal dominant arteriopathy with subcortical infarcts and leukoencephalopathy is a well-recognized form of inherited vascular dementia associated with stroke, TIA, migraine with aura, and mood disorders. Less precisely defined dementias are associated with large or multiple cerebral infarctions of virtually any cause. Current neuropsychological and cerebral imaging techniques allow distinction between Alzheimer-type dementia and vascular dementia.[75] Even though stroke and, by inference, carotid disease may cause dementia, the role of carotid disease in more subtle cognitive impairment and the potential for reversal of such impairment by treatment of carotid disease remain highly controversial. No studies have convincingly linked carotid stenosis to cognitive decline. Similarly, although most carotid surgeons can point to a few cases in which endarterectomy seemed to result in cognitive and behavioral improvement, no large-scale trials have convincingly demonstrated a consistently beneficial effect.

Recently, however, some studies have linked carotid stenosis to cognitive decline. Johnston and colleagues performed serial Modified Mini-Mental State Examinations and serial duplex scans in a large cohort of neurologically asymptomatic patients over a 5-year period. Left carotid stenosis of 75% or greater was associated with cognitive impairment (OR, 6.7; 95% CI, 2.4 to 18.1) and progressive cognitive decline (OR, 2.6; 95% CI, 1.1 to 6.3), even after correction for the presence of right-sided disease.[76] Similarly, in a Scandinavian neuropsychological study, subjects with asymptomatic carotid stenosis were found to perform more poorly than subjects without carotid disease on tests of attention, psychomotor speed, memory, and motor functioning.[77] Of note is that MRI study of these subjects revealed no difference in performance between those with and without "silent" cortical infarcts.[77] Also of note and apropos of the preceding discussion of lacunar infarcts is that in this study silent lacunar infarcts were statistically significantly more common in the cohort with asymptomatic carotid stenosis ($P = .03$).[77]

Some data suggest that in selected patients, carotid endarterectomy might improve cognitive function. In a study of patients before and after endarterectomy, Fearn and coworkers found that patients who had exhausted cerebrovascular reserve to inhaled carbon dioxide before endarterectomy showed marked improvement postoperatively in attention, reaction time, and other measures of cognitive function. Subjects with preserved cerebrovascular reserve showed much less improvement in their tests.[78] Although studies such as these are provocative and anecdotal experiences suggest that some

patients do derive cognitive and behavioral benefit from endarterectomy, proof of a predictable, quantifiable effect is lacking. Still, by far the most compelling indication for the treatment of cerebrovascular disease is prevention of stroke.

Vertebrobasilar Insufficiency

The manifestations of vertebrobasilar disease are more varied and often more subtle. Still, ischemia of the regions of the brain supplied by the vertebral arteries and their branches causes distinctive symptoms that should lead to appropriate diagnosis and treatment.

The vertebrobasilar system's built-in redundancy (two vertebral arteries merging to form a single basilar artery) provides some protection against ischemia related to occlusion of a single vertebral artery. In addition, unlike internal carotid artery flow, vertebral artery flow can be reconstituted, in the event of proximal stenosis or occlusion, from collaterals related to the external carotid artery, the thyrocervical trunk, and multiple small branches of the cervical vertebral artery. However, the vertebrobasilar circulation is much more variable than the carotid circulation. In 45% of patients the left vertebral artery is larger than the right, in 21% the right is larger than the left, and in only 34% are the arteries approximately the same size.[79] Occasionally, one vertebral is atretic and the other large. Because of this variability, the protective redundancy of the vertebrobasilar system is often incomplete. Furthermore, because the vertebral arteries pass through the bony canals through the transverse processes of the first through sixth cervical vertebrae, they are subject to repetitive trauma or compression from osteophytes or other lesions forming in and around these usually protective structures. Such repetitive trauma or compression may lead to atherosclerosis or thrombosis. The most frequent symptoms and signs of vertebrobasilar or posterior circulation ischemia are shown in Box 92-4.[80]

Although the symptoms and signs of vertebrobasilar disease can be complex and confusing, affected patients tend to have distinctive clinical syndromes based on the location of their posterior circulation lesion. Perhaps most common are patients with subclavian steal physiology related to occlusion or tight stenosis of a subclavian vessel proximal to the vertebral origin. In these patients, the most frequent symptom is arm pain with exercise. Often, however, arm fatigue, tightening, and discomfort are associated with neurologic complaints. The most frequent neurologic symptom in these patients is dizziness or vertigo. Some patients also complain of diplopia, bilateral visual blurring, and occasionally, an inability to focus.[80] Motor or sensory symptoms, as commonly seen in carotid territory ischemia, are very rare with subclavian steal syndrome and almost always indicate the presence of concomitant carotid disease. Neurologic findings are rare in patients with subclavian steal syndrome. Posterior circulation stroke in these patients is unusual, and when strokes do occur in such patients, they are almost always related to atherosclerotic lesions elsewhere.

Box 92-4 Clinical Manifestations of Vertebrobasilar Ischemia

SYMPTOMS
- Dizziness or vertigo
- Diplopia
- Inability to stand
- Bilateral limb weakness
- Alternating bilateral weakness
- Bilateral numbness
- Crossed weakness
- Crossed paresthesias or numbness
- Bilateral visual loss
- Tinnitus or deafness
- Poor memory
- Difficulty seeing to one side
- Gait ataxia

SIGNS
- Nystagmus
- Vertical gaze palsy
- Dysconjugate gaze
- Ophthalmoplegia
- Ocular skew
- Bilateral limb weakness
- Crossed weakness (left face/right body or vice versa)
- Crossed sensory loss
- Unilateral gaze palsy
- Palsy of nerves VI and VII
- Amnesia
- Hemianopia, bilateral hemianopia

From Caplan LR, Wityk RJ. Transient ischemic attacks and stroke in the distribution of the vertebrobasilar system: clinical manifestations. In: Moore WS, ed. *Surgery for Cerebrovascular Disease*. 2nd ed. Philadelphia, PA: WB Saunders; 1996:78-95.

Box 92-5 Signs and Symptoms of Lateral Medullary Infarction

- Ipsilateral facial pain, numbness, sensory loss
- Vertigo with nystagmus
- Ipsilateral ptosis and meiosis
- Loss of pinprick and temperature sensation on the contralateral trunk and limbs
- Dysphagia
- Hoarseness
- Ipsilateral clumsiness
- Loss of balance
- Tachycardia
- Blood pressure lability
- Nausea and vomiting

Patients with lesions at the origin of the vertebral artery have neurologic symptoms similar to those seen in patients with subclavian steal syndrome, but of course without the arm pain with exertion. Because the vertebral artery can be reconstituted distally by collateral flow, tight stenoses or occlusions proximally do not usually lead to vertebral thrombosis, so although transient symptoms may be caused by these lesions, stroke is unusual. Even though vertebral lesions are generally thought to be less likely to embolize than carotid plaque and although vertebrobasilar territory symptoms, when compared with carotid territory symptoms, are less commonly related to emboli, such plaque can be the source of emboli. When they are, the symptoms are more typical of distal cervical vertebral or intracranial branch vessel occlusion.

Distal vertebral and intracranial vessel occlusion is most often associated with symptoms and signs related to ischemia or infarction of the cerebellum or lateral medulla. Cerebellar symptoms almost always include gait ataxia and less frequently finger-to-nose ataxia and intention tremor.[80] Ischemia or infarction of the lateral medulla may lead to a wide variety of symptoms because many cranial nerve nuclei and other critical structures are concentrated there. Potential symptoms and signs related to lateral medullary infarction are shown in Box 92-5.

Cerebellar and lateral medullary symptoms and signs are most often related to distal vertebral occlusion. This can be seen with atherosclerotic occlusion or tight stenosis, with spontaneous or traumatic vertebral dissection, and less commonly with embolization from a more proximal source. Vertebral dissection can be related to chiropractic manipulation.

Clinical syndromes associated with embolization to the basilar artery or to other intracranial branches of the vertebrobasilar system are equally distinctive.

Management of vertebrobasilar disease is discussed in Chapters 94 (Cerebrovascular Disease: Decision Making and Medical Treatment) and 102 (Vertebral Artery Disease).

■ BASIC CLINICAL ASSESSMENT

Although the essentials of vascular history taking and physical examination are discussed in the initial section of this textbook, there are elements of the history and physical examination that are especially important when evaluating patients with cerebrovascular disease. The history of present illness should include a careful neurologic and vascular history. The patient should be asked to describe in detail all neurologic events or symptoms. A precise description of the nature of the symptoms is most important. Rapidity of onset, presence or absence of a preceding aura, duration of symptoms, and rapidity of resolution are important features of the history. In patients with carotid territory TIA, the typical symptoms (see Box 92-2) are usually sudden in onset without a preceding aura and 1 to 10 minutes in duration (although longer is possible) with complete resolution over a period of a few minutes or less. Patients who complain of an aura or prodrome, whose symptoms are not those listed in Box 92-2, or whose history deviates in other ways from the norm may have atypical migraine, atypical seizures, or cardiogenic presyncope. The neurologic symptoms often associated with conditions other than carotid disease are listed in Box 92-3. Vertebrobasilar symptoms can be more varied and subtle, but the essential features of TIA (rapid onset without aura, short duration, localizing symptoms, and prompt complete resolution) are common to both vertebrobasilar and carotid events. It is also important to get information on past neurologic events such as strokes, seizures, head injuries, and neurosurgical procedures.

A thorough vascular history should follow the neurologic history. Previous myocardial infarction, previous stroke, presence of peripheral arterial disease, and presence of aneurysmal disease may all influence the evaluation and management of patients with cerebrovascular disease. Vascular risk factors (smoking, hyperlipidemia, diabetes, hypertension, family history) must be recorded accurately. All medications should be recorded. It is important to note whether the patient's risk factors are under active and satisfactory management. Is the patient taking aspirin or another coagulation modifier, reductase inhibitor, beta blocker, or insulin? Previous surgical procedures, especially those related to the nervous or vascular system, should be recorded.

A thorough review of systems is an important component of the initial evaluation. Special attention should be given to symptoms suggesting angina, congestive heart failure, chronic lung disease, kidney disease, or liver disease. Elderly patients with vascular disease are at risk for a variety of common cancers, and the review of systems should include questions on bowel and bladder habits, breast masses, and respiratory status.

Physical examination of a patient with cerebrovascular disease starts with determination of the pulse rate and blood pressure. Blood pressure should always be recorded in both arms for comparison. Palpation of the carotid pulses is essential because an absent or diminished carotid pulse indicates significant proximal carotid disease that might be missed on routine duplex examination. Carotid auscultation should be carried out at the mandibular angles and supraclavicular regions bilaterally. Bruits loudest at the mandibular angle are usually associated with bifurcation disease, whereas those loudest at the clavicles are often associated with more proximal common carotid disease or with radiating aortic stenosis murmurs. Bruits should be graded according to pitch and duration. In general, the higher the pitch and the longer the duration of the bruit, the worse the stenosis. It should be kept in mind that truly preocclusive lesions may slow flow enough that no bruit is audible. Moreover, bruits may be associated with external carotid stenosis, aortic valvular stenosis, and subclavian stenosis, so the finding of a bruit does not necessarily imply clinically significant carotid disease. After the neck examination, the remainder of the vascular examination is completed. One useful but often neglected assessment is funduscopic examination. All patients with visual symptoms should undergo a funduscopic examination to evaluate for Hollenhorst plaque or other retinal findings characteristic of atherosclerosis, hypertension, or diabetes.

All patients with cerebrovascular disease should undergo a neurologic examination because the presence of abnormal neurologic findings requires brain imaging studies and usually consultation with a neurologist before endarterectomy or stenting. Mental status and speech can be assessed during the history. Difficulty with word finding or articulation should prompt further evaluation. Facial expression, symmetry, and movement are easily assessed, as are extremity strength and

sensation. Gait offers an easy means to evaluate for lower extremity ataxia, and having patients write their name or fill out a health questionnaire will allow assessment for ataxia of the dominant arm. Visual fields are assessed by the direct confrontation technique, and gross visual acuity can be evaluated by several different techniques. Although it is not expected that the vascular surgeon's neurologic examination skills will be as detailed and well honed as a neurologist's, a thorough history and physical examination should be reveal virtually all relevant neurologic findings that would indicate a need for brain imaging or more detailed clinical assessment by a neurologist. Only after a detailed history and physical examination can the vascular surgeon choose the most appropriate imaging studies, laboratory studies, and specialty consultations for the patient.

SELECTED KEY REFERENCES

Centers for Disease Control and Prevention (CDC). Stroke facts and statistics. 2/9/2007. Available at http://www.cdc.gov/stroke/stroke_facts.htm.
Excellent source of epidemiologic data about stroke in the United States.

Chambers BR, Norris JW. Outcome in patients with asymptomatic neck bruits. *N Engl J Med.* 1986;315:860-865.
This classic paper gives the natural history of asymptomatic carotid disease.

El Barghouty N, Geroulakos G, Nicolaides A, Androulakis A, Bahal V. Computer assisted carotid plaque characterization. *Eur J Vasc Endovasc Surg.* 1995;9:389-393.
This paper correlates head computed tomography (CT) findings with the carotid plaque gray-scale median to demonstrate that more echolucent plaque is associated with CT-detected embolic infarcts.

Mathiesen EB, Waterloo K, Joakimsen O, Bakke SJ, Jacobsen EA, Bønaa KH. Reduced neuropsychological test performance in asymptomatic carotid stenosis: the Tromsø Study. *Neurology.* 2004;62:695-701.
This study demonstrates reduced performance on psychometric tests in patients with "asymptomatic" carotid stenosis, again raising the question of the role of carotid disease in the overall cognitive and behavioral decline associated with aging.

Roederer GO, Langlois YE, Jager KA, Primozich JF, Beach KW, Phillips DJ, Strandness DE Jr. The natural history of carotid arterial disease in asymptomatic patients with cervical bruits. *Stroke.* 1984;15:605-613.
This paper explores the effect of carotid plaque progression on outcomes in asymptomatic patients.

Takaya N, Yuan C, Chu B, Saam T, Underhill H, Cai J, Tran N, Polissar NL, Isaac C, Ferguson M, Garden GA, Cramer SC, Maravilla KR, Hashimoto B, Hatsukami TS. Association between carotid plaque characteristics and subsequent cerebrovascular events. *Stroke.* 2006;37:818-823.
The authors use magnetic resonance technology to evaluate carotid plaque fibrous cap thickness and integrity and relate these characteristics to the clinical course.

Tejada J, Diez-Tejedor E, Hernandez-Echebarria L. Does a relationship exist between carotid stenosis and lacunar infarction? *Stroke.* 2003;34:1404-1411.
This provocative paper points to a possible association between lacunar infarctions and carotid bifurcation atherosclerosis.

REFERENCES

The reference list can be found on the companion Expert Consult Web site at *www.expertconsult.com.*

CHAPTER 93

Cerebrovascular Disease: Diagnostic Evaluation

A. Ross Naylor and George Markose

Preceding chapters have described the methodology, diagnostic criteria, and limitations of each of the principal investigative modalities. The aim of this chapter is to provide the reader with a more pragmatic guide for planning safe and reliable evaluation of patients with cerebrovascular disease. The ultimate choice cannot be uncritically standardized because it will inevitably reflect (1) access to state-of-the-art or older technology, (2) experience, (3) opinion regarding what now constitutes the "gold standard," (4) (rapid) availability, (5) cost, (6) robustness in sensitivity analyses, (7) the particular measurement method being used (North American versus European; see Chapter 15: Vascular Laboratory: Arterial Duplex Scanning), (8) whether discrimination between 50% to 69% and 70% to 99% internal carotid artery (ICA) stenosis is desired, and (9) matching to current requirements for performing carotid endarterectomy (CEA) or carotid artery stenting (CAS) because planning for CEA and CAS is completely different.

Several important themes will emerge, but none is more important than the need for rapid investigation in symptomatic patients. The Carotid Endarterectomy Trialists Collaboration (CETC) combined data from the European Carotid Surgery Trial (ECST), North American Symptomatic Carotid Endarterectomy Trial (NASCET), and Veteran's Administration Trial (having remeasured all 6000 prerandomization angiograms with the NASCET method) and then performed subgroup analyses on the effect of delay in surgery[1] (Table 93-1). As is apparent, any delay significantly reduces the long-term benefit conferred by CEA. Accordingly, any imaging modality that incurs undue delay (e.g., waiting list pressure,

image processing time, reporting) will reduce overall clinical effectiveness, even if it might also prove to be the most accurate on sensitivity analyses. This paradox must be considered when planning the most appropriate investigative strategy.

DUPLEX ULTRASOUND

Indications

There are a variety of clinical scenarios in which duplex ultrasound (DUS) examination can provide useful information for the practitioner (see Chapter 15: Vascular Laboratory: Arterial Duplex Scanning).

Carotid Artery Disease

In 2006,[2] the U.K. Health Technology Assessment (HTA) published a meta-analysis of studies evaluating the accuracy of noninvasive imaging (but not including multidetector computed tomographic angiography [MDCTA]) and concluded that although contrast-enhanced magnetic resonance angiography (CEMRA) was the most accurate imaging modality overall (Table 93-2), its clinical effectiveness was limited by inaccessibility, unavailability, and delays. In light of this, the HTA concluded that color DUS remained the preferred first-line imaging modality for identifying patients with 70% to 99% ICA stenosis because of (1) low cost, (2) the much higher number of strokes likely to be prevented in the long term (because patients are identified and scheduled rapidly for surgery), (3) its robustness in sensitivity analyses (see Table

Table 93-1 Effect of Delay in Surgery on Overall Benefit Conferred by Carotid Endarterectomy*

Stenosis Group (%)	Delay (wk)[†]	ARR[‡] (%)	NNT[§]	Strokes Prevented per 1000 Carotid Endarterectomies at 5 Years[ǀ]
50-69	<2	14.8	7	148
	2-4	3.3	30	33
	4-12	4.0	25	40
	>12	−2.9	nil	nil
70-99[¶]	<2	30.2	3	302
	2-4	17.6	6	176
	4-12	11.4	9	114
	>12	8.9	11	89

*Data recalculated from the Carotid Endarterectomy Trialists Collaboration.[1]
[†]Delay indicates time from randomization to surgery. The mean delay from the onset of symptoms to randomization was 7 days.
[‡]Absolute risk reduction in 5-year risk for ipsilateral stroke conferred by carotid endarterectomy over best medical therapy.
[§]Number needed to treat to prevent one ipsilateral stroke at 5 years.
[ǀ]Number of ipsilateral strokes prevented at 5 years by performing 1000 carotid endarterectomies.
[¶]Excludes patients with near-occlusion.

Table 93-2 Results of a Meta-analysis of the Accuracy of Noninvasive Imaging for All Stenosis Groups and Imaging Modalities

Stenosis Group (%)	Imaging	Sensitivity (95% CI)	Specificity (95% CI)
70-99	US	0.89 (0.85-0.92)	0.84 (0.77-0.89)
	CTA	0.77 (0.68-0.84)	0.95 (0.91-0.97)
	MRA	0.88 (0.82-0.92)	0.84 (0.76-0.90)
	CEMRA	0.94 (0.88-0.97)	0.93 (0.89-0.96)
50-69	US	0.36 (0.25-0.49)	0.91 (0.87-0.94)
	CTA	0.67 (0.30-0.90)	0.79 (0.63-0.89)
	MRA	0.37 (0.26-0.49)	0.91 (0.78-0.97)
	CEMRA	0.77 (0.59-0.89)	0.97 (0.93-0.99)
0-49, 100	US	0.83 (0.73-0.90)	0.84 (0.62-0.95)
	CTA	0.81 (0.70-0.88)	0.91 (0.74-0.98)
	MRA	0.81 (0.70-0.88)	0.88 (0.76-0.95)
	CEMRA	0.96 (0.90-0.99)	0.96 (0.90-0.99)

CEMRA, contrast-enhanced magnetic resonance angiography; CI, confidence interval; CTA, computed tomographic angiography; MRA, magnetic resonance angiography; US, ultrasound.
Reproduced with permission from Wardlaw JM, Chappell FM, Stevenson M, et al. Accurate, practical and cost-effective assessment of carotid stenosis in the UK. Health Technology Assessment 2006. Vol 10, No. 30. Available at: http://www.hta.ac.uk/fullmono/mon1030.pdf.

93-2), and (4) its ability to match the needs of current surgery (i.e., patients were selected for surgery through attendance at single-visit clinics incorporating DUS imaging with a low probability of the surgeon's encountering unexpected findings at surgery that might otherwise compromise patient safety).[3] The HTA did, however, highlight concerns about the accuracy of DUS in diagnosing 50% to 69% stenosis (see Table 93-2; sensitivity, 0.36; specificity, 0.91).[2] Because the benefit conferred by CEA in patients with 50% to 69% stenosis falls significantly with any delay in surgery (see Table 93-1), the HTA recommended that if 4 weeks or more had elapsed after the index event, it would be advisable to perform corroborative imaging (CEMRA or MDCTA) to confirm the severity of stenosis. If, however, DUS was performed within 4 weeks of the index event, the HTA thought it reasonable to proceed with CEA (on the basis of DUS alone) because the number of strokes prevented by rapid access to surgery then exceeded the risk that patients with less than 50% stenosis will undergo inappropriate surgery.

Vertebrobasilar Disease

Extracranial DUS offers only basic information about flow dynamics in the vertebral arteries (VAs) and nothing about the basilar system (feasible with color transcranial DUS). It is not always possible to image the VA origins, and only sections running between the transverse processes can be imaged higher up. Accordingly, if a patient is suspected of having vertebrobasilar symptoms, DUS assessment is helpful (if only to exclude coexistent carotid disease), but some other form of imaging (probably MDCTA) is mandated. DUS is, however, useful for demonstrating complete/partial VA flow reversal and thus suggesting the possibility of proximal subclavian or innominate artery disease.

Role in Screening

Whereas the Society for Vascular Surgery actively advocates screening in patients older than 55 years with cardiovascular risk factors, the 2007 U.S. Preventive Services Task Force actively recommends against it.[4] A reluctance to screen also exists in Canada, the United Kingdom, and Scandinavia. For those committed to screening, DUS is the first-line modality. Portable DUS machines are available, but data about their accuracy are limited. Accordingly, those who use portable machines to screen asymptomatic populations are strongly advised to undertake a corroborative DUS study in an accredited vascular laboratory (or use MDCTA/CEMRA) should a greater than 50% stenosis be suspected and should CEA or CAS be considered. DUS is also the preferred screening modality before coronary artery bypass graft surgery. Screening everyone is not cost-effective (5% yield for 80% to 99% stenosis),[5] but the yield is increased in selected patient cohorts (those with left mainstem disease, carotid bruit, previous stroke/transient ischemic attack [TIA]). Any patient being considered for coronary artery bypass grafting with the internal mammary artery and who has weak/absent radial pulses should undergo assessment of the subclavian arteries, innominate arteries, and VAs. When inflow disease or VA flow reversal is suspected, further imaging (MDCTA or CEMRA) is required and the cardiac surgeon should be warned that unless a subclavian or innominate artery lesion is corrected, subsequent use of the ipsilateral internal mammary artery (as a conduit) could cause postoperative coronary steal syndrome (Fig. 93-1).

Role in Trauma

DUS provides a useful screening and surveillance role in patients with zone II injuries to the carotid artery (between the cricoid cartilage and angle of the mandible), especially intimal irregularities or small false aneurysms being treated conservatively. However, DUS is less reliable in zone I injuries (clavicle to cricoid cartilage) or zone III injuries (angle of the mandible to base of the skull). In the past, DUS was used to select patients for angiography. After the advent of MDCTA, however, many would argue that this is now the investigation of choice because vascular imaging can be combined with evaluation of bony and soft tissue injuries.

Evaluation of Carotid Body/ Glomus Vagale Tumors

Because of their vascularity, DUS is ideally suited for excluding the possibility of carotid body tumors (CBTs) or glomus vagale tumors (GVTs), both closely related to the carotid system. Given the rapid availability of DUS, it would probably be unwise to biopsy a "lymph node" in the jugulodigastric region without having undertaken such a simple screening investigation. Once a tumor is suspected, MDCTA or magnetic resonance angiography (MRA) should be performed to exclude bilateral lesions (5% incidence) and to image the

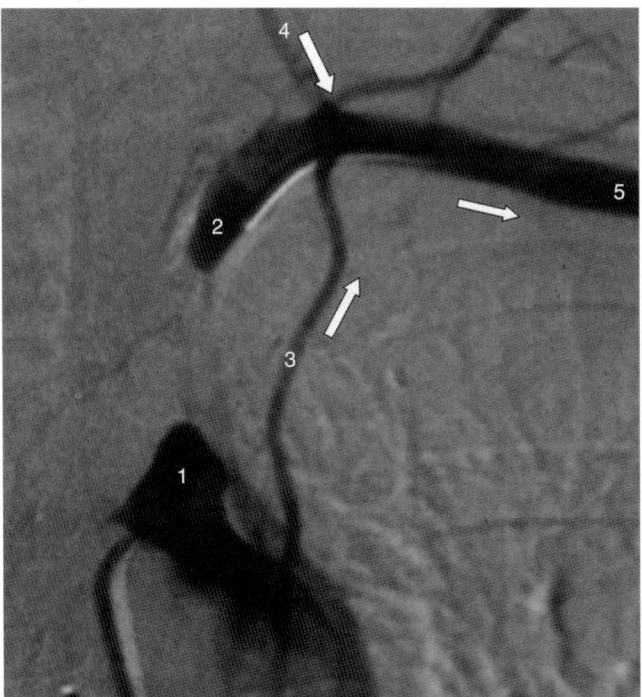

Figure 93-1 Intra-arterial digital subtraction arteriography in a patient with coronary steal syndrome who had previously undergone coronary bypass with the left internal mammary artery. There is occlusion of the proximal left subclavian artery (1), which refills distally (2, 5) via reversed flow in the left vertebral (4) and internal mammary artery (3). It was treated successfully by angioplasty.

upper and lateral extent of the lesion. Large, highly placed lesions require a different operative strategy from that for smaller, lower lesions that must be anticipated preoperatively (temporomandibular subluxation cannot be performed once the operation is under way). DUS can also warn the surgeon that a GVT might be present (Fig. 93-2), thus enabling the patient to be counseled in advance about the possibility of having to resect the vagus nerve, which can result in hoarseness or swallowing difficulties. CBTs cause splaying of the carotid bifurcation. GVTs do not splay the bifurcation, but they do cause displacement of the upper ICA. In addition, GVTs tend to have vascular serpiginous feeding vessels tracking down the proximal vagus nerve. These vessels can be seen to lie separate from the bifurcation, internal jugular vein, and common carotid artery.

Role in the Planning of Carotid Endarterectomy and Carotid Angioplasty with Stenting

In many centers, up to 95% of CEA procedures are currently undertaken on the basis of DUS alone,[3] and there is no evidence that reliance on ultrasound compromises patient safety or operability. Most importantly, patients can be identified and scheduled for surgery faster than with any other imaging modality, thereby optimizing the long-term benefit conferred by surgery (see Table 93-1). There are, however, important caveats with this protocol. First, the vascular labo-

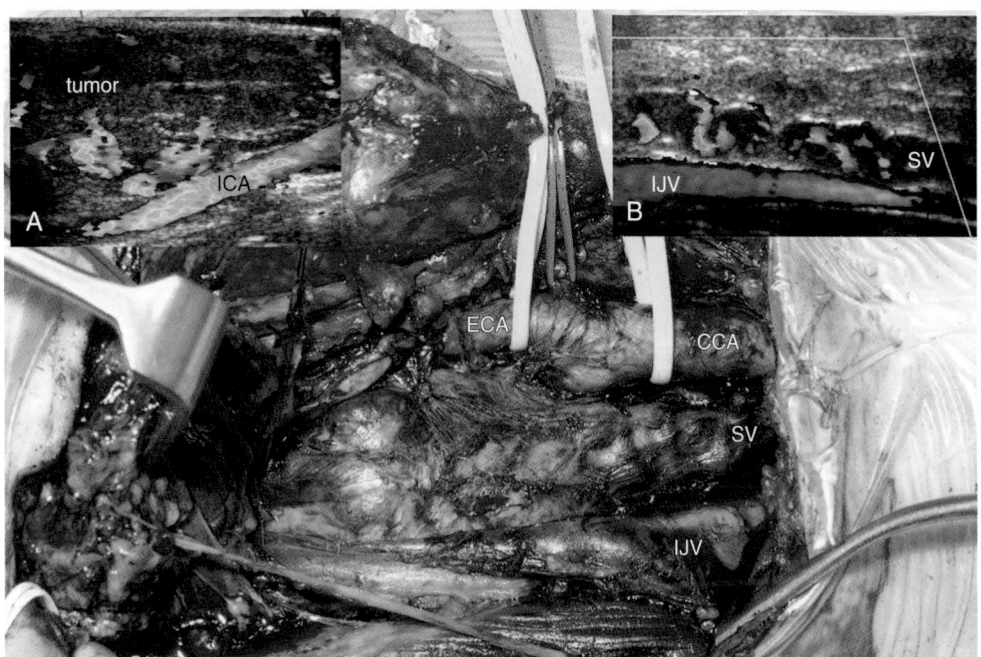

Figure 93-2 Glomus vagale tumor (GVT, main picture). This does not splay the bifurcation but displaces the distal internal carotid artery (ICA) (duplex image, **A**). Occasionally, preoperative ultrasound features can suggest that this is a GVT and not a carotid body tumor. Note the serpiginous feeding vessels extending down the vagus nerve (SV: main picture and duplex ultrasound scan [**B**]). These are separate from the common carotid artery (CCA) and internal jugular vein (IJV).

ratory should be accredited and have clear and validated criteria for measuring carotid stenosis. Second (and not relevant to North America), European vascular units must be absolutely clear which measurement method is being used (NASCET versus ECST; see Chapter 15: Vascular Laboratory: Arterial Duplex Scanning). Recent evidence suggests that there may be considerable confusion.[6] Third is awareness of DUS findings that suggest tandem inflow/outflow problems or subocclusion. In each of these situations, corroborative imaging is mandated (MDCTA, CEMRA, or intra-arterial digital subtraction arteriography [IADSA]). In practice, one of the most frequent pathologic lesions missed with DUS is a coiled distal ICA (see Chapter 99: Carotid Artery: Dissection and Other Disorders). In most situations this does not present any undue problems for the surgeon, but it can be a cause of shunt failure (and intraoperative hemodynamic stroke) should the distal shunt tip occlude against the distal loop and not be recognized. This problem can be avoided by using intraoperative transcranial Doppler (TCD) to assess for adequate shunt flow. DUS can also be useful in warning of unusual causes of cerebrovascular symptoms, such as the ICA "stump syndrome" (Fig. 93-3). In this rare condition, an occluded ICA stump (identifiable on DUS) acts as a reservoir for fresh thrombus, which can then embolize up the external carotid artery (ECA) into the brain via retrograde flow through the supraorbital and infraorbital vessels.

By contrast, CAS cannot be planned on the basis of DUS alone. Table 93-3 details anatomic and morphologic features that either are associated with an adverse outcome after CAS or might influence the choice of cerebral protection device (CPD) or stent. For example, the choice of CPD will depend on factors such as patency of the ECA, integrity of the circle of Willis, and whether there is a straight enough and nontortuous distal ICA. Stent selection will depend on varying combinations of vessel tortuosity and plaque friability. As can be seen, DUS can demonstrate the presence of an appropriate ipsilateral stenosis, ECA patency, the extent of contralateral disease, and localized tortuosity around the bifurcation, and it can advise on plaque morphology and warn that there may be coexistent inflow and outflow problems. However, DUS cannot provide information regarding (1) the type of aortic arch, (2) the extent of calcification at the origins of the great vessels, (3) proximal tortuosity (common carotid artery), (4) the availability of an adequate distal landing zone for a filter CPD, or (5) the status of the circle of Willis. If, for example, the circle of Willis is not intact (Fig. 93-4), CAS practitioners tend not to deploy the flow reversal type of CPD. This type of information can be provided only by MDCTA, CEMRA, or IADSA. However, this unavoidable reliance on additional imaging will inevitably introduce delays in planning the management of symptomatic patients. If such delays are likely to be excessive (i.e., >2 weeks), some patients may be better treated by CEA.

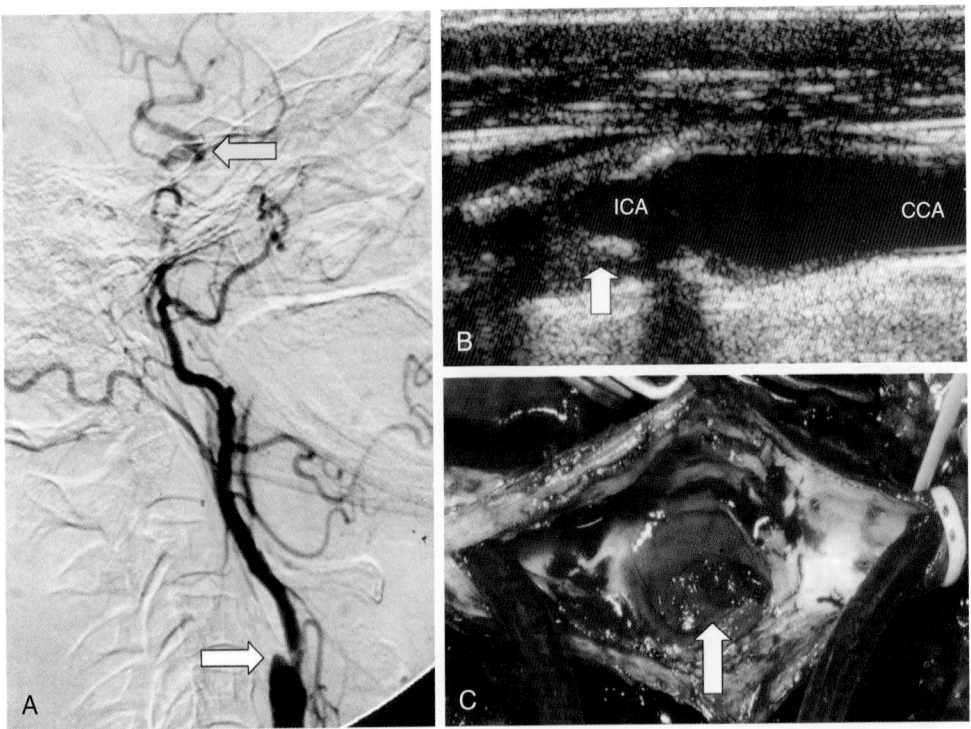

Figure 93-3 Internal carotid artery (ICA) stump syndrome. **A,** Selective intra-arterial digital subtraction arteriography with delayed imaging confirms the presence of an occluded ICA with a small stump (*white arrow*). The external carotid artery (ECA) is an important source of collateral flow because there is refilling of the distal ipsilateral carotid syphon (*yellow arrow*). **B,** B-mode ultrasound image of the ICA stump in this patient (*arrow*). **C,** Operative image with a shunt inserted between the common carotid artery (CCA) and the ECA. Note the extensive fresh thrombus within the ICA stump (*arrow*).

Table 93-3 Anatomic and Morphologic Features Associated with Adverse Outcomes after Carotid Artery Stenting or That Might Influence the Choice of Protection Device or Stent and Relationship with Imaging Modalities

Vessel Affected	Feature	Modality			
		US	CEMRA	MDCTA	IADSA
Aortic arch	Ulceration	X	+	++	++
	Excessive calcification	X	X	++	+
	Bovine arch variants	X	++	++	++
	Type III arch	X	++	++	++
Great vessels	Ulceration	X	+	++	+
	Tortuosity/kinking	X	++	++	++
	Excessive calcification	X	X	++	+
	Anatomic anomalies	X	+	++	+
	Severe inflow stenosis	X	+	++	++
Common carotid	Diffuse disease	+	++	++	++
	Coiling/kinking	+	++	++	++
	Excessive calcification	+	X	++	+
Carotid bifurcation	Excessive calcification	X	X	++	+
	Angulation	++	++	++	++
Ipsilateral external carotid artery	Occlusion/severe stenosis	++	++	++	++
Ipsilateral internal carotid artery	Excessive calcification	X	X	++	+
	Distal tortuosity/coiling	X	++	++	++
	Plaque characterization	++	++	+	X
	Fresh thrombus	+	+	+	X
	Preocclusive stenosis	++	++	++	++
	Long lesion (>3 cm)	+	+	++	++
Contralateral internal carotid artery	Stenosis >50%	++	++	++	++
Incomplete circle of Willis		X	++	++	+

X, not really suited for imaging; +, basic information provided; ++, highly suitable for imaging.
CEMRA, contrast-enhanced magnetic resonance angiography; IADSA, intra-arterial digital subtraction angiography; MDCTA, multidetector computed tomographic angiography; US, ultrasound.

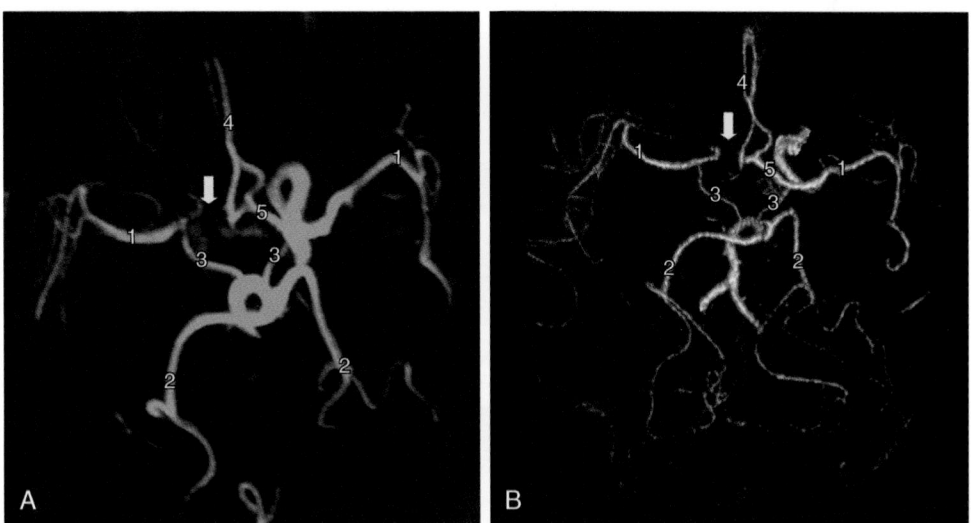

Figure 93-4 Circle of Willis imaged by contrast-enhanced magnetic resonance angiography (**A**) and multidetector computed tomographic angiography (**B**). There are normal middle cerebral arteries (1), posterior cerebral arteries (2), posterior communicating arteries (3), and A2 segments of the anterior cerebral arteries (4). The A1 segment of the anterior cerebral artery is intact on one side (5) but absent on the other (*arrow*). Recognition of this abnormality does not influence the performance of carotid endarterectomy but might influence the choice of protection device during carotid artery stenting (i.e., a filter may be preferred instead of a flow reversal device).

Role in Evaluating Plaque Morphology

Ultrasound provides a basic (but relatively subjective) interpretation of plaque morphology (Table 93-4) that has generated conflicting opinions with regard to its potential usefulness in guiding clinical practice.[7,8] In the Asymptomatic Carotid Surgery Trial (ACST), there was no evidence that the Gray-Weale classification (see Table 93-4) predicted outcome in medically treated asymptomatic patients,[9] but the Asymptomatic Carotid Stenosis and Risk of Stroke (ACSRS) study showed that if "image normalization" was performed beforehand, 94% of the strokes destined to occur in a cohort of 1000 asymptomatic patients with 50% to 99% stenosis had Geroulakis type 1 to 3 plaque[8,10] (see Table 93-4). The weakness of DUS plaque morphology studies has been its lack of objectivity. This shortcoming has now been partially addressed by the development of gray-scale median (GSM) measurement,[11] in which high-resolution B-mode images are combined with quantitative computer-assisted measurement of plaque echogenicity (Fig. 93-5). The GSM is a numerical measure representing the overall echogenicity of the plaque (low values are observed in predominantly echolucent plaque, whereas higher values are observed in more sclerotic fibrous lesions). Evidence from the Imaging in Carotid Angioplasty and Risk of Stroke (ICAROS) study suggested that a GSM of less than 25 was associated with a 7.1% stroke rate after CAS (this risk was not reduced by the use of protection devices) versus a 1.5% rate in patients with a GSM higher than 25.[12] This study was one of the first to suggest that objective assessment of plaque morphology could be used to plan management (i.e., when one might avoid CAS, especially for less experienced practitioners), and it could evolve a role in selecting patients at higher risk for stroke, especially in asymptomatic cohorts. In practice, few centers currently incorporate DUS evaluation of plaque morphology in the planning of patient management.

Perioperative Roles

DUS is often repeated immediately before surgery if an interval has elapsed since the initial DUS. This ensures that the ICA has not occluded (i.e., CEA is now unnecessary), provides a final opportunity to warn of distal disease extension (i.e., the last chance for a surgeon to consider temporomandibular subluxation), and fulfils an important quality control function because it permits internal validation of DUS machines and

Table 93-4 Plaque Characterization with Duplex Ultrasound

Gray-Weale Classification[7]		Geroulakis Classification[8]	
Type	Description	Type	Description
Type 1	Echolucent	Type 1	Uniformly echolucent Bright echoes occupy <15% of plaque
Type 2	Predominantly echolucent	Type 2	Mainly echolucent Bright echoes occupy 15%-50% of plaque
Type 3	Predominantly echogenic	Type 3	Mainly echogenic Bright echoes occupy 50%-85% of plaque
Type 4	Echogenic	Type 4	Uniformly echogenic Bright echoes occupy >85% of plaque
		Type 5	Calcified cap (>15% of cap) with acoustic shadow

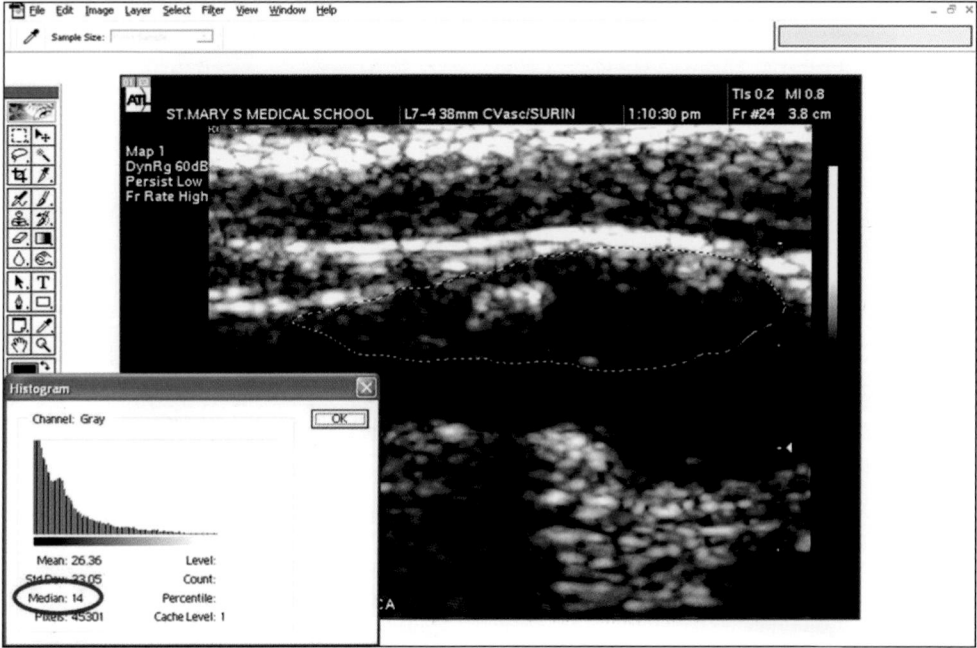

Figure 93-5 Gray-scale median (GSM). A B-mode image of the carotid bifurcation has been image-normalized and a region of interest drawn around the plaque, which shows areas of blackness (low GSM value) and bright areas (higher GSM score). After computerized analysis, an average GSM score (14) is recorded (*red circle*). (*Courtesy of Professor Andrew Nicolaides.*)

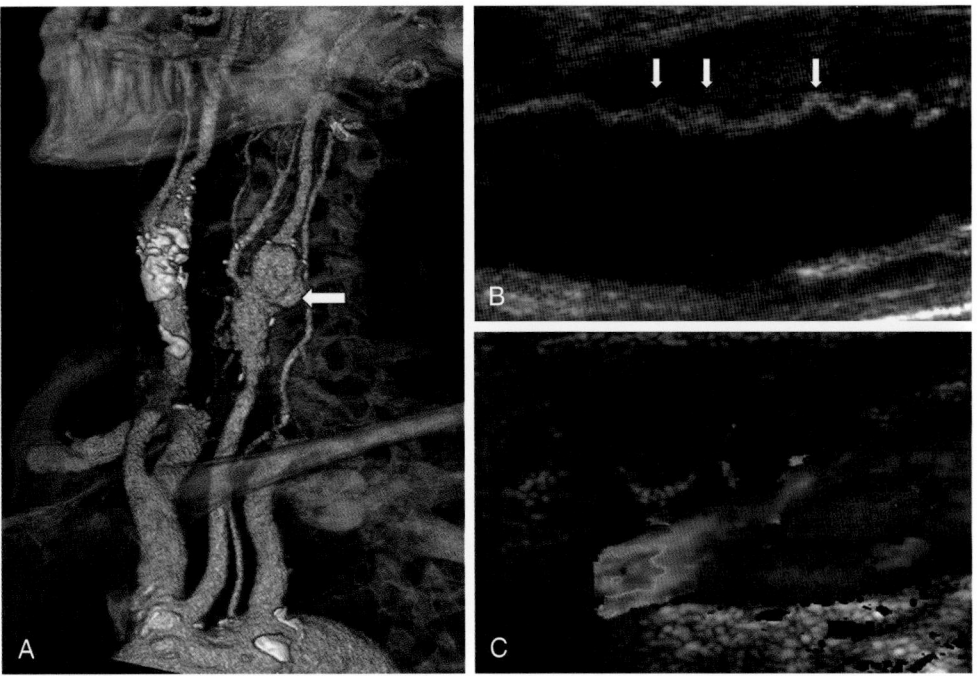

Figure 93-6 Prosthetic patch infection 15 years after carotid endarterectomy. Multidetector computed tomographic angiography (**A**) shows a false aneurysm (*arrow*) at the left carotid bifurcation. **B,** Corrugation of the polyester patch on B-mode ultrasound imaging (*arrows*). **C,** Color duplex ultrasound showing jets of blood into a false aneurysm secondary to patch infection (not the same patient).

operators. Intraoperatively, DUS is a simple means of performing completion assessment after restoration of flow by looking (specifically) for residual filling defects (luminal thrombus), undue turbulence, and evidence of intimal flaps or residual stenosis (see Chapter 95: Carotid Artery Disease: Endarterectomy). No randomized trial has evaluated whether completion assessment reduces procedural risk. A recent overview has suggested that it makes no difference,[13] but this study needs to be interpreted with caution because all events (fatal cardiac events, intraoperative/postoperative strokes, all causes of stroke) were combined in the analysis.

Postoperative Roles

Because of its versatility, DUS is invaluable in guiding the management of patients with a postoperative neurologic deficit. These deficits often occur when other imaging modalities are unavailable, and DUS can be brought to the patient's bedside rapidly. Air in the deep tissues can interfere with insonation early after surgery, but it is usually possible to exclude thrombosis. Diagnosing the exact cause of the deficit can be difficult, and the role of DUS is enhanced if combined with TCD. The role of serial DUS surveillance after CEA and CAS remains controversial. As with screening, it is rarely undertaken in the United Kingdom and Scandinavia but is common practice in North America, Australasia, and mainland Europe. Advocates of DUS surveillance can find anecdotal reports supporting their position, but a critical review of restenosis rates and risk for ipsilateral stroke in patients who were randomized in trials in which surveillance strategies were planned from the outset does bring into question

whether screening confers any long-term benefit.[14] On a practical note, those who offer DUS surveillance after CAS must be aware that stents change the physical properties of the carotid artery such that different diagnostic criteria are required.[15]

DUS is, however, useful in warning about the possibility of late prosthetic patch infection (Fig. 93-6). It is the first-line investigation undertaken in patients returning with pulsatile neck swelling, draining sinus tracts, or neck pain, and recognition of patch "corrugation" usually precedes the onset of clinical symptoms by up to a year (i.e., recognition of this phenomenon can alert the surgeon to the possibility of patch infection early and to start antibiotics).[16] DUS should also identify "leaks" into early false aneurysms (see Fig. 93-6).

Contraindications

There are no specific contraindications to carotid ultrasound examination. However, the examination should be undertaken only by an operator who has been adequately trained (see Chapter 15: Vascular Laboratory: Arterial Duplex Scanning).

Accuracy and Limitations in Clinical Practice

The most important determinant of the diagnostic accuracy of DUS is the experience and skill of the operator. There is an important learning curve, and this has to be anticipated. Surgical units cannot simply start operating on the basis of DUS without a careful review of practice and personnel. Second is the wide array of stenosis thresholds being used in individual centers (>50%, >60%, >70%) and the wide range of peak systolic velocity and velocity ratios currently being used to classify stenosis subgroups. This variability has been lessened by publication of North American DUS consensus criteria,[17] and a similar consensus group will be reporting shortly in the United Kingdom. Third is knowledge of whether the operator is using ECST or NASCET measurement criteria. This is less of a problem in North America, but experience in the United Kingdom suggests that many vascular laboratories remain unsure.[6] Interestingly, the North American consensus document makes no reference about how one should grade a large carotid bulb that contains large amounts of atherothrombotic material. This could be scored 0% with the NASCET measurement method but 70% stenosis with the ECST method. Future guideline makers must address this anomaly. Fourth is situations in which caution must be exercised when interpreting DUS findings. Such situations include (1) an inability to clearly image high bifurcations, (2) an inability to image above the plaque, (3) damped waveforms in the proximal common carotid artery (suggesting inflow stenosis), (4) high-resistance flow in the distal ICA (suggesting a distal tandem lesion), (5) increased peak systolic velocity in the contralateral ICA (secondary to hyperemic collateralization) in the presence of a contralateral occlusion or very severe stenosis (leading to the potential for overestimating the degree of ipsilateral stenosis), (6) excessive calcification (which prevents accurate velocity measurement because of acoustic shadowing), and (7) suspicion of near-occlusion. The latter condition has aroused considerable controversy. Though previously considered to be a marker for increased stroke risk, the CETC has now shown that near-occlusion (i.e., severe ICA stenosis that does not open into a normal-caliber lumen) is not a high-risk predictor for stroke and that CEA does not appear to confer long-term benefit.[1] Finally, color transcranial DUS can provide additional information regarding the integrity of the circle of Willis. However, this is unnecessary before CEA, and CEMRA and MDCTA provide more accurate images should this type of information be required (e.g., before CAS).

The Need for Corroborative Imaging

Corroborative imaging is necessary whenever there is uncertainty about the duplex findings, whenever intervention is planned in cases with borderline benefit based on the severity of stenosis (e.g., symptomatic patients with 50% to 69% stenosis, especially when more than 4 weeks have elapsed since the initial consultation), whenever new technologists are undertaking DUS assessment, and in any patient undergoing CAS.

■ MAGNETIC RESONANCE IMAGING/ANGIOGRAPHY

Indications

MRA has been available since 1996, but only recently (after the introduction of CEMRA) has it been considered a legiti-

mate rival to angiography (see Chapter 22: Magnetic Resonance Imaging). One of its main advantages is that it avoids any exposure to radiation. Because of the way images are acquired, bony structures are not present on the image, thus avoiding the need for complicated postprocessing. Unfortunately, however, the surrounding soft tissue structures are also not visualized unless additional magnetic resonance imaging (MRI) is performed, and calcium within plaque is not well defined.

Role in Carotid Disease

MRA is playing an increasingly important role in the evaluation of patients with carotid artery occlusive disease. Table 93-2 summarizes the principal sensitivity analyses from the HTA systematic review for time-of-flight (TOF) MRA and CEMRA. The sensitivity and specificity for diagnosing 70% to 99% stenosis with TOF MRA are identical to that for DUS and similarly poor for diagnosing 50% to 69% stenosis. Two-dimensional (2D) TOF MRA provides strong vascular signals, even when flow is low (thus making it good for differentiating occlusion from near-occlusion), whereas three-dimensional (3D) TOF MRA offers better spatial resolution for measuring the degree of stenosis and also enables assessment of flow directionality (useful in evaluating steal phenomena). However, to minimize the very long acquisition times and artifacts (flow related, motion, and boundary), its field of view has to be restricted. Accordingly, although it is possible to image both carotid bifurcations at the same time, two further sets of data acquisition are required to image the aortic arch/great vessels and the circle of Willis with TOF. This greatly limits its overall versatility and accessibility and means that for the most part, it offers little in addition to DUS.

However, CEMRA is assuming a much more important role in imaging patients with cerebrovascular disease (Fig. 93-7). CEMRA uses the paramagnetic agent gadolinium, and images are obtained more rapidly than with TOF MRA. Each individual acquisition period may take only 20 seconds, but given the requirement for correct patient and listening coil positioning, the total time will be closer to 20 minutes. CEMRA offers fewer flow-related artifacts and a much greater field of view that allows high-resolution imaging from the aortic arch (see Fig. 93-7) up to the circle of Willis (see Fig. 93-4) while retaining the ability to evaluate flow directionality. The HTA systematic review and meta-analysis (see Table 93-2) concluded that CEMRA is now the best (noninvasive) imaging modality (although MDCTA was not evaluated) and has superseded TOF MRA. However, as was noted by the HTA, many centers still do not have rapid access to CEMRA. Accordingly, if it is going to take several weeks for the CEMRA scan to be performed, symptomatic patients will gain greater clinical benefit by undergoing expedited CEA on the basis of DUS alone (see Table 93-1). Another advantage of TOF MRA and CEMRA is that they can be combined with functional MRI of the brain, although (unlike MDCTA) this requires an additional period of data acquisition.

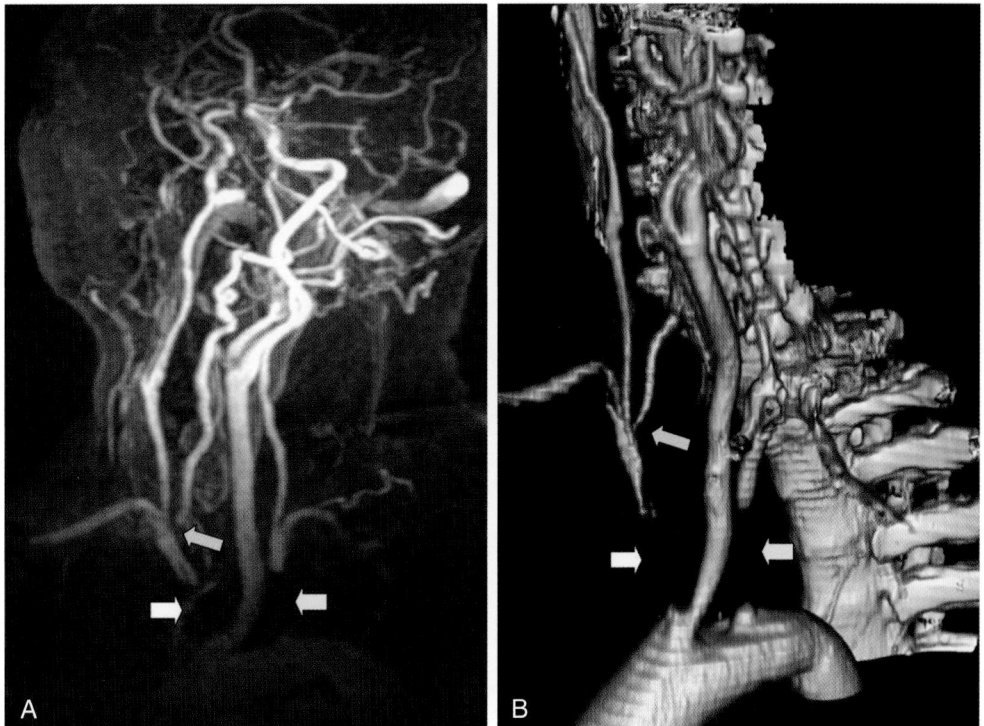

Figure 93-7 Sixty-year-old woman with a vertebrobasilar stroke and recurring unsteadiness of gait imaged by contrast-enhanced magnetic resonance angiography (CEMRA) (**A**) and multidetector computed tomographic angiography (MDCTA) (**B**). There is complete occlusion of the innominate artery (*white arrow*) and left subclavian artery (*yellow arrow*). The right vertebral artery has a stenosis at its origin (*blue arrow*). CEMRA and MDCTA have shown identical features, but MDCTA is probably easier to interpret because of venous contamination in the CEMRA image.

Role in Vertebrobasilar Disease

One of the main advantages of both TOF MRA and CEMRA is that they provide information regarding flow directionality, which is useful in evaluating steal phenomena (subclavian, coronary). Both, however, are limited by an increased likelihood of encountering artifacts at the VA origins because of vessel tortuosity, respiratory motion, and cardiac pulsation. In practice, MDCTA is probably the preferred (noninvasive) investigation for evaluating patients with suspected vertebrobasilar symptoms, although it cannot provide information on flow directionality.

Role in Screening

MRA currently has no role as a screening modality. Most importantly, it is not cost-effective.

Role in the Evaluation of Trauma

MRI and MRA are seldom undertaken in trauma patients, largely because of logistic issues such as scanner location (in relation to the emergency department or operating room), prolonged acquisition times, and poor access to an unstable patient for monitoring. In practice, MDCTA offers a better modality, principally because of its rapid acquisition times (5 seconds for the aortic arch to the circle of Willis) and its ability to image adjacent bony and soft tissue structures (including the brain) with a single scan. This is important because patients with serious arterial trauma tend to have other injuries as well.

Role in the Evaluation of Carotid Body/ Glomus Tumors

MRA and CEMRA provide basic angiographic information that can be useful in planning surgical management and excluding contralateral lesions (Fig. 93-8). However, CEMRA is limited by the fact that there are no bony landmarks retained on the image. Therefore, MDCTA is probably the better imaging modality in this situation, mainly because of the high-resolution axial images that can detail the full extent of the lesion and its relationship to adjacent structures.

Role in the Planning of Carotid Endarterectomy and Carotid Angioplasty with Stenting

Surgeons who believe that the vast majority of CEAs can be performed on the basis of DUS alone will be unlikely to find an additional role for CEMRA and will have little or no use for TOF MRA techniques in routine clinical practice. In the event that DUS studies are nondiagnostic, MDCTA is

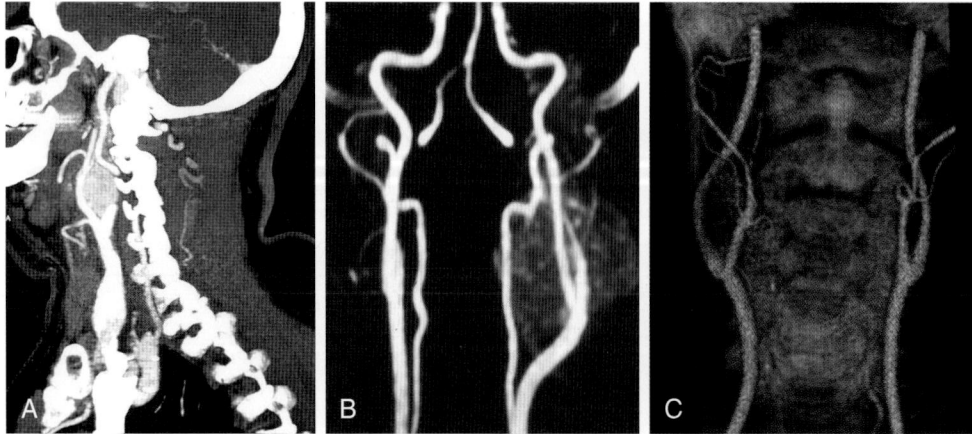

Figure 93-8 Carotid body tumors. **A,** Multidetector computed tomographic angiography (MDCTA) maximum intensity projection (MIP) image. **B,** Contrast-enhanced magnetic resonance angiography MIP image. **C,** MDCTA volume rendition image.

probably preferable to CEMRA. However, CAS requires much more imaging information during the planning process than CEA does (see Table 93-3). Accordingly, the choice of using CEMRA, MDCTA, or digital subtraction angiography (DSA) will inevitably reflect resources, clinician preferences, and local expertise. CEMRA is preferable to computed tomographic angiography (CTA) (by conventional spiral computed tomography [CT]), whereas MDCTA is now generally accepted to be superior because of its ability to combine the anatomic imaging of CEMRA (arch to the circle of Willis) with identification of calcification, vessel tortuosity, and vascular anomalies, as well as the ability to perform functional brain imaging during one period of data acquisition. CEMRA can identify vessel anomalies, but if the vessels are occluded, they can sometimes be missed because of the way in which the images are acquired. As is apparent from Table 93-3, the main limitation of CEMRA is its inability to display calcification. Documenting the extent of calcification in the arch and origins of the great vessels is not a major problem during planning for CEA, but with increasing age, the arch and great vessels become more tortuous and calcified. These features make CAS more challenging (especially for less experienced practitioners) and are also associated with an increased procedural risk.[18] A further problem with CEMRA is the tendency for multiple vessels to be included in the final image (some venous), which can lead to difficulties in overall interpretation of the image (see Fig. 93-7).

Role in Evaluating Plaque Morphology

Most management algorithms use degree of stenosis as the principal determinant of who should be considered for CEA and CAS. The last decade has witnessed increasing interest in evaluating more sophisticated imaging modalities that specifically look for subtle changes in plaque morphology that may help identify a subgroup of patients who may be at higher risk for suffering a stroke if left untreated (see Chapter 92: Cerebrovascular Disease: General Considerations and Chapter 94:

Cerebrovascular Disease: Decision Making and Medical Treatment). In this respect, MR offers considerable potential, although it requires even more periods of data acquisition (i.e., plaque morphology data cannot be acquired during vessel or brain imaging studies). MR is probably the best modality for visualization of the fibrous cap[19] and lipid core,[20] whereas MR spectroscopy (still very much a research tool) can image inflammatory molecules within the plaque. Considerable interest has focused on the ability of MR to diagnose intraplaque hemorrhage (IPH), thought by many to be one of the most important predictors of increased stroke risk. In a series of projects, Altaf and colleagues showed that an MR diagnosis of IPH was significantly associated with (1) spontaneous embolization in recently symptomatic patients, (2) embolization during operative carotid dissection in symptomatic patients undergoing CEA, (3) an increased prevalence of white matter hyperintense lesions (leukoaraiosis), and (4) a much higher risk for ipsilateral recurrent stroke/TIA in symptomatic patients with 70% to 99% stenosis awaiting CEA and in recently symptomatic patients with 30% to 69% stenosis managed medically.[21-24] These studies suggest a potentially important role for MR imaging of plaque morphology in the future, but there is an important anomaly that still needs to be addressed. Although an MR diagnosis of IPH in symptomatic patients was associated with the various adverse outcomes just indicated, the presence of IPH in the asymptomatic, contralateral ICA was not associated with an increased risk for late stroke.[23,24] This suggests a much lower likelihood that this type of technology could be used to identify patients at high risk for stroke within large asymptomatic cohorts. One possible explanation for this anomaly is that an MR diagnosis of IPH may also include some patients with overlying plaque thrombus, a feature known to be relatively common in recently symptomatic patients.[25]

Perioperative Roles

There is no role presently for MR in the perioperative setting.

Postoperative Roles

Although new hyperintense white matter lesions (attributed to microembolization) have been well documented in the early period after CEA and particularly CAS,[26] there is no evidence that awareness of this phenomenon influences early management or late prognosis. Accordingly, this feature is primarily of research interest at this time but could be used to develop better CPDs in the future. Similarly, MRI/MRA does not offer a practical role in the investigation of patients suffering a procedural stroke after CEA or CAS beyond what can be achieved with the much more easily performed MDCTA (which combines vascular and functional imaging in a single scan). The exception is a patient suspected of having had a hyperperfusion stroke in which CT suggests that there is an evolving ischemic infarct (usually in the posterior circulation). Perfusion MRI will usually demonstrate that this area of the brain remains well perfused and that the area of low attenuation seen on CT does not represent an evolving brain infarct but is due to vasogenic as opposed to cytotoxic edema.[27] This pathology will be considered further in the section on CT. Finally, CEMRA does not offer a practical role in surveillance after CEA and CAS because it is not cost-effective and because of the effect of some of the metallic stents.

Contraindications

Contraindications to MR evaluation include patients with (1) selected metallic implants (cardiac pacemakers, implantable defibrillators, metallic stents, joint replacements), (2) claustrophobia, and (3) obesity. Caution should also be exercised in patients with evidence of chronic renal impairment because they may be predisposed to the development of nephrogenic systemic fibrosis after exposure to gadolinium.[28]

Accuracy and Limitations in Clinical Practice

Diagnostic accuracy is largely related to the available technology and expertise. For reasons alluded to earlier, 2D and 3D TOF MRA was vulnerable to inaccuracies (especially a tendency to overestimate the degree of stenosis), needed multiple data acquisitions to image the inflow and outflow vessels accurately, and was prone to artifact (motion, flow related). These problems have now been significantly reduced after the development of CEMRA, although the contraindications listed earlier still apply. The relative inability to image calcification makes it less attractive for evaluating patients for CAS, and its lower spatial resolution can lead to difficulty identifying subtle tandem lesions. In addition, anomalous vessels that have occluded may not be apparent on CEMRA. In clinical practice, however, the main limitations of CEMRA are availability and lack of rapid access. As alluded to earlier, any delay in performing CEMRA will further delay referral for CEA or CAS and thus reduce overall stroke prevention in the long term (see Table 93-1).

■ POSITRON EMISSION TOMOGRAPHY

Indications

Unlike other diagnostic modalities described in this chapter, positron emission tomography (PET) has a limited role in the evaluation of patients with cerebrovascular disease.

Role in Carotid Artery Disease

PET has no role in the routine evaluation of patients being considered for CEA or CAS. However, because of its ability to measure cerebral blood flow and the oxygen extraction fraction, PET remains the gold standard for evaluating the hemodynamic effect of extracranial disease,[29] particularly autoregulatory failure and impaired cerebrovascular reserve. In reality, measurement of perfusion reserve has never found a role in the investigation of patients with classic thromboembolic carotid disease, but it could evolve an important role in selecting patients with carotid occlusion, hemodynamic failure, or recurrent carotid territory symptoms who might benefit from extracranial-intracranial bypass. This is currently being evaluated in prospective studies.

Role in Evaluating Plaque Morphology

PET scanners offer very good spatial resolution (2 mm), and many are now combined with a CT scanner to allow tomographic radionuclide imaging (with anatomic correlation). This raises the possibility that a number of inflammatory processes could be targeted within carotid plaque (inflammation, macrophages, apoptosis, angiogenesis, protease enzyme function[30]). The ability to link metabolic activity with plasma biomarkers and plaque imaging could have important implications for the future (selecting patients, monitoring drug therapy). However, despite considerable research enthusiasm, there remains little evidence that it will alter practice in the near future.

Other Roles

PET scanning plays no role currently in the evaluation of vertebrobasilar disease, as a screening modality, in the evaluation of trauma, in perioperative management, or in the evaluation of carotid body/glomus tumors.

Accuracy and Limitations in Clinical Practice

PET is limited by its inaccessibility, high cost, and lack of relevance to current clinical practice. To many surgeons it is primarily of research interest. Only time will tell whether evaluation of hemodynamic reserve can reliably target patients for extracranial-intracranial bypass or whether PET will prove superior to DUS, MRA, or CT in interpretation of plaque morphology.

COMPUTED TOMOGRAPHIC ANGIOGRAPHY

Indications

CTA has proved to be a valuable modality in the evaluation of patients with cerebrovascular disease (see Chapter 21: Computed Tomography).

Role in Carotid Artery Disease

CTA has the advantage of being less susceptible than MRA to the risk of overestimating the severity of stenosis. In the 2006 HTA systematic review and meta-analysis of noninvasive imaging modalities summarized in Table 93-2, only CTA with spiral CT was evaluated. The published data suggest little overall advantage over DUS and TOF MRA with regard to diagnosing surgically important (and irrelevant) carotid disease. Accordingly, centers with this older type of CT technology will prefer to use CEMRA should DUS provide discordant findings. When neither CEMRA nor MDCTA is available, formal DSA may be the only way of resolving any lingering diagnostic issues.

Subsequent to the HTA report in 2006, 64-slice MDCTA has become more widely available, and it is soon to be joined by 256- and 320-slice MDCTA, which will increase temporal resolution. MDCTA has revolutionized the role of CTA because (1) it is extremely fast (5 seconds to perform a scan from the aortic arch to the circle of Willis (Fig. 93-9); (2) it is less expensive than CEMRA; (3) it offers submillimeter spatial resolution[31] (0.3-mm spatial resolution versus 0.8 mm for CEMRA and 0.2 mm for DSA); (4) sophisticated imaging workstations enable the production of high-quality 2D and 3D reformatted images from the aortic arch to the circle of Willis that are easy to interpret (see Figs. 93-4 and 93-7); (5) it provides faster processing times; (6) it has the ability to visualize soft tissue, bone, and vessel at the same time; (7) its ability to rapidly demonstrate vascular anomalies is not compromised by the vessels being occluded (Fig. 93-10); and (8) it has the ability to indicate the extent of vessel calcification, especially in the aortic arch (Fig. 93-11). Because of these characteristics, imaging of extracranial and intracranial vascular anatomy and functional brain imaging are possible during one period of data acquisition. Stenoses (NASCET or ECST) can be measured directly with electronic microcallipers. Recent work suggests that a residual luminal diameter of 1.3 mm corresponds to a NASCET 70% stenosis whereas a 2.2-mm lumen equates to a 50% stenosis.[32]

Role in Vertebrobasilar Disease

Imaging the VAs has always presented a challenge (see Fig. 93-9). The VAs have a tortuous course, a thick bony covering, adjacent veins, and large variation in normal vessel caliber, and it is not unusual to find that one is hypoplastic. MDCTA provides better images of the extracranial and intracranial vertebrobasilar system than CEMRA does, although CEMRA is preferable to CTA using conventional spiral CT. An important advantage of MDCTA is that it retains important bony landmarks (see Fig. 93-9) and vessel coverings (which can then be "virtually dissected off" if required). Vessel tortuosity is easily demonstrated, and there is no problem with artifact at the VA origins. Accordingly, MDCTA can provide rapid imaging of the complete vertebrobasilar system, as well as vascular anomalies. MDCTA cannot, however, provide information regarding flow directionality. When this information

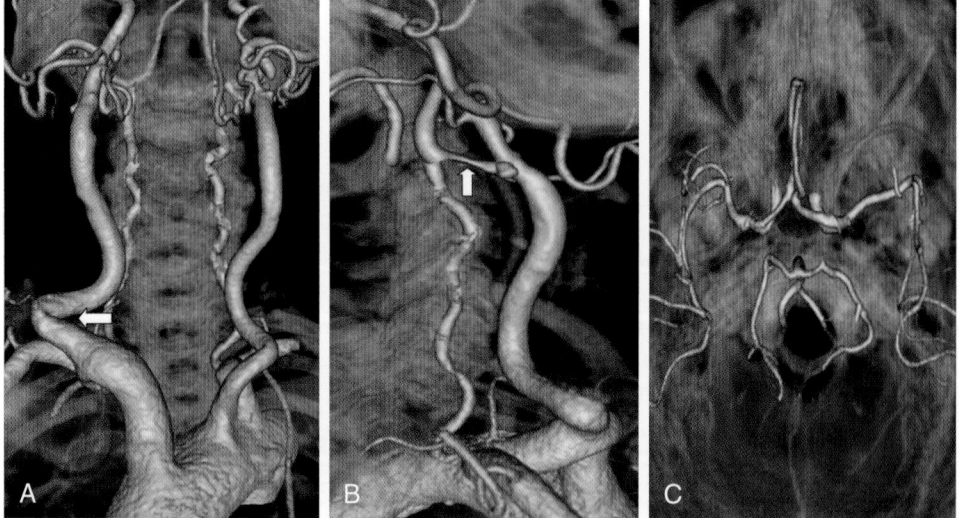

Figure 93-9 Multidetector computed tomographic angiography of the aortic arch and great vessels (**A**), carotid and vertebral arteries (**B**), and circle of Willis (**C**). This scan took 10 seconds to acquire. Note the acutely angled right common carotid artery (CCA) (**A,** *arrow*), which would pose a significant challenge to safe passage of a wire and sheath for carotid artery stenting. The left CCA is less angulated and would not pose such a problem. A severe, relatively smooth stenosis is seen in the internal carotid artery (**B,** *arrow*).

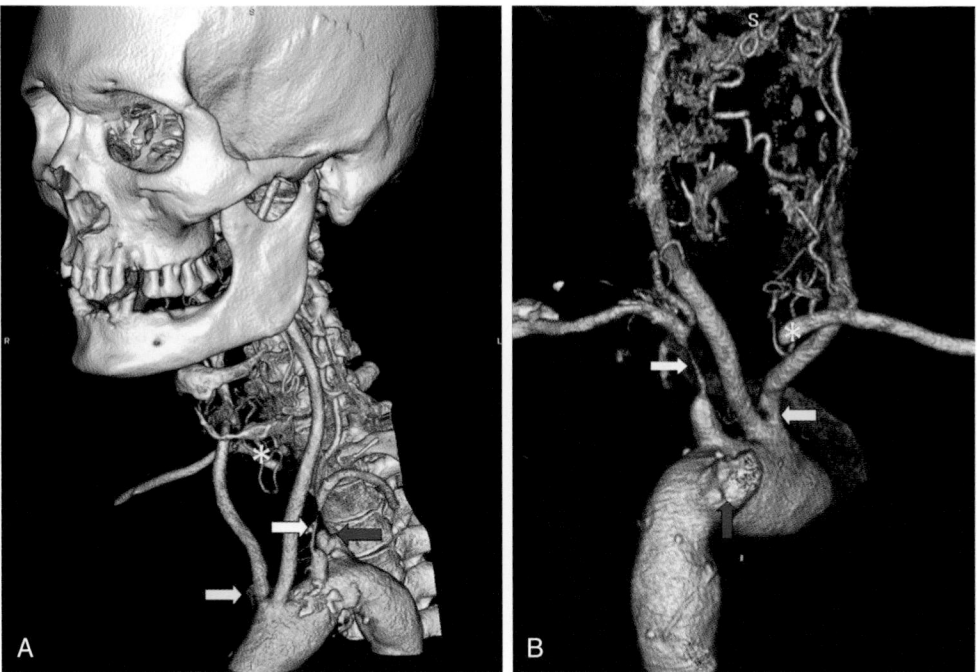

Figure 93-10 Multidetector computed tomographic angiography showing an unexpected anomaly of the great vessels of the aortic arch. **A,** Arch viewed from its anterior aspect. **B,** Arch viewed from its posterior aspect. Both common carotid arteries arise from a joint origin (*yellow arrow*), and there is a long, severe stenosis of the proximal left subclavian artery (*white arrow*). The right subclavian artery arises from an aberrant position and is occluded just beyond its origin (*red arrow*) with refilling distally (*asterisk*). The *red arrow* marks the "diverticulum of Kommerl."

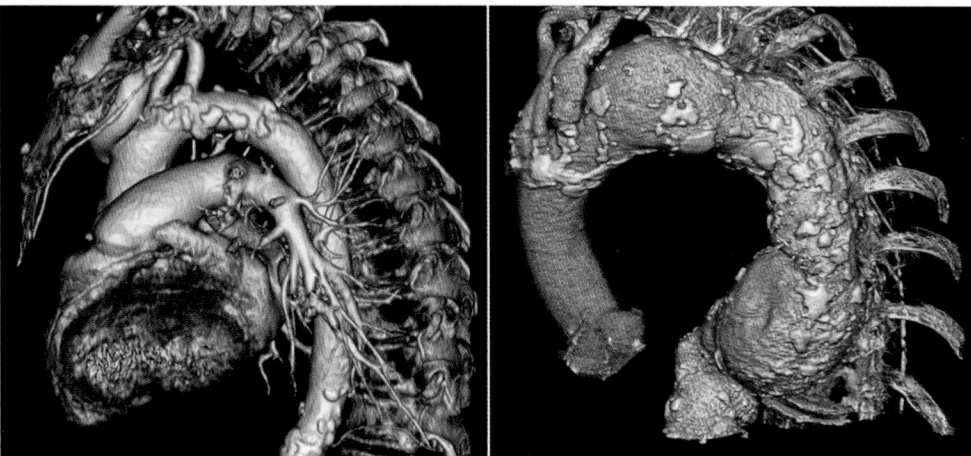

Figure 93-11 Volume rendition multidetector computed tomographic angiography showing calcification in the thoracic aorta, aortic arch, and origins of the great vessels.

is required (subclavian, coronary steal phenomena), CEMRA (or DUS) should be undertaken.

Role in Screening

There is currently no role for CTA as a screening tool. It is not cost-effective, and the patient is exposed to unnecessary radiation.

Role in the Evaluation of Trauma

MDCTA has an important role in this challenging situation, largely because it can rapidly provide anatomic vascular images from the arch to the circle of Willis, together with bony, soft tissue, and functional brain imaging during a single scan, even in a ventilated patient. Neither of these features can be provided by CEMRA without extra MRI acquisition sequences and time.

Role in the Evaluation of Carotid Body/ Glomus Tumors

Because of its better spatial resolution and easy interpretation, MDCTA is probably the optimum imaging modality for evaluating tumor circulation (see Fig. 93-8), the extent of the tumor, whether it is bilateral, and the relationship between tumor and adjacent soft tissue structures. These image data are usually more than enough to plan a safe surgical resection and can generally warn when a high and difficult dissection might be encountered, enabling the surgeon to plan in advance for temporomandibular subluxation as required.

Role in the Planning of Carotid Endarterectomy and Carotid Angioplasty with Stenting

As with CEMRA, most CEAs can be performed safely without the need for MDCTA, but if there is evidence of inflow/outflow disease or excessive calcification on DUS, MDCTA can reliably and safely provide the additional information required to plan management. MDCTA, however, is currently the optimal noninvasive imaging modality for determining whether CAS can be undertaken safely (see Table 93-4), partly because of the production of 3D (easily interpretable) images from the aortic arch to the circle of Willis (see Fig. 93-9) but also because of the ease of demonstrating vessel tortuosity, abnormalities of the circle of Willis (see Fig. 93-4), patterns of calcification in the aortic arch (see Fig. 93-11), and the status of the origins of the great vessels (see Fig. 93-7). Unlike CEMRA, MDCTA is unaffected by occluded anomalous vessels arising from the arch (see Fig. 93-10). Procedural risks after CAS increase in elderly patients (>80 years), which is thought to be related to the progressive degeneration and calcification/tortuosity of the arch and great vessels that occur with age. This can lead to difficulty accessing the carotid arteries with guide wires, sheaths, and other devices (see Fig. 93-11). Although many of the adverse features detailed in Table 93-4 may not deter an experienced interventionist, they should help a less experienced operator identify an unsuitable or suboptimal patient for CAS.

Role in Evaluating Plaque Morphology

At present, the role of CT in evaluating plaque morphology is largely of research interest, but there is considerable potential. With axial imaging, MDCT can be used to divide carotid plaque into one of three subgroups based on plaque density measurement (measured in Hounsfield units [HU]). Other visualization or postprocessing tools such as maximum intensity projection, multiplanar reformatting, and volume rendition are less effective (especially maximum intensity projection) in evaluating plaque components. A "soft" plaque (<50 HU) usually has a soft lipid-rich core and is more likely to be associated with symptoms and perhaps higher procedural risk after CAS. At the other extreme is "calcified"

plaque (>120 HU), which seems to be associated with a reduced risk for symptoms. In between is "intermediate" plaque (50 to 119 HU).[33,34] In practical terms, the ability of CT to image heavily calcified plaque confers an important advantage over DUS and CEMRA. This is potentially a very important attribute in selecting the optimal imaging modality when considering patients for CAS because the presence of heavy calcification, especially in the aortic arch and carotid bifurcation, is associated with an increased risk for procedural stroke.

As has been alluded to earlier, several imaging modalities have been used to evaluate plaque morphology in an attempt to identify cohorts of patients at higher risk for stroke. The available evidence suggests that MRI is better than CT for looking at thrombus, the fibrous cap, and its rupture (largely because MRI is better than CT at differentiating soft tissue structures), but there is emerging evidence that MDCTA may be better at identifying plaque ulcers.[35,36] IPH (provided that it is >1 mm in diameter) can be visualized indirectly on MDCTA but is not as reliably predicted as with MRI. Ongoing research in this important area will probably lead to more clinical application of these techniques in the future, including GSM DUS.

Perioperative Roles

There is no role in contemporary practice for CTA in the perioperative management of patients with cerebrovascular disease.

Postoperative Roles

MDCTA has a potentially important role in the evaluation of patients suffering a stroke or other neurologic problems in the postoperative period after CEA and CAS (Fig. 93-12). In the first 12 hours the chance of encountering an intracranial hemorrhage is remote. Accordingly, the patient should generally be considered for re-exploration, which should not be delayed to perform a CT scan in most circumstances. However, because MDCTA can often be performed very rapidly, it may be useful in selected patients with early postoperative neurologic deficits, especially if completion DUS or DSA was normal and intracranial embolism is suspected. After 12 hours have elapsed, there is an increasing possibility that the stroke may be due to intracranial hemorrhage or hyperperfusion syndrome. In this situation it is important to avoid an unnecessary (and potentially dangerous) return to the operating room. An emergency CT scan will exclude hemorrhage but may also demonstrate some features associated with hyperperfusion syndrome (Fig. 93-13). In the latter condition, middle cerebral artery (MCA) velocities are generally elevated (frequently in association with hypertension), and it is not unusual for the CT scan to display areas of low attenuation that can sometimes be misinterpreted as an evolving infarct.[27] Diffusion-weighted MRI studies have shown that the white matter edema seen in patients with hyperperfusion syndrome on CT is actually vasogenic (if it were an evolving infarct it

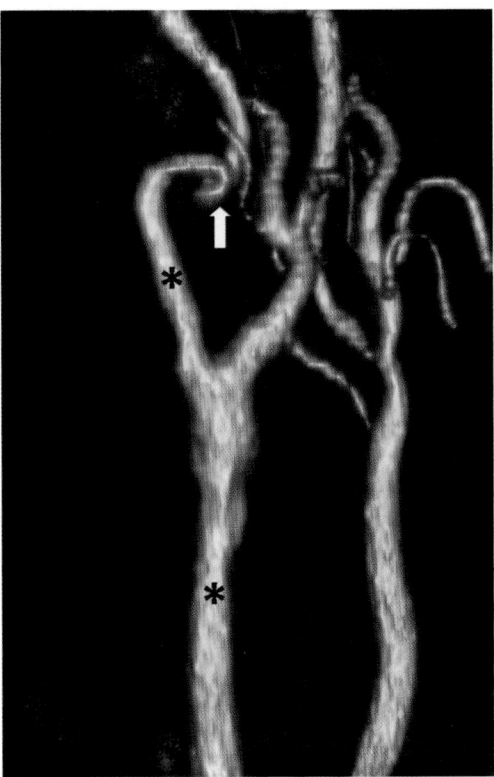

Figure 93-12 Multidetector computed tomographic angiography performed less than 45 minutes after completing an uneventful carotid endarterectomy. In the recovery room, the patient became hypertensive (265/170 mm Hg) and developed seizures. He was reintubated and transferred to the CT scanner to exclude an intracranial hemorrhage. Subsequent volume rendition images of the reconstructed internal carotid artery (ICA) showed no significant luminal abnormality (the upper and lower limits of the patched endarterectomy zone are indicated by *asterisks*). Note also the distal loop in the ICA (*arrow*), which had been missed on preoperative ultrasound imaging.

would be cytotoxic), whereas perfusion studies show that there is no loss of blood supply.[37] Why hyperperfusion syndrome causes vasogenic edema in the posterior circulation has not been explained.

If intracranial hypertension and hyperperfusion syndrome have been excluded, there remains the possibility that the neurologic deficit was thromboembolic in origin (see under "Transcranial Doppler/Duplex"). DUS of the carotid bifurcation can be difficult to interpret in the early postoperative period (air in the deeper tissues, edema, overlying hemostatic gauze), and it may not be possible to exclude an intraluminal filling defect. In this situation, MDCTA will quickly provide high-quality images of the extracranial circulation (see Fig. 93-12), which will not unduly delay the patient's return to surgery if deemed necessary.

Finally, MDCTA does not have a routine role in serial surveillance after CEA and CAS. This is better achieved with DUS. However, when used in conjunction with DUS, it can be useful in evaluating and planning management in the very rare patient with prosthetic patch infection after CEA (see Fig. 93-6).

Contraindications

A history of allergy or reaction to iodinated contrast agents may be a contraindication to CTA, although in milder cases parenteral steroid therapy may allow safe completion of the test. The risk of anaphylaxis (1 in 500 to 5000 procedures) is higher in patients with a history of asthma and food allergies. Caution must be exercised in those with impaired renal function; such patients require intravenous hydration beforehand.

Limitations in Practice

MDCTA has now superseded all previous CT technologies and is headed toward being considered the overall new gold standard. By implication, therefore, older CT technology will not be able to answer as many of the clinical questions posed in this section. Notwithstanding this important caveat, MDCTA is limited by the need for intravenous contrast material. Also, there is a potential risk for contrast medium–related nephropathy (hence the need for hydration), MDCTA cannot provide information on flow directionality (DUS or CEMRA is required), and there is the inevitable exposure to radiation. Newer CT scanners, however, have automatic exposure control systems that continuously modulate the x-ray tube (based on patient size and tissue density), thereby allowing potential reductions in radiation dose. Finally, there do remain occasional situations in which MDCTA (and CEMRA) cannot reliably provide accurate and diagnostic imaging information in selected complex patients, especially those with tandem syphon disease or stenoses within coiled segments of the ICA (Fig. 93-14). In this case, high-quality selective carotid DSA remains the gold standard (see under "Digital Subtraction Angiography").

■ DIGITAL SUBTRACTION ANGIOGRAPHY

Indications

For many, conventional catheter angiography still remains the undisputed gold standard for imaging the extracranial and intracranial circulation (see Chapter 18: Arteriography). Used in four of five of the main randomized trials comparing CEA with best medical therapy, its easily interpreted images of the arch, carotid arteries, and VAs, as well as the siphons and intracranial circulation, found considerable favor among surgeons and neurologists. However, although the performance of angiography enforced a standardized discipline of having to measure the degree of stenosis with either the NASCET or ECST measurement method, reliance on routine angiography came at a price. Approximately 1% to 2% of patients undergoing angiography suffer a neurologic deficit,[38] and angiographic stroke accounted for 50% of the procedural risk after CEA in the Asymptomatic Carotid Atherosclerosis Study (ACAS).[39] Evidence suggests that the risk for angiographic stroke is highest in symptomatic patients (especially those initially seen with a stroke), in those with increasing degrees of stenosis (especially if less severe disease is screened

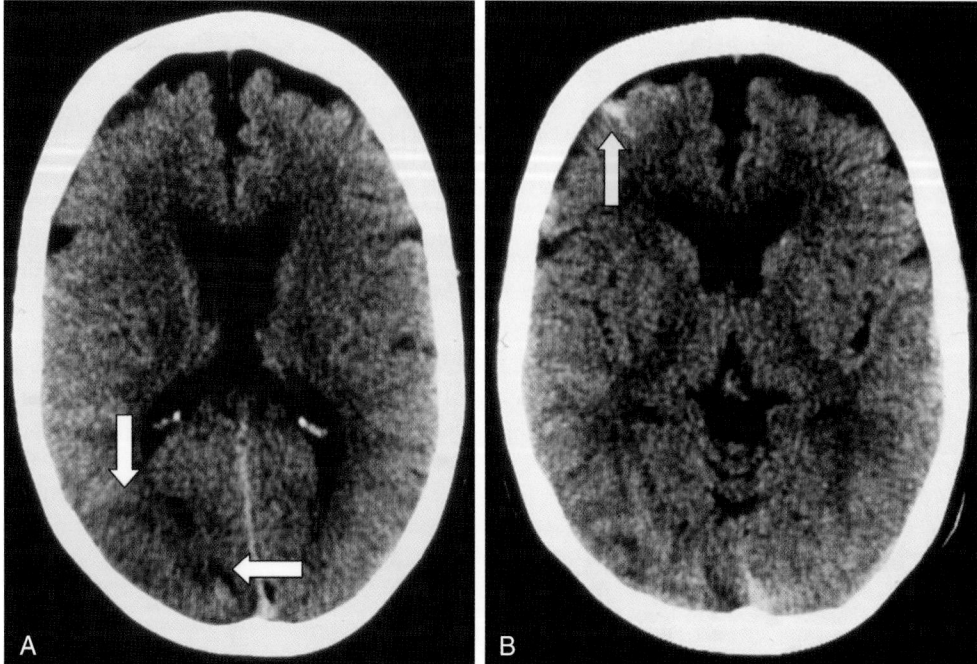

Figure 93-13 CT scan in a patient who underwent right carotid endarterectomy and was seen 5 days later with seizures, hypertension, and left-sided weakness. The CT scan revealed an area of white matter edema in the right posterior circulation (**A,** *arrows*) and a focal petechial hemorrhage in the right frontal region (**B,** *arrow*). White matter edema in the posterior circulation is not an uncommon finding in this syndrome and is often mistaken for an evolving infarct. *(Reproduced with permission from Naylor AR, Evans J, Thompson MM, et al. Seizures after carotid endarterectomy: hyperperfusion, dysautoregulation or hypertensive encephalopathy? Eur J Vasc Endovasc Surg. 2003;26:39.)*

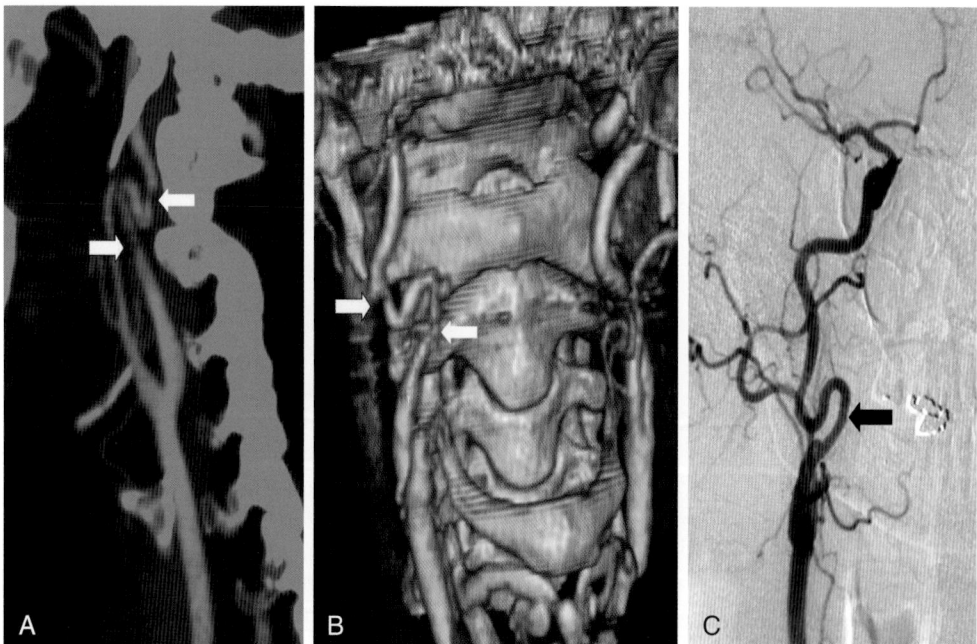

Figure 93-14 Image processing in patients with distal internal carotid artery (ICA) loops can lead to the creation of artifacts that can be interpreted as clinically important stenoses. **A,** Multidetector computed tomographic angiography (MDCTA) maximum intensity projection; note the normal bifurcation and a distal looped ICA with apparent inflow and outflow stenoses (*arrows*). **B,** Three-dimensional volume rendition MDCTA in the same patient suggesting that the stenoses were real (*arrows*). **C,** Selective intra-arterial digital subtraction arteriography showing the looped ICA but no stenoses. The "stenoses" identified on **A** and **B** were caused during image processing.

out with DUS), and after selective common carotid artery catheterization. The risk appears to decrease with seniority and experience of the operator, with newer catheter technologies, and with injection of contrast material into the arch, although the latter is associated with poorer quality images.

Role in Carotid Artery Disease

Conventional angiography has now been rendered obsolete by IADSA, and even though newer 2D and 3D rotational angiography now offers the prospect of computer-enhanced rotational 3D images, it is incontestable that the era of recommending formal angiography in all patients being considered for CEA has passed. By contrast, in the last decades, diagnostic angiography was essential in the evaluation of patients being considered for CAS, but even this is now increasingly being considered unnecessary in the majority of patients (see Table 93-3). In practice, most potential CAS patients undergo a screening DUS examination followed by CEMRA or MDCTA (depending on local resources and preferences). A formal diagnostic angiogram is usually performed only in conjunction with the planned CAS or in those in whom diagnostic uncertainty persists.

However, there are still situations when it is important to perform IADSA. Improvements in CEMRA and (especially) MDCTA now mean that it is rarely necessary to undertake IADSA to look at the origins of the great vessels (see Figs. 93-7 and 93-10). Similarly, MDCTA can provide valuable imaging information in patients with heavily calcified plaque in the arch or great vessel origins (see Fig. 93-11). However, both CEMRA and MDCTA can provide misleading information in patients with severe distal ICA disease (Fig. 93-15) and in patients with marked coiling of the ICA in the upper reaches of the neck (see Fig. 93-14). In the former, slow flow through a tiny lumen can be missed. In the latter, unless extreme care is taken with image processing (i.e., ensuring that the axial measurements are in a true perpendicular cross-sectional plane), it is possible that an artifact introduced during image processing can lead to the surgeon's or interventionist's being persuaded that significant carotid disease exists.

Role in Vertebrobasilar Disease

Until the advent of CEMRA and MDCTA, IADSA remained the gold standard for imaging the vertebrobasilar circulation. This no longer holds true, and these less invasive imaging modalities can now usually identify most patients who might benefit from intervention. As with CAS, most patients being considered for vertebral angioplasty will currently undergo a formal diagnostic angiogram only as the initial part of the planned interventional procedure.

Role in Screening

There is presently no role for DSA as a screening tool. The risks of angiographic stroke and the extent of radiation exposure make this an unethical screening technique.

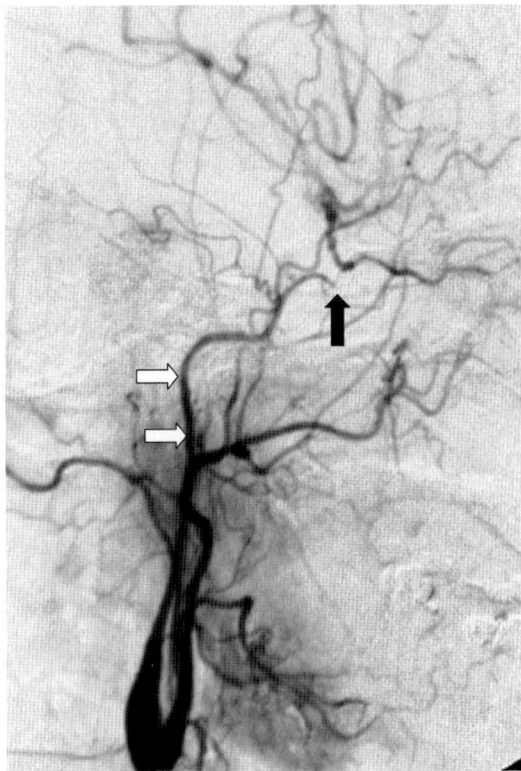

Figure 93-15 Selective intra-arterial digital subtraction arteriography (IADSA) in a 38-year-old woman with stroke (middle cerebral territory infarct on CT scan). Duplex ultrasound showed slow, high-resistance flow in the carotid artery but a normal bifurcation. Contrast-enhanced magnetic resonance angiography suggested a subocclusion but could not image the distal internal carotid artery (ICA). This delayed IADSA image shows a normal-caliber carotid bifurcation with a narrow-caliber ICA in its midsection (*white arrows* where flow was extremely slow). In the very distal ICA (*black arrow*), vessel diameter dwindles toward complete occlusion. The images are probably consistent with acute dissection and compression of the true lumen by thrombus in the false lumen.

Role in Trauma

Angiography was previously the first-line imaging modality in patients suspected of having an extracranial arterial injury. Once again, this role has largely been superseded by MDCTA, which can perform a diagnostic study from the arch to the circle of Willis in 5 seconds. However, IADSA still remains an important secondary option in situations in which image quality is compromised or difficult to interpret. Furthermore, angiography retains the distinction of allowing one to proceed with endovascular interventions (coil/balloon occlusion, insertion of a covered stent).

Role in the Evaluation of Carotid Body/ Glomus Vagale Tumors

There is no need for IADSA in the routine evaluation of patients being considered for resection of CBTs and GVTs. It provides no information on the overall extent or operability of the lesion. However, preoperative embolization of ECA feeding vessels is thought by some to reduce perioperative bleeding, whereas insertion of a covered stent into the ECA can significantly reduce bleeding in patients with very large tumors.[40]

Role in the Planning of Carotid Endarterectomy/Carotid Angioplasty with Stenting

As alluded to earlier, most centers now carry out the majority of CEAs without performing preoperative IADSA. Large studies suggest that reliance on such a strategy does not compromise patient safety and that the surgeon very rarely encounters operative scenarios that cannot be dealt with safely.[3] Safe performance of CEA does not depend on preoperative imaging of inflow or distal vessels (unless the DUS scan suggests an abnormality there), and there is no evidence that imaging the intracranial circulation alters outcome. The preceding discussion ("Digital Subtraction Angiography, Role in Carotid Artery Disease") does, however, summarize situations in which performing a diagnostic IADSA would be advisable.

By contrast, some CAS practitioners have been reluctant to dispense with a separate diagnostic IADSA as part of the routine evaluation of their patients. Advocates of this strategy must remember that the need for a preliminary diagnostic angiogram (in place of or in addition to CEMRA/MDCTA) will inevitably delay treatment and therefore potentially reduce the overall effectiveness of any procedure (see Table 93-1), in addition to subjecting the patient to two catheterization procedures. The advent of CEMRA and (especially) MDCTA, together with the current drive toward expedited treatment, has probably rendered this practice obsolete. In practical terms, this could mean that on very rare occasion, a patient may be evaluated for CAS solely on the basis of CEMRA/MDCTA, only to have the procedure abandoned after the diagnostic IADSA that immediately precedes the planned CAS procedure. In reality, this is unlikely to happen often because of excellent pre-interventional imaging and planning.

Role in Evaluating Plaque Morphology

DSA has no role in evaluating plaque morphology other than demonstrating surface irregularity. Angiography is not particularly good at identifying intraluminal thrombus.[41] Although NASCET and ECST showed that plaque irregularity (diagnosed on angiography) was associated with an increased risk for stroke in medically treated patients and an increased risk for major cardiac events during follow-up,[41] this is insufficient evidence to justify recommending routine IADSA for evaluation of plaque morphology given other better modalities.

Perioperative Roles

Intraoperative completion angiography can identify important technical errors (intimal flaps, luminal thrombus, residual stenosis) after restoration of flow, but it has largely been

superseded by color DUS (facilitated by dedicated small L-shaped probes) or angioscopy. Completion angiography can be cumbersome, it requires the presence of a C-arm and radiology technician in the operating room, and (for most patients) it represents an unnecessary exposure to radiation.

Angiography does, however, retain a useful diagnostic role in the rare patient who has a stroke as a result of carotid thrombosis or acute distal dissection in the early postoperative period after CEA and CAS (Fig. 93-16). After CEA, the key to ensuring the best outcome is early re-exploration (preferably within 1 hour). At re-exploration it is not uncommon to find a "pulse" in the ICA (suggesting to an unwary surgeon that the vessel is still patent). In this situation it is important to avoid undue manipulation of the bifurcation because this can precipitate major embolism. Despite the apparent pulsation, it is not unusual for the angiogram to demonstrate complete occlusion (see Fig. 93-16). Angiography can also identify the very rare case of acute distal dissection that may follow shunt trauma. In the latter situation, the diagnostic angiogram can be followed by insertion of a stent or covered stent into the true lumen, whereas embolic occlusion of intracranial vessels can be treated by intra-arterial, low-dose thrombolysis or catheter-directed retrieval of emboli.

Thromboembolic stroke in the first few hours after CAS raises the possibility of in-stent thrombosis (Fig. 93-17). For a detailed discussion of CAS and prevention/management of complications, see Chapter 96 (Carotid Artery: Stenting).

Postoperative Roles

There is no role for IADSA in the serial surveillance of patients after CEA or CAS.

Contraindications

An important contraindication is previous allergic reaction to iodinated contrast media. IADSA should not be performed by incompletely trained personnel or on poorly compliant patients. The presence of infrarenal aortic occlusion (i.e., preventing Seldinger access via the common femoral artery) can be overcome by using the brachial artery for access.

Accuracy and Limitations in Clinical Practice

IADSA is now largely relegated to the role of supporting the newer, less invasive modalities because of its use of radiation, the inevitable delays in performing studies, and the risk for procedural stroke. In addition, formal angiography is associated with a small but important risk for access complications (bleeding, dissection, thromboembolism) and contrast-induced nephropathy.

The Need for Corroborative Imaging

DSA can image only what is outlined by the contrast agent. It therefore cannot provide any information regarding

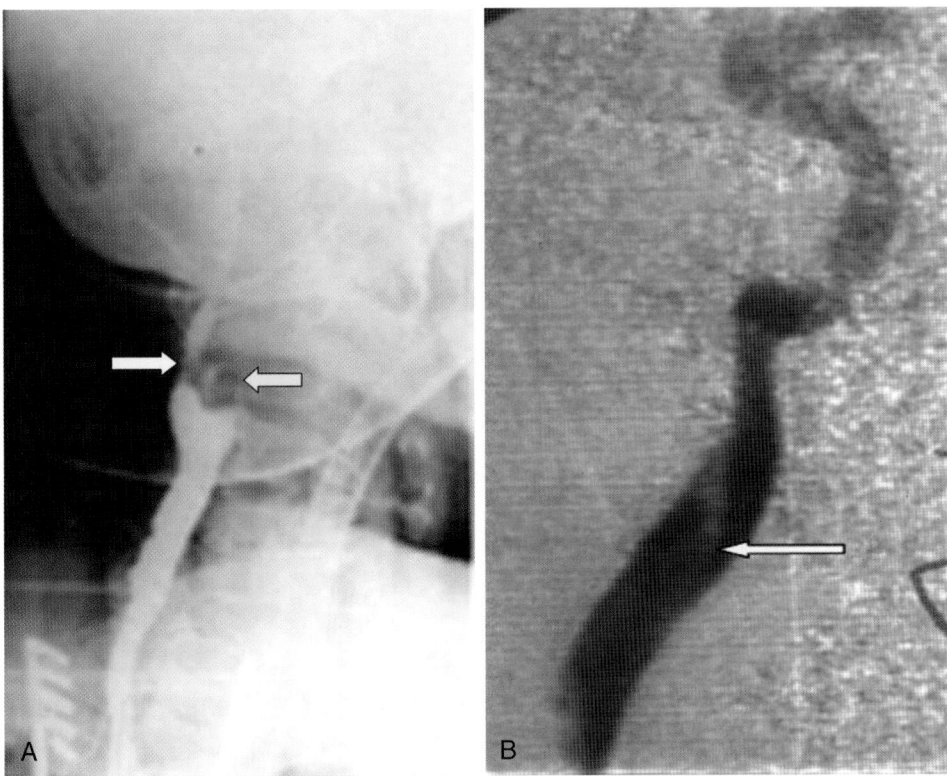

Figure 93-16 A, On-table conventional carotid angiogram in a patient who underwent re-exploration after the onset of a dense neurologic deficit following uneventful carotid endarterectomy. The external carotid artery (*white arrow*) has a partial filling defect. The internal carotid artery (ICA) is completely occluded (*yellow arrow*). This case was treated before routine postoperative transcranial Doppler (TCD) monitoring was used to prevent this complication from taking place. **B,** On-table intra-arterial digital subtraction arteriogram in a patient who recovered from anesthesia with a new neurologic deficit. TCD showed flow rates consistent with carotid occlusion, but there had been no preceding embolization. At re-exploration, dissection of the distal ICA extended to the base of the skull (stenting at the *arrow*).

surrounding soft tissues or direct visualization of processes affecting the vessel wall. Accordingly, the original true lumen of the vessel cannot be assessed. MRI or CT will be required if extrinsic compression is suspected on the angiogram.

TRANSCRANIAL DOPPLER/DUPLEX

Indications

Though not part of the routine evaluation of most patients with cerebrovascular disease, TCD can provide useful diagnostic information in selected cases. For a discussion of the details of Doppler or DUS for this application, see Chapter 14 (Vascular Laboratory: Arterial Physiologic Assessment) and Chapter 15 (Vascular Laboratory: Arterial Duplex Scanning).

Role in Carotid Artery Disease

TCD has no role in imaging carotid disease, but it can provide a simple evaluation of the hemodynamic effect of a stenosis by measuring the proportional increase in MCA velocity in response to the intravenous administration of acetazolamide

(cerebral vasodilator). TCD is, however, the only modality capable of diagnosing in vivo embolization. This is because the larger embolus reflects more backscattered signal than red cells do, and despite initial skepticism, there are now well-accepted and validated criteria for diagnosing embolization and excluding artifact.[42] Embolization is more commonly encountered in the MCA ipsilateral to a symptomatic carotid stenosis and is generally thought to be indicative of unstable plaque. Recognition of this phenomenon should prompt the surgeon to expeditiously undertake CEA, and although it seems obvious that these patients might be suboptimal candidates for CAS, this assumption has never been properly evaluated. Of practical importance (for the future) is whether TCD-diagnosed embolization can identify a cohort of patients with asymptomatic carotid disease who are at high risk for stroke.[43]

Role in Vertebrobasilar Disease

One practical role for TCD in the vertebrobasilar circulation relates to the cohort of patients reporting isolated dizziness and other symptoms after head movements. In the past, many have been labeled as having "vertebrobasilar TIAs" secondary

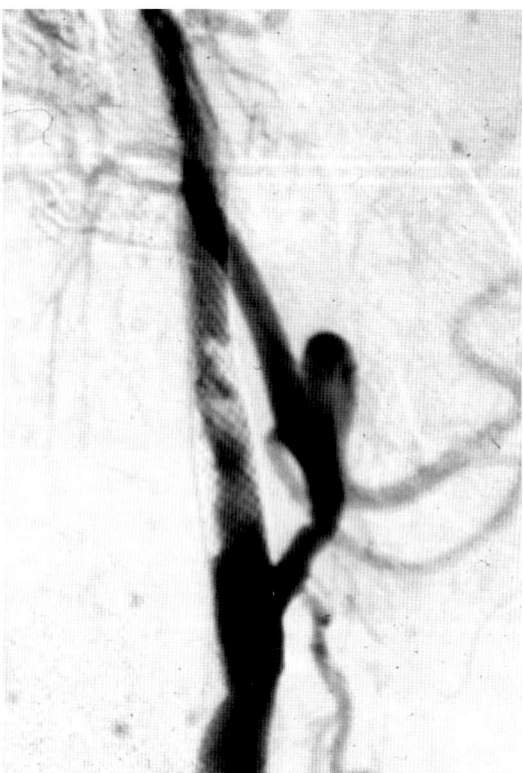

Figure 93-17 Selective intra-arterial digital subtraction arteriography in a patient who had undergone uneventful stenting of an extensive symptomatic plaque at the origin of the internal carotid artery. He was readmitted on day 5 with extensive hemiplegia. This image shows extensive in-stent thrombosis.

to compression of the VAs within the transverse processes of the upper cervical vertebrae during neck movement. In the Leicester unit, a protocol combines extracranial duplex and intracranial duplex with the head rotated into provocative positions. In a series of 40 patients (unpublished data), no one has demonstrated flow reversal or flow reduction, thus suggesting that most cases are probably being misdiagnosed. In reality, most such patients probably have inner ear pathology.

Role in the Evaluation of Trauma

TCD has no role in the management of trauma other than being used to monitor the effect of carotid ligation/endovascular balloon occlusion in an unconscious patient should reconstruction prove impossible. Provided that mean MCA velocity is greater than 15 cm/sec, most will tolerate carotid ligation (balloon occlusion) without having a stroke. Clearly, however, this type of intervention should be considered only an option of last resort.

Role in Intraoperative Monitoring

The main reason why monitoring and quality control assessment have failed to gain wider acceptance is failure to ask the right questions.[44] TCD warns of embolization (allowing the surgeon to modify the technique), but it cannot be expected to prevent a stroke caused by embolization of luminal thrombus after restoration of flow; some other form of quality control assessment is required for that (Fig. 93-18). Accordingly, the Leicester unit asks only four questions of TCD during CEA[45]: (1) Is there spontaneous embolization during operative carotid dissection (i.e., warning the surgeon of unstable plaque and thereby allowing modification of the dissection technique)? (2) Is the shunt working (3% of shunts malfunction after insertion[46])? (3) Is MCA velocity greater than 15 cm/sec (if not, flow can be increased by pharmacologic elevation of blood pressure)? (4) Is this patient one of the very rare ones destined for thrombosis of the carotid artery before the operation is even completed (Fig. 93-19)? TCD has been used during CAS, but there is a practical problem in that embolization can be both particulate and gaseous. At present, the role of TCD monitoring during CAS has not been clarified, but the potential to answer some of the questions posed earlier during CEA could also be relevant for CAS.

Role in Evaluating Postoperative Stroke

TCD has a useful (but unexploited) role in determining the cause of intraoperative and postoperative stroke when used in conjunction with extracranial DUS. Intraoperative strokes follow inadvertent technical error; hemodynamic failure accounts for only 20% of intraoperative events, with the remainder being thromboembolic.[45] In a large, prospective audit, intraoperative stroke was virtually abolished by using completion angioscopy.[45] Although intimal flaps were occasionally diagnosed, 3% to 4% of patients had retained luminal thrombus (despite venting and irrigation) that was derived from transected vasa vasorum (see Fig. 93-18). For those without recourse to angioscopy and other modalities, a patient wakening with a new neurologic deficit poses a considerable management dilemma. However, if TCD-derived MCA velocity is now the same as observed during carotid clamping, it is highly likely that the carotid artery has thrombosed (see Fig. 93-19). If MCA velocity is satisfactory but embolization is ongoing, it is likely that there is an evolving thrombus within the endarterectomy zone. Both these scenarios warrant immediate reoperation.

However, the etiology of postoperative stroke is multifactorial. After 24 hours has elapsed, most strokes result from intracranial hemorrhage or hyperperfusion syndrome. Unfortunately, no TCD protocol has been developed to reliably anticipate and prevent either of these conditions. In the first 24 hours after CEA, postoperative carotid thrombosis remains the most frequent cause of stroke.[47] Previously considered unpredictable, there is now growing evidence that it is probably related to patient-mediated factors (e.g., increased platelet sensitivity to adenosine diphosphate[48]) and is preventable. Numerous studies have now shown that a patient destined to have a stroke because of postoperative carotid thrombosis has a 1- to 2-hour period of increasing embolization before the neurologic deficit develops.[49] The Leicester unit currently

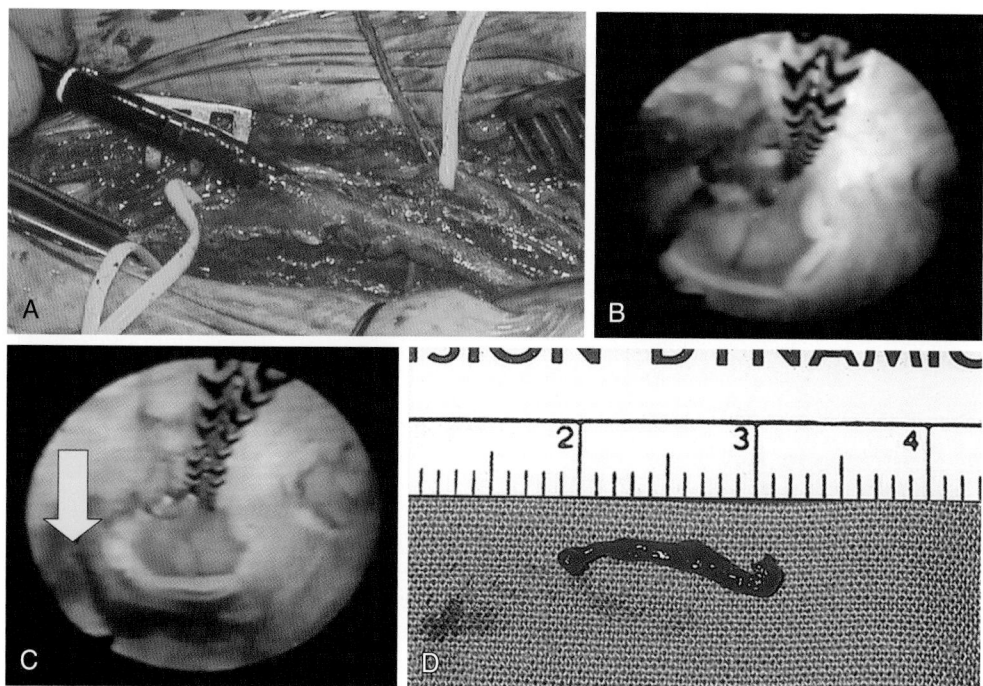

Figure 93-18 Completion angioscopy (using a hysteroscope) in a patient undergoing an interposition vein bypass between the common carotid artery (CCA) and internal carotid artery. **A,** Angioscope inserted into vein graft immediately after removal of the shunt. **B,** Large thrombus adherent to the proximal CCA/endarterectomy zone region. **C,** The source of the thrombus is bleeding from transected vasa vasorum. **D,** Extent of the thrombus after removal.

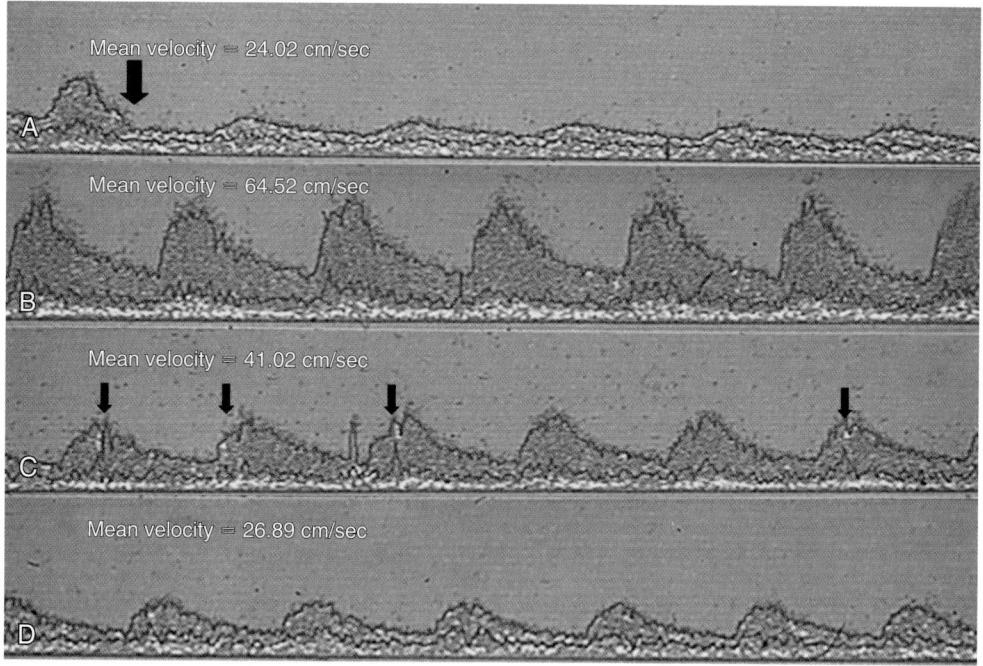

Figure 93-19 Transcranial diagnosis of on-table carotid thrombosis. **A,** Last cardiac cycle (*arrow*) before a carotid clamp is applied. After clamping, middle cerebral artery (MCA) velocity falls to 24.02 cm/sec. **B,** MCA waveform after restoration of flow (i.e., after endarterectomy). MCA velocity is now 64.52 cm/sec. **C,** Increasing embolization is detected within 12 minutes of restoration of flow (*arrows*) associated with a gradual decline in MCA velocity. **D,** Within 23 minutes of restoration of flow, the internal carotid artery is occluded, as demonstrated by the fact that MCA velocity (26.89 cm/sec) is now virtually identical to that noted during carotid clamping (**A**).

monitors CEA patients with TCD for up to 2 hours postoperatively[45] and administers incremental doses of intravenous dextran to patients who have more than 25 emboli detected in any 10-minute period. This combination of intraoperative TCD and completion angioscopy has been associated with a 60% reduction in operative risk. In particular, the use of TCD-directed dextran therapy has abolished progression to postoperative carotid thrombosis.[45] In practical terms, this is probably the single most useful role for TCD after CEA. Interestingly, this strategy has also been adopted for patients with a neurologic deficit and high-grade embolization after CAS.[50]

Accuracy and Limitations in Clinical Practice

The Achilles' heel of TCD is its total reliance on operator experience. This improves with time, and most experienced technologists can identify an accessible cranial window in about 90% of patients undergoing CEA. Common pitfalls include a lack of knowledge about intracranial anatomy (about 40% of circles of Willis are incomplete) and unfamiliarity with practical tips on how to proceed if the initial study suggests an inaccessible window. Elderly women are the cohort in whom the failure rate is highest. In addition, increasing experience reduces the likelihood that the wrong artery is being insonated. On a practical note, the most common reason for failing to find the MCA signal intraoperatively is not having identified it beforehand.

■ LABORATORY INVESTIGATIONS

All patients should undergo a number of relatively simple but important laboratory investigations at the initial consultation.

Baseline Evaluation

Provision of "best medical therapy" involves more than just recommending stopping smoking, checking the blood pressure, and starting aspirin and a statin. A full blood count will exclude (1) thrombocytopenia (potential bleeding risk; i.e., be careful about the choice and dose of antiplatelet agent), (2) thrombocytosis (prothrombotic tendency), (3) anemia (possible neoplasm), (4) polycythemia (prothrombotic tendency; consider therapeutic phlebotomy because of the increased risk for postoperative thrombosis), and (5) sickle cell disease (important in susceptible patient groups). Baseline biochemistry should identify the extent of any chronic renal impairment (important if CAS is being considered because procedural risks increase) and exclude undiagnosed diabetes. Fasting total cholesterol and triglyceride levels should be checked along with high-density lipoprotein cholesterol, low-density lipoprotein cholesterol, and the total lipoprotein–high-density lipoprotein ratio. Finally, simple measurement of plasma viscosity or the erythrocyte sedimentation rate may warn of the possibility that there may be an underlying vasculitis rather than atherosclerosis.

Secondary Evaluations

This category of blood testing is reserved for selected patients (usually the younger age group) who exhibit specific clinical or demographic features that warrant further investigation, usually because there is a significant possibility that a nonatheromatous or prothrombotic disorder is responsible. A full thrombophilia screen (including lupus anticoagulant) and fasting homocysteine levels should be undertaken in young patients (<50 years) who suffer an ischemic stroke or TIA or have a personal (or strong family) history of thrombosis. Similarly, a full autoantibody screen should be performed in any patient with an elevated erythrocyte sedimentation rate or plasma viscosity or a clinical history suggestive of an autoimmune disorder (e.g., telangiectatic facial rash, arthralgias, purpura). It is also important to remember that drug abuse (especially cocaine and methamphetamines) is an important cause of stroke and TIA, especially in younger patients.

There may also be a role in the future for measuring plasma biomarkers (e.g., high-sensitivity C-reactive protein[51] and matrix metalloproteinase-9[52]), especially in patients with asymptomatic carotid disease. Here the aim will (hopefully) be to use elevated levels of biomarkers to select patients at high risk for stroke and thus optimize clinical and cost-effective use of resources. To date, however, most of these biomarker parameters are of research interest only.

A further subject of considerable importance for the future is the issue of antiplatelet resistance. Currently, most clinicians start their patients on a standard dose of aspirin (or clopidogrel), irrespective of the patient's age, gender, or body weight. Unfortunately, between 5% and 10% of patients will be resistant to aspirin and more than 20% will exhibit only a partial response to aspirin.[53] Similarly, clopidogrel resistance may affect up to 31% of patients at 5 days and 15% at 30 days,[54] with little evidence that increasing the dose reduces the prevalence of resistance. The clinical relevance of testing for clopidogrel resistance has not been extensively evaluated in patients with carotid artery disease, but parallels may be drawn from the cardiac literature. In a series of patients with non–ST segment myocardial infarction undergoing percutaneous coronary interventions, 40% of patients falling within the lowest quartile of responders to clopidogrel (i.e., resistant) had a recurrent cardiovascular event. This compares with only 6.7% of patients in the second quartile and 0% of patients in the third and fourth quartiles (i.e., more/most sensitive to clopidogrel).[55] In the future, testing for resistance to aspirin or clopidogrel might enable targeting of the most appropriate antiplatelet therapy.

SELECTED KEY REFERENCES

Biasi GM, Froio A, Diethrich EB, Deleo G, Galimberti S, Mingazzini P, Nicolaides AN, Griffin M, Raithel D, Reid DB, Valsecchi MG. Carotid plaque echolucency increases the risk of stroke in carotid stenting: the Imaging in Carotid Angioplasty and Risk of Stroke (ICAROS) Study. *Circulation.* 2004;110:756.
One of the first studies to use a computerized method for scoring carotid plaque echogenicity and show how it might be used to select (reject) a patient for CAS.

Grant EG, Benson CB, Moneta GL, Alexandrov AV, Baker JD, Bluth EI, Carroll BA, Eliasziw M, Gocke J, Hertzberg BS, Katanick S, Needleman L, Pellerito J, Polak JF, Rholl KS, Wooster DL, Zierler RE. Carotid artery stenosis: gray-scale and Doppler US diagnosis: Society of Radiologists in Ultrasound Consensus Conference. *Radiology.* 2003;229:340.

In the current era where ultrasound is not being compared with angiography, this group has developed consensus criteria for diagnosing the degree of carotid stenosis with ultrasound.

Nicolaides AN, Kakkos SK, Griffin M, Sabetai M, Dhanjil S, Thomas DJ, Geroulakos G, Georgiou N, Francis S, Ioannidou E, Doré CJ; Asymptomatic Carotid Stenosis and Risk of Stroke (ACSRS) Study Group. Effect of image normalisation on carotid plaque classification and the risk of ipsilateral ischemic events: results from the Asymptomatic Carotid Stenosis and Risk of Stroke Study. *Vascular.* 2005;13:211.

Using the ACSRS database (>1000 asymptomatic patients), this group showed that by normalizing the B-mode image before ascribing it to one of five categories, it was possible to predict which patients had the highest and lowest risks for stroke while being treated medically.

Rothwell PM, Eliasziw M, Gutnikov SA, Warlow CP, Barnett HJ; Carotid Endarterectomy Trialists Collaboration. Endarterectomy for symptomatic carotid stenosis in relation to clinical subgroups and timing of surgery. *Lancet.* 2004;363:915.

All of the individual patient data from NASCET, ECST, and the Veterans Administration Trial (>6000 patients) have been combined after remeasuring the degree of stenosis via the NASCET measurement method. This paper shows that delay in surgery significantly reduces the long-term benefit in terms of stroke reduction.

Schneider PA, Kasirajan KK. Difficult anatomy: what characteristics are critical to good outcomes of either CEA or CAS? *Semin Vasc Surg.* 2007;20:216.

Overview of the anatomic features that make CAS more difficult and that therefore need to be actively looked for during evaluation for CAS.

Wardlaw JM, Chappell FM, Stevenson M, et al. Accurate, practical and cost-effective assessment of carotid stenosis in the UK. *Health Technology Assessment.* 2006;10. Available at: http://www.hta.ac.uk/fullmono/mon1030.pdf.

Very large systematic review and meta-analysis of studies evaluating the various noninvasive imaging modalities (but excluding MDCTA).

REFERENCES

The reference list can be found on the companion Expert Consult Web site at *www.expertconsult.com.*

Cerebrovascular Disease: Decision Making and Medical Treatment

Timothy F. Kresowik and Harold P. Adams, Jr.

The evidence base for decisions about intervention for atherosclerotic occlusive disease of the carotid bifurcation is extensive. In no other clinical area encountered by the vascular surgeon are the quality and breadth of evidence as strong. It is essential that the vascular surgeon be well versed in the details of this evidence base. Proper selection of patients for intervention is as important a contributor to achieving overall patient benefit as technical skill in performance of the procedure.

■ CAROTID BIFURCATION DISEASE

The most important determinant of both adverse events associated with intervention and the likelihood of patient benefit is the preintervention symptomatic status of the patient (see Chapter 92: Cerebrovascular Disease: General Considerations). Unfortunately, various definitions have been used for defining symptomatic versus asymptomatic disease in trials supporting intervention and in clinical practice.

Asymptomatic Patients

It would seem that the most straightforward classification of patients with carotid bifurcation disease should be the asymptomatic classification. However, in this case the term *asymptomatic* can refer to absence of symptoms in the carotid hemisphere ipsilateral to the carotid disease, the anterior circulation, or any brain/brainstem origin. It is important to understand the definitions used for valid comparison of randomized trials and other studies.

Definition

In the Asymptomatic Carotid Atherosclerosis Study (ACAS), patients met eligibility criteria as long as they had no previous symptoms in either the ipsilateral cerebral hemisphere or the vertebrobasilar circulation.[1] Patients who had either transient symptoms or stroke in the cerebral hemisphere contralateral to the carotid artery of interest were still eligible for ACAS. In the European Asymptomatic Carotid Surgery Trial (ACST), patients were eligible for entry as long as it was deemed that the "stenosis had not caused any stroke, transient cerebral ischemia, or other relevant neurological symptoms in the past 6 months."[2] In a population-based report of carotid endarterectomy (CEA) outcomes obtained through complete abstraction of individual hospital medical records (multistate Medicare), patients were classified as asymptomatic only if they had no previous history of symptoms or events in either the carotid or the vertebrobasilar distribution.[3] Patients with only dizziness or lightheadedness were considered asymptomatic in all studies.

Carotid Endarterectomy Trial Outcomes

Both the ACAS and the ACST demonstrated a benefit of CEA with medical therapy (aspirin and atherosclerotic risk factor reduction) over medical therapy alone for patients with carotid stenosis in the 60% to 99% range. The 5-year results from ACAS and ACST are provided in Figure 94-1 and Table 94-1. The trials showed a similar absolute and relative reduction in risk for stroke of approximately 5% and 50%, respectively, at 5 years for CEA over medical therapy.[1,2] The endpoints of the two trials were different, with ACAS reporting ipsilateral stroke and ACST reporting all strokes. Both trials included perioperative death or any perioperative stroke in the surgical group event rate.

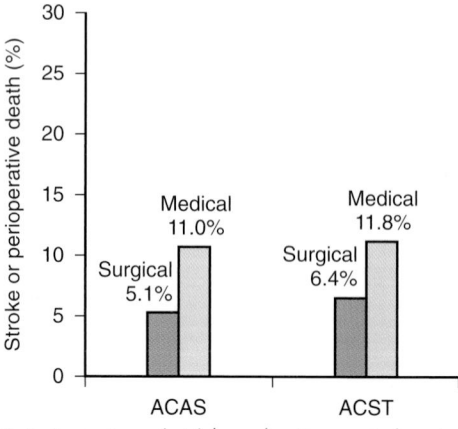

Figure 94-1 Asymptomatic trial results, 5-year stroke rate. ACAS, Asymptomatic Carotid Atherosclerosis Study; ACST, Asymptomatic Carotid Surgery Trial.

Table 94-1 Asymptomatic Patient Carotid Endarterectomy Trial Results, 5-Year Stroke Rate

Study	Degree of Stenosis (%)	Number of Patients	Endpoint	Medical Event Rate (%)	Surgical Event Rate (%)	Absolute Risk Reduction (5 Year) (%)	Relative Risk Reduction (5 Year) (%)
ACAS[1]	60-99	1662	Ipsilateral stroke	11.0	5.1	6.1	53
ACST[2]	60-99	3120	Any stroke	11.8	6.4	5.4	46

ACAS, Asymptomatic Carotid Atherosclerosis Study; ACST, Asymptomatic Carotid Stenosis Trial.

Both ACAS and ACST used duplex ultrasound criteria for determining the degree of carotid stenosis. ACAS had standardized duplex velocity criteria, whereas ACST used "locally validated criteria."[4] ACAS required arteriographic confirmation in all patients randomized to CEA but ACST did not. The angiographic standard for ACAS was the same as the North American Symptomatic Carotid Endarterectomy Trial (NASCET), whereas the corresponding reference for ACST was not specified, but typically European centers used the European Carotid Surgery Trial (ECST) methodology (see discussion of NASCET and ECST angiographic criteria under "Results of Randomized Trials"). The large number of centers in ACST probably created considerable variation in the degree of determination of stenosis because of the "locally validated criteria" standard.[5] However, the wide range of stenosis (60% to 99%) that describes the population that benefited from CEA in both ACAS and ACST most likely makes differences in criteria somewhat less critical because the majority of the patients would still fall within the 60% to 99% range in both studies except at the lower end of the range.

ACAS provides the best benchmark for outcomes associated with CEA in asymptomatic patients. Thirty-day outcomes were verified by mandatory follow-up visits and examinations with standardized definitions. Although the reported surgical group intention-to-treat 30-day combined event rate was 2.3%, the actual event rate in the patients who underwent CEA was 1.5% (10 nonfatal strokes and 1 death in 724 patients). The reported 2.3% rate includes in the denominator 101 patients who did not undergo CEA after randomization, and the numerator includes three events in patients prior to CEA and five strokes (one fatal) directly related to angiography prior to CEA. The five events in 414 patients who underwent the required arteriogram after randomization prior to CEA correspond to a 1.2% combined event rate attributable to angiography. Avoiding preoperative intra-arterial angiography increases the benefit of CEA over medical therapy alone. Because intra-arterial diagnostic arteriography is rarely necessary with current noninvasive technology (see Chapter 93: Cerebrovascular Disease: Diagnostic Evaluation), it is not necessary to include angiography-related events in the expected adverse event rate for CEA decision making.

Community Results

Some have questioned the relevance of the ACAS adverse event rates to community practice by citing the "rigorous"

selection criteria used for eligibility of participating surgeons. They would suggest that the ACAS results represented best practice rather than typical or average adverse event rates across the spectrum of surgeons performing CEA in the community. Figure 94-2 and Table 94-2 compare the perioperative CEA outcomes for ACAS, ACST, and the multistate Medicare report. In the multistate Medicare report the overall adverse event rate in asymptomatic patients was 3.9%.[3] It must be recognized that in this population-based report the patients were older than those in ACAS because the report included all Medicare patients (generally >64 years of age with no upper limit), whereas ACAS excluded patients older than 79 years. Patients in ACAS were also excluded if they had experienced recent cardiac events or were thought to have a shortened life expectancy. These criteria did not necessarily apply to patients in the multistate Medicare report.

The ACST perioperative combined event rate was higher than that in ACAS, and perioperative mortality was identical to that observed in the asymptomatic multistate Medicare study (1%). The demonstrated benefit of CEA over medical therapy in ACST with a perioperative combined event rate only slightly lower than what was observed in the multistate Medicare experience would suggest that there was still overall net patient benefit from CEA in the multistate Medicare

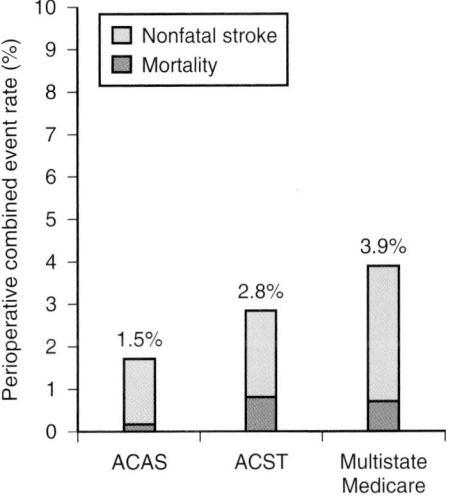

Figure 94-2 Asymptomatic patient surgical outcomes. ACAS, Asymptomatic Carotid Atherosclerosis Study; ACST, Asymptomatic Carotid Surgery Trial.

Table 94-2 Asymptomatic Patient Carotid Endarterectomy Surgical Outcomes

Study	Study Type	Time Period	Number of Procedures	Mortality (30 Day) (%)	Combined Event Rate (30 Day) (%)
ACAS[1]	Randomized trial	1987-1993	721	0.1	1.5
ACST[2]	Randomized trial	1993-2003	1405	1.1	2.8
Multistate Medicare[3] (asymptomatic)	Medical record review	1995-1999	7984	1.0	3.9

ACAS, Asymptomatic Carotid Atherosclerosis Study; ACST, Asymptomatic Carotid Stenosis Trial.

patients. It is also worth noting that ACST included patients and surgeons from 30 different countries, which certainly suggests that the results also reflect a "community" experience.

Although the overall asymptomatic patient CEA combined event rate in the multistate Medicare report was 3.9%, there was significant variability among states, and in at least one state the overall statewide combined event rate in all Medicare patients was the same as the rate in ACAS (1.5%). These data, in combination, would suggest that a 1.5% combined event rate is an achievable benchmark for the entire population of asymptomatic patients undergoing CEA. Unfortunately, the fact that this benchmark is not uniformly achieved demonstrates the continued need for surgical quality improvement.

Natural History

The relatively benign natural history of asymptomatic carotid stenosis is an important take-home message from ACAS and ACST. The overall stroke risk in patients managed with medical therapy alone is on the order of 2%/yr. This means that although CEA was shown to be of benefit, the benefit is relatively small and dependent on patient selection. Patients should be at low risk for perioperative adverse events and have a reasonable life expectancy (at least 5 years or longer). If perioperative combined event rates are higher than 3%[6,7] or if patients with limited life expectancy undergo intervention (or both), it is likely that more strokes could be caused than prevented by intervention. The relatively benign natural history of asymptomatic carotid stenosis must be emphasized to patients as part of the informed consent process in discussing intervention.

Severity of Stenosis

Other important observations from ACAS include the lack of a difference in stroke risk in the medical group between patients with 60% to 79% stenosis and those with 80% to 99% stenosis. The lack of association of stroke risk with higher degrees of stenosis is contrary to what has been observed in the symptomatic trials.[8-10] A lack of correlation between the degree of stenosis (>60%) and stroke risk in medically treated asymptomatic patients was also observed in ACST.

Existing symptoms are likely to indicate the presence of unstable plaque, and the severity of stenosis thus predicts

higher risk within the unstable-plaque subset. The lack of correlation between higher degrees of stenosis and risk in asymptomatic patients should give pause to a more aggressive approach in patients with increased surgical risk or limited life expectancy just because of the finding of a very high-grade stenosis.

Plaque Morphology

Although the discrepant observations in asymptomatic versus symptomatic patients with respect to the degree of stenosis and risk for stroke seem paradoxical, there may be differences in their carotid lesions that could explain the observations. As is true for the coronary vessels, acute events are sometimes associated with sudden plaque expansion or rupture from intraplaque hemorrhage.[11,12] Moderate stenoses are at risk for sudden expansion. Other criteria (e.g., heterogeneity, echolucency, presence of a lipid core, ulceration, observed progression) may be more relevant indicators of future events in asymptomatic patients than the degree of stenosis[13,14] (see Chapter 92: Cerebrovascular Disease: General Considerations).

Progressing Stenosis

There does seem to be a relationship between observed progression of a carotid stenosis and the risk for stroke.[15,16] This would suggest that patients with asymptomatic carotid stenosis and observed progression merit stronger consideration for intervention. However, it should be noted that observed progression of a carotid stenosis is a risk factor not only for stroke but also for all cardiovascular events (myocardial infarction, vascular death).[16] Progressive carotid stenosis is a marker for a more aggressive atherosclerotic process. These patients are probably a higher-risk population for adverse procedural events and lower long-term survival. Thus, overall risk assessment remains critical in determining a recommendation for intervention, even in patients with observed progression.

Symptomatic Patients

The benefit of CEA in patients with recent ipsilateral carotid territory symptoms and moderate to severe carotid stenosis is much greater than the benefit of CEA in asymptomatic patients. Yet there is no question that symptomatic patients are at higher risk than asymptomatic patients for perioperative adverse events.

Results of Randomized Trials

If the surgical results from ACAS are compared with those from NASCET, the results indicate that symptomatic patients have a fourfold higher risk for perioperative stroke or death than do asymptomatic patients (6.5% versus 1.5%).[1,17] However, the natural history of patients with high-grade symptomatic stenosis treated by medical therapy alone is much worse than that of asymptomatic patients. The results of two phases of NASCET and ECST are presented in Figure 94-3 and Table 94-3.[8-10] The trials did differ somewhat in methodology, and the major endpoint was reported at different intervals: 2 years for NASCET 70% to 99% stenosis, 3 years for ECST, and 5 years for NASCET 50% to 69% stenosis. Medical treatment in the symptomatic trials was aspirin as first-line therapy, but more aggressive anticoagulation (i.e., warfarin) could have been used at the discretion of the treating physician. Both these trials were performed before the widespread use of ticlopidine or clopidogrel.

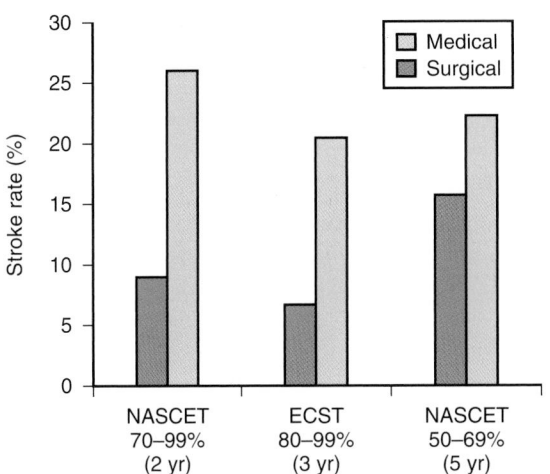

Figure 94-3 Symptomatic trial event rates. ECST, European Carotid Surgery Trial; NASCET, North American Symptomatic Endarterectomy Trial. "Symptomatic" is defined as ipsilateral hemispheric or ocular transient ischemic attack or stroke within 120 days (NASCET) or 180 days (ECST) before trial entry.

NASCET and ECST also differed in the angiographic determination of stenosis. In NASCET (as well as ACAS), the degree of stenosis on angiography was determined by comparing the residual lumen at the narrowest point of stenosis with the lumen of the internal carotid artery (ICA) distal to the carotid bulb (i.e., distal to the point where the walls of the ICA first become parallel). ECST used estimated bulb diameter as the denominator for determination of stenosis, which will overestimate the degree of stenosis relative to the ACAS/NASCET distal internal carotid methodology. The stenosis category reported in Figure 94-3 and Table 94-3 for ECST of 80% to 99% should be roughly comparable to the NASCET 70% to 99% phase. When indirect measurement methodologies are used to determine the degree of stenosis (e.g., absolute velocities or velocity ratios from duplex ultrasound examinations), the velocity criteria should correspond to reference angiographic stenoses based on the distal ICA denominator methodology.[18]

In NASCET, the medically treated group with 70% to 99% stenosis had a 26% risk for ipsilateral stroke within 2 years. The 17% absolute stroke risk reduction at 2 years achieved by CEA in symptomatic patients with greater than 70% stenosis should be contrasted with the 6% absolute stroke risk reduction at 5 years observed in ACAS. This suggests that unlike asymptomatic patients, symptomatic patients could be considered for intervention even if they have serious co-morbid conditions and a shortened life expectancy. Most patients fear the disability associated with stroke more than they fear death.

It is important to precisely define what constituted symptomatic disease in the clinical trials that support intervention. In NASCET and ECST, only patients who had either transient or permanent ipsilateral cerebral hemispheric or ocular symptoms were eligible for entry. The symptoms had to have occurred relatively recently with respect to trial entry (within 120 days for NASCET and 180 days for ECST). Patients who exhibited only lightheadedness, dizziness, or even syncope were not considered to be symptomatic. As time from transient symptoms or stroke increases, the risk of another event's occurring decreases.[19] Therefore, the results of the symptomatic trials should not be used to estimate the benefit versus risk of CEA in patients who have a history of remote events or nonhemispheric/ocular symptoms. It is appropriate to view these patients more like asymptomatic patients with respect

Table 94-3 Symptomatic* Patient Carotid Endarterectomy Trial Event Rates

Study	Degree of Stenosis (%)	Number of Patients	Endpoint (Time and Event)	Medical Event Rate (%)	Surgical Event Rate (%)	Absolute Risk Reduction (%)	Relative Risk Reduction (%)
NASCET[8]	70-99	659	2-yr ipsilateral stroke	26.0	9.0	17.0	65
ECST[9]	80-99	576	3-yr ipsilateral stroke	20.6	6.8	13.8	67
NASCET[10]	50-69	858	5-yr ipsilateral stroke	22.2	15.7	6.5	29

*Symptomatic is defined as ipsilateral hemispheric or ocular transient ischemic attack or stroke within 120 days (NASCET) or 180 days (ECST) before trial entry.
ECST, European Carotid Surgery Trial; NASCET, North American Symptomatic Carotid Endarterectomy trial.

to issues of life expectancy and co-morbid diseases when considering intervention. Patients with ocular symptoms alone have a lower risk (approximately half) for a subsequent hemispheric stroke than do those with hemispheric symptoms.[19] All these factors should be taken into account when considering the risks and benefits of intervention.

Severity of Stenosis

In contradistinction to the asymptomatic trials, stenosis severity was correlated with the risk for stroke in medically treated patients in the symptomatic trials. NASCET was prematurely halted for patients who had 70% to 99% stenosis because the observed benefit of CEA reached statistical significance earlier than the planned trial duration.[8] NASCET continued for patients with stenosis in the 30% to 69% range. When the trial was completed, there was a significant benefit for patients with stenosis in the 50% to 69% range, but the benefit was less than that for those with higher degrees of stenosis.[10] Patients with less than 50% stenosis did not benefit from CEA. Because of differences in the method of stenosis measurement between NASCET and ECST, there was some initial difficulty in comparing the trial results with respect to the degree of stenosis. A reanalysis of the ECST results was performed by conversion to the distal internal carotid artery methodology used in NASCET.[20] This analysis demonstrated some consistency in the ECST and NASCET findings in that no benefit was found for CEA in patients with less than 50% stenosis. The benefit was greater in medically treated patients with stenosis in the 70% or greater range because of a much higher stroke risk than in those with 50% to 69% stenosis. A consistent finding in the randomized trials is that the degree of ipsilateral stenosis is not predictive of higher surgical risk for perioperative stroke or death.[1,2,17,20]

Community Results

The surgical results with respect to perioperative stroke or death were similar in NASCET and ECST (Fig. 94-4 and Table 94-4), and very similar findings for perioperative outcomes were observed in the overall multistate Medicare review, in which the definition of symptoms was ipsilateral hemispheric or ocular transient events or stroke within 90 days before the procedure. This suggests that the results of ECST and NASCET can be extrapolated to the community.

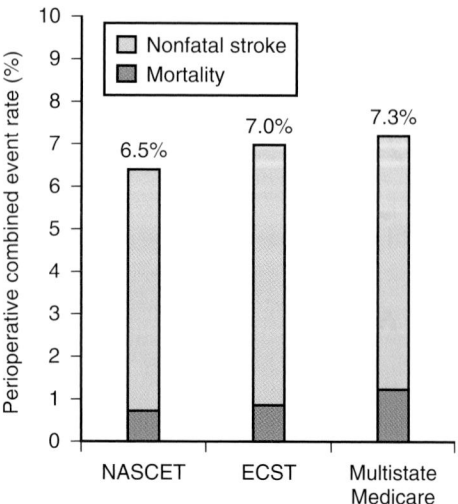

Figure 94-4 Symptomatic patient surgical outcomes. ECST, European Carotid Surgery Trial; NASCET, North American Symptomatic Endarterectomy Trial. "Symptomatic" is defined as ipsilateral hemispheric or ocular transient ischemic attack or stroke within 120 days (NASCET) or 180 days (ECST) before trial entry or 90 days before carotid endarterectomy (multistate Medicare).

On the other hand, there was significant variation even among statewide results, with very high adverse event rates observed in some cases.

Completed Stroke

Another observation from NASCET and ECST was that patients who had a completed hemispheric stroke as their "symptom" meeting the entry criteria gained benefit from CEA that was comparable to or possibly greater than that in patients with only transient symptoms.[19] At the time of the trial the prevailing surgical wisdom was that CEA should be delayed at least 4 to 6 weeks after a completed stroke to avoid worsening because of reperfusion and hemorrhagic conversion of a bland infarct. The observation in NASCET and ECST that the highest risk for stroke or recurrent stroke was early after the index "symptom" led to re-examination of the approach to patients with stroke and high-grade ipsilateral carotid stenosis.[19,21] There is evidence that CEA can be performed safely early (<3 weeks) after a completed stroke.[22]

Table 94-4 Symptomatic* Patient Carotid Endarterectomy Surgical Outcomes

Study	Study Type	Time Period	Number of Procedures	30-Day Mortality (%)	30-Day Combined Event Rate (%)
NASCET[17]	Randomized trial	1987-1996	1415	1.0	6.5
ECST[9]	Randomized trial	1981-1994	1745	1.3	7.0
Multistate Medicare[3] (symptomatic)	Medical record review	1995-1999	4193	1.7	7.3

*Symptomatic is defined as ipsilateral hemispheric or ocular transient ischemic attack or stroke within 120 days (NASCET) or 180 days (ECST) before trial entry or 90 days before carotid endarterectomy (multistate Medicare).
ECST, European Carotid Surgery Trial; NASCET, North American Symptomatic Carotid Endarterectomy trial.

Most studies have focused on patients who do not have large infarcts or hemorrhagic transformation seen on imaging studies before considering intervention. These imaging findings are still considered reasons to delay intervention for at least 4 to 6 weeks.

Timing of Intervention

It has been suggested that a much more aggressive approach (i.e., within 48 hours) is necessary for symptomatic patients with respect to timing of intervention to achieve maximum benefit.[21,23] Population-based studies with complete follow-up of patients with transient ischemic attack (TIA) or stroke suggest that the risk for a new or recurrent stroke may approach 7% in 2 days and 10% within 7 days of the initial event.[24] Operative risk is probably elevated with very early intervention.[21,25] However, the risk of stroke occurring without intervention appears to outweigh the increased operative risk.

Some caution still seems warranted in pushing the envelope for early intervention because the procedure is usually preventive rather than therapeutic. There is no evidence that restoring flow in a patient with a truly completed stroke is likely to hasten or change the ultimate degree of recovery. The risk of harm with intervention is balanced against the risk of another stroke in the period before a delayed intervention. The available data suggest that there is no reason to insist on a fixed amount of time after a stroke in all patients before performing intervention for an ipsilateral high-grade carotid stenosis. There is potential harm (new or recurrent stroke) associated with "delay." In patients who are medically stable and have relatively small or no infarcts seen on imaging studies, it seems reasonable to perform early intervention (i.e., within 48 hours) after a stroke.

Crescendo Transient Ischemic Attacks

Patients with multiple or crescendo (increasing frequency) symptoms and high-grade carotid stenosis should be considered for urgent intervention. The decision to intervene may be influenced by the patient's baseline antithrombotic regimen when the symptoms developed and the response to medical therapy. Patients who were taking no antiplatelet medications at the initial consultation should have aspirin given immediately. Patients already receiving antiplatelet therapy or with evidence of intraluminal thrombus adjacent to a high-grade stenosis probably benefit from full anticoagulation with heparin.

Although emergency intervention seems warranted, it should be apparent that patients with crescendo symptoms from carotid stenosis have unstable plaque. These unstable lesions probably increase the risk for embolization at the time of intervention.[26,27] Patients whose symptoms cease with institution of medical therapy may benefit from at least a brief delay (e.g., 48 to 72 hours) of intervention.[27,28] Intraluminal thrombus may stabilize or regress after anticoagulation and thus allow an intervention to be performed with less risk.[26,29]

Stroke in Evolution

Another clinical scenario that may indicate an urgent need for intervention is a so-called stroke in evolution or progressive stroke. These are patients in whom new or worsening neurologic deficits develop after initial evaluation. These situations require careful assessment and thought about the etiology of the worsening symptoms. Obviously, patients whose progressive symptoms are a result of hemorrhagic transformation or edema are unlikely to benefit from and may experience harm with revascularization. In contrast, patients who have watershed ischemic areas around an infarct may benefit from early revascularization. The collateral flow (status of the contralateral carotid, vertebral arteries, and circle of Willis) to the potentially ischemic areas in the distribution of the carotid artery being considered for intervention should influence the decision. Some patients may have ischemic but not yet infarcted areas isolated to the distribution of the stenotic carotid because of absent or compromised collaterals. Early intervention could be extremely beneficial in limiting disability in these patients.

Patients with Nonhemispheric or Remote Symptoms

The high-level (i.e., randomized trial) evidence base for CEA decision making is largely confined to either asymptomatic patients or those with recent hemispheric or ocular symptoms. There are many patients who do not fall into these two categories. As many as 30% to 40% of patients undergoing carotid intervention have vertebrobasilar, global, contralateral, or remote ipsilateral symptoms (nonspecific symptoms).[3] These patients appear to have a surgical risk intermediate between patients who are completely asymptomatic and those with recent, ipsilateral, hemispheric, or ocular symptoms (Fig. 94-5). What is lacking is solid evidence of the natural history of this group of patients with medical therapy alone. Obviously, the heterogeneity of this nonspecific group and the small numbers in the individual subgroups make the likelihood of randomized trial–level evidence in the future extremely low.

The absence of high-level evidence is not uncommon in many areas of contemporary medical practice. In these situations we have to use lower levels of evidence or logical extrapolation from related evidence, or both. Pooled data from the randomized trials suggest that symptomatic patients whose last symptom occurred more than 12 weeks previously have a much lower benefit from intervention.[19] It may be more appropriate to consider patients with remote symptoms similar to asymptomatic patients for intervention decision making. Patients with global symptoms (e.g., recurrent near-syncope or syncope with widespread cerebrovascular disease, a high-grade carotid stenosis amenable to intervention, and absence of other clear causes of the symptoms) should probably be strongly considered for intervention. On the other hand, a patient with the same clinical findings but with only a single stenotic internal carotid (i.e., with uncompromised

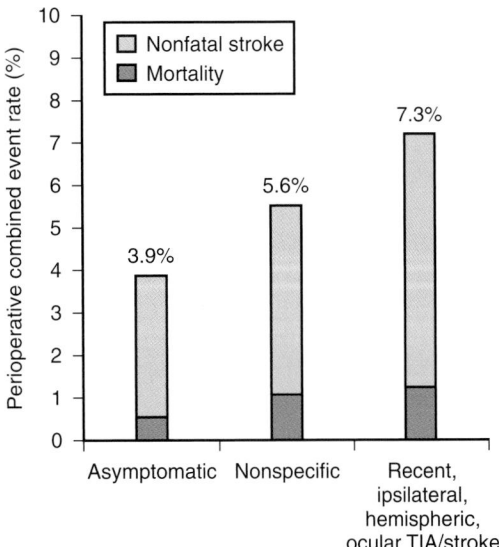

Figure 94-5 Carotid endarterectomy (CEA) outcomes by preoperative symptom status. Thirty-day stroke or mortality rates were based on complete medical record review of 19,690 CEA procedures (excluding CEA/coronary artery bypass grafting [CABG] or "redo" procedures for recurrent stenosis) in Medicare patients randomly sampled from 10 states between 1995 and 1999.[3] "Asymptomatic" refers to no previous history of transient ischemic attack [TIA] or stroke in either the cerebral hemisphere or vertebrobasilar distribution; "nonspecific" refers to a history of remote (>90 days before CEA), contralateral, vertebrobasilar, or global symptoms; "recent" means last symptom <90 days before CEA.

contralateral carotid, vertebral, and intracerebral vessels) should probably be considered the same as an asymptomatic patient for counseling regarding the benefit of intervention.

Age, Gender, and Other Considerations

Age

ACAS and the early phase of NASCET excluded patients older than 79 years. ACST and ECST did not arbitrarily exclude older patients, although the number of patients 80 years or older was small. Age is an inconsistent indicator of increased surgical risk, especially when associated comorbidity is accounted for. A subgroup meta-analysis using combined data from NASCET and ECST (after adjustment for stenosis) was published.[19] In symptomatic patients, age older than 75 years was associated with a higher risk for stroke with medical therapy than was age younger than 65 years, comparable surgical risks, and thus overall greater benefit of CEA in older patients.

This increased benefit should not necessarily be extrapolated to asymptomatic patients. The subset older than 75 years in ACST did not show significant benefit with CEA versus medical therapy, and ACAS excluded patients older than 79.[1,2] The long-time survival necessary to achieve a benefit of prophylactic CEA in asymptomatic patients would

Table 94-5 Patient Characteristics and Outcome for Intervention Decision Making

Characteristic	Outcome*
Female gender	Lower risk for stroke with medical therapy Higher risk for stroke or death with CEA
Age >75	Higher risk for stroke with medical therapy in symptomatic patients
Increasing degree of stenosis over 50%	Higher risk for stroke with medical therapy in symptomatic patients
Contralateral carotid occlusion	Higher risk for stroke or death with CEA
Increasing time from TIA/stroke	Lower risk for stroke with medical therapy
Ocular symptoms only	Lower risk for stroke with medical therapy Lower risk for stroke with CEA

*Based on significant associations determined in randomized trial subset analyses.
CEA, carotid endarterectomy; TIA, transient ischemic attack.

suggest conservatism in patients older than 80 years unless they are in good health.

Gender

The benefit of CEA in women versus men has been questioned. The randomized trials included a majority of men, and the individual trial subset analyses by gender have not always had enough women to draw firm conclusions. There does seem to be a consistent pattern in that the overall benefit of CEA for women is less than that for men in both symptomatic and asymptomatic patients.[1,2,8-10,19] The lesser benefit appears to be predominantly due to a lower stroke risk in women treated medically than in men. There is also some evidence suggestive of a higher perioperative stroke risk in women with CEA.[1,19] The higher stroke risk with CEA has been at least partially attributed to smaller vessels in women than in men. There was no demonstrated benefit of CEA in ACAS for women, but only 568 women (34% of patients) were enrolled. The larger ACST did suggest a benefit of CEA for women, but it was less than that for men. The combined NASCET and ECST analysis demonstrated a benefit for women with 80% to 99% symptomatic stenosis but not for those in the 50% to 79% group. Women should probably be treated more conservatively than men with respect to carotid intervention. Table 94-5 describes some the evidence-based relationships between patient characteristics and outcomes from medical and surgical management that should be taken into account in intervention decision making.

Individual Surgeon Outcomes

For the benefit to patients demonstrated in the randomized trials to be realized in the surgical community at large, surgical outcomes need to be at least comparable to those observed in the trials. This is especially critical for asymptomatic patients because the benefit of intervention over medical therapy alone is not large. Ideally, surgeons should be citing their own complication rates in discussions with patients rather than rates from the literature. One's own perioperative stroke or mortality rate can be contrasted with the medical natural history observed in the randomized trials.

Case Mix

Given the vast difference in surgical risk between symptomatic and asymptomatic patients observed in the randomized trials, symptom status needs to be taken into account when analyzing individual results. A complete analysis probably needs to have at least three strata: asymptomatic, recent hemispheric or ocular symptoms (NASCET/ECST criteria), and nonspecific/other (contralateral, remote, vertebrobasilar, or global symptoms). In practice, because the numbers in the subgroups can be small for an individual surgeon, the perioperative event rate for the asymptomatic subgroup is probably the most important to determine. Another advantage at looking at the surgical event rate in asymptomatic patients is that there is no need for risk adjustment for co-morbid conditions or age. Identifying neurologically asymptomatic patients who are at low risk for surgery is an important component of surgical judgment. Previous consensus statements have suggested a 3% threshold for the combined event rate in asymptomatic patients.[6,7] The 3% rate should be viewed as an upper limit of acceptability because a rate of 1.5% is an achievable benchmark and should be the goal. Table 94-6 provides some suggested outcome benchmarks, stratified by preoperative patient symptom status, for individual surgeon comparison.

Surgical Volume

There is currently a great deal of interest in public reporting of outcomes to encourage provider accountability and informed choice by patients. There is no standardized data collection methodology in widespread use that would provide a valid perioperative 30-day combined event rate for CEA with appropriate adjustment for symptom status. The limitations of existing administrative (claims) data make in-hospital mortality the only valid outcome available from this source. Standard claims data also do not allow appropriate stratification by symptom status.

Table 94-6 Recommended Benchmark Carotid Endarterectomy Combined Event Rates* by Preoperative Symptom Status

Preoperative Symptom Status	Mortality (%)	Combined Event Rate (%)
Asymptomatic	0.1	1.5
Nonspecific—remote, contralateral, global, vertebrobasilar symptoms	1.0	3.0
Recent (within 90 days), ipsilateral, hemispheric, or ocular transient ischemic attack or stroke	1.0	5.0

Authors' estimates of achievable surgical outcomes from the results of randomized trials or large population-based medical record review.
*Combined event rates (stroke or mortality within 30 days after a procedure).

In the absence of meaningful outcome data, there has been a focus on using surrogate measures such as an annual procedure rate to select surgeons. There are several problems with the use of an annual procedure rate in lieu of outcome data. An annual rate does not necessarily reflect the totality of an individual's "experience" and does not always correlate with benchmark outcomes.[30,31] Most importantly, the use of annual procedure rates as an index of quality creates a perverse incentive. There are a limited number of symptomatic patients but a large number of asymptomatic patients with at least some carotid occlusive disease. Rather than encouraging careful patient selection and counseling in the asymptomatic cohort, annual procedure rate thresholds or comparisons encourage the performance of more procedures to reach or exceed the threshold.

It is in the best interest of both the public and high-quality surgeons that comparison data for public reporting be valid and meaningful. It is also essential that perverse incentives be avoided.

Proximal Vessel Disease and Intracerebral Tandem Lesions

When duplex ultrasound alone was first being considered sufficient for evaluation of carotid stenosis before CEA, one of the issues used to justify arteriography was the possibility of proximal brachiocephalic arterial disease or intracerebral disease. However, the incidence of unsuspected concomitant lesions is relatively low, and their presence rarely influences the decision to intervene.[32-34] A consensus developed that imaging of the carotid bifurcation was adequate in the majority of patients before CEA, and many surgeons began performing CEA based on duplex findings alone.[35-37] Subsequent developments in less invasive methods of both identifying concomitant lesions (using magnetic resonance or computed tomographic angiography) and treating them (using endovascular modalities) have eliminated the need for higher-risk arteriography in almost all patients (see Chapter 93: Cerebrovascular Disease: Diagnostic Evaluation).

Proximal Vessel Disease

Although the availability of imaging modalities that do not have the same risk for morbidity as intra-arterial angiography makes routine imaging of the aortic arch and intracerebral vessels more attractive, there are still cost considerations. It is hard to justify imaging studies that do not change management. Significant lesions in the aortic arch vessels proximal to the neck can be suspected by qualitative examination of the carotid pulse, examination of the common carotid waveform and velocities on duplex ultrasound, and bilateral arm blood pressure readings. Abnormalities in any of these examinations could suggest a need for imaging of the arch. Physical examination is obviously not useful for screening for intracerebral lesions. A high-resistance flow pattern in the ICA on duplex ultrasound is an indication for evaluation of the distal internal carotid circulation (see Chapter 93: Cerebrovascular Disease: Diagnostic Evaluation).

In the absence of any these findings, asymptomatic patients probably do not need imaging of the arch or intracerebral vessels. Arch and intracerebral imaging should be considered in symptomatic patients with moderate carotid bifurcation disease (e.g., 50% to 70%) before CEA to look for other lesions that might be a more likely cause of the symptoms. An argument could be made that symptomatic patients with high-grade carotid stenosis but without abnormalities on physical examination or duplex as previously described could undergo CEA without arch or intracerebral imaging.[32] The carotid bifurcation disease is likely to require treatment irrespective of the other disease.[38,39] Any patient with continued symptoms after successful CEA would of course require further imaging.

Although imaging of the arch or intracerebral vessels may not be necessary, many patients are initially seen by the surgeon after having had these studies performed. The question of how the presence of stenoses in these vessels should influence the decision to intervene for carotid bifurcation stenosis remains unanswered. Because of the paucity of high-level evidence, extrapolation from other evidence is necessary. If there is a high-grade stenosis (e.g., associated with pulse reduction or a significant drop in pressure) proximal to a carotid lesion undergoing intervention, it may be reasonable to consider concomitant intervention for the proximal lesion. Direct or extra-anatomic surgical reconstruction is a consideration, but CEA with intraoperative retrograde endovascular stenting of the proximal lesion seems to offer the lowest-risk alternative with respect to cerebral protection (e.g., by clamping or creating flow reversal in the internal carotid during stenting).[40-42] A retrograde endovascular approach through an exposed carotid in the neck also avoids the complicated access issues that often accompany a fully endovascular approach to both lesions.

Intracerebral Lesions

The issue of treatment of intracerebral lesions concomitant with carotid bifurcation disease seems less clear. If the carotid bifurcation lesion is high grade, it should be treated even if no intervention is planned for the intracerebral disease.[38,39] In a subanalysis of NASCET, patients with tandem intracranial stenosis had a higher risk for stroke with medical therapy, and this risk was reduced by CEA.[39] There is no reason to avoid treatment of the carotid bifurcation because of distal disease unless there is high resistance to runoff, which might increase the chance of perioperative thrombosis of the reconstruction. Improving flow through the ICA would seemingly lessen the possibility of events related to the intracerebral disease. In contrast, if the intracerebral lesion is thought to require treatment because of its nature or suspicion that it is the more likely cause of symptoms, a fully endovascular approach to both the carotid bifurcation and intracerebral disease may be the best option. Imaging requirements and operator access for optimal treatment of intracerebral disease would make concomitant treatment in an operating room through the carotid incision less attractive than endovascular treatment of the proximal disease.

Severe Contralateral Carotid Disease

The presence of severe contralateral carotid stenosis or occlusion has been found to be a predictor of an increased adverse event rate with CEA.[19,43-45]

Contralateral Carotid Occlusion

The presence of severe bilateral carotid occlusive disease is a marker for more widespread atherosclerotic disease and especially coronary artery disease. The increased risk associated with bilateral carotid occlusive disease is probably more a reflection of this generalized increased risk for morbidity/mortality than a specific indicator of an increased risk for stroke with the procedure. The decision to treat a high-grade symptomatic stenosis should not be influenced by the presence of contralateral high-grade stenosis or occlusion.[19]

In asymptomatic patients there is often a presumption that patients with stenosis and contralateral occlusion would be at higher risk for future stroke than those with a patent contralateral ICA. In a subgroup analysis of ACAS, patients with contralateral carotid occlusions did not benefit from CEA over medical therapy alone.[46] This difference was almost exclusively due to a surprisingly low event rate in medically treated patients with contralateral occlusion in ACAS. However, ACAS was not sufficiently powered to support these observations with a high level of confidence, and the contralateral occlusion subgroup did show benefit from CEA in ACST.[2] The endpoint difference between ACAS and ACST may explain the contradictory findings. The endpoint of ipsilateral stroke was used in ACAS, and all stroke in ACST. It is certainly plausible that having a high-grade stenosis and contralateral occlusion may increase the overall risk for stroke, but not necessarily in the hemisphere ipsilateral to the patent vessel. These observations would suggest that patients should not be denied CEA because of contralateral occlusion. On the other hand, the finding of a contralateral occlusion in an asymptomatic patient should not be seen as a mandate for intervention in a poor-risk patient.

Contralateral Severe Carotid Stenosis

Assessing a patient with bilateral high-grade asymptomatic carotid stenosis introduces other considerations. What is the stroke risk with medical therapy alone in a patient with bilateral disease relative to a patient with unilateral stenosis? What is the relative benefit of unilateral versus staged bilateral intervention? Because most strokes associated with carotid bifurcation stenosis are thought to be related to embolic events, there is reason to consider the risks associated with each of the two stenoses as independent and thus additive for the patient. This suggests that in a good-risk patient, staged bilateral reconstruction should provide the optimum reduction in stroke risk. Unilateral repair probably reduces overall stroke risk by no more than 50%. The presence of bilateral disease is generally indicative of more widespread atherosclerotic disease and thus may be associated with increased procedural risk or a shortened life expectancy from coronary artery disease. In asymptomatic poor-risk patients the presence of bilateral stenosis should not compel a surgeon to at least perform unilateral repair. There is no valid mechanism to determine which side is more likely to be a source of future stroke, and unilateral repair probably does not influence the risk for stroke from the contralateral stenosis.

This same logic would not apply to a patient with a symptomatic stenosis and a contralateral asymptomatic stenosis. Even if the asymptomatic stenosis were more severe, the known stroke risk of the symptomatic stenosis (assuming that it is at least >50%) would indicate initial repair of the symptomatic side. Unilateral repair of the symptomatic stenosis may still be appropriate in a patient with serious co-morbidity suggesting increased procedural risk or shortened life expectancy (or both). The decision to perform a subsequent staged repair of the asymptomatic side should be based on an independent assessment of the risks and benefits without necessarily being influenced by the prior contralateral symptomatic stenosis.

Recurrent Carotid Stenosis

Management of recurrent carotid stenosis is influenced by the length of time from the index procedure to the recurrent stenosis and the presence or absence of symptoms. Early recurrent stenosis is almost always due to intimal hyperplasia. Although early restenosis is typically defined as recurrence that becomes manifested within the first 2 years after CEA, the process is usually apparent to some degree within the first 3 to 6 months.[47-50] Early recurrent stenosis from intimal hyperplasia is generally very smooth and homogeneous and thus less prone to spontaneous disruption or embolization.[51-53] This suggests that the risk for stroke is less than that with typical atherosclerotic plaque. Intimal hyperplasia may stabilize or even regress, but in some cases it can progress to occlusion.[54-56]

Patients with clear symptoms in the territory of an early recurrent stenosis in the 50% or greater range should be considered for repeat intervention. If the recurrence is moderate (50% to 70%), careful evaluation to exclude other sources of symptoms (e.g., proximal or intracerebral lesions) should probably precede intervention given the typical nature and thus the low embolic risk associated with intimal hyperplasia. Patients who are asymptomatic and have moderate recurrent stenosis should be observed and intervention considered only if they continue to progress to a high-grade (e.g., >80%) level. The risks and benefits of intervention must be balanced as for any patient without symptoms. There is certainly no evidence that asymptomatic patients with early recurrent stenosis are at higher risk for stroke with medical therapy alone than are patients with primary disease.

Information to guide decision making in the treatment of recurrent stenosis in an asymptomatic patient may be obtained from the initial procedure. A documented need for shunting based on intraoperative monitoring during the previous CEA would seem to indicate an ipsilateral cerebral hemisphere with poor collateral flow. This would suggest a more aggressive approach to a high-grade recurrent stenosis even in an asymptomatic patient.

Patients with restenosis years after CEA often have more typical atherosclerotic plaque.[53] The risk for stroke with medical therapy alone is akin to that of patients with primary disease, and the decision to intervene should be similar.

Recurrent stenosis after CEA is usually treated more conservatively than primary disease because of a perceived increased risk associated with reoperation. However, if symptomatic status is taken into account, it is not clear that patients undergoing CEA for recurrent stenosis are more likely to experience perioperative stroke or death.[3,48,55,57-60] Patients who are undergoing repeat CEA are more likely to experience local complications.[58,60] There is a higher incidence of cranial nerve dysfunction with dissection in a scarred field, and more distal dissection of the ICA is typically needed because of stenosis at the previous distal endpoint. Carotid artery stenting (CAS) may have advantages over CEA in the treatment of recurrent stenosis (see later under "Open versus Endovascular Treatment").

Combined Carotid and Coronary Disease

Patients with significant disease in both the carotid and coronary distributions are not uncommon.[61] Stroke is a feared complication of coronary artery bypass grafting (CABG). Patients with severe carotid bifurcation disease who are undergoing CABG do appear to be at higher risk for stroke or death than those without carotid disease.[62,63] It is not clear, however, that this increased risk for stroke is directly related to events arising from the carotid bifurcation disease. Patients without carotid bifurcation or intracerebral vessel disease do experience stroke with CABG.[64] Emboli arising from clamping and other manipulation of the aortic arch, as well as particulates or air introduced from the pump oxygenator circuit, are probably major sources of adverse neurologic events.[65] It seems plausible that patients with compromised cerebral flow from occlusive disease would at least have a theoretical risk for low-flow ischemia while being maintained on a pump oxygenator because the perfusion pressure waveform is different from that in a normal heart. There is no good reason, however, to think that undergoing CABG should necessarily increase the risk for embolization from the carotid bifurcation disease itself.

An intervention that would reduce the incidence of stroke associated with CABG would be attractive to both cardiac surgeons and patients. Some have therefore suggested carotid revascularization before or concomitant with CABG as a useful approach to reduce neurologic adverse events associated with CABG. Although many published single-institution series suggest that CEA and CABG can be performed concomitantly without excessive morbidity/mortality, this does not appear to hold true across the community because of very high adverse events reported for the combined procedure.[66-73] The 30-day stroke or mortality rate was 17.7% in the CEA/CABG subset of the multistate Medicare study.[72] However, patients undergoing the combined procedure are likely to be at higher risk because of the extent of their disease and would be expected to have more adverse events even if the procedures were not combined.[62,67] The real issue is whether there is any risk reduction associated with the combined procedure and whether performing them concomitantly adds risk.

Symptomatic Carotid Disease

Decision making for patients with combined coronary and carotid disease should be influenced by the symptom status and severity of disease in the respective circulations (Table 94-7). Clearly, patients with recently symptomatic high-grade carotid occlusive disease and stable symptomatic coronary artery disease need to have the carotid occlusive disease treated either before or concomitant with coronary revascularization. Symptomatic carotid disease should typically be considered an urgent problem, and stable symptoms from coronary artery disease more elective. Most patients with stable symptoms from coronary artery disease can tolerate CEA with good medical management of their coronary disease (beta blockade, aspirin, statin therapy). CEA can also be performed in most patients under local anesthesia or regional block. Although there is no high-level evidence that local/regional anesthesia for CEA is associated with significantly reduced cardiac events, the apparently lower incidence of perioperative hemodynamic instability under local/regional anesthesia suggests an advantage.[74,75] In addition, general anesthesia does appear to increase the risk for overall thrombotic events over regional/local anesthesia.[76]

Table 94-7 Decision Making for Combined Coronary and Carotid Disease

Clinical Scenario	Recommended Staging
Symptomatic carotid stenosis with indications for elective CABG	CEA preceding or concurrent with CABG
Asymptomatic patient with unilateral carotid high-grade stenosis and indications for elective CABG	CABG followed by CEA
Asymptomatic patient with bilateral high-grade carotid stenosis/contralateral occlusion or significant vertebrobasilar compromise and indications for elective CABG	CEA preceding or concurrent with CABG
Symptomatic carotid stenosis with a patent drug-eluting coronary stent placed within 1 year previously	CAS

Based on the authors' interpretation and logical extrapolation from best available current evidence.
CABG, coronary artery bypass grafting; CAS, coronary artery stenting; CEA, carotid endarterectomy.

Asymptomatic Carotid Disease

Patients with asymptomatic carotid occlusive disease can usually have treatment deferred in the presence of increased cardiac risk when ongoing coronary ischemia requires treatment. After treatment of their coronary disease and hopefully improvement in their cardiac risk and long-term survival, it may be more appropriate to consider intervention for asymptomatic carotid disease. Exceptions to this approach might include patients with severely compromised cerebrovascular perfusion (e.g., high-grade ICA stenosis in the presence of contralateral carotid occlusion or contralateral stenosis and subclavian/vertebral artery disease). These patients might theoretically be at risk for low-flow ischemia while on pump for CABG and should be considered for CEA, either before or concomitant with CABG.

Although most patients with unilateral asymptomatic carotid stenosis could have CEA deferred, another exception might be a patient with a truly preocclusive stenosis (i.e., >95%). The coagulation changes that occur around the time of any major procedure might predispose to thrombosis, although this must be considered logical speculation rather than a high evidence–based decision.

The issue of staging of CEA/CABG has an extensive literature base without adequate randomized trial evidence or consistent nonrandomized evidence.[77] The major problem with trying to determine the answer to the staging-versus-concomitant question from retrospective clinical studies is the inability to capture true intent. Patients who undergo isolated CABG or CEA with the intent to undergo a subsequent staged procedure but who experience a serious adverse event (death, severe stroke, complete carotid thrombosis) may never proceed to the intended second-stage procedure. These patients never appear in the staged cohort and therefore inappropriately reduce the complication rate ascribed to staging. Additionally, although it is possible to determine the adverse event rate associated with combined CEA/CABG procedures, in most series there is no way to determine the patient selection process for the various approaches, which introduces a significant potential bias.

Although it is certainly likely that adding CEA to CABG does not increase the risks related to CABG, it is not clear that the converse is true. CABG procedures are associated with coagulopathy, which is likely to increase the possibility of neck hematoma, a potentially life-threatening condition. The coagulopathic alterations are not limited to increased bleeding risk. Prothrombotic states can result from the pump oxygenator circuit or perioperative pharmacologic/blood product treatment of a bleeding diathesis. This could increase the risk of thrombosis or embolism arising from the fresh endarterectomy site. It would seem wise to avoid the combined procedure unless it is clear that the approach poses less risk to the patient than a staged procedure does. The role of CAS in patients with combined coronary and carotid disease is discussed later in the section on open versus endovascular treatment.

VERTEBROBASILAR INSUFFICIENCY

Decision making in the area of vertebrobasilar insufficiency suffers from a lack of randomized trial evidence, as well as issues arising from definitions and causes of symptoms.[78,79] The collateral overlap with the anterior circulation introduces additional complexity. Symptoms sometimes ascribed to a vertebrobasilar etiology, such as syncope, near-syncope, or dizziness, more often have a noncerebrovascular etiology. It is certainly important that other causes of hypoperfusion, such as neurogenic postural hypotension, cardiac arrhythmias, vasovagal reactions, and others, be "ruled out" before considering intervention for subclavian or vertebral artery occlusive disease (see Chapter 92: Cerebrovascular Disease: General Considerations and Chapter 102: Vertebral Artery Disease). In patients who have global symptoms thought to be related to cerebral perfusion and concomitant high-grade carotid bifurcation occlusive disease, it is reasonable to initially consider intervention for the carotid disease because of the better established risk-to-benefit profile.[80] Even in the presence of proximal vertebral artery disease, the collaterals to the posterior circulation may be adequate to preclude the need for direct vertebrobasilar intervention.

Subclavian Steal

A specific cause of vertebrobasilar symptoms is the subclavian steal syndrome.[81,82] The syndrome exists when a patient has compromised upper extremity blood flow as a result of high-grade stenosis or occlusion in the corresponding subclavian artery proximal to a patent vertebral artery, which develops reversed flow to supply the arm. Subclavian steal symptoms occur if vertebrobasilar territory symptoms (e.g., syncope or presyncope) develop because of "steal" of blood from the posterior cerebral circulation down the vertebral artery to supply the arm. Disease of the brachiocephalic (innominate) trunk on the right can cause a similar phenomenon secondary to altered vertebral or carotid flow, or both. Revascularization of the upper extremity should eliminate the steal. In addition, the presence of anatomic reversed flow in the vertebral artery on angiography or duplex ultrasound imaging at rest or during stress is sometimes referred to as subclavian steal but does not dictate the need for revascularization in the absence of symptoms. There is no evidence that the presence of subclavian steal without symptoms—or for that matter with symptoms—is an indicator of a high risk for stroke in the vertebrobasilar territory without revascularization.[83] Again, it may be reasonable to initially consider carotid intervention in patients with global symptoms and severe carotid bifurcation disease.

Coronary Subclavian Steal

Use of the internal mammary artery for coronary revascularization may result in another form of subclavian steal syndrome in the presence of a proximal subclavian stenosis or occlusion.[84-86] The drop in pressure associated with proximal subclavian stenosis can result in a reduction in perfusion of the internal mammary graft and subsequent coronary ischemia. Unlike subclavian-vertebral steal, it may be reasonable to consider subclavian revascularization in the presence of an internal mammary graft and subclavian/innominate occlusion or stenosis significant enough to cause a drop in pressure, even without clear coronary ischemic symptoms.

OPEN VERSUS ENDOVASCULAR TREATMENT

The general considerations for decision making regarding an endovascular versus open approach to arterial disease are similar irrespective of the arterial bed of interest. The most important considerations are the risk for complications associated with the respective approaches and the long-term effectiveness. The severity of both early and late complications should be weighed. The patient's co-morbid conditions, as well as predicted longevity, will obviously influence the importance of procedural risks versus durability. As for any procedure, the ultimate decision maker should be a well-informed patient, but surgeons have a large influence on this decision based on how the "facts" are presented.

In the current health care environment, cost should also be an important consideration. Cost-effectiveness considerations must take into account not only the direct procedural cost but also the resources required for periprocedural care, the cost of complications, and the cost associated with follow-up and any repeat procedures required to maintain effectiveness. Currently, cost-effectiveness deliberations are more appropriate at the population/health plan level than at the individual level.

Carotid Bifurcation Disease

The choice of CEA versus CAS is limited by a lack of adequate evidence. CEA is a much more mature procedure with an established record in both prospective trials and community-wide, population-based studies with surgeons of various backgrounds (see Chapter 95: Carotid Artery: Endarterectomy). CAS is still an evolving procedure, and there are limited data with respect to results across the large numbers of practitioners who could potentially offer the procedure (see Chapter 96: Carotid Artery: Stenting). There are no good data regarding the adverse event rate of CAS appropriately stratified by patient symptom status for the typical patients who have been undergoing CEA. It is hoped that ongoing trials, particularly the National Institutes of Health–sponsored Carotid Revascularization Endarterectomy versus Stent Trial (CREST), will provide a more rigorous evidence base for decision making.[87]

The published trials of CAS versus CEA have not yet established CAS as an equivalent procedure to CEA with respect to the risk for periprocedural stroke (see Chapter 96: Carotid Artery: Stenting).[88-90] It can also be said that the data do not unequivocally establish CEA as a superior procedure in the patient groups that have been studied. Many of the trials to date have focused on patients who are thought to be at "high risk" for CEA. Unfortunately, this high-risk group has commingled both patients who are considered to be medically at high risk because of co-morbid conditions (cardiac, pulmonary, renal) and patients who have anatomic considerations (recurrent stenosis, high bifurcations or distal ICA lesions, hostile neck) that are associated with an increased risk for surgical site complications with CEA. The distinction between medical high risk and anatomic high risk has important implications for decision making.

Asymptomatic Disease

Many of the CEA-versus-CAS high-risk trials have included a large number of asymptomatic patients. A review of the adverse event rates for either CAS or CEA reveals results suggesting that there may not have been benefit of either procedure over medical therapy alone. The long life expectancy that was necessary to demonstrate surgical benefit in asymptomatic patients is important when considering intervention for patients who would be predicted to have a shortened life expectancy. It is important not only that CAS be at least equivalent to CEA in terms of procedural risk but also that the risk be low enough so that the outcomes are superior to those of medical therapy alone. It should be recalled that in ACAS the risk for stroke with angiography alone was comparable to the perioperative stroke risk with CEA (1.2% versus 1.5%). The strokes associated with cerebral angiography are probably related to embolism secondary to catheter manipulation in the diseased aortic arch. The increased manipulation required to gain access to the intended carotid for CAS and cross the lesion to place a cerebral protection device can only add to this risk. Extrapolating published results from the literature for asymptomatic patients, it is hard to make a case that CAS is justified for asymptomatic patients who are at typical risk with CEA. The data also suggest that asymptomatic patients who are at significantly increased risk with CEA because of serious medical co-morbidities are better treated with medical therapy alone.

One of the perceived advantages of CAS over CEA in patients who have increased medical risk for surgery is the suggestion that medical complications are less likely. In the Stenting and Angioplasty with Protection in Patients at High Risk for Endarterectomy (SAPPHIRE) trial, the rate of myocardial infarction defined by routine periprocedural serial troponin monitoring was significantly higher in the CEA group (6.6%) than in the CAS group (1.9%).[91]

It is important to recognize that the vast majority of patients who underwent CEA as part of the SAPPHIRE trial had the procedure performed under general anesthesia, whereas CAS was almost exclusively performed under local anesthesia. Because hemodynamic instability can frequently accompany CAS as well as CEA, it is at least reasonable to postulate that the increased rate of myocardial damage in the CEA group versus the CAS group may be due to the difference in anesthetic approaches. The question remains whether

a symptomatic patient with increased cardiac risk is better served by CAS or by CEA performed under local/regional anesthesia.

Anatomic High-Risk Factors for Carotid Endarterectomy

Patients who have anatomic factors that increase the risk associated with CEA warrant separate consideration. The available literature to date does suggest that CAS can be performed with a complication rate low enough to justify a preference over CEA when the risk for complications at the surgical site is clearly increased.[88-90] These anatomic factors should include lesions that present problems for access during CEA because of a high carotid bifurcation or distal ICA extent of disease. Even if the lesion is accessible for CEA, the increased risk for cranial nerve injury and other complications associated with high dissection in the neck may indicate an advantage for CAS. Other anatomic risk factors that would suggest a preference for CAS over CEA include a hostile neck because of previous surgery or radiation therapy or increased risk for infection (i.e., presence of a tracheostomy).

Patients with symptomatic disease and significant anatomic high risk for CEA should generally undergo CAS. It cannot be said at this time that CAS is superior to medical therapy alone for all asymptomatic patients with anatomic high-risk factors for CEA. In asymptomatic patients who are good risk other than anatomic factors, it would seem that offering CAS over CEA is a reasonable approach.

Previous Carotid Endarterectomy

One of the major advantages of CAS over repeat CEA is absence of the potential complication of cranial nerve injury. In addition, the nature of early recurrent stenosis suggests that the embolic risk associated with stenting would be lower than for typical atherosclerotic plaque. The hemodynamic consequences that occur with balloon dilatation of the carotid bulb and stimulation of the carotid baroreceptors appear to be less with treatment of recurrent stenosis than with treatment of primary disease.[92] This has been attributed to denervation of the carotid bulb associated with CEA. The absence of risk for cranial nerve injury with CAS, as well as the probably lower embolic and hemodynamic risks associated with stenting for the treatment of recurrent stenosis versus primary disease, suggests that CAS treatment of recurrent carotid stenosis after CEA has advantages over redo CEA.

Increased Risk with Carotid Artery Stenting

Anatomic high-risk and medical high-risk factors for CAS can also influence the decision to elect CAS. Aortic arch anatomy and the extent of disease, the nature of the carotid bifurcation lesion, the tortuosity of the distal ICA's interfering with placement of protection devices, and difficult arterial access may preclude safe CAS (see Chapter 96: Carotid Artery: Stenting). These anatomic risk factors should be considered

Table 94-8 Endovascular versus Open Surgical Decision Making for Carotid Bifurcation Disease

Clinical Scenario	Recommended Approach
Asymptomatic or nonspecific symptoms in a patient with high medical risk or limited life expectancy	Medical therapy
Asymptomatic or nonspecific symptoms in a patient with low or typical medical risk	Medical therapy or CEA
Asymptomatic or nonspecific symptoms in a patient with high anatomic risk* and low or typical medical risk	Medical therapy or CAS
Symptomatic patient with low or typical risk	CEA
Younger symptomatic patient with high medical risk	CAS or CEA under local/regional anesthesia
Older symptomatic patient with high medical risk	CEA under local/regional anesthesia
Symptomatic patient with high anatomic risk*	CAS

Based on the authors' interpretation and logical extrapolation from best available current evidence.
*Anatomic risk for CEA (high bifurcation or distal extent of disease; previous surgery in the carotid field, e.g., "redo" CEA or neck nodal dissection; previous radiation to neck or risk of infection, e.g., tracheostomy).
CAS, carotid artery stenting; CEA, carotid endarterectomy.

in decision making for CAS versus CEA. Advanced age is associated with a higher risk for neurologic adverse events with CAS,[93] probably because the configuration and extent of atherosclerotic disease of the aortic arch in older individuals increase the embolic risks related to obtaining access to the carotid artery for CAS. In contrast, when adjusted for comorbid conditions, it is not clear that CEA-associated risks are significantly elevated in older individuals. Advanced age may be a medical risk factor that suggests a preference for CEA. Table 94-8 summarizes CEA versus CAS considerations in decision making.

Costs

Another consideration predominantly at the health system or payer level is the cost of the respective procedures. A valid cost-effectiveness analysis is complex because it would have to take into account not only the procedural cost but also the rate and cost of complications. Relative effectiveness in terms of durability, likelihood of future stroke, and need for subsequent procedures should be considered in the analysis. Because there are limited data in many of these areas for CAS, most of the cost-effectiveness analyses have included assumptions and have come to varied conclusions.[94-96] Even calculation of the direct costs related to procedures is highly dependent on assumptions about preprocedure diagnostic evaluations (e.g., imaging, cardiac evaluation) and resource use periprocedurally (e.g., length of hospital stay, utilization of intensive care). It is not hard to imagine how, depending on assumptions, cost-effectiveness analyses could come to widely divergent conclusions.

Using the literature as a guide, one could make the assumption that in many of these areas, optional resource utilization could be considered comparable (i.e., anesthetic costs, need for intensive care, hospital length of stay). If the assumption was made that complication rates and long-term effectiveness were equivalent, a cost comparison could be made on the nonoptional procedure-related costs. With these assumptions there is no question that CAS would be more expensive than CEA.[94,95] The cost of single-use devices such as stents, catheters, wires, and protection devices, as well as the capital costs associated with imaging facilities, would far outweigh the equivalent costs (suture, prosthetic patch) typically associated with CEA. CAS would have to be superior rather than just "noninferior" to CEA in terms of complications or long-term effectiveness to justify the increased cost.

Combined Carotid and Coronary Artery Disease

Patients with combined coronary artery disease and carotid occlusive disease are worthy of special attention with respect to a decision to recommend CAS versus CEA. This may be especially important in patients being considered for or having recently undergone intervention for their coronary artery disease. Of major importance in decision making are the antithrombotic regimens required for optimal results associated with the respective procedures. In a patient in whom it is thought appropriate or necessary to intervene for carotid bifurcation occlusive disease before CABG, CAS and CEA are alternative approaches to be considered. If a patient requires urgent CABG, CEA before or concomitant with CABG is probably preferable because optimal results with CAS would suggest a need for at least short-term (e.g., 30 days) antithrombotic therapy with clopidogrel. Clopidogrel is probably associated with an increased bleeding risk during CABG surgery. In a patient who requires urgent treatment of carotid occlusive disease and in whom a coronary drug–eluting stent has recently been placed, clopidogrel should not be stopped to reduce the bleeding risk associated with CEA. In such patients, CAS may be preferable.

Vertebrobasilar Insufficiency

Patients with vertebrobasilar insufficiency also may be considered for both endovascular and open approaches to their disease (see Chapter 100: Brachiocephalic Artery: Surgical Treatment and Chapter 101: Brachiocephalic Artery: Endovascular Treatment). A relative increased overall morbidity and need for other than local/regional anesthesia differentiate most vertebrobasilar open procedures (vertebral endarterectomy or bypass, carotid/subclavian bypass) from CEA, thus favoring endovascular approaches when feasible. In addition, endovascular approaches to proximal subclavian artery disease (e.g., stenting) do not necessarily complicate a subsequent open procedure (e.g., carotid subclavian bypass) in the event of early or late failure. Although complete occlusions do not preclude endovascular therapy, close anatomic proximity of a subclavian occlusion or stenosis to the origin of the vertebral or internal mammary graft may be associated with a high complication rate and should dictate an open approach in most cases. Other anatomic issues such as severe calcification and unfavorable arch anatomy would also argue for open repair.

■ MEDICAL MANAGEMENT

Medical management of patients with atherosclerotic cerebrovascular disease is multifaceted and depends on the patient's clinical characteristics. Surgical interventions to treat carotid artery disease should be considered complementary to medical interventions, including measures to treat risk factors for accelerated atherosclerosis and antithrombotic therapy (Table 94-9). The goals of medical therapy are to prevent arterial occlusion and artery-to-artery embolization. Several medical therapies of proven utility are available. Treatment is selected on a case-by-case basis and is influenced by certain variables, including plans for surgical treatment, concomitant diseases, previous therapies, and specific contraindications such as medication allergies. All patients with symptomatic carotid artery atherosclerosis should undergo screening for hyperlipidemia and hyperglycemia. In addition, the evaluation should include tests to screen for concomitant heart diseases such as atrial fibrillation.

Risk Factor Modification

Current guidelines for the prevention of stroke in patients with previous neurologic symptoms include recommendations for treatment of risk factors.[97] Recommendations for lifestyle changes include weight loss, increased exercise, limitation of alcohol use, and smoking cessation. In addition, besides reducing caloric intake, dietary modifications to limit consumption of sodium and increased use of foods high in potassium are advised.

Hypertension

These lifestyle changes are complemented by the administration of medications to treat the patient's risk factors. There is abundant evidence that lowering blood pressure is an effective method of reducing the risk for stroke (see Chapter 29: Atherosclerotic Risk Factors: Hypertension).[98] Clinical trials have tested the utility of several antihypertensive medications given alone or in combination for lowering the risk for stroke. In addition to lowering blood pressure, angiotensin-converting enzyme inhibitors and angiotensin receptor blockers may slow the progression of atherosclerotic disease.[99,100] Other factors, such as the presence of renal artery stenosis, renal dysfunction, diabetes mellitus, or heart disease, may also affect decisions about the selection of specific antihypertensive medications.[97] Aggressive management of hypertension may be especially important in patients with diabetes mellitus.

Table 94-9 Medical Measures to Lower the Risk for Stroke in Patients with Symptomatic Carotid Artery Disease and Treatment of Risk Factors for Stroke

Disease	Parameter		Treatment
	Systolic BP (mm Hg)	**Diastolic BP (mm Hg)**	
Hypertension			
Prehypertension	120-139	80-89	Lifestyle changes
Stage 1	140-159	90-99	Lifestyle changes Thiazide diuretics ACEI, beta blocker ARB, CCB
Stage 2	>159	>99	Same as above, usually two medications

	Goals	Treatment
Hyperlipidemia		
	LDL cholesterol <100 mg/dL (2.59 mmol/L) HDL cholesterol >50 mg/dL (1.30 mmol/L)	Lifestyle changes Statins Other medications*
Diabetes Mellitus		
	Hemoglobin A_{1c} <7%	Lifestyle changes Oral agents Insulin
	Normalize blood pressure LDL cholesterol <70 mg/dL (1.813 mmol/L)	See above See above
Smoking		
	Stop smoking	Lifestyle changes Nicotine products Bupropion Varenicline

Antithrombotic Agents	
Medication	*Dosage*
Aspirin	81-325 mg/day
Aspirin/dipyridamole	25/200 mg twice a day
Clopidogrel	75 mg/day
Ticlopidine	250 mg twice a day

ACEI, angiotensin-converting enzyme inhibitor; ARB, angiotensin receptor blocker; BP, blood pressure; CCB, calcium channel blocker; HDL, high-density lipoprotein; LDL, low-density lipoprotein.
*Other medications include ezetimibe, niacin, gemfibrozil, pioglitazone, and metformin.
Adapted from Sacco RL, Adams R, Albers G, et al. Guidelines for prevention of stroke in patients with ischemic stroke or transient ischemic attack: a statement for healthcare professionals from the American Heart Association/American Stroke Association Council on Stroke: Co-Sponsored by the Council on Cardiovascular Radiology and Intervention: The American Academy of Neurology affirms the value of this guideline. *Stroke.* 2006;37: 577-617.

Hyperlipidemia

Hyperlipidemia causes accelerated cerebrovascular atherosclerosis just as it does for coronary artery disease. Management of hyperlipidemia is considered a quality-of-care indicator in patients hospitalized with stroke. Statins have been effective in lowering the risk for ischemic stroke in patients with coronary artery disease.[101,102] Statins slow progression of carotid artery disease.[103] The Stroke Prevention Aggressive Reduction of Cholesterol Levels (SPARCL) trial tested the efficacy of atorvastatin in addition to medical measures in preventing stroke in patients with recent TIA or ischemic stroke.[104] Atorvastatin lowered the risk for stroke by 16% during a 5-year follow-up period. Statins given periprocedurally may also decrease the adverse events associated with CEA or CAS.[105] Besides lowering lipid levels, statins may stabilize the arterial wall; these effects could explain some of the benefit of the medications in patients with arterial disease. Statins do have side effects, including muscle pain and liver dysfunction (see Chapter 28: Atherosclerotic Risk Factors: Hyperlipidemia) If a patient cannot tolerate a statin or if adjunctive medications to treat hyperlipidemia are needed, gemfibrozil, ezetimibe, or niacin may be prescribed.

Diabetes Mellitus

Patients with diabetes mellitus have a high risk for both large-artery atherosclerosis and microvascular disease affecting the brain. Dietary modifications and medications to achieve near-normoglycemic levels for patients with ischemic cerebrovascular disease are advised.[97] Besides treating hyperglycemia, aggressive management of hypertension and hyperlipidemia is also important. In diabetic patients the goal for low-density lipoprotein cholesterol is to achieve a level of 70 mg/dL (1.8 mmol/L). Because angiotensin-converting enzyme inhibitor and angiotensin receptor blocker therapy may be effective in limiting some of the renal complications that may accompany diabetes, these antihypertensive agents are often preferred in patients with diabetes (see Chapter 27: Atherosclerotic Risk Factors: Diabetes).

Smoking

Smoking is an important risk factor for atherosclerotic cerebrovascular disease, particularly in younger persons. Even passive exposure to cigarette smoke is associated with an increased risk for stroke.[106] Smoking cessation rapidly reduces the risk for ischemic events. Within 5 years of smoking cessation, the overall risk for stroke declines to levels seen in persons who have never smoked. Patients should be encouraged to participate in a smoking cessation program. Options include counseling and the use of nicotine replacement products (gum, patch), bupropion, and varenicline (see Chapter 26: Atherosclerotic Risk Factors: Smoking).

Antiplatelet Therapy

Antiplatelet agents are the desired antithrombotic medications for prevention of thromboembolic events in patients with atherosclerotic extracranial or intracranial disease.[107] These medications are effective in preventing ischemic stroke, myocardial infarction, and vascular death in men and women of all age groups. The presence of diabetes mellitus or hypertension does not alter the efficacy of antiplatelet agents. Because of their effectiveness, antiplatelet agents are the standard against which other medications and surgical interventions are compared. The choices of antiplatelet agents are aspirin, aspirin combined with extended-release dipyridamole, clopidogrel, and ticlopidine (see Chapter 34: Antithrombotic Agents).

Aspirin in daily doses of 30 to 1300 mg is effective in preventing ischemic stroke in high-risk patients.[107-110] The combination of aspirin and extended-release dipyridamole has been shown to be more effective than aspirin monotherapy in preventing recurrent ischemia in patients with cerebrovascular disease.[108,111] The combination is not associated with an increased risk for bleeding. The most common side effect of dipyridamole is headache. In general, patients with a past history of migraine do not tolerate this combination.

Ticlopidine was tested in several clinical trials with mixed results. Two trials showed that the medication was superior to aspirin for the prevention of recurrent stroke or vascular death, but a third trial, which enrolled only African Americans, did not demonstrate any difference in outcomes between patients taking aspirin or ticlopidine.[112-114] Because of its side effects, use of ticlopidine has declined. The most frequent complications are abdominal distress, diarrhea, skin eruptions, neutropenia, and thrombotic thrombocytopenic purpura.

Clopidogrel has pharmacologic effects similar to those of ticlopidine. Although rare cases of thrombotic thrombocytopenic purpura and other serious side effects are reported with the use of clopidogrel, in general the agent appears to be much safer than ticlopidine.[115] Clopidogrel has been tested in patients with different types of ischemic vascular disease.[116] Overall, clopidogrel was found to be superior to aspirin, but most of the difference is found in patients with symptomatic lower extremity arterial disease. Even though clopidogrel did lower the risk for ischemic events in patients with symptomatic cerebrovascular disease, its superiority over aspirin was not statistically significant. The combination of aspirin and clopidogrel has been compared with either aspirin or clopidogrel monotherapy. In one trial that enrolled patients with recent TIA or stroke, the combination of aspirin and clopidogrel was not more effective than treatment with clopidogrel alone in the reduction of vascular events (stroke, vascular death, myocardial infarction).[117] However, the combination was associated with an increased bleeding risk. In another trial, the combination of clopidogrel and aspirin was compared with aspirin treatment alone in a broad variety of patients with coronary artery disease, cerebrovascular disease, peripheral vascular disease, or the presence of risk factors for atherosclerosis.[118] Overall, no major differences were noted between the two treatment groups, although there was a trend for fewer ischemic events in patients who received the combination of aspirin and clopidogrel.[119] Another study measured the frequency of microembolic signals detected by transcranial Doppler ultrasonography and found that the combination of clopidogrel and aspirin was superior to aspirin alone.[120] Another pilot study found that the combination of clopidogrel and aspirin might be effective in preventing early recurrent stroke in high-risk patients with recent TIA.[121] This observation needs additional testing.

Although clopidogrel or the combination of aspirin and extended-release dipyridamole has been shown to be more effective than aspirin monotherapy, many physicians often prescribe aspirin first. Clopidogrel and aspirin/extended-release dipyridamole appear to have similar benefits with respect to prevention of stroke.[122] Current guidelines do not recommend one of these medications over the other.[97] Selection of antiplatelet agents continues to be made on a case-by-case basis.

Anticoagulant Therapy

Although oral anticoagulants are effective in preventing stroke in patients with cardiac sources of emboli, including those with atrial fibrillation, there is little evidence of efficacy of these agents for prevention of stroke or recurrent stroke in persons with extracranial or intracranial atherosclerosis.[123-126] Based on these negative studies, oral anticoagulation is not indicated for prevention of stroke caused by carotid artery disease. Oral anticoagulants are of established utility in lowering the risk for stroke in patients with cardiac sources of embolism, including patients with atrial fibrillation.[97] For most indications, the desired level of anticoagulation is an international normalized ratio of 2 to 3. Anticoagulants may also be prescribed to some patients with prothrombotic diseases or as a measure to prevent deep venous thrombosis or pulmonary embolism.

Even though anticoagulants such as unfractionated and low-molecular-weight heparin have been administered for the emergency management of patients with ischemic cerebrovascular disease, including those with recent TIA or an acute stroke, clinical trials have not been able to demonstrate efficacy of this therapy. These medications do not improve neurologic outcomes or lower the risk for early recurrent stroke and are associated with an increased risk for serious intracranial bleeding.[127] Recent guidelines do not recommend the use of anticoagulants as part of the emergency management of patients with acute ischemic stroke.[128] The role of anticoagulation in patients with high-grade carotid stenosis and crescendo TIAs or intraluminal thrombus is discussed earlier under the heading "Crescendo Transient Ischemic Attacks."

Treatment of Acute Stroke

Despite advances in medical and surgical interventions to lower the risk for stroke in high-risk persons, including those with carotid artery disease, many patients continue to have serious, potentially disabling or fatal ischemic strokes. Other patients may have a life-threatening or life-changing stroke as the first manifestation of their cerebrovascular disease. Thus, treatment of patients having a stroke remains crucial. Management of patients with stroke is multifaceted and involves measures to limit the neurologic injury, prevent or control acute or subacute medical or neurologic complications, initiate rehabilitation, maximize recovery, and prevent recurrent stroke. Most of this management, which primarily involves medical interventions, is beyond the scope of this chapter. However, it is important to consider emergency treatment of the acute ischemic stroke itself, which is summarized by the term "brain attack." This term reflects the current treatment of patients with acute ischemic stroke, modeled on the management of patients with acute myocardial ischemia. Just as "time is myocardium," "time is brain."

Stroke and myocardial infarction are the two leading nontraumatic causes of sudden death. Both are accompanied by life-threatening medical and neurologic complications. The key to success is to restore perfusion as quickly as possible. In most instances therapy focuses on thrombolytic agents and endovascular interventions, but surgery may be needed in some cases. The strategy for brain attack involves early recognition, speedy transport to a hospital that has the resources and expertise to treat stroke, urgent evaluation, and rapid treatment with reperfusion therapy. Guidelines for the treatment of patients with acute ischemic stroke are available for clinicians.[128] In an effort to improve the management of patients with acute stroke, primary and comprehensive stroke centers have been designated and certified across the United States.[129,130] An integrated approach that involves emergency medical services, hospital emergency departments, and physicians of several specialties is being advocated.

Emergency evaluation of patients with suspected stroke includes a limited number of tests (Box 94-1).[128] The goals of the initial evaluation are to exclude causes other than ischemic stroke as the source of the patient's symptoms, screen for acute complications of the stroke or severe co-morbid diseases, and determine eligibility for emergency treatment with reperfusion therapy. The panel of tests is readily available on an emergency basis in most community hospitals. The goal is to complete evaluation within 1 hour of the patient's arrival in the emergency department. Computed tomography (CT) is the most important diagnostic study because it helps exclude the most important alternative diagnosis—intracranial hemorrhage. In addition, it provides information about the presence of ischemic stroke or other brain diseases. Magnetic resonance imaging is an alternative to CT but is less readily available. However, it may detect the first changes of stroke within minutes of the onset of the ischemia. It is also superior

---

Box 94-1 Emergency Evaluation of Patients with Suspected Acute Ischemic Stroke

- Non–contrast-enhanced computed tomography or magnetic resonance imaging of the brain
- Blood glucose, serum electrolytes, and renal function tests
- Markers of acute cardiac ischemia
- Complete blood count and platelet count
- Activated partial thromboplastin time
- Prothrombin time (international normalized ratio)
- Oxygen saturation
- Electrocardiogram

to CT for detection of smaller ischemic lesions, particularly in the brainstem and cerebellum. Other studies, including vascular imaging, are not required for general emergency treatment of ischemic stroke, but they are important if intra-arterial administration of thrombolytic agents or endovascular treatment is planned. A number of recommendations for general emergency treatment of patients with recent stroke, including administration of antihypertensive medications, are included in the guidelines.[128]

Thrombolytic Therapy for Acute Stroke

Intravenous thrombolysis is an important recent advance in emergency stroke care.[131] Based on the results of a pivotal study, the U.S. Food and Drug Administration approved the use of intravenous alteplase (recombinant tissue plasminogen activator [rt-PA]) for the treatment of carefully selected patients. The approved dose of rt-PA is 0.9 mg/kg (maximum dose, 90 mg); 10% of the dose is given as a bolus and the remainder is infused over a 1-hour period. The medication must be started within 3 hours of the onset of acute ischemic stroke. The success of emergency treatment with rt-PA has been reproduced by clinical experience.[132] At present, intravenous rt-PA is the desired intervention in patients with acute ischemic stroke. Other thrombolytic agents have been tested, but to date, none have been established as safe and effective. Criteria for screening a patient for possible treatment with rt-PA are presented in Box 94-2. Ancillary care includes close follow-up and observation with frequent assessment of blood pressure and neurologic status, aggressive management of hypertension, and delay in the placement of catheters or other devices that may cause bleeding. Neither antiplatelet agents nor anticoagulants are started within 24 hours of treatment with rt-PA. The most important complication of intravenous thrombolysis is symptomatic hemorrhagic transformation of the infarction. The risk is increased by a factor of approximately 10, and hemorrhagic transformation is most likely in patients with large multilobar infarctions.[131,133] Emergency thrombolysis does not increase the risk for death in seriously ill patients, even if hemorrhage does occur, because the chance of dying from a malignant brain infarction is high in those not treated with thrombolysis.

Intra-arterial administration of thrombolytic agents is an alternative to intravenous therapy. Although evidence supporting the use of intra-arterial therapy is not as strong as for intravenous rt-PA, it is an option for the treatment of selected patients with major stroke of less than 6 hours' duration in whom major intracranial arteries are occluded.[128,134] This intervention is less readily available than intravenous therapy. In general, patients need to be transferred to a comprehensive stroke center that has immediate access to cerebral arteriography and physicians who have expertise. Intra-arterial thrombolysis may also be an alternative treatment of patients with acute ischemic stroke who cannot be treated with intravenous rt-PA; for example, a patient who has recently undergone surgery might be treated. Endovascular interventions are also used to treat patients with acute ischemic stroke. Choices

---

Box 94-2 Screening Criteria for the Emergency Administration of Recombinant Tissue Plasminogen Activator for the Treatment of Acute Ischemic Stroke

Onset of symptoms
- Treatment started within 3 hours of the onset of symptoms
- If previous transient ischemic attack, the patient may be treated
- If symptoms longer than 3 hours but recent worsening, the patient is not treated
- If symptoms present on awakening and the time of onset is not known, the patient is not treated

Presence of a co-morbid disease that increases bleeding risk and precludes treatment
- Head injury or stroke in the last 3 months
- Myocardial infarction in the last 3 months
- Gastrointestinal or genitourinary hemorrhage in the last 3 weeks
- Major surgery in the last 2 weeks
- Arterial puncture at a noncompressible site in the last week
- History of previous intracranial hemorrhage

Findings on examination that affect bleeding risk
- Active bleeding or acute trauma on examination
- Elevated blood pressure (>185 mm Hg systolic or >110 mm Hg diastolic)—blood pressure can be lowered so that the patient can be treated

Findings on evaluation that may preclude treatment
- International normalized ratio >1.7
- Prolonged activated partial thromboplastin time
- Platelet count <100,000
- Blood glucose concentration <50 mg/dL (2.8 mmol/L)
- Imaging demonstrating hemorrhage
- Imaging demonstrating other neurologic cause of the symptoms

Patient and/or family understands the risks associated with treatment

---

include angioplasty and stenting, devices to mechanically disrupt the clot, and devices to extract the thrombus. Such interventions are often given in conjunction with intra-arterial administration of thrombolytic agents. Two clot extraction devices have been approved by the Food and Drug Administration for use in restoring blood flow in occluded intracranial arteries, and additional devices will probably be approved in the future.[135,136] The issues related to intra-arterial pharmacologic thrombolysis are the same as those for the implementation of strategies to use mechanical interventions.

SELECTED KEY REFERENCES

Adams HP Jr, del Zoppo G, Alberts MJ, Bhatt DL, Brass L, Furlan A, Grubb RL, Higashida RT, Jauch EC, Kidwell C, Lyden PD, Morgenstern LB, Qureshi AI, Rosenwasser RH, Scott PA, Wijdicks EF. Guidelines for the early management of adults with ischemic stroke: a guideline from the American Heart Association/American Stroke Association Stroke Council, Clinical Cardiology Council, Cardiovascular Radiology and Intervention Council, and the Atherosclerotic Peripheral Vascular Disease and Quality of Care Outcomes in

Research Interdisciplinary Working Groups: The American Academy of Neurology affirms the value of this guideline as an educational tool for neurologists. *Stroke*. 2007;38:1655-1711.
Multidisciplinary guideline for the early management of ischemic stroke.

Barnett HJ, Taylor DW, Eliasziw M, Fox AJ, Ferguson GG, Haynes RB, Rankin RN, Clagett GP, Hachinski VC, Sackett DL, Thorpe KE, Meldrum HE, Spence JD. Benefit of carotid endarterectomy in patients with symptomatic moderate or severe stenosis. North American Symptomatic Carotid Endarterectomy Trial Collaborators. *N Engl J Med*. 1998;339:1415-1425.
The final report from NASCET, which established the benefit of CEA plus medical therapy over medical therapy alone in symptomatic patients with at least 50% carotid stenosis.

Beneficial effect of carotid endarterectomy in symptomatic patients with high-grade carotid stenosis. North American Symptomatic Carotid Endarterectomy Trial Collaborators. *N Engl J Med*. 1991; 325:445-453.
The initial report of NASCET, which demonstrated the benefit of CEA plus medical therapy over medical therapy alone in symptomatic patients with 70% to 99% stenosis.

Brahmanandam S, Ding EL, Conte MS, Belkin M, Nguyen LL. Clinical results of carotid artery stenting compared with carotid endarterectomy. *J Vasc Surg*. 2008;47:343-349.
Recent meta-analysis of trials comparing CAS with CEA.

Endarterectomy for asymptomatic carotid artery stenosis. Executive Committee for the Asymptomatic Carotid Atherosclerosis Study. *JAMA*. 1995;273:1421-1428.
The North American randomized trial of asymptomatic patients that established the benefit of CEA plus medical therapy over medical therapy alone in patients with at least 60% carotid stenosis.

Kresowik TF, Bratzler DW, Kresowik RA, Hendel ME, Grund SL, Brown KR, Nilasena DS. Multistate improvement in process and outcomes of carotid endarterectomy. *J Vasc Surg*. 2004;39: 372-380.
The largest community-wide (more than 20,000 procedures from 10 states) report of 30-day outcomes of CEA with stratification by procedural indication. The report is derived from complete hospital medical record review rather than query of an administrative/claims database.

Prevention of disabling and fatal strokes by successful carotid endarterectomy in patients without recent neurological symptoms: randomized controlled trial. *Lancet*. 2004;363:1491-1502.
The final results of the European trial in asymptomatic patients demonstrating the benefit of CEA.

Randomised trial of endarterectomy for recently symptomatic carotid stenosis: final results of the MRC European Carotid Surgery Trial (ECST). *Lancet*. 1998;351:1379-1387.
The European trial establishing the benefit of CEA in symptomatic patients.

Rothwell PM, Eliasziw M, Gutnikov SA, Warlow CP, Barnett HJ. Endarterectomy for symptomatic carotid stenosis in relation to clinical subgroups and timing of surgery. *Lancet*. 2004;363:915-924.
Report of pooled results from NASCET and ECST (5893 patients with 33,000 patient-years of follow-up). This report provides the best available data on subgroups of symptomatic patients.

Sacco RL, Adams R, Albers G, Alberts MJ, Benavente O, Furie K, Goldstein LB, Gorelick P, Halperin J, Harbaugh R, Johnston SC, Katzan I, Kelly-Hayes M, Kenton EJ, Marks M, Schwamm LH, Tomsick T. Guidelines for Prevention of Stroke in Patients with Ischemic Stroke or Transient Ischemic Attack: A Statement for Healthcare Professionals From the American Heart Association/American Stroke Association Council on Stroke: Co-Sponsored by the Council on Cardiovascular Radiology and Intervention: The American Academy of Neurology affirms the value of this guideline. *Stroke*. 2006;37:577-617.
Multidisciplinary guideline for the secondary prevention of stroke after TIA or stroke.

REFERENCES

The reference list can be found on the companion Expert Consult Web site at *www.expertconsult.com*.

CHAPTER 95

Carotid Artery Disease: Endarterectomy

Glen S. Roseborough and Bruce A. Perler

The era of carotid surgery began in 1954 when Eastcott, Pickering, and Rob published a case report documenting the first successful reconstruction of the carotid artery to treat symptomatic carotid occlusive disease in a woman with recurrent transient ischemic attacks (TIAs).[1] Her treatment included excision of the carotid bifurcation, ligation of the external carotid artery (ECA), and reconstruction with direct anastomosis of the common carotid artery (CCA) to the internal carotid artery (ICA). Michael DeBakey had performed a successful carotid endarterectomy (CEA) the year before but did not publish his experience until 1959 in a paper that encompassed surgical management of occlusive disease of the carotid, vertebral, and aortic arch vessels.[2] In this remarkably prescient paper he documented numerous approaches to managing carotid occlusive disease, including eversion endarterectomy, patch angioplasty, and even shunting.

Performance of CEA experienced remarkable growth in the 1970s and 1980s after several natural history studies demonstrated that carotid stenosis was an ominous risk factor for disabling stroke and death[3-6] and after a randomized multicenter trial published in 1969 showed that carotid surgery reduced the incidence of stroke from symptomatic carotid lesions.[7] However, other studies showed that complication rates were often high, thus compromising the potential benefit of CEA.[8] Randomized controlled studies performed in the 1990s established the safety and efficacy of CEA and its superiority over the best medical management of patients with symptomatic and asymptomatic carotid disease.[9-12]

◼ EPIDEMIOLOGY

Incidence

Cerebrovascular disease is the second leading cause of death worldwide and is responsible for approximately 9.5% of all deaths.[13,14] At least 750,000 stokes occur annually in the United States. Approximately 15% of strokes are fatal, 15% to 20% are severely disabling, and another 15% to 20% of stroke patients who recover will have a subsequent disabling stroke in the future (see Chapter 92: Cerebrovascular Disease: General Considerations).

Etiology

Approximately 80% of strokes are ischemic, and carotid disease accounts for about two thirds of these strokes as a consequence of embolization of carotid artery bifurcation plaque to the intracranial vessels, usually to the middle cerebral artery (MCA) in the anterior circulation, or as a consequence of low flow. These strokes can also result from lesions in the CCA or in the distal or intracranial portion of the ICA (see Chapter 92: Cerebrovascular Disease: General Considerations).

◼ INDICATIONS FOR CAROTID ENDARTERECTOMY

Indications for CEA are covered in detail in Chapter 94 (Cerebrovascular Disease: Decision Making and Medical Treatment). Appropriate indications for intervention have been solidified by level I evidence derived from several randomized prospective clinical trials (Table 95-1).

Symptomatic Disease

The main risk factors for stroke secondary to carotid atherosclerotic disease are the presence of symptoms and the degree of carotid stenosis. In 1991, the North American Symptomatic Carotid Endarterectomy Trial (NASCET) demonstrated a clear benefit of CEA and best medical management over best medical management alone for symptomatic patients with high-grade (70% to 99%) carotid stenosis. The benefit of CEA was so significant that the trial was stopped prematurely.[9,17] The same year, the European Carotid Surgery Trial (ECST) demonstrated a similar but smaller benefit in symptomatic patients with 70% to 99% stenosis.[10] Analysis of a

Table 95-1 Benefit of Carotid Endarterectomy: Randomized Trials

Trial	Indication	Perioperative CVA/Death	Risk Reduction	P Value
NASCET	Sx: ≥70%	5.8%	16.5%/2 yr	<.001
	Sx: 50%-69%	6.7%	10.1%/5 yr	<.05
ECST	Sx: 70%-99%	7.5%	9.6%/3 yr	<.01
ACAS	Asx: ≥60%	2.3%	5.9%/5 yr	.004
ACST	Asx: >60%	3.1%	5.4%/5 yr	<.0001

ACAS, Asymptomatic Carotid Atherosclerosis Study; ACST, Asymptomatic Carotid Surgery Trial; Asx, asymptomatic; CVA, cardiovascular accident; ECST, European Carotid Surgery Trialists; NASCET, North American Symptomatic Carotid Endarterectomy Trial; Sx, symptomatic.
Data from references 9-12, 15, 16.

second cohort of symptomatic patients with moderate (50% to 69%) stenosis in NASCET demonstrated a smaller but statistically significant benefit as well.[18] Interim and late analysis of patients in ECST did not show a benefit of treating patients with moderate stenosis because of higher perioperative morbidity and mortality rates.[12,15] In addition, their methodology for measuring the degree of stenosis was different such that ECST overestimated the degree of stenosis in comparison to NASCET.

Asymptomatic Disease

The Asymptomatic Carotid Atherosclerosis Study (ACAS) demonstrated a significant benefit of CEA and best medical management over best medical management alone for patients with asymptomatic stenosis of 60% to 99%.[11] These findings have been confirmed in the Asymptomatic Carotid Surgery Trial (ACST) in Europe.[16]

◼ PREOPERATIVE IMAGING

Documentation of carotid disease with appropriate imaging is critical before performing CEA. Standard options for imaging the carotid artery include duplex ultrasound and digital subtraction angiography (DSA), whereas more recently, computed tomographic angiography (CTA) and magnetic resonance angiography (MRA) have been used successfully for this purpose. The literature concerning these imaging modalities is thoroughly reviewed in Chapter 94 (Cerebrovascular Disease: Decision Making and Medical Treatment). There is no consensus on the most accurate noninvasive imaging modality for evaluation of carotid artery disease, with some series suggesting that duplex ultrasound and others indicating that either MRA or CTA is the most accurate.[19-25] There is some evidence that CTA underestimates and MRA overestimates the degree of stenosis.[23] Each practitioner should assess the relative accuracy of these imaging modalities in his or her own institution. Clearly, if the patient is found to have an intermediate stenosis and is asymptomatic, one should perform at least another noninvasive test to confirm this finding before recommending CEA. If there is discordance between these studies, one should either obtain a third noninvasive test or resort to angiography, which in today's practice is safe.

◼ PERIOPERATIVE MEDICAL MANAGEMENT

Antiplatelet Therapy

The medical management of carotid disease has evolved and improved significantly over the last decade, and this topic is covered in Chapter 94 (Cerebrovascular Disease: Decision Making and Medical Treatment). Similarly, perioperative medical management of patients undergoing CEA has also improved. Foremost among these improvements is the aggressive perioperative use of antiplatelet therapy. Meta-analyses of antiplatelet therapy trials published by the U.K. Antithrombotic Trialist Group in 1994 and 2002 concluded that antiplatelet therapy significantly reduces the incidence of stroke in high-risk patients, with a resultant 25% reduction in strokes overall.[26,27] The majority of these studies included aspirin or aspirin plus another antiplatelet agent. The benefit of acetylsalicylic acid (ASA) in reducing postoperative stroke and death after CEA was first shown in a secondary analysis from NASCET in 1991. NASCET was a randomized controlled trial (RCT) that demonstrated the benefit of CEA in symptomatic patients with at least 50% ICA stenosis.[9] In that trial, patients were prescribed up to 1300 mg ASA daily if tolerated. A subsequent association was found between perioperative stroke and death and the amount of ASA taken before surgery. The risk for perioperative stroke and death was 1.8% in patients taking 650 to 1300 mg ASA daily versus 6.9% in patients taking 0 to 325 mg daily. An RCT was subsequently conducted in which 232 patients undergoing CEA were randomized to receive either ASA 75 mg or placebo preoperatively and for 6 months postoperatively.[28] Stroke at 30 days and at 6 months occurred in 0 and 2 ASA-treated patients, respectively, versus 7 and 11 placebo patients, respectively ($P < .01$), with no difference in bleeding complications.

To determine the optimal daily dose of preoperative ASA in reducing stroke and death associated with CEA, the ASA and Carotid Endarterectomy (ACE) trial randomized 2849 patients to ASA doses of 81, 325, 650, or 1300 mg started preoperatively and continued for 3 months.[29] The combined endpoint of 30-day stroke, death, or myocardial infarction after CEA occurred in 5.4% in the low-dose groups (81 and 325 mg) versus 7.0% in the high-dose groups ($P = .03$). In an efficacy analysis focusing on patients not previously taking high-dose ASA, the combined endpoint was seen in only 3.7% of the low-dose groups versus 8.2% of the high-dose group at 30 days ($P = .002$). Fewer hemorrhagic complications were also seen in the low-dose ASA groups, but this difference was not significant. Note that a placebo group was not deemed appropriate for this study because of the widely accepted benefit of ASA in preventing stroke.

Other antiplatelet agents have not been as extensively studied in terms of their benefit in stroke reduction after CEA, but recent studies of clopidogrel provide evidence that perioperative embolization is decreased. In a recent trial, 100 patients undergoing CEA who were taking 150 mg ASA daily were randomized to receive in addition either clopidogrel 75 mg or placebo the night before surgery.[30] The number of emboli detected by transcranial Doppler (TCD) within 3 hours of CEA was the main outcome measure. There was a 10-fold reduction in the number of patients who experienced more than 20 microemboli in that period (odds ratio, 10.2; 95% confidence interval, 1.3 to 83.3; $P < .01$) in the group taking clopidogrel combined with ASA. No increase in bleeding complications or transfusion requirements was noted. The embolization rate was used as a surrogate for stroke because stroke occurs infrequently, and the embolization rate has been well correlated with stroke risk during CEA. Other antiplatelet agents such as ticlopidine and glycoprotein IIb/IIIa antagonists, though demonstrated to reduce stroke risk in nonsurgical patients, have not been specifically studied during CEA and generally have a higher risk profile than ASA or clopidogrel. Based on this level I evidence, it is possible to recommend either ASA or clopidogrel, or both, for use before and after CEA.

Surprisingly, a recent meta-analysis found that antiplatelet therapy was not effective in preventing stroke and other vascular events *after* CEA.[31] It is difficult to reconcile these seemingly conflicting results. Nevertheless, based on the weight of evidence supporting the efficacy of aspirin in primary and secondary stroke prevention and its overall cardiovascular benefits, we believe that all patients should receive antiplatelet therapy at the time of and after CEA.

Heparin

Heparin has been administered as therapy for acute stroke or crescendo TIAs to patients before undergoing CEA. The International Stroke Trial did not find any benefit of routine heparin administration for acute stroke because of increased numbers of hemorrhagic stroke and fatal extracranial bleeding.[32] However, a report from the Oregon Health Sciences University found that urgent crescendo TIAs could be controlled with intravenous heparin, thereby allowing urgent CEA to be delayed in these patients.[33]

Unfractionated heparin is routinely used intraoperatively to prevent carotid thrombosis despite a lack of level I evidence to support this practice. The combination of aspirin and intraoperative heparin administration appears to be especially effective in preventing thrombosis.[34] The University of Rochester group found that low-dose intraoperative heparin is safe and can obviate the need for protamine to reverse heparin intraoperatively.[35]

Protamine Administration

Numerous publications have examined whether reversing heparin with protamine during CEA is safe. The only randomized trial that looked at this question was a small study consisting of just 64 patients. This trial demonstrated significantly reduced wound drainage with protamine but a trend toward an increased rate of stroke and death from carotid thrombosis.[36] Treiman and colleagues retrospectively compared their experience with 328 patients who received protamine versus 369 who did not over a 5-year period and found no difference in stroke rates but a significantly higher incidence of wound hematomas in those who did not receive protamine.[37] Similar results were reported in a retrospective study of 407 CEAs by Levison and coauthors.[38] However, in another retrospective study of 348 patients, Mauney and associates found a significantly higher stroke rate with protamine (2.6% versus 0%, $P < .045$) and no significant increase in bleeding rate in patients who did not receive protamine.[39] In a recent publication of observations of protamine use during

the GALA trial (General Anesthesia versus Local Anesthesia for carotid surgery), protamine was not found to be associated with stroke.[40]

Dextran

Dextran is a polysaccharide that inhibits platelet aggregation.[41] It has been used to control embolic episodes both preoperatively and postoperatively. British investigators in 1997 showed that a 6-hour dextran infusion effectively controlled postoperative embolic events as measured by TCD, with a 0% stroke and mortality rate in a series of 100 patients.[42] In a follow-up study they found that a 3-hour infusion was just as effective as a 6-hour infusion.[43] In a study of 19 patients with recurrent or crescendo TIAs and high-grade carotid stenosis, dextran was used effectively preoperatively to control both clinical symptoms and embolic events, as measured by TCD, before undergoing CEA.[44] The same investigators showed dextran infusion and TCD to be cost-effective in preventing stroke.[45] We favor dextran infusion after CEA to control platelet aggregation on the endarterectomy site and potential microembolization.

Statins

The potential benefits of statins in patients with carotid artery disease are severalfold. A reduction in cholesterol levels with statins may be associated with plaque regression (see Chapter 28: Atherosclerotic Risk Factors: Hyperlipidemia).[46-54] For example, the Asymptomatic Carotid Artery Progression Study (ASAPS) demonstrated that lovastatin was associated with reduced carotid artery intima-media thickness and also a lower rate of combined cardiovascular events, although not the stroke rate.[55,56]

However, numerous trials conducted over the past decade have demonstrated statin medications to be highly effective in primary and secondary stroke prevention.[57-61] Furthermore, it appears that the stroke prevention benefits of statins are related to the pleiotropic effects of statin medications rather than their cholesterol-lowering effects. In addition, several studies have demonstrated that statins are associated with a reduced rate of perioperative cardiac morbidity and overall mortality in patients undergoing major vascular surgical procedures.[62-65]

The demonstrated benefit of statins in primary and secondary stoke prevention and its positive impact on the incidence of perioperative cardiac complications and mortality in patients undergoing major vascular surgery stimulated our group to investigate the potential influence of statin medications specifically on the outcome of CEA. In a series of nearly 1600 patients undergoing CEA, we found that statins were associated with a reduced 30-day incidence of stroke (1.2% versus 4.5%, $P < .01$), TIA (1.5% versus 3.6%, $P < .01$), and mortality (0.3% versus 2.1%, $P < .01$).[66] In another report, Kennedy and coauthors, in a population-based analysis from Canada, reported a significantly lower rate of perioperative stroke and death in symptomatic patients who were taking statin medications at the time of CEA.[67] Furthermore, Lamuraglia and coworkers reported that lipid-lowering agents were associated with significant protection against recurrent carotid stenosis or late anatomic failure after CEA.[68]

OPERATIVE TECHNIQUE

Anesthesia

A fundamental consideration in the conduct of CEA is selection of the anesthetic method. CEA may be performed under general anesthesia (GA), under regional anesthesia (RA) with deep or superficial cervical block, and even under pure local anesthesia (LA). Although early reports suggested a reduced length of hospital stay associated with CEA performed under RA, comparable lengths of stay are routinely documented today in patients who undergo surgery under GA. The majority of studies comparing the two techniques have reported improved perioperative cardiac stability with RA, but this does not necessarily result in a reduced incidence of myocardial infarction.[69,70]

Disadvantages of RA include patient discomfort or anxiety, risk of seizure or allergic reaction, anxiety for the operating surgeon, and compromise of technique in a teaching setting. A meta-analysis by Tangkanakul and associates,[71] as well as one by Rerkasem and colleagues,[70] showed no clear benefit for CEA performed under LA. The GALA trial, a large prospective European multicenter study of more than 3500 patients, was designed to definitively determine whether one technique is superior to the other. It demonstrated no difference in outcomes between GA and LA.[72] The main benefit of LA is that it facilitates efficient selective shunting if that is the surgeon's preference. However, the benefit of selective shunting is unclear (see under "Shunting").

Patient Positioning

Careful positioning of the patient is important to ensure patient comfort and adequate operative exposure (Fig. 95-1). Positioning begins with placing a roll behind the scapulae to achieve some hyperextension of the neck. A padded ring is placed under the head to prevent neck injury from extreme hyperextension. If GA is used, the endotracheal tube should be taped to the corner of the mouth opposite the surgical field. If LA or RA is used, a Mayo stand is placed over the patient's head to suspend the surgical drapes away from the patient's face to prevent sensations of claustrophobia. It is our practice to tape the fan for a "Bare Hugger" warmer on the underside of the Mayo stand because blowing air on the patient's face relieves discomfort. If GA is used, it is induced before placement of additional lines. A radial artery catheter is inserted for continuous blood pressure monitoring, and a Foley catheter is placed. The patient is placed in the flexed position with the table rotated to expose the side of the neck to be operated on.

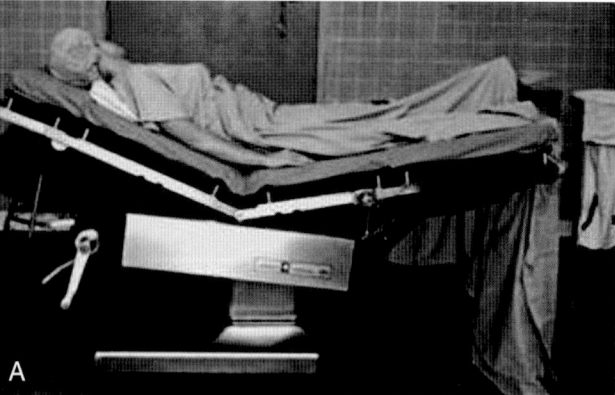
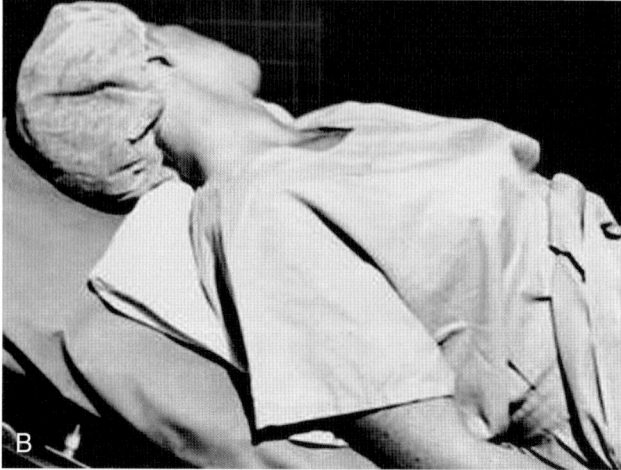

Figure 95-1 Patient positioning for carotid endarterectomy. **A,** The table is placed in the reversed Trendelenburg position with the patient's legs elevated. **B,** The patient's head is turned to the contralateral side with a roll placed under the shoulders to extend the neck.

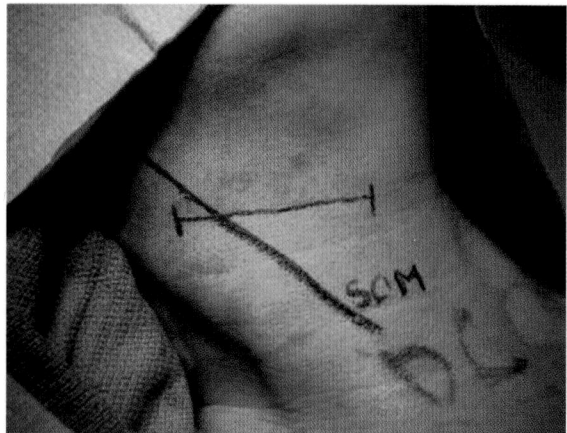

Figure 95-2 Longitudinal and transverse skin incisions for carotid endarterectomy.

Skin Incision

One of two skin incisions may be used (Fig. 95-2). The standard incision is a longitudinal incision parallel to the medial border of the sternocleidomastoid muscle. The upper portion of the incision is angled posterior to the earlobe if cephalic exposure above the angle of the jaw is required. An alternative method is to place the incision in an appropriately located skin crease, usually 1 to 2 cm inferior to the angle of the jaw. This incision provides excellent cosmesis postoperatively; frequently, the resulting scar is all but invisible. However, if the incision is made in a suboptimal location, it is difficult to obtain more cephalic and caudal exposure in the wound. Therefore, if the surgeon is not experienced with a skin crease incision, it is best to make a skin crease incision based on the location of the carotid bifurcation, known either from preoperative DSA, CTA, or MRA or from intraoperative Duplex examination, or to use a longitudinal incision. With experience the surgeon will become more comfortable making the incision based on the location of the carotid pulse, although this can be misleading at times. If the incision is made too low, more cephalic exposure can be obtained by extending the skin crease incision posteriorly. If the incision is made too high, more caudal exposure can be obtained by extending the incision more anteriorly.

Conventional versus Eversion Endarterectomy

There are two basic surgical techniques for CEA: conventional and eversion. Regardless of which method is used, meticulous surgical technique is paramount for a successful operation. Manipulation of the carotid artery should be minimized because intraoperative embolization can result from careless handling. Any blood in the field should be carefully aspirated.

The dissection is begun by dividing the platysma and mobilizing the medial border of the sternocleidomastoid muscle. The external jugular vein lies deep to the platysma and should be sought in this plane to avoid injury or to retrieve it if it is needed for patching. It is more commonly encountered with an oblique skin crease incision than with a longitudinal incision. The other structure located at this level is the greater auricular nerve; injury to this nerve leads to numbness of the earlobe, which is bothersome to patients, especially those who wear earrings (see later under "Cutaneous Sensory Nerves"). The medial border of the platysma is mobilized and retracted laterally with self-retaining retractors. The carotid sheath is entered and the medial border of the jugular vein dissected. The facial vein is identified crossing medially in the base of the wound and divided; sometimes it has an early bifurcation or trifurcation, and multiple branches need to be ligated. The jugular vein is then retracted laterally. The vagus nerve is identified at this point in the carotid sheath, usually located posteriorly between the jugular vein and carotid artery, although in a minority of patients it may lie anteriorly. Dissection is continued down onto the distal CCA and is controlled circumferentially with an umbilical tape and a Rumel tourniquet. At this point the ansa cervicalis nerve should be identified; it usually lies medial to the distal CCA. Identifying this nerve facilitates safe dissection of the carotid bifurcation and avoids injury to the hypoglossal nerve, which crosses medially from a superior to an inferior location.

As the surgeon dissects superiorly along the ansa cervicalis, the dissection should be continued along the posterior edge of this nerve. As one follows the nerve cephalad and encounters its junction with the hypoglossal nerve, the surgeon will continue the dissection safely along the posterior border of the hypoglossal nerve with minimal risk of injury; if one dissects along the anterior border of the ansa, it is possible to inadvertently transect the hypoglossal nerve in the crotch of the junction of these two nerves before the hypoglossal nerve is identified (Fig. 95-3).

At this point the carotid bifurcation is carefully exposed. The superior thyroid artery is identified coming off the medial border of the carotid bifurcation or proximal ECA and controlled with a tie or plastic vessel loop. Dissection continues cephalad on the medial edge of the bifurcation until the origin of the ECA is identified. It is exposed and controlled circumferentially with a vessel loop. Finally, the ICA is exposed coming off the lateral side of the bifurcation. Extreme care must be taken during this part of the dissection. The artery should be controlled in a location that is above the plaque and completely free of disease; in this location the artery has a typical bluish appearance because of translucency of the vessel. During dissection of the carotid bifurcation and its branches, one should avoid dissecting in the crotch of the carotid bifurcation to avoid injuring the carotid body because such dissection can result in hemodynamic instability and troublesome bleeding. If hemodynamic instability results, the carotid body can be gently injected with 1% lidocaine.

Before clamping, the patient is administered 70 to 100 U/kg of heparin, which is allowed to circulate for 3 minutes. The ICA is clamped first to prevent the embolization that can result when the CCA or ECA is clamped. Care should be taken to make sure that the ICA is clamped on a

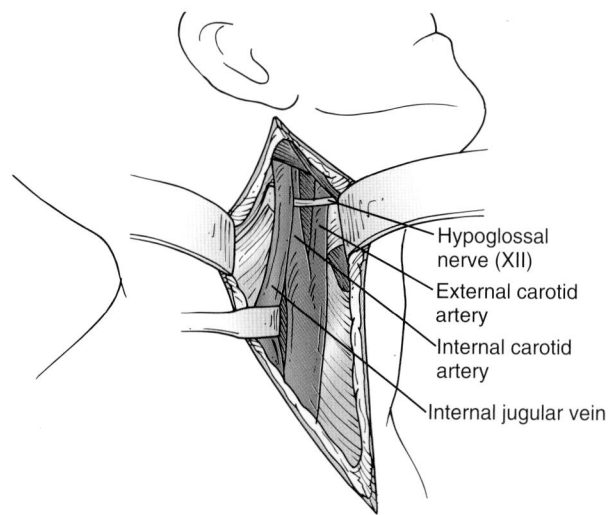

Figure 95-3 Operative field. Note the internal jugular vein mobilized posteriorly after ligation of the anterior facial branch and the hypoglossal nerve crossing the vessels superior to the bifurcation.

Hypoglossal nerve (XII)
External carotid artery
Internal carotid artery
Internal jugular vein

normal portion of the artery distal to the plaque. There is typically a bluish discoloration of the artery in this location.

If LA or intraoperative electroencephalography is used for selective shunting, a test clamp on the distal ICA should be applied for at least 3 minutes to check for changes in the neurologic examination or electroencephalographic (EEG) pattern. If such changes occur, the artery should be unclamped to allow reperfusion before reclamping and opening the carotid bifurcation; opening the bifurcation and placing a shunt may take 2 to 3 minutes and should not be performed while the brain is already ischemic. However, unclamping the ICA introduces the potential for embolization from disrupted plaque.

If carotid stump pressure is to be measured, clamps are placed on the CCA and ECA, and a needle connected to a pressure line is placed into the distal CCA below the carotid bifurcation. Both clamping the CCA and placing the needle into the artery introduce the potential for embolization.

Conventional Endarterectomy

The conventional technique for CEA consists of a vertical arteriotomy and closure by patch angioplasty. In this case a vertical arteriotomy is begun on the CCA and continued through the carotid bifurcation into the ICA. One should avoid making the incision too close to the flow divider at the ECA origin because this can distort the anatomy and make the closure more difficult. If a shunt is used, it is placed in the distal ICA and backbled before the proximal end is placed into the CCA. Two commonly used shunts are the Pruitt-Inahara and Javid shunts. A third shunt that we prefer is a simple vinyl tube, originally described by Collins and associates (Fig. 95-4).[73] Because this shunt lies entirely within the artery, it allows the surgeon to almost completely finish closing the arteriotomy before the shunt is removed. Its small diameter permits atraumatic placement in even small ICAs, whereas its short length offers less resistance to blood flow such that physiologic flow in the ICA is maintained. Wilkinson and colleagues compared the Pruitt-Inahara and Javid clamps in a randomized trial.[74] Using TCD, they found that the Pruitt shunt was less likely to maintain physiologic flow in the MCA, whereas the Javid shunt was associated with a higher incidence of cerebral embolism at declamping.

The endarterectomy is begun in the CCA in the plane between the media and the adventitia. The proximal endpoint in the distal CCA is established and the plaque is trimmed in that location in a beveled manner. The endarterectomy is continued into the orifice of the ECA, first with a Freer elevator and then with a fine clamp that is passed up into the ECA in the plane of the endarterectomy. The clamp is spread apart to further mobilize the plaque away from the adventitia in the 6-, 9-, and 12-o'clock positions; it is usually hard to pass the clamp in this plane at the 3-o'clock position next to the flow divider. The vessel loop on the ECA is released transiently while the plaque is everted from within the ECA. The endpoint of the plaque is inspected; an ideal endpoint is gradually tapering and feathered (Fig. 95-5). In our practice, all loose

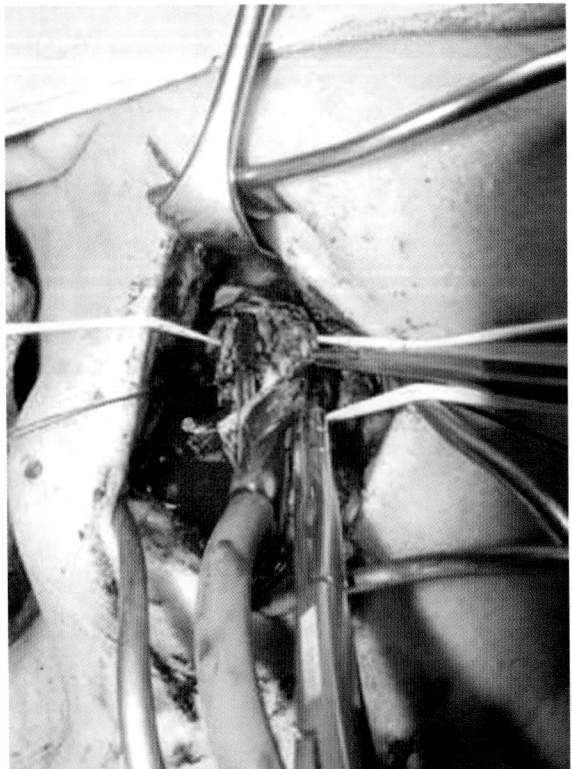

Figure 95-4 Operative field after the arteriotomy has been made and the shunt placed (*arrow*). Note how the shunt lies within the vessel.

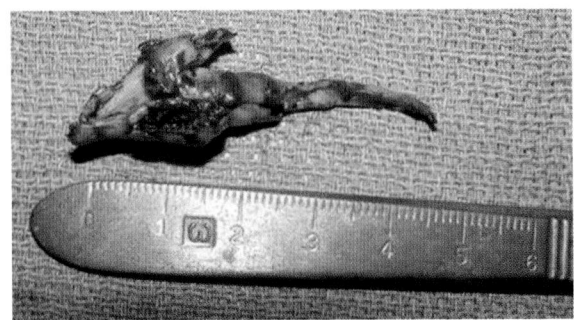

Figure 95-5 Carotid endarterectomy specimen. Note the smooth endpoints of the distal plaque from the internal and external carotid arteries (shorter extent of plaque).

bits of intima and media in the orifice of the ECA are removed to perform complete endarterectomy of the ECA. However, Ascher and coworkers have found in a large series that endarterectomy of the ECA may be neglected without compromising results.[75]

The endarterectomy is continued up into the ICA. A technically perfect endpoint in the ICA is critical to avoid perioperative stroke and recurrent stenosis. In our experience, it is virtually always possible to achieve a satisfactory endpoint in the ICA, although special maneuvers may be required to expose the distal ICA and make an extended arteriotomy in this vessel to facilitate extraction of a long endarterectomy specimen, as seen in Figure 95-5. Tacking sutures at the distal endpoint should be avoided unless absolutely necessary; such suturing is problematic and associated with an increased perioperative stroke rate.[76] The endarterectomy should be terminated in normal ICA with a gradual, tapered transition to normal intima; this is best accomplished by pulling the plaque transversely away from the artery with lateral traction. One should avoid pulling out or down on the plaque, which is more likely to result in a stepoff that can be difficult to correct without traumatizing the artery.

We believe that repairing the arteriotomy with a patch angioplasty represents the standard of care in contemporary practice (Fig. 95-6). The patch is sewn in with running non-absorbable suture. A variety of patch materials are available for use, including autologous vein, polytetrafluoroethylene (PTFE), woven polyester (Dacron), and bovine pericardium. Some studies have suggested that autologous vein may be superior to synthetic patches, but of the prosthetic patches, no material appears to be clearly superior to another (see under "Patch Closure").

Options for autologous vein include the external jugular and saphenous veins. The external jugular vein can be harvested through the same surgical incision and is generally used as a double-layer patch after inverting an intact tubular segment of vein without filleting open the vein. Care must be taken to keep the inverted tube flattened out as a rectangular patch while it is being sewn onto the artery. If this is not done, the edges can sometimes roll over or under and lead to a tapered, asymmetric, or severely deformed patch. It is our practice to always start the suture line at the superior end of the arteriotomy in the ICA, which is typically the most difficult—and critical—part of an anastomosis. As the patch material is sewn to one side of the artery, the artery must be stretched out with gentle tension so that an appropriate length of patch is used before it is trimmed; otherwise, there may not be enough patch material available to sew to the other side of the artery in the arteriotomy.

When the suture line is nearly completed, the CCA and ICA are reclamped and the shunt is removed. Both clamps are briefly released to flush air or debris (or both) out of the arteries. The clamps should be placed proximal and distal to the patch or endarterectomized surface of the artery because these surfaces can be thrombogenic. The carotid bifurcation is flushed vigorously with heparinized saline and inspected again for debris or intimal flaps before the arteriotomy is finally closed. Once again the clamp on the ICA is briefly released to fill the bifurcation with blood. It is then replaced while the clamps on the CCA and ECA are released so that any remaining air or debris will be flushed up the territory of the ECA rather than the ICA. At this point the ICA clamp is removed.

Any bleeding from the suture line is addressed at this time. However, a final important technical point in this step again relates to the thrombogenicity of stagnant blood in contact with the patch material or endarterectomized surface of the carotid bifurcation. One should avoid reclamping unless absolutely necessary to control bleeding at this stage and avoid the risk for formation of thrombus or a fibrin-platelet aggregate on the patch or endarterectomized vessel. This phenomenon should not be underestimated; in 2002, AbuRahma and colleagues noted a 5% carotid thrombosis rate with Dacron patches in a prospective trial with a resultant 7% perioperative stroke rate.[77] As a result of that trial, the makers of the Dacron patch re-engineered to patch to make it less thrombogenic.

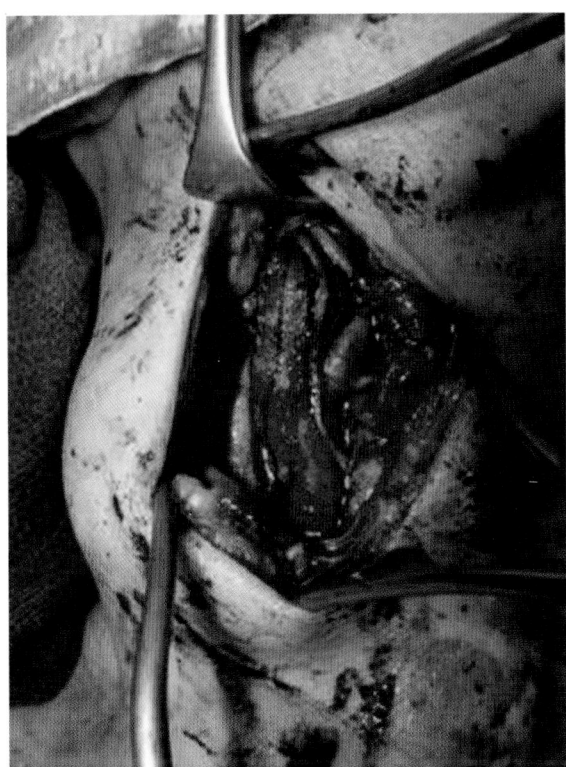

Figure 95-6 Patch closure of the arteriotomy for carotid endarterectomy. Dacron was used in this case. Note the ansa cervicalis coursing along the vessel, the vagus nerve posteriorly, and the hypoglossal nerve at the apex of the incision.

Eversion Endarterectomy

Eversion endarterectomy is an excellent alternative technique that is practiced successfully in many centers throughout the world. Two different versions of eversion endarterectomy are performed. DeBakey originally described eversion endarterectomy with partial transection of the anterior portion of the carotid bifurcation.[2] Etheredge improved on DeBakey's technique with complete transection of the bifurcation,[78] which allowed the origins of both the ICA and ECA to be everted for a longer distance. The endarterectomy is performed by mobilizing the entire circumference of the carotid adventitia off the plaque (described as a "circumcision" by Etheredge) and then everting the adventitia and mobilizing it upward while gentle caudad traction is applied to the plaque. This maneuver is performed distally into the orifices of the ICA and ECA and then proximally into the CCA. Once the endarterectomy is complete, the divided bifurcation is reunited with a simple end-to-end anastomosis.

Advantages of this technique are that the anastomosis can be performed rapidly and it is not prone to restenosis, and therefore patching is not required. Disadvantages of this technique are that more extensive dissection is sometimes necessary to mobilize the vessels during the eversion, the procedure does not lend itself readily to shunting (although shunting is not precluded by this technique), and it can be difficult to visualize the endpoint in the ICA after the plaque has been removed; the artery tends to retract as soon as the plaque pulls away from the adventitia, and it can be difficult to expose and reinspect this area of the artery again. Therefore, in our opinion, a completion study should be performed with this technique.

Kieney and coworkers introduced a modification of eversion endarterectomy in 1985 in which the origin of the ICA is excised obliquely off the carotid bifurcation, the ICA is inverted on its own, and endarterectomy of the CCA and ECA is performed through an arteriotomy in the side of the carotid bifurcation.[79] With this technique it is easier to manipulate the ICA by itself, so eversion of the ICA is less cumbersome. The ICA is reanastomosed to the carotid bifurcation primarily (Fig. 95-7). This technique allows rapid plaque extraction, the anastomosis is not prone to restenosis, and no prosthetic material is required.

This technique is particularly effective for dealing with redundant, coiled, or kinked ICAs. The ICA can be pulled down and straightened and the redundant portion excised. The remaining portion of the ICA is spatulated and reattached to the arteriotomy on the carotid bifurcation. Although this procedure typically is not performed with a shunt, the technique does not preclude shunt use. Less dissection is required than with transection of the bifurcation. However, exposure for thorough endarterectomy of the CCA and ECA may be suboptimal with this approach.

Comparison of Conventional and Eversion Carotid Endarterectomy

Numerous studies have compared standard CEA plus patching with eversion CEA. Perhaps the most important is the EVEREST (EVERsion carotid Endarterectomy versus Standard Trial study), a randomized prospective multicenter study performed in Italy that was published in 1997.[80] More than 1400 patients were randomized to eversion or standard CEA, with shunting and patching done at the discretion of the operating surgeon. There were no statistically significant differences in outcomes between the two techniques, although a slightly higher incidence of perioperative complications was noted with eversion CEA and a slightly higher incidence of restenosis with standard CEA. In a subsequent publication in 2000, however, longer term follow-up in the EVEREST trial demonstrated that patients who underwent eversion CEA had a lower incidence of restenosis than did those who underwent standard CEA (patch and primary closure), but standard CEA with patch angioplasty had the lowest incidence of neurologic complications and the lowest rate of restenosis—1.5% —versus 2.8% for eversion CEA and 7.9% for standard CEA with primary closure.[81] Other studies have shown better outcomes with eversion CEA,[82,83] and yet others have shown no difference between the two techniques.[84,85] Thus, there

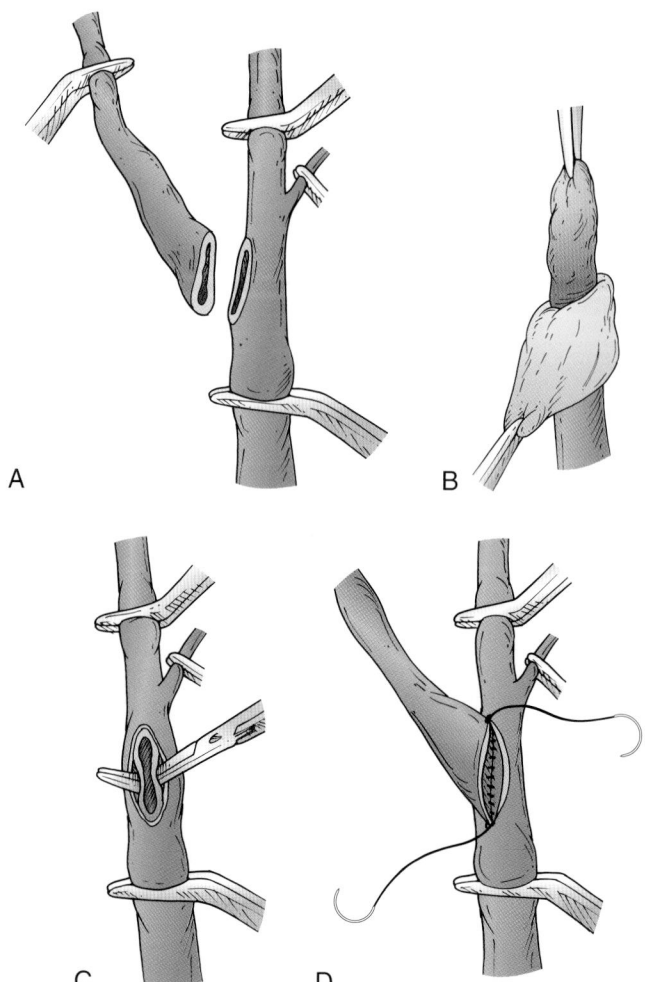

Figure 95-7 Eversion endarterectomy. **A,** Internal carotid artery transected from the bifurcation. **B,** Adventitia teased back off the internal carotid artery plaque. **C,** Plaque endarterectomized from the common carotid and origin of the external carotid artery. **D,** Reanastomosis of the internal carotid artery to the bifurcation. *(Redrawn from Saratzis N, Saratzis A, Milaras S, et al. Eversion carotid endarterectomy illustrated: tips and tricks of the procedure. Surg Rounds. August 2006. http://www.hcplive.com/general/publications/surgical-rounds/2006/2006-08)*

is no clear consensus that one technique is superior to the other.

Exposure for High Lesions

The carotid bifurcation can be located anywhere between the second and seventh cervical vertebrae, and a bifurcation located high in the neck poses technical challenges that can increase perioperative risk for stroke and cranial nerve injury. Ideally, one will recognize a high bifurcation on the preoperative imaging study. This is a potential advantage of CTA, in which bony anatomy is always included in the images. A conscious effort must be made to locate the bony anatomy with DSA if unsubtracted images are not provided with the study, but the anatomy can still be defined from subtracted images. Bony landmarks are never provided with carotid duplex imaging, but an astute vascular technologist will note a high bifurcation and should record it in the report.

Nasotracheal Intubation

Several methods can be used to gain additional cephalic exposure of a high carotid bifurcation. The easiest of them—and the initial approach—is to start the operation with nasotracheal intubation. With the patient's mouth closed, the vertical ramus of the mandible is displaced anteriorly 1 to 2 cm relative to its position when the mouth is open with an oral endotracheal tube. The additional few millimeters of exposure afforded by this maneuver will often be the difference in achieving a suitable endarterectomy endpoint in the distal ICA.

Division of the Digastric Muscle

The next step to enhance distal exposure is to divide the posterior belly of the digastric muscle (Fig. 95-8). This muscle takes the same diagonal course through the wound as the hypoglossal nerve, but it is located superficial to the nerve. Therefore, this nerve should be carefully identified and protected before the muscle is divided. Two other nerves that can be injured high in the neck are the spinal accessory nerve, which enters the tendinous portion of the sternocleidomastoid muscle, usually in the upper third of the muscle, and the glossopharyngeal nerve, which lies deep to the digastric muscle.

Resection of the Styloid Process

The final maneuver that can be extremely effective in gaining cephalic exposure is resection of the styloid process. The insertions of the muscles on the styloid process are excised with a scalpel with either a No. 15 blade or a Beaver blade, and the styloid process is carefully resected with a rongeur. In

our experience with four cases in which resection of the styloid process was necessary, this maneuver alone permitted exposure of the ICA all the way to the skull base.

Anterior Subluxation of the Mandible

Two other options can be used to improve distal exposure of a high bifurcation, both of which require preoperative planning and coordination with an oral or plastic surgeon. Anterior subluxation of the mandible requires placing the mandible in temporary intermaxillary fixation. An even more aggressive approach involves the use of a complete vertical osteotomy through the vertical ramus of the mandible and separation of the mandible to expose the ICA.

■ CEREBRAL PROTECTION AND MONITORING

Shunting

One of the long-standing debated issues related to the performance of CEA concerns the use of intravascular shunts: routine nonuse of shunts, selective use of shunts, and routine use of shunts. The simplest way to perform CEA is to just clamp the carotid bifurcation and perform CEA without a shunt, and several large series have documented excellent results of CEA without shunts.[86-88] However, all these studies report at least a small incidence of stoke, and in at least some cases the etiology of the stroke is intraoperative cerebral ischemia during carotid artery clamping.

Alternatively, some operators routinely shunt in all cases of CEA, and excellent results have been reported in several large series.[89-92] However, all these studies document an incidence of stroke, and in some of these cases the cause of the stroke was attributed to technical problems related to use of the shunt (Fig. 95-9).

A third option, founded on the notion that shunting is inherently risky, is to use shunts selectively in patients who would be at high risk for ischemic stroke if a shunt were not used. However, accurate identification of the small group of patients who require shunts has been difficult. Several techniques have been used to identify patients who truly need a shunt. In a patient under GA, such techniques include intraoperative measurement of carotid "stump pressure" after the CCA and ECA have been clamped, intraoperative neurologic monitoring of the patient's electroencephalogram or somatosensory evoked potentials (SSEP), measurement of MCA flow by TCD, and monitoring with cerebral oximetry. An alternative method is to perform CEA under RA, with selection of patients for shunting based on alterations in the neurologic examination that develop after the carotid artery is clamped.

The etiology of intraoperative stroke may be ischemic or embolic. Ischemic stroke results solely from inadequate cerebral perfusion related to clamping of the carotid artery. Embolic stroke can occur during manipulation of the carotid artery before clamping, during the actual process of clamping

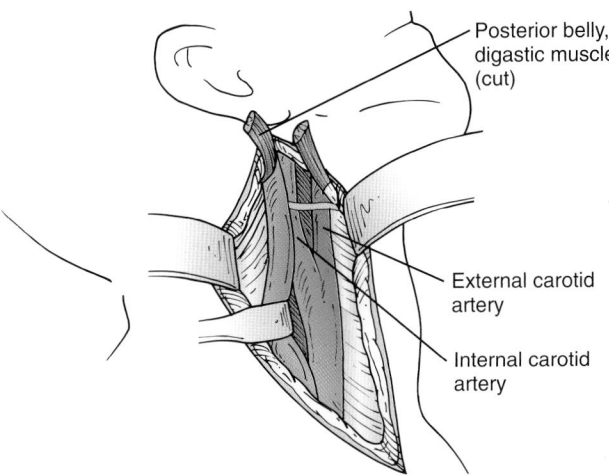

Figure 95-8 Division of the digastric muscle to facilitate distal carotid artery exposure.

Posterior belly, digastic muscle (cut)

External carotid artery

Internal carotid artery

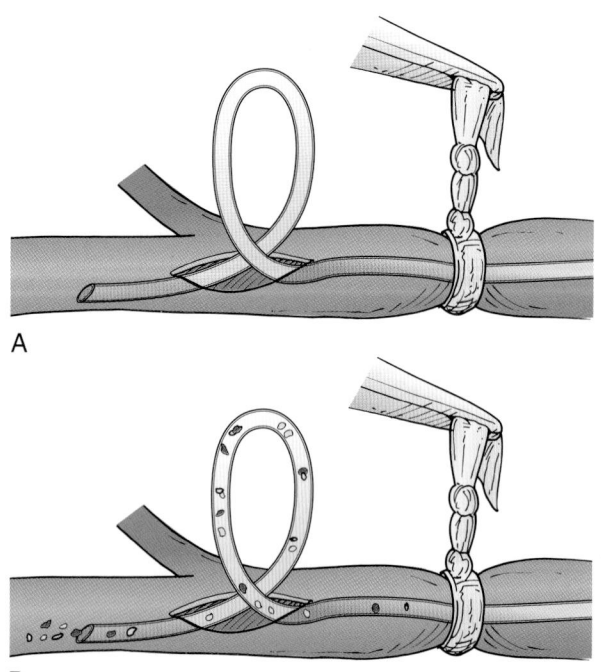

A

B

Figure 95-9 Pitfalls of carotid shunt placement. **A,** Potential traumatic injury to the distal internal carotid artery intima. **B,** Potential for embolization of atherosclerotic debris or air.

of the carotid artery, and during reperfusion—either after placing a shunt or after unclamping the carotid bifurcation as the endarterectomy is completed. Embolic stroke can also occur as a result of technical defects in the endarterectomy site or adjacent vessels related to damage from a clamp or a shunt or as a result of a technically inadequate endarterectomy. This latter situation can lead to intraoperative stroke or (delayed) postoperative stroke. All the adjuncts described in the preceding paragraph are designed to detect intraoperative cerebral ischemia, whereas TCD has the added advantage of detecting intraoperative embolism.

Placing a shunt has the capacity only to prevent ischemic stroke, and it could actually increase the risk for embolic stroke if performed poorly. Intraoperative cerebral ischemia is actually a relatively uncommon cause of intraoperative stroke.[93-95] This would support the argument of the routine nonshunters, who believe that cerebral ischemia is a rare cause of stroke and that shunting may do more harm than good (by causing embolic complications) such that even selective shunting is never justified. However, there is no denying that when cerebral ischemia does occur, it can lead to perioperative stroke.[96-98]

It is clear that cerebral ischemia can be completely relieved by placement of a shunt. This should translate into prevention of stroke in these patients if embolic complications related to shunt placement are minimized. In fact, there is evidence that the benefits of shunting outweigh the risks in these patients.[99-101]

From a medical-legal point of view, routine nonshunting under GA would be hard to defend in the case of a patient who suffered an intraoperative stroke during CEA. Consequently, routine nonuse of shunts cannot be advocated, although it is still practiced by those who favor eversion endarterectomy,[102] in which placement of a shunt is technically more difficult but not impossible.

Cerebral Monitoring

Selective shunting is dependent on using a technique to identify patients with intraoperative ischemia. The majority of CEAs are performed today under GA, and strategies to assess cerebral ischemia include stump pressure measurement; EEG, TCD, and SSEP monitoring; and measurement of regional blood and cerebral oxygen saturation. The problem is that none of these techniques is completely accurate. They do not uniformly predict the occurrence of intraoperative ischemia, nor do they prevent the unnecessary use of shunts. Finally, the selective use of shunting may actually increase the risk for an ischemic or embolic stroke that would not otherwise occur with routine shunting.

Stump Pressure

Measurement of carotid stump pressure was the first method used to predict intraoperative ischemia.[103] In patients with measured stump pressures lower than 50 mm Hg, Hays and colleagues noted a 50% neurologic event rate in those who were not shunted versus a 10% rate in those who were in a series of 297 patients.[104]

With the advent of other adjuncts to detect cerebral ischemia, such as intraoperative electroencephalography and TCD, studies were performed to validate carotid stump pressure measurement. Kelly and coworkers measured stump pressure with concurrent EEG monitoring in 289 patients[105] and performed shunting only in those with evidence of ischemia by EEG criteria. They found that 6% of patients with stump pressure higher than 50 mm Hg had ischemia by EEG criteria. Stump pressure correlated well with EEG findings in patients with completed strokes but had a false-negative rate of 77% in patients with vertebral artery disease. In another report using electroencephalography as a "gold standard," Harada and associates found that a stump pressure lower than 50 mm Hg had a positive predictive value of only 36%.[106] In this series, 11% of patients with ischemia by EEG criteria would not have received shunts and 64% of patients with a stump pressure lower than 50 would have received them unnecessarily by stump pressure criteria. Similarly, Brewster and coworkers found that 11 of 17 patients with ischemic EEG findings would not have been shunted by stump pressure criteria and 7 of 63 would have unnecessary shunts.[107] Finocchi and colleagues used TCD to verify stump pressure and found that stump pressure did not correlate well with ischemia by TCD criteria in patients with postoperative deficits.[108] Clearly, even in the setting of what appears to be a satisfactorily high stump pressure, there may still be regions of the brain that are relatively hypoperfused.

Electroencephalographic and Somatosensory Evoked Potential Monitoring

Intraoperative EEG monitoring is the most widely used method of intraoperative cerebral monitoring. It can be performed by using 8, 12, or 16 leads, with the 16-lead configuration being standard. Standard criteria for intraoperative ischemia are at least a 50% decrease in fast background activity, increase in delta wave activity, or complete loss of EEG signals. By using these criteria, shunt use can be minimized.[109,110] In some of these studies the decreased use of shunts resulted in improved neurologic outcome,[111,112] whereas in others, neurologic outcome was unchanged or even worse.[109,110] A common finding in all these studies is that electroencephalography is overly sensitive—positive in 10% to 40% of patients with unilateral carotid disease and positive in as many as 69% with bilateral carotid disease,[113,114] thereby overestimating the number of people who require shunts. Blume and coworkers observed postoperative strokes in only 9% of patients with abnormal EEG findings in whom shunts were not placed.[115]

Furthermore, several series have documented neurologic events that occurred in the absence of EEG abnormality when shunting was not used.[110,116] Tempelhoff and associates found that 5 of 6 patients with postoperative deficits in a series of 103 patients showed EEG changes only late in the operation, when shunting was no longer feasible.[116]

Similarly, there are multiple published studies on the use of SSEP suggesting that it is a useful adjunct to detect ischemia.[117-121] However, in a meta-analysis of 15 studies, Wober and colleagues found that SSEP monitoring is not a reliable means of detecting ischemia and predicting neurologic outcome.[122]

Transcranial Doppler

Transcranial Doppler was introduced by Schneider and coworkers in 1988.[123] Visser and coauthors reported that with normal TCD findings one could safely avoid shunting in a third of patients but that abnormal findings on TCD predicted ischemia by EEG criteria only 60% of the time.[124] TCD has the unique advantage of detecting microemboli intraoperatively, which may alert the surgeon to avoid further manipulation that may cause a stroke.[125,126] However, Belardi and associates also reported that TCD (as well as stump pressure) was not accurate in predicting cerebral ischemia.[127]

Awake Carotid Endarterectomy with Regional or Local Anesthesia

In view of these findings, performing CEA under RA is the most reliable method of predicting the need for selective shunting. It can be done with either a cervical plexus block or purely local anesthesia. In this case the decision to shunt is based solely on the development of hemispheric or global neurologic symptoms after the carotid artery is clamped. This criterion is considered the gold standard for selective shunting by which all other adjuncts should be compared. Shunt rates are consistently lower than with other modalities, on the order of 5% to 15%.[127-134] In two recent prospective trials in which both stump pressure and EEG measurements were recorded before performing endarterectomy under RA but in which the need to shunt was ultimately determined by neurologic changes, both EEG findings and stump pressure were found to inaccurately predict the need for shunting.[135,136] In the study by Calligaro and Dougherty published in 2005, a cost analysis found that RA saved more than $3000 per case by avoiding EEG measurements.[135]

In addition to its benefit in predicting the need for shunting, it has been suggested that there are other potential benefits of performing CEA on awake patients. One study has demonstrated a lower rate of myocardial infarction with RA that was statistically significant,[137] whereas others have not confirmed this benefit.[132,138,139] Bowyer and colleagues showed a statistically significant decrease in the neurologic event rate with RA, but not all patients were selectively shunted in this study, and no other study has duplicated this finding.[139] Three studies have shown decreased length of stay with RA,[131,137,138] but in two of them the length of stay in the GA group was not reflective of modern practice, approximately 5 days.[131,138] This does not necessarily translate into decreased cost,[140] but RA is probably the only adjunct for selective shunting that does not increase cost over routine shunting; there is not a single study in the literature that demonstrates cost-effectiveness of any form of selective shunting over routine shunting. Finally, as mentioned earlier in this chapter, the recently published GALA trial, the definitive study of RA versus GA in CEA that included more than 3500 patients in Europe, failed to show any significant benefit of performing CEA under RA.[72]

The disadvantages of RA are that not all anesthesiologists, surgeons, or patients are comfortable with performing CEA under RA. Cervical block is an advanced RA technique that requires considerable skill on the part of the anesthesiologist. Many surgeons find it stressful to have an awake patient who can behave unpredictably during the procedure. Some patients tolerate RA poorly because of claustrophobia or inadequate anesthesia with just a regional or local block. There is a small risk of seizure or cardiac arrhythmia with inadvertent administration of local anesthetic into the carotid artery or jugular vein.

Routine Shunting

One flaw in the strategy of selective shunting is that neurologic events in the shunted group may be attributable to the shunt itself secondary to embolism or ischemia and may not occur with routine shunting. Specifically, selective shunting, regardless of the adjunct used, always involves a test clamp. In the case of stump pressure measurement, instrumenting the carotid artery with a needle introduces the added risk of embolism. When a test clamp is positive, there are two options. One is to unclamp the vessels and reperfuse the brain while preparations are made to shunt. This maneuver exposes the patient to the risk of embolization. The other option is to proceed with the endarterectomy and placement of a shunt. In this instance, the brain is ischemic when the test clamp becomes positive and is exposed to an additional period of ischemia while the shunt is being placed, whereas during routine shunting, shunt placement can usually be accomplished in 2 to 3 minutes after clamping, before the brain becomes ischemic. The additional period of ischemia after a positive test clamp can be detrimental. Templehoff and coauthors reported that five of six postoperative neurologic deficits occurred in patients who had ischemic times longer than 9 minutes by EEG criteria,[116] and Hays and associates noted that in patients who were shunted on the basis of low stump pressure, all those who experienced neurologic events had ischemic times longer than 2½ minutes.[104] It is therefore not fair to compare shunted with nonshunted patients in a group of selectively shunted patients. A better evaluation would be comparison of the outcomes of all selectively shunted patients with an nonshunted group of patients in the same study, with an intent-to-treat analysis for *selective shunting* rather than the placement of a shunt. To date, no such study has been published.[69,70,141]

The routine use of carotid shunts eliminates these concerns. It allows CEA to be performed in a consistent manner, which eliminates surgeon and patient anxiety, without the added cost or complexity of monitoring equipment. It is easy to do and facilitates performing CEA in a teaching environment. All studies consistently show that carotid shunting with either the Javid or Pruitt-Inahara shunt completely relieves the intracerebral ischemia caused by clamping, whether measured by neurologic status, EEG changes, MCA flow on TCD, or cerebral blood flow. There is no evidence that placement of a shunt increases embolic complications or causes arterial injury leading to more subacute or chronic complications. There is evidence, however, that placing a shunt in the setting of severe ischemia decreases the stroke rate.[142] As noted earlier, minimizing ischemic time to the brain by routine shunt placement has the theoretical advantage of limiting ischemia-reperfusion injury. Parrson and associates have shown that carotid shunting diminishes the inflammatory response of ischemic brain injury, as demonstrated by the production of various inflammatory mediators.[143] This may be an important mechanism in the occurrence of delayed postoperative strokes, which can account for up to 70% of perioperative strokes.[94] There are numerous large series that document excellent results with the use of routine shunting in CEA. Thompson demonstrated superb results over a 15-year period spanning the 1960s and 1970s, with a stroke rate of 1.4% in 1107 CEAs.[90] Javid and coauthors reported similarly excellent results in a series of more than 1800 patients from the same era.[91] In 1997, Hertzer and colleagues reported a series of over 1900 CEAs at the Cleveland Clinic, virtually all of which were shunted routinely, with a perioperative stroke rate of 1.8%.[92] Hamdan and associates published a series of 1001 consecutive patients in whom routine shunting was used most of the time, with a combined stroke

and death rate of 1.6%.[89] In contrast, there is only one series of comparable magnitude for selective shunting—the published experience of Sundt and coauthors, who reported a 1% stroke rate in 1145 patients.[144]

In our practice, routine carotid shunting during CEA is the preferred operative technique because it best accommodates anesthesiologists, surgeons, and patients without compromising results. Despite acceptable results in some individuals' hands, routine nonuse of shunts cannot be advocated in view of the abounding evidence that intraoperative ischemia can be a source of stroke that is preventable with shunts. Selective shunting based on stump pressure, TCD, or neurophysiologic monitoring does not accomplish the goal of improving results through decreased shunt use and only adds to the cost and complexity of the procedure. The only form of selective shunting that is truly reliable is that based on neurologic examination during RA; all other forms are imperfect.

In some instances placement of a shunt has the potential to damage the ICA, such as in patients with narrow or tortuous vessels (see Fig. 95-9). An absolute requirement for safe shunt placement is that the superior end of the plaque be positively identified and adequately exposed through the arteriotomy so that the distal end of the shunt does not "snow-plow" into the plaque when it is placed and cause embolization or dissection. We therefore advocate "super selective shunting": routine shunting except in situations in which shunting is associated with high risk.

ARTERIOTOMY CLOSURE

When CEA is performed through a longitudinal arteriotomy, an important consideration is how the arteriotomy is closed. It has been known for decades that primary closure of a longitudinal arteriotomy can result in significant stenosis of the vessel, yet this is the simplest and most efficient way to close an arteriotomy. However, considerable experience indicates that patch closure yields superior clinical and anatomic outcomes.

Patch Closure

Saphenous Vein Patches

Before the advent of synthetic patches, the surgeon's choices for patch material included saphenous vein or external jugular vein. Imparato used vein patching routinely as early as 1965, but no rigorous comparison of the results of patch angioplasty and direct closure was made until more than 20 years later.[145] Saphenous vein patching has been used extensively with good results, but problems specific to saphenous vein patching include wound complications at the harvest site, potential compromise of a valuable conduit for later bypass procedures, and the devastating complication of patch rupture, which has been reported to occur in 0.5% to 4% of cases.[146-150] Because most of these were ankle veins, several investigators recommended harvesting the great saphenous vein (GSV) from above the knee. Lord and coworkers also noted that aneurysmal expansion of saphenous vein patches can occur in up to 17% patients.[151]

Archie and Green investigated the relationship of GSV diameter and rupture pressure and found that GSVs with diameters less than 3.5 mm were more prone to rupture.[152] Their group also noted that women were three times more likely to have a GSV measuring less than 3.5 mm. Applying this knowledge to their practice, Archie found that by using a GSV with a distended vein diameter of greater than 3.5 mm and maintaining a carotid bulb diameter of less than 13 mm, patch rupture was completely avoided in a series of 534 patients over an 8-year period.[153]

Synthetic Patches

As synthetic patch materials became available, they were incorporated into practice to avoid the pitfalls of saphenous vein patching. Synthetic materials that are commonly used for this purpose include PTFE, woven polyester (Dacron), and bovine pericardium. Studies on the influence of the type of carotid closure have therefore not only compared carotid patching with primary closure but also analyzed outcomes with different patch materials.

Comparative Analyses

The British Joint Vascular Research Group RCT compared 104 patients undergoing primary closure with 109 patients treated by patch closure with either autologous vein or Dacron.[154] Six strokes occurred in the primary closure group and two in the patch group, and six perioperative thromboses were noted in the primary closure group versus none in the patched group. At 1 year there were 17 occlusions of greater than 50% stenosis in the primary closure group versus 6 in the patch group. In 1994, Katz and coauthors reported on 100 CEAs randomized to primary closure (n = 51) or patch closure with PTFE (n = 49) and found no significant difference in outcomes, although there was a trend toward higher neurologic morbidity in the primary closure group.[154] AbuRahma and colleagues randomized 74 patients with bilateral carotid stenoses to primary closure followed by patch closure or patch closure followed by primary closure to eliminate systemic factors that might confound results in different patients, such as female gender, smoking, hyperlipidemia, young age, diabetes mellitus, hypertension, and disseminated atherosclerosis.[155] They found a significantly higher perioperative stroke rate for primary closure than for patching (4% versus 0%), as well as a higher stroke/TIA rate for primary closure than for patching (12% versus 1%). All the strokes in the primary closure group were due to perioperative thrombosis of the carotid bifurcation. With long-term follow-up to 5 years, there was also a statistically significant difference in the rate of repeat carotid surgery, 14% in the primary closure group versus 1% in the patch group.

Pooled data from meta-analyses and large databases unequivocally support the use of patching over primary closure. Meta-analyses by Counsell and associates in 1997 and

Bond and colleagues in 2004 found that all short-term (30 day) and long-term endpoints were significantly improved with patching versus primary closure. Comparison of vein patches with prosthetic patches in these studies demonstrated no significant difference in the major endpoints.[156,157] Rockman and coworkers used a state database in New York to review outcomes with primary closure versus patch angioplasty or eversion endarterectomy in 1972 CEAs at six regional hospitals. Perioperative stroke was significantly more common with primary closure than with eversion or patching (5.6% versus 2.2%, no difference between eversion and patching), as well as higher perioperative stroke rates and death with primary closure than with eversion or patching (6% versus 2.5%). There were no differences in any outcomes between eversion and patching.[158] Finally, Kresowik and coauthors reported the outcomes of more than 10,000 CEAs performed in several states and found that use of a patch, in particular a prosthetic patch, was a statistically significant indicator for improved outcomes.[159] Based on these findings, the U.S. Centers for Medicare and Medicaid Services adopted patching of conventional CEA as a physician quality measure for 2009.

After these studies were published, Al-Rawi and coworkers reported no differences between primary closure and patching with a collagen-coated polyester patch in a fairly large RCT that included 328 patients. Of note, primary closure was performed by a single surgeon using microvascular techniques. There were no statistically significant differences in outcomes, but a trend toward a higher combined stroke and death rate was noted in the patched group.[160] Therefore, primary closure with microvascular technique may be the only instance in which it might be justified.

Optimal Patch Material

The optimal patch material remains to be defined. Grego and colleagues compared the results of patching with external jugular vein and PTFE in a randomized trial of 160 CEAs and reported no difference in stroke-free survival at 12, 30, and 60 months and no difference in recurrent stenosis rates, but a trend toward improved results with vein patch.[161] Marien and associates performed an RCT in which bovine pericardium was compared with Dacron in 95 CEAs performed in 92 patients and observed significantly less suture line bleeding with bovine pericardium than with Dacron (4% versus 30%) and no difference in neurologic outcomes.[162] Goldman and coworkers compared saphenous vein and internal jugular vein with knitted Dacron in 275 CEAs and found no significant differences in perioperative morbidity, mortality, or early restenosis between any of these groups.[163]

In a small trial comparing internal jugular vein, GSV from the thigh, and knitted Dacron, Jacobowitz and coworkers found a higher death rate in the jugular vein group (8% versus 0% with GSV and 1.1% with knitted Dacron), as well as a higher stroke rate that was not statistically significant (4% versus 1.3% and 1.1%, respectively).[164] AbuRahma and colleagues examined the outcomes of primary closure versus patching with GSV, jugular vein, and PTFE.[165] They found that perioperative neurologic event rates were significantly higher with primary closure than with all patch methods. Event rates were slightly higher with jugular vein patches, and recurrent stenosis was also higher in this group than in the GSV or Dacron patch group and similar to primary closure. In a follow-up study 2 years later, they reported that primary closure had a higher incidence of restenosis and need for reoperation, especially in women who had smaller carotid arteries.[166]

Finally, in a small RCT comparing Dacron with PTFE, AbuRahma and associates found a higher stroke rate with Dacron that was largely due to perioperative thrombosis.[167] As a result of this trial the manufacturer of the Dacron patch re-engineered it, which AbuRahma's group studied in a follow-up trial.[168] This investigation showed no difference in outcomes between the two patches. The cause of this difference in outcomes in the original trial was not clear because as long ago as 1996, Margovsky and coworkers found in an animal model that platelet accumulation was not significantly different between gelatin-sealed Dacron and PTFE, whereas platelet accumulation was much lower on vein patches than on either of these prosthetic patches.[169]

Selective Patching

It has been suggested that carotid patching may not be necessary in all patients, and the technique does have some drawbacks, such as longer operative time, greater potential for bleeding from longer suture lines, and increased cost. To avoid these pitfalls while preventing the increased morbidity associated with primary closure, some surgeons use a policy of selective patching. Golledge and associates studied selective patching based on intraoperative measurement of the outer diameter of the ICA and found that selective patching was safe in arteries measuring at least 6 mm.[170] Similarly, Cikrit and colleagues demonstrated no difference in outcomes between primary closure and patching in a small study of selectively patched patients.[171] Pappas and associates based their decision to patch on whether the ICA could be closed without tension over a Javid shunt. Using this criterion, they actually found a higher stroke rate in the patch group in a small retrospective series.[172] Other work has clearly identified other risk factors for recurrent carotid stenosis and indications for selective patching, including female gender, elevated cholesterol level, and possibly cigarette smoking and hypertension[120] (see "Recurrent Carotid Stenosis").

■ COMPLETION STUDIES

Although there are several potential causes of perioperative stroke in patients who undergo CEA, a preventable cause is thromboembolism or carotid artery thrombosis resulting from technical imperfections in repair of the carotid artery. To minimize this risk, intraoperative completion studies have been used, including continuous wave Doppler, duplex ultrasound, and intraoperative angiography.

Continuous Wave Doppler

Continuous wave Doppler analysis is a purely qualitative method in which a hand-held Doppler probe is used to confirm patency of the carotid vessels; an experienced operator can also identify areas of stenosis by the high pitch associated with a stenosis. However, it is insensitive to small intimal flaps or more subtle stenoses, and its accuracy is operator dependent.

Duplex Ultrasound

Duplex ultrasound is a much more sensitive tool that provides detailed anatomic imaging, as well real-time physiologic information regarding blood flow through the carotid vessels. However, the data obtained from the study are also operator dependent, and there can be technical limitations in placing the Doppler probe in the wound to achieve an adequate examination.

Intraoperative Angiography

Intraoperative angiography has been considered the gold standard of completion studies. The quality of the information obtained from an angiogram, however, may vary significantly depending on the technique used; options for angiography include "single-shot" exposure on a flat plate of x-ray film performed through a needle in the CCA or fluoroscopic studies with a portable C-arm or even a fixed fluoroscopy unit, if available, performed through a needle in the CCA or through a catheter navigated through the aortic arch into the CCA, with contrast material injected through a power injector.

Results of Completion Studies

Several studies have demonstrated the utility of completion studies to identify technical defects, with subsequent improvement of results.[173,174] On the other hand, not all technical imperfections, such as minor intimal flaps and especially ECA lesions, will cause strokes. In addition, attempts to revise significant lesions may not be successful and can carry with them additional morbidity from repeat manipulation of the carotid system and a further risk for ischemia, embolism, thrombosis, or bleeding. For example, in the EVEREST trial, in which all patients had some form of completion study performed and major defects were found in 4% of cases, revision of these defects produced little improvement in outcomes and was highly predictive of stroke (odds ratio, 11.5; $P = .0002$). The only significant risk factor for a major defect found in this study was plaque extension greater than 2 cm into the ICA (odds ratio, 1.5; $P = .03$). One of the unanswered questions about completion studies is the extent of abnormality (either flap length or stenosis severity) that warrants intervention.

Rockman and Haim performed a large review of patients who underwent CEA from a New York State database to investigate the usage patterns and outcomes of intraoperative completion studies.[175] They found no significant benefit with any form of completion study. This study suggests that if a technically perfect operation can be achieved, completion studies are not necessary. However, this relies on complete exposure of the carotid plaque through a long vertical arteriotomy in the ICA. If there is any doubt about the condition of the endpoint, though, a completion study should be obtained. During eversion endarterectomy one may have only a fleeting glimpse of the endarterectomy endpoint before the artery retracts when the plaque separates from the artery, or none at all. Therefore, completion studies are more likely to be useful in this procedure. Such studies may also be beneficial for inexperienced surgeons who are early in their career and gaining experience with CEA.

PERIOPERATIVE STROKE MANAGEMENT

In a detailed study of the etiology of perioperative stroke associated with CEA in patients in all clinical classes, more than 20 mechanisms were delineated.[96] In general, however, these mechanisms can be grouped in decreasing order of frequency as postoperative arterial thrombosis and embolization, cerebral ischemia during carotid clamping, and intracerebral hemorrhage. Perioperative carotid arterial thrombosis most often results from technical imperfection in performance of the operation, such as disruption of the intima during placement of the intraluminal shunt, residual intimal flaps or atheromatous disease, or residual luminal thrombus. Completion imaging studies, as described in the previous section, will help identify technical imperfections and can reduce the incidence of neurologic complications.

Maximizing the chance for neurologic recovery is most dependent on early recognition of the deficit and immediate institution of proper therapy. Because not all deficits result from causes that are surgically correctable, accurate diagnosis is critical to implementing appropriate therapy. Establishing the correct diagnosis is dependent on the time of onset of symptoms with respect to the operative procedure and is supported by selected noninvasive vascular laboratory or radiologic studies.

Intraoperative

A patient undergoing CEA under GA should be awakened in the operating room immediately after wound closure, and a neurologic examination performed. If a new focal central neurologic deficit is identified, the artery should be immediately re-evaluated. The incision is opened, and the ICA is checked for a pulse and flow with Doppler. If flow appears to be present, the surgeon should perform duplex ultrasonography or arteriography to identify a potential correctable etiology. Intracranial imaging should be included if no cause is found at the endarterectomy site because a distal embolus is potentially treatable by thrombolysis or extractable via microcath-

eter techniques (see "Postoperative"). Examining a patent artery with duplex or arteriography avoids the need to reclamp the artery for blind exploration and potentially aggravating the neurologic deficit. However, if the ICA does not have flow or if duplex/arteriography identifies a local defect, the endarterectomy must be re-explored. If acute thrombosis of the endarterectomy site is identified, meticulous search for a technical defect, such as a distal intimal ledge, should be performed after careful thromboembolectomy. It is best not to clamp the distal ICA initially in the case of thrombosis and to extract the clot in the bulb and visible ICA so that backpressure may extrude any more distal ICA thrombus. If there is no back flow, a balloon catheter can be used, but care must be taken to prevent distention in the distal ICA to avoid causing a carotid artery–cavernous sinus fistula.[176] If there is a local flap, platelet accumulation, or other problem within the endarterectomy, it should be corrected. Correction may involve extending the endarterectomy, performing a patch angioplasty if not initially carried out, or resecting the vessel and replacing it with a bypass graft, depending on the operative findings. In the setting of re-exploration, if a shunt was used initially, great care must be taken if a shunt is reinserted to be sure that the distal endpoint is not injured and a flap created with insertion of the shunt.

If at re-exploration the vessel is found to be patent without a local defect, the most likely cause is either ischemia during carotid clamping or, much more likely, intraoperative embolization. Risk for intraoperative embolization can be minimized by the administration of aspirin preoperatively, minimizing vessel manipulation before clamping, and instituting an intravenous low-molecular-weight dextran drip at completion of the procedure. Nevertheless, in a small minority of patients, excessive platelet deposition may occur acutely on the endarterectomy site and predispose to distal embolization or even acute thrombosis of the vessel. In this case, we favor resection of the endarterectomy segment, replacement of the graft, and institution of an intravenous heparin drip (assuming that the possibility of heparin-induced thrombocytopenia has been eliminated; see Chapter 37: Hypercoagulable States). Conversely, if the vessel appears normal at re-exploration, thus suggesting that the patient experienced either embolization during vessel dissection before clamping or ischemia during clamping, treatment is medical (namely, close attention to hemodynamic monitoring, oxygenation, and blood pressure stability postoperatively) or thrombolysis/microcatheter embolus extraction in institutions with such capability.

Postoperative

If the patient awakens neurologically intact in the operating room and then a new deficit develops in the recovery room or later postoperatively, the differential diagnosis is more complex. Initially, the patient should undergo Duplex ultrasound if it can be performed rapidly. If this testing indicates occlusion of the vessel or abnormal flow velocities suggestive of an intimal flap or other anatomic deficit, the patient should be immediately taken to the operating room for re-exploration. Timing is crucial because most neurologic deficits are significantly reversible if flow is restored within 1 to 2 hours after vessel thrombosis. If the noninvasive studies are negative and thus suggest a patent vessel, head computed tomography (CT) should be performed immediately to rule out a cerebral hemorrhage. If negative, carotid angiography should be performed to identify any technical defect requiring revision at the operative site or a possible intracerebral embolus.

The availability of intracerebral catheter-directed thrombolysis has provided another tool for neurologic salvage in a patient who experiences an embolic event associated with CEA. In a report from the Johns Hopkins Hospital, we documented the first successful case of immediate postoperative thrombolytic therapy with urokinase in a patient who underwent CEA for a high-grade stenosis, had angiographically documented fresh intraluminal thrombus, and awakened with hemiplegia and aphasia. An embolus to the MCA was confirmed on postoperative arteriography, and it was lysed completely via catheter-directed administration of 500,000 units of urokinase, with complete neurologic recovery.[177] In addition, catheter-based thrombectomy of ICA and MCA emboli has been accomplished successfully in the setting of acute ischemic stroke and as "neurorescue" for carotid thrombosis complicating carotid artery stenting (CAS).[178-184] This technique may prove advantageous in the future because the higher clot burden of an ICA thrombosis seems to be more resistant to successful treatment with thrombolysis alone.[185]

■ SURGICAL RESULTS

The sole purpose of CEA is prevention of stroke. Therefore, the incidence of this complication perioperatively and in long-term follow-up is a paramount determinant of its efficacy. The considerable clinical experience reported over the last 3 decades indicates that CEA can be performed with low rates of perioperative complications and that it substantially reduces the risk for subsequent stroke in patients with significant symptomatic as well as asymptomatic extracranial carotid atherosclerotic lesions.[186-191]

Randomized Trials

Symptomatic Disease

The National Institutes of Health (NIH)-funded NASCET included investigations of both high-grade (70% to 99%) and moderate-grade (50% to 69%) stenosis (see Table 95-1). Among the series of 1415 patients, 30-day mortality, disabling stroke, and nondisabling stroke rates were 1.1%, 0.9%, and 4.5%, respectively.[9,18] In the NASCET high-grade stenosis investigation, 659 patents with symptomatic ICA stenosis (70% to 99%) were randomized to optimal medical management versus CEA and optimal medical management. At the 2-year follow-up there was a highly significant reduction in ipsilateral stroke incidence (9% versus 26%) in patients who underwent CEA.[9] This benefit became apparent within 3

months of randomization and has persisted through 8 years of follow-up.

In the moderate-stenosis limb of the investigation, 865 patients with 50% to 69% ICA stenosis were randomized. At 5 years of follow-up, the ipsilateral stroke incidence was 22.2% in medical patients and 16.7% in surgical patients (P = .045), and this benefit has persisted through 8 years of follow-up.[18]

Asymptomatic Disease

Management of asymptomatic carotid disease has been more controversial because the long-term risk for stroke is not as high in asymptomatic as in symptomatic patients. In the NIH-funded ACAS, 1600 patients with greater than 60% asymptomatic stenosis were randomized to optimal medical management versus CEA and optimal medical management (see Table 95-1). The 30-day stroke/death rate was 2.3% in the surgical cohort by intent-to-treat analysis. However, there were seven strokes and two deaths preoperatively, so the actual perioperative stroke rate was 1.3% and mortality rate was 0.1%. At the 5-year follow-up, stroke and death rates were 5.1% in the CEA group and 11% in the medical management group (P = .004).[11]

The ACST was recently concluded in Europe; it had randomized 3200 patients with greater than 60% asymptomatic ICA stenosis and had an outcome comparable to that of ACAS. The 5-year stroke and death rates were 6.4% for CEA and 11.8% for medically managed patients (P < .0001) (see Table 95-1).[11,192]

Institutional Experience

Since publication of the NASCET and ACAS results, the safety and efficacy of CEA have been confirmed in institutional reports. For example, in one of the largest individual institutional series reported to date, 2236 CEAs were performed between 1989 and 1999 at the Massachusetts General Hospital with a 5.5% overall perioperative complication rate. The perioperative stroke and death rate was only 1.4%.[193] The most commonly reported complication was neck hematoma (1.7%). In a report from the Johns Hopkins Hospital, 1440 CEAs were performed from 1994 through 2004. The 30-day rates of stroke and death were 2.5% and 0.8%, respectively.[66]

Population-Based Experience

In recent years several population-based analyses have demonstrated excellent results of CEA in community practice, comparable to the outcomes in tertiary referral centers and randomized trials.

Statewide Experience

A statewide study from North Carolina examined the outcome of 11,973 CEAs performed between 1988 and 1993 in 70 of the 157 hospitals in the state. The perioperative stroke rate was 1.7% and the mortality rate was 1.2%, for a combined stroke and death rate of 2.7%.[194] Likewise, in a similar analysis of 9308 CEAs performed by 482 surgeons in 167 hospitals in New York State from 1998 through 1999, the perioperative mortality rate was 1.1% and the nonfatal stroke rate was 2.9%, for a combined perioperative stroke and death rate of 4.0%.[195] Another study compared the outcomes of CEA in both Maryland and California. Retrospective review of the Maryland Health Services Cost Review Commission database identified 23,237 CEAs performed between 1994 and 2003 by 437 surgeons in 47 nonfederal acute care hospitals in the state, only 2 of which were university hospitals. Over this 10-year period, the in-hospital stroke rate was 0.7% and the stroke and death rate was 1.3%. The stroke rate also decreased over the duration of the study.[196] Likewise, the California Office of Statewide Health Planning and Development database was queried for all CEAs performed in that state between 1999 and 2003. During that time 51,331 CEAs were performed with an in-hospital stroke rate of 0.5% and an overall mortality rate of 0.5%. Also similar to the Maryland results, the stroke rate in California decreased over the study period.[196] Of note, approximately 85% of the operations in both Maryland and California were performed for asymptomatic carotid disease, which may have contributed to the superior results.[196] Another recent study compared the outcomes of 7089 CEAs performed between 1997 and 2002 in Veterans Administration and nonfederal hospitals in Connecticut. There were no significant differences in the rates of perioperative stroke (1.4% and 0.3%), death (1.4% and 0.9%), and combined stroke and death (2.8% and 1.2%) in the two hospital groups, respectively.[197]

Medicare Experience

The outcomes of CEA have also been confirmed in several Medicare database analyses as well. For example, a retrospective review of 1945 CEAs performed on Medicare patients in the state of Georgia in 1993 revealed a 30-day mortality of 1.9% and moderate to severe stroke rate of 1.8%.[198] It has been argued by some that these large administrative databases underreport subtle strokes, thus minimizing the true surgical morbidity rates. Therefore, it is instructive to focus on operative mortality as a metric in assessing operative risk. Two independent studies involving Medicare patients have shown a progressive decrease in mortality over time in patients undergoing CEA.[199,200] For example, in an analysis of the outcome of CEA performed on more than 3000 Medicare beneficiaries across the United States from 1990 through 2000, median perioperative mortality declined from 1.9% in 1990, to 1.5% in 1995, to 0.9% in 2000, results reflecting a dramatic improvement in perioperative outcomes.[200] At the same time, Medicare data have also shown that significant variations in the outcome of CEA do exist between hospitals. In a study by Wennberg and colleagues it was found that hospitals that participated in NASCET and ACAS had as much as a 43% reduction

in mortality when compared with hospitals that did not participate in those trials.[201]

National Registries

The National Surgical Quality Improvement Program (NSQIP) database was queried for all CEAs performed between 2000 and 2003 at 123 Veterans Affairs and 14 private sector academic medical centers. During the study period, 13,622 CEAs were performed, with a combined stroke and death rate of just 3.4%.[202] Similarly, the Nationwide Inpatient Sample was recently examined to compare in-hospital stroke and death rates in patients undergoing CEA and CAS. In this analysis of 259,080 carotid revascularization procedures performed in the United States in 2003 and 2004, there was an overall stroke rate of 0.9% and a mortality rate of 0.4% with CEA.[203]

Long-term Results of Carotid Endarterectomy

CEA has proved able to provide excellent long-term clinical and anatomic results. For example, in a series of 135 patients, 92% were stroke free at 5 years by life-table analysis. The overall survival rate was 82%, with no deaths being due to cerebrovascular disease.[204] In a similar analysis of 374 patients undergoing 391 eversion CEAs, 5- and 10-year survival rates were 96.3% and 85.7%, and stroke-free survival rates were 95.6% and 84.8%, respectively. Diabetes mellitus and cardiac disease were independent predictors of reduced long-term survival in multivariate analysis.[205] Healey and associates observed that the annual stroke rate after CEA depended on the original indication for the operation: the mean stroke incidence was 2.8% per year in patients whose indication for CEA was TIA, 6.2% per year in patients with stroke, and only 0.65% per year in asymptomatic patients.[206] The recurrent stroke rate in patients who undergo CEA with a contralateral ICA occlusion does not appear to be especially high, 0.6% per year in one study.[207]

■ COMPLICATIONS

Cardiac

Myocardial infarction is responsible for 25% to 50% of all perioperative deaths after CEA.[208-210] Furthermore, more late deaths are due to myocardial infarction than to stroke or other causes.[208,209,211] These observations reflect the systemic nature of arteriosclerosis in general and, specifically, the prevalence of coronary artery disease (CAD) in patients with significant carotid lesions. At least 40% to 50% of patients who undergo CEA have symptomatic CAD.[26-28,212-214] In a prospective angiographic study, severe surgically correctable CAD was identified in 20% of patients about to undergo treatment of carotid disease.[215]

However, despite the prevalence of CAD in patients undergoing CEA, as noted earlier, operative mortality has declined significantly over the past 2 decades. In large measure this decreased mortality has resulted from a significant reduction in the incidence of major cardiac complications. For example, in a recent large institutional series that included 2236 CEAs, the incidence of cardiac complications was 0.5%.[196] At the Johns Hopkins Hospital, in a series of 1440 patients undergoing isolated CEA over the last 10 years, the 30-day incidence of myocardial infarction was 1.5%.[66] The reduction in cardiac morbidity in patients undergoing CEA reflects improvements in screening, as well as perioperative medical management of this patient population (see Chapter 30: Preoperative Management and Chapter 31: Intraoperative Management).

Cranial Nerve Injury

Incidence

Cranial nerve dysfunction is the most common neurologic complication of CEA and clearly one of the more troublesome for many patients. The incidence of postoperative dysfunction of cranial nerves ranges from 5% to 20% in several retrospective series, and a variety of nerves may be affected (Table 95-2).[216-225] The wide discrepancy in the incidence of this complication is a reflection of how aggressively various authors have attempted to document cranial nerve dysfunction in their patients because many deficits may not be easily discernible on routine physical examination. In other words, retrospective reviews, which constitute much of the published literature in this area, may significantly underestimate the true incidence of cranial nerve dysfunction after CEA. It also depends on when nerve function is assessed because most cranial nerve injuries resolve (see "Anatomic and Clinical Considerations"). In a prospective study of patients undergoing 450 CEA procedures and who also underwent postoperative otolaryngologic examination, 72 cranial nerve injuries were identified in 60 (13%) patients. Approximately a third of the patients with documented deficits were asymptomatic and would have been missed by cursory clinical examination.[225] In another prospective study of 139 patients who underwent 169 CEA procedures and in which formal evaluation was performed preoperatively and postoperatively,

cranial nerve injury was documented after 20% of the operations. This reflected a much higher incidence of nerve injury than noted in a retrospective analysis from this institution.[218] In a more recent prospective study of 183 consecutive CEAs, 26 (14%) cranial nerve injuries were identified in 26 patients.[219] In another prospective study of this problem, Evans and coauthors reported a 16% incidence of cranial nerve dysfunction based on clinical examination after 128 CEA procedures performed on 116 patients. However, when the patients underwent formal testing and examination by speech pathologists, the incidence of deficits rose to 39%. The majority of these deficits were uncovered by more detailed evaluation of superior recurrent laryngeal nerve function.[220] In the vast majority of cases the clinical deficit is transient, with complete resolution noted within weeks to months after the procedure. In one prospective study, all injuries resolved within 5 months.[221] In another prospective study, almost all nerve deficits resolved within 12 months after CEA, although it was noted that two patients with recurrent laryngeal nerve dysfunction regained normal function at 20 and 50 months after CEA, respectively.[219]

Based on a review of outcomes of the ECST randomized prospective investigation, it was noted that the risk for permanent nerve injury was 0.5%.[221] In another report, the incidence of permanent cranial nerve injury was only 1.1%.[219] The disability resulting from cranial nerve injury varies from minimal to severe, depending on the nerve involved and mechanism of the operative insult.

Anatomic and Clinical Considerations

Iatrogenic injury to the cranial nerves results from the close anatomic proximity of these structures to the carotid bifurcation (Fig. 95-10). Most deficits are due to direct blunt injury during dissection, stretch trauma from excessive retraction, electrocoagulation damage, inexact placement of ligatures, or pressure injury secondary to postoperative hematoma formation. Cranial nerve injury is much more likely during reoperative surgery because of excessive scar formation.[217] In one recent detailed analysis, the incidence of cranial nerve dysfunction correlated with the duration of surgery. Specifically, there was a significantly higher incidence of nerve injury when the duration of CEA exceeded 2 hours.[221]

The incidence of cranial nerve injury is listed in Table 95-2 for the individual nerves described in the following paragraphs.

Hypoglossal Nerve. Hypoglossal nerve dysfunction, manifested by ipsilateral tongue weakness and deviation to the affected side with protrusion and difficulty masticating, is the most frequent cranial nerve deficit documented in most reports (see Table 95-2). The structure descends from the hypoglossal canal (anterior condylar foramen) medial to the ICA and then courses lateral to the ECA, usually several centimeters distal to the carotid bifurcation, although in rare cases it may cross at the carotid bifurcation.[225] In this situa-

Table 95-2 Incidence of Cranial Nerve Dysfunction after Carotid Endarterectomy

Nerve	Reported Incidence of Dysfunction (%)
Hypoglossal	4.4-17.5
Recurrent laryngeal	1.5-15
Superior laryngeal	1.8-4.5
Marginal mandibular	1.1-3.1
Glossopharyngeal	0.2-1.5
Spinal accessory	<1.0

Data from references 216-225.

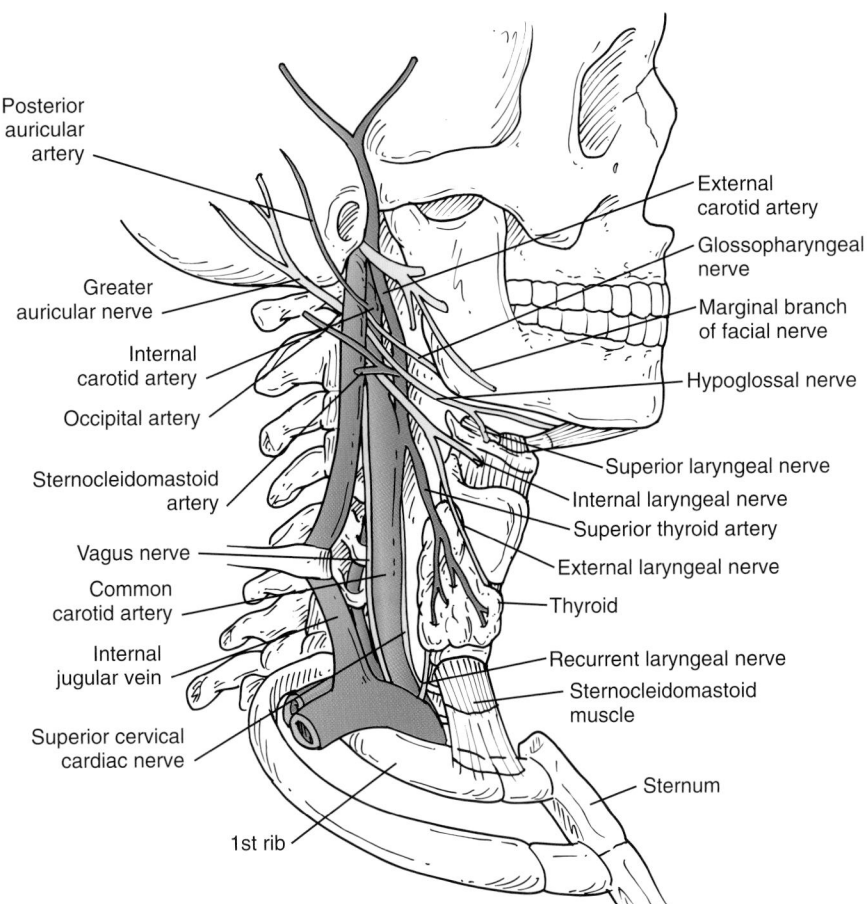

Figure 95-10 Relationship of the cranial nerves and their major branches to the common, internal, and external carotids in the neck. *(Reproduced from Eisele DW, Smith RV, eds.* Complications in Head and Neck Surgery. *Philadelphia, PA: Elsevier; 2009.)*

tion, if a patient has an unusually high carotid bifurcation or if atheromatous plaque extends well past the origin of the ICA, cephalad mobilization of the nerve is usually required for adequate operative exposure. In most cases mobilization can be accomplished safely without morbidity by division of the ansa hypoglossi. In other cases, division of tethering branches of the ECA or internal jugular vein is required, which increases the likelihood of transient injury. Although unilateral hypoglossal nerve injury is rarely serious, bilateral deficits have been associated with serious articulation and swallowing difficulty and upper airway obstruction requiring tracheotomy.[226] Therefore, it is important to assess the functional integrity of this nerve after CEA in a patient who is scheduled for early contralateral CEA.[220]

Vagus Nerve. The vagus nerve is easily identified within the carotid sheath posterior to the CCA, although in the occasional patient it may lie anterior to the carotid and be mistaken for the ansa hypoglossi. Before division of the latter structure, therefore, the vagus nerve should first be clearly identified. The recurrent laryngeal branch usually originates from the vagus within the mediastinum, loops around the subclavian artery on the right or the aortic arch on the left side, and passes cephalad in the tracheoesophageal groove

behind the strap muscles. In most cases this nerve is not in close proximity to the operative field and not likely to be directly injured. Typically, recurrent laryngeal nerve dysfunction results from vagus nerve trauma. In rare cases, the recurrent laryngeal nerve arises from the vagus at the level of the carotid bifurcation, the so-called nonrecurrent recurrent laryngeal nerve, and enters the larynx posterior to the CCA. Careful arterial dissection and clamp application should minimize the likelihood of vagus or recurrent laryngeal nerve injury, which results in paralysis of the ipsilateral vocal cord in the paramedian position and is manifested as hoarseness and loss of an effective cough mechanism. In occasional patients the vagus and hypoglossal nerves will be in apposition in the upper portion of the operative field, and no effort should be made to separate these structures to minimize the risk for injury. Patients who have previously undergone contralateral carotid, thyroid, or parathyroid surgery should have a careful examination of their vocal cords before CEA if there is any suggestion of recurrent laryngeal nerve injury because bilateral vocal cord paralysis may cause postoperative airway obstruction.

Superior Laryngeal Nerve. The superior laryngeal nerve originates from the vagus near the jugular foramen and passes obliquely to the larynx posterior to the ECA and ICA, where it divides into internal and external branches. It is not usually visualized during routine dissection for CEA and may be injured by injudicious clamping of the ICA or ECA. Injury to the external branch of the superior laryngeal nerve primarily results in loss of tensioning of the ipsilateral vocal cord and may be manifested clinically by early fatigability of the voice and difficulty with voice modulation at the high registers. Conversely, injury to the internal branch may result in decreased sensation at the laryngeal inlet and mild swallowing difficulty.[219]

Facial Nerve: Marginal Mandibular Branch.

Injury to the marginal mandibular branch of the facial nerve causes drooping of the ipsilateral lower lip. Although this may be cosmetically bothersome to the patient, it is of little functional significance. This nerve courses from the anterior border of the parotid gland between the platysma and deep cervical fascia across the masseter muscle and ramus of the mandible. It may be drawn into the operative field as the patient's head is turned to the opposite side and the chin is extended for exposure of the carotid bifurcation. Injury is usually due to excessive stretch from self-retaining retractors in a transverse cervical incision. When a longitudinal incision is used for CEA, angling the superior aspect of the incision posteriorly toward the mastoid process below the angle of the mandible will minimize the risk of injury to the nerve.[227]

Glossopharyngeal and Spinal Accessory Nerves.

Injury to the glossopharyngeal and spinal accessory nerves is exceedingly uncommon during CEA because of their anatomic location at the upper extent of the operative field. In rare cases in which excessive mobilization or division of the digastric muscle is required for distal ICA exposure, however, either nerve may be encountered and traumatized. The glossopharyngeal nerve provides sensory and motor innervation to the larynx. Symptoms of glossopharyngeal nerve injury range from mild dysphasia to recurrent aspiration.[219,222]

The spinal accessory nerve exits the jugular foramen, runs posterior to the stylohyoid muscle, and enters the most cephalic extent of the sternocleidomastoid muscle. Injury is manifested as shoulder droop and pain, scapular winging, and difficulty abducting the shoulder because of weakness of the trapezius muscle.[219,223]

Cutaneous Sensory Nerves.

Two important cutaneous sensory nerves that are not infrequently injured during the performance of CEA are the greater auricular and transverse cervical nerves. In one prospective study, the incidence of greater auricular and transverse cervical nerve injury was 60% and 69%, respectively, 1 week after CEA.[228] The greater auricular nerve courses along the most superior and the transverse cervical nerve along the most inferior area of the typical CEA longitudinal incision. Injury to the greater auricular nerve is manifested as numbness of the angle of the mandible and the lower part of the ear, and injury to the transverse cervical nerve is manifested as anesthesia of the anterior neck

skin. The latter outcome, though common, usually resolves over a 6- to 12-month period.

Hemodynamic Instability

Incidence and Etiology

If hypotension occurs after CEA, it usually does so within the first 2 hours after CEA, is generally associated with bradycardia, and most likely results from disordered baroreceptor function.[229-231] The carotid sinus baroreceptors, located in the outer muscle layer of the artery at the carotid bifurcation, transmit impulses through the carotid sinus nerve to the vasomotor center within the medulla. Carotid sinus stimulation inhibits central nervous system sympathetic activity with a subsequent reduction in heart rate and blood pressure.[232] Considerable evidence suggests that endarterectomy of fixed atheromatous plaque at the bifurcation, with its chronic dampening effect on pulse pressure, creates a heightened sensitivity of the baroreceptor mechanism that results in reduced central nervous system sympathetic activity with resultant hypotension or bradycardia, or both.[229,230,233,234] This theory is supported by the clinical observation that injection of the carotid sinus with local anesthetic reduces the incidence of this complication.[231] This reflex hypotension persists until the carotid sinus mechanism has been reset.[232]

Others have suggested that preoperative hypovolemia may be responsible in some cases.[233] Recent evidence suggests that patients with significant contralateral carotid disease have reduced baroreceptor reserve and therefore manifest more pronounced baroreceptor dysfunction and hemodynamic lability after CEA.[234]

Although the development of hypertension after CEA is closely correlated with preoperative hypertension, especially inadequately controlled hypertension, its mechanism remains poorly understood. Baroreceptor dysfunction as a result of enervation of the carotid bulb is commonly assumed to be responsible, although considerable evidence is accumulating to refute this hypothesis.[231,235] The association between preoperative hypertension and severe hypertensive episodes after CEA suggests that other possible mechanisms may be responsible, including elevated cerebral norepinephrine or renin production.[274,275] In at least 80% of patients this hypertensive response normalized within the first 24 hours, and in approximately 60% of patients it did so within the first 16 hours after surgery.[188]

Treatment

The episodic and generally unpredictable nature of post-CEA hypotension or hypertension is one of the more cogent reasons for observing the patient in a monitored unit after CEA, at least initially, with an indwelling radial artery catheter for systemic blood pressure monitoring. Hypotension should initially be treated by infusion of colloid solutions while a careful evaluation is conducted for any other causes of hypotension, including cardiac evaluation. Once normovolemia has been achieved, if hypotension persists with no other cause, we favor supporting blood pressure with an intravenous infusion of phenylephrine (Neo-Synephrine), an α-adrenergic agent, under the assumption that the hypotension is baroreceptor mediated. The dosage should be adjusted to maintain systolic blood pressure within at least 20 mm Hg of the preoperative level. In almost all cases the patient may be weaned from this vasoconstricting agent during the first postoperative day.

Conversely, in our opinion, postoperative hypertension is most effectively and safely treated with intravenous sodium nitroprusside, a direct relaxer of arterial smooth muscle. Its effect is immediate, and it is quickly dissipated by stopping the infusion, which makes it an ideal agent after CEA, when abrupt blood pressure fluctuations frequently occur. The agent should be titrated to maintain systolic pressure within 20 mm Hg of the preoperative level while avoiding sudden marked drops in pressure. If myocardial ischemia is associated with these hypertensive episodes, intravenous nitroglycerin should also be administered. Other cardiac issues might require different treatment, such as beta blockade when hypertension is accompanied by tachycardia. Most patients are able to resume their preoperative oral antihypertensive agents on the evening of surgery or within the next 12 hours, and this often obviates the need for further and more prolonged intravenous therapy.

Cerebral Hyperperfusion Syndrome

Cerebral hyperperfusion syndrome usually occurs several days after CEA and is often associated with severe hypertension, and the acute neurologic deficit is frequently preceded by severe headache. Intracerebral hemorrhage represents the most devastating manifestation of hyperperfusion syndrome that can occur after CEA and is clearly the most devastating etiology of stroke. The reported incidence of cerebral hyperperfusion syndrome ranges from 0.4% to 7.7% after CEA.[236,237] This complication is now also being recognized after CAS procedures as well.[238,239] Symptoms include a migraine-like headache progressing to seizures and, in its most severe manifestation, intracerebral hemorrhagic stroke. Though an infrequent complication of CEA and CAS, it is associated with a very high mortality rate that approaches 75% to 100% in some series.[240,241]

The cause of hyperperfusion syndrome appears to be increased regional cerebral blood flow secondary to disordered intracerebral autoregulation after relief of a high-grade carotid stenosis in the setting of severe contralateral carotid disease.[238] Recognition of patients at increased risk for intracerebral hemorrhage after CEA is easier than its prevention. Systemic hypertension appears to be an important risk factor. Therefore, strict attention to postoperative blood pressure control is paramount, especially in a patient who undergoes CEA for a high-grade stenosis contralateral to complete ICA occlusion or severe stenosis. There may be some association with the use of anticoagulants and antiplatelet agents, but this evidence is speculative at best. If cerebral hemorrhage occurs, neurosurgical consultation is required to determine the neces-

sity for craniotomy. Danish investigators have found that hyperperfusion syndrome can be predicted by a significant drop in pressure (>25%) across the carotid stenosis and that it is related to temporary loss of cerebral autoregulation as evidenced by a transient increase in mean arterial velocity of the ipsilateral MCA after CEA.[242-244] A study by Ascher and colleagues confirmed this latter finding and also found that CEA performed less than 3 months after contralateral CEA was associated with a higher risk for hyperperfusion syndrome.[245]

Other Complications

Infections

Unlike most peripheral vascular reconstructive procedures, in which chronic ischemia compromises wound healing and predisposes to infection, the vascular supply to the neck is rich, even in patients with severe atherosclerotic disease. Therefore, CEA is rarely associated with infectious complications. Difficulty in primary healing is occasionally seen when this operation is performed in a previously irradiated field but is almost nonexistent in the absence of this complicating factor.[217] The reported incidence of wound infection, generally cellulitis, ranges from 0.09% to 0.15%.[246,247]

The increasing use of synthetic patches to repair the arteriotomy after CEA raises potential concern about an increased incidence of infectious complications. However, although the true incidence of patch infection has not been established, it must be extremely rare and essentially a case report type of complication. In several studies not a single case of patch infection was documented.[247-249] In another comprehensive review of the literature, 57 carotid pseudoaneurysms were identified, and 40 were associated with carotid patches. However, only four (10%) were infectious in etiology.[249]

Bleeding

Postoperative hemorrhage is a relatively uncommon yet important complication of CEA. The reported incidence ranges from 0.7% to 3.0%.[212,233,250-252] Most cases result from diffuse capillary oozing secondary to administration of heparin during the procedure and the concomitant administration of antiplatelet drugs. Though not systematically studied, at least anecdotally this degree of oozing appears to be greater in patients who are taking the antiplatelet agent clopidogrel at the time of surgery. Nevertheless, if there are indications for the administration of this agent, such as a recent coronary stent procedure or symptomatic carotid disease, we would not stop clopidogrel before surgery. In general, unless bleeding appears excessive at surgery, we do not favor reversal of the heparin effect with protamine sulfate at completion of the procedure, but this practice varies widely (see "Protamine Administration").

If the neck incision has been closed over a suction drain, the acute onset of drainage of bright red blood postoperatively is suggestive of suture line disruption and is an indication for urgent re-exploration. Similarly, the development of a hematoma in the neck, often caused by inadequate function of the drain, may compress the trachea and is an indication for re-exploration of the wound. More gradual development of a neck hematoma usually results from inadequate ligature of facial veins or other muscle arterioles or venules.[217]

Recurrent Carotid Stenosis

One of the more important arterial complications of CEA is the development of recurrent carotid stenosis. The incidence of this complication depends on the definition of recurrent stenosis, method of diagnosis, and duration of follow-up. It has been estimated to occur in 5% to 22% of patients in several published institutional series, although only approximately 3% of these lesions were symptomatic.[68,253-256] In a meta-analysis of 55 reports, the overall incidence of recurrent carotid stenosis after CEA was 6% to 14%, which reflected an annual incidence of restenosis or occlusion of 1.5% to 4.5%.[257] In another analysis of the MEDLINE database, the rate of restenosis was 10% within the first year, 3% in the second, and 2% in the third year after CEA, thus suggesting that the rate of restenosis is clearly not a linear process biologically.[258]

Within the first 36 months after CEA, recurrent stenosis usually results from intimal hyperplasia. Evidence from serial duplex evaluation suggests that at least some of these lesions regress with time, and in part this regression may be responsible for some variability in the reported rates of recurrent stenosis. An occasional "recurrent" stenosis in fact represents residual arteriosclerotic disease after the endarterectomy. Lesions that develop more than a few years after CEA generally result from progressive or new arteriosclerotic disease.

Recurrent stenoses develop more frequently in women, in patients who continue to smoke, and in hypercholesterolemic, diabetic, and hypertensive individuals.[254] It has also been suggested that intraoperative injury secondary to arterial clamping, insertion of an intraluminal shunt, or placement of tacking sutures within the vessel may also predispose to early myointimal hyperplastic lesions.[253] As noted earlier, there is compelling evidence that closure of the arteriotomy with a patch will reduce the incidence of recurrent stenosis, although the optimal patch material remains to be identified.

Long-term follow-up of 950 CEAs performed at the Massachusetts General Hospital demonstrated that reintervention was required in 3.8% of patients with a cumulative follow-up of 4.5 years. There was no difference in restenosis rates between patients who underwent patch closure and eversion endarterectomy.[85] In another series that included 1150 patients, 98.8% were free of occlusion or restenosis greater than 70% at a mean follow-up of 74 months after CEA.[259] In the EVEREST trial, the only large randomized trial to compare eversion and standard endarterectomy, life-table estimates of the cumulative risk for restenosis at 4 years after eversion, patch closure, and primary closure were 3.5%, 1.7%, and 12.6%, respectively.[81] The difference in restenosis rates between eversion and patch closure was not statistically significant.

Repeat Carotid Endarterectomy

Repeat carotid endarterectomy presents additional challenges with dissection and reconstruction that can increase the risk over that associated with a primary procedure, but with careful planning and technique, excellent results can be achieved in this situation as well. Early recurrent stenosis usually develops within 2 years of CEA and typically results from intimal hyperplasia, an inflammatory response that produces a firm, rubbery plaque rich in fibroblasts and smooth muscle cells surrounded by dense accumulation of collagen and acid mucopolysaccharide, and it typically develops within the endarterectomy bed (see Chapter 5: Intimal Hyperplasia). It is much less prone to ulceration or thromboembolic complications. Regression of these lesions is not uncommon and is observed in as many as a third or more of cases.[260,261] Later restenoses typically have features of atheromatous plaque and are more widely distributed along the carotid artery. There are no prospective randomized trials to support repeat CEA, but most available evidence supports treatment of symptomatic and very high grade asymptomatic recurrent stenosis.[253,262]

Scarring typically makes the dissection more technically difficult such that a higher incidence of cranial nerve injury and hematoma has been reported.[263] In addition, the more extensive disease within the carotid artery may necessitate carotid artery replacement with an interposition graft. This is technically more difficult, may preclude shunting, and could be associated with longer periods of cerebral ischemia, possibly leading to higher perioperative stroke rates.[263] However, repeat endarterectomy is often possible, even after eversion endarterectomy.[264]

Carotid Artery Stenting versus Repeat Carotid Endarterectomy

The increased technical difficulty and higher complication rate anticipated with repeat CEA has led some to advocate CAS as an alternative to CEA for recurrent stenosis. However, AbuRahma and coauthors reported lower perioperative stroke rates with repeat CEA than with CAS for recurrent stenosis, as well as significantly lower rates of recurrent stenosis after CEA; at 48 months, 100% of patients were free of restenosis after CEA versus 52% after CAS.[265] Similarly, Bowser and associates reported lower stroke and death rates in 27 repeat CEAs than in 52 CAS procedures performed for recurrent stenosis (3.7% versus 5.7%), although this difference was not statistically significant.[266] In fact, during the last decade several centers have reported excellent results with repeat CEA. Stoner and colleagues recently reported their experience with 153 repeat CEAs over a 14-year period: no mortality or myocardial infarction, a 1.9% incidence of stroke, a 1.3% incidence of cranial nerve injury, and a 3.2% incidence of hematoma.[267] Two thirds of patients who underwent reoperation had their carotid artery closed primarily during their first CEA. Similarly excellent results have been reported by Archie[268] and by Cho and coworkers[269] in smaller series of patients.

In summary, repeat CEA is a viable therapeutic option that should be considered for symptomatic and asymptomatic high-grade recurrent stenosis. Although one should anticipate increased technical difficulty with dissection and reconstruction, including possibly the need for an interposition graft, good results can be expected.

SPECIAL CONSIDERATIONS

Combined Carotid Endarterectomy/ Cardiac Surgery

Significant carotid disease occurs in approximately 3% to 14% of patients undergoing cardiac surgery, and prospective studies of patients undergoing cardiac surgery conducted in the 1980s demonstrated that significant carotid disease (>50% stenosis) conveyed a higher risk for perioperative stroke and mortality,[270] as well as long-term stroke and mortality,[271] than in those without significant carotid disease. Carotid occlusions in particular are associated with increased perioperative events, and the extent of disease in the contralateral artery correlates directly with the risk for perioperative mortality; the presence of a high-grade (>60%) stenosis contralateral to a carotid occlusion may be associated with perioperative stroke rates as high as 25%.[272] Between 1970 and 2000, Naylor and colleagues found that the risk for stroke after coronary artery bypass grafting (CABG) was 2% overall—less than 2% in patients without carotid disease, 3% in asymptomatic patients with unilateral 50% to 99% stenosis, 5% in those with bilateral 50% to 99% stenosis, and 7% to 11% in patients with carotid occlusion. However, the authors noted that 50% of CABG patients who experienced a stroke did not have significant carotid disease and that 60% of territorial infarctions on CT scan/autopsy could not be attributed to carotid disease alone. They estimated that CEA could prevent only about 40% to 50% of perioperative strokes in this patient population.[273]

Simultaneous Carotid Endarterectomy and Coronary Artery Bypass Grafting

A strategy pursued to reduce the risk for stroke has been to perform simultaneous CEA and CABG. A prospective randomized trial performed at the Cleveland Clinic demonstrated a significantly lower stroke risk in patients undergoing combined CEA/CABG versus staged CABG followed by CEA, a stroke rate of 14% versus 2.8%, respectively, although mortality was not significantly different. The stroke rate was much higher if CEA was performed early after CABG than at later intervals.[274] Numerous other published studies have shown good results by applying combined CEA/CABG in appropriately selected patients, with perioperative stroke and mortality rates as low as 2% to 5%,[275-282] as well as good long-term freedom from stroke.[278,280]

In contrast, other studies have documented increased morbidity from combined CEA/CABG. Coyle and associates found that combined CEA/CABG had a perioperative stroke/

mortality rate of 26% versus 6.6% with delayed coronary bypass.[283] Similarly, Giangola and coworkers found that CABG should precede CEA instead of combining the procedures.[284] In addition, a recent study that presumably included modern medical management of cardiovascular disease did not show any disadvantage with CABG alone in patients with carotid disease versus staged CEA followed by CABG.[285] A study at the Johns Hopkins Hospital found little utility in combined CEA/CABG but did find value in selective carotid screening.[286]

Furthermore, meta-analyses have also suggested that combined CEA/CABG does not confer any advantage. Borger and coauthors reviewed 16 studies consisting of 1764 patients, two of which showed statistically higher morbidity with combined CEA/CABG, and overall there was a trend toward higher risk for the endpoints of stroke and death; the crude event rates for stroke were 6.0% versus 3.2% for combined versus staged procedures, 4.7% versus 2.9% for death, and 9.5% versus 5.7% for stroke or death, respectively.[287] Naylor and colleagues reviewed 97 published studies and found no significant difference in outcomes for staged and synchronous procedures.[288] Mortality was highest in patients undergoing synchronous CEA/CABG (4.6%; 95% confidence interval, 4.1 to 5.2). Reverse staged procedures (CABG-CEA) were associated with the highest risk for ipsilateral stroke (5.8%) and any stroke (6.3%). Perioperative myocardial infarction was lowest after the reverse staged procedure (0.9%) and highest in patients undergoing staged CEA-CABG (6.5%). The risk for death with or without any stroke was highest in patients undergoing synchronous CEA-CABG (8.7%) and lowest after staged CEA/CABG (6.1%). The risk of death/ stroke or myocardial infarction was 11.5% after synchronous procedures versus 10.2% after staged CEA and then CABG. In a related paper they found that the risk for death/stroke appeared to significantly diminish in studies published after 1993.[289] Patients with severe bilateral carotid disease were significantly more likely to suffer death or stroke (or both) than were patients with unilateral disease. Similarly, patients with a previous history of stroke/TIA were significantly more likely to suffer a further stroke than were asymptomatic patients. In one series including 834 patients, combined CEA/ CABG had a combined stroke/mortality rate of 4.3% in patients with asymptomatic and 6.1% in those with symptomatic carotid disease.[290]

Reviewing community-wide outcomes of randomly selected patients from a U.S. Medicare database that included 10 states and more than 10,000 CEAs, Brown and associates found that the combined stroke and death rate for 226 patients who underwent combined CEA/CABG was 17.7% (25 nonfatal strokes, 2 fatal strokes, and 13 non–stroke-associated deaths). Eighty percent of the nonfatal strokes were disabling. Proximal aortic arch atherosclerosis and symptomatic carotid stenosis were associated with stroke ($P < .05$). Female gender, emergency surgery, repeat CABG, blood pressure on pump, total pump time, presence of left main disease, and the number of diseased coronary arteries were associated with mortality ($P < .05$). Most strokes were not limited to the hemisphere ipsilateral to the CEA. The community-wide outcomes of combined CEA/CABG in the Medicare population are inferior to those reported in many single-institution reviews.[291]

In addition, off-pump coronary artery bypass (OPCAB) has been introduced as an alternative method for coronary bypass, and outstanding results have been published on combined CEA/OPCAB, with combined stroke and mortality rates of 0% to 1.2%.[277,292]

Carotid Artery Stenting before Coronary Artery Bypass Grafting

The introduction of CAS has provided another therapeutic option for managing coexisting carotid and cardiac disease (see Chapter 96: Carotid Artery: Stenting). Ziada and coworkers found that performing CAS followed by cardiac surgery was associated with a significantly lower incidence of stroke or myocardial infarction than after combined procedures (5% versus 19%, $P = .02$).[293] However, Abassi and colleagues did not find an advantage with staged CAS and CABG versus combined CEA/CABG.[294] A review of six studies by Guzman that included 227 patients found that morbidity and mortality were still high.[295] Specifically, the incidence of stroke and death associated with the stent procedure was 4.7%, the incidence of stroke with CABG was 2.2%, and the overall combined 30-day event rate after CABG, including all events during CAS, was as follows: minor stroke, 2.9%; major stroke, 3.2%; mortality, 7.6%; and combined death and any stroke, 12.3%.

Using the National Inpatient Sample database, Timaran and colleagues found CAS-CABG safer than CEA/CABG.[296] During a 5-year period, 27,084 concurrent carotid revascularization and CABG procedures were performed; 96.7% of the procedures were CEA/CABG, whereas only 3.3% (887 patients) were CAS-CABG. Patients undergoing CAS-CABG had fewer major adverse events than did those undergoing CEA-CABG, with a lower incidence of postoperative stroke (2.4% versus 3.9%) and combined stroke and death (6.9% versus 8.6%) than in the combined CEA/CABG group ($P < .001$). In-hospital death rates were similar (5.2% versus 5.4%). After risk stratification, CEA/CABG patients had a 62% increased risk for postoperative stroke when compared with patients undergoing CAS before CABG, but no differences in the risk for combined stroke and death were observed. Patients who undergo CAS-CABG have experienced significantly lower in-hospital stroke rates than have patients undergoing CEA/CABG but similar in-hospital mortality.

Summary

In summary, combined CEA/CABG should be used only in centers with good results to justify this approach. Otherwise, a staged approach with CEA followed by CABG, combined CEA/OPCAB, or CAS followed by CABG may provide safer carotid revascularization options for patients who require CABG.

Advanced Age

The prevalence of stroke increases exponentially with advancing age, and the elderly population is the fastest growing segment of the population. Therefore, one would assume that it is the elderly who can most benefit from CEA. In fact, patients 80 years and older were excluded from NASCET and ACAS, and it has therefore been assumed that advanced age represents a high-risk factor for CEA and that such patients might thus be optimally treated by CAS. However, compelling evidence accumulated over the past 2 decades has confirmed the safety of CEA in elderly individuals. In a recent meta-analysis that included more than 20 institutional series and over 3000 elderly patients with a minimum age of 75 or 80 who underwent CEA, the perioperative stroke rate was 2.2% and the mortality rate was 1.5%.[297] In a population-based analysis of CEA in the state of Maryland from 1990 through 1995, the outcome in octogenarians was the same as in younger patient cohorts (perioperative stroke and death rate of 2.6%).[298] In another study the perioperative mortality rate was higher in nonagenarians than octogenarians, although there was no difference in neurologic outcomes.[299] However, because CEA is a prophylactic operation designed to prevent stroke, it will be most beneficial in patients with long life expectancy such that the lower future stroke risk overcomes the initial operative morbidity and mortality. However, studies have shown that long-term results in octogenarians can be surprisingly good. In an Italian study of 345 CEAs performed on 269 octogenarians, although the operative mortality of 1.4% was significantly higher than that in younger patients, it was still acceptable, and 6-year overall and stroke-free survival rates were 86% and 76%, respectively.[300] A Canadian study similarly reported a 5-year survival rate of 72% and a 90% stroke-free survival rate.[301] Meanwhile, a study of 182 CEAs in octogenarians from the Cleveland Clinic compared less favorably—5-year survival and stroke-free survival rates were just 45% and 42%, respectively.[302] These differences suggest that CEA can be an effective operation in the elderly if patients are selected appropriately.

Gender

There are conflicting reports of the impact of gender on the outcome of CEA. In ACAS, for example, women received less benefit in terms of stroke prevention than did men in that they had more strokes in both the perioperative period and long-term follow-up.[11] Other studies have shown no difference in outcomes between men and women.[303] One population-based study examined 14,095 CEAs performed in Virginia between 1997 and 2001 and demonstrated that female gender was not an independent predictor of a higher stroke or death rate.[304] Likewise, investigators in Ontario found no difference in perioperative complication rates between men and women in a review of 6038 CEA patients, 35% of whom were women.[305] Even though female gender has not been shown to increase the risk associated with CEA in large population-based studies such as these, consideration of anatomic (i.e., smaller arteries) and physiologic (i.e., later age at initial consultation) factors is prudent when performing CEA on women.

Race

The study of the impact of race on CEA outcomes has also demonstrated conflicting results. Lucas and associates examined national Medicare data to determine postoperative mortality after eight specific cardiovascular and cancer operations between 1994 and 1999. African American patients in this study had crude mortality rates higher than 20% in seven of the eight procedures, including CEA. The study suggests multiple reasons for this finding, including more frequent emergency operations and residence in low-income areas. Additionally, African Americans were more likely to receive care in lower volume hospitals and hospitals with overall higher mortality.[306] Likewise, a 2002 meta-analysis demonstrated a 40% greater likelihood of short-term death after CEA for African Americans than for whites undergoing CEA.[307] In our review of the Maryland state database, African American patients undergoing CEA had an increased incidence of in-hospital stroke, longer hospital stays, and higher hospital charges. This research noted that African American patients were more likely to undergo CEA in low-volume hospitals and less likely to be treated by higher volume surgeons.[308]

However, Horner and colleagues' review of the NSQIP data revealed similarly low stroke and death rates between African American and white patients in the VA system. In patients with TIA, though, Hispanic males experienced significantly worse outcomes in terms of stroke and death when compared with white patients.[309] An institutional review from Henry Ford Hospital revealed similar stroke and death rates between African American and whites, as well as acceptable protection from ipsilateral stroke without racial variation. African American patients in this study did, however, have a higher incidence of all strokes in the long term than did white cohorts.[310]

The influence of race on the outcome of CEA merits further research. It is not clear at this time whether race or associated limitations in access to care are more robust factors influencing outcomes. Nevertheless, there is strong evidence that CEA can be performed safely on African American patients in the United States in contemporary practice.

External Carotid Endarterectomy

It has been recognized for more than 30 years that in the setting of ICA occlusion, atherosclerotic disease of the ipsilateral ECA can result in embolic stroke through the various collateral pathways that exist between the external carotid and intracranial circulation.[311] Numerous authors have reported small series of patients treated successfully for symptomatic ECA stenoses with ECA endarterectomy.[312-319] In larger series the perioperative stroke rate has varied from 0% to 10%[318,320] but was as high as 33% to 38% in patients with contralateral disease and previous stroke or if ECA endarterectomy was combined with adjunctive procedures. On long-term follow-up with angiography or duplex ultrasonography, Rush and coworkers found that two thirds of ECAs closed primarily occluded or developed significant stenoses versus none with patch angioplasty.[321] The best results were seen in patients with monocular amaurosis fugax related to microembolism from the ECA.

In a review of 195 ECA endarterectomies and 23 ECA bypasses, resolution of symptoms was seen in 83% of patients, with another 7% showing marked improvement. The perioperative mortality rate was 3%, mostly secondary to stroke, and the overall neurologic complication rate was 5%. A diseased contralateral carotid artery was associated with higher neurologic morbidity, whereas disease in the vertebral arteries had no impact on outcome. The best results were obtained when surgery was performed to relieve specific hemispheric or retinal symptoms as opposed to nonspecific neurologic complaints or previous stroke.[321] There is no evidence that ECA endarterectomy should be performed prophylactically for asymptomatic disease. Therefore, it remains a rarely performed operation that is reserved for symptomatic patients only.

Impact of Radiation Therapy

An uncommon but challenging clinical problem is presented by a patient with carotid stenosis who has undergone cervical irradiation. Several small surgical series dealing with this topic have been published, the largest of which is the most recently published French series of Lesèche and associates, which consisted of 30 cases.[322] They summarized their experience along with 77 cases published by other authors; the overall stroke and mortality rate for this entire cohort was 2%. Restenosis and recurrent stroke were not commonly encountered. The mean interval between cervical irradiation and CEA was 10 years in the French series. Bypasses from either the CCA or the subclavian artery were required to reconstruct the carotid artery in a third of their cases; in their experience it was not necessary to use any kind of tissue advancement flaps to achieve wound healing. In the only other sizable surgical series, the University of California, Los Angeles, experience published in 1999 (26 cases), bypasses were rarely performed, whereas tissue flaps were used more frequently.[323] The mean time interval between irradiation and CEA in that series was even longer, 17 years. Therefore, it would appear that radiation-induced carotid stenosis is mostly an issue in long-term survivors after cervical irradiation, and it can be effectively managed with carotid surgery.

Hospital/Surgeon Volume

In contemporary practice many have advocated regionalization of specialized care or high-risk procedures (or both) to higher volume centers. In this regard, some have proposed that CEA, like many other high-risk cardiovascular procedures, should be performed exclusively at centers with higher volume. Likewise, proponents of regionalization argue that CEA is performed best by high-volume surgeons. A meta-analysis published in 2007 suggests that the stroke and death rate is significantly lower in high-volume centers, with a critical volume threshold of 79 CEAs per year. Interestingly, this study demonstrated that patients undergoing operations performed by lower volume surgeons operating in higher volume centers also experienced lower stroke and death rates, thus suggesting that the hospital infrastructure and available resources rather than surgeon experience were more important in lowering complication rates.[324] Other population-based studies have shown similar trends of mortality being inversely proportional to volume. In California between 1982 and 1994, mortality rates decreased for CEA, lower extremity bypass, and unruptured abdominal aortic aneurysm repair, and higher hospital volume was found to be an important determinant of outcome.[325]

However, conflicting data exist regarding volume and outcomes. A retrospective review of CEAs performed in Oregon over a 2-year period examined the outcomes between two low-volume institutions (total of 156 CEAs) and one high-volume institution (404 CEAs). In this study there was no significant difference in 30-day stroke and death rates between the low- and high-volume centers.[326] This was observed despite the fact that the low-volume centers had significantly older patients, more smokers, and fewer asymptomatic patients. This paper makes a legitimate point that an individual surgeon in a low-volume institution may perform more individual high-risk procedures than another individual surgeon at a higher volume center.

Ultimately, it should be recognized that it is surgeons and not hospitals that perform surgery. Furthermore, the ideal break point to define a suitably "high-volume" caseload remains to be defined. It was recognized 15 years ago that the efficacy of CEA depends on good surgical outcomes, which led the American Heart Association to publish consensus guidelines in 1995 stating that CEA should not be performed unless the combined risk of stroke and mortality was less than 6% in symptomatic patients and 3% in asymptomatic patients.[327] Therefore, each surgeon must strive to use careful surgical technique and good judgment in patient selection to achieve such results. Since that time, the large amount of data that have been published on CEA outcomes from institutional series, as well as massive hospital and government databases, much of which has been summarized in this chapter, would suggest that vascular surgeons both individually and as a group have been tremendously successful in achieving these goals. As a result, CEA continues to be an effective treatment of carotid disease more than 50 years after it was introduced by Eastcott, Pickering, and Rob and

is the treatment with which all future therapies must be compared.

SELECTED KEY REFERENCES

Barnett HJ, Taylor DW, Eliasziw M, Fox AJ, Ferguson GG, Haynes RB, Rankin RN, Clagett GP, Hachinski VC, Sackett DL, Thorpe KE, Meldrum HE, Spence JD. Benefit of carotid endarterectomy in patients with symptomatic moderate or severe stenosis. *N Engl J Med.* 1998;339:1415-1425.
NIH-funded multicenter prospective randomized trial that demonstrated the superiority of CEA and best medical therapy over best medical therapy alone for patients with moderate-grade (50% to 69%) symptomatic internal carotid stenosis.

Beneficial effect of carotid endarterectomy in symptomatic patients with high-grade carotid stenosis. North American Symptomatic Carotid Endarterectomy Trial Collaborators. *N Engl J Med.* 1991;325:445-453.
NIH-funded multicenter prospective randomized trial that demonstrated the superiority of CEA and best medical therapy over best medical therapy alone for patients with high-grade (70% to 99%) symptomatic internal carotid stenosis.

Cao P, Giordano G, De Rango P, Zannetti S, Chiesa R, Coppi G, Palombo D, Peinetti F, Spartera C, Stancanelli V, Vecchiati E. Eversion versus conventional carotid endarterectomy: late results of a prospective multicenter randomized trial. *J Vasc Surg.* 2000;31:19-30.
Long-term follow-up of a randomized prospective clinical trial comparing eversion CEA with standard CEA and either primary closure or patch closure; the trial demonstrated that eversion endarterectomy is safe and effective and provides anatomic outcomes equivalent to those of standard CEA with patch closure.

Executive Committee for the Asymptomatic Carotid Atherosclerosis Study. Endarterectomy for asymptomatic carotid artery stenosis. *JAMA.* 1995;273:1421-1428.
NIH-funded multicenter prospective randomized trial that demonstrated the superiority of CEA and best medical management over best medical management alone for patients with asymptomatic 60% to 99% internal carotid stenosis.

GALA Trial Collaborative Group. General anaesthesia versus local anaesthesia for carotid surgery (GALA): a multicentre, randomised controlled trial. *Lancet.* 2008;372:2132-2142.
Multicenter controlled trial of 3526 patients with symptomatic or asymptomatic carotid stenosis randomized to either general or local anesthesia for CEA; the trial failed to show a benefit of either anesthetic method.

Halliday A, Mansfield A, Marro J, Peto C, Peto R, Potter J, Thomas D; MRC Asymptomatic Carotid Surgery Trial (ACST) Collaborative Group. Prevention of disabling and fatal strokes by successful carotid endarterectomy in patients without recent neurological symptoms: randomised controlled trial. *Lancet.* 2004;363:1491-1502.
European multicenter randomized prospective clinical trial that confirmed the ACAS findings, namely, the superiority of CEA and best medical management over best medical management alone for patients with asymptomatic 60% to 99% internal carotid stenosis.

Naylor AR, Cuffe RL, Rothwell PM, Bell PRF. A systematic review of outcomes following staged and synchronous carotid endarterectomy and coronary artery bypass. *Eur J Vasc Endovasc Surg.* 2003;25:380-389.
A comprehensive review of staged versus synchronous CEA and CABG.

REFERENCES

The reference list can be found on the companion Expert Consult Web site at *www.expertconsult.com.*

CHAPTER 96

Carotid Artery Disease: Stenting

Piergiorgio Cao and Paola De Rango

In 1977 and 1980, Mathias and colleagues[1,2] and Kerber and coauthors[3] reported successful results with percutaneous angioplasty for carotid stenosis by using technology derived from peripheral arterial angioplasty. The technique developed rapidly during the subsequent years. Balloon-expandable stents were first deployed in the carotid artery in 1989 but were prone to extrinsic compression and had a high rate of major adverse events.[4-6] These issues were resolved by using self-expanding mesh wire Elgiloy carotid stents and later nitinol stents.[7] Prevention of embolic stroke was the major concern that limited early enthusiasm for endovascular treatment of carotid arteries. The first report on the use of cerebral protection devices (CPDs) was attributed to Theron and associates in 1990, who used an occlusive balloon in the distal carotid artery,[8] after which antiembolic protection technology developed rapidly.

In recent years, proponents have stressed the apparent simplicity of carotid artery stenting (CAS) in comparison to carotid endarterectomy (CEA). Its feasibility in nonsurgical settings has accelerated use of the procedure as an alternative to surgery. However, the future role of CAS is still debated and will hopefully be determined by several ongoing randomized clinical trials (RCTs).

■ CASE SELECTION

Recommendations for carotid revascularization are based primarily on symptoms and the severity of the carotid stenosis.[9,10]

There is a large body of evidence available for CEA but not for CAS. To what extent the selection criteria derived for carotid surgery can be applied to carotid stenting is widely debated, with detractors excluding any endoluminal treatment in the carotid territory and the most enthusiastic interventionists arguing that all indications for carotid surgery can be extended to CAS.

Clearly, minimizing the incidence of complications and improving outcomes of CAS depend on how patients are selected to undergo the procedure and identification of factors that have been associated with increased periprocedural risk.[11-13]

Clinical Considerations

In some clinical situations, such as severe cardiac or pulmonary co-morbidity, CEA might be considered risky, and CAS appears to be more suitable. However, none of these conditions are absolute, and they should be balanced against other unfavorable risk factors for endovascular treatment.

Symptomatic Patients and Timing

It is well accepted that candidates for carotid surgery include patients with symptoms associated with carotid stenosis ranging from 70% to 99% and in selected cases from 50% to 70%, provided that perioperative risk is less than 6%.[9] Two recent European RCTs have compared CAS and CEA (the Endarterectomy versus Stenting in Patients with Symptomatic Severe Carotid Stenosis [EVA-3S] and Stent-Supported Percutaneous Angioplasty of the Carotid Artery versus Endarterectomy [SPACE] trials), and both suggest higher risk with CAS in symptomatic patients.[14,15] In particular, the French EVA-3S study reported a twofold increase in relative risk associated with CAS as opposed to CEA.

Analysis of pooled data from RCTs on carotid surgery has shown that the benefit from CEA is higher when it is performed within the first 2 to 4 weeks after the appearance of symptoms.[16] The benefits of CEA decline rapidly with delay and are reduced by half when surgery is postponed beyond 2 weeks, with an even greater reduction after 4 weeks. Data are conflicting whether this decline in benefit applies to CAS.[17,18] Topakian and coworkers analyzed the effect of timing in 77 CAS patients and identified old age and treatment within 2 weeks as the only predictors of increased risk for 30-day complications; they reported an unacceptable stroke and death rate of 26% versus 1.9% in those treated later.[17] In a series of 57 patients undergoing CAS between 24 and 48 hours of the last transient ischemic attack (TIA) or between 14 and 30 days after minor stroke, Setacci and coauthors reported a 30-day adverse event rate as low as 1.7%, with only one death and no strokes.[18] Management of patients by CAS in the first 2 weeks after the onset of stroke is a challenge to be resolved by larger studies.

Asymptomatic Patients

The results of RCTs comparing CEA with medical treatment in patients without symptoms during the previous 6 months suggested a reduction in risk for stroke with surgery as opposed to a very low incidence of neurologic events with the best medical treatment. Therefore, it is generally accepted that CEA should be offered to patients with severe vessel stenosis, provided that their perioperative risk is below 3%.[9,10] The decision to treat these asymptomatic low-risk patients with CAS is still vigorously debated and depends on a very low periprocedural complication rate. Essentially, comprehensive evaluation of patient co-morbid conditions and case-by-case selection should be undertaken.

Age

One of the most challenging age groups with respect to clinical decision making is patients older than 80 years. Epidemiologic studies have shown that the risk for stroke increases with advanced age and is approximately 22.4% in octogenarians.[19] Because these patients have a relatively short life expectancy, any benefit from revascularization may be limited by increased medical co-morbid diseases. Although CAS is a less invasive approach, older patients frequently have extensive atherosclerotic disease that translates into more frequently encountered vessel tortuosity, diffuse calcification, "shaggy" arches, and impaired cerebrovascular reserve. Most of the data indicate that the rate of complications after CAS is higher in patients older than 80 years. In the lead-in phase of the largest ongoing multicenter RCT comparing CAS and CEA (the Carotid Revascularization Endarterectomy versus Stenting Trial [CREST]), the 30-day risk for stroke or death in 1479 patients undergoing CAS was directly related to age: 2.2% in those 60 to 69 years, 5.4% in those 70 to 79 years, and 11.3% in those older than 80 years. Today, there are compelling data supporting CEA rather than CAS in the treatment of octogenarians.[20] A post hoc analysis of potential risk factors for stroke and death within 30 days in patients randomized in the SPACE trial showed that age was the only variable that significantly increased risk in the CAS group. In particular, patients older than 75 years had an event rate of 10.9% as compared with 2.1% in patients younger than 62 years.[21]

Conversely, younger patients may have a more favorable natural history, longer life expectancy, and lower CAS periprocedural risk. Shortcomings involve the durability of CAS and its efficacy in preventing stroke because no data are yet available with follow-up lengths comparable to those with CEA.

Women

Women are less likely than men to benefit from CEA according to RCTs on symptomatic and asymptomatic patients. These poorer results are due to higher perioperative stroke and death rates, which are nearly twice as high in women compared with men (10.4% versus 5.8%, respectively, according to the European Carotid Surgery Trial [ECST]; 3.6% versus 1.7% according to the Asymptomatic Carotid Atherosclerosis Study [ACAS]),[22,23] and lower stroke risk reduction in the long term: in asymptomatic women the 5-year relative reduction in risk was 17%, versus 66% in men in the ACAS, and the absolute reduction in risk was 4.08%, versus 8.21%

in men according to the Asymptomatic Carotid Surgery Trial [ACST].[23,24]

Whether these results in women after CEA are applicable to CAS remains a subject of investigation because studies addressing this issue exclude any significant differences in outcome between genders.[21,25]

Combined Coronary Artery Disease

Approximately 50% of patients undergoing CEA have clinically relevant coronary artery disease, and cardiac death is the most common cause of mortality in patients with carotid stenosis.[26,27] Data from the North American Symptomatic Carotid Endarterectomy Trial (NASCET), which excluded patients with unstable angina and recent myocardial infarction (MI), showed an overall cardiovascular complication rate of 8.1% after CEA; this rate may be underestimated and hide an even higher rate of complications in common practice.[28] As an alternative and because it is less invasive, CAS has been evaluated in patients with severe cardiac co-morbidity. The randomized Stenting and Angioplasty with Protection in Patients at High Risk for Endarterectomy (SAPPHIRE) trial compared CEA with CAS in 334 patients at high risk for open surgery and reported lower rates of the composite endpoint (stroke, death, and MI) with CAS than with CEA at 1 year (12% versus 20%; $P = .053$). However, this favorable outcome in CAS was due to the rates of MI (3.0% versus 7.5%) more than the rates of stroke (6.2% versus 7.9%).[29]

The relationship between coronary disease and carotid stenosis is also emphasized by the high prevalence of carotid disease (9% to 28%) in patients referred for coronary artery bypass grafting (CABG).[30-34] Combined or staged performance of CABG and CEA has been associated with an increased likelihood of perioperative stroke, death, and MI when compared with solitary CEA.[33-35]

In this regard, conflicting results have been reported in patients undergoing CAS immediately before CABG. Ziada and associates reported a lower incidence of adverse events in patients undergoing CAS and heart surgery than in those undergoing combined CEA and cardiac surgery (5% versus 19%, respectively).[36] Similar results were reported by Van der Heyden and colleagues in a single-center experience of 356 patients undergoing CAS and CABG (6.7% rate of stroke/death and MI) without a control group.[37] However, a cumulative 30-day stroke and death rate as high as 12%, similar to that in studies on CEA and CABG, was found in a meta-analysis by Guzman and collaborators, who evaluated pooled data from 277 patients after undergoing staged CAS and CABG.[38]

Important issues in the strategy of performing carotid and cardiac revascularization include (1) minimizing the delay between CAS and open heart surgery to reduce the risk for cardiac death in unstable patients and (2) avoiding the risk of increased bleeding at the time of CABG from the dual antiplatelet regimen after CAS.

Management of these patients can be summarized as follows:

- Patients with chronic stable angina undergoing CAS should have cardiac surgery delayed for 3 to 4 weeks and should continue dual antiplatelet therapy until 5 days before the procedure.
- Patients who require urgent coronary revascularization may undergo CABG after successful CAS regardless of dual antiplatelet treatment[37,39-43] if only aspirin is used and clopidogrel is started immediately after surgery[41,42] or if short-acting glycoprotein IIb/IIIa inhibitors are used during CAS and CABG is delayed for 4 to 6 hours.[38,40]

Other Subgroups

Decreased Cerebral Reserve. Poor cerebral reserve has been recognized as another unfavorable factor that increases the risk associated with CAS. Indeed, although carotid revascularization is associated with some degree of cerebral embolization, the rate and extent of embolism are significantly higher with CAS than with CEA, although most of the time the embolism remains silent.[44-46] Microembolization is well tolerated in patients with good cerebral reserve, but the consequence can be amplified in the presence of a hemisphere lacking good collateral support. Therefore, patients with previous strokes, lacunar infarcts, or dementia of varying stages may be more likely to experience neurologic deficits after CAS.[13]

Chronic Renal Insufficiency. In patients with asymptomatic carotid stenosis, chronic renal insufficiency (CRI) is a known risk factor for the occurrence of a first-time stroke.[47,48] A higher rate of periprocedural complications in patients with CRI has been shown after CAS, as well as after CEA. Therefore, the presence of CRI should increase the threshold for intervention, particularly in asymptomatic patients. Preoperative intravenous hydration with renal-protective pharmacotherapy (acetylcysteine, sodium bicarbonate) and dilution of contrast material with saline have been suggested to reduce the incidence of contrast-induced nephropathy in these patients. In general, severe CRI represents a contraindication to CAS.

Contraindication to Antiplatelet Agents. Patients intolerant of antiplatelet agents or at risk for hemorrhagic complications (active peptic ulcer disease or history of gastrointestinal bleeding) can be managed safely with CEA, as can patients in need of an open surgical procedure within 3 weeks after CAS.

Diabetes. Data suggest that diabetes confers a threefold increase in risk for ischemic stroke. Management of these patients is difficult because their vascular disease is usually more extensive, and a more complex procedure with increased risk for complications may be required. However, no data show increased morbidity from CAS in these patients. The indication for treatment should be balanced with other co-morbid conditions and the benefits of treatment.

Anatomic Features

Anatomic issues tend to influence the selection process for endovascular or surgical treatment of carotid stenosis. Important anatomic structures are contained within the surgical field of CEA. Although the incidence of cranial nerve injury, infection, and bleeding is very low in the typical patient, the risk may not be negligible in certain situations, such as patients who had previous neck surgery, irradiation, or tracheostomy, and this makes CAS an attractive alternative.

The working field for CAS includes the remote puncture site, vascular access to the target vessel, the carotid bifurcation, and the intracranial vasculature. It is imperative to have thorough knowledge on how all these anatomic issues may influence the outcome of the procedure.

Preprocedural assessment of patients for CAS is generally based on duplex ultrasound, which provides morphologic information, as well as velocity measurements—useful data for evaluating the severity of stenosis and eligibility of the patient for treatment. However, in patients with diffuse vascular disease it is advisable to obtain full supra-aortic vessel imaging with magnetic resonance angiography or computed tomographic angiography before planning the intervention. This allows careful evaluation of aortic arch morphology, the origin and possible tortuosity of all supra-aortic trunks, the severity of stenosis, and information on the intracranial circulation. It is also mandatory to evaluate all arteries, including calcification and thrombotic or soft atheromas, to define the morphology and length of the target lesion and to make accurate measurements of the diameter of the common carotid artery (CCA) and internal carotid artery (ICA) for selection of the appropriate size of devices to be used.

Aortic Arch

Arch morphology can be variable and becomes more elongated and tortuous with advancing age. With age, the upper inner aspect of the arch becomes a fulcrum; with increasing tortuosity the ascending aorta and the transverse arch can elongate and push the aortic valve and the origins of the innominate artery and left CCA downward. As the arch becomes more tortuous, the origins of the major branches become more difficult to select by remote endoluminal access. The shape and curvature of the aortic arch can be categorized into three types, depending on the position of the innominate artery as defined by two horizontal lines drawn across the highest point of the outer and inner curvatures of the arch. In a type I aortic arch, the great vessels arise above or in the same horizontal plane as the outer curvature of the arch (Fig. 96-1). In a type II aortic arch, the origin of the innominate artery lies between the horizontal planes of the outer and inner curvatures of the aortic arch. In a type III arch, the innominate artery lies below the horizontal plane of the inner curvature of the arch. The more inferior the origin of the supra-aortic vessels (type II or III arch), the greater the difficulty in gaining access to the carotid arteries. Indeed, with each increase in aortic arch level, catheter guidance and

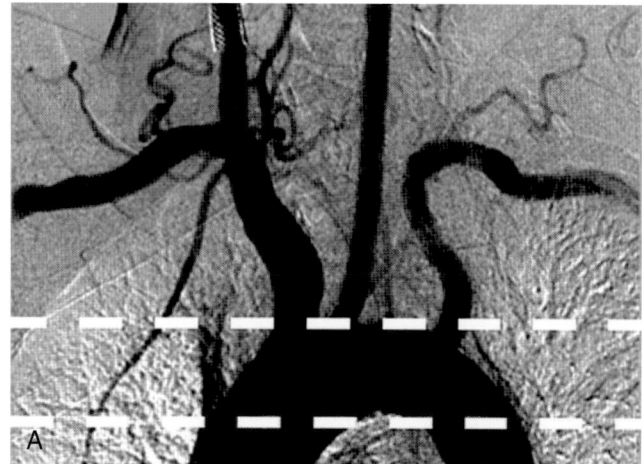

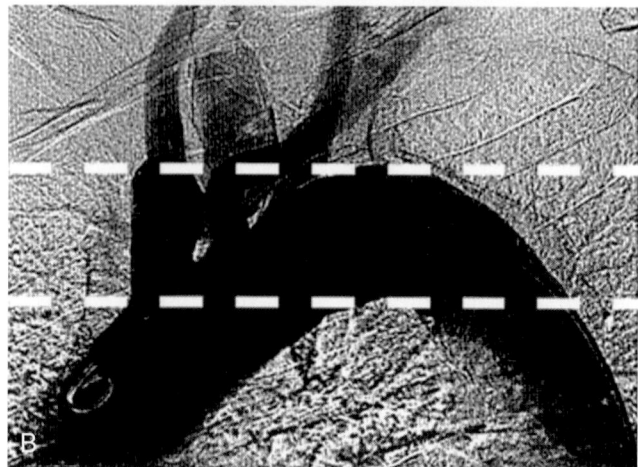

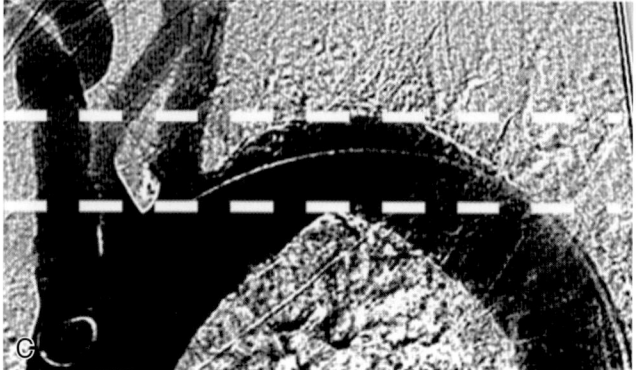

Figure 96-1 Aortic arch classification: **A,** Type I: the great vessels arise above or in the same horizontal plane of the outer curvature of the arch. **B,** Type II: the origin of innominate artery lies between the horizontal planes of the outer and inner curvatures of the aortic arch. **C,** Type III: the innominate artery lies below the horizontal plane of the inner curvature of the arch.

exchange become more difficult. Because of the acute angle between the arch and the origin of the left CCA, a type III aortic arch may lead to prolonged catheter manipulation in accessing the inferiorly dislocated origin of the CCA, with a possible risk for aortic plaque embolization.

In addition to these arch configurations, some congenital variations in the origin of the great vessels are relatively common. The so-called bovine arch, present in up to 27% of

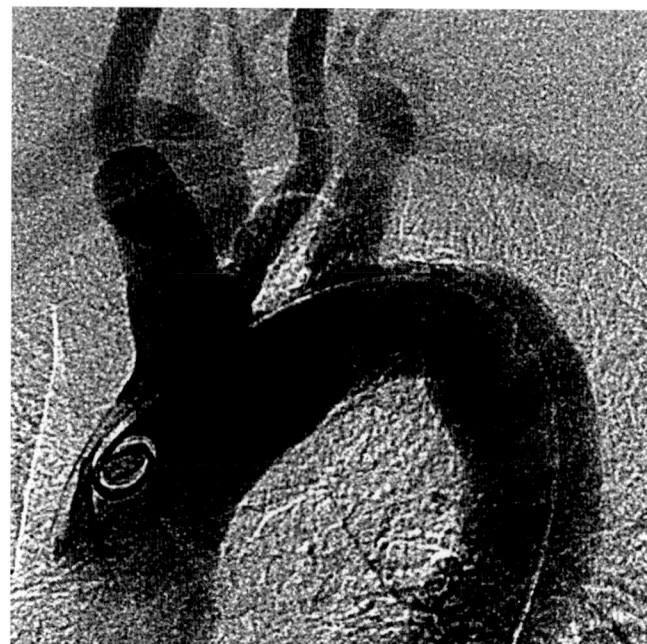

Figure 96-2 Type 2 bovine aortic arch. There is a common ostium between the innominate artery and the left common carotid artery.

patients,[49] may take two different anatomic patterns: the more frequent, type 2 (8% to 10% of cases), is when the innominate artery and left CCA share a common origin (Fig. 96-2); the other is when the common carotid branch takes off from the innominate artery. A "pure" bovine arch, extremely rare, occurs when there is a common arterial trunk originating from the arch and branching into three separate trunks: right subclavian, common carotid (right and left), and left subclavian.[49]

Factors involving the aortic arch that may limit patient suitability for CAS include the presence of extensive aortic wall irregularities (shaggy aorta) or severe aortic calcification (eggshell aorta). First, a patient with a shaggy aorta is at very high risk for massive atheroembolism and may have an absolute contraindication to CAS. Second, the presence of loose, squashy atherosclerotic debris (a rare condition) can cause catastrophic distal embolism not only to the brain but also to the viscera and lower extremities, with major ischemic consequences. Third, an eggshell aorta is associated with a risk for intimal disruption and embolism because of lack of compliance while directing guide wires or catheters. Furthermore, the stiffness of the origin of the vessels may decrease the torqueability of wires and catheters and cause resistance to progression of a long sheath or stent delivery system to the target lesion.

Carotid Tortuosity, Calcification

Any heavy circumferential calcification along the carotid vessels may decrease procedural success, particularly when severe calcifications are associated with vessel tortuosity, which increases the difficulty of accessing the lesion and inserting the device. Severe ICA tortuosity distal to the bifurcation, even without relevant calcification, may prevent positioning of the distal embolic protection system with a landing zone sufficient for stent deployment and may predispose to severe vascular spasm at the end of the procedure. When a kink is located at the distal end of carotid plaque, stent deployment may change the conformation of the vessel and cause distal angulation. Occasionally, extreme tortuosity may preclude a patient from undergoing intervention.

Finally, extensive calcification in the area of the stenosis may make stent delivery more difficult and may lead to insufficient expansion after deployment or recoiling of the dilated stenosis after deflation of the balloon.

Plaque Morphology

Quantitative and qualitative carotid plaque analysis, primarily achieved with duplex ultrasound, has been suggested as an important parameter for assessing the risk for stroke during CAS. Plaque echogenicity is the most important ultrasound parameter for identifying the so-called vulnerable plaque. Plaque echogenicity, defined in comparison to the echodensity of the surrounding media, is classified as hyperechoic or echodense (bright on ultrasound and indicative of harder or calcified plaque) versus hypoechoic or echolucent (dark on ultrasound and indicative of high lipid-rich–containing or blood-containing soft plaque).[50] There appears to be higher potential for embolism during CAS in the presence of hypoechoic lipid-containing plaque.[51-54] However, the definition of plaque echogenicity is operator dependent and difficult to classify in terms of different grades of severity. Novel computerized ultrasound technology such as the gray-scale median score has been proposed, with a low score being consistent with hypoechoic and unstable plaque.[53] However, its validation and reproducibility are not universally accepted, and this methodology is not ready for routine use in clinical practice. In general, the reliability of ultrasound evaluation and correlation with pathologic specimens remain under study.[55]

The timing of transformation from stable carotid plaque to unstable plaque is unpredictable. Identification of the biomechanisms of plaque instability remains an active area of investigation. Several local or systemic factors that have been implicated include proteolytic enzymes, intercellular adhesion molecule-1, growth factors, matrix metalloproteinases, fibrinogen, high-sensitivity C-reactive protein, genetic polymorphisms, and oxidant/antioxidant imbalance as a result of oxidized low-density lipoprotein.[56-62] However, the clinical applicability of these observations for triaging patients to CAS versus CEA await more solid confirmation.

According to the recommendations of Narins and colleagues and the Expert Consensus Document on Carotid Stenting of the American College of Cardiology (American College of Cardiology Foundation [ACCF]/Society for Cardiovascular Angiography and Interventions [SCAI]),[11,12]

1. CEA should be *recommended* for patients older than 80 years and in those with shaggy aortas.

Table 96-1 Case Selection for Carotid Artery Stenting

CAS Worse	CAS Better
Clinical Features	
Advanced age (≥80 yr)	COPD
Intolerance of antiplatelet agents	CHD with an abnormal cardiac stress test, unstable angina, or myocardial infarction <1 month
Severe renal dysfunction	Valvular heart disease
	Congestive heart failure (EF <30%)
	Contralateral recurrent laryngeal nerve dysfunction
	Severe obesity
Anatomic Features	
Access related	Previous neck irradiation
Shaggy aorta	Previous radical neck surgery
Eggshell aorta	Tracheostomy
Severely angulated type III aortic arch	Neck immobility
Aortoiliac occlusive disease	Recurrent stenosis
Target vessel related	High lesions (above C2)
Heavy calcification	Contralateral carotid occlusion
Severe tortuosity	
String sign	
Fresh thrombus	
Unstable plaque	

CAS, carotid artery stenting; COPD, chronic obstructive pulmonary disease; CHD, coronary heart disease; EF, ejection fraction.

2. CEA should be *preferred* for patients with a difficult arch, excessive vessel tortuosity, heavy calcification, or difficult vascular access.
3. CAS should be *recommended* for patients with previous neck radiation, radical neck surgery, or tracheostomy.
4. CAS should be *preferred* in patients with recurrent stenosis, neck immobility, a high carotid bifurcation, or contralateral occlusion but also in those with clinical conditions associated with high surgical risk, such as severe cardiac or pulmonary disease.

A complete outline for case selection for CAS is shown in Table 96-1.

PERIPROCEDURAL MEDICAL MANAGEMENT

Several developments in medical treatment before, during, and after CAS have evolved since the 1990s, including newer antiplatelet agents, statins, and the recognized benefits of lowering blood pressure.

Antiplatelet Drugs

The occurrence of rapid thrombus formation and potential embolization immediately after CAS provides the rationale for double antiplatelet therapy. Aspirin, the most studied antiplatelet agent, causes irreversible inhibition of platelet cyclooxygenase by decreasing production of thromboxane A_2. Doses of 75 to 150 mg daily are as effective as higher doses.[63-66]

For survivors of an ischemic stroke or TIA, aspirin reduces serious vascular events by about 25%.[64,66] However, there is interpatient variability in the response of platelets to aspirin, as well as occasional resistance to the drug.[67] Thienopyridine derivatives, such as ticlopidine and clopidogrel, which act as adenosine diphosphate receptor antagonists via a separate pathway from inhibition of cyclooxygenase, have recently been considered a valid alternative or adjunctive treatment to aspirin.[68,69]

Clinical evidence supporting the use of double antiplatelet treatment to prevent vascular events is derived mainly from studies involving coronary interventions.[70-77] RCTs indicate that dual therapy is associated with a favorable benefit in preventing major vascular events in patients at high risk, such as those with acute coronary syndromes and after coronary stenting.[70-77]

The benefit is less clear when dual treatment is applied to patients who had ischemic stroke or TIA.[78] The recently published MATCH trial (Management of AtheroThrombosis with Clopidogrel in High-risk patients with recent TIA or ischemic stroke) found only a nonsignificant 6.4% reduction in the relative risk for primary endpoints (stroke, MI, vascular death, rehospitalization) with a dual antiplatelet regimen.[79] Similar results were obtained in the CHARISMA trial (Clopidogrel for High Atherothrombosis Risk and Ischemic Stabilization, Management and Avoidance). The benefit of combination therapy became marginally significant in high-risk subgroups, such as patients with symptoms or demonstrated vascular disease (relative risk reduction of 12%, $P = .046$); conversely, the related risk of bleeding obviated the benefits of treatment in low-risk subgroups such as asymptomatic patients.[80,81]

Studies using transcranial Doppler in patients with symptomatic carotid stenosis found a reduced number of microembolizations when clopidogrel was added to aspirin (Clopidogrel and Aspirin for the Reduction of Emboli in Symptomatic carotid Stenosis study [CARESS]).[82]

Despite conflicting information regarding the effectiveness of dual antiplatelet treatment in preventing cerebrovascular ischemic events, there is consensus that patients undergoing CAS should receive a regimen similar to those undergoing coronary stenting, as recommended by guidelines from the American College of Cardiology (ACC)/American Heart Association (AHA)[83,84] and European Society of Cardiology.[85] The standard regimen includes aspirin, 81 to 325 mg/day for 4 days, and clopidogrel, 300- to 600-mg loading dose and 75 mg/day for 4 days before the procedure.[11] Alternatively, a loading dose of clopidogrel (300 to 600 mg) at least 4 to 6 hours before the procedure is advocated.

Today, most centers administer aspirin and clopidogrel for up to 4 weeks after carotid stenting because of the vulnerability of carotid plaque through the stent struts during this period, as suggested by studies documenting the occurrence of adverse events during the first 24 to 48 hours and up to 30 days after the procedure.[86]

Longer treatment may be warranted in patients at high risk for restenosis or stroke, such as diabetics or patients with coronary disease.[69,83,84] In these cases a lower dose of aspirin may be considered for long-term dual therapy.

Regarding the potential risk of increased bleeding in patients scheduled for staged carotid and cardiac or noncardiac major surgery, the ACC/AHA guidelines recommend stopping clopidogrel therapy at least 5 days (preferably 7 days) before CABG.[87]

Anticoagulation

Few studies have compared antiplatelet with *anticoagulant* therapy after CAS. In a small RCT that included 47 patients undergoing CAS, the 30-day neurologic complications rate was 0% with clopidogrel and aspirin versus 25% ($P = .02$) with aspirin plus heparin. The unacceptable level of complications in the anticoagulant group resulted in early termination of the study.[88]

Warfarin is recommended for primary and secondary prevention of stroke in patients with atrial fibrillation.[89,90] Based on these trials, warfarin is indicated in patients with carotid stenosis and a concurrent risk for cardioembolic stroke. In these patients it is reasonable to maintain the antithrombotic therapy without adjunctive antiplatelet drugs to avoid the increased hemorrhagic risk. Warfarin is converted to intravenous heparin before the procedure.

Statins

Statins (3-hydroxy-3-methylglutaryl coenzyme A reductase inhibitors) have been found to be highly effective in preventing primary and secondary stroke in patients with cardiovascular disease. A recent review of studies analyzing the effect of statins in patients undergoing vascular surgery showed significant improvement in postoperative outcomes.[91] This benefit appears to be largely independent of the cholesterol-lowering effect of the drug but is due to its so-called pleiotropic effects. Statins have been shown to stabilize atherosclerotic plaque and exert anti-inflammatory, antithrombogenic, antiproliferative, and anti–leukocyte adhesion effects.

A number of studies have focused on the effect of statin therapy on outcomes of carotid surgery.[91-94] The early experience suggests benefit in patients undergoing CEA, thus raising the question of whether similar pleiotropic effects would affect the outcomes of CAS, but few studies have addressed this issue. In a single-center experience, the incidence of cardiovascular events after CAS was 4% in statin users versus 15% in those not taking statins ($P < .05$).[95] Based on these data, it is reasonable to prescribe statins early before the procedure but also monitor liver function and creatine kinase levels thereafter to detect potential side effects of the drug (AHA guidelines).[10]

Intraprocedural Drugs
Adequate Fluid Administration. Adequate administration of fluids is the first fundamental step in reducing the risk for contrast-induced nephropathy and intraprocedural hypotension in preparing patients for CAS.

Anticoagulation. As in any vascular procedure, heparin administration is essential with carotid stenting. Heparin, 70 U/kg (or 100 U/kg), is administered after gaining arterial access and before manipulation of catheters in the aortic arch. An activated clotting time not longer than 250 to 300 seconds is recommended to avoid the risk for intracerebral hemorrhage from reperfusion. Heparin is rarely reversed at the end of the procedure. Given that the half-life of heparin is about 90 minutes, the procedure is usually finished before the anticoagulant effect of the initial dose has completely worn off.

Atropine. Intravenous atropine (0.4 to 1 mg) is recommended before stent deployment and balloon inflation to suppress the hemodynamic response to stretching of carotid baroreceptors. Hypotension associated with marked bradycardia is a common feature after balloon dilatation, especially in elderly patients with heavily calcified stenoses.[96-98] In the case of a severe hemodynamic response, aggressive volume expansion and an additional dose of atropine or vasopressors, including intravenous phenylephrine and dopamine infusion, may be necessary. Moderate hypotension may last from 24 to 48 hours before the carotid sinus adapts to the radial force of the self-expanding stents, and pharmacologic support is occasionally required. The hemodynamic response may be exaggerated in patients with baseline bradycardia or those taking beta blockers or digoxin, whereas patients with a denervated carotid sinus because of previous CEA or with pacemakers are at lower risk. During the early years of carotid stenting, temporary pacing guide wires were advocated to prevent severe bradycardia.[99-102] This approach has its own set of complications, and pacemaker insertion is rarely indicated today.

Vasodilators. In the distal ICA, spasm may appear at the end of the procedure, especially in the presence of vessel tortuosity, as a result of manipulation of guide wires or distal protection devices. Most cases of spasm will resolve in a few minutes. However, when spasm is severe and persistent, administration of vasodilators may be required. Commonly, nitroglycerin (100 µg) is administered directly into the ICA through the carotid sheath (500 µg diluted in 10 mL and 2 mL). Additional doses may be administered every 3 to 5 minutes. The patient must be observed for possible exaggerated hypotension.

■ PERIPROCEDURAL MONITORING

One important aspect of performing CAS safely is ensuring that the patient is adequately monitored before, during, and a few hours after the procedure. Continuous electrocardiographic, pulse oximetry, and intra-arterial monitoring through the side arm of the arterial access site introducer sheath is necessary.

The level of alertness, speech, and motor function must be continuously evaluated by asking the patient to answer simple questions and to squeeze a plastic toy in the contralateral hand. However, because more subtle ischemic neurologic changes may be overlooked, more accurate assessment is advisable after completion of the procedure.

Transcranial Doppler is a useful adjunctive technique to monitor the patient during and immediately after CAS. Indeed, it is known that cerebral embolic events may occur in any step of the procedure, but mainly during CPD deployment, stent delivery, balloon dilatation, and CPD recovery. High-intensity transient signals can be detected as warning signs.[103] Because reflection of ultrasound power depends on both the size and composition of the embolus, the use of multifrequency transcranial Doppler has been suggested for automatic recognition of high-intensity transient signals and differentiation between particulate emboli and air bubbles or artifacts.[103-105] Nevertheless, sources of error are frequent, and the ability of transcranial Doppler to differentiate emboli with relevant clinical consequences is questionable.[53,54,106-114] When symptoms of focal neurologic injury develop during CAS, it is best to complete the procedure, retrieve the catheters, and reassess the patient.

Mild sedation may be offered, but in most cases the procedure should be performed with local anesthesia and patient reassurance. Avoidance of sedatives enhances neurologic monitoring and limits hypotension.

Noninvasive hemodynamic monitoring should be maintained until the following morning. Ultrasound evaluation to assess the morphology of the treated vessel, inspection of the arterial access site, and laboratory chemistry evaluation to rule out renal damage are suggested before discharge.

Because a number of embolic complications have been reported to occur up to several days after the procedure, the double antiplatelet regimen is continued for at least 1 month. At discharge the patient should be instructed to comply with the follow-up schedule and inform the practitioner in the event of any new neurologic symptoms.

■ TECHNICAL DETAILS
Procedural Steps

The CAS procedure widens the stenotic zone by dilatation and attempts to prevent future embolization by scaffolding the ruptured plaque against the vessel wall with a stent. The specific technique may vary according to operator experience. However, some steps are widely accepted in standardized protocols.

Access. Retrograde right femoral access followed by a 5 to 8 Fr introducer access sheath is the most convenient catheter manipulation by a right-handed operator. The left common femoral and brachial arteries are second choices if the right femoral route is not available. Insertion of guide wires and catheters should follow the method for any endovascular procedure.

Aortic Arch Angiogram. At the beginning of the procedure, the suitability of the aortic arch should be evaluated with an angiogram performed via a pigtail catheter. Arch angiograms are performed in a 45- to 60-degree left oblique

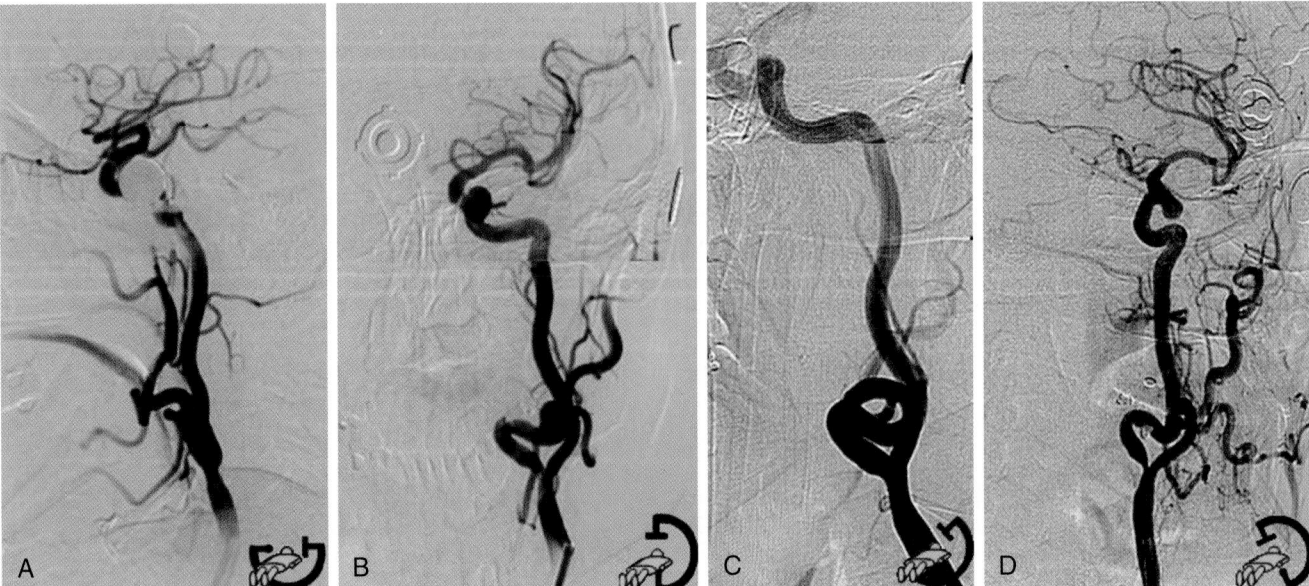

Figure 96-3 Standard projections showing mild to moderate stenosis. The projection selected with rotational angiography shows severe stenosis. **A,** Laterolateral. **B,** Anteroposterior. **C,** Left anterior oblique. **D,** Right anterior oblique.

projection to better visualize the arch type and the origin of the arch vessels. Vessels that originate below the apex of the aortic arch are more difficult to cannulate, and catheter insertion and exchange become increasingly difficult with a type II or III aortic arch. As a general rule, the fewer the manipulations in the arch and epiaortic vessels, the lower the risk for an embolic event.

Selective Common Carotid Cannulation. Selective cannulation is a critical step. Two main techniques for advancing the catheter into the CCA are used. In the "sheath-based platform," preshaped 5 Fr catheters, such as the Judkins 4, Head Hunter, Simmons 1, or other models, may be used for CCA cannulation according to the preference of the operators. Through these catheters an exchange-length stiff 0.035-inch guide wire is placed in the terminal branches of the external carotid artery (ECA), and a 6 Fr 90-cm sheath (e.g., Shuttle, Cook, Inc.; Destination, Terumo Interventional systems) with its dilator is then advanced over the wire and positioned with a pull-and-push maneuver in the distal CCA a few centimeters below the bifurcation. Care must be taken to identify the tip of the dilator because it should be kept away from the carotid bulb. Otherwise, a 125-cm curved catheter premounted into the sheath is used for cannulation and advancement of the guide wire and sheath (telescopic technique). The "telescopic" method is preferable in patients with a calcified and tortuous aortic arch because the catheter and guide wire assembly provides additional support. One possible disadvantage is the mismatch between the size of the catheter (5 Fr) and the sheath, which may cause the tip of the sheath to scrape the arterial wall ("snowplowing") and result in distal embolization.

With the alternative "guiding catheter–based platform" technique, CCA access is achieved directly with a preshaped guiding catheter (e.g., multipurpose curve, vertebral or reverse-angle Vitek catheter) with a 7 to 8 Fr external diam-

eter that is left at the proximal CCA level for the entire procedure. In case of difficult stent advancement, a high-support 0.014-inch coronary "buddy wire" placed into the ECA may be necessary to stabilize the guiding catheter. This technique is useful in patients with a difficult arch and tortuous origin of the CCA because buddy wires, available in various tip shapes, provide better torque control. Once in place, the sheath side arm is intermittently irrigated or attached to a slow continuous infusion of heparinized saline to avoid stagnation of blood in the sheath and is then connected to monitor blood pressure.

A selective angiogram of the carotid bifurcation through the sheath shows the area of the lesion and the intracranial carotid circulation. Usually, an anteroposterior or lateral projection is needed to obtain minimal overlap of the ICA and ECA and optimal visualization of the target lesion. Occasionally, when differentiation between the two carotid branches is not easily obtained with two projections, rotational angiography may be useful to select the optimal projection to accomplish the procedure (Fig. 96-3).

Crossing the Internal Carotid Stenosis. The stenosis is crossed with a 0.014-inch guide wire that is a component of the CPD in use, usually with a roadmapping technique. Distal filters should be deployed into the ICA, just before its petrous (C3) segment at the skull base; the position must be checked throughout the entire procedure. It is important not to advance the tip of the device any further because the intracranial portion of the carotid artery is highly prone to dissection with guide wire manipulation.

Predilatation. When the stenosis is extremely severe, predilatation with a 2.5- or 4.0-mm coronary balloon at relatively low inflation pressure (4 to 6 atm) may prevent difficulty in stent deployment.

Stent Delivery. The stent is deployed under roadmapping control or by using the vertebral bones as landmarks. Usually, the stent is placed across the bifurcation because most of the time the plaque extends to the bulb area. A self-expanding stent is used; a variety of diameters (6 to 10 mm), lengths (2 to 4 cm), and shapes (cylindrical or tapered) are available. The diameter of the stent must be sized to the largest portion of the vessel, typically the distal CCA, and stent diameter should be approximately 1 mm larger than CCA diameter. Different models of stents can be used to better adapt to the vessel in the event of tortuosity and to avoid bending the ICA at the end of the stent.

Postdilatation. After stent deployment, short (2 cm) 5- to 6-mm balloons are used to dilate the narrowest portion of the stent. Balloon diameter should never exceed the diameter of the distal ICA. The balloon is always maintained within the stent. Higher pressure might be needed for heavily calcified plaque, which has a tendency to recoil.

Retrieval of the Cerebral Protection Device and Completion Angiography. A completion angiogram of the carotid bifurcation and intracranial carotid vessels is performed before removing the protection device to ensure the accuracy of deployment and assess for any dissection. ICA spasm may occur, particularly when the CPD has been allowed to move up or down during guide wire manipulations. Typically, watchful waiting and occasionally the administration of small doses of nitroglycerin (100 to 200 μg) through the guiding sheath allow resolution of the problem.

After retrieval of the guide wire and CPD, a final completion angiogram of the cervical carotid and intracranial circulation is performed.

Access Hemostasis. Heparin's action is not usually reversed. Access site hemostasis may be achieved with a percutaneous closure device.

Cerebral Protection Devices

The debate concerning routine use of CPDs during carotid stenting is open because of different results reported in the studies available. In a survey of 53 centers worldwide, Wholey and coauthors reported a 5.29% stroke and death rate in 6753 patients without a CPD versus 2.23% in 4221 patients with CPDs.[115] The EVA-3S trial provided strong support for the use of a CPD: a 30-day risk of stroke of 7.9% with protected CAS versus 25% with unprotected CAS.[14] On the other hand, the SPACE trial found the same rate of events in both groups (7% versus 7%).[15] In a meta-analysis by Kastrup and associates that included a total of 2537 unprotected CAS and 896 protected CAS procedures, the combined stroke rate at 30 days was as low as 1.8% with use of a CPD versus 5.5% in patients without protection ($P < .001$).[116] On the contrary, dissenting comments have been raised concerning the specific risk for stroke from improper placement of the CPD, and these investigators therefore argue for selective use.[86,113,117-121] Only one small RCT has compared CAS with CPD versus no

CPD; just 36 patients were enrolled (18 assigned to CPD and 18 to no CPD), and the study provided conflicting data.[122] Two strokes occurred in each group, with the only major stroke occurring in the nonprotected group. Astonishingly, the rate of cerebral lesions detected by diffusion-weighted magnetic resonance imaging was higher in the group with CPD than in the group without CPD (72% versus 44%; $P = .9$).[122]

Finally, the ACCF/SCAI/Society for Vascular Medicine and Biology (SVMB)/Society of Interventional Radiology (SIR)/American Society of Interventional & Therapeutic Neuroradiology (ASITN) consensus document stated that the "availability of CPD appears to be important in reducing the risk of stroke during CAS" and that "it seems unlikely that major CAS trials will be performed without CPD."[11]

Today, there are a large variety of CPD models with different mechanisms that extend its applicability to disparate anatomic conditions. Three conceptually different methods, each with advantages and drawbacks, have been developed:
- Distal filter
- Flow reversal (proximal occlusion)
- Distal occlusion balloon

Distal Filter. Filter-type CPDs are the most widely used devices.[120,121,123-126] Distal filter systems function like an umbrella that is opened in the ICA between the target lesion and the brain to capture any debris during the CAS procedure (Fig. 96-4). Filters can be mounted either on a guide wire or with their own dedicated delivery system and are placed in the distal ICA after crossing the lesion. After successful angioplasty and stent placement, the distal filter containing the debris is then removed with a dedicated retrieval system. The main advantages of these CPDs are maintenance of blood flow to the brain and the availability of angiographic control throughout the procedure. The main drawbacks are the need to cross the ICA lesion before delivery of the protective filter, difficulty crossing very tight and tortuous lesions, and the uncertainty of maintaining complete arterial wall apposition so that all debris can be captured. Occasionally, a filter can be occluded by debris; prompt completion of the procedure and quick removal of the device may clear any neurologic symptoms should they develop.

Flow Reversal (Proximal Occlusion). Flow reversal devices are characterized by two compliant balloons, one placed in the CCA and the other in the ECA. Reversed flow from the ICA is then attained by continuous arteriovenous shunting through the side arm of the introducer connected to a separate access in the femoral vein (Gore Neuro Protection System)[127,128] or by active syringe aspiration after the stenting and ballooning phases, which are performed with blocked flow (Mo.Ma system, Invatec).[129] The main advantage of these systems is that they allow cerebral protection before crossing the lesion and can be used to treat very friable and tight lesions in tortuous vessels where filters cannot be deployed or may be ineffective. However, proximal occlusion devices usually require larger introducers and may be more techni-

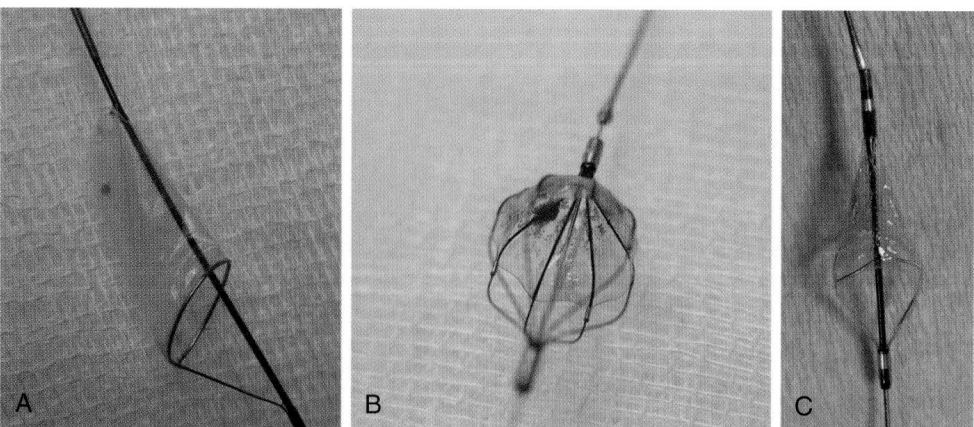

Figure 96-4 Different types of filters containing debris after retrieval. **A,** EPI FilterWire. **B,** Angioguard. **C,** Emboshield. *(A, courtesy of Boston Scientific, Natick, MA; B, courtesy of Cordis, Somerville, NJ; C, courtesy of Abbott Vascular, Redwood City, CA.)*

cally demanding. Furthermore, interruption or reversal of flow through the ICA is not tolerated by all patients, particularly those with reduced cerebral reserve or contralateral occlusion.

Distal Occlusion Balloon. Though introduced many years ago, distal occlusion balloons are not frequently used today.[8,130] Protection is obtained by occluding the distal ICA above the lesion with an inflated balloon and flushing and suctioning after stent deployment. Their main disadvantages include the need to cross the lesion without protection as with filters, endoluminal occlusion of the ICA, and risk for distal spasm or wall damage as a result of balloon inflation.

The available literature on CPDs does not support superiority of the different models.[131-134] Preference should be based on operator experience and morphology of the lesion and vessels. Operators should be familiar with at least two different classes of CPDs so that the technique can be tailored to each individual case.[11]

Stent Selection

The self-expandable carotid stents used today are composed of either stainless steel (a cobalt alloy) or nitinol (a nickel-titanium alloy). Flexibility (the ability to conform to vessel tortuosity) and scaffolding (the amount of support given to the vessel wall) are the two main characteristics that drive stent choice. In the case of tortuous anatomy, a rigid stent may create a kink at the distal end of deployment (Fig. 96-5). Insufficient scaffolding might cause squeezing of plaque material through the stent strut and produce distal embolization (Fig. 96-6). In general, nitinol stents have higher radial force, which is useful in counteracting recoiling of severely calcified plaque.

An important technologic feature of stents for the carotid artery has been the development of two main configurations: "closed cell," where all stent struts are interconnected, and "open cell," where not all struts are interrelated (Fig. 96-7; also see Fig. 96-5). It has been suggested that closed-cell stents with a smaller free cell area and a greater percentage

of wall coverage may contain the fractured and dilated plaque better after CAS, thereby resulting in a lower rate of post-procedural embolization compared with the open-cell structure.[135] However, this finding has produced conflicting observations. In a multicenter experience of 3179 CAS procedures, Bosiers and colleagues reported a 1.3% adverse event rate in patients with closed-cell stents and 3.4% in those with open-cell stents, mainly in symptomatic patients.[135] In another multicentric study of 1648 patients, Schillinger and collaborators reported a similar stroke and death rate: 3.1% (95% confidence interval [CI], 2.3 to 3.9) for closed-cell stents versus 2.4% (95% CI, 1.7 to 3.1) for open-cell stents (*P* = .077, *P* = 0.38).[136]

The main advantage of the open-cell design is that it allows better flexibility and adaptability in tortuous vessels (see Fig. 96-7). Stents with a mixed or hybrid configuration (closed-cell design in the midsegment and open-cell design at the distal ends) have recently been introduced (Cristallo-Ideale, Invatec, Roncadelle, Italy).

Another important advance in carotid stent technology is the development of tapered stents; such stents are useful in patients with a marked discrepancy in size between the CCA and ICA, which occurs in about 10% to 15% of cases. Tapered stents can be either conical (e.g., Acculink Sinus 5F, Xact, Cristallo Ideale) or shouldered (e.g., Protégé). In the former there is a gradual decrease in diameter from the proximal to the distal end, whereas the latter has a short transition zone in the midsegment of the stent.

However, it should be emphasized that no randomized studies have yet been performed in which different stents are compared, and any conclusion regarding the safest stent configuration is not supported by data. Different configurations and models may increase the applicability of CAS in different anatomy, and careful assessment is required to select the most suitable stent for each patient.

Procedural Complications

Details on types of neurologic complications and options for their management after CAS are summarized in Table 96-2.

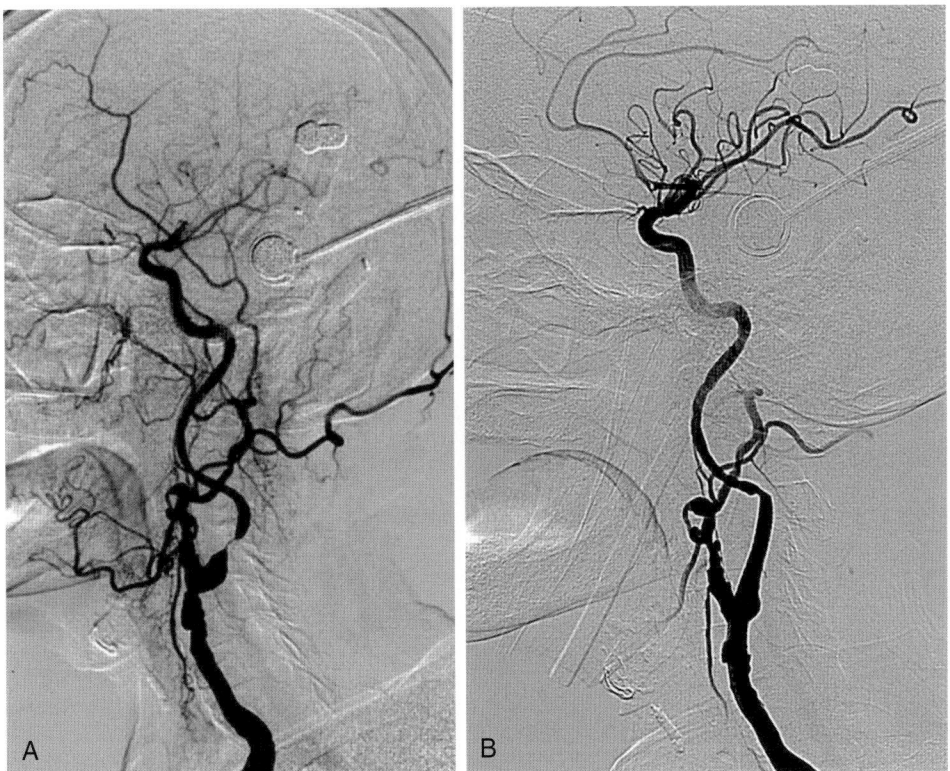

Figure 96-5 Severe symptomatic carotid stenosis in a patient with a tracheostomy (**A**) treated by carotid stenting with a closed-cell stent (**B**) (Wallstent, Boston Scientific Corp, Natick, MA). A kink is apparent in the distal stent.

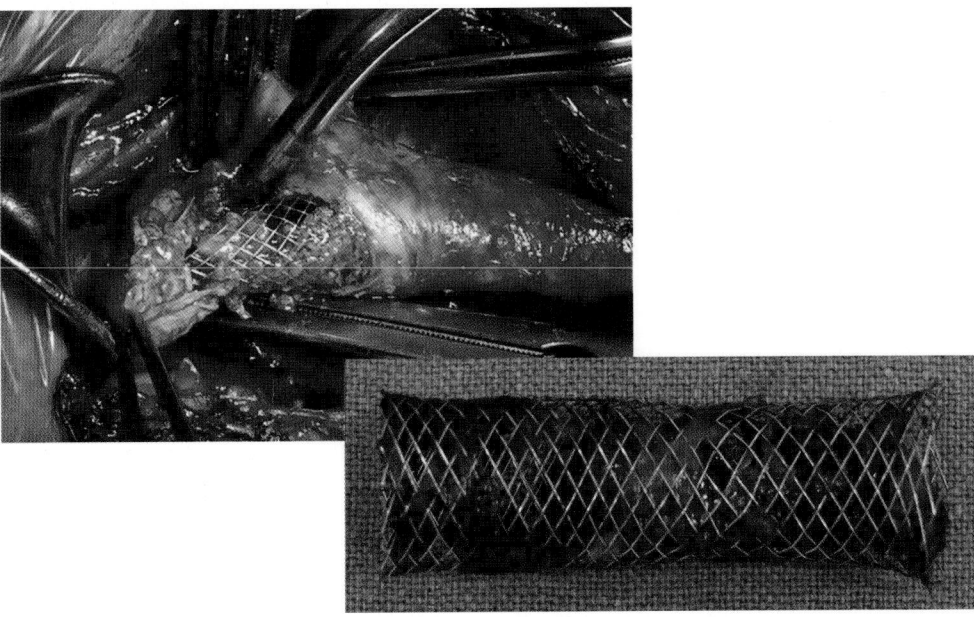

Figure 96-6 Postprocedural conversion because of a transient ischemic attack. Plaque can be seen prolapsing through the stent strut.

Embolization from atherosclerotic plaque or catheter-generated thrombus is the most common and serious complication reported after CAS. The incidence varies and is dependent on operator experience and patient selection.[137,138] Advanced age, difficult arch, and the presence of long or multiple lesions have been implicated as predictors of embolic stroke.[12]

The consequences of distal embolization can vary from silent cerebral infarction, to TIA, to stroke of varying severity. Although studies with transcranial Doppler showed varying and at times high rates of intraprocedural embolization with different plaque compositions and size, most of these signals are not associated with acute clinical consequences.[113,114]

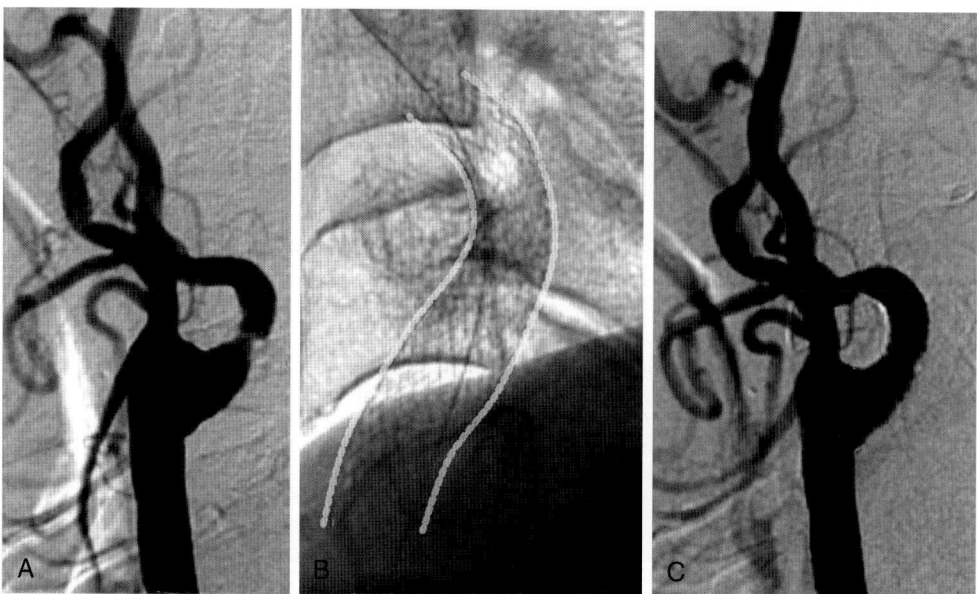

Figure 96-7 Stenting of an angulated segment of internal carotid artery with an open cell system. Before (**A**), during (**B**), and after (**C**) system release. *(Courtesy of PRECISE Carotid Stent, Cordis, Warren, NJ.)*

Table 96-2 Management of Carotid Artery Stenting Complications

Complication	Management
Stent thrombosis	Immediate conversion to CEA
Kinking after stenting	Observation vs. additional stent vs. surgery
Carotid dissection	Anticoagulation/antiplatelet vs. additional stent
Distal embolization	Neurorescue techniques
	• Catheter-directed thrombolysis (t-PA or UK) vs. IIa/IIIb inhibitor, intravenous/intra-arterial
	• Thrombus maceration
	• Aspiration thrombectomy
	• Capture and removal of embolus
Bubbles emboli	No treatment
Internal carotid artery spasm	No treatment vs. nitroglycerin
Thrombosed filter	CPD retrieval
Arch injury	Stenting vs. surgery
Hyperperfusion	Hypotensive drug

CEA, carotid endarterectomy; CPD, cerebral protection device; t-PA, tissue plasminogen activator; UK, urokinase.

When neurologic symptoms occur and intracranial arterial occlusion is visible on the angiogram, a number of neurorescue maneuvers have been suggested for retrieval of distal emboli, including catheter-directed chemical thrombolysis with urokinase or tissue plasminogen activator, thrombus maceration, aspiration thrombectomy, snare removal, or glycoprotein IIb/IIIa receptor inhibitor administration, all with variable results. Presently, prevention remains the best option to avoid the disastrous consequences of distal cerebral embolization.[136-139]

Acute stent thrombosis requires immediate surgical exploration, stent removal, and performance of CEA.

Arch trauma with local vessel injury or cerebral embolization, carotid dissection, and even perforation of intracranial vessels because of misplacement of a large-profile CPD have been described.[138]

Cerebral hyperperfusion with seizures and intracranial hemorrhage has been reported, particularly in patients with severe stenoses and poor cerebrovascular reserve. This complication may occur within the first 2 weeks after CAS and may be triggered by poorly controlled hypertension.[140-142]

Finally, local complications can develop at the access site, with or without the use of dedicated closure devices. Such complications include hematoma, false aneurysm, infection, thrombosis, and arteriovenous fistula, although they are reported relatively infrequently in published series.[137-139]

Systemic complications such as severe bradycardia and hypotension from stretching of the carotid bulb rarely lead to serious cardiac rhythm or ischemic disorders. Congestive heart failure in patients with reduced cardiac output can be provoked by the osmotic load associated with the administration of contrast agents. Another adverse sequela of contrast administration after CAS is deterioration of renal function.

RESULTS OF CAROTID ARTERY STENTING

Since its introduction, percutaneous treatment of carotid stenosis has been extensively investigated but is still awaiting more definitive evaluation by comparison with outcomes after CEA, which should come from ongoing RCTs.

The results of CAS can be divided in two main periods because of substantially changed approaches and techniques.

Period 1: Early carotid endovascular period (1979-1995)
Period 2: Modern carotid endovascular period (after 1995)

Early studies were limited by poor technology and lack of CPD, and patient outcomes were unpredictable. The results are therefore no longer relevant to the current treatment method. The transition from the early age to the modern age was not sharp because of reluctance in acceptance of evolving techniques. However, technologic innovations became largely disseminated after 1995 and to a greater extent after 2002. Advancements that allowed shifting from period 1 to period 2 consisted essentially of the routine use of stents versus simple balloon angioplasty and the introduction of CPD and dedicated materials. Furthermore, the development of imaging technology and new pharmacologic treatments allowed further improvement.

Carotid Artery Stenting in Period 1

A limited number of RCTs evaluated CEA versus CAS performed during this interval and focused mainly on symptomatic or high-risk patients.[143-147] These RCTs were designed early and the results are not relevant to current CAS because of the obsolete technology used, regardless of the publishing date. The first randomized (Leicester), single-center study on CAS was stopped by the safety monitoring committee after only 17 patients were randomized because of an excessive (70%) periprocedural stroke rate in the stenting arm.[143] Another multicenter study (Wallstent) was also stopped after more than 200 patients were randomized because of a high incidence of stroke and death in the stenting group (12.1% versus 4.5%; P = .049), and it remains unpublished.[144]

The largest study of this period (Carotid Artery and Vertebral Artery Transluminal Angioplasty Study [CAVATAS]) randomized more than 500 patients, 90% of whom were symptomatic, to CAS versus CEA and used simple balloon angioplasty without stenting in 74% of cases. The trial found no significant differences, but periprocedural rates of stroke and death, approximately 10%, similar in both arms, were higher than the NASCET-recommended rates. Long-term follow-up (>5 years) is ongoing.[145]

Finally, a small single-center trial (Kentucky) that included 104 patients with greater than 70% stenosis, as well as an asymptomatic group of 85 patients with greater than 80% carotid stenosis, found comparable and small complication rates in both arms.[146,147]

Carotid Artery Stenting in Period 2

Four main innovations contributed to dramatic changes in CAS technique over time:
- Routine use of stents
- Introduction of CPD
- Use of long introducers or guiding catheters advanced in the CCA and used as a working channel throughout the procedure
- Use of low-profile guide wires with a monorail technique that allows a much shorter wire than used previously and

enables the operator to maintain more precise and faster control of any device exchange during the procedure

Case Series and Reviews

Some of the most recent and largest series published since 1996 are listed in Table 96-3[86,113,115,117,123,124,132,135,136,148-166] (see the Expert Consult Web site). Roubin and coworkers reported on 528 consecutive patients over a 5-year period with both balloon-expandable and self-expanding stents, with and without CPDs.[7] When divided into yearly intervals, the risk of stroke and death reached a maximum of 12.5% and fell to a minimum of 3.2% at the end of the period. According to the authors, this rather dramatic change in results reflected technologic improvements as well as improved skills of the investigators to select appropriate patients for intervention.

Phatouros and associates reviewed 11 case series published after 1996, including a total of 929 procedures.[167] The overall reported procedure-related mortality rate was 4.5%, the minor stroke rate was 6.5%, and the major stroke rate was 4.5%.

After 2002, new technologic advances were more widely used, and large case series and multicenter experiences with more than 100 patients each and more than 12,000 in total have been published (see Table 96-3 on the Expert Consult Web site).

In a review article including 20 series and more than 24,000 procedures, Goodney and colleagues found an average 30-day stroke rate of 3% and a combined rate of stroke, MI, and death of 4%.[168]

Burton and coworkers performed a review of CAS studies, all using CPD. Data from 3091 procedures showed estimated average 30-day stroke and death rates of 2.4% ± 0.3%, minor stroke rates of 1.1% ± 0.2%, and major stroke rates of 0.6% ± 0.2%. However, these outcomes should be interpreted with caution because of the high variability in different studies, with the minor stroke rate ranging from 0% to 6%, the major stroke rate from 0% to 3%, and death from 0% to 7%.[169]

Registries

In addition to these series, the vast majority of nonrandomized studies on CAS in period 2 consist of a number of independent and industry-sponsored registries (Table 96-4 [see the Expert Consult Web site]; see also Table 96-3 on the Expert Consult Web site).[129,170-180]

The Carotid Revascularization using Endarterectomy or Stenting System (CaRESS; sponsored by Boston Scientific Corp., Natick, MA, and Medtronic AVE, Santa Rosa, CA) trial was designed as a prospective, multicenter, nonrandomized cohort study in which investigators were allowed to enter patients in a broad-risk population with symptomatic and asymptomatic carotid stenosis into either the CAS or CEA arm. The advantage of the CaRESS methodology is that it allows direct comparison between treatments in a concurrent series of patients. The drawbacks include investigator and patient selection bias because there is no randomization.

Results from the CaRESS trial on 397 CAS procedures showed no significant differences in combined death/stroke rates (see Table 96-4 on the Expert Consult Web site) at 1 year (13.6% versus 10% with CEA versus CAS, respectively).[170]

Four industry-sponsored studies (ARCHeR [Acculink for Revascularization of Carotids in High-Risk Patients], CABERNET [Carotid Artery Revascularization Using the Boston Scientific EPI FilterWire EX/EZ and the EndoTex NexStent], CREATE [Carotid Revascularization with ev3 Arterial Technology Evolution], and SECuRITY [Study to Evaluate the Neuroshield Bare Wire Cerebral Protection System and X-Act Stent in Patients at High Risk for Carotid Endarterectomy] registries) leading to device approval by the U.S. Food and Drug Administration included only patients at high risk for CEA. Stroke rates at 30 days varied from 2% to 7%, and combined stroke, death, and MI rates varied from 3% to 8%.[181] Most data are not published in peer review journals (see also http//www.fda.gov/cdrh/mda/docs/p040038.html). Other sponsored studies are listed in Table 96-4 (see the Expert Consult Web site).

Randomized Controlled Trials

Three RCTs have been completed during period 2 (Table 96-5): SAPPHIRE, EVA-3S, and SPACE.[14,15,29,182] These published trials reached different conclusions on the safety of CAS versus CEA and failed to provide strong evidence supporting the best option for treatment.

SAPPHIRE. This study, sponsored by the Cordis Corporation (Johnson & Johnson Company, Warren, NJ), was initially published in 2004 and then updated in 2008 with long-term results (3-year).[29,182] The study design tested the hypothesis of noninferiority of stenting versus CEA. The primary endpoint was the cumulative incidence of death, stroke, or MI within 30 days and death or ipsilateral stroke within 1 year. The study enrolled patients with symptomatic carotid artery stenosis of at least 50% or asymptomatic stenosis of at least 80% at high surgical risk for either anatomic reasons or co-morbid conditions. An ancillary registry included patients ineligible for randomization. All patients undergoing CAS were treated with a nitinol stent (SMART [Second Manifestations of ARTerial disease] or PRECISE [Phase III Randomized Evaluation of Convection Enhanced Delivery of IL 13-PE38QQR Compared to GLIADEL Wafer With Survival Endpoint in Glioblastoma Multiforme Patients at First Recurrence]) with the routine use of CPD (Angioguard). The trial was stopped earlier than planned because of slow enrollment: 334 patients were randomized to CAS (n = 167) and CEA (n = 167), and an additional 406 patients had been included in the registry. The 1-year cumulative major primary endpoint was lower in the stenting group than in the CEA group (12.2% versus 20.1%; P = .05 for superiority, P = .004 for noninferiority). This nonsignificant difference became even less evident at 3 years (26.2% versus 30.3%; P = .71).[182]

The results of the SAPPHIRE trial have been somewhat controversial; it was cited as supportive of CAS by its enthusiasts and criticized by CEA proponents. A major criticism relates to the concern that 67% of the patients had asymptomatic stenosis and experienced a perioperative risk of death, stroke, and MI of 5.4% with CAS versus 10.2% with CEA. Furthermore, differences in adverse events were largely due to the lower incidence of MI in the CAS group than in the CEA group (2.5% versus 8.1%; P = .03). Inclusion of MI as an endpoint was controversial because MI was not considered as an endpoint in published CEA trials. Finally, all CAS patients received clopidogrel, whereas CEA patients did not. This diversity in treatment regimen may have played a role in the reduced incidence of MI in the stented group.

EVA-3S. Both the EVA-3S and SPACE trials, the two most recently published randomized trials comparing CEA and CAS, were powered to show noninferiority outcomes of CAS versus CEA in patients with symptomatic carotid stenosis.[14,15,21]

In the EVA-3S study, 259 patients were assigned to CEA and 261 to CAS within 2 weeks after study randomization. CPDs were not routinely used in all CAS patients. Dual antiplatelet therapy was recommended but not uniformly administered to CAS patients.[14] The study was stopped prematurely because of a significant 2.5-fold higher risk for 30-day stroke and death in the CAS group than in the CEA group (9.6% versus 3.9%). Similar results were reported at 6 months (11.7% versus 6.1%; P = .02). The conclusion was that "in patients with symptomatic carotid stenosis of 60% or more, stroke and death rates at 1 and 6 months were lower with endarterectomy than with stenting."

SPACE. The SPACE trial randomized 1196 patients to either CAS (n = 607) or CEA (n = 589). The rate of death or ipsilateral ischemic stroke was 6.9% (95% CI, 5.0 to 9.2) in the CAS group and 6.5% in the CEA group (95% CI, 4.6 to 8.7). The study did not prove noninferiority of CAS in comparison to CEA with regard to the periprocedural complication rate (absolute difference, 0.5). The investigators concluded that widespread use of CAS is not justified in the short term for the treatment of carotid artery stenosis.[15,21]

Criticism of the SPACE trial results focused on the incomplete learning curve of the interventionists, which might have contributed to the high stroke and death rates in the CAS arm. In the EVA-3S trial the participating centers were required to perform 12 CAS procedures or 35 supra-aortic stenting procedures, with at least 5 in the carotid artery, under the supervision of a tutor.[14,183] In the SPACE trial the minimum requirement was generically defined as 25 successful consecutive angioplasty or stent procedures.[15] On the other hand, there is general agreement today that requirements for training in CAS are higher than in other anatomic regions.[137,139,140]

Meta-analysis. A recent Cochrane meta-analysis of all available RCTs on CAS, including 12 RCTs with 3227

Table 96-5 Randomized Controlled Trials on Carotid Artery Stenting in Period 2 (Alphabetical Order)

Trial	Sample Size	Population	Study Design— CAS:CEA	Primary Endpoints	Stent	CPD	Results CAS	CEA	Status
ACT-I, 2005	1858	Asymptomatic, >80% stenosis Standard surgical risk	Multicentric— 3:1	30-day stroke Death MI 1-yr ipsilateral stroke	X-Act	Emboshield	N/A		Enrolling
ACST-2, 2006	5000	Asymptomatic high-grade stenosis Standard surgical risk	Multicentric— 1:1	30-day stroke Death MI 5-yr stroke and death	Any CE marked	Optional (only CE marked)	N/A		Enrolling
CREST, 2000	2500	Symptomatic, >50% stenosis Asymptomatic, >70% stenosis Standard surgical risk	Multicentric— 1:1	30-day stroke Death MI 4-yr ipsilateral stroke	Rx Acculink	Rx Accunet	N/A		Enrolling
ICCS, 2001	1500	Symptomatic, >70% stenosis Standard risk	Multicentric European	30-day stroke Death—MI, TIA Cranial nerve palsy—QoL Hematoma— restenosis	Not specified	Optional Not specified	N/A		Enrolling
EVA-3S, 2006[14]	527 (872 planned)	Symptomatic, >60% stenosis Standard surgical risk	Multicentric French noninferiority	30-day stroke Death	Not specified	Optional Not specified	30-day stroke/death 9.6% 3.9% 6-mo stroke/death 11.7% 6.1%		Completed
SAPPHIRE, 2004,[29] 2008[182]	334 (2400 planned)	Symptomatic, >50% stenosis Asymptomatic, >80% stenosis High surgical risk	Multicentric noninferiority	30-day stroke Death—MI 1-yr ipsilateral stroke and death	SMART Precise	Angioguard	1-yr stroke/death/MI 12% 19% 3-yr stroke/death/MI 26.2% 30.3%		Completed
SPACE, 2006[15]	1196 (1900 planned)	Symptomatic, >70% stenosis Standard surgical risk	Multicentric noninferiority	30-day ipsilateral stroke Death	Not specified	Optional Not specified	30-day ipsilateral stroke/death 6.9% 6.5%		Completed
TACIT	3700	Asymptomatic, >60% stenosis Standard surgical risk	3-armed trial: CAS:CEA: medical 1:1:1	30-day stroke and death 5-yr stroke and death Neurocognitive decline	Not specified	Not specified	N/A		Enrolling

CAS, carotid artery stenting; CEA, carotid endarterectomy; CPD, cerebral protection device; MI, myocardial infarction; N/A, not available; QoL, quality of life; TIA, transient ischemic attack.

patients, concluded that there was no significant difference in pooled outcomes at 30 days for any stroke or death, although the trend favored surgery. Cranial nerve injury rates significantly favored CAS.[184] However, this meta-analysis was severely affected by high heterogeneity because of the inclusion of RCTs performed during period 1 and period 2, and the authors concluded that there was no strong message to change current clinical practice.

In the near future other clinical trials may provide new insight with regard to the clinical efficacy of CAS in standard patients with carotid stenosis. Specifically, the U.S. National Institutes of Health CREST[20] trial recruited 2522 symptom-

atic and asymptomatic patients, who were then randomly assigned to either CEA or CAS in a 1:1 ratio. The randomized phase was completed on July 18, 2008. Follow-up is ongoing. Several other RCTs comparing CAS, CEA, and best medical treatment of symptomatic or asymptomatic patients are planned or ongoing (see Table 96-5).[185-189]

In conclusion, CAS and CEA will probably play a complementary role in patients with occlusive carotid disease. However, at present it remains unclear which patients will benefit more from one intervention versus the other.

Based on the published literature, two important observations should be emphasized further:

- CAS has not been definitively proved to be superior or even equivalent to CEA.
- CAS is technically feasible in the majority of cases, but outcomes are related to the interventionist's experience level, patient selection, and possible technologic improvement.

TECHNOLOGIC REQUIREMENTS

In the optimal setting, carotid intervention should be performed in angiosuites specifically equipped with a sterile environment and all the facilities necessary for an operating room, as in the so-called hybrid operating rooms (Fig. 96-8).[137,190]

Generally, specific minimum requirements are the following:

- Appropriate equipment and sufficient space to allow positioning of patient monitoring and anesthesia equipment while preserving the sterile field
- High-resolution image intensifier with the ability to acquire and store high-quality images with the lowest radiation exposure
- Adequate physiologic monitoring system and prompt access to surgical and medical emergency support

It has been suggested that a bank of three monitors be used to show simultaneous working and reference images, as well as hemodynamic data. The monitors should be positioned in front of the operator to allow thorough understanding of patient conditions and progress of the procedure.

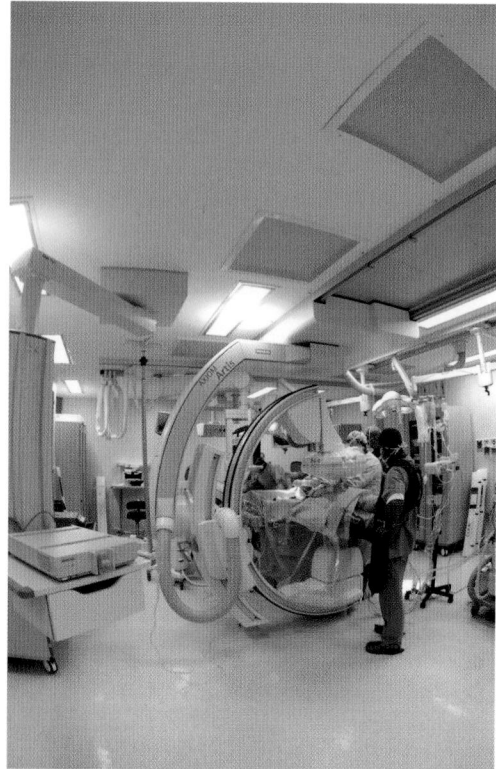

Figure 96-8 Hybrid operating room with a fixed angiographic system (Siemens Axiom Artis dTA).

Prompt availability of a large inventory of endovascular supplies, as well as any emergency equipment and medication, is critical for a successful carotid stent program.

TRAINING ISSUES

A number of studies have demonstrated that increased operator experience with CAS decreases the incidence of stroke.[139,140,191,192] Although there are no formal training requirements for CAS or universally accepted standards, different proposals have been set by several multispecialist societies. The SCAI/SVMB/Society for Vascular Surgery (SVS) multidisciplinary consensus document of 2005 supported a minimum of 30 cervicodiagnostic angiograms and 25 carotid interventions before performing CAS independently.[193,194] The other U.S. multidisciplinary document (ASITN/ASNR/Congress of Neurological Surgeons [CNS]/SIR) of 2005 defines 100 supervised cerebral angiograms and either 10 supervised CAS procedures or 25 noncarotid stent placements, 4 supervised carotid stent placements, and 16 hours of continued medical education with acceptable results as a minimum requirement.[162] The document from interventional cardiologists, neuroradiologists, vascular and endovascular surgeons, and radiologist societies in Europe (ICCS-SPREAD [Italian Concensus Carotid Stenting/Stroke PRevention and Educational Awareness Diffusion]) set higher minimum standards: at least 150 supra-aortic vessel angiographies (>100 as the primary operator) and at least 75 CAS procedures (>50 as the primary operator) were required for the acquisition of competence and an additional 50 CAS procedures per year for maintenance of competence.[137]

The use of virtual training simulators for reproducing the procedure and interacting with the operator may represent first-line training but is not intended as a substitute for live experience. As a second step, a number of tutoring or training programs or device-specific programs offered by industry are widely available and recommended to improve skills and shorten the training phase while preserving patient safety.

Each institution should have a clearly designed program for carotid stent procedures and for assessing outcomes with independent postprocedural neurologic assessment.

LONG-TERM RESULTS

After CAS all patients should be evaluated in a regular follow-up protocol that includes duplex scanning and clinical assessment. As for all endovascular approaches, a main concern is the durability of the procedure, which is defined as effectiveness in preventing stroke and restenosis.

Stroke Prevention

Most information regarding stroke prevention comes from case series. Setacci and colleagues, in a 6-year experience on 1027 CAS procedures, reported overall stroke/death rates at 1 and 3 years of 2.8% and 7.4%, respectively, by life-table analysis.[162] In 261 CAS procedures, Ouriel and associates found that the cumulative 1-year risk (Kaplan-Meier) of any major adverse clinical events was 10.9% ± 2.0%; no new major ipsilateral strokes occurred between 30 days and 1 year.[165] Gröschel and collaborators performed a systematic review of midterm results in 3814 patients and found an extremely low ipsilateral stroke rate associated with restenosis ranging from 0% to 2%.[195] However, according to the same authors, the disparate case mix, accuracy of follow-up, and potential selection bias made the results questionable. The only long-term results from RCTs are provided by the updated results of SAPPHIRE at 3 years.[182] Accordingly, 92.0% of patients in the stenting group and 93.3% in the endarterectomy group were free of stroke at 3 years (*P* = NS). There were 15 strokes in each of the two groups (117 CEA and 143 CAS procedures), 11 of which in the stenting group and 9 in the endarterectomy group were ipsilateral.

Restenosis

Besides the uncertainty of the benefit in late stroke prevention, another limiting factor in the wider application of CAS was the perceived problem of carotid restenosis regardless of the association with late stroke. In CAVATAS, an alarming restenosis rate of 14% in the endovascular versus 1% in the surgical group at 1 year was reported, even though the risk of stroke/death at 3 years was similar in the two arms of the study (14.3% versus 14.2%).[145] However, it should be stressed that in this trial the majority of the procedures were performed only with balloon angioplasty without stenting.

In more recent studies with routine use of stenting, the incidence of restenosis appears to be low. In the SAPPHIRE trial, the 12-month restenosis rate was 0.6% for CAS and 4% for CEA[29]; unfortunately, the updated results of the trial did not provide careful information on restenosis at 3 years and reported only the "target vessel revascularization" rate, which was not significantly lower in the CAS and CEA groups, 3.0% versus 7.1%.[182]

Recent data from clinical series on restenosis rates after CAS are shown in Table 96-3 (see the Expert Consult Web site)[153,196] and appear to be comparable to CEA (from 0.6% to 18%).[197] Unfortunately, not all the authors used life-table estimates to give reliable information on the issue. In the review article by Gröschel and colleagues that included 34 studies reporting on restenosis rates after CAS over a median of 13 months (6 to 31 months), the cumulative restenosis rate was 6% at 1 year and 7.5% at 2 years for the studies using a threshold of 50%, and 4% for the studies using a threshold of greater than 70%.[195]

The risk for restenosis might be increased in patients treated for recurrent stenosis after CEA or previous neck irradiation or cancer.[160,198,199] In an experience by Skelly and coworkers that included 101 patients, the rate of freedom from greater than 60% restenosis after CAS was as low as 27% ± 17% in patients with neck cancer versus 88% ± 6% in those without.[199] There are also data suggesting that patients in whom restenosis develops after CEA are also more prone to the development of restenosis after CAS.[198,200,201]

Care should be taken in the diagnosis of in-stent restenosis. There is increasing evidence that the ultrasound criteria are different from those used in nonstented arteries. It has been suggested that stent placement can alter the biomechanical properties of the carotid territory by decreasing vessel compliance. The enhanced stiffness of the stent–arterial wall complex renders the flow-pressure relationship of the carotid artery closer to that observed in a rigid tube, and as a consequence the degree of stenosis may be overestimated. Although standardized velocity criteria are not well established for patients with carotid stents, new modified criteria have been proposed. Peak systolic velocity as high as 300 cm/sec or greater or an ICA/CCA peak systolic velocity ratio of 4.3 have been defined as thresholds for detection of greater than 70% restenosis.[202-206] Further studies should clarify this issue.

After CAS, restenosis is frequently asymptomatic, but larger experiences to assess its clinical relevance are needed. The decision with respect to re-treatment should involve rapid progression or the onset of symptoms, as in restenosis after CEA. The majority of in-stent restenoses are manageable by repeated balloon dilatation or with cutting balloons, although occasionally additional stenting may need to be performed.[207]

Based on these data, accurate and prolonged surveillance after CAS is advisable. Duplex ultrasonography should be performed during the same admission and baseline velocities recorded to serve as a basis for comparison with future assessments. The examination should be repeated every 6 months for the first 2 years, when the incidence of restenosis secondary to intimal hyperplasia is higher, and then annually thereafter.

SELECTED KEY REFERENCES

American College of Cardiology Foundation; American Society of Interventional & Therapeutic Neuroradiology; Society for Cardiovascular Angiography and Interventions; Society for Vascular Medicine and Biology; Society of Interventional Radiology, Bates ER, Babb JD, Casey DE Jr, Cates CU, Duckwiler GR, Feldman TE, Gray WA, Ouriel K, Peterson ED, Rosenfield K, Rundback JH, Safian RD, Sloan MA, White CJ. ACCF/SCAI/SVMB/SIR/ASITN 2007 clinical expert consensus document on carotid stenting: a report of the American College of Cardiology Foundation Task Force on Clinical Expert Consensus Documents (ACCF/SCAI/SVMB/SIR/ASITN Clinical Expert Consensus Document Committee on Carotid Stenting). *J Am Coll Cardiol.* 2007;49:126-170.
Clinical expert consensus documents on carotid stenting from the American College of Cardiology.

Ederle J, Featherstone RL, Brown MM. Percutaneous transluminal angioplasty and stenting for carotid artery stenosis. *Cochrane Database Syst Rev.* 2007;4:CD000515.
Met-analysis of RCTs comparing CAS and CEA from the Cochrane collaboration.

Gurm HS, Yadav JS, Fayad P, Katzen BT, Mishkel GJ, Bajwa TK, Ansel G, Strickman NE, Wang H, Cohen SA, Massaro JM, Cutlip DE, for the SAPPHIRE Investigators. Long-term results of carotid stenting versus endarterectomy in high-risk patients. *N Engl J Med.* 2008; 358:1572-1579.
Late results of the SAPPHIRE trial: 3-year stroke and restenosis rates.

Hobson RW 2nd, Howard VJ, Roubin GS, Brott TG, Ferguson RD, Popma JJ, Graham DL, Howard G, CREST Investigators. Carotid artery stenting is associated with increased complications in octogenarians: 30-day stroke and death rates in the CREST lead-in phase. *J Vasc Surg.* 2004;40:1106-1111.
Lead-in data from the largest ongoing RCT comparing CAS and CEA that provide the strongest evidence on CAS risk in older patients.

Kastrup A, Gröschel K, Krapf H, Brehm BR, Dichgans J, Schulz JB. Early outcome of carotid angioplasty and stenting with and without cerebral protection devices: a systematic review of the literature. *Stroke.* 2003;34:813-819.
The largest available meta-analysis comparing CAS with cerebral protection versus CAS without cerebral protection.

Mas JL, Chatellier G, Beyssen B, Branchereau A, Moulin T, Becquemin JP, Larrue V, Lièvre M, Leys D, Bonneville JF, Watelet J, Pruvo JP, Albucher JF, Viguier A, Piquet P, Garnier P, Viader F, Touzé E, Giroud M, Hosseini H, Pillet JC, Favrole P, Neau JP, Ducrocq X, EVA-3S Investigators. Endarterectomy versus stenting in patients with symptomatic severe carotid stenosis. *N Engl J Med.* 2006; 355:1660-1671.
The French randomized trial on carotid stenting versus endarterectomy showing that CAS in symptomatic patients carries a higher risk for periprocedural complications than does CEA.

SPACE Collaborative Group, Ringleb PA, Allenberg J, Brückmann H, Eckstein HH, Fraedrich G, Hartmann M, Hennerici M, Jansen O, Klein G, Kunze A, Marx P, Niederkorn K, Schmiedt W, Solymosi L, Stingele R, Zeumer H, Hacke W. 30 day results from the SPACE trial of stent-protected angioplasty versus carotid endarterectomy in symptomatic patients: a randomised non-inferiority trial. *Lancet.* 2006;368:1239-1247.
The largest randomized trial published on carotid stenting versus endarterectomy.

Wholey MH, Al-Mubarek N, Wholey MH. Updated review of the global carotid artery stent registry. *Catheter Cardiovasc Interv.* 2003;60: 259-266.
The first and largest worldwide registry of CAS with new technology; it included 12,392 CAS procedures with or without cerebral protection.

Yadav JS, Wholey MH, Kuntz RE, Fayad P, Katzen BT, Mishkel GJ, Bajwa TK, Whitlow P, Strickman NE, Jaff MR, Popma JJ, Snead DB, Cutlip DE, Firth BG, Ouriel K. Stenting and Angioplasty with Protection in Patients at High Risk for Endarterectomy Investigators. Protected carotid-artery stenting versus endarterectomy in high-risk patients. *N Engl J Med.* 2004;351:1493-1501.
The first randomized trial comparing carotid stenting and endarterectomy with a single brand of new-generation of cerebral protection devices and stents in a high-risk patient population.

REFERENCES

The reference list can be found on the companion Expert Consult Web site at *www.expertconsult.com.*

CHAPTER 97

Carotid Artery Disease: Fibromuscular Dysplasia

Peter A. Schneider

Based in part on chapters in the previous edition by Peter A. Schneider, MD; James C. Stanley, MD; and Thomas W. Wakefield, MD.

Fibromuscular dysplasia (FMD) is a nonatheromatous degenerative process that involves long, unbranched segments of medium-sized conduit arteries such as the renal artery, the internal carotid artery, and others (see Chapter 144: Renovascular Disease: Fibrodysplasia).[1-3] Although FMD is a systemic process of unknown etiology, it is usually described in terms of the artery in which it occurs and causes the clinical manifestations. This chapter focuses on FMD of the extracranial cerebral arteries.

■ EPIDEMIOLOGY

FMD has been found on 0.25% to 0.68% of consecutive cerebral arteriograms.[4,5] The incidence of carotid FMD was 0.42% in 3600 patients undergoing cerebral arteriographic examination.[6] Many of these examinations were performed for suspected cerebrovascular disease, and thus the true frequency of carotid FMD in the general population is probably lower. In one series of 2000 carotid operations, FMD was the identified pathology in 3.4% of cases.[7] In another sizable series of carotid operations, dilatation for FMD was performed in less than 1%.[8] Carotid FMD is bilateral in 39% to 86% of reported cases.[1,4,9,10] Women predominate in most series, constituting 60% to 90% of patients.[1,7,9,11] A patient may have evidence of FMD in a single artery or in multiple vascular beds. Carotid FMD is associated with cerebral aneurysms and FMD involving the renal arteries. These associations are detailed later in this chapter and are also discussed in Chapter 144 (Renovascular Disease: Fibrodysplasia).

■ PATHOGENESIS

Arterial fibrodysplasia consists of a heterogeneous group of nonatherosclerotic diseases manifested by both occlusive and aneurysmal morphology. The pathology of FMD is discussed further in Chapter 144 (Renovascular Disease: Fibrodysplasia). Although the etiology of FMD is not known, there are several theories, each with partial supporting evidence (Box 97-1). Complications occurring with carotid FMD include encroachment on the arterial lumen causing reduced perfusion, formation and distal embolization of thrombus, and dissection and rupture. These complications occur in less than 10% of cases. Progression of carotid FMD is not well

---

Box 97-1 Factors That May Share in the Etiology of Fibromuscular Dysplasia

- Ischemia—sparsity of vasa vasorum
- Hormonal—predominance in women
- Antitrypsin deficiency—possible contributing factor
- Genetic—occasional familial association of a rare condition
- Tissue hypoxia—association in some cases with smoking
- Infectious-immunologic—immunoglobulin deposition within the intimal tissues of stenotic vessels
- Healed or partially healed arteritis—may be responsible for some atypical cases

---

defined.[2,6,12,13] Most cases of asymptomatic carotid FMD are known to remain clinically silent, and there is no optimal method of noninvasive follow-up of these lesions to reliably grade progression. Among the four types of FMD, the internal carotid artery is most often affected by medial fibroplasia, which results in an arteriographic appearance resembling a "string of beads" (Fig. 97-1), seen in 80% to 95% of the lesions.[4,7,11,14] In one large series, medial fibroplasia was found in 89%, with fusiform narrowing in 7% and an eccentric septum-like lesion in 4%.[4] The arterial segments involved tend to be more distal than occurs with arteriosclerosis and are located in the mid and distal segments of the extracranial internal carotid artery without any appearance of disease at the carotid bifurcation. The serial stenoses are frequently evident on examination of the external surface of the artery (Fig. 97-2). The artery is often elongated and tortuous, and kinking occurs in approximately 5% of cases (Fig. 97-3). Similar disease of the external carotid artery or the intracerebral arteries is rare.

Concurrent lesions that frequently complicate the management of carotid FMD include (1) atherosclerotic occlusive disease at the carotid bifurcation, (2) extracranial carotid artery aneurysms, (3) carotid artery dissection, (4) vertebral artery FMD, (5) intracranial aneurysms and occlusive disease, and (6) renal artery FMD.

Atherosclerotic Occlusive Disease

Ipsilateral atherosclerosis of the carotid bifurcation is present in as many as 20% of individuals with carotid FMD,[7,15] but it

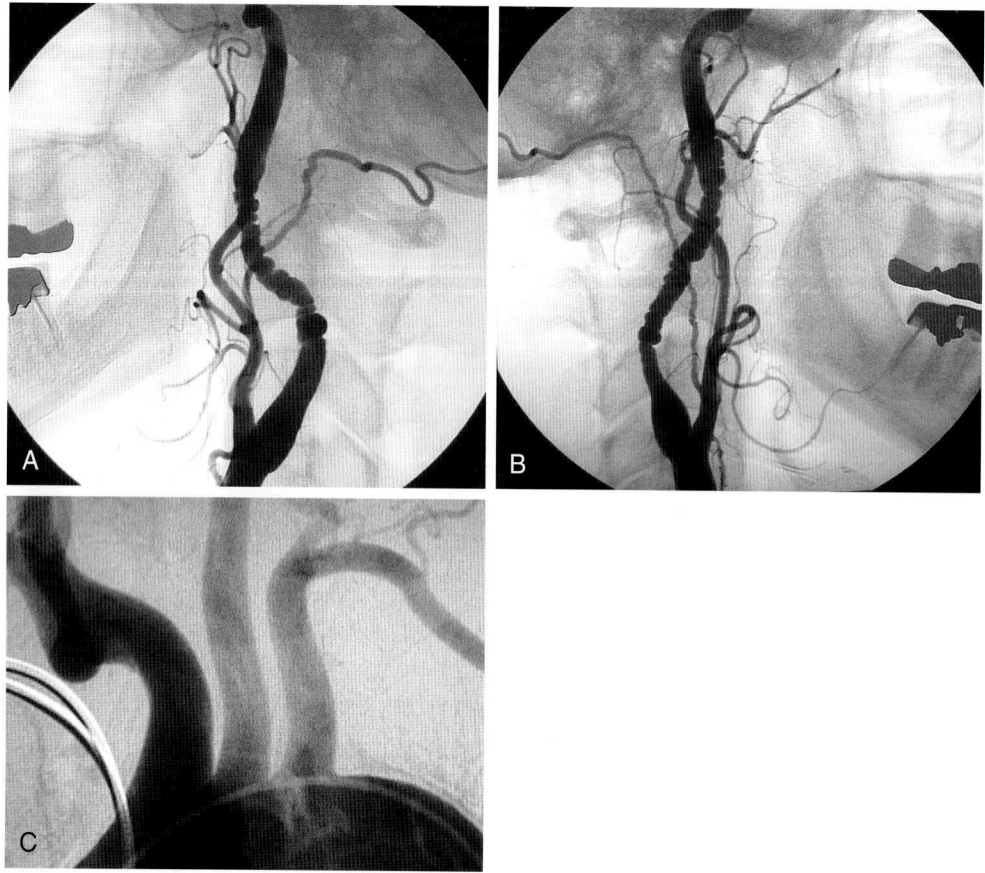

Figure 97-1 A and **B,** Carotid arteriograms demonstrating the classic appearance of fibromuscular dysplasia in the usual location opposite the C1-3 vertebral bodies and intervening disks. Note the low bifurcation and long internal carotid artery. The lesions are present bilaterally in this 43-year-old woman. **C,** The aortic arch shows no evidence of disease, and the arch branches originate near the top of the arch.

may not be possible to attribute cerebral symptoms to one lesion or the other. When atherosclerotic and fibromuscular dysplastic lesions occur together in the same symptomatic artery, they are usually treated simultaneously. In a series of 72 operations for extracranial FMD, carotid endarterectomy was performed as part of a combined procedure in 14 patients (19%).[7]

Extracranial Carotid Artery Aneurysms

Extracranial carotid artery aneurysms are uncommon, and those associated with FMD are rare. Among 130 extracranial carotid aneurysms in one literature review, 2.3% were associated with FMD.[16] In a single-institution series of 15 carotid aneurysms, a third were thought to be caused by or at least associated with FMD, and most were successfully managed by resection and replacement grafting.[17]

Carotid Artery Dissection

FMD may play a role in the development of spontaneous dissection of the carotid artery. This often catastrophic event is responsible for up to 4% of strokes and is associated with

fibrodysplasia in approximately 15% of cases.[18-20] In a series of 50 patients undergoing surgery for carotid dissection, 12% had FMD as the cause and were treated by either graduated rigid dilatation or vein graft replacement.[21] In seven consecutive patients with carotid dissection that was managed by carotid stent placement, five had FMD as the cause.[19] FMD should be considered among the potential etiologic mechanisms of spontaneous carotid dissection.[14,22-24] However, reports of spontaneous dissection occurring subsequent to the identification of asymptomatic carotid FMD are not available. The structural abnormality of the arterial wall in FMD and its association with spontaneous dissection suggest that dilatation of the artery may pose an increased risk for perioperative dissection. Nevertheless, dissection is an unusual complication of dilatation.[1,7,25]

Vertebral Artery Fibromuscular Dysplasia

Vertebral artery FMD is identified in 7% to 38% of those with carotid lesions and is occasionally an isolated finding.[7,12,25] The vertebral artery disease is usually located at the level of the C2 vertebral body and does not extend intracranially.[11]

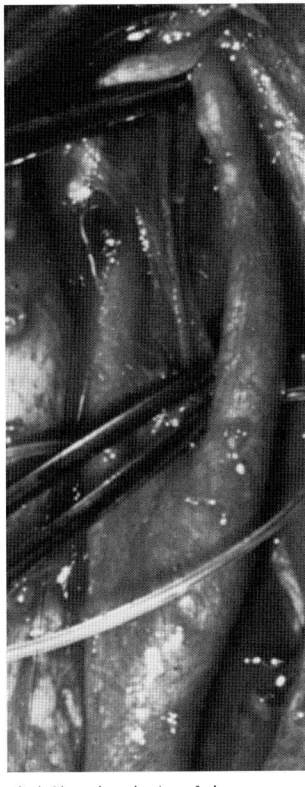

Figure 97-2 Medial fibrodysplasia of the extracranial internal carotid artery. Operative exposure of the artery reveals an external beaded appearance as a result of serial narrowing.

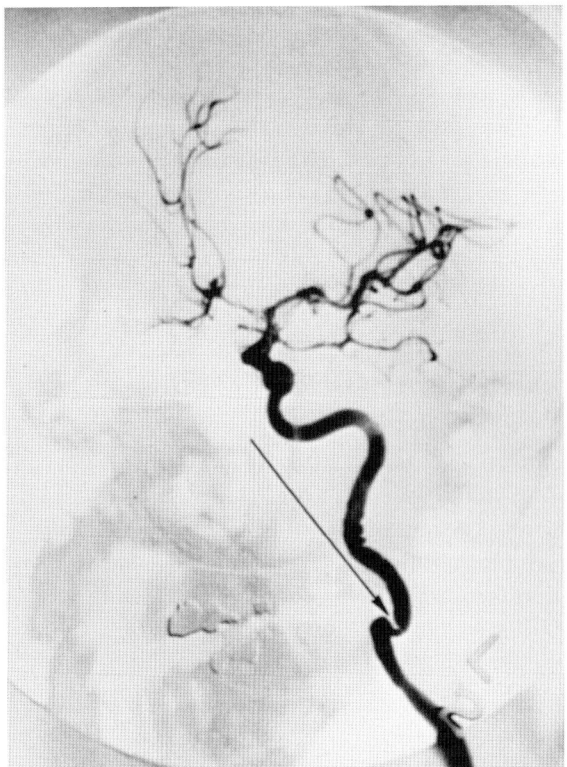

Figure 97-3 Medial fibrodysplasia of the extracranial internal carotid artery with angulation (*arrow*) affecting a tortuous elongated segment. *(From Stanley JC, Fry WJ, Seeger JF, et al. Extracranial internal carotid and vertebral artery fibrodysplasia. Arch Surg. 1974;109:215-222.)*

FMD has been associated with vertebral artery dissection after neck or spine manipulation.[26] Fortunately, it is rarely responsible for symptoms and does not usually complicate management of the internal carotid lesion. One series reported 32 patients with vertebrobasilar transient ischemic attack (TIA) and stroke as a result of vertebral artery FMD.[25] Among 12 vertebral artery reconstructions performed, half were for isolated vertebral FMD and half were performed at the time of rigid dilatation of a carotid lesion. The most frequently used operative approach was a vein bypass to the distal vertebral artery (see Chapter 102: Vertebral Artery Disease).

Intracranial Aneurysms and Occlusive Disease

Intracranial aneurysmal disease is another important expression of the dysplastic process. It is found in at least 10% of patients with FMD in general and as many as 51% of patients with internal carotid FMD in particular (20% on average).[9,12] Solitary intracranial aneurysms are present in 80% of these patients, but multiple aneurysms occur in the remaining 20%. These aneurysms tend to be on the same side as the extracranial carotid FMD.[9] They pose an independent threat of rupture and hemorrhage, and their natural history has the potential to be worsened by relief of a proximal stenosis. In one series, intracranial aneurysms and extracranial FMD each caused half the symptoms, and in another series, half of the strokes were due to aneurysm rupture.[9,27] In most studies,

however, intracranial aneurysms were responsible for a quarter to a third of the neurologic symptoms caused by the cervical carotid lesion.[2]

Nonetheless, intracranial aneurysms should be treated on their own individual merits (e.g., size, initial symptoms). Furthermore, the presence of a small, asymptomatic intracranial aneurysm should not dissuade the vascular surgeon from repairing a threatening cervical lesion. The supraclinoid vasculature may also be affected by occlusive disease that suggests FMD as the etiology. This occurs rarely and primarily in young and middle-aged women without other apparent etiologic factors. There may be associated evidence of FMD of the cervical internal carotid artery.[28]

Renal Artery Fibromuscular Dysplasia

Renal artery FMD coexists with carotid FMD in 8% to 40% of patients.[2,7,29] It is an additional threat in patients with intracranial aneurysms in that it is often accompanied by severe hypertension. Because renal artery FMD generally responds well to percutaneous balloon angioplasty, the possibility of coexistent renal artery involvement should be considered before the treatment of carotid stenosis, especially if the patient has hypertension that is difficult to control (see Chapter 144: Renovascular Disease: Fibrodysplasia).

Table 97-1 Initial Symptoms in Patients with Extracranial Fibromuscular Arterial Dysplasia

		Symptom (%)			
Series	Number of Patients	Hemispheric TIA	Hemispheric Stroke	Amaurosis Fugax	Vertebrobasilar TIA or Stroke
Schneider et al.[29]	115	42	23	22	NA
Chiche et al.[25]	70	36	27	NA	45
Moreau et al.[7]	58	31	12	28	22

NA, not available; TIA, transient ischemic attack.

CLINICAL FINDINGS

More than 90% of patients with medial fibroplasia are women, and the disease is diagnosed most often during the fourth and fifth decades of life. Bilateral disease has been reported to occur in 35% to 85% of patients with these lesions. This lesion is rare in African Americans. Although medial fibrodysplasia is considered to be a systemic arteriopathy, clinically overt arterial involvement is usually limited to the renal, extracranial internal carotid, and external iliac vessels.[6,13,25,27]

History and Physical Examination

Extracranial cerebral artery FMD may be either an incidental finding without symptoms or the cause of neurologic events. Symptomatic manifestations in large, contemporary series of treated patients included TIA, stroke, and disability (Table 97-1). Stroke was the initial finding in 12% to 27% of patients. Hemispheric TIA occurred in 31% to 42%, and amaurosis fugax was present in 22% to 28%.[6,15,16] Several other series have confirmed this distribution of symptoms.[12,30,31]

Other than this process occurring in a relatively young, mostly female population, the history and physical examination may be notable for the absence of other identifying factors. There may be no particular history or inciting factors. The presence of atherosclerotic risk factors is variable. On physical examination there may be bruits in other locations.

DIAGNOSTIC EVALUATION

Duplex Ultrasound

Most asymptomatic patients with a carotid bruit and those with hemispheric or nonfocal neurologic symptoms undergo carotid duplex scanning (see Chapter 93: Cerebrovascular Disease: Diagnostic Evaluation). Duplex may reveal elevated velocity as a result of FMD, but the lesion may be missed because it is located more distally than the usual atherosclerotic plaque.[11,32] If the lesion is detected, the duplex study may not be able to evaluate the artery distal to the lesion because FMD may involve the artery all the way to base of the skull.

Arteriography

Catheter-based contrast-enhanced arteriography continues to be the best method for clearly delineating the anatomic features of FMD of the extracranial cerebral arteries (see "Mechanical Repair"). Many cases of carotid FMD are discovered during arteriography.[11]

Computed Tomographic and Magnetic Resonance Angiography

Computed tomographic angiography (CTA) may replace standard catheter-based arteriography in the evaluation of carotid FMD when enough experience has been gained for clinical and anatomic correlation, just as CTA has done in other vascular beds and disease processes. When carotid FMD is identified, the intracranial vascular anatomy should be evaluated to check for the presence of intracranial aneurysms, as well as contralateral carotid stenosis and vertebral artery disease. Magnetic resonance angiography (MRA) has not been particularly useful in the diagnostic evaluation of carotid FMD because of the tendency for signal dropout with tight lesions and the propensity to produce a "beaded" appearance in normal conduit arteries that may be confused with FMD. MRA may be beneficial for follow-up of known FMD.[33] Patients with carotid FMD should undergo computed tomography or magnetic resonance imaging of the brain to look for evidence of infarction, as well as the presence of cerebral aneurysms.

SELECTION OF TREATMENT

Natural History

Our understanding of the natural history of FMD of the carotid circulation is not complete. Many series have documented the potential for carotid FMD to cause symptoms, as discussed earlier, but the natural history of asymptomatic lesions is less well documented. In one series of 79 patients, most of whom were found to have carotid FMD incidentally on cerebral angiography (0.6% of the total), only 3 patients (4%) subsequently suffered a cerebral ischemic event during an average follow-up of 5 years.[13] When small groups of asymptomatic patients were studied prospectively, less than 10% went on to experience new neurologic symptoms.[2,9,13] Roughly a third of carotid FMD lesions demonstrate significant angiographic progression with time.[2,12] None of these studies, however, have included a significant number of high-grade asymptomatic stenoses, the group in which the risk for stroke would be expected to be higher.

Most reported cases of symptomatic carotid FMD have been treated by dilatation of the responsible artery. There is no study in which a large number of patients with carotid FMD and focal cerebral ischemic events were treated medically. In one series, 13 patients with either TIA (10 patients) or stroke (3 patients) did not undergo surgical correction of carotid FMD. Only one patient remained symptomatic.[33] Some have suggested that even symptomatic lesions should not be considered for surgery until their natural history is better understood.[27,34] At present, we are left with a rare cause of focal cerebral ischemic events caused by extracranial carotid stenosis that can be repaired with a fairly simple open operation or by percutaneous balloon dilatation.

Therapeutic Challenges

Because of the lack of sophisticated data on carotid FMD, the following challenges frequently arise in its management and must be considered during the treatment-planning stage.

1. One of the key driving factors in the treatment of atherosclerosis of the carotid bifurcation, the degree of stenosis, is not possible to determine with any reliability in carotid FMD. This makes the severity of the disease in a given patient extremely difficult to assess. The indication for mechanical treatment is driven primarily by the development of cerebral ischemia. This factor also compromises the follow-up of asymptomatic patients.

2. It is not always possible to determine which of two concurrent lesions is causing the cerebral symptoms, as is the case with coexistent carotid FMD and significant atherosclerotic disease of the bifurcation. These lesions are usually treated simultaneously. Carotid FMD may also be associated with a coexistent cerebral aneurysm and present the same dilemma of competing suspect lesions.

3. When symptomatic carotid FMD is treated, it can be a challenge to decide how to manage a contralateral severe but asymptomatic lesion. Although asymptomatic lesions seem to have a generally benign course, such may not be the case in a patient who suffered a stroke on the contralateral side because of the same pathology.

4. Patients with carotid FMD often have nonfocal symptoms, some of which may be due to global ischemia. The indications for intervention in this situation are ambiguous.

5. The presence of an intracranial aneurysm may alter the treatment sequence or the surgical approach.

6. The presence of hypertension secondary to renal artery FMD may complicate any procedure performed for carotid FMD.

Clinical Considerations

Because of the relative safety and effectiveness of mechanical intervention (see "Mechanical Repair"), dilatation of the artery is appropriate for lesions causing focal ischemic events (hemispheric or ocular) or episodes of cerebral hypoperfusion. A lesion causing a focal cerebral ischemic event should be considered for treatment because it remains a significant

threat. Hypoperfusion is rare but can occur in the setting of critical bilateral carotid FMD or even unilateral disease when there is a significant defect in the circle of Willis. Percutaneous transluminal angioplasty (PTA) has been successful in the treatment of renal artery FMD, and carotid angioplasty with stenting has a growing role in the management of carotid disease; however, the results and durability of balloon angioplasty for carotid FMD, with or without stent placement, are not known. Symptomatic patients at high surgical risk should be considered for percutaneous balloon angioplasty, especially if the anatomy allows the use of cerebral protection devices.

Anatomic Considerations
Cerebral Protection

The lesion requiring treatment in carotid FMD is usually a series of webs with intervening pockets, in between which platelet thrombi and cellular debris have accumulated. Disruption of the webs, whether by balloon dilatation or rigid dilatation, produces potentially embolic debris. Some type of cerebral protection is warranted. Carotid FMD tends to involve the carotid artery for several centimeters distal to the bifurcation and may affect the length of the artery to the base of the skull, thus precluding a landing zone for an embolic filter during the procedure. Most distal filters require a few centimeters of straight, healthy artery proximal to the petrous portion of the carotid artery to be functional and safely placed. At some point in the future, protection with a reversed-flow device and proximal occlusion may be the best method of protection during percutaneous intervention.

Stents

It is not clear whether carotid balloon angioplasty should be accompanied by stent placement in FMD. Stent placement is not usually required after PTA in renal artery FMD because the results are excellent without stents, and the patients are usually otherwise young and healthy with good life expectancies. However, stents are routinely placed when atherosclerotic stenosis of the carotid bifurcation is treated percutaneously, and there is some likelihood that stent placement after PTA helps stabilize flaps and disrupted dysplastic tissue. Experience with PTA for carotid FMD is limited, and there are even fewer cases of carotid stent placement for FMD. In light of this paucity of cases, more time will be required to determine the role of PTA with or without stenting in the treatment of patients with carotid FMD.

■ TREATMENT
Medical Management

Patients with asymptomatic carotid stenosis secondary to FMD should be placed on a regimen of antiplatelet agents. Diagnostic evaluation should be undertaken to rule out other arterial pathology. If associated conditions are identified, either in the carotid circulation (e.g., carotid aneurysm) or in other vascular beds (e.g., renal artery stenosis), they should be treated as needed.

Carotid FMD should be monitored at intervals of 6 months with noninvasive studies such as duplex ultrasound, CTA, or MRA. If duplex follow-up is used, the internal carotid artery must be interrogated as distally as possible. If symptoms develop or there is a significant change in the pathologic lesion (e.g., dissection), mechanical repair of the artery should be considered. There is no established role for anticoagulation or for anti-inflammatory medications such as steroids. Chiropractic manipulation of the neck should be avoided, as well as sports that are likely to produce whiplash-type neck injuries.

Mechanical Repair

Methods of mechanical intervention for the treatment of carotid FMD include the following:
1. Open surgical graduated rigid dilatation
2. Open access for transluminal balloon dilatation with proximal clamping and backbleeding
3. PTA (with or without stent placement or cerebral protection devices)

Open Surgical Dilatation

The usual fibrodysplastic lesion encountered in the internal carotid artery responds to mechanical dilatation. Over the past several decades such treatment has been performed with relative success and safety by means of rigid dilators of progressively enlarging size passed antegrade into the internal carotid artery with arterial control.[1,7,25,29,30] This approach permits gentle disruption of the obstructive webs while allowing associated debris to be flushed out of the artery and has been shown over the years to produce reasonable results.

The main disadvantage of this approach is that it is performed without imaging of the luminal surface. The length of the arterial segment to undergo treatment must be estimated. Kinks and coils must be managed by "feel" without direct guidance. There is no simple method of assessing the results of treatment in real time, the way interval arteriography can guide a procedure during percutaneous treatment. The other disadvantage is the need for a neck incision and arterial exposure.

Exposure for the open approach is similar to that for carotid endarterectomy except that higher internal carotid artery exposure is usually required to ensure that dilatation is carried out under direct vision and that the extracranial carotid artery can be safely straightened during passage of the dilator (see Chapter 95: Carotid Artery Disease: Endarterectomy). The posterior belly of the digastric muscle may be divided, but subluxation of the mandible is rarely required. If the distal internal carotid artery is not accessible, balloon angioplasty should be considered (see under "Open-Access Balloon Dilatation"). The normal arterial segment above the

highest point of involvement is apparent by direct inspection, and the internal carotid artery is encircled at this point.

The surgeon should take care to not manipulate the intervening segment of the internal carotid artery as it is gently exposed throughout its length. Determination of stump pressure or electroencephalographic monitoring is not ordinarily needed for this brief procedure but may be indicated if a more extensive procedure is planned (e.g., bifurcation endarterectomy, correction of redundancy, or interposition grafting). Except in such unusual circumstances, a shunt is unnecessary.

Heparin is administered (75 to 100 U/kg) before interrupting flow. Dextran 40, 25 mL/hr beginning at the time of surgery and continued during the immediate postoperative period, may help prevent early deposition of thrombotic material on the inner surfaces of the arteriotomy and the fractured septa. The common carotid artery is cross-clamped. Traction on a Silastic "sling" placed around the internal carotid artery just above the bifurcation is performed to straighten the artery. A short arteriotomy is made in the internal carotid artery at the base of the bulb. Graduated metal dilators are then gently passed up the straightened internal carotid artery, beginning with a 1.5-mm-diameter probe and progressing up to a 3.5-mm- or, occasionally, a 4.0-mm-diameter probe (Fig. 97-4). A series of "giving" sensations are usually felt as each septal stenosis is gently fractured for the first time, but such sensations are not felt thereafter.

The procedure is terminated after the segment has been gently stretched to full diameter throughout its course. This can usually be observed under direct vision. It is important not to exceed this gentle stretching and, therefore, not to proceed beyond a 4-mm diameter. Backbleeding after passage of the dilators should be thorough because large debris is sometimes retrieved. The short arteriotomy is closed rapidly with a simple running suture of 6-0 polypropylene. Careful interrogation of the entire segment with a Doppler probe or duplex scanner after restoration of flow ensures patency without turbulence or residual defect.

Poor candidates for this operation include patients with lesions that are too distal to be adequately exposed and patients who have contraindications to open surgery. In such cases the options are open exposure for PTA with outflow control or, more likely, transfemoral PTA with a cerebral protection device (if possible) and a stent if dissection occurs.

Results. The results of three large, contemporary series of surgically managed patients are presented in Tables 97-2 and 97-3. These reports consist primarily of patients undergoing rigid carotid dilatation but also include some instances of carotid replacement and vertebral revascularization.[7,25,29] The incidence of perioperative stroke during surgical treatment in these series ranged from 1.4% to 2.6%. TIA occurred in 1.4% to 7.7%, and perforation occurred twice in 318 operations (0.6%).[7,29] Cranial nerve injuries, most of which were transient, resulted from extensive distal operative exposure of the

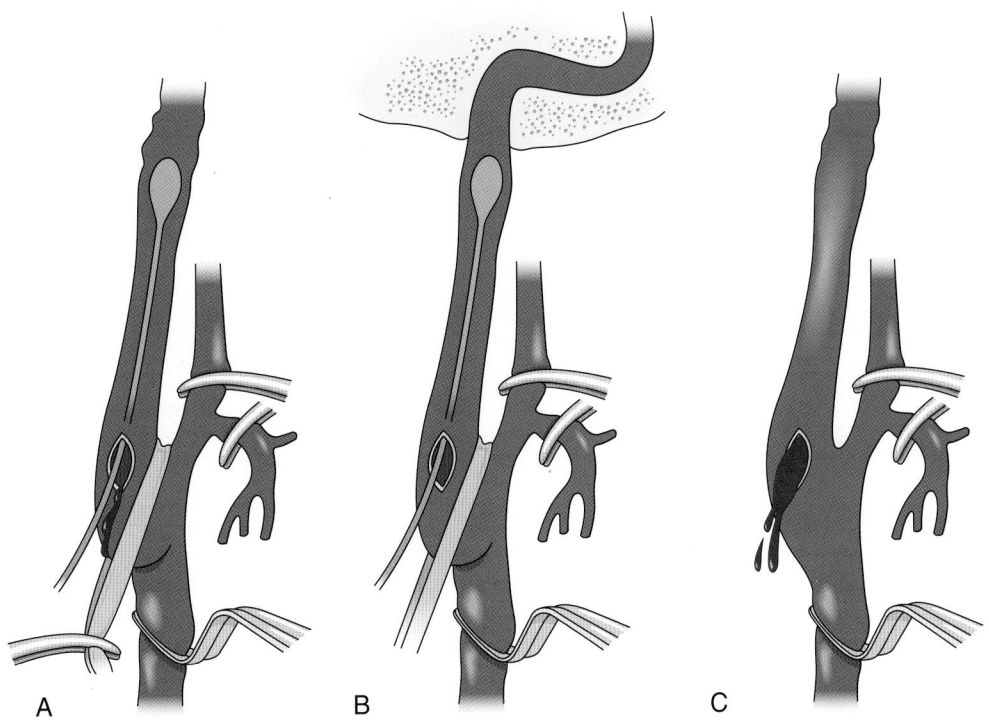

A   B   C

Figure 97-4 Drawings showing the main features of the open surgical technique. **A,** Straightening of the carotid artery with downward traction on a Silastic sling. **B,** Gentle, graduated dilatation of the internal carotid artery from 2 to 4 mm. Passage of the dilator to the bony canal at the base of the skull is shown. **C,** Backbleeding of the artery to remove dislodged debris. *(From Wylie EJ, Stoney RJ, Ehrenfeld WK, Effeney DJ. Nonatherosclerotic diseases of the extracranial carotid arteries. In: Manual of Vascular Surgery. New York, NY: Springer-Verlag; 1986:184-185.)*

Table 97-2 Results of Surgical Treatment of Extracranial Fibromuscular Arterial Dysplasia

Series	Number of Patients	Number of Operations	Result (%)		
			Operative Stroke	*Operative TIA*	*Operative Death*
Schneider et al.[29]	115	168	1.7	6.0	0
Chiche et al.[25]	70	78	2.6	7.7	1.3
Moreau et al.[7]	58	72	1.4	1.4	0

TIA, transient ischemic attack.

Table 97-3 Late Follow-up after Surgical Treatment of Extracranial Fibromuscular Arterial Dysplasia

Series	Number of Patients	Mean Years of Follow-up (Range)	Results (%)			
			Recurrent Stenosis	*Late Occlusion*	*Late Stroke*	*Death, Other Causes*
Schneider et al.[29]	115	1-17	2.3	0.6	1.2	NA
Chiche et al.[25]	70	7 (1-15)	0	0	2.9	8.6
Moreau et al.[7]	58	13 (6-22)	0	2.8	3.8	13.2

NA, not available.

internal carotid artery and were reported to occur in 5.1% to 16.7% of cases.[7,25]

Excellent long-term follow-up data are available (see Table 97-3). Late stroke developed in 1.2% to 3.8% of patients, and nearly all late deaths (up to 22 years) were due to non-neurologic causes. In one series, 94% of patients underwent duplex scanning (mean follow-up, 7 years).[25] Actuarial rates of primary patency, survival, and stroke-free survival were 94%, 96%, and 94%, respectively, at 5 years and 94%, 82%, and 88%, respectively, at 10 years. When follow-up angiography is performed, it usually demonstrates a normal-sized lumen (Fig. 97-5).

Open-Access Balloon Dilatation

When the length of the diseased internal carotid artery extends too far distally to be dissected and ensure adequate control of manual dilatation, some authors have advised balloon angioplasty combined with open arterial control, as described in "Open Surgical Dilatation."[35-38] The benefit of this approach is the opportunity for controlled dilatation with interval arteriography while maintaining the ability to back-bleed the artery and avoid embolization of debris from the dilated lesion. Among a small number of patients in several reports, it appears that early results with this approach may be comparable to those of rigid dilatation.

Percutaneous Transluminal Angioplasty

PTA may be a reasonable approach for more proximal internal carotid artery FMD.[39-43] The rationale for this approach is based on the success of PTA in the treatment of renal artery FMD and dramatic improvement in the technology, which supports balloon angioplasty and stenting of the atherosclerotic carotid bifurcation. Balloon angioplasty is associated with fewer complications than open surgery of the renal artery for FMD and provides reasonable long-term results.

Technique

Diagnostic evaluation for carotid FMD is likely to include an arch aortogram and carotid and cerebral arteriograms, as noted earlier. These are valuable tools in planning carotid PTA. Arteriography will provide important information with respect to the optimal strategy that should be pursued based on the demonstrated anatomy. Lesions that have signs of aneurysm formation should not be considered for endovascular management. They may be better treated by open arterial replacement. On the other hand, lesions that show some evidence of dissection should be considered for stent placement, and care should be taken to avoid overdilatation and possibly rupture.

If significant kinking of the distal artery at the diseased segment is noted, there are additional considerations. Kinks are not favorable for stent placement because the stent can make the kinks worse. During open, rigid dilatation, the

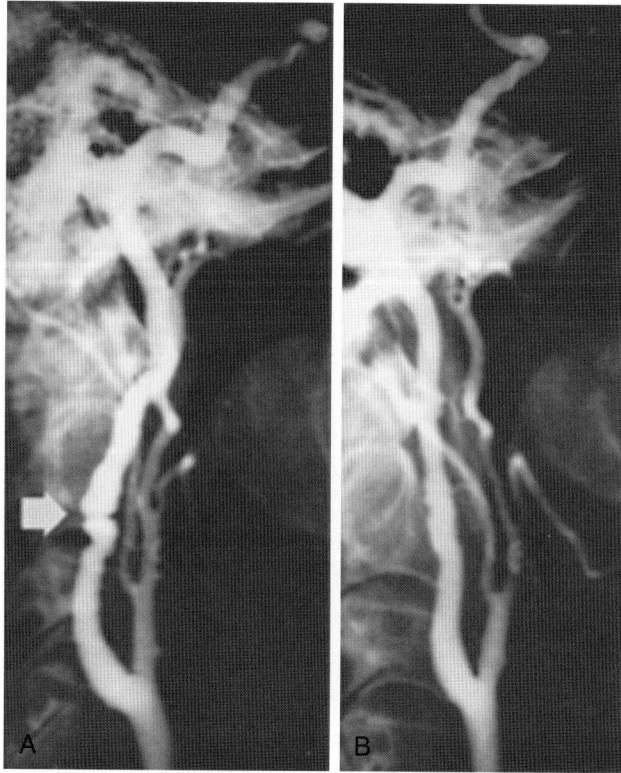

Figure 97-5 A, Preoperative right carotid arteriogram showing a localized zone of fibromuscular dysplasia characterized by an intraluminal diaphragm (*arrow*). **B,** Postoperative right carotid arteriogram after graduated intraluminal dilatation. The carotid lumen is now widely patent.

artery is dissected and straightened before treatment, and surgical shortening of the artery may be required. Such shortening obviously cannot be done during balloon angioplasty.

It is not always possible to tell where the lumen is located when using angiography to help with passage of the guide wire, and patience and persistence may be required to safely cross the lesion. Having the sheath tip close by to use as a stable platform is helpful. In addition, an angled catheter may be used to support and direct the guide wire as it traverses the weblike internal carotid artery lesions, which sometimes have only pinhole openings. As the guide wire passes through each lesion, the responsiveness and directionality of the guide wire decrease.

Heparin is administered to provide an activated clotting time in excess of 250 seconds. Most patients with carotid FMD are young, and they are much more likely than other vascular patients to have an arch favorable for percutaneous carotid artery access, one with less tortuosity and less ectopic vascular disease. The carotid arteries frequently arise from the superior aspect of the arch rather than on the upslope of the proximal arch (see Fig. 97-1). The carotid artery sheath may be placed in the distal common carotid artery because the bifurcation is not usually diseased (Fig. 97-6). The external carotid artery is generally normal in appearance and can be used as a place to anchor the stiff exchange guide wire for sheath placement.

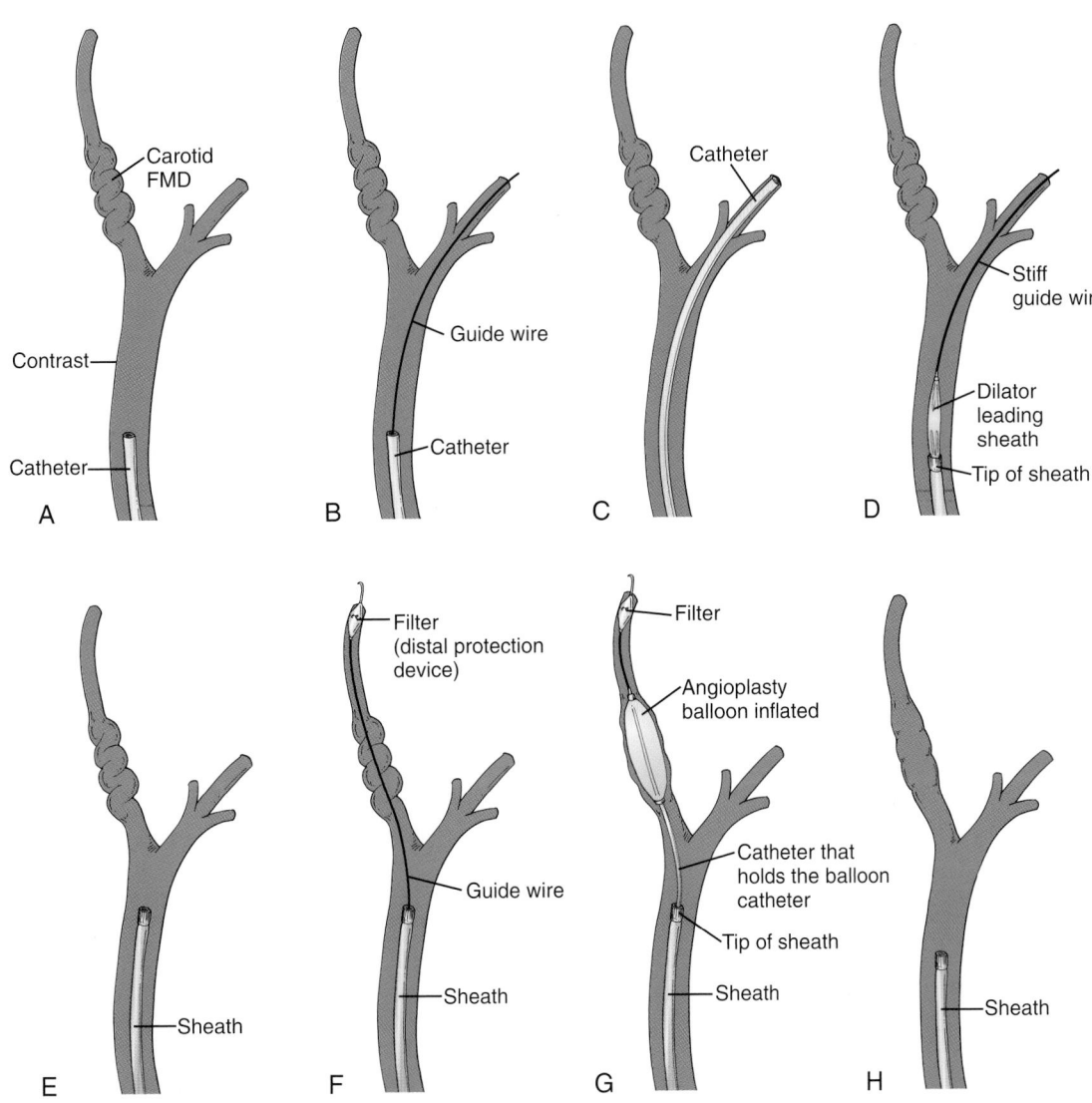

Figure 97-6 Endovascular technique. **A,** Internal carotid artery narrowed by fibromuscular dysplasia (FMD). An arteriogram was performed through a carotid catheter. **B,** Guide wire placed in the external carotid artery by using a roadmap of the carotid bifurcation. **C,** Cerebral catheter advanced into the external carotid artery. **D,** Stiff guide wire advanced into the external carotid artery. The carotid access sheath is advanced over the exchange guide wire. **E,** Carotid sheath in place with the tip of the sheath in the distal common carotid artery. **F,** Cerebral protection device in place in the distal internal carotid artery. **G,** Balloon angioplasty of the fibromuscular lesion in the internal carotid artery. **H,** After balloon angioplasty, the lumen has improved significantly.

After the stiff exchange guide wire is placed, the carotid sheath is advanced. Once the sheath is in place, its position is confirmed with an arteriogram and the bifurcation is road-mapped. Because internal carotid artery lesions may extend to the base of the skull, the image intensifier must be placed so that the operator can observe the distance from the tip of the sheath inferiorly to the area distal to the lesion superiorly. Use of some type of cerebral protection is highly desirable but not always possible, as discussed previously. If there is no safe landing zone for a distal protection device, it is better to perform the procedure without it. The distal filter or occlusion balloon may move slightly during the procedure, even when performed with meticulous technique. Therefore, the distal protection device must be placed at least 1.5 to 2 cm distal to the lesion. If stent placement is anticipated, the nose cone on the stent delivery catheter typically requires at least 2 cm of clearance. Care must also be taken to avoid guide wire interactions with any associated intracranial pathology that may be present.

If a distal occlusion balloon or filter is used, placement is likely to be in the petrous carotid or above so that it is distal to the disease. This segment of the internal carotid artery is more prone to spasm and dissection than the extracranial segment, so caution should be exercised. The distal protection device with the shortest landing zone is the distal occlusion balloon. Proximal occlusion devices, with or without reversed flow, may be a reasonable future alternative for cerebral protection in those with distal internal carotid artery lesions and no safe filter landing zone.

FMD generally covers a longer distance of the internal carotid artery than does carotid atherosclerosis and may therefore require a longer balloon (4 cm). It is best to dilate the entire lesion with one inflation. The balloon should be undersized slightly with regard to the intended diameter of the artery to help avoid dissection or rupture.

Fortunately, the most frequently encountered extracranial carotid FMD pathologic lesion is medial fibroplasia, which is amenable to dilatation and less likely to include aneurysmal dilatation. For FMD lesions that contain aneurysmal segments, PTA is probably not advisable.

Carotid stent placement may be challenging in patients with carotid FMD because many of these patients have redundancy, kinks, and coils of the cervical internal carotid artery. The segments involved by FMD tend to be longer than those involved by atherosclerosis, where almost all lesions are shorter than 2 cm, and experience with stent placement near the base of the skull is limited. In addition, no one knows the implications of stent placement in patients with a life expectancy of many decades, as is the case with many FMD patients.

Given a track record of success with PTA of FMD lesions in other locations, primary stent placement is probably not warranted. In addition, FMD tends to occur in a younger group of patients with a reasonable long-term life expectancy, and the performance of carotid stents over decades is not known. However, if dissection, residual stenosis, or flaps are evident on completion arteriography, a stent should be considered. Smaller stents are used than is normally the case with bifurcation disease because self-expanding stents are sized for the distal internal carotid artery (5 or 6 mm) rather than the common carotid artery (8 or 10 mm). The minimum length of artery required to cover the disease should be stented because stents confer stiffness and create compensatory bends or even kinks in the more relaxed, nonstented segment of artery. Preexisting kinks, coils, and redundancy are common in FMD. These configurations present unique challenges for stenting. Stent placement in a kink should be performed cautiously because the extra curvature is usually transferred to another segment of the artery and may exacerbate a kink in that area. Stent placement in a coil should be avoided altogether.

Cerebral Protection Devices

The development of distal cerebral protection devices has made the percutaneous approach to carotid FMD conceptually much more appealing. However, it is not clear whether this approach can be readily applied to carotid FMD. The emboli produced by PTA may consist of disrupted tissue and can be large. Balloon angioplasty may cause dissection.

Results

Unfortunately, it is not possible at present to provide a comprehensive assessment because few data are available regarding perioperative complications or longer-term success. Since 1981, a few dozen patients have been reported in the literature as having undergone PTA for carotid FMD, usually as part of larger series of angioplasty patients.[40-43] In one case report, postangioplasty carotid dissection resulted in stroke; in other reports, however, no specific mention was made of periprocedural complications.[44] No follow-up is available beyond the perioperative period.

■ COEXISTENT FIBROMUSCULAR DYSPLASIA AND CAROTID ATHEROSCLEROSIS

When significant associated atherosclerosis of the bifurcation is present, concomitant endarterectomy or a carotid bifurcation stent may be performed. If an open approach is planned, the initial arteriotomy is longitudinal. If severe elongation and kinking are present and the kinking cannot be ruled out as a cause of hypoperfusion episodes (particularly position-related syncope), an oblique arteriotomy, initially placed anteriorly at the base of the carotid bulb at the bifurcation, can be extended circumferentially after the dilatation procedure; it is then carried longitudinally down the common carotid artery to allow the internal carotid to be translocated downward until it is straightened and anastomosed at this lower position. Another option is to resect or imbricate a segment of artery to remove the redundancy.

SELECTED KEY REFERENCES

Slovut DP, Olin JW. Fibromuscular dysplasia. *N Engl J Med.* 2004;350: 1862-1871.
Recent and comprehensive summary of fibromuscular dysplasia and its manifestations.

Moreau P, Albat B, Thevenet A. Fibromuscular dysplasia of the internal carotid artery: long-term results. *J Cardiovasc Surg.* 1993;34: 465-472.
Best long-term follow-up of treated patients available.

Chiche L, Bahnini A, Koskas F, Kieffer E. Occlusive fibromuscular disease of the arteries supplying the brain: results of surgical treatment. *Ann Vasc Surg.* 1997;11:496-504.
Large and thoroughly evaluated surgical series with good long-term data on patency and stroke prevention.

REFERENCES

The reference list can be found on the companion Expert Consult Web site at *www.expertconsult.com.*

CHAPTER 98

Carotid Artery Disease: Aneurysms

Marvin D. Atkins and Ruth L. Bush

Based in part on a chapter in the previous edition by Jerry Goldstone, MD, FACS, FRCS.

Aneurysms of the extracranial carotid arteries can occur as a result of atherosclerotic degeneration, traumatic injury, dissection, or local infection or as a complication after carotid endarterectomy (CEA). Extracranial carotid artery aneurysm (ECAA) is an uncommon but important clinical entity. Carotid aneurysms are extremely rare when compared with atherosclerotic occlusive disease of the same location. These aneurysms are also rare in comparison to aneurysms involving the *intracranial* carotid arteries and their branches. The reported incidence of incidental intracranial aneurysms discovered in autopsy studies ranges from 0.8% to 18%.[1,2] The incidence of ECCA is largely unknown, but it represents only 1% to 1.5% of procedures performed for extracranial cerebrovascular disease at major referral centers.[3-5] The true incidence of ECAA is well less than 1% of all carotid pathologies.

Experience with endovascular carotid interventions for occlusive disease has produced technologies that have increasingly been used as a minimally invasive alternative to conventional surgical treatment of ECAAs. This chapter updates the contemporary management of ECAAs, including both open surgery and the evolving experience with endovascular therapy.

■ DEFINITION

The normal carotid bifurcation is typically 40% greater in diameter than the more distal internal carotid artery (ICA). The accepted definition of most arterial aneurysms is "an artery having at least a 50% increase in diameter compared to the expected normal diameter of the artery."[6] Given this definition, it does not require much dilatation of the carotid bulb to reach this threshold, which has led to disagreement about what constitutes an ECAA. deJong and colleagues proposed that ECAA be defined as bulb dilatation greater than 200% of the diameter of the ICA or 150% of the diameter of the common carotid artery.[7] This strict definition is used in many of the contemporary reports of ECAA and is helpful given the normal physiologic dilatation of the carotid bulb.

■ HISTORICAL REVIEW

Sir Astley Cooper is credited with the first both unsuccessful and successful operations for ECAA in London in 1806 and 1808, respectively.[8] Because direct surgical reconstruction was not possible, ligation of the common carotid artery was the sole treatment. Winslow reported an exhaustive review of 124 reported cases through 1925.[9] In that review, 82 patients treated by carotid ligation had a mortality rate of 28%. By the 1970s, direct arterial reconstruction or autogenous vein grafting (or both) had supplanted carotid ligation. With the introduction of endovascular therapies for carotid occlusive disease, this strategy was first applied to ECAAs beginning in the 1990s.

■ EPIDEMIOLOGY
Population Affected

The population affected and age at diagnosis are directly related to the cause of the aneurysm. The relative frequency of the various potential causes of ECAA has changed over the years. Syphilis, tuberculosis, and middle ear and tonsillar infections were the most frequent causes of carotid artery aneurysms before the advent of antibiotics. In Winslow's review, the majority of these early cases were pseudoaneurysms related to trauma or "erosions" from middle ear infections and tonsillitis rather than true atherosclerotic aneurysms.[9] Therefore, the majority of patients were between 20 and 40 years of age, and the surgical morbidity and mortality associated with treatment were excessive.

In modern practice, atherosclerotic degeneration, dissection, trauma, and previous carotid surgery have supplanted infection as the most frequent causes of ECAA, so the age at initial evaluation tends to mirror that of patients with carotid occlusive disease (Table 98-1).[3,10-22] Increasing use of antibiotics for head and neck infections has significantly reduced the incidence of mycotic arterial infections involving the carotid artery from local extension of a septic process. ECAAs have also occurred in patients who have undergone extensive surgery and radiation therapy for head and neck cancer.[23]

Blunt trauma, dissection, and penetrating injury to the neck can result in a carotid pseudoaneurysm. These are typically encountered in a younger population. False aneurysms after CEA performed for occlusive disease usually affect individuals in their sixth and seventh decades of life.

True degenerative carotid aneurysms affect men twice as often as women,[13,24] and there does not seem to be a predilection for the right or left side. Most patients are older than 60 years, but true degenerative carotid artery aneurysms have been reported in children.[25] There does not seem to be a specific racial distribution of true degenerative carotid aneurysms. Earlier reports suggested that the incidence of ECAAs

Table 98-1 Data from the 14 Largest Single-Center Experiences with Extracranial Carotid Artery Aneurysms Since 1950

Series	Year Range	Total Number of Carotid Procedures	Number of ECCA Cases	% of Total	ASO	PA	Trauma	Dissection	FMD	Infection	Other	Bilateral
Bower et al.[10]	1950-1990	NA	25	NA	3	2	8	6	3	2	1	0
Welling et al.[11]	1952-1982	1104	41	3.7	21	3	0	16	0	1	0	5
McCollum et al.[12]	1956-1977	4000	37	0.93	16	19	2	0	0	0	0	3
Zwolak et al.[13]	1957-1983	NA	24	NA	24	0	0	0	0	0	0	3
Rhodes et al.[14]	1959-1975	NA	23	NA	16	3	4	0	0	0	0	4
Pratschke et al.[15]	1960-1979	1047	28	2.67	13	1	9	0	1	2	2	1
Krupski et al.[16]	1960-1982	NA	22	NA	8	1	10	0	0	1	3	1
El-Sabrout and Cooley[3]	1960-1995	4991	67	1.34	23	38	6	0	0	0	0	2
Moreau et al.[17]	1961-1985	2000	38	1.9	12	0	6	6	8	1	5	3
Faggioli et al.[18]	1974-1995	1324	24	1.8	9	2	1	0	12	0	0	4
Sundt et al.[19]	1978-1985	1250	20	2	4	0	7	6	2	1	0	1
Schievink et al.[20]	1980-1993	NA	22	NA	0	0	11	11	0	0	0	0
Pulli et al.[21]	1982-1995	2138	21	0.98	10	5	0	0	6	0	0	0
Zhou et al.[22]	1984-2004	NA	42	NA	22	15	5	0	0	0	0	0
Totals	**1950-2004**	**17,854**	**434**	**2.4**	**181**	**89.3**	**69**	**45**	**32**	**8**	**11**	**27**

Adapted from El-Sabrout R, Cooley DA. Extracranial carotid artery aneurysms: Texas Heart Institute experience. *J Vasc Surg.* 2000;31:702-712.
ASO, atherosclerotic origin; FMD, fibromuscular dysplasia; NA, not available; PA, pseudoaneurysm.

coexisting with other aneurysmal disease ranged from 14% to 25%.[9,11] Most modern series, however, have not reported similar findings.

Incidence/Prevalence

A 1979 report of a search of the world's literature from 1687 to 1977 found only 853 ECAAs.[4,5] Pooled data from the 13 largest single-center series from 1960 to 1995 demonstrated 392 aneurysms involving the extracranial carotid arteries. Including only series that reported CEA volume during that same time period, 17,854 carotid procedures were performed, 276 of which were for ECAA, for a relative incidence of 1.54%. The largest single-center series reported, that by El-Sabrout and Cooley from the Texas Heart Institute, included 67 ECAAs treated between 1960 and 1995.[3] During the same period, 7394 peripheral aneurysm and 4991 carotid operations were performed at the same institution. This 1.31% relative incidence is mirrored in several other published series.[12,26] These single-center series are from large referral centers, so the true incidence of ECAAs is probably less than 1% of all carotid pathologies. Because these aneurysms are rare, it is impossible to define their true incidence or to determine whether their frequency is increasing. However, advances in vascular and soft tissue imaging have contributed to increased recognition of them, especially in victims of trauma.[27]

PATHOGENESIS

Etiology

Degenerative/Atherosclerotic

Currently, degenerative (or atherosclerotic) is the most frequently reported pathology associated with ECAAs (40% to 70% of cases). These are "true aneurysms" (see Chapter 126:

Arterial Aneurysms: General Considerations). The histologic features are typically atherosclerotic (often termed degenerative), with disruption of the internal elastic lamina and thinning of the media. Although most true carotid aneurysms exhibit arteriosclerosis, it is considered a secondary event rather than a primary etiologic factor. Grossly, these aneurysms tend to be fusiform rather than saccular and are most commonly located at the bifurcation of the common carotid artery or the proximal ICA, where atherosclerotic plaque is common. Atherosclerotic aneurysms that do not involve the carotid bifurcation are frequently saccular and occur in patients with severe arterial hypertension. Most bilateral, nontraumatic ECAAs are of the saccular type.

Post-traumatic Causes

Penetrating Injury. Penetrating injuries involving the extracranial carotid arteries can lead to two important vascular sequelae: arteriovenous fistula and false aneurysm formation. The incidence of carotid artery injury in civilian trauma series ranges from 12% to 17% of the total penetrating neck injuries. The jugular vein appears to be more frequently injured in most reports. When compared with military injuries, civilian carotid injury tends to be caused by blunt or stabbing mechanisms. Data from the Vietnam vascular registry suggest that most penetrating carotid injuries involve the common carotid artery.[28] The incidence of false aneurysm development after penetrating carotid injury is not known. The vast majority of injuries require immediate surgical intervention. Delays in treatment can result in the development of a false aneurysm. What is not known, however, is the number of penetrating injuries that eventually heal without sequelae.

Iatrogenic injury to the carotid artery during attempted placement of a catheter in the internal jugular vein is another frequent cause of false aneurysms, with the wall of the aneurysm being composed of the surrounding fascial and soft tissue structures (see Chapter 126: Arterial Aneurysms: General Considerations).

Blunt Cervical Injury and Carotid Dissection. Blunt
cervical carotid injury, though rare, can be a devastating injury. Blunt carotid injuries typically involve the distal cervical segment of the ICA at the skull base. These injuries present a unique set of challenges because they often occur in the setting of multisystem trauma, particularly head injuries, and symptoms are frequently attributed to traumatic brain injury. Unfortunately, because the vast majority of these injuries are diagnosed after the development of symptoms from central nervous system ischemia, neurologic morbidity rates of up to 80% and associated mortality of up to 40% have been reported. Blunt injury to the carotid or vertebral vessels is diagnosed in approximately 1 in 1000 (0.1%) patients hospitalized for trauma in the United States. When asymptomatic patients are screened for blunt cerebrovascular injury, the incidence rises to 1% of all blunt trauma patients. These injuries are considered further in Chapter 99 (Carotid Artery Disease: Dissection and other Disorders).

Blunt trauma to the cervical carotid arteries produces a spectrum of injury that includes vasospasm, intimal and medial tears, thrombosis, and partial or complete transection of the artery. Of the four main mechanisms associated with blunt cervical carotid injury, the most common involves hyperextension and rotation of the head and neck. The lateral articular processes and pedicles of the upper three cervical vertebrae project more anteriorly than C4-C7, so the distal cervical ICA is prone to stretch injury during hyperextension. The styloid process has also been implicated in the pathophysiology of these injuries because it rotates independently with the skull on the dens, as opposed to the artery, which moves with the cervical spine.[29] Other mechanisms of injury include a direct blow to the artery or compression between the mandible and vertebral body associated with severe hyperflexion. Basilar skull fractures involving the sphenoid or petrous bones can lacerate the artery from sharp fragments. In addition, intraoral trauma can directly injure the artery and lead to a traumatic pseudoaneurysm.

Blunt traumatic injuries to the carotid arteries can also lead to dissection and intramural hematoma, which can cause various degrees of luminal obstruction. Carotid dissection can occur spontaneously or as consequence of "minor trauma" such as chiropractic manipulation, shaving, sneezing, vomiting, and a host of other innocuous activities. Biffl and coworkers proposed an injury grading scale to classify blunt carotid and vertebral artery injuries (Box 98-1).[30] Injury grade III refers to traumatic pseudoaneurysms and represents disruption of the continuity of the arterial wall with the development of a false aneurysm. A periarterial hematoma contained by the fascial planes and surrounding soft tissue structures is formed. This cavity, which contains blood and laminated thrombus, is in continuity with the arterial lumen and has the potential for embolization, as well as expansion and rupture.

Box 98-1 Classification of Blunt Carotid Injuries

- Grade I—intimal irregularity with <25% narrowing
- Grade II—dissection or intramural hematoma with >25% narrowing
- Grade III—pseudoaneurysm
- Grade IV—occlusion
- Grade V—transection with extravasation

As proposed by Biffl WL, Moore EE, Offner PJ, et al. Blunt carotid arterial injuries: implications of a new grading scale. *J Trauma*. 1999;47:845-853.

Fabian and colleagues reported a large single-center experience with traumatic carotid artery injuries.[31] Heparin was the only factor independently associated with improved neurologic outcome. When heparin anticoagulation is possible in a traumatized patient, it is the initial treatment of choice. In patients unable to tolerate anticoagulation, antiplatelet therapy is recommended. Endovascular treatment with a carotid stent in an attempt to tack down the intima, exclude the pseudoaneurysm from the circulation, and prevent distal embolization and rupture is gaining acceptance as the treatment of choice in patients with a persistent traumatic pseudoaneurysm. Some authors have suggested that a traumatic pseudoaneurysm present beyond a week warrants intervention.[32]

Postendarterectomy Aneurysms

CEA-related pseudoaneurysms are some of the most frequently reported aneurysms of the extracranial carotid arteries. El-Sabrout and Cooley demonstrated that 57% of their 67 cases were a result of previous CEA.[3] Zhou and associates, in a more recent series from the Baylor College of Medicine, found post-CEA pseudoaneurysm to be the principal etiology in 15 (36%) of 42 cases.[22] The development of post-CEA pseudoaneurysm is related to either suture line failure or infection. El-Sabrout and Cooley reported seven patients in whom the silk sutures used for patch angioplasty before the advent of monofilament sutures degenerated. Infection complicates approximately a third of all post-CEA pseudoaneurysms. These patients typically have local signs and symptoms of infection, including pain and erythema at the operative site or draining neck sinuses. Infection of the synthetic patch is identified at the time of removal, with *Staphylococcus* species being the most commonly cultured causative organism.

Arterial Dysplasia

Arterial dysplasia, usually a fibromuscular variant, was the most frequent pathologic cause of ECAAs reported in the series by Faggioli and colleagues and also by others.[18,26,33] However, this finding has not been the experience documented in most other reported large series. The arteries of patients with fibromuscular dysplasia typically display a beaded appearance (alternating stenotic webs and dilatations). These dysplastic lesions may lead to ICA dissection and false aneurysm formation.

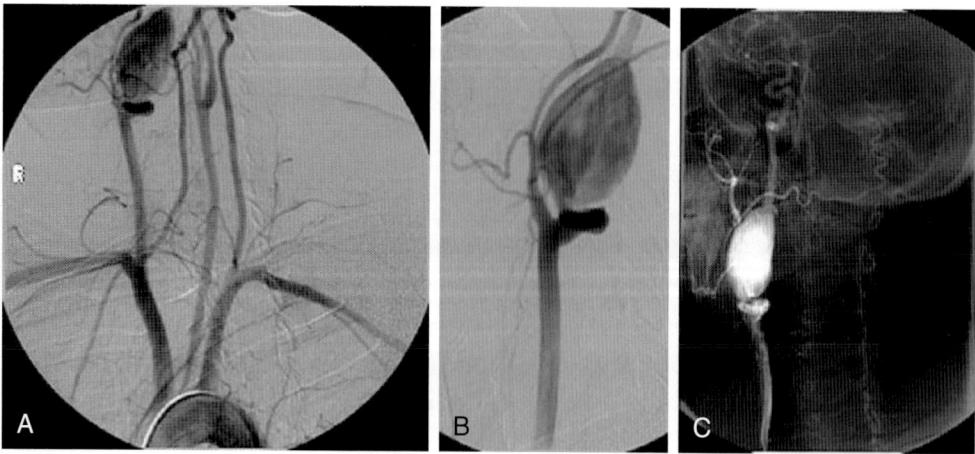

Figure 98-1 A-C, Arch and right carotid arteriograms showing a large extracranial carotid artery aneurysm involving the proximal internal carotid artery.

Pathology

Most primary ECCAs are secondary to a degenerative process that causes true aneurysms. Though frequently associated with atherosclerotic pathologic changes, the pathologic process is much more complex (see Chapter 8: Arterial Aneurysms). There is an enormous disparity in the incidence of carotid occlusive disease and aneurysmal disease in the extracranial carotid artery. The rarity of primary carotid artery aneurysm versus the hundreds of thousands of patients with carotid occlusive disease makes it difficult to accept atherosclerosis as the sole cause. Histologic study of carotid artery aneurysms, however, does reveal many of the findings seen in atherosclerotic specimens: fragmentation of the elastic lamina, lipid-laden foam cells, extracellular accumulation of cholesterol, deposition of hemosiderin, degeneration of the media, and neoangiogenesis. Thinning of the media and fragmentation of the internal elastic lamina are also seen, as in aging arteries. Just as many propose for abdominal aortic aneurysms, atherosclerosis is a coexisting finding but may not be the primary cause.[34,35]

The location of aneurysms involving the extracranial carotid artery depends on the underlying pathology. True atherosclerotic aneurysms typically involve the carotid bifurcation (Fig. 98-1). Penetrating traumatic injuries typically involve the common carotid artery, whereas blunt traumatic injuries typically involve the distal ICA. No predisposition exists for right- or left-sided involvement in patients with unilateral aneurysms.

◼ CLINICAL FINDINGS

Physical Features/Symptoms

Pulsatile Mass

The symptoms of ECAAs vary according to their location, size, and etiology. The most common symptom is a pulsatile neck mass, which was the initial symptom in 93% of patients in the series by Zhou and coworkers.[22] Small internal carotid aneurysms may be asymptomatic, but most cervical carotid aneurysms are identified by finding a pulsating mass in the neck just below the angle of the mandible. These aneurysms may be painful, tender, or asymptomatic. Tenderness and overlying erythema, especially if associated with fever, should raise suspicion for an infected aneurysm.

ICA aneurysms are occasionally recognized as a pulsating mass in the tonsillar fossa or pharynx with little or no manifestation of their presence externally in the neck. The classic analytic study by Shipley and Winslow emphasized that aneurysms of the ICA are directed inward into the throat, whereas those of the common carotid are directed outward into the neck.[36] The absence of cervical swelling in the former is attributed to the dense, deep cervical fascia and muscles attached to the styloid process anteriorly and the cervical vertebrae posteriorly that crowd the gradually dilating aneurysm inward toward the tonsillar fossa, where the thin superior pharyngeal constrictor muscle and mucous membrane offer only minimal resistance to inward protrusion. The level at which the common carotid bifurcates also influences the point of appearance. When the carotid bifurcation is low, an internal carotid aneurysm can be visible and palpable externally in the neck.

Aneurysms that arise at or proximal to the carotid bifurcation are readily palpable and usually pose no diagnostic difficulty. Those arising from the internal carotid near the base of the skull can and do cause diagnostic problems. A chronic unilateral swelling of the posterior pharynx should raise the level of suspicion, especially when other physical signs are lacking, bizarre, or atypical. Otolaryngologists are often the first to see these lesions. A high index of suspicion usually leads to computed tomography angiography (CTA), magnetic resonance angiography (MRA), or catheter-based angiography, which are nearly always diagnostic when an aneurysm is present.

Neurologic Symptoms

Many series report hemispheric neurologic events as the initial symptom of carotid artery aneurysms. In Cooley's

Texas Heart Institute series, 28 of the 65 patients (43%) had neurologic symptoms, including amaurosis fugax and transient hemispheric ischemic attacks.[3] Three of the 28 patients suffered a stroke preoperatively. Zhou reported six patients (14%) with transient ischemic attack, stroke, or Horner's syndrome.[22] Most neurologic events are secondary to embolization of thrombotic material from within the aneurysm wall, but some could be potentially related to diminished flow and compression of the ICA from the mass effect of large aneurysms. Transient ischemic attacks appear to occur twice as often as completed strokes.[11,13,37]

Cranial Nerve Dysfunction

Distal ICA aneurysms are more frequently associated with cranial nerve dysfunction than are aneurysms located more proximally, but clearly this is also dependent on the size of the aneurysm. The ICA enters the cranium through the foramen lacerum and traverses the carotid canal in the petrous portion of the temporal bone. Accompanying the ICA are the sympathetic nerve fibers of the carotid plexus. Compression of these fibers can result in Horner's syndrome, which includes ptosis, miosis, anhidrosis, enophthalmos, and vasodilatation affecting the facial and cervical skin. Aneurysms located more proximally can result in hoarseness from compression of the vagus or recurrent laryngeal nerves. Compression of the facial nerve can cause severe facial pain. Compression of the fifth (trigeminal) and sixth (abducens) cranial nerves has been reported as well.

Dysphagia

Occasionally, the mass of a large aneurysm can cause difficulty swallowing. Protrusion of the aneurysm into the pharyngeal constrictor muscles can produce the sensation of dysphagia, as well as compression of the nerves involved in the swallowing mechanism. On occasion these aneurysms are discovered during evaluation for dysphagia.

Hemorrhage and Rupture

Fortunately, hemorrhage and rupture are now infrequent manifestations of carotid artery aneurysms. There have been descriptions of "herald bleeds" or multiple smaller bleeding episodes before massive rupture. These episodes are similar to the bleeding associated with aortoenteric fistula. When these aneurysms do rupture into the oropharynx, the bleeding is profound and death is usually due to suffocation and aspiration. Mycotic aneurysms are especially susceptible to rupture and bleeding, but with the advent of antibiotics, they are exceedingly rare.

Another group of patients at risk for the so-called carotid blowout syndrome[23] are those who have received extensive head and neck radiation therapy and those undergoing extensive surgery for head and neck cancer. Lesley and coauthors reported their experience with 16 carotid ruptures or impending ruptures in 12 patients.[23] Ten of these patients had undergone extensive treatment of head and neck cancer. Risk factors identified for the development of carotid blowout as a complication of treatment of head and neck cancer included thrombosis of the vasa vasorum secondary to wound infection, direct exposure and desiccation of the carotid artery, stripping of the carotid sheath, exposure of the artery to saliva, adjacent tissue necrosis, pharyngeal fistula formation, and previous irradiation.

Differential Diagnosis

The differential diagnosis for a pulsatile neck mass is extensive. The most common cause is a tortuous, kinked, or coiled carotid artery. Duplex ultrasound and occasionally CTA are required to help differentiate this finding from an ECAA. See Chapter 99 (Carotid Artery Disease: Dissection and Other Disorders) for further details of kinks/coils involving the carotid arteries. Other diagnoses in the differential include a prominent carotid bifurcation in a thin neck, cervical lymph nodes overlying the carotid bifurcation, carotid body tumors, glomus jugulare tumors, cervical metastatic disease, branchial cleft cysts, and cystic hygromas.

■ DIAGNOSTIC EVALUATION

Duplex ultrasound is the initial diagnostic imaging modality of choice for the evaluation of ECAAs emanating low enough in the neck to be evaluated by this modality. Aneurysms located high in the distal ICA, such as those related to blunt cervical carotid dissection, are notoriously missed by ultrasound. Such aneurysms require further imaging with CTA or MRA. MRA has the advantage of being able to distinguish old from recent thrombus, which is particularly helpful in cases of carotid dissection. Knowledge of the strengths and weaknesses of the imaging modalities at one's institution should direct the next noninvasive imaging study chosen (see Chapter 93: Cerebrovascular Disease: Diagnostic Evaluation).

CTA has the benefit of providing the relationships of bony anatomic landmarks, which is critical in deciding whether a lesion is considered "surgically inaccessible" and requires an endovascular intervention (Fig. 98-2). MRA, when obtained in conjunction with head and brain imaging, provides indispensable information regarding the circle of Willis and collateral cerebral circulation. CTA can also provide similar intracranial imaging views; however, this is dependent on the institution. We have found it useful to obtain both studies at our institution to provide such complementary information.

Catheter-based angiography was previously considered mandatory in the evaluation of ECAAs to obtain the detailed vascular anatomy necessary for planning surgical treatment.[38] We currently find this practice unnecessary and reserve catheter-based angiography for endovascular interventions because of the potential stroke risk associated with this invasive diagnostic procedure.

The utility of diagnostic angiography in the current management of ECAAs involves the rare case in which open or endovascular reconstruction is not considered an option and

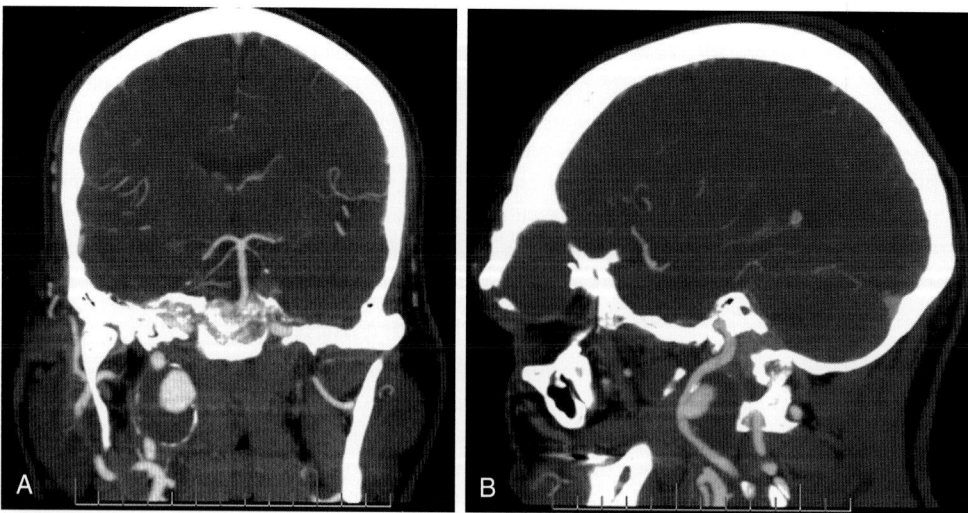

Figure 98-2 A and **B,** CT angiograms of a 4-cm distal internal carotid artery aneurysm. *(Courtesy of Steven Oweida, MD, and John Parp Jones, MD.)*

carotid ligation may be necessary. Combined preprocedure noninvasive imaging of the circle of Willis anatomy and a balloon occlusion test of the ipsilateral ICA have been recommended before ligation. This study involves a period of occlusion with an end-hole balloon occlusion catheter in patients who are awake, anticoagulated, and at their baseline blood pressure. The end-hole catheter also allows measurement of carotid artery "stump" pressure or backpressure. A stump pressure greater than 50% of mean systemic pressure indicates adequate cerebral blood flow during the carotid balloon occlusion test.[39] Occlusion of the ICA is typically performed for 30 minutes, and the awake patient is assessed for neurologic changes. Blood pressure is also pharmacologically lowered to assess tolerance of hypotension. Several reports have detailed the inadequacy of the balloon occlusion test to accurately predict tolerance of carotid occlusion in 10% to 20% of patients.[40,41] In patients in whom ipsilateral hemispheric neurologic events developed after carotid occlusion, thromboembolic events secondary to disturbed flow were thought to be the cause. These reports stress the importance of anticoagulation with warfarin for 6 weeks to 3 months after carotid ligation (see "Ligation" and "Morbidity" under "Open Surgical Repair").

NATURAL HISTORY

The natural history of ECAAs managed by observation is poorly defined. No single institution has a large clinical experience. The largest reported series is 67 aneurysms in 65 patients from the Texas Heart Institute.[11] Only estimates of natural history can be made because they are based on multiple case reports, small series, and collected reviews. These series typically include aneurysms of all types and causes, and because the numbers are small, it is difficult to correlate results with specific aneurysm etiology. Typically, only aneurysms requiring medical attention are reported in the literature. Therefore, it is impossible to determine the number and clinical outcome of asymptomatic, incidentally found ECAAs

that are managed by observation. Although routine autopsy studies suggest that the incidence of ECAA is low, the available literature would suggest that the natural history of these lesions is unfavorable. Winslow's 1926 report showed a 71% mortality rate from rupture, thrombosis, or distal embolization in 35 untreated patients,[9] but this and other early reported series had a preponderance of mycotic aneurysms, which are thought to be associated with a higher risk for rupture and probably do not represent current experience. However, in a more contemporary report from the University of Michigan, 13 of the 19 patients with carotid aneurysms had amaurosis fugax, transient ischemic attack, stroke, or vague neurologic symptoms.[14] Given the likelihood of symptoms and risk for permanent adverse neurologic events, a conservative approach to ECAAs cannot be justified in the vast majority of cases.

TREATMENT

Treatment of ECAAs has evolved with the specialty of vascular surgery. The primary objective in the treatment of such aneurysms is to prevent the permanent neurologic deficits that can arise from atheroembolism and thromboembolism. This is best accomplished by exclusion of the aneurysm from the arterial circulation and restoration of antegrade flow. The choice of therapy must be tailored to the individual and based on the location, size, and cause of the aneurysm, as well as consideration of the overall condition of the patient.

Open Surgical Repair

Ligation

History. In 1552, Ambroise Paré published the first account of operative ligation of the common carotid artery to control hemorrhage caused by a laceration of the artery. Unfortunately, this resulted in aphasia and contralateral hemiplegia.[42] Sir Astley Cooper performed the first common carotid ligation for the treatment of an aneurysm in 1806. Hemiplegia resulted on the eighth postoperative day and the patient died 13 days later. Two years later he successfully ligated a carotid artery with good clinical outcome. Proximal ligation, coupled occasionally with distal ligation and resection, was the mainstay of treatment of carotid artery aneurysms until Matas developed the technique of endoaneurysmorrhaphy.

The subsequent development of modern reconstructive vascular techniques has eliminated ligation as a standard therapy for ECAAs. Ligation was performed in just 1 of the 65 patients with carotid aneurysms treated at the Texas Heart Institute over a 35-year period.[11] Aneurysms extending to the skull base, once thought to be nonreconstructible because of an inability to achieve distal control, have been treated by special maneuvers to improve distal exposure, such as drilling away portions of the petrous and mastoid bones.[26] Ligation of the carotid may still be necessary in emergency situations of arterial rupture, especially if infection is the cause.

Morbidity. Ligation typically results in thrombosis from the level of interruption up to the first major intracranial arterial branch, usually the ophthalmic artery. As shown by Cooper's first attempt in 1806, the risk for major stroke is significant, and it is estimated to occur in 30% to 60% of patients, half of whom die as a result of such strokes.[43,44] Stroke in these patients is due to acute cerebrovascular insufficiency secondary to inadequate collateral circulation or clot propagation and distal embolization. The fact that many strokes occur in a delayed fashion after carotid ligation adds evidence in support of the latter mechanism. It is recommended that patients undergoing carotid ligation be placed on warfarin anticoagulation for a period to prevent distal embolization. The duration of treatment is not standardized, but several groups have recommended a 2-week to 3-month course of therapy.[45,46]

Balloon Occlusion Test. If a carotid ligation procedure is being considered, preoperative evaluation with the carotid balloon occlusion test and stump pressure measurement, as described earlier, is necessary. This may be the only reasonable option when faced with a nonreconstructible ECAA after extensive neck irradiation and radical neck resection in patients with head and neck cancer. An endovascular alternative to open surgical ligation may have utility in patients with a hostile surgical field. Coil embolization and detachable permanent balloon occlusion are useful endovascular techniques for this difficult situation (see "Endovascular Treatment").

Adjunctive Measures. In patients who fail the balloon occlusion test and in whom carotid ligation is required, consideration should be given to extracranial-to-intracranial bypass. This procedure is seldom performed, however, because of results of the EC-IC Bypass study, which failed to show improved outcome with surgical treatment of internal carotid occlusion or intracranial occlusive lesions.[47] However, it may be useful in selected patients, even though the technique is limited in modern neurosurgical practice. Candon

and associates described the novel technique of a saphenous vein bypass graft tunneled through the lumen of the distal ICA aneurysm and anastomosed to the petrous portion of the ICA for the treatment of a very distal ICA aneurysm.[48]

Other historical attempts at aneurysm repair, such as wrapping of the aneurysm with fascia lata or prosthetic material, are mentioned only to be condemned. Wrapping may control the growth of the aneurysm and limit the risk for rupture, but it does nothing to reduce the more significant risk for distal embolization or thrombosis.

Resection

Resection of the aneurysm with restoration of antegrade flow has been the conventional standard for treatment of ECAAs in contemporary practice (Fig. 98-3). This surgical option is applicable to lesions involving the common carotid and proximal third of the ICA. Aneurysms involving distal portions of the ICA require further adjuncts to gain distal exposure and control (see "Open Surgical Repair" under "Treatment Technique").[26,49] Aneurysms involving the external carotid artery alone are typically ligated without reconstruction.

History. The first report of resection of a carotid aneurysm with primary anastomosis was described by Shea in 1955. The first successful procedure of this type was performed by Dimitza in 1952.[50] When inadequate length of vessels precludes primary anastomosis, an interposition graft must be used. Beall and coworkers performed the first prosthetic graft replacement for this lesion in 1959.[51] Prosthetic and autogenous (artery or vein) grafts have been used with equally good result; however, an autogenous conduit is preferred whenever the possibility of infection exists.

Morbidity. Complete excision of large carotid aneurysms risks injury to the cranial nerves, including the facial, vagus, spinal accessory, hypoglossal, and glossopharyngeal nerves. Profound disturbances in swallowing can occur as a result of injury to the pharyngeal muscular branches arising from the vagus, superior laryngeal, and glossopharyngeal nerves. Although these deficits are usually temporary, they cause considerable morbidity and concern for the patient. To minimize these problems, the surgeon must use extreme care when dissecting these structures. Use of the bipolar cautery for hemostasis has been advocated by some. The surgeon should always handle the aneurysm gently to prevent dislodgement and distal embolization of a mural thrombus.

Reconstruction Options. After resection of a carotid artery aneurysm, several reconstruction options are available. Small saccular aneurysms with narrow necks can be resected and the artery closed primarily or with a patch. Mobilization of a tortuous carotid artery can occasionally allow resection with primary end-to-end anastomosis. Another option that has previously been described for penetrating injuries of the ICA involves transposition of the external carotid after branch vessel ligation.

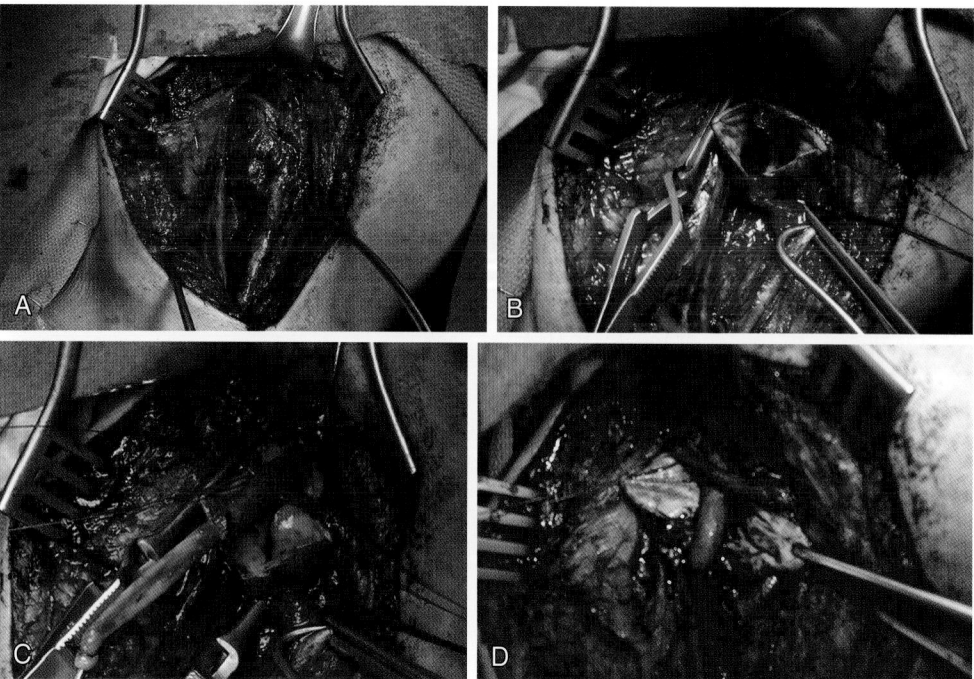

Figure 98-3 A-D, Open repair of the extracranial carotid artery aneurysm seen in Figure 98-1 via reversed-segment saphenous vein interposition.

Pseudoaneurysm Repair after Previous Carotid Endarterectomy. Patch angioplasty during CEA has become routine in an effort to decrease the restenosis rates seen after primary closure of the arteriotomy. Materials currently used for patch angioplasty include Dacron, polytetrafluoroethylene, and bovine pericardium. Callow reported his early experience with 22 patients in whom pseudoaneurysms developed after patch closure, including 12 in whom external jugular vein was used.[52] He also described similar experience with patches made of saphenous vein harvested at the ankle. These vein patches lack the tensile strength to withstand pulsatile arterial pressure and are prone to aneurysmal degeneration. If an autologous conduit is to be used, as in cases of infection, saphenous vein from the groin should be used whenever possible. In current practice, patch pseudoaneurysms after CEA are more frequently related to infection than degeneration of the patch.

Clinical Experience

Primary repair by direct closure, patch angioplasty, or resection and end-to-end primary anastomosis without grafting was used in 50 of the 67 aneurysms treated at the Texas Heart Institute.[11] Most of the patients (n = 38, 58%) had pseudoaneurysms related to Dacron patches that had been applied at the time of CEA, including 7 in which silk sutures had been used and another 13 that were infected. Hertzer, in his invited review of the Texas Heart Institute experience, noted the authors' preference for partial aneurysm excision and patch angioplasty, even in cases of true atherosclerotic aneurysms (9 of 23, 39%).[53] One would suspect that leaving residual

aneurysmal tissue behind could predispose to the formation of a recurrent aneurysm. However, follow-up in 20 of the 23 patients (at an average of 6 years) revealed no further pseudoaneurysms. Follow-up in this study consisted of duplex ultrasound at 3 months and then when clinically indicated. In other words, it is possible that recurrent aneurysms might have been missed, particularly if they were very small.

In cases of true ECAA, it would seem intuitive to replace the entire aneurysmal segment to prevent the risk for further aneurysmal degeneration with partial excision. In the treatment of patch pseudoaneurysm, resection back to normal arterial wall plus patch angioplasty with autologous conduit is an acceptable alternative to interposition grafting.

Adjunctive Measures

Methods of cerebral monitoring and protection during carotid cross-clamping are the same as those used during conventional CEA and include electroencephalographic waveform analysis, selective shunting based on carotid stump pressure, and routine shunting (see Chapter 95: Carotid Artery Disease: Endarterectomy). General anesthesia is usually recommended over cervical block regional anesthesia because of the difficult exposure and longer operative times for aneurysm repair than for CEA. As part of our usual practice, we routinely use shunting during CEA in patients under general anesthesia. This approach is recommended during carotid aneurysm repair as well. Hertzer and colleagues recommended the use of an in-line straight shunt, as opposed to the Javid type, during vein interposition to tailor the vein graft to the appropriate length so that kinking could be avoided.[24] In such cases, the vein interposition graft is telescoped over a straight shunt. After the distal anastomosis is performed, the vein graft is pulled to length over the shunt and trimmed accordingly. The shunt is then removed just before completion of the proximal anastomosis, and flushing maneuvers are performed in the usual fashion. We routinely use intraoperative duplex ultrasound to evaluate carotid reconstructions.

Endovascular Treatment

Endovascular management of ECAAs offers the advantage of avoiding a potentially difficult dissection and eliminating the need for high cervical exposure, thus reducing the risk for cranial nerve injuries and other procedure-related complications. Although most cranial nerve dysfunction is temporary, the incidence of such injuries is significant and has reached 20% in some series.[22]

Several endovascular techniques for the treatment of ECAAs have been reported, including bare-metal stents with and without trans-stent coiling (Fig. 98-4),[54] placement of double stents,[55] autogenous vein graft–covered stents,[56] endovascular coil or balloon occlusion,[57] and placement of covered stent-grafts (Fig. 98-5).[58]

Percutaneous injection of thrombin under ultrasound guidance has become the treatment of choice for traumatic pseudoaneurysms of the common femoral artery. Holder and coauthors reported successful thrombosis of a traumatic carotid pseudoaneurysm by balloon occlusion of the neck of the aneurysm followed by percutaneous injection of thrombin after inadvertent central venous catheter puncture.[59] We have

had no personal experience with this technique and have concerns about the risk for embolization once the balloon is deflated.

In 2006, the Baylor College of Medicine group reported their evolution in the treatment of such aneurysms, including 14 patients managed by endovascular means.[22] Stent-grafts were used in seven patients, carotid stenting with trans-stent coiling in six, and endovascular balloon occlusion in one. In most series of endovascular treatment of carotid artery aneurysms a variety of endovascular therapies have been used, and thus the small numbers in each group have precluded any meaningful comparison of the various treatments.

In patients with prohibitive operative risk, endovascular therapy is preferable to observational therapy given the high risk associated with the natural history of such aneurysms.

Suspicion of infection or the presence of a known mycotic aneurysm is generally a contraindication to endovascular therapy. Although there has been a report of successful endovascular treatment of an infected carotid aneurysm combined with suppressive antibiotic therapy,[60] this approach cannot be recommended except in the most extenuating circumstances.

Selection of Treatment

The location and size of a carotid aneurysm also play a critical role in determining which therapy to offer. Large aneurysms and those involving the distal ICA, given the difficult surgical exposure and significant morbidity, are probably best managed with endovascular techniques. On the other hand, the

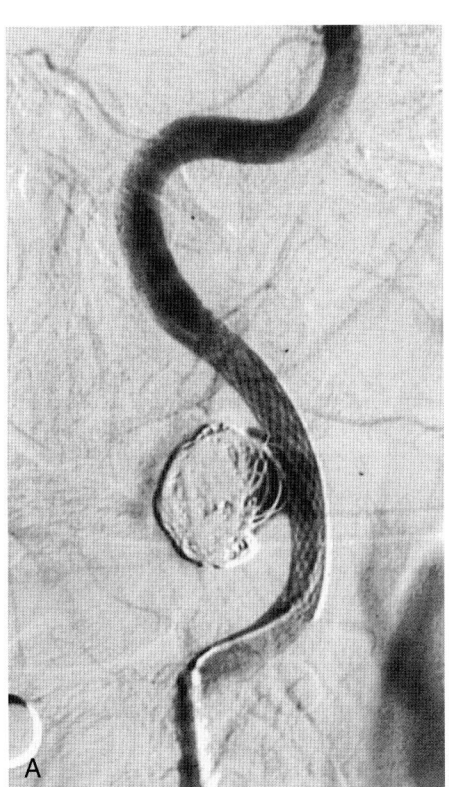 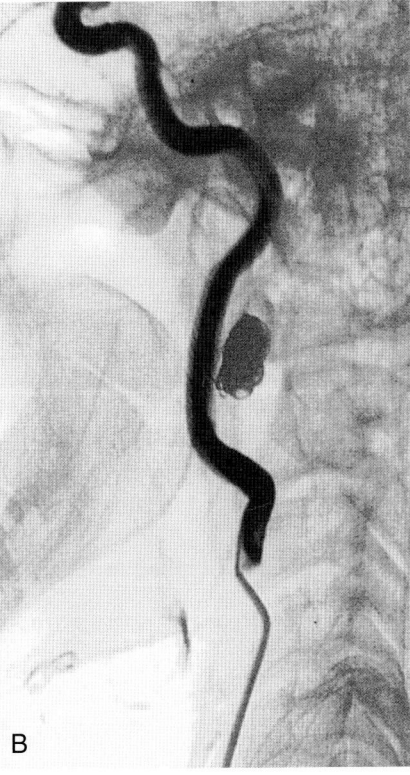

Figure 98-4 After placement of a self-expanding stent across the neck of the aneurysm, a microcatheter is used to introduce coils into the aneurysm sac. **A,** Completion arteriogram documented a patent internal carotid artery (ICA) with aneurysm exclusion. **B,** Arteriography after 5 months showed excellent flow through the ICA with exclusion of the pseudoaneurysm. *(From Bush RL, Lin PH, Dodson TF, et al. Endoluminal stent placement and coil embolization for the management of carotid artery pseudoaneurysms. J Endovasc Ther. 2001;8:53-61.)*

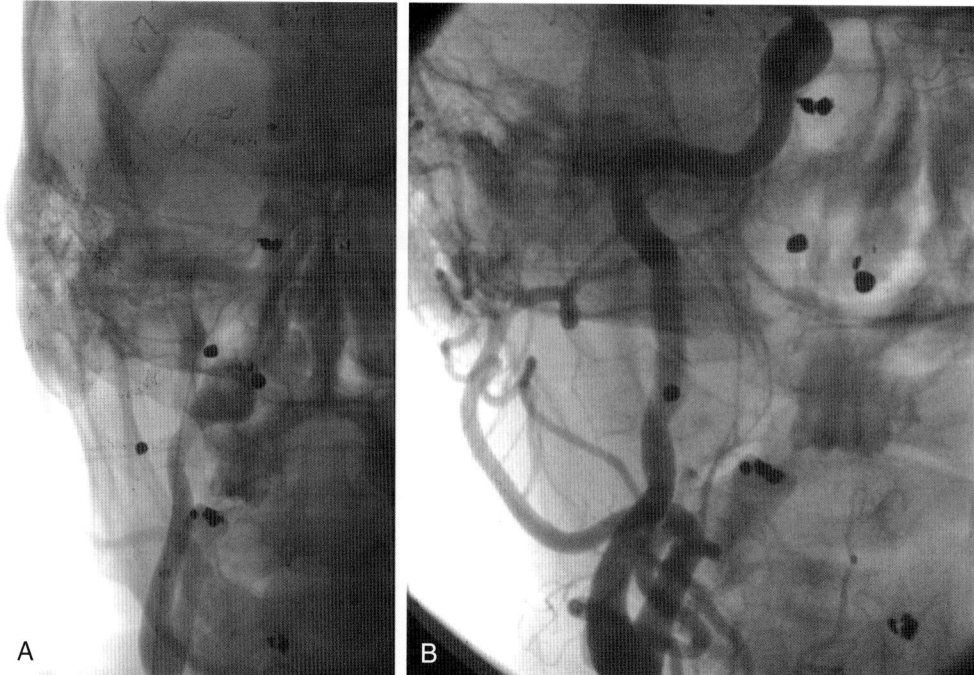

Figure 98-5 A, Selective right carotid arteriogram revealing the distal right internal carotid artery aneurysm demonstrated in Figure 98-2. **B,** Placement of a 5-mm × 2.5-cm Gore Viabahn (Flagstaff, AZ) covered stent-graft for treatment of the distal right internal carotid artery aneurysm seen in **A** and Figure 98-2.

presence of unstable-appearing thrombus within an aneurysm or pseudoaneurysm may be considered a relative contraindication to endovascular repair. Aneurysms in very tortuous carotid arteries are also a relative contraindication to endovascular therapy because of the difficulty of stent tracking and conformability to the artery wall. In fact, tortuous arteries lend themselves to aneurysm excision and primary end-to-end repair of the artery.

TREATMENT TECHNIQUE
Open Surgical Repair

Large aneurysms and aneurysms extending to the most distal ICA are technically challenging. Several techniques can be used to improve distal operative exposure, including the following:

1. The first step in obtaining distal exposure should always be extension of the incision to curve in a posterior fashion behind the ear to the mastoid process.
2. Divide the ansa cervicalis to allow gentle retraction on the hypoglossal nerve.
3. Divide the posterior belly of the digastric muscle.
4. Divide the occipital artery and adjacent venous branches.
5. Divide the ascending pharyngeal artery.
6. Divide the sternocleidomastoid muscle from its mastoid attachment and elevate or resect the parotid gland. Careful dissection of the facial nerve and its branches is mandatory.
7. Remove the styloid process and its attached muscles.

8. Subluxate the mandible to increase the width of exposure at the skull base by approximately 1 cm.
9. Drill and remove portions of the inferior surface of the petrous portion of the temporal bone. This usually requires a multidisciplinary approach, including nonvascular surgeons with experience in skull base surgery.
10. Use of intraluminal balloons, usually as part of a shunt, to control distal internal carotid backbleeding can be a useful adjunct when distal control is difficult.

Once proximal and distal control is obtained, the decision must be made for complete aneurysm exclusion or partial resection. With true atherosclerotic aneurysms we typically replace the entire aneurysm with a saphenous vein interposition graft harvested from the groin (see "Pseudoaneurysm Repair after Previous Carotid Endarterectomy"). This is typically done with an endoaneurysmorrhaphy technique so that the cranial nerves are not injured during excision of the aneurysm wall. As with repair of abdominal aortic aneurysms, the sac of the aneurysm is used to cover the interposition graft. Use of a prosthetic graft in this situation has been reported. No large series have compared use of the two conduits, but a prosthetic graft is a reasonable alternative.

In situations of prosthetic patch pseudoaneurysm, El-Sabrout and Cooley have reported good results with resection of the pseudoaneurysm back to normal arterial wall and repeat patch angioplasty.[3] In such circumstances we would also recommend autologous material to patch the artery because infection is frequently encountered in this situation.

We recommend the use of an in-line straight shunt, as opposed to the Javid type, during vein interposition to tailor

Table 98-2 Endovascular Stent-Grafts Available in the United States in 2009

Company	Device	Material	Introducer Sheath	Stent Diameter	Stent Length
Gore	Viabahn	Nitinol/ePTFE	7 Fr 8 Fr	5, 6 mm 7, 8 mm	25, 50, 100, 150 mm
Atrium	iCast	Stainless steel/ePTFE	6 Fr 7 Fr	5, 6 mm 7, 8, 9, 10 mm	16, 22, 38, 59 mm 16, 22 mm only for 7-mm stent
Bard	Fluency	Nitinol/ePTFE	8, 9 Fr	6, 7, 8, 9 mm	40, 60, 80 mm
Boston Scientific	Wallgraft	PET-covered Elgiloy	9, 10 Fr	6, 7, 8, 9, 10 mm	Various

ePTFE, expanded polytetrafluoroethylene; PET, polyethylene terephthalate.

the vein graft to the appropriate length to avoid kinking. In such cases, the vein interposition graft is telescoped over a straight shunt. The distal anastomosis is performed, and the vein graft is pulled to length over the shunt and trimmed accordingly. The shunt is then removed just before completion of the proximal anastomosis, and flushing maneuvers are performed in the usual fashion. We routinely use intraoperative duplex ultrasound to evaluate carotid reconstructions.

Endovascular Therapy

Applications of noninvasive endovascular treatment of carotid occlusive disease and improvements in technology specific for the carotid circulation have been noteworthy. The technique of obtaining sheath access to the carotid arteries from a femoral approach is described further in Chapter 96 (Carotid Artery Disease: Stenting). Long hydrophilic sheaths designed for carotid stenting procedures have decreased in size since their original introduction. We currently use a 6 Fr Cook Shuttle Sheath (Bloomington, IN) in the majority of carotid interventions performed from a femoral approach. If one is contemplating the use of a covered stent, such as the Gore Viabahn (Flagstaff, AZ) or Atrium iCast (Hudson, NH), larger sheaths may be needed (Table 98-2). We typically use a 0.014-inch wire to cross the aneurysm and have used a distal embolic protection device as long as there is reasonable length to land such a device above the aneurysm neck.

Trans-stent Coil Embolization

The technique of trans-stent coiling involves initially crossing the neck of a saccular aneurysm with a self-expanding stent. If a distal embolic protection device is deployed on the 0.014-inch wire, there is adequate room to introduce a second wire ("buddy wire") to track a 3 Fr Rapid Transit microcatheter (Cordis Endovascular) into the aneurysm sac between the stent interstices. Coil embolization of the entire aneurysm sac is performed with detachable or platinum coils. The stent prevents migration of the coils into the distal carotid circulation.

Stent-Graft Coverage

In patients with a fusiform aneurysm without a discrete neck, a stent-graft prosthesis is a better treatment option as long as

there is adequate length of artery for proximal and distal sealing. How much proximal and distal seal zone is considered adequate, however, is unknown. Typically, a larger introducer sheath is required for a stent-graft prosthesis (see "Endovascular Therapy"). The stents are oversized to the artery per the instructions for use of the individual device. The shortest length stent-graft that will have adequate seal is chosen so that a distal kink is not created in the carotid artery. We balloon minimally and try to keep the angioplasty balloon within the stent-graft and away from the normal proximal and distal intima of the carotid artery.

Hori and coworkers described a novel double-stent technique in which overlapping stents are placed within each other.[55] The increased surface area coverage of the two stents is thought to increase the chance of immediate aneurysmal thrombosis through decreased flow into the sac. We have no personal experience with this technique but are concerned that if aneurysm sac flow is persistent, it may be impossible to track a catheter across the double latticework of stents to place coils.

TREATMENT OUTCOME

Early Results

Open Surgical Repair

With modern vascular surgical techniques, correction of most ECAAs should be possible with a high rate of success and an acceptable rate of neurologic complications. Results vary widely depending on the type, size, and location of the aneurysm. Carotid ligation was previously associated with a 30% to 60% risk for stroke, and half of such patients died after stroke.[9,43,44] In El-Sabrout's review of the 13 largest single-center series since 1950, the combined stroke/death rate associated with carotid ligation had decreased to 12%.[3] This probably represents improvements in anesthetic technique and medical management, as well as an understanding of the importance of anticoagulation after carotid ligation. Carotid ligation is currently reserved in current surgical practice for the unusual circumstance of a nonreconstructible carotid artery.

In general, surgical reconstruction is associated with a combined stroke and mortality rate of about 10%.[3] This rate is obviously higher than that associated with the treatment of occlusive carotid bifurcation atherosclerosis. Transient cranial nerve dysfunction occurs in about 20% of patients.[3] Pooled data from El-Sabrout, including 392 cases of ECAA, showed a combined stroke and death rate of 21% in those managed nonoperatively, 12% in those treated by carotid ligation, and 9% in those treated by surgical reconstruction (Table 98-3).[3,10-22]

Endovascular Therapy

The early results of endovascular repair of ECAAs appear favorable when compared with open surgical repair. Most of the small case series report no strokes associated with the procedure. As one would expect, endovascular therapy does not lead to cranial nerve dysfunction. There may, however, be selection bias in the published literature concerning ECAAs because negative results are not frequently reported, but the data available are promising. Multiple successful single case reports abound, but there are limited series with more than a few patients.

Saatci and coauthors reported using stent-grafts to treat 25 distal ICA pseudoaneurysms, the majority of which were post-traumatic.[61] Endoleak, which occurred in two patients, resolved spontaneously in one and required placement of a bare-metal stent in the other. Twenty-three aneurysms were immediately excluded from the circulation after stent-graft placement. No technical adverse events occurred, including vessel dissection, vessel perforation, or thromboembolism. No mortality or morbidity developed during or after the procedure or during the follow-up period. Follow-up angiography in 21 patients showed reconstruction of the ICA with no aneurysm recanalization. All symptoms resolved after treatment in patients who initially had mass effect complications.

Coldwell and colleagues reported their results in 14 patients with traumatic pseudoaneurysms after blunt cerebrovascular injury.[32] In their protocol, all patients with evidence of blunt carotid dissection underwent anticoagulation with heparin for 7 days, followed by repeat arteriography. Those with flow-limiting dissections or pseudoaneurysm formation were treated with self-expanding Wallstents and warfarin anticoagulation. In the follow-up period of 2.5 years, no strokes occurred and repeat arteriography showed all lesions to have healed by 4 months.

Zhou and associates recently updated the Baylor College of Medicine series and compared two different treatment periods: 22 cases all treated by open repair before 1995 and 20 cases treated after 1995.[22] Of the 20 more recent cases, 14 underwent endovascular therapy by a variety of techniques as listed earlier. They found that in the second treatment period, hospital length of stay was significantly shorter, cranial nerve injury was diminished, and 30-day combined stroke/death rates were lower (14% versus 5%, $P < .004$). No strokes occurred in the endovascular group at 30 days. At a mean follow-up of 4.6 years, 11 of 16 deaths were thought be related to cardiovascular causes, and continued aneurysm exclusion was confirmed in all patients.

Treatment of Carotid Blowout

Lesley and coauthors reported a series of 16 carotid blowout events occurring in 12 patients, the majority of whom had undergone radiation therapy or surgery (or both) for head and neck cancer.[23] All the patients were deemed to be at high risk for cerebral ischemic complications because of a failed balloon occlusion test or known incomplete circle of Willis. These patients were managed with a variety of stent devices and techniques. Adjunctive embolization of carotid pseudoaneurysms with platinum coils or acrylic glue was performed in five of these patients. Hemostasis was achieved in all cases, although one patient with traumatic carotid blowout and three patients with aggressive head and neck cancer–related carotid blowout syndrome required re-treatment with endovascular therapy. Recurrent carotid blowout rates were similar to those reported in other studies using percutaneous balloon occlusion. Overall, no treatment-related strokes or deaths occurred.

Late Results

Open Surgical Repair

The long-term results of open surgical reconstruction for ECAAs are generally very good. Recurrent true aneurysms or pseudoaneurysms are rare after operative repair. There have been reports of delayed infection complicating the repair of carotid artery aneurysms. For example, there were six such patients noted in El-Sabrout and Cooley's series.[3] They were managed by a variety of techniques, including carotid ligation (one patient), autologous patch closure (one patient), and prosthetic patch closure (three patients) with reportedly good long-term results. Use of prosthetic patch material in the presence of an infected previous repair cannot generally be recommended except in extenuating circumstances.

Endovascular Therapy

The midterm results of endovascular therapy for ECAAs show that it is a feasible and durable alternative to conventional open repair. Based on the available evidence from small case series of endovascular repair for carotid artery aneurysms, the combined stroke and death rates appear to be at least equivalent to the reported results of open surgery. Obviously, there is probably significant publication bias in the limited small case series, but such promising results warrant further investigation. Long-term follow-up is necessary if the results of endovascular therapy are to be compared with those of open surgical repair.

■ MEDICAL MANAGEMENT

Antithrombotic Therapy

Medical management after open repair or endovascular treatment of carotid artery aneurysms has not been standardized.

Table 98-3 Management and Outcomes for the 14 Largest Single-Center Experiences with Extracranial Carotid Artery Aneurysms Since 1950

Series	Ligation — Number of Cases	Ligation — Stroke/Death (%)	Nonoperative — Number of Cases	Nonoperative — Stroke/Death (%)	Management — Graft	Patch	EEA	Primary Closure	EC-IC	Other	Major Stroke	Death	Outcome — Combined Results for Major Stroke and Death (%)	CN Dysfunction (%)
Bower et al.[10]	5	1 (20)	0	0	10	0	7	2	0	1	1	0	1 (5)	7 (35)
Welling et al.[11]	0		20	1 (5)	19	0	0	1	1	0	2	0	2 (9.5)	NS
McCollumet al.[12]	4	1 (25)	9	3 (33)	6	18	0	0	0	0	2	1	3 (12.5)	0
Zwolak et al.[13]	0		6	3 (50)	8	2	6	2	0	0	1	0	1 (5.6)	5 (22)
Rhodes et al.[14]	1	0	2	0	8	3	8	1	0	0	2	0	2 (10)	1 (5)
Pratschke[15]	8	0	5	2 (40)	8	2	0	4	1	0	2	1	3 (20)	0
Krupski et al.[16]	4	1 (25)	1	0	5	6	5	0	0	0	2	0	2 (13)	6 (15)
El-Sabrout and Cooley[3]	1	0	1	0	9	39	10	1	0	6	4	1	6 (9)	4 (6)
Moreau et al.[17]	1	0	0	0	12	0	11	14	0	0	0	1	1 (3)	26 (66)
Faggioli et al.[18]	0	0	0	0	10	3	9	2	0	0	2	0	2 (8)	5 (21)
Sundt et al.[19]	3	0	0	0	7	0	5	0	4	1	1	0	1 (6)	5 (25)
Schievink et al.[20]	5	0	0	0	11	0	1	1	4	0	2	0	2 (12)	12 (55)
Pulli et al.[21]	0		0	0	10	6	4	0	0	0	3	0	3 (14)	2 (10)
Zhou et al.[22]*	5	NS	0	0	17	6	0	0	0	14*	1	3	4 (9.5)	4 (9.5)
Totals	**37**	**3 (8.1)**	**44**	**9 (20)**	**140**	**85**	**66**	**28**	**10**	**23**	**25**	**7**	**33 (9.8)**	**77 (17.8)**

*Series included 14 patients who underwent endovascular treatment.
CN, cranial nerve; EC-IC, extracranial-intracranial bypass; EEA, end-to-end anastomosis; NS, not specified.

After carotid ligation there is consensus for anticoagulation with warfarin to prevent distal embolization of the distal ICA thrombosis up to its first intracranial branch. There are no specific data to help guide the length of treatment, but most authors have recommended 2 to 12 weeks.[45,46] Most patients who have undergone open reconstruction with primary repair, patch angioplasty, or interposition grafting have been treated with aspirin alone.

Patients being considered for elective endovascular therapy are typically started on clopidogrel therapy at least 5 days preoperatively. In urgent or emergency situations, therapeutic levels of clopidogrel can be reached by loading patients with 300 mg of Plavix after endovascular therapy. After endovascular repair, dual antiplatelet therapy with aspirin and clopidogrel (Plavix, 75 mg/day) has been suggested by many to facilitate re-endothelialization of the treated surface.[62] The duration of administration is not standardized, but we have typically kept patients who underwent stent placement in the carotid circulation on a regimen of clopidogrel for 6 weeks and aspirin for life. Based on lack of evidence, no additional recommendation can be made for additional treatment in those undergoing endovascular stent-grafting as opposed to stenting alone.

Statins

A recent series from the Johns Hopkins Hospital examined the use of statin therapy perioperatively after CEA.[63] The authors found that perioperative use of statins decreased the risk for stroke threefold, the risk for death fivefold, and length of hospitalization by a day. Kennedy and colleagues reviewed 3360 CEAs performed throughout western Canada and found a 75% reduction (odds ratio [OR], 0.25; 95% confidence interval [CI], 0.07 to 0.9) in the odds for death and a 45% reduction (OR, 0.55; 95% CI, 0.32 to 0.95) in the odds for ischemic stroke or death in symptomatic patients.[64] Groschel and coworkers reported a series of 180 patients undergoing carotid artery stenting for high-grade symptomatic carotid artery stenoses and examined the use of statins.[65] As seen with CEA, statin use significantly decreased the rates of stroke, myocardial infarction, and death.

These data suggest that statins have an acute neuroprotective benefit during the perioperative period, the mechanism of which is not entirely clear. Proposed mechanisms include anti-inflammatory effects, plaque stabilization, and effects on thrombosis and coagulation. Given these data, it would seem reasonable to extrapolate that perioperative administration of statins is justified in the management of carotid artery aneurysms, although this is purely speculative.

Mycotic Aneurysms

Medical management of suspected or known mycotic carotid aneurysms involves the perioperative administration of antibiotics specific for the organism or organisms responsible. *Staphylococcus aureus* and *Staphylococcus epidermidis* are the most frequently encountered organisms. Gram-positive coverage

with either vancomycin or linezolid is recommended until definitive culture and susceptibility results are available. *Escherichia coli*, *Klebsiella* species, *Corynebacterium* species, *Proteus mirabilis*, and *Yersinia enterocolitica* have also been reported. Therefore, initial broad gram-negative coverage is warranted as well. Once the standards for treating vascular infection have been completed, including graft removal, autologous reconstruction, débridement of perigraft tissue, muscle flap coverage, and drainage, a course of parenteral antibiotics is recommended. There are no clinical trial data on which to base recommendations for the length of antibiotic therapy, but patients are typically treated with parenteral culture-specific antibiotics for 4 to 6 weeks followed by oral antibiotics for 3 to 6 months or for life (see Chapter 41: Local Complications: Graft Infection).

■ SPECIAL CONSIDERATIONS
Pediatric Patients

Pourhassan and coworkers recently reviewed their experience and the available reports of ECAAs in children.[25] Their review cited 27 case reports of ECAAs occurring in the pediatric population within the past 25 years. The etiology of these aneurysms included infectious (such as peritonsillar abscess), traumatic (including penetrating, blunt, and post-tonsillectomy injury), and congenital causes. Fourteen of the 27 cases were categorized as mycotic pseudoaneurysms with an associated antecedent serious oropharyngeal infection. Six were thought to be congenital or a manifestation of a systemic disease process (i.e., Behçet's disease or type IIb hyperlipoproteinemia). Five infected pseudoaneurysms were thought to be secondary to surgical trauma after recent tonsillectomy. This emphasizes the anatomic proximity of the carotid artery to the tonsillar fossa. As seen in adults, the majority of aneurysms involved the common carotid artery or the ICA. If the external carotid artery is involved, it usually represents a pseudoaneurysm secondary to trauma or infection.

The usual initial symptom of carotid artery aneurysm in children is a pulsatile mass in the neck. Rupture of a carotid artery aneurysm is seen more frequently in children than in adults. In Pourhassan and colleagues' review, 42% of patients were initially evaluated for either hematemesis or epistaxis. The increased frequency of rupture seen in children is probably a manifestation of the etiology. Traumatic and mycotic aneurysms seem to have the highest risk for rupture, and these causes represent the majority of cases occurring in childhood.

Operative intervention is clearly recommended for all symptomatic carotid aneurysms with manifestations of cerebral ischemic events and local discomfort. Given the higher rates of rupture seen in children, aggressive surgical intervention is warranted. Multiple carotid reconstructions have been proposed, depending on the size, location, and etiology of the aneurysm. As in adults, resection plus interposition grafting is the treatment of choice. In the pediatric population, resection of the aneurysm should be followed by interposition grafting with saphenous vein. An autologous conduit is recommended because of the infectious etiology in many cases. It also allows longitudinal growth of the vessels as the child ages.

SELECTED KEY REFERENCES

Bush RL, Lin PH, Dodson TF, Dion JE, Lumsden AB. Endoluminal stent placement and coil embolization for the management of carotid artery pseudoaneurysms. *J Endovasc Ther.* 2001;8:53-61.
Provides a description and rationalization for the technique of stent placement followed by coil embolization for the treatment of extracranial carotid artery aneurysm.

Coldwell DM, Novak Z, Ryu RK, Brega KE, Biffl WL, Offner PJ, Francoise RJ, Burch JM, Moore EE. Treatment of posttraumatic internal carotid arterial pseudoaneurysms with endovascular stents. *J Trauma.* 2000;48:470-472.
A large series of traumatic blunt carotid pseudoaneurysms treated by endovascular stents. It includes a discussion of the initial medical management of such injuries and presents a decision protocol to recommend treatment of persistent pseudoaneurysms.

El-Sabrout R, Cooley DA. Extracranial carotid artery aneurysms: Texas Heart Institute experience. *J Vasc Surg.* 2000;31:702-712.
The largest single-center experience with extracranial carotid artery aneurysms.

Saatci I, Cekirge HS, Ozturk MH, Arat A, Ergungor F, Sekerci Z, Er U, Turkoglu S, Ozcan OE, Ozgen T. Treatment of ICA aneurysms with a covered stent: experience in 24 patients with mid-term follow-up results. *AJNR Am J Neuroradiol.* 2004;25:1742-1749.
The largest series to date using covered stents for ICA aneurysms.

Zhou W, Lin PH, Bush RL, Peden E, Guerrero MA, Terramani T, Lubbe DF, Nguyen L, Lumsden AB. Carotid artery aneurysm: evolution of management over two decades. *J Vasc Surg.* 2006;43:493-496; discussion, 497.
Description of the evolving experience with endovascular therapy for carotid artery aneurysms and comparison to the large series of open surgery at the same institution.

REFERENCES

The reference list can be found on the companion Expert Consult Web site at *www.expertconsult.com.*

Carotid Artery Disease: Dissection and Other Disorders

T. Johelen Carleton and Karl A. Illig

Patients with nonatherosclerotic carotid disease are encountered very infrequently, and these unusual problems continue to challenge our evidence-based practice. Treatment decisions are often guided by case reports, small trials, or anecdotal experiences. This chapter summarizes the current state of knowledge about these uncommon but important disease entities.

■ CAROTID ARTERY DISSECTION

Arterial dissection occurs when disruption of the intima allows blood to extravasate between layers of the vessel wall. The resulting intramural hematoma usually extends distally and can lead to acute stenosis or occlusion (Fig. 99-1) and later to aneurysmal change with an increased risk for thromboembolic events. Dissection of the carotid artery either is spontaneous or has a precipitating mechanical event (traumatic or iatrogenic). Although each type of dissection is relatively uncommon, both are important clinically because they can be a source of stroke and occur particularly in young people. Cervical carotid artery dissections are responsible for only 2% of all ischemic strokes but account for 10% to 20% of strokes in young and middle-aged patients.[1] Spontaneous and traumatic carotid dissections differ in their pathophysiology and will be reviewed separately.

Spontaneous Carotid Artery Dissection

Epidemiology

The overall incidence of clinically apparent spontaneous carotid dissection is reported to be between 1.7% and 2.6%.[2,3] Spontaneous cervical carotid artery dissection occurs most frequently in the third through the fifth decades of life, and the mean age at diagnosis is 45 years. There is no gender predilection for spontaneous dissection, but women are affected at an average of 5 years younger than men.[4,5]

Pathogenesis

Spontaneous dissection can occur in any artery but is more likely to occur in the extracranial carotid and vertebral arteries than in other vessels of similar size. These arterial segments are mobile and can potentially come into contact with the bony structures of the head and neck.[4] A history of antecedent minor trauma is often elicited in patients with "spontaneous

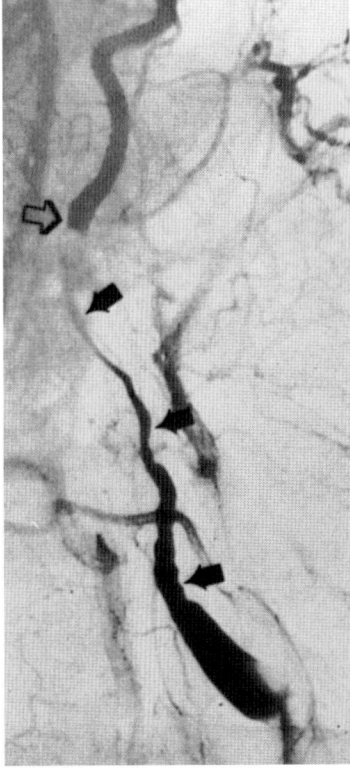

Figure 99-1 Dissection of the cervical segment of the internal carotid artery. Note the elongated, narrowed, and tapered luminal stenosis (*solid arrows*), a finding frequently seen in association with extracranial dissections. Another common feature of this entity, fairly abrupt reconstitution of the carotid lumen at the base of the skull (*open arrow*), is also shown. (*From Mokri M. Dissection of the cervical and cephalic arteries. In: Meyer FB, ed.* Sundt's Occlusive Cerebrovascular Disease. *Philadelphia, PA: WB Saunders; 1994:51.*)

dissection," but the significance of these events is unclear and the course is distinctly different from dissection caused by definite and severe trauma.[5] Chiropractic manipulation has been implicated as an etiology of "spontaneous" dissection of the carotid and vertebral arteries, but a true relationship is elusive because 25% of these patients also have connective tissue disorders and neck pain, which may or may not be related to the dissection.[4,6]

Atherosclerosis and other known risk factors for vascular disease such as smoking, diabetes, hypercholesterolemia, and oral contraceptive use are usually absent in patients with spontaneous dissection. These patients do have a higher incidence of hypertension, and a migraine disorder has also been shown to have an independent association with spontaneous dissection.[7,8] Spontaneous cervical carotid artery dissection occurs more frequently in the winter, and recent infection is present in up to 58% of patients. There is a preponderance of respiratory infections, but mechanical factors such as coughing, sneezing, and vomiting do not seem to be independent risk factors.[9] Winter peaks in hypertension and infection may contribute to seasonal variability.[10]

Underlying abnormalities of the vasculature have been implicated in spontaneous cervical carotid artery dissection, including fibromuscular dysplasia, Ehlers-Danlos syndrome, cystic medial necrosis, Marfan's syndrome, autosomal dominant polycystic kidney disease, and osteogenesis imperfecta type I.[4] Associated vascular anomalies implicated in spontaneous dissection include arterial redundancy, intracranial aneurysms, aortic root dilatation, and increased arterial distensibility.[11] Familial occurrences of spontaneous carotid dissection are also described, which further supports the possibility of an inherited disorder,[8] but definitive proof is lacking.

Clinical Findings

The most common initial symptom in patients with spontaneous dissection of the carotid artery is headache, whereas "classic" patients have a partial Horner's syndrome. Nausea occurs more often with vertebral dissections, and hemispheric symptoms more often with carotid dissections.[12] Patients with cervical carotid artery dissection also suffer from neck pain, amaurosis fugax, anisocoria, pulsatile tinnitus, and cranial nerve palsy.[4,12] Cranial nerves IX through XII and in particular the hypoglossal nerve are most commonly involved.[13]

The classic clinical description of patients with spontaneous carotid dissection is ipsilateral head or neck pain, ipsilateral partial Horner's syndrome (also referred to as oculosympathetic palsy), and cerebral or retinal ischemia. Oculosympathetic palsy refers to miosis and ptosis caused by involvement of the sympathetic fibers accompanying the internal carotid artery but does not include the facial anhidrosis of Horner's syndrome, which is mediated by sympathetic fibers running along the external carotid artery. The onset of cerebral or retinal ischemia can occur hours or days after the initial symptoms. The classic triad of symptoms is present in less than a third of patients with spontaneous carotid dissection, and the diagnosis must obviously be considered in patients with more subtle manifestations and isolated symptoms.[4]

Traumatic Carotid Artery Dissection

Epidemiology

The incidence of traumatic carotid artery dissection in all patients seeking medical care after blunt traumatic injury is 0.08%,[14] but it is higher in patients with specific patterns of injury.[15] After blunt head and neck trauma the incidence of internal carotid dissection is 0.86%,[16] and patients with head

and neck injury and an altered level of consciousness have a reported incidence of carotid injury of up to 3.2%.[17]

Improved imaging modalities and increased awareness of cervical carotid arterial injury may have contributed to an apparent rise in incidence over the past decade. It is suggested that cervical carotid artery dissection is underdiagnosed, and several groups have reported a much higher incidence than was previously noted when all patients with severe head and cervical spine injuries are screened.[17,18] Screening may have particular value in trauma patients because neurologic deficits can have a delayed manifestation or be attributed to associated injuries, and some data suggest that early anticoagulation in asymptomatic patients with blunt carotid injury detected by screening leads to improved neurologic outcome.[19,20]

Pathogenesis

Traumatic cervical carotid artery dissection can occur after blunt or penetrating trauma, and both direct and indirect forces contribute to injury. The most common mechanism of injury is extreme cervical hyperextension or lateral hyperflexion associated with severe blunt head and neck trauma caused by a motor vehicle collision.[15,16]

Clinical Findings

Most series reporting patients who experienced traumatic dissection are small or retrospective, describe clinical manifestation that vary from exclusively asymptomatic patients to patients with lateralizing symptoms appearing after a latent period of 4 hours to 75 days, and combine outcomes for injury and dissection of all cervical vessels.[15,17,21] Head and neck pain, hemiparesis, hemiplegia, dysphasia, aphasia, Horner's syndrome, lateralizing transient ischemic attack, and stroke have all been described as initial symptoms of traumatic cervical carotid artery dissection. Some advocate routine screening (ultrasonography) in all patients with head and neck trauma.[17,18] Mandatory diagnostic evaluation is advocated for active bleeding in the head and neck, expanding neck hematomas, cervical bruits in patients older than 50 years, imaging suggesting acute brain infarction, central or lateralizing neurologic deficits, Horner's syndrome, head or neck pain, cervical spine fracture, Glasgow Coma Scale score less than 6, petrous bone fracture, diffuse axonal injury, basilar skull fracture, Le Fort II or III fracture, or any combination of these findings.[16,21]

Diagnostic Evaluation

Diagnostic modalities are the same for spontaneous and traumatic carotid artery dissection. Although ultrasound is readily available and thus commonly used as the initial test, four-vessel selective cerebral angiography remains the "gold standard." Angiography allows visualization of the arterial lumen and characterization of the lesion. An intimal flap or double lumen is pathognomonic for dissection. The internal carotid stenosis caused by dissection is usually irregular, originates 2

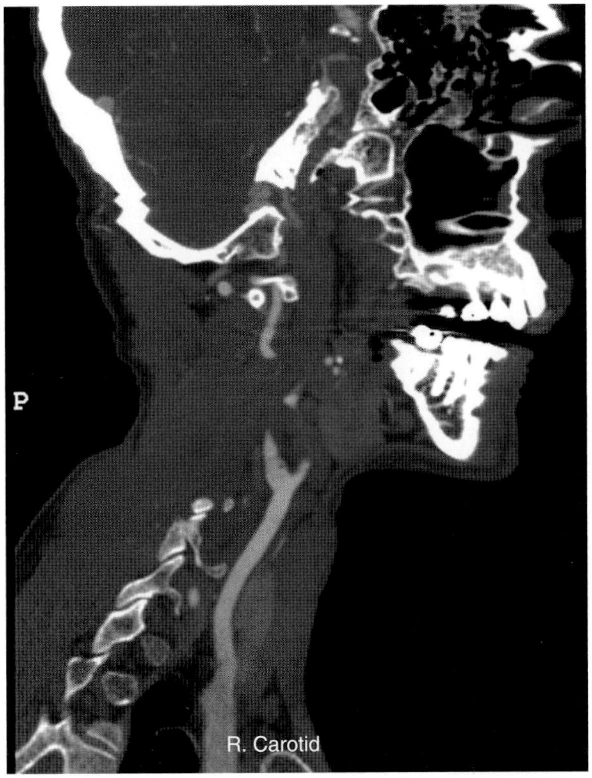

Figure 99-2 CTA (centerline trace, right carotid artery) of a patient with a spontaneous dissection. Note the tapered occlusion with reconstitution near the skull base.

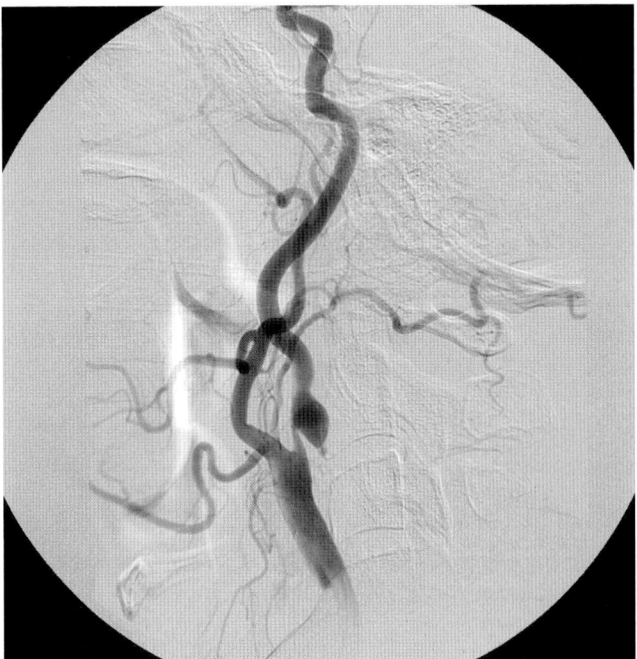

Figure 99-3 Angiogram showing residual stenosis and proximal pseudoaneurysm formation after traumatic carotid dissection.

to 4 cm distal to the bulb, and has a long tapering stenosis that usually ends before the internal carotid artery enters the petrous portion of the temporal bone.[4,22] Occlusions are characteristically tapered and have a flamelike appearance (Fig. 99-2), whereas aneurysms, often a later development, are usually fusiform and most commonly occur in the distal subcranial segment, although more proximal saccular pseudoaneurysms are also seen (Fig. 99-3). Angiography carries a 1% to 2% risk of hematoma or pseudoaneurysm at the access site, a 1% to 2% risk of contrast-induced nephropathy, and a 1% risk of stroke,[23] but it may also provide opportunities for endovascular intervention or surgical planning.

Computed tomographic angiography (CTA), magnetic resonance angiography (MRA), and ultrasound are increasingly used noninvasive alternatives for diagnosing and monitoring carotid artery dissection. CTA and MRA are particularly attractive for diagnosis because their resolution approaches that of conventional angiography in detecting direct signs of vascular injury, such as irregular vessel margins, filling defects, changes in caliber, extravasation of contrast material, and occlusion,[24] and they are superior to angiography for evaluation of intramural hematoma and injury to surrounding structures. It should be noted that the initial results from two prospective studies in the trauma literature comparing CTA and MRA with angiography were disappointing and showed poor sensitivity and specificity.[25,26] CTA technology has improved, however, and more recent studies show 97.7% sensitivity and 100% specificity for 16-slice CTA in the diag-

nosis of blunt carotid and vertebral artery injuries.[27] These results suggest that CTA is a reliable, safe, fast, and cost-effective means of diagnosing cerebral artery dissections. Potential problems with CTA include artifact from metal (including projectiles) and bone, effective timing of the administration of contrast material, and the high doses of contrast material needed.

In addition to demonstrating the hyperintense crescent-shaped mural hematoma and eccentric flow typical of dissection, MRA shows a characteristic evolution of signal intensity over time and is the modality able to detect ischemic changes in the brain the earliest. Disadvantages of MRA are lack of availability, longer time required for imaging, and interference from extrinsic structures such as external fixation devices in trauma patients. Nephrogenic systemic fibrosis is a potential complication in patients with renal insufficiency who receive gadolinium for MRA.

Ultrasound does not evaluate the surrounding tissue or define the actual site of dissection as well as other noninvasive modalities do, but it does effectively detect resulting flow abnormalities. In experienced hands it is up to 95% sensitive in the diagnosis of carotid dissection when extracranial Doppler, transcranial Doppler, and duplex ultrasonography are appropriately combined.[28] Advantages of ultrasound are accessibility and convenience, which are particularly valuable in an acutely injured patient and for purposes of monitoring disease progression and resolution over time.

Natural History

Cerebral infarction is documented in 42% of spontaneous carotid dissections, and 58% of patients have persistent neurologic deficits.[12] Higher incidences of stroke appear in earlier reports,[13] and this may be the result of improved diagnosis and treatment.[4] More recently, studies of blunt traumatic carotid injury report mortality rates of up to 30% (in many cases related to associated injuries) and rates of permanent severe neurologic deficits of up to 20%.[19,20]

In patients with spontaneous dissection managed medically, the incidence of recurrent dissection is 0.3% to 1.4%, and recurrent dissection is more frequent in the first month and more common in patients with connective tissue disease or a family history of cervical carotid artery dissection. The annual risk of recurrent stroke ranges from 0.3% to 3.4%. Dissection is the most common cause of extracranial internal carotid aneurysm, but two thirds of carotid aneurysms resolve, and complications related to aneurysm are rare.[29]

The prognosis is worse for traumatic carotid dissection. Patients with traumatic dissection are more likely to develop aneurysms and progress to occlusion and are less likely to show improvement or resolution of aneurysms and stenoses than are patients with spontaneous dissection.[30] The prognosis after stroke caused by dissection is worse than the prognosis after stroke caused by atherosclerosis. Dissection patients have more global middle cerebral artery involvement and severe clinical impairment.

Patients with strokes caused by dissection are younger with fewer vascular risk factors.[31] Although the overall functional prognosis in patients with stroke caused by dissection may be the same in young patients with stroke from other causes,[29] the overall implications of permanent impairment are greater because younger people are involved.

Treatment

Medical Therapy

Carotid artery dissection is thought to cause stroke as a result of ischemic stenosis or embolism from the site of the intimal tear. Microemboli have been detected acutely after dissection and correlate with the presence of stroke in patients with spontaneous and traumatic dissections.[32] Because of these factors, antithrombotic therapy has logically been the mainstay of medical treatment of carotid artery dissection. Concerns regarding anticoagulation include possible worsening of intramural bleeding at the site of dissection, bleeding from associated injuries in the case of trauma, and bleeding from unrelated sources. A Cochrane Database Systematic Review in 2003 unfortunately found no randomized trials that compared antiplatelet drugs with anticoagulants or either type of agent with controls for the treatment of dissection. Although nonrandomized studies do not show a difference in mortality between patients receiving antiplatelet medications and patients receiving anticoagulation, the intracranial hemorrhage rate of anticoagulated patients is 0.5%, as opposed to 0% in those receiving antiplatelet medications alone.[33] An ongoing prospective trial is currently comparing antiplatelet therapy with anticoagulation for the treatment of acute cervical carotid artery dissection. The primary endpoint is ipsilat-

eral stroke or death within 3 months of randomization, and secondary endpoints include any transient ischemic attack or stroke, major bleeding, and residual stenosis.[34]

Despite the lack of level I evidence, most patients with spontaneous or traumatic dissection are treated with systemic heparin followed by warfarin for 3 to 6 months. Therapy after this is typically individualized and depends on vascular imaging.[32]

Surgical Treatment

Indications for surgical treatment of acute carotid artery dissection are fluctuating or deteriorating clinical neurologic symptoms despite medical treatment, compromised cerebral blood flow, contraindications to antithrombotic therapy, and a symptomatic or expanding aneurysm.[35-37] Indications for surgery after 6 months of medical treatment are persistent high-grade stenosis and a new or persistent aneurysm greater than twice the diameter of the normal internal carotid segment.[35] Aneurysms rarely (if ever) enlarge or rupture but may be a source of distal thromboembolization.[38] A cerebral embolus is an appropriate indication for repair, but there are no data regarding the need for repair in an asymptomatic patient with an aneurysm.

Exposure of the internal carotid artery for treatment of dissection is more difficult than exposure for atherosclerotic disease because lesions are more distal. Most dissections are superior to the bulb in the transition zone, where the artery becomes elastic rather than muscular. Distal exposure is discussed in detail in Chapter 95 (Carotid Artery Disease: Endarterectomy) and can require maneuvers that include division of the digastric muscle, mandibular subluxation, fracture of the styloid bone, and subtotal petrosectomy. Reports of distal balloon control in this setting could not be found, but it might be considered. Once exposure is obtained, surgical options include carotid ligation, interposition saphenous vein graft to a cervical or intracranial segment, and patch angioplasty. Ligation is considered safe, if necessary, in patients with systolic stump pressure greater than 70 mm Hg,[39] and the response to preoperative temporary balloon occlusion is also helpful in predicting whether ligation will be tolerated.

Postoperative complications are common after surgery for carotid dissection. In one group's experience, mortality was 2%, ipsilateral stroke occurred in 8%, 20% of reconstructions did not have primary patency at discharge, and 58% of patients experienced cranial nerve dysfunction (although 41% had a cranial nerve palsy preoperatively).[35] Another group reported a 9% rate of postoperative stroke and a high rate of cranial nerve palsy after high cervical exposure but no sequelae at a mean follow-up of 6.2 years.[38] Most providers continue antithrombotic medication postoperatively if there are no contraindications, but confirmatory data do not exist.

Endovascular Therapy

Two trials have compared intravenous thrombolysis and stent-assisted intra-arterial thrombolysis for symptomatic middle cerebral artery occlusion secondary to carotid dissection. The larger series (N = 18) showed no difference between the groups at 3 months,[40] and the smaller series (N = 10) showed a better outcome at 3 months with endovascular treatment.[41] The authors of both papers agree that larger randomized controlled trials are needed.

Endovascular treatment is increasingly being applied to a number of acute cerebrovascular conditions, including stroke secondary to atherosclerosis or dissection,[42] carotid "blowout" syndrome, aneurysm, stenosis,[43] and arteriovenous fistulae.[44] Endovascular treatment of cervical carotid artery dissection is also being explored, and multiple case reports have documented encouraging outcomes.[45-47] An early small series from 1999 reported the results of carotid stents placed for four acutely symptomatic traumatic dissections and one spontaneous dissection.[48] There were no procedural complications, all patients improved clinically within the first 24 hours, and all remained well at follow-up. Another group reported placement of stents in seven patients with acute and chronic spontaneous carotid dissection. All patients exhibited improvement or resolution of symptoms, and the patency rate was 100% on follow-up imaging.[36] The only complication was an asymptomatic intraprocedural dissection (one patient died after heart transplantation 4 months after stent placement). All patients were pretreated for at least 4 days with clopidogrel and aspirin, received heparin intraoperatively, and took clopidogrel for at least 6 weeks postoperatively and aspirin indefinitely. All procedures were performed under local anesthesia without the use of cerebral protection devices. Equally favorable results have been reported for the treatment of traumatic dissection[37] and in series combining patients with traumatic and spontaneous dissection.[49] Given the morbidity and mortality associated with open procedures, preliminary results describing endovascular treatment of carotid dissection seem promising.

Selection of Treatment

At present, there are no randomized trials comparing open and endovascular treatment of patients with acute or late sequelae of carotid dissection and no clear indications regarding when either approach might be preferred. There is concern that endovascular interventions at the skull base could be compromised by bony resistance to stent deployment or bending and rotational forces at the point where the skull constrains the vessel. Although the early results from recent endovascular series are promising, the case numbers are small and do not conclusively support endovascular intervention over open repair or medical management.

■ CAROTID BODY TUMORS

The carotid body is a chemoreceptor located at the bifurcation of the common carotid artery in the posterior medial adventitia and is part of the extra-adrenal paraganglia system derived from neural crest cells. The carotid body is critical for acute adaptation to hypoxia and releases neurotransmitters in response to changes in oxygen levels, carbon dioxide levels, and proton concentration.[50,51] Tumors arising from this tissue are interchangeably called carotid body tumors, paragangliomas, chemodectomas, and glomus tumors. Paraganglioma is a current general term that refers to any extra-adrenal neuroendocrine tumor, with the added reference to anatomic location (e.g., carotid paraganglioma) to yield a clear description.

Epidemiology

Carotid body tumors are so rare that the literature does not cite a specific incidence, but they are the most common paraganglioma of the head and neck and account for 65% of these tumors.[51] A recent review reports that many major vascular centers do not have experience with carotid body tumors, but those that report their experience document a mean age at diagnosis of 55 years (range, 18 to 94) and a male-female ratio of 1:1.9. Fifty-seven percent of tumors were on the right, 25% were on the left, 17% were bilateral, only one tumor was functional, and 4.3% were malignant.[52] A retrospective study from Mexico found an overwhelming predominance in women, thus suggesting that Hispanic females may be at higher risk than the general population for carotid body tumors.[53] A female preponderance is consistent with earlier epidemiologic data.[54]

Pathogenesis

One proposed risk factor for carotid body tumors is hypoxemia, which can be the result of chronic obstructive pulmonary disease or living at high altitude. Both hyperplasia and neoplasia of the carotid body have been associated with chronic hypoxic states.[52,53,55-57] Carotid body tumors can occur sporadically but are also seen as part of syndromes, including Carney's triad (gastric stromal sarcoma, pulmonary chondroma, and paraganglioma), von Hippel-Lindau disease (pheochromocytoma, spinal hemangioblastoma, and paraganglioma), neurofibromatosis type 1, and multiple endocrine neoplasia type 2. Approximately 20% of carotid body tumors are familial and have a pattern of autosomal dominant transmission, although a paternally derived gene has been proposed.[55] Seventy-eight percent of familial paragangliomas are multicentric, whereas only 23% of nonfamilial paragangliomas are multicentric.[58]

Specific mutations that have an association with paragangliomas have been identified. Succinate dehydrogenase is a mitochondrial enzyme complex with roles in oxidative phosphorylation and intracellular oxygen sensing and signaling. Mutations of the subunits SDHB on chromosome 1p35-36 and SDHD on chromosome 11q23 result in loss of gene product function and give rise to paragangliomas and pheochromocytoma. Patients with SDHD mutations have a higher prevalence of head and neck paragangliomas, whereas patients with SDHB mutations have a higher rate of malignancy.[59]

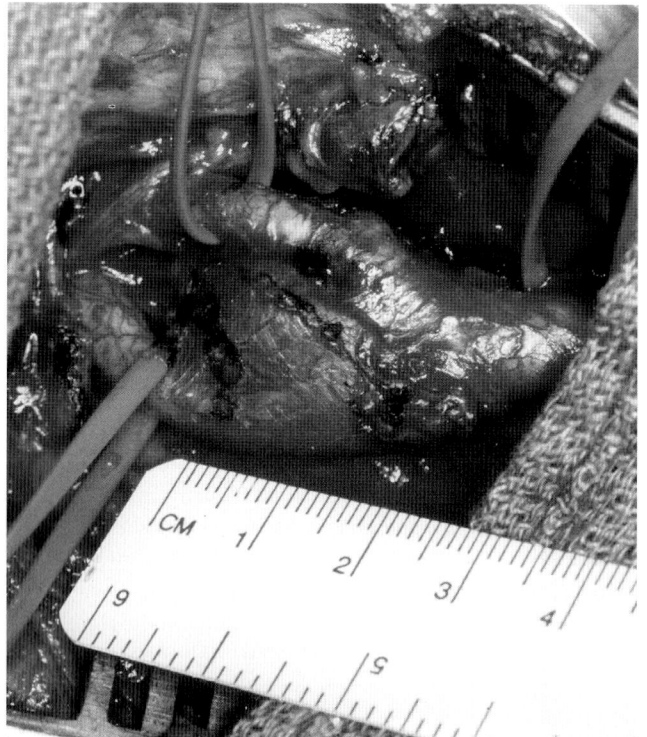

Figure 99-4 Operative photograph taken during resection of a small carotid body tumor. Vessel loops encircle the common (*right*), external (*left upper*), and internal (*left lower*) carotid arteries.

Malignancy in carotid body tumors is not well defined and is diagnosed according to clinical behavior rather than histologic appearance. Almost all carotid body tumors show microscopic capsular invasion, but the rate of "clinical malignancy" is reported to be less than 5%.[60] Even locally invasive tumors are not definitely malignant, and it is generally accepted that carotid body tumors are malignant only if they have metastasized to non-neuroendocrine tissue such as the cervical lymph nodes, lung, liver, and skin.[61]

Grossly, carotid body tumors are brownish, ovoid or round, and lobulated with thin-walled vessels on the outer surface and a thin fibrous capsule (Fig. 99-4). Microscopically, the tumors reproduce the architecture of the normal carotid body, which is composed of granular epithelioid chief cells and sustentacular supporting cells that form clusters called Zellballen or cell balls. The cell balls are highly vascular and surrounded by extensive vascular sinusoids (Fig. 99-5).[62,63] The median doubling time of paragangliomas is 4.2 years, and both small and large tumors grow more slowly than intermediate-sized tumors.[64]

Clinical Findings

The majority of carotid body tumors are slow-growing, asymptomatic lateral neck masses that may be associated with a thrill or a bruit. Because the tumor is fixed to the carotid, it is mobile horizontally but not vertically (Fontaine's sign).

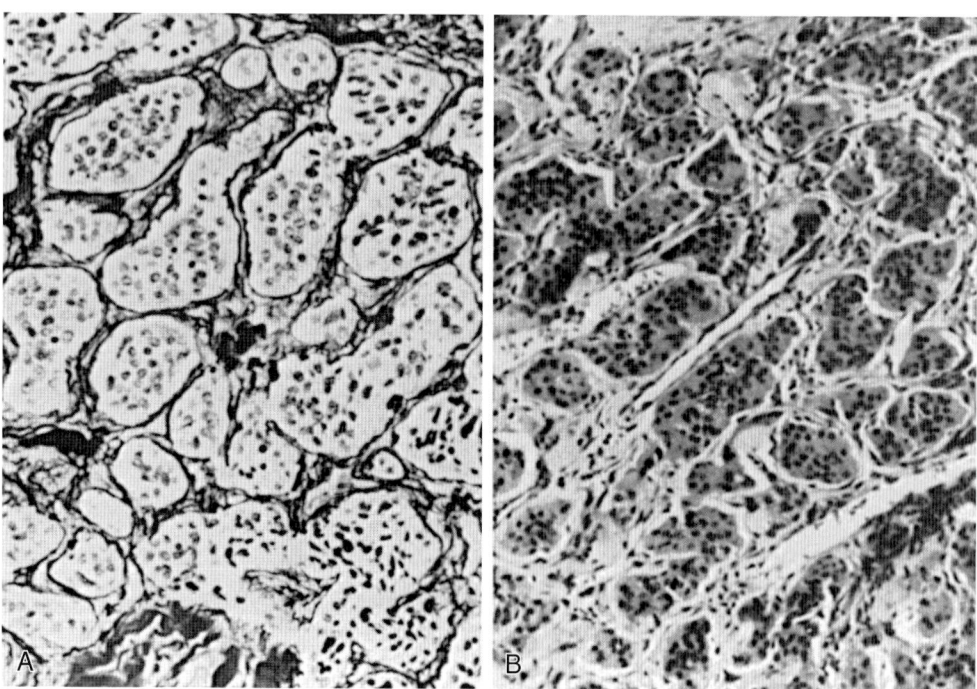

Figure 99-5 Cross-sectional photomicrographs of a carotid body tumor. **A,** Reticulin stains accentuate the characteristic Zellballen (cell balls). Clusters of darkly stained red blood cells mark numerous small blood vessels. **B,** On hematoxylin-eosin staining, the cell balls are shown to be separated by fibrous septa containing numerous small vascular spaces. The tumor cells have moderately abundant, finely granular eosinophilic cytoplasm, indistinct cell borders, and round to oval nuclei (×125). (*From Krupski WC, Effeney DJ, Ehrenfeld WK, Stoney RJ. Cervical chemodectoma: technical considerations and management options. Am J Surg. 1982;144:215-220.*)

As size increases, associated symptoms such as neck pain, dysphonia, hoarseness, stridor, dysphagia, odynophagia, jaw stiffness, or sore throat (or any combination of these symptoms) may be present. Ten percent to 22% of patients have preoperative cranial nerve deficits.[52,54] The rare functional tumor can cause palpitations, tachycardia, and hypertension.

Diagnostic Evaluation

Carotid body tumors are usually detected by clinical examination, and the diagnosis is confirmed by basic imaging. Diagnostic biopsy is avoided because paragangliomas are so highly vascular, rarely malignant, and easily diagnosed with routine imaging modalities. Ultrasound, computed tomography (CT), and magnetic resonance imaging (MRI) are all effective for diagnosis; bilateral imaging is advocated to rule out multicentricity. On ultrasound examination, carotid body tumors usually appear as solid, well-defined, hypoechoic, hypervascular masses that characteristically splay the carotid bifurcation (Fig. 99-6).[65] MRI and CT show a hypervascular tumor that does not invade the carotid. Positron emission tomography is being used to diagnose paragangliomas with a diameter of less than 1 cm and may be helpful in diagnosing small or multicentric tumors.[66]

Some clinicians and investigators believe that preoperative angiography is mandatory for lesions at the carotid bifurcation both to confirm the diagnosis and to provide accurate preoperative information about the blood supply to the lesion (Fig. 99-7).[67] In Europe, however, noninvasive testing is increasingly being used as the sole test before surgery, and a recent review reports that angiography was used for diagnosis

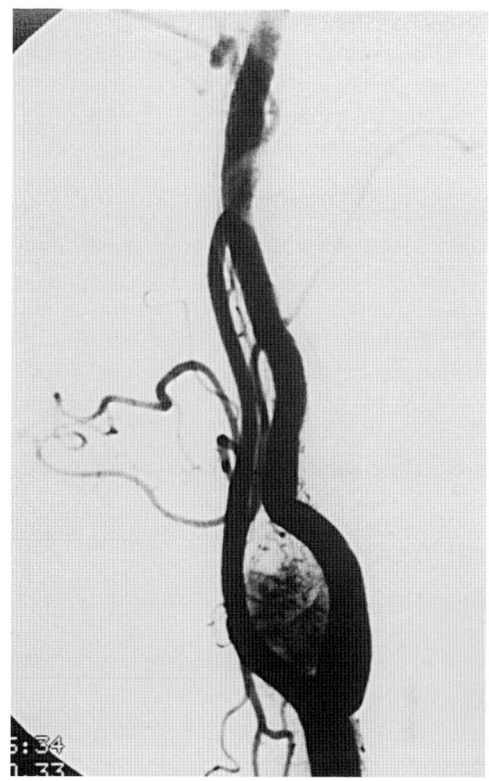

Figure 99-7 Selective carotid angiogram demonstrating the classic characteristics of a carotid body tumor. The bifurcation is widened by the tumor; note the contrast density of the "tumor blush," which illustrates the highly vascular nature of these tumors.

and preoperative assessment in only 20% of patients.[52] Angiography does carry the risk of procedural complications, and the rare functional tumor can secrete catecholamines during catheter manipulation and give rise to a hypertensive crisis. Some authors recommend measuring urinary catecholamines before angiography for a suspected carotid body tumor.[68] Patients with a positive family history and carriers of succinate dehydrogenase mutations should also undergo urinalysis for catecholamines and imaging of sites with a predilection for these tumors.[59,69]

An advantage of diagnostic angiography is the opportunity for concomitant preoperative embolization. The goals of embolization are to minimize blood loss, decrease tumor size, and facilitate excision of the carotid body tumor in a periadventitial plane.[67] The first case reports describing preoperative embolization of carotid body tumors were presented in 1983 and 1987. The authors of these papers reported decreased tumor mass, decreased vascularity, and increased ease of surgical resection after embolization.[70,71] Since that time, the advantages of preoperative embolization have been controversial. A more recent retrospective series demonstrated no difference in blood loss or perioperative morbidity between embolized and nonembolized groups.[72] Another modern series documented no statistical difference in operative blood loss between embolized and nonembolized groups for carotid body tumors less than 3 cm in diameter.[68] The larger and presumably more technically challenging tumors were embolized preoperatively.

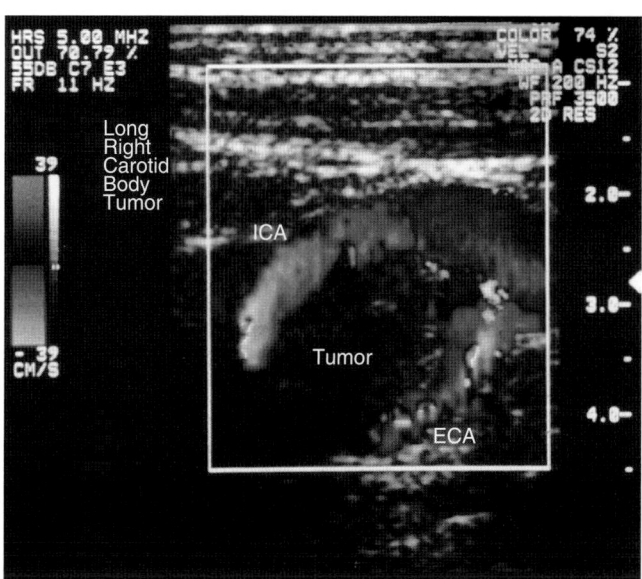

Figure 99-6 Characteristic duplex color-flow image of a carotid body tumor. The internal (ICA) and external (ECA) carotid arteries are splayed open by the tumor mass. The tumor itself may exhibit a very active mixed signal pattern representing the extensive vascularity of the tumor. *(From Krupski WC. Uncommon disorders affecting the carotid arteries. In: Rutherford RB, ed.* Vascular Surgery. *6th ed. Philadelphia, PA: Elsevier Saunders; 2005:2070.)*

The major risk associated with embolization of carotid body tumors is reflux of particulate material into the cerebral or ophthalmic circulation. One series documented stroke in one of six embolized patients. These authors pointed out that the benefits of embolization must be weighed against the risk for stroke and suggest limiting embolization to tumors greater than 5 cm in diameter.[63] Others suggest a smaller tumor diameter (>2 cm) as the threshold for embolization,[67] but the use of new surgical technologies, such as the ultrasonic aspirator, may lead to better outcomes in large tumors without preoperative embolization. Improving diagnostic modalities may also contribute to early identification of carotid body tumors and thus lead to the opportunity for repair at a smaller size. Operations should be performed within 48 hours of embolization to avoid any resulting inflammatory response.[67]

Surgical Treatment

Surgical resection is the preferred treatment of carotid body tumors. Excision of carotid body tumors is notoriously difficult because of anatomic distortion caused by the tumor bulk, high vascularity, and adherence to the carotid arteries and cranial nerves. Shamblin introduced a classification scheme that reflects the degree of technical challenge in tumor excision. Type I tumors are small, are attached to the carotid, and can be removed without difficulty (Fig. 99-8). Type II tumors

are larger, have moderate arterial attachment, and can be removed with care. Type III tumors are large, incarcerate the carotid and nerves, and should be approached with great care; vessel replacement should be considered.[62]

Operative considerations are similar to those for carotid endarterectomy. A thorough cranial nerve examination should be performed and documented preoperatively. Surgery may be performed with the patient awake or under general anesthesia, and the potential for blood loss should prompt consideration of the use of cell-saving technologies for larger tumors. The patient is positioned supine with the neck rotated to expose the operative side, and a site for saphenous vein harvest is prepared in case carotid resection is necessary. The incision is made along the anterior border of the sternocleidomastoid muscle, and the common, internal, and external carotid arteries are controlled. In most cases the blood supply to the tumor is from the external carotid artery. The hypoglossal and vagus nerves are identified and preserved. The superior laryngeal nerve may be involved posteriorly at the bulb, and the marginal mandibular branch of the facial nerve may be near tumors extending superiorly. Nasotracheal or orotracheal intubation facilitates upward displacement of the floor of the mouth if mandibular retraction or resection is necessary, whereas a modified radical neck T incision helps in exposure of large tumors.[54] The tumor is mobilized circumferentially at the inferior margin, and the dissection proceeds cephalad

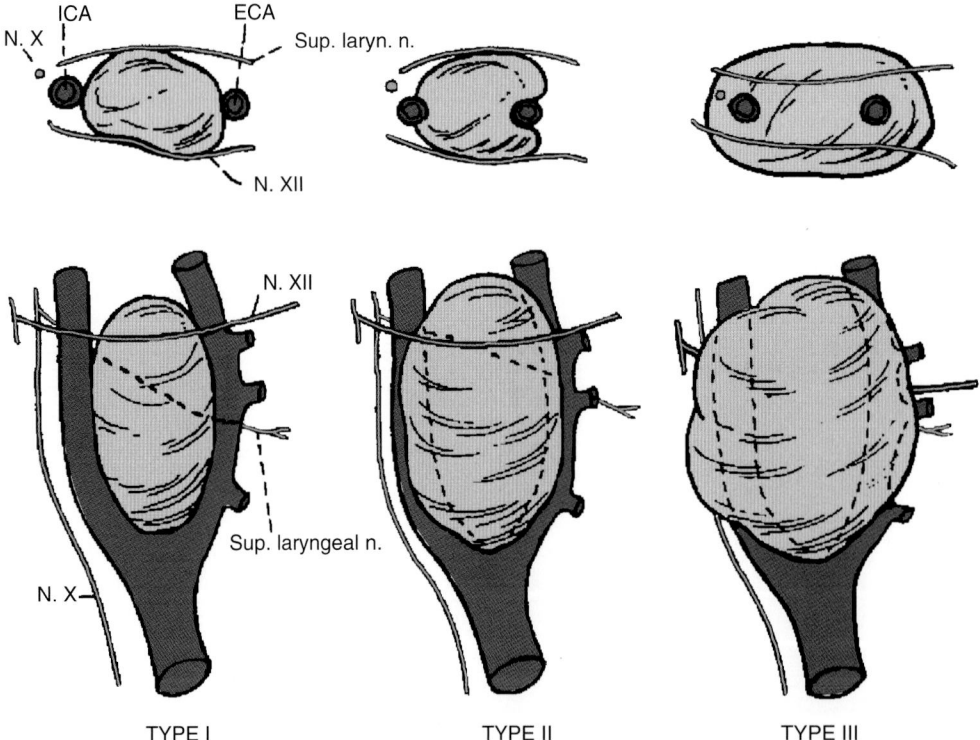

TYPE I   TYPE II   TYPE III

Figure 99-8 Shamblin's classification of carotid body tumors based on the degree of difficulty of resection. Type I tumors are localized and easily resected. Type II tumors include tumors adherent to or partially surrounding vessels. Type III tumors intimately surround or encase the vessels and nerves. ECA, external carotid artery; ICA, internal carotid artery. (*Redrawn from Hallet JW. Trends in neurovascular complications of surgical management for carotid body and cervical paragangliomas: a fifty-year experience with 153 tumors. J Vasc Surg. 1988;7:284-291.*)

in the periadventitial plane. The external carotid artery may be ligated. Reconstruction of the internal carotid artery with saphenous vein may be required. Prosthetic grafts, shunts, and patches should be available.

Results

Resection of carotid body tumors has historically been associated with high morbidity and mortality and a risk for nonfatal stroke. A recent review of the literature describes mortality rates between 0% and 3%, stroke rates between 0 and 8%, and cranial nerve palsy in less than 1% to 49% of patients.[52] Cranial nerve palsy is the most frequent complication after resection of a carotid body tumor, but most are stretch injuries that resolve with time.[52]

Although radiation therapy is used for the treatment of patients who are not operative candidates and in many patients with recurrent cervical paragangliomas, surgery is the preferred treatment of recurrent carotid body tumors.[73]

■ CAROTID SINUS SYNDROME

The carotid sinus is a collection of sensory nerve endings embedded in elastic tissue at the bifurcation of the distal common carotid artery. The carotid sinus is distinct from but frequently collocated with the carotid bulb, which is the fusiform dilatation of the proximal internal carotid artery, and the carotid body, which is a chemoreceptor located at the bifurcation. The glossopharyngeal nerve gives rise to the nerve of Hering, also called the carotid sinus nerve, which travels down the surface of the internal carotid artery or between the internal and external carotid arteries and functions as the afferent tract for the baroreflex. The carotid artery baroreceptors respond to stretch (evolutionarily to pressure) by increasing transmission of impulses through the glossopharyngeal and vagus nerves. These nerves deliver signals to the nuclei tractus solitarii of the medulla, where parasympathetic nuclei become activated and sympathetic nuclei are inhibited, thereby resulting in decreased heart rate, vascular tone, and blood pressure.[74] Both the carotid sinus and the carotid bulb are supplied by the nerve of Hering.

Epidemiology

The term *carotid sinus syndrome* (CSS) is used to refer to patients experiencing excessive bradycardia (cardioinhibitory CSS), hypotension (vasodepressor CSS), or both (mixed CSS) in response to stimulation of the carotid sinus. Effective stimuli include carotid massage, neck suction, and cervical movement.[75] CSS is a disease of the elderly. Depending on definition and severity criteria, CSS is present in 10% of the elderly population but occurs in up to 48% of patients older than 65 years who suffer from dizziness, falls, or syncope.[76] CSS has been associated with other risk factors for vascular disease, including hypertension, coronary artery disease, atherosclerosis, and diabetes.[77] Some authors consider CSS a marker for widespread atherosclerotic disease rather than a

distinct clinical entity.[75] There is a male preponderance and correlation with the use of digitalis, methyldopa, and beta blockers.[75]

CSS has historically been treated by carotid sinus denervation (by means of surgery or irradiation), but the majority of cases are now treated by cardiac pacing and medications. In patients with severe symptoms who do not respond to conventional treatment, carotid sinus denervation by periarterial stripping can be considered. The glossopharyngeal nerve should not be sacrificed because this causes anesthesia of the posterior part of the tongue and pharynx and impaired swallowing.[78]

Carotid Sinus Stimulation

The ability to decrease blood pressure by stimulation of the carotid sinus has important clinical implications. An implantable medical device that stimulates the carotid sinus with electrodes implanted on the external surface of the carotid artery, activates the baroreflex, and produces sustainable decreases in blood pressure is currently undergoing human clinical trials and is showing promise for the treatment of resistant hypertension.

Epidemiology

Hypertension is defined as systolic blood pressure greater than 140 mm Hg or diastolic blood pressure greater than 90 mm Hg, or both. At the turn of the 21st century at least 65 million adults (31.3%) in the United States had hypertension, and the prevalence is rising.[79] A subset of these patients have uncontrolled or resistant hypertension. Patients who are not compliant with medications, are on suboptimal regimens, or are resistant to treatment have what is termed *uncontrolled hypertension*. *Resistant hypertension* is defined as blood pressure that remains above goal despite the concurrent use of optimal doses of three antihypertensive agents in different classes, one of which is a diuretic.[80]

The prevalence of truly resistant hypertension is not known. Data from the Antihypertensive and Lipid Lowering Treatment to Prevent Heart Attack Trial (ALLHAT) are thought to provide a reasonable estimate of the prevalence of resistant hypertension because the medication was free of cost and closely monitored according to study protocol.[80] In this trial 34% of participants' hypertension remained uncontrolled with an average of two medications at 5-year follow-up. At study completion approximately 50% of participants would have required three or more medications for blood pressure control.[80,81]

The prevalence of resistant hypertension increases with the severity of hypertension,[82] and these patients have an increased absolute cardiac risk and a higher prevalence of target organ damage.[83] For every 20 mm Hg systolic or 10 mm Hg diastolic increase in blood pressure, there is a doubling of mortality from both ischemic heart disease and stroke.[84] These data suggest that clinically relevant improvements need to be made in the treatment of hypertension.

Pathophysiology

The carotid baroreflex is generally accepted as a system that responds to short-term fluctuations in blood pressure by changing autonomic efferent output.[74] The role of the carotid baroreflex in long-term blood pressure control has been questioned because the baroreflex resets within 48 hours after a sustained increase in blood pressure[85] and because baroreceptor deafferentation does not produce a sustained increase in arterial pressure.[86] Long-term blood pressure regulation by the baroreflex appears to be more complex than resetting or deafferentation imply, however, because a sustained decrease in blood pressure is easily achieved with electrical carotid sinus stimulation. In a canine model, chronic unloading of the baroreceptor by proximal ligation of the common carotid artery produced sustained hypertension, thus demonstrating that changes in pressure are perceived differently from denervation by the baroreflex.[87] In another canine model, an implanted device electrically activated the baroreflex and successfully produced a sustained decrease in blood pressure over a period of 7 days without evidence of habituation. Heart rate also decreased, but the changes were not as pronounced (Fig. 99-9).[88]

The effects of the baroreflex on the renin-aldosterone-angiotensin system (RAAS) are also relevant. A recent study measured the effects of the baroreflex on the sympathetic nervous system and the RAAS in canines.[89] All dogs received an implantable device to stimulate the baroreflex. Mean arterial pressure, plasma norepinephrine levels, and plasma renin activity were measured before and after the device was turned on. After 7 days of stimulation, mean arterial pressure and norepinephrine concentrations were decreased, but plasma renin activity was unchanged. These findings support the hypothesis that electrical baroreflex stimulation decreases blood pressure by reducing sympathetic nervous system activity and prevents activation of the RAAS.[90]

Clinical Applications. In a paper published in 1923, Hering described the nerve carrying the afferent signals of the baroreflex to the medulla.[91] Early work from McCubbin and colleagues demonstrated fewer impulses from the carotid sinus nerve in hypertensive subjects than in normotensive subjects, thus implying that the baroreflex resets with chronic hypertension.[92] Work done in 1958 showed that electrical stimulation of the carotid sinus produces a reduction in blood pressure in humans,[93] and in 1967, the first series of eight patients successfully treated for resistant hypertension with an implanted carotid sinus stimulator was described by Schwartz and coauthors.[94] This line of treatment was abandoned, however, probably because the devices were cumbersome and the concomitant advances in medical therapy were effective and attractively noninvasive.[95]

As described earlier, however, resistant hypertension continues to be a significant public health problem. For patients with severe hypertension treated with many medications, the addition of another drug often increases side effects with minimal improvement in blood pressure (Fig. 99-10). Because of these circumstances, the concept of carotid baroreflex stimulation has re-emerged as a treatment option. Modern work done by Lohmeier and associates in canine models validated and refined electrical stimulation of the carotid sinus for the treatment of hypertension,[88,89,96] and a commercial device has been created to reproduce this effect in humans.

A phase II feasibility trial using the Rheos Baroreflex Hypertension Therapy System (CVRx, Maple Grove, MN) to activate the baroreflex and decrease blood pressure in patients with resistant hypertension has reported early results.[90,95] The study was performed from 2005 to 2006 in Europe and the United States. In the first 10 American patients participating in the Rheos feasibility trial, stimulation in the operating room reduced systolic pressure by 37 mm Hg

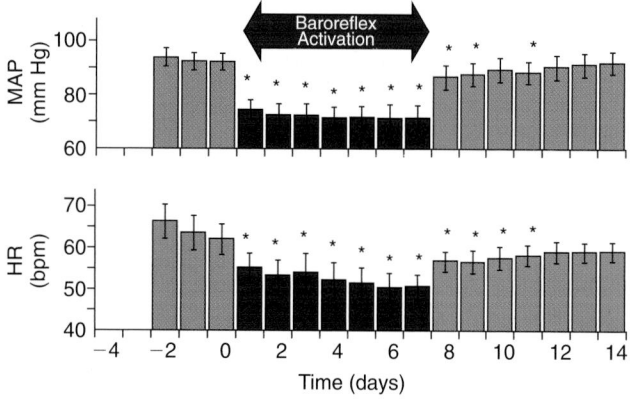

Figure 99-9 Baroreflex activation in the normal canine. Note the drop in mean arterial blood pressure (MAP) and heart rate (HR) produced by electrical stimulation of the carotid sinus (*asterisks* denote P < .05) and the fact that this response is sustained for a week with no evidence of habituation. (*Modified from Lohmeier TE, Irwin ED, Rossing MA, et al. Prolonged activation of the baroreflex produces sustained hypotension.* Hypertension. *2004;43:306-311; courtesy of CVRx, Inc., Minneapolis, MN.*)

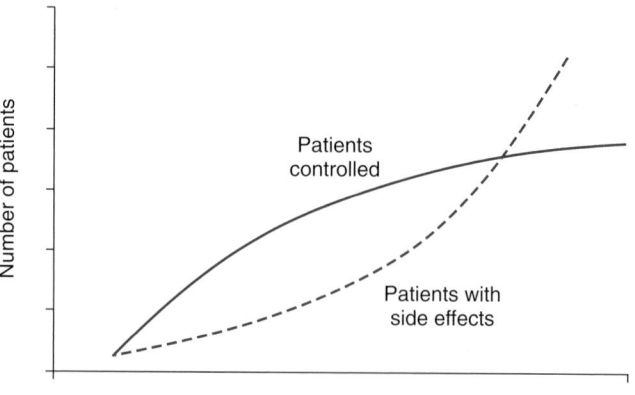

Figure 99-10 Schematic diagram illustrating the qualitative relationship between control of hypertension (HTN) and side effects as a function of increasing the number of antihypertensive medications. In general, although the first few medications will often control blood pressure with relatively manageable side effects, as more and more medications are added, incremental blood pressure control becomes less and side effects disproportionately increase. (*Courtesy of CVRx, Inc., Minneapolis, MN.*)

(170 to 133 mm Hg). In awake patients, on postoperative day 1 systolic blood pressure was reduced by 41 mm Hg (180 to 139 mm Hg). Data from the parallel European feasibility study (DEBut-HT [Device Based Therapy in Hypertension Trial]) conducted in six clinical centers demonstrated a sustained dose-response curve at 4 months after implantation[95] and a sustained 39 mm Hg decrease in systolic blood pressure after 1 year of therapy.[97] At present a phase III prospective randomized trial is under way at 30 centers in Europe and the United States, with planned enrollment of 300 patients.

■ VASCULITIS

Inflammation of the aorta and great vessels can be seen in a number of disorders, including Kawasaki's syndrome, Behçet's syndrome, rheumatoid arthritis, syphilis, and tuberculosis. However, the most common large-vessel arteritides are Takayasu's arteritis and giant cell arteritis. Although the epidemiology of these diseases differs, they share similar cellular immune responses, and neither has evidence of an autoantibody component.[98]

Takayasu's Arteritis

This section addresses features of Takayasu's disease pertinent to carotid pathology. For a full discussion, see Chapter 78 (Takayasu's Disease). Takayasu's arteritis is a rare vasculitis of unknown etiology that causes stenoses or aneurysms in affected arteries, with a predilection for the aorta and its major branches. Stenoses are seen in 98% of patients and aneurysms in 27%.[99] The disease occurs more frequently in females and is most prevalent in Japan, Southeast Asia, and Mexico.[100] Takayasu's arteritis usually develops in the second or third decade of life with a range of clinical findings from asymptomatic to catastrophic stroke. The most common clinical finding is a bruit.[99]

Treatment

Immunosuppression is the mainstay of treatment of Takayasu's arteritis, and there are no established indications for surgery. In one study, indications for surgery in patients with cerebrovascular stenosis were clinical features of ischemia or stenoses greater than 70% (or both) in at least three cerebral vessels.[99] Nine patients had bypass grafts placed for carotid stenosis, with the ascending aorta being the most frequently used vessel for proximal anastomosis. One postoperative stroke was reported. Restenosis occurs commonly after surgical or endovascular intervention in patients with Takayasu's arteritis and may be related to the inflammatory nature of the disease. Results from a 2005 meta-analysis indicate a 20% to 30% average rate of restenosis or occlusion after any bypass at any location.[101] The few series on endovascular treatment also show a high rate of restenosis or occlusion.[99,102,103]

Current recommendations (and the modern standard of care) are to treat patients with lesions in the active, inflammatory phase with steroids, avoid surgery or endovascular intervention at all cost, and consider intervention only in patients with chronic, noninflammatory lesions ("pulselessness" phase) that are highly symptomatic. If bypass in these patients is considered, it is important to start and finish in areas that are statistically unlikely to be affected by progressive disease—the hallmark example being to use the ascending aorta rather than another brachiocephalic vessel as inflow in patients with arch disease.

The authors of a case series on repair of extracranial carotid aneurysms caused by Takayasu's arteritis advocate repair of all these lesions.[104] Anastomotic aneurysm is a possible complication after any surgical treatment of Takayasu's arteritis and is described after repairs with either prosthetic material or autologous vein.[104,105] The risk for de novo and anastomotic aneurysms makes surveillance crucial in the management of these patients.

Giant Cell Arteritis

Giant cell arteritis is reviewed thoroughly in Chapter 76 (Vasculitis and Other Arteriopathies) and is discussed here with a specific focus on its predilection for branches of the internal and external carotid arteries. Involvement of these vessels leads to the classic manifestations of blindness, headache, scalp tenderness, and jaw claudication. Giant cell arteritis is also predominant in women, but unlike Takayasu's arteritis, it occurs in people older than 50 years. Although transmural inflammation leads to intimal hyperplasia and luminal narrowing in giant cell arteritis, occlusion and aneurysmal change are less frequently seen than in Takayasu's arteritis.[98]

Treatment

Immunosuppression is also the mainstay of treatment of giant cell arteritis, but some occlusive lesions may progress despite medical therapy. Minimal literature exists on the surgical treatment of carotid stenoses caused by giant cell arteritis, but one series does report the results of angioplasty in the upper extremities of 10 symptomatic patients.[106] The primary patency rate was 65.2% and the secondary patency rate was 82.6%, which led the authors to conclude that despite a tendency for restenosis, angioplasty in conjunction with ongoing medical management is an efficient treatment of extracranial giant cell arteritis. A smaller and earlier series showed no significant recurrent stenosis after angioplasty. The authors speculate that their positive outcomes were related to the postprocedural continuation of steroids and aspirin.[107]

Radiation Arteritis

Radiation therapy is commonly used in the treatment of head and neck cancer and is known to cause arterial radiation damage. Large arteries are affected the least, and the resulting damage resembles atherosclerotic changes. The morphology of chronic arterial lesions suggests a distinct disease process or abnormally accelerated and severe localized atherosclerotic degeneration, and unusual, multiple, and—when appropriate

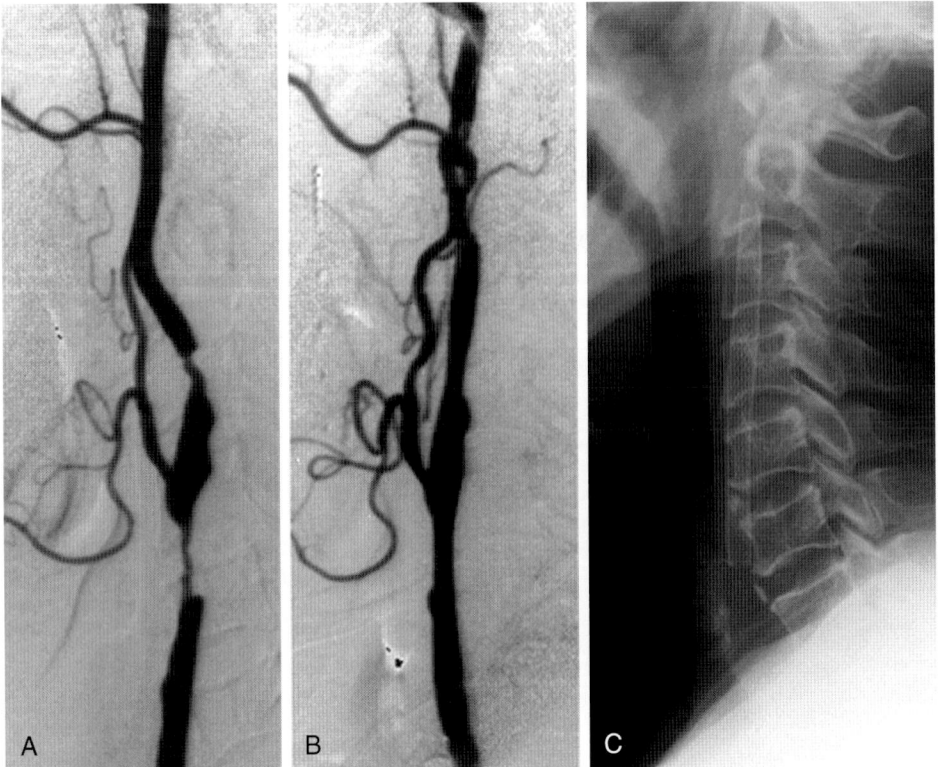

Figure 99-11 A–C, CTA (three-dimensional reconstruction) of a patient who had received radiation therapy for Hodgkin's lymphoma 10 years before. Note the severe diffuse disease process.

in terms of radiation fields—bilateral segments are often involved (Fig. 99-11).[108,109] Arterial rupture after exposure to radiation is rare and occurs most commonly in patients who have also been treated surgically.[110]

Regardless of the mechanism, cervical irradiation is a risk factor for carotid artery stenosis. In prospective screening studies using duplex ultrasonography, patients who had undergone head and neck radiation therapy had an approximately 40% incidence of internal carotid artery stenosis greater than 50%.[111,112] In a similarly designed study, the incidence of internal or common carotid artery stenosis of 70% or greater was 16%.[113]

There are shared risk factors between atherosclerotic disease and cancer of the head and neck, such as tobacco use, but this overlap does not appear to confound the relationship between carotid stenosis and neck irradiation. A retrospective review of duplex ultrasound examinations compared a group of patients with a history of radiation therapy and a group of randomly chosen age-matched controls from the same cohort.[114] No statistically significant difference between the groups was detected in smoking status, coronary artery disease, hypertension, cholesterol levels, diabetes mellitus, or peripheral vascular disease. The irradiated group had a 21.7% incidence of advanced carotid disease (70% to 99% stenosis) versus a 4% incidence in the control group.

Because the prevalence of carotid stenosis is higher in patients who have undergone neck irradiation, several authors have advocated routine carotid duplex surveillance.[112-114] Current recommendations from the 2007 American Society

of Neuroimaging are to start screening all patients after unilateral or bilateral irradiation of the neck 10 years after treatment.[115] The authors acknowledge that this recommendation is derived from data that include patients who received doses larger than 45 Gy. They do not recommend screening before radiation treatment, and the optimal interval for repeat imaging is unclear.

Natural History

Carotid stenoses caused by radiation may have a natural history different from those caused by atherosclerosis, but irradiated patients do have a higher stroke rate. A retrospective review compared the actuarial risk of stroke in 413 patients irradiated for head and neck cancer and the expected risk from population-based data.[116] The 5-year actuarial risk was 12%, which corresponded to a relative risk of 2.09. The authors emphasized that although the relative risk for stroke is increased with radiation therapy, the absolute risk is modest in comparison to recurrence of cancer. A pediatric case series described five cancer survivors between the ages of 17 and 36 who had 80% to 100% carotid stenosis after neck irradiation, thus emphasizing the need for careful surveillance in these patients.[117]

Treatment

Open carotid surgery has been used successfully to treat stenosis in patients with a history of cervical irradiation. Several retrospective series show that this population does not have a higher risk for perioperative stroke or death related to carotid surgery or recurrent stenosis than patients treated for atherosclerotic disease.[118-121] Open carotid repair for stenosis caused by radiation is more technically demanding than repair for atherosclerosis. Technical issues of concern after treatment of head and neck cancers include frequent involvement of the common carotid artery, obliteration of the endarterectomy plane by radiation-induced fibrosis, the presence of previous reconstructions, and generalized tissue abnormality, which may impair wound healing and preservation of cranial nerves during dissection.

For these reasons, neck irradiation became one of the major inclusion criteria in the Stenting and Angioplasty with Protection in Patients at High Risk for Endarterectomy (SAPPHIRE) trial and an accepted indication for carotid artery stent placement. One recent study compared patients undergoing carotid angioplasty and stent placement for atherosclerotic and radiotherapy-induced occlusive disease.[122] The authors found no statistically significant difference between the groups with regard to all-cause mortality, adverse events, and 3-year neurologic event–free rate. Only patients in the irradiated group had late symptomatic occlusions. Three-year patency was worse in the irradiated group, which had a higher rate of reintervention. The authors concluded that stenting may not be preferable to open surgery for radiation-induced stenosis and that if stenting is performed, closer postoperative surveillance is required.

OTHER CONDITIONS
Carotid Artery Kinks and Coils

Coiling is elongation of the internal carotid artery in a restricted space that results in a C- or S-shaped curvature. Kinks, a variant of coils, are defined as angulation between vessel segments of 90 degrees or less or the formation of a loop (Fig. 99-12).[123] Unlike coils, kinks are often associated with stenosis.[124] Possible causes of these conditions include developmental abnormalities, fibromuscular dysplasia, age-related degeneration, atherosclerosis, post–carotid endarterectomy changes,[125,126] and normal morphologic variation.

Epidemiology

The prevalence of carotid artery kinks and coils is not definitely known. Most patients are asymptomatic and thus are never identified as having these conditions. In addition, much of the available epidemiologic literature is old. For example, an autopsy series from 1924 described a 30% prevalence of "tortuosity."[127] A large angiographic series of symptomatic patients from 1965 reported a 35% incidence of "tortuosity," a 6% incidence of coils (53% of which were bilateral), and a 5% incidence of kinks (27% of which were bilateral).[128] A female preponderance is reported[126] and confirmed by data from a recent randomized controlled trial.[124]

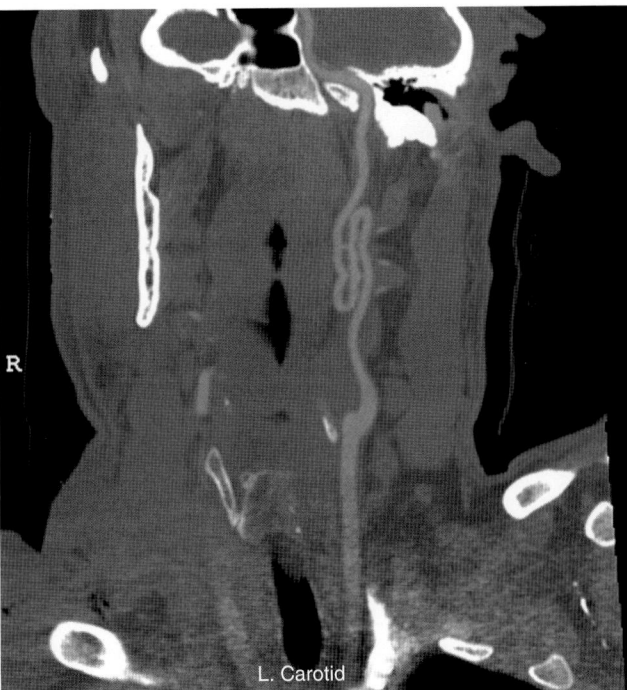

Figure 99-12 CTA (centerline trace, left carotid artery) of an extreme case of a redundant, coiled internal carotid artery. This was an incidental finding in an asymptomatic patient.

Management

The indications for treatment in patients with carotid kinks and coils are elusive because there is not always a clear association between the lesion and symptoms, which can be frustratingly vague. Dizziness, gait instability, syncope, blurry vision, and bilateral paresthesias are examples of complaints that cannot be considered lateralizing.

The recent literature does support surgical management of patients with hemispheric symptoms. In 2005, the first randomized controlled trial comparing surgical and medical treatment of carotid artery kinks and coils in 182 symptomatic patients was published.[124] Patients were considered for the trial if they reported hemispheric symptoms or symptoms impairing daily activity that persisted after 3 months of antiplatelet therapy and no vertebral pathology was present. Patients with previous carotid surgery, patients with existing carotid stenosis, patients managed with long-term anticoagulation or aspirin, and patients intolerant of aspirin were excluded. Patients were randomized to treatment with aspirin or surgical treatment. A single surgeon performed all operations with a uniform technique that included general anesthesia, electroencephalographic monitoring, transection of the internal carotid artery at the bulb, straightening of the internal carotid after division of any fibrous attachments, dilatation of the artery, and end-to-side reimplantation of the internal carotid on the lateral wall of the common carotid (Fig. 99-13). Specimens from the common and internal carotid were sent for pathology.

No perioperative strokes or deaths occurred. No patient in the surgical group had a late stroke or occluded carotid artery, but 6.6% of the patients treated with aspirin alone had

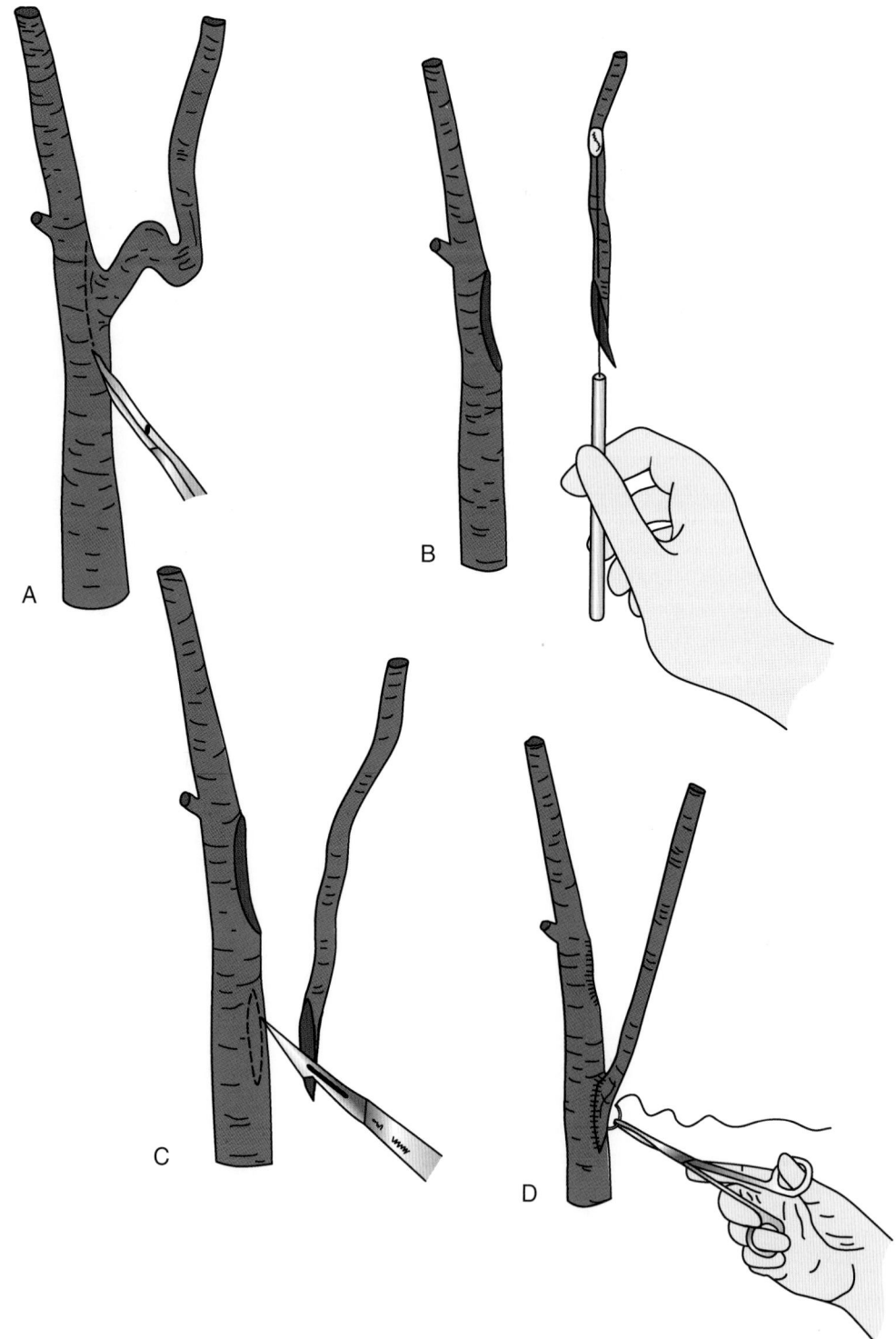

Figure 99-13 Management of highly redundant internal carotid artery. **A,** Transection of the internal carotid artery from the bulb. **B,** Transluminal dilatation of any internal webs or fibrous bands. **C** and **D,** Reimplantation of the internal carotid artery lower on the common carotid artery with repair of the original orifice. (*From Ballotta E, Thiene G, Baracchini C, et al. Surgical vs medical treatment for isolated internal carotid artery elongation with coiling or kinking in asymptomatic patients: a prospective randomized clinical study.* J Vasc Surg. *2005;42:838-846.*)

a late stroke, 2.2% of which were fatal. Late carotid occlusion occurred in 5.5% of the medically treated group. Late mortality was similar between the groups and was primarily due to cardiac events. All nonhemispheric symptoms resolved in the surgical group, and all patients in the medical group reported worse or persistent symptoms, with 41.1% of the medical group crossing over to surgical treatment for new or worsening symptoms. All arterial specimens were abnormal and displayed degeneration of the media, hyperplasia of the media, or fibromuscular dysplasia. The authors concluded that surgical management is better than medical management for relief of symptoms and prevention of stroke and that kinks and coils

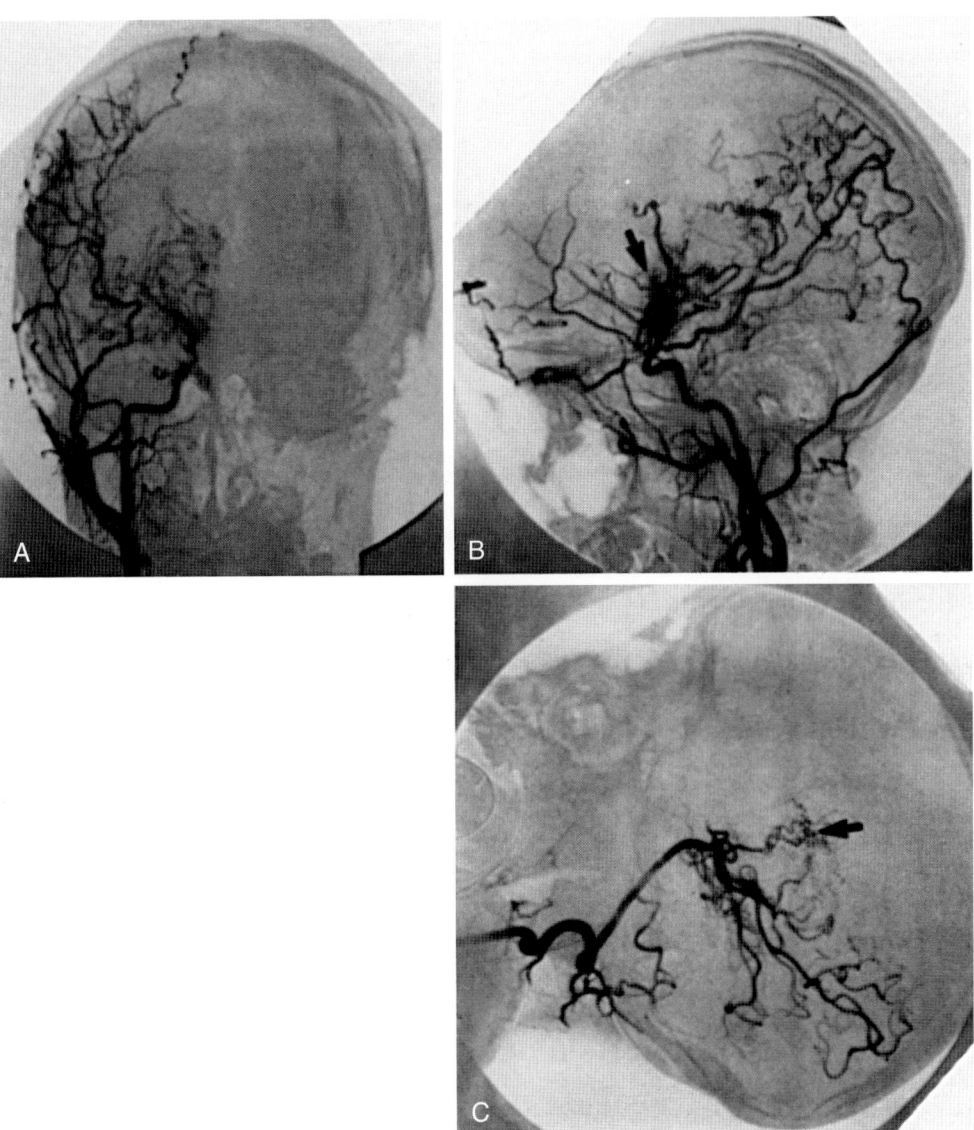

Figure 99-14 A-C, Angiograms of moyamoya disease.

are associated with nonatherosclerotic, noninflammatory change in the arterial wall.[124]

A second series of 81 patients with carotid kinks who underwent surgical treatment of persistent hemispheric symptoms despite antiplatelet therapy reported a postoperative stroke rate of 1%, a primary patency rate of 89%, a neurologic symptom–free rate of 92%, and a 5-year survival rate of 71%.[129] The surgical techniques in this series include shortening and reimplantation of the internal carotid artery on the common carotid artery, transposition of the internal carotid artery to the external carotid artery, and insertion of a bypass graft. Both these studies strongly support the concept that symptomatic carotid artery kinks and coils should be treated surgically.

Moyamoya Disease

Moyamoya disease is a rare condition characterized by progressive stenosis of the cerebral vessels, particularly the distal intracranial internal carotid, middle cerebral, and anterior

cerebral arteries. As the circle of Willis becomes occluded, there is concomitant development of a collateral network at the base of the brain.[130] The "smoky" angiographic appearance of these collaterals is the origin of the name moyamoya, which means puffy, obscure, or vague in Japanese (Fig. 99-14).[131]

Epidemiology and Pathogenesis

Moyamoya disease predominantly affects Japanese and other Asian populations. In Japan the incidence is one per million, the majority of cases occur in children younger than 10 years, and the female-male ratio is 1.7:1.[131] Ten percent of cases have a familial association and linkage to specific loci on chromosomes 2, 3, 6, 17, and 25.[130] Moyamoya syndrome refers to the pattern of cerebral vasculopathy in the context of known systemic disease, and associations with lupus, CREST syndrome (calcinosis cutis, Raynaud's phenomenon, esophageal dysfunction, sclerodactyly, and telangiectasia), neurofibromatosis type 1, Down's syndrome, hypercoagulable states, radiation exposure, and cocaine abuse have all been described.[130]

Clinical Findings

Children with moyamoya disease frequently have transient ischemic attacks induced by effort-related activities such as running. Its signs and symptoms can be unilateral or bilateral, depending on the severity or location of the involved vasculature, and there can also be subtle behavioral or cognitive changes. Adults are more likely than children to have permanent ischemic deficits and intracranial hemorrhage (which carries a worse prognosis). It is not clear whether the more severe manifestation in adults represents advanced disease or a qualitatively different phenomenon.

Diagnosis

Moyamoya disease is diagnosed by its characteristic angiographic findings. Criteria include stenosis or occlusion of the distal internal carotid artery, proximal middle cerebral artery, or proximal anterior cerebral artery (or any combination of the three), usually bilateral, along with abnormal collaterals in the region of arterial narrowing. CT and MRI can also demonstrate the characteristic vessel abnormalities. Because vessel appearance may not reflect the hemodynamic impact of moyamoya disease, functional imaging with CT, electroencephalography, MRI, and PET is used to evaluate the clinical implications of hypoperfusion.

Treatment

Surgical indications for moyamoya disease are not well established, but surgery is usually performed for some manifestation of cerebral hypoperfusion. Surgical treatment of moyamoya disease is either direct or indirect bypass (which can be performed together). Direct bypass is performed from the superficial temporal artery to the middle cerebral artery (sometimes the anterior cerebral artery). This operation is technically challenging in children because of the small size of the arteries. Indirect bypass refers to the apposition of vascularized tissue to the ischemic brain to foster the development of collaterals. Tissue sources include dura, temporalis muscle, superficial temporal artery, and galea. An indirect bypass has the disadvantage of delayed efficacy and continued ischemia while collaterals develop. Children can be treated by indirect bypass or symptomatically managed with antiplatelet agents and calcium channel blockers if direct bypass is not technically possible.[130]

Results

As recently as 1994 a Japanese study found no statistically significant therapeutic difference between patients managed medically and those managed surgically. These results may have been confounded by mild cases receiving medical management and severe cases receiving surgical management.

Unfortunately, no randomized trial has compared the treatments.[131] A recent review of the surgical pediatric moyamoya literature reported that 73% of cases were indirect procedures, 23% of which were performed in combination with direct procedures. Preoperative stroke occurred in 4.4% of patients, and 6.1% had reversible ischemic events. Eighty-seven percent of patients had symptomatic benefit from surgery, although no significant differences were seen in the indirect, direct, and combined groups. Direct or combined procedures did result in significantly better collateral formation.[132]

Incidental Intracranial Lesions

Intracranial carotid pathology presents a number of surgical challenges. Operative indications are not well defined, the types of possible interventions are evolving rapidly, including endovascular approaches, and open surgery is technically demanding. This section reviews the literature pertinent to intracranial carotid stenosis and aneurysm.

Intracranial Carotid Stenosis

An extracranial-intracranial (EC-IC) bypass joins the superficial temporal artery to the middle cerebral artery to treat occlusive disease of the distal internal carotid artery or the middle cerebral artery. In 1985, the EC-IC Bypass Study reported the results from a randomized trial comparing EC-IC bypass with best medical care.[133] The researchers randomized 1377 patients with recent hemispheric stroke, retinal infarction, or transient ischemic attacks who had atherosclerotic narrowing or occlusion of the ipsilateral internal carotid or middle cerebral artery into treatment groups consisting of surgery or best medical therapy. Although the postoperative bypass patency rate was 96%, nonfatal and fatal stroke occurred more frequently in the operative group. No subgroup showed benefit from surgery, and the authors concluded that their study failed to show that EC-IC bypass is effective in preventing cerebral ischemia in patients with atherosclerotic arterial disease in the carotid and middle cerebral arteries.

Criticisms of the EC-IC bypass trial are indicative of the difficulty involved in patient selection for operative treatment of intracranial stenosis or occlusion. In the EC-IC bypass trial it is not clear which patients were symptomatic from hypoperfusion as opposed to thromboembolic events, and the degree of intracranial stenosis had no correlation with hemodynamic status.[134] Functional imaging has improved since the trial, and CT, MRI, or PET can now be performed with concomitant chemical challenge to cerebral perfusion. These advanced imaging techniques may be helpful in identifying patients with clinically significant stenoses or occlusions. There are currently trials in the United States and Japan using functional imaging to address which intracranial lesions are hemodynamically important or amenable to surgery (or both).[135,136]

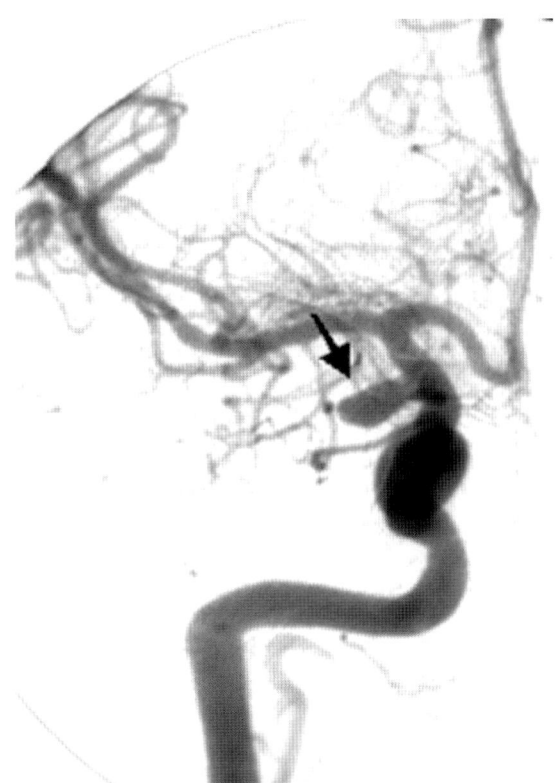

Figure 99-15 Right internal carotid angiogram demonstrating a right posterior communicating artery aneurysm (*arrow*). *(From Tirakotai W, Sure U, Yin Y, et al. Surgery of intracranial aneurysms previously treated endovascularly. Clin Neurol Neurosurg. 2007;109:744-752.)*

Intracranial Aneurysm

The incidence of unruptured cerebral aneurysms ranges from 1% to 5%.[137-139] Approximately 33% of intracranial aneurysms are found in the internal or cavernous carotid artery.[138] Management of these aneurysms is controversial. In the recent past, the risk of rupture was thought to be low and did not exceed the risk associated with surgery if the aneurysm was less than 10 mm in diameter and there was no previous history of ruptured intracranial aneurysm at a different location.[138] In addition, clipping of unruptured aneurysms less than 10 mm in diameter with no history of subarachnoid hemorrhage could not be justified on actuarial grounds.[140] The most recent guidelines have addressed concerns regarding patient selection in earlier studies and have integrated advances in microsurgical and endovascular techniques. The current neurosurgical recommendations are repair of all symptomatic aneurysms, conservative management of incidental aneurysms smaller than 5 mm, serious consideration of surgical treatment of aneurysms larger than 5 mm in patients younger than 60 years, surgical treatment of nearly all incidental aneurysms larger than 10 mm in patients younger than 70, and clipping rather than coiling in low-risk patients (Fig. 99-15).[139]

SELECTED KEY REFERENCES

Ballotta E, Thiene G, Baracchini C, Ermani M, Militello C, Da Giau G, Barbon B, Angelini A. Surgical vs medical treatment for isolated internal carotid artery elongation with coiling or kinking in symptom-atic patients: a prospective randomized clinical study. *J Vasc Surg.* 2005;42:838-846.
  Randomized trial comparing medical and surgical treatment of symptomatic carotid elongation with coiling or kinking.

Baumgartner RW. *Handbook on Cerebral Artery Dissection.* Basel, Switzerland: Karger; 2005.
  Comprehensive resource on cervical artery dissection.

Both M, Aries PM, Müller-Hülsbeck S, Jahnke T, Schäfer PJ, Gross WL, Heller M, Reuter M. Balloon angioplasty of arteries of the upper extremities in patients with extracranial giant-cell arteritis. *Ann Rheum Dis.* 2006;65:1124-1130.
  Recent series evaluating patency after balloon angioplasty of upper extremity arteries in patients with giant cell arteritis. The results might be of help if considering carotid intervention.

Edgell RC, Abou-Chebl A, Yadav JS. Endovascular management of spontaneous carotid artery dissection. *J Vasc Surg.* 2005;42:854-860; discussion 860.
  One of the few recent case series evaluating the safety and efficacy of carotid stenting for the treatment of spontaneous dissection after failed medical therapy.

Failure of extracranial-intracranial arterial bypass to reduce the risk of ischemic stroke. Results of an international randomized trial. The EC/IC Bypass Study Group. *N Engl J Med.* 1985;313:1191-1200.
  Seminal trial comparing surgical and medical therapy for symptomatic intracranial carotid stenosis or occlusion. The results showing worse outcomes with surgery have not been refuted in the modern literature.

Illig KA, Levy M, Sanchez L, Trachiotis GD, Shanley C, Irwin E, Pertile T, Kieval R, Cody R. An implantable carotid sinus stimulator for drug-resistant hypertension: surgical technique and short-term outcome from the multicenter phase II Rheos feasibility trial. *J Vasc Surg.* 2006;44:1213-1218.
  Short-term results from a multicenter Food and Drug Administration–monitored trial assessing the response of patients to an implantable carotid sinus stimulator for control of drug-resistant hypertension.

Komotar RJ, Mocco J, Solomon RA. Guidelines for the surgical treatment of unruptured intracranial aneurysms: the first annual J. Lawrence Pool Memorial Research Symposium—controversies in the management of cerebral aneurysms. *Neurosurgery.* 2008;62:183-193.
  Literature review on the management of unruptured cerebral aneurysms with associated treatment guidelines.

Litle VR, Reilly LM, Ramos TK. Preoperative embolization of carotid body tumors: when is it appropriate? *Ann Vasc Surg.* 1996;10:464-468.
  One of the few papers on preoperative embolization of carotid body tumors.

Nissim O, Bakon M, Ben Zeev B, Goshen E, Knoller N, Hadani M, Feldman Z. Moyamoya disease—diagnosis and treatment: indirect cerebral revascularization at the Sheba Medical Center. *Isr Med Assoc.* 2005;7:661-666.
  Literature review and case series examining surgical treatment of moyamoya disease.

Steele SR, Martin MJ, Mullenix PS, Crawford JV, Cuadrado DS, Andersen CA. Focused high-risk population screening for carotid arterial stenosis after radiation therapy for head and neck cancer. *Am J Surg.* 2004;187:594-598.
  Prospective screening showing increased clinically significant carotid stenosis in previously irradiated patients.

REFERENCES

The reference list can be found on the companion Expert Consult Web site at *www.expertconsult.com.*

CHAPTER 100

Brachiocephalic Artery Disease: Surgical Treatment

David L. Lau and Hazim J. Safi

The branches of the transverse aortic arch most commonly consist of the innominate, left common carotid, and left subclavian arteries. These arteries supply the upper extremities and brain and are thus commonly referred to as the brachiocephalic arteries. When these arteries are affected by atherosclerosis, symptoms can result from both flow-limiting stenoses and distal embolism. Single-vessel disease may be manifested as stroke, transient ischemic attacks, upper extremity ischemia, and vertebrobasilar insufficiency from subclavian steal syndrome. Multivessel disease is more often accompanied by symptoms of vertebrobasilar insufficiency from generalized low flow but can also exhibit single-vessel symptoms. Other diseases affecting the brachiocephalic arteries include aneurysmal degeneration, dissection, vasculitides (e.g., Takayasu's disease and giant cell arteritis), and infection, as can radiation therapy. Although lesions involving the brachiocephalic arteries are uncommon, they pose a major risk for morbidity and mortality because of the vascular beds that they supply. In this chapter we describe surgical reconstruction of the brachiocephalic arteries for the treatment of arterial occlusive disease, as well as its application in hybrid procedures involving endovascular aortic aneurysm repair.

ANATOMY

Anatomically, the ascending aorta and transverse arch can be divided into three segments (Fig. 100-1): (1) the aortic root houses the aortic valve, three sinuses, and the two main coronary arteries; (2) the tubular portion of the ascending aorta lies between the supracoronary ascending aorta and the innominate artery; and (3) the transverse arch is the area between the innominate artery and the left subclavian artery. The brachiocephalic arteries arise from the dorsal aspect of the transverse arch.

The most common configuration is three separate trunks, with the innominate artery giving rise to the right subclavian and right common carotid arteries, the left common carotid in close proximity, and the left subclavian artery originating posterior to and to the left of the left common carotid artery. The most common variant is a bovine arch (16% to 24%), in which the left common carotid artery either shares a common ostium with the innominate artery or arises from it. An aortic origin of the vertebral artery (6%) typically involves the left vertebral artery arising between the left common carotid and left subclavian arteries (Fig. 100-2). An aberrant right subcla-

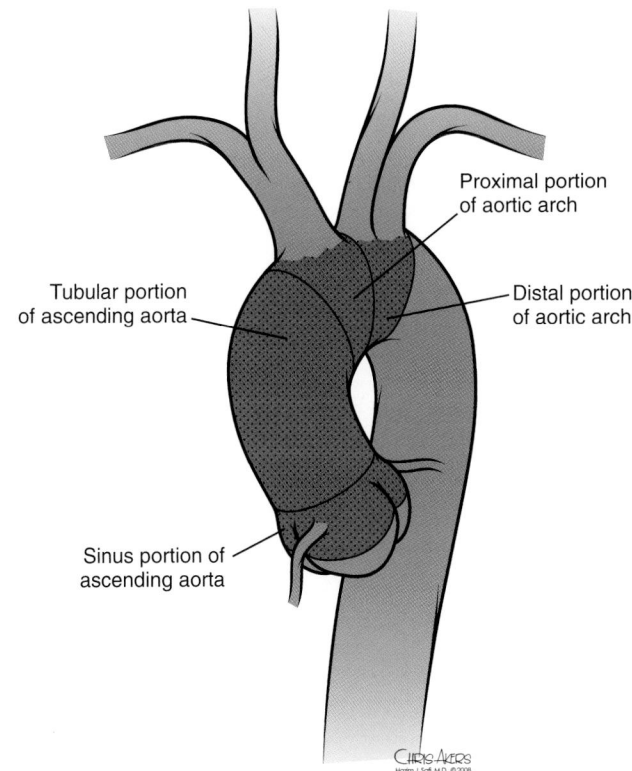

Figure 100-1 Normal anatomy of the ascending and arch aorta.

vian artery (0.5% to 1%) occurs when the right subclavian artery arises distal to the left subclavian artery (Fig. 100-3).[1]

CLINICAL FINDINGS

The clinical manifestations of lesions involving the brachiocephalic arteries depend on the etiology of the disease, the presence of single-vessel or multivessel disease, and anatomic location. Atherosclerosis is the most common disease affecting the brachiocephalic arteries. Severe disease is defined as stenosis greater than 75% of the vessel's diameter. Deep ulcerated plaque or thrombus within the arterial lumen is also considered a severe lesion. Atherosclerotic disease can be unifocal, multifocal, single vessel, or multivessel. In Berguer's series of 282 transthoracic and transcervical brachiocephalic revascularizations, there was a 40% incidence of multivessel disease (Fig. 100-4).[2,3]

Single-vessel atherosclerotic occlusive disease typically causes symptoms as a result of hemispheric or upper extremity

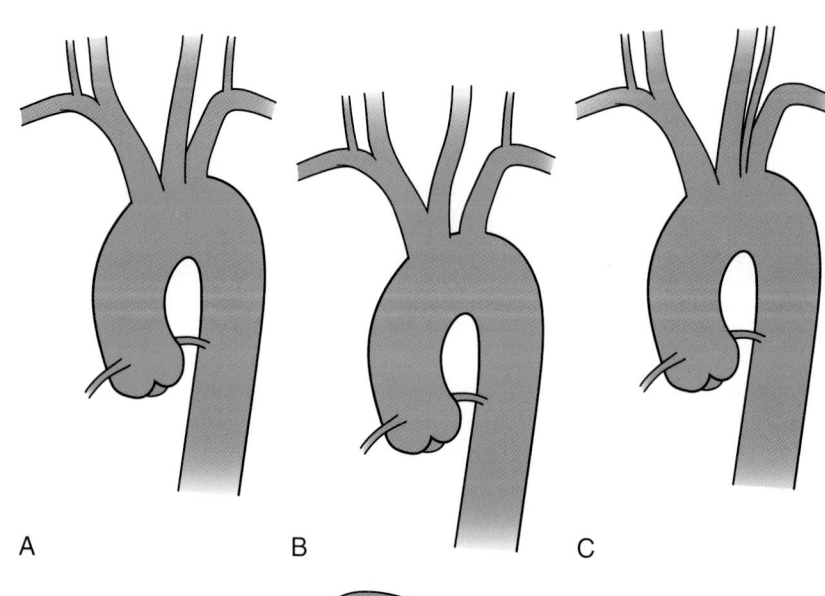

Figure 100-2 Normal arch (**A**), bovine arch (**B**), and arch origin (**C**) of the left vertebral artery.

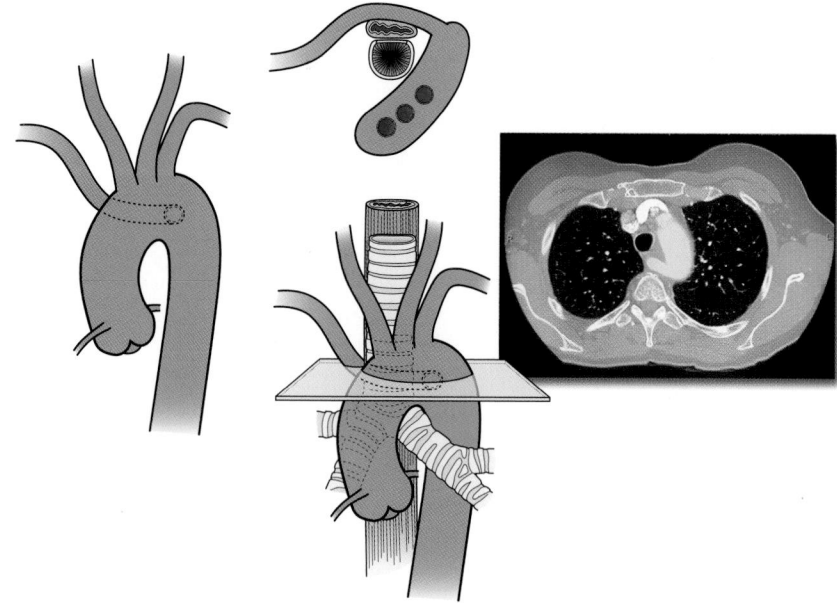

Figure 100-3 Aberrant right subclavian artery with a retroesophageal course.

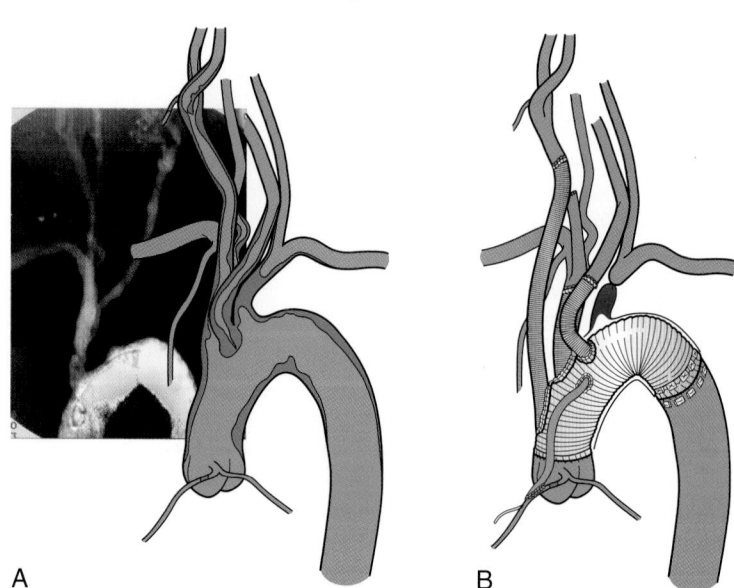

Figure 100-4 A, Severe multivessel atherosclerotic disease with involvement of the ascending and arch aorta. **B,** Replacement of the ascending and arch aorta with individual brachiocephalic bypasses.

emboli. When the innominate artery is involved, patients may suffer from stroke, transient ischemic attack, or upper extremity ischemia (or any combination of the three). Isolated common carotid disease is typically manifested as stroke or transient ischemic attack. Single-artery occlusion involving the origin of the subclavian artery can cause subclavian-vertebral steal.[4] Reversal of flow in the ipsilateral vertebral artery to provide blood supply to the arm results in vertebrobasilar insufficiency with resultant vertigo, nausea, vomiting, imbalance, and diplopia (Fig. 100-5) (see Chapter 92: Cerebrovascular Disease: General Considerations). In patients who have previously undergone coronary artery bypass with the internal mammary artery, angina may recur because of flow reversal in the bypass and can lead to myocardial ischemia (subclavian-coronary steal).[5] Occlusion of the innominate artery can be manifested as subclavian-carotid steal, with reversal of flow in the ipsilateral carotid artery causing anterior cerebral symptoms (aphasia, hemiparesis).[6] Disease involving multiple

vessels usually results in vertebrobasilar insufficiency secondary to a low-flow state.[7-9]

Infectious processes (including syphilis and tuberculosis) can lead to aneurysmal degeneration of the brachiocephalic arteries (Fig. 100-6) and in particular the subclavian artery.[10] These are rare causes of proximal (intrathoracic) aneurysm. Blunt traumatic injuries can also lead to proximal aneurysm formation, usually involving the origin of the innominate artery.[11] Penetrating trauma may affect the brachiocephalic vessels in any location (Fig. 100-7) (see Chapter 152: Vascular Trauma: Head and Neck and Chapter 153: Vascular Trauma: Thoracic). Distal (extrathoracic) subclavian artery aneurysms are commonly related to a cervical rib causing arterial thoracic outlet syndrome (Fig. 100-8) (see Chapter 124: Thoracic Outlet Syndrome: Arterial). The pathogenesis of the aneurysm is thought to be related to post-stenotic dilatation.[12,13] The clinical consequences of aneurysmal degeneration are usually related to the distal embolism's causing arm claudication, pain at rest, and digital ulcerations. Compressive symptoms involving the recurrent laryngeal nerve (hoarseness) and brachial plexus (upper extremity weakness, pain) and rupture can also occur.[14]

Takayasu's disease frequently involves all three brachiocephalic arteries proximally (Fig. 100-9) (see Chapter 78: Takayasu's Disease). The disease is characterized by an acute inflammatory phase and a "burned-out" sclerotic phase. The inflammatory process leads to fibrosis and thickening of the arterial wall. Symptoms are typically related to vertebrobasilar insufficiency once the disease has progressed to multivessel occlusion. Chronic disease can also be manifested as aneurysmal degeneration with embolic potential.[15]

DIAGNOSTIC EVALUATION

Physical examination is the mainstay of screening for lesions of the brachiocephalic arteries. Careful assessment of the upper extremity pulses, individual upper extremity blood pressure measurements, and auscultation of the carotid and subclavian arteries for bruits are all effective tools that may lead one to suspect the presence of significant disease. Duplex

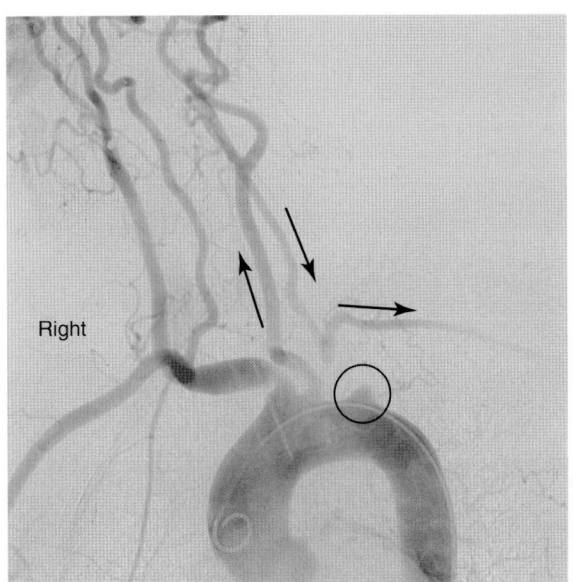

Figure 100-5 Mechanism of subclavian steal in a patient with an occluded proximal left subclavian artery.

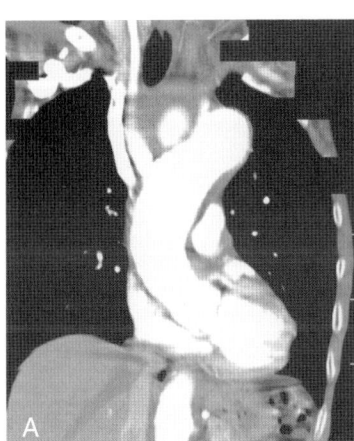
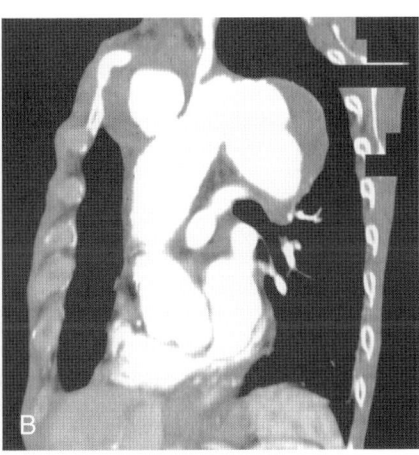

Figure 100-6 A, CT scan of a syphilitic aneurysm. **B,** CT scan of a syphilitic aneurysm with left carotid artery occlusion.

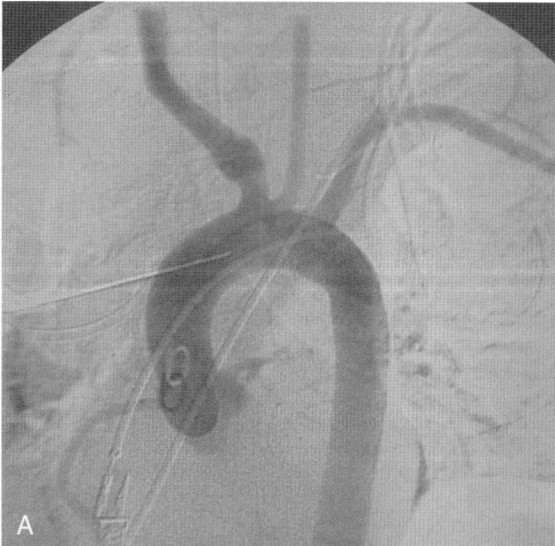

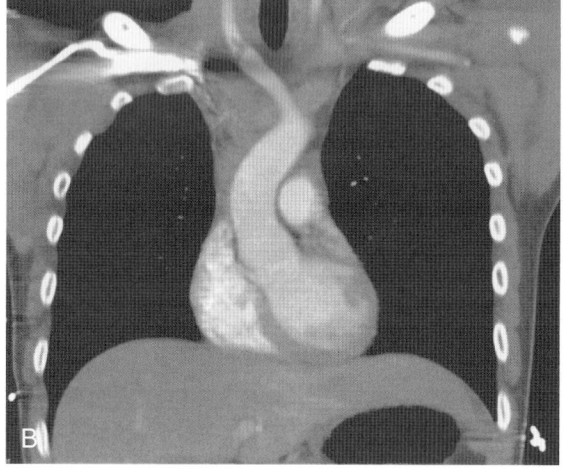

Figure 100-7 A, Aortogram demonstrating blunt traumatic injury to the innominate artery. **B,** CT scan demonstrating an intimal flap in the innominate artery after blunt traumatic injury.

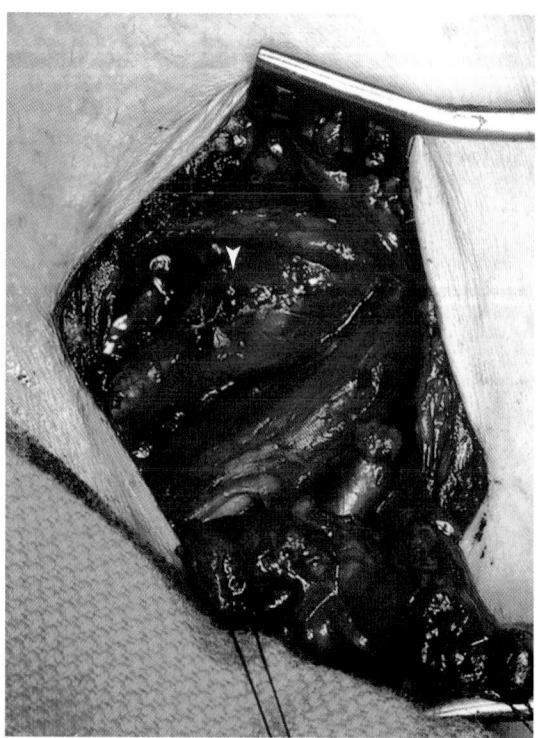

Figure 100-8 Distal subclavian artery aneurysm in a patient with arterial thoracic outlet syndrome.

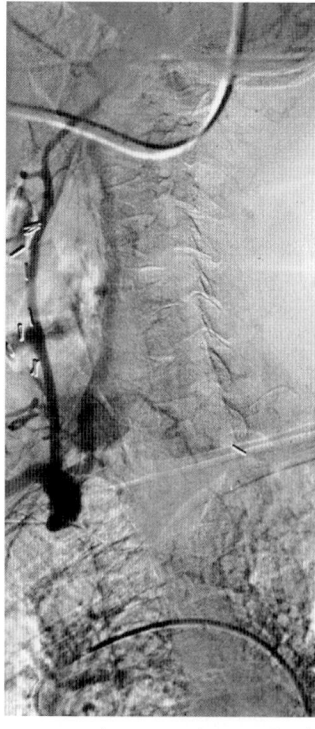

Figure 100-9 Aortogram demonstrating proximal occlusion of the brachiocephalic arteries in a patient with Takayasu's arteritis.

ultrasound of the aortic arch has been described[16] but is of limited utility because of the overlying bony structures. Duplex ultrasound can be useful in identifying reversal of flow in the vertebral arteries and excluding significant disease of the extracranial carotid arteries (see Chapter 93: Cerebrovascular Disease: Diagnostic Evaluation).[17]

Once the presence of a brachiocephalic lesion is suspected, noninvasive imaging with magnetic resonance imaging (MRI) or computed tomography (CT) can provide excellent imaging of the aorta and great vessels (see Chapter 93: Cerebrovascular Disease: Diagnostic Evaluation). Some patients may not be able to tolerate MRI because of claustrophobia or the presence of metallic implants. Body habitus also affects the quality of images for both CT and MRI. Metallic implants may create an artifact that interferes with accurate imaging of the vessels by CT and MRI. CT or MRI of the brain should also be performed before any planned revascularization. Identification of any recent infarcts should prompt caution because these lesions may be more susceptible to reperfusion injury.[18]

Aortography remains the definitive test if noninvasive imaging is inconclusive. Disadvantages of aortography include local arterial trauma, risk for stroke, and nephrotoxicity from iodinated contrast material. Because the incidence of concomitant coronary atherosclerosis approaches 40%, cardiac evaluation should also be performed, especially if transthoracic revascularization is planned.[19] We routinely obtain a transthoracic echocardiogram and 12-lead electrocardiogram. Patients with a low ejection fraction (<50%) or ischemic changes on their electrocardiogram are referred for additional evaluation with a stress test or coronary angiography.[20]

Transesophageal echocardiography (TEE) is another important diagnostic tool because of its ability to accurately identify atherosclerotic disease in the proximal ascending and descending thoracic aorta.[21] Disadvantages of TEE are that accurate evaluation requires an experienced sonographer and that the patient usually needs conscious sedation during the procedure. If transthoracic revascularization is planned, the proximal ascending aorta should be devoid of any atheromatous plaque or dissection. If accurate preoperative or intraoperative TEE is not available, a hand-held ultrasound probe (epiaortic ultrasound) can be used intraoperatively once the aorta is exposed to rule out the presence of atheromatous plaque in the ascending aorta.[22]

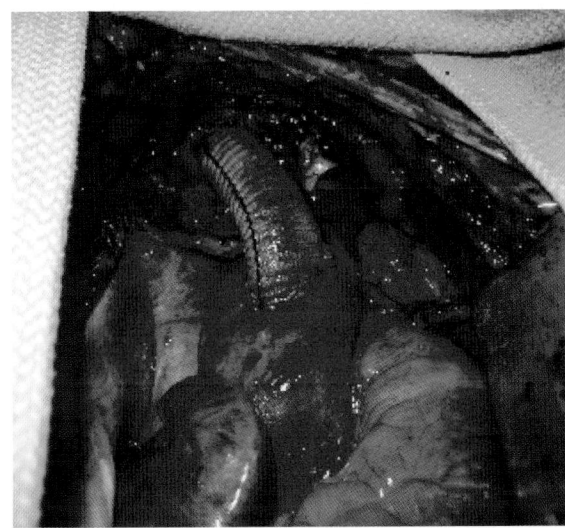

Figure 100-10 Completed aorta-innominate bypass in a patient with blunt traumatic injury to the proximal innominate artery.

REVASCULARIZATION

Indications

General indications for brachiocephalic revascularization include all symptomatic lesions (hemispheric, low flow, or upper extremity). Hemispheric symptoms are predominately stroke and transient ischemic attack. Low-flow states result in symptoms of vertigo, nausea, and imbalance, consistent with vertebrobasilar insufficiency. Steal syndromes, related to proximal occlusion of the innominate and subclavian arteries, can result in vertebrobasilar insufficiency, myocardial ischemia, and anterior cerebral symptoms of hemiparesis and aphasia. Arm pain with exercise or digital ischemia from distal embolization may occur. There are few natural history data to guide decision making for patients with asymptomatic brachiocephalic disease. Some suggest that asymptomatic patients with severe (>75%) stenosis of the innominate or common carotid artery should undergo revascularization if they have reasonable surgical risk.[23] There is agreement, however, that revascularization of severe (>75%) asymptomatic stenosis of the subclavian artery should be performed if coronary artery bypass with the ipsilateral internal mammary artery is planned.[24] A significant number of patients with proximal subclavian stenoses may demonstrate reversal of flow in the vertebral artery without displaying symptoms of vertebrobasilar insufficiency. These patients can be safely observed until symptoms develop.[25]

Options

Anatomic (transthoracic) revascularization is preferred for good-risk patients with multivessel disease. Proximal innominate and subclavian aneurysms and traumatic injuries are also best treated by direct arterial reconstruction, which is typically accomplished with a bypass from the ascending aorta to the involved brachiocephalic arteries (Fig. 100-10).

Extra-anatomic (cervical) revascularization is ideal for single-vessel subclavian disease or for patients at prohibitive risk for median sternotomy. Cervical revascularization is increasingly being used in combination with endovascular treatment of thoracic aortic aneurysms. Transposition of the left subclavian artery or carotid-subclavian bypass can extend the proximal landing zone to the left carotid artery. A right-to-left carotid bypass can further extend the proximal landing zone to the level of the innominate artery (see Chapter 133: Thoracic and Thoracoabdominal Aneurysms: Endovascular Treatment and Chapter 134: Aortic Arch Aneurysms and Dissection).

Anatomic Revascularization

The ascending aorta and transverse aortic arch are approached through a median sternotomy. Incision of the pericardium exposes the heart, aorta, innominate vein, and brachiocephalic arteries. Anatomic revascularization of the brachiocephalic arteries can be accomplished by either endarterectomy or bypass.

Endarterectomy. Endarterectomy is an effective strategy for focal lesions involving the midsection of the proximal innominate or common carotid artery. When the atherosclerotic lesion is located at the orifice of the brachiocephalic trunk, the transverse arch is usually involved in this process. Endarterectomy in this setting can be fraught with the danger of embolization, incomplete endarterectomy, and aortic dissection. Patients with disease involving a bovine arch (left common carotid artery arising from the innominate artery) are also unsuitable for endarterectomy because clamping of the innominate artery would cause ischemia in both cerebral hemispheres.

Bypass Grafts. Bypasses can be constructed from the ascending aorta to the brachiocephalic arteries if the ascending aorta is free of atherosclerotic disease (Fig. 100-11). The presence of atheroma can be confirmed by intraoperative

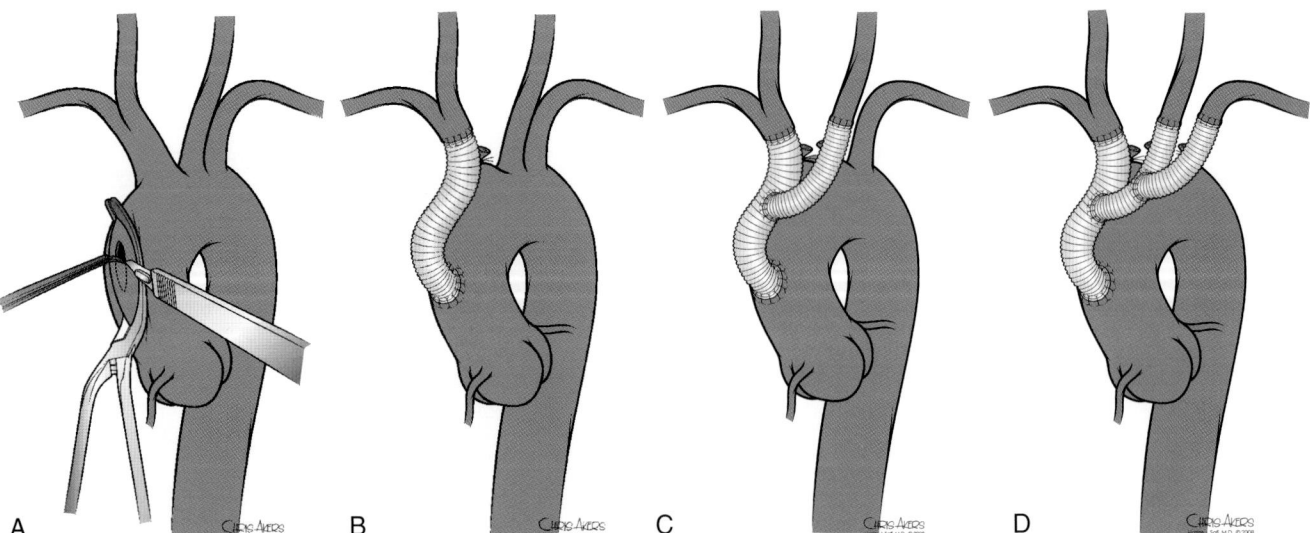

Figure 100-11 A, Partial-occluding clamp placed on the ascending aorta with creation of a punch arteriotomy. **B,** Creation of an aorta-innominate bypass. **C,** Sidearm graft to the left carotid artery. **D,** Sidearm graft to the left subclavian artery.

TEE or epiaortic ultrasound.[21] The patient is heparinized with 1 mg/kg (body weight) (90 units/kg) of intravenous heparin. A partial-occluding clamp is applied after heparinization (see Fig. 100-11), and a 12- to 14-mm woven Dacron tube graft impregnated with collagen or gelatin is sewn to the ascending aorta in end-to-side fashion with 4-0 polypropylene suture. The partial-occluding clamp is released with the patient in the Trendelenburg position and a clamp is placed distally on the graft. The innominate artery is then transected distal to the diseased portion and the proximal stump is oversewn with 4-0 polypropylene suture. The distal anastomosis is completed end to end with 4-0 or 5-0 polypropylene suture.

When the left common carotid artery is involved, we avoid the use of a bifurcation graft because the volume of this graft creates difficulty when closing the sternotomy. We use a separate sidearm graft hand sewn to the innominate bypass graft in an end-to-side fashion with 4-0 polypropylene suture. This graft is then sewn end to end to the left common carotid artery with 5-0 polypropylene suture.

If the left subclavian artery also has a proximal lesion, a separate bypass is constructed in similar fashion. There is a misperception that the left subclavian artery cannot be exposed with a median sternotomy. Actually, exposure of the proximal left subclavian artery is achieved by downward pressure retraction on the ascending aorta and the transverse arch. This maneuver allows transection of the left subclavian artery and end-to-end anastomosis. After completion of all anastomoses, the anticoagulated state is reversed with protamine sulfate. We insert two large (32 or 36 Fr) chest tubes in the mediastinum for drainage.

Patients with severe atheromatous plaque involving the ascending and transverse arch aorta have a significant risk for stroke from atheroembolic debris with any manipulation of the vessel (i.e., clamping). In such patients who need anatomic reconstruction, we replace the ascending and arch aorta and reconstruct the brachiocephalic arteries with a prefabricated branched graft (Fig. 100-12). This is accomplished with the assistance of cardiopulmonary bypass, profound hypothermia, and cardiocirculatory arrest. Nasopharyngeal temperature is maintained below 20° C so that the electroencephalogram is isoelectric. We use the same protocol for conventional open repair of aneurysms involving the ascending and arch aorta. This approach yields low mortality and neurologic morbidity, even in patients deemed to be at "high risk."[26]

Operative Results. DeBakey and associates performed the first aorta-innominate bypass in 1957.[27] Crawford and coworkers subsequently examined the initial results of direct brachiocephalic revascularization (combining endarterectomy and bypass) in 1962 and reported a 30-day mortality of 7.5%.[28] In 1983, these authors reported their own series of brachiocephalic revascularization, with stroke and 30-day mortality rates of 6.9% and 4.7%, respectively, after thoracic bypass.[29] Since that time there have been several reports of excellent initial and long-term results after transthoracic revascularization of the brachiocephalic arteries. Kieffer and coauthors reported 2.9% stroke, 1.5% myocardial infarction, and 5.2% mortality rates, with 5- and 10-year patency rates of 98.4% and 96%, respectively.[19] Rhodes and colleagues reported 7% stroke, 3% myocardial infarction, and 3% mortality rates, with a 5-year patency rate of 80%.[30] Berguer and associates reported 8% stroke, 3% myocardial infarction, and 8% mortality rates, with 5- and 10-year patency rates of 94% and 88%, respectively (Table 100-1).[2,19,28-31]

Postoperative Management. In the immediate postoperative period, patients are observed in a monitored unit for the first 24 hours. Mediastinal drains are removed once the drainage is less than 200 mL/day. Patients are discharged

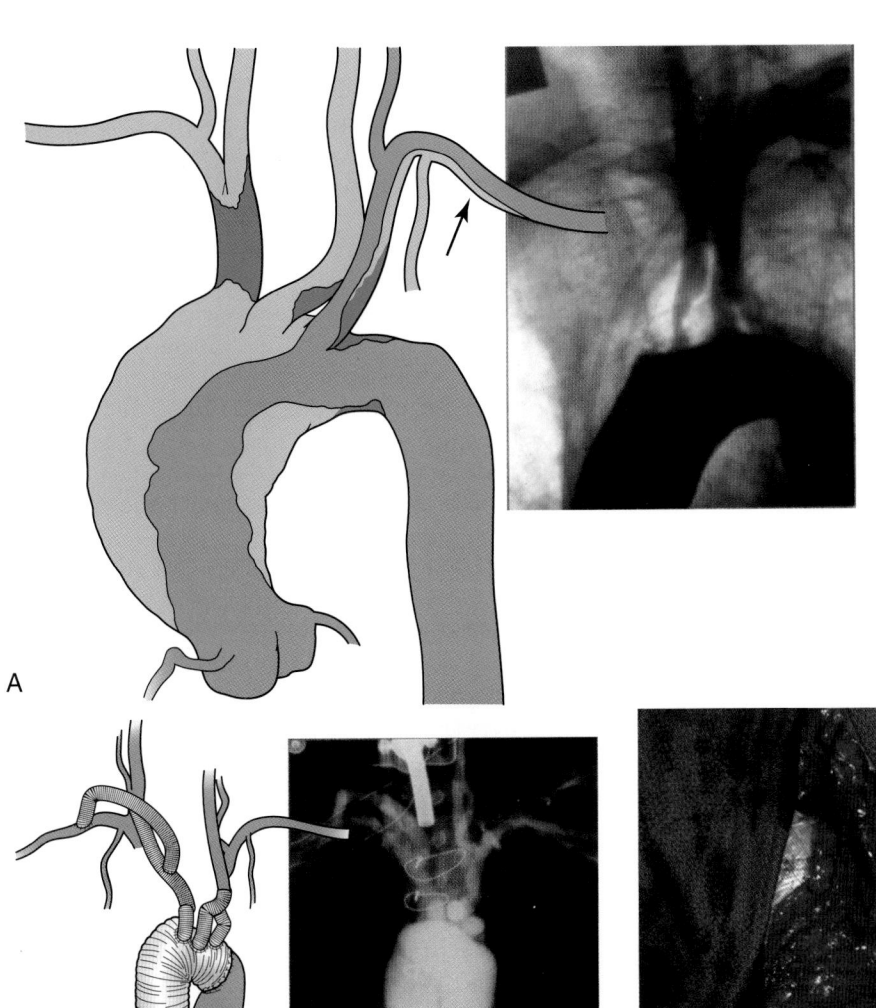

A

B

C

Figure 100-12 A, Illustration and preoperative aortogram of patient with multivessel ascending aorta, arch, and brachiocephalic atherosclerosis (*arrow*).
B, Illustration and postoperative aortogram after replacement of the ascending aorta and aortic arch with individual bypasses to the brachiocephalic arteries.
C, Completed replacement of the ascending aorta and aortic arch with individual bypasses to the brachiocephalic arteries.

Table 100-1 Results of Transthoracic Revascularization

| | | | | | | Results | | | |
| | | | | | | Survival | | Patency | |
Series	Year	Number of Patients	Mortality	Stroke	MI	5-Yr	10-Yr	5-Yr	10-Yr
Crawford et al.[28]	1962	67	7.5	2.9	NA	NA	NA	NA	NA
Crawford et al.[31]	1969	122	13 (10.8*)	NA	NA	NA	NA	NA	NA
Crawford et al.[29]	1983	43	4.7	6.9	NA	NA	NA	NA	NA
Kieffer et al.[19]	1995	135	5.2	2.9	1.5	77.5	51.9	98.4	96
Berguer et al.[2]	1998	100	8	8	3	87	81	94	88
Rhodes et al.[30]	2000	92	3	7	3	88	NA	80	NA

MI, myocardial infarction; NA, not available.
*Incidence for bypass procedures alone.

with strict post-sternotomy precautions. After the initial post-operative visit, we monitor patients with duplex ultrasound of the extracranial carotid system and the graft itself every 6 months for the first year, followed by yearly scans.

Extra-anatomic Revascularization

Extra-anatomic reconstructions are suitable for patients with single-vessel disease or very high-risk patients in whom median sternotomy poses a risk for death. A bypass can be constructed between the carotid and subclavian, bilateral carotid, bilateral subclavian, or bilateral axillary arteries. The most common finding is isolated subclavian artery stenosis,[3] and there are several options for revascularization.

Carotid-Subclavian Transposition. Direct subclavian-carotid transposition carries the advantage of avoiding prosthetic material; however, it does require more extensive dissection of the proximal subclavian artery and individual isolation of the vertebral and internal mammary arteries

(Fig. 100-13). When performing a transposition, a transverse supraclavicular incision starting between the two heads of the sternocleidomastoid muscle provides exposure of the common carotid and subclavian arteries. The omohyoid muscle is divided and the common carotid artery is circumferentially dissected and mobilized medially. The internal jugular vein and vagus nerve are retracted laterally. Exposure of the sub-clavian artery and its proximal branches proceeds after division of the vertebral vein. Once the vertebral and internal mammary arteries are controlled, the patient is heparinized and the proximal subclavian artery is transected. It is crucial to maintain control of the proximal stump and securely oversew it because a transected stump lost in the thoracic cavity can be disastrous. The inflow artery is then clamped and an end-to-side anastomosis is performed with 5-0 or 6-0 polypropylene suture. Transposition is contraindicated in patients with an early origin of the vertebral artery and in patients with patent internal mammary–coronary artery bypass grafts (Table 100-2).[32-34]

Carotid-Subclavian Bypass. Carotid-subclavian bypass is a straightforward procedure with excellent results (Fig. 100-14, Table 100-3).[29,31,35-40] It does not require extensive dissection of the proximal subclavian artery; however, a conduit (usually prosthetic) must be used. A transverse supra-

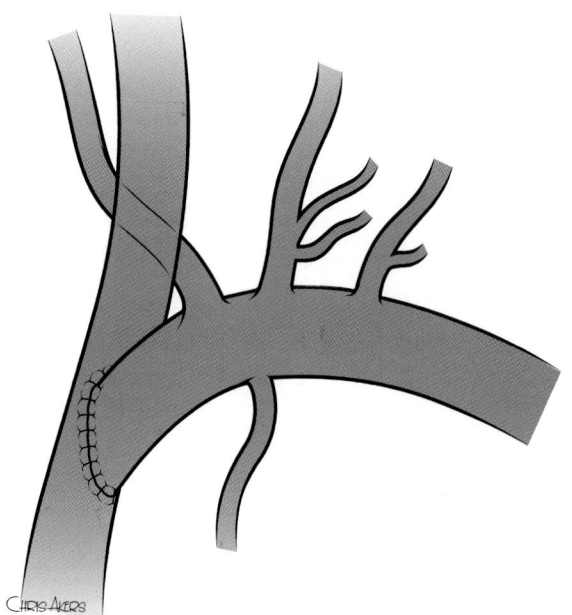

Figure 100-13 Subclavian-carotid transposition.

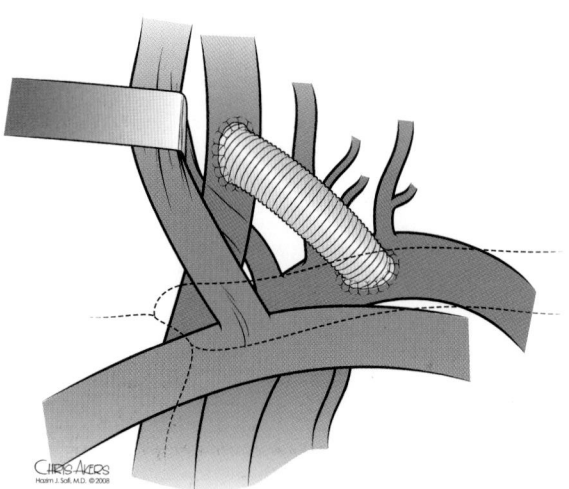

Figure 100-14 Carotid-subclavian bypass.

Table 100-2 Results of Carotid-Subclavian Transposition

| | | | | | | Results | | | |
| | | | | | | Survival | | Patency | |
Series	Year	Number of Patients	Mortality	Stroke	MI	5-Yr	10-Yr	5-Yr	10-Yr
Edwards et al.[32]	1994	178	2.2	1	0	NA	NA	NA	NA
Schardey et al.[33]	1996	108	0	0	1	83	NA	100	NA
Cinà et al.[34]	2002	27	0	0	0	NA	NA	NA	NA

MI, myocardial infarction; NA, not available.

Table 100-3 Results of Carotid-Subclavian Bypass

Series	Year	Number of Patients	Mortality	Stroke	MI	Survival 5-Yr	Survival 10-Yr	Patency 5-Yr	Patency 10-Yr
Diethrich et al.[36]	1967	125	4.8	1.6	2.4	NA	NA	NA	NA
Crawford et al.[31]	1969	177	2.2	NA	NA	NA	NA	NA	NA
Perler and Williams[38]	1990	28	0	NA	NA	88	48	92	NA
Salam et al.[39]	1994	28	0	0	0	NA	NA	82	NA
Vitti et al.[40]	1994	124	0.8	NA	NA	83	59	95	95
Law et al.[37]	1995	51	0	2	0	100	NA	88	NA
AbuRahma et al.[35]	2000	51	0	0	2	86	57	96	92

MI, myocardial infarction; NA, not available.

clavicular incision extending lateral to the clavicular head of the sternocleidomastoid muscle provides exposure for both the carotid and subclavian arteries. The platysma is divided and the sternocleidomastoid is retracted medially. The jugular vein is dissected free and also retracted medially to expose the common carotid artery, which is encircled and mobilized sufficiently to obtain proximal and distal control. The subclavian artery is exposed by dividing the inferior insertion of the anterior scalene muscle (on the first rib). Care must be taken to identify and protect the phrenic nerve. Meticulous attention should be given to careful ligation of the thoracic duct and all its tributaries. The thyrocervical trunk can be divided for further mobilization of the subclavian artery. Once sufficient length is obtained for control of the artery and space for an arteriotomy, the patient is heparinized. We perform the subclavian anastomosis first in an end-to-side fashion with 5-0 or 6-0 polypropylene suture. The graft is passed under the jugular vein, flushed, and cut to the appropriate length. Carotid clamps are then applied and a clamp is placed on the graft near the subclavian anastomosis. The carotid anastomosis is completed in end-to-side fashion with 5-0 or 6-0 polypropylene suture (see (Fig. 100-14). If the procedure is being done for proximal common carotid artery disease involving ulcerated plaque, we transect the carotid artery distal to the plaque and perform an end-to-end anastomosis with the graft. Our preference is to use 8-mm woven Dacron, although the use of autologous vein and polytetrafluoroethylene has also been described. Prosthetic conduit appears to have superior patency.[37,41]

Moore and colleagues initially examined their experience in the choice of conduit for carotid-subclavian bypass in 1986.[41] Their series consisted of 36 revascularizations, 18 of which were bypasses with a prosthetic graft, 13 were bypasses with autogenous vein, and 5 were transpositions. The prosthetic graft patency rate at 5 years was 94.1%, whereas the vein graft patency rate at 5 years was 58.3% ($P < .01$). Based on this initial experience, the authors subsequently adjusted their practice by decreasing their use of autogenous vein as conduit. They reported their series in 1995,[37] which consisted of 60 revascularizations, 25 with polytetrafluoroethylene (5-year patency rate, 95.2% ± 4.6%), 15 with Dacron (5-year

patency rate, 83.9% ± 10.5%), 11 with autogenous vein (5-year patency, 64.8 ± 16.5%), and 9 transpositions (5-year patency rate, 100%). Prosthetic grafts again demonstrated an advantage in patency over autogenous vein, but because the 5-year patency rate for all revascularizations was 87.5%, it was not statistically significant.

Axilloaxillary and Subclavian-Subclavian Bypass. A third option to revascularize the subclavian artery is axilloaxillary bypass (Fig. 100-15). The axillary artery is exposed bilaterally by transverse infraclavicular incisions along the lateral third of the clavicle. The pectoralis major is split along its fibers, and the axillary artery is identified just inferior to the clavicle, posterior to the deep pectoral fascia. A subcutaneous tunnel is created between the two arteries, and an end-to-side anastomosis with prosthetic graft is performed bilaterally. Although good results have been reported (Table 100-4),[42-44] the potential risks of graft infection and skin erosion and the need for possible future sternotomy have limited widespread use of this technique. A subclavian-subclavian bypass can be used, and most would prefer it over an axilloaxillary bypass if required by the patient's anatomy.

Carotid-Carotid Bypass. Occasionally, no ipsilateral source artery is suitable for bypass. In these situations the

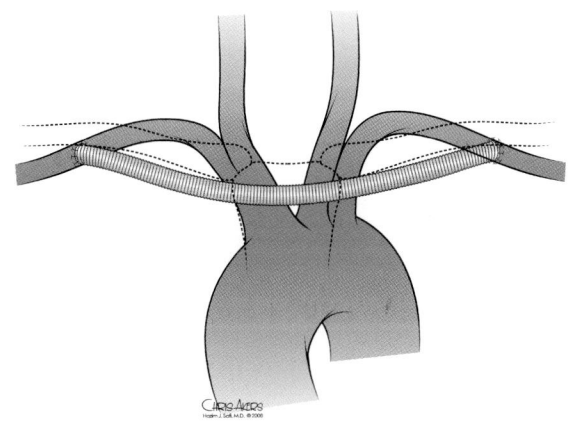

Figure 100-15 Axilloaxillary bypass.

Table 100-4 Results of Axilloaxillary Bypass

Series	Year	Number of Patients	Mortality	Stroke	MI	Survival 5-Yr	Survival 10-Yr	Patency 5-Yr	Patency 10-Yr
						Survival		**Patency**	
						5-Yr	10-Yr	5-Yr	10-Yr
Chang et al.[43]	1997	39	0	0	0	NA	NA	NA	87.8
Mingoli et al.[44]	1999	61	1.6	0	0	NA	NA	90	NA

MI, myocardial infarction; NA, not available.

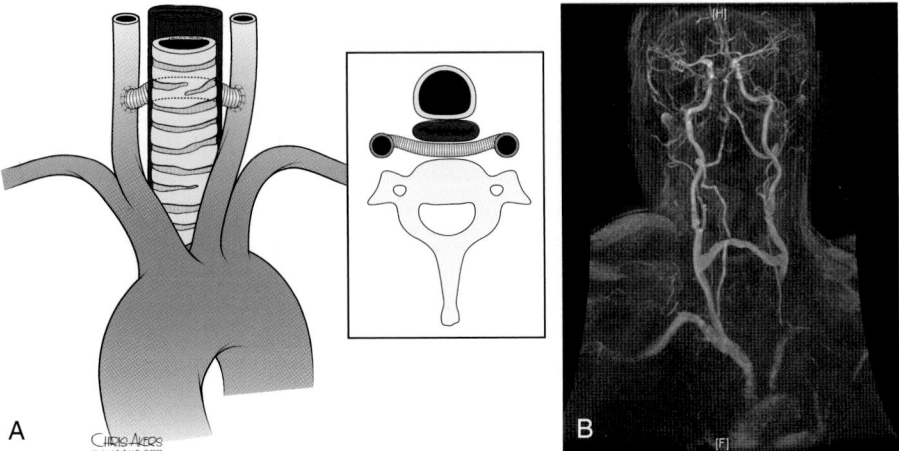

Figure 100-16 A, Retropharyngeal carotid-carotid bypass. **B,** Completion arteriogram after carotid-carotid bypass.

contralateral carotid artery can provide inflow for either carotid or subclavian revascularization (Fig. 100-16). Exposure of the carotid artery bilaterally is achieved through a longitudinal incision overlying the anterior border of the sternocleidomastoid muscle on each side. The carotid sheath is opened and the common carotid artery is dissected free bilaterally. The pharynx is identified medially, and blunt dissection is used to create a tunnel posterior to the pharynx and anterior to the prevertebral fascia. This retropharyngeal tunnel, as described by Berguer and Gonzalez,[45] eliminates the risk of skin erosion, enables transposition of the carotid artery, and places any graft safely away from possible future tracheostomy. Once the tunnel is created, the patient is heparinized and the inflow carotid artery clamped proximally and distally. An arteriotomy is created and a prosthetic graft is sewn end to side with 5-0 or 6-0 polypropylene suture. The graft is passed through the tunnel, the carotid clamps released, and the graft clamped. The target carotid is then clamped, and an end-to-side anastomosis with 5-0 or 6-0 polypropylene suture is performed (see Fig. 100-16). If the proximal plaque on the target carotid artery is ulcerated, we transect the artery distal to the plaque. The proximal stump is oversewn, and an end-to-end anastomosis to the graft is performed with 5-0 or 6-0 polypropylene suture (Table 100-5).[45,46]

Carotid–Contralateral Subclavian Bypass. If the target vessel is the contralateral subclavian artery, exposure of the subclavian artery is performed as described earlier for subclavian transposition and the graft is sewn end to end with 5-0 or 6-0 polypropylene suture. If transposition is contraindicated, the graft can be sutured end to side at a more distal location on the subclavian artery.

Table 100-5 Results of Carotid-Carotid Bypass

Series	Year	Number of Patients	Mortality	Stroke	MI	Survival 5-Yr	Survival 10-Yr	Patency 5-Yr	Patency 10-Yr
						Survival		**Patency**	
						5-Yr	10-Yr	5-Yr	10-Yr
Berguer and Gonzalez[45]	1994	16	0	6.2	0	87.5	NA	94	NA
Ozsvath et al.[46]	2003	24	0	4.1	0	NA	NA	70	NA

MI, myocardial infarction; NA, not available.

Table 100-6 Results of Cervical Reconstructions

Series	Year	Number of Patients	Mortality	Stroke	MI	Survival 5-Yr	Survival 10-Yr	Patency 5-Yr	Patency 10-Yr
Crawford et al.[29]	1983	99	1	2	NA	NA	NA	NA	NA
Salam et al.[47]	1993	31	0	0	0	NA	NA	NA	NA
Salam et al.[39]	1994	41	0	0	0	NA	NA	73	NA
Berguer et al.[3]	1999	182	0.5	3.8	3	72	41	91	82
Byrne et al.[48]	2007	143	0.7	1.4	4.3	NA	NA	92	NA

MI, myocardial infarction; NA, not available.

Operative Results. The short-term outcome of cervical brachiocephalic revascularization is excellent. Diethrich and colleagues' review of carotid-subclavian bypass in 1967 demonstrated 1.6% stroke, 2.4% myocardial infarction, and 4.8% mortality rates and greatly promoted the use of extra-anatomic bypass for isolated subclavian (or common carotid) artery disease.[36] Crawford and associates updated this series in 1969 and then reviewed their own series in 1983, which demonstrated 1% stroke and 2.2% mortality rates.[29,31] More recently, Vitti and coauthors reported a mortality rate of 0.8% with 5- and 10-year patency rates of 95%.[40] Schardey and coworkers reported in 1996 that subclavian transposition carries no additional risk for stroke or death and has superior 5-year patency rates approaching 100%.[33]

Chang and colleagues in 1997 and Mingoli and associates in 1999 demonstrated that axilloaxillary bypass could be done safely with combined stroke, myocardial infarction, and mortality rates of 0% and 1.6%, respectively. Chang and colleagues also reported a 10-year patency rate of 88%, whereas Mingoli and coauthors reported a 5-year patency rate of 90% (see Table 100-4).[43,44]

The efficacy of carotid-carotid bypass was demonstrated by Berguer and Gonzalez in 1994. Their series reported no deaths and a 6.2% incidence of stroke. The 5-year patency rate was 94%.[45] Others have reported similar results.

Berguer and coworkers reviewed a large series of varied cervical reconstructions in 1999. Stroke, myocardial infarction, and mortality rates were 3.8%, 3%, and 0.5%, respectively. Five- and 10-year survival rates were 72% and 41%, with 5- and 10-year patency rates of 91% and 82%.[3] Most recently, Byrne and coauthors reported a series of 143 patients in 2007, with stroke, myocardial infarction, and mortality rates of 1.4%, 4.3%, and 0.7%, respectively. The 5-year patency rate was 92% (Table 100-6).[3,27,39,47,48]

Postoperative Management. The physiologic stress after extra-anatomic revascularization is less than that after direct revascularization. The primary postoperative concern is the presence of neurologic deficits (in patients in whom the carotid artery was clamped). All patients are observed in the operating room for gross motor function before transfer to a recovery room for a 1-hour period of observation. If patients do not exhibit any neurologic changes, we observe them for 24 hours on a telemetry floor before discharge. After the initial postoperative visit, patency is monitored by duplex ultrasound examination of the graft every 6 months for the first year, followed by yearly scans.

HYBRID PROCEDURES

The adoption of endovascular treatment of thoracic aortic aneurysms increases the potential need for reconstruction of the brachiocephalic artery. Specifically, the various combinations of supra-aortic reconstructions with thoracic stent-grafts allow a "hybrid" treatment of thoracic aortic aneurysms that would otherwise be anatomically unsuitable for endovascular management. Reconstruction of the aortic arch branch vessels, whether transthoracic or extrathoracic, can be done safely with minimal morbidity and has proven durability.

The choice of open brachiocephalic surgical procedure is dependent on the required proximal landing zone for the endograft and the medical fitness of the patient. Although the majority of reports describing hybrid procedures refer to the use of endografts to treat the distal and transverse aortic arch, the incidence of left subclavian artery coverage during treatment of descending thoracic aortic aneurysms approaches 20%.[49] There is increasing evidence that coverage of the left subclavian artery during endovascular repair of the descending thoracic aorta is associated with an increased risk for perioperative stroke and paraplegia when the artery is not revascularized.[50,51] Staged subclavian-carotid transposition or carotid-subclavian bypass should be considered when proximal sealing of a descending thoracic aortic stent-graft requires coverage of the left subclavian artery.

When the entire arch is treated, a transthoracic aorta-innominate bypass with a separate branch to the left carotid and a left carotid–subclavian bypass/transposition is required (Fig. 100-17). This technique allows landing of the graft in the distal ascending aorta. If the innominate artery is not covered by the graft, the left common carotid artery is revascularized by right-to-left carotid-carotid bypass followed by left carotid–subclavian bypass (Fig. 100-18). The majority of series report staged treatment, with initial "debranching" of the brachiocephalic vessels, followed by placement of the stent-graft via a femoral or iliac conduit approach.

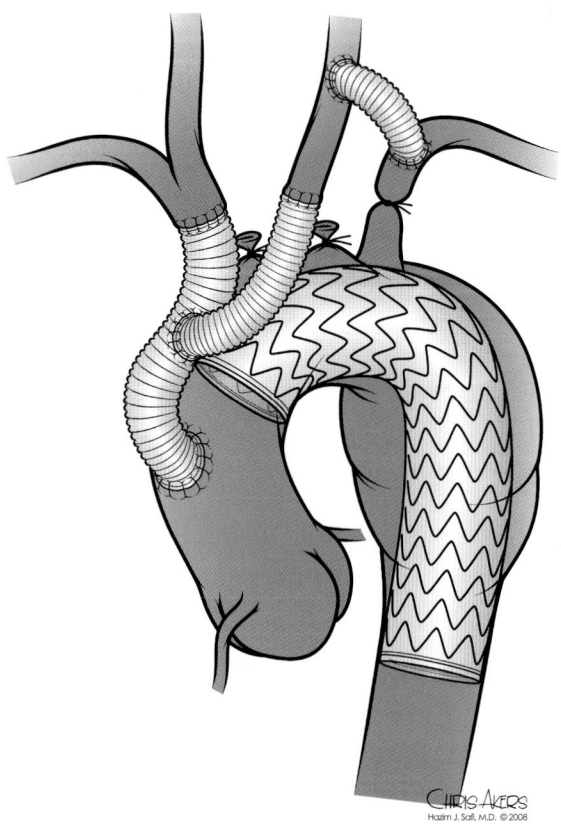

Figure 100-17 Hybrid repair of a distal arch and descending thoracic aortic aneurysm with debranching of the innominate, left carotid, and left subclavian arteries.

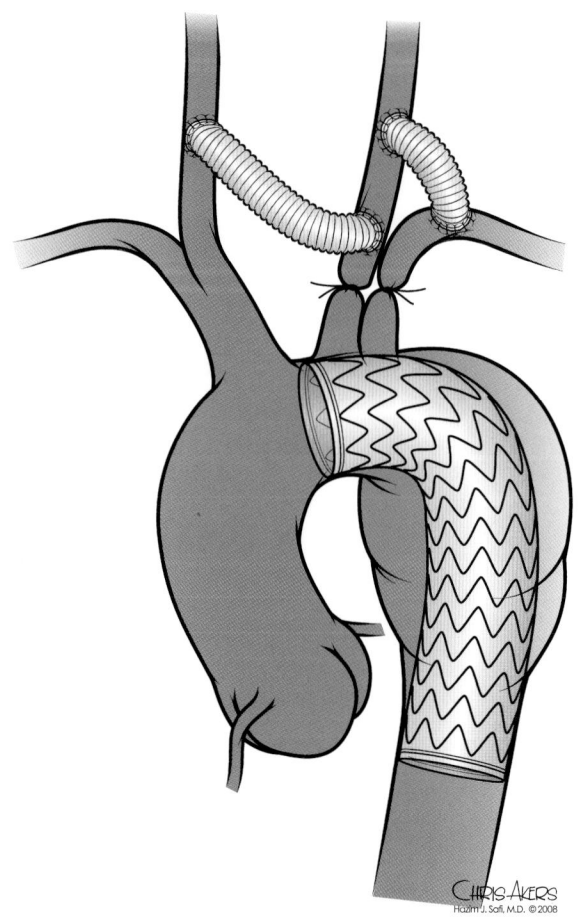

Figure 100-18 Hybrid repair of a distal arch and descending thoracic aortic aneurysm with debranching of the left carotid and left subclavian arteries.

Conversely, there are some reports of one-stage hybrid procedures that entail construction of an aorta-innominate-carotid bypass, followed by delivery of the stent-graft via the main trunk of the bypass under fluoroscopy.[52] Initial reports have shown mixed results regarding effective treatment of arch aneurysms. When performed in an elective setting, Bergeron and coauthors reported the incidence of postoperative stroke, myocardial infarction, and death to be 7.7%, 0%, and 7.7%, respectively. There was a 7.7% incidence of endoleak and a 2-year survival rate of 88.5%.[53] Saleh also reported excellent results, with no patients suffering stroke, myocardial infarction, or death and a 1-year survival rate of 93%.[54,55] Schu-

macher and coworkers reported their results in 25 patients considered to be at prohibitive risk for cardiopulmonary bypass. Postoperative stroke, myocardial infarction, and death rates were 5%, 5%, and 20%, respectively. Endoleak was observed in 20% of patients.[56] Szeto and colleagues' series of eight patients, including more emergency situations, reported stroke, myocardial infarction, and death rates to be 25%, 12.5%, and 12.5%, respectively.[57] Czerny and coauthors reported midterm results in a series of 27 patients.[58] The incidence of stroke, myocardial infarction, and death was 0%, 3.7%, and 7.4%, respectively. Endoleaks were noted in 18% of the patients. The 3-year survival rate was 72% (Table 100-7).

Table 100-7 Results of Hybrid Procedures

Series	Year	Number of Patients	Mortality	Stroke	MI	Survival (2-Yr)	Patency (1-Yr)	Endoleak
Leurs[49]	2004	5	0	0	0	NA	100	0
Bergeron et al.[53]	2005	27	7.7	7.7	0	88.5	NA	7.7
Szeto et al.[57]	2007	8	12.5	25	12.5	NA	NA	0
Saleh and Inglese[55]	2006	16	0	0	0	93	100	0
Schumacher et al.[56]	2006	25	20	5	5	NA	NA	20
Czerny et al.[58]	2007	27	7.4	0	3.7	72	NA	18

MI, myocardial infarction; NA, not available.

The role of hybrid procedures should be considered within the context of the outcomes of conventional open surgical repair of the ascending aorta and aortic arch in contemporary practice. For example, we recently reviewed our series of 1107 conventional ascending aorta and aortic arch repairs. Of these patients, 357 underwent repair of the transverse aortic arch. The overall 30-day mortality was 10.4%; for patients with arch involvement, 30-day mortality was 11.8%. The incidence of stroke was 2.8%.[59] Prior reviews of our series demonstrated the efficacy of our protocol in preventing stroke, with an incidence of postoperative stroke of less than 4%.[60,61] Our current review also examined the effect of preoperative estimated creatinine clearance. Patients with an estimated preoperative creatinine clearance of greater than 100 mL/min (234 patients) had a 30-day mortality rate of 4.7%. If the estimated preoperative creatinine clearance was 76 to 100 mL/min (222 patients), the 30-day mortality rate was 8.6%.[26]

Acknowledgment

We wish to thank G. Ken Goodrick for editing and Chris Akers for providing illustrations.

SELECTED KEY REFERENCES

Berguer R, Kieffer E. *Surgery of the Arteries to the Head*. New York, NY: Springer-Verlag; 1992.
Textbook of techniques to revascularization of the arteries to the head.

Berguer R, Morasch MD, Kline RA. Transthoracic repair of innominate and common carotid artery disease: immediate and long-term outcome for 100 consecutive surgical reconstructions. *J Vasc Surg*. 1998;27:34-41.
This presented a large series of transthoracic innominate revascularization.

Crawford ES, Stowe CL, Powers RW Jr. Occlusion of the innominate, common carotid, and subclavian arteries: long-term results of surgical treatment. *Surgery*. 1983;94:781-791.
This provides long-term results of brachiocephalic arterial reconstruction.

DeBakey ME, Morris GC Jr, Jordan GL Jr, Cooley DA. Segmental thrombo-obliterative disease of branches of aortic arch; successful surgical treatment. *JAMA*. 1958;166:998-1003.
This was the first description of treatment of the atherosclerotic brachiocephalic arteries.

Kieffer E, Sabatier J, Koskas F, Bahnini A. Atherosclerotic innominate artery occlusive disease: early and long-term results of surgical reconstruction. *J Vasc Surg*. 1995;21:326-337.
This was a large series of innominate artery revascularization.

REFERENCES

The reference list can be found on the companion Expert Consult Web site at *www.expertconsult.com*.

CHAPTER 101

Brachiocephalic Artery Disease: Endovascular Treatment

Daniel G. Clair

Occlusive disease of the arch vessels can have a dramatic impact on a patient with this condition. The neurologic consequences of disease in these vessels have been recognized for some time, but there are also other issues that can be affected by occlusive disease of the arch vessels, including loss of the ability to use the upper extremities to perform basic tasks and an inability to simply monitor blood pressure in the upper extremities. This last effect can have significant health implications because it can be nearly impossible to adequately evaluate central blood pressure, and the impact of therapeutic strategies for treating blood pressure in these patients cannot be easily assessed.

Initial treatments were surgical and involved either revascularization with a prosthetic graft[1] or endarterectomy of the arch vessels themselves[2] (see Chapter 100: Brachiocephalic Artery: Surgical Treatment). Although early reports of open repair demonstrated excellent results, the technical skills required and the potential need to deal with problems related to intraoperative misadventure stimulated search for a less invasive method to treat these patients. Initial reports of endovascular interventions in the arch vessels consisted of small numbers of patients treated with angioplasty and limited follow-up.[3-6] However, it was clear from these studies that the option of endovascular therapy for arch vessel disease was reasonable. Since the initial descriptions, stents have been added to the interventional armamentarium, and endovascular therapy has gained widespread acceptance as the primary form of therapy for occlusive disease of the arch vessels. In skilled hands, the risks are low and the morbidity minimal. However, it is one of the more complex endovascular interventions performed, and the consequences of poor technique can be devastating for the patient.

■ PROCEDURE PLANNING

Planning for these interventions requires detailed understanding of the anatomy of the arch of the aorta itself along with clarity regarding the positions of the vessel origins. The most common cause of stenosis of the arch vessels is atherosclerosis, but even atherosclerotic stenoses in these vessels occur relatively infrequently. In evaluations for carotid occlusive disease, only about 5% to 15% of patients are found to have disease in the arch vessels.[7-10] The incidence in patients without cerebrovascular disease is lower, but it is not insignificant in the general population, with an incidence of about 1.5% to 2.0%.[11,12] Furthermore, in patients with coronary

disease, it can be as high as 4% to 7%,[13,14] with increasing incidence (up to 11%) in patients with more significant coronary disease. Most of the disease in these vessels occurs in the left subclavian artery, with less than 30% affecting the innominate artery and a similar percentage affecting the left common carotid artery.[8,15] Other causes of arch vessel disease include Takayasu's arteritis, radiation-induced injury, aneurysm, and dissection.

A great deal of the information on patients with occlusive disease of the arch vessels comes from surgical series of patients,[16-19] and although much of the demographic information can be gleaned from these series, they also offer insight into the risks related to surgical reconstruction, including both direct anatomic and extra-anatomic approaches. A thorough understanding of the nature of the disease being addressed is just as important as a thorough assessment of the anatomic situation of the arch.

Imaging Studies

Computed Tomographic and Magnetic Resonance Angiography

The most commonly used methods for assessing the anatomy of the aortic arch are computed tomographic angiography (CTA) and magnetic resonance angiography (MRA), along with standard angiography (see Chapter 93: Cerebrovascular Disease: Diagnostic Evaluation). Advantages of CTA and MRA include the ability to gain information on the arch itself while not placing catheters or wires within the arch or arch vessels, the ability to assess disease within the aortic arch itself, and the ability to determine whether the arch is affected by aneurysmal disease. These studies can also assess the extent of calcification at the origins of the vessels and, when the imaging region includes the brain, can define the intracranial circulation as well. In most instances the source images can be reformatted into three-dimensional models of the aortic arch and its branches to allow excellent visualization of the anatomy both within and above the arch (Fig. 101-1). The information obtained from these studies can often allow complete procedural planning before performing conventional angiography.

The normal anatomic situation in the aortic arch involves three arch vessels: the innominate or brachiocephalic artery, which normally gives rise to the right subclavian and right common carotid artery; the left common carotid artery; and

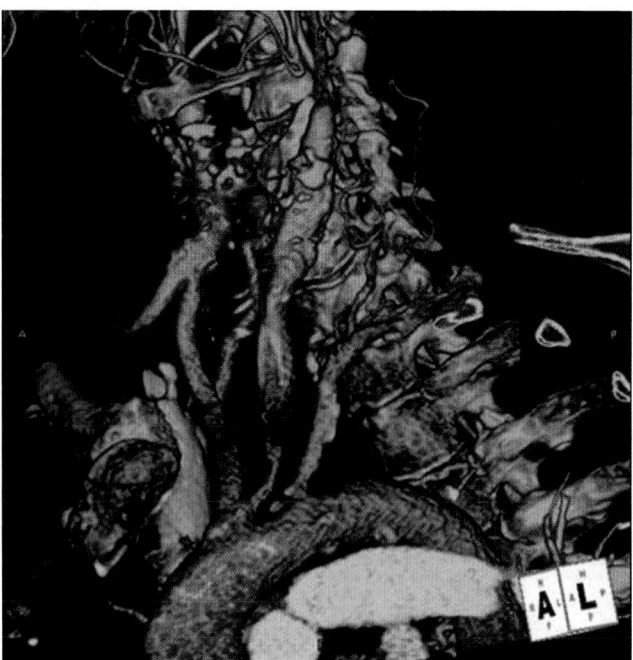

Figure 101-1 CTA three-dimensional surface rendering of arch vessel disease.

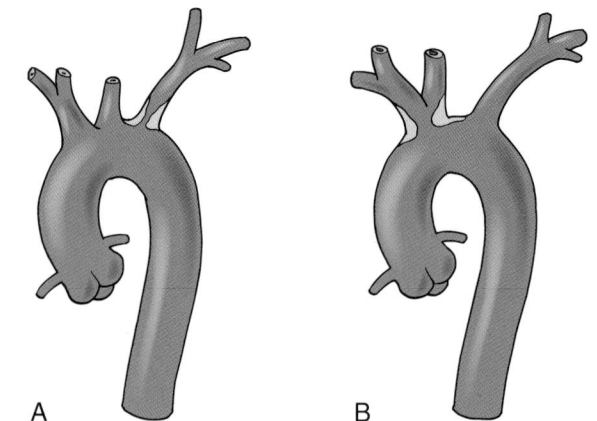

Figure 101-2 A, Normal aortic arch anatomy. **B,** Bovine arch anatomy.

the left subclavian artery. However, in up to 20% of individuals the left common carotid artery may originate from the innominate artery, thus leaving only two main trunks off the aortic arch (Fig. 101-2).[20] In as many as 6% of individuals, the left vertebral artery may originate from the aortic arch directly, in between the left common carotid and left subclavian arteries. A clear understanding of the precise anatomy is important when treating patients with these lesions, and imaging with CTA and MRA provides this information before the performance of formal angiography.

Arteriography

Arch angiography is usually the next step in imaging to assess the arch vessels and the extent of disease. Care must be taken when performing this procedure because the occlusive process in the vessels usually extends into the aortic arch and debris can be dislodged by simply placing a wire across the arch. Flush aortography is generally performed with a pigtail or halo catheter rather than a straight flush catheter because a straight catheter can cause dissection when high-pressure injections are performed with the catheter through the arch. The imaging is best performed in the left anterior oblique projection so that the arch can be "opened up" on the imaging screen. Frequently, it is helpful to rotate the imaging acquisition arm with a wire in place across the arch so that the optimal projection to fully open the arch can be identified. The images obtained from this aortogram are used to help assess the location of the vessel origins, the degree of vessel stenosis, and the type of catheter or guide that will be necessary to access and image the vessel origin.

Angiographic imaging of the origins of the right common carotid and right subclavian arteries is best obtained with selective catheterization of the innominate artery origin and imaging in the right anterior oblique projection at approximately 20 degrees. This particular orientation will open up the origins of the innominate branches to afford ideal visualization for treating either origin. Comparison of CT-rendered three-dimensional images and angiography gives a better understanding of the information that can be gained from the imaging performed before angiography is completed (Fig. 101-3).

Transesophageal Echocardiography

An additional method that has been used to image the arch but is not frequently used in planning arch interventions is transesophageal echocardiography.[21] This imaging modality in particular can give real-time information regarding the presence and extent of dissection in this region and the mobility of atheromatous plaque near the arch vessel origins. Though it is not commonly thought of as an imaging method that is necessary for these procedures, this study can provide important information, especially in the setting of complex arch disease.

Anatomic Considerations

With an understanding of normal anatomy and common variants and the information that is obtained from pre-interventional diagnostic studies with respect to the severity and extent of disease, a plan can be formulated for treatment. Among the variety of preoperative imaging modalities available, preference should be given to the best available method at the practitioner's facility. CTA offers better anatomic information and can allow assessment of the extent of calcification in the arch vessel origins.

Normal arch anatomy places the origins of the arch vessels at the most superior aspect of the arch. In this configuration the easiest of the arch branches to access is the left subclavian artery and the most difficult is often the innominate artery. In the setting of a common origin of the left common carotid

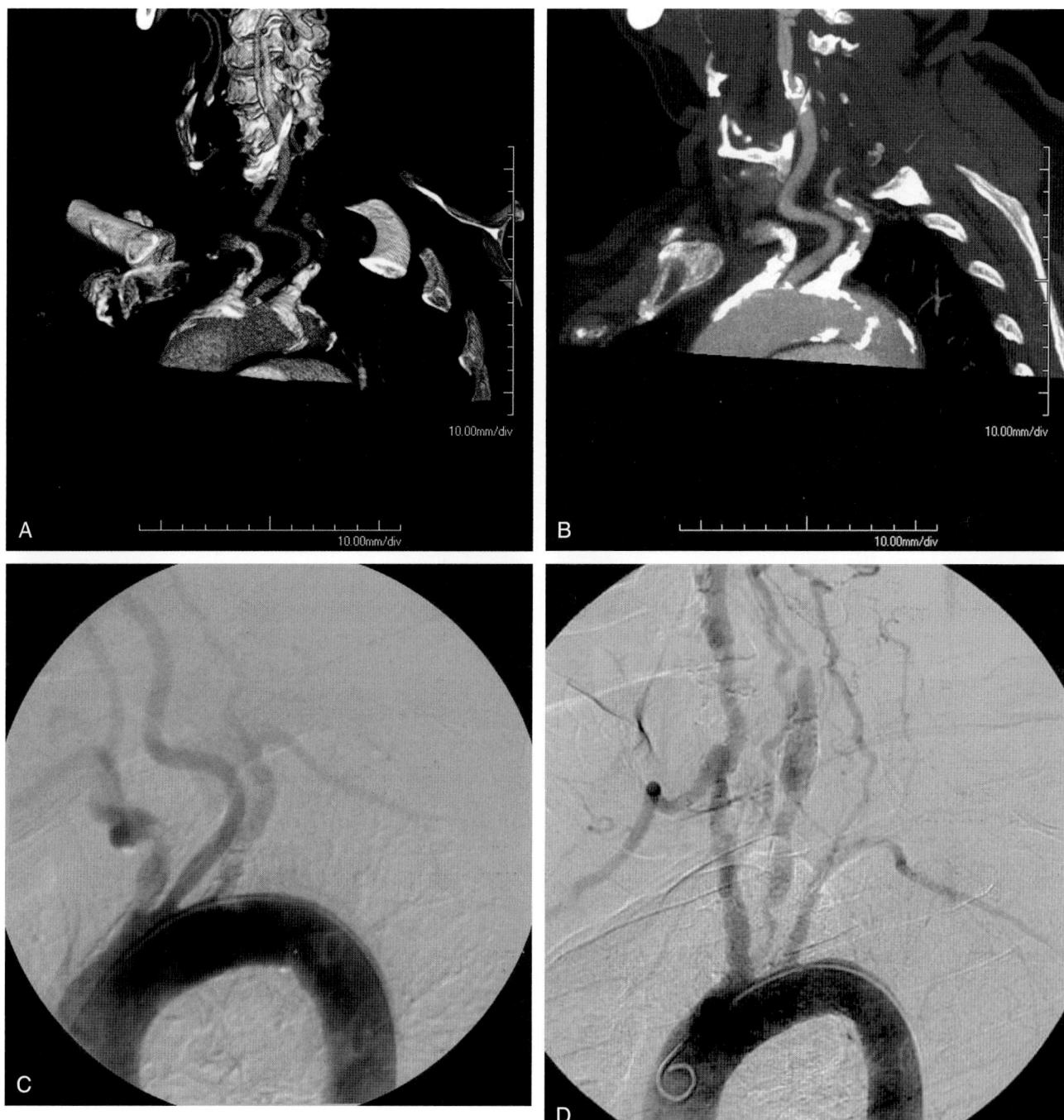

Figure 101-3 A, CT three-dimensional surface rendering of the aortic arch showing severe calcific disease of the origins of the innominate and left subclavian arteries. **B,** Maximum intensity projection images of the same patient reconstructed from the CT scan. **C,** Angiogram of the same patient. Note the extensive calcification at the origins of the innominate and left subclavian arteries. **D,** Angiogram of the patient from Figure 101-1. Once again, note the extensive calcification at the vessel origins.

artery and the innominate artery, access to the left common carotid artery can be more challenging. Additionally, rotation of the vessel origins around the arch toward the ascending aorta can make access and intervention much more challenging and in some instances may make surgical treatment of the disease preferable (Fig. 101-4). Features that make performance of the intervention easier are highlighted in Box 101-1. Conversely, long, occlusive lesions of the arch vessels with

proximity to the vertebral or carotid origins pose significant challenges to intervention.

One advantage of intervention in this vascular distribution is the potential for an alternative access site for treatment. Brachial access for intervention in the subclavian arteries and the innominate artery can provide an approach to open an obstructive lesion that might otherwise prove impossible to treat from the femoral access route. These other access routes

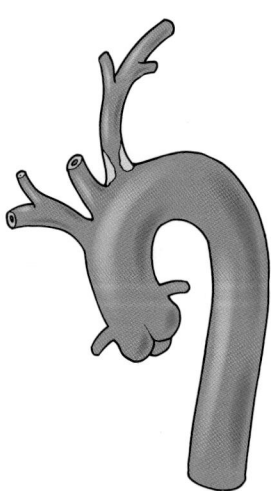

Figure 101-4 Proximal rotation of the aortic arch makes access to the arch vessels difficult.

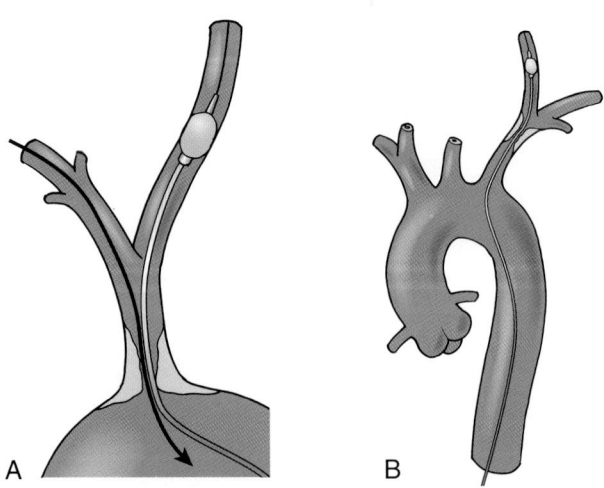

Figure 101-5 A, Left brachial access can provide a method to insert a protection device. **B,** Protection in the right common carotid artery delivered via a femoral approach during treatment of the innominate artery.

Box 101-1 Anatomic Determinants of Risk with Arch Vessel Endovascular Therapy

ANATOMIC LESIONS FAVORABLE TO INTERVENTION
- Stenosis
- Concentric lesions
- Nonostial lesions
- Lesions with vessel origin distal in the arch
- Noncalcified lesions
- Nonulcerated lesions

ANATOMIC LESIONS UNFAVORABLE TO INTERVENTION
- Occlusion
- Eccentric lesions
- Lesions with proximal rotation of the vessel origin
- Calcification
- Ulceration
- Symptomatic lesions
- Lesions near the vertebral artery origin

---

also provide alternative methods for imaging or insertion of protection devices while trying to intervene for treatment of stenotic lesions (Fig. 101-5).

Disease Distribution

A complete understanding of the extent of disease within the vessels is important when planning arch interventions. Complete occlusion of these vessels has proved difficult to recanalize in a significant number of patients, with published series reporting failure rates ranging from 0% to 40% when trying to recanalize occluded subclavian arteries.[22-25] In addition, it is important to understand how the arch itself is affected by occlusive disease affecting the vessel origins and the relationship of critical branches to the lesion being treated. For the left subclavian artery, it is imperative that an understanding of the origin of the left vertebral artery and its proximity to the disease be obtained, whether directly off the arch near the subclavian origin or from the normal anatomic position off

the proximal subclavian artery. Additionally, it is essential to understand that intervention in the origin of any of these vessels can have an impact on the orifice of closely neighboring vessels (Fig. 101-6). This is particularly important when treating the origin of an innominate artery near the left common carotid artery; the origin of either the right common carotid artery or the right subclavian artery, because treatment of one can affect the patency of the other; and the left subclavian artery near the arch origin of the left vertebral artery. All these situations are best addressed by understanding the anatomy ahead of time and planning appropriately.

OPTIONS FOR ENDOVASCULAR THERAPY

Angioplasty

Initial descriptions of endovascular interventions in the supra-aortic trunks involved angioplasty alone.[3-6,26-30] In the majority of these patients, initial success rates were in the range of 80% to 95%, and recurrence rates were acceptable and varied from 8% to 25% at 1 to 2 years in those in whom immediate technical success was achieved. Impressively, these results were achieved without the use of stents and with very early interventional equipment. Frequently, technical failure was not a function of an inability to cross the lesion with a wire but instead an inability to cross the lesion with the dilating balloon. New lower profile balloons make this problem very unusual, and more recent reports of technical success rates in crossing occlusions indicate that technical failure occurs in less than 10% of cases.[25,31]

Stents

The introduction of stents for treating arch vessel occlusive disease began in the 1990s, and they have become the primary mode of therapy for most surgeons treating this disease with

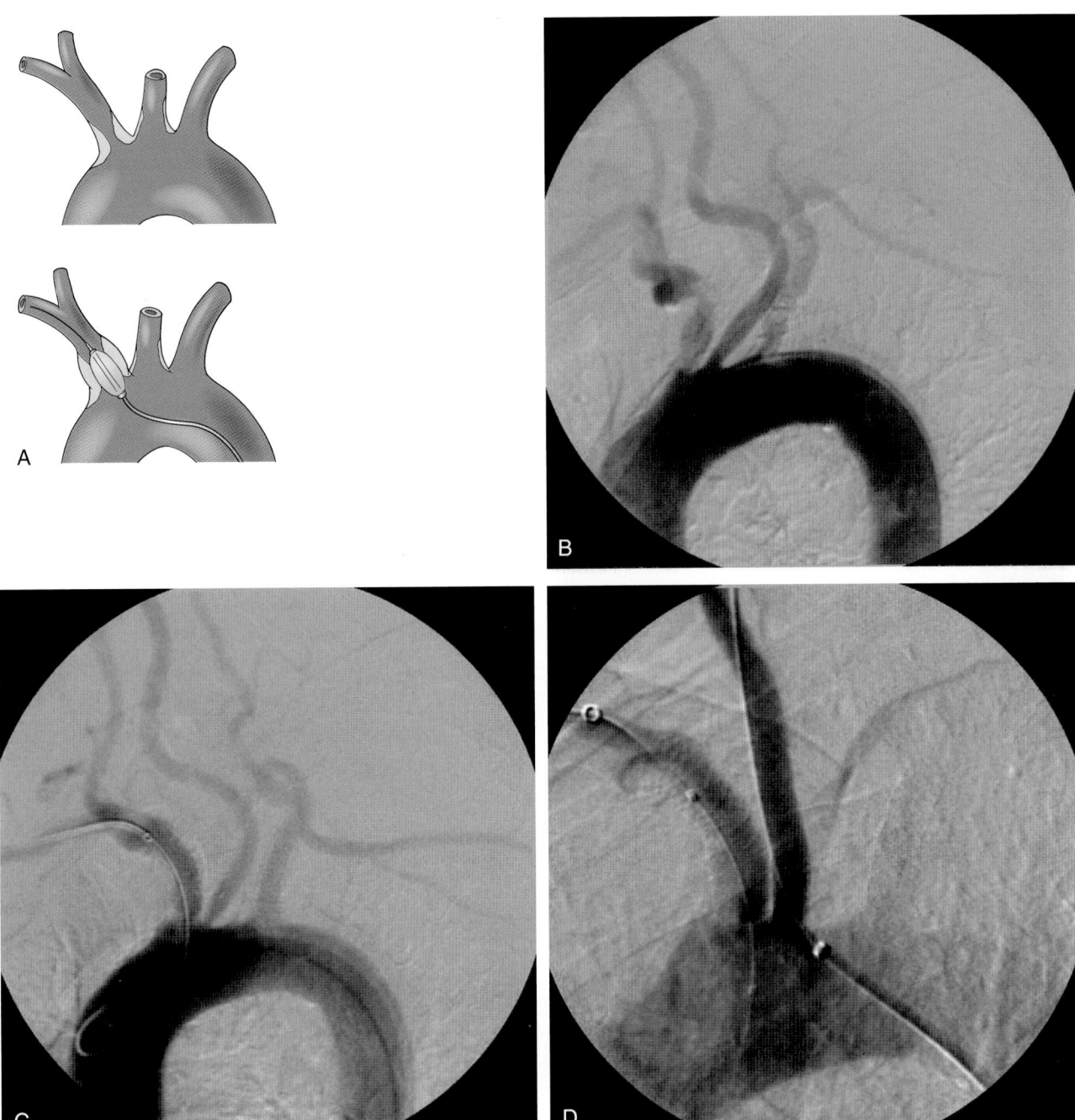

Figure 101-6 A, Treatment of a neighboring arch vessel can force other vessels off the aortic arch. **B,** After treatment of the innominate artery, the left common carotid is impinged on by a shift of aortic plaque, thus necessitating intervention in the left common carotid origin. **C,** A successfully treated innominate artery has shifted aortic plaque, which resulted in stenosis at the origin of the left common carotid artery. **D,** Treatment of the common carotid origin and simultaneous protection of the innominate artery's stented origin.

an interventional approach.[23,32-37] These authors report technical success rates from 91% to 100%, with failures occurring only in patients with occlusions that were unable to be crossed. Follow-up in the larger of these series has demonstrated patency rates of 77% to 100% over an 18- to 24-month period. It remains unclear whether primary stenting of all arch vessel lesions is clearly beneficial, and some authors have suggested that a selective approach to stenting may be a better alternative.[38,39] The most common approach reported today involves the routine use of stents in treating these vessels, and it appears that when treating occlusions or complex stenoses,

primary stenting should be the preferred approach. There is currently limited reported use of medicated stents for the treatment of supra-aortic trunk[40] occlusive disease, and no medicated stents are designed for this use.

Covered Stents

Covered stents for the treatment of arch vessel disease have been reported in the setting of aneurysm and traumatic injury,[41-44] but no meaningful data are available to date on the use of these devices for the treatment of occlusive disease. These reports document excellent acute success of these devices in this setting, and patency of these devices has been maintained, although repeat interventions have been necessary at times for treatment of either kinks or angulation within the prosthesis. It may be that the use of these devices for occlusive disease may prove especially helpful in reducing the incidence of neointimal hyperplastic recurrent stenosis, but at present there is inadequate information to make a recommendation for their use in this setting.

Perioperative Medical Management

Antiplatelet Agents

There are few data regarding the use of antiplatelet therapies for intervention in the supra-aortic trunk. Much of what is recommended is based on inference from the use of these agents in patients with peripheral and cerebrovascular disease and their use in carotid bifurcation intervention (see Chapter 34: Antithrombotic Agents). The benefit of the use of aspirin in patients with peripheral vascular disease is well documented, and it is recommended that all patients with peripheral or cerebrovascular disease be maintained on aspirin.[45] In the setting of acute intervention the routine use of aspirin is mandatory, and for interventions in the aortic arch it should be considered part of standard therapy. The use of clopidogrel for the treatment of patients with atherosclerotic vascular disease has also been well documented, and it provides a reduction in risk when compared with aspirin use in this population.[46] The combination of this agent with aspirin for the treatment of symptomatic carotid disease is beneficial in reducing embolic episodes, as documented by transcranial Doppler examination,[47] and the combination of aspirin and clopidogrel has shown benefit when used as the antiplatelet regimen in carotid stenting.[48,49] The addition of glycoprotein IIb/IIIa inhibitors to the dual antiplatelet regimen of aspirin and clopidogrel has not been shown to reduce embolic events and may significantly increase intracranial hemorrhagic complications.[50-52] Based on this information, aspirin and clopidogrel without additional antiplatelet therapy is recommended as the standard antiplatelet therapy for arch intervention.

Intraprocedural Heparin

Heparin is normally used as the intraoperative anticoagulant for intervention in the arch vessels, and at present there are no meaningful data assessing alternative anticoagulant strategies in this clinical setting.[53] The use of bivalirudin in carotid interventions has been reported,[54] and this approach may prove to be a safe alternative to the routine use of unfractionated heparin, but without additional data routine use of bivalirudin cannot be recommended. Currently, heparin administration adequate to maintain activated clotting times of greater than 250 to 300 seconds is recommended, and reversal of the heparin with protamine after intervention is reasonable.

■ TECHNICAL DETAILS

After angiography of the arch, selective catheterization must be performed to gain adequate imaging of the arch vessels and allow performance of the intervention. In most instances this is best achieved with a forward-facing catheter with minimal angulation. Options for this initial access include the vertebral, Headhunter, and angled Glide catheters. These less complex catheters allow simple access to the vessels, and if advancement of the catheter is necessary, it may be performed easily. When the angulation of the vessel origin mandates an increased angle on the catheter, alternatives include the C2, JR4, and internal mammary catheters. The use of complex or reverse-curve catheters necessitates formation of the catheter within the aorta, which can increase embolic potential and may complicate access to these vessels. Nevertheless, use of these reverse-curve catheters may be essential because of the angulation of the vessel origin. Once selective access has been obtained, the vessel can be imaged and the intervention performed.

Left Subclavian Artery Intervention

Many of the techniques described here are applicable to interventions in the other vessels in this distribution and can be helpful to keep in one's armamentarium. The other arch vessels less frequently undergo intervention because they are less often affected by occlusive disease. However, because of the increased angulation noted at the origin of these vessels, these interventions can prove to be more challenging, especially when performed from a groin approach.

Access to the left subclavian artery off the arch is usually the easiest of the three vessels to obtain. Often only a mild angled catheter is required, and most interventions can be performed with a sheath rather than an angled guide catheter. Typically, after arch aortography with either a 4 or 5 Fr flush catheter, an exchange is made for a selective catheter. After accessing the origin of the vessel, a 0.035-inch Glidewire (Terumo Cardiovascular Systems, Ann Arbor, MI) is passed across the lesion into the distal vessel. If a stiff Glidewire is used, it can be left in place and a long 6 Fr sheath advanced from the groin over this wire. If the Glidewire used has less support, wire exchange for either a Rosen or Storq wire can be performed and the sheath then advanced over this wire. The sheath is positioned just at the origin of the vessel and just below the disease. The vessel origin and the area of disease are positioned within the center of the imaging field to minimize distortion from parallax. Predilatation with a 4- to 6-mm angioplasty balloon allows determination of size and will ensure free passage of the stent. Frequently, this predilatation is performed with a balloon that is longer than the lesion itself to allow fixation of the balloon at either end of the stenosis. The balloon diameter chosen for predilatation should be slightly smaller than the vessel distally so that dissection of the distal vessel is not induced. This will limit the potential for damage to the origin of the vertebral artery. This technique also allows imaging of the distal extent of the lesion to gauge the involvement of the vertebral and internal mammary artery origins because preservation of these origins is critical, especially the vertebral artery origin. The length and diameter of the stent selected should be sufficient to ensure that the lesion is covered fully and the vessel is expanded to its true size and not that of a post-stenotic dilated segment. The stent should not extend beyond the origin of the vertebral artery origin. Ideally, for lesions located proximally in the vessel, the stent should extend some 1 to 2 mm into the aortic lumen. If the balloon-expandable stent is undersized, it will allow further expansion by dilatation with a larger balloon. It is important to know the limits of expansion of the stent while still retaining the strut architecture that provides adequate radial resistance to compression. After adequate dilatation of the stent in the vessel, if the proximal extent of the stent has been positioned partially in the aorta, it is helpful to "flare" this end of the stent by dilating it with an oversized balloon. This will further open the origin of the vessel and reduce protrusion of the stent into the aortic lumen, which can sometimes be an impediment to future interventions in the vascular system either in the arch vessels or in the coronary arteries.

Vertebral Artery Protection

When the lesion approaches the origin of the vertebral artery and does not directly involve the origin of the subclavian artery, it is important to "protect" the vertebral artery origin. This can be done in two ways. The first is to use a slightly larger sheath and insert a second wire into the origin of the vertebral artery. If there is concern that the origin of the vessel may need to be partially covered, once the sheath is within the subclavian artery, the 0.035-inch wire can be exchanged for a 0.014-inch wire placed antegrade out the axillary artery. A second 0.014-inch wire can then be positioned in the vertebral artery. If a balloon-expandable stent is used in this region, it may be possible to place a 0.035-inch system over both wires and position the stent over both wires. This ensures that the origin of the vertebral artery will be protected. In this region a self-expanding stent may be preferable because some vessel torsion and flexion occur outside the thorax. The delivery system of a self-expanding stent will not allow proximate placement to the vertebral origin if the delivery system is inserted over both wires. Therefore, the stent delivery system must be placed over the wire in the axillary artery. Placing this system on the wire in the vertebral artery poses a significant risk of dissecting the origin of the vertebral artery.

It is imperative in this situation to be able to adequately visualize the vertebral origin as the stent is being deployed, and for this reason, brachial access should be considered. Ultrasound guidance can be used to obtain micropuncture access to the brachial artery, which is cannulated in a retrograde direction with a 5 Fr sheath. A straight catheter can be positioned in the proximal vessel just beyond the vertebral origin, and retrograde imaging via this catheter will allow

precise visualization of the origin and positioning of the stent. An additional degree of safety can be afforded if a longer sheath (30 to 45 cm) is inserted into the brachial artery and wire access into the vertebral artery is obtained via this access. This will allow continuous angiographic imaging of the vertebral origin and protective wire access at the same time.

Embolic protection of the vertebral artery system has been described,[55] but its routine use cannot be advocated because the risk of embolic problems with intervention in this region is very low and the risks related to insertion of embolic protection devices remain undefined. Complex lesions proximal to the origin of the vertebral artery pose an increased risk, and therefore care should be taken when crossing and treating these lesions. In the setting of subclavian steal, it is clear that normalization of flow takes some time to occur and there is inherent protection from vertebral embolization in this setting.[56] In some situations the interventionalist may choose to place the stent "protected" through the lesion. To do so, the sheath and dilator are passed through the lesion and the sheath remains within the lesion. Typically, for origin disease of the vessel, a balloon-expandable stent is positioned just at the origin of the vessel, and if the stent has been placed in protected fashion, the sheath is withdrawn to expose the stent within the lesion. When using this approach, the interventionalist must ensure that the stent is positioned appropriately before complete withdrawal of the sheath. This positioning can sometimes be difficult to achieve and thus is not often the principal approach used.

Brachial Access

Retrograde brachial access can be important for traversing proximal occlusions in the left subclavian artery. With flush occlusion of the vessel origin, it can be impossible to position a catheter at the origin to allow traversal of the occlusion. Here, retrograde recanalization from the brachial artery may be the only method by which traversal of the lesion can be achieved. In certain difficult situations, through-and-through access may be necessary to ensure access across the lesion and adequate purchase within the vessel to allow delivery of the device. Access to the brachial artery is similarly obtained as noted earlier, and a long 5 or 6 Fr sheath is positioned in the vessel just distal to the extent of the occlusion. A Glidewire is used in conjunction with either a straight or mildly angled catheter (vertebral or angled Glide catheter) to traverse the occlusion. It is important to ensure reentry into the aorta because it is relatively easy to enter a dissected plane within the arch of the aorta. Once it appears that the wire is traversing through the arch or the descending aorta, the catheter can be introduced, and with the wire removed, blood should exit the catheter freely. In the absence of free flow of blood, the catheter can be assumed to be in the plane outside the vessel lumen and a different path needs to be created to achieve access into the aortic lumen. Once access into the aortic lumen has been obtained, treatment of the lesion can be completed from the brachial approach. In this situation it is imperative that the stent be positioned 1 to 2 mm into the aorta because this is an ostial lesion and the stent must extend across the lesion. When positioning the stent, imaging can be difficult from the brachial sheath. In this situation, the groin access that has been obtained for arch aortography can be extremely helpful. The wire is positioned within the flush catheter around the aortic arch. This wire then creates a fluoroscopic marker for the aortic wall so that the location of the subclavian artery origin can be identified. This technique can be used to assist in identifying the level of the origin of any of the arch vessels but is particularly helpful when performing a retrograde intervention.

Innominate Artery Interventions

Interventions in the innominate artery expose the patient to a risk for embolization in both the carotid and vertebral distributions because the right subclavian and right common carotid arteries originate from this vessel. However, the risk of embolization should be low. There are options to minimize the potential for embolization, including protection during the intervention (see "Carotid Protection"), but in most circumstances, interventions completed from the groin in this vessel do not involve the use of protection devices.

In treating innominate artery disease, it is important to understand where the origins of the branches of this vessel are in relation to the disease process. Frequently, one will need to image the vessel in the left anterior oblique projection to image the origin of the innominate artery from the arch of the aorta and also image the vessel in the right anterior oblique projection to isolate the origins of the innominate branches. It may be necessary to add either caudad or cephalad angulation to the right anterior oblique projection to isolate the origins of these branches. However, it is imperative to ensure that the distal aspect of the stent placement be understood in relation to the bifurcation of the innominate artery (Fig. 101-7).

Access

Access to the innominate artery from the groin is the most challenging of the arch vessels in the normal anatomic distribution. In the situation in which the left common carotid originates from the innominate artery as well, there is the additional possibility of exposure of the left anterior cerebral circulation to the potential for embolization. One must also ensure that the origin of the left common carotid artery is not compromised by stent placement across the origin of the innominate artery. In some instances it may be better to perform extra-anatomic revascularization of the left common carotid artery and then treat the innominate vessel as needed with an interventional approach. This option will avoid the possibility of "jailing" the left common carotid artery with stent placement.

Because the innominate artery often has the most difficult angulation off the arch of the aorta, it can sometimes be very difficult to engage the orifice of the innominate artery adequately to allow interventional access. Here again, as with the left subclavian artery, access via the brachial artery on

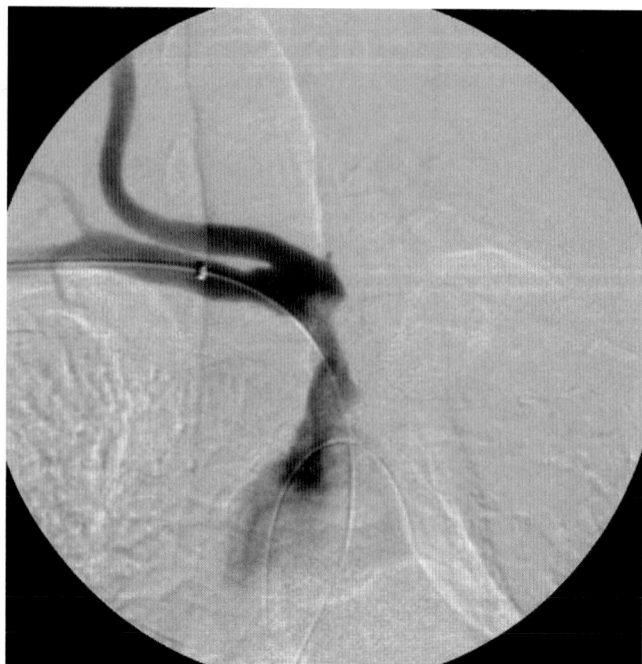

Figure 101-7 Right anterior oblique projection with caudal angulation to isolate the innominate branches and assess the extent of innominate plaque distally before treatment. Note the arch wire, which will allow identification of the vessel origin when injection is performed from the right subclavian artery access.

this side can allow excellent interventional access and visualization of the distal aspect of the plaque. Access via a through-and-through technique can also be used here by snaring the wire and bringing it through the alternative access site. In some instances it may be helpful to have a second access so that a protection device can be used to protect the right common carotid distribution. Normally, if access from the groin has not been achieved easily within 15 to 20 minutes of initiating this attempt, brachial access should be used. Extensive attempts in patients with significant disease at the origin expose them to unnecessary risk when there is an easy alternative site for interventional access. In most situations when the brachial approach is used, the distal brachial wire is left in the ascending aorta so that the angle of stent placement is closer to the angle of blood flow within the proximal aorta and the innominate artery.

Carotid Protection

If there is concern about the need for protection in the carotid distribution and access from the groin has proved challenging, the wire from the arm can be snared and brought out through the femoral access. This will allow a catheter to be brought through the lesion from below and a guide to be positioned at the origin of the vessel. The through-and-through wire can be used to provide support to hold the guide in place, a protection device can be placed from either the brachial or femoral approach to within the right carotid distribution, and the lesion can then be treated from the groin. If the protection device has been placed from the groin, the intervention should be performed over the protection device wire. This will allow

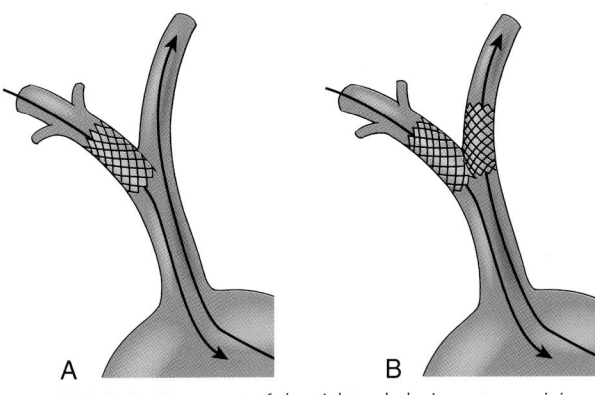

Figure 101-8 A, Treatment of the right subclavian artery origin can result in "jailing" the origin of the right common carotid artery. **B,** Treatment of the innominate artery branch origins with a kissing-stent technique to preserve both origins.

capture and removal of the protection device through the stent rather than around it.

In most instances, however, there is a low risk of embolization and the lesion can be treated using the simplest approach, without protection. As discussed earlier, when access from the arm is used, the femoral wire can be left around the arch to assist in identifying the origin of the arch vessel.

Innominate Branches

Disease in branches of the innominate artery usually occurs at the vessel origins and in many instances will require a kissing-stent technique to avoid impingement of the origin of the other vessel (Fig. 101-8). This approach can be performed from a single access in the groin but requires a larger sheath for the introduction of two stent delivery systems. An alternative approach involves access from the groin and the arm to allow separate introduction of the devices. From the groin, wire access to the carotid artery is obtained, and from the arm, access through the proximal subclavian artery is obtained. Simultaneous positioning of stents in the origin of each vessel can be achieved, and imaging from the sheaths in both places allows excellent visualization of the proximal and distal aspect of the occlusive lesion. Simultaneous deployment of the stents allows preservation of the ostia of both vessels.

Left Common Carotid Artery Interventions

Interventions in the left common carotid artery most commonly involve the origin of the vessel as it arises from the arch of the aorta but may be necessitated by disease at the origin of the vessel as it arises from the innominate artery. When the vessel originates from the arch, the intervention is performed similar to that described earlier for a femoral approach to the left subclavian artery. Access to the vessel is obtained with the least angled catheter possible, and a decision is made regarding the use of either a guide catheter or sheath to deliver the stent device. In some instances, access to the origin of this vessel is tenuous because of its angle off the aorta, and in this situation one can use a "buddy wire"

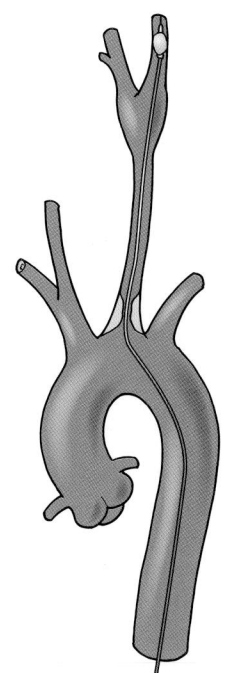

Figure 101-9 Use of a "buddy wire" to stabilize the guide at the origin of the carotid artery.

positioned in the external carotid artery distally to maintain the position of the guide or sheath at the origin of the vessel (Fig. 101-9). A protection device is then advanced and deployed within the internal carotid artery and the intervention is performed over the protection device wire, which can then be captured and removed. The "buddy wire" is removed last to ensure that the access sheath or guide remains stable throughout the treatment.

When access to the origin of this vessel proves difficult, the interventionalist must make a decision whether to attempt retrograde interventional access through open exposure and an incision in the common carotid artery or to proceed to surgical revascularization. A number of factors contribute to this decision, including the amount of disease in the other arch vessels, in particular the left subclavian artery; the status of the ipsilateral carotid bifurcation, which may be addressed at the same time by carotid endarterectomy and retrograde intervention; and a history of previous operations or radiation therapy to the neck. When attempting intervention in this vessel, it is important to remember that changing to an alternative approach may be safer than persisting in attempting access in a very diseased arch.

RESULTS

The initial descriptions of endovascular treatment of arch vessel disease involved limited numbers of patients treated with angioplasty alone.[3,4,57,58] Since that time, however, extension of the experience of these and other authors has increased the information available regarding perioperative complications and longer-term outcomes.[24,59,60] These authors note a low complication rate with reasonable initial success and acceptable long-term results. In these patients, stents were applied selectively.

Table 101-1 Technical Success Rates and Stent Use in Endovascular Treatment of Arch Occlusive Disease

| Series | Year | Number of Patients (Lesions) | Technical Success | | Number of Stents Used (%) |
			Stenosis (%)	Occlusion (%)	
Mathias et al.[38]	1993	46 (46)		38/46 (83)	7/38 (18)
Motarjeme[60]	1996	112 (151)	135/138 (98)	6/13 (46)	1/135 (0.7) stenosis
					2/6 (33.3) occlusion
De Vries et al.[59]	2005	110 (110)	88/89 (99)	13/21 (62)	51/89 (57) stenosis
					8/13 (62) occlusion
Przewlocki et al.[24]	2006	75 (76)	58/58 (100)	13/18 (72)	62/71 (87)
Rodriguez-Lopez et al.[37]	1999	69 (70)	55/58 (95)	15/15 (100)	Primary stenting
Sullivan et al.[36]	1998	83 (87)	76/77 (99)	6/10 (60)	Primary stenting
Al-Mubarak et al.[33]	1999	38 (38)	34/34 (100)	2/4 (50)	Primary stenting
Bates et al.[32]	2004	91 (91)	83/83 (100)	6/8 (75)	Primary stenting
Brountzos et al.[23]	2004	48 (49)	42/42 (100)	5/7 (71)	Primary stenting

The introduction of stents has markedly changed the interventional options available for treating lesions, and they have more commonly been used as a primary method of treating occlusive lesions in this region. Initial technical success rates with these two approaches are presented in Table 101-1. The results noted here do not clearly demonstrate a need for primary stenting when treating these lesions, although in the majority of instances primary stenting is now the preferred approach.

Complication rates in these trials have ranged from 0% to 20%, with the majority of complications consisting of access-related problems, including hematoma or bleeding, pseudo-aneurysm formation, and vessel thrombosis. Importantly, there were very few neurologic sequelae in these series, with two strokes occurring in a single series[36] and both during the performance of combined carotid endarterectomy and retrograde common carotid stent placement. Three additional strokes occurred throughout these series, for an extremely low overall incidence of neurologic morbidity of less than 1%. Additionally, three deaths were noted in the periprocedural period in all these reports. These deaths were related to additional operations performed during the initial 30 days after the interventions, except in one instance in which a patient with an occlusion of the subclavian artery had a hemorrhagic stroke during attempts to cross a subclavian artery occlusion.

Patency

From the reported series published to date, endovascular patency rates appear to be lower than those reported for surgical reconstruction in these vessels. In the reports noted earlier, long-term patency rates are not routinely available, but for studies that have these results available, the data are summarized in Table 101-2. One-year patency rates vary from 88.5% to 97%, and 5-year patency rates vary from 77% to 89%. Importantly, recurrent stenosis can be treated by reintervention, with improvement in primary patency rates as noted by Rodriguez-Lopez and associates.[37] These investigators reported a 36-month secondary patency rate of 90%, which is comparable to data from surgical bypass series.

There are currently three retrospective assessments that have compared the results of endovascular therapy for subclavian occlusive disease with outcomes from surgical reconstruction.[61-63] In the first of these studies, AbuRahma and colleagues compared data on procedures performed over a 13-year period at a single institution. During this period, 121 patients underwent intervention with angioplasty and stenting for subclavian artery occlusive disease, whereas 51 patients underwent operative reconstruction via carotid-subclavian bypass grafting. Patients had arm pressure measurements and duplex ultrasonography performed to determine patency after both procedures, and the diagnosis of restenosis was based on the presence of an arm pressure differential along with duplex criteria for stenosis. In the endovascular group, two completely occlusive lesions could not be crossed. Complication rates were 5.9% in the bypass group versus 14.9% in the endovascular group. Bypass complications included two phrenic nerve injuries, from which both patients recovered within several months, and one nonfatal myocardial infarction. Endovascular complications included two distal embolic events treated by intervention, congestive heart failure, brachial artery thrombosis treated by thrombectomy, reperfusion

Table 101-2 Long-term Arch Vessel Patency after Endovascular Therapy

| Series | Patency Measure | Patency (%) | | | | |
		1-Yr	2-Yr	3-Yr	4-Yr	5-Yr
deVries et al.[59]	Duplex (>50%) and clinical symptoms	94	89	89	89	89
Przewlocki et al.[24]	Duplex (>50%), clinical symptoms, and arm pressure	88.5	83.6	N/A	N/A	77.2
Rodriguez-Lopez et al.[37]	Duplex (>50%)	92	82	73		
		100*	96*	90*		
Bates et al.[32]	Arm pressure	97	91	83	N/A	77

N/A, not available.
*Secondary patency.

arm edema, pseudoaneurysm, procedure-related dissection/thrombosis treated by thrombolysis and stenting, and 11 minor complications (8 hematomas not requiring transfusion, 2 instances of headache/syncope, and 1 superficial wound infection), resulting in a major complication rate of 5.8%, which is very similar to the major complication rate of surgical bypass. Primary patency rates for bypass at 1, 3, and 5 years were 100%, 98%, and 96%, respectively, versus 93%, 78%, and 70%, respectively, for endovascular therapy.

The second of these studies compared the outcomes of 114 patients who underwent 137 procedures for subclavian artery stenosis treated by either primary stent placement (67 lesions) or carotid-subclavian bypass grafting (70 lesions).[62] Among the 67 lesions that underwent endovascular therapy, 62 were successfully treated. The five patients with failed attempts underwent bypass therapy. Primary patency rates in the interventional patients were 78%, 72%, and 62%, respectively, at 1, 3, and 5 years, with assisted-primary patency rates at the same time points of 84%, 76%, and 76%. For patients undergoing surgical therapy, 1-, 3-, 5-, and 10-year patency rates were 95%, 92%, 90%, and 90%, respectively, and primary-assisted patency rates at the same time points were 97%, 97%, 95%, and 95%, respectively. There was no mortality in either group, and complication rates were similar in the two groups: 20% in the open surgery group and 10% in the endovascular group. Furthermore, no cerebrovascular events occurred in either group.

In a report from Great Britain by Modarai and coworkers, 76 patients treated over a 20-year period at a single institution were evaluated.[63] Of these patients, 35 underwent surgical reconstruction with bypass and 41 had attempted angioplasty. Patency was determined by duplex or digital subtraction angiography in both groups. The surgical group had a total of four complications, including an early graft occlusion treated by thrombectomy, two brachial plexus neurapraxias that resolved fully, and one hematoma in the neck, with no perioperative neurologic events and no deaths. The 5-year secondary patency rate in this group was 97%. In the endovascular group there were eight failed attempts at treatment. Six of these failures occurred in nine subclavian occlusions, and one failure occurred in the setting of the development of a cerebellar infarct, at which point further interventional attempts were abandoned. There were four complications in these patients, including the one cerebellar infarct noted earlier, two subclavian artery dissections requiring stenting (which may not necessarily be viewed as a complication), and one covered stent protruding into the aorta that necessitated surgical removal of the stent. The primary patency rate of successfully treated lesions was 82% at 4 years.

It appears notable from these reports that long-term patency seems to be better with open surgical reconstruction than with endovascular therapy (see Chapter 100: Brachiocephalic Artery Disease: Surgical Treatment). However, the option of endovascular therapy is not unreasonable because it offers extremely low risk at the time of intervention, rapid recovery with hospitalizations that are normally no longer than 1 to 2 days, and early resumption of normal activities.

ARCH INTERVENTION IN INFLAMMATORY CONDITIONS

Interventional therapy for inflammatory diseases (e.g., Takayasu's arteritis) of these vessels mandates an understanding of the nature of the inflammatory process (see Chapter 78: Takayasu's Disease). For stenosis of an arch vessel that is severe enough for symptoms to develop, the inflammatory disease process must have been active for some time. In most instances, treatment with anti-inflammatory medications is aimed at reducing the inflammatory state and not at decreasing the amount of stenosis in the vessel. It is the exception that anti-inflammatory therapy corrects vessel stenosis, and in most instances, significant residual stenosis is still present.

Because all revascularization procedures in these disease states are hampered by cell overgrowth and neointimal hyperplasia, it is important to ensure that the patient's disease is quiescent before vascular reconstruction by any route. This should include normalization of serum markers of inflammation, as well as improvement in systemic symptoms of the inflammatory process, such as the absence of fevers and malaise. The inflammatory state may take some time to correct. There are times when the cerebral ischemic symptoms that develop mandate acute attention to revascularization, even in the setting of an increased inflammatory state. Ideally in this setting, reconstruction with autogenous material carries the lowest risk of recurrence. However, stenting in the setting of short-segment stenosis may have recurrence rates of less than 10% over a period of 3 to 5 years, thus making this approach justifiable for these specific lesions. With longer, more complex lesions, surgical intervention appears to be a better option.

Once the inflammatory state has diminished, the lesion in question should be assessed. Better endovascular outcomes are obtained with the treatment of short focal stenoses. Stent placement appears to have a distinct advantage over angioplasty alone. For complex lesions, especially long occlusions, it would appear that autogenous reconstruction via arch vessel transposition, if possible, offers recurrence rates that are about half those of endovascular therapy. Little information is available regarding the use of either covered stents or medicated stents in this setting, but it would seem likely that they might play a more significant role in treating these problems in the future.

LONG-TERM MANAGEMENT

Long-term management of this patient population includes appropriate medical therapy to address the underlying atherosclerotic process in an attempt to limit their overall risk for cardiovascular complications. This will involve appropriate medical therapy for their co-morbid conditions, including hypertension, hyperlipidemia, and diabetes. Obviously, smoking cessation should be a major component of therapy aimed at reducing this risk as well (see Chapter 26: Atherosclerotic Risk Factors: Smoking).

Medical Therapy

Medical therapy for patients treated by stenting for arch vessel disease should include antiplatelet therapy, which should be initiated before any procedure as noted earlier. The antiplatelet therapy is continued for at least 1 month as a combination of both aspirin, 325 mg, and clopidogrel, 75 mg, with a transition normally to clopidogrel alone after 1 month. However, there are currently no data to objectively define the optimal time frame for continuing aggressive antiplatelet therapy.

Surveillance Protocol

After intervention in the arch distribution, it is important to maintain continued follow-up. These patients have on average a 15% to 25% risk for recurrent stenosis within the first 3 to 5 years, and it would appear that about half these recurrences will be symptomatic. Follow-up should consist of an office evaluation with a focused history and physical examination that should at the very least consist of bilateral arm pressure determination. In many instances, recording of segmental arm pressure and pulse volume recordings give important information regarding the symmetry of perfusion to both arms and the possibility of recurrent disease. In addition to these basic evaluations, duplex assessment of the origins of the arch vessels should be done every 6 months for the first 18 to 24 months, with annual evaluation thereafter. Duplex evaluation should allow an assessment of the degree of restenosis based on the velocities obtained by Doppler evaluation near the origins of the arch vessels.

In some instances, duplex examination will be unable to assess the degree of stenosis within these vessels because of the difficulty that can be encountered when trying to insonate at this depth behind the bony anatomy of the chest. In this situation, CTA can be helpful in assessing the degree of stenosis. Although CTA is more invasive than ultrasound testing, when imaging with ultrasound is difficult, this modality may be useful to assess the vessel origins for the presence of restenosis. Repeat evaluations are recommended at 6-month intervals for the first 2 years after intervention and then a reduction in the rate of follow-up to assessment on an annual basis. This recommendation is based on the fact that recurrent stenosis in a number of the previously published studies appears to occur at significantly diminished frequency more than 2 years after interventional therapy.

SELECTED KEY REFERENCES

AbuRahma AF, Bates MC, Stone PA, Dyer B, Armistead L, Scott Dean L, Scott Lavigne P. Angioplasty and stenting versus carotid-subclavian bypass for the treatment of isolated subclavian artery disease. *J Endovasc Ther.* 2007;14:698-704.
A retrospective comparison of concurrent patients treated at a single institution by open and endovascular revascularization, including long-term (5-year), life-table–derived patency.

Bates MC, Broce M, Lavigne PS, Stone P. Subclavian artery stenting: factors influencing long-term outcome. *Catheter Cardiovasc Interv.* 2004;61:5-11.
Review of long-term outcomes and variables affecting these outcomes in symptomatic patients undergoing subclavian artery stenting.

Berguer R, Morasch MD, Kline RA, Kazmers A, Friedland MS. Cervical reconstruction of the supra-aortic trunks: a 16 year experience. *J Vasc Surg.* 1999;29:239-246.
Review of outcomes in more than 180 patients with extra-anatomic reconstruction of aortic arch vessels, including 5- and 10-year patency data.

Palchik E, Bakken AM, Wolford HY, Saad WE, Davies MG. Subclavian artery revascularization: an outcome analysis based on mode of therapy and presenting symptoms. *Ann Vasc Surg.* 2008;22: 70-78.
A retrospective comparison of concurrent patients treated at a single institution by open and endovascular revascularization.

Przewlocki T, Kablak-Ziembicka A, Pieniazek P, Musialek P, Kadzielski A, Zalewski J, Kozanecki A, Tracz W. Determinants of immediate and long-term results of subclavian and innominate artery angioplasty. *Catheter Cardiovasc Interv.* 2006;67:519-526.
A review of determinants for recurrent stenosis in percutaneous arch vessel interventions.

Shadman R, Criqui MH, Bundens WP, Fronek A, Denenberg JO, Gamst AC, McDermott MM. Subclavian artery stenosis: prevalence, risk factors, and association with cardiovascular diseases. *J Am Coll Cardiol.* 2004;44:618-623.
Review of four cohort populations to determine the prevalence of subclavian artery stenosis and association with other cardiovascular risk factors.

REFERENCES

The reference list can be found on the companion Expert Consult Web site at *www.expertconsult.com.*

CHAPTER 102

Vertebral Artery Disease

Mark D. Morasch

Based in part on a chapter in the previous edition by Mark D. Morasch, MD, and Ramon Berguer, MD, PhD.

Atherosclerosis and other vasculopathies involving the vertebrobasilar system are known to cause symptoms of posterior circulation ischemia. Approximately 25% of ischemic strokes occur in the vertebrobasilar territory. The posterior circulation, or the vertebrobasilar system, supplies blood to the brainstem, cerebellum, and occipital lobes via paired vertebral arteries. Brainstem ischemia, most often the result of atherosclerotic disease involving the vertebrobasilar arteries, remains poorly understood, and misdiagnosis is common. In contradistinction to the clear focal symptoms of anterior circulation ischemia, the symptoms associated with brainstem ischemia can be multiple, varied, and vague. Furthermore, a number of medical conditions may mimic vertebrobasilar ischemia, thus confounding the selection of patients in need of posterior circulation intervention (see Chapter 92: Cerebrovascular Disease: General Considerations). Consequently, clinicians appear to be reluctant to aggressively pursue diagnosis or recommend treatment for many of the surgically correctable lesions that may be responsible for these syndromes.

Vertebrobasilar ischemia is less common than internal carotid artery disease, yet it must be diagnosed appropriately because it is a treatable vasculopathy. Significantly, 50% of patients will initially be evaluated for stroke and 26% for transient ischemic symptoms rapidly followed by stroke.[1] For patients who experience vertebrobasilar transient ischemic attacks, disease in the vertebral arteries portends a 22% to 35% risk for stroke over a 5-year period.[2-4] The mortality associated with a posterior circulation stroke is 20% to 30%, significantly higher than that for an anterior circulation event.[5-7]

PATHOGENESIS

One reason that the pathophysiology of vertebrobasilar ischemia is less well understood than carotid/anterior hemispheric ischemia is that the peculiar anatomy of the vertebral artery makes it less accessible to surgical reconstruction and postmortem examination. The surgical anatomy of the paired vertebral arteries has traditionally been divided into four segments: V1, the origin of the vertebral artery arising from the subclavian artery to the point at which it enters the C6 transverse process; V2, the segment of the artery buried deep within intertransversarium muscle and the cervical transverse processes of C6 to C2; V3, the extracranial segment between the transverse process of C2 and the base of the skull before it enters the foramen magnum; and V4, the intracranial

portion beginning at the atlanto-occipital membrane and terminating as the two vertebrals converge to form the basilar artery (Fig. 102-1).

Ischemia affecting the temporo-occipital areas of the cerebral hemispheres or segments of the brainstem and cerebellum characteristically produces bilateral symptoms. The classic symptoms of vertebrobasilar ischemia are dizziness, vertigo, drop attacks, diplopia, perioral numbness, alternating paresthesia, tinnitus, dysphasia, dysarthria, and ataxia. When patients have two or more of these symptoms, the likelihood of vertebrobasilar ischemia is high (Box 102-1). Posterior circulation strokes occur most commonly in relation to large-artery occlusive diseases (Table 102-1). The vertebral artery is the most common large vessel to be involved with an occlusive lesion that leads to stroke (Table 102-2).

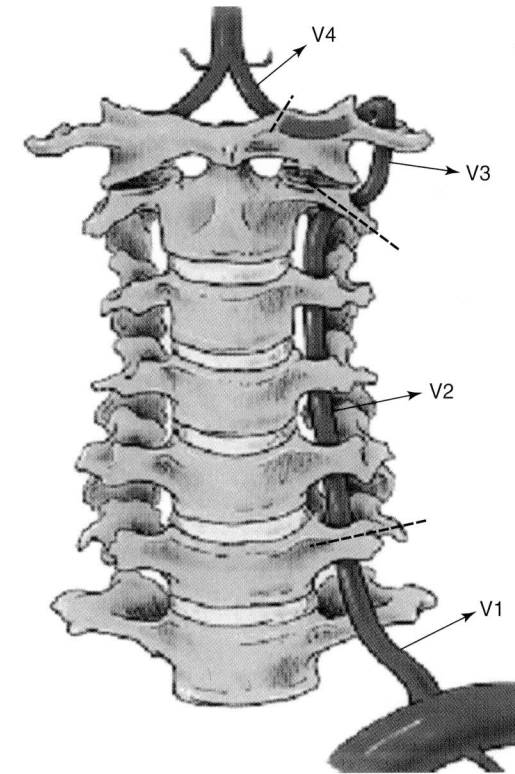

Figure 102-1 The four segments of the vertebral (V) artery. *(From Berguer R. Surgical management of the vertebral artery. In: Moore WS, ed. Surgery for Cerebrovascular Disease. New York, NY: Churchill Livingstone; 1986.)*

Box 102-1 Symptoms Associated with Vertebrobasilar Ischemia

- Disequilibrium
- Vertigo
- Diplopia
- Cortical blindness
- Alternating paresthesia
- Tinnitus
- Dysphasia
- Dysarthria
- Quadriplegia
- Drop attacks
- Ataxia
- Perioral numbness

Table 102-1 Mechanisms of Posterior Circulation Stroke or Transient Ischemic Attack in 407 Patients

Mechanism	Number (%)
Large-artery occlusive disease	132 (32)
Embolism—cardiac source	99 (24)
Embolism—arterial source	74 (18)
Penetrating artery disease	58 (14)
Vasospasm/migraine	10 (2)
Other causes	34 (8)

Adapted from Caplan LR, Wityk RJ, Glass TA, et al. New England Medical Center Posterior Circulation registry. *Ann Neurol.* 2004;56:389-398.

Table 102-2 Frequency of Symptomatic Vascular Occlusive Lesions in 417 Patients

Lesion	Number
Innominate artery	2
Subclavian artery	5
Extracranial vertebral artery	131
Intracranial vertebral artery	132
Basilar artery	109
Posterior cerebral artery	38

Adapted from Caplan LR, Wityk RJ, Glass TA, et al. New England Medical Center Posterior Circulation registry. *Ann Neurol.* 2004;56:389-398.

The most common disease affecting the vertebral artery is atherosclerosis. Less common pathologic processes include trauma, fibromuscular dysplasia, Takayasu's disease, osteophyte compression, dissections, aneurysms, and other arteritides.

Ischemic Mechanisms

In general, the ischemic mechanisms can be broken down into those that are hemodynamic and those that are embolic. The low-flow hemodynamic mechanism of ischemia is better recognized and more frequent than the embolic one.

Low Flow

Patients with low-flow hemodynamic ischemia have transient symptoms in the territory of the basilar artery because they lack appropriate inflow from the vertebral artery and have inadequate compensation from the carotid territory. Hemodynamic symptoms occur as a result of transient end-organ (brainstem, cerebellum, occipital lobes) hypoperfusion and can be precipitated by postural changes or a transient reduction in cardiac output. Ischemia from hemodynamic mechanisms rarely results in infarction. Rather, symptoms are short lived, repetitive, and more of a nuisance than a danger. Some patients may be prone to traumatic injuries from loss of balance. For hemodynamic symptoms to occur in direct relation to the vertebrobasilar arteries, significant occlusive disease must be present in both of the paired vertebral vessels or in the basilar artery. In addition, compensatory contribution from the carotid circulation via the circle of Willis must be incomplete. Alternatively, hemodynamic ischemic symptoms may result from proximal subclavian artery occlusion and the syndrome of subclavian/vertebral artery steal.

Embolic

Embolic causes of vertebrobasilar ischemia may not be as well recognized. Symptoms may be due to microembolization from the heart or aortic arch or, more frequently, from vessels directly leading to the basilar artery. Arterial-to-arterial emboli can arise from atherosclerotic lesions, from intimal defects caused by extrinsic compression or repetitive trauma, and rarely from fibromuscular dysplasia, aneurysms, or dissections. Although fewer patients suffer from embolic phenomena than from hemodynamic mechanisms, actual infarctions in the vertebrobasilar distribution are most often the result of embolic events. When compared with the hemodynamic mechanisms of ischemia, emboli are much more likely to cause fatal events or dangerous or debilitating infarcts. It is estimated that up to a third of vertebrobasilar ischemic episodes are caused by distal embolization from plaque or mural lesions of the subclavian, vertebral, or basilar arteries (or any combination of these vessels).[8] These patients may have transient ischemic attacks or strokes in the territory supplied by the basilar artery. The importance of the embolic mechanism as a cause of vertebrobasilar symptoms has been emphasized in clinical and anatomicopathologic studies. This information has been derived from autopsy studies and magnetic resonance imaging (MRI), which have identified small infarcts in the brainstem and cerebellum and shown their source, via arteriography, to be lesions in the subclavian or vertebral arteries. As opposed to patients with hemodynamic symptomatology, multiple and multifocal infarcts in the brainstem, cerebellum, and occasionally the posterior cerebral artery territory often develop in patients with embolic ischemia.[9,10]

■ PATIENT SELECTION FOR VERTEBRAL ARTERY RECONSTRUCTION

Anatomic Considerations

In vertebral artery reconstructions performed for hemodynamic symptoms, the minimal anatomic requirement to justify vertebral artery reconstruction is stenosis greater than 60% diameter in both vertebral arteries if both are patent and complete or the same degree of stenosis in the dominant vertebral artery if the opposite vertebral artery is hypoplastic, ends in a posteroinferior cerebellar artery, or is occluded. A single, normal vertebral artery is sufficient to adequately perfuse the basilar artery, regardless of the patency status of the contralateral vertebral artery. Unlike carotid artery disease, the mere presence of vertebral artery stenoses in an asymptomatic patient is rarely an indication for reconstruction because these patients are well compensated from the carotid circulation through the posterior communicating vessels.

Etiologic Considerations

Low Flow

For patients with hemodynamic symptoms, it is essential to rule out systemic causes of ischemia before advising evaluation of the vertebrobasilar arteries as the source of symptoms. In the later years of life, vertebral artery stenosis is a frequent arteriographic finding, and dizziness is a common complaint. The presence of both cannot necessarily be assumed to have a cause-effect relationship. The indication for intervention in patients with hemodynamic symptoms depends on the ability to demonstrate insufficient blood flow to the basilar artery. Other common systemic causes of hemodynamic ischemia, aside from vascular occlusion, include orthostatic hypotension, poorly regulated antihypertensive therapy, arrhythmias, heart failure, malfunction of pacemakers, and anemia.

Embolic

In contrast to individuals with low-flow states among patients with posterior circulation ischemia secondary to microembolism and appropriate lesions in a vertebral or subclavian artery, the potential source of the embolus needs to be eliminated regardless of the status of the contralateral vertebral artery. Patients with symptomatic vertebrobasilar ischemia secondary to emboli are candidates for surgical correction of the lesion irrespective of the condition of the contralateral vertebral artery. However, surgical intervention is not indicated in asymptomatic patients who harbor suspicious radiographic findings.

Global Ischemia

Another indication for vertebral artery reconstruction pertains to patients who have extensive extracranial disease with one or both internal carotid arteries occluded and global manifestations of cerebrovascular ischemia. In these patients the carotid arteries may be occluded or involved with severe siphon stenosis, thus making direct revascularization via the internal carotid arteries impossible or inadvisable, and reconstruction of the vertebral artery may offer the best option for re-establishment of adequate cerebral blood flow. In patients with global ischemia, the vertebral arteries are important pathways for cerebral revascularization when they are critically stenosed or occluded. Demonstration of normal-sized posterior communicating arteries increases the likelihood of successfully correcting global ischemic symptoms by vertebral artery reconstruction. Once the diagnosis of vertebrobasilar ischemia (or global ischemia requiring vertebral revascularization) has been confirmed and significant pathology identified radiographically, endovascular or surgical correction may be considered.

Differential Diagnosis

Identifying patients who can benefit from vertebral artery reconstruction begins with an accurate assessment of the symptom complex, followed by efforts to exclude other causes of the symptoms (Box 102-2). These other medical conditions include inappropriate use of antihypertensive medications, cardiac arrhythmias, anemia, brain tumors, and benign vertiginous states. A thorough investigation consists of ruling out (1) inner ear pathology, (2) cardiac arrhythmias, (3) internal carotid artery stenosis/occlusion, and (4) inappropriate use of medications (Box 102-3).

Box 102-2 Routine Testing for the Potential Diagnosis of Vertebrobasilar Ischemia

- Cardiology consultation
- Echocardiography
- Holter monitoring
- Medication review
- Serum electrolytes
- Neurology consultation
- Thyroid function tests
- Audiology/ear, nose, throat evaluation
- Magnetic resonance imaging

Box 102-3 Nonvascular and Cardiac Conditions That Cause or Mimic Vertebrobasilar Ischemia

- Cardiac arrhythmia
- Pacemaker malfunction
- Cardioemboli
- Labyrinthine dysfunction
- Tumors of the cerebellopontine angle
- Use of antihypertensive medications
- Cerebellar degeneration
- Myxedema
- Electrolyte imbalance
- Hypoglycemia

Evaluation of patients with posterior circulation ischemia should include assessment of the precise circumstances associated with the development of symptoms. Symptoms often appear on standing in older individuals with poor sympathetic control of their venous tone, which causes excessive pooling of blood in the veins of the leg. This is particularly common in patients with diabetes who have diminished sympathetic venoconstrictor reflexes. A 20 mm Hg drop in systolic pressure on rapid standing is a criterion for a diagnosis of orthostatic hypotension causing low flow in the vertebrobasilar system. In these cases the drop in pressure triggers the symptoms of posterior circulation ischemia.

Any systemic mechanism that decreases the mean pressure of the basilar artery may be responsible for hemodynamic symptomatology, and affected individuals may or may not have concomitant vertebral artery stenosis or occlusion. Because certain prescription medications can mimic vertebrobasilar ischemia, patient medications require thorough review. In fact, excessive use of antihypertensive medications is the most common etiology of posterior circulation symptoms and can also cause hemodynamic posterior circulation ischemia by decreasing perfusion pressure and inducing severe orthostatic hypotension.

A cardiac source is the next most common cause of brainstem ischemia, especially in the elderly, and thorough evaluation should include 24-hour Holter monitoring for arrhythmias and echocardiography to assess heart valve function. Arrhythmias are another common cause of symptoms as a result of decreased cardiac output. Patients with ischemia secondary to arrhythmias often report the association of palpitations with the appearance of symptoms. In addition, transesophageal echocardiography may be useful in patients with a suspected embolic mechanism of ischemia to rule out a cardiac source.

In some patients, the cause of the drop in mean arterial pressure can be corrected simply by readjusting their antihypertensive regimen, by the administration of antiarrhythmic drugs, or by inserting a cardiac pacemaker. In patients with orthostatic hypotension, the problem may not respond to medical treatment, and only reconstruction of a diseased or occluded vertebral artery will render the patient asymptomatic in the presence of persistent oscillations in blood pressure.

Investigation must also be undertaken to exclude inner ear pathology, including rare cerebellopontine-angle tumors. In addition, neurologic evaluation to rule out benign vertiginous states should be considered.

Because patients are often initially seen with a combination of anterior and posterior hemispheric symptoms, investigation of the great vessels and the carotid circulation is usually warranted. An important aspect of the history is identifying triggering events such as positional or postural changes. This is followed by a thorough physical examination, which includes palpation, auscultation, pulse examination, and comparative arm blood pressures (recumbent and standing).

Physical examination can alert the physician to the possibility of subclavian steal in patients with differences in brachial blood pressure greater than 25 mm Hg or with diminished or absent pulses in one arm. The diagnosis of reversal of vertebral artery flow can be made accurately by noninvasive indirect methods and demonstrated directly by duplex imaging of the reversal of flow in the vertebral artery (see Chapter 92: Cerebrovascular Disease: General Considerations and Chapter 94: Cerebrovascular Disease: Decision Making and Medical Treatment).

Patients may relate their symptoms to turning or extending their head. These dynamic symptoms usually appear when turning the head to one side. Symptoms are caused by extrinsic compression of the vertebral artery, usually the dominant or the only one, by arthritic bone spurs.[11] To differentiate this mechanism from dizziness or vertigo secondary to labyrinthine disorders that appear with head or body rotation, the patient should attempt to reproduce the symptoms by turning the head slowly and then repeating the maneuver, but this time briskly, as when shaking the head from side to side. In labyrinthine disease, the sudden inertial changes caused by the latter maneuver result in immediate symptoms and nystagmus. Conversely, with extrinsic vertebral artery compression, a short delay occurs before imbalance develops.

Diagnostic Tests

Once a suspicion of vertebrobasilar ischemia has been entertained, only a few diagnostic tests are available to clearly ascertain the vertebral anatomy (see Chapter 93: Cerebrovascular Disease: Diagnostic Evaluation).

Duplex Ultrasonography

Although duplex ultrasound is an excellent tool for detecting lesions in the carotid artery, it has significant limitations when used to detect vertebral artery pathology. Direct visualization of the second portion of the vessel is difficult because of its intraosseous course through the transverse processes of C2 to C6. The usefulness of duplex ultrasound lies in its ability to confirm reversal of flow within the vertebral arteries and detect changes in flow velocity consistent with a proximal stenosis.[12] In addition, ultrasound imaging can diagnose great-vessel pathology and confirm subclavian steal.

Computed Tomography and Magnetic Resonance Imaging

MRI is another modality that provides a safe, noninvasive, detailed evaluation of both the extracranial and intracranial vasculature, as well as structures within the posterior fossa. Contrast-enhanced magnetic resonance angiography (MRA) with three-dimensional reconstruction and maximum image intensity techniques provides full imaging of the vessels, including the supra-aortic trunks and the carotid and vertebral arteries (Fig. 102-2).

In contrast to traditional computed tomography (CT) scans, transaxial MRI can readily diagnose both acute and chronic posterior fossa infarcts (Fig. 102-3). Brainstem infarc-

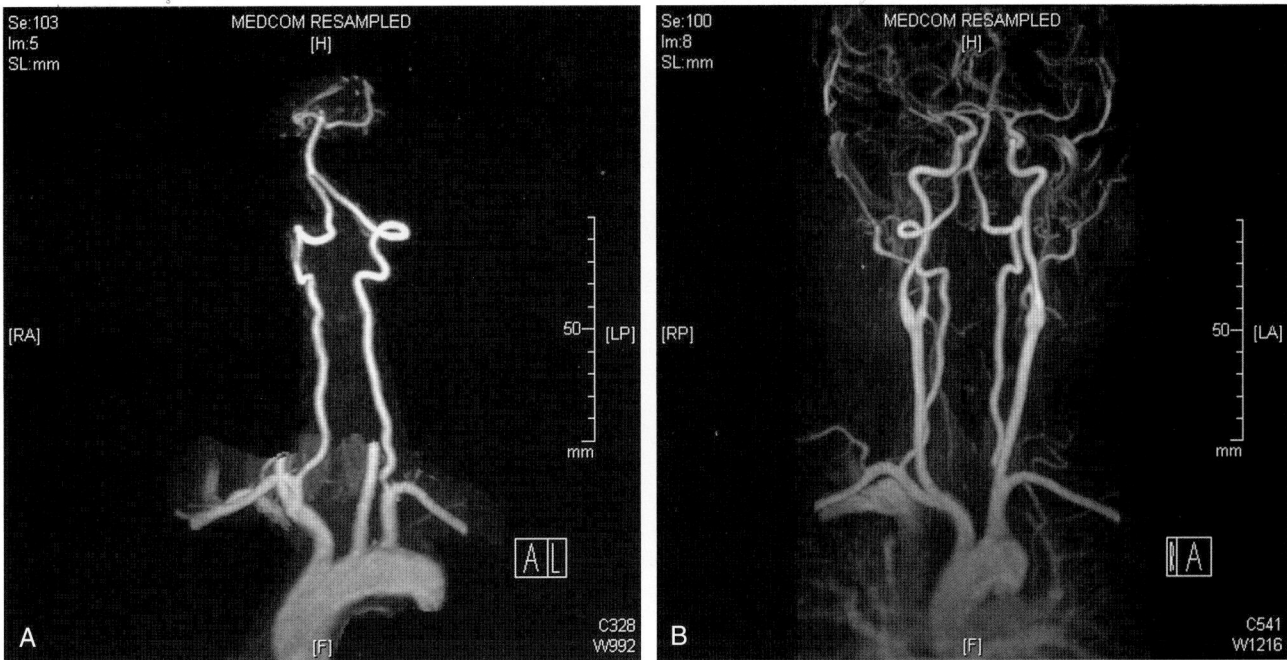

Figure 102-2 A, Vertebral MRA (with the carotid image subtracted). **B,** Arch and four-vessel MRA.

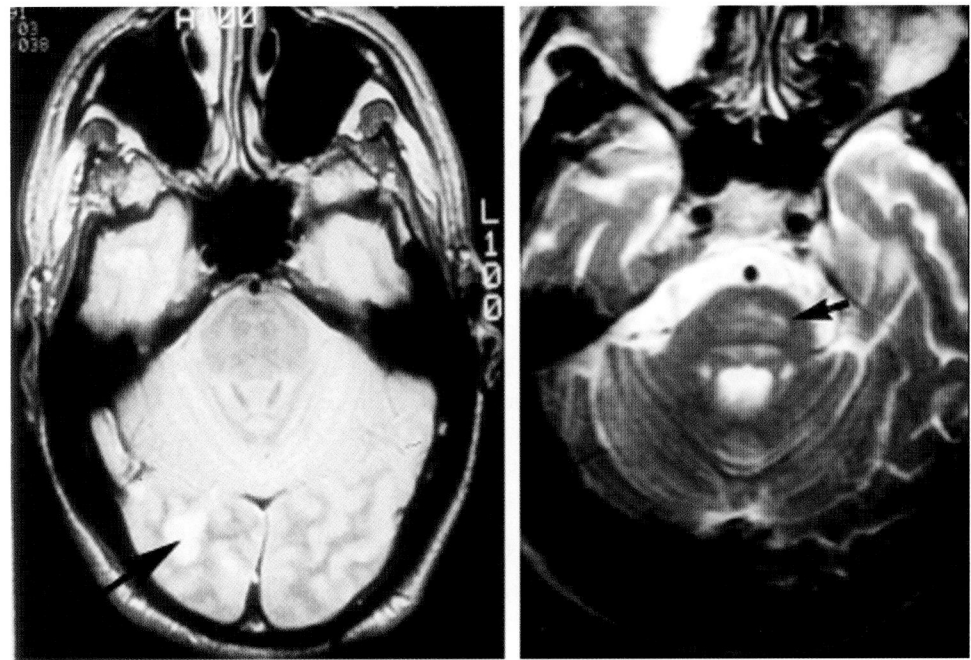

Figure 102-3 MRI-defined posterior fossa strokes (*arrows*).

tions are often missed by CT because they tend to be small and the resolution of CT in the brainstem is poor. In patients who are candidates for vertebral artery reconstruction, brain MRI is performed preoperatively to ascertain whether infarctions have taken place in the vertebrobasilar territory. Transaxial MRI is particularly important in patients suspected of having suffered embolic infarction in the distribution of the posterior circulation.

Arteriography

Despite the technologic advances in MRI and CT evaluation, selective subclavian and vertebral angiography remains the "gold standard" for preoperative evaluation of patients with vertebrobasilar ischemia. Some surgeons still consider angiography mandatory before endovascular intervention or surgical reconstruction. The most common site of disease, the vertebral artery origin, may not be well imaged with

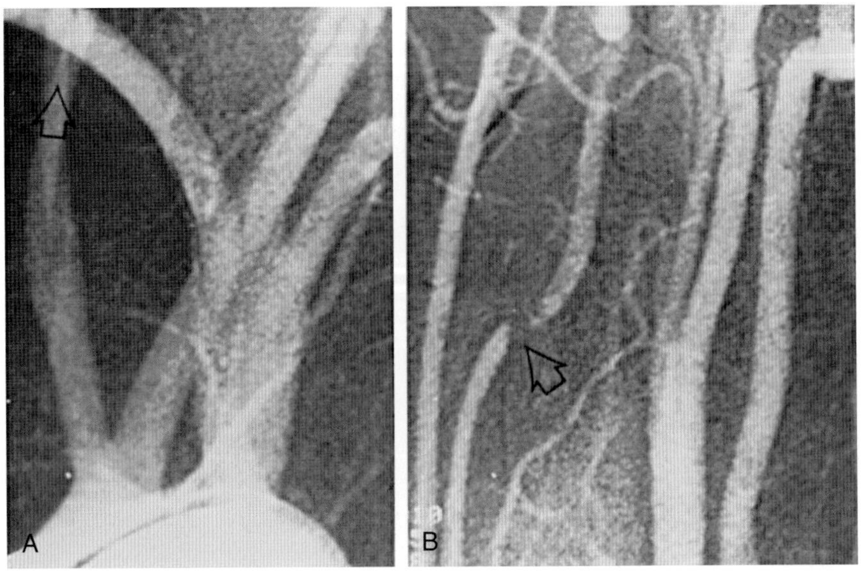

Figure 102-4 Arch injection in a 33-year-old woman with vertebrobasilar ischemia. **A,** The right vertebral artery and the right external carotid artery arise from a long common right carotid trunk (*arrow*). The right internal carotid artery is congenitally absent. The right subclavian arises as the last branch of the aorta. **B,** The right vertebral artery, which has an anomalous origin, enters the spine at a high level (C4) and is severely compressed (*arrow*) at this level with head rotation.

ultrasound or MRA and, in fact, can often be displayed only with oblique projections that are not part of the standard aortic arch evaluation. Patients with suspected vertebral artery compression should undergo dynamic angiography, which incorporates provocative positioning. Finally, delayed imaging should be performed to demonstrate reconstitution of the extracranial vertebral arteries through cervical collaterals.

Arteriographic investigation of vertebral artery pathology necessitates systematic positions and projections to evaluate the vertebrobasilar system from its origin to the top of the basilar artery. Arteriographic evaluation begins with an arch view, which determines the presence or absence of a vertebral artery on each side. Angiography shows whether one vertebral is dominant (generally the left) and can clearly define aberrant vessel anatomy. The most common anomalous origin involves the left vertebral artery, which can originate from the aortic arch in 6% of patients. A much rarer variant involves the right vertebral artery, which can be seen to arise from the innominate or right common carotid artery (Fig. 102-4). This anatomy usually occurs in patients with an aberrant retroesophageal right subclavian artery. Arch views must be obtained in at least two projections: right and left posterior oblique views. Usually these two projections will sufficiently display the first segment (V1) of the vessel from its subclavian origin up to the transverse process of C6.

Disease Distribution

V1 Segment

The most common atherosclerotic lesion of the vertebral artery is stenosis of its origin. The prevalence of such lesions is approximately 20% to 40% in patients with cerebrovascular disease.[8] This lesion may be missed in standard arch views because of superimposition of the subclavian artery over the

first segment of the vertebral artery. Additional oblique projections may be needed to "throw off" the subclavian artery to obtain a clear view of the origin of the vertebral artery (Fig. 102-5). The presence of a post-stenotic dilatation in the first centimeter of the vertebral artery suggests that there may be a significant stenosis at its origin hidden by an overlying subclavian artery. Redundancy and kinks are common, but only very severe kinks associated with post-stenotic dilatations can be responsible for hemodynamic symptoms.

V2 Segment

Visualization of the second segment (V2) of the vertebral artery, from C6 to the top of the transverse process of C2, is accomplished in the oblique arch views in conjunction with selective subclavian injections. A point should be made to attempt to angiographically identify the point of entry of the vertebral arteries into the transverse processes of the spine. Whether a patient has an abnormally low entry at the level of C7 instead of C6 should be noted. This finding is associated with a short V1 segment of the artery. In this circumstance, the short extraosseous length can create challenges for reconstruction at the V1 level. In addition, extrinsic compression by musculotendinous structures is common in vertebral arteries with an abnormally high level of entry into the spine, usually C4 or C5 (see Fig. 102-2). Such compression is due to the sharp angulation resulting from the abnormal level of entry. The level of entry into the spine is best determined on unsubtracted views.

The most common pathology of the V2 segment is extrinsic compression of the vertebral artery by osteophytes,[11] but compression can also be caused by the edges of the transverse foramina (Fig. 102-6) or the intervertebral joints. Positional changes or rotation or extension of the neck usually triggers compression of the vertebral artery in this segment. Arteriog-

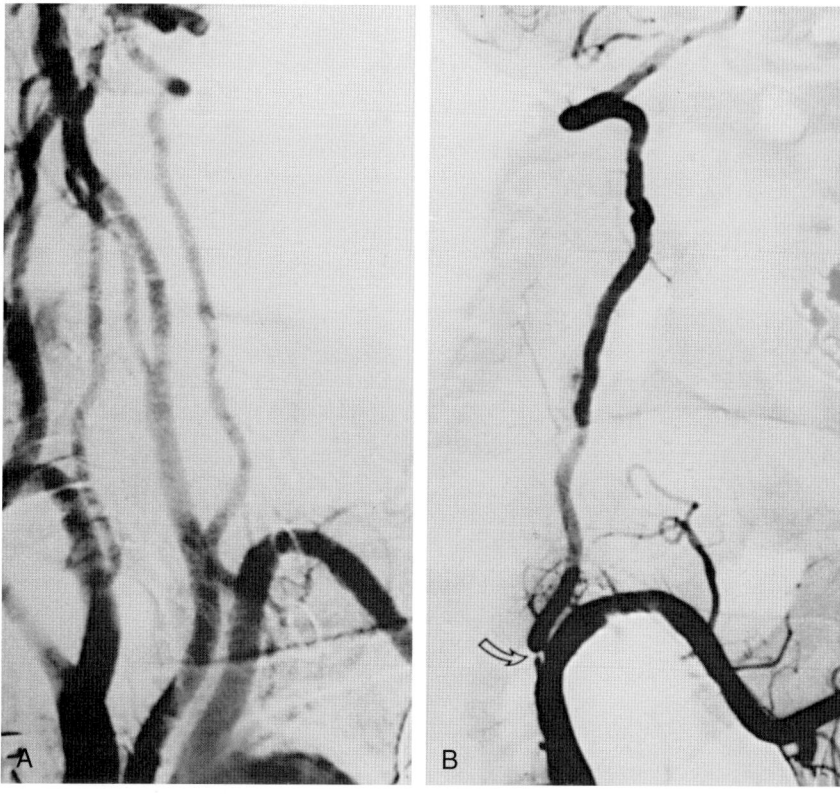

Figure 102-5 A, Arch arteriogram on anteroposterior projection. **B,** Severe stenosis (*arrow*) of a dominant left vertebral artery seen only after additional oblique rotation of the patient (*right*). *(From Berguer R. Role of vertebral artery surgery after carotid endarterectomy. In: Bergan JJ, Yao JST, eds.* Reoperative Arterial Surgery. *Orlando, FL: Grune & Stratton; 1986:555-564.)*

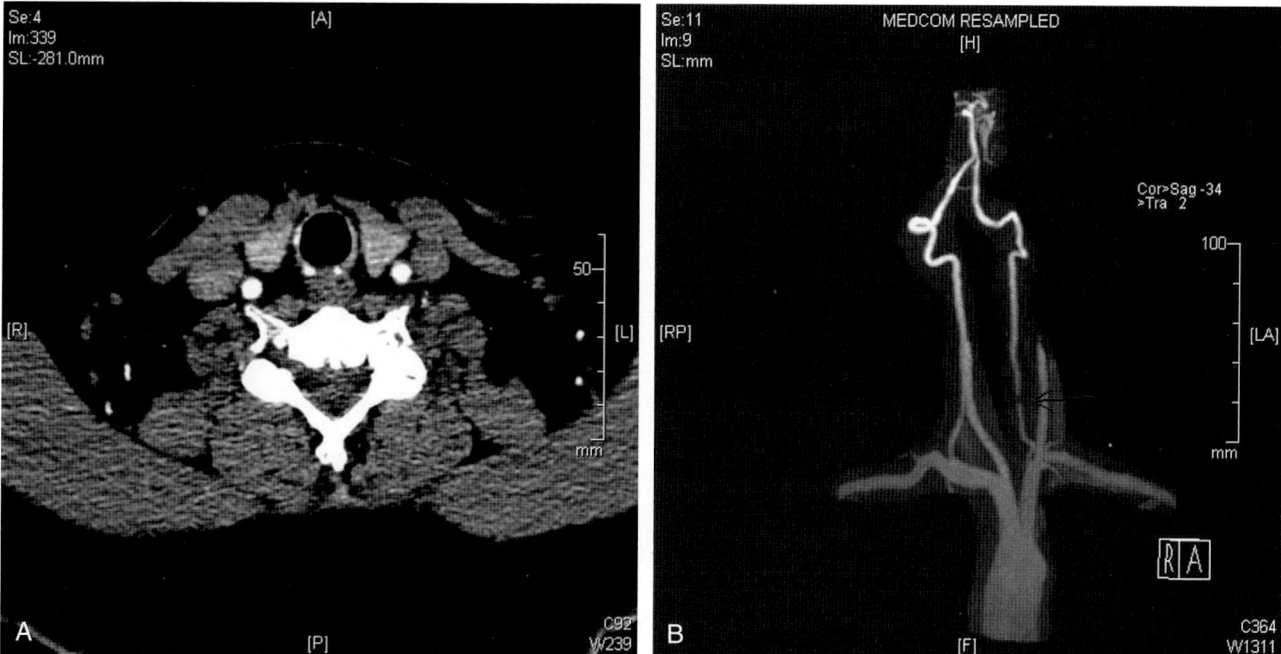

Figure 102-6 CT (**A**) and MRA (**B**) images demonstrating large osteophytes occluding the vertebral artery at C5.

raphy is required to demonstrate extrinsic dynamic compression of the vertebral artery. This is performed either with the patient sitting up, by means of bilateral brachial injections, or if the transfemoral approach is used, with the patient supine in the Trendelenburg position with the head resting against a block. The reason to position the patient either sitting up or in a 25-degree Trendelenburg position is to mimic the effects of the weight of the head on the spine. With the patient standing, the weight of the head acting on the cervical spine changes its curvature and decreases the distance between C1 and C7. This longitudinal compression of the spine often enhances the extrinsic compression effects caused

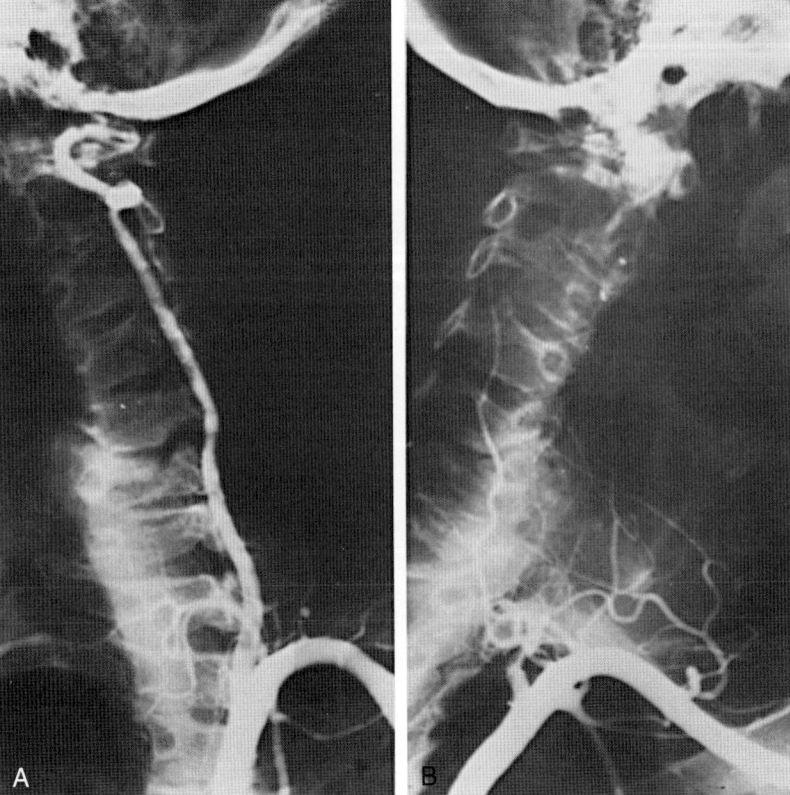

Figure 102-7 A patient with a single vertebral artery showing minimal extrinsic compression (**A**) when the neck is rotated to the right and occlusion (**B**) when the neck is rotated to the left. *(From Berguer R. Surgical management of the vertebral artery. In: Moore WS, ed.* Surgery for Cerebrovascular Disease. *New York, NY: Churchill Livingstone; 1986.)*

by osteophytic spurs. In these positions, intended to exert axial compression on the cervical vertebrae, the angiographer should obtain the specific rotation or extension of the head that provokes the symptoms. When the patient is rendered symptomatic, arteriographic injection should demonstrate the extrinsic compression that developed with the head rotation or extension.[13] The vertebral artery may be normal in one projection and occluded by extrinsic compression in the other (Fig. 102-7). The agent of compression may be bone (an osteophyte) or tendon (longus colli).

The V2 segment is a frequent site for the development of traumatic or spontaneous arteriovenous fistulae, which should easily be identified with angiography. Fistulae occur commonly in the V2 segment because fixation of the adventitia of the vertebral artery to the periosteum of the foramina makes the former vulnerable to luxation/subluxation of the vertebrae or to fractures of their lateral mass. The close proximity of the artery to its surrounding venous plexus results in an arteriovenous fistula whenever the artery and the vein are damaged in continuity. The vertebral artery may tear completely or incompletely (dissection) as a consequence of stretch injury after brisk rotation or hyperextension of the neck.

The V2 segment is also the most common site of aneurysmal degeneration (Fig. 102-8), fibromuscular disease, and embolizing atherosclerotic plaque. Disease in the second segment of the vertebral artery can result in extracranial occlusion or stenotic lesions in the intraforaminal segment, which commonly give rise to emboli.

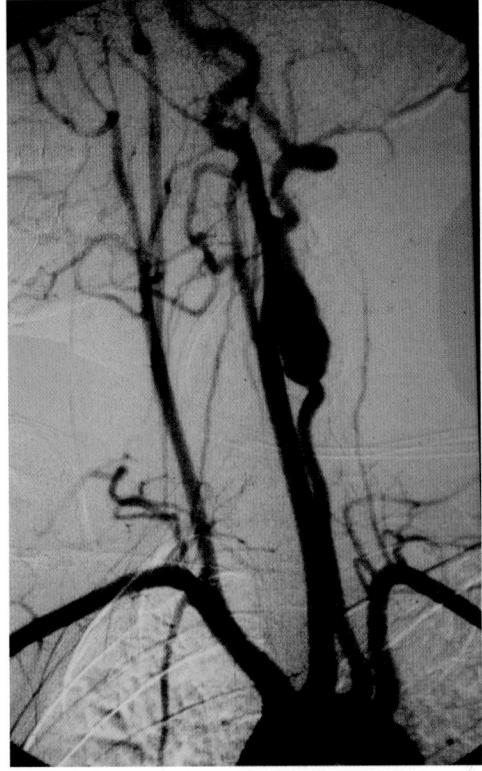

Figure 102-8 V2 segment aneurysm.

V3 Segment

The third segment of the vertebral artery (V3) extends from the top of the transverse process of C2 to the atlanto-occipital membrane. After crossing this membrane, the artery enters the foramen magnum at the base of the skull and becomes intradural. The first two cervical vertebrae are the most mobile of the spine. About 50% of neck rotation occurs between C1 and C2. The vertebral artery is redundant at this level to allow the arc of displacement of the transverse process of the atlas (80 degrees) to which the vertebral artery is attached. Imaging of V3 is not complete without stressed views in rotation when this segment is fully patent in a neutral position.

The most common problems at the V3 level are related to trauma and arterial dissection and include occlusive lesions, arteriovenous fistulae, and pseudoaneurysms. Dissection may be associated with fibromuscular dysplasia or occur in a normal artery after seemingly trivial trauma (Fig. 102-9). Dissection of a vertebral artery may result in stenosis, thrombosis, distal embolization, and pseudoaneurysmal dilatation (Fig. 102-10). An arteriovenous fistula results from rupture of the wall of the vertebral artery into its surrounding venous plexus. In long-standing fistulae, the pulsatile mass formed by the fistula and its dilated venous channels is called an arteriovenous aneurysm. The vertebral artery may be compressed in the pars atlantica of the third segment between the occipital ridge and the arch of the atlas. In these patients the symptoms of low-flow posterior circulation systems are usually precipitated by head extension or rotation.

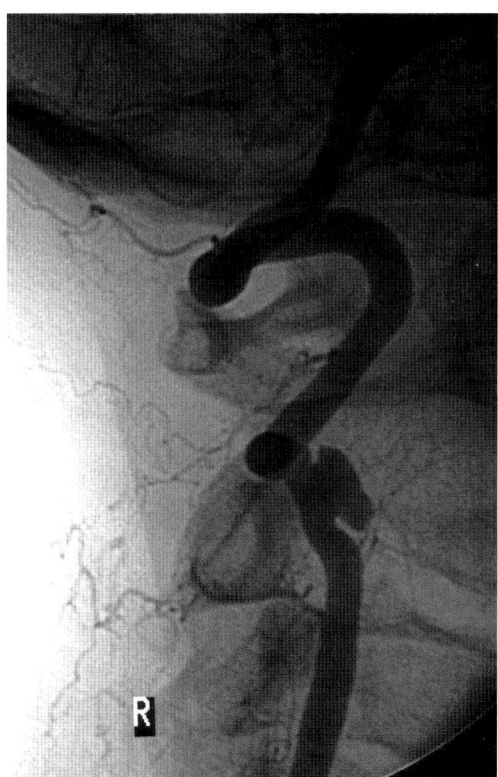

Figure 102-10 Distal V2 segment pseudoaneurysm resulting from dissection.

When the vertebral artery is occluded proximally, it usually reconstitutes at the V3 segment by collateral blood vessels from the external carotid via the occipital artery (Fig. 102-11) or by collaterals from the ipsilateral subclavian artery via branches of the thyrocervical trunk (Fig. 102-12).[14] Because of this collateral network, the distal vertebral and basilar arteries usually remain patent despite a proximal vertebral artery occlusion. This anatomic finding is crucial for developing surgical strategy. Delayed angiographic views are of the utmost importance in identifying a patent V3 segment that can be exploited as a distal target for reconstruction.

V4 Segment

The fourth segment (V4) is infrequently affected by atherosclerosis. At this level the vertebral artery is vulnerable to direct trauma and stretch injuries that can lead to intimal damage, thrombosis, embolization, and dissection. This segment is also prone to arteriovenous fistula formation and aneurysmal degeneration. Finally, the basilar artery should be seen clearly in a lateral projection. Subtracted views are needed to eliminate the temporal bone density in the lateral projection. In the Towne anteroposterior view, routinely used in neuroradiology, the basilar artery is foreshortened and therefore the resolution is poor. Advanced atherosclerotic disease of the basilar artery is a contraindication to reconstruction of vertebral artery lesions.

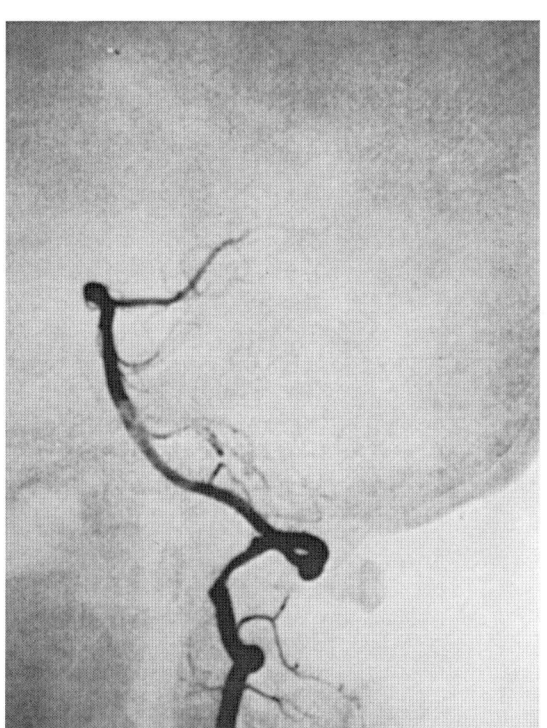

Figure 102-9 Intramural dissection of the vertebral artery at the V3 segment in a 40-year-old woman with Klippel-Feil syndrome and subluxation of the atlantoaxial joint.

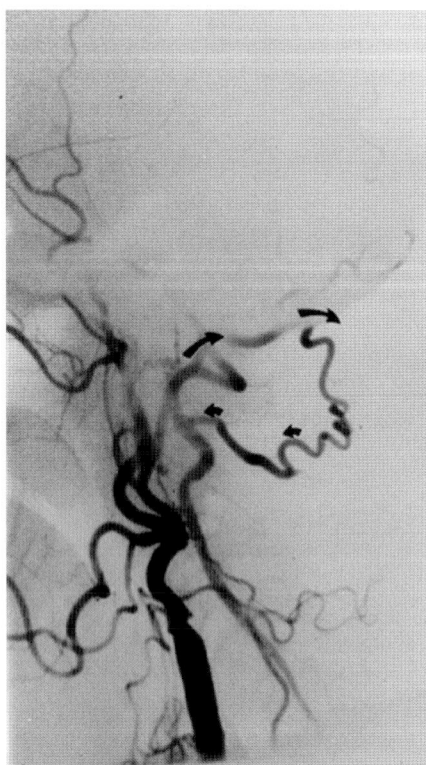

Figure 102-11 The distal vertebral and basilar artery being fed by an occipital collateral in a patient with proximal vertebral artery occlusion.

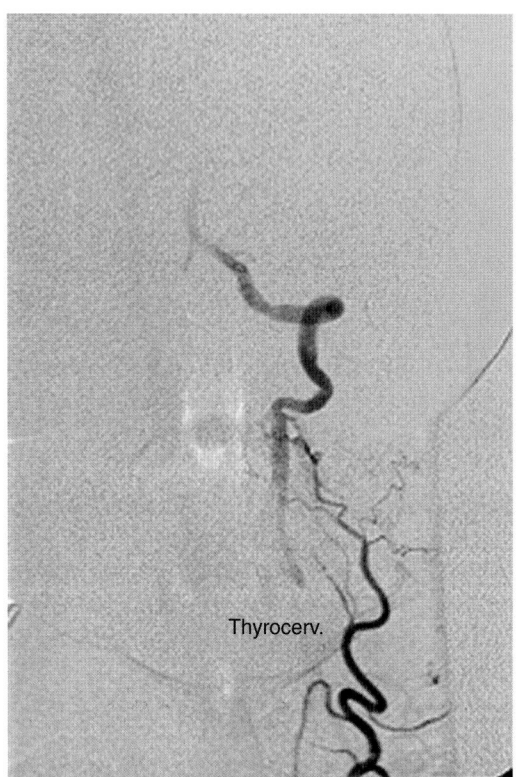

Thyrocerv.

Figure 102-12 The distal vertebral and basilar artery fed by a thyrocervical collateral in a patient with proximal vertebral artery occlusion.

■ VERTEBRAL ARTERY RECONSTRUCTIVE PROCEDURES

Accumulated experience has shown that with appropriate surgical intervention, predictable resolution of hemodynamic symptoms and cessation of embolic events can occur.

Disease Location

The location of disease will dictate the type of surgical reconstruction that is required. With rare exceptions, most reconstructions of the vertebral artery are performed to relieve an orificial stenosis (V1 segment) or stenoses, dissection, or occlusion of its intraspinal component (V2 and V3 segments).[15]

V1 Segment

A number of operations have been described for treating stenosing ostial lesions in V1.[16,17] Transposition of the proximal vertebral artery onto the adjacent carotid artery is the most common reconstruction. Less commonly, a bypass using either saphenous vein or expanded polytetrafluoroethylene can be performed from either the common carotid artery or the adjacent subclavian artery.[18,19] Alternatively, a subclavian-vertebral artery endarterectomy can be preformed, but this operation is fraught with technical challenges.

V2 Segment

The second segment of the vertebral artery, the portion that ascends within the foramina of the cervical vertebrae, is the site of a wide variety of pathologic conditions. Rarely, however, is the V2 segment accessed surgically because of its mostly interosseous position. The most common indication for exposure of the V2 segment is for control of hemorrhage, which is best relieved by proximal and distal ligation of the artery. This has not been associated with worsening neurologic sequelae. After complete V2 occlusion, patency of the distal extracranial segment is often maintained by collaterals from the external carotid or subclavian artery. Ligation (at the C1-C2 level) and bypass to the distal (V3 segment) vertebral artery may be indicated for embolizing V2 pathology.

V3 Segment

Reconstruction of the distal (V3 segment) vertebral artery is usually performed at the C1-C2 level. The technique most often used to reconstruct the distal vertebral artery includes great or small saphenous vein bypass from the common carotid, subclavian, or proximal vertebral artery.[14,16] Alternatively, the radial artery can be used as a conduit in the absence of suitable vein. Transposition of the external carotid or hypertrophied occipital artery into the distal vertebral artery, as well as transposition of the distal vertebral artery into the side of the internal carotid artery, has also been described.

Suboccipital Segment

For more distal pathology, the vertebral artery can also be accessed surgically above the level of the transverse process of C1. Surgical exposure at the suboccipital segment requires resection of the C1 transverse process and part of its posterior arch. Reconstruction at this level is limited to saphenous vein bypass from the distal internal carotid artery. Bypasses above the level of C1 (suboccipital) are technically demanding and have been required in only 4% of cases of distal vertebral artery reconstruction.

Transposition of the Proximal Vertebral Artery into the Common Carotid Artery

The approach to the proximal vertebral artery is the same as the approach for a subclavian-to-carotid transposition. The incision is placed transversely about a fingerbreadth above the clavicle and directly over the two heads of the sternocleidomastoid muscle (Fig. 102-13). Subplatysmal skin flaps are created to provide adequate exposure. Dissection is carried down directly between the two bellies of the sternocleidomastoid, and the omohyoid muscle is divided. The internal jugular vein and vagus nerve are retracted laterally and the carotid sheath entered. The carotid artery should be exposed proximally as far as possible, which is facilitated if the surgeon temporarily stands at the head of the patient and looks down into the mediastinum.

After the carotid artery is mobilized, the sympathetic chain is identified running behind and parallel to it. On the left side, the thoracic duct is divided between ligatures while avoiding transfixion sutures, which will result in lymph leaks. The proximal end of the thoracic duct is doubly ligated. Accessory lymph ducts—often seen on the right side—are identified,

ligated, and divided. The entire dissection is confined medial to the prescalene fat pad that covers the scalenus anticus muscle and phrenic nerve. These latter structures are left unexposed lateral to the field. The inferior thyroid artery runs transversely across the field, and it is ligated and divided.

The vertebral vein is next identified emerging from the angle formed by the longus colli and scalenus anticus and overlying the vertebral artery and, at the bottom of the field, the subclavian artery. Unlike its sister artery, the vertebral vein has branches. It is ligated in continuity and divided. Below the vertebral vein lies the vertebral artery. It is important to identify and avoid injury to the adjacent sympathetic chain. The vertebral artery is dissected superiorly to the tendon of the longus colli and inferiorly to its origin in the subclavian artery. The vertebral artery is freed from the sympathetic trunk resting on its anterior surface without damaging the trunk or the ganglionic rami. Preserving the sympathetic trunks and the stellate or intermediate ganglia resting on the artery usually requires freeing the vertebral artery from these structures, and after dividing its origin, the latter is transposed anterior to the sympathetics.

Once the artery is fully exposed, an appropriate site for reimplantation in the common carotid artery is selected. The patient is given heparin systemically. The distal portion of the V1 segment of the vertebral artery is clamped below the edge of the longus colli with a microclip placed vertically to indicate the orientation of the artery and to avoid axial twisting during its transposition. The proximal vertebral artery is closed by transfixion with 5-0 polypropylene suture immediately above the stenosis at its origin. The artery is divided at this level, and its proximal stump is further secured with a hemoclip. The artery is then brought to the common carotid artery and its free end is spatulated for anastomosis.

The carotid artery is then cross-clamped. An elliptical 5- to 7-mm arteriotomy is created in the posterolateral wall of the

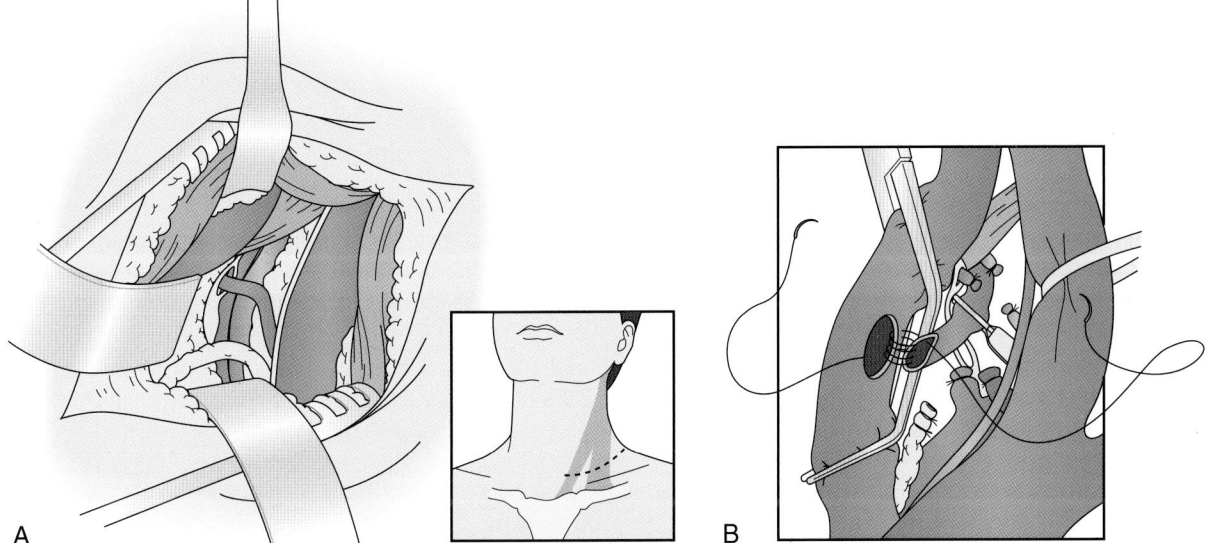

Figure 102-13 A, Access to the proximal vertebral artery between the sternocleidomastoid muscle bellies. **B,** Transposition of the proximal vertebral artery to the posterior wall of the common carotid artery. *(From Berguer R, Kieffer E. Surgery of the Arteries to the Head. New York, NY: Springer-Verlag; 1992.)*

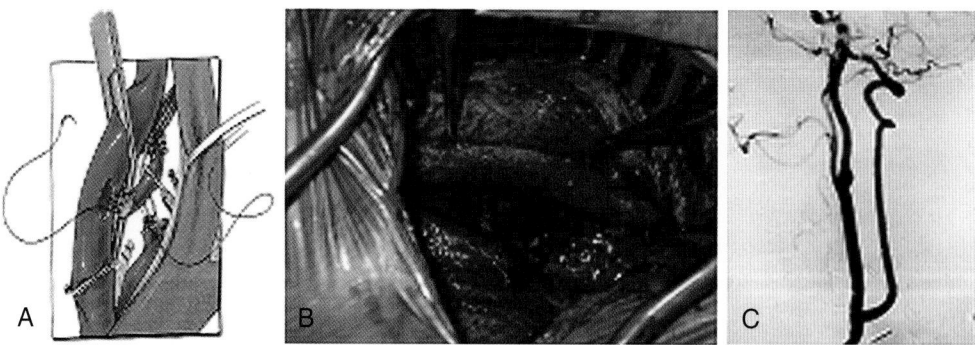

Figure 102-14 A–C, Proximal vertebral–to–common carotid transposition.

common carotid artery with an aortic punch. The anastomosis is performed in open fashion with continuous 6-0 or 7-0 polypropylene suture while avoiding any tension on the vertebral artery, which tears easily. Before completion of the anastomosis, any slack in the suture is tightened appropriately with a nerve hook, standard flushing maneuvers are performed, and the suture is tied to re-establish flow (Fig. 102-14).

When simultaneous carotid endarterectomy is planned, the vertebral artery is approached through the standard carotid incision extended inferiorly to the head of the clavicle. With this approach, the sternocleidomastoid muscle is lateral and the field is a bit narrower than when the vertebral artery is approached between the heads of the sternocleidomastoid. The remaining steps of the operation are performed as described previously.[20]

Distal Vertebral Artery Reconstruction

Common Carotid–Vertebral Artery Bypass

Reconstruction of the distal vertebral artery is generally done at the C1-C2 level. Rarely, the reconstruction is done between C1 and the base of the skull via a posterior approach. Although various techniques can be applied to revascularize the vertebral artery in its V3 segment (between the transverse processes of C1 and C2), the approach to the vertebral artery at this level is the same for all procedures.[14,21]

The incision is made anterior to the sternocleidomastoid muscle, the same as for a carotid operation, and is carried superiorly to immediately below the earlobe (Fig. 102-15). The dissection proceeds between the internal jugular vein and the anterior edge of the sternocleidomastoid to expose the spinal accessory nerve. The nerve is followed distally as it joins the jugular vein and crosses in front of the transverse process of C1, which can easily be felt by the operator's finger. This necessitates freeing and retracting the digastric muscle upward or dividing it.

The next step involves identification of the levator scapulae muscle by removal of the fibrofatty tissue overlying it. With the anterior edge of the levator scapulae identified, the surgeon searches for the anterior ramus of C2. With the ramus as a guide, a right-angle clamp is slid over the ramus

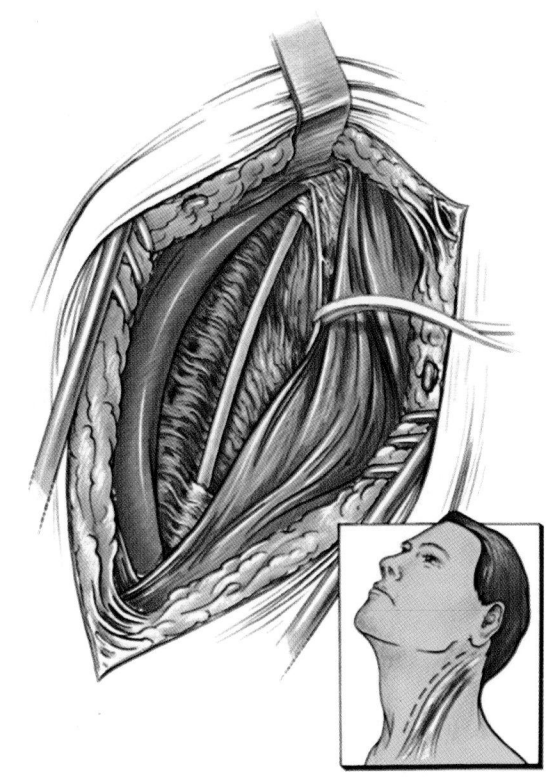

Figure 102-15 Retrojugular approach and isolation of the spinal accessory nerve. *(From Berguer R, Kieffer E.* Surgery of the Arteries to the Head. *New York, NY: Springer-Verlag; 1992.)*

to elevate the levator scapulae, which is transected from its origin (Fig. 102-16). The proximal stump of the levator is excised up to its insertion on the C1 transverse process. The C2 ramus divides into three branches after crossing the vertebral artery. The artery runs below, in contact with the nerve and perpendicular to it. The surgeon cuts the ramus (Fig. 102-17) before its branching; underneath it, the vertebral artery can be identified.

Dissection of the artery at this level is best accomplished with loupe magnification, advisable for all vertebral artery reconstructions. The artery is freed from the surrounding veins with extreme care because hemorrhage is difficult to control at this level. Before encircling the artery with fine silicone vessel loops (Fig. 102-18), one must ensure that a

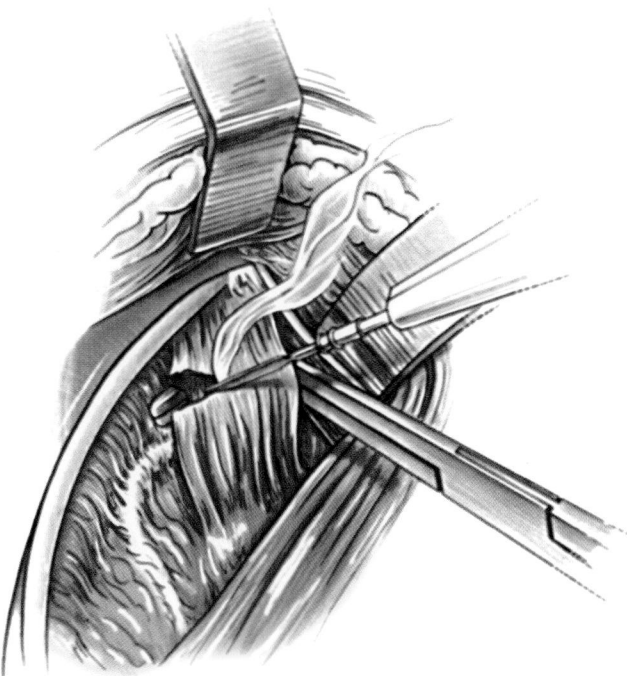

Figure 102-16 Dividing the levator scapulae over the C2 ramus. The vagus, internal jugular vein, and internal carotid artery are anterior to the muscle. *(From Berguer R, Kieffer E. Surgery of the Arteries to the Head. New York, NY: Springer-Verlag; 1992.)*

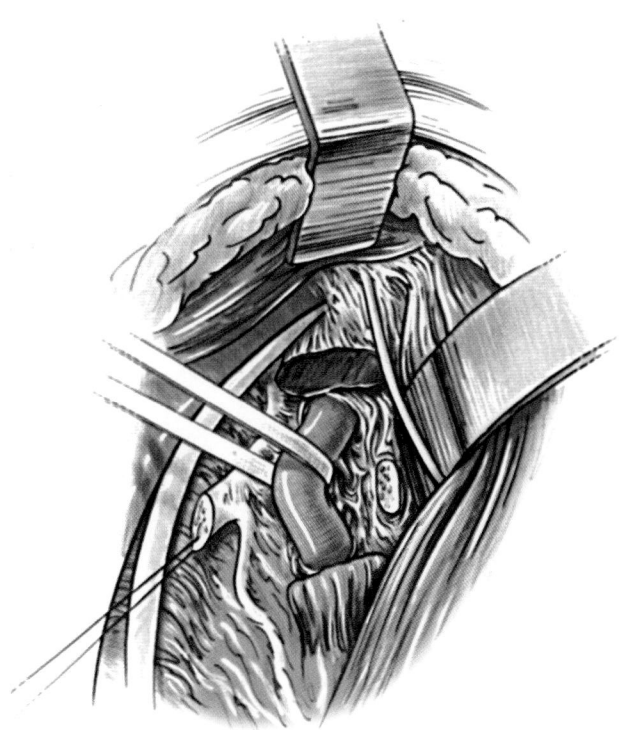

Figure 102-18 After the vertebral venous plexus is dissected away, the vertebral artery is slung with a polymeric silicone (Silastic) loop for clamping and anastomosis. *(From Berguer R, Kieffer E. Surgery of the Arteries to the Head. New York, NY: Springer-Verlag; 1992.)*

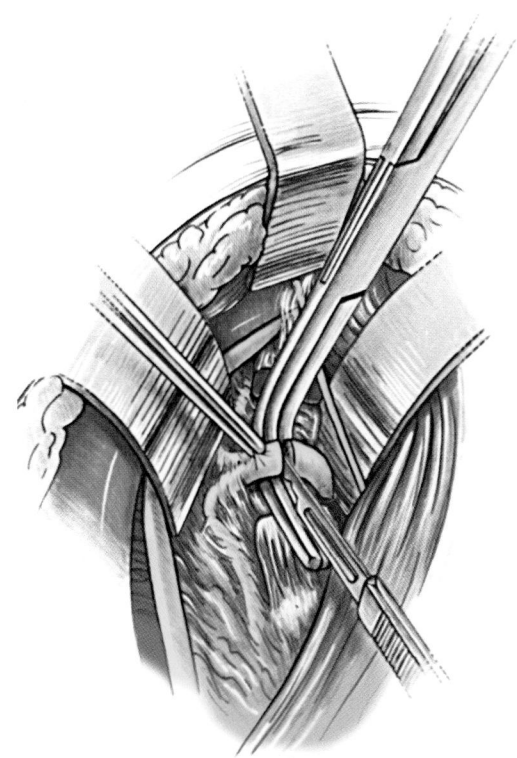

Figure 102-17 Dividing the anterior ramus of C2 to expose the underlying vertebral artery running perpendicular to the anterior ramus. *(From Berguer R, Kieffer E. Surgery of the Arteries to the Head. New York, NY: Springer-Verlag; 1992.)*

branch from the occipital collateral artery does not enter the posterior aspect of the vertebral artery at the location at which the surgeon is dissecting. Tearing of this important collateral vessel complicates preparation of the distal vertebral artery unnecessarily. Once the vertebral artery is encircled, the distal common carotid artery is dissected and prepared to receive a saphenous vein graft. There is no need to dissect the carotid bifurcation. The location selected for the proximal anastomosis of the saphenous vein graft on the common carotid artery should not be too close to the bifurcation because cross-clamping at this level may fracture any underlying atheroma.

A saphenous vein graft or other suitable conduit of appropriate length is harvested from the thigh and prepared. A valveless segment facilitates backbleeding of the vertebral artery after completion of the distal anastomosis. The patient is given intravenous heparin. The vertebral artery is elevated by gently pulling the loop and is occluded with a small J-clamp to isolate this segment for an end-to-side anastomosis. The vertebral artery is opened longitudinally with a coronary knife for a length adequate to accommodate the spatulated end of the vein graft. The end-to-side anastomosis is performed with continuous 7-0 polypropylene and fine needles. The distal anastomosis is assessed for backflow, and if satisfactory, a Heifitz clip is placed in the vein graft proximal to the anastomosis to restore flow through the vertebral artery.

The proximal end of the graft is passed beneath the jugular vein and in proximity to the side of the common carotid

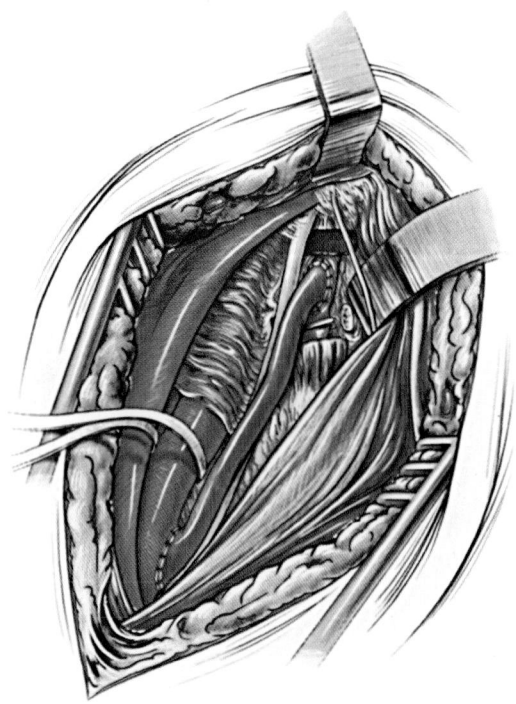

Figure 102-19 A completed common carotid artery–to–distal vertebral artery bypass using the saphenous vein. *(From Berguer R, Kieffer E. Surgery of the Arteries to the Head. New York, NY: Springer-Verlag; 1992.)*

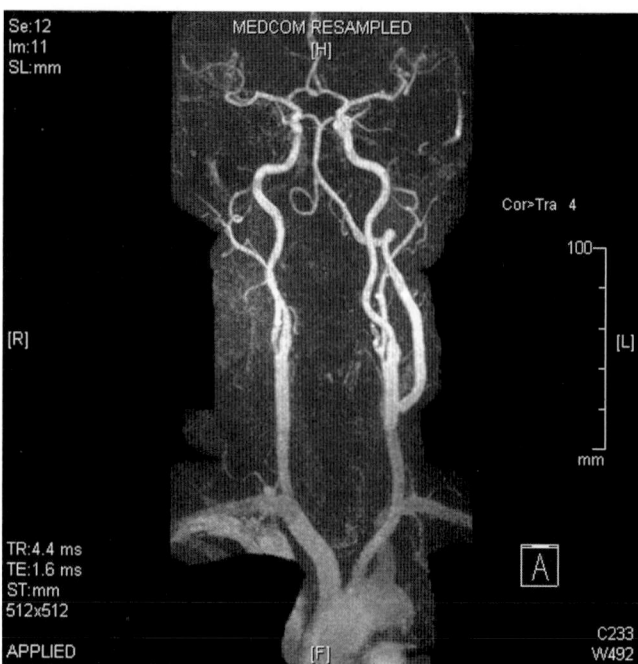

Figure 102-20 Follow-up MRA showing a patent distal vertebral bypass.

artery. The common carotid artery is then cross-clamped, an elliptical arteriotomy is made in its posterior wall with an aortic punch, and the proximal vein graft is anastomosed end-to-side to the common carotid artery with continuous 6-0 polypropylene (Figs. 102-19 and 102-20). Before the anastomosis is completed, standard flushing maneuvers are performed, the suture is tied, and flow is re-established. Next, the vertebral artery is occluded with a clip immediately below the anastomosis so that competitive flow or the potential for recurrent emboli is avoided. In the absence of suitable common carotid artery, the ipsilateral subclavian artery can be used as a donor vessel.

External Carotid–Vertebral Artery Transposition

The distal vertebral artery may also be revascularized via the external carotid artery (ECA) either directly by means of transposition of the ECA to the distal vertebral artery or by anastomosis of the proximal end of a graft to the ECA. Transposition of the ECA to the distal vertebral artery (Figs. 102-21 and 102-22) requires a carotid bifurcation free of disease and a long ECA trunk. ECAs that divide early are often too small to match the caliber of the vertebral artery. If the trunk of the ECA is of adequate size and length to reach the vertebral artery, the ECA is skeletonized by dividing all its branches. The ECA is then rotated over the internal carotid artery and beneath the internal jugular vein to construct an end-to-side anastomosis to the distal vertebral artery at the C1-C2 level.

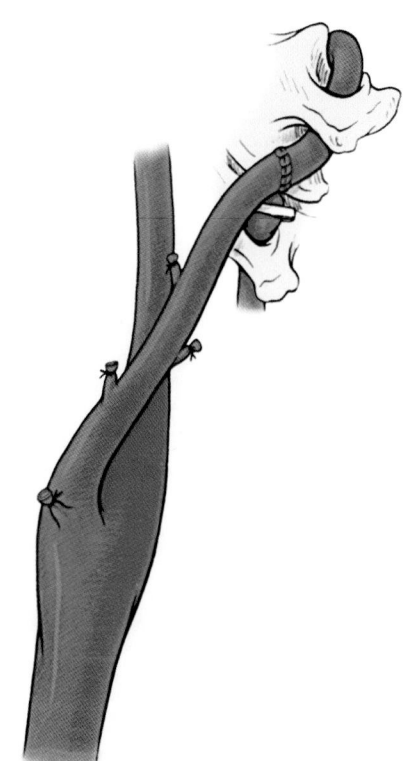

Figure 102-21 Transposition of the external carotid artery to the distal vertebral artery. *(From Berguer R, Kieffer E. Surgery of the Arteries to the Head. New York, NY: Springer-Verlag; 1992.)*

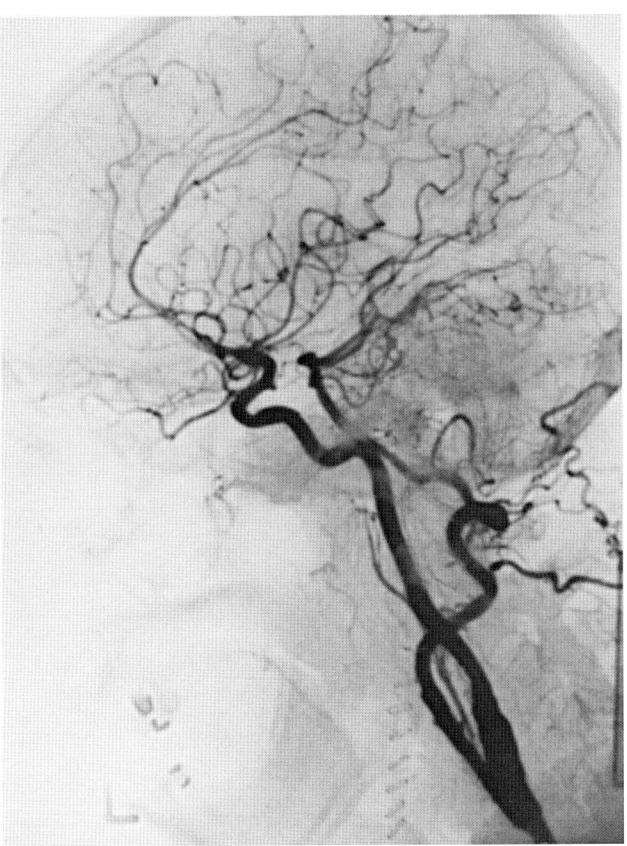

Figure 102-22 Arteriogram of a transposition of the external carotid artery to the distal vertebral artery. This patient had previously undergone internal carotid endarterectomy. *(From Berguer R, Kieffer E. Surgery of the Arteries to the Head. New York, NY: Springer-Verlag; 1992.)*

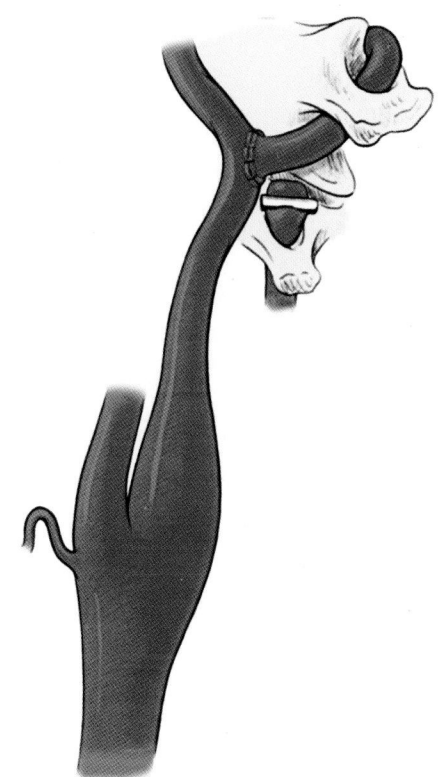

Figure 102-23 Transposition of the distal vertebral artery into the cervical internal carotid artery. *(From Berguer R, Kieffer E. Surgery of the Arteries to the Head. New York, NY: Springer-Verlag; 1992.)*

After completion of this anastomosis, the vertebral artery is permanently occluded with a clip immediately below the anastomosis.

External Carotid–Vertebral Artery Bypass

A patient may have a segment of saphenous vein that is of appropriate diameter but insufficient length to bridge the distance between the common carotid artery and the distal vertebral artery. In this case the proximal ECA can be used as the inflow source for the vein graft. This technique is particularly useful when the contralateral internal carotid artery is occluded and one wishes to avoid clamping the common carotid supplying the only patent internal carotid artery. If a vein bypass graft is used between the ECA and the distal vertebral artery, it should be placed with the proper amount of tension and assessed with the neck rotated back to the neutral position to avoid kinking.

Vertebral Artery–Internal Carotid Artery Transposition

Another method of revascularization of the distal vertebral artery is transposition of this vessel into the distal cervical internal carotid artery below the transverse process of C1 (Fig. 102-23). This technique is particularly applicable for patients with inadequate saphenous vein or in whom the ECA cannot be used because of unsuitable anatomy or disease of the carotid bifurcation. This is a straightforward end-to-side anastomosis between the distal vertebral artery and the distal cervical internal carotid artery. This procedure, however, is contraindicated in patients with contralateral internal carotid artery occlusion, in whom the risk for cerebral ischemia during the anastomosis would be prohibitive.

A small group of patients have disease that extends up to the level of C1 and require revascularization in the most distal segment of the extracranial vertebral artery.[22,23] To accomplish this, the vertebral artery must be exposed in its pars atlantica, where the artery runs parallel to the lamina of the atlas before entering the foramen magnum.

Posterior Suboccipital Vertebral Artery Bypass

The approach to the suboccipital segment of the distal vertebral artery is posterior.[24] The patient lies prone in the "park bench" position. The incision is racket shaped, with a horizontal segment below the occipital bone from the midline laterally to the level of the sternocleidomastoid. There, the incision becomes oblique and follows the posterior belly of the sternocleidomastoid muscle. The superficial nuchal muscle layer (splenius capitis and semispinalis) is transected (Fig. 102-24). The accessory spinal nerve is isolated laterally

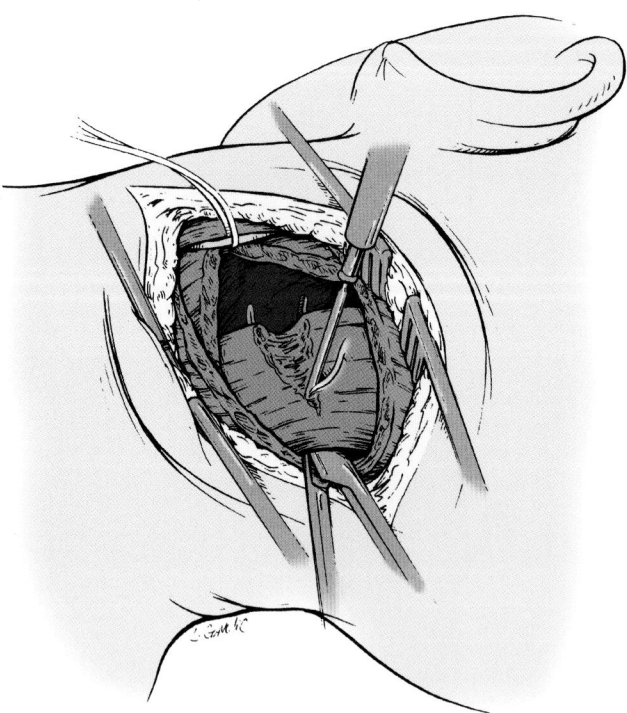

Figure 102-24 Posterior approach to the suboccipital segment of the distal vertebral artery: division of the splenius capitis and semispinalis.

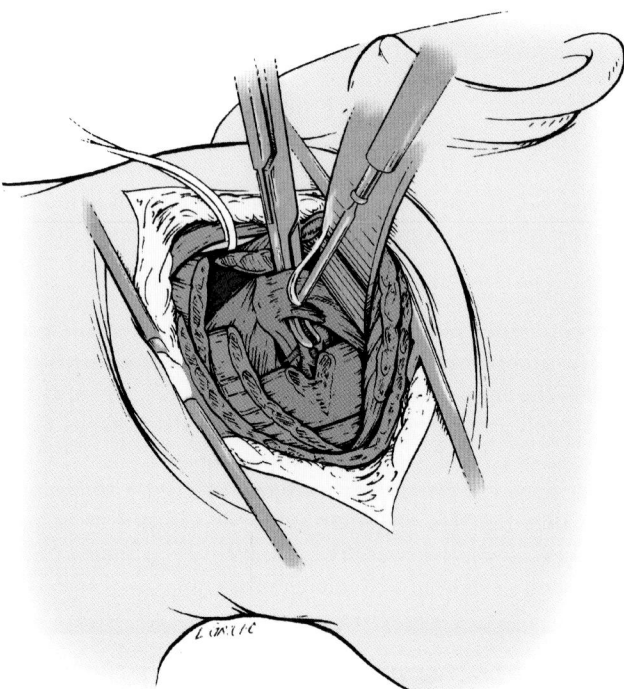

Figure 102-25 Posterior approach to the suboccipital vertebral artery: division of the obliquus and rectus capitis.

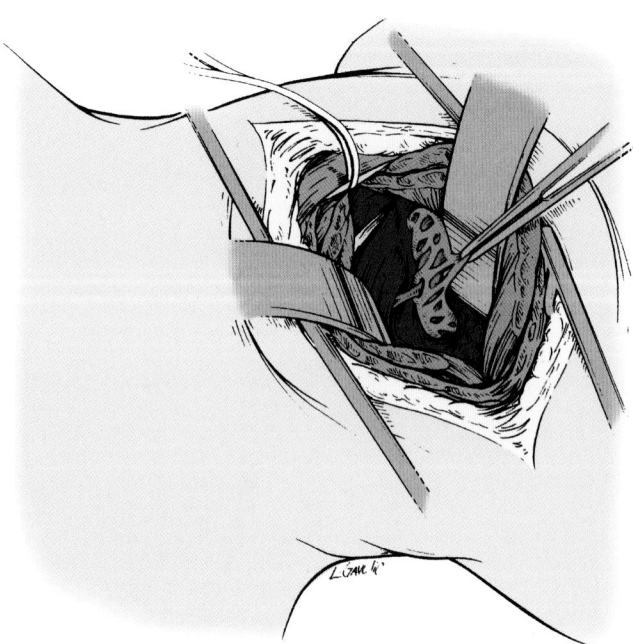

Figure 102-26 The pars atlantica of the distal vertebral artery exposed and surrounded by a dense venous plexus.

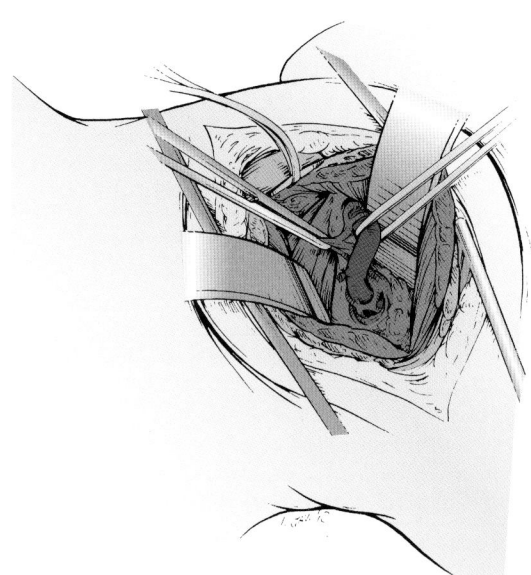

Figure 102-27 Exposure of the pars atlantica of the vertebral artery from its exit from the transverse foramen of C1 to its entrance into the dura mater.

below the sternocleidomastoid muscle. The transverse process of C1 is located by palpation. The short posterior muscles between the atlas and occipital bone (obliquus capitis and rectus capitis posterior major) are divided (Fig. 102-25). The artery can now be seen enveloped by a dense venous plexus

(Fig. 102-26), from which it is extricated by bipolar coagulation and microligature of these veins. The artery can be exposed from its emergence at the top of C1 to the dura mater (Fig. 102-27). Through the same posterior approach, the internal carotid artery can be isolated posterior and medial to the sternocleidomastoid after mobilization and retraction of the hypoglossal and vagus nerves, which at this level cover its posterior wall. The distal anastomosis of the vein graft to the vertebral artery is performed first. The vein is allowed to distend over the lamina of the atlas and into its site of anastomosis at the posterior wall of the internal carotid artery (Figs. 102-28 and 102-29).

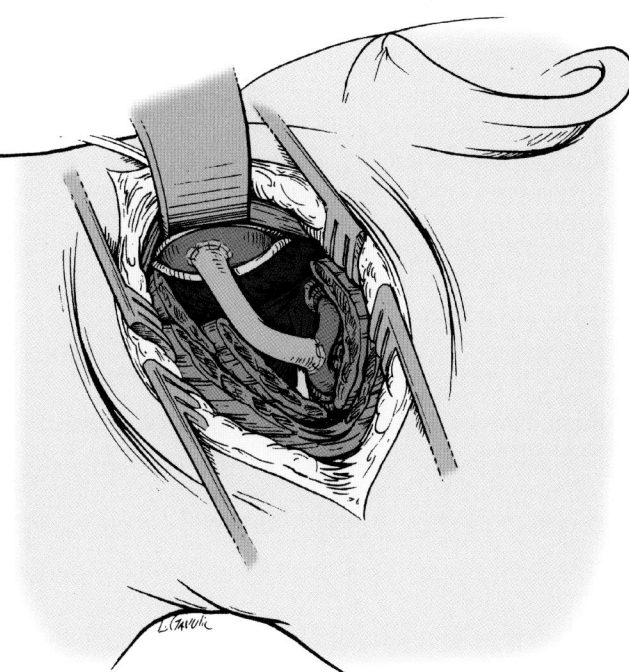

Figure 102-28 Distal cervical internal carotid–to–suboccipital vertebral bypass.

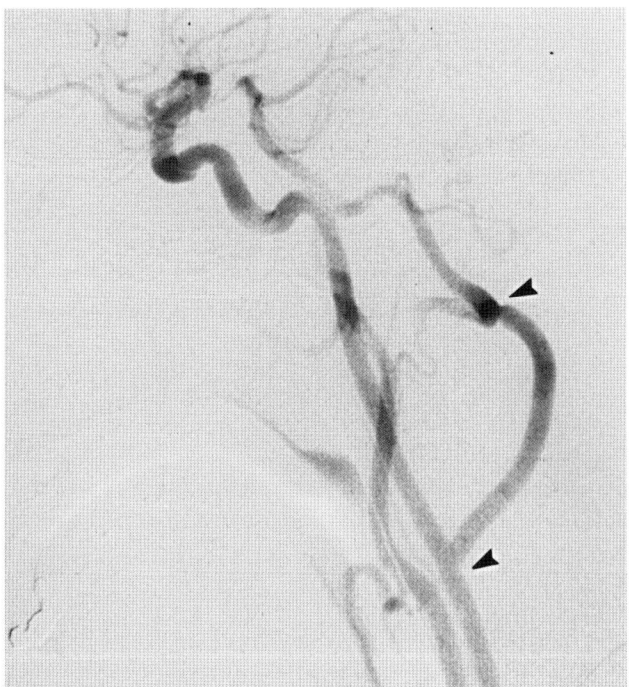

Figure 102-29 Bypass from the midcervical internal carotid artery to the suboccipital vertebral artery (*arrowheads*).

■ OPERATIVE RESULTS

Perioperative

Perioperative complication rates differ for proximal versus distal vertebral artery repairs. Perioperative complications that can follow any reconstruction include stroke, bleeding, thrombosis, and nerve injury. Intraoperative completion

imaging with digital angiography is useful and should be considered for all types of vertebral artery reconstruction. A significant number of reparable technical flaws may be identified, and repair can prevent reconstruction failure.

Proximal Reconstructions

The technically easier proximal operations have been reported to have a combined stroke and death rate of 0.9%.[12] Among patients undergoing proximal operations in one report, there were no deaths or strokes in those who underwent only a vertebral reconstruction. When the proximal vertebral artery reconstruction was combined with a carotid operation, the observed stroke and death rates increased to 5.7% in that same report.[12] Berguer and coauthors reported four instances of immediate postoperative thrombosis (1.4%). Three of the four patients had vein grafts interposed between the vertebral artery and the common carotid because of a short V1 segment. The grafts kinked and thrombosed. Other complications that are particular to proximal reconstruction include vagus and recurrent laryngeal nerve palsy (2%), Horner's syndrome (8.4% to 28%), lymphocele (4%), and chylothorax (0.5%).

Distal Reconstructions

Operations on the distal vertebral artery carry higher stroke and death rates than do operations on the proximal vertebral artery. Distal reconstructions have a combined stroke and death rate of 3% to 4%.[25] The immediate graft thrombosis rate has been reported at 8%, and spinal accessory nerve injury occurs in 2% of patients.[26] Among 141 distal operations, there were seven strokes, five of which resulted in death: three patients had brainstem strokes and deaths related to the procedure, and two died of a large hemispheric infarction.

Long-term Outcomes

Results after both proximal and distal vertebral artery reconstruction are generally equal to or better than those reported in series reviewing other forms of extracranial cerebrovascular reconstruction.[25,27] Proximal vertebral artery reconstruction is attended by fewer ischemic complications and has long-term results equal to or better than those after carotid surgery. Long-term patency of the reconstructions is excellent. After proximal vertebral–to–common carotid transposition, patency rates at 5 and 10 years equal or exceed 95% and 91%, respectively. When selected appropriately, more than 80% of patients will have relief of their symptoms after proximal surgical reconstruction.[27]

For distal bypass reconstruction, patency rates of 87% and 82% should be expected at 5 and 10 years.[25,27] Seventy percent of patients undergoing distal vertebral artery reconstruction are dead at 5 years' follow-up, mostly from cardiac disease, whereas 97% of survivors are free of stroke at 5 years. Symptoms are expected to be cured in 71% of patients and improved in 16%.[25,27]

ENDOVASCULAR THERAPY

Vertebral and basilar artery angioplasty, with or without adjuvant stent placement, has been performed in some centers for a number of years. A growing number of case reports and small nonrandomized case series suggest that endovascular intervention in the posterior circulation may be safe and technically feasible.[28-39] Patients are pretreated with antiplatelet medications. Most cases are performed from a femoral approach, although the brachial route has also been used. The stenotic lesions are crossed and treated with a 0.014- or 0.018-inch wire platform and small coronary-diameter balloons and stents. In contrast to intervention on the extracranial carotid artery, vertebral artery angioplasty with stenting is usually performed without the assistance of embolic protection. Periprocedural risks include but are not limited to stent malposition, vessel rupture, thrombosis, arterial dissection, and discrete embolization.

Vertebral artery angioplasty alone, especially when used for the treatment of disease at the origin of the vessel, appears to have an unacceptably high rate of restenosis. Adjuvant stent placement adds to the technical challenge but is associated with improved durability. A recently published Cochrane review identified 313 endovascular interventions for vertebral artery stenosis, with just over half of the interventions using stent placement as part of the treatment. The technical success rate was 95%, and the 30-day stroke and death rate was 6.4%.[40] A subset of 16 patients treated within the Carotid and Vertebral Artery Transluminal Angioplasty Study (CAVATAS 2001) represents the only report of a randomized controlled trial comparing endoluminal therapy with best medical care for symptomatic vertebral stenosis. There were no 30-day strokes or deaths in either group, although two of eight patients who underwent endoluminal therapy experienced transient ischemic symptoms. Furthermore, with a mean follow-up of 4.5 years, there were no posterior circulation strokes noted in either group. The Cochrane group concluded that although angioplasty with stenting for vertebral artery stenosis is technically feasible, there is currently insufficient evidence to support its routine application.[40]

SELECTED KEY REFERENCES

Berguer R, Flynn LM, Kline RA, Caplan L. Surgical reconstruction of the extracranial vertebral artery: management and outcome. *J Vasc Surg*. 2000;31:9-18.
Retrospective review of a large series of all types of surgical vertebral reconstruction.

Berguer R, Morasch MD, Kline RA. A review of 100 consecutive reconstructions of the distal vertebral artery for embolic and hemodynamic disease. *J Vasc Surg*. 1998;27:852-859.
Retrospective review of the largest series of distal vertebral reconstructions to date.

Caplan LR, Wityk RJ, Glass TA, Tapia J, Pazdera L, Chang HM, Teal P, Dashe JF, Chaves CJ, Breen JC, Vemmos K, Amarenco P, Tettenborn B, Leary M, Estol C, Dewitt LD, Pessin MS. New England Medical Center Posterior Circulation registry. *Ann Neurol*. 2004; 56:389-398.
Comprehensive review of the natural history of posterior circulation lesions.

Coward LJ, Featherstone RL, Brown MM. Percutaneous transluminal angioplasty and stenting for vertebral artery stenosis. *Cochrane Database Syst Rev*. 2005;2:CD000516.
Cochrane meta-analysis of the literature on endoluminal therapy for vertebral disease.

REFERENCES

The reference list can be found on the companion Expert Consult Web site at *www.expertconsult.com*.

Lower Extremity Arterial Disease | *Section* **15**

Joseph L. Mills, Sr.

CHAPTER 103

Lower Extremity Arterial Disease: General Considerations

John V. White

Based in part on chapters in the previous edition by Mark R. Nehler, MD; Heather Wolford, MD; John V. White, MD; Robert B, Rutherford, MD, FACS, FRCS (Glasg.); and Kaj Johansen, MD, PhD.

Walking is a fundamental human requirement. Chronic lower extremity ischemia, also known as peripheral arterial disease (PAD), is the most common cause of loss of normal walking ability seen by the vascular specialist. In addition to affecting the legs, it is associated with high systemic morbidity and mortality. This constellation of disorders stems from atherosclerotic stenoses or occlusions within the lower extremity arterial tree, causing a reduction in blood flow to the leg. The manifestations of chronic lower extremity ischemia usually include some type of pain (Table 103-1) and are produced by varying degrees of muscle ischemia; they range from no symptoms to intermittent claudication to critical limb ischemia (CLI). The challenge for the vascular specialist is to recognize the presence of lower extremity ischemia, quantify the extent of local and systemic disease, identify and control risk factors, and establish a comprehensive treatment program.

■ CLASSIFICATION

Claudication

Intermittent claudication is one of the most common reasons for referral to a vascular specialist. The typical patient with intermittent claudication experiences calf symptoms ranging from fatigue to aching while walking. Pain or discomfort may also occur in the thigh or buttock. The pain sensation results from ischemic neuropathy involving small unmyelinated A delta and C sensory fibers and a local intramuscular acidosis from anaerobic metabolism enhanced by the release of substance P. The symptoms of intermittent claudication are alleviated by a brief period of rest, after which the patient can resume walking. Initially the symptoms do not occur with regularity; they occur intermittently when walking, and the distance walked before symptoms are noticed is generally similar on different outings. As the process progresses, symptoms occur more frequently, and the distance walked before the onset of discomfort lessens.

Asymptomatic patients with a reduced ankle-brachial index (ABI) but no symptoms while walking have a prognosis similar to those with intermittent claudication. Among 460 patients with PAD and a reduced ABI, 91 had no symptoms; of these, 28 were less active and appeared to control their symptoms through a reduction in walking speed and distance, while 63 remained active, walking more than 6 blocks a week.[1] When subjected to a 6-minute walking test, the 63 active

patients performed in a manner similar to claudicants, walking slightly farther but with a slower maximal velocity. These data suggest that even when mild, apparently asymptomatic PAD reduces distal blood flow sufficient to impair leg function and ambulatory ability when tested objectively, patients can reduce or eliminate symptoms by reducing their walking distance, speed, or both, thereby masking the presence of PAD.

Disease Location

Claudication generally results from a single level of arterial occlusion, such as the iliac artery or the superficial femoral artery. Collateral vessels can reconstitute the artery distal to a single site of occlusion and provide distal flow. Symptoms of claudication associated with PAD usually manifest in the muscle groups below the site of hemodynamically significant stenosis or occlusion. There are three major patterns of arterial obstruction: inflow disease, outflow disease, and a combination of the two. Inflow disease refers to lesions in the suprainguinal vessels, most commonly the infrarenal aorta and iliac arteries, that limit blood flow to the common femoral artery. Outflow disease consists of occlusive lesions in the lower extremity arterial tree below the inguinal ligament, from the common femoral artery to the pedal vessels. Patients with a combination of inflow and outflow disease may have broad symptoms of intermittent claudication affecting the buttock, hip, thigh, and calf. These symptoms frequently begin in the buttock and thigh and then involve the calf muscles with continued ambulation; however, they may appear in reverse order if the distal disease is more severe than the inflow disease. Severe combined inflow-outflow disease may result in limb-threatening ischemia.

Inflow Disease. Occlusive lesions of the infrarenal aorta or iliac arteries commonly lead to buttock and thigh claudication. In men, if the stenoses or occlusions are bilateral and are proximal to the origins of the internal iliac arteries, vasculogenic erectile dysfunction may be present as well. Although buttock and thigh claudication may be the first symptoms, with continued ambulation, these patients may exhibit classic symptoms of intermittent calf claudication resulting from inadequate perfusion of the entire leg while walking. Acute infrarenal aortic occlusion may cause profound leg ischemia; however, when chronic atherosclerotic occlusive disease of the infrarenal aorta and iliac vessels results in a single segment

Table 103-1 Vascular Pain Syndromes

Condition	Etiology	Character of Pain	Location/Presentation
Intermittent claudication	Arterial perfusion inadequate to meet demands of working skeletal muscle metabolism	Burning, cramping, aching	Buttocks, hips, thighs, calves Occurs with walking, exercise; relieved by rest
Neurogenic claudication	Lumbosacral neurospinal nerve root compression	Diffuse, deep aching or burning May be associated with distal paresthesias or numbness	Extends from buttocks to feet Occurs with walking; relieved by sitting or bending over while walking
Venous claudication	Proximal venous occlusion	Bursting	Engorgement of exercising extremity
Compartment syndromes	Arterial insufficiency resulting from venous congestion and compartment tissue hypertension	Localized	Anterolateral aspect of leg (calf)
Aorta and large-artery pain	Dissection or hematoma resulting from direct trauma, shear, or stretch	Tearing, ripping, boring along line of dissection, with possible distal ischemia	Substernal, interscapular (aorta) initially; then also from ischemic organs (bowel, kidneys, legs)
	Aortic rupture Vasculitic inflammation	Sudden, burning, penetrating Diffuse, aching, poorly localized	Peritoneal, retroperitoneal, pleural Midback (aorta), tenderness over affected artery
Nondiabetic rest pain	Chronic ischemic neuropathy Positional malperfusion of sensory nerves	Diffuse, poorly localized, aching, burning	Distal foot Initially presenting in recumbent position, dissipating in dependent position
Nondiabetic ulcer	Ischemic necrosis of sensory nerves	Unremitting, severe, aching, burning	Shallow, nonhealing pallid erosion of skin of distal foot
Gangrene	Tissue destruction	Paradoxical decrease in pain, insensate, anesthetic	Initially toes or heel
Diabetic foot	Nonischemic diabetic neuropathy Structural changes of foot	Chronic pain in lower extremity and foot Widespread loss of sensation in distal leg and foot	Nonhealing ulceration and toe gangrene Soft tissue bacterial infection
Atheroembolization (blue toe syndrome)	Distal embolization from proximal source	Aching, burning	Cyanosis, ischemic changes in toes or distal foot secondary to digital or branch artery occlusion
Pain after stroke	Ischemia secondary to hemorrhage or tumor	Intracranial	Ipsilateral to neurologic deficit
Small-artery erythromelalgia (Raynaud's syndrome— vasospastic form)	Vasoconstriction/vasodilatation Abnormal arterial reactivity	Dull, aching digital pain with vasoconstriction Reperfusion or vasodilatation produces "fiery" burning pain	Coolness, pallor, numbness, cyanosis, hyperemia
Small-artery Raynaud's phenomenon (vaso-occlusive form)	Vasoconstriction/vasodilatation Digital and palmar artery occlusion resulting from autoimmune conditions	Severe, unremitting distal digital pain; may be refractory	Fingertip ulceration or necrosis
Small-vessel Buerger's disease (thromboangiitis obliterans)	Nonatherosclerotic necrotizing process involving arteries, veins, and nerves Excellent arterial inflow with poor collateralization	Severe, unremitting, aching, burning, agonizing	Upper and lower extremities
Venous disorders Post-thrombotic syndrome	Prior lower extremity deep venous thrombosis	Mild itching, burning; localized ulcer pain	Lower extremity edema, secondary varicosities, hyperpigmentation, stasis ulcer formation
Varicosities	Incompetent valvular system	Diffuse aching or burning	Lower extremities
Superficial phlebitis	Chemical irritation of peripheral vein or infection	Well-localized tenderness along vein	Inflammation, palpable "cord" along course of vein
Lymphatic disease	Idiopathic, iatrogenic, or resulting from infection Pain develops secondary to cellulitis or lymphangitis	Localized	Site of inflammation
Postamputation pain Acute	Wound-related and secondary to obligatory section of major nerves Neuropathic phenomena	Incisional Ranging from mild itching sensation to severe, incapacitating pain	Amputation site/stump Phantom limb
Late	Ill-fitting prosthesis, progressive stump ischemia, deep venous thrombosis, neuroma	Localized	Amputation stump

Adapted from Norgren L, Hiatt WR, Dormandy JA, et al. TASC II Working Group. Inter-Society Consensus for the Management of Peripheral Arterial Disease (TASC II). *J Vasc Surg.* 2007;45 Suppl S :S5-67; and Johansen K. Vascular pain. In: Rutherford RB, ed. *Vascular Surgery.* 6th ed. Philadelphia: WB Saunders; 2005.

of arterial occlusion, this most commonly produces claudication rather than limb-threatening ischemia.

Outflow Disease. Below the inguinal ligament, superficial femoral artery stenosis or occlusion is the most common lesion associated with intermittent claudication. This lesion leads to calf discomfort with ambulation and relief with rest. No specific thigh or foot symptoms are associated with superficial femoral artery occlusion. Because the deep femoral artery provides collateral circulation to and reconstitution of the popliteal artery, isolated superficial femoral artery occlusion without distal disease is rarely the cause of more advanced forms of ischemia. Popliteal and tibial artery occlusions are more commonly associated with limb-threatening ischemia owing to the paucity of collateral vascular pathways beyond these lesions. As isolated lesions, they are usually not the cause of intermittent claudication and are associated with vascular disease in patients with diabetes.

Nonatherosclerotic Causes of Claudication

Intermittent claudication in younger individuals may be caused by popliteal artery entrapment syndrome (see Chapter 111: Nonatheromatous Popliteal Artery Disease) or chronic compartment syndrome (see Chapter 159: Compartment Syndrome). The pain of popliteal entrapment, produced by extrinsic compression of the popliteal artery by the gastrocnemius muscle during leg movement, is similar to that of intermittent claudication and has the same pathophysiologic mechanism as that associated with atherosclerotic lower extremity arterial occlusive disease.[2] Chronic compartment syndrome causes exercise-related discomfort only in the anterolateral aspect of the calf. The cellular basis for the anterior muscle compartment pain associated with chronic compartment syndrome is ischemia resulting from diminution of the muscular arteriovenous pressure differential owing to venous congestion and compartment tissue hypertension.[3]

Critical Limb Ischemia

The natural history of CLI differs significantly from that of claudication. CLI is associated with a high risk of limb loss in the absence of revascularization, whereas claudication rarely progresses to the point of requiring amputation. The common major manifestations of CLI are rest pain and ischemic ulceration or gangrene of the forefoot or toes, representing a reduction in distal tissue perfusion below resting metabolic requirements. The clinical diagnosis is objectively confirmed by a fall in ankle pressure to less than 50 mm Hg, toe pressure to less than 30 mm Hg, or ABI to less than 0.40. Rest pain is often described as burning or as an uncomfortable coldness or paresthesias of sufficient intensity to interfere with sleep. The discomfort is worsened by leg elevation due to loss of the gravitational pull of blood to the foot; it is relieved by placing the limb in a dependent position, such as dangling it off the side of the bed.

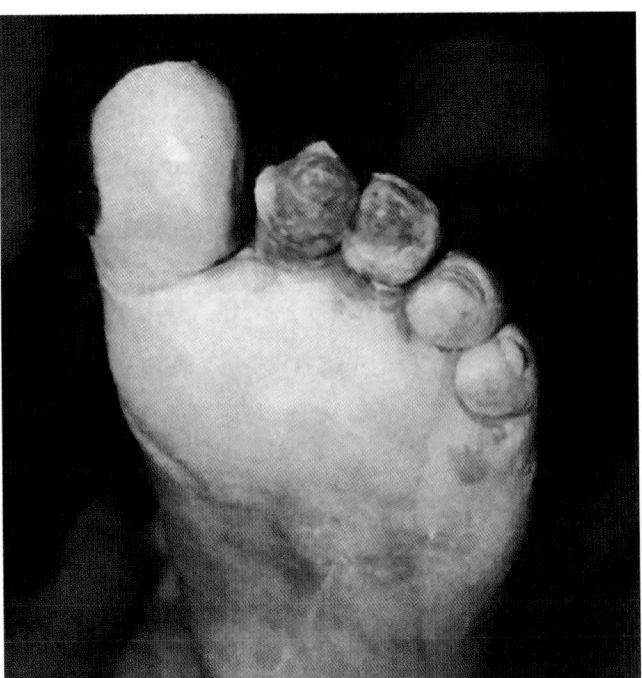

Figure 103-1 Ischemic ulceration of the distal foot.

Ischemic ulcers represent the effect of soft tissue trauma, often very mild in degree, with erosion of the overlying skin. Skin repair is hampered by inadequate tissue perfusion, oxygenation, and cellular replication. Arterial ulceration in a nondiabetic patient is characterized by a shallow, nonhealing, pallid erosion of the skin in the distal foot—in a distribution similar to that of rest pain (Fig. 103-1). The pain of such ulcerations, described as aching or burning, is often unremitting and severe and is occasionally refractory to even high-dose oral narcotic analgesics. It is the result of not only chronic, severe ischemic neuropathy but also actual exposure of the sensory nerves in the skin at the site of the ulcer.

Ischemic gangrene occurs when resting limb blood flow is insufficient to maintain cellular viability. Tissue death inexorably extends to the junction of threshold blood flow for tissue viability. Initially the pain may be severe, resulting from not only ischemic neuropathy but also ischemic injury of the skin and subcutaneous sensory nerves, osteomyelitis, and ascending infection. As the course of ischemic necrosis progresses, pain may actually decrease owing to complete ischemic death of the nerves and other pain-producing tissues.

CLI usually requires the presence of severe arterial occlusive disease at two or more levels, the additive effects of which severely limit flow through collateral beds and result in profound distal ischemia. The pattern of occlusion often affects sequential vascular beds, such as femoropopliteal and infrapopliteal occlusions, but it may affect parallel beds, such as superficial femoral and deep femoral artery occlusions. Both patterns prevent collateralization and reconstitution of the more distal arterial tree.

EPIDEMIOLOGY

The prevalence of PAD has been the subject of numerous investigations over the past several decades.[4-7] Widely varying results have been reported because of methodologic differences in the documentation of this disorder. Many investigators have relied on the presence of symptoms or the assessment of peripheral pulses, whereas others have used data collected from patients referred to vascular clinics. Under- or overestimation of the prevalence of PAD may result from a lack of standardized detection methods or selection bias in the study population. Additionally, prevalence varies with the risk factor profile of the study population. The best method of assessing the percentage of patients with chronic lower extremity arterial occlusive disease is to record the ABI and correlate it with risk factors. The ABI correlates well with the mortality risk associated with PAD, regardless of whether symptoms are present. Although this relationship has been known for more than a decade, it was recently confirmed in a longitudinal study of 3209 subjects followed for 8 years after recording baseline resting and postexercise ABIs. In this study, lower resting ABI values, lower postexercise ABI values, and a greater drop in resting ABI over the study period were associated with a higher incidence of death.[8]

To appropriately establish the prevalence of PAD, the ABI must be obtained in a large, randomly selected segment of the population. In the United States, the most comprehensive effort using such methodology was undertaken in the National Health and Nutrition Examination Survey (NHANES) from 1999 to 2000.[9] This study involved interviewing 9000 individuals aged 40 years or older to obtain demographic and risk factor information. ABIs were recorded for 2381 study subjects, and a complete data set was available for analysis in 2174 participants. The overall prevalence of PAD (defined as an ABI < 0.90) was 4.3% (95% confidence interval [CI], 3.1% to 5.5%). Although there was a slightly higher prevalence in men than in women, the prevalence dramatically increased with age, rising from 0.9% in those younger than 50 years to 14.5% in those 70 years or older (Fig. 103-2). Statistically

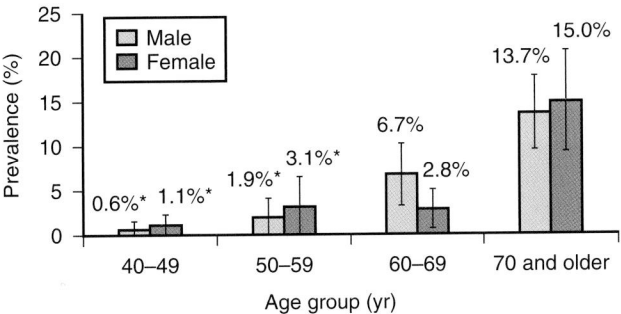

Figure 103-2 Prevalence of peripheral arterial disease by age and gender in adults 40 years and older, United States, 1999–2000 (n = 2174). *(Redrawn from Selvin E, Erlinger TP. Prevalence of and risk factors for peripheral arterial disease in the United States: results from the National Health and Nutrition Examination Survey, 1999-2000. Circulation. 2004;110:738-43.)*

significant associations between PAD and the common risk factors of hypertension, diabetes, hypercholesterolemia, and smoking were also noted.

The relationships of PAD to age, gender, race, and ethnicity have been confirmed by several other studies. In a primary care setting, 403 patients stratified by race and gender were evaluated with ABIs to determine the prevalence of lower extremity arterial occlusive disease.[10] Study subjects included white, African American, and Hispanic women and men. No gender differences were noted, but as with the NHANES data, African American women had a statistically significant greater prevalence of PAD than did white or Hispanic women. A follow-up study using NHANES data from 1999 to 2004 re-evaluated the prevalence of PAD in the general population and ethnic subpopulations. As in the earlier study, a relationship between age and the prevalence of lower extremity arterial occlusive disease, confirmed by ABI, was established. For those aged 60 to 69 years, the prevalence was 7.0% (95% CI, 5.6% to 8.4%); it increased to 12.5% (95% CI, 10.4% to 14.6%) for those 70 to 79 years of age and to 23.2% (95% CI, 19.8% to 26.7%) for individuals 80 years or older. The impact of ethnicity has also been documented.[11] Overall, non-Hispanic black men and women (19.2% prevalence) and Mexican American women (19.3% prevalence) had a higher prevalence of PAD than did non-Hispanic white men and women (15.6% prevalence).

These studies and many others clearly demonstrate that there is a high prevalence of lower extremity PAD in the United States. It is higher in some ethnic subpopulations and in those with uncontrolled risk factors, including hypertension, smoking, hypercholesterolemia, diabetes, and renal failure. Because of its high prevalence and substantial mortality risk, even in the absence of symptoms, the identification and treatment of affected patients are essential.

NATURAL HISTORY
Asymptomatic Disease

Patients with asymptomatic PAD may eventually develop symptoms of claudication or may demonstrate little progression of their disease. The Edinburgh Artery Study found that patients with asymptomatic PAD had no statistically significant drop in ABI over the 5 years of observation.[12] Regardless of whether symptoms are present, individuals with lower extremity PAD, identified by an ABI less than 0.90, have higher morbidity and mortality risks than age-matched controls with normal ABIs. The risks are inversely related to the amount of physical activity the patient undertakes each day. Evaluating the natural history of 460 patients with ABI-proved PAD, investigators noted that reduced physical activity correlated with increased mortality and cardiovascular events.[13] Therefore, patients who attempt to control or eliminate their lower extremity PAD symptoms by reducing their walking efforts actually worsen their risk of myocardial infarction (MI), stroke, and death. This group of patients should be evaluated and treated in the same way as those with intermittent claudication.

Intermittent Claudication

Impact on Extremity

The natural history of intermittent claudication is marked by slow progression to shorter walking distances, but it rarely reaches the level of rest pain and limb-threatening ischemia. This is especially true if risk factors are controlled. Of 224 nondiabetic patients with intermittent claudication followed for 6 years, only 8% of those who stopped smoking progressed to rest pain, whereas 79% of those who continued to smoke developed signs of limb-threatening ischemia.[14] Similarly, in a long-term study of 1244 claudicants, only insulin-requiring diabetes, low initial ABI, and high pack-years of smoking predicted progression to ischemic rest pain and ischemic ulceration.[15] It is far more common for intermittent claudication to remain a disorder that impairs walking than to advance to limb-threatening ischemia. The risk of major amputation is small; over a 5-year period, the rate of amputation was less than 5%.[12]

The limitation of independent mobility and the discomfort imposed by intermittent claudication profoundly impact the patient's quality of life. The Short Form (36) Health Survey (SF-36), a generic quality of life instrument that includes eight domains to assess physical and emotional function, has been used extensively to document the effect of claudication on quality of life.[16] In a study of 68 claudicants, scores in all eight domains were reduced compared with nonclaudicants, especially physical function and role limitations due to emotional impact.[17] These findings were extended in a community-based study of 53 patients with documented intermittent claudication and 327 controls without claudication.[18] Using the Rose Intermittent Claudication Questionnaire and the SF-36, the investigators noted reductions in physical function, role limitations due to physical dysfunction, role limitations due to emotional dysfunction, and changes in bodily pain, energy, and general health perception. Only social function and mental health appeared to be unaffected. The adverse impact of claudication appears to be directly related to walking ability. Limitations on ambulation give rise to broad physical and emotional effects, as documented in a study of 80 claudicants evaluated with the Walking Impairment Questionnaire, SF-36, ABI, and 6-minute walking test.[19] The results of the 6-minute walking test correlated well with quality of life scores. Patients with shorter walking distances during the walking test had worse scores in the physical function and role limitations owing to physical dysfunction subscales of the SF-36.

Association with Systemic Atherosclerosis

The presence of PAD as documented by an ABI less than 0.90 is also a strong marker for the presence of coronary artery and cerebrovascular disease. This relationship was documented in the PAD Awareness, Risk, and Treatment: New Resources for Survival (PARTNERS) study, which assessed 6979 patients aged 70 years or older or aged 50 to 69 years with diabetes or a history of smoking. Symptomatic coronary artery or cerebrovascular disease was identified in 16% of study subjects with an ABI less than 0.90.[20] Multiple large community studies have also confirmed the increased risk of cardiovascular death. The Edinburgh Artery Study evaluated the incidence of cardiovascular events over a 5-year period in 1490 randomly selected volunteers aged 55 to 74 years.[12] In this random sample, there were 73 patients with intermittent claudication and 105 with asymptomatic PAD documented by an ABI less than 0.90 and a further decrease in ABI with hyperemic testing. During the observation period, claudicants and those with asymptomatic reductions in ABI had a statistically significant increase in cardiovascular death compared with normal controls. More recently, the fate of 2777 male claudicants was documented over a 15-year period, and mortality rates of 42% and 65% at 5 and 10 years, respectively, were noted.[21] MI accounted for 66% of the deaths among the 1363 claudicants who died during the study period. The risk of cardiac or cerebrovascular disease increases with lower ABI values, as confirmed by the Atherosclerotic Risk in Communities Study of 13,678 individuals followed for a median of 13.1 years.[22] Thus, the natural histories of asymptomatic PAD and intermittent claudication are similar and marked by a significantly elevated risk of fatal cardiac and cerebrovascular events, despite the rather small risk of progression to limb-threatening peripheral ischemia.

Critical Limb Ischemia

Impact on Extremity

The natural history of CLI is grim, remarkable for the high risk of major amputation and death (Fig. 103-3). Patients with CLI appear to have a more aggressive form of PAD, with involvement of several segments of the lower extremity arterial tree, especially infrapopliteal vessels. Not all patients with

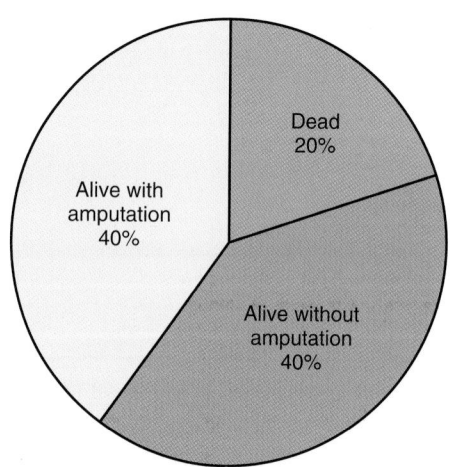

Figure 103-3 Diagrammatic summary of the outcome of patients with critical limb ischemia 6 months after diagnosis. *(Redrawn from Norgren L, Hiatt WR, Dormandy JA, et al. TASC II Working Group. Inter-Society Consensus for the Management of Peripheral Arterial Disease (TASC II). J Vasc Surg. 2007;45:S9A.)*

CLI progress through stages of worsening claudication before advancing to the severely ischemic level. This was clearly demonstrated in a study of 100 consecutive patients presenting with a new onset of CLI.[23] After a careful interview of each patient, investigators noted that 37 had no antecedent symptoms of claudication, and an additional 12 had only a remote history of intermittent claudication and no symptoms at the time of the appearance of CLI. Therefore, interruption of the disease process before the development of CLI is not always possible.

In several studies of patients with CLI due to unreconstructable arterial occlusive disease, the major amputation rate ranged from 14.3% to 46.4%.[24-27] The risk of major amputation appears to be inversely proportional to the ABI, as documented in a prospective study of 56 patients who had symptoms suggestive of stable claudication but significantly reduced toe pressures and ABIs.[28] Over a mean observation period of 31 ± 4 months, 19 patients (34%) deteriorated and developed clear symptoms and signs of CLI. The mean ABI of those who experienced deterioration was 0.38 ± 0.2, compared with 0.44 ± 0.2 in those who remained stable. The relationship between ABI and amputation was also noted in a prospective study of 142 patients harboring 169 severely ischemic limbs with ulceration who could not undergo revascularization.[29] At the end of 1 year, only 15% of patients with an ABI greater than 0.50 required major amputation, whereas 34% of those with an ABI less than 0.50 sustained major limb loss. This abysmal natural history of CLI propels most vascular specialists to attempt to interrupt the course of the disease by improving distal flow to reduce the risk of limb loss.

Association with Systemic Atherosclerosis

As would be expected given the systemic nature of atherosclerosis, severe PAD is often associated with advanced coronary artery and cerebrovascular disease. This results in an exceedingly high mortality from MI and stroke among patients presenting with CLI. A review of major series reporting the fate of patients with CLI by Wolfe and Wyatt noted that 26% died within 1 year of diagnosis.[30] The Trans-Atlantic Inter-Society Consensus Working Group reviewed numerous series and confirmed an overall 1-year mortality rate of 20%.[31] The major cause of death in CLI patients is cardiovascular disease. In a study of 574 patients with CLI, 31.6% of the study subjects had died at the end of the 2-year observation period, the majority from cardiovascular causes.[32] Thus, the symptoms and signs of CLI are clear indicators of severe systemic vascular disease. Without aggressive treatment, a significant number of patients will die from this disease within 1 year, and a significant number of survivors will undergo major amputation.

Clearly, the significant morbidity and mortality associated with chronic lower extremity ischemia, whether manifested by intermittent claudication or limb-threatening ischemia, mandates early diagnosis and aggressive risk factor modification to slow the systemic atherosclerotic process.

■ DIAGNOSIS

History

Health history information should be directed toward the delineation of pertinent symptoms and the presence of atherosclerotic risk factors. This information is valuable not only for documenting the presence of problems but also for following the benefits of treatment at future visits.[33] In the classic presentation of intermittent claudication, the patient experiences calf symptoms ranging from fatigue to aching while walking. These symptoms are alleviated by a brief period of rest. With more proximal levels of arterial occlusion, pain may be felt in the buttocks, thighs, or both. Initially the symptoms are intermittent, interspersed with the ability to walk well beyond the distance at which pain sometimes begins. Patients with CLI generally complain of rest pain localized to the forefoot or toes. It is often intermittent at the onset and associated with elevation of the foot to the level of the heart, as occurs with bed rest. Relief can be achieved by placing the foot in a dependent position. Symptoms of chronic lower extremity ischemia can be well defined through a series of simple questions (Box 103-1).

Precise definition of the symptom complex is helpful in distinguishing vasculogenic claudication from other causes of similar calf discomfort (Table 103-2); however, it does not establish the underlying cause. Several other disorders produce symptoms that may mimic arterial occlusive disease. Of these, perhaps the most challenging to differentiate is peripheral nerve pain from nerve root compression by a herniated disk or osteophytic bone growth encroaching on its exit from the spinal canal. Although spinal stenosis also causes leg pain while standing or walking and can mimic symptoms of intermittent claudication, there are clinical distinctions that may assist the physician in differentiating these two disorders. Neurogenic claudicants frequently complain of diffuse discomfort extending from the buttock to the foot and find relief by walking bent forward to decompress nerve roots. When the pain is too severe to continue walking, patients find relief only by sitting or lying down to

---

Box 103-1 Relevant History for the Evaluation of Intermittent Claudication

- Where is the pain or discomfort located?
- How long do the symptoms last?
- Has the pain worsened or improved with time? Has conservative therapy had an effect?
- How far can the patient walk before (1) experiencing discomfort and (2) being forced to stop?
- How long after stopping exercise is the pain relieved?
- What type of rest or position (standing at rest, sitting, lying) relieves the pain?
- Does the pain return after the same time and distance if exercise is then resumed?

Adapted from Dormandy JA, Rutherford RB. Management of peripheral arterial disease (PAD). TASC Working Group. TransAtlantic Inter-Society Consensus (TASC). *J Vasc Surg.* 2000;31(1 Pt 2):S1-S296.

Table 103-2 Differential Diagnosis of Intermittent Claudication

Condition	Location	Prevalence	Characteristic	Effect of Exercise	Effect of Rest	Effect of Position	Other Characteristics
Calf IC	Calf muscles	3%-5% of adult population	Cramping, aching discomfort	Reproducible onset	Quickly relieved	None	May have atypical limb symptoms on exercise
Thigh and buttock IC	Buttock, hip, thigh	Rare	Cramping, aching discomfort	Reproducible onset	Quickly relieved	None	Impotence May have normal pedal pulses with isolated aortoiliac disease
Foot IC	Foot arch	Rare	Severe pain on exercise	Reproducible onset	Quickly relieved	None	Also may present as numbness
Chronic compartment syndrome	Calf muscles	Rare	Tight, bursting pain	After significant exercise (e.g., jogging)	Subsides very slowly	Relief with elevation	Typically affects heavily muscled athletes
Venous claudication	Entire leg, worse in calf	Rare	Tight, bursting pain	After walking	Subsides slowly	Relief speeded by elevation	History of iliofemoral deep venous thrombosis, signs of venous congestion, edema
Nerve root compression	Radiates down leg	Common	Sharp lancinating pain	Induced by sitting, standing, or walking	Often present at rest	Improved by change in position	History of back problems Worse with sitting Relief when supine or sitting
Symptomatic Baker's cyst	Behind knee, down calf	Rare	Swelling, tenderness	With exercise	Present at rest	None	Not intermittent
Hip arthritis	Lateral hip, thigh	Common	Aching discomfort	After variable degrees of exercise	Not quickly relieved	Improved when not weight bearing	Symptoms variable History of degenerative arthritis
Spinal stenosis	Often bilateral buttocks, posterior leg	Common	Pain and weakness	May mimic IC	Variable relief, but can take a long time to recover	Relief by lumbar spine flexion	Worse with standing and spine extension
Foot/ankle arthritis	Ankle, foot arch	Common	Aching pain	After variable degrees of exercise	Not quickly relieved	May be relieved by not bearing weight	Variable; may relate to activity level and present at rest

IC, intermittent claudication.
Adapted from Norgren L, Hiatt WR, Dormandy JA, et al. TASC II Working Group. Inter-Society Consensus for the Management of Peripheral Arterial Disease (TASC II). *J Vasc Surg.* 2007;45 Suppl S:22A.

further reduce the load on the spine. Claudicants can usually simply stop and stand still until perfusion matches muscle needs and the pain resolves. Careful characterization of the specific pattern of symptom onset and elucidation of factors that provoke, exacerbate, and relieve symptoms can greatly aid the vascular specialist in identifying patients whose problems are the result of arterial occlusive disease. Although atherosclerosis is the most common cause, other forms of arterial pathology may interrupt distal blood flow through luminal narrowing or extrinsic arterial wall compression (Box 103-2).

A comprehensive health history also provides an opportunity to identify significant co-morbid conditions. The physician's initial baseline assessment of a patient with vascular disease is an important step in the identification of overall health, risk factors, and impact of vascular impairment. Only by incorporating all these data into the diagnostic and therapeutic plan can the vascular specialist begin to improve the patient's quality and, perhaps, quantity of life.

Box 103-2 Nonatherosclerotic Causes of Intermittent Claudication

- Thromboangiitis obliterans
- Popliteal aneurysm
- Aortic coarctation
- Fibromuscular dysplasia
- Takayasu's disease
- Pseudoxanthoma elasticum
- Remote trauma or radiation injury
- Thrombosis of persistent sciatic artery
- Peripheral emboli
- Arteritis
- Popliteal entrapment
- Primary vascular tumor
- Adventitial cyst of popliteal artery
- Endofibrosis of external iliac artery (iliac artery syndrome in cyclists)

Modified from Norgren L, Hiatt WR, Dormandy JA, et al. TASC II Working Group. Inter-Society Consensus for the Management of Peripheral Arterial Disease (TASC II). *J Vasc Surg.* 2007;45 Suppl S:22.

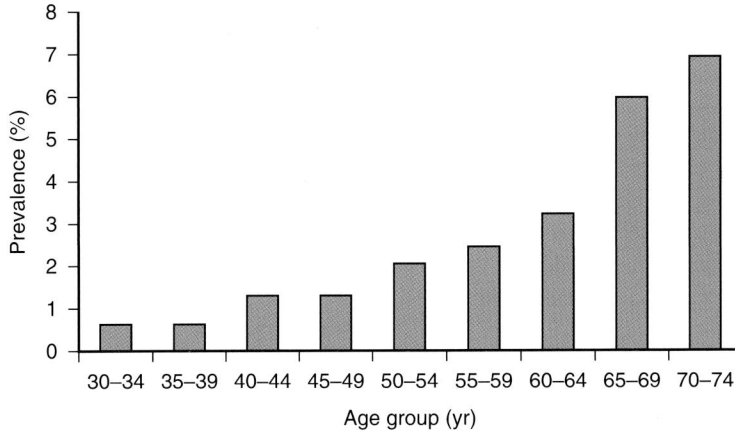

Figure 103-4 Weighted mean prevalence of intermittent claudication (symptomatic peripheral arterial disease) in large population-based studies. *(Redrawn from Norgren L, Hiatt WR, Dormandy JA, et al. TASC II Working Group. Inter-Society Consensus for the Management of Peripheral Arterial Disease (TASC II). J Vasc Surg. 2007;45:S7A.)*

Box 103-3 Risk Factors for Atherosclerosis

- Advanced age
- Race (non-Hispanic blacks)
- Male gender
- Hyperfibrinogenemia
- Diabetes mellitus
- Hyperhomocysteinemia
- Smoking
- Hypercoagulability
- Hypertension
- Elevated C-reactive protein
- Dyslipidemia
- Chronic renal insufficiency

Adapted from Norgren L, Hiatt WR, Dormandy JA, et al. TASC II Working Group. Inter-Society Consensus for the Management of Peripheral Arterial Disease (TASC II). *J Vasc Surg.* 2007;45 Suppl S:S7-S9.

Risk Factor Assessment

Atherosclerosis is a pathologic process related to human aging. There is a stepwise increase in the incidence of intermittent claudication with each passing decade of age (Fig. 103-4). Many other risk factors also seem to accelerate the development and growth of atherosclerotic lesions (Box 103-3). The classic risk factors, including hypertension, diabetes mellitus, and cigarette smoking, as well as other less frequently recognized factors, must be identified and defined during the health history documentation. It is essential to control modifiable risk factors to slow the progression of atherosclerosis and enhance the benefits of any eventual vascular intervention (see Section 3: Atherosclerotic Risk Factors). Hypertension increases the risk of developing symptoms of intermittent claudication 2.5-fold in men and 3.9-fold in women.[34,35] The relationship between diabetes and intermittent claudication has also been well documented.[34-36] When all other variables are controlled, claudication is more common in patients with diabetes than in those without. Similarly, cigarette smoking is a long-established stimulus for atherosclerosis and increases the risk that PAD will develop in men and women.[34,36] The stoichiometry is straightforward: the severity of arterial occlusive disease is proportional to the

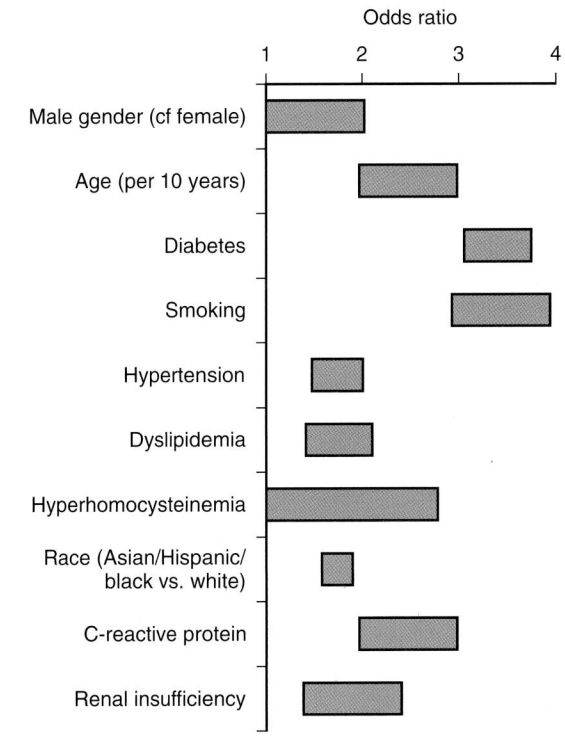

Figure 103-5 Approximate odds ratios for risk factors for symptomatic peripheral arterial disease. *(Redrawn from Norgren L, Hiatt WR, Dormandy JA, Nehler MR, et al. TASC II Working Group. Inter-Society Consensus for the Management of Peripheral Arterial Disease (TASC II). J Vasc Surg. 2007;45:S9A.)*

number of cigarettes smoked.[37] Each additional risk factor independently increases the risk of developing symptomatic PAD (Fig. 103-5).

The absence of commonly recognized risk factors; a sudden symptom onset, especially in younger individuals; or a more rapidly progressive form of PAD should raise suspicion of unrecognized and uncontrolled risk factors for accelerated atherosclerosis, such as hyperhomocysteinemia or hypercoagulability. McCully examined the autopsy results of 194 consecutive patients and correlated the extent of atherosclerosis with serum cholesterol and other risk factors.[38]

Section **15** Lower Extremity Arterial Disease

The mean serum cholesterol of patients who died of complications from arterial occlusive disease was not extremely high (187 mg/dL [4.84 mmol/L]); 65% had a total serum cholesterol level less than 200 mg/dL (5.18 mmol/L), and 92% had a total serum cholesterol level less than 250 mg/dL (6.48 mmol/L). In 66% of patients with severe systemic atherosclerosis, elevated serum cholesterol, hypertension, and diabetes were absent. This study strongly supports the effort to actively search for other, less common risk factors. An elevated homocysteine level, which is often not measured during routine health assessments, may increase the patient's likelihood of developing PAD nearly sevenfold.[39] Hypercoagulable states are more common in patients who require vascular reconstruction for the treatment of lower extremity arterial occlusive disease.[40] Unless these risk factors are identified and controlled, invasive therapies for the treatment of lower extremity arterial occlusive disease are merely palliative and provide no long-term health benefits for patients.

Physical Examination

When the history is completed, a full physical examination should be undertaken. This examination should not be limited to a peripheral pulse assessment because atherosclerosis is a systemic disorder and most often affects many end-organs. The examination should include vital signs, with blood pressure and pulse recorded in both arms. Conjunctivae and sclerae may provide insight into the presence of severe hyperlipidemia, liver dysfunction, or anemia. For a diabetic patient, visual impairment may indicate vascular retinopathy and point toward associated intrinsic renal disease. The presence of thyroid nodules may explain changes in skin texture. Pulmonary examination may further delineate the impact of smoking. A cigarette smoker with repeated episodes of pneumonia over a short span of time may be harboring an occult lung cancer. Palpation of an abdominal aortic aneurysm may explain the sudden onset of symptoms of peripheral ischemia. A neurologic assessment may reveal degenerative disk disease or peripheral neuropathy.

The appearance of the lower extremities provides an indication of the extent and severity of PAD. Loss of skin hair distally, thinning and dry skin, and nail thickening all suggest the presence of chronic, advanced ischemia. Calf, ankle, and pedal edema may indicate a sedentary lifestyle or dependent positioning of the legs to relieve rest pain. Ulcers located on the forefoot and toes are frequently a manifestation of severe PAD, whereas ulcers located in the area of the medial malleolus are more common with venous insufficiency.

The essence of a vascular examination is pulse palpation. Combined with information obtained in the history and other parts of the physical examination, it may help rule in or rule out a vascular cause for the patient's complaints and may help localize the diseased vascular segment. Although palpation of all pulses is essential, when lower extremity arterial occlusive disease is suspected, femoral, popliteal, dorsalis pedis, and posterior tibial pulses should be palpated for a sufficient length of time to determine their presence, strength, and character. Strength of the pulse is generally graded on a scale in which 2 denotes a normal pulse, 1 a diminished pulse, and 0 an absent pulse. A grade of 3 is sometimes used to describe a pathologically prominent pulse, such as the water-hammer pulse of severe aortic insufficiency or the pulse immediately proximal to an acutely occluded vessel. The character of the pulse refers to upstroke, downstroke, and presence of thrills. In stiffened vessels or in vessels with high outflow resistance, the upstroke or radial expansion of the vessel may be slowed. In the presence of low outflow resistance, such as proximal to a traumatic arteriovenous fistula, downstroke may be significantly reduced. Absent pulses suggest a proximal critical stenosis or occlusion. After palpation of the pulses, auscultation permits the detection of bruits, frequent indicators of an adjacent or upstream stenosis.

Correlation of the pulse examination with the history and clinical symptoms often identifies the presence, site, and hemodynamic significance of arterial occlusive lesions.[41] Once a complete history and physical examination have been performed, the physician can choose from a variety of diagnostic studies to confirm the clinical impression if such information will affect patient management.

■ DIAGNOSTIC STUDIES

Hematologic Studies

At initial presentation, a patient with manifestations of PAD should undergo a battery of basic hematologic studies to characterize risk factors and identify end-organ involvement (Box 103-4). The hemoglobin and hematocrit levels yield potential information about blood hemorheology and other forms of distal perfusion inhibitors, such as secondary polycythemia from cardiopulmonary disease. Elevated platelet counts may suggest the risk of thrombotic occlusions. A fasting blood glucose or hemoglobin A_{1c} level is an important test for all patients who initially present with PAD because diabetes is such a significant risk factor for claudication and more advanced forms of ischemia. Increased serum creatinine levels may indicate the presence of intrinsic renal disease, especially in the presence of diabetes.

Box 103-4 Initial Hematologic Evaluation of Claudicants

- Complete blood count, including white blood cells and platelets
- Fasting blood glucose
- Serum creatinine
- Fasting lipid profile
- Urinalysis

Adapted from Dormandy JA, Rutherford RB. Management of peripheral arterial disease (PAD). TASC Working Group. TransAtlantic Inter-Society Consensus (TASC). *J Vasc Surg.* 2000;31(1 Pt 2):S1-S296..

Lipid Profile

A fasting lipid profile, consisting of total cholesterol, high-density lipoprotein, low-density lipoprotein, and triglyceride concentration, is an important part of patient screening and risk stratification. This assessment should be done at the patient's initial presentation for the evaluation of vascular disease. The lipid profile evaluates the possibility that lipid abnormalities underlie the progression of atherosclerosis to claudication or limb-threatening ischemia. Although the impact of elevated cholesterol or low-density lipoproteins on the course of atherosclerosis has thus far been more clearly defined in patients with coronary artery disease than in those with PAD, it is likely that lipids accelerate PAD as well.[42] The impact of diabetes on the progression of atherosclerosis may be worsened in the setting of lipid abnormalities.[43] Careful lipid control may reduce the risk of coronary, cerebral, and peripheral artery morbidity and mortality.[44]

Fibrinogen

The fibrinogen level may be of value in detecting hypercoagulable states. Additionally, this value may be more predictive of cardiac morbidity than cholesterol in patients older than 60 years. When a fibrinogen level cannot be readily obtained, an erythrocyte sedimentation rate can serve as an acceptable surrogate marker. The increased fibrinogen content in the blood causes rouleaux formation and accelerates red blood cell sedimentation. Erythrocyte sedimentation rate is also helpful in assessing the presence of collagen vascular disease, which may be a cause of lower extremity ischemia.

C-Reactive Protein

A C-reactive protein (CRP) level should be obtained to evaluate the patient's inflammatory status. There is an increasing body of evidence that atherosclerosis is an inflammatory process with an elevation in inflammatory markers. Of the many markers that can be easily assayed, CRP has a strong correlation with a reduced ABI. CRP levels were evaluated in 370 patients with an ABI less than 0.90 and compared with levels in 231 patients with an ABI greater than 0.90.[45] Levels of this inflammatory marker were associated with ABI in patients with cardiac and cerebrovascular disease. CRP was not associated with ABI in patients without arterial occlusive disease in these vascular beds (P = .026). Subsequently, the Edinburgh Artery Study reported the results of a longitudinal study conducted over 12 years to evaluate CRP as a predictor of progressive lower extremity arterial occlusive disease.[46] CRP demonstrated a statistically significant inverse correlation with ABI over time. Thus, this easily measured inflammatory marker serves as an indicator not only of worsening lower extremity arterial occlusive disease but also of increased risk of cardiac and cerebrovascular disease.

Box 103-5 Secondary Hematologic Evaluation Based on Clinical Suspicion

- Thrombin, prothrombin times
- Activated partial thromboplastin time
- Protein S, protein C assays
- Factor V Leiden assay
- Lupus anticoagulant assay
- Heparin-induced platelet antibodies
- Platelet adhesiveness, aggregability
- Fibrinogen, plasminogen levels
- Antithrombin III activity
- Anticardiolipin antibody assay

Modified from Dormandy JA, Rutherford RB. Management of peripheral arterial disease (PAD). TASC Working Group. TransAtlantic Inter-Society Consensus (TASC). *J Vasc Surg.* 2000;31(1 Pt 2):S1-S296..

Hypercoagulable States

An evaluation for hypercoagulable states should be undertaken when such a condition is suspected clinically on the basis of prior thrombotic events or a familial history. Despite the plethora of tests available for the specific diagnosis of hypercoagulable states, the best screening test is a carefully performed patient history. Random thrombotic events without a specific cause should raise the suspicion of a clotting disorder. Hypercoagulable states can be identified in a significant proportion of patients with arterial occlusive disease.[40] When such a condition is suspected, a broad range of testing may be required (Box 103-5).

The discovery of protein C deficiency is especially important in patients who will be treated with warfarin (Coumadin); when this drug is administered to patients with low levels of protein C without heparin, the possibility of skin necrosis is increased. Heparin-induced thrombocytopenia is increasingly identified in patients who manifest not only acute thrombotic occlusions but also diffuse distal arterial occlusive disease and accelerated graft failure. This disorder should be suspected in patients who present with a sudden onset of PAD symptoms and no other significant risk factors. The likelihood of heparin-induced platelet aggregation is greater in patients with a decrease in platelet count after the administration of heparin for venous thrombosis or other reasons.

Homocysteine

Patients who develop manifestations of PAD at an early age, without other identifiable risk factors, should have a plasma homocysteine level documented. High levels of homocysteine indicate hyperhomocysteinemia, which may accelerate atherosclerosis through a variety of mechanisms.[47,48] High levels of this amino acid may be toxic to endothelial cells and reduce their ability to generate and release nitric oxide. Excessive concentrations of homocysteine also may promote medial smooth muscle cell proliferation and arterial wall inflammation and increased levels of plasminogen activator inhibitor. As a result, arterial wall atherosclerotic plaque formation may be increased and thromboresistance decreased. Patients with hyperhomocysteinemia may develop clinically apparent vascular disease and coronary artery occlusive disease at a young age in the absence of other risk factors.[49]

The relationship between increased levels of homocysteine and vascular disease in older patients is not as well defined. Taylor and colleagues evaluated homocysteine levels in 214 patients with symptomatic arterial occlusive disease and tracked ABIs over time.[50] They found a more rapid progression of occlusive disease in patients with elevated homocysteine levels, after correction for other variables. Other authors failed to identify a similar impact, however. Valentine and associates performed a case-control study of the impact of lipoprotein, homocysteine, and hypercoagulable states on the presentation of symptomatic arterial occlusive disease in younger men.[51] These investigators found no significant difference in homocysteine levels between men with and without peripheral arterial occlusive disease. In Germany, a study of 6880 primary care patients found only a slightly enhanced degree of arterial occlusive disease, as evidenced by ABI measurements, in patients with high levels of homocysteine compared with patients with low levels.[52] Nonetheless, because treatment of hyperhomocysteinemia with the oral administration of folate and other vitamins and nutrients is relatively simple, many vascular specialists believe that evaluation for this potential cause of accelerated atherogenesis should be undertaken.[53]

Other laboratory tests may be necessary to more clearly define and control risk factors for progressive atherosclerosis. These tests need not be included in the initial evaluation of a patient presenting with lower extremity arterial occlusive disease.

Cardiac and Cerebrovascular Evaluation

The importance of evaluating the extent of cardiac and cerebrovascular disease in patients with manifestations of PAD is being clarified. The systemic nature of atherosclerosis has a significant impact on all vascular beds to a greater or lesser extent. The presence of coronary artery and cerebrovascular disease must be assessed in all patients with a new onset of manifestations of PAD who have not undergone such studies. Indeed, the presence of any form of lower extremity arterial occlusive disease, even if asymptomatic, is associated with an elevated risk of MI and stroke.

Cardiac Disease

Hooi and associates found that asymptomatic patients with even a mild reduction in ABI had a risk of ischemic heart disease equivalent to those with symptoms of claudication.[54] In a study of 66 consecutive patients who had percutaneous interventions for the treatment of symptomatic PAD, Mukherjee and colleagues noted that at the time of discharge and at 6-month evaluation, few patients had control of risk factors for atherosclerosis.[55] Of the 66 patients, 12 experienced MI, stroke, or death within 6 months.

In a study comparing the presence of angina, prior MI, or resting electrocardiogram (ECG) abnormalities in 300 consecutive claudicants with 100 age-matched controls, Sonecha and Delis detected coronary artery disease in 47% of the claudicants but only 6% of controls.[56] Stress ECG detected coronary artery disease in 46% of claudicants and 11% of controls. Of the claudicants who had no symptoms of angina, prior MI, or resting ECG abnormalities, 28% had significant coronary artery disease.

Patients undergoing peripheral vascular surgery are at high risk (>5% likelihood) of having a perioperative MI, and they frequently manifest more than one of the clinical predictors of MI, heart failure, or death (Box 103-6). The evaluation of patients for cardiac disease should be directed toward identifying the presence of disease and determining its severity. This evaluation can be done most effectively in a stepwise manner. The guidelines for patient assessment developed by the American Heart Association and the American College of Cardiology provide a framework for this aspect of patient care.[57] Algorithms for the perioperative management of cardiovascular disease are based on clinical markers, functional capacity, and surgery-specific risk (Fig. 103-6). Resting left ventricular function alone is not a specific indicator of perioperative MI.[58]

Box 103-6 Clinical Predictors of Increased Perioperative Cardiovascular Risk

- Unstable coronary syndromes
  - Unstable or severe angina (CCS class III or IV)*
  - Recent MI†
- Decompensated HF (NYHA functional class IV; worsening or new-onset HF)
- Significant arrhythmias
  - High-grade atrioventricular block
  - Mobitz II atrioventricular block
  - Third-degree atrioventricular block
  - Symptomatic ventricular arrhythmias
  - Supraventricular arrhythmias (including atrial fibrillation) with uncontrolled ventricular rate (HR > 100 beats/minute at rest)
  - Symptomatic bradycardia
  - Newly recognized ventricular tachycardia
- Severe valvular disease
  - Severe aortic stenosis (mean pressure gradient >40 mm Hg, aortic valve area <1.0 cm², or symptomatic)
  - Symptomatic mitral stenosis (progressive dyspnea on exertion, exertional presyncope, or HF)

*May include "stable" angina in patients who are unusually sedentary.
†The American College of Cardiology National Database Library defines a recent MI as one occurring more than 7 days ago but less than or equal to 1 month ago (within 30 days).
CCS, Canadian Cardiovascular Society; HF, heart failure; HR, heart rate; MI, myocardial infarction; NYHA, New York Heart Association.
Adapted from Fleisher LA, Beckman JA, Brown KA, et al. Executive summary. A report of the American College of Cardiology/American Heart Association Task Force on Practice Guidelines [Writing Committee to revise the 2002 Guidelines on Perioperative Cardiovascular Evaluation for Noncardiac Surgery]. *J Am Coll Cardiol.* 2007;50:1707-1732.

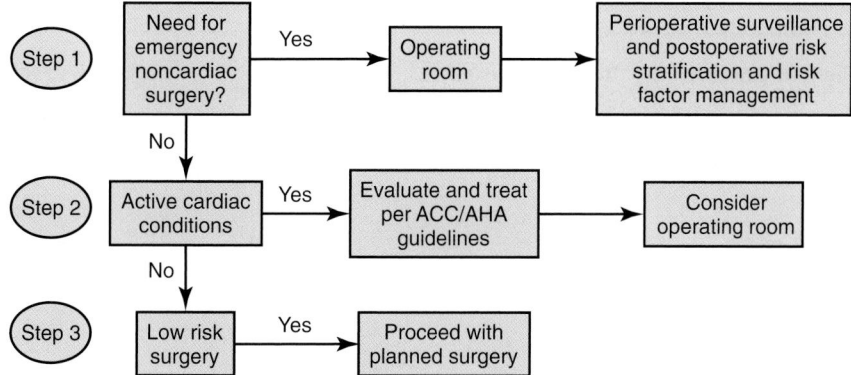

Figure 103-6 Cardiac evaluation for noncardiac surgery based on active clinical conditions, known cardiovascular disease, or cardiac risk factors in patients aged 50 years or older. For clinical risk factors, see Box 103-3. For active clinical conditions, see Box 103-6. ACC/AHA, American College of Cardiology/American Heart Association. *(Redrawn from Fleisher LA, Beckman JA, Brown KA, et al. Executive summary. A report of the American College of Cardiology/American Heart Association Task Force on Practice Guidelines [Writing Committee to revise the 2002 Guidelines on Perioperative Cardiovascular Evaluation for Noncardiac Surgery]. J Am Coll Cardiol. 2007;50:1707-1732.)*

Cerebrovascular Disease

Patients with lower extremity ischemia also have an increased incidence of carotid artery stenosis. In a prospective study of 225 patients undergoing infrainguinal bypass for either claudication or limb threat who were screened for carotid artery disease with duplex imaging, Gentile and colleagues noted hemodynamically significant stenoses in 28.4%.[59] More than 12% had a stenosis of 60% or greater, and 4% had a greater than 80% stenosis requiring surgery. Similarly, De Virgilio and associates noted that 11 of 89 patients (12%) with symptomatic lower extremity arterial occlusive disease who were prospectively screened for carotid artery stenosis had greater than 75% diameter reduction.[60] Patients had no symptoms of cerebrovascular disease at the time of diagnosis. Newly presenting patients or patients with progressive PAD should undergo carotid artery duplex imaging.

Exclusion of Associated Aneurysms

There is a growing body of information that supports screening patients with PAD for the presence of infrarenal abdominal aortic aneurysms. Using B-mode ultrasonography to evaluate the abdominal aortas of 475 patients undergoing assessment of PAD, Wolf and colleagues noted aneurysms of 4 cm or greater in 8.8% of men older than 65 years who smoked, compared with 3.2% in the overall population screened.[61] A subsequent meta-analysis using an aortic diameter greater than 2.5 cm for determining the presence of an aneurysm confirmed that men with PAD had a higher prevalence of aortic aneurysms (odds ratio 2.5) than the general population.[62] More recently, the relationship between aortic aneurysm and arterial occlusive disease was examined in a Swedish study of 5924 patients undergoing duplex imaging for the evaluation of stenoses and aortic aneurysms.[63] The prevalence of aneurysms was 7.3% in men older than 60 years

with occlusive disease of a major artery (carotid, renal, or lower extremity), compared with 4.0% in the absence of such stenoses. Although the aneurysms detected in each of these studies were generally well below the threshold for intervention, the low risk of screening men older than 60 with clinically significant PAD seems to justify doing so.

Vascular Laboratory and Imaging Studies

The decision to recommend surgical or percutaneous intervention for a patient with lower extremity arterial occlusive disease is based on many factors, including symptoms, comorbid conditions, and location and severity of occlusive lesions. In addition, the anatomic pattern of the disease may have a significant impact on the type of procedure that can be used to improve distal perfusion. A clear understanding of the extent of PAD is required before a therapeutic plan can be established.

Vascular Laboratory

Disease Severity. In most patients with lower extremity ischemia, the initial vascular laboratory measurement of segmental arterial pressure and the calculation of ABI are sufficient to identify the presence of arterial occlusive disease and localize the segment involved. Pressures and pressure gradients are not sufficient indicators of patency and occlusion because of the variable presence of calcium within the arterial walls of patients with PAD. A high or even supranormal ABI can be recorded in patients with severe calcific arterial occlusive disease. Pressures and indices must be correlated with pulse volume recording and waveform analysis and, in certain instances, toe pressures to clearly identify and quantify the presence of arterial occlusive disease and indicate the segment

Table 103-3 Stages of Chronic Limb Ischemia

Fontaine Grade	Rutherford Category	Clinical Description	Objective Criteria
0	0	Asymptomatic	Normal treadmill or reactive hyperemia test
	1	Mild Claudication	Completes treadmill exercise*; AP after exercise >50 mm Hg but at least 20 mm Hg lower than resting value
I	2	Moderate Claudication	Between categories 1 and 3
	3	Severe Claudication	Cannot complete standard treadmill exercise*; AP after exercise <50 mm Hg
II[†]	4	Ischemic Rest Pain	Resting AP <40 mm Hg; ankle or metatarsal PVR flat or barely pulsatile; TP <30 mm Hg
III[†]	5	Minor Tissue Loss	Resting AP <60 mm Hg; ankle or metatarsal PVR flat or barely pulsatile; TP <40 mm Hg
	6	Major Tissue Loss[‡§]	Same as 5

*Five minutes at 2 miles per hour on a 12% incline.
[†]Grades II and III correspond to critical limb ischemia.
[‡]Nonhealing ulcer or focal gangrene with diffuse pedal ischemia.
[§]Extending above transmetatarsal level, or foot no longer salvageable.
AP, ankle pressure; PVR, pulse volume recording; TP, toe pressure.
From Rutherford RB, Baker JD, Ernst C, et al. Recommended standards for reports dealing with lower extremity ischemia: revised version. *J Vasc Surg.* 1997;26(3):517-538.

in which the disease is located. For patients with palpable pulses but disproportionately disabling symptoms or those capable of undergoing an exercise therapy program, exercise testing in the vascular laboratory can be helpful.[64]

There are numerous regimens for performing an exercise test. Commonly, after the recording of ankle pressures at rest, a patient walks at 3.5 km/hr on a treadmill at a 12% incline until the onset of claudication-like symptoms. At that time, ankle pressures are measured again. A more than 20% decrease in ankle pressures for more than 3 minutes after the cessation of exercise indicates vascular claudication[65] No decrease or a small decrease in pressure after exercise suggests a nonvascular cause of symptoms, even in the presence of decreased peripheral pulses. Other regimens measure the distance walked per unit time or maximal walking distance. Although each of these methods has proponents, perhaps the most important factor is the use of a consistent methodology to follow patients. The combination of ankle pressure and exercise response can also be used to classify the patient's degree of ischemia (Table 103-3).

Disease Location. Such hemodynamic information is valuable and is generally sufficient for screening, for establishing an exercise therapy program for patients with claudication, and for monitoring the results of peripheral interventions. However, the segmental arterial Doppler study, calculation of ABI, and exercise testing cannot identify the anatomic locations of hemodynamically significant lesions. These modalities are of little direct benefit in planning intervention in either the claudicant or the patient with CLI. Currently, color-guided duplex imaging, gadolinium-enhanced magnetic resonance imaging (MRI), computed tomographic angiography (CTA), and intra-arterial subtraction angiography are the most frequently used imaging modalities for the delineation of arterial anatomy. All these modalities are capable of iden-

tifying the site and severity of infrainguinal arterial occlusive disease, but each has intrinsic limitations.

The improved resolution of duplex imaging has made this diagnostic modality a suitable alternative to contrast angiography in some patients. A significant advantage of this noninvasive modality is that it yields both anatomic and blood flow information, providing an assessment of the hemodynamic effect of arterial occlusive lesions without the use of nephrotoxic contrast agents. Current devices offer significantly improved image quality. Combined with an assessment of peak systolic velocity ratios, duplex imaging can characterize arterial anatomy and detect hemodynamically significant lesions with an accuracy similar to that of conventional contrast angiography. Cossman and associates compared color duplex imaging with contrast angiography in 61 patients.[66] These authors found that duplex imaging had a sensitivity of 99% and a specificity of 87% for the detection of lesions causing greater than 50% stenosis, and it had a sensitivity of 99% and a specificity of 81% for occlusions. These findings were supported by the report of Aly and colleagues, who compared duplex imaging and contrast angiography in 90 patients.[67] These investigators found an overall sensitivity of 92% and a specificity of 99% for the detection of arterial occlusive disease and a sensitivity of 89% and a specificity of 98% for the assessment of lesion length. In 1999, Wain and associates documented that in 41 patients undergoing infrainguinal bypass, color duplex imaging correctly predicted the suitability of the popliteal artery for the distal anastomosis in 90%; however, it identified the appropriate tibial site in only 24%.[68] Ascher and colleagues reviewed their experience with preoperative duplex arterial mapping in 466 patients undergoing distal reconstruction for claudication or limb-threatening ischemia and noted that the study was adequate in all but 36 cases.[69] Additional imaging studies were necessary in the presence of extensive ulcers that prevented an adequate assessment of the underlying vessel, extensive arterial wall calcification, severe edema, and poor runoff.

Arteriography

Conventional contrast intra-arterial subtraction angiography continues to be the most commonly used imaging modality for planning bypass surgery and percutaneous interventions. Complete visualization of the arterial tree is accomplished easily and rapidly. This is especially true of the inflow segments, the infrarenal aorta and iliac arteries, and the renal and visceral vessels, which frequently are not well visualized by duplex imaging.[70] Biplanar angiograms provide detailed information not only in the anteroposterior axis but also in the mediolateral axis to identify eccentric plaques. Hemodynamic measurements are also beneficial in establishing the impact of a stenosis on distal flow.[71] Additionally, when used in conjunction with arterial duplex imaging, selective angiography can be performed, minimizing contrast loads to reduce the likelihood of contrast-induced renal failure in patients with borderline renal function.

Because there is no image loss induced by arterial wall calcium, angiography is complementary to color duplex imaging in patients in whom the distal vasculature cannot be completely evaluated. Angiography is associated with higher morbidity and mortality risks, however, than other imaging modalities. There is an estimated 0.1% risk of a significant reaction to the contrast medium, a 0.16% risk of mortality, and a 0.7% risk of a serious complication adversely affecting planned therapy.[72,73] Angiography should be undertaken in patients with PAD only when the need for and possibility of intervention have been established.

Magnetic Resonance Angiography

Gadolinium-enhanced magnetic resonance angiography (MRA) is gaining acceptance for the evaluation of patients with lower limb ischemia because it can visualize the entire arterial tree, including pedal vessels, without the use of arterial puncture or standard ionic contrast agents. In a study of 24 patients with diabetes and limb-threatening ischemia, Kreitner and colleagues used MRA and intra-arterial digital subtraction angiography to assess the appearance of vessels in the distal calf and foot.[74] The investigators noted that in 38% of the studies, MRA revealed a patent pedal vessel suitable for grafting that was not seen on conventional angiography. This finding led them to conclude that MRA is superior for the visualization of patent distal vessels. Exaggeration of the degree of stenosis within a vessel has been noted, but this can be minimized by using multiple data sets for the evaluation of each vascular segment. Lundin and associates prospectively evaluated 39 patients with symptomatic lower extremity arterial occlusive disease using time-of-flight and contrast-enhanced MRI and digital subtraction angiography.[75] They found that when only time-of-flight information was used to evaluate the vasculature, the sensitivity was 81% and the specificity was 91%, but the degree of stenosis and lesion

length were overestimated. Contrast-enhanced MRI had a sensitivity of 81% and a specificity of 92%. When these images were used in conjunction with the time-of-flight images, accuracy was improved. More recently, a meta-analysis of MRA for the evaluation of lower extremity arterial occlusive disease revealed that gadolinium-enhanced, three-dimensional studies were accurate for the assessment of the abdominal aorta, iliac vessels, and lower extremity and pedal arteries.[76]

MRA is not completely free of patient-related difficulties, however. Patients with newly placed metallic implants are frequently not candidates for exposure to the magnetic field. Others may require sedation because of claustrophobia or difficulty lying flat for a long time. Additionally, although gadolinium is only mildly nephrotoxic, it may adversely affect renal function in patients with preexisting renal insufficiency. In a study of 260 patients undergoing MRA, 195 with chronic renal insufficiency had gadolinium administered for the visualization of distal vessels. Sam and colleagues noted a worsening of renal function in 3.5%.[77] The prestudy creatinine clearance and amount of contrast agent used did not predict which patients would have renal deterioration. More recently, there have been reports of nephrogenic systemic fibrosis related to the administration of gadolinium to patients with a glomerular filtration rate less than 30 mL/min. The incidence may be highest in those with end-stage renal failure who require hemodialysis. The odds ratio for the development of nephrogenic systemic fibrosis in patients with renal failure is 6.671 after a single exposure and 44.5 after multiple exposures.[78] Although this complication is infrequent overall, in view of the large number of gadolinium-enhanced magnetic resonance angiograms performed each year, nephrogenic systemic fibrosis is associated with significant disability and mortality. Therefore, MRA should be incorporated into a thoughtful diagnostic and therapeutic plan to ensure that the potential benefit of the information obtained outweighs the small risk of complication and discomfort.

Computed Tomographic Angiography

With improvements in computed tomography technology, such as the development of the 64-slice multidetector scanner, CTA has become another frequently used imaging modality for viewing even the small distal tibial vessels. The studies are obtained quickly, requiring no more than a few minutes to scan from the proximal abdominal aorta to the feet, which minimizes issues related to patient noncompliance. The three-dimensional reconstruction of images provides the physician not only with views of angiographic quality but also with the ability to rotate images along vertical and horizontal axes to obtain a 360-degree assessment of the vessels. A recent meta-analysis of multidetector CTA for the evaluation of the lower extremity arterial tree confirmed the value of this modality.[79] This analysis revealed that CTA has an overall sensitivity and specificity of 92% and 93%, respectively. These values were slightly higher in vessels above the knee—96% sensitivity and 97% specificity—than in those below the knee—90% sensitivity and 85% specificity. Although the meta-analysis did not discover a statistically significant relationship between the number of detectors and sensitivity and specificity, the best results for sensitivity (96%), specificity (97%), and interobserver variability (kappa = 0.84 to 1.0) were achieved in a study that used a 16-slice scanner.[80]

Despite these excellent results, there are limitations to the widespread use of CTA for the evaluation of lower extremity ischemia. Of major concern is the requirement for an intravenous bolus of more than 100 mL of iodinated contrast in the average adult. This high contrast load limits the use of CTA to patients with normal renal function, unless medical necessity indicates otherwise. Additionally, in the presence of significant amounts of arterial wall calcium, especially in smaller vessels, cross-sectional images must be carefully reviewed and compared with the reconstructed three-dimensional images. Because the reconstruction software chooses the bright-flow surface images, small arteries that are occluded with calcified plaque may be misconstrued as patent.[81,82] Finally, blooming metal artifact may obscure images in patients with metal implants or surgical clips in their legs. Nonetheless, CTA is a valuable imaging modality, especially for patients who are not candidates for MRA because of the presence of a pacemaker or other metallic implant not suitable for the magnetic field, those who are unable to lie in the supine position for long periods, and those with other exclusion criteria.

Imaging Modality Selection

Patients with borderline renal function, especially those who are diabetic, present a special challenge to the vascular specialist. Because of the risks of renal failure associated with iodinated contrast agents and nephrogenic systemic fibrosis induced by gadolinium, the decision to proceed to advanced imaging of lower extremity inflow and outflow vessels for the planning of intervention can be problematic. Improvements in image processing have renewed the interest in carbon dioxide angiography, a modality that can clearly delineate both large, high-flow vessels and smaller, distal vessels (Fig. 103-7). The gas infusion is well tolerated and has no adverse effect on renal function, although it may be difficult to clear in patients with severe chronic obstructive pulmonary disease.[83]

The optimal choice of arterial imaging studies depends on the type of anticipated intervention. Visser and colleagues performed a Markov analysis to determine the best testing strategies for the evaluation of claudicants.[84] Using test sensitivity, incidence and type of complications associated with the test, implications of a missed lesion, and the cost of overtreatment based on test results, the authors evaluated the cost-effectiveness of duplex imaging, MRA, and digital subtraction conventional angiography. They found that if treatment considerations were limited to angioplasty in patients suspected of having suitable lesions, MRA was more cost-effective than conventional angiography. Likewise, digital subtraction angiography proved superior to duplex ultrasound

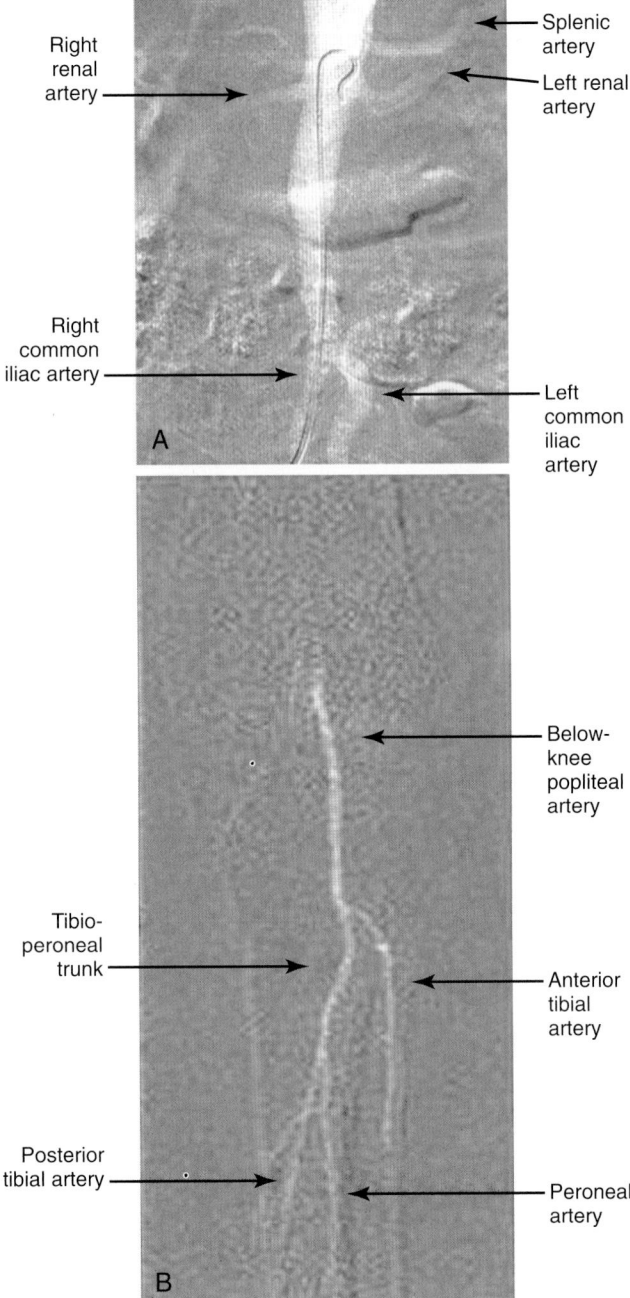

Figure 103-7 Carbon dioxide angiogram demonstrating the detail achievable with current imaging technology in both large vessels, such as the aorta (**A**), and small vessels, such as the tibial arteries (**B**). *(Courtesy of Drs. Andy Park and Richard Messersmith, Department of Radiology, Advocate Lutheran General Hospital, Park Ridge, IL.)*

and MRA if surgery was anticipated. Although the difference in overall cost of these diagnostic modalities was small (<$1800 lifetime costs), the results of the study indicate that the pretreatment evaluation of claudicants is generally simple, and the need for multiple imaging studies is uncommon.

A comprehensive systematic review comparing duplex ultrasound, MRA, and computed tomography for the diagnosis of lower extremity ischemia concluded that contrast-enhanced MRA has better overall accuracy than the other imaging modalities when evaluating the entire arterial segment from abdominal aorta to foot.[85] As noted by Visser and colleagues, this systematic review also confirmed that when a single arterial segment of the leg above or below the knee is to be evaluated, two-dimensional time-of-flight MRI is the most cost-effective study.

Although the vascular specialist has the ability to visualize specific portions of the arterial tree with increasing detail and ease, diagnostic tests beyond the standard vascular laboratory assessment should be reserved for patients in whom a percutaneous or open intervention is planned.

◼ TREATMENT

The decision of when and how to treat intermittent claudication or CLI can be difficult and is the subject of Chapter 104 (Lower Extremity Arterial Disease: Decision Making and Medical Treatment). Nonetheless, in view of the high risk associated with systemic atherosclerosis, all patients should attempt to control cardiovascular risk factors and implement risk-reduction strategies to decrease the risk of MI and stroke.

Antiplatelet Therapy

The mainstay of cardiovascular risk reduction is antiplatelet therapy (see Chapter 34: Antithrombotic Agents). Numerous studies have demonstrated that aspirin in doses ranging from 75 to 325 mg/day significantly lowers the risk of MI and stroke.[86,87] Clopidogrel is a suitable alternative to aspirin for risk reduction. In very high risk patients, a combination of aspirin and clopidogrel may be beneficial. A statistically significant benefit, documented by a reduction in MI, stroke, or death, was noted in patients with symptomatic lower extremity ischemia treated with aspirin and clopidogrel compared with those who received aspirin and placebo.[88] Despite the plethora of evidence supporting the benefit of antiplatelet therapy for the reduction of adverse cardiovascular events in patients with PAD, many remain untreated.

Smoking Cessation

Smoking cessation is also critical for reducing atherosclerotic risk and is central to the medical management of patients with PAD. Smoking is associated with progression of atherosclerosis, an increased incidence of death due to coronary artery disease, and accelerated graft failure after lower extremity revascularization.[89,90] Smoking cessation reduces death from coronary heart disease in both men and women (see Chapter 26: Atherosclerotic Risk Factors: Smoking).[89-91]

Treatment of Hyperlipidemia

The treatment of hyperlipidemia with a statin to achieve a cholesterol level less than 100 mg/dL (2.59 mmol/L) is recommended for all patients with PAD, symptomatic or not, to reduce the risk of MI. This recent recommendation from the Adult Treatment Panel III of the National Cholesterol Education Program is based on the fact that patients with lower extremity ischemia are at high or very high risk for cardiac events (see Chapter 28: Atherosclerotic Risk Factors: Hyperlipidemia).[92]

Treatment of Hypertension

Control of hypertension to achieve a systolic blood pressure less than 140 mm Hg and a diastolic pressure less than 90 mm Hg in nondiabetic, non–renal failure patients should be implemented. β-Adrenergic blockers are an excellent class of drugs for this purpose. Although there has been theoretical concern that a reduction in systolic pressure might worsen symptoms of lower extremity ischemia, this does not appear to occur. A meta-analysis of six major studies addressing this issue concluded that beta blockade does not reduce walking distance or worsen the pain of intermittent claudication.[93] Other drug classes, such as angiotensin-converting enzyme inhibitors, are also of benefit (see Chapter 29: Atherosclerotic Risk Factors: Hypertension).

Treatment of Diabetes and Other Risk Factors

Careful management of diabetes is also essential to reduce the likelihood of adverse cardiovascular events and the progression of PAD (see Chapter 27: Atherosclerotic Risk Factors: Diabetes). Other risk factors, such as dietary indiscretion and inactivity, should be identified and addressed. Each patient with chronic lower extremity ischemia must have a comprehensive treatment plan for the control of risk factors as soon as the diagnosis of PAD is established. Once this is done, the patient will be better prepared for any subsequent intervention that might be required for limb salvage and improvement in walking ability and quality of life.

SELECTED KEY REFERENCES

Dormandy JA, Rutherford RB. Management of peripheral arterial disease (PAD). TASC Working Group. Trans-Atlantic Inter-Society Consensus. *J Vasc Surg.* 2000;31:S1-S296.
Excellent compendium of information and references regarding PAD. Divided into sections on epidemiology, intermittent claudication, acute limb ischemia, and critical limb ischemia, this document is unique in its analysis of the literature, reviewing all major references prior to 1999. It identifies areas of diagnosis and treatment for which there is adequate information and provides clear recommendations.

Fleisher LA, Beckman JA, Brown KA, Calkins H, Chaikof E, Fleischmann KE, Freeman WK, Froehlich JB, Kasper EK, Kersten JR, Riegel B, Robb JF. ACC/AHA. 2007 Guidelines on Perioperative Cardiovascular Evaluation and Care for Noncardiac Surgery: Executive Summary: A Report of the American College of Cardiology/American Heart Association Task Force on Practice Guidelines (Writing Committee to Revise the 2002 Guidelines on Perioperative Cardiovascular Evaluation for Noncardiac Surgery) Developed in Collaboration With the American Society of Echocardiography, American Society of Nuclear Cardiology, Heart Rhythm Society, Society of Cardiovascular Anesthesiologists, Society for Cardiovascular Angiography and Interventions, Society for Vascular Medicine and Biology, and Society for Vascular Surgery. *J Am Coll Cardiol.* 2007;50:1707-1732.

These recent guidelines provide excellent recommendations and algorithms for the assessment and treatment of cardiac disease in patients who require intervention for vascular disease.

Garg P, Tian L, Criqui MH, Ferrucci L, Guralnik JM, Tan J, McDermott MM. Physical activity during daily life and mortality in patients with peripheral arterial disease. *Circulation.* 2006;114:242-248.

This longitudinal epidemiologic study followed 460 patients for more than 4 years to confirm the relationship between higher activity levels and longer life span, underscoring the need to design treatment strategies for PAD patients that permit an increased level of activity.

Hirsch AT, Haskal ZJ, Hertzer NR, Bakal CW, Creager MA, Halperin JL, Hiratzka LF, Murphy WR, Olin JW, Puschett JB, Rosenfield KA, Sacks D, Stanley JC, Taylor Jr LM, White CJ, White J, White RA, Antman EM, Smith SC Jr, Adams CD, Anderson JL, Faxon DP, Fuster V, Gibbons RJ, Hunt SA, Jacobs AK, Nishimura R, Ornato JP, Page RL, Riegel B. American Association for Vascular Surgery; Society for Vascular Surgery; Society for Cardiovascular Angiography and Interventions; Society for Vascular Medicine and Biology; Society of Interventional Radiology; ACC/AHA Task Force on Practice Guidelines Writing Committee to Develop Guidelines for the Management of Patients With Peripheral Arterial Disease; American Association of Cardiovascular and Pulmonary Rehabilitation; National Heart, Lung, and Blood Institute; Society for Vascular Nursing; TransAtlantic Inter-Society Consensus; Vascular Disease Foundation. ACC/AHA 2005 Practice Guidelines for the management of patients with peripheral arterial disease (lower extremity, renal, mesenteric, and abdominal aortic): a collaborative report from the American Association for Vascular Surgery/Society for Vascular Surgery, Society for Cardiovascular Angiography and Interventions, Society for Vascular Medicine and Biology, Society of Interventional Radiology, and the ACC/AHA Task Force on Practice Guidelines (Writing Committee to Develop Guidelines for the Management of Patients With Peripheral Arterial Disease): endorsed by the American Association of Cardiovascular and Pulmonary Rehabilitation; National Heart, Lung, and Blood Institute; Society for Vascular Nursing; TransAtlantic Inter-Society Consensus; and Vascular Disease Foundation. *Circulation.* 2006;113:e463-e654.

These guidelines represent an extension of the original Trans-Atlantic Inter-Society Consensus document. A broader approach is taken, with significant emphasis on atherosclerosis involving the carotid, coronary, and peripheral arteries. This document provides evidence-based recommendations for the diagnosis and treatment of PAD as well as its associated disorders.

Hooi JD, Stoffers HE, Kester AD, Rinkens PE, Kaiser V, van Ree JW, Snotterus JA. Risk factors and cardiovascular diseases associated with asymptomatic peripheral arterial disease. The Limburgh PAOD study. *Scand J Prom Health Care.* 1998;16:177-182.

This longitudinal study established that asymptomatic patients with a reduced ABI have an incidence of cardiovascular disease comparable to those with a reduced ABI and intermittent claudication. This and other similar reports confirmed that the presence of PAD, whether symptomatic or not, is an indicator of systemic atherosclerosis.

Weatherley BD, Nelson JJ, Heiss G, Chambless LE, Sharrett AR, Nieto FJ, Folsom AR, Rosamond WD. The association of the ankle-brachial index with incident coronary heart disease: the Atherosclerotic Risk in Communities (ARIC) study, 1987-2001. *BMC Cardiovasc Disord.* 2007;7:3.

This excellent longitudinal epidemiologic study confirmed the strong relationship between ABI and risk of an adverse cardiovascular event. This and similar studies reinforced the need to comprehensively treat all patients with evidence of PAD, regardless of whether the disease is symptomatic.

REFERENCES

The reference list can be found on the companion Expert Consult Web site at *www.expertconsult.com.*

CHAPTER 104

Lower Extremity Arterial Disease: Decision Making and Medical Treatment

John W. York and Spence M. Taylor

The management of lower extremity peripheral arterial disease (PAD) represents one of the most challenging problems for the vascular specialist. Moreover, as the population ages, a profound increase in the number of patients with lower extremity PAD is inevitable. Lower extremity PAD affects more than 10 million individuals in the United States, including an estimated 4.3% of adults older than 40 years and 14.5% of those older than 70.[1,2] Each year, more than 100,000 of these patients will undergo some form of arterial revascularization. Decisions regarding the management of lower extremity PAD pose a unique challenge owing to the complex interplay of factors that must be considered, including the underlying pathology, anatomic defect, degree of ischemia, co-morbid conditions, functional status, ambulation potential, and suitability of anatomy for successful revascularization. Appropriate management of lower extremity PAD requires a firm understanding of these factors and good decision making.

Patients with lower extremity ischemia are typically divided into two groups—those with intermittent claudication and those with critical limb ischemia (CLI)—depending on symptoms at presentation. Claudication and CLI are managed differently because of major differences in their natural histories and expected clinical outcomes after treatment. In general, there is more consensus among clinicians regarding decision making for CLI because the natural history of untreated CLI more frequently leads to limb loss than does claudication. Appropriate decision making requires a basic understanding of the systemic nature of the disease. Patients with CLI often have severe associated cardiovascular co-morbidities and are generally older and in poorer health than those with claudication. Treatment must therefore be structured accordingly. In contrast, patients with claudication typically seek treatment for the relief of lifestyle-limiting pain with ambulation. These patients exhibit a more benign natural history with respect to limb viability, with amputation rates of 1% to 7% at 5 years and clinical deterioration of the limb in only 25%.[3-5] As with CLI, claudication is a marker of significant systemic atherosclerosis, with associated cardiovascular mortality rates at 1, 5, and 10 years as high as 12%, 42%, and 65%, respectively.[3-5] All patients with PAD require medical management and often benefit from interventional or surgical treatment, as discussed later.

MEDICAL MANAGEMENT

Because atherosclerosis is a systemic disease, the initial treatment of lower extremity PAD should include risk factor modification in an effort to limit progression of the atherosclerotic process. Pharmacologic treatment geared toward the relief of symptoms and the stabilization of existing atherosclerosis is also essential. Patients presenting with PAD are at significantly increased risk for premature cardiovascular events, including myocardial infarction (MI), stroke, and death.[6,7] Detection of occult PAD is an important indirect marker for systemic atherosclerosis.[8] Any patient older than 40 years who is found to have an ankle-brachial index (ABI) of less than 0.90 has significant PAD, even in the absence of symptoms.[9] An ABI of less than 0.90 is 95% sensitive in identifying angiographically confirmed PAD (Fig. 104-1).[10,11] Interestingly, more than 50% of patients with an abnormal ABI fail to show typical symptoms of claudication or CLI owing to the coexistence of other major co-morbidities, a condition sometimes referred to as "chronic subclinical lower extremity ischemia."[12] Risk factor modification is indicated for

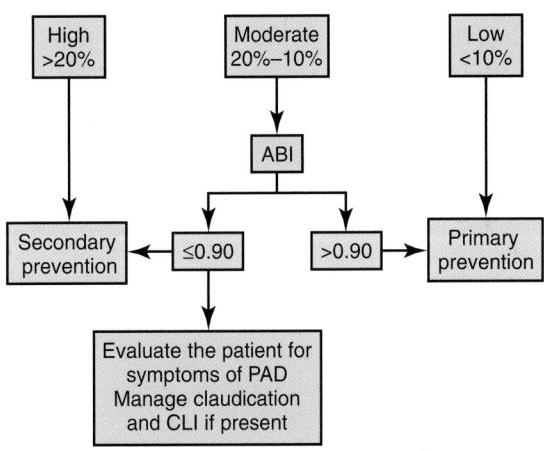

Figure 104-1 Cardiovascular 10-year risk score. Algorithm using the ankle-brachial index (ABI) to assess systemic cardiovascular risk. CLI, critical limb ischemia; PAD, peripheral arterial disease. *(Redrawn from Norgren L, Hiatt WR, Dormandy JA, et al. TASC II Working Group. Inter-Society Consensus for the Management of Peripheral Arterial Disease (TASC II). J Vasc Surg. 2007;45(Suppl S):S5-S61.)*

any patient with significant lower extremity PAD, regardless of symptom presence or severity.

Risk Factor Modification

Other than age—the incidence of PAD increases 1.5- to 2-fold for every decade of life[13-15]—the most common risk factors for the development of PAD include smoking, diabetes mellitus, hypertension, hypercholesterolemia, abnormalities of homocysteine metabolism, elevated serum C-reactive protein, and decreased estrogen levels following menopause (Fig. 104-2).[16] All patients with the diagnosis of PAD require appropriate risk factor modification, regardless of whether more aggressive therapy is also being contemplated. Risk factor modification is discussed in detail in Section 3: Atherosclerotic Risk Factors and is summarized here, given that this is such a key component of PAD treatment.

Smoking

Smoking has been associated with lower extremity ischemia since the early 1900s and arguably remains the most important risk factor for its development. Smoking cessation has been shown to reduce the risk of MI and death in patients with PAD and to delay the progression of lower extremity symptoms from claudication to CLI and limb loss.[17-19] The physiologic effects of smoking are incompletely understood; however, several pathologic processes have been implicated. Nicotine inhalation has been demonstrated to reduce high-density lipoprotein (HDL) levels, increase platelet aggregation, decrease prostacyclin, increase levels of thromboxane, and promote vasoconstriction.[20] Each of these effects contributes to the development and progression of atherosclerotic disease.

Although the beneficial effects of smoking cessation have been clearly demonstrated,[21] the role of smoking cessation in the treatment of intermittent claudication is less clear. Treadmill studies have demonstrated an increase in pain-free ambulation distances in some but not all patients following smoking cessation.[22] Nonetheless, smoking cessation should be the goal in all patients with lower extremity ischemia to reduce their risk of cardiovascular events and limit the progression of lower extremity PAD. The importance of smoking cessation extends to patients who have undergone lower extremity revascularization because there is a threefold increased risk of graft failure in smokers compared with nonsmokers.[23]

The role of the physician is to educate patients about the consequences of this high-risk behavior, provide emotional support, and prescribe pharmacologic aids aimed at treating the addiction. Structured smoking cessation programs have demonstrated a 22% cessation rate at 5 years, compared with 5% in patients who attempt to stop smoking independently.[21] The addition of pharmacologic agents such as bupropion have increased smoking cessation rates in randomized studies of patients with PAD, achieving 3-, 6-, and 12-month abstinence rates of 34%, 27%, and 22%, respectively, compared with 15%, 11%, and 9% in control groups.[23] More recently, varenicline has been approved for use in the United States, with remarkable early results. This pharmacologic agent acts as a partial agonist of the $\alpha_4\beta_2$ nicotine acetylcholine receptor and was developed for the sole purpose of treating tobacco addiction. It stimulates the release of dopamine in sufficient quantities to reduce nicotine craving while minimizing the effects of withdrawal. Randomized studies of varenicline have shown continuous abstinence rates of 44% and 22% at 12 and 52 weeks, respectively, versus 17% and 8% in controls.[24] Despite the promise of these new pharmacologic agents, the prognosis for smoking cessation in most patients continues to be poor. Tobacco addiction tends to be inexorable and is characterized by frequent relapses and poor long-term cessation rates. The best way to prevent tobacco addiction is to avoid initial exposure. (See Chapter 26: Atherosclerotic Risk Factors: Smoking.)

Diabetes Mellitus

The association between diabetes mellitus (DM) and atherosclerotic vascular disease is well documented.[25-28] Diabetes is widely prevalent among patients with lower extremity ischemia. It has been estimated that each incremental 1% increase in glycosylated hemoglobin is associated with a 28% increase in risk for PAD.[10] Atherosclerosis in individuals with DM occurs as a consequence of arterial wall degeneration due to alterations in nitric oxide availability to endothelial cells and the stimulation of proatherogenic activity in vascular smooth muscle cells by the reduction of phosphatidylinositol-3 kinase. Diabetes also alters blood component activity via enhanced platelet aggregation, increased blood viscosity, and elevation of fibrinogen levels.[29]

Whereas the microvascular complications of diabetic retinopathy and nephropathy appear to be a consequence of uncontrolled DM, the effect of intensive blood glucose control on macrovascular complications is unclear. The Diabetes Control and Complications Trial evaluated 1441 patients with type 1 diabetes and compared conventional to intensive insulin therapy. Tighter glucose control regimens

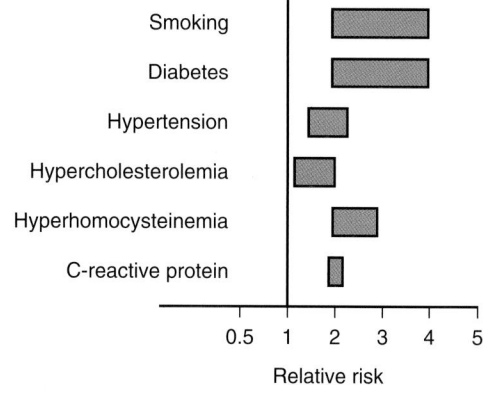

Figure 104-2 Odds ratios for risk factors for symptomatic peripheral arterial disease. *(Redrawn from Norgren L, Hiatt WR, Dormandy JA, et al. TASC II Working Group. Inter-Society Consensus for the Management of Peripheral Arterial Disease (TASC II). J Vasc Surg. 2007;45(Suppl S):S5-S61.)*

exhibited only a non–statistically significant trend toward a reduction in cardiovascular events and had no demonstrable effect on the incidence of PAD.[30] Additional studies have demonstrated similar findings; strict glucose control reduced microvascular complications but failed to significantly decrease macrovascular complications.[31,32] Despite these findings, many experts continue to believe that strict glucose control in PAD patients is important to prevent further atherosclerotic complications. The current American Diabetes Association guidelines recommend hemoglobin A_{1c} levels less than 7% as a treatment goal for all patients with DM. They further suggest that the goal of therapy should be to maintain glucose control as close to normal as possible (hemoglobin A_{1c} <6%) without inducing significant hypoglycemia. (See Chapter 27: Atherosclerotic Risk Factors: Diabetes.)[33]

Hypertension

The Framingham Offspring Study showed, and other studies confirmed, that hypertension is associated with a two- to threefold increased risk of PAD.[34,35] Hypertension is also a risk factor for stroke, coronary artery disease, congestive heart failure, and chronic renal insufficiency. Current guidelines recommend a target blood pressure of less than 140/90 mm Hg in high-risk groups, such as those with documented PAD, and less than 130/80 mm Hg in patients who also have diabetes or renal insufficiency.[36,37]

The specific pharmacologic agent chosen for blood pressure control is less important than the maintenance of a normotensive state.[38] All drugs that are effective at reducing systemic blood pressure decrease the risk of cardiovascular events. Most patients require multiple agents for adequate blood pressure control. Angiotensin-converting enzyme (ACE) inhibitors are particularly beneficial, as shown in the Heart Outcomes Prevention Evaluation (HOPE) study. Patients with adequate blood pressure control using the ACE inhibitor ramipril experienced a reduction in subsequent stroke, MI, and vascular-related mortality.[39] Subgroup analysis of 4046 patients with PAD found a 22% risk reduction in patients randomized to ramipril compared with placebo. This finding was independent of the absolute reduction in blood pressure, leading the Food and Drug Administration (FDA) to approve ACE inhibitors as a cardioprotective drug in high-risk groups. (See Chapter 29: Atherosclerotic Risk Factors: Hypertension.)

Hyperlipidemia

Total serum cholesterol levels greater than 200 mg/dL (5.18 mmol/L) are associated with an increased risk of cardiac-related events, especially in combination with a low HDL fraction (<40 mg/dL [1.04 mmol/L] in men; <50 mg/dL [1.30 mmol/L] in women) and an elevated low-density lipoprotein (LDL) level (>130 mg/dL [3.37 mmol/L]).[40-42] Lipid-lowering agents, specifically 3-hydroxy-3-methylglutaryl coenzyme A (HMG-CoA) reductase inhibitors ("statins"), have been shown to decrease the risk of MI-related death in high-risk patients.[43] The beneficial effects of statin therapy are pleomorphic and appear to be independent of their lipid-lowering properties; they work by stabilizing existing atherosclerotic plaques, decreasing oxidative stress, and reducing vascular inflammation.[44] Statin therapy may also protect against thrombosis by altering the lipid content of platelets, thereby decreasing platelet aggregability.

The direct benefits of statin therapy on cardiac-related events have been demonstrated in multiple well-designed studies.[45-47] Until recently, however, the effects of lipid management on PAD had been studied only in subgroup analyses of larger comprehensive coronary artery disease trials. For example, subgroup analysis of high-risk patients with PAD enrolled in the Heart Protection Study and treated with simvastatin found significant reductions in cardiovascular events (MI, stroke, vascular-related death).[43] Perhaps more significantly, Feringa and associates demonstrated in their cohort study of 1374 patients with lower extremity PAD that intense statin therapy (target LDL levels <70 mg/dL [1.81 mmol/L]) was independently associated with improved survival over a mean follow-up period of 6 years.[48]

The modulation of HDL cholesterol, though less well studied, is also believed to play an important role in hyperlipidemia management in patients with PAD.[42] Well-designed studies have found that adding niacin to conventional statin therapy results in regression of atherosclerotic plaques in patients with femoral artery stenosis and a decrease in the intima or media thickness of carotid artery plaques.[49] These beneficial effects were in addition to a pronounced reduction in progression of coronary artery disease. These PAD-specific benefits occur independently of lipid control. Improvements in leg function, ABI, walking performance, symptoms of claudication, and perioperative and long-term mortality have been demonstrated.[50]

Currently, the American College of Cardiology–American Heart Association (ACC/AHA) guidelines recommend an LDL cholesterol level of less than 100 mg/dL (2.59 mmol/L) in patients with PAD and an even lower level (<70 mg/dL [1.8 mmol/L]) in high-risk patients with more generalized atherosclerosis. In patients with PAD who have elevated triglycerides, precluding the accurate calculation of serum LDL levels, a non-LDL cholesterol level less than 130 mg/dL (3.37 mmol/L) is recommended (Table 104-1). (See Chapter 28: Atherosclerotic Risk Factors: Hyperlipidemia.)[51-54]

Homocysteinemia

The important influence of homocysteine metabolism on premature atherosclerosis was suspected in the 1990s when a distinct group of young patients with advanced atherosclerosis and no other established risk factors was investigated.[55] Plasma levels of homocysteine are regulated in part by B vitamins, and vitamin supplementation lowers plasma homocysteine levels.[56] Thus, low levels of folate and vitamin B_6 are also associated with the risk of PAD, perhaps through the modulation of homocysteine levels.[57] Elevated circulating homocysteine results in endothelial dysfunction and injury, followed

Table 104-1 TASC II Recommendations for Lipid Control in Patients with Peripheral Arterial Disease

Patient Characteristics	Recommendation
Symptomatic PAD	Lower LDL cholesterol level to <100 mg/dL (2.59 mmol/L)
PAD and a history of vascular disease in other beds (e.g., coronary artery disease)	Lower LDL cholesterol level to <70 mg/dL (1.81 mmol/L)
Asymptomatic PAD and no other clinical evidence of cardiovascular disease	Lower LDL cholesterol level to <100 mg/dL (2.59 mmol/L)
Elevated triglyceride levels and LDL cannot be accurately calculated	Measure LDL level directly and treat to achieve values listed above Alternatively, calculate non-HDL cholesterol level, with a goal of <130 mg/dL (3.36 mmol/L); in high-risk patients, the level should be <100 mg/dL (2.59 mmol/L)
All symptomatic PAD	Dietary modification—initial intervention to control abnormal lipid levels Statins—primary agents to lower LDL to reduce risk of cardiovascular events
PAD and abnormal lipid fractions	Consider fibrates, niacin, or both to raise HDL levels and lower triglyceride levels

HDL, high-density lipoprotein; LDL, low-density lipoprotein; PAD, peripheral arterial disease; TASC, Trans-Atlantic Inter-Society Consensus for the Management of Peripheral Arterial Disease.
Adapted from Norgren L, Hiatt WR, Dormandy JA, et al. TASC II Working Group. Inter-Society Consensus for the Management of Peripheral Arterial Disease (TASC II). *J Vasc Surg.* 2007;45(Suppl S):S5-S61.

by platelet activation and thrombus formation. Other effects of hyperhomocysteinemia include the production of hydrogen peroxide, which mediates endothelial injury; increases in factors XII and V; decreases in protein C; and inhibition of thrombomodulin and heparan sulfate. Early studies found elevated homocysteine to be an independent risk factor for coronary artery disease and stroke.[58] More recently, however, studies such as the Vitamin Intervention for Stroke Prevention Trial have questioned the actual impact of abnormal homocysteine metabolism on premature atherosclerosis, failing to show a benefit of high-dose folic acid therapy on stroke prevention.[59] Other randomized controlled trials by Liem and coworkers[60] and Wrone and colleagues[61] failed to show a beneficial impact of folic acid administration on cardiovascular endpoints in patients with stable coronary artery disease and end-stage renal disease.

Despite these recent reports, serologic evaluation for elevated homocysteine levels is still recommended for patients with family histories of multiple thrombotic events, patients with premature cardiovascular symptoms in the absence of conventional risk factors, and selected patients with coronary artery disease, PAD, stroke, deep venous thrombosis, and pulmonary embolism. Supplemental B vitamins or folic acid therapy may be worthwhile; however, level I data showing a benefit in the prevention of cardiovascular disease are lacking (see Chapter 25: Atherosclerotic Risk Factors: General Considerations).[33]

Platelets and Thrombosis

Antiplatelet therapy is now widely accepted among physicians for the treatment of cardiovascular disease, and it has been shown to reduce the risk of nonfatal MI, ischemic stroke, and vascular-related death. It should be used in all patients with PAD. The Antiplatelet Trialists' Collaboration included 102,459 patients with cardiovascular disease (MI, stroke, PAD, or other vascular disease) and concluded that the risk of fatal or nonfatal cardiovascular events in patients treated with antiplatelet therapy was 9.5%, compared with 11.9% in the untreated control group.[62] Subgroup analysis of patients with claudication in this study revealed an 18% to 23% reduction in cardiovascular-related events.

Clopidogrel is the only antiplatelet agent approved by the FDA for the secondary prevention of atherosclerotic vascular disease, including PAD. The primary supporting data were derived from the findings of the Clopidogrel versus Aspirin in Patients at Risk of Ischemic Events (CAPRIE) trial, which randomized more than 19,000 patients with known cardiovascular disease to receive either daily clopidogrel (75 mg) or aspirin (325 mg). Endpoints of stroke, MI, or death were examined. Clopidogrel was associated with an overall 8.7% reduction in the composite endpoint. In a subgroup analysis of 6452 PAD patients, a relative cardiovascular risk reduction of 24% was found in the clopidogrel group compared with the aspirin group. Clopidogrel is well tolerated, with few adverse effects.[63]

A third antiplatelet drug, picotamide, has been studied for the treatment of cardiovascular disease. Picotamide is an inhibitor of thromboxane A_2 synthase and thromboxane-endoperoxide receptors. The Drug Evaluation in Atherosclerotic Vascular Disease in Diabetics (DAVID) study demonstrated that picotamide was more effective than aspirin alone in reducing overall mortality at 24 months in patients with PAD and type 2 diabetes.[64]

Exercise Therapy for Claudication

Multiple reports have clearly demonstrated improvements in pain-free ambulation and overall walking performance with structured exercise training.[5,65-67] Data from more than 20 randomized trials have confirmed that exercise therapy is the best initial treatment of intermittent claudication.[67] The benefits of exercise extend beyond improvement in the symptoms of claudication. Regular aerobic exercise reduces cardiovascular risk by lowering cholesterol and blood pressure and by improving glycemic control. In most patients, claudication initiates a downward spiral of cardiovascular deconditioning that can result in an annual mortality rate as high as 12%.[67] Ambulation distance can decline at a rate of 8.4 m/yr beginning with symptom onset.[68] This cycle can be impressively reversed with exercise training. In a recent report from Japan, Sakamoto and colleagues showed that the implementation of structured exercise resulted in a 5-year cardiovascular event–free survival rate of 80.5% in patients with PAD, compared with 56.7% in untreated matched controls.[69]

Box 104-1 Key Components of a Structured Exercise Program for Claudication

ROLE OF THE PRIMARY CLINICIAN

- Establish the diagnosis of PAD using the ABI or other objective vascular laboratory evaluations.
- Determine that claudication is the major symptom limiting exercise.
- Discuss the risks and benefits of therapeutic alternatives, including pharmacologic, percutaneous, and surgical interventions.
- Initiate systemic atherosclerosis risk modification.
- Perform treadmill stress testing.
- Provide formal referral to a claudication exercise rehabilitation program.

EXERCISE GUIDELINES FOR CLAUDICATION*

- Include warm-up and cool-down periods of 5 to 10 minutes each.

Types of Exercise

- Treadmill or track walking is the most effective exercise for claudication.
- Resistance training may be beneficial for individuals with other forms of cardiovascular disease, and its use (as tolerated) for general fitness is complementary to but not a substitute for walking.

Intensity

- Initially, set the treadmill to a speed and grade that elicits claudication symptoms within 3 to 5 minutes.

- Patients walk at this workload until they experience claudication of moderate severity, at which point they take a brief rest period, either standing or sitting, to permit symptoms to resolve.

Duration

- The exercise-rest-exercise pattern should be repeated throughout the exercise session.
- The initial duration usually consists of 35 minutes of intermittent walking. This should be increased by 5 minutes each session until 50 minutes of intermittent walking can be accomplished.

Frequency

- Perform treadmill or track walking three to five times per week.

ROLE OF DIRECT SUPERVISION

- As walking ability improves, the exercise workload should be increased by modifying the treadmill grade or speed (or both) to ensure the stimulus of claudication pain during the workout.
- As walking ability improves, it is possible that cardiac signs and symptoms (e.g., dysrhythmia, angina, ST-segment depression) may appear. These events should prompt physician re-evaluation.

*These general guidelines should be individualized and based on the results of treadmill stress testing and the patient's clinical status. A full discussion of the exercise precautions for persons with concomitant diseases can be found elsewhere for diabetes (Ruderman N, Devlin JT, Schneider S, Kriska A. *Handbook of Exercise in Diabetes*. Alexandria, VA: American Diabetes Association; 2002), hypertension (ACSM's Guidelines for Exercise Testing and Prescription. In: Franklin BA, ed. Baltimore, MD: Lippincott, Williams & Wilkins; 2000), and coronary artery disease (Guidelines for Cardiac Rehabilitation and Secondary Prevention/American Association of Cardiovascular and Pulmonary Rehabilitation. Champaign, IL: Human Kinetics; 1999).
From Stewart KJ, Hiatt WR, Regensteiner JG, et al. Exercise training for claudication. *N Engl J Med.* 2002;347:1941-1951.

The current ACC/AHA guidelines support supervised exercise for the treatment of intermittent claudication as a level IA recommendation.[70] The guidelines suggest that exercise training, in the form of walking, should be performed for a minimum of 30 to 45 minutes per session, three to four times per week, for a period not less than 12 weeks. During each session, the patient should be encouraged to walk until the limit of lower extremity pain tolerance is reached, followed by a short period of rest until pain relief is obtained, then a return to exercise. This cycle should be followed for the duration of the session. As the pain-free interval of ambulation increases, the level of exercise should be increased (Box 104-1).[65]

Although exercise therapy appears to be easy to implement, effectiveness is often limited by poor patient compliance. Studies have shown the superiority of clinic-based exercise programs over home-based programs.[5] However, effective exercise training is not possible in up to 34% of patients because of co-morbid medical conditions, and an additional 30% of patients simply refuse to participate in exercise training.[71] In addition, supervised exercise training programs are usually not covered by third-party insurance plans, including Medicare. Therefore, even though exercise therapy in motivated patients offers proven benefits, its effec-

tiveness is applicable to only about one third of patients presenting with intermittent claudication.

Pharmacologic Treatment of Claudication

Pharmacologic therapy for intermittent claudication has been the subject of intense research for more than 30 years. To date, only two drugs (pentoxifylline and cilostazol) have achieved FDA approval for the treatment of intermittent claudication in the United States. However, a number of other medications have been investigated, with varying degrees of evidence supporting their efficacy. The following is a survey of the most widely studied pharmacologic agents for symptomatic lower extremity ischemia.

Pentoxifylline

In 1984, pentoxifylline (Trental) became the first drug approved by the FDA for the treatment of intermittent claudication. It is a methylxanthine derivative that is thought to improve oxygen delivery owing to its rheolytic effect on red blood cell wall flexibility and deformability, ultimately reducing blood viscosity. Pentoxifylline is also believed to inhibit platelet aggregation and to increase fibrinogen levels.[72] Early trials of pentoxifylline were promising and showed that maximal treadmill walking distances in patients with claudication were improved by 12% compared with placebo.[73] Although walking distances improved, patient discomfort with walking typically persisted. Porter and coworkers evaluated the efficacy of pentoxifylline in a multicenter double-blinded study and demonstrated modest improvements in pain-free ambulation distance and maximal walking distance after pentoxifylline administration compared with controls.[73] These findings were reproduced in several well-designed studies.[74,75]

Although pentoxifylline has produced a very modest improvement in walking distance in clinical trials of patients with claudication, this improvement appears to be more statistically significant than clinically significant. In clinical practice, some patients experience substantial long-term symptom relief with pentoxifylline, but others do not, and it is impossible to predict patient response without a trial of the drug. Whether these observed improvements are a consequence of a placebo effect is unclear.

Pentoxifylline is well tolerated, safe, and relatively inexpensive. Although its clinical impact has been modest, pentoxifylline represents one of the earliest successful pharmacologic advances for the treatment of claudication. Dosing recommendations for pentoxifylline begin at 400 mg orally three times a day and can be increased as tolerated up to 1800 mg/day. Pentoxifylline can interfere with blood clotting, especially if taken with sodium warfarin. Pentoxifylline has rarely been associated with nausea, headache, anxiety, insomnia, drowsiness, and loss of appetite. Increased blood pressure can occur, so blood pressure should be monitored.[73-75]

Cilostazol

Cilostazol (Pletal) gained FDA approval in 1999 for the treatment of intermittent claudication. Oral administration of this phosphodiesterase III inhibitor increases cyclic adenosine monophosphate (cAMP) and results in a variety of physiologic effects, including the inhibition of smooth muscle cell contraction and platelet aggregation. Cilostazol is also thought to decrease smooth muscle cell proliferation, a process that has been implicated in coronary artery restenosis following percutaneous transluminal angioplasty.[76] Finally, cilostazol has a beneficial effect on plasma lipid concentrations, resulting in a decrease in serum triglycerides and an increase in HDL. Although the precise mechanism by which cilostazol improves the symptoms of intermittent claudication is unknown, it is likely a combination of these effects.

Several controlled clinical trials, including a meta-analysis, have confirmed the efficacy of cilostazol.[74,77,78] Results have shown increased maximal walking distances up to 50%, as well as significant improvements in quality of life (QoL) measures.[77] There is also increasing evidence that cilostazol may modulate the synthesis of vascular endothelial growth factor (VEGF), potentially stimulating angiogenesis in patients with chronic lower extremity ischemia.[79]

The benefits of cilostazol in the treatment of intermittent claudication were compared with those of pentoxifylline in a randomized controlled trial performed by Dawson and associates.[74] They found that cilostazol therapy significantly increased maximal walking distance by 107 m (54% increase), compared with a 64-m improvement in the pentoxifylline group (30% increase). There was no difference in maximal walking distance improvement between the pentoxifylline and placebo groups.

Cilostazol has a moderate but notable adverse-effect profile that includes headache, diarrhea, and gastrointestinal discomfort. Its use is contraindicated in patients with congestive heart failure, and high plasma drug levels may result when taken in combination with other medications metabolized by the liver via the cytochrome-450 pathway.

The adverse effects of cilostazol can be minimized by initiating a progressive treatment regimen, starting at 50 mg/day for 1 week, increasing to 50 mg twice a day the following week, and finally achieving the standard dose of 100 mg twice a day in week 3. Of the pharmacologic agents used to treat claudication, cilostazol has the most data supporting its clinical use.

Naftidrofuryl

Naftidrofuryl is a serotonin antagonist thought to improve aerobic metabolism in ischemic tissue by stimulating the entry of carbohydrate and fat into the Krebs cycle at the mitochondrial level, as well as by promoting peripheral vasodilatation. It has been widely available in Europe for the treatment of claudication for more than 20 years. Several trials have demonstrated a clinical benefit ranging from 15% to 100% improvement in pain-free walking distance, but with no significant effect on maximal walking distance.[80,81] The primary adverse effects of naftidrofuryl include minor gastrointestinal symptoms, flatulence, and abdominal discomfort. Naftidrofuryl is not currently approved for use in the United States.

Levocarnitine

Levocarnitine is a naturally occurring carrier molecule involved in the transport of long-chain fatty acids across the inner mitochondrial membrane. It does not affect blood flow to ischemic tissue, as other agents do; rather, it increases the availability of substrate for energy production at the cellular level of skeletal muscle metabolism. Encouraging results have been demonstrated in patients with claudication; in one study, levocarnitine improved maximal walking distance and pain-free walking distance by 54% when compared with placebo.[82] Carnitine supplements are commonly available without prescription, although dosing recommendations for the treatment of claudication have not been established.

HMG-CoA Reductase Inhibitors (Statins)

As discussed earlier, the benefits of lipid-lowering drugs for patients with PAD include decreased risk of stroke, MI, and cardiac-related deaths. However, statin therapy also improves walking distances in patients with claudication.[83] This beneficial effect was demonstrated in a randomized study in which the pain-free walking time increased 63% in patients treated with 80 mg of atorvastatin versus those receiving placebo (81 seconds versus 39 seconds).[84] However, there was no difference in maximal walking time after 12 months of treatment. The exact mechanism of action is unknown, but it is theorized that statins improve vasomotor blood flow and possibly stimulate angiogenesis.[84] These considerations supplement the already compelling evidence for the use of statin therapy in patients with PAD.

Buflomedil

Buflomedil is a vasoactive drug that has α_1- and α_2-adrenolytic properties causing vasodilatation. It also inhibits platelet aggregation and improves red cell deformability, actions analogous to those of cilostazol. Limited evidence is available regarding the clinical benefits of buflomedil; marginal improvements in pain-free walking distance have been shown in randomized controlled trials, representing an increase of 59% (77 m; 95% confidence interval [CI], 32 to 121). Similarly, a 75% increase in maximal walking distance (113 m; 95% CI, 28 to 198) was seen with buflomedil 600 mg/day in two divided doses versus placebo.[85,86] Further studies are necessary to define the role of buflomedil in the treatment of claudication.

L-Arginine

Arginine is the amino acid precursor of endothelium-derived nitric oxide and indirectly modulates the vasodilatation of vascular smooth muscle. Nitric oxide and its precursors have been the focus of investigation for a variety of ischemic disorders, including claudication. Arginine has been shown to confer only minimal benefit in the treatment of claudication, as evidenced by an increase in pain-free distance without improvement in overall walking distance.[87] A single study of intravenous arginine administration demonstrated increases in pain-free walking distance as well as maximal walking distance; however, achieving similar plasma levels of arginine would be prohibitive with an oral dose equivalent.[88] Owing to its lack of convincing benefit, arginine has not been recommended for the treatment of claudication outside of investigational studies.

Ketanserin

Ketanserin is a selective serotonin (S2) antagonist with vasodilatory properties as well as antiplatelet effects that lower blood viscosity. Unlike other serotonin agonists such as naftidrofuryl, no clinical benefit for this class of drugs has been shown in randomized, double-blinded, placebo-controlled trials performed in Europe.[89] The use of ketanserin in patients receiving diuretics is associated with increased mortality. Currently, data are insufficient to recommend ketanserin for the treatment of intermittent claudication.

Prostaglandins

The primary focus of prostaglandin therapy for PAD has been for the treatment of CLI; however, there is evidence that prostaglandins may also improve symptoms of claudication.[90] The effects of prostaglandin analogues on vasodilatation and platelet aggregation are hypothesized to be of benefit in patients with lower extremity ischemia. Prostaglandin E_1 is the most studied and was shown in one prospective trial to increase maximal walking distance and pain-free interval.[90,91] This trial used an intravenous delivery protocol that is not readily applicable to the general patient population. In this trial, maximal walking distance was increased a median of 28 m after 4 weeks of treatment, compared with a median improvement of 4.5 m in the placebo group. Similarly, the pain-free walking distance was significantly improved in the treatment group (median increase of 19.5 m) compared with the placebo group (median increase of 9 m).[90] Subsequently, an oral preparation of prostaglandin I_2 (beraprost) was studied in a European trial in which 424 patients with intermittent claudication were randomized to receive 40 μg three times a day or placebo for 6 months. There was a significant increase in pain-free walking distance at 6 months in the beraprost group—an average increase of 36 m—compared with the placebo group (81% versus 52.5% increase; P = .001). The treatment group also realized a significant increase in maximal walking distance compared with the placebo group, with a mean increase of 70 m (60% versus 35% increase; P = .004).[92] However, Mohler and associates found no improvement in claudication symptoms in a large randomized study of 762 patients using the same beraprost dose versus placebo.[93] The available data are therefore conflicting with respect to the benefit of prostaglandin therapy. Prostaglandins and their analogues are currently not approved by the FDA for the treatment of claudication. Study of the potential benefit of prostaglandin therapy is ongoing.

Antiplatelet Drugs

Although beneficial overall for patients with PAD, antiplatelet therapy does not improve walking performance in patients with claudication. Currently, there is no evidence to support its use in this capacity. However, antiplatelet therapy is of value in enhancing graft patency after lower extremity revascularization. In the Antiplatelet Trialists' Collaboration meta-analysis of 3000 patients who underwent peripheral artery bypass, patients treated with aspirin had a 16% graft occlusion rate, compared with 25% in the control group (P < .00001).[62] The Dutch Bypass Oral Anticoagulants or Aspirin Study compared the effects of aspirin and warfarin on bypass graft patency (autologous and prosthetic conduit). In this large randomized trial, 2690 patients undergoing infrainguinal bypass, regardless of conduit or indication (claudication versus CLI), were randomized to aspirin 80 mg/day or warfarin total systemic anticoagulation (international normalized ratio 3.0 to 4.5). Although there was no difference in the primary endpoint of bypass patency at 21 months, there was a difference when subgroups were examined according to bypass conduit. Vein graft patency was found to be better with warfarin, whereas prosthetic bypass patency was found to be better with aspirin.[94] Despite the limitations of subgroup analysis, the findings of this trial confirm the efficacy of antiplatelet therapy in the maintenance of prosthetic infrainguinal bypass graft patency. At face value, a recommendation for systemic anticoagulation with warfarin in patients with infrainguinal vein bypass grafts seems justified; however, this recommendation must be weighed against the relative risk of major bleeding, which occurred nearly twice as frequently in anticoagulated patients compared with controls in this trial.

In summary, antiplatelet therapy should be recommended for all patients with PAD. Although there is no evidence supporting its use for the primary treatment of claudication, the benefits of reducing overall cardiovascular events are compelling. Antiplatelet therapy should be initiated before lower extremity revascularization. Trials using different antiplatelet agents in combination are currently under way, with no conclusive evidence to date.

Other Drugs

A wide variety of agents have been employed to treat lower extremity claudication, including defibrotide, ethylenediaminetetraacetic acid (EDTA) chelation, vitamin E, inositol, omega-3 fatty acids, *Ginkgo biloba*, testosterone, and niacinate. None of these substances has any proven clinical benefit, and they cannot be recommended for the treatment of lower extremity PAD.[95]

Intermittent Pneumatic Compression for Claudication

Intermittent pneumatic compression (IPC) in combination with appropriate risk factor modification may be a viable method of treatment for patients with unreconstructable vascular disease or who are physiologically unfit for surgical intervention or those with intermittent claudication who do not want invasive treatment. IPC involves sequential inflation and deflation of pneumatic pressure cuffs positioned at the foot or calf. Inflation-deflation rates vary according to the system used, each applying a pressure up to 120 mm Hg for 2 to 3 seconds before deflating. This sequence is continued at a rate of three cycles per minute throughout the treatment session. The physiologic effects of IPC are thought to be a consequence of three mechanisms: an increase in the arteriovenous pressure gradient, reversal of vasomotor paralysis, and enhanced release of nitric oxide.[96]

Sporadic reports of IPC's favorable effects on lower extremity ischemia date from the 1960s. However, several recently published studies have described the clinical benefit of IPC for the treatment of intermittent claudication and CLI.[96-98] In one of these reports, 48 patients with CLI were randomized to receive IPC plus stringent wound care versus

stringent wound care alone. With a follow-up period of 18 months, the investigators observed limb salvage in 58% of those treated with IPC, compared with 17% receiving stringent wound care alone (*P* < .01).[98] These studies show that although the role of IPC is not completely defined for the treatment of PAD, it may be beneficial in high-risk patients with limited treatment options.

Improvements in limb salvage have also been demonstrated using IPC. Kavros and colleagues examined the effects of IPC on patients with chronic CLI or tissue loss for whom limb revascularization was thought to be impossible. These investigators achieved limb salvage with complete wound healing in 14 of 24 patients (54%) receiving IPC, compared with 4 of 24 patients (17%) who received equivalent wound care but no IPC.[98] This treatment method appears to have significant benefits in patients with CLI when combined with dedicated medical management and wound care, particularly in those with limited revascularization options.

Angiogenesis for Peripheral Arterial Disease

The modulation of growth factors to stimulate angiogenesis is an area of focus in the treatment of lower extremity PAD, particularly in patients who are not candidates for surgical or interventional techniques. Therapeutic angiogenesis is defined as the growth of new blood vessels from preexisting blood vessels to treat ischemic disease. This modality is under clinical investigation for the treatment of both ischemic heart disease and CLI. The putative concept by which angiogenesis improves limb perfusion is the growth of new blood vessels and possible direct stimulation of wound healing by growth factors. Therapeutic angiogenesis can be accomplished by gene therapy or stem cell therapy. Preclinical animal models, such as the rabbit hind limb ischemia model, have clearly shown that angiogenic gene therapy can improve limb perfusion compared with placebo-treated animals. Growth factors act as mitogens that stimulate endothelial cell proliferation in response to local tissue ischemia, but the mechanism has not been completely delineated.[99]

Many different growth factors involved in angiogenesis have been individually tested in clinical trials.[100,101] Because the half-life of the recombinant protein is short, most trials have used gene therapy to allow for a more prolonged expression of the protein. Growth factors that have been studied include various VEGF isoforms, fibroblast growth factor (FGF), hepatocyte growth factor, and the transcription factor hypoxia-inducible factor-1α. Gene therapy has usually been delivered in either a plasmid or an adenovirus via intramuscular injection into the ischemic limb. Although several trials have evaluated the effect of gene therapy on claudication, the major emphasis has been on the CLI patient population. The Therapeutic Angiogenesis with Recombinant Fibroblast Growth Factor-2 for Intermittent Claudication (TRAFFIC) study was the first randomized clinical trial to show a positive effect of growth factor therapy in limb ischemia.[102] In this study, patients with intermittent claudication were treated with 30 μg/kg of recombinant FGF-2 via bilateral femoral artery infusions; both maximal walking time and ABI increased at 90 days. Unfortunately, these encouraging results were offset by the adverse effects of proteinuria and lower extremity edema. Two placebo-controlled, randomized, prospective multicenter trials have been completed in patients with CLI. The Therapeutic Angiogenesis Leg Ischemia Study for the Management of Arteriopathy and Nonhealing Ulcer (TALISMAN) trial demonstrated that intramuscular injection of FGF-1 resulted in a twofold decrease in major amputation compared with placebo.[103] There was no difference in hemodynamics or wound healing between the groups. The Study to Assess the Safety of Intramuscular Injection of Hepatocyte Growth Factor Plasmid to Improve Limb Perfusion in Patients with Critical Limb Ischemia (HGF-STAT) demonstrated a doubling of the transcutaneous oxygen tension ($tcPo_2$) from baseline in the hepatocyte growth factor gene therapy group compared with the placebo group.[104] In that trial, 80% of the gene therapy patients had a $tcPo_2$ greater than 30 mm Hg at the 6-month endpoint, compared with 39% of the placebo-treated patients. Because of the heterogeneous nature of the CLI population, these trials have demonstrated the necessity of incorporating a placebo control arm in the clinical trial design. These trials have also demonstrated that angiogenic gene therapy can improve perfusion in ischemic limbs. Thus far, angiogenic gene therapy has proved to be safe. Potential side effects of gene therapy, such as the progression of diabetic retinopathy or the development of malignancy, have not been observed. There are currently several larger pivotal trials under way to assess the efficacy of angiogenic gene therapy on the clinically relevant endpoint of amputation-free survival.

Stem cell therapy is another developing technique to induce therapeutic angiogenesis. This technique has used bone marrow mononuclear cells or endothelial progenitor cells obtained from bone marrow harvest or, less frequently, from circulating peripheral blood stem cells. Endothelial progenitor cells can be identified by cell sorting for CD34-positive, VEGF receptor-2–positive cells. Once concentrated, the cells can be injected into the ischemic limb to induce angiogenesis. The mechanisms by which stem cell therapy induces angiogenesis are unclear. Tateishi-Yuyama and coworkers, in a randomized prospective trial, showed that injection of bone marrow–derived mononuclear cell injections resulted in a significant increase in ABI and $tcPo_2$ compared with controls.[105]

It is too early to determine what role, if any, therapeutic angiogenesis will have in the future care of patients with vascular disease. Early results from clinical trials are encouraging, but much work needs to be done to determine whether this will prove effective as a stand-alone therapy for patients with ischemic vascular disease or, more likely, it will serve as an adjuvant treatment to current forms of revascularization.

Future Developments

Similar to other fields, such as oncology, the mapping of the human genome promises to advance therapeutic approaches to the treatment of lower extremity PAD. Future decision making will undoubtedly be impacted by these advances. Alternative strategies for the pharmacologic treatment of vascular disease are under investigation. Paramount are strategies aimed at the neovascularization of ischemic tissue and the prevention of intimal hyperplasia. Stem cell transfer and implantation of progenitor bone marrow mononuclear cells are theorized to promote neovascularization.[99] Such therapies may be particularly valuable for the treatment of CLI in patients with physiologic or anatomic contraindications for revascularization. Preliminary findings, to date, are encouraging.

Perhaps the most promising area for substantial progress in the treatment of lower extremity PAD involves gene therapy. Investigations of immune modulation therapy, targeting the inflammatory component of vascular disease in an effort to decrease the development and progression of atherosclerosis and possibly angioplasty-associated intimal hyperplasia, are encouraging. Other areas of research aimed at advancing our understanding of vascular disease include viral-directed gene transfer, targeted antibiotic therapy, and alternative circulating cell–free oxygen delivery vectors.

INTERVENTIONAL AND SURGICAL DECISION MAKING

Patients with lower extremity PAD present with a wide spectrum of symptoms. Patients may be asymptomatic, may experience only minor exertional leg pain, may suffer significant walking impairment, or may present with gangrene. The first critical step in decision making for the treatment of PAD, therefore, is to confirm that PAD is indeed responsible for the patient's symptoms (see Chapter 103: Lower Extremity Arterial Disease: General Considerations). Once the symptom complex is determined to be secondary to PAD, decision making depends on whether the symptoms are from acute or chronic lower extremity ischemia. The following discussion relates to chronic lower extremity ischemia; acute ischemia is discussed in Chapter 157 (Acute Ischemia: Evaluation and Decision Making) and Chapter 158 (Acute Ischemia: Treatment).

Trans-Atlantic Inter-Society Consensus Guidelines

In January 2000, the Trans-Atlantic Inter-Society Consensus for the Management of Peripheral Arterial Disease (TASC) published a document authored by a working group of representatives from 14 surgical vascular, cardiovascular, and radiologic societies.[106] An upgraded document (TASC II) was published in January 2007. These important works compiled and interpreted evidence-based data concerning the treatment of lower extremity PAD and offered a series of treatment recommendations based on presentation. A decision-making summary for the treatment of chronic lower extremity PAD, based on TASC II, is shown in Figure 104-3.[107]

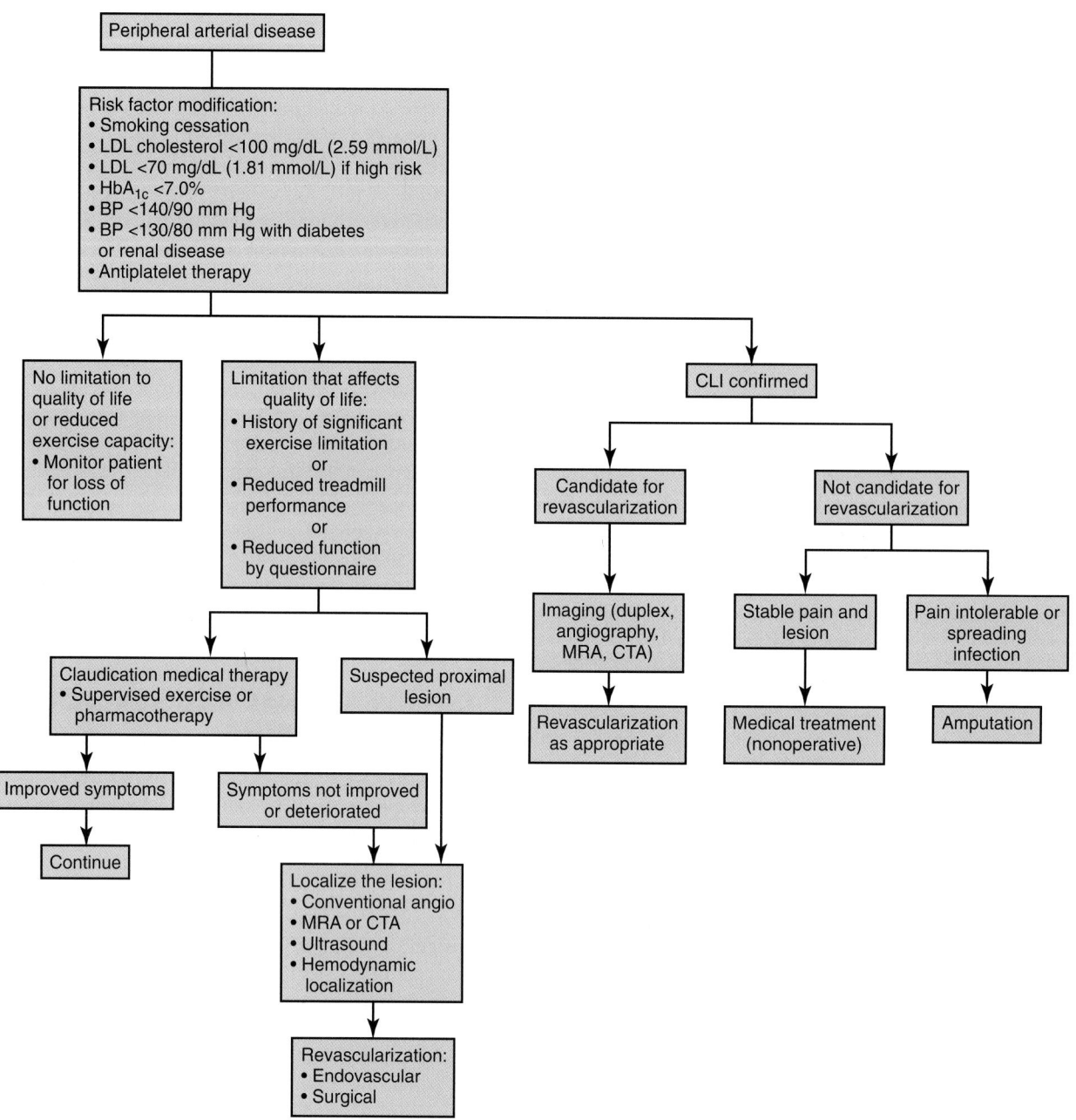

Figure 104-3 Overview of the management of lower extremity peripheral arterial disease according to TASC II. angio, angiography; BP, blood pressure; CLI, critical limb ischemia; CTA, computed tomographic angiography; HbA$_{1c}$, hemoglobin A$_{1c}$; LDL, low-density lipoprotein; MRA, magnetic resonance angiography. *(Redrawn from Norgren L, Hiatt WR, Dormandy JA, et al. TASC II Working Group. Inter-Society Consensus for the Management of Peripheral Arterial Disease (TASC II). J Vasc Surg. 2007;45(Suppl S):S5-S61.)*

Claudication

Traditional treatment recommendations for intermittent claudication have balanced the risk of intervention against the natural history of the disease. It has long been appreciated that claudication is a marker for more serious potential manifestations of systemic atherosclerosis. With the goal of preserving life and limb, experts have decided that the best strategy is to initiate systemic medical therapy aimed at reducing cardiac morbidity. This strategy is based on the low relative risk of limb loss in patients with claudication compared

with the significant relative risk of stroke, MI, and death. The ACC/AHA guidelines suggest that the risk of major limb amputation for a patient with intermittent claudication is approximately 1% per year, whereas the risk of cardiac death is approximately 3% to 5% per year (Fig. 104-4).[70,108,109,110] Treatment strategies have therefore stressed cardiovascular risk factor modification and medical therapy as the best initial treatment for patients with PAD symptoms limited to intermittent claudication. Revascularization is recommended only in cases of severe claudication, and only after medical therapy

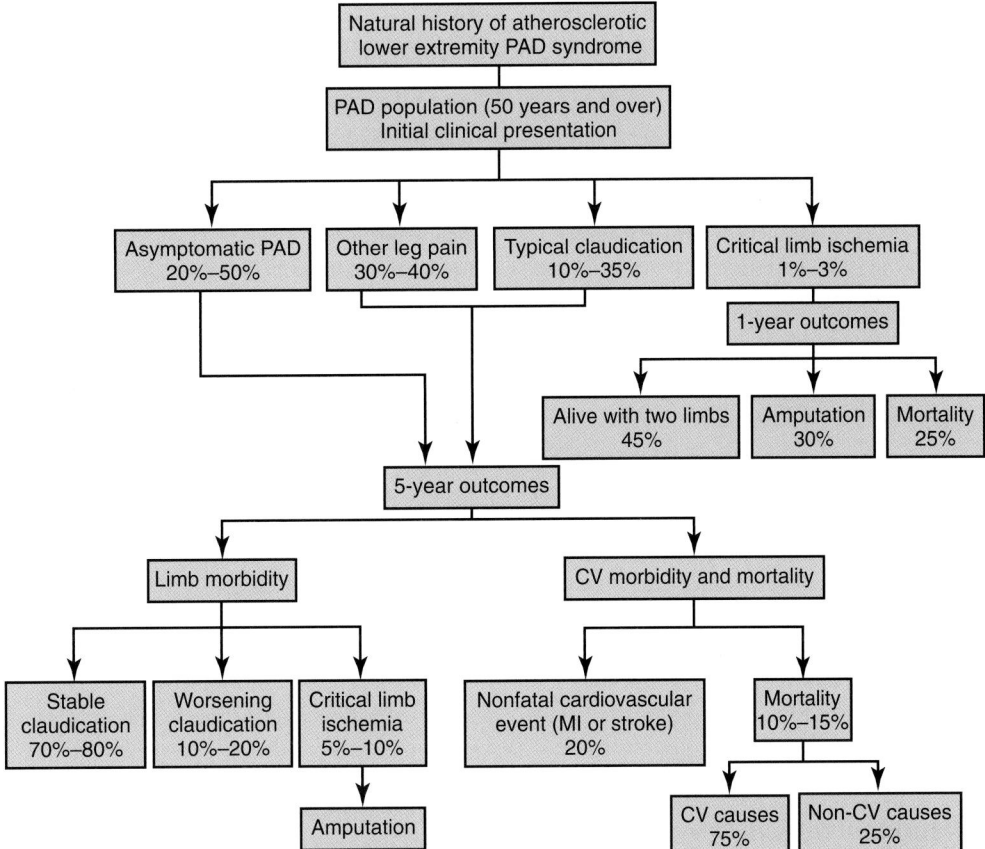

Figure 104-4 Fate of the patient with claudication over 5 years (adapted from American College of Cardiology–American Heart Association guidelines). CV, cardiovascular; MI, myocardial infarction; PAD, peripheral arterial disease. *(Redrawn from Norgren L, Hiatt WR, Dormandy JA, et al. TASC II Working Group. Inter-Society Consensus for the Management of Peripheral Arterial Disease (TASC II). J Vasc Surg. 2007;45(Suppl S):S5-S61.)*

has failed. Medical treatment for intermittent claudication consists of smoking cessation, exercise training, and pharmacologic therapy, as described earlier.

Medical versus Interventional Treatment

The role of smoking cessation in treating the symptoms of claudication is not clear. Although studies have shown that smoking cessation can improve walking distance in some cases, these findings are not universal.[111] The association between tobacco use cessation and the reduction of subsequent cardiovascular events is undisputed, however. The rationale for smoking cessation is therefore based on reducing patient mortality and slowing the overall atherosclerotic disease process.

Currently available pharmacologic agents for claudication have already been discussed (see "Pharmacologic Treatment of Claudication"). The ACC/AHA guidelines recommend, in addition to routine antiplatelet therapy, a therapeutic trial of cilostazol (100 mg two times a day) as an effective method for increasing overall ambulation (class I recommendation). This agent is limited to patients with PAD and intermittent claudication and no history of congestive heart failure, because cilostazol is a phosphodiesterase-3 inhibitor capable of exac-

erbating ventricular dysfunction.[70] Unfortunately, adverse effects prevent the routine use of cilostazol in up to 15% of patients.[74,77] As an alternative to cilostazol, pentoxifylline (400 mg three times a day) may be of benefit in selected patients. Although this drug is well tolerated, data supporting its effectiveness are marginal.

When comparing medical to interventional therapy, there are abundant data supporting the efficacy of medical therapy. For instance, the Edinburgh walking study consisted of a randomized trial to determine outcome differences in patients with intermittent claudication treated with angioplasty and stent versus medical management (daily low-dose aspirin, lifestyle modification) after 2 years. These investigators found no difference in maximal walking distance, treadmill distance until onset of claudication, and QoL measures between the two groups.[112]

Interventional therapy has traditionally been recommended only after all attempts at medical therapy have failed. In large part, this was based on the historical morbidity of open surgical treatment. However, contemporary results of endovascular therapy for intermittent claudication suggest that interventional treatment should have a more prominent role. In a recent series of 669 patients (1000 limbs) with claudication who underwent interventional therapy, Taylor and coworkers found that more than 60% of limbs could be treated using endovascular therapy.[113] Symptomatic relief occurred in 78% of patients, early death occurred in less than 1%, and there were no early limb amputations. Five-year secondary patency was 94%, limb salvage was 99%, and survival was 77%. This modern series demonstrates the potential benefit of endovascular therapy, with its lower morbidity than surgery, for the treatment of claudication. Indeed, endovascular therapy has tipped the risk-to-benefit ratio toward intervention in many cases, especially in the treatment of aortoiliac occlusive disease. The TASC II document recommends percutaneous intervention before extensive exercise training for patients who present with claudication and in whom a proximal lesion is suspected.[114]

In summary, when deciding between medical therapy and revascularization for the treatment of intermittent claudication, the risk-to-benefit ratio favors initial medical therapy in most cases. However, medical therapy may be effective in as few as 30% of patients because of noncompliance and drug intolerance. Modern intervention has become predominantly endovascular owing to its reduced procedural risks compared with open surgery. It is important to recognize the potential of interventional therapy for patients with claudication, especially those in whom a proximal arterial lesion is suspected.

Interventional Treatment versus Open Surgery

Ultimately, the selection of the best method of revascularization for an individual with claudication is based on a balance between the risks of the specific intervention and the degree and durability of improvement that can be expected from the intervention.[115] Because the natural history of vasculogenic claudication is relatively benign, that balance usually does not favor open surgery. In contrast, its relatively low morbidity and mortality make endovascular therapy particularly attractive,[115] and when it is anatomically feasible, endovascular therapy is generally preferred to open surgery for most cases of claudication.[112]

Anatomy is a supremely important consideration when selecting the best interventional modality for patients with claudication as well as those with CLI. Prospective studies dating to the 1980s have characterized the arterial lesions and anatomy most conducive to long-term patency after angioplasty. Johnston and colleagues demonstrated in a prospective analysis that the arterial anatomy and clinical presentation most amenable to long-term patency and success using angioplasty were focal arterial lesions in large-diameter vessels with adequate outflow.[116] Outcomes were more favorable in nondiabetic patients presenting with claudication than in those with CLI. The arterial segment best managed with percutaneous transluminal angioplasty is thus the common iliac artery, a vessel with all the favorable anatomic characteristics identified by Johnston's study. Atherosclerotic lesions in this segment are usually focal and possess good outflow. Angioplasty patency rates at 5 years generally exceed 70%.[113] Conversely, long-segment arterial disease, such as a long superficial femoral artery occlusion, is probably best treated with open

bypass. Diffuse multisegmental disease, more common with CLI, can present a therapeutic dilemma.

TASC Guidelines. Recognizing the importance of the pathologic anatomy for decision making, the TASC working group has classified anatomic patterns of disease involvement (types A through D) for both the aortoiliac (Fig. 104-5) and femoropopliteal (Fig. 104-6) segments, based on recommended treatment (angioplasty versus open surgery). We believe that sufficient evidence exists to recommend angioplasty for TASC type A lesions and open surgery for TASC type D lesions. There is insufficient evidence concerning TASC type B and C lesions to definitively recommend one modality over the other; however, type B lesions are probably best treated with angioplasty, and type C lesions are probably best treated with surgery.[115]

Lower Extremity Grading System. Although the TASC recommendations offer broad treatment guidelines, they fall short of providing the best treatment modality based on outcomes. The Lower Extremity Grading System (LEGS) was proposed in 2002 (Table 104-2).[117] The LEGS score is a standardization tool for the interventional treatment of lower extremity arterial disease; it was created by a group of experienced surgeons using the best available data. We advocate using the LEGS score, which is applicable to patients with either claudication or CLI, once the decision to intervene has been made. The score considers five objective criteria—angiographic pattern of disease, presenting complaints, functional status of the patient, medical co-morbidities, and technical factors—to recommend the most appropriate interventional therapy—angioplasty, open surgery, or major limb amputation. The LEGS score has been studied prospectively, and outcomes in those treated according to and contrary to the LEGS algorithm have been compared retrospectively. Using arterial reconstruction patency, limb salvage, maintenance of ambulation, and maintenance of independent living as endpoints, patients treated according to LEGS had significantly better reconstruction patency, limb salvage, and maintenance of ambulation than those treated contrary to LEGS.[118,119] Although the merits of using this specific algorithm are debatable, the LEGS score speaks to the importance of decision analysis algorithms in general and illustrates the potential to facilitate cost-efficient care by using structured decision-making protocols.

Critical Limb Ischemia

CLI is defined as chronic lower extremity PAD and ischemic rest pain or the ischemic skin changes of nonhealing ulcers and gangrene (see Chapter 103: Lower Extremity Arterial Disease: General Considerations). Typically, symptoms have to be present for more than 2 weeks and associated with an ankle pressure less than 50 mm Hg or a toe pressure less than 30 mm Hg.[112] Although far fewer patients present with CLI than with intermittent claudication, CLI patients consume the vast majority of treatment resources. A surprisingly small

TYPE A LESIONS

- Unilateral or bilateral stenoses of CIA
- Unilateral or bilateral single short (≤3 cm) stenosis of EIA

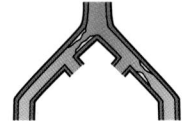

TYPE B LESIONS

- Short (≤3 cm) stenosis of infrarenal aorta
- Unilateral CIA occlusion
- Single or multiple stenoses totaling 3–10 cm involving the EIA not extending into the CFA
- Unilateral EIA occlusion not involving the origins of internal iliac or CFA

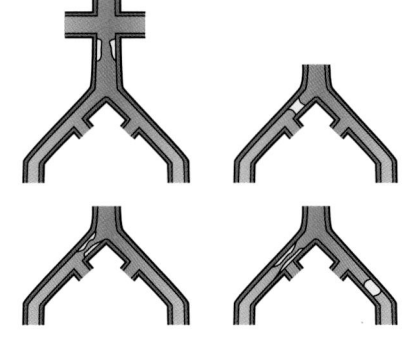

TYPE C LESIONS

- Bilateral CIA occlusions
- Bilateral EIA stenoses 3–10 cm long not extending into the CFA
- Unilateral EIA stenosis extending into the CFA
- Unilateral EIA occlusion that involves the origins of internal iliac and/or CFA
- Heavily calcified unilateral EIA occlusion with or without involvement of origins of internal iliac and/or CFA

TYPE D LESIONS

- Infrarenal aortoiliac occlusion
- Diffuse disease involving the aorta and both iliac arteries requiring treatment
- Diffuse multiple stenoses involving the unilateral CIA, EIA, and CFA
- Unilateral occlusions of both CIA and EIA
- Bilateral occlusions of EIA
- Iliac stenoses in patients with AAA requiring treatment and not amenable to endograft placement or other lesions requiring open aortic or iliac surgery

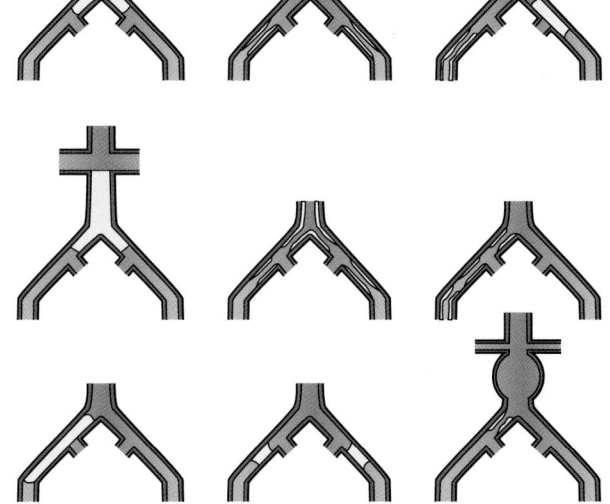

Figure 104-5 TASC classification of aortoiliac lesions. AAA, abdominal aortic aneurysm; CFA, common femoral artery; CIA, common iliac artery; EIA, external iliac artery. *(Redrawn from Norgren L, Hiatt WR, Dormandy JA, et al. TASC II Working Group. Inter-Society Consensus for the Management of Peripheral Arterial Disease (TASC II). J Vasc Surg. 2007;45(Suppl S):S5-S61.)*

fraction of patients (<5%) with intermittent claudication progress to CLI. Patients with "chronic subclinical ischemia"—those with low perfusion and ankle pressures but who are asymptomatic for a variety of reasons—are also at risk for the development of limb ischemia.[112]

Prognosis for CLI is considerably worse than for intermittent claudication; as many as 25% of CLI patients progress to major limb amputation within 1 year, and 25% die of cardiovascular complications within 1 year.[117] Decision making for CLI commonly poses three dilemmas: whether to treat medically or with intervention; if treating with intervention, whether to amputate or revascularize; and if revascularizing, whether to employ balloon angioplasty or open surgery.

Medical versus Interventional Treatment

The natural history of untreated CLI is poorly understood because most functional patients receive some type of revas-

cularization. However, limb loss and cardiac death are common. One-year mortality ranges from 20% to 30%, with cardiac deaths outnumbering noncardiac deaths four to one.[120] The best information regarding the natural history of nonrevascularized limbs in patients with CLI comes from the placebo arms of pharmacotherapy trials of patients with unreconstructable vascular disease. Results suggest that this subgroup has a dismal prognosis, with nearly 40% of limbs progressing to amputation at 6 months.[121] Therefore, in functional patients, some type of revascularization is almost always preferable to medical therapy.

Medical therapy for CLI is not without some noteworthy successes, however. Indeed, wound care centers have become common adjuncts to many vascular surgical practices (see Chapter 81: Wound Care). Ischemic ulcer healing rates of 55% have been reported from dedicated centers using modern wound care methods such as negative-pressure wound therapy,

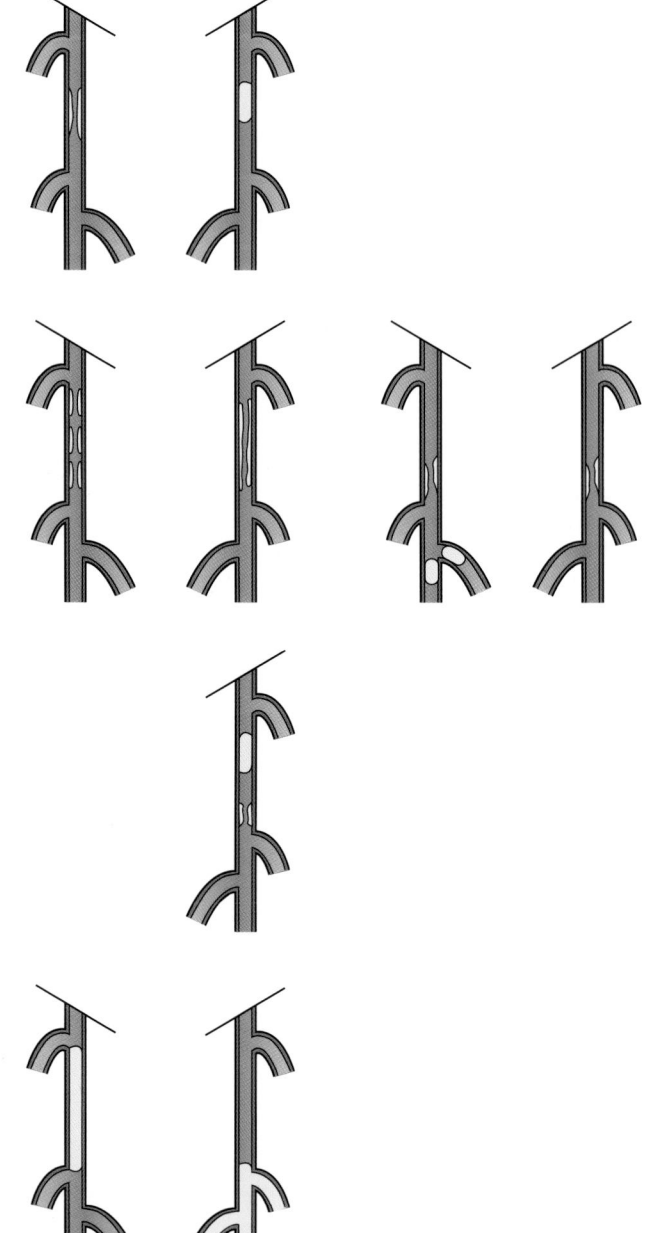

TYPE A LESIONS

- Single stenosis ≤10 cm in length
- Single occlusion ≤5 cm in length

TYPE B LESIONS

- Multiple lesions (stenoses or occlusions), each ≤5 cm
- Single stenosis or occlusion ≤15 cm not involving the infrageniculate popliteal artery
- Single or multiple lesions in the absence of continuous tibial vessels to improve inflow for a distal bypass
- Heavily calcified occlusion ≤5 cm in length
- Single popliteal stenosis

TYPE C LESIONS

- Multiple stenoses or occlusions totaling >15 cm with or without heavy calcification
- Recurrent stenoses or occlusions that need treatment after two endovascular interventions

TYPE D LESIONS

- Chronic total occlusions of CFA or SFA (>20 cm, involving the popliteal artery)
- Chronic total occlusion of popliteal artery and proximal trifurcation vessels

Figure 104-6 TASC classification of femoropopliteal lesions. CFA, common femoral artery; SFA, superficial femoral artery. *(Redrawn from Norgren L, Hiatt WR, Dormandy JA, et al. TASC II Working Group. Inter-Society Consensus for the Management of Peripheral Arterial Disease (TASC II). J Vasc Surg. 2007;45(Suppl S):S5-S61.)*

intense débridement, and antibiotic therapy.[122] However, wound healing in such situations is often a slow, laborious, and unpredictable process. To date, pharmacotherapy for CLI has failed to yield any breakthrough therapy. The routine use of prostanoids, vasodilators, antiplatelet agents, and even hyperbaric oxygen for the treatment of ischemic ulcers remains of unproven benefit.[122]

In summary, revascularization is an essential component in the relief of CLI. Although medical adjuncts geared at risk factor modification may be important to slow the progression of systemic atherosclerotic disease, they play a secondary role

in the treatment of the ischemic limb. In those rare cases in which vascular disease is truly unreconstructable, a trial of intensive wound care, preferably at a wound care center, may yield satisfactory healing rates for motivated patients with superficial ulcerations, or it may avoid major limb amputation in high-risk patients who are approaching the end of life.

Limb Amputation versus Revascularization

For the overwhelming majority of patients with CLI, revascularization is the interventional treatment of choice.

Table 104-2 Lower Extremity Grading System (LEGS) Score

Arteriographic Findings	Score	Presentation	Score	Functional Status	Score	Co-morbidities	Score	Technical Factors	Score
Aortic		Claudication	5	Ambulatory	0	Obesity	2	All cases	
<3 cm aortic stenosis/ occlusion or 3 to 5 cm stenosis of aortoiliac bifurcation	8							"Redo" surgery	2
>3 cm aortic stenosis/ occlusion or >5 cm stenosis of aortoiliac bifurcation	0	Limb-threatening ischemia	2	Ambulatory at home only	2	High-risk coronary artery disease	3	"Redo" angioplasty	−2
Iliac				Nonambulatory/ transfer only	5	Age >70 yr	1	Infrainguinal cases	
TASC type A or B	8			Nonambulatory	20	Age >80 yr	2	Blind segment target	2
TASC type C	2							No venous conduit	6
TASC type D	0							No vein with foot infection	8
Femoral-popliteal-tibial									
<5-cm occlusion/ stenosis	5								
>5-cm occlusion with distal target	0								
Isolated common or deep femoral stenosis	0								
>5-cm occlusion without distal target	6								
Possible score	**0-8**	**Possible score**	**2 to 5**	**Possible score**	**0 to 20**	**Possible score**	**0 to 7**	**Possible score**	**−2 to 12**

Recommended Treatment

Sum of total score from each column:*
  0 to 9 = open surgery
  10 to 19 = endovascular treatment
  ≥20 = primary amputation

*If a heel ulcer and end-stage renal disease are present, double the score.
TASC, Trans-Atlantic Inter-Society Consensus.
Adapted from Kalbaugh CA, Taylor SM, Cull DL, et al. Invasive treatment of chronic limb ischemia according to the Lower Extremity Grading System (LEGS) score: a 6-month report. *J Vasc Surg.* 2004;39:1268-1276.

However, primary limb amputation continues to be required in 10% to 40% of CLI patients owing to overwhelming infection or unreconstructable vascular disease.[123] Unreconstructable vascular disease accounts for nearly 60% of patients requiring secondary amputation.[122] In many of these cases, revascularization has failed owing to progression of disease, recurrent ischemia, or persistent infection or necrosis despite a patent revascularization.

Though counterintuitive, limb amputation and prosthetic rehabilitation can be an excellent option, offering an expedient return to a useful QoL in selected cases. Maintenance of ambulation can exceed 70%, and maintenance of independence can exceed 90% in young, good-risk patients after below-knee amputation.[124] Clearly, amputation should be considered a tool capable of extending functionality and not a failure of treatment in these cases. If there is the potential for some degree of rehabilitation, the limb amputation should be performed at the lowest possible level at which healing can be expected, because the work of walking increases dramatically as the level of amputation becomes more proximal. Typically, patients with well-controlled medical co-morbidities, a pal-

pable femoral pulse, a warm calf, and no signs of infection are likely to heal after a below-knee amputation (see Chapter 115: Lower Extremity Amputation: Techniques and Results).

Patients too sick or infirm to realize the benefit of limb revascularization should undergo palliative primary above-knee amputation. However, judging patients "too sick or infirm" can be difficult. Obviously, a nonambulatory elderly nursing-home patient with knee contractures and neuropathic heel ulcers would qualify for a palliative above-knee amputation. Patients who are minimally ambulatory and who have multiple medical co-morbidities pose a particularly difficult clinical dilemma. Judgment is required to determine whether these patients will be better served by primary amputation or limb revascularization. In a recent single-institution study of 1000 consecutive revascularizations for CLI, the patient's preoperative functional performance status was the most important predictor of postoperative functional outcome—even more important than limb salvage itself.[125] This finding strongly suggests that there is a definite subset of patients who are too sick or debilitated to realize the functional benefits of revascularization. Although more work is needed to better define such patients, this cohort is likely best suited for primary amputation.

With these caveats, revascularization remains the cornerstone of treatment for CLI. The aforementioned series of 1000 consecutive limbs typifies the modern results achievable through aggressive revascularization; the reported 5-year limb salvage rate was 72%, maintenance of ambulation was 71%, maintenance of independence was 81%, and survival was 46%.[125]

Interventional Treatment versus Open Surgery

For many years, the classic treatment approach for CLI has been open surgery. CLI is usually associated with multilevel arterial disease that is not ideally suited to percutaneous intervention. Diffuse, extensive PAD causing CLI in both aortoiliac and femoropopliteal locations (see Figs. 104-5 and 104-6) is best treated by surgical bypass according to TASC.[126] However, the primacy of surgical bypass for CLI management has been challenged in recent years and has become the subject of intense debate. Those who favor open surgery for the treatment of CLI often cite superior reconstruction patency and increased durability.[127-129] However, open surgery is usually associated with higher perioperative morbidity and longer hospitalization (Table 104-3).[130] Expensive and tedious long-term postoperative graft surveillance is necessary to maintain a patent infrainguinal bypass, although well-performed studies in both Europe and North America suggest that such surveillance is economically justified by preventing vein graft occlusion and late amputation.[131,132] A re-intervention rate of 20% to 30% to treat failing grafts due to intrinsic vein graft stenoses is usually necessary to maintain the increased durability attributed to open surgery.[131,133] Last, successful surgery depends on the presence of a suitable venous conduit for bypass.[134,135] Those who favor interventional treatment cite the low morbidity and mortality associated with a procedure that is usually performed on an outpatient basis.[136] Though proponents acknowledge the limited reconstruction patency rates associated with interventional treatment, especially for the high-risk lesions often encountered in CLI,

they argue that restenosis rarely jeopardizes subsequent surgery.[136-138]

Situational Perfusion Enhancement. Proponents of percutaneous intervention frequently cite the phenomenon of situational perfusion enhancement and its role in the treatment of CLI. They argue, correctly, that there is a population of asymptomatic patients with subclinical lower extremity ischemia and very low perfusion pressures. These patients become symptomatic only when they develop incidental foot ulceration and do not have the circulatory reserve to heal. A boost in arterial perfusion, even transiently, usually allows healing of the ulcer. Once the ulcer is healed, maintenance of enhanced perfusion is not critical, and recurrent ischemia is usually well tolerated as the patient resumes the subclinical ischemic state. Percutaneous intervention proponents therefore argue that inferior reconstruction patency rates after such interventions are inconsequential. Although the phenomenon of situational perfusion enhancement has been observed and reported anecdotally, it should be accepted with caution. If the patient's ulceration is a sporadic event (e.g., the result of minor incidental trauma), a situational boost to perfusion should be sufficient to accomplish healing. However, if the ulcer is the result of neuropathic changes in the foot, in which case ulcer recurrence is the rule rather than the exception, a more durable reconstruction is probably indicated. The role of situational perfusion enhancement in patients who develop ischemic rest pain is likewise unclear.

BASIL Trial. There is a striking paucity of level I data to guide decision making for interventional treatment versus open surgery. In the United Kingdom, the Bypass versus Angioplasty in Severe Ischemia of the Legs (BASIL) study represents one of the only randomized controlled multicenter trials comparing angioplasty to open surgery for severe limb ischemia.[139] In this study of nearly 450 patients randomized to bypass or balloon angioplasty for the initial treatment of infrainguinal disease, the findings support much of what is known about the two modalities and underscore several important caveats. Using amputation-free survival as the primary endpoint, the authors found that patients treated with bypass first had comparable outcomes to patients treated with balloon angioplasty first at 6 months (amputation or death = 21% with bypass first versus 26% with balloon angioplasty first; P = not significant). Although the early mortality was similar in both treatment groups, surgery was associated with higher morbidity. Crossover treatment after initial therapy (surgery to angioplasty or angioplasty to surgery) was common in both treatment groups, with more than half the angioplasty arm and approximately one third of the surgical arm requiring further intervention. At the end of 5 years, 55% of patients were alive without amputation, 8% were alive with amputation, 8% were dead after amputation, and 29% were dead without amputation. After 2 years, both amputation-free survival (hazard ratio 0.37; P = .008) and overall survival (hazard ratio 0.34; P = .004) were better in the surgical arm.

Table 104-3 Morbidity after Infrainguinal Bypass for Claudication and Critical Limb Ischemia

	First Year	3-5 Years
Time for healing	15-20 wk	—
Wound complications	15%-25%	—
Persistent lymphedema	10%-20%	Unknown
Graft stenosis	20%	20%-30%
Graft occlusion	10%-20%	20%-40%
Major amputation	5%-10%	10%-20%
Graft infection	1%-3%	—
Perioperative death	1%-2%	—
All death	10%	30%-50%

Adapted from Norgren L, Hiatt WR, Dormandy JA, et al. TASC II Working Group. Inter-Society Consensus for the Management of Peripheral Arterial Disease (TASC II). *J Vasc Surg.* 2007;45(Suppl S):S5-S61.

The BASIL trial re-enforces several principles. It clearly supports the phenomenon of situational perfusion enhancement. Patients who have lower extremity ulceration that would be expected to heal with conventional wound therapy and enhanced perfusion within 6 months are good angioplasty candidates. The TASC document currently recommends angioplasty over open surgery when the desired outcomes of the two modalities are comparable.[126] However, angioplasty is probably not appropriate when recurrent ulceration and persistent ischemic symptoms are expected to exceed 6 months. The advantage of having surgery first becomes apparent at 2 years. If it appears that the patient's life expectancy or the course of the disease will exceed 2 years, surgery is probably the more appropriate first intervention. Finally, the degree of treatment crossover in the BASIL trial was arguably its most remarkable finding. It stresses that angioplasty and open surgery are not "either-or" therapies but are complementary. It underscores the importance of training surgeons who manage lower extremity ischemia so that they possess both open and endovascular skill sets.[140]

LEGS Score and TASC Classification. Interestingly, the LEGS score (see Table 104-2) is more applicable to decision making for the treatment of CLI than of claudication. Inspection of the algorithm shows that many of the principles reinforced in the BASIL trial are incorporated in the scoring system. Also, the TASC classifications (see Figs. 104-5 and 104-6) underscore the anatomic considerations that are important in decision making, something not considered in the BASIL trial. Other factors to be considered when deciding between interventional treatment and open surgery are the degree of ischemia and the extent of tissue loss. Open surgery is preferred when ischemia and tissue loss are severe. Conventional wisdom has advocated the presence of in-line flow and a palpable pedal pulse for severe cases of foot ischemia. Unfortunately, objective data correlating the extent of revascularization required to heal specific degrees of tissue loss are lacking.

■ DEFINING TREATMENT SUCCESS
Clinical versus Functional Outcome

It has been recognized that traditional clinical measures of success—namely, reconstruction patency, limb salvage, and mortality—do not fully address the functional concerns of most patients who present with lower extremity PAD. Bypass patency after revascularization matters little to the patient or the patient's family if progressive disability, limb loss, or death occurs over the ensuing months. A better understanding of patient expectations after treatment and patient-oriented endpoints of success is clearly needed.

Critical Limb Ischemia

Leaders in the vascular surgery field recently identified functional outcome after treatment for CLI as a critical area

in need of research. A better understanding of such patient-oriented measures of success will have a profound impact on decision making for the treatment of lower extremity PAD.[141] Considering physician-oriented endpoints only, reconstruction patency rates of 60% to 80% and limb salvage rates of 70% to 90% have consistently been reported after the treatment of CLI, implying that with appropriate treatment methods, the problem of lower extremity PAD has largely been solved.[126] However, in the late 1990s the vascular surgery group from the Oregon Health Sciences Center published a series of studies examining outcomes after lower extremity revascularization from the patient's perspective. They concluded that superior results in terms of graft patency and limb salvage only partially defined success, and more often than not, patient function was not improved.[142-144] Patients who present with CLI are often consumed by their disease and are condemned to a course of prolonged recovery with multiple reoperations and hospital admissions, findings confirmed independently by the vascular group at the University of Arizona.[145] The Oregon group reported that only 14% of patients undergoing revascularization had uncomplicated operations, symptom relief, wound healing, and no reoperation and maintained their original level of function. In contrast, the remaining 86% required ongoing treatment in some fashion for the remainder of their lives. Based on such observations, it is apparent that clinically oriented endpoints, such as bypass graft patency and limb salvage, fail to accurately represent successful outcome after revascularization for CLI. However, the benefits of graft patency in terms of QoL, wound healing, and relief of chronic ischemic pain should not be discounted.

Claudication

Simultaneously, reports from Northwestern University and others challenged the traditional approach to patients with claudication.[146,147] As implied earlier in this chapter, surgeons have traditionally defined successful treatment for claudication using graft patency and limb salvage, and classically, nonoperative therapy has been recommended because claudication rarely progresses to CLI and limb loss. However, the group at Northwestern, using the Short Form (36) Health Survey (SF-36), found that reassurances about the benign natural history of their condition did little to alleviate patients' symptoms. Intervention for claudication improved QoL scores considerably. Improvements were similar to those found after coronary artery bypass surgery for angina and were half as beneficial as hip replacement surgery. In a more recent series, Taylor and coworkers reported significant symptomatic improvement after intervention for claudication in nearly 80% of treated patients.[113] Interventional treatment in this series was exceedingly safe, with no early amputations and a 99% limb salvage rate at 5 years. These reports show that, as with CLI, surgeon-oriented endpoints of success often fail to correlate with patient satisfaction or patient-perceived success.

Quality of Life Assessment

Although it is accepted that revascularization is not appropriate in every case, there is clear evidence that QoL is improved by revascularization in most instances.[148-151] Indeed, the recent focus on patient-oriented endpoints has stimulated new research in the objective measurement of QoL for patients undergoing lower extremity revascularization. Various questionnaires have emerged as tools to measure QoL. Unfortunately, there is no consensus on the ideal questionnaire to use for the evaluation of patients with CLI. The two most commonly used surveys are the SF-36 and the Nottingham Health Profile.[152,153] These questionnaires assess overall QoL and sometimes fail to consider disease-specific issues. Morgan and colleagues developed the Vascular QoL Questionnaire as a disease-specific survey capable of assessing QoL in patients with CLI.[154] To date, the largest study performed assessing QoL in patients with CLI is the PREVENT III (Prevention of Recurrent Venous Thromboembolism) trial, which used the Vascular QoL Questionnaire to study QoL as a secondary endpoint in 1404 patients undergoing infrainguinal bypass.[155] This study and others demonstrated significant improvement in QoL after bypass and also found that QoL correlated directly with bypass graft patency.[150-153,155,156] In addition, prolonged patency is required in many patients to eventually achieve healing. A significant number of patients with CLI take longer than 6 months to heal[147]; nevertheless, they have their limbs and are at home, wound care is simplified, and ischemic pain is relieved. In addition, severe ischemia and extensive infection or soft tissue necrosis can be major factors in selecting tibial or pedal bypass over percutaneous transluminal angioplasty for patients with TASC type C and D disease (see Chapter 109: Infrainguinal Disease: Surgical Treatment); such patients are likely to require maximal and durable foot perfusion to achieve and maintain a healed foot.[144,147,153]

■ FUTURE TRENDS

Patient Selection

Decision making in the treatment of lower extremity PAD has focused on *how* to treat patients. In the future, as the financial condition of the health care system continues to deteriorate, decision making will focus on *whom* to treat. It is naive to believe, for instance, that all patients who present with CLI will benefit from aggressive intervention. Indeed, in the BASIL study cited earlier, an independent data-monitoring committee overseeing patient enrollment in this trial found that half the patients with severe limb ischemia were regarded as unsuitable or unfit for any form of revascularization. The authors concluded that patients eligible for revascularization represent the tip of an iceberg, the true dimensions of which remain incompletely defined.[139] Interventional treatment cannot and should not be offered to everyone. The true task, then, is to refine definitions of success and construct tools using evidence-based data to help

Table 104-4 Probability of Failure after Bypass* When the Clinical Condition Is Present at Presentation

Predictor Variable	Probability of Failure (%)	Odds Ratio (95% CI)
Impaired ambulation	58	6.4 (2.9, 14.4)
Infrainguinal disease	46	3.9 (1.6, 9.8)
ESRD	35	2.5 (1.2, 5.4)
Gangrene	34	2.4 (1.5, 4.0)
Hyperlipidemia	11	0.6 (0.34, 0.93)

*Defined as patent bypass until healed, limb salvage for 1 year, maintenance of ambulation for 1 year, and survival for 6 months.
ESRD, end-stage renal disease.
From Taylor SM, Cull DL, Kalbaugh CA, et al. Critical analysis of clinical success after surgical bypass for lower extremity ischemic tissue loss using a standardized definition combining multiple parameters: A new paradigm of outcome assessment. *J Am Coll Surg.* 2007;204:831-839.

distinguish patients who will benefit from therapy from those who will not.

To that end, Taylor and colleagues recently studied 331 consecutive patients treated for Rutherford class 5 and 6 ischemia (tissue loss).[156] A bypass was deemed clinically successful if all four outcome criteria were met: (1) bypass patency until wound healing occurred, (2) limb salvage for at least 1 year, (3) maintenance of ambulatory status for at least 1 year, and (4) survival for at least 6 months. The authors found acceptable results when examining these components separately, including a graft patency rate of 72% and a limb salvage rate of 73% at 36 months. However, the clinical success rate, defined as the achievement of all four criteria, was only 44%. Furthermore, patients who presented with impaired ambulatory status, end-stage renal disease, gangrene, and infrainguinal disease (each independent statistical predictors) were especially prone to failure (Table 104-4).[156] Prospects for a successful outcome became progressively dismal as the number of independent negative predictors increased. Patients harboring two of these independent predictors of failure experienced roughly a 33% probability of success; those with three predictors, a 10% probability of success; and those with all four independent predictors of failure, less than a 5% probability of success. Similar studies using consensus definitions of success are needed to help guide decision-making regarding who should receive intervention and who should not.

Cost Considerations

As health care costs continue to rise, decision making will increasingly be influenced by governmental and third-party payers. There is conflicting evidence regarding the most cost-efficient methods of treating lower extremity PAD. Although there is evidence that revascularization is more cost-effective than primary amputation,[134,157-160] the cost differential is attributed to the expense of rehabilitation in most series.[158] Indeed, primary amputation for patients forgoing rehabilitation (as might occur in a nursing-home patient) is cheaper than revascularization. Therefore, economic decision making depends on the patient's postoperative rehabilitation potential, which is often determined by preoperative functional status.[125] Despite the debate concerning the economic merits of one treatment over another, most would agree that the current financial system can ill afford to pay for multiple revascularizations of a single ischemic limb. The scenario becomes even more cost-prohibitive if, after multiple revascularizations, major limb amputation results anyway. Future economic decision making will therefore require the identification of the most cost-effective single treatment for patients who present with PAD and, more specifically, CLI.

Other Changes

The acquisition of endovascular skills by vascular surgeons has drastically influenced treatment patterns for lower extremity PAD over the past decade. As an illustration, Sullivan and associates examined the change in treatment patterns at a single institution shortly after vascular surgeons who had previously referred cases to interventional radiology began performing their own endovascular interventions. They found that the volume of open surgery dropped 5%, endovascular therapy increased by more than 400%, and referrals to interventional radiology essentially ceased (Fig. 104-7).[161] Third-party payers in our current health care system will increasingly insist on the delivery of evidence-based care. Quality will be defined, increasingly monitored, and financially linked to compliance with Medicare All-Care measures. Care for lower extremity PAD will increasingly become protocol driven, placing a premium on value and durability. Traditional surgeon-oriented endpoints of success such as graft patency often have little value to patients. An increasing focus on patient-oriented outcomes is emerging and promises to have a profound effect on surgical decision making.[141] Last, the definitive treatment of lower extremity PAD has traditionally been

interventional therapy. Through the mapping of the human genome, angiogenesis and other genetically driven therapies hold great promise in providing meaningful medical solutions and may render many interventions unnecessary.

SELECTED KEY REFERENCES

Bradberry AW. BASIL Trial Participants. Bypass versus angioplasty in severe ischemia of the leg (BASIL): multicenter, randomized controlled trial. *Lancet.* 2005;366:1925-1934.
This rare randomized, controlled multicenter trial concluded that surgery and angioplasty have similar amputation-free survival at 6 months (thus favoring angioplasty as the best first approach), but surgery has better amputation-free survival after 2 years. This study stressed the complementary nature of the two treatment approaches.

Feinglass J, McCarthy WJ, Slavensky R, Manheim LM, Martin GJ. Functional status and walking ability after lower extremity bypass grafting or angioplasty for intermittent claudication: results from a prospective outcomes study. *J Vasc Surg.* 2000;31:93-103.
This study of more than 500 patients was one of the first to suggest that traditional outcome measures, such as reconstruction patency and limb salvage, are insensitive endpoints of success after intervention for claudication and that functional assessment is needed.

Hirsch AT, Haskal ZJ, Hertzer NR, Bakal CW, Creager MA, Halperin JL, Hiratzka LF, Murphy WR, Olin JW, Puschett JB, Rosenfield KA, Sacks D, Stanley JC, Taylor LM Jr, White CJ, White J, White RA, Antman EM, Smith SC Jr, Adams CD, Anderson JL, Faxon DP, Fuster V, Gibbons RJ, Halperin JL, Hiratzka LF, Hunt SA, Jacobs AK, Nishimura R, Ornato JP, Page RL, Riegel B. American Association for Vascular Surgery, Society for Vascular Surgery, Society for Cardiovascular Angiography and Interventions, Society for Vascular Medicine and Biology, Society for Interventional Radiology, ACC/AHA Task Force on Practice Guidelines, American Association of Cardiovascular and Pulmonary Rehabilitation, National Heart, Lung and Blood Institute, Society for Vascular Nursing, TransAtlantic Inter-Society Consensus, Vascular Disease Foundation. ACC/AHA 2005 guidelines for the management of patients with peripheral arterial disease (lower extremity, renal, mesenteric and abdominal aortic): executive summary a collaborative report from the American Association for Vascular Surgery, Society for Vascular Surgery, Society for Cardiovascular Angiography and Interventions, Society for Vascular Medicine and Biology, Society for Interventional Radiology and the ACC/AHA Task Force on Practice Guidelines (Writing Committee to Develop Guidelines for the Management of Patients with Peripheral Arterial Disease) endorsed by the American Association of Cardiovascular and Pulmonary Rehabilitation; National Heart, Lung and Blood Institute; Society for Vascular Nursing; TransAtlantic Inter-Society Consensus; and Vascular Disease Foundation. *J Am Coll Cardiol.* 2006;47:1239-1312.
This consensus document is similar to others but has a greater focus on the medical treatment of PAD.

Landry GJ. Functional outcome of critical limb ischemia. *J Vasc Surg.* 2007;45:141A-148A.
This review article outlines the future emphasis on patient-oriented rather than physician-oriented outcomes after the treatment of lower extremity PAD.

Norgren L, Hiatt WR, Dormandy JA, Nehler MR, Harris KA, Fowkes FG; TASC II Working Group. Inter-Society Consensus for the Management of Peripheral Arterial Disease (TASC II). *J Vasc Surg.* 2007;45(Suppl S):S5-S67.
The TASC II document updates TASC and represents the latest evidence-based data on the natural history and treatment of lower extremity PAD.

TASC. Management of Peripheral Arterial Disease (PAD) Transatlantic Inter-Society Consensus (TASC). *J Vasc Surg.* 2000;31:S1-S287.
Multidisciplinary task force review of evidence pertaining to lower extremity PAD, including recommendations based on current

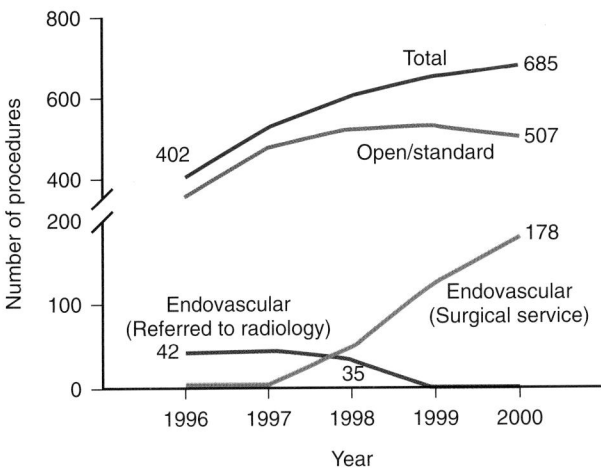

Figure 104-7 Impact of integrating an endovascular surgery program into a mature vascular practice in which angioplasty (previously referred to interventional radiology) is performed by vascular surgeons. *(Redrawn from Sullivan TM, Taylor SM, Blackhurst DW, et al. Has endovascular surgery reduced the number of open vascular operations performed by an established surgical practice?* J Vasc Surg. 2002;36(3):514-519.)

evidence. This is one of the most important sources of data on lower extremity PAD.

Taylor SM, Cull, DL, Kalbaugh CA, Cass AL, Harmon SA, Langan EM 3rd, Youkey JR. Critical analysis of clinical success after surgical bypass for lower extremity ischemic tissue loss using a standardized definition combining multiple parameters: a new paradigm of outcome assessment. *J Am Coll Surg.* 2007;204:831-839.
This study defined successful outcome after lower extremity bypass for tissue loss as graft patency until wound healing, limb salvage and ambulatory ability for 1 year, and survival for 6 months. It identified end-stage renal disease, the need for an infrainguinal bypass, gangrene, and impaired preoperative ambulatory status as independent predictors of failure.

Taylor SM, Kalbaugh CA, Blackhurst DW, Cass AL, Trent EA, Langan EM 3rd, Youkey JR. Determinants of functional outcome after revascularization for critical limb ischemia: an analysis of 1000 consecutive vascular interventions. *J Vasc Surg.* 2006;44:747-756.

Though retrospective, this large series demonstrated that functional performance after intervention for CLI is often determined by factors other than limb salvage. Postoperative functional outcomes were most profoundly impacted by the patient's preoperative medical condition and functional status.

Wixon CL, Mills JL, Westerband A, Hughes JD, Ihnat DM. An economic appraisal of lower extremity bypass graft maintenance. *J Vasc Surg.* 2000;32:1-12.
This study is an example of the growing body of evidence that cost is a factor in treatment decision making.

REFERENCES
The reference list can be found on the companion Expert Consult Web site at *www.expertconsult.com.*

CHAPTER 105

Aortoiliac Disease: Direct Reconstruction

Matthew T. Menard and Michael Belkin

Based in part on a chapter in the previous edition by David C. Brewster, MD.

The clinical manifestation of atherosclerosis involving the abdominal aorta and iliac arteries is one of the most common therapeutic challenges encountered by vascular surgeons. British anatomist and surgeon John Hunter first appreciated the implications of arterial occlusive disease of the aortic bifurcation in the late 1700s. His dissection specimens remain on view at the Hunterian Museum in London and laid the groundwork for Leriche's later appreciation of the disease process that bears his name.[1]

The modern era of surgical reconstruction for complex atherosclerotic occlusive disease began in 1947 with the successful endarterectomy of a heavily diseased common femoral artery (CFA) by Portuguese surgeon dos Santos.[2] Wylie and coworkers in San Francisco extended this new technique to the aortoiliac (AI) level 4 years later,[3] but it would be another 10 years before synthetic grafts were regularly used for aortic bypass grafting. Early preference for aorta–to–iliac artery grafting would eventually be supplanted by the more durable aortobifemoral bypass (ABFB) procedure.

In recent years, tremendous advances in our understanding of the biology of atherosclerosis and in our ability to treat arterial occlusive disease percutaneously have dramatically impacted the treatment algorithms for peripheral arterial disease as a whole and for AI disease in particular. The growing range of treatment options allows us to tailor therapy to the particular clinical situation, and ongoing improvements in graft material, surgical technique, and perioperative management have contributed to a steady decline in postoperative morbidity and mortality. Given the advent of less invasive therapeutic options, traditional aortobifemoral grafting is increasingly being performed for more complex patterns of disease or as a secondary or tertiary procedure in the setting of recurrent disease.[4] High levels of patient satisfaction and excellent long-term outcomes, however, remain the hallmark of aortobifemoral surgical revascularization. This chapter reviews the role of direct operative reconstruction in the current surgical management of AI arterial occlusive disease.

PATHOLOGY AND CLINICAL PRESENTATION

Pathology

AI disease typically begins at the aortic terminus and common iliac artery origins and slowly progresses proximally and dis-

tally over time.[5] Progression is variable but may ultimately result in total aortic occlusion (Fig. 105-1). In the setting of adequate collateralization, patients can tolerate their levels of claudication and can be successfully managed nonoperatively for many years. Approximately one third of patients operated on for symptomatic AI occlusive disease have significant orificial profunda femoris occlusive disease, and more than 40% have significant superficial femoral artery (SFA) disease. Disease can also extend to the level of the renal arteries (see Fig. 105-1). Although early reports indicated that up to one

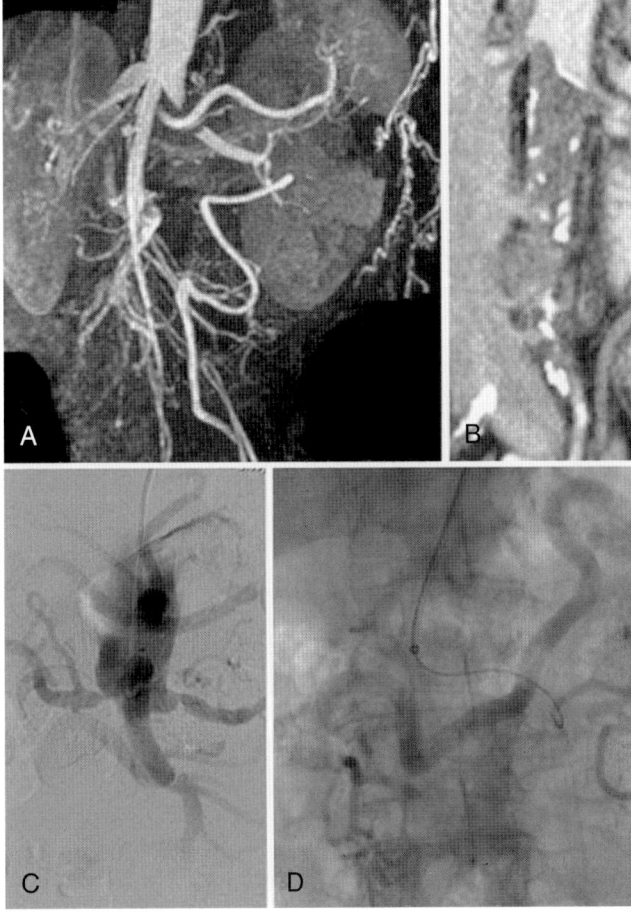

Figure 105-1 Two patients with total aortic occlusion extending to the level of the renal arteries. **A** and **B,** Coronal CT images in one patient demonstrate propagation of thrombus into the renal arteries. **C** and **D,** The second patient also has associated renal artery occlusive disease. Meandering mesenteric arteries are demonstrated in both patients.

third of patients with aortic occlusion went on to develop renal artery thrombosis over a period of 5 to 10 years,[6] later prospective studies failed to demonstrate a similar degree of compromise of the renal vessels in this population.[7] Involvement of the renal or mesenteric vessels to a degree warranting concurrent repair is seen in only a minor proportion of patients with AI disease.

Collateral Circulation

Although atherosclerotic disease limited to the AI region commonly gives rise to claudication of varying degrees, it is rarely associated with critical limb ischemia (CLI). This is largely the result of abundant collateralization around the point of obstruction, which reconstitutes the infrainguinal system with sufficient flow to ensure adequate resting tissue perfusion (Fig. 105-2). The primary compensatory networks develop from the lumbar and hypogastric feeding vessels and connect to circumflex iliac, hypogastric, femoral, and profunda recipients. Additional collaterals that arise in more

extreme degrees of obstruction include the internal mammary artery–to–inferior epigastric connection and the superior mesenteric artery–to–inferior mesenteric artery and hemorrhoidal artery pathway. The latter connection comprises the arc of Riolan and the meandering mesenteric artery (Fig. 105-3); it is important to recognize the presence of such a large and important collateral because it should be preserved during surgical reconstruction.

Embolism

Two well-recognized exceptions to the general observation that isolated AI occlusive disease does not result in CLI arise in the context of embolic disease. Large thromboemboli that arise from a cardiac or other proximal source and lodge at the aortic bifurcation, referred to as saddle emboli, can lead to profound acute bilateral lower extremity ischemia. The so-called blue toe syndrome, in contrast, occurs when atherosclerotic debris breaks free from an aortic or iliac plaque and embolizes to the distal vessels.[8,9] Wire manipulation during

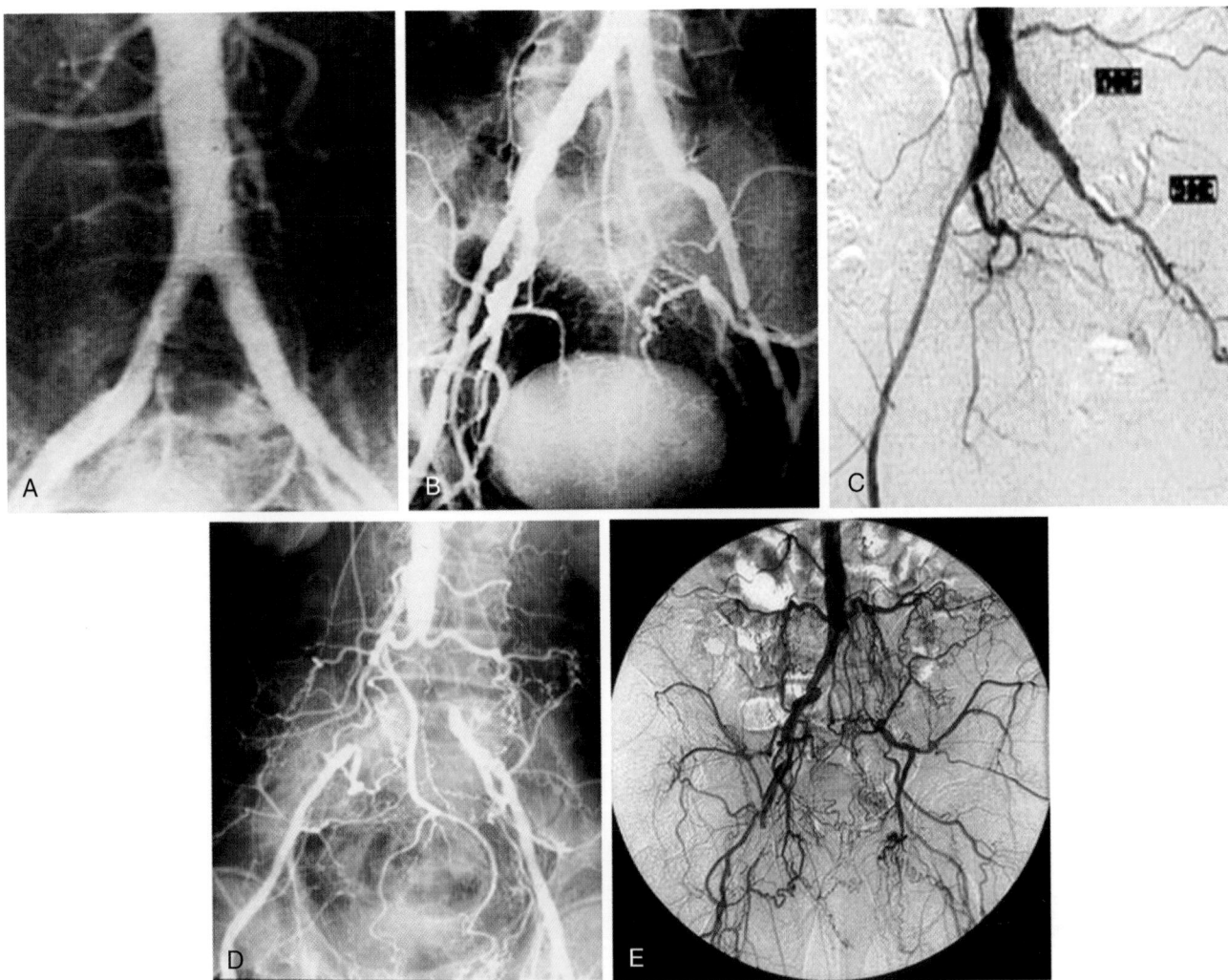

Figure 105-2 A–E, Aortoiliac occlusive disease of increasing severity, with a progressively well-developed pattern of iliolumbar to hypogastric and femoral circumflex collateralization. Male patients with a disease distribution illustrated in **B–E** may be impotent secondary to compromised hypogastric perfusion.

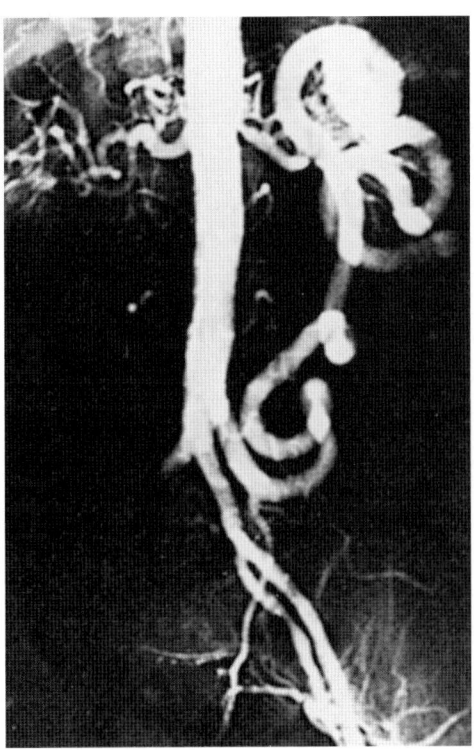

Figure 105-3 Large meandering mesenteric artery associated with total superior mesenteric and celiac artery occlusion. Aortobifemoral bypass with an end-to-side proximal anastomosis would best preserve both mesenteric and pelvic perfusion.

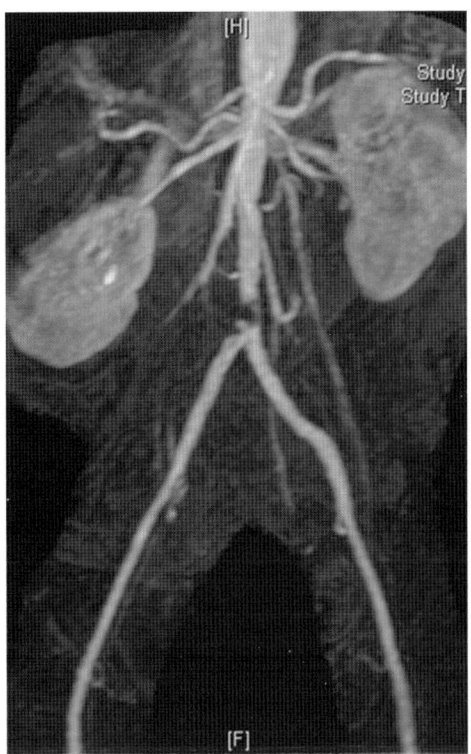

Figure 105-4 Short-segment stenoses localized to the distal aorta are particularly common in young female smokers and are amenable to endarterectomy.

coronary or peripheral angiographic procedures or surgical cross-clamping across a calcific aortic plaque can trigger such emboli. The terminal targets of the microembolic particles, composed of cholesterol crystals, calcified plaque, thrombus, or platelet aggregrates, are typically the small vessels of the toes or heel. The syndrome is typically characterized by palpable pedal pulses in the presence of patchy ischemia (livedo), but more severe ischemia or gangrene of the proximal or distal forefoot may occur.

Epidemiology

The majority of patients presenting with atherosclerotic occlusive disease of the aorta and iliac vessels have diffuse disease involving multiple levels of the peripheral vasculature tree; in most cases, AI occlusive disease is found in combination with femoropopliteal or infrageniculate occlusive disease. Patients with isolated AI disease are generally younger and have a higher relative incidence of smoking and hypercholesterolemia as associated vascular risk factors.[10] They are nearly as likely to be female as male and typically have a normal life expectancy.[11] In contrast to this pattern, patients with more progressive multilevel disease are commonly older, more frequently have diabetes and hypertension, and are more likely to be male and to have concomitant cerebrovascular, coronary, and visceral atherosclerosis.[10] Not surprisingly, patients with diffuse, multisegment disease often present with ischemic rest pain or more severe perfusion impairment, leading to tissue loss or gangrene as opposed to isolated claudica-

tion.[12] Such patients manifest a significant reduction in life expectancy compared with their age-matched counterparts.[11]

A particularly virulent form of atherosclerotic arterial disease is often found in young women who smoke.[13,14] Radiographic imaging in this subset of patients typically reveals atretic, narrowed vasculature with diffusely calcific atherosclerotic changes. Frequently, a focal stenosis is found posteriorly at or proximal to the aortic bifurcation (Fig. 105-4). In the setting of this particular disease distribution and characteristic patient profile, the term *small aortic syndrome* or *hypoplastic aortic syndrome* is used.[15] Such patients invariably have an extensive smoking history but may be without other typical risk factors for atherosclerosis. The diminutive size of the aorta and iliac vessels has important treatment implications; the durability of either endovascular intervention or local endarterectomy is generally inferior in such patients, particularly in the presence of continued cigarette use.

Presenting Symptoms

Chronic obliterative atherosclerosis of the distal aorta and iliac arteries commonly manifests as symptomatic arterial insufficiency of the lower extremities, producing a range of symptoms from mild claudication to more severe levels of CLI. Disease limited to the AI segment is seen in a minority of cases; more often, it is present in combination with occlusive disease of the femoropopliteal arteries (Fig. 105-5) or other arterial beds. Patients with hemodynamic impairment limited to the AI system may have intermittent claudication

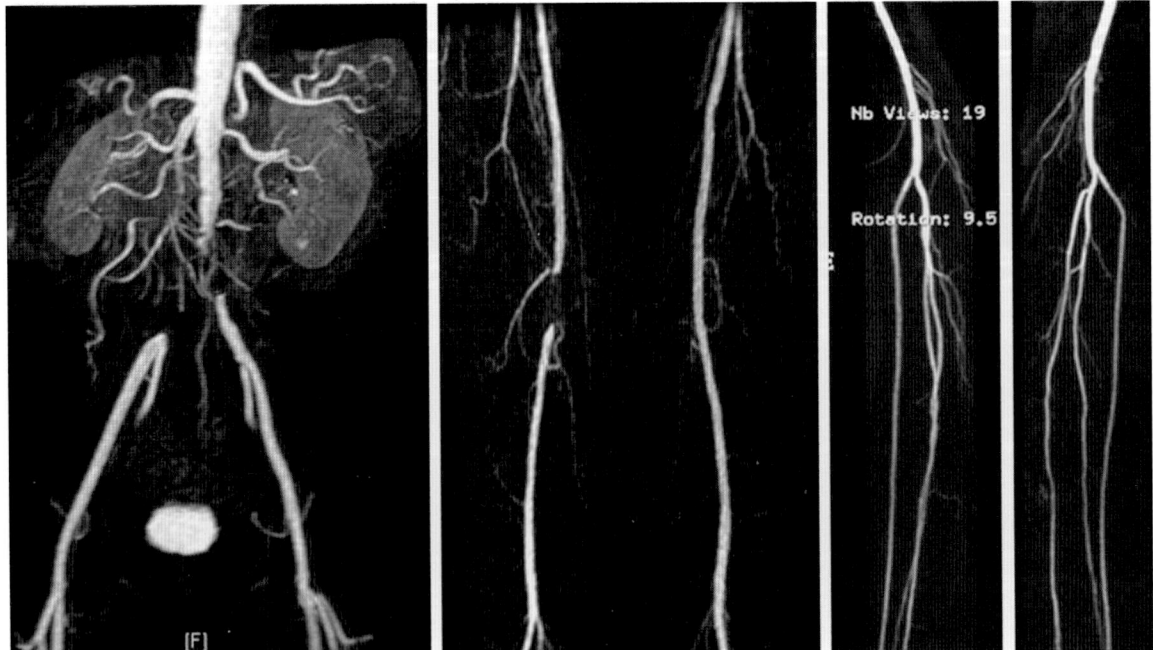

Figure 105-5 Aortoiliac occlusive disease is frequently seen in combination with more distal disease. Here, there is a short-segment occlusion of the right superficial femoral artery.

of the calf muscles alone or involvement of the thigh, hip, or buttock; patients with CLI usually have multilevel disease of the AI and infrainguinal arteries. Those presenting with claudication secondary to AI disease are, on average, nearly a decade younger than those with claudication stemming from infrainguinal occlusive disease.[13] Up to 30% of male patients may have difficulty achieving and maintaining an erection owing to inadequate perfusion of the internal pudendal arteries.[16] In men, the well-characterized constellation of symptoms and signs known as Leriche syndrome, associated with terminal aortic occlusion, includes thigh, hip, or buttock claudication; atrophy of the leg muscles; impotence; and reduced femoral pulses.[17] The equivalent impact of impaired pelvic perfusion in women remains poorly understood but has recently attracted investigative attention.[18]

DIAGNOSIS

History and Physical Examination

The diagnosis of AI occlusive disease can usually be made following a careful history and physical examination (see Chapter 103: Lower Extremity Arterial Disease: General Considerations). For a patient with multiple vascular risk factors; hip, buttock, or thigh claudication; and absent femoral pulses, the diagnosis of AI disease is straightforward. In other patients, symptoms of claudication can sometimes be difficult to distinguish from those of hip arthritis or nerve root irritation stemming from lumbar disk disease or spinal stenosis.[19]

The variability of presenting signs and symptoms in patients with AI disease sometimes leads to diagnostic confusion. Although proximal claudication is most common, patients with AI occlusive disease in isolation or those with combined infrainguinal disease may present exclusively with calf claudication. Although the involved muscle groups may be atrophic from disuse in patients with claudication, the lower extremities frequently appear well perfused at rest. Palpable femoral and even pedal pulses may be detectable at rest, reflecting the presence of robust collateral networks; pulses may become diminished or absent only following a trial of exercise. Similarly, a palpable thrill or audible bruit may initially be absent at the lower abdominal or groin level but become detectable after exertion. Conversely, femoral bruits or diminished femoral pulses arising from CFA or profunda femoris stenotic disease can mistakenly be attributed to AI inflow disease.

Noninvasive Hemodynamic Assessment

Noninvasive arterial testing in the form of segmental systolic blood pressure measurements and pulse volume recordings can be helpful in confirming a clinical diagnosis of peripheral arterial disease and further defining the level and extent of obstruction (see Chapter 14: Vascular Laboratory: Arterial Physiologic Assessment and Chapter 103: Lower Extremity Arterial Disease: General Considerations).[20] A difference of at least 20 mm Hg between the brachial pressure and the proximal thigh pressure reflects a significant stenosis in the aorta or iliac arteries, but it may be confused by proximal SFA occlusion. A further reduction in pressure between the thigh and ankle level is consistent with concomitant SFA, popliteal, or tibial outflow disease. Because patients with disabling symptoms occasionally demonstrate normal or near-normal ankle-brachial indices, repeating the pressure measurements following provocative graded exercise treadmill testing can be particularly useful if clinical suspicion of AI disease persists.

Combined with a careful history and physical examination, noninvasive hemodynamic arterial studies usually provide sufficient data to select patients for revascularization. Only after establishing the diagnosis of AI disease and reaching the clinical decision to intervene is further imaging warranted.

Imaging

Duplex Ultrasound

Duplex assessment of the AI, renal, and visceral arteries is labor-intensive and time-consuming and requires an institution with dedicated protocols and vascular laboratory personnel. Nevertheless, a number of institutions routinely obtain information of sufficient quality to be useful in preprocedure planning.[21] In the absence of overlying bowel gas, obesity, or vessel tortuosity, the precise anatomic location of stenoses can be determined and their severity quantified. Indirect techniques to assess the resistive index are of some value in overcoming the commonly encountered limitations in renal arterial analysis and can be of utility in deciding whether a given lesion warrants concomitant revascularization at the time of aortic reconstruction.[22] Duplex ultrasound is particularly beneficial in patients with renal insufficiency, in whom the avoidance of contrast agents is advantageous. As the technology continues to be refined, as operator skill and training improve, and as novel adjunctive duplex imaging agents evolve, this modality will likely play an increasing role in the management of patients with visceral and AI disease.[23] At present, however, it remains inferior to other imaging techniques for preoperative planning and has not gained wide acceptance.

Axial Imaging

With new acquisition techniques, shorter acquisition times, and high-quality three-dimensional postprocessing capabilities, magnetic resonance angiography (MRA) has become particularly well suited to evaluating the aorta and renal and mesenteric vessels. Indeed, several series have reported 100% sensitivity and specificity in detecting origin stenoses of the visceral vessels.[24,25] In many centers, MRA has supplanted contrast angiography as the initial imaging study of choice (see Chapter 22: Magnetic Resonance Imaging and Chapter 103: Lower Extremity Arterial Disease: General Considerations). Advances have solved many of the technical limitations of earlier studies, and reliable roadmaps to guide percutaneous or operative planning are now obtainable and reproducible (Fig. 105-6). MRA continues to occasionally overestimate the degree of renal artery stenosis, albeit much less so than previously.

In some institutions, computed tomographic angiography (CTA) is favored over MRA as a more clinically useful noninvasive alternative to standard angiography (see Chapter 21: Computed Tomography and Chapter 103: Lower Extremity Arterial Disease: General Considerations). Current-generation multislice technology has overcome many of the earlier

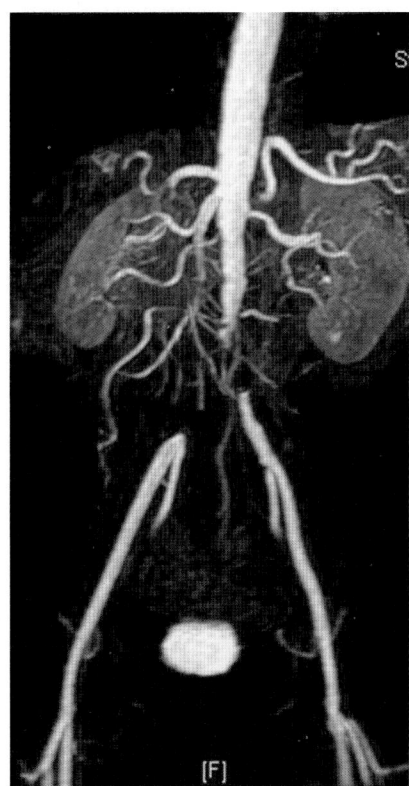

Figure 105-6 Total aortic occlusion demonstrated by MRA of sufficient quality to support surgical planning and obviate the need for formal angiography.

limitations of computed tomography (CT),[26,27] and images of exceptional clarity and submillimeter spatial resolution are now routinely available for the aortic and iliac arterial segments (Fig. 105-7). The recent development of 320-slice scanners, and those on the horizon that combine angiography and CT technology, will likely push this modality closer to the forefront in the near future.

Arteriography

When a lesion in the aorta or iliac arteries amenable to percutaneous therapy is identified on MRA, CT, or duplex imaging, arteriography is then pursued. If good-quality imaging is obtained with MRA or CTA and the clinical situation or anatomic pattern is unfavorable to a percutaneous approach, AI reconstruction can frequently be planned directly from the information obtained by MRA or CTA, obviating the need for traditional subtraction angiography.[28,29] Although duplex ultrasound, CTA, and MRA have significantly impacted preoperative planning algorithms for patients with AI disease, invasive contrast angiography remains the "gold standard" imaging modality if anatomic questions remain. Technical advances in catheters, contrast agents, radiographic equipment, and image processing have led to greatly improved safety and image quality (see Chapter 18: Arteriography). In cases in which the decision has been made to proceed with surgical revascularization, angiography may be undertaken to obtain a final detailed roadmap of the

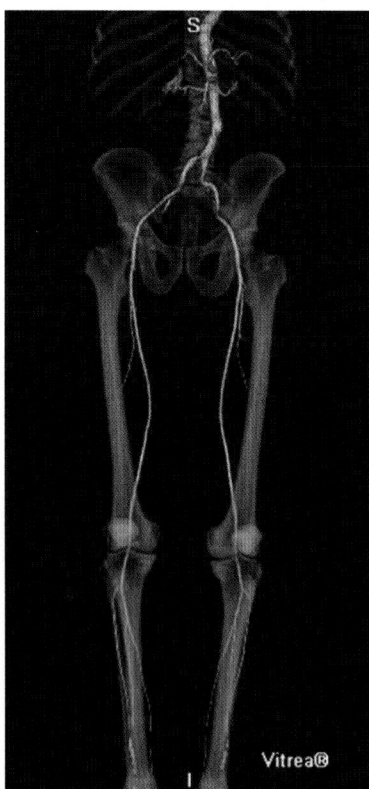

Figure 105-7 Aortic CTA with three-dimensional reconstruction provides sufficient detail to guide percutaneous or operative planning.

relevant anatomy. Although a transbrachial approach is sometimes required,[30] more often than not a standard retrograde femoral approach is possible, despite long-segment near-occlusive or occlusive aortic or biiliac disease. Supplemental lateral and oblique views of the abdominal aorta are advised to delineate possible concomitant mesenteric or renal artery occlusive disease. Specific attention should be directed to the inferior mesenteric artery; a large patent inferior mesenteric artery, particularly in the presence of superior mesenteric artery or hypogastric artery occlusive disease, may require preservation during aortic reconstruction to avoid potentially disastrous bowel ischemia. Multiple projections of the iliac and femoral bifurcations are essential to clarify the extent of disease in these regions, because involvement of the hypogastric and external iliac arteries has significant implications when choosing the operative approach. Full runoff views of the lower extremities are also needed to assess the presence or absence of femoropopliteal or crural disease. In ambiguous cases, pullback pressure measurements, both before and after the administration of a systemic vasodilator such as papaverine or nitroglycerine or the application of a tourniquet to induce reactive hyperemia, can be useful in documenting the hemodynamic significance of a particular stenotic segment.[31] A resting systolic gradient of approximately 5 to 10 mm Hg or a change in the systolic pressure greater than 15% following pharmacologic vasodilatation is a reliable indicator of disease warranting inflow revascularization.[32]

INDICATIONS FOR SURGICAL INTERVENTION

Impact of Endovascular Treatment

A significant paradigm shift has occurred in the treatment of atherosclerotic arterial disease.[19,33] Angioplasty and stenting have become first-line therapy for most patients with AI, renal, subclavian, and coronary occlusive disease.[34] Whereas percutaneous treatment of the aorta and iliac arteries was previously limited to short-segment, Trans-Atlantic Inter-Society Consensus (TASC) type A or B iliac lesions, wire-based technology has now been successfully applied to even long-segment (TASC type D) occlusions extending for the length of the iliac arteries. In no other vascular territory has the shift from open surgery to interventional treatment been more apparent than in the AI segment. Using the Nationwide Inpatient Sample, one recent report documented an 850% increase in the use of percutaneous transluminal angioplasty and stenting for AI occlusive disease from 1996 to 2000, along with a simultaneous decrease of 16% in the rate of aortobi-femoral grafting.[34] Further reflecting this transformation in management strategy, in anatomically favorable circumstances, concomitant renal or mesenteric artery stenosis might be treated percutaneously as a staged initial procedure, even when subsequent open surgical AI reconstruction is planned.[35] Decision making for surgical versus endovascular treatment is discussed in detail in Chapter 104 (Lower Extremity Arterial Disease: Decision Making and Medical Treatment).

In the current era, in which direct reconstruction for AI disease has been relegated to a second- or even third-line therapy, open bypass is increasingly undertaken in patients in whom endovascular treatment has been technically unsuccessful or in those with such extensive disease that an endovascular approach is deemed inadvisable. These shifting demographics have been reflected in reports documenting the increasing complexity of aortobifemoral grafting, with a higher incidence of suprarenal clamping, adjunctive visceral revascularization, simultaneous operative inflow and outflow disease, and "redo" grafting.[4,36] Patients with a combination of more proximal aneurysmal disease and common or external iliac occlusive disease continue to be good candidates for open reconstruction, although this group will continue to diminish with ongoing technologic advancements. Patients with extensive calcification at the aortic bifurcation thought to be at risk for rupture with balloon angioplasty and those with disease extending to the CFA are additional examples of patients who were once, but no longer, considered unsuitable for an endovascular approach. The incidence of rupture has proved low in the former group, and the introduction of low-profile covered stents and techniques of primary stenting will likely further increase the safety of endovascular treatment in this clinical setting. The second subgroup of patients can potentially be managed with a hybrid approach, whereby the CFA plaque is treated with a traditional endarterectomy and patch repair and the iliac component is concurrently addressed with endovascular techniques.[37]

Patients with early recurrence of AI disease following angioplasty or stenting represent a growing group for whom open surgical repair may be indicated. Patients with significant renal failure in whom endovascular therapy entails a prohibitive risk of triggering dialysis dependence are also considered better suited for operative repair. Complications of endovascular treatment, including dissection and vessel rupture, are infrequent indications for surgical reconstruction. At the advent of the endovascular era, there were significant fears that endoluminal therapy would accelerate the disease process or adversely impact available surgical options. Although these concerns have not been realized to any great extent in clinical practice to date, there are no doubt cases in which focal aortic disease has been rendered unsuitable for subsequent endarterectomy following stent placement. Similarly, some degree of stent explantation may be necessary to successfully complete aortofemoral reconstruction in patients who have previously undergone stent placement to the level of the renal arteries or in those who imprudently had stenting of their CFAs or profunda femoris arteries.

Claudication

The traditional indications for surgical reconstruction for symptomatic AI occlusive disease are disabling claudication, ischemic rest pain, or tissue loss. Claudication is a relative indication for intervention, given the natural history of the disease. Multiple reports, among them the Framingham Heart Study, indicate that patients with claudication have increased rates of cardiovascular mortality but an overall low risk of associated limb loss.[5,38] The majority of claudicants demonstrate a stable pattern of disease throughout their lifetimes or have an improvement in symptoms as a result of risk factor modification, whereas 20% to 30% require operation within 5 years as a result of disease progression. The annual rates of mortality and limb loss in patients with claudication have historically been reported as 5% and 1%, respectively.[39] Of relevance to a discussion of the appropriate threshold for intervention for claudication, Rutherford has taken issue with these commonly quoted estimates. Citing evidence based on objective hemodynamic confirmation of the diagnosis rather than clinical assessment alone, he believes the actual annual rate of limb loss for claudicants is closer to 5%, particularly in those with ankle-brachial indices in the range of 0.4 to 0.6.[40] Others have offered evidence that claudicants with AI disease are more likely to progress to CLI.[41]

In any case, the degree of disability a particular level of claudication represents remains a subjective assessment by both the patient and the surgeon. For example, two-block claudication in a younger patient whose livelihood depends on walking tolerance constitutes a more significant disability than the same degree of claudication in an older, retired individual who can attend to his or her daily affairs without significant consequence. The anticipated benefit of therapy—that is, improvement in functional quality of life—must be carefully weighed against the specific limitations imposed by concomitant cardiac impairment, pulmonary disease, and musculoskeletal conditions in a given patient.

As the associated risks of AI balloon angioplasty and stenting have fallen and the relative success rates have risen in recent years, the threshold for offering endovascular treatment to patients with claudication at all points along the spectrum of occlusive disease has significantly decreased. Indeed, patients once considered appropriate only for risk factor modification, exercise therapy, and medical treatment are now increasingly being offered percutaneous revascularization as a primary treatment option. As a corollary trend, balloon technology is increasingly being applied to hypogastric arterial disease, primarily for buttock or hip claudication, to a degree not previously seen and to a degree not paralleled by an increase in surgical revascularization.[42]

The indications to proceed to surgical reconstruction for claudication have not shifted appreciably during this same period. Given the relatively benign natural history of the disease, a conservative treatment approach continues to be appropriate for many patients with claudication. Unlike the scenario in patients with CLI, it has been argued that an overly aggressive approach might place patients without limb-threatening conditions at unnecessary risk for adverse outcomes. The majority of claudicants remain stable for years, allowing time for collateral pathways to develop; this often results in sufficient improvement, making intervention unnecessary.[43] In contrast, for patients who are good surgical risks and have disease limited to the aortobifemoral segment, surgical bypass is an appropriate option. With current levels of perioperative morbidity and mortality, bypass grafting can be undertaken safely and with the expectation of excellent long-term patency rates.

Critical Limb Ischemia

CLI is associated with likely amputation and significant suffering unless revascularization is undertaken. As such, the presence of ischemic rest pain, frank ulceration, or digital gangrene is a well-accepted and unambiguous indication for surgical correction of AI disease. As mentioned, patients manifesting pregangrenous or gangrenous skin changes typically have hemodynamically significant infrainguinal as well as AI occlusive disease.[12] Thus, whereas patients treated for claudication or rest pain usually require only a single-stage inflow operation, simultaneous or staged inflow and outflow revascularization should be considered in patients with tissue loss (see under "Multilevel Occlusive Disease").

Patients with an aortic or iliac source of distal emboli, typically from an ulcerated atheromatous plaque or so-called shaggy aorta, represent another group in which operative reconstruction is clearly indicated.[44] Such patients may be without symptoms of claudication, and the culprit lesion or lesions may be hemodynamically insignificant. In these cases, the goal of intervention is usually not to relieve obstruction per se but to prevent recurrent distal embolization.

Recent studies have documented the generally excellent outcomes of aortobifemoral grafting in elderly patients, suggesting that in older patients who are otherwise good surgical risks, surgical therapy should not be withheld.[45] Conversely, lower long-term patency rates with aortic bypass in younger patients or those with smaller aortic diameters suggest that caution should be applied to early surgical intervention in these patient populations.[45]

SURGICAL TREATMENT

The modern therapeutic armamentarium for treating arterial occlusive diseases is barely half a century old. Its development has been marked by several landmark advances, among them the discovery of the anticoagulant heparin by Best in the early 1930s, the advent of arteriography in 1927, the first application of arterial homografts by Gross in 1948 and prosthetic grafts by Voorhees in 1952, and the introduction of balloon angioplasty by Gruntzig in 1974 and of stenting by Puel and Sigwart in 1986. Continual improvements in surgical instrumentation and suture materials to facilitate vascular reconstruction and general advances in perioperative management, including cardiopulmonary care, infection control, and blood product utilization, have further contributed to the dramatic progress made. Historically, the surgical options for AI occlusive disease have included AI endarterectomy, aortobiiliac bypass, ABFB, and extra-anatomic bypass in the form of iliofemoral, femorofemoral, or axillofemoral grafting (see Chapter 106: Aortoiliac Disease: Extra-anatomic Bypass). Given its superior long-term patency rates, aortobifemoral grafting is currently considered the revascularization procedure of choice unless the patient is a poor candidate for major open surgery.

Preoperative Preparation

Careful assessment of the factors that influence operative risk and postoperative complications is an important component of the surgical management of aortic occlusive disease. Patient selection should be based on an objective evaluation of the patient's co-morbidities, functional limitations, and life expectancy. Particular attention should be paid to those patients with the identified risk factors of cardiac, renal, or pulmonary disease (see Chapter 38: Systemic Complications: Cardiac; Chapter 39: Systemic Complications: Respiratory; and Chapter 40: Systemic Complications: Renal). The patient's cerebrovascular, hepatic, and hematologic status should also be reviewed, with further attention given to those with a personal or family history of hypercoagulability (see Chapter 37: Hypercoagulable States).

In patients with known renal insufficiency, elective AI surgery should not immediately follow the diagnostic angiogram; if possible, it should be delayed to allow recovery from the nephrotoxic effects of the contrast load. Similarly, preoperative fluid status should be optimized to the extent possible, with the avoidance of extremes of hypovolemia or fluid overload to minimize the risk of further postoperative renal compromise or congestive heart failure. This is particularly important if concomitant renal revascularization is being considered, which necessitates a period of renal ischemia and

confers additional risk in the form of potential emboli or perioperative renal hypoperfusion. Patients with significant pulmonary dysfunction can usually be identified by history and physical examination, making routine pulmonary function testing unnecessary. If compromised pulmonary reserve is present, an aggressive regimen of preoperative pulmonary rehabilitation in the form of steroid and bronchodilator therapy may be beneficial to optimize the perioperative status.[46] Smoking cessation is critical, and preoperative weight loss in obese patients is of further value in this regard. Perioperative pulmonary risk can also be reduced by the use of postoperative epidural analgesia and by strict adherence to protocols aimed at preventing postoperative deep venous thrombosis and pulmonary embolism.

Coronary Artery Disease

Nearly half of patients proceeding to surgery for AI occlusive disease have significant coronary artery disease.[47] The reduced perioperative mortality and morbidity seen with AI surgery in recent years is largely due to advances in the management of concomitant coronary disease (see Chapter 38: Systemic Complications: Cardiac). Specifically, better preoperative identification of the small number of patients in need of initial coronary revascularization, awareness of the benefit of a waiting period between coronary stenting and major noncoronary vascular surgery, improved perioperative pharmacologic management of patients with impaired myocardium, and more focused efforts to tailor operative and postoperative fluid administration to the individual patient's myocardial reserve are all well-recognized advances.[48,49] Nevertheless, myocardial infarction remains the leading perioperative and long-term complication of AI surgery. For this reason, much energy has been devoted to identifying patients at particular risk for adverse coronary events stemming from the stress of surgery.[50] The American Heart Association has recently updated its consensus recommendations regarding preoperative cardiac assessment in patients with peripheral arterial disease, reflecting the latest investigative results.[50] Although the trend has clearly swung toward less extensive preoperative cardiac evaluation, it is not unreasonable to assume that all patients undergoing AI reconstructive surgery have some degree of coronary disease and would likely benefit from basic preventive measures. For instance, the routine use of perioperative beta blockade is probably the most important practice (see Chapter 38: Systemic Complications: Cardiac).[51] Although the administration of aspirin was routinely discontinued in the past, the cardioprotective value of continuing aspirin through the time of AI reconstruction has now been clearly documented.[52] In contrast, although lower extremity, carotid, and even coronary revascularization is increasingly being performed without stopping clopidogrel, its use is still thought to be prohibitive in major cardiovascular surgery, given the associated bleeding risk.[50,53] The use of mechanical bowel preparations and bowel sterilizing oral antibiotics was previously common practice, but this is no longer routine. Finally, all patients should be administered appropriate preoperative intravenous antibiotics, typically either cefazolin or vancomycin, to ensure adequate tissue levels at the time of the skin incision.

Aortoiliac Endarterectomy

Dos Santos's successful endarterectomy of an atherosclerotic CFA lesion was serendipitous, in that he had not originally intended to remove any intima or media. His success, after multiple failed attempts, was attributed to the novel use of heparin.[2] Wylie and coworkers soon extended this technique to the AI level,[3] and during the 1950s and 1960s, endarterectomy was the standard therapy for severe AI occlusive disease. Enthusiasm for the procedure dimmed, however, with the introduction of prosthetic graft material 10 years later, which was in turn largely replaced by aortic bypass grafting.

Patient Selection

An obvious benefit of endarterectomy is the elimination of the need for a prosthetic graft, making it an appealing alternative in the setting of infection and removing the possibility of myriad late graft-related complications. Advocates have likewise pointed to the advantages of endarterectomy for younger patients or those with small vessels who are less than ideal candidates for endovascular therapy or aortobifemoral grafting.[54] Patients with erectile dysfunction attributable to proximal segment hypogastric occlusive disease are also well suited to this therapeutic option. Such patients can be expected to have a greater degree of improved pelvic perfusion following thorough endarterectomy of their AI and hypogastric segments compared with those undergoing ABFB grafting, and high rates of restored sexual function have been reported.[54,55]

Endarterectomy is most feasible and durable when applied to focal stenotic lesions in large-caliber, high-flow vessels. Indeed, the technique has proved particularly efficacious in patients with localized disease limited to the distal aorta or proximal iliac arteries (see Fig. 105-4), and excellent long-term patency rates, on a par with aortic bypass grafting, have been reported.[54,56-58] In distinction, results in cases of long-segment disease involving the entire infrarenal aorta and extending into the external iliac arteries have been disappointing.[59] In current practice, endarterectomy is now rarely performed for AI disease, having fallen into disfavor owing to its relative technical difficulty, potential for significant blood loss, and poor durability, as well as the clear advantages of bypass grafting in this location. The increasing popularity of endovascular therapy is further eroding the already small proportion of patients considered suitable for this reconstructive approach. As a result, the number of vascular surgeons who are comfortable and facile with this technique is limited; those who maintain their familiarity with endarterectomy and appreciate its benefits will be best positioned to serve the needs of their patients.

Technique

Endarterectomy is a direct disobliterative, debulking technique that takes advantage of the pathologic localization of atherosclerosis to the intima and media. Typically, a cleavage plane is easily developed between the plaque and the outer layers of the vessel wall, with the exact location dependent on the size, location, and muscular content of the involved artery. Haimovici has characterized the three cleavage planes encountered in the operative setting as subintimal, transmedial, and subadventitial; in his view, the latter two planes are preferable because the subintimal plane predisposes to subsequent thrombosis.[60] The residual outer layer is generally of sufficient mechanical strength to hold surgical sutures and resist disruption or progressive enlargement when newly subjected to arterial pressure. In atypical circumstances, the residual adventitia may be attenuated to such a degree that reconstruction of the wall with a patch or, in extreme cases, an interposition graft proves necessary. In practice, this most often occurs when the plaque is extensively calcified.

The various techniques all involve blunt separation of the plaque, termination by spontaneous tapering or sharp division, and careful attention to the endpoints (Fig. 105-8). Tacking sutures should be used when necessary, particularly to secure the distal endpoint, which must be firmly adherent to resist dissection or flap elevation leading to thrombosis. The simplest approach from a technical standpoint is the so-called open method, which employs a longitudinal arteriotomy that allows direct visualization of both endpoints as well as the entire endarterectomized surface; this technique is most commonly used for disease limited to the aorta and common iliac arteries. If primary closure is rendered problematic by the small or marginal caliber of the vessel, patch angioplasty using a vein, synthetic material, or bovine pericardial patch material should be undertaken.

Extraction, eversion, and semiclosed methods are variations that can be helpful in specific anatomic situations. The last technique, useful to treat the external iliac arteries, involves arteriotomies at both the proximal and distal extents of the plaque and the initiation of plaque excision at the endpoints, similar to that undertaken in the open technique. A ringed stripper is then advanced between the endpoints to complete the plaque disengagement, obviating the need for full exposure of the treated segment. In the early 1970s, Inahara[61] modified the technique of eversion endarterectomy first described by Harrison and colleagues,[62] whereby the circumferentially dissected iliofemoral arterial segment is transected distally and passed proximally under the inguinal ligament into the pelvis before being endarterectomized and later reattached.

Aortobifemoral Bypass

Adequate intravenous access, intra-arterial pressure monitoring, Foley catheter placement, and preoperative antibiotics to minimize the risk of prosthetic and wound infection are routine aspects of aortic replacement surgery. Although the use of cell-saver technology is advantageous in patients with relative anemia, its cost-effectiveness has not been firmly established in routine cases.[63] Attention should be paid to maintaining normothermia throughout the procedure to reduce the significant organ dysfunction and operative mor-

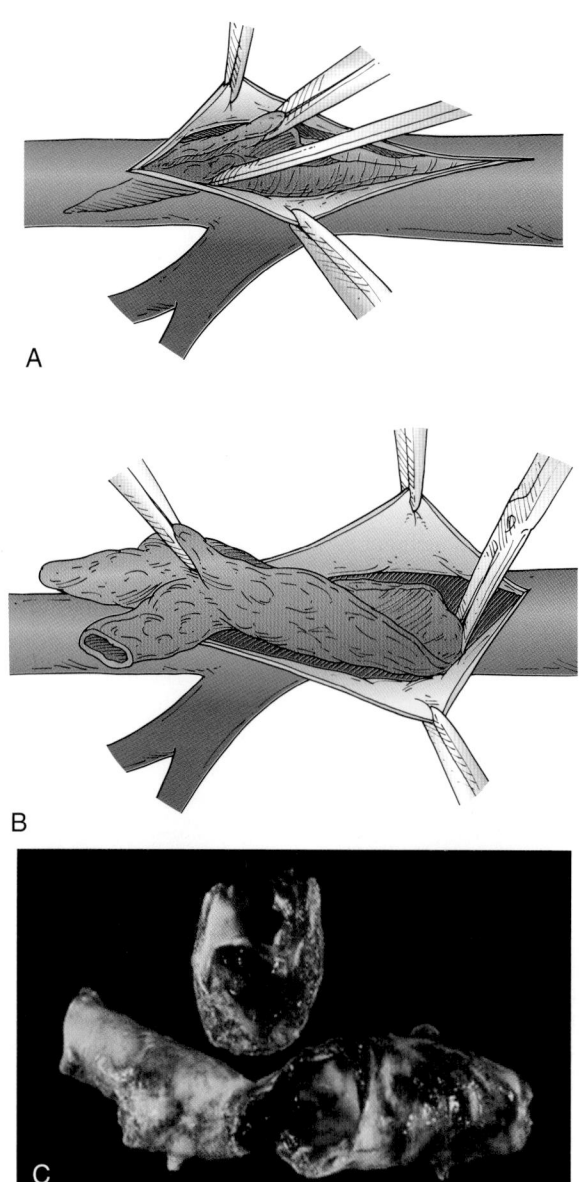

Figure 105-8 A, The technique of endarterectomy involves the initial separation of plaque in the appropriate cleavage plane, with mobilization facilitated by a fine spatula. **B,** Ideally, the endarterectomy is terminated by feathering to a tapered endpoint. **C,** Photograph of an operative specimen removed by endarterectomy.

tality associated with intraoperative hypothermia.[64] This is typically achieved with the use of forced-air body warming devices. ABFB grafting is performed under general endotracheal anesthesia. An epidural catheter is usually placed for postoperative pain control.

Exposure

The initial vascular exposure and proximal and distal vessel control are attained before the institution of systemic anticoagulation, in an effort to minimize blood loss. The femoral vessels are typically exposed first through bilateral longitudinal, oblique incisions to reduce the time during which the

abdomen is open and the viscera exposed. The extent of exposure is dictated by the severity of disease and the level of reconstruction planned at the CFA and its bifurcation. In general, the distal extent of the dissection involves circumferential control of the proximal SFA and profunda femoris arteries; the inferior epigastric and circumflex iliac branches at the anatomic transition from the external iliac to the CFA mark the proximal extent of the dissection. A circumflex femoral arterial branch frequently arises from the posterior aspect of the distal CFA and must be controlled to avoid troublesome backbleeding. The inferior aspects of the retroperitoneal tunnels through which the graft limbs will course to reach the femoral region are begun with blunt digital dissection posterior to the inguinal ligament, which can be partially divided posteriorly to prevent graft limb compression. The tunnels should track directly along the anterior aspect of the external iliac artery, with care taken to elevate all soft tissues to ensure that the ureters remain anterior. A crossing vein normally present beneath the inguinal ligament must be ligated or carefully avoided to prevent bleeding during the tunneling process.

Infrarenal aortic exposure is often performed through a transperitoneal approach via a longitudinal midline laparotomy, although some prefer a transverse incision. The midline incision typically extends from below the xyphoid process to just inferior to the umbilicus; as such, it is shorter than the incision normally employed for abdominal aortic aneurysm repair. The abdomen is explored for any intra-abdominal abnormalities, and the stomach is palpated to ensure proper positioning of the nasogastric tube. The transverse colon is retracted cephalad, and the small bowel is shifted to the patient's right side. The ligament of Treitz is then taken down, and the duodenum is mobilized to the right, allowing access to the infrarenal aorta. A self-retaining fixed retractor is placed to aid in exposure, with care taken to protect the displaced bowel from retractor blade injury. The retroperitoneal tissue overlying the aorta is dissected superiorly to the level of the left renal vein, and the larger lymphatic vessels encountered within the retroperitoneal lymphatic network are ligated. If renal artery reconstruction is not planned, the dissection can often be limited to the region between the renal arteries and the inferior mesenteric artery. Extensive dissection anterior to the aortic bifurcation and proximal left iliac artery should be avoided because the autonomic nerve plexus regulating erection and ejaculation in men sweeps over the aorta in this region. If exposure in the area of the plexus proves necessary, dissecting along the right lateral aspect of the infrarenal aorta and reflecting rather than transecting the tissue overlying the terminal aorta and proximal iliac arteries can minimize the risk of iatrogenic neurogenic sexual dysfunction.

Should thrombus or significant aortic calcification extend to the level of the renal arteries, it may be necessary to continue the proximal aortic dissection to the suprarenal level to allow for safe proximal clamp placement. Alternatively, proximal control may be obtained by intraluminal balloon deployment or supraceliac clamping via the gastrohepatic ligament.

In all cases, it is important to extend the reconstruction close to the level of the renal arteries to minimize the risk of failure secondary to disease progression in the remnant infrarenal aortic neck. If end-to-side repair is planned, exposing and controlling all relevant lumbar or accessory renal arteries before performing the aortotomy helps avoid backbleeding, which can be challenging to control with cross-clamps in place and the aorta compressed. The superior aspects of the graft limb tunnels are completed with further digital manipulation from above and below, again taking care to maintain a course anterior to the iliac vessels but posterior to the ureters. On the left side, the tunnel passes beneath the sigmoid mesentery and slightly more laterally in an effort to avoid disruption of the autonomic nerve plexus. Moist umbilical tapes or Penrose drains are passed with a smooth aortic clamp to mark the tunnels. With vessel exposure and tunnel creation complete, but before vascular occlusion, a standard dose of heparin sodium anticoagulation is given as an intravenous bolus. The half-life of heparin is between 60 and 90 minutes in most patients, and repeated doses may be necessary, depending on the length of the operation and the requirement for additional periods of flow occlusion. Measurement of the activated clotting time is readily accomplished using standard equipment available in most cardiovascular operating suites, and this facilitates appropriate heparin dosing during longer procedures. For peripheral vascular operations, the initial dose typically ranges between 70 and 100 units/kg, and an activated clotting time in the 250- to 350-second range is adequate.

Clamp Placement

Using noncontrast CTA guidance (when available) to delineate sites of heavy calcification, the aorta is carefully palpated to identify the optimal sites for application of the cross-clamps. In the event of asymmetric plaque, the technique of clamping soft plaque against hard plaque minimizes the risk of emboli. It also lessens the risk of a traumatic clamp injury, which can be a formidable technical problem in a heavily calcified aorta. Anterior to posterior clamping may be necessary in the presence of a soft anterior but calcified posterior aortic wall. Appropriate atraumatic vascular clamps are

selected, and after allowing sufficient time for the heparin to circulate, the aorta is clamped first proximally or distally at the site of least disease to avoid dislodgement and potential distal embolization of plaque. The distal clamp is usually placed above or below the inferior mesenteric artery. The proximal clamp is placed just below the renal arteries if the disease pattern does not obligate suprarenal clamping, with as little dissection of the renal artery origins as possible.

If an end-to-end anastomosis is planned, the aorta is transected several inches below the proximal clamp, and the distal aorta is oversewn in two layers with running monofilament suture or stapled with a surgical stapler (Fig. 105-9A). A short segment of the distal aortic cuff is excised to allow better exposure of the aortic neck and more precise proximal reconstruction. This maneuver also allows the graft to lie more flatly against the vertebral column rather than in an anterior orientation and facilitates retroperitoneal coverage (Fig. 105-10). If necessary, it is important to carry out a complete thromboendarterectomy of the infrarenal neck (Fig. 105-9B). Removal of all thrombotic debris and calcified plaque facilitates both suture placement and creation of a widely patent proximal anastomosis. Brief repositioning of the proximal clamp to the suprarenal position or the application of digital pressure sufficient to temporarily occlude the suprarenal aorta may be helpful to ensure the thorough removal of all intraluminal debris (Fig. 105-9C). Mobilization and cephalad or caudad retraction of the left renal vein can facilitate adequate exposure of the juxtarenal aorta. Division of the left renal vein is usually unnecessary but acceptable if additional exposure is required, provided that the adrenal, lumbar, and gonadal collateral branches are preserved. If suprarenal clamping is undertaken, concurrent clamping of the renal arteries is advisable to prevent the potentially adverse effects of inadvertent emboli.

A minority of patients present with an aortic occlusion extending to the level of the renal arteries. These patients are best managed by controlling the renal arteries and then thrombectomizing the infrarenal cuff, without placement of an infrarenal proximal aortic clamp, which could displace thrombotic material proximally. The aortic plug encountered at this location is often soft, propagated, secondary thrombus

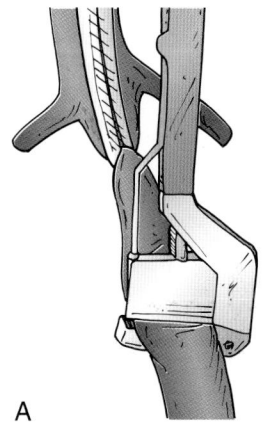

A

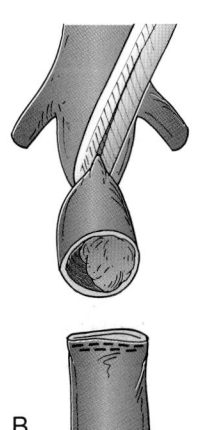

B

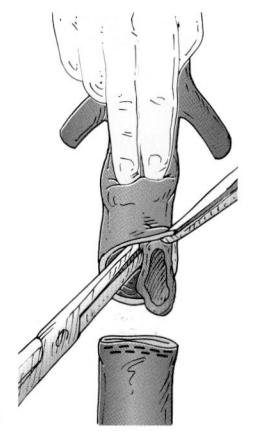

C

Figure 105-9 A, The end-to-end proximal anastomosis for aortofemoral reconstruction can be initiated with the infrarenal aorta cross-clamp placed in an anteroposterior direction, as close to the origin of the renal arteries as possible. The aorta is then stapled or occluded with a second clamp just proximal to the origin of the inferior mesenteric artery. **B,** After excising a short segment of aortic cuff, a complete thromboendarterectomy of the remaining proximal cuff is carried out. **C,** Brief digital or clamp control of the juxtarenal aorta may prove necessary to complete the thromboendarterectomy.

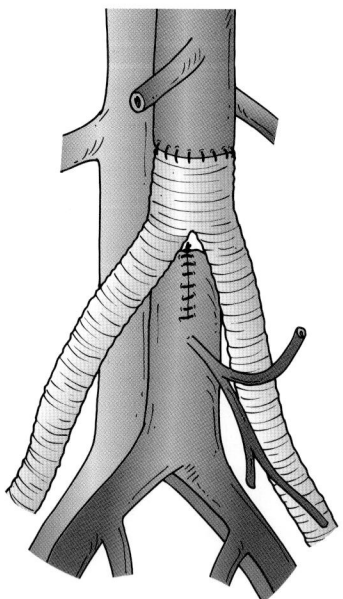

Figure 105-10 The end-to-end proximal anastomotic configuration for aortofemoral reconstruction allows the graft to lie flat against the vertebral column and results in less turbulent flow.

that can be easily removed with a Kelly clamp. After aortic pressure is used to flush out the remaining plug, suprarenal control is briefly utilized. Remnant debris is cleared from the infrarenal cuff, the aorta is flushed again, the renal arteries are backbled, and an infrarenal clamp is placed.

Graft Selection

A bifurcated graft appropriately sized to match the aorta and femoral vessels is selected. Although some surgeons prefer polytetrafluoroethylene (PTFE) grafts, knitted polyester (Dacron) grafts are more commonly used. Current low-porosity knitted versions have excellent handling and hemostatic properties and a proven track record of durability (see Chapter 88: Prosthetic Grafts). They also develop a more stable pseudointima than earlier woven grafts, although their tendency to slowly dilate over time has been documented.[65] Woven polyester grafts can also be used and may tend to dilate less during long-term follow-up. Greater appreciation of the importance of sizing the graft to the runoff vessels followed an early experience with limb thrombosis believed to be secondary to sluggish flow from oversizing.[66,67] Bifurcated grafts measuring 18 by 9 mm or 16 by 8 mm are typically chosen for male patients; grafts measuring 14 by 7 mm or even 12 by 6 mm are usually suitable for female patients.

Anastomoses

One of the technical considerations related to ABFB grafting that has prompted considerable debate involves the type of proximal anastomosis. The published literature has established that both end-to-end and end-to-side techniques are acceptable and effective. Despite strong preferences expressed by various surgeons, neither approach has demonstrated

overall superiority, but each may be preferred in certain circumstances.

End to End. Those favoring an end-to-end configuration claim that it facilitates a more comprehensive thromboendarterectomy of the proximal stump and allows for a better in-line flow pattern, with less turbulence and more favorable hemodynamic characteristics (see Fig. 105-10).[68] Lower rates of proximal suture line pseudoaneurysm and better long-term patency rates reported in some series lend support to this view.[69] Stapling or oversewing of the distal aorta with the end-to-end technique also has the benefit of reducing the risk of clamp-induced emboli to the lower extremities following release of the distal clamp compared with the end-to-side option. Further, those in favor of this approach assert that because the graft lies flatter in the retroperitoneum, this enhances the ability to close the retroperitoneum over the graft, resulting in a lower rate of late graft infection and aortoenteric fistulae; there is, however, little direct evidence to support this claim. Finally, creation of an end-to-side anastomosis can be technically challenging in a heavily diseased aorta, particularly if partially occluded by a side-biting clamp (favored by some surgeons). In the setting of concomitant aneurysmal disease or complete aortic occlusion extending up to the level of the renal arteries, an end-to-end approach should be used.

End to Side. There are certain circumstances when an end-to-side proximal anastomosis is advantageous. The most common indication is in patients with occluded or severely diseased external iliac arteries but patent common and internal iliac arteries, in whom the interruption of forward aortic flow may result in the loss of critical pelvic perfusion. Without the retrograde flow through the external iliac arteries normally present in an end-to-end configuration, pelvic ischemia, ranging from mild hip claudication to severe buttock rest pain or ulceration, may result.[70,71] Additional ischemic complications, such as erectile dysfunction in males and rarely seen paraplegia secondary to cauda equina syndrome,[72] can potentially be avoided with an end-to-side approach. Preservation of either a large inferior mesenteric artery, sometimes necessary to avert colonic or mesenteric ischemia, or an important accessory renal artery arising from the distal aorta or an iliac artery can more easily be accomplished with an end-to-side technique. Alternatively, these vessels can be re-implanted onto the side of an end-to-end graft.

Technique. For end-to-end proximal anastomoses, the main body of the graft is shortened to minimize graft redundancy and allow the graft limbs to straddle rather than override the transected aortic stump (see Fig. 105-10). The anastomosis is performed with running 3-0 polypropylene suture. If an end-to-side anastomosis is to be performed, a beveled anastomosis is fashioned after an approximately 3-cm longitudinal aortotomy is created as close to the renal arteries as practical (Fig. 105-11). Care is taken to remove all loose debris and mural thrombus from the excluded portion of the

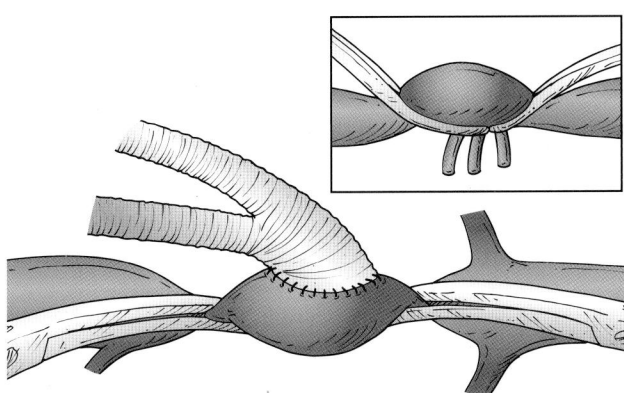

Figure 105-11 An end-to-side proximal anastomosis for aortofemoral grafting is required to preserve antegrade pelvic perfusion in situations in which retrograde flow would be compromised owing to heavily diseased or occluded external iliac arteries.

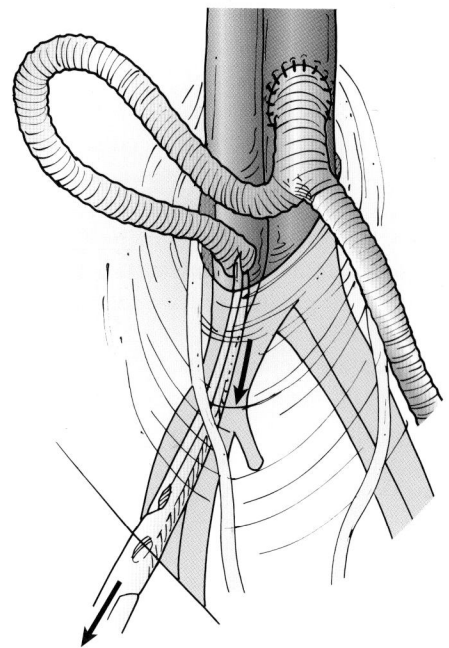

Figure 105-12 Aortobifemoral graft limbs are carefully tunneled beneath the ureters to avoid kinking.

aorta, and a particular effort is made to ensure adequate back-flushing of clot and debris before re-establishing forward flow in the native aorta and graft. Side-biting clamps are best avoided when performing an end-to-side anastomosis because they compress the aortic sidewalls, rendering both adequate thromboendarterectomy and accurate suture placement more difficult (see Fig. 105-11).

After completion of the abdominal portion of the procedure, the graft limbs are clamped with soft-jaw insert clamps and flushed with heparinized saline. They are then passed through the retroperitoneal tunnels, taking care to prevent twisting and to eliminate excess redundancy (Fig. 105-12), and attention is turned to the distal anastomoses. Proximal femoral control is typically obtained with either a soft-jaw clamp or a Satinsky clamp placed from a lateral direction, and distal control is usually achieved with vessel loops or atraumatic bulldog or profunda clamps. For those patients with normal femoral and distal runoff, a longitudinal arteriotomy limited to the distal CFA is sufficient. More commonly, extension of the arteriotomy across the profunda femoris artery origin and profundaplasty will prove necessary (see "Adjunctive Profundaplasty"). The distal anastomoses are completed in a beveled end-to-side fashion using 5-0 polypropylene, again carrying out retrograde and antegrade flushing maneuvers before completing the anastomoses and restoring flow. It is important to alert the anesthetic team before clamp release, given the expected blood pressure drop with reperfusion.

Closure

Before wound closure, the surgeon must confirm adequate distal perfusion and ensure that no distal embolization has occurred. The quality of the pulses and Doppler signals just beyond the distal anastomosis and at the pedal level is assessed, as is the color, temperature, and general appearance of the feet. If the revascularization is deemed satisfactory and no further distal reconstruction is to be undertaken, the effects

of heparin can be reversed by administering protamine sulfate (1 mg/100 units of circulating heparin) at the surgeon's discretion to help attain hemostasis. Once hemostasis is sufficient, the abdomen is irrigated and the retroperitoneum is closed over the proximal anastomosis and graft behind the duodenum to the extent possible. If adequate retroperitoneal coverage is not possible, particularly with an end-to-side proximal anastomosis, a sleeve of omentum should be fashioned to cover any exposed segment of the anastomosis and to separate the graft from the adjacent bowel. It is important to tack down this omental apron to prevent small bowel herniation. The groin wounds are copiously irrigated with antibiotic solution, and the deeper tissue is closed in several layers using absorbable Vicryl sutures.

Adjunctive Profundaplasty

The important role of profundaplasty in preserving the long-term patency of anatomic or extra-anatomic inflow grafts in patients with AI disease has been widely established.[11,59,73-76] As mentioned, for those patients with normal proximal SFAs and profunda femoris arteries, the distal anastomosis of an aortobifemoral graft can be performed to the CFA. However, most patients with AI disease severe enough to warrant aortofemoral bypass in the endovascular era have both profunda and SFA disease that limits outflow and reduces the likelihood of graft thrombosis. In patients with severe AI, SFA, and profunda disease causing CLI, a concomitant profundaplasty may be sufficient to sustain the patency of the inflow graft and salvage the limb, particularly if there is good profunda collateral circulation to a patent popliteal artery. Some authors have even recommended that the aortofemoral bypass graft limb should be extended to the profunda in every case of SFA occlusion, even in the absence of orificial profunda disease, arguing that a "functional" obstruction on the order of 50% stenosis is present in these patients.[77] Although this position has not been universally adopted, it is now common practice to extend the hood of the distal anastomosis over the origin of the profunda femoris artery to enhance the graft outflow, particularly if the SFA is occluded or severely diseased. In the presence of significant CFA or profunda femoris origin plaque, an endarterectomy or profundaplasty is almost always indicated (Fig. 105-13). The need for adjunctive profundaplasty should be determined at the time of preoperative angiography. Although anatomic variations are not uncommon, the profunda typically arises as a posterolateral branch off the terminal CFA. As such, proper visualization requires dedicated oblique views, because subtle disease can easily be obscured by the overlying SFA in the anteroposterior projection.

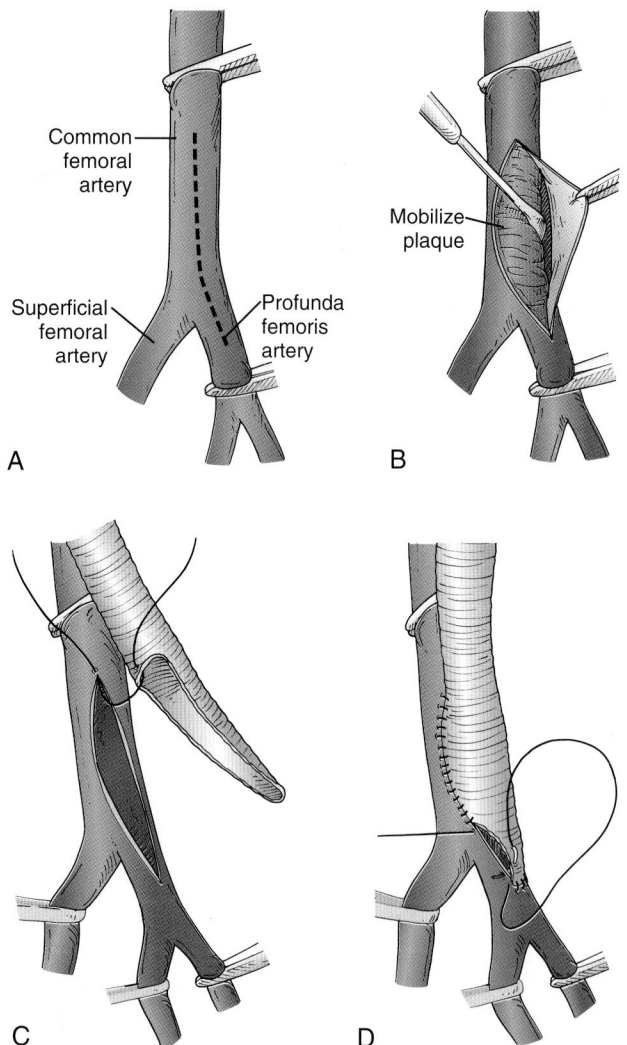

Figure 105-13 A–D, In the setting of superficial femoral artery and orificial profunda femoris artery disease, extending the common femoral arteriotomy to the origin of the profunda and performing a profundaplasty before completing the distal anastomosis of the aortobifemoral bypass can improve outflow and maximize graft patency.

Technique

The profunda is usually exposed by distal extension of the dissection used to access the CFA, although a lateral approach through a fresh tissue plane with medial retraction of the sartorius can be used to avoid a scarred or infected groin. Every effort should be made to spare all collateral branches arising from the CFA and profunda femoris artery, because they may prove vital to preserving lower extremity perfusion in the event of later graft thrombosis. Once exposed, the CFA and profunda femoris should be palpated to gauge the degree of atherosclerotic plaque present, particularly given angiography's well-known tendency to underestimate the extent of disease. Profunda arterial plaque not uncommonly ends at the first or second major branch point. The profunda orifice can be visually inspected after incising the CFA, and its lumen can be further assessed by noting the quality of backbleeding and by gentle interrogation with a series of sizing metal probes. The dissection is continued along the anterior aspect of the artery as necessary; the extent is guided by the location of a suitable endpoint as identified by palpation, inspection, and reference to the preoperative angiogram. The lateral femoral circumflex vein coursing deep to the SFA and crossing anteriorly over the proximal profunda must be ligated in most cases. Isolated orificial plaque can sometimes be entirely removed using an eversion technique through the CFA. If it becomes necessary to extend the arteriotomy to the profunda, care should be taken to avoid incising the crotch of the superficial and deep femoral arteries. The endarterectomy is performed as described earlier. In the event an extensive endarterectomy proves necessary, it may be preferable to close the endarterectomy site with a vein or bovine pericardial patch, onto which the distal anastomosis can then be attached, rather than creating a long profunda patch with the graft limb.[73] If an outflow bypass is to be performed, this can be taken off either the distal patch or the graft limb.

Other Operative Considerations
External Iliac Anastomosis

Early in the operative experience for AI occlusive disease, the tendency was to place the distal anastomosis of aortic bypass grafts at the iliac level. With time came a growing appreciation of the benefits of extending the distal anastomosis to the femoral level; creation of the distal anastomosis is technically easier at the groin level, and long-term patency rates for aortobifemoral grafts are notably improved compared with AI grafts.[78] In addition, with meticulous surgical technique and improvements in graft materials, the feared increase in graft infection caused by moving the distal dissection to the femoral level has not proved to be a significant problem in the majority of patients.[79] There are certain circumstances, however, when performing an aortobiiliac bypass remains advantageous. Patients with hostile groin creases from prior surgery or radiation therapy, for example, are likely to be better served by this option, as are obese, diabetic patients with an intertriginous rash at the inguinal crease and patent external iliac arteries. Excellent preoperative imaging and intraoperative confirmation of suitable anatomy are necessary if one chooses this reconstructive alternative.

Multilevel Occlusive Disease

The optimal management of patients with multilevel occlusive disease is often difficult to determine. The question frequently arises whether, or under what circumstances, concomitant versus staged outflow procedures should be performed in association with an inflow operation. Of relevance, the impact of synchronous SFA disease on the results of AI revascularization remains undefined in the current literature: some reports have indicated similar patency rates between patients with and without SFA occlusion,[36] while others have reported lower long-term patency rates in this setting.[80,81] If an atretic or prohibitively diseased profunda is present in addition to a severely diseased SFA, infrainguinal bypass grafting is likely necessary to ensure sufficient outflow for graft patency and perfusion of the foot. A recent investigation that specifically addressed the impact of diabetes concluded that diabetic patients with multilevel occlusive disease were no more likely to require subsequent infrainguinal revascularization following an inflow reconstruction than were nondiabetics.[82] Further, although up to 80% of patients with claudication and both inflow and outflow disease manifest symptomatic improvement following aortofemoral bypass grafting alone,[12,83] some studies indicate that as many as two thirds have some degree of persistent claudication.[84]

No single criterion mandates a combined procedure; however, the severity of distal ischemia is probably the most important factor to be considered. If significant tissue loss is present, concurrent inflow and outflow procedures are likely warranted if limb salvage is to be achieved. In deciding whether a staged approach is appropriate, the patient's ability to tolerate a prolonged operative procedure must be weighed against the potential risk of wound and graft infection resulting from redissection in the groin and the risk of progressive tissue loss during the initial recuperative period. When performed with several teams operating simultaneously, concurrent inflow and outflow revascularization can be completed in a timely and safe manner. Indeed, several recent reports found no significant differences in perioperative mortality or morbidity in patients undergoing multilevel reconstruction and those having a major inflow procedure alone.[85,86]

Associated Renal or Mesenteric Artery Occlusive Disease

In recent decades, the introduction of potent new antihypertensive drugs and the growing application of percutaneous interventions have significantly impacted the treatment algorithms for renal artery occlusive disease. Balloon angioplasty and stenting are likewise playing an increasing role in mesenteric occlusive disease. The decision whether to address coexisting renal or mesenteric disease at the time of aortic

reconstruction is a challenging one that warrants careful consideration of multiple individual factors, as well as the obligatory increase in operative time and complexity and the greater operative mortality and morbidity. In the setting of multidrug-refractory hypertension or ischemic nephropathy believed to have a potentially reversible functional component based on a thorough diagnostic assessment, simultaneous repair of significant renal occlusive disease may be indicated. Combined repair is also appropriate when accessory renal arteries arise from the diseased aortic segment. Simultaneous revascularization is more controversial when the functional significance of the renal artery stenosis is less certain or is thought to be clinically silent.

Advocates of an aggressive treatment approach cite the clinical deterioration seen with the progression of untreated renal artery occlusive disease and the increasing safety of combined aortic and renal reconstruction. Those who favor a more conservative position believe that the increased surgical risk does not offset the potential clinical gain. Perioperative mortality rates for patients undergoing simultaneous aortic and renal repair have consistently been in the 5% to 6% range,[87-89] in comparison to rates of 1.7% and 0.7% for those undergoing renal or aortic reconstruction alone, respectively.[87] A favorable response to hypertension has been reported in 60% to 70% of patients undergoing combined revascularization, and improvement in renal excretory function has been reported in up to 33% of patients.[87,88] The most common reconstruction approach is aortorenal bypass from the aortic graft, using either saphenous vein or prosthetic graft. In select cases, in situ thromboendarterectomy, endarterectomy with re-implantation onto the aortic graft, or extra-anatomic splenorenal or hepatorenal grafting may prove preferable (see Chapter 142: Renovascular Disease: Open Surgical Treatment). With regard to visceral artery occlusive disease, strict attention to preserving the inferior mesenteric artery usually suffices to prevent postoperative mesenteric ischemia, and simultaneous revascularization of the celiac or superior mesenteric arteries is rarely required. Staged open or percutaneous revascularization of the renal or mesenteric arteries is another option in specific circumstances, although the role of simultaneous renal reconstruction versus angioplasty before or after surgery remains unclear.[90,91]

Retroperitoneal Approach

Although the retroperitoneal approach to the infrarenal aorta is a well-accepted alternative to the more standard transperitoneal technique in the setting of aneurysmal disease, it is also favored by some surgeons in select patients with occlusive disease.[92,93] This option may be advantageous in patients with a history of multiple prior abdominal operations, abdominal wall stoma, concurrent renal or mesenteric arterial disease requiring a more suprarenal exposure, or severe cardiopulmonary disease. Stated benefits of reduced pulmonary morbidity and lower rates of postoperative ileus have not been consistently supported by the literature.[94] Clear disadvantages of the retroperitoneal approach include the attendant difficulty in accessing the right renal and iliac arteries and the right groin, particularly in obese patients.

The technique involves placing the patient on an inflatable beanbag in the partial right lateral decubitus position, with flank extension. The hips are rotated as far posteriorly as possible to maximize exposure to the right femoral arteries. An oblique incision is created from the left lateral border of the rectus abdominis to the posterior axillary line, and the lateral third of the 11th rib is excised. The retroperitoneal plane is identified, and the peritoneal contents are mobilized anteriorly to reveal the left iliac artery and infrarenal aorta (see Chapter 128: Abdominal Aortic Aneurysms: Open Surgical Treatment).

Minimally Invasive Approaches

Reflecting widespread trends toward more minimally invasive approaches in other areas of surgery, the technique of performing aortofemoral bypass grafting through a shorter midline incision has recently been reported.[95] The described minilaparotomy is less than 10 cm long, and the procedure is undertaken without displacement of the small bowel. As with laparoscopic aortic replacement (see Chapter 107: Aortoiliac Disease: Laparoscopic Reconstruction),[96,97] enthusiasm for the technique remains limited.

■ RESULTS

The short- and long-term results of both endarterectomy and ABFB have generally been excellent, particularly in more recently published series. When endarterectomy is performed for disease limited to the distal aorta and proximal iliac segments, 5-year patency rates of 95% and 10-year rates between 85% and 90% are consistently achieved.[61,57-59] In contrast to the nearly 7% perioperative mortality rates reported in the early experience of endarterectomy, more recent reports reflect improvements in patient selection and perioperative management, with rates as low as 1%.[56-59]

Two large meta-analyses evaluating the comprehensive experience with ABFB grafting from its inception in the mid-1950s through the 1980s indicated similar overall 30-day mortality rates of 4.0% and 4.4%.[98,99] Several recent single-institution series more representative of the current era reported an operative mortality of 1%,[36,45,82,100] on a par with that of elective abdominal aortic aneurysm repair. Increasing age, chronic pulmonary disease, and a low-volume hospital setting predict higher perioperative mortality (Table 105-1).

The accumulated experience to date has shown that 5-year primary patency rates between 85% and 90% and 10-year rates between 75% and 85% can be expected with aortobifemoral grafting (see Table 105-1).[36,45,80,82,98-101] Age has proved to be a significant predictor of outcome; in one report, primary patency rates at 5 years were greater than 95% for patients older than 60 years but only 66% for those younger than 50 years (Fig. 105-14).[45] Although it is not clear why younger patients have inferior long-term patency rates, one could speculate that they have a more aggressive form of atherosclerosis or are at a different point in disease evolution than their older counterparts.

The reported influence of gender on graft patency has been more inconsistent, with some studies indicating less favorable outcomes in females and others demonstrating equivalent long-term patency rates in males and females.[36,45,80,98] Similarly, conflicting results have been documented with regard to the impact of preexisting SFA occlusion, with some but not all reports suggesting improved late patency when a simultaneous outflow procedure is performed at the time of aortobifemoral grafting.[36,80,81] In contrast, the benefits of combining profundaplasty with the inflow procedure have been unambiguously demonstrated.[11,59,73-76] Of note, no major differences in aortobifemoral graft durability have been noted between the transperitoneal and retroperitoneal approaches,

Table 105-1 Outcomes of Aortobifemoral Bypass: Operative Mortality and Long-term Patency Rates

| Series | Year | Number of Patients | Results | | | | |
			Operative Mortality (%)	5-Year PP (%)	5-Year SP (%)	10-Year Patency (%)	15-Year Patency (%)
de Vries et al.[98]*	1997	1429	4.4	88-91		82-87	75-82
de Vries et al.[98]†	1997	1429	4.4	80-86		72-79	63-72
McDaniel et al.[99]‡	1997	2689	4	82-92		74-78	69
Ballard et al.[80]	1998	54	1.9	93§			
Onohara et al.[100]	2000	38	0	89	97	94	
Farie et al.[82]	2001	370	0	93			
Mingoli et al.[101]	2001	130	4.6	81	87		
Dimick et al.[102]	2003	3073	3.3				
Reed et al.[45]	2003	281	1	85	93		
Back et al.[4]	2003	107	3.7				
Hertzer et al.[36]	2007	224	1.2	88		81	71

*Meta-analysis of 23 studies between 1975 and 1996, limb based.
†Meta-analysis of 23 studies between 1975 and 1996, patient based.
‡Meta-analysis of 18 reports between 1985 and 1992.
§42-month PP.
PP, primary patency; SP, secondary patency.

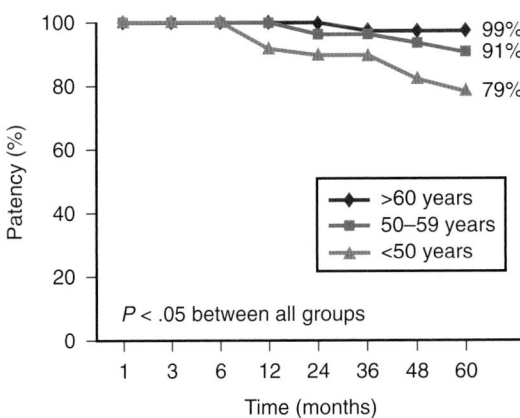

Figure 105-14 Overall 5-year cumulative secondary patency rates in a recent cohort of patients undergoing aortobifemoral bypass grafting, indicating an inverse relationship between age and graft patency.[34]

Table 105-2 Complications of Aortobifemoral Bypass

Complication	Percentage
Early (Perioperative)	
Hemorrhage	1-2
Renal failure	<5
Acute limb ischemia	1-3
Bowel ischemia	2
Groin complications (lymphocele, lymphocutaneous fistula, wound infection, hematoma)	3-15
Sexual dysfunction	≤25
Ureteral injury	<1
Spinal cord ischemia	0.25
Pneumonia	<7
Myocardial infarction	1-5
Death	0-4
Late	
Graft thrombosis	5-30
Graft infection	0.5-3
Aortoenteric fistula	<3
Anastomotic pseudoaneurysm	1-5

between end-to-end and end-to-side anastomotic techniques, or between the indications of claudication and CLI.[36,45,93,94,98]

In general, patients with occlusive disease limited to the AI region can expect to have excellent relief of symptoms following aortobifemoral grafting; those with multilevel disease generally have a lesser degree of symptom reduction. In one study, more than 80% of patients reported satisfaction with their result 5 years after undergoing ABFB.[103] Similarly, although 10-year survival rates are as low as 50% in patients with diffuse disease, those with more localized AI disease have a life expectancy not appreciably different from that of their normal age- and sex-matched counterparts.[11,104,105]

Early Complications

Reported overall morbidity rates range from 17% to 32% following aortic surgery for occlusive disease (Table 105-2).[4,36,45,80-82,101,103,106] Cardiac complications are the most common cause of mortality[36,83] and result from the hemodynamic stress associated with major vascular surgery and the obligatory fluid shifts during the early postoperative period. Pulmonary complications are also common and are most likely to occur in the elderly or those with chronic obstructive pulmonary disease, a significant smoking history, or poor preoperative nutritional status.[107] Adequate pain control, appropriate diuresis, and strict attention to pulmonary toilet are important measures to prevent the development of pneumonia and the progression of relatively benign alveolar collapse to more extreme degrees of pulmonary collapse.

Acute renal failure following aortic reconstruction for occlusive disease is relatively uncommon in patients with normal preoperative renal function, even when a period of suprarenal clamping proves necessary. Ensuring adequate hydration and avoiding repetitive aortic cross-clamping and perioperative hypotension are valuable prophylactic maneuvers; less clear is the benefit of the adjunctive use of mannitol and furosemide (Lasix) prior to aortic cross-clamping to trigger diuresis. Our limited ability to alter the natural history of acute tubular necrosis or the effects of atheroemboli

results in some inevitable progression to dialysis dependence; those patients with a preoperative creatinine greater than 1.8 mg/dL [159 μmol/L] are at much higher risk for this complication.[108]

Injury to the ureters during dissection, graft tunneling, or retroperitoneal closure can usually be avoided with careful surgical technique and diligence, as discussed previously. Spinal cord ischemia is a particularly devastating complication of infrarenal aortic surgery and one that is thought to be potentially preventable. The central component of prophylaxis is careful preservation of hypogastric perfusion; however, the use of gentle technique to minimize the risk of atheroemboli and the avoidance of peri- and postoperative hypotension have also proved to be important preventive measures.[109] Fortunately, this complication is uncommon, occurring in only 0.3% (4 of 1209) of AI reconstructions for occlusive disease in one series.[110]

Hemorrhage

Bleeding complications associated with endarterectomy, particularly when the treated segments were extensive, were partly responsible for the waning popularity of this technique for AI occlusive disease. With modern-day suture and patch materials and the less extensive disease typically repaired in the current era, bleeding associated with endarterectomy has become less problematic. For patients undergoing aortobifemoral grafting, postoperative hemorrhage is a relatively rare event, occurring in 1% to 2% of cases.[106] This rarity is due in part to a greater awareness of bleeding disorders, better intraoperative anticoagulation and blood product management, and the improved hemostatic properties of the grafts used (see Chapter 36: Coagulopathy and Hemorrhage).

Bleeding points in the anastomotic suture line following a test release of the aortic or femoral clamps are usually effectively managed with repair sutures re-enforced with felt pledgets. It is important to replace the clamp before placing any necessary repair stitches, because attempted placement under tension risks extending the defect and worsening the bleeding. In cases in which the walls of the infrarenal aortic cuff are particularly thin following thromboendarterectomy, a previously positioned sleeve of graft advanced over the aortic suture line can act as a prophylactic bolster. Intraoperative venous injuries can occur during dissection between the aorta and vena cava or from a tear in a lumbar vein; such injuries can often be controlled with judicious tamponade. A number of sealants, glues, and thrombin-based hemostatic adjuncts are now available to help control troublesome diffuse oozing and persistent needle hole bleeding.

Bleeding may present in a delayed fashion if the postoperative blood pressure is appreciably higher than the pressure at the time of closure. Blood products, including platelets and fresh frozen plasma, are the preferred replacement fluid in most cases during the early postoperative period, particularly if intraoperative blood loss was significant and the patient is considered at risk for dilutional coagulopathy. Careful postoperative monitoring of the abdominal girth, hematocrit, bladder pressure, coagulation parameters, and hemodynamic status is paramount to identify ongoing bleeding significant enough to require urgent reoperation (see Chapter 32: Postoperative Management).

Intestinal Ischemia

Intestinal ischemia following aortic reconstruction has been reported in 2% of cases.[111] The involved segment is usually the rectosigmoid, and the cause is multifactorial. Although sacrifice of either the primary or the main collateral source of perfusion to the colon during reconstruction is the most common causative event, perioperative hypotension leading to insufficient perfusion and atheroemboli are other possible contributors. If compromised bowel perfusion is recognized intraoperatively following the creation of an end-to-end anastomosis, inferior mesenteric artery re-implantation is indicated. Although some surgeons advocate routine re-implantation of all patent inferior mesenteric arteries as the safest means to avoid colonic malperfusion,[112] this practice has not been universally adopted. Intraoperative detection of ischemia can be difficult, and all of the various techniques of doing so have their limitations. In addition to direct visual assessment, interrogation of Doppler flow along the antimesenteric border, measurement of the inferior mesenteric artery stump pressure, and the use of intravenous fluorescein have been used. Given the frequency of delayed presentation, maintaining a high index of suspicion and having a low threshold for performing sigmoidoscopy during the early postoperative period are critical in the effort to avoid potentially catastrophic colonic perforation.

Late Complications

Late complications following aortobifemoral grafting include graft limb thrombosis, aortoenteric fistula, graft infection, and anastomotic pseudoaneurysm (see Table 105-2).

Graft Thrombosis

Graft thrombosis is the most frequently encountered late complication (see Chapter 44: Local Complications: Graft Thrombosis). It occurs in as many as 30% of cases in some series in which the grafts were observed for 10 years or longer.[113] Occlusion of the entire graft is relatively rare and usually stems from placing the proximal anastomosis inappropriately low in relation to the renal arteries, with subsequent progression of proximal atherosclerosis. A more commonly encountered scenario is unilateral limb thrombosis, which most often reflects progressive intimal hyperplasia at the distal anastomosis or progression of outflow disease. Flow can frequently be restored with aggressive efforts using special thrombectomy catheters designed to remove the chronically adherent fibrinoid thrombus typically encountered. If inflow is successfully restored, revising the distal anastomotic site with a profundaplasty or extension of the graft may prove necessary. If more extensive progression of outflow disease is identified, or if extraction of a distally propagating thrombus is unsuccessful, the addition of an outflow graft may be needed to ensure patency of the revascularized limb. A femorofemoral or axillofemoral graft usually suffices as a secondary source of inflow when an aortobifemoral limb is not successfully reopened.

False Aneurysm

Anastomotic false aneurysms are far less common in modern practice compared with the early experience of aortic grafting, but they continue to be seen as a late complication in 1% to 5% of cases (see Chapter 43: Local Complications: Anastomotic Aneurysms).[106,114] They arise secondary to a weakening in the suture line as a result of structural fatigue or fabric degeneration. Undue tension, poor suturing technique, and focal weakening of the recipient arterial wall following endarterectomy have been implicated as causative factors. Infection undoubtedly plays a role in many cases, despite the frequent absence of any obvious clinical signs; *Staphylococcus* species are the predominant organisms identified in culture. Femoral anastomotic false aneurysms are most common and typically present as a slowly enlarging, asymptomatic groin bulge. Proximal anastomotic false aneurysms are often discovered incidentally during radiographic evaluation for other reasons or come to attention when they rupture. Given the potential complications of thrombosis, embolization, or rupture, repair is generally recommended for femoral false aneurysms larger than 2 cm or aortic false aneurysms greater than 50% of the graft diameter. Treatment usually consists of débridement of the degenerated tissue and placement of a short interposition graft.

Graft Infection

Prosthetic graft infection is a particularly feared complication of aortic reconstruction, given its high associated morbidity and mortality (see Chapter 41: Local Complications: Graft

Infection).[115] The diagnosis is typically reached by a combination of clinical suspicion and CT or isotope-labeled leukocyte scanning, with the groin being the most common site of presentation. On occasion, exploration is needed to confirm or refute the diagnosis. Prevention through strict adherence to sterile technique, particularly in the setting of septic distal ulcerations, and the timely administration of preoperative antibiotics is critical. Graft contamination at the time of implantation is difficult to prove but is believed to be common. Once infection is diagnosed, graft excision is usually indicated.

Aortoenteric Fistula

Aortoenteric fistula is another relatively rare but potentially devastating late complication associated with aortobifemoral grafting (see Chapter 42: Local Complications: Aortoenteric Fistulae).[116] The most common pathophysiologic process is erosion of the proximal aortic suture line through the third or fourth portion of the duodenum, although fistulae between the iliac anastomoses into the small bowel or colon are also well described. The diagnosis can be challenging and typically involves some combination of CT scanning, endoscopy, and angiography. The classically described triad of gastrointestinal bleeding, sepsis, and abdominal pain is present in only a minority of patients. Far more commonly, a small, self-limited "herald bleed" presages a large gastrointestinal bleed, which can be massive in nearly a third of cases. In many respects, treatment is similar to that for graft infection; extra-anatomic bypass and graft removal are usually required, in addition to repair of the involved gastrointestinal tract. Dedicated efforts to ensure adequate tissue coverage between the graft and the overlying bowel before abdominal wall closure are important in preventing this highly lethal complication.

ISOLATED PROFUNDAPLASTY

The last 3 decades have been marked by an increased awareness of the critical role played by the deep femoral artery in achieving successful lower extremity revascularization. Profunda circulation is frequently spared, even in the setting of severe obliterative disease of both the AI and femoropopliteal arterial segments. When present, profunda occlusive disease is often limited to the orifice or proximal segment (Fig. 105-15). This has important implications for the profunda's unique role in maintaining collateral perfusion, because even in the presence of proximal profunda disease, the more distal segments beyond the obstruction can continue to support key anastomotic networks. In extreme cases, these pathways can serve as the sole limb-sustaining bridge between pelvic or abdominal wall inflow vessels proximally and geniculate connections distally. In some diabetic patients, however, profunda disease is more diffuse, and distal collaterals are minimal.

The value of the profunda in supplying sufficient distal perfusion in the setting of SFA occlusion has been known since the early 1960s. Although isolated profundaplasty is less common in the current era of more aggressive percutaneous and open surgical reconstruction for lower extremity occlusive disease, it can be an effective alternative to either balloon angioplasty or surgical bypass of the SFA. It is particularly

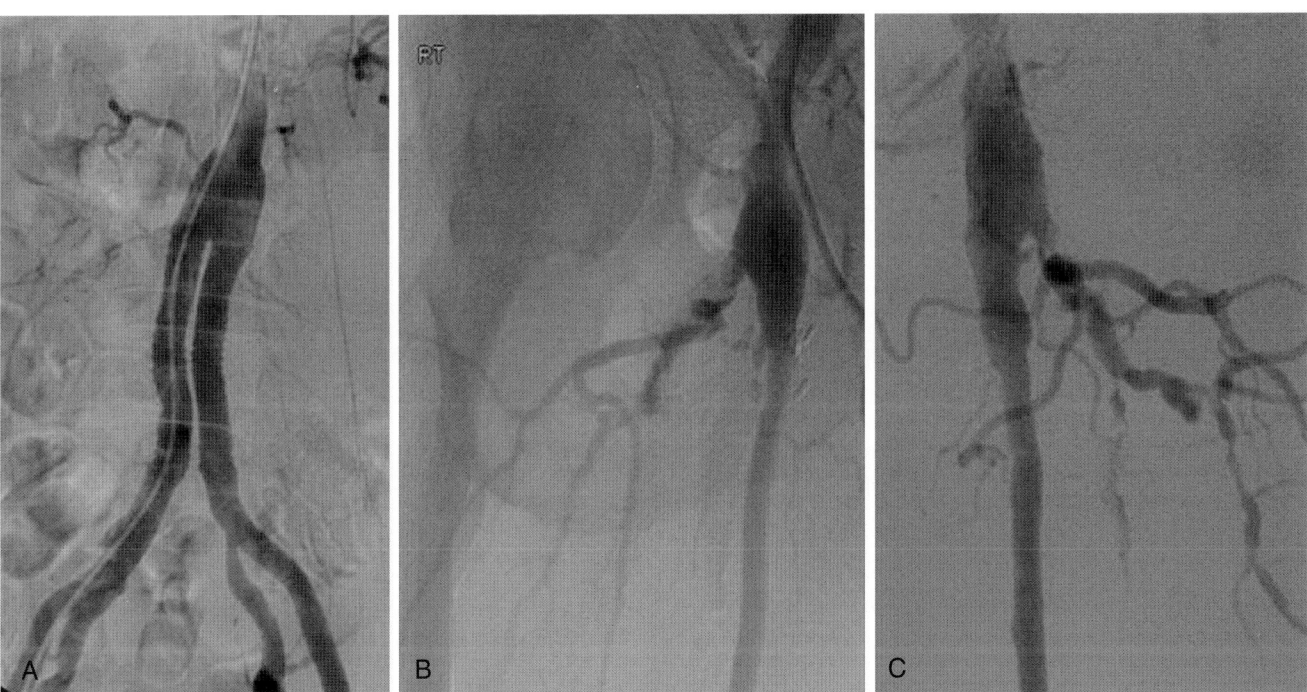

Figure 105-15 A patient with widely patent aortobifemoral and bilateral femoroperoneal bypass grafts (**A**) developed limiting bilateral thigh claudication secondary to profunda femoris occlusive disease (**B** and **C**). Symptoms resolved following bilateral staged isolated profundaplasties.

useful when infected infrainguinal grafts require removal or in the setting of failed bypass grafts when suitable autogenous conduit is absent and "redo" surgery is less appealing. It may also allow healing of a below-knee amputation in situations in which distal bypass is no longer an option.

Although profunda femoris occlusive disease can be detected with duplex ultrasound, CT, and MRA, formal angiography remains the diagnostic gold standard. The optimal conditions for an isolated profundaplasty are widely patent inflow and good distal profunda runoff beyond a diseased proximal profunda; longer diseased segments are more amenable to profunda bypass. Hemodynamic criteria assessing the resistance across the knee joint have also proved useful in predicting the clinical success of profundaplasty in particular patients. The operative technique is as described earlier for adjunctive profundaplasty. Associated mortality and morbidity are low, with the latter most commonly related to a lymphatic leak or other groin-related issues. Three-year limb salvage rates in the range of 75% have been reported in patients with critical ischemia, and 5-year patency rates of 88% have been achieved when isolated profundaplasty was performed for claudication.

SELECTED KEY REFERENCES

de Vries SO, Hunink MGM. Results of aortic bifurcation grafts for aortoiliac occlusive disease: a meta-analysis. *J Vasc Surg.* 1997;26:558.
Meta-analysis of aortobifemoral grafting results up to 1996.

dos Santos JC. Sur la desobstion des thromboses arterielles anciennes. *Mem Acad Chir.* 1947;73:409.
First description of endarterectomy technique.

Hertzer NR, Bena JF, Karafa MT. A personal experience with direct reconstruction and extra-anatomic bypass for aortobifemoral occlusive disease. *J Vasc Surg.* 2007;45:527.
Large single-surgeon experience with surgical treatment of aortofemoral occlusive disease.

Inahara T. Evaluation of endarterectomy for aortoiliac and aortoiliofemoral occlusive disease. *Arch Surg.* 1975;110:1458.
Descriptive summary of endarterectomy results from an expert in the technique, from a period when that procedure was the leading surgical therapy for aortoiliac occlusive disease.

Leriche R, Morel A. The syndrome of thrombotic obliteration of the aortic bifurcation. *Ann Surg.* 1948;127:193.
First description of the constellation of symptoms now known as Leriche syndrome.

McDaniel MD, Macdonal PD, Haver RA, Littenberg B. Published results of surgery for aortoiliac occlusive disease. *Ann Vasc Surg.* 1997;11:425.
Meta-analysis of aortobifemoral grafting results up to 1996.

Reed AB, Conte MS, Donaldson MC, Mannick JA, Whittemore AD, Belkin M. The impact of patient age and aortic size on the results of aortobifemoral bypass grafting. *J Vasc Surg.* 2003;37:1219.
Representative institutional series from the current era, describing notably inferior results with aortobifemoral grafting in younger patients.

Zannetti S, L'Italien GJ, Cambria RP. Functional outcomes after surgical treatment for intermittent claudication. *J Vasc Surg.* 1996;24:65.
One of few studies reporting functional outcomes following aortobifemoral grafting.

REFERENCES

The reference list can be found on the companion Expert Consult Web site at *www.expertconsult.com.*

CHAPTER 106

Aortoiliac Disease: Extra-anatomic Bypass

Joseph R. Schneider

The term *extra-anatomic bypass* refers to any bypass graft, autologous or otherwise, that is placed in a site different from that of the arterial segment being bypassed. The term is imprecise at best, because many common procedures—for example, femorotibial bypass with in situ great saphenous vein or carotid artery–to–subclavian artery bypass—might be considered extra-anatomic. However, the term *extra-anatomic bypass* generally refers to procedures addressing disease of the aortoiliac and femoral arterial systems and includes the basic procedures discussed in this chapter: femorofemoral bypass, axillofemoral bypass, obturator bypass, and thoracofemoral and supraceliac-to-iliofemoral bypass.

GENERAL CONCEPTS

Extra-anatomic bypass procedures were developed to treat patients at unusually high risk for direct aortoiliac replacement (coronary artery atherosclerosis or other severe medical co-morbidities) and those with "hostile" abdomens (previous surgery or infection with adhesions, intestinal stomas, active intra-abdominal infection, or otherwise contaminated fields), infected prosthetic intra-abdominal vascular grafts, aortoenteric fistulae, and infected inguinal and infrainguinal arterial bypass grafts or other groin sepsis. These problems became apparent almost as soon as aortic and femoropopliteal vascular reconstructions were first performed in the 1950s and 1960s. Thus, all the basic procedures were developed during that era. Although questions remain and data are contradictory regarding several aspects of the outcomes associated with these extra-anatomic bypass procedures, the basic techniques are "mature."

With respect to aortoiliac atherosclerotic occlusive disease, rapid advances in endovascular therapy include techniques that may be effective in patients who previously would have been treated with extra-anatomic bypass. However, younger patients with aortoiliac atherosclerosis, who would have been treated with direct aortofemoral bypass in the past, tend to have more discrete disease,[1-3] and patients with more discrete disease tend to enjoy the best results with endovascular therapy. Older patients with more advanced co-morbidities tend to have more diffuse atherosclerosis and for that reason have less favorable results with endovascular therapy.[4-9] Such older, higher risk patients are more likely to require open surgical therapy, so extra-anatomic techniques would be expected to represent an increasing fraction of open surgical therapies for aortoiliac atherosclerosis. However, endovascular techniques continue to improve and are being applied to a rapidly increasing fraction of patients treated for iliac arterial occlusive disease, and they may be applicable to a larger proportion of patients with diffuse aortoiliac disease in the future.[10-12] Thus, although the procedures themselves may be considered mature, their role and relative importance in the care of arterial problems are likely to continue to evolve.

History

Freeman and Leeds appear to have been the first to describe femorofemoral bypass,[13] although a similar (ilioiliac) operation may have been performed earlier as part of a secondary procedure for iliac limb thrombosis after homograft repair for aortic bifurcation thrombosis and reported later by Oudot and Beaconsfield.[14] Vetto's 1962 report provided the first comprehensive description of a series of patients undergoing prosthetic femorofemoral bypass using techniques similar to those still performed today.[15] Lewis[16] described a truly remarkable subclavian artery–to–distal aortic homograft bypass as part of the reconstruction in a patient with both a ruptured infrarenal aortic aneurysm and what was likely a type B aortic dissection.[17] The first use of the axillary artery for inflow in an axillofemoral extra-anatomic bypass appears to have been performed virtually simultaneously by Blaisdell and Hall[18] and Louw.[19] Blaisdell in particular continued to write about axillofemoral reconstruction and associated outcomes.[20,21] Shaw and Baue included what are probably the first three cases of obturator bypass in an article describing approaches to a number of infected arterial graft problems,[22] although Courbier and Monties had suggested the possibility of a transobturator graft route 3 years earlier.[23] The first use of the thoracic aorta as the inflow for an extra-anatomic bypass was described by Stevenson and coworkers.[24] Axillofemoral and descending thoracic aorta–to–iliofemoral bypass (which hereafter will be called thoracofemoral bypass, for simplicity) rapidly became important options for aortic prosthetic graft infection. For example, Fry and Lindenauer in 1967 reported the application of a number of these procedures, including at least one axillofemoral, one thoracofemoral, and one supraceliac aorta–to–femoral bypass, to cases of aortic graft infection.[25] Each of these procedures has been refined, and the experience with them is now sufficient to derive some general conclusions about their applicability and results.

Indications

The indications for extra-anatomic bypass are diverse and vary by the specific procedure contemplated. Femorofemoral and axillofemoral bypass are appropriate for patients with unilateral or bilateral chronic or acute arterial occlusive processes (most commonly atherosclerosis) whose disease is not amenable to endovascular treatment and for whom aortofemoral bypass would be a high-risk procedure. Outcomes are particularly poor in patients with critical limb ischemia (CLI)[26] who do not undergo arterial revascularization of some sort.[27] Therefore, even high-risk patients with CLI due to aortoiliac occlusive disease are, in most cases, suitable candidates for some sort of reconstruction, and femorofemoral and axillofemoral bypass are certainly among the interventions to be considered in such patients. These procedures may also be appropriate for revascularization in patients with active intra-abdominal infections (including "mycotic" aortic aneurysms or infected aortic prostheses), aortoenteric fistulae, or otherwise hostile abdomens that would be unusually difficult to treat with aortofemoral bypass. Obturator bypass is most commonly employed for femoral arterial reconstruction in patients with groin sepsis, including primary vascular infection; for example, it is used in patients with femoral mycotic aneurysms after puncture for a diagnostic or therapeutic endovascular procedure or recreational drug use, in those requiring removal of an infected arterial prosthesis in the groin, or in patients with otherwise hostile groins (e.g., after radiation therapy or previous surgery). Thoracofemoral and supraceliac aorta–to–iliofemoral bypass are most often employed to avoid reoperation in the infrarenal aorta after failure of aortofemoral bypass or after removal of infected prosthetic aortic grafts.

Contraindications

Femorofemoral and axillofemoral bypass are contraindicated in patients with extreme medical risks for surgery or with unusually short life expectancies. Obturator bypass with vein is a formidable procedure, comparable to or even more invasive than femorofemoral or axillofemoral bypass (or conventional femoropopliteal bypass), but the indications for obturator bypass are such that the only alternative may be to ligate the arteries in the groin and accept a substantial risk of major amputation. Consequently, obturator bypass may be necessary, even if the patient is at high risk. Thoracofemoral and supraceliac-to-iliofemoral bypass are formidable procedures that are at least as invasive as conventional aortofemoral bypass; they are inappropriate for patients at high risk for open abdominal or thoracic surgery. With respect to femorofemoral, axillofemoral, thoracofemoral, and supraceliac aorta–to–iliofemoral bypass, aortofemoral bypass remains the standard against which all other methods of reconstruction for iliac artery occlusive disease must be measured.[28-33]

■ FEMOROFEMORAL CROSSOVER BYPASS

Basic Concepts, Indications, and Patient Selection

Femorofemoral bypass depends on the capacity of one iliac arterial system to supply adequate blood flow to support both legs, and it is one possible reconstructive alternative for patients with symptoms related to unilateral stenosis or occlusion of a common or external iliac artery. Hemodynamic studies (see "Hemodynamic Considerations") confirm that one iliac artery can support both legs, at least at rest, in the absence of flow-limiting lesions in the planned donor iliac arterial system. Even a diseased donor iliac arterial system may be improved with endovascular techniques to allow a less invasive yet effective femorofemoral bypass when a more invasive procedure would otherwise be required.

One attractive alternative to femorofemoral bypass is direct (ipsilateral) iliofemoral bypass. Kretschmer and colleagues found no difference between femorofemoral bypass and unilateral iliofemoral bypass with respect to patency,[34] but virtually all other published studies have found that iliofemoral bypass yields somewhat better patency than femorofemoral bypass, assuming the presence of an appropriate common iliac artery for inflow to the graft.[35-44] Indeed, van der Vliet and associates, in a truly remarkable study, compared the results of 184 unilateral iliac reconstructions (62% based on iliac artery inflow) to 350 contemporaneous patients undergoing aorta–to–bilateral iliac or femoral reconstruction over a 10-year period and found no difference in patency between the groups, implying that iliofemoral bypass yields results comparable to the "benchmark" aortofemoral bypass.[45] However, iliofemoral bypass is more invasive than femorofemoral bypass, and the latter may be preferred by some surgeons for that reason. Femorofemoral bypass may also be used as a component of endovascular repair of aortic aneurysms.[46-56]

Technique and Graft Configuration

Femorofemoral bypass is performed with the patient positioned supine. Although the operation can be performed with local infiltration anesthesia, spinal or general anesthesia is usually used. The abdomen is prepped along with the groins and anterior thighs to allow access to the abdomen in case of unexpected findings during surgery. Longitudinal incisions are generally used to expose and control the femoral arteries on both sides. Oblique incisions (parallel to the groin creases) can be used, but they are somewhat less versatile if exposure must be extended much beyond the femoral artery bifurcation. General geometric considerations, discussed later, may affect the site selected for the arterial anastomoses.[57]

Femorofemoral bypass is certainly an operation of less magnitude than aortofemoral bypass, and many surgeons consider the technique simple. However, femorofemoral bypass, both as a stand-alone procedure and as part of an axillofemo-

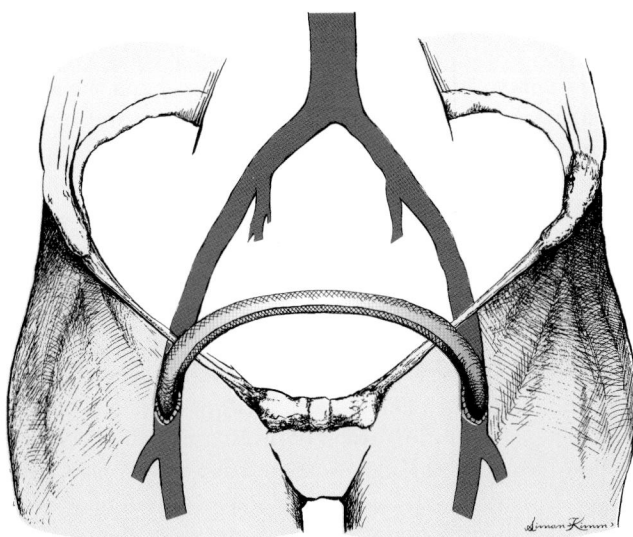

Figure 106-1 Standard "inverted C" (perhaps better termed "inverted U") configuration of a femorofemoral bypass graft.

ral, thoracofemoral, or other bypass procedure, presents unique technical (geometric) challenges. The graft is tunneled from one groin incision to the other within the abdominal wall superior to the pubis (Fig. 106-1). The tunnel is created bluntly with fingers, a large clamp, or a tubular tunneler. The prefascial subcutaneous plane is the appropriate location for the graft tunnel in most patients; however, a preperitoneal position may be selected or may be appropriate if unfavorable conditions exist in the abdominal wall, such as prior surgery, radiation-damaged skin or other skin changes, an unusually thin subcutaneous fat layer, or obesity predisposing to unfavorable graft geometry.[58,59] A preperitoneal tunnel position may be associated with injury to the bowel or urinary bladder and must be used with great caution, especially if there has been previous abdominal surgery.[60,61] However, inflow for crossover bypasses may be provided in some cases by a contralateral iliac artery,[35,62-67] and these iliac origin crossover grafts are usually most conveniently placed in the preperitoneal position. With the exception of Ng and coworkers,[68] most authors have found the patency of iliofemoral crossover bypasses to be comparable to or perhaps slightly better than that of femorofemoral bypasses. The outflow of such crossover grafts may be the popliteal or even tibial arteries,[69-71] or there may be sequential grafts with an intermediate anastomosis to the femoral system in the groin as well as a popliteal or other distal anastomosis to address both inflow (aortoiliac) and outflow (femoropopliteal) disease, especially in the setting of CLI due to multilevel disease.[72,73] Even more unusual presentations may be addressed using a transperineal graft route.[74-79] Readers are directed to the original publications for more detailed descriptions of these approaches.

The graft is roughly confined to a plane that is tipped forward superiorly from the coronal plane to an extent that varies considerably with patient habitus. Anastomoses are made to some component of the femoral arterial system; these are end-to-side anastomoses in nearly all cases, so that the graft is directed roughly longitudinally at the anastomoses.

Whether the graft is configured as an "inverted C" (perhaps better termed "inverted U" and preferred by most surgeons; see Fig. 106-1)[80] or a "lazy S,"[81] it makes two abrupt changes in direction within the plane described earlier. The likelihood of kinking can be reduced by using a slight excess of graft material, which reduces the graft's tendency to kink at the heel of the anastomoses, and by making the tunnel a continuous curve between the groin incisions and an area several centimeters superior to the proposed anastomoses, to try to increase the radii of the graft curves transitioning from a roughly longitudinal direction to a transverse direction coursing from one groin to the other.

The graft's tendency to kink within the sagittal plane is a separate concern. A protuberant abdomen presents a problem not encountered in an aortofemoral graft that parallels the distal external iliac artery and emerges from beneath the inguinal ligament. The more obese the patient or the more protuberant the abdomen, the more the plane of the graft is tipped forward from the coronal plane within the sagittal plane. This causes the angle between the graft and the native artery to become less acute and thereby causes a standard-length end-to-side anastomosis (roughly three times the graft diameter) to kink in the sagittal plane. This can usually be prevented by making a shorter femoral arteriotomy (and anastomosis) or by making the anastomosis to a more distal part of the femoral arterial system, which has the effect of bringing the graft and the femoral artery into a more parallel (and desirable) relationship. Extending the anastomosis at least partially onto the deep femoral artery may also help reduce the graft's tendency to kink in both the sagittal and coronal planes.

Systemic heparin is administered after the completion of dissection and tunneling. Endarterectomized superficial femoral artery was used in Freeman and Leeds's first femorofemoral bypass,[13] and autologous vein grafts were common and even preferred conduits in some surgeons' early experience with femorofemoral bypass.[82-84] A prosthetic graft is now used in nearly all cases, although almost every reported series of femorofemoral grafts includes a few constructed of vein or other autologous vessel, generally used when there is substantial concern about infection.[13,59,85-89] Another alternative, especially in the presence of infection, is to use the femoral popliteal vein. D'Addio and colleagues recently reported excellent results with femoral popliteal vein conduits in 54 patients, 16 of whom were undergoing femorofemoral bypass as the sole procedure.[90] Either anastomosis can be performed first when using prosthetic conduits, but I perform the donor anastomosis first when using venous conduits so that the presence of one or more competent valves in the conduit does not interfere with flushing just before completion of the second (recipient) anastomosis. Great care must be taken to allow some redundancy in the graft, as noted earlier. It is important to confirm enhancement of flow in the recipient vessels and continued flow in the outflow vessels beyond the donor-side anastomosis using continuous-wave Doppler or another suitable test after the anastomoses are completed and all clamps are removed.

Results

The perioperative mortality associated with femorofemoral bypass is highly dependent on patient selection but should be well under 5% in elective operations. Patients undergoing femorofemoral bypass are likely to have somewhat less advanced co-morbidities and thus are likely to enjoy longer survival than patients undergoing axillofemoral bypass. For example, my colleagues and I estimated 3-year survival rates of 71% for patients undergoing femorofemoral bypass, versus 35% for those having axillofemoral bypass.[91,92] Furthermore, far more patients undergo femorofemoral than axillofemoral bypass procedures; for example, there were more than four times as many femorofemoral bypasses than axillofemoral bypasses in Johnson and Lee's prospective study.[93] Consequently, reports including 5-year results are much more common for femorofemoral bypass, allowing a more confident assessment of long-term performance. The sixth edition of this textbook suggested that primary and secondary patency rates for femorofemoral bypass at 3 to 5 years should be about 60% and 70%, respectively.[91,94-96] Ricco and Probst recently updated a multicenter comparison of femorofemoral to direct (aortofemoral or iliofemoral) bypass and tabulated the results of previously published studies of femorofemoral bypass that included at least 40 patients, follow-up of at least 5 years, and life-table estimates of graft patency at 5 years.[44] Table 106-1 is a modification of that tabulation; it includes only reports that also provided the number of grafts at risk at 5 years, as well as some additional precedent articles that qualify.[30,34,40,44,88,93-95,97-105] These data allow the calculation of a weighted-average estimate of 5-year primary patency of 66%. As Table 106-1 demonstrates, there is some variation in the patency estimates among these studies, but it should be noted that these studies are diverse with respect to the fraction of patients with CLI and failed previous aortofemoral bypass, which can significantly affect the patency of femorofemoral grafts; this variation is much less than that seen with axillofemoral bypass (see in "Axillofemoral Bypass" under the heading "Results").

Causes of Failure

The cause of failure of extra-anatomic bypass grafts is elusive but likely includes progression of disease in both inflow and outflow arteries. Although some early authors may have viewed femorofemoral bypass as a durable procedure not vulnerable to disease progression,[106,107] and da Gama actually suggested that the donor artery enlarges over time after placement of an extra-anatomic bypass,[108] others viewed femorofemoral bypass to be at risk from progression of disease in the donor iliac system.[109,110]

Surveillance

The role of noninvasive surveillance of femorofemoral and other extra-anatomic bypass grafts remains unclear, but Stone and coworkers presented a unique exploration of the possible predictive value of duplex scan surveillance. They concluded that if duplex scanning estimated a peak systolic velocity greater than 300 cm/sec in the inflow artery or a midgraft peak systolic velocity less than 60 cm/sec, this was predictive of impending graft thrombosis.[111] Early experience in our own practice since adopting this approach seems to confirm Stone's findings, although these findings have not been confirmed by others.

Effect of Surgical Indications and Patient Characteristics

Pursell and associates noted a trend toward better patency in claudicants, consistent with observations in virtually every other arterial intervention.[103] In contrast, Brener and colleagues (in one of the largest, longest, and most completely followed series of femorofemoral bypasses)[94] and Criado and coworkers[95] noted no apparent difference in femorofemoral bypass patency when comparing claudicants and patients with CLI. A previous investigation actually suggested a trend toward reduced patency in claudicants compared with patients with CLI, although the trend was not significant and would be difficult to explain except as a result of random error.[91]

Femorofemoral bypass is one of many methods of treating patients with symptomatic occlusion of one limb of a previously placed aortobifemoral graft.[64,112,113] Although most authors have reported inferior results in this situation compared with primary femorofemoral bypass,[86,91,94,99,114-116] others have described more favorable results.[117-121] Most patients who experience thrombosis of an aortobifemoral graft limb

Table 106-1 Femorofemoral Bypass Patency

Series*	Year	Primary Patency at 5 Years (%)	Number of Grafts at Risk at 5 Years
Plecha and Plecha[97]	1984	72	39
Lamerton et al.[98]	1985	60	12
Rutherford et al.[99]	1987	62	5
Piotrowski et al.[30]	1988	55	5
Farber et al.[100]	1990	82	21
Self et al.[102]	1991	42	5
Perler et al.[101]	1991	57	2
Kretschmer et al.[34]	1991	52	3
Harrington et al.[40]	1992	64	31
Criado et al.[95]	1993	60	21
Brener et al.[94]	1993	55	54
Johnson and Lee et al.[93]	1999	49	51
Mingoli et al.[88]	2001	70	89
Pursell et al.[103]	2005	74	20
Kim et al.[104]	2005	65	27
Mii et al.[105]	2005	83	38
Ricco and Probst[44]	2008	72	51
Weighted average		**66**	

*Previously reported studies of femorofemoral bypass including at least 40 patients, follow-up of at least 5 years, and life-table estimates of 5-year primary patency that appear to be compliant with current reporting standards.[241,242]

Modified from Ricco J-B, Probst H. Long-term results of a multicenter randomized study on direct versus crossover bypass for unilateral iliac artery occlusive disease. *J Vasc Surg.* 2008;47:45-54.

are symptomatic and require urgent intervention.[112,122-125] Femorofemoral bypass is one option, and the surgeon and patient may need to accept the greater risk of later failure in exchange for more expedient reperfusion of the leg. There is also a trend toward an inverse relationship between age and patency for femorofemoral bypass.[91] However, there is a similar trend after aortobifemoral bypass, and this may represent the effect of more aggressive atherosclerosis in patients who require intervention at a younger age.

Femorofemoral bypass was first used in patients considered unfit for aortofemoral bypass. However, the relative ease of the procedure and the substantially lower level of physiologic insult prompted many to extend the procedure to better risk patients who would be candidates for aortofemoral bypass.[94,99,116,126-130] Femorofemoral bypass may also be preferred by some patients and surgeons because the risk of erectile dysfunction in men is likely lower than after aortofemoral bypass.[66,86,91,131-133] I am aware of no randomized prospective comparisons of femorofemoral versus aortofemoral bypass, and even contemporaneous case-control studies are unusual. My colleagues and I compared the results of patients who would have been candidates for aortofemoral bypass but who underwent femorofemoral bypass instead with the results of patients undergoing aortofemoral bypass during the same period in the same institution. The results of femorofemoral bypass even in these good-risk patients were clearly inferior to the results of aortofemoral bypass.[91] However, Mingoli and coworkers retrospectively reviewed and compared femorofemoral and aortofemoral bypass in two institutions between 1973 and 1993 and found no differences.[134] This latter study must be considered unique because other studies of femorofemoral bypass consistently report inferior patency compared to contemporaneous studies of aortofemoral bypass. Furthermore, many of the patients undergoing aortofemoral bypass in the past would now be more appropriately treated with transluminal balloon angioplasty or iliofemoral bypass, and it is unlikely that such a study could be repeated in a single institution today. In practice, it is rare that patient characteristics and arterial anatomy leave only two alternatives—femorofemoral or aortofemoral bypass—but when this is the case, I continue to recommend femorofemoral bypass for poor-risk patients and aortofemoral for good-risk patients.

In addition to its use for occlusive disease, femorofemoral bypass may be part of endovascular aneurysm repair with aortouniiliac systems.[46-56] Local femoral wound complications have been a concern in several publications. However, patency of the femorofemoral graft in such patients has been excellent and is clearly better than in patients treated for occlusive disease. These results are described in more detail in Chapter 129 (Abdominal Aortic Aneurysms: Endovascular Treatment).

Effect of Graft Material and External Support

Most femorofemoral grafts have been constructed of prosthetic material. Dacron (polyester) was used virtually exclusively until expanded polytetrafluoroethylene (ePTFE)

became available. It is difficult to determine whether either of these classes of materials dominates femorofemoral bypasses today. I could find no convincing evidence that ePTFE or externally supported PTFE (xPTFE) is superior to polyester grafts in terms of patency and hemodynamic performance. I am aware of no published data regarding PTFE grafts with support within the wall (Gore Intering, W. L. Gore and Associates, Flagstaff, AZ) for this application. At least one study found a trend toward inferior patency for ePTFE femorofemoral grafts.[95] However, the remainder of published articles reported comparable patency results using PTFE and polyester grafts for this application.[44,88,93,135,136] Thus, surgeons can choose either polyester or PTFE grafts and expect similar outcomes.

It is certainly plausible that external or internal support could improve the performance of femorofemoral and other subcutaneous bypass grafts. However, with the exception of Mingoli and coworkers, who found external support to be advantageous in a retrospective study of both polyester and PTFE grafts,[88] I am aware of no clear evidence that external support provides superior outcomes in this application. Indeed, Kim and coworkers[104] recently reported results with mostly unsupported ePTFE grafts that are indistinguishable from Mingoli's[88] results with xPTFE (Kim, personal communication with respect to the use of unsupported PTFE grafts). Pursell and associates reported excellent results using unsupported polyester grafts (Galland, personal communication with respect to the use of unsupported polyester grafts).[103] Finally, in a series that examined 6-, 7-, 8-, and 10-mm-diameter ePTFE grafts, there was no relationship between diameter and hemodynamic performance or patency,[91] findings recently confirmed by Ricco and Probst.[44] Consequently, I use 6-mm-diameter xPTFE or Intering PTFE grafts for convenience and because of the potentially decreased infection risk when performing femorofemoral bypass; however, the hemodynamic performance and patency profiles of the available prosthetic grafts are probably indistinguishable in this application.

Hemodynamic Considerations

Many surgeons have expressed the concern that one iliac artery cannot adequately supply blood flow to both legs or that the femorofemoral graft might "steal" from the donor limb and produce new or worse symptoms of ischemia in the donor limb.[84,85,110,137] Ehrenfeld and colleagues showed that the capacity of a healthy iliac artery in an animal model far exceeds the resting flow requirements of both legs.[137] Several authors have investigated the hemodynamic performance of femorofemoral grafts in patients and have concluded that there is no significant deleterious effect on the donor limb and that the recipient limb is well reperfused as long as there is no hemodynamically significant lesion in the donor iliac arterial system.[59,126,138,139] The conclusions of these authors have dominated the thinking about femorofemoral graft hemodynamics to the present day. However, some authors have detected a slight fall in the mean resting ankle pressure on the donor side, a finding subsequently duplicated by others.[59,91,139-141] Investigators for Veterans Affairs Cooperative Study 141 noted that the combination of hemodynamic deterioration and clinical symptoms of steal were present in only 3% of patients, although a much higher fraction of patients developed hemodynamic evidence of donor limb steal at rest, and angiographic findings did not predict the occurrence of donor limb steal.[142] Harris and coworkers made the remarkable observation that 45% of patients suffered deterioration in donor limb hemodynamics under exercise conditions, despite normal resting donor limb hemodynamics after femorofemoral bypass.[143] However, on balance, the evidence supports the contention that although there is some fall in donor limb pressure after femorofemoral bypass, donor limb function is not adversely affected by placement of a femorofemoral bypass, as long as there is no hemodynamically significant lesion in the donor iliac arterial system.

Significance of Iliac Artery Inflow Lesions.

The hemodynamic significance of angiographically detected stenoses in the prospective donor iliac arteries has also been a topic of great interest in patients being considered for femorofemoral bypass. Angiography alone is unreliable.[81,139,144,145] The increased flow in a donor arterial system after bypass may unmask previously hemodynamically occult lesions.[144,146] Sako was probably the first to report the use of directly measured femoral artery pressures at rest and after the injection of papaverine, a potent arterial vasodilator, to assess the capacity of the iliac arterial inflow to support a significant increase in flow.[147] This test was subsequently evaluated by Flanigan and colleagues.[148] As described by Flanigan, the test is performed by directly measuring both the systemic pressure and the arterial pressure in the proposed donor femoral artery before and after the injection of 30 mg of papaverine into the femoral artery. These measurements have been used to predict whether an angiographically detected iliac lesion is of clinical importance when selecting inflow versus outflow reconstructive procedures and to determine whether an iliac artery will support a femorofemoral bypass. Flanigan's group found that femoral pressures more than 15% less than radial or brachial pressures are associated with an unsatisfactory outcome.

The concept of a physiologic test to predict how a potential donor iliac arterial system will behave under the stress of supporting two legs instead of just one is appealing. However, as Archie has pointed out,[81] Flanigan's is the only study that has examined the predictive value of the papaverine test.[148] Furthermore, the technique has not been standardized. Papaverine tests are often performed with a vasodilator other than papaverine, typically nitroglycerin or tolazoline. I have been unable to find literature confirming that tests performed with other vasodilators are valid. I have also observed the test being performed without a separate radial artery or other catheter to measure systemic pressure. This may cause a false-positive result, because systemic pressure often falls briefly but significantly during the 1 or 2 minutes immediately after papaverine is injected into the femoral artery. Finally, Flanigan and colleagues stressed the importance of Doppler con-

firmation of increased flow in the proposed donor femoral arteries after papaverine injection, an often neglected portion of the test.[148] Absence of such an increase in flow implies a technical problem with the test or significant occlusive disease limiting femoral outflow on the donor side and is likely to lead to a false-negative test.

Archie has reported the largest and most detailed study of papaverine testing and its value in femorofemoral bypass.[81] He found that the test had inadequate sensitivity and specificity to be reliable. Despite these concerns, Archie's work focused on the value of papaverine test data to predict patency and hemodynamic results as assessed in the noninvasive vascular laboratory. The value of papaverine testing as a predictor of symptom relief after femorofemoral bypass has not been so carefully examined. Thus, I continue to use papaverine testing as one element of decision making in femorofemoral bypass, particularly when balloon angioplasty of the donor iliac system is employed, although I have discounted the test's importance in view of Archie's work.

Hemodynamic Results.

The ability of femorofemoral bypass to normalize perfusion of the recipient limb is questionable. Recipient limb perfusion is predictably improved by technically successful femorofemoral bypasses with appropriate anatomy.[141] However, many surgeons have noted a significant number of clinical failures, as measured by persistent claudication, rest pain, or failure to heal gangrenous lesions.[140,149] The Veterans Affairs Cooperative Study 141 included more than 300 patients, making it the largest study of femorofemoral hemodynamics to date, but these researchers presented no information about exercise testing of these patients.[142] My colleagues and I previously examined the postoperative resting hemodynamics of femorofemoral bypass in 91 patients and concluded that recipient limb pressures would not be normal even at rest with completely normal femoral and other infrainguinal outflow vessels; this finding was independent of the diameter of the graft used.[91] Despite a less than complete normalization of hemodynamics, femorofemoral bypass in most cases provides adequate improvement in perfusion to maintain the limb in patients with CLI.[132,150] Many surgeons view femorofemoral bypass to be a satisfactory treatment for claudication,[94,131,151] but given the persistent resting hemodynamic abnormalities in the recipient limb, it seems likely that femorofemoral bypass would perform poorly under exercise conditions. Given this likelihood and the potentially unsatisfactory patency profile, I have been reluctant to offer this procedure to claudicants.[91,116,143]

Angioplasty of Donor Iliac Artery before Femorofemoral Bypass

Successful femorofemoral bypass is highly dependent on a hemodynamically satisfactory donor iliac arterial system. Endovascular intervention for selected iliac artery lesions provides excellent short- and long-term results in terms of hemodynamic improvement and patency (see Chapter 108: Aortoiliac Disease: Endovascular Treatment). It is not surprising that endovascular procedures to improve suboptimal donor iliac arteries might be considered prior to or concomitant with femorofemoral bypass. Porter and coworkers[152] described two patients who underwent graduated dilatation (as previously described by Dotter [Porter's coauthor] and Judkins[153]) of the donor iliac artery before femorofemoral bypass, with satisfactory early results in both. This procedure was performed before the development of balloon angioplasty by Grüntzig[154,155] and others. Several authors have reported experience with transluminal balloon angioplasty prior to or concomitant with femorofemoral bypass.[91,94,95,156-163] With rare exceptions,[38,94] the results of these studies generally support the view that donor iliac artery balloon angioplasty with stenting in selected cases is associated with a satisfactory hemodynamic outcome and patency rate. Furthermore, the results of balloon angioplasty have probably improved since the initial studies were published.[163] On balance, it appears that as long as the donor iliac lesion would be considered favorable for angioplasty apart from the proposed femorofemoral bypass (ideally, a short, minimally calcified lesion of the common iliac artery), it is reasonable to proceed with angioplasty of the donor iliac artery and femorofemoral bypass.

Effect of Outflow Disease

Vascular surgeons recognized the importance of outflow and particularly of the deep femoral artery very early in the experience with aortofemoral reconstruction.[164-166] This principle is almost certainly applicable to extra-anatomic bypass as well. As with other operations for iliac arterial occlusive disease, many surgeons have suspected that disease of the femoral outflow arteries has a major impact on long-term femorofemoral bypass patency.[30,39,44,59,99,167] However, many authors have found that the patency of the superficial femoral artery has no detectable impact on long-term patency.[86,91,94,95,168] Ensuring outflow to at least one healthy artery—either the superficial femoral or, more often, the deep femoral artery—appears to provide adequate outflow to support patency, as is the case with direct aortofemoral bypass.[91,169,170] Some have argued that routine profundaplasty is indicated in inflow operations, including femorofemoral, axillofemoral, and aortofemoral bypass,[171] but this probably has no impact on hemodynamic performance or patency in the absence of significant deep femoral origin stenosis.[33] The ability to pass a 3.5-mm-diameter probe into the outflow artery after completing the "toe" portion but before completing the anastomosis is reassuring with respect to the adequacy of outflow, and I have always confirmed that this maneuver can be accomplished before completing any inflow operation. On balance, despite my previous observations, I believe that the quality of outflow may impact patency, but I also believe that maneuvers to ensure the best possible outflow are likely to minimize this effect.

Complications

Complications of femorofemoral bypass are those common to nearly all arterial operations, including those discussed in

Section 6 (Complications) of this text. Complications that are relatively specific to femorofemoral bypass include possible perforation of the bladder or intraperitoneal viscera during creation of the graft tunnel, particularly when a preperitoneal tunnel is used.[60,61] Transvesical and transbowel passage of conventional aortofemoral grafts has also been reported.[172]

AXILLOFEMORAL BYPASS

Basic Concepts, Indications, and Patient Selection

Axillofemoral bypass depends on the ability of a healthy axillary artery to supply adequate blood to the ipsilateral arm and one or both legs, at least at rest. With the exception of occasional use as treatment for aortic coarctation,[173-175] axillofemoral bypass is employed almost exclusively as treatment for primary or secondary disease of the infrarenal aorta or iliac arteries. Like any other method of intervention for primary or secondary infrarenal aortoiliac disease, axillofemoral bypass must be judged against aortofemoral bypass.[29,31-33] Axillofemoral bypass is an essential tool for the treatment of many patients with infected aortic or prosthetic arterial grafts or aortoenteric fistulae,[176-184] although in situ alternatives (discussed in Section 6: Complications and elsewhere in this text) have been proposed even for these patients.[185-189] Early experience demonstrated that axillofemoral bypass is an excellent choice for frail, elderly patients with bilateral iliac artery occlusions and those with other co-morbidities such as multiple prior abdominal operations, abdominal stomas, or prior radiation therapy.[85,128,141,190-203] However, the choice between aortofemoral and axillofemoral bypass is often less than clear. The definition of "high risk" is highly subjective, and the threshold for choosing axillofemoral over aortofemoral bypass is likely to vary significantly among surgeons. For example, approximately 25% of our open reconstructions for bilateral iliac artery occlusive disease were axillofemoral bypasses (and we were criticized for this high ratio when we presented our work in 1991),[92,204] whereas Hepp and colleagues performed axillofemoral bypass about 10 times as often as aortofemoral bypass.[205] This has led to markedly different profiles of patient samples in published series of axillofemoral bypass (a topic that is further explored later).

Technique and Graft Configuration

Axillofemoral bypass is nearly always performed with general anesthesia.[206] I have on rare occasions performed the entire operation with local anesthesia and sedation, but exploration of the axillary artery and tunneling of the axillofemoral graft segment are difficult to perform under these circumstances. The operation may be expedited by the use of two operating teams, especially for axillobifemoral bypass. Either axillary artery can be an appropriate donor unless there is disease in the subclavian or axillary artery; however, the right side is preferred in cases of aortic infection because subsequent remedial operations may involve left flank or thoracic exposures. I have approached this question by measuring blood pressures in both arms and recording continuous-wave Doppler waveforms in the brachial arteries. The axillary artery on the side with the higher blood pressure is chosen if there is a 10 mm Hg or greater systolic pressure discrepancy between the arms. I insist on a triphasic Doppler waveform in the brachial artery in the proposed donor limb. Some authors have recommended routine preoperative arch and subclavian arteriography, citing a substantial frequency of occult disease in the axillosubclavian arterial system of patients considered for axillofemoral bypass.[207] If both axillary arteries appear to be hemodynamically adequate to support axillofemoral bypass, I generally choose the arm ipsilateral to the patient's more ischemic lower extremity, even when performing axillobifemoral bypass. However, the contralateral axillary artery may be used as the inflow, even for axillounifemoral bypass, if required by the circumstances. It may occasionally be necessary to place bilateral axillounifemoral or axillodistal grafts to avoid infected wounds.[208] These choices are often based on other practical issues, such as avoiding stomas or other pathology or avoiding placing the graft on the side preferred by the patient for sleeping. I discourage placement of an axillofemoral graft on the side of a patent arteriovenous hemodialysis fistula, although I am unaware of any objective examination of the results of such procedures. Intraoperative arterial pressure–monitoring catheters should generally be placed in the nondonor arm.

Some surgeons perform the operation with the donor-side arm at the patient's side, but I prefer a supine position with the arm abducted to 90 degrees on the donor side. I also place a rolled towel under the patient on that same side to lift the torso several centimeters from the operating table deck. These maneuvers improve exposure of the most medial portion of the axillary artery and allow visualization of the flank and lateral chest wall while passing the graft tunneler. The 65-cm Gore tunneler (W. L. Gore and Associates, Flagstaff, AZ) allows easy passage of the axillofemoral graft limb without an intermediate incision in the flank. Femorofemoral limbs are positioned using the same approach used for isolated femorofemoral bypass (see under "Technique and Graft Configuration"). I always drape with wide exposure to allow thoracotomy, sternotomy, or celiotomy to manage intraoperative bleeding or other complications that would dictate these approaches (Fig. 106-2), although I have never found it necessary to perform any of these maneuvers.

Axillary Anastomosis

A transverse infraclavicular incision is carried through the clavipectoral fascia, exposing the pectoralis major muscle. The pectoralis major muscle fibers are pushed superiorly and inferiorly, exposing the deep fascia and, beneath that, the fat containing the axillary vein, artery, and brachial plexus elements. The axillary artery is exposed from the clavicle medially to the pectoralis minor muscle laterally, often requiring the ligation of crossing veins or small arterial branches. The axillosubclavian arteries are considerably more fragile than

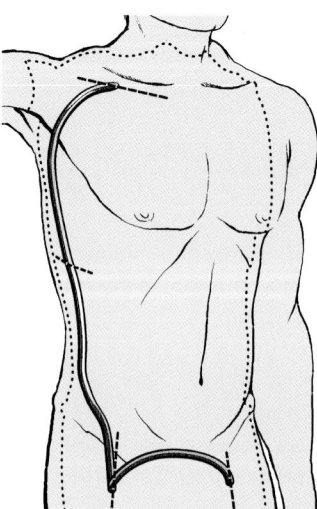

Figure 106-2 Typical area of exposure for an axillobifemoral bypass graft. The right axillary artery is the donor artery in this case. The intermediate incision in the right lower chest or upper flank is generally unnecessary if an appropriate tunneler is used.

the femoral arteries, and care must be taken not to injure them or the adjacent veins and brachial plexus elements during dissection or the placement of retractors or vascular clamps. Similarly, care must be taken when performing anastomoses to the axillary arteries, because sutures are much more likely to pull through these more fragile vessels. Conventional longitudinal or oblique groin incisions are used for femoral artery exposure.

Some early adopters of axillofemoral bypass recommended proximal anastomosis to the third portion of the axillary artery (lateral to the pectoralis minor muscle) because that portion of the artery is so accessible.[190,196,200,209] However, Blaisdell[20,210] and others since that time have stressed medial placement of the axillary anastomosis on the first portion of the axillary artery (medial to the pectoralis minor muscle) to avoid tension. I generally place the graft posterior to the pectoralis major muscle unless the patient has had prior axillary surgery, but placement of the axillary end of the graft anterior or posterior to the pectoralis minor muscle is probably unimportant with respect to results. It is far more important to place the axillary graft anastomosis as medially as possible to avoid tension on the axillary anastomosis when the arm is abducted.[211] Furthermore, medial placement of the axillary anastomosis eliminates the need to divide the pectoralis minor muscle in most cases. Leaving an excess length of graft in the axilla has also been advocated to reduce the likelihood of tension on the anastomosis.[212,213] The axillofemoral graft must be tunneled in the midaxillary line to prevent kinking of the graft with torso flexion or kinking over the costal margin, which tends to be more prominent anteriorly than in the midaxillary line. Care must also be taken to avoid injury to the neurovascular structures of the axilla during tunneling.

Femoral Anastomoses

Systemic heparin is given after the tunnels have been completed. The anastomosis of the proximal end of the graft to

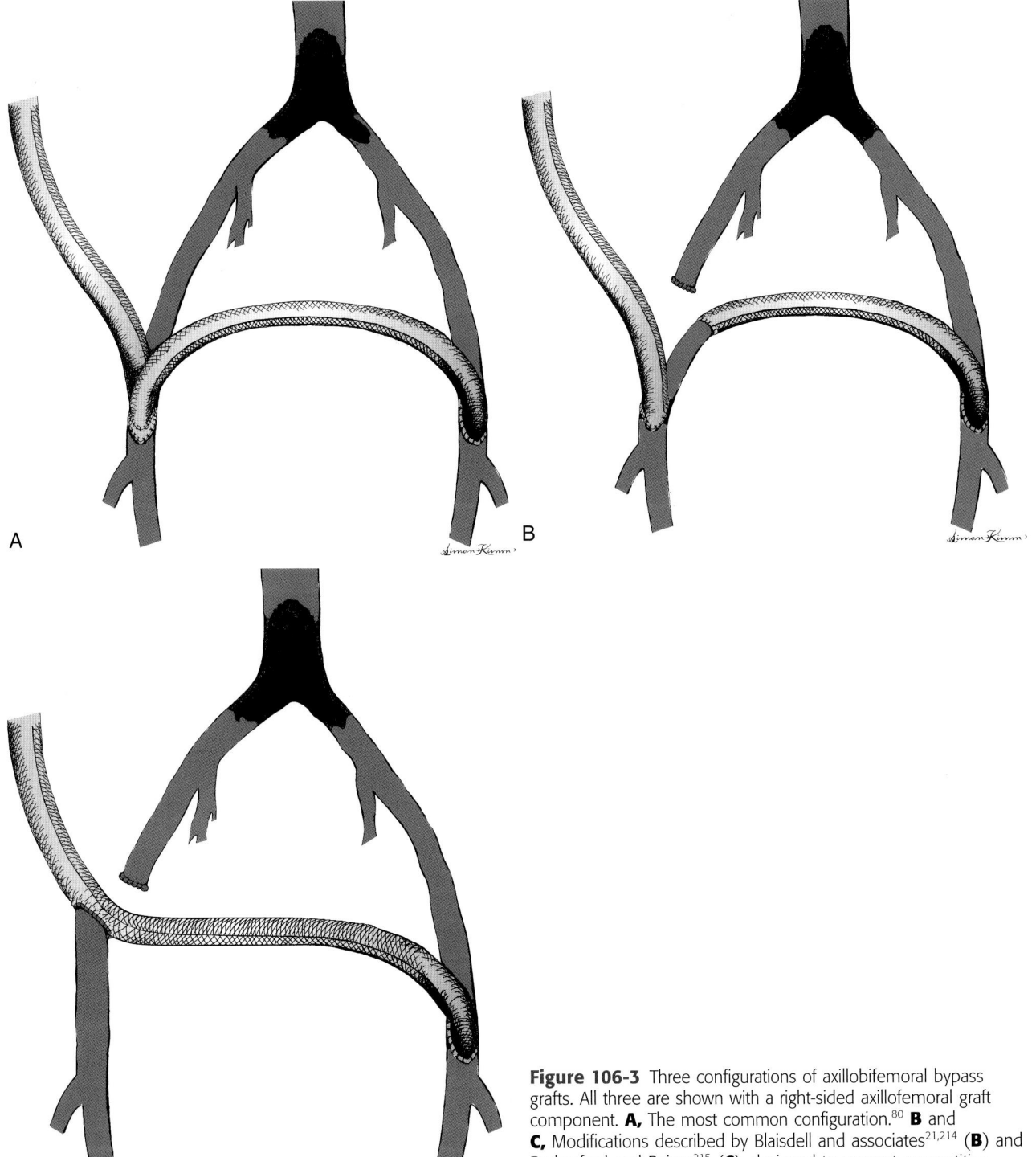

Figure 106-3 Three configurations of axillobifemoral bypass grafts. All three are shown with a right-sided axillofemoral graft component. **A,** The most common configuration.[80] **B** and **C,** Modifications described by Blaisdell and associates[21,214] (**B**) and Rutherford and Rainer[215] (**C**), designed to prevent competitive inflow from a patent ipsilateral iliac system.

the side of the axillary artery is generally performed first. The order of distal anastomoses for axillobifemoral grafts may vary, depending on whether there are one or two surgeons. The distal anastomosis is conventionally performed end to side to an appropriate artery in the groin. It is important to ensure adequate outflow. In the case of an axillobifemoral configuration, the femorofemoral component may be placed by "piggybacking" the femorofemoral graft onto the distal

anastomotic hood of the axillofemoral graft (Fig. 106-3A). Alternatively, the femorofemoral graft may be placed first (as described earlier), and the distal anastomosis of the axillofemoral component may be piggybacked onto the ipsilateral femorofemoral graft anastomotic hood. Either of these two variations qualifies as an inverted U femorofemoral component and maintains maximal flow throughout the axillofemoral component, a desirable characteristic with respect to graft patency. Femorofemoral graft components should be placed using the principles described earlier.

Blaisdell and associates[21,214] and Rutherford and Rainer[215] have described alternative configurations that theoretically prevent competitive inflow from the native iliac arterial system on the side of the distal axillofemoral anastomosis and may thereby decrease the risk of graft thrombosis due to stasis (Fig. 106-3B and C). In Figure 106-3B, the common femoral artery is divided superior to the distal axillofemoral anastomosis, and the femorofemoral graft component is anastomosed end to end to the distal common femoral artery. In Figure 106-3C, the common femoral artery is divided in the same manner, but the common femoral artery is anastomosed to the side of the axillofemoral graft, which is then continued from the right groin to the left groin for the left femoral anastomosis. This latter configuration has the potential advantage of reducing the total number of anastomoses from four to three.

Another alternative approach has been advocated by Wittens and coworkers.[216] These authors examined a variety of grafts with manufactured bifurcations for axillobifemoral reconstructions and found that a graft with a flow divider similar to that in bifurcated aortobifemoral grafts provided both superior hemodynamic performance and superior patency; however, I could not identify any published confirmatory data except for Wittens's later doctoral thesis.[217] Thus, I consider this approach potentially useful but unconfirmed at this time. Indeed, this configuration appears to be similar to that first used by Sauvage and Wood[192] but later described as "incorrect" by the same group.[80] These grafts appear to have long ipsilateral and contralateral distal limbs beyond the graft bifurcation, contrary to the typical strategy. Furthermore, such a configuration seems to require either a much longer ipsilateral groin incision or a counterincision on the ipsilateral flank to avoid kinking of the contralateral distal graft limb.

It is very important to confirm enhancement of flow in the recipient vessels using continuous-wave Doppler or another suitable test after the anastomoses are completed and all clamps are removed. It is also essential to ensure adequate blood flow in the donor arm beyond the axillary anastomosis by confirming a good radial pulse or satisfactory oxygen saturation (as indicated by pulse oximetry) in the hand with both the axillofemoral graft and axillary outflow vessels unclamped.

Results

Effects of Surgical Indications and Patient Characteristics

Early Literature. Early series of axillofemoral bypass made it clear that this procedure provided acceptable patencies in high-risk patients.[194-196,218] However, the emergence and adoption of life-table methods for patency estimates allowed more meaningful comparisons between axillofemoral bypass and aortofemoral bypass and between series of axillofemoral

bypass. An examination of reports of axillofemoral bypass yields perhaps the broadest range of long-term patencies of any arterial reconstructive procedure.[99,219] A prior review of pertinent articles on axillofemoral bypass, confined primarily to patients with chronic lower extremity arterial occlusive disease and published between 1960 and 1993, yielded 3-year primary patency estimates as low as 39% and as high as 85%.[220] A 1996 report from Passman and associates cited a 5-year estimated primary patency rate of 74%.[221]

There are many potential explanations for these discrepancies. Patients undergoing axillofemoral bypass as part of the treatment for infection of the aorta or an aortic prosthesis or for aortoenteric fistula tend to have high perioperative morbidity and mortality. However, with the exception of Oblath and colleagues,[222] most investigators report that survivors are likely to have better patency than those with chronic severe arterial occlusive disease.[99,184,223] Series including substantial numbers of such patients generally report a more favorable patency experience. In contrast, it is likely that patients undergoing emergent axillofemoral bypass for acute lower extremity ischemia suffer substantially more early and late complications than do those undergoing elective surgery.[224,225] Results after primary operations, including axillofemoral bypass, can be expected to be superior to those for secondary operations.[99] Patient characteristics and surgical indications influence outcome and must be considered when reading published reports. In addition, axillofemoral bypass was initially proposed only for high-risk patients,[192,193,197,198] but by the mid to late 1970s, some authors advocated extending these procedures to other patients and in some cases even advocated axillofemoral bypass as the procedure of choice for all but the youngest and healthiest of patients, when the anatomy allowed.[126] Many surgeons were strongly influenced by three specific favorable reports,[80,226,227] but the experience reported in these articles may have been influenced by the characteristics of the patients reported and the approach to patency reporting.

Claudication versus Critical Limb Ischemia. Claudicants generally have better patency than patients with CLI for virtually every type of arterial reconstruction for chronic lower extremity arterial disease (with the possible exception of femorofemoral bypass). Furthermore, claudicants tend to live longer than patients with CLI and thus tend to contribute to patency life-tables longer than those with CLI. As a result, series with substantial numbers of low-risk claudicants tend to report a disproportionately favorable patency experience compared with those restricted to high-risk patients with CLI.[228] If analysis is confined to high-risk patients, then most patients are likely to have CLI, patency is likely to be poorer, and late mortality is likely to be high. These issues have probably not changed significantly over time. For example, Bliss and Barrett reported estimated survival of only 43% at 28 months after axillofemoral bypass,[196] Devolfe and coworkers observed an approximately 35% 3-year survival 10 years after Bliss,[201] and my colleagues and I reported 35% 3-year estimated survival 20 years after Bliss.[91]

Secondary Patency. Finally, some of these favorable reports were based on what is currently termed "secondary patency." Nearly all authors have noted that axillofemoral bypass grafts are more likely than aortofemoral grafts to thrombose, and the favorable secondary patency of the former was at the expense of a significantly more frequent requirement for graft thrombectomy. Some reports have also considered the axillofemoral and femorofemoral components of axillobifemoral grafts as two distinct grafts, thus doubling the total number of "observed" grafts. Using this approach, thrombosis of one component has only half as much impact on patency calculations than if the entire graft were considered as a unit. I consider this approach misleading because patients find little consolation in the persistent patency of half the graft when they are told they require amputation because of thrombosis of the other component of the graft.

Recent Literature. The published literature addressing axillofemoral bypass for chronic lower extremity ischemia in the 30 years since those earlier favorable reports has generally been much less optimistic. The exceptions are the uniquely favorable experiences of Ray and associates and El-Massry and colleagues from the same group in Seattle and that reported by a group at the Oregon Health Sciences University.[80,221,229,230] It is intriguing to examine these reports after stratification by operative indication. For example, Corbett and colleagues reported 38% secondary patency at 2 years in a series composed of only patients with CLI,[231] whereas Ray and associates' roughly contemporary series, which included 59% claudicants, reported 79% primary patency at 3 years.[80] Dé and Hepp had to perform at least one and as many as five explorations for thrombosis in half of 131 axillofemoral bypass grafts.[232] K.A. Harris and coworkers reported only a 53% 3-year patency,[233] whereas E.J. Harris and colleagues reported 78% 5-year primary patency in roughly the same era.[229] Urayama and associates noted markedly reduced primary patency for extra-anatomic bypass compared with direct aortofemoral reconstruction, but the former group was older, was more likely to have CLI, and had markedly lower survival rates 10 years after the procedure.[234]

Systematic Review. Table 106-2 represents the results of a prior review,[220] including reports that appeared to adhere to current reporting standards,[80,92,221,226,229,230,235-240] with the addition of data from Passman and colleagues.[221] I selected articles that provided adequate information about indications for axillofemoral bypass, co-morbidities, and late mortality and that clearly used life-table methods to calculate patency, as defined by the Society for Vascular Surgery criteria.[241,242] In some articles it was unclear whether patency was calculated by the number of graft limbs or the number of patients. These studies are arranged in Table 106-2 in order of ascending primary patency. None of the primary reports of axillofemoral bypass published since that by Passman's group[221] qualified for inclusion in Table 106-2 based on these criteria, although there seems to be a trend toward lower operative mortality in these more recent reports.[243-246] With the exception of the

report of Donaldson and associates,[238] the series included in Table 106-2 are fairly easily separated into those with few claudicants (six of the first seven series listed) and those that included significant numbers of claudicants (Donaldson plus the last five citations in the table). Thus, it appears that the inclusion of as few as 20% claudicants has a potentially dramatic impact on the patency experience of axillofemoral bypass. Operative and late (3-year) mortality, when reported, were also lower in series with larger numbers of claudicants, thus enhancing patency predictions by the aforementioned mechanisms. Finally, there is a wide range of co-morbidities in patients undergoing axillofemoral bypass, re-enforcing the contention that the definition of "high risk" differs among institutions. Jämsén and associates also provided an excellent description of their results, but failure to distinguish claudicants from those with CLI disqualified that series' inclusion in the table.[243] However, a review of their results showed them to be generally consistent with those described by others and included in Table 106-2.

I have identified no prospective randomized comparisons of axillofemoral and aortofemoral bypass, and I am aware of only five reports using the case-control approach to analyzing outcome in contemporaneous patient cohorts treated with axillofemoral and aortofemoral bypass in a single institution.[92,221,226,244,247] Johnson and colleagues compared primary axillofemoral bypass to contemporaneous results with aortofemoral bypass in the same institution and observed 76% (axillofemoral) versus 77% (aortofemoral) estimated secondary graft patency at 5 years.[226] My experience was substantially different, yielding 63% (axillofemoral) versus 85% (aortofemoral) estimated primary patency at 3 years for contemporaneous patients in a study with only 6% claudicants in the axillofemoral group.[92] Inspection of the life-table patency graph provided by Mason and coworkers suggests significantly lower patency for axillofemoral bypass compared with aortobifemoral bypass.[247] Passman and associates reported 5-year estimated primary patency of 74% (axillofemoral) versus 80% (aortofemoral), a difference that was not statistically significant.[221] The discrepancy in results is almost certainly related to significant differences in the patient mix, the use of secondary patency in Johnson's work and primary patency in mine, and the fact that my review included both primary and secondary axillofemoral and aortobifemoral bypass procedures. The results reported by Passman and associates remain impressive, even after this type of scrutiny. Despite the enthusiasm for axillofemoral bypass among a few authors, most continue to view this operation as most appropriate for patients at very high risk for aortofemoral bypass who cannot be treated with iliac endovascular techniques, or as part of the treatment for infection of the native aorta or previously placed aortic prostheses.[245] A more recent publication from the same institution as Passman did not report life-table estimates of patency, but a review of the material suggests that patency rates in patients treated more recently are not as favorable as those reported previously and are more consistent with others' experience.[248] Finally, Onohara and coworkers performed a multivariate analysis of patients

Table 106-2 Indications, Patient Characteristics, and Mortality Associated with Axillofemoral Graft Patency

Series	Year	Number of Patients	Mean Age (yr)	Chronic Limb Threat (%)	Chronic Claudication (%)	Acute Ischemia (%)	Other Indication (%)	Smoking History (%)	Coronary Artery Disease (%)	Hypertension (%)	COPD; Lung Disease (%)	Diabetes Mellitus (%)	Operative Mortality (%)	3-Year Mortality (%)	3-Year Primary Patency (%)	3-Year Secondary Patency (%)
Eugene et al.[235]	1977	59	66	64	12	0	24	—	76 ("heart disease")	41	61	19	8	53*	39*	—
Allison et al.[236]	1985	94	61	88	5	0	7	80	45	55	40	—	6.4	44	43	—
Ascer et al.[237]	1985	56	69	95	0	5	0	68	≥41	41	—	32	5	40* (57 at 5 yr)	47	85*
Donaldson et al.[238]	1986	100	67	64	19	0	17	—	51 ("cardiac disease")	38	44	19	8	38	54	72
Schneider et al.[92]	1992	34	70	88	6	6	0	100	91	68	74	56	18	65	63	74
Kalman et al.[239]	1987	90	67	67	6	0	27	—	—	—	—	20	9	50	68	—
Naylor et al.[240]	1990	38	68	95	0	5	0	—	82	50	—	13	11	66 (at 5 yr)	71	79
Johnson et al.[226]†	1977	56	63	78	22	0	0	—	—	—	—	—	1.8	21* (33 at 5 yr)	—	76 (at 5 yr)
Passman et al.[221]	1996	108	68	80	20	0	0	86	84 ("heart disease")	—	13	29	3	57	74 (at 3 and 5 yr)	—
Ray et al.[80]	1979	54	67	31	59	0	10	72	22	37	11	22	3.7	—	79	—
Harris et al.[294]	1990	76	65	—	—	—	26	93	68	57	—	30	4.5	—	85	—
El-Massry et al.[230]	1993	79	69	59	38	0	3	77	58	62	35	16	5	33*	85 (78 at 5 yr)	88*

*Not quoted for 3 years but estimated from life-table graphs in the original article.
†Method of patency calculation in this article appears consistent with Society for Vascular Surgery definition of secondary patency.[241]
‡Included because of unusually high graft patency despite lack of adequate information regarding indications for surgery and late mortality. Subsequent update of this series showed 78% 3-year primary patency.[261]
COPD, chronic obstructive pulmonary disease.
Modified from Schneider JR, Golan JF. The role of extranatomic bypass in the management of bilateral aortoiliac occlusive disease. *Semin Vasc Surg.* 1994;7:35-44.

undergoing axillofemoral and aortofemoral bypass, hoping to adjust for several possible predictors of patency.[244] Their analysis suggests that axillofemoral bypass patency is comparable to that for aortofemoral bypass after adjustment for other factors. Such a conclusion is intriguing, but larger sample sizes and validation by others would be required before it could be generally accepted.

Limb Salvage. Limb salvage may be the best criterion to assess operations for limb-threatening ischemia, but appropriate life-table estimates of limb salvage are unusual in published reports of axillofemoral bypass. Limb salvage may also include results in claudicants or other patients whose surgical indications did not include CLI. An examination of reports in which life-table methods were clearly used in patients suffering predominantly from CLI or in which separate results were tabulated for patients whose initial presentation was CLI yields 3-year limb salvage estimates ranging from 69% to slightly more than 80%, a much narrower range than that for patency.[92,239,240,249] Most important, although axillofemoral bypass does not provide complete hemodynamic normalization, it appears to achieve limb salvage in most patients whose initial indication for reconstruction is CLI, and it is an excellent compromise when confronted with patients at extreme risk for direct aortic reconstruction.[246]

Surveillance. The role of noninvasive surveillance of axillofemoral grafts is questionable. Sanchez and coworkers[250] and Calligaro and associates[251] found duplex scanning to be of some utility but did not distinguish between axillofemoral and other graft positions. Musicant and colleagues were unable to identify a clear duplex scan–derived threshold predictive of impending axillofemoral graft failure.[248] Thus, routine surveillance of axillofemoral grafts cannot be justified at this time.

Effect of Graft Material and External Support

The first axillofemoral bypasses were performed when only saphenous vein or other autologous grafts and unsupported prosthetic (polyester or textile PTFE) grafts were available.[19,209,252] Autologous grafts may be appropriate in some circumstances,[252,253] but prosthetic grafts are used almost exclusively today. Externally supported polyester,[254,255] ePTFE,[200,256] and xPTFE[229] have subsequently become available, and each has been touted as superior to its predecessors. Each of these materials is mechanically durable, and material failures are extremely rare.[257,258]

Several retrospective studies comparing polyester and PTFE detected no differences in patency.[202,214,259,260] Published studies that suggest better results with a new graft material suffer from the problem of comparison to historical controls. Harris and coworkers reported excellent results with xPTFE when compared with the same group's prior results with unsupported grafts of unspecified material.[229] A subsequent update of this series produced a downward revision of patency, although the results remain impressive.[261] However,

the number of claudicants was not specified in that study, and my group observed much less favorable results with the identical xPTFE graft placed during roughly the same period in a high-risk group consisting almost exclusively of patients with limb-threatening ischemia and severe outflow disease.[92] El-Massry and colleagues reported excellent results with externally supported polyester grafts in a series with 38% claudicants,[230] but these results were only marginally better than those with unsupported polyester prostheses reported by Ray and coworkers from the same group 14 years earlier.[80] Indeed, Ray's group reported one of the highest axillofemoral graft patencies ever, despite the fact that the report is now 30 years old (see Table 106-2). Finally, hemodynamic studies attempting to assess the importance of external compression as a potential cause of graft thrombosis have yielded conflicting results,[262,263] and the basic assumptions that graft compression is a cause of failure or that external support prevents compressive occlusion of the graft remain unconfirmed.

Johnson and Lee, in the only randomized prospective comparison of externally supported polyester versus xPTFE axillofemoral bypass grafts, demonstrated no detectable difference between the two.[93] PTFE, collagen-impregnated polyester, and gelatin-coated polyester grafts are all convenient, avoiding the requirement for preclotting and the possibility of bleeding within the subcutaneous tunnel; any of these can be used with similar outcome expectations. Thus, although many have concluded that the value of external support is unquestionable in axillofemoral bypass,[132,229,261] a critical review of the literature does not support this conclusion. The concept of external support has "face validity," and I continue to use externally supported grafts, although this is not based on solid evidence. The development of new prosthetic grafts may alter our preferences in the future.

Axillounifemoral versus Axillobifemoral Configuration, Graft Diameter, and Other Hemodynamic Considerations

The average resting flow in the axillofemoral limb of an axillobifemoral graft is on the order of 600 to 900 mL/min (somewhat less in axillounifemoral grafts) when measured intraoperatively with an electromagnetic flowmeter[80,227,264] or when using duplex scan–derived estimates of volume flow.[92] This is consistent with the estimated resting flow of 300 to 400 mL/min in each normal common femoral artery,[265] and it is comparable to the average estimated flow in upper extremity arteriovenous dialysis fistulae. Thus, it is not surprising that axillofemoral bypass can provide adequate flow to support the legs. However, despite the observation that one axillary artery can accommodate the "entire cardiac output,"[20] axillofemoral bypass may not provide a normal hemodynamic result, probably owing to resistance posed by the long graft length. There is some clinical evidence that axillofemoral bypass does not result in complete improvement in claudication symptoms.[99] Previously, my colleagues and I noted that axillofemoral bypass resulted in a predicted ankle-brachial index of only about 0.7 with normal outflow vessels, much inferior to the results obtained with conventional aortofemoral bypass. We also noted a trend toward less satisfactory improvement as measured by the ankle-brachial index in patients with greater estimated graft flow, implying that the axillofemoral graft itself may be flow limiting.[92] Given the length and diameter of the grafts used for axillofemoral bypass in particular, it is not surprising that these reconstructions do not provide a hemodynamically normal result.[266] Nevertheless, as is the case with femorofemoral bypass, axillofemoral bypass provides sufficient enhancement of perfusion to allow limb salvage in most patients.[132]

Axillofemoral bypass was originally described as a unilateral (unifemoral) procedure. Sauvage and Wood were probably the first to suggest that the patency of axillobifemoral grafts would be superior to that of axillounifemoral grafts because of the increased blood flow in the former.[192] The majority opinion for more than 20 years was that axillobifemoral graft patency was superior to that of axillounifemoral grafts and that axillofemoral bypass should virtually always be performed in a bifemoral configuration.[80,99,199,205,226,239,267,268] Recent evidence suggests that this dogma may be flawed. The diameter of graft components is not stated in all published reports. Ray and coworkers suggested an increased rate of thrombosis for 8-mm-diameter grafts when flow is less than 240 mL/min.[80] Published estimates of flow in axillounifemoral grafts are only slightly more than this threshold, whereas estimated flows are roughly twice as high in axillobifemoral grafts,[92,227] thus providing a plausible theoretical explanation for the alleged superior patency of the axillobifemoral configuration. Ray's work also implies that larger diameter grafts are at risk of thrombosis at even higher minimum flow rates, suggesting that axillofemoral grafts should be no more than 8 mm in diameter and that 10- and 12-mm-diameter grafts would be at very high risk of thrombosis in an axillounifemoral configuration.

Despite these observations and the theoretical arguments, other authors have found no difference[92,201,235,237,269,270] or no more than an insignificant trend toward improved patency[238] for axillobifemoral grafts compared with axillounifemoral grafts. In some cases, this may reflect the use of smaller diameter grafts, consistent with the aforementioned arguments. For example, Ascer and colleagues used 6-mm-diameter components for axillounifemoral and axillobifemoral grafts and observed no discrepancy in patency between these configurations.[237] Ray's work suggests a thrombosis threshold of substantially less than 240 mL/min for a 6-mm graft.[80] It is also ironic that the highest reported patency for axillofemoral grafts came from a series dominated by axillounifemoral grafts and performed by the group that originally championed the axillobifemoral configuration (all uni- and bifemoral grafts were 8-mm-diameter externally supported polyester).[230] Thus, it appears that axillounifemoral bypass performed with a 6- or 8-mm-diameter graft will perform as well as axillobifemoral bypass performed with an 8-mm axillofemoral component. I prefer an 8-mm xPTFE axillofemoral component and a 6-mm xPTFE femorofemoral component for axillobifemoral grafts. I generally use an 8-mm xPTFE graft for axillounifemoral grafts unless the patient is small, in which case I choose a 6-mm xPTFE graft.

Effect of Outflow Disease

As with femorofemoral bypass, superficial femoral artery patency has been found by some authors to be an important determinant of axillofemoral graft patency,[20,80,99,227] whereas others have found it has no impact.[92,221,237] It is often necessary to perform local procedures to ensure good outflow, usually to the deep femoral artery, in a substantial fraction of cases—certainly more frequently than in aortofemoral bypass.[92,167,170,216] I use the same principles as in aortofemoral and femorofemoral bypass, including passage of a 3.5-mm probe into either the superficial or deep femoral artery, to ensure adequate outflow. Thus, the inability to demonstrate a difference between patients with patent and those with occluded superficial femoral arteries may reflect the effect of an aggressive approach to ensure adequate deep femoral arterial outflow.

Axillopopliteal Bypass

Axillofemoral bypass has occasionally been extended to the popliteal artery, primarily for cases in which there is groin sepsis and the superficial femoral artery is an unacceptable distal target vessel or when the surgeon believes that foot perfusion will not be adequately enhanced by a bypass to the groin because of infrainguinal occlusive disease. Bastounis and coworkers noted very poor patency among patients undergoing axillopopliteal or axillotibial bypass,[271] but groups led by McCarthy,[272] Ascer,[273] and Keller[274] all noted the acceptable performance of this configuration. However, these authors all found that patency was inferior to that expected with more conventional reconstructions. This finding is not surprising, given the long graft length and the requirement to cross at least one flexion point. Indeed, it is surprising that any of these compromised grafts remain patent. Nevertheless, this technique is occasionally the only reasonable approach to patients with groin sepsis, those who are unacceptable risks for more conventional reconstructions, and those whose arterial occlusive anatomy is not amenable to either an inflow or an outflow procedure alone. Readers are directed to the original publications for more information on these rarely required procedures.

Complications

Although axillofemoral bypass is subject to the same complications as other arterial operations discussed in Section 6 (Complications), several complications are unique to axillofemoral bypass, including brachial plexus injuries, axillary pullout syndrome (disruption of the axillary artery–to–graft anastomosis), and thromboembolic risks to the donor arm and recipient legs following thrombosis of the graft.[167,211,275-284] Taylor and associates have provided an excellent review of the literature on axillary pullout syndrome and have proposed a modification of the technique that allows some redundancy of the graft to prevent this complication.[213,285] Axillary pullout most likely occurs owing to tension on the anastomosis with abduction of the arm when the axillary artery–to–graft anastomosis has been placed too far laterally on the axillary artery or because the reconstruction has failed to provide some graft redundancy (as recommended earlier). Mannick and coworkers cautioned against placing grafts with tension on the axillary anastomosis and cited this as a possible cause of axillary thrombosis.[195] We have observed three cases of thromboembolic complications in three episodes in all three involved extremities in a patient with a thrombosed axillofemoral graft.

Reports of these complications are unusual, and I was unable to find any recent ones, suggesting that they may have become less common as the technique evolved and surgeons gained experience with it. Infection of axillofemoral bypass grafts poses unique problems because these patients have often been treated for failure of prior reconstructions; often have multiple co-morbidities, making them extremely poor candidates for additional reconstructive surgery to deal with this problem; and have extremely limited anatomic options for revascularization.[188,286,287]

■ OBTURATOR BYPASS AND OTHER EXTRA-ANATOMIC ALTERNATIVES TO DIRECT FEMORAL ARTERY BYPASS

Indications and Patient Selection

Shaw and Baue first described obturator bypass as a strategy to avoid frankly contaminated fields during reconstruction after the removal of infected grafts in the groin.[22] This indication accounted for a large fraction of patients requiring obturator bypass in the past,[288-292] but obturator bypass can also be used for reconstruction in patients after the removal of infected ePTFE dialysis access grafts based on the femoral arteries; in patients with infected femoral pseudoaneurysms after diagnostic or therapeutic femoral arterial access or recreational drug use[293,294]; in those with groin neoplasms requiring en bloc removal of tumor and artery, with a residual soft tissue defect that would expose an in situ reconstruction[295-297]; and in patients who have undergone therapeutic radiation in the groin.[295,298-300] With respect to the risk of persistent infection and hemorrhage and concerns about the injection of recreational drugs into bypass grafts placed for infected femoral pseudoaneurysms, the most conservative approach is to simply débride and ligate the arteries in the groin, although this is associated with a significant risk of limb loss.[293,301] The question of whether one should routinely perform reconstruction in addition to local débridement and ligation for femoral mycotic aneurysms and other vascular infections in the groin has aroused significant debate[294,301-304] and is addressed in Chapter 139 (Infected Aneurysms).

The term *obturator bypass* is imprecise at best; alternative terms such as *transobturator foramen bypass* would be preferable, but the former is in common usage. The original grafts employed polyester, but ePTFE, xPTFE, saphenous vein in various configurations, autologous deep vein, and human umbilical vein have all been used.[292,305-308] The presence of an infected prosthetic aortofemoral graft limb on the side to be reconstructed is a relative contraindication for obturator bypass, particularly if there is frank pus adjacent to the graft limb. Preoperative imaging studies may indicate involvement of the aortofemoral graft limb, and in such cases, other techniques such as axillopopliteal bypass may be the only alternative.

Technique and Graft Configuration

Guida and Moore have provided an excellent review of the anatomic principles and technique of obturator bypass,[309] although few surgeons would use the third (upper thigh) incision originally recommended by those authors (and by Courbier and Monties in their original cadaver study[23]) to facilitate tunneling. The operation is typically performed with general anesthesia. The patient is placed supine, and the abdomen is prepped. The leg to be reconstructed is prepped circumferentially to allow manipulation during the operation. Infected wounds are excluded from the field to the extent possible. The donor artery is most often exposed using an oblique, curvilinear, lower quadrant incision and a retroperitoneal approach, although a transperitoneal approach may be used. The common or external iliac artery can serve as the donor artery. As noted earlier, an aortofemoral graft limb can serve as the donor vessel if this portion of the graft is uninvolved with infection.[310-312] This alternative requires that the graft be divided and the distal infected portion excluded from the operative field until the bypass has been completed and the wounds closed before exploring the groin wound to remove infected prosthetic material and native tissue. None of my patients has had a prosthetic inflow source, and I have not had occasion to use this approach. The obturator foramen is approached from this same incision by dissection medial to the external iliac vein and posterior to the pubic ramus and blunt dissection of the obturator internus muscle away from the obturator membrane (Fig. 106-4). The obturator artery and nerve perforate this membrane posterolaterally, so it is safest to avoid these structures by passing the graft through the anteromedial aspect of the obturator foramen. The membrane is extremely strong and cannot be perforated bluntly without the risk of injuring adjacent structures and must be opened sharply or with electrocautery.

Target Artery and Tunneling

The target vessel is often the popliteal or distal superficial femoral artery, but it may also be the deep femoral artery.[313,314] Although approaching the deep femoral artery from the posteromedial side is technically possible, doing so risks entry into the infected groin and should be avoided unless there is no alternative target artery. In such a case, an incision is made along the mid to upper medial thigh, taking care not

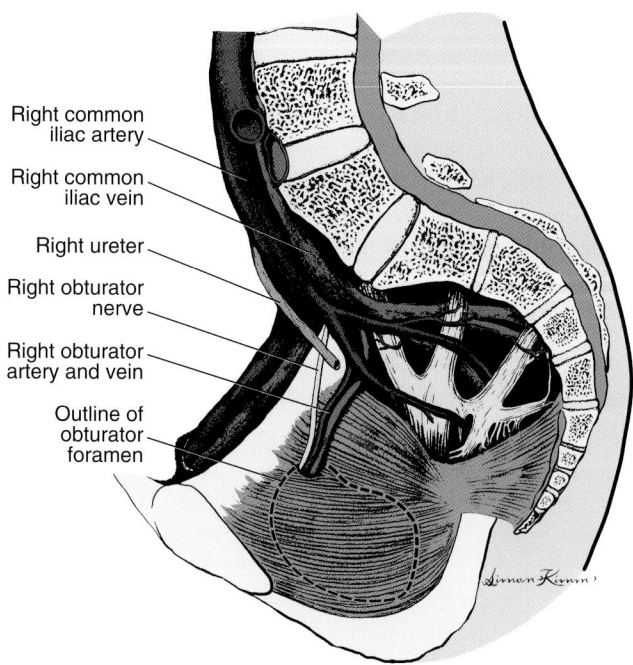

Right common iliac artery

Right common iliac vein

Right ureter

Right obturator nerve

Right obturator artery and vein

Outline of obturator foramen

Figure 106-4 Approach to the obturator foramen with adjacent iliac vessels, as viewed from the medial side of the pelvis.

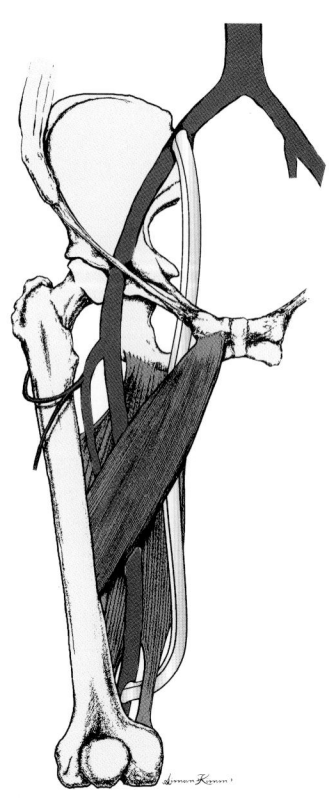

Figure 106-5 Typical course of the obturator bypass graft. It originates from the most proximal portion of the right external iliac artery, passes through the obturator foramen, and terminates at the popliteal artery.

to enter the contaminated area of the groin. The tunnel between the inflow and target arteries is usually made in the potential space between the adductor longus and brevis muscles anteriorly and the adductor magnus muscle posteriorly, which leads directly to the obturator foramen (Fig. 106-5).[307] However, some authors recommend that the tunnel be maintained posterior to the adductor magnus to reduce the risk of entry into the contaminated groin.[309] Others recommend passing the tunneling device from superior to inferior, but I find it easier to pass it from inferior to superior,[315,316] especially when the iliac exposure is limited by factors such as obesity, stomas, or the noncompliant lower abdominal wall observed in patients after radiation. The superficial femoral artery is easily identified and controlled in the plane of the tunnel anterior to the adductor magnus muscle. However, if the popliteal artery is the target, the graft must be either tunneled through the tendinous portion of the adductor magnus (as the native superficial femoral artery does at the adductor hiatus) or brought around the adductor tendon (as a conventional femoropopliteal graft would be). The proximal and distal anastomoses are then completed using standard techniques, usually end to side to both donor and target arteries. The surgeon may wish to ligate the external iliac artery downstream from the proximal anastomosis to reduce blood loss during the subsequent femoral artery exploration. Once the reconstruction has been completed, the surgical incisions are closed and excluded before the groin is explored to remove any infected prosthetic or native material and ligate vessels as necessary to prevent hemorrhage. It is critical to débride sufficient artery to permit oversewing of grossly noninfected segments of the femoral arteries proximally and distally.[317]

Thigh Perfusion

The thigh may be "isolated" and ischemic after obturator bypass with ligation of the femoral arteries.[318] Consequently, I always ligate the superficial femoral artery as high as possible in the thigh; on occasion, I have anastomosed the superficial femoral artery to the deep femoral artery after débridement of the common femoral artery, thus allowing blood at systemic pressures to reach the deep femoral artery by retrograde flow when the superficial femoral artery is patent.[305,318] This was done only in cases in which the sepsis was well controlled, the arteries were débrided back to grossly healthy tissue, and the infecting organism was an antibiotic-sensitive *Staphylococcus aureus*. I do not recommend this practice with gram-negative organisms, especially *Pseudomonas* species.[319]

Results

As with all extra-anatomic bypasses, results vary from one report to another. Van Det and Brands estimated 80% patency (likely primary patency as currently defined) at 6 years in their personal series of 13 obturator bypasses and compared this to a number of previous reports.[300] Sautner and associates provided an excellent review of mortality, graft patency, and limb salvage in patients undergoing obturator bypass.[320] Estimated patency rates of 73% and 57% at 1 and 5 years, respectively, and a limb salvage rate of 77% at 5 years are somewhat less than would be expected with conventional femoropopliteal bypass, but these figures are better than those expected with simple excision of infected graft material and local measures, including muscle flap treatment,[321] or nonoperative treatment. However, Nevelsteen and colleagues[305] and Kretschmer and associates[322] presented substantially less optimistic estimates of 5-year patency, and the surgeon can expect the need for revision or new reconstruction in a significant number of patients. Despite its technical demands and the relative difficulty of creating the tunnel, transobturator grafts appear to provide good hemodynamic performance and seem relatively insensitive to hip movement.[295]

Graft Material

Most early obturator bypasses were performed with prosthetic grafts,[22,290,295,299,311,323-325] but placing prosthetic grafts in the setting of active infection, even if one can exclude the operative field from frank infection, carries a substantial risk of secondary infection of the newly placed prosthesis.[302] Indeed, Shaw and Baue placed polyester grafts in their original three patients, and two of these prosthetic grafts ultimately became infected.[22] However, Patel and coworkers described a series of prosthetic obturator bypass grafts (eight PTFE, four polyester) without an apparent case of infection of the new graft.[312] Others, including my own group, have used autologous vein in all cases and have had no problems with persistent infection.[288,291,292,306,307] On balance, I believe that obturator bypass should be performed with autologous vein whenever possible because the risk of infectious complications is much less when autologous conduit is used. Second choices for conduit include superficial femoral or popliteal vein or cephalic or basilic veins from the arm. Benjamin and colleagues described eight patients with infected pseudoaneurysms, five of whom had femoral pseudoaneurysms due to recreational drug use; autologous deep vein conduit was used to construct obturator bypasses, with control of sepsis and limb salvage in all five patients.[308] Bell and associates used superficial femoral-popliteal veins in 11 cases, 4 of which were placed in a transobturator foramen position to reconstruct infected femoral pseudoaneurysms.[326] One may be willing to use prosthetic conduit in cases without infection (e.g., in irradiated groins), but the long-term patency advantage of autologous conduit almost certainly parallels that in conventional femoropopliteal bypass, where autogenous great saphenous vein is clearly superior to current prosthetic conduits.

Alternatives to Standard Obturator Bypass

In some cases it may be possible to route bypass grafts lateral to the groin wound, anterior to the pelvis, and sufficiently remote from an infected groin to a popliteal, superficial femoral, or deep femoral arterial target, thus obviating the more difficult transobturator tunnel.[308,317,326-330] Certain situations may dictate other extra-anatomic bypass routes, such as one through the iliac bone.[330-332] Finally, a number of variations have been described, including a subscrotal transperi-

neal crossover graft route (see earlier under "Femorofemoral Crossover Bypass") that obviates the need to pass through the obturator foramen.

In situ replacement of the femoral artery in the presence of active infection, even with autologous arterial or venous grafts, is associated with a substantial risk of graft or anastomotic disruption and likely exsanguination. Obturator bypass is the most conservative approach and should be considered the favored method in patients with infection involving the femoral artery who require reconstruction and are considered appropriate candidates for obturator bypass.[322] However, in situ replacement with autologous material may be appropriate in highly selected patients with limited local inflammation and limited autologous conduit or whose medical co-morbidities place them at very high risk for an operation as large as obturator bypass with autologous vein.[333]

Complications

The most serious complications of obturator bypass are those of persistent or recurrent infection, including generalized sepsis and hemorrhage from the groin vessels. As noted earlier, the use of autogenous conduit seems to reduce the risk of infection of the obturator bypass graft and the operative sites associated with grafting. The risk of hemorrhage is higher in the presence of persistent infection or nutritional or other immunocompromise,[334] and it is likely reduced by generous débridement of infected and necrotic tissue, secure closure in healthy portions of the groin vessels, and coverage with well-vascularized adjacent tissue, such as the sartorius muscle[335] or gracilis muscle flap.[336] Injury to the obturator nerve and artery is possible, especially if the tunnel is not kept in the anteromedial portion of the obturator fossa. Even more unusual complications of transvaginal[320] and transvesical[337] passage of the graft have been reported, although the latter has also been described as a complication of aortofemoral bypass.[172]

THORACOFEMORAL AND SUPRACELIAC-TO-ILIOFEMORAL BYPASS

Indications and Patient Selection

These procedures have most often been applied to patients with failure or infection of previous infrarenal aortic reconstructions, previous abdominal surgery for other than aortic pathology, prior radiation treatment, or other reasons that would make a conventional transperitoneal or retroperitoneal approach to infrarenal aortic surgery difficult or impossible and who are not candidates for endovascular intervention. Blaisdell's original patient actually had a thoracofemoral graft placed during the same operation in which the infected infrarenal aortic graft was removed; he died of sepsis 1 month after thoracofemoral bypass, although the thoracofemoral graft did not appear to be infected at autopsy.[338] Nevertheless, placement of a thoracofemoral graft in the presence of simultaneous active infection elsewhere is associated with a significant risk of infection of the graft, so this is probably not a reasonable indication for this procedure.[339,340] Repeat aortic replacement with conventional infrarenal aorta–to–graft anastomosis may be possible after a suitable delay following the removal of infected aortic prostheses,[341-343] but most surgeons would likely view a previously undissected supraceliac or descending thoracic aorta as a preferable inflow source in such patients.

The first known use of thoracofemoral bypass was to treat a patient with prior abdominal surgery and failed infrarenal aortic replacement[24]; shortly thereafter, a similar technique was employed to treat a patient with an infected aortic prosthesis.[338] These remain the primary indications for thoracofemoral bypass today. However, results of thoracofemoral bypass have been so encouraging that some groups have advocated thoracofemoral bypass as a primary treatment in selected patients with aortoiliac occlusive disease, at least when the disease extends into the visceral segment of the abdominal aorta.[344,345] The procedure is formidable—certainly more so than axillofemoral bypass. Thus, the procedure is most applicable to patients who are physiologically appropriate for thoracotomy.

Exposure and control of the supraceliac aorta were probably first proposed as a method of aortic control during the repair of ruptured abdominal aortic aneurysms.[346] However, exposure and control of the supraceliac aorta developed into an important technique for the treatment of juxtarenal aortic aneurysms[347-349]; operations on the visceral segment of the aorta and its branches[266,350,351]; "redo" aortic surgery, including "redo" aortofemoral bypass[352-356]; and as an alternative approach to aortodistal bypass by using the generally less diseased supraceliac aorta in patients with extensive disease of the perirenal and visceral segment of the aorta.[357,358]

Technique and Graft Configuration

The ascending aorta is favored for inflow in the repair of many complex anomalies of the aortic arch; it has also been used successfully as an inflow source for lower extremity arterial reconstruction.[359,360] However, this is a very invasive procedure requiring median sternotomy, and graft positioning and tunneling may be difficult. Such a procedure is generally reserved for situations in which access to the descending thoracic or supraceliac aorta would be difficult.

Use of Descending Thoracic Aorta for Inflow

Several authors since Stevenson[24] have described techniques for thoracofemoral bypass based on the descending aorta.[339,344,345,358,361-384] The following technique should be considered a composite of those descriptions, but readers are directed to the original publications for alternatives. The operation is performed using general endotracheal anesthesia. Some authors have recommended the use of a dual-lumen endotracheal tube to allow collapse of the left lung to facilitate surgery (my preference),[339,345,363,378,383] but others do not con-

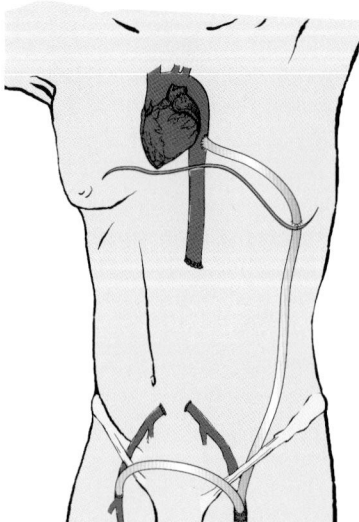

Figure 106-6 Typical course of the thoracofemoral bypass graft. This illustrates a single graft from the descending aorta to the left common femoral artery, with a left-to-right femorofemoral graft. Other approaches, some involving the use of a bifurcated graft, are possible (see text).

sider this to be essential.[376,377,379,382] The pelvis is kept as horizontal as possible while the left chest is elevated to approximately 45 degrees off the horizontal. This is usually facilitated by the use of a "beanbag" to stabilize the patient's position while simultaneously reducing the risk to any dependent pressure points during surgery.[383] The left arm is positioned anteriorly and supported with a Mayo stand or other appropriate device. A left thoracotomy is performed through the seventh, eighth, or ninth intercostal space or with removal of the seventh or eighth rib, allowing exposure and control of an adequate portion of the mid to distal descending thoracic aorta (Fig. 106-6). The inferior pulmonary ligament is generally divided to facilitate this exposure. Distal anastomoses are typically made to the femoral arteries; however, they may be made to the iliac or other arteries, as dictated by the anatomy and the presence of infection. Standard exposures of these vessels are achieved with groin incisions or retroperitoneal incisions. The graft must be tunneled from the chest into the extraperitoneal abdominal space. Some authors recommend carrying the intercostal incision across the costal margin[379] or even making a formal thoracoabdominal incision,[366] allowing access to the peritoneal, retroperitoneal, or anterior extraperitoneal space. Using this approach, the graft can be tunneled extraperitoneally from the left hemithorax to the left femoral arteries in the anterior axillary line, using only a small peripheral incision in the diaphragm and an incision in the left inguinal ligament to gain access to the extraperitoneal space from an inferior direction. Tunneling the graft in the retroperitoneum posterior to the left kidney may require a separate incision in the mid to lower left abdominal wall to gain access to the retroperitoneum[345,376] or an extension of the thoracotomy incision across the costal margin to allow access to the retroperitoneum,[344,371,379] but this facilitates exposure of the left iliac arteries when one of these is the proposed target.

DeLaurentis,[339] Schellack and coworkers,[374] Bowes and colleagues,[375] and Kalman[382] have described techniques whereby the graft can be tunneled blindly from the left groin, anterior or posterior to the left kidney and up to the left posterior diaphragmatic attachments, without complete exposure of the retroperitoneum. Branchereau and colleagues[376] described a technique that includes a flank incision to gain access to the retroperitoneum; they and others have used it,[339,370,372,373,375] and Branchereau believes it is "simpler" than the approach of McCarthy and coworkers,[371,379] although it does not appear simpler to me.

The graft may be a straight graft from the descending aorta to the left iliofemoral arteries, with a crossover graft from left to right as necessary, or it may be a standard bifurcated graft. The former approach is particularly useful when converting a femorofemoral graft or an axillobifemoral graft with a patent femorofemoral component to a thoracobifemoral graft because the crossover component is already in place. The right limb of a standard bifurcated graft is usually too short and must be extended to reach the right groin; also, it may have a tendency to kink if brought out under the left inguinal ligament and then turned to the right in the subcutaneous suprapubic space, as with a conventional femorofemoral bypass. Thus, it is probably better placed in the preperitoneal space of Retzius,[382] although the creation of this preperitoneal tunnel may be difficult and hazardous in patients with previous midline laparotomies for aortofemoral bypass or other surgery.

Once the inflow and target arteries have been controlled and the graft has been tunneled, the patient is given heparin, and the operation is performed using standard vascular surgical techniques. The aorta is generally clamped completely proximally and distally during performance of the proximal side aorta–to–end graft anastomosis. The graft is clamped and the aortic clamps are removed as early as possible to reperfuse intra-abdominal viscera and, possibly, the spinal cord during performance of the distal anastomoses. McMillan and McCarthy have described a thoracoscopic approach to the thoracic portion of the operation.[385]

Use of Supraceliac Aorta for Inflow

The supraceliac aorta is generally less likely than the infrarenal aorta to be affected by atherosclerotic disease.[355] The supraceliac aorta can be exposed and controlled from an anterior transperitoneal approach,[353,355,358] from a thoracoabdominal approach,[354,386] or from the left flank retroperitoneal (extrathoracic) approach for repeat or primary surgery of the abdominal aorta and its branches.[342,351,354,356,387] Williams and coworkers[351] and O'Mara and Williams[387] have convincingly demonstrated that a totally retroperitoneal approach without thoracotomy is adequate for nearly all procedures involving the visceral segment and supraceliac portion of the aorta. They, along with Sicard and Reilly,[388] have provided excellent general descriptions of the approaches to positioning and

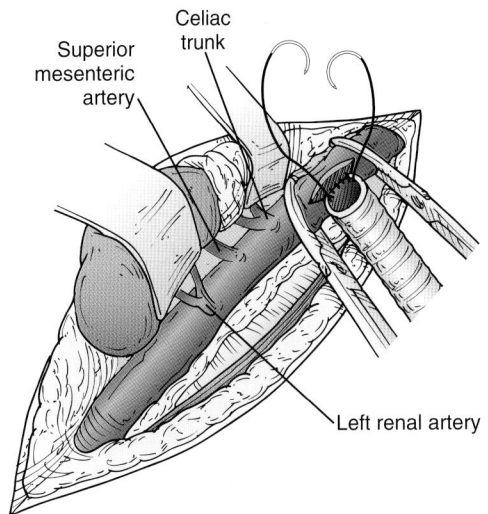

Figure 106-7 Exposure of the supraceliac aorta from the left retroperitoneal approach. Sufficient exposure can generally be obtained to clamp the supraceliac aorta, allow anastomosis to a suitable graft, and perform a bypass to the iliac or femoral arteries distally, just as is possible with thoracic aortic inflow. This exposure may also facilitate the reconstruction of celiac, superior mesenteric, and left renal branches.

incisions. Mills and colleagues have also provided a clear description of an extrathoracic retroperitoneal approach (Fig. 106-7), with extension into the 11th intercostal space without entering the pleural cavity; they used this approach to perform supraceliac aorta–to–femoral bypass in 11 patients, with very good results.[356] This approach avoids adhesions, which could be problematic from a transperitoneal approach, and it allows dissection in a previously undissected area in patients who have had prior exposure and control of the aorta; this is an especially difficult exposure after the previous removal of infected aortic grafts and ligation of the aorta. Another possible advantage of this approach is avoidance of a thoracotomy. Finally, graft tunneling is facilitated compared with thoracofemoral bypass because the entire left common and external iliac arteries are easily exposed (and controlled, if desired) from this approach. This exposure also provides good access to the celiac, superior and inferior mesenteric, and left renal arteries in most patients.

As with thoracofemoral bypass, graft configurations may include aorta–to–left femoral bypass with left-to-right femorofemoral bypass; alternatively, it may be possible to use a conventional bifurcated graft. Tunneling of the right limb of a bifurcated graft may be difficult in the area of a previously placed aorta–to–right femoral graft limb, risking injury to the right ureter, iliac veins, and colonic cecum in particular, and an anterior preperitoneal tunnel may be used, as with thoracofemoral grafts. Distal target arteries may be the iliac or femoral arteries; rarely, the target may be some other vessel, such as the popliteal artery,[389] based on patient characteristics. This approach may be applicable in patients in whom it would be difficult to expose and control the infrarenal aorta.

Results

The patency of thoracofemoral bypass approaches that of aortofemoral bypass—a remarkable observation, given that most of these operations are performed after the failure of one or more conventional reconstructions.[383] McCarthy and coworkers reported no thromboses prior to 49 months in their series of 21 grafts.[379] Passman and colleagues reported a 5-year primary patency rate of 79% in 50 patients.[345] Carrel and associates reported no failures in eight thoracofemoral grafts followed for an average of 2.7 years.[380] Branchereau and colleagues reviewed publications prior to 1993 and concluded that the results in series including 10 or more patients suggest a mortality approaching 10%,[376] although these publications include patients with infections or other problems that are clearly associated with an increased mortality risk. The mortality risk in uninfected patients undergoing elective procedures is generally much lower. Five of the largest series of these operations reported a combined total of 3 perioperative deaths out of 112 patients.[345,369,375,377,379] Intensive care unit and total hospital stays tend to be longer than those for standard aortofemoral bypass, reflecting the fact that this is a formidable procedure.

Results in patients undergoing supraceliac-to-iliofemoral bypass have been encouraging. Canepa and associates performed supraceliac-to-distal bypass in seven patients, with no mortality, one graft thrombosis, and one graft removed for infection.[354] Mills and colleagues reported no deaths and three graft thromboses, two of which were salvaged with thrombectomy, in a series of 11 supraceliac-to-iliofemoral bypasses.[356] Thus, supraceliac-to-iliofemoral bypass is a good reconstructive option for this group of patients.

Acknowledgments

Julie Stielstra, MLS, provided invaluable literature research support.

SELECTED KEY REFERENCES

Brener BJ, Brief DK, Alpert J, Goldenkrantz RJ, Eisenbud DE, Huston J, Parsonnet V, Creighton D, Cross F. Femorofemoral bypass: a twenty-five year experience. In: Yao JST, Pearce WH, ed. *Long-term results in vascular surgery*. East Norwalk: Appleton & Lange; 1993:385-393.
  One of the largest, longest, and best-followed series of femorofemoral bypass from a group that has published extensively on this topic.

Criado E. Descending thoracic aorta to femoral artery bypass: surgical technique. *Ann Vasc Surg.* 1997;11:206-215.
  Good description of indications, technique, and results from an author with significant interest in and multiple publications on this topic.

Johnson WC, Lee KK. Comparative evaluation of externally supported Dacron and polytetrafluoroethylene prosthetic bypasses for femorofemoral and axillofemoral arterial reconstructions. Veterans Affairs Cooperative Study #141. *J Vasc Surg.* 1999;30:1077-1083.
  Best-designed and best-conducted study with level I evidence comparing two commonly used prosthetic graft materials in axillofemoral and femorofemoral bypass.

McCarthy WJ, Mesh CL, McMillan WD, Flinn WR, Pearce WH, Yao JS. Descending thoracic aorta-to-femoral artery bypass: ten years' experience with a durable procedure. *J Vasc Surg.* 1993;17:336-348.
  Description of technique and long-term follow-up from another group with a long interest in and multiple publications on this topic.

Mills JL, Fujitani RM, Taylor SM. The retroperitoneal, left flank approach to the supraceliac aorta for difficult and repeat aortic reconstructions. *Am J Surg.* 1991;162:638-642.
  Clearest description of technique and outcomes for this valuable procedure.

Passman MA, Taylor LM, Moneta GL, Edwards JM, Yeager RA, McConnell DB, Porter JM. Comparison of axillofemoral and aortofemoral bypass for aortoiliac occlusive disease. *J Vasc Surg.* 1996;23:263-271.
  One of many excellent publications on this topic from a group with a uniquely positive experience with axillofemoral bypass.

Sautner T, Niederle B, Herbst F, Kretschmer G, Polterauer P, Rendl KH, Prenner K. The value of obturator canal bypass. A review. *Arch Surg.* 1994;129:718-722.
  Excellent review of results from the authors' institution as well as a literature review.

Schneider JR, Besso SR, Walsh DB, Zwolak RM, Cronenwett JL. Femorofemoral versus aortobifemoral bypass: outcome and hemodynamic results. *J Vasc Surg.* 1994;19:43-57.
  Contemporaneous case-control comparison of femorofemoral bypass to aortofemoral bypass, with multivariate exploration of possible predictors of outcome.

Stone PA, Armstrong PA, Bandyk DF, Keeling WB, Flaherty SK, Shames ML, Johnson BL, Back MR. Duplex ultrasound criteria for femorofemoral bypass revision. *J Vasc Surg.* 2006;44:496-502.
  Excellent long-term observation and exploration of the possible role of noninvasive surveillance.

REFERENCES

The reference list can be found on the companion Expert Consult Web site at *www.expertconsult.com*.

CHAPTER 107

Aortoiliac Disease: Laparoscopic Reconstruction

Marc Coggia and Olivier Goëau-Brissonnière

The Trans-Atlantic Inter-Society Consensus (TASC) and American College of Cardiology–American Heart Association (ACC/AHA) guidelines suggest that treatment of extensive aortoiliac occlusive disease (AIOD) should remain aortofemoral bypass (AFB) as opposed to complex endovascular procedures.[1,2] For many years, AFB was performed through a midline or flank incision. Mortality was less than 3%, but 30% of systemic and local complications were related to the surgical approach.[3,4] As in other specialties, the primary aim of laparoscopy in aortic surgery is to reduce surgical trauma due to abdominal or lumbar incisions. The underlying concept of laparoscopic AIOD repair is to combine the advantages of minimally invasive surgery with the well-known results of AFB. The feasibility of treating AIOD laparoscopically is now well established (Table 107-1).[5-13] However, laparoscopic aortic bypass is a major technical challenge for vascular surgeons, most of whom had no experience with this procedure during their surgical training. Moreover, the increasing use of endovascular techniques to treat AIOD and the paucity of indications for laparoscopic ABF make it difficult for surgeons to overcome the learning curve. The initial requirements for vascular surgeons who want to set up laparoscopic aortic surgery programs are (1) a basic knowledge of the instruments, (2) practice to gain skills in laparoscopic suturing, and (3) proctored training in laparoscopic procedures.

LAPAROSCOPIC EQUIPMENT

Basic Equipment

Basic equipment for laparoscopic aortic surgery includes gas insufflators, optical instruments and fiberoptics, and a video camera and monitor. Operating suites designed for laparoscopic surgery that include all the requisite equipment are now available.

Gas Insufflators

Carbon dioxide (CO_2) insufflation induces pneumoperitoneum, distends the abdominal cavity, and creates the working space for laparoscopic procedures. The system incorporates pressure, flow, and volume indicators. High-flow insufflators are essential in vascular surgery to compensate for vigorous suction, which evacuates pneumoperitoneum, and the immediate loss of visualization. Insufflators with preheated gas are useful for laparoscopic aortic procedures to prevent hypothermia.

Optical Instruments and Fiberoptics

The eyes of the laparoscopic vascular surgeon are the endoscope. Endoscopes provide excellent, bright, high-resolution

Table 107-1 Reports of Total Laparoscopic Aortofemoral Bypass for Aortoiliac Occlusive Disease

Series	Year	Number of Patients	Conversion to Open Repair (%)	Results Mortality (%)	Morbidity (%)
Said et al.[20]	1999	7	0	1 (14.3)	0
Alimi et al.[13]	2000	15	1 (6.7)	1 (6.7)	2 (13.3)
Barbera et al.[10]	2001	30	5 (16.6)	0	4 (13.3)
Dion et al.[12]	2004	49	4 (8.2)	1 (2)	3 (6.1)
Olinde et al.[7]	2005	22	2 (9)	1 (4.5)	4 (18.2)
Rouers et al.[8]	2005	30	6 (20)	0	11 (36.7)
Remy et al.[9]	2005	21	1 (4.7)	0	5 (23.8)
Cau et al.[5]	2006	72	2 (2.7)	0	3 (4.2)
Dooner et al.[6]	2006	13	3 (23)	0	1 (7.7)
Di Centa et al.[29]	2008	150	5 (3.3)	4 (2.7%)	21 (14)

images and allow an appreciation of operative field depth. Endoscopes are classified according to their caliber and optical axis. Scope caliber for aortic surgery is preferentially 10 mm because of the increased brightness. Angulated endoscopes (30 or 45 degrees) are essential in aortic surgery to provide a circumferential view of vascular structures and to vary the visual field.

Fiberoptics connect the light source to the endoscope. Cold light from halogen provides adequate illumination of the operative field.

Video Camera and Monitor

Video cameras are based on charge-coupled devices (CCDs), with either single-CCD or three-CCD systems available. Three-CCD video cameras provide higher-resolution images with definition up to 600 to 700 lines, compared with 400 to 500 lines with a single-CCD system. Video cameras are equipped with automatic focus and zoom. A television monitor and recorder complete the video tower.

Surgical Instruments

Basic laparoscopic surgical instruments for aortic procedures include Veres needles and trocars, dissecting and cutting instruments, suturing instruments, suction-irrigation devices, retractors, and clamps (Fig. 107-1A).

Veres Needles and Trocars

The Veres needle is used to create the pneumoperitoneum with the "blind" technique. It allows a low insufflation flow of less than 2 L/min, which is preferable at the beginning of the procedure to avoid an acute increase in pneumoperitoneum pressure. The trocars most commonly used are 5- to 10-mm diameter, either disposable or reusable. Trocars without blades are preferable for aortic surgery to avoid injury to abdominal wall vessels.

Dissecting and Cutting Instruments

A variety of grasping forceps and scissors are designed with either straight or curved jaws and blades. Insulated electric cables are used for hemostasis and electrocoagulation. The harmonic scalpel can be used, especially in obese patients with dense fat and ganglia around the aorta.

Suturing Instruments

Needle holders and clip and staple applicators are essential in laparoscopic aortic surgery. Needle holders are designed with straight or curved jaws and handles. Large-diameter (10 mm) and medium-diameter (5 mm) sheaths are used for anastomoses and suturing, depending on the thickness and degree of calcification of the aortic wall. Clip and staple applicators used in general surgery are also commonly used in aortic surgery for small-vessel hemostasis. For aortic and iliac occlusion, the

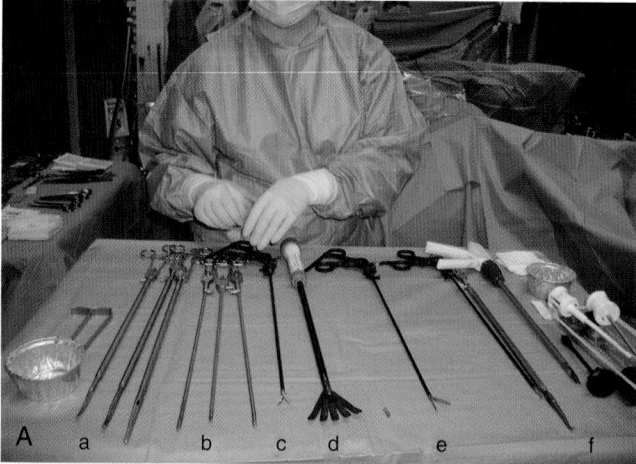

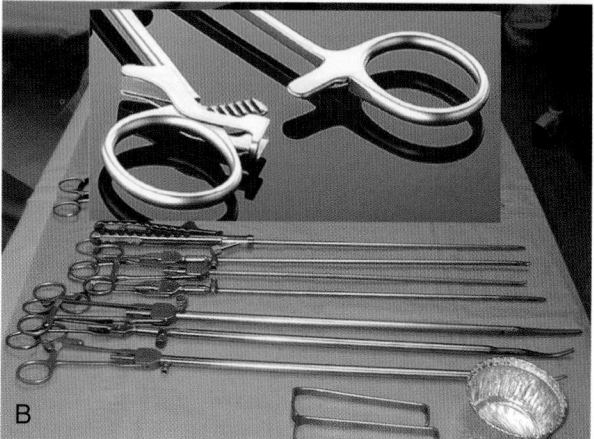

Figure 107-1 A, Basic instruments for laparoscopic aortic surgery: aortic clamps (a), needle holders (b), scissors (c), endoretractor (d), forceps (e), and clip applicator (f). **B,** Laparoscopic aortic clamps with double-locking security.

EndoGIA stapler (Multifire Powered EndoGIA 60, Autosuture, Norwalk, CT) can be used, but only if there is no severe calcification.

Specific laparoscopic stapling devices for aortoiliac occlusion and aortic-prosthetic sutures are still experimental and not yet available for human use.

Suction-Irrigation Devices and Retractors

A suction-irrigation device is key in laparoscopic aortic surgery because maintenance of a clear surgical field unobscured by blood is essential. Irrigation and suction are connected to a single handle. Irrigation with heparinized serum is useful to clean the operative field whenever ongoing bleeding has resulted in clot formation. Mechanical pumps are available to create high-pressure flow.

Intestinal retractors are commonly used in laparoscopic aortic surgery. A variety of laparoscopic intestinal retractors have been described, using either nets or blades. These instruments are useful for laparoscopic approaches to the aorta and are mandatory during transperitoneal direct and retroperitoneal procedures.

Laparoscopic Clamps

Different shapes and sizes of laparoscopic aortic clamps are available. Detachable clamps are also used. The strength of the jaws allows effective clamping of a moderately calcified aorta, but as in open surgery, a heavily calcified aorta is unclampable and poses the potential risk of aortic rupture. We always use double-locking aortic clamps (Fig. 107-1B). The redundant security of double-locking clamps is important in laparoscopic aortic surgery because of the closed nature of the approach and the catastrophic complications that can occur with equipment failure.

■ TRAINING PROGRAM

Practice to gain videoscopic skills is particularly important for vascular surgeons because they generally lack such training and experience. Although training in videoscopic suturing is essential, thorough training in a broad range of videoscopic skills is a prerequisite for performing laparoscopic aortic surgery. The equipment needs are simple: (1) videoscope, camera, and monitor (a compact system, Medipack, is manufactured by Storz France-SA, Paris, France; a homemade video system can also be used with a simple camcorder); (2) needle holder, grasping forceps, and scissors; (3) laparotrainer with ergonomics comparable to those for human aortic procedures; and (4) prostheses and sutures. Training consists of performing end-to-end and end-to-side anastomoses similar to those required in human procedures, with the same preparation of stitches. Such training is possible in the office, in the operating room, or at home. We recommend regular, daily training for at least 3 months before embarking on one's first human procedure. Once initial expertise is gained, training can be continued periodically, depending on the surgeon's skill level. Long-term training is essential, however, because vascular surgeons generally lack the opportunity to regularly perform simple laparoscopic procedures, such as cholecystectomy, that allow the maintenance of expertise.

Training on animals or cadavers is also an important means of gaining expertise in all steps of videoscopic aortic procedures. Such training is usually organized during courses and workshops.

For surgeons who want to set up a laparoscopic program, proctorship is essential to avoid pitfalls and complications during one's initial procedures.

■ INDICATIONS AND CONTRAINDICATIONS

Indications for Laparoscopic Aortofemoral Bypass

Indications for laparoscopic AFB are identical to those for open surgery. According to the recently published TASC recommendations and ACC/AHA guidelines,[1,2] patients with severe AIOD or associated abdominal aortic aneurysm (AAA) are candidates for surgery rather than endovascular repair. The choice of open or laparoscopic technique depends on the surgeon's skill set and does not alter the indications for AFB. For unilateral AIOD, a choice between crossover femorofemoral and laparoscopic aorto-unifemoral bypass is necessary. Advantages of laparoscopic bypass include the ability to perform a direct aortic repair with better long-term patency rates,[3] the requirement of only one groin incision, and the avoidance of laparotomy. The major disadvantages of laparoscopic bypass are the potential risks of direct aortic repair and aortic cross-clamping and a higher risk of complications, including sexual dysfunction.

Contraindications for Laparoscopic Aortofemoral Bypass

Technical Issues

With growing experience, the contraindications for laparoscopic AFB are now limited to (1) inability to safely expose the abdominal aorta owing to retroperitoneal fibrosis; (2) unsuitable abdominal aorta due to heavy, circumferential calcification; (3) associated severe, diffuse renal or visceral occlusive lesions not amenable to endovascular repair; and (4) aortic infection. Preoperative computed tomography (CT) without contrast enhancement is essential to examine the aortic wall and identify potential venous anomalies.

Patient Status

Criteria for patient selection require the objective balancing of risks and benefits, as well as close collaboration between surgeons and anesthetists.

Patient status is determined in accordance with the American Society of Anesthesiologists (ASA) classification. In addition, all patients should undergo stress echocardiography and pulmonary, hepatic, and renal function tests. Coronary arteriography is reserved for patients with abnormal stress echocardiograms. Contraindications to laparoscopic aortic reconstruction are ASA class V patients and patients with major cardiac, hepatic, or renal dysfunction.

Criteria for high-risk open aortic surgery also apply to laparoscopic aortic bypass and include (1) advanced coronary artery disease with unreconstructable coronary lesions, (2) critical aortic valve stenosis, (3) severe cardiac insufficiency, (4) left ventricular ejection fraction less than 40%, (5) renal insufficiency with serum creatinine level greater than 2.2 mg/dL (194 μmol/L), and (6) cirrhosis. Unlike open aortic surgery, severe chronic obstructive pulmonary disease is not an absolute contraindication for laparoscopy but deserves careful consideration. Reducing the pneumoperitoneum pressure or choosing a retroperitoneal approach should be strongly considered in such patients.

Contraindications to CO_2 pneumoperitoneum are not absolute, but particular caution is advised in the presence of (1) severe hypertension, (2) hypovolemia and dehydration, (3) severe arrhythmias, (4) bullous pulmonary dystrophy, (5) severe emphysema with blebs, (6) history of spontan-

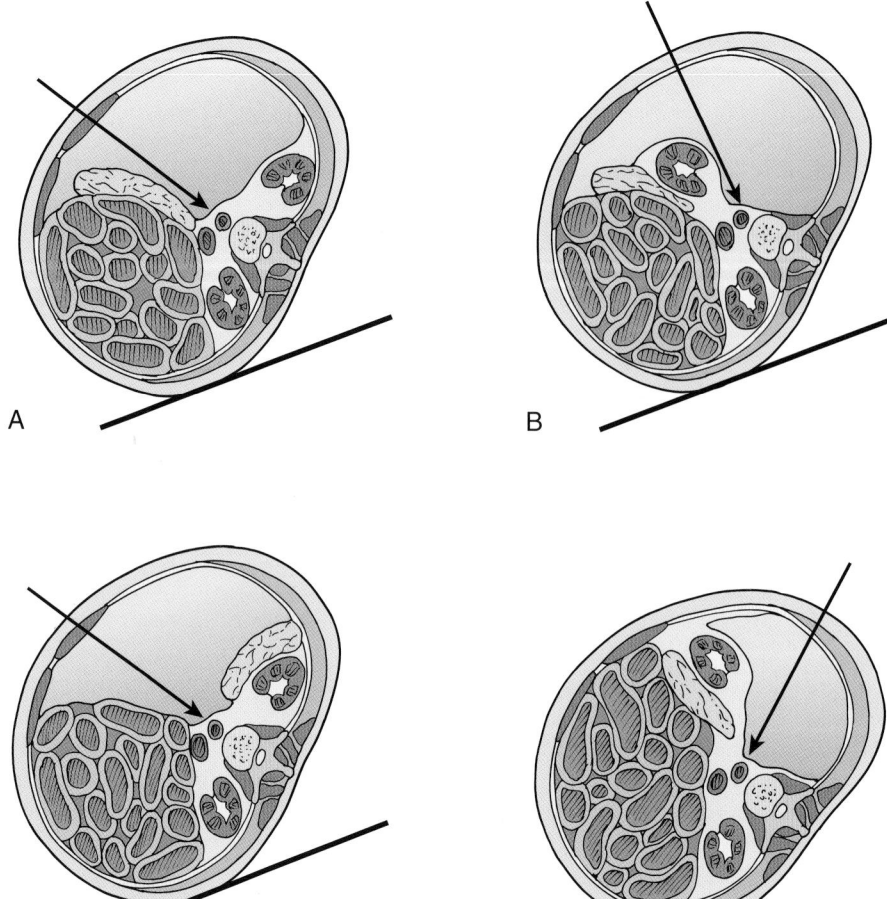

Figure 107-2 Transverse sections show the four different videoscopic approaches to the abdominal aorta. **A,** Transperitoneal left retrocolic. **B,** Transperitoneal left retrorenal. **C,** Transperitoneal direct. **D,** Retroperitoneal.

eous pneumothorax, and (7) intracranial and intraocular hypertension.

■ TECHNIQUE

Laparoscopic aortic reconstructions for AIOD proceed with the following reproducible steps: (1) laparoscopic approach to the abdominal aorta, (2) laparoscopic aortobifemoral bypass, and (3) closure.

Preoperatively, the patient should undergo effective bowel preparation. This reduces the volume of bowel in the abdomen and eases the task of maintaining bowel retraction during surgery.

Videoscopic bypasses for AIOD are not performed when the abdominal aorta is unusable or unsuitable. In such cases, bypasses would originate from either the ascending or descending thoracic aorta; these procedures are beyond the scope of this chapter.

Laparoscopic Approaches to the Abdominal Aorta

A laparoscopic approach to the abdominal aorta is performed after groin exposure. Videoscopic approaches to the abdomi-

nal aorta use the same anatomic landmarks and surgical dissection planes as open surgery. Four different approaches have been described (Fig. 107-2): transperitoneal retrocolic (TPRC), transperitoneal retrorenal (TPRR), transperitoneal direct (TPD), and retroperitoneal (RP).

Different techniques have been described to achieve and maintain a stable aortic exposure. Dion and Gracia reported the peritoneal apron technique in 1997.[14] In this technique, the patient is slightly tilted to the right, and the operating surgeon stands to the patient's left. A peritoneal apron is made with the left parietal peritoneum sutured to the right abdominal wall. After creation of the peritoneal apron, the aorta is approached and exposure is obtained through a left retroperitoneal route. The kidney is freed only on its inferior and lateral surface, and its lower pole is mobilized cephalad. In 2003, Dion and colleagues modified this approach using the apron technique with a TPRC approach.[15] More recently, Stadler and associates described the use of the apron technique for the TPD approach.[16] They make the apron with the peritoneum lying on the left mesocolon. Alimi,[17] Barbera,[18] and Cau[19] and their respective coauthors described a variety of intestinal retractors to facilitate the TPD approach. In the technique described by Barbera, the patient is placed in the Trendelenburg position, and the small bowel is retracted upward. In contrast, Alimi and Cau use intestinal retractors to maintain the small bowel in the right part of the abdomen; the patient is tilted slightly to the right, and the operator stands on the left. In 1999, Said and coworkers, in a cadaver study, used a TPRC approach with retractors to maintain the left mesocolon.[20] In this technique, the patient is tilted slightly to the right, and the surgeon stands on the patient's left. In 2002, we described the use of an 80-degree right lateral decubitus (RLD) position to drop the viscera out of the operative field.[21] With this technique, the operating surgeon stands on the patient's right, and there is no need for additional maneuvers to maintain the exposure. We described the use of the RLD position for TPRC,[21] TPRR,[22] and TPD[23] approaches. The RP approach to the aorta was first reported by Edoga.[24] It requires no special devices or techniques to maintain exposure. Edoga first used this approach for videoscopic-assisted AAA repair. We reported on the RP approach for total AAA and AIOD repair in 2005.[25]

Transperitoneal Approaches

The patient is placed in a dorsal decubitus position, with an inflatable pillow (Pelvic-Tilt, O. R. Comfort, Glen Ridge, NJ) behind the left flank. Insufflation of the pillow provides 50 to 60 degrees of rotation of the abdomen. Maximal right rotation of the operating table affords an abdominal slope of 80 degrees. The operator faces the patient's abdomen. The video tower is viewed distally on the left side of the patient. The camera assistant stands in front of the surgeon on the opposite side of the patient. The first assistant stands on the right of the operating surgeon (Fig. 107-3). Anesthetic management is similar to that for open aortic surgery, with at least two peripheral venous access lines and an arterial line. The patient is under ventilatory support. A nasogastric tube and a Foley catheter are routinely placed. Intraoperative transesophageal echocardiography is used when indicated.

The procedure begins with a conventional open exposure of the femoral arteries. On the right side, the retroperitoneal tunnel is initiated from the groin and conducted as far proximally as possible on top of the iliac artery. On the left side, the tunnel is not prepared yet because gas leakage would occur.

We usually use a blind technique to create the pneumoperitoneum. A Veres needle is introduced 3 cm below the costal margin in the left midclavicular line, and the pneumoperitoneum is insufflated up to 14 mm Hg. In cases of previous abdominal scars, the first trocar is positioned using an open technique 2 cm medial to the anterior superior iliac spine. This trocar is used to create the pneumoperitoneum and introduce the endoscope (Storz-France SA, Paris, France).

Retrocolic Approach.

In the TPRC approach, trocar positioning depends on the type of aortoiliac lesion. We use only 10-mm trocars because large instruments are required to perform the procedure. For patients with AIOD, the first trocar (trocar 1) is positioned 3 cm below the costal margin in the anterior axillary line. It is introduced with graspers

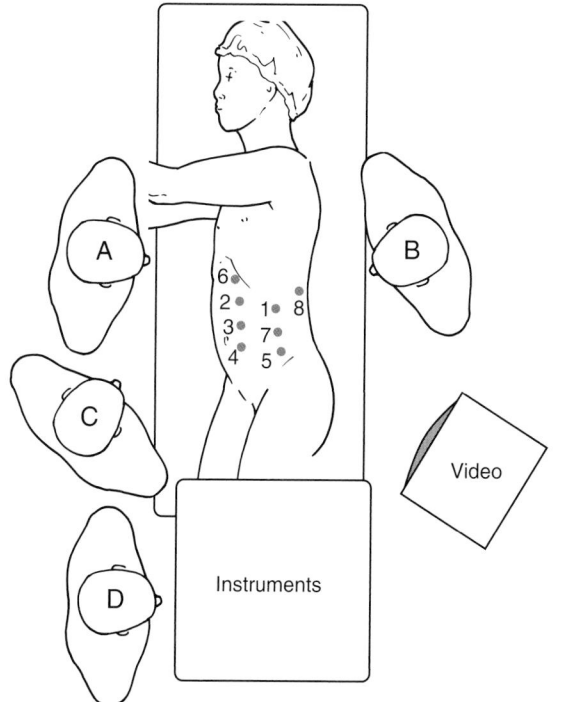

Figure 107-3 Basic operating room setup: operating surgeon (A), assistant for laparoscope (B), assistant for instrumentation (C), nurse (D). Laparoscopic ports: 10-mm port for laparoscope (1); 10-mm ports for operator instruments (2 and 3); 10-mm ports for assistant instrumentation (4 and 5); 10-mm port for endoretractor or proximal laparoscopic clamp (6); 10-mm port for large aneurysms, used for assistant instrumentation, laparoscope, or operator instruments (7); and 10-mm port for proximal laparoscopic clamp in cases of suprarenal clamping or associated abdominal aortic aneurysm (8).

using a hybrid open-blind technique, until the peritoneum is opened. This technique avoids muscle wounds and abdominal injuries. Two trocars (trocars 2 and 3) are placed about 8 cm apart at the supraumbilical and left paramedian level to insert the operating instruments. Trocar 4 is positioned below the navel to introduce the assistant's instruments and the distal aortic clamp. Trocar 5 is placed in the left lower abdomen 2 cm medial to the anterior superior iliac spine and is used for the assistant's instruments. Finally, trocar 6 is placed beneath the xiphoid. It has two functions: (1) at the beginning of the procedure, an endoretractor (Endoretract II, Autosuture Company, Elancourt, France) is introduced through this trocar to maintain retraction of the left mesocolon; and (2) during aortic repair, this trocar is used to introduce the proximal aortic clamp. For associated AAA repair, trocar 1 is placed just below the costal margin, especially if the aortic neck is short or angulated. Once the first trocar is placed, pneumoperitoneum pressure is decreased to 14 mm Hg. An additional trocar (trocar 7) is introduced between trocars 1 and 5 to insert instruments or the endoscope.

A peritoneal incision is made in the left paracolic gutter up to the splenic flexure. By elevating and displacing the left colon, the avascular plane of the Toldt fascia is entered and developed medially to reach the internal edge of the kidney. The left gonadal vein provides an important landmark because

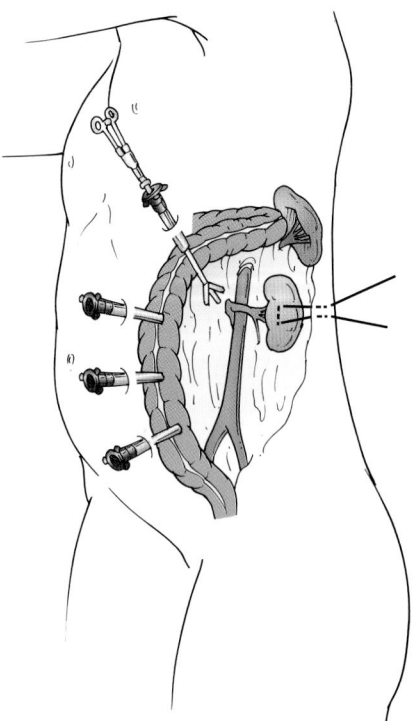

Figure 107-4 Two major steps of the transperitoneal retrocolic approach: an endoretractor is positioned through port 7 to maintain the left mesocolon, and a stitch is placed in Gerota's fascia and pulled out through the left abdominal wall.

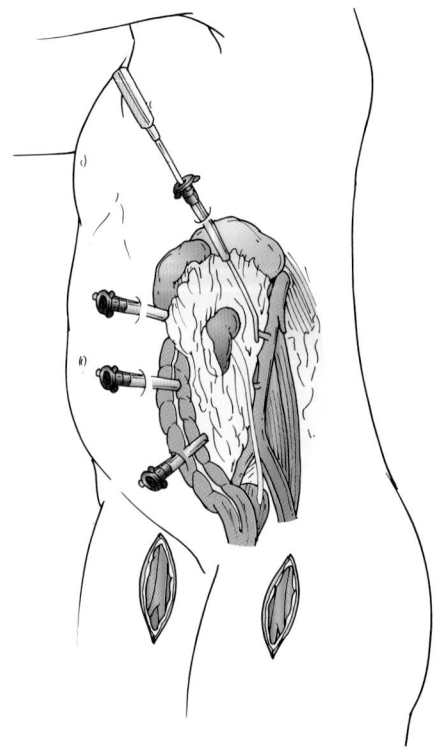

Figure 107-5 Exposure of the infrarenal aorta via the transperitoneal retrorenal approach. An endoretractor is placed through port 7 to maintain control of the viscera.

it leads to the left renal vein. After the left renal vein is visualized, we always perform two steps to maintain the exposure: (1) we place an endoretractor through trocar 7 to contain the left mesocolon, and (2) we place a stitch in Gerota's fascia and pull it out through the left abdominal wall (Fig. 107-4). Traction on this stitch allows retraction of the kidney and opens the operative field in front of the preaortic ganglia. The RLD position allows the small bowel and left mesocolon to drop into the right part of the abdomen. Dissection of the aorta is then conducted craniad to level of the left renal artery and caudad to the left iliac artery. The inferior mesenteric artery is dissected toward the mesocolon. The final step is exposure of the right common iliac artery in preparation for graft limb tunneling. For this step, we always perform the same maneuvers: The assistant introduces the endoretractor through trocar 4 and the suction device through trocar 5; he or she points these two instruments toward the common iliac artery and retracts the left mesocolon. The operating surgeon conducts the dissection as far as possible with this assistance—beyond the right ureter, if possible. Once the dissection is completed, exposure of the aorta is maintained by traction on additional stitches placed in the para-aortic fat.

Retrorenal Approach. In the TPRR approach, trocar 1 is positioned 2 cm medial to the line of the anterior superior iliac spine. Other trocars are positioned the same as for the TPRC approach, but translated slightly laterally. We do not place trocar 6 at the beginning of the procedure; instead, we

wait for positioning of the spleen after completion of the medial visceral rotation. A peritoneal incision is made in the left paracolic gutter up to the diaphragm. We enter the retroperitoneal plane in the iliac fossa and visualize the left ureter and iliac artery. Left retrorenal dissection is conducted craniad and medially from the psoas muscle after incision of the retrorenal fascia. We perform a complete right medial visceral rotation because it allows a larger working space. Owing to the RLD position, the small bowel, left mesocolon, left kidney, and spleen drop into the right part of the abdomen. We place a stitch in the left perirenal fat and pull it out through the right abdominal wall to maintain visceral retraction. The aorta is dissected craniad from the left iliac to the left renal artery. We transect the left lumbar splanchnic nerve, which overlies the left side of the aorta. Just below the left renal artery, the renal-azygos-lumbar venous trunk often crosses the left side of the aorta. Its transection provides complete retraction of the kidney, without the risk of bleeding, and improves the dissection and exposure of the juxtarenal aorta. If necessary, we develop the dissection cranially, proximal to the left renal artery, to the level of the left diaphragmatic crus. Its division provides exposure of the aortic visceral segment. After completing the dissection, subcostal trocar 6 is carefully placed, avoiding iatrogenic injury to the spleen. Through this trocar we introduce an endoretractor to contain the left kidney. The retractor tip is placed just below the left renal artery and stabilizes exposure of the juxtarenal aorta (Fig. 107-5). Exposure of the right iliac artery is conducted as in the TPRC approach.

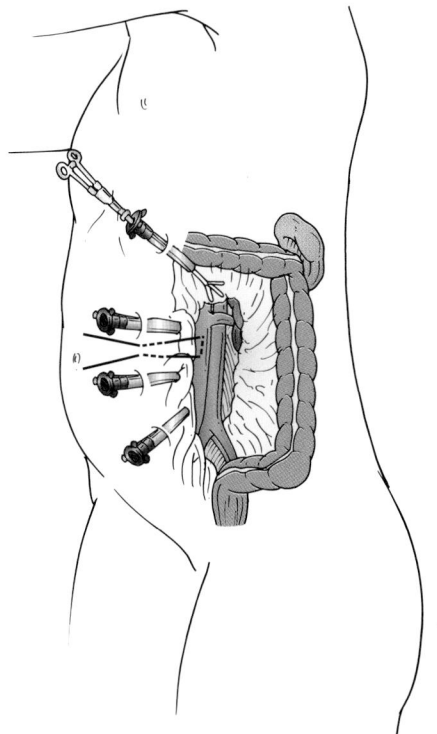

Figure 107-6 Exposure of the infrarenal aorta via the transperitoneal direct approach.

Direct Approach. In the TPD approach, trocar positioning is similar to that described for the TPRC approach. After abdominal exploration, the transverse mesocolon is elevated with a stitch pulled out through the left subcostal abdominal wall. The retroperitoneum is longitudinally incised overlying the anterior aortic wall, just to the left of the mesentery. This incision is extended down to the iliac arteries. Another stitch is placed on the posterior peritoneum, near the duodenum, and pulled out through the right abdominal wall. If necessary, an additional trocar is used to maintain retraction of the small bowel with an endoretractor introduced in the left flank or the pelvis, in the right paramedian line. Intestinal retractors can also be used to maintain small bowel retraction. The aortic periadventitial plane is freed, and circumferential aortic dissection is performed from the iliac arteries up to the left renal vein (Fig. 107-6). After aortoiliac dissection is achieved, the pillow is deflated and the operating table is rotated to the left, which enables conventional approaches to the femoral arteries. The patient is then returned to the RLD position for aortoiliac videoscopic reconstruction.

Retroperitoneal Approach

The patient receives general anesthesia and is placed in a dorsal decubitus position with an inflatable pillow behind the left flank, which provides 30 degrees of rotation of the abdomen. The surgeon stands on the patient's left side, and the video monitor is viewed distally on the right side. The trocar used to introduce the 45-degree endoscope is positioned using an open technique midway between the costal margin and the anterior superior iliac spine. Retroperitoneal blunt dissection is performed first, to prepare the working space. After gas insufflation, dissection begins with the endoscope. The psoas muscle is the first anatomic landmark. The left kidney is then identified. Two operating trocars are placed in the left flank, between the iliac crest and the rib cage. Two 10-mm trocars are inserted in the left iliac fossa for assistant instrumentation and retraction. After the left retrorenal fascia is incised, the left lower pole of the kidney is dissected free and retracted cephalad and medially. The left common iliac artery is visualized. The infrarenal aorta is then dissected craniad until the left renal artery is encountered. The renal-azygos-lumbar venous trunk is divided to provide exposure of the juxtarenal aorta. The peritoneal sac and left kidney are maintained out of the operative field with a retractor. The anterior surface of the right common iliac artery is dissected over 3 to 5 cm if necessary. As in conventional open surgery, ligation of an occluded inferior mesenteric artery improves the exposure of the right common iliac artery. After the dissection is complete, the pillow is deflated, which allows a conventional approach to the femoral arteries if necessary.

Choice of Approach

The choice of approach depends primarily on anatomic and patient factors. Adequate workspace is essential, and this is usually achieved with a positive-pressure pneumoperitoneum.

The TPRR approach is our first choice. It allows wide exposure, especially when control of the juxtarenal aorta is needed. The suprarenal or celiac aorta is dissected in line on the left side of the aorta after division of the diaphragmatic crus. Unlike with the TPRC or TPD approach, neither the kidney nor the mesocolon obscures the exposure of the left side of the aorta. This is particularly important for control of the lumbar arteries during AAA repair. At the end of the procedure, the viscera are allowed to fall back into place, providing optimal coverage of the prosthesis.

The TPRR approach is contraindicated in cases of perisplenic adhesions or a retroaortic left renal vein. In such cases, we use the TPRC approach; this approach is also indicated for concomitant left renal or superior mesenteric videoscopic bypass.[26] In cases of an extremely hostile abdomen, we use the RP approach. However, workspace is reduced, either externally for the placement of trocars or internally behind the peritoneal sac. For AAA repair, the RP approach is feasible but exceptionally difficult; in such cases, conversion to open repair is often necessary. For these reasons, the RP approach is rarely indicated, and even in cases of previous abdominal scars, we often try to enter the peritoneal cavity to perform a transperitoneal approach.

Finally, in a few cases we use the TPD approach. Theoretically, TPD is the simplest approach because it relies on common landmarks that are familiar to vascular surgeons. However, this approach requires careful dissection close to the intestine. Upward retraction of the transverse mesocolon is not always simple and may require two or more stitches.

Exposure of the juxtarenal aorta is then difficult, especially for AAAs with short or angulated necks. Use of a variety of maneuvers is essential to avoid repetitive prolapse of bowel loops in the operative field. The main drawback of the TPD approach is difficulty providing adequate coverage of the prosthesis, especially in thin patients. For these reasons, we use the TPD approach only in cases of previous left nephrectomy, when retrorenal and retrocolic dissection planes are blocked.

Laparoscopic Aortofemoral Bypass

Before aortic repair, we prepare specific stitches for laparoscopic anastomoses with either polypropylene (3-0 or 4-0 Prolene) or polytetrafluoroethylene (PTFE) sutures. Stitches for running sutures are between 18 and 22 cm long and knotted on 10- by 10-mm Teflon or prosthetic pledgets. Stitches for single sutures are between 8 and 12 cm long and knotted on small pledgets. Technical variation depends on laparoscopic approaches and aortic lesions.

Transperitoneal Retrorenal Approach

Once the aortic and femoral exposures are complete, the vascular prosthesis is beveled to allow an end-to-end or end-to-side aortic-prosthetic anastomosis. A knot is placed as a landmark on the left limb. Before introducing the prosthesis into the abdomen, a clamp is placed in the right graft limb tunnel from the groin. The assistant exposes the right common iliac artery with an endoretractor in his or her left hand (trocar 4) and a suction device in the right hand (trocar 5). Using this exposure, the operating surgeon introduces an aortic clamp from the groin and conducts its tip over the right common iliac artery under abdominal videoscopic control (Fig. 107-7). Once the clamp is positioned, the vascular prosthesis is introduced into the abdomen through one of the trocars, and the right limb is easily brought to the groin incision. The left prosthetic limb is also brought down with the help of an aortic clamp introduced through the left groin. Unlike the right side, the left tunnel is short and widely open because the organs have fallen away toward the right side of the peritoneal cavity. The diameter of the left graft limb tunnel should be minimized to reduce the risk of gas leakage.

Aortic clamping is performed with videoscopic clamps (see Fig. 107-1). Proximal and distal videoscopic clamps are positioned through trocars 6 and 4, respectively. Clamps stabilize the viscera in position during performance of the aortic-prosthetic anastomosis (Fig. 107-8A). When suprarenal clamping is needed, or in the case of an associated AAA, we introduce the proximal clamp through an additional trocar placed in the left flank (trocar 8; see Fig. 107-3). With this configuration, the retractor is in trocar 6 and maintains the viscera (Fig. 107-8B). To perform an end-to-end aortic-prosthetic anastomosis, the operator transects the aorta with videoscopic scissors in the left hand. An important technical point is to avoid oblique transection of the aorta. Closure of a noncalcified distal aorta can be done with a mechanical stapler (Multifire

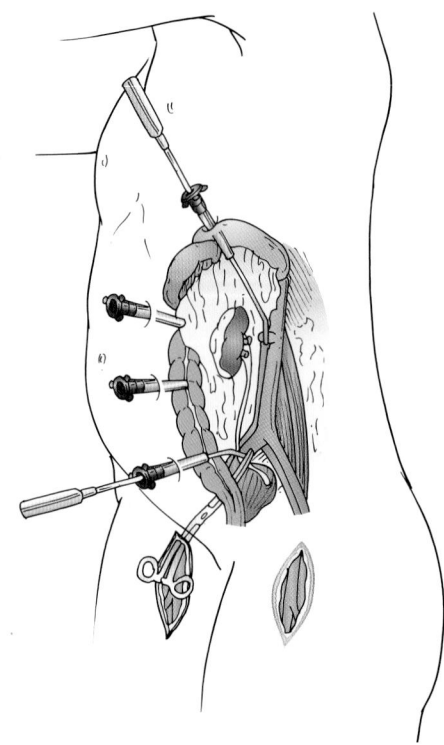

Figure 107-7 Placement of an aortic clamp in the right graft limb tunnel under videoscopic control before the prosthesis is introduced into the abdomen.

EndoGIA 30, Autosuture Company, Elancourt, France). For calcified aortas, we prefer to use 2-0 or 3-0 polypropylene or PTFE double running sutures. For end-to-side aortic-prosthetic anastomosis, aortotomy is performed according to the length of the prosthetic spatula. We use either standard videoscopic scissors or a videoscopic lancet and Potts scissors.

Aortic-prosthetic anastomoses are begun with a single stitch and then performed with two hemicircumferential running sutures (using the sutures previously knotted on pledgets) tied together intracorporeally (Fig. 107-9). After unclamping, the suture line is checked, and additional stitches are placed if needed for hemostasis.

Measurement of the aortic clamping time for AIOD repair depends on the proximal aortic-prosthetic anastomosis. For an end-to-side anastomosis, aortic clamping time is measured until unclamping of the aorta when the aortic-prosthetic anastomosis is completed. For an end-to-end anastomosis, aortic clamping time is defined as the time between proximal aortic clamping and unclamping of the first prosthetic limb. For laparoscopic AIOD repair, median aortic clamping time is 45 minutes (range, 15 to 130 minutes), and blood loss is 500 mL (range, 100 to 3900 mL).

After an end-to-end aortic-prosthetic anastomosis, thorough videoscopic surveillance ensures suture line hemostasis of the distal aortic stump. We also inspect the left colon videoscopically to assess its viability. Intraoperative Doppler ultrasound (Ultrasonic Doppler Flow Detector model 811b, Parks Medical Electronics, Aloha, OR) is used to assess the adequacy of blood flow to the left mesocolon. If reimplantation of the inferior mesenteric artery is needed, it can

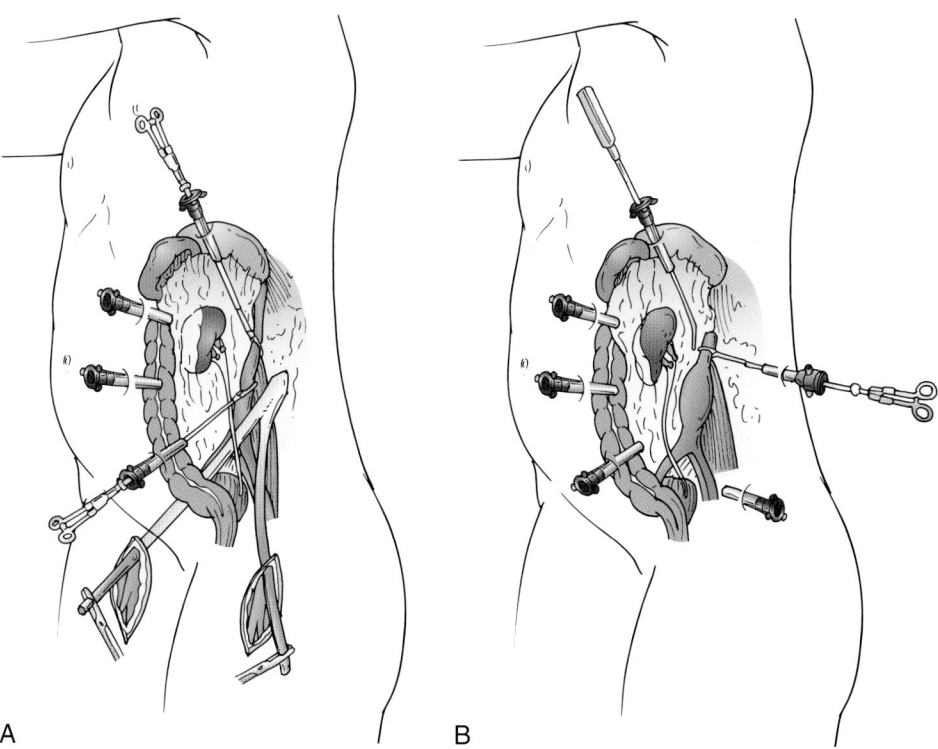

Figure 107-8 Positioning of laparoscopic clamps during the transperitoneal retrorenal approach. The proximal clamp is introduced through either a subxiphoid (**A**) or a flank (**B**) port.

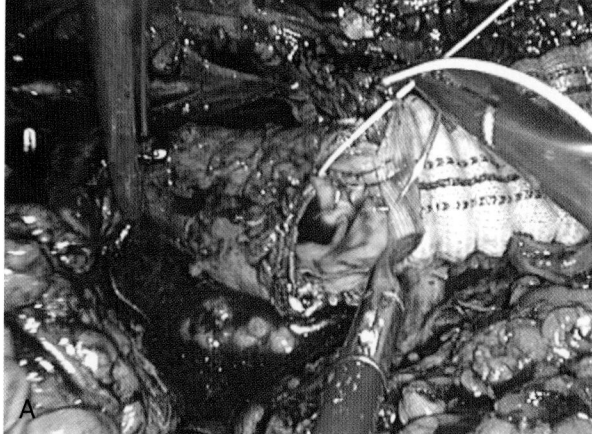

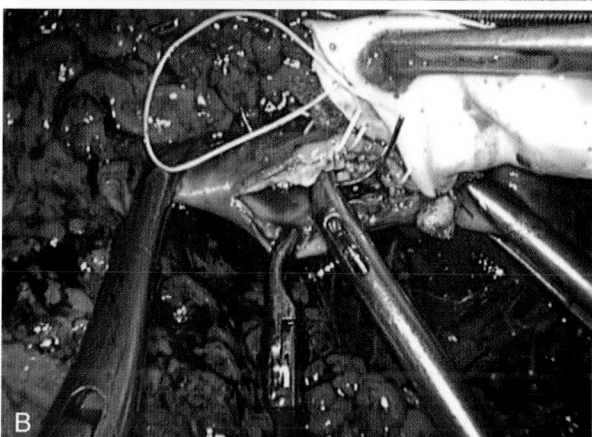

Figure 107-9 Operative views showing end-to-end (**A**) and end-to-side (**B**) aortic-prosthetic anastomoses with PTFE sutures.

be performed videoscopically or via a short laparotomy. On closure, a suction drain is positioned near the prosthesis. There is no need to reattach the edge of the peritoneum because the viscera fall back into place once the patient is returned to a dorsal decubitus position. Abdominal fascia trocar holes and groin incisions are closed with absorbable suture. The median operative time is 260 minutes (range, 120 to 520 minutes), including the learning curve and the training of fellows and young vascular surgeons.

Technical Variations

Transperitoneal Retrocolic and Direct Approaches.

Aortic repair through TPRC and TPD approaches uses the same steps as the TPRR approach. The main differences are clamp positioning and graft limb tunneling. Positioning of the proximal aortic clamp uses the subxiphoid trocar (trocar 6) after removal of the endoretractor. This clamp stabilizes the left mesocolon (Fig. 107-10). Tunneling of the graft limbs for aortobifemoral bypass grafts is similar for both TPRC and TPRR approaches. On the right side it is identical. On the left side, as part of the TPRC approach, the operator advances the clamp from the groin toward the aorta under videoscopic control, passing the tip beneath the ureter, which overlies the iliac artery bifurcation. When performing a TPD approach, tunneling of the left graft limb is more demanding. Video-scopic dissection along the anterior aspect of the left iliac artery is blinded by the left mesocolon, and there is insuffi-cient exposure to ensure that the tunnel is strictly behind the ureter. We recommend a short peritoneal incision in the left iliac fossa with retroperitoneal dissection and exposure of the

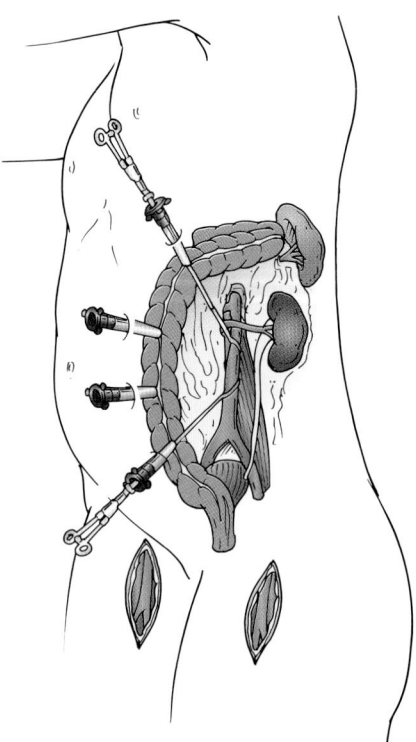

Figure 107-10 Placement of laparoscopic clamps during the transperitoneal retrocolic approach. Note that the clamps stabilize the left mesocolon.

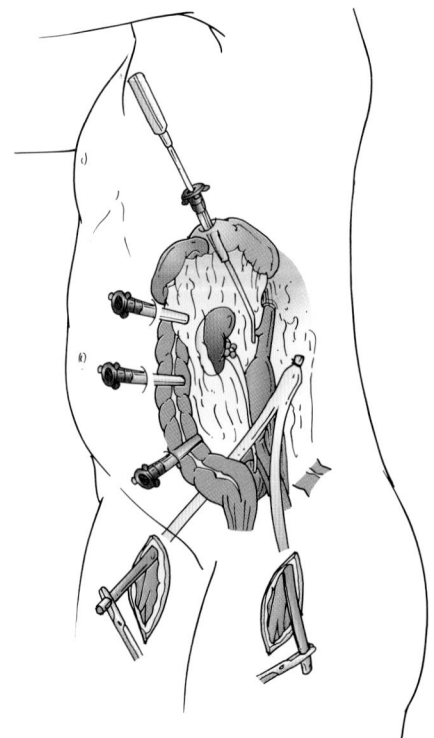

Figure 107-11 Aortoiliac occlusive disease and associated abdominal aortic aneurysm. Demonstrated is the proper positioning of a bifurcated graft before performing the distal anastomoses.

distal common iliac artery. With such exposure, tunneling is simple, and the operator can pass the clamp behind the ureter under strict videoscopic control.

Retroperitoneal Approach. The proximal clamp is introduced through a sixth trocar placed above the left 12th rib. The distal clamp is positioned through a seventh trocar placed in the left iliac fossa. Aortic-prosthetic anastomoses are based on the same principles but are performed in a reverse fashion compared to transperitoneal exposures.

Juxtarenal Thrombosis. When aortic thrombus extends up to the level of the renal arteries, suprarenal clamping is needed to ensure complete thrombectomy without risk of renal impairment. As mentioned earlier, dissection is conducted proximal to the renal arteries through either a TPRR or a TPRC approach. We use sequential steps for suprarenal clamping to decrease renal ischemic time. The suprarenal clamp is positioned but left unclamped during transection and thrombectomy of the infrarenal aorta. When the juxtarenal thrombectomy is nearly finished, the suprarenal clamp is applied. If the target zone of the proximal anastomosis below the renal arteries is of sufficient length, we clamp the infrarenal aorta through trocar 2 and move the suprarenal clamp below the renal arteries. As with open surgery, this maneuver reduces renal ischemic time to the amount needed for thrombectomy. If preparation of the infrarenal aorta does not allow enough length to move the clamp after thrombectomy,

we perform the proximal anastomosis with suprarenal clamping.

Associated Abdominal Aortic Aneurysm. Decreasing aortic cross-clamp time is important when placing aortobifemoral grafts during laparoscopic AAA repair. Whenever possible, once the graft limbs have been tunneled to the groins, the distal femoral anastomoses are performed first (Fig. 107-11). Using such an approach, the total aortic cross-clamp time is only that required for aneurysmorrhaphy and creation of the proximal anastomosis. Blood flow to the internal iliac arteries is ensured by either retrograde perfusion or re-implantation.

Conversion to Open Repair

Conversion to open direct repair through a short incision should not be considered a failure; it is a safe and reasonable strategy when difficulties arise during total videoscopic procedures. Such a decision is sometimes difficult for surgeons, especially early in the learning curve. An ongoing dialogue with the anesthesia team is essential to determine the appropriate conversion time. Typical indications for open conversion are (1) difficult reconstruction with prolonged aortic cross-clamp time; (2) extensive calcification with an unclampable aorta; (3) difficult or unstable exposure of the abdominal aorta (especially during the RP approach) because of small abdominal cavities, unexpected dense adhesions, and excessive

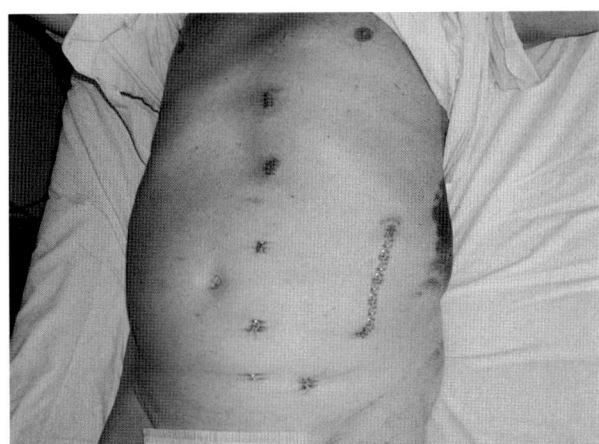

Figure 107-12 Postoperative clinical photograph of a patient after conversion to open repair.

dilatation of the small bowel; (4) injuries to structures adjacent to the aorta, such as the small bowel, inferior vena cava, or iliac veins; and (5) systemic disturbances due to pneumoperitoneum pressure or RLD positioning of the patient. Relative indications for conversion include the need for inferior mesenteric artery re-implantation and inadequate exposure or visibility to control bleeding.

When converting to open repair, the patient remains in the RLD position while the surgeon performs a short vertical laparotomy between the laparoscope and the assistant's trocars (trocars 1 and 5; Fig. 107-12). This laparotomy can be performed rapidly in an emergency situation without changing the patient's position, and if necessary it can be extended. Exposure through the initial direct, retrocolic, or retrorenal route is maintained with autostatic retractors or valves. Completion of the procedure is based on the same principles as for conventional open direct repair. Sometimes it is useful to use laparoscopic clamps, which are less cumbersome than conventional aortic clamps. Another useful maneuver is the percutaneous introduction of clamps.

Postoperative Management and Recovery

In the majority of cases, we attempt to remove the patient from mechanical ventilation and extubate at the end of the procedure. Patients are taken to the intensive care unit immediately after the procedure and returned to their rooms as soon as hemodynamic, respiratory, and biologic parameters have normalized. A liquid diet is introduced on day 1. Soft and general diets are usually introduced on days 2 and 4, respectively.

■ RESULTS

Clinical outcomes of laparoscopic procedures are comparable to those of open surgery in terms of mortality and morbidity (see Table 107-1). Severe systemic complication rates compare favorably with those of open surgery, but there is a low inci-

dence of pulmonary and gastrointestinal complications. This potential benefit of laparoscopy relates to several factors, including avoidance of a large abdominal incision, reduced pain, and more rapid return of gastrointestinal motility. Most patients are ambulatory by the third day and experience minimal wound discomfort. Median intensive care unit and hospital stays are 24 hours and 7 days, respectively. Technically challenging laparoscopic AIOD repair is not usually associated with prolongation of the postoperative course. The incidence of complications decreases after the initial learning curve, which is about 20 cases.

Midterm results demonstrate the reliability of laparoscopic AIOD repair, with patency rates similar to those achieved with open surgery.[27-29] In our series, primary and secondary cumulative patency rates were 93% and 95.6%, respectively, at 3 years.[29] As stated earlier, laparoscopic bypass techniques are based on the proven AFB, and we can expect excellent long-term results. However, longer follow-up is necessary to confirm these impressions.

Other patient benefits reported in other specialties are also valid for laparoscopic AIOD repair.[5-13] Laparoscopy allows an uneventful recovery in the majority of patients, reduces postoperative pain, and allows a more rapid return to a regular diet and full ambulation. Moreover, as observed in our series, a major advantage of laparoscopy is the avoidance of abdominal wall hernia, which occurs following 10% to 15% of open AIOD repairs.[30,31] Because it eliminates the need for laparotomy, laparoscopy reduces the incidence of surgery for laparotomy-related complications and hospitalization for bowel obstruction.[32]

■ COMPLICATIONS

Major laparoscopy-related complications have been described in general surgery and can occur during laparoscopic aortic procedures. Major complications specifically related to laparoscopic AIOD repair are rare, but their incidence will be better defined when the results of large series become available.

Vascular Complications

Vascular complications can occur during the setup phase of laparoscopy (76.5%), related to the early maneuvers required for entry into the peritoneal cavity, or they may result from the surgical dissection required for specific laparoscopic procedures (23.5%).[33] The incidence of major vascular complications during laparoscopic surgery is between 0.05% and 0.25%.[33,34]

Vascular Injuries of Retroperitoneal Vessels

Major vascular injuries related to entering the peritoneal cavity can occur with the blind insertion of the Veres needle and primary trocar.[33,34] Factors that predispose to visceral and vascular injuries are (1) adhesions between the viscera and the abdominal wall, resulting from previous inflammation or surgery; (2) a thin abdominal wall; and (3) poor technique or surgical inexperience.

An alternative is to use an open technique to create the pneumoperitoneum. With this technique, the peritoneal cavity is opened under direct vision, and a blunt-tipped trocar is introduced. Although the open technique appears to be safer than the closed technique, most surgeons prefer the closed technique because it is faster, requires a smaller incision, and is not associated with the leakage of CO_2. We currently use an "open modified technique" whereby the pneumoperitoneum is created through a Veres needle. The abdominal cavity is then entered with forceps until gas loss can be felt; then the first trocar is safely introduced. The comparative study performed by Bonjer and coworkers showed that the incidence of vascular injury associated with closed laparoscopy is significantly greater than that with open laparoscopy.[34]

Vascular injuries secondary to Veres needle insertion usually result in small 2- to 3-mm puncture lacerations. These can be repaired primarily with the placement of a few interrupted vascular sutures to obtain adequate hemostasis.

Major vascular injuries caused by the primary trocar occur by the same mechanism as Veres needle insertion. Vascular injury is recognized immediately in most cases and prompts emergency laparotomy to repair the lacerated vessel.

During laparoscopic aortic surgery, a major risk factor is the presence of a large aortic aneurysm, which renders use of the blind technique to enter the abdominal cavity hazardous. Conversion to open repair and control of bleeding after aortic injury are less challenging for vascular surgeons.

To prevent perforation of viscera or blood vessels, disposable trocars with safety shields were developed.[34] The safety shield is supposed to shoot forward after the peritoneum has been penetrated. However, the shield can be held back for a considerable distance, particularly in the case of loss of the pneumoperitoneum. This leaves the stylet of the trocar unprotected in the peritoneal cavity; this can easily cause vascular injuries, especially when the patient is thin, the abdominal cavity is small or not sufficiently elevated, or the AAA is large.

The incidence of major vascular injury is 0.4 per 1000 interventions; the associated mortality is approximately 10%.[25] Delay in diagnosis is probably the most significant contributor to morbidity and mortality.

As in open surgery, other injuries involving retroperitoneal vessels can occur during the various steps of the procedure, due to either tears or electrocoagulation.

Some authors have reported conversion to open repair for venous injuries.[6,35] To avoid vena cava injury during aortic repair, the posterior aortic wall should be kept intact for end-to-end anastomoses. Moreover, because laparoscopic clamps are heavy and their tips are sharp, they must be placed with care and attention to the iliac vein to avoid venous injury.

Vascular Injuries of Abdominal Wall Vessels

The use of multiple trocar sites makes injury to epigastric vessels or abdominal wall vessels increasingly likely.[36] Laparoscopic AIOD procedures carry a higher risk of abdominal wall vessel injuries because of the presence of potentially large arterial collaterals. These injuries can be recognized by the dripping of blood down the trocar sleeve into the abdomen or by hematoma formation around the trocar insertion site. It is important to avoid these injuries by placing the trocar after lighting the abdominal wall videoscopically and identifying the epigastric vessels, especially in thin patients. Undiagnosed injuries to the epigastric artery can lead to an expanding intramuscular hematoma or hemoperitoneum, especially in patients who are anticoagulated. Care must be taken at the end of the procedure to diagnose bleeding when removing trocars. In our experience, intramuscular hematoma after trocar insertion represents less than 0.5% of cases.

Clamping Problems

Aortic clamping can be challenging during laparoscopic surgery, especially when the infrarenal aorta is extensively calcified. During laparoscopy, surgeons lack tactile feedback when placing clamps; review of the preoperative CT scan is thus essential to assess the location and extent of aortic calcifications. Whenever the infrarenal aorta is unclampable, we first place a suprarenal clamp through a TPRR or TPRC approach. This allows a forceps endarterectomy of the infrarenal aorta, after which the cross-clamp is moved to below the renal arteries. If significant backbleeding occurs from an unclampable distal aorta, balloon occlusion can be used. In our series,[29] proximal aortic clamping was always feasible, either infrarenal or suprarenal. Two patients (<1%) needed balloon occlusion of unclampable distal aortas. No patients experienced postoperative complications related to aortic clamping.

Hemorrhagic Complications

Major hemorrhagic complications during laparoscopic AIOD repair can be due to clamp release, an unclampable aorta, and vascular injuries. In these cases, conversion to open repair is mandatory. We have not personally observed proximal clamp release, but this is probably a catastrophic complication, considering the closed nature of the approach.

Minor blackbleeding from either an unclampable aorta or tissue dissection is easily overcome with effective suction and does not preclude the performance of laparoscopic aortic repair for experienced surgeons.

A major difficulty may be obtaining hemostasis in the operative field at the end of the procedure. The lack of effective tamponade makes it difficult to obtain a dry field. Moreover, intraperitoneal pressure limits backbleeding from dissected fields, especially from small veins, causing additional difficulty in obtaining hemostasis. The use of thrombin glue is often useful to achieve hemostasis.

Anastomotic Difficulties

Aortic anastomotic complications are directly dependent on the surgeon's training and experience. However, because tactile feedback is reduced during laparoscopy, assessment of aortic wall quality is more difficult than during open surgery. It is important to choose the clamping site with the help of CT and to evaluate arterial walls with grasping forceps before proceeding. Dion,[35] Alimi,[37] and Cau[5] and their respective coauthors have reported conversion to open repair for difficult anastomoses to a calcified aorta. We also observed a case in which oversewing of the distal aortic stump was difficult, requiring conversion. Dion and colleagues reported a technical error during the aortic anastomosis in which the stitch included only aortic plaque, without adventitia.[35] Subtotal occlusion of the proximal anastomosis is always a concern, usually secondary to a stitch that grasps the opposite suture line.

To avoid these problems, one must take special care during preparation of the target zones for aortic anastomoses. Moreover, all stitches must be performed with precise control of the suture line. Insufficiently tensioned running suture is common during laparoscopic anastomoses, likely owing to the lack of tactile feedback. Simple techniques to overcome this problem include applying traction on the initial pledget or the suture line or placing an additional stitch to maintain suture-line tension.

Nonvascular Complications

Complications of Pneumoperitoneum

CO_2 pneumoperitoneum may cause a significant decrease in splanchnic vessel blood flow.[38,39] The decrease in visceral blood flow is due to a drop in cardiac output (–30%), direct mechanical compression of intra-abdominal blood vessels or humoral mechanisms, and mesenteric vasoconstriction due to hypercapnia (transperitoneal absorption of CO_2). Moreover, CO_2 pneumoperitoneum at pressures above 15 mm Hg may cause visceral vasoconstriction as a result of the intraoperative release of vasopressin, increasing portal vein pressure owing to retained CO_2. Use of halothane may also contribute to the reduction in visceral vessel blood flow.[39] Such a decrease in splanchnic vessel blood flow may be catastrophic in patients with certain preexisting conditions, especially impairment of splanchnic vessels and hypercoagulable states. In this case, it is important to keep intra-abdominal pressure as low as possible throughout the procedure; it should always be maintained below 15 mm Hg. Minute volume insufflations should be maintained at an adequate level to avoid hypercapnia (<8 L/min).

Gas embolism is a rare but often fatal complication of laparoscopy. It is caused by direct injection of more than 25 to 30 mL/kg per minute of CO_2 into blood vessels, especially the vena cava or its branches. The incidence of gas embolism is 0.001% with the closed technique but is highly unlikely during open laparoscopy. Delay in diagnosis leads to cardiocirculatory collapse or cardiac arrest, which is often fatal.

Others serious complications of CO_2 pneumoperitoneum are pneumothorax due to ventilatory barotrauma in patients with preexisting pulmonary dystrophy, CO_2-induced pneu-

mothorax due to diffusion of intra-abdominal pneumoperitoneum, and pneumomediastinum. The last is extremely rare if the inferior mediastinum is not opened.

Visceral Injuries

Visceral injuries during laparoscopic aortic procedures may result from trocar insertion; accidental tears with instruments, especially grasping forceps and scissors; and electrocoagulation. Visceral injuries may involve the intestine, spleen, ureter, liver, and pancreas. The nature of the lesion determines the severity of the immediate adverse consequences, its intraoperative management, and the late effects on the patient. Additional factors influencing the outcomes of these iatrogenic injuries are the timing of their recognition and the repair technique.

During laparoscopic AIOD repair, spleen injury can also occur during retraction of the viscera to the right side. This medial visceral rotation can lead to tears, decapsulation, or subcapsular hematoma. The choice of laparoscopic approach is critical to avoid spleen injuries, and care must be taken during retraction of the viscera.

SELECTED KEY REFERENCES

Alimi YS, Di Molfetta L, Hartung O, Dhanis AF, Barthelemy P, Aissi K, Giorgi R, Juhan C. Laparoscopy-assisted abdominal aortic aneurysm endoaneurysmorrhaphy: early and mid-term results. *J Vasc Surg.* 2003;37:744-749.
  Midterm results of laparoscopic aortofemoral reconstructions for AIOD using either an assisted or total laparoscopic technique.

Cau J, Ricco JB, Marchand C, Lecis A, Habbibeh H, Guillou M, Febrer G, Bossavy JP. Total laparoscopic aortic repair for occlusive and aneurysmal disease: first 95 cases. *Eur J Vasc Endovasc Surg.* 2006;31: 567-574.
  Report of a large experience (72 patients) with total laparoscopic AIOD repair.

Coggia M, Bourriez A, Javerliat I, Goeau-Brissonniere O. Totally laparoscopic aortobifemoral bypass: a new and simplified approach. *Eur J Vasc Endovasc Surg.* 2002;24:274-275.
  Description of a new laparoscopic approach to the abdominal aorta using a simple maneuver—placing the patient in the RLD position.

Coggia M, Di Centa I, Javerliat I, Colacchio G, Goeau-Brissonniere O. Total laparoscopic aortic surgery: transperitoneal left retrorenal approach. *Eur J Vasc Endovasc Surg.* 2004;28:619-622.
  Description of the transperitoneal left retrorenal approach to the abdominal aorta, which is the technique of choice for laparoscopic AIOD and AAA repair.

Coggia M, Javerliat I, Di Centa I, Colacchio G, Leschi JP, Kitzis M, Goeau-Brissonniere OA. Total laparoscopic bypass for aortoiliac occlusive lesions: a 93 cases experience. *J Vasc Surg.* 2004;40: 899-906.
  To date, the largest series of total laparoscopic AIOD repair; the results are short term.

Di Centa I, Coggia M, Cerceau P, Javerliat I, Alfonsi P, Beauchet A, Goeau-Brissonniere O. Total laparoscopic aortobifemoral bypass: short- and middle-term results. *Ann Vasc Surg.* 2008;22:227-232.
  Largest reported series of total laparoscopic AIOD repair, including midterm results. One major conclusion is that patency is the same as with open repair.

Dion YM, Gracia CR. A new technique for laparoscopic aortobifemoral grafting in occlusive aortoiliac disease. *J Vasc Surg*. 1997;26:685-692.
Pioneering work in total laparoscopic aortic surgery. Dion describes the first laparoscopic approach to the abdominal aorta—the apron technique.

Dion YM, Griselli F, Douville Y, Langis P. Early and mid-term results of totally laparoscopic surgery for aortoiliac disease: lessons learned. *Surg Laparosc Endosc Percutan Tech*. 2004;14:328-334.
Midterm results of laparoscopic aortofemoral reconstructions for AIOD using either an assisted or total laparoscopic technique.

Kolvenbach R, Puerschel A, Fajer S, Lin J, Wassiljew S, Schwierz E, Pinter L. Total laparoscopic aortic surgery versus minimal access techniques: review of more than 600 patients. *Vascular*. 2006;14:186-192.
Clinical report by a pioneer's team in laparoscopic aortic surgery, including an interesting overview of the field and important considerations concerning total and assisted laparoscopic techniques.

Remy P, Deprez AF, D'hont CH, Lavigne JP, Massin H. Total laparoscopic aortobifemoral bypass. *Eur J Vasc Endovasc Surg*. 2005;29:22-27.
Extensive experience with total laparoscopic AIOD repair reported by a Belgian team. They emphasize the importance of creating a cohesive, dedicated surgical team, which is essential to the achievement of reproducible results.

REFERENCES

The reference list can be found on the companion Expert Consult Web site at *www.expertconsult.com*.

CHAPTER 108

Aortoiliac Disease: Endovascular Treatment

Richard J. Powell and Eva M. Rzucidlo

As endovascular techniques develop, it is crucial for vascular surgeons to keep apprised of the latest approaches to treating aortoiliac occlusive diseases, bearing in mind that treatment should be tailored to the individual patient's symptoms and co-morbidities, as well as the location and extent of disease. This chapter highlights the most recent developments in the endovascular management of aortoiliac occlusive disease.

■ BACKGROUND

The advent of endovascular surgery has resulted in a dramatic shift in the treatment of patients with aortoiliac occlusive disease. In the early stages of development, however, surgeons viewed endovascular approaches to the treatment of aortoiliac occlusive disease with suspicion. In many respects, this was justified because of relatively high complication rates and poor durability. However, early pioneers such as Dotter and Gruntzig persisted and moved the field forward.[1] Because of their early work in the development of balloon angioplasty systems and subsequent work in stent development by Palmaz, these techniques slowly gained traction in the treatment of patients with peripheral vascular disease.[2-4] As improvements in technology such as higher resolution imaging, lower profile systems, premounted balloon-expandable stents, and self-expanding stents resulted in better outcomes, vascular surgeons began to incorporate these treatment modalities into their practices. Today the majority of patients with aortoiliac occlusive disease can be safely treated with percutaneous endovascular procedures. As the technology further evolves, it is likely that even patients with more advanced aortoiliac occlusive disease will be candidates for endovascular therapy by means of stent-grafts and hybrid open-endovascular approaches.

■ INDICATIONS

There are both patient- and lesion-specific indications for aortoiliac intervention. Patient-specific indications for treatment include lifestyle-limiting claudication, rest pain, and tissue loss. Less frequent indications include vasculogenic impotence and atheroembolization to the lower extremities. As for all vascular reconstructions, the expected benefits of the proposed procedure must be weighed against its potential risks in view of patient co-morbidities.

Limb Ischemia

Patients with hip, buttock, thigh, or calf claudication constitute the largest group of patients who undergo aortoiliac endovascular revascularization. Patients with critical limb ischemia (CLI) manifesting as either rest pain or tissue loss frequently have multilevel occlusive disease. In this patient population, the aortoiliac disease is commonly diffuse and complex, often extending into the common femoral arteries (CFAs) and associated with infrainguinal occlusive disease. Patients in whom CFA occlusive disease does not cause significant obstruction can typically be treated with percutaneous approaches that improve perfusion to the lower extremities sufficiently to resolve the rest pain or heal ischemic ulceration. In patients with a significant CFA disease burden, combined femoral artery endarterectomy and patch angioplasty with simultaneous aortoiliac stenting or stent-grafting often provides adequate perfusion to treat CLI.

Younger Patients

Patients younger than 50 years have worse outcomes following aortoiliac endovascular therapy. However, the same is true for open surgical approaches such as aortobifemoral bypass.[5-8] Many younger patients cannot be absent from work for the 6- to 8-week recovery period required after open aortic surgery, and as a result they opt for the less invasive endovascular approach. In addition, many men are concerned about the relatively high incidence of erectile dysfunction that can occur following open aortobifemoral bypass surgery and thus choose an endovascular approach.

Embolization

Less frequently encountered are patients who present with spontaneous embolization to the lower extremity, or so-called blue toe syndrome, who may benefit from endovascular therapy. This is a controversial indication for endovascular therapy and usually involves placement of a bare or covered stent to trap the underlying pathogenic atherosclerotic lesion and prevent embolization during treatment.[9-11] Endovascular intervention is typically not indicated for patients whose atheroembolization is a result of arterial catheterization procedures. In the absence of subsequent catheterization procedures, the risk of recurrent embolization is low.

Improving Inflow for Concomitant Procedures

Endovascular therapy for aortoiliac disease is frequently required as an adjunct to various open procedures to provide adequate inflow. It may be performed simultaneously with lower extremity bypass or in conjunction with femorofemoral bypass. Indications for treatment in this setting include a resting systolic pressure gradient proximal to the intended infrainguinal bypass procedure of greater than 10 mm Hg or a vasodilator-enhanced gradient of greater than 20 mm Hg.

■ CONTRAINDICATIONS

There are no absolute contraindications to the endovascular treatment of aortoiliac occlusive disease. Relative contraindications are largely anatomic and include juxtarenal aortic occlusion, circumferential heavy (>1 mm) calcification, hypoplastic aortic syndrome, and juxtaposition to aneurysmal disease. Renal insufficiency is also a relative contraindication owing to potential contrast-induced nephropathy, although preventive regimens and minimal contrast techniques have reduced the impact of this complication.[12-14]

■ RELEVANT ANATOMY: TASC CLASSIFICATION

Lesion-specific indications for the endovascular therapy of aortoiliac occlusive disease can be guided by the Trans-Atlantic Inter-Society Consensus (TASC) guidelines. The TASC classification system (Fig. 108-1) was recently revised to offer more current guidelines on the use of endovascular therapy based on lesion anatomy.[15] In general, endovascular therapy is the recommended first-line therapy for TASC A and B lesions and increasingly for TASC C lesions as endovascular techniques improve. Good-risk patients with TASC type C disease can also be treated with open surgery, depending on patient preference. Surgery is usually recommended for TASC D lesions, but advanced endovascular approaches are now being applied in these lesions as well, with good results.[16] High-risk patients with TASC C and D disease, CLI, and advanced co-morbidities such as severe chronic obstructive pulmonary disease, unreconstructable coronary artery disease, or a low cardiac ejection fraction may be treated with endovascular therapy, acknowledging that this approach will be less durable than open surgical options.

■ PATIENT EVALUATION AND OPERATIVE PLANNING

Primary Evaluation

Once a decision has been made that intervention is indicated (see Chapter 104: Lower Extremity Arterial Disease: Decision Making and Medical Treatment), information must be gath-

ered to determine the location and extent of the atherosclerotic occlusive disease. This begins with a history and physical examination to determine whether the aortoiliac segment is involved. A history of hip, thigh, or buttock claudication; impotence; the presence of a lower quadrant abdominal or CFA bruit; and diminished femoral pulses are all suggestive of aortoiliac occlusive disease. Patients should undergo non-invasive physiologic arterial studies, such as ankle-brachial index (ABI) and toe pressure measurements, if indicated. In patients with a history suggestive of vasculogenic claudication but a normal pulse exam or resting ABI, treadmill testing may help differentiate vascular from neurogenic symptoms.

Noninvasive Imaging

Just as when planning for an open aortobifemoral bypass, additional diagnostic studies are indicated before endovascular intervention to assess the location and extent of arterial occlusive disease and the degree of calcification. The use of arteriography as a purely diagnostic tool is now rarely indicated because of the widespread availability of less invasive imaging modalities that provide anatomic detail without the risks of an invasive procedure. Imaging modalities currently used to evaluate the aortoiliac segment include duplex arterial mapping, magnetic resonance angiography (MRA), and computed tomographic angiography (CTA). All these modalities have benefits and drawbacks.

Duplex Arterial Mapping

Duplex arterial mapping of the aortoiliac segment and CFAs can adequately assess the location of hemodynamically significant lesions (Fig. 108-2). This modality is especially useful in patients with renal insufficiency who are at risk for contrast-induced renal dysfunction.[17] Drawbacks of duplex arterial mapping are that it provides only a semiquantitative assessment of the degree of iliac calcification, it may not adequately image the iliac system in certain patients owing to overlying bowel gas or body habitus, and it requires a significant time commitment and a highly trained vascular technologist.[18,19] These constraints have prevented duplex arterial mapping from becoming a more widely adopted imaging modality.

Magnetic Resonance Angiography

MRA can reliably assess the aortoiliac arterial segment, although there continues to be institutional variability in its accuracy. The major drawback to MRA is its failure to provide an accurate assessment of the degree of calcification of aortoiliac lesions.

Computed Tomographic Angiography

The presence of severe calcification has significant implications for operative or interventional planning. Circumferential calcification thicker than 1 mm is a relative contraindication to aortoiliac angioplasty and stenting because of the potential

TYPE A LESIONS

• Unilateral or bilateral stenoses of CIA
• Unilateral or bilateral single short (≤3 cm) stenosis of EIA

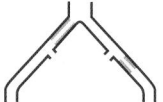

TYPE B LESIONS

• Short (≤3 cm) stenoses of infrarenal aorta
• Unilateral CIA occlusion
• Single or multiple stenoses totaling 3–10 cm involving the EIA not extending into the CFA
• Unilateral EIA occlusion not involving the origins of internal iliac artery or CFA

TYPE C LESIONS

• Bilateral CIA occlusions
• Bilateral EIA stenoses 3–10 cm long not extending into the CFA
• Unilateral EIA stenosis extending into the CFA
• Unilateral EIA occlusion that involves the origins of internal iliac artery and/or CFA
• Heavily calcified unilateral EIA occlusion with or without involvement of origins of internal iliac artery and /or CFA

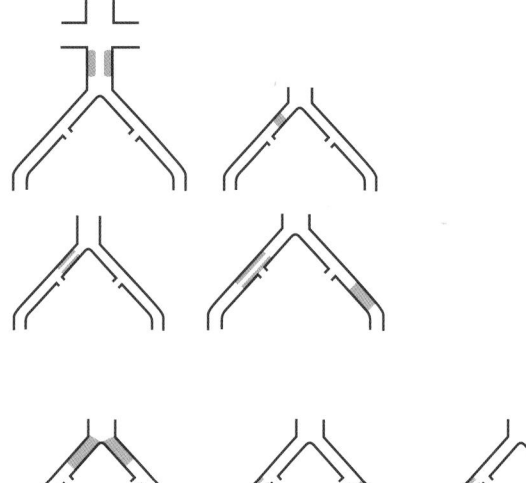

TYPE D LESIONS

• Infrarenal aortoiliac occlusion
• Diffuse disease involving the aorta and both iliac arteries requiring treatment
• Diffuse multiple stenoses involving the unilateral CIA, EIA, and CFA
• Unilateral occlusions of both CIA and EIA
• Bilateral occlusions of EIA
• Iliac stenoses in patients with AAA requiring treatment and not amenable to endograft placement or other lesions requiring open aortic or iliac surgery

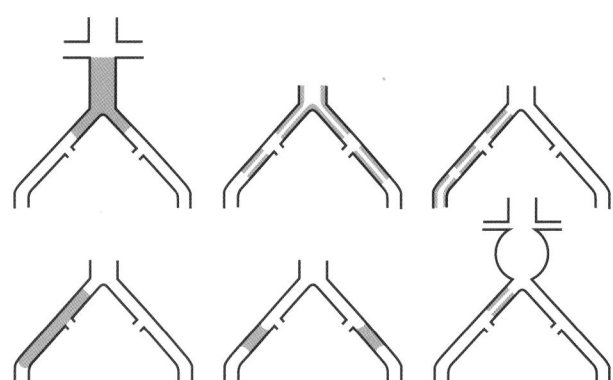

Figure 108-1 TASC classification of aortoiliac lesions. AAA, abdominal aortic aneurysm; CFA, common femoral artery; CIA, common iliac artery; EIA, external iliac artery. (*Redrawn from Norgren L, Hiatt WR, Dormandy JA, et al. TASC II Working Group. Inter-Society Consensus for the Management of Peripheral Arterial Disease (TASC II). J Vasc Surg. 2007;45(Suppl S):S5-S7.*)

risk of fracture and rupture of the iliac artery. In patients with significant co-morbidities in whom intervention is mandated by CLI, use of a stent-graft may be considered in an attempt to limit the incidence of clinically significant arterial perforation. In this setting, CTA has been used with success to assess calcification of the aortoiliac segment before intervention. The major disadvantages of this imaging modality include exposure to ionizing radiation and the need for iodinated contrast agent, with the risk of contrast-induced renal dysfunction. In appropriate patients, CTA can accurately assess lesion location and extent and degree of calcification. Based on CTA, the severity of aortoiliac and femoral disease can be classified according to TASC; this additional information regarding anatomy and severity of calcification allows the formulation of an appropriate procedural plan and the selection of either open or endovascular therapy.

Evaluation for Common Femoral Artery Disease

The determination whether to proceed with percutaneous endovascular therapy or an open femoral approach is based

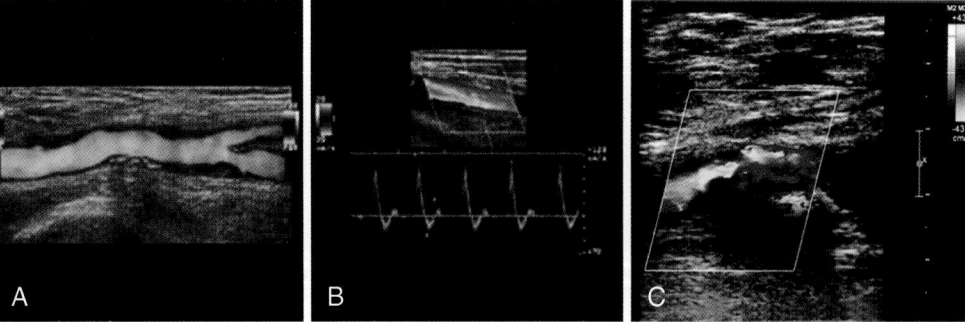

Figure 108-2 Duplex mapping of the common femoral artery. **A,** Longitudinal view of the common femoral artery (power imaging) and the bifurcation of the superficial and deep femoral arteries. **B,** Doppler spectral waveform from a normal right femoral artery. The Doppler signal was obtained from a longitudinal view with the Doppler sample volume placed in the middle of the lumen. The characteristic triphasic Doppler signal shows a brisk upstroke to peak systole, reversal of blood flow during early diastole, and a forward flow component during late diastole. **C,** Longitudinal view of the common femoral artery with greater than 50% stenosis due to posterior plaque.

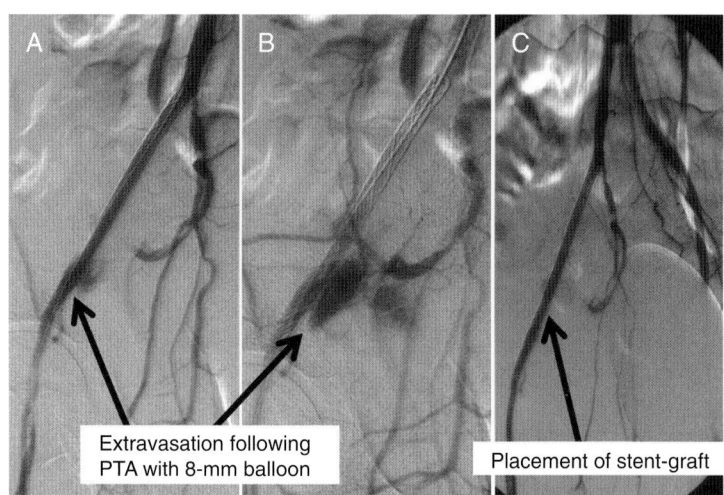

Extravasation following PTA with 8-mm balloon

Placement of stent-graft

Figure 108-3 Ruptured external iliac artery treated with a stent-graft. **A** and **B,** After placement of bare metal stents and dilatation with an 8-mm balloon. **C,** Stent-graft placed to achieve hemostasis.

on the presence of significant CFA disease. Patients with greater than 50% CFA stenosis on duplex arterial mapping, MRA, or CTA are usually treated with a hybrid approach that entails open femoral endarterectomy, patch angioplasty, and simultaneous stent or stent-graft placement. In patients with less severe CFA disease, a percutaneous approach can be undertaken. Depending on the location and extent of disease as determined by preoperative imaging, an ipsilateral retrograde, contralateral, bilateral femoral, or brachial approach can be planned. In patients with extensive calcification of the aortoiliac segment who are poor candidates for open surgery, consideration should be given to use of a stent-graft. This is especially true when treating elderly women for occlusive disease in the external iliac artery segment because of the increased risk of arterial rupture. Potential advantages of stent-graft therapy in this setting are decreased risk of bleeding from or rupture of the iliac artery and the ability to more aggressively dilate the iliac segment (Fig. 108-3).[20] These

considerations may be offset by the disadvantage of the larger arterial sheath required for stent-graft placement, although smaller delivery sheaths are becoming available.

Concomitant Aortic Disease

Aortic angioplasty and stenting for lesions proximal to the aortic bifurcation warrant special consideration because these lesions are frequently exophytic and calcific. When treating such lesions, emphasis should be placed on obtaining an adequate hemodynamic response; acceptance of an imperfect angiographic completion image is critical to avoid aortic rupture. Because of the exophytic nature of these lesions, primary stent placement to trap potential atheroembolic debris should be considered. Primary stenting should also be considered for lesions suspected of being the source of atheroembolization to minimize the potential for embolic complications.

TECHNIQUE

Pretreatment Considerations

Before the intervention, the patient's history and all pertinent imaging studies are reviewed, and informed consent is obtained. Laboratory tests of coagulation status and renal function are essential.

Avoiding Contrast Nephropathy

Contrast-induced nephropathy, defined as an increase in serum creatinine greater than 25%, or >0.5 mg/dL (44.2 µmol/L) within 3 days of intravascular contrast administration in the absence of an alternative cause, is the third most common cause of new-onset acute renal failure in hospitalized patients.[21,22] The incidence may be as high as 25% in patients with preexisting renal impairment or certain risk factors such as diabetes, congestive heart failure, advanced age, and concurrent administration of nephrotoxic drugs.[23] Preprocedural volume loading and the use of low-osmolar or iso-osmolar contrast agents can decrease the risk of contrast-induced nephropathy.[24-26] However, the risk is not eliminated in some patients, even when an iso-osmolar contrast agent is used.[27,28] Many studies have evaluated the use of N-acetylcysteine (NAC), theophylline, fenoldopam, and other agents to prevent contrast-induced nephropathy; the results have been heterogeneous and are difficult to compare across the different treatment regimens. A recent meta-analysis of 41 randomized trials found that preprocedural treatment with NAC effectively reduced the risk of contrast-induced nephropathy.[29] NAC significantly decreased the risk of contrast-induced nephropathy compared with saline alone (relative risk, 0.62; 95% confidence interval, 0.44 to 0.88; $P < .0001$). Because free radicals are postulated to mediate contrast-induced nephropathy,[30] alkalinizing renal tubular fluid with sodium bicarbonate[31] has been shown to reduce injury. Merten and coworkers reported a single-center randomized controlled trial comparing the infusion of sodium chloride versus sodium bicarbonate as the hydration fluid to prevent renal failure in patients with stable renal insufficiency undergoing diagnostic or interventional procedures requiring radiographic contrast agent.[14] The absolute risk reduction of contrast-induced nephropathy (defined as 25% change in serum creatinine) using sodium bicarbonate compared with sodium chloride was 11.9%, resulting in a number-needed-to-treat of 8.4 patients to prevent 1 case of renal failure. Briguori and colleagues hypothesized that a combination of different antioxidant compounds may provide additive benefits in preventing contrast-induced nephropathy.[12] They tested this hypothesis by performing a prospective, double-blinded, randomized study comparing different combinations of antioxidant compounds in patients at medium to high risk for contrast-induced nephropathy undergoing iso-osmolar contrast agent administration during coronary or peripheral procedures. Contrast-induced nephropathy occurred in 11 of 111 patients (9.9%) in the saline plus NAC group, in 2 of 108 (1.9%) in the bicar-

bonate plus NAC group ($P = .019$ by Fisher exact test versus the saline plus NAC group), and in 11 of 107 (10.3%) in the saline plus ascorbic acid plus NAC group ($P = 1.00$ versus the saline plus NAC group).

Patients with a baseline serum creatinine greater than 1.5 mg/dL (133 µmol/L) should therefore receive both NAC and bicarbonate. The initial intravenous bolus is 3 mL × kg^{-1} × h^{-1} (154 mEq/L sodium bicarbonate in dextrose and water) for 1 hour immediately before contrast injection, followed by continuous administration of the same fluid at a rate of 1 mL × kg^{-1} × h^{-1} during the period of contrast exposure and for 6 hours thereafter.[14] All patients receive NAC orally at a dose of 1200 mg twice daily on the day before and the day of contrast administration (total of 2 days).[13] Diuretics should be routinely withheld on the day of contrast injection.

Determination of Approach

Common iliac artery (CIA) disease is generally treated through an ipsilateral, retrograde approach. If the CIA is occluded, contralateral flush catheter placement should be considered so that a complete diagnostic study can be performed before any intervention; this technique also provides access to protect the contralateral CIA from injury during ipsilateral CIA intervention. A complete diagnostic arteriographic examination includes a study of the aorta to exclude abdominal aortic aneurysm, oblique pelvic imaging of the iliac bifurcations to determine internal iliac artery patency and origin, and adequate views to evaluate CFA bifurcation disease. In general, the contralateral oblique projection shows the iliac artery bifurcations, whereas the ipsilateral oblique projection best displays the profunda origins at the femoral artery bifurcations. Finally, complete imaging of the infrainguinal runoff is requisite before inflow intervention. If imaging of the runoff is done only after completion of the intervention, differentiating preexisting distal occlusive lesions from emboli may be problematic. External iliac disease is generally better approached from the contralateral side because it permits more extensive treatment of the external iliac artery (EIA) into the proximal portion of the CFA if needed (Fig. 108-4).

The procedure begins with placement of an arterial sheath to facilitate catheter exchanges. The lesion is crossed with the use of a catheter–guide wire combination. An angle-tip catheter with a floppy-tipped guide wire is used to cross the lesion first, followed by the catheter. In difficult cases, hydrophilic guide wires may be used (see Fig. 108-4B). After advancing the catheter across the lesion, the wire is removed, and free aspiration of blood ensures that the catheter tip is intraluminal.

Determination of Hemodynamically Significant Lesion

Pressure measurements across the lesion should be obtained by connecting the hub of the catheter and the side arm of the vascular sheath to the intra-arterial pressure monitor.

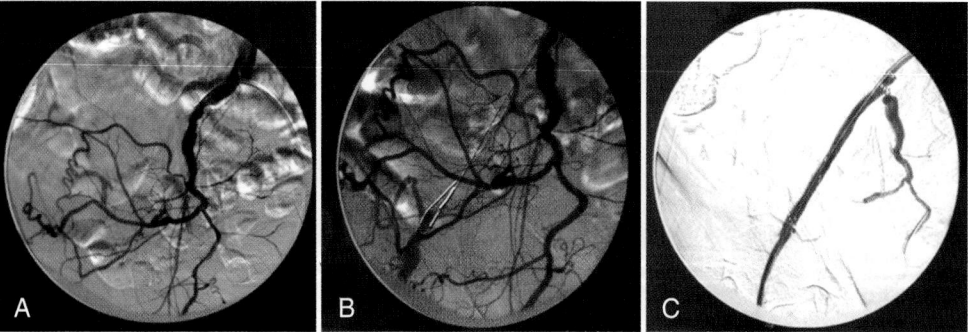

Figure 108-4 A, External iliac artery occlusion approached through the contralateral common femoral artery. **B,** Subintimal crossing of the complete occlusion with a reentry catheter. **C,** Contralateral placement of a bare metal stent into the external iliac artery, allowing for placement in the proximal portion of the common femoral artery.

The catheter should be at least 1 Fr smaller than the sheath; however, this measurement technique is not uniformly reliable. Other options include the "pullback method," in which an end-hole catheter is withdrawn from proximal to distal across the lesion over a 0.014-inch wire. Most consider a peak-to-peak systolic pressure gradient of 10 mm Hg or greater at rest to be hemodynamically significant. In the absence of a resting gradient, intra-arterial nitroglycerin (100 to 200 µg) or papaverine (25 mg) can be administered distally to reveal the significance of a lesion. The maximal increase in pressure gradient occurs 20 to 40 seconds after vasodilator injection. If the mean pressure gradient increases to above 10 mm Hg, the lesion may be considered for treatment.

Technique to Recanalize Occluded Iliac Arteries

Contralateral Approach

When attempting to recanalize an occluded iliac artery in a retrograde fashion, the guide wire frequently follows a subintimal path. Once this has occurred, it may be difficult to redirect the guide wire into the lumen. An antegrade approach from the contralateral CFA is frequently successful, especially if there is a stump and the CIA is not flush-occluded. A hooked catheter is used to probe the occlusion. The lesion can then be crossed in most cases with the use of hydrophilic guide wires. As soon as the guide wire has crossed the obstructive lesion and lies within the ipsilateral EIA lumen, it is snared from the ipsilateral CFA. A short catheter is then inserted in a retrograde fashion over the wire end into the abdominal aorta proximal to the lesion. Intra-arterial catheter placement is confirmed through aspiration of blood from the aortic catheter. The hydrophilic guide wire is then removed, and a working guide wire is inserted to facilitate the intervention.

Brachial Approach

In the presence of a flush CIA occlusion, a contralateral femoral approach to cross the lesion is generally unsuccessful;

transbrachial or ipsilateral femoral approaches are more likely to achieve success. A brachial approach reduces the risk of creating or extending an aortic dissection and provides better "pushability." The presence of significant subclavian artery occlusive disease obviously limits this approach, as does the unavailability of catheters and stents of sufficient working length.

Reentry Catheters

The recent development of reentry catheters has greatly increased the technical success of crossing complete arterial occlusions. The Outback reentry catheter (LuMend Inc., Redwood City, CA) is a single-lumen catheter designed to facilitate access and positioning of a guide wire within the peripheral vasculature from a remote vascular entry site (Fig. 108-5). The Pioneer catheter (Medtronic, Minneapolis, MN) contains an intravascular ultrasound probe in the distal portion that assists in orienting the reentry needle toward the flow lumen. The hydrophilic guide wire is exchanged for a 300-cm-long, 0.014-inch guide wire using a hydrophilic catheter. The guide catheter is then removed, and a reentry catheter is advanced into the level of the aortic bifurcation under continuous fluoroscopy. An angiogram is performed via the contralateral access to confirm traversal of the occlusion and positioning of the lateral exit port of the catheter at the aortic bifurcation proximal to the occlusion. The precise location and orientation of the lateral exit port are confirmed by aligning the fluoroscopic guide. The orientation of the catheter's lateral exit port relative to the intima, as visualized by the radiopaque marker band under fluoroscopy, is aided by using an angled catheter in the distal aorta, passed up from the contralateral side. This technique minimizes the number of angiographic runs needed to verify a satisfactory position. The nitinol cannula is then advanced forward through the lateral exit port under continuous fluoroscopy. Applying firm but guarded forward pressure while deploying the cannula may contribute to a successful puncture. Free passage of the 0.014-inch wire indicates true lumen access, which is confirmed by contrast injection through the catheter. The catheter is then exchanged for a 3-mm-diameter angioplasty

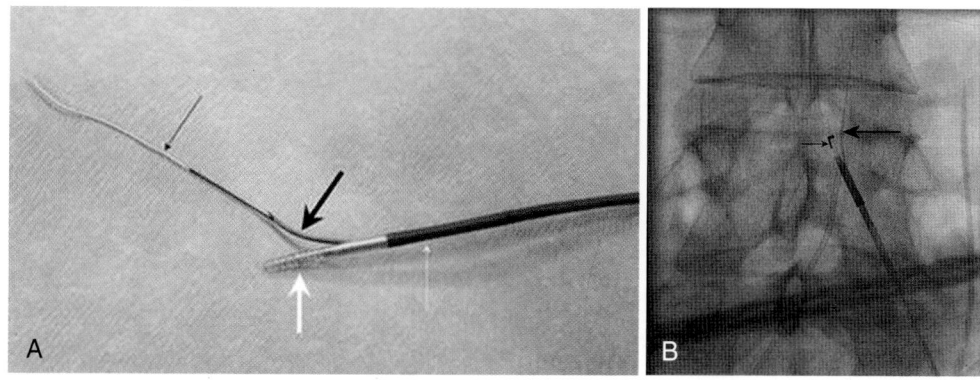

Figure 108-5 Reentry catheters. **A,** Outback LTD catheter. The cannula (*large black arrow*) is deployed, and the 0.014-inch guide wire (*small black arrow*) is advanced through it. The nosecone (*large white arrow*) has the radiopaque "LT" orientation marker. The catheter shaft is indicated by the *small white arrow*. **B,** Outback catheter. The cannula is deployed (*large arrow*), with free passage of the guide wire into the true lumen of the aorta. Note the "L" configuration (*small arrow*).

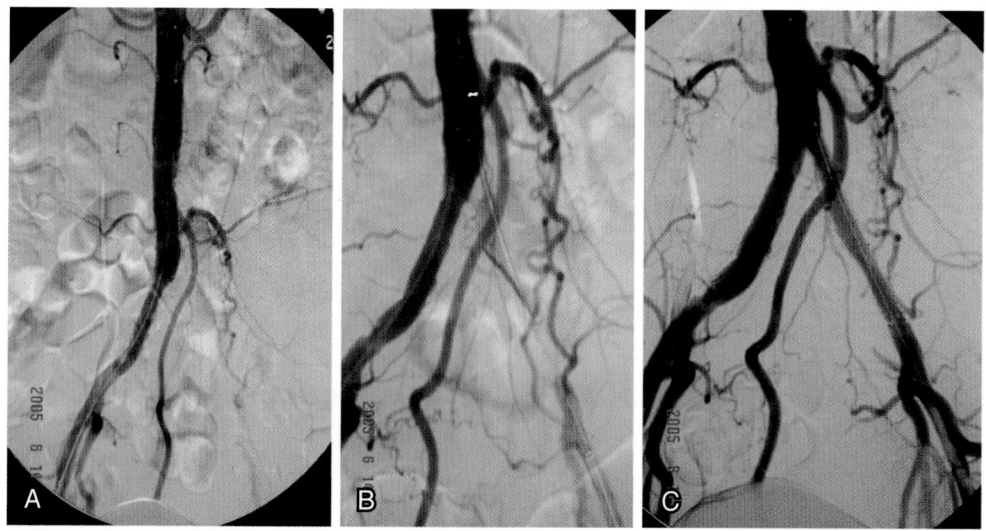

Figure 108-6 Results using a reentry catheter. **A,** Pelvic arteriogram showing complete occlusion of the left common and external iliac arteries. **B,** Glide catheter advancement into the aorta after reentry at the aortic bifurcation. **C,** Retrograde stent-graft placement into the common iliac artery. Note the contralateral bare metal common iliac stent.

balloon that is used to dilate the intimal puncture site. This step enables a catheter to pass and allows exchange for a standard 0.035-inch guide wire to facilitate stenting. Stenting can then be performed in a conventional manner (Fig. 108-6).

Aortic Bifurcation Lesions

Technical Approach

Lesions at the aortic bifurcation are traditionally treated using the "kissing balloons" technique. Simultaneous balloon dilatation at the origins of both CIAs is advocated, even in the presence of a unilateral lesion, to protect the contralateral CIA from dissection, plaque dislodgement, or subsequent embolization. A retrospective review of patients undergoing

percutaneous treatment for unilateral CIA occlusive lesions by Smith and associates challenged this long-established practice.[32] In this report, 175 patients with unilateral ostial iliac artery lesions were treated with percutaneous transluminal angioplasty (PTA) or stenting without contralateral protection; in only 2 patients did the contralateral unprotected CIA develop mild stenosis (17% and 24%, respectively). The authors concluded that protection of the contralateral CIA during PTA or stenting of the ipsilateral proximal CIA is not mandatory.

Aortic Bifurcation Advancement

Because calcified lesions at the aortic bifurcation are not amenable to balloon dilatation alone, the "kissing stents" or "aortic reconstruction" technique is applied (see Fig.

108-6C).[33] The aortic bifurcation reconstruction technique is technically successful; however, some have expressed fear that extension of the proximal ends of the stents into the distal aorta ("aortic advancement") may serve as a nidus for thrombus formation or cause hemolysis.[33] This fear has not been realized, as demonstrated by the low complication rates of this procedure.

Concomitant Femoral Endarterectomy

As previously discussed, patient evaluation through duplex ultrasound, CTA, or MRA can help determine which CFA should be used for percutaneous access; in addition, if such studies identify significant CFA disease, an open femoral approach with combined endovascular iliac therapy and femoral endarterectomy should be strongly considered (Fig. 108-7A).[34] The CFA is exposed from the circumflex femoral branches down to the femoral bifurcation. The CFA is punctured under direct vision, and the iliac lesion is crossed prior to endarterectomy. This technique allows complete assurance of intraluminal wire placement distally at the endarterectomy site. For cases in which retrograde guide wire passage is not possible, a percutaneous approach from the contralateral femoral artery or brachial artery can be used to cross the iliac lesion. The guide wire can then be brought out through the femoral artery. Wire access is left in place, proximal and distal control is obtained, and a longitudinal arteriotomy is created, allowing for standard endarterectomy and patch angioplasty. Before completion of the patch angioplasty, the center of the patch is punctured with an 18-gauge needle, and the guide wire is brought out through the needle. Patch closure is then completed, and flow is restored. An appropriate sheath can then be passed over the wire to allow iliac stenting. Stents may be extended down to the proximal endpoint of the endarterectomy and patch if necessary (Fig. 108-7B).

Stent Sizing

Selection of the appropriate balloon or stent diameter is of utmost importance for a successful intervention. Slight oversizing of 5% to 10% is recommended, except in the case of heavily calcified lesions that may rupture. The optimal vessel diameter can be estimated from the adjacent normal arterial segment or by comparison to the same vessel on the contralateral side. A calibrated catheter inserted into the vessel allows measurement of the artery. The length of the balloon or stent should cover the diseased area without damaging the normal vessel. If in doubt when balloon-dilating a lesion, it is wise to undersize. A larger balloon can be used if the initial result is not satisfactory. With stenting, this rule does not apply, because an undersized stent usually cannot be exchanged for an optimal one. Balloon inflation should be gradual to avoid trauma to the adjacent normal vessel. A waist on the balloon indicates the lesion location; the waist disappears after successful dilatation. Mild pain during dilatation is acceptable and indicates stretching of the adventitia; excessive or persistent pain may indicate arterial rupture (see Fig. 108-3A and B). The technical success of the intervention is judged not only by the angiographic appearance but also, and more importantly, by the measurement of any residual pressure gradient. Less than 20% residual stenosis and a less than 10 mm Hg systolic pressure gradient is considered a technical success. The determination of the angioplasty's success should be based on the translesional pressure gradient measurement; angiographic criteria are not reliable.[35,36]

Stent Selection

Commercially available stents are numerous and fall into two main categories: balloon-expandable and self-expanding (see Chapter 91: Nonaortic Stents and Stent-Grafts). Features of

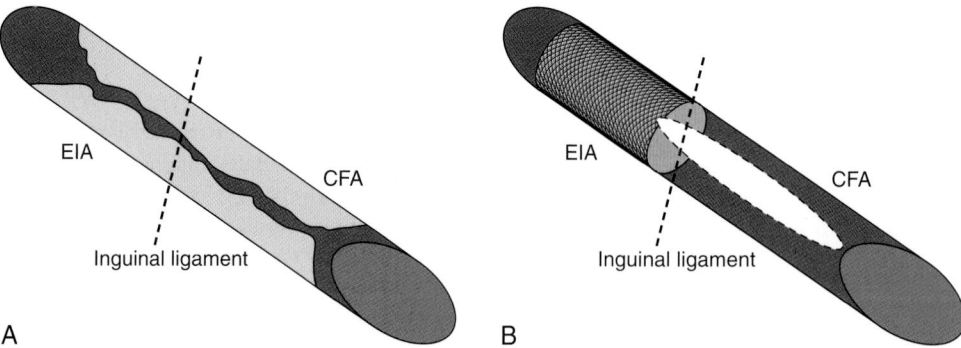

Figure 108-7 Operative technique for an open femoral approach to the diseased common femoral artery (CFA) and external iliac artery (EIA). **A,** The common femoral artery is exposed from the circumflex femoral branches, distal to the femoral bifurcation. The common femoral artery is punctured under direct vision, and the iliac lesion is crossed before endarterectomy. Wire access is left in place, and a standard subintimal endarterectomy with patch angioplasty is performed. Before completion of the patch angioplasty, the patch is punctured in the center with an 18-gauge needle, and the guide wire is brought out through the center of the patch. After patch angioplasty is complete and flow is restored, a short sheath can be placed over the wire and through the center of the patch. **B,** Iliac stenting can be performed such that the distal endpoint of the stent is just proximal to the endarterectomy and patch angioplasty.

balloon-expandable stents include precision of placement, high radiopacity, and high hoop strength. However, they are less flexible than self-expanding stents and become permanently deformed if external force is directly applied to them. The development of new stent designs has somewhat blurred these distinctions.

Placement of a balloon-expandable stent generally requires the sheath to be advanced beyond the lesion, especially in severe stenoses, to avoid dislocation of the stent on the balloon. The stent mounted on the balloon is inserted into the sheath and positioned across the lesion using bone landmarks or roadmapping. The sheath is then retracted, and the balloon is inflated to expand the stent. Self-expanding stents are mounted on a carrier device and constrained by an outer sheath. The introducer sheath does not need to cross the lesion. Stent deployment is achieved by holding the carrier device with one hand and retracting the outer sheath with the other. Selection of an iliac artery stent depends on availability and the operator's familiarity with specific devices. In addition, iliac artery tortuosity, introducer sheath diameter, and intrinsic lesion characteristics influence the selection of an appropriate stent type. Short, eccentric, calcified lesions, typically occurring at the aortic bifurcation, are best treated with balloon-expandable stents owing to the ability to place them with great precision. In contrast, whenever the stent must follow a tortuous path or is to be placed from the contralateral side over the aortic bifurcation, self-expanding stents are recommended because of their flexibility.

RESULTS

Percutaneous Angioplasty versus Selective Stenting

PTA of focal iliac artery stenoses has demonstrated acceptable success rates (Table 108-1).[37] The reported 4-year success rates for iliac angioplasty are approximately 44% to 65%. Complications associated with angioplasty include vessel dissection, abrupt closure, spasm, and thrombus formation.

Moreover, several studies evaluating the use of PTA for total iliac artery occlusions showed a significant embolization incidence, which led some to question the usefulness of PTA in this patient subset.[38,39] In another study of 106 patients, kissing iliac stents showed good results in aortic bifurcation disease (a location that can be problematic for balloon angioplasty), with primary and secondary patency rates of 78% and 98%, respectively, at 3 years.[40]

Several randomized studies have compared stenting with stand-alone PTA. The Dutch Iliac Stent Trial Study Group performed a randomized comparison of primary balloon-expandable stent placement with primary angioplasty followed by selective stent placement in patients with iliac artery occlusive disease. Iliac patency ranged from 97% (122 of 126 patients) at 3 months to 83% (90 of 109 patients) at the final mean follow-up of 5 years in the patients with primary stent placement; it ranged from 94% (113 of 120 patients) to 74% (67 of 90 patients) in the patients treated with PTA and selective stent placement. This difference was not significant. The study also showed that selective stent placement was more cost-effective than primary stenting of iliac artery stenosis.[35,41] However, nearly half the patients (43%) randomized to balloon angioplasty underwent stent placement for a suboptimal result during the primary procedure. Twenty-five of 143 patients (17%) treated with primary stent placement needed re-intervention in the iliac artery segment because of the development of symptomatic or hemodynamic (by noninvasive testing) restenosis. In the PTA and selective stent placement group, 28 of 136 patients (21%) needed re-intervention. Complication rates were nearly double (4% versus 7%) in the angioplasty group.[41]

Primary Stenting versus Selective Stenting

Other randomized trials have shown primary stenting to be superior to selective stent placement in terms of both hemodynamic parameters and Rutherford classification (see Table 108-1). These include a meta-analysis comparing the results

---

Table 108-1 Review of Outcomes in Interventional Treatment of Aortoiliac Occlusive Disease

Series	Year	Number of Patients	Indication	Type of Intervention	Primary Patency (%)
Parsons et al.[37]	1998	45		PTA	74 (5-yr)
Klein[41]	2006	279		Primary stenting vs. selective stenting	83 (5-yr)
Bosch and Hunink[42] (meta-analysis)	1997	1300	Claudication vs. CLI	Selective stenting vs. primary stenting	70 (5-yr)
	1997	1300		Primary stenting	77 (4-yr) 67 (4-yr)
Murphy[43] (meta-analysis)	1998	2058		Primary stenting	73 (5-yr)
Schurmann et al.[44]	2002	110	93% claudication	Primary stenting	66 (5-yr)
Galaria and Davies[45]	2005	276	TASC A and B	Primary stenting	71 (10-yr)
Leville et al.[16]	2006	92	TASC C and D	Primary stenting	76 (3-yr)
Rzucidlo et al.[20]	2005	34	TASC B, C, and D	Stent-grafting	80 (5-yr)

CLI, critical limb ischemia; PTA, percutaneous transluminal angioplasty; TASC, Trans-Atlantic Inter-Society Consensus.

of PTA versus stent placement for iliac occlusive disease.[42] This meta-analysis of more than 1300 patients compared selective to primary iliac artery stenting and found significantly higher initial technical success (>90%) and improved primary patency rates (>70% at 2 and 5 years) in both claudicants and those with limb-threatening ischemia among patients treated with primary stenting.[42] Because critical ischemia was considered an independent risk factor for failure, the authors stratified patency rates for claudication versus critical ischemia. The 4-year primary patency rate for claudication, with technical failures excluded, was 68% (range, 65% to 74%) after PTA, compared with 77% (range, 72% to 81%) after stenting. The 4-year primary patency rate for critical ischemia, with technical failures excluded, was 55% (range, 48% to 63%) after PTA, versus 67% (range, 55% to 79%) after stenting. The authors concluded that stent placement reduced the risk of long-term failure by 39% compared with PTA alone. Disease severity (claudication versus critical ischemia) was an independent predictor of long-term failure. However, whenever initial success was achievable, no statistically significant difference in long-term patency was found between stenoses and occlusions.

Long-term Results

Murphy summarized the results of 18 published studies of primary iliac artery stent placement in a total of 2058 limbs (see Table 108-1).[43] Using weighted averages, the technical success rate was 97%, the complication rate was 6%, and the 5-year primary and secondary patency rates were 73% and 85%, respectively. Although iliac stent treatment has been in clinical use for more than 15 years, few reports of long-term patency are available. Schurmann and colleagues published a 10-year follow-up of 110 patients with iliac arterial occlusive disease who underwent implantation of self-expanding stents.[44] The mean patient age was 57 years, and 93% were claudicants. Based on angiographic or color duplex imaging follow-up in 105 patients and clinical follow-up in 5 patients, primary cumulative stent patency rates were 66% ± 5 after 5 years and 46% ± 6 after 10 years; secondary patency rates were 79% ± 4 and 55% ± 6.3, respectively. Mean follow-up time was 5.7 years. Restenosis occurred in 51 of 126 (41%) lesions after a mean of 3.9 years. Seventeen patients (16%) underwent surgical bypass of the aortoiliac segment that had been stented—14 because of stent restenosis, and 3 because of stenosis in other iliac arterial segments (Fig. 108-8).

Patency Based on TASC Classification

TASC Types A and B Lesions

Outcomes of iliac intervention depend on TASC lesion classification. Galaria and associates examined reported 10-year patency results for patients with TASC types A and B lesions.[45] Indications for intervention were claudication (77%) or critical ischemia (23%). Altogether, 276 patients (all men; average age, 64 ± 11 years; range, 32 to 87 years) underwent 394

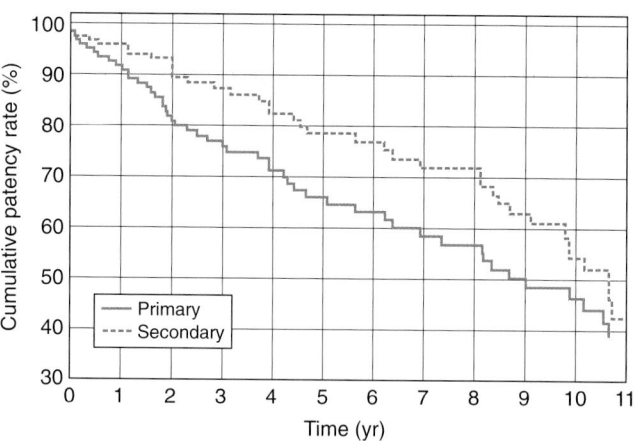

Figure 108-8 Long-term primary and secondary patency rates in 126 iliac lesions treated with stent placement. *(From Schurmann K, Mahnken A, Meyer J, et al. Long-term results 10 years after iliac arterial stent placement.* Radiology. *2002;224:731-738.)*

interventions. Sixty-two percent of the lesions were TASC type A, and the remainder were type B. Of the 394 primary interventions, 51% included the placement of stents. Technical success (defined as <30% residual stenosis) was achieved in 98% of treated vessels. The procedure-related mortality rate was 1.8% at 30 days and 4.7% at 90 days; the procedure-related complication rate was 7%. Hemodynamic success (defined as a rise in the ABI >0.15) was achieved in 82%. The average Society for Vascular Surgery symptom score was 3.4 ± 0.9 before intervention; this improved to 1.9 ± 0.8 following intervention. Within 3 months, 84% of patients demonstrated clinical improvement. The cumulative assisted patency rate was 71% ± 7 at 10 years. The presence of two-vessel femoral runoff, two or more patent tibial vessels, or both was associated with improved patency. Limb salvage rates were 95% ± 2 and 87% ± 9 at 5 and 10 years, respectively. By Cox proportional hazards analysis, hypertension, hypercholesterolemia, and chronic renal insufficiency were associated with increased risk of primary failure, whereas the presence of immediate hemodynamic improvement was associated with increased long-term patency. Use of a stent did not influence outcome. These results approach those reported for surgical aortoiliac bypass grafting. For comparison, in a meta-analysis of 23 studies of aortoiliac or aortofemoral bypass grafts published between 1970 and 1996, de Vries and Hunink calculated limb-based patency rates of 91% and 86.8% at 5 and 10 years, respectively, for patients with claudication, and patency rates of 88% and 82%, respectively, for patients with critical ischemia (Fig. 108-9).[46]

TASC Types C and D Lesions

Although iliac angioplasty and stenting of TASC types A and B common iliac lesions achieve a patency similar to that of open surgical reconstruction, patients with diffuse aortoiliac occlusive disease (TASC types C and D lesions) have markedly inferior patency with bare metal stenting when compared with aortobifemoral bypass. Recently, several authors have

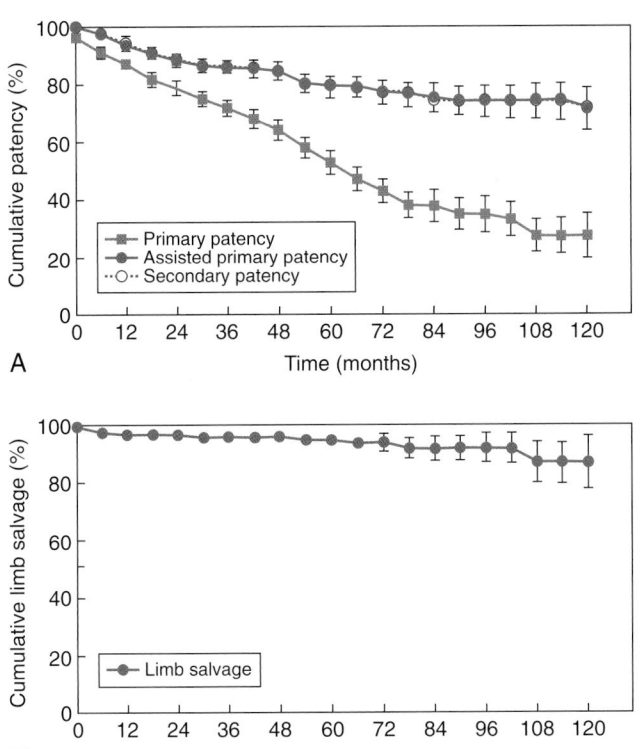

Figure 108-9 A, Cumulative primary patency, assisted primary patency, and secondary patency (superimposed in assisted primary patency) intervals for all vessels. **B,** Cumulative limb salvage for all patients. In both **A** and **B**, the values are the mean ± a standard error less than 10% for all data points by life-table analysis. *(From Galaria II, Davies MG. Percutaneous transluminal revascularization for iliac occlusive disease: long-term outcomes in Trans-Atlantic Inter-Society Consensus A and B lesions. Ann Vasc Surg. 2005;19: 352-360.)*

documented more promising results in the treatment of more complex TASC types C and D iliac lesions. Review of the data published since 1995 reveals that 2-year primary patency ranges from 69% to 76%, with secondary patency rates of 85% to 95%.[47-50] In a series of 212 patients with chronic iliac occlusions, successful recanalization was accomplished in nearly 90% of patients, with marked clinical improvement in the vast majority.[51] The primary patency at 4 years was 75.7%. Leville and coworkers recently reported late results of the treatment of complex iliac occlusive disease.[16] Three-year primary patency, secondary patency, and limb salvage rates were 76%, 90%, and 97%, respectively; progression of infrainguinal disease led to late limb loss in two patients. Diabetes was associated with a significantly decreased primary patency rate (57% versus 83%; *P* = .049). Critical ischemia at presentation was also associated with decreased patency (*P* = .002), but TASC classification did not significantly alter patency.

Patency with Concomitant Common Femoral Artery Disease

Chang and colleagues recently reported their long-term results of combined endovascular and open treatment of ilio-

femoral occlusive disease. One hundred seventy-one patients underwent 193 CFA endarterectomies and iliac stent or stent-graft placement. Indications were rest pain (32%), tissue loss (22%), and claudication (46%). EIA lesions were present in 39%, combined CIA and EIA lesions were seen in 61%, and complete CIA-EIA occlusions were present in 41% of patients. Stent-grafts were used in 41% of patients. Technical success was reported in 98%, and clinical improvement was seen in 92% of patients. Five-year primary, primary assisted, and secondary patency rates were 60%, 97%, and 98%, respectively. Endovascular re-intervention was required in 14% of patients; inflow surgical procedures were required in 10%. By logistic regression analysis, use of stent-grafts compared with bare stents was associated with significantly higher primary patency (87% ± 5 versus 53% ± 7; *P* < .01).[52]

Predictors of Failure

Extension of disease into the EIA increases procedural complexity and decreases the durability of the intervention. The presence of external iliac disease is a powerful predictor of decreased primary and primary assisted patency rates.[45,53-55] In a study by Powell and coworkers, patients with severe EIA disease treated with bare metal stents had a 1-year primary patency rate of only 47%.[53,54] These patients also had poor rates of hemodynamic and clinical improvement after intervention. Many required surgical inflow procedures or subsequent endovascular re-intervention to maintain aortoiliac patency. Other reported predictors of worse outcome after iliac artery angioplasty are female gender,[56] renal insufficiency, and CLI.[55] Timaran and associates concluded that women with EIA stents had the poorest outcomes.[55] Other groups have noted that small vessel diameter and female gender are factors predictive of failure.[57]

Stent-Grafting

Stent-grafting has been used to treat patients with severe aortoiliac occlusive disease, especially those with small calcified EIAs, who are not candidates for open surgical intervention. Covered stents are generally reserved for the treatment of isolated iliac aneurysms, iatrogenic perforations or ruptures, and arteriovenous fistulae. There have been limited studies in patients with peripheral arterial occlusive disease. These devices are stainless steel, nickel-cobalt-titanium-steel alloy (Elgiloy), or nitinol stents covered with Dacron or polytetrafluoroethylene (PTFE).[20,58,59] In theory, covered stents should reduce in-stent restenosis by excluding the diseased segment from the circulation; however, experimental data suggest that they may induce more neointimal overgrowth at the end of the stent-graft compared with bare stents.[59]

Stent-Graft Patency

Stent-graft treatment of patients with severe aortoiliac occlusive disease (85% TASC types C and D lesions) was reported by Rzucidlo and colleagues.[20] The use of stent-grafts increased the primary and primary assisted patency at 1 year to 70% and 88%, respectively, compared with patients treated with stents alone, and led to 100% early hemodynamic and clinical success. There was a trend toward improved primary iliac artery patency in patients who underwent concomitant common femoral endarterectomy compared with patients who did not. At 6 and 12 months, the primary patency rates in patients who underwent concomitant common femoral endarterectomy were 94% and 94%, respectively, compared with 79% and 53% in patients who did not undergo endarterectomy.

Long-term results of stent-grafts for the treatment of complex aortoiliac occlusive disease have recently been reported. At 3 and 5 years after intervention, the primary patency rates of the iliac segment were 80% and 80%, respectively; corresponding primary assisted patency rates were 95% and 95% (Fig. 108-10). Primary patency using stent-grafts differed significantly depending on TASC classification. Patients with TASC type B iliac lesions had a 100% 5-year patency rate. Those with TASC type C iliac lesions had the lowest 5-year primary patency—significantly lower than TASC type D iliac lesions when type B lesions were removed from the log-rank analysis (61% versus 85%; $P = .04$; unpublished data).

Others have reported the use of stent-grafts to treat diffuse iliac occlusive disease. Cynamon and associates used homemade stent-grafts (6-mm PTFE grafts sewn to 294 Palmaz stents).[60] Eighteen grafts were placed to treat iliac occlusive disease in 17 patients with limb-threatening ischemia and significant CFA disease. These authors reported a primary patency rate of 81% at 2 years. Nevelsteen and coworkers placed 29 stent-grafts in 24 patients to treat claudication (n = 7) or limb-threatening ischemia (n = 17).[61,62] Mean primary and secondary cumulative patency rates after 1 year were 85%

and 95%, respectively. All patients in this series underwent outflow procedures—that is, profundaplasty or femoral distal grafting. Krajcer and colleagues reported preliminary results of a comparative study of Wallstents (Boston Scientific, Natick, MA) versus Wallgrafts (Boston Scientific).[63] Ten patients received six Wallgrafts and nine Wallstents. At 1-month follow-up, marked improvement was noted in claudication symptoms in four of five patients who received the Wallgrafts. In the Wallstent group, symptoms improved in one patient; in another patient, symptoms improved in one limb and worsened in the other limb; and the remainder of patients demonstrated no improvement in symptoms.

Predictors of Failure for Stent-Grafting

CFA disease was a significant predictor of failure at long-term follow-up.[20] The 5-year primary patency rate was 88% for patients who had concomitant CFA endarterectomy and iliac stent-grafting, versus 66% for stent-grafting alone ($P = .04$; relative risk, 8). This finding has prompted more intense evaluation of the CFA plaque burden before proceeding with iliac intervention (Fig. 108-11).

Mortality

It has been estimated that the life expectancy of patients with peripheral arterial disease, especially those with intermittent claudication, is reduced by about 10 years compared with the general population.[64-66] The main cause of death in patients with peripheral arterial disease is cardiac disease, accounting for 40% to 60%.[64-66] The overall mortality rates from all causes in patients with intermittent claudication are approximately 30% after 5 years, 50% after 10 years, and 70% after 15 years.[67] About 10% to 20% of patients die of cerebrovascular disease, and about 10% die of other vascular causes,

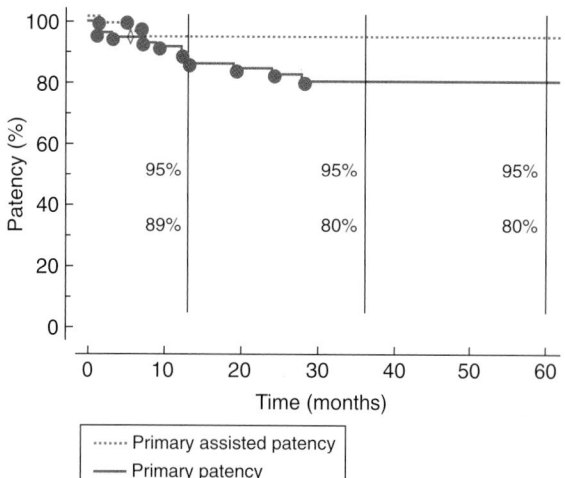

Figure 108-10 Kaplan-Meier curve estimate for primary and primary assisted stent-graft patency of severe occlusive iliac artery disease for all patients. Primary patency was 80% and primary assisted patency was 95% at 60 months, with a standard error less than 10%.

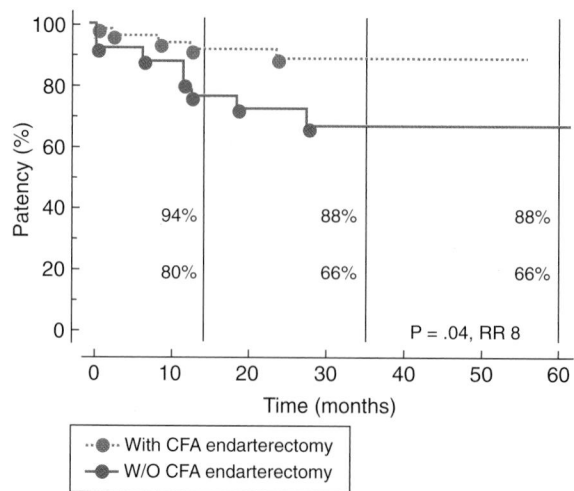

Figure 108-11 Kaplan-Meier primary patency curves for patients with common femoral artery (CFA) disease as a variable. Patients with concomitant CFA endarterectomy had significantly better patency than those without (W/O) endarterectomy (88% versus 66% at 60 months; $P = .04$). RR, relative risk.

mainly ruptured aortic aneurysms. Nonvascular causes account for about 20% to 30% of deaths, with the most frequent probably being cancer.[67] In a prospective follow-up study of more than 550 patients with CLI, 21.9% of patients were deceased after 1 year, and 31.6% after 2 years.[68] The overall incidence of cardiovascular death was 34.5%, compared with 8.5% of deaths resulting from nonvascular causes. These numbers, based on large series, are well reflected in the small population studies of patients undergoing endovascular treatment for iliac occlusive disease. Long-term mortality rates reported by Schurmann and associates for patients treated with iliac stents were 17% after 5 years and 36% after 10 years.[44] Galaria and colleagues reported that patient survival by life-table analysis was 38% at 10 years for patients with TASC types A and B lesions treated with angioplasty and stenting of the iliac arteries.[45] It can be hypothesized that successful treatment of claudication might prolong survival time; however, there are no study findings proving this hypothesis.

COMPLICATIONS

Bypass surgery has the best long-term durability, with 5-year patency in excess of 80%, but it has been associated with a perioperative complication rate of up to 30%.[69-73] Recovery from aortobifemoral bypass typically requires weeks of absence from work, a financial burden that many patients cannot absorb. Thus, less invasive endovascular treatment for aortoiliac occlusive disease has largely supplanted aortobifemoral bypass because focal iliac disease is well treated with angioplasty or stent placement. These less invasive options are not without complications, however. These complications can be categorized as contrast related, sheath site related, and remote.

Contrast Related

Patients with preprocedure renal insufficiency are at greatest risk for postprocedure nephropathy. As previously discussed, patients with serum creatinine greater than 1.5 mg/dL (133 μmol/L) should be treated with NAC and sodium bicarbonate infusion.[14,29-31] In addition, contrast volume should be limited. Patients with creatinine greater than 2.5 mg/dL (221 μmol/L) are treated with a combination of intravascular ultrasound and pre-and postprocedure pressure measurements.

Sheath Site Related

The incidence of local wound complications related to sheath insertion is 1% to 3%, but this can be reduced by accurate placement of the puncture site in the CFA, avoiding high and low punctures. Most sheath sites can be closed with suture-type closure devices to decrease the incidence of hematoma and CFA pseudoaneurysm.[74]

Iliofemoral arteriography is performed, and if the femoral artery is less than 7 mm or significant calcification is present,

the sheath is removed after the activated clotting time has decreased to less than 200 seconds and manual pressure is applied. If CFA disease is not well defined before intervention, posterior plaque disruption by means of the initial needle puncture can cause acute CFA occlusion. Femoral artery occlusion is obvious on physical examination by the loss of color and pulses; immediate operative intervention with groin exploration is necessary.

Remote

Arterial Rupture

Arterial rupture is an uncommon (<1%) but potentially serious complication. In most instances, arterial rupture occurs in the setting of angioplasty or stenting of small, heavily calcified EIAs. When the procedure is performed under local anesthesia, patients typically have significant flank or back pain before the artery ruptures. If such pain occurs, further dilatation should not be performed. Patients under regional or general anesthesia do not exhibit these symptoms. Arterial rupture can usually be treated with the placement of stent-grafts to seal the ruptured iliac artery (see Fig. 108-3A to C). A balloon occlusion catheter may be needed to stabilize hypotensive patients. This must often be placed from the contralateral femoral artery to allow for upsizing of the ipsilateral femoral sheath to a size sufficient to allow placement of a stent-graft.

Arterial Dissection

Arterial dissection has been described as a complication of PTA. Proximal or distal progression of iliac dissection can occur beyond the site of intervention. The typical cause is overdilatation of a small calcified artery. Treatment consists of the extension of stenting to stop flow-limiting occlusion due to the dissection.

Embolization

Distal embolization is uncommon in the absence of aggressive dilatation prior to iliac stent placement. Appropriate assessment by pre- and postprocedural arteriography, physical examination, and Doppler evaluation is important to detect this complication.

POSTOPERATIVE MANAGEMENT

There are well-accepted criteria for reporting procedural success, clinical improvement, and patency, and the proper use of these standards for outcomes is critical. Initiation of a program of ongoing care to monitor and treat modifiable risk factors is also an important aspect of postoperative management. Risk factor management is critical and is discussed in Chapter 104 (Lower Extremity Arterial Disease: Decision Making and Medical Treatment).

Criteria for Reporting Significant Change in Clinical Status

Clinical assessment expressed grossly in terms of "symptomatic relief" is notoriously unreliable because it lacks objectivity. Combining standard clinical categories with objective noninvasive testing can overcome this weakness. For reporting purposes, the designation "clinically improved" requires an upward shift by at least one clinical category (see Chapter 103: Lower Extremity Arterial Disease: General Considerations, Table 103-3), except for those with actual tissue loss (category 5), who must move up at least two categories and reach a level of claudication to be considered improved. In addition, to claim a cause and effect and attribute the improvement to treatment, some objective evidence of hemodynamic improvement must be documented; an increase of more than 0.10 in ABI is recommended. In patients in whom the ABI cannot be accurately measured (e.g., those with diabetes and medial calcinosis), the systolic toe pressure (which is less commonly affected by vessel incompressibility) or any measurable pressure distal to the revascularization can be substituted.

Criteria for Patency

The determination of patency for iliac stents should be based on objective findings. Although physical examination can detect the presence of a palpable femoral pulse, iliac stent patency should be demonstrated by an accepted vascular imaging technique such as arteriography, duplex ultrasound color-flow scan, or magnetic resonance imaging. A diameter reduction within the stented segment of greater than 50% indicates significant restenosis. A biphasic or triphasic Doppler waveform should be noted at the CFA level. No clear duplex criteria for the iliac segment exist; however, most would consider a doubling of the peak systolic velocity indicative of restenosis, especially with an ABI drop greater than 0.1.

Quality of Life Outcomes

Few trials have looked at quality of life outcomes after the treatment of iliac occlusive disease with stents. The Dutch Iliac Stent Trial Study Group reported that at early follow-up, all RAND 36-Item Health Survey scores increased substantially in both patients treated with angioplasty alone and patients treated with selective stenting.[75] Quality of life assessments (consisting of the RAND 36, time tradeoff, standard gamble, rating scale, health utilities index, and EuroQol-5D) were completed by 254 patients in telephone interviews performed before treatment and after 1, 3, 12, and 24 months. When the two treatments were compared, no significant difference was observed ($P > .05$). All measurements showed a significant improvement in quality of life after treatment ($P < .05$). The RAND 36-Item Health Survey, which measures physical functioning, role limitations caused by physical problems, and bodily pain, and the EuroQol-5D were most sensitive to the impact of revascularization. Compared with the external patient group (i.e., patients with intermittent claudi-

cation who participated in an exercise program), patients in the trial had lower quality of life values before revascularization and higher values after revascularization. The proportion of trial patients with pre-revascularization values below the 95% confidence interval of the reference values among the exercise group ranged from 21% (standard gamble) to 67% (RAND 36 physical functioning). After revascularization, these proportions decreased significantly. At 2-year follow-up, the proportion of trial patients with health values equal to or higher than the upper 95% confidence limit of the reference values among the exercise group ranged from 62% (EuroQol-5D) to 78% (RAND 36, bodily pain). At 5 years after treatment, all scores, except that for general health perception, were still markedly higher than the pretreatment scores in both groups.[41] Survival analyses showed no differences in RAND 36 scores between the two treatment groups over the follow-up period.

When we compared the quality of life scores of the two treatment groups 5 years after treatment with data from age-matched controls in the literature, the scores of patients treated with PTA and selective stent placement were as high as the scores of age-matched controls in all dimensions. However, the scores of patients treated with primary stent placement were substantially lower for physical functioning, physical role functioning, vitality, bodily pain, and general health perception, whereas the scores for emotional role functioning, social functioning, mental health, and health change were equivalent to those in age-matched controls.[41] The authors therefore concluded that cost rather than effectiveness may be the decisive factor in the choice of percutaneous treatment.

SELECTED KEY REFERENCES

Bosch JL, Hunink MG. Meta-analysis of the results of percutaneous transluminal angioplasty and stent placement for aortoiliac occlusive disease. *Radiology.* 1997;204:87-96.
Large meta-analysis that determined that stent placement and PTA yield similar complication rates, but the technical success rate is higher after stent placement and the risk of long-term failure is reduced.

Briguori C, Airoldi F, D'Andrea D, Bonizzoni E, Morici N, Focaccio A, Michev I, Montorfano M, Carlino M, Cosgrave J, Ricciardelli B, Colombo A. Renal Insufficiency Following Contrast Media Administration Trial (REMEDIAL): a randomized comparison of 3 preventive strategies. *Circulation.* 2007;115:1211-1217.
Randomized controlled trial showing the benefit of adding sodium bicarbonate to NAC prophylaxis.

de Vries SO, Hunink MG. Results of aortic bifurcation grafts for aortoiliac occlusive disease: a meta-analysis. *J Vasc Surg.* 1997;26:558-569.
Large meta-analysis of aortoiliac or aortofemoral bypass graft procedures in aortoiliac occlusive disease that provides a benchmark for comparing endovascular results.

Galaria II, Davies MG. Percutaneous transluminal revascularization for iliac occlusive disease: long-term outcomes in TransAtlantic Inter-Society Consensus A and B lesions. *Ann Vasc Surg.* 2005;19:352-360.
Large retrospective study that used multivariate analysis to define factors associated with worse results after iliac endovascular treatment.

Klein WM, van der Graaf Y, Seegers J, Moll FL, Mali WP. Long-term cardiovascular morbidity, mortality, and reintervention after endovascular treatment in patients with iliac artery disease: The Dutch Iliac Stent Trial Study. *Radiology.* 2004;232:491-498.
This study compared cardiovascular morbidity, mortality, and re-intervention for patients randomized to primary stent placement versus primary PTA and found no difference in the number of re-interventions 5 years after treatment.

Leville CD, Kashyap VS, Clair DG, Bena JF, Lyden SP, Greenberg RK, O'Hara PJ, Sarac TP, Ouriel K. Endovascular management of iliac artery occlusions: extending treatment to TransAtlantic Inter-Society Consensus class C and D patients. *J Vasc Surg.* 2006;43:32-39.
This study demonstrated the efficacy of PTA stenting for more advanced TASC lesions and found that diabetes and CLI but not TASC type C classification negatively affected outcome.

Merten GJ, Burgess WP, Gray LV, Holleman JH, Roush RS, Kowalchuk GJ, Bersin RM, Van Moore A, Simonton CA 3rd, Rittase RA, Norton HJ, Kennedy TP. Prevention of contrast-induced nephropathy with sodium bicarbonate: a randomized controlled trial. *JAMA.* 2004; 291:2328-2334.
Prospective, single-center, randomized trial showing that hydration with sodium bicarbonate before contrast exposure is more effective than hydration with sodium chloride for the prophylaxis of contrast-induced renal failure.

Powell RJ, Fillinger M, Bettmann M, Jeffrey R, Langdon D, Walsh DB, Zwolak R, Hines M, Cronenwett JL. The durability of endovascular treatment of multisegment iliac occlusive disease. *J Vasc Surg.* 2000;31:1178-1184.
This paper demonstrated the effective endovascular treatment of multisegment iliac occlusive disease but found that re-intervention was frequently needed and that external iliac involvement was a predictor of worse outcome.

Rzucidlo EM, Powell RJ, Zwolak RM, Fillinger MF, Walsh DB, Schermerhorn ML, Cronenwett JL. Early results of stent-grafting to treat diffuse aortoiliac occlusive disease. *J Vasc Surg.* 2003;37: 1175-1180.
This study found that stent-graft placement to treat diffuse aortoiliac occlusive disease produced better patency than stenting alone. Concomitant CFA endarterectomy also improved the patency of stent-graft treatment.

REFERENCES

The reference list can be found on the companion Expert Consult Web site at *www.expertconsult.com.*

Section 15 Lower Extremity Arterial Disease

CHAPTER 109

Infrainguinal Disease: Surgical Treatment

Joseph L. Mills, Sr.

Lower extremity arterial reconstruction is most commonly performed in patients with moderate to severe limb ischemia due to atherosclerotic peripheral arterial disease (PAD). Although the techniques described herein may also be applied to patients with traumatic, aneurysmal, and nonatherosclerotic conditions, this chapter focuses exclusively on patients with PAD. *Infrainguinal bypass* is defined as any major arterial reconstruction using a bypass conduit, either autogenous or prosthetic, that originates at or below the inguinal ligament. Inflow sites therefore include the common, deep, or superficial femoral arteries, as well as the popliteal or even tibial arteries. The bypass insertion site may be the femoral, above- or below-knee popliteal, tibial, peroneal, or pedal artery. Over the past 2 decades, progress in patient evaluation and selection and in the conduct of infrainguinal bypass operations has resulted in a more aggressive and generally more successful approach to distal arterial reconstructions, especially for patients with critical limb ischemia (CLI) who would otherwise face major limb amputation. Although graft patency and limb salvage rates have demonstrated parallel improvements, there remains a critical need for detailed clinical studies examining the cost-effectiveness of infrainguinal bypass as well as patient quality of life outcomes to ensure the appropriate use of these procedures and to permit meaningful comparison with less invasive endovascular therapies.

■ INDICATIONS

The two primary indications for infrainguinal bypass are claudication and CLI.

Claudication

Patients who are significantly disabled by claudication, such that they are unable to perform their primary occupations or comfortably carry out the activities of daily living, or those whose lifestyles are significantly limited are potential candidates for infrainguinal bypass. A trial of smoking cessation, lifestyle modification, and exercise, with or without medical therapy, is usually indicated before operative intervention (see Chapter 104: Lower Extremity Arterial Disease: Decision Making and Medical Treatment). There is consensus that bypass is preferable to angioplasty in patients with Trans-Atlantic Inter-Society Consensus (TASC) type D lesions—that is, complete common femoral artery (CFA) or superficial

femoral artery (SFA) occlusions or complete popliteal and proximal trifurcation occlusions; however, it may also be applied to patients with types B and C lesions (see Chapter 104: Lower Extremity Arterial Disease: Decision Making and Medical Treatment).[1] Operation should be offered only if the benefit-to-risk ratio is high and if anatomic characteristics suggest a favorable and durable result. The primary reason for intervention in claudicants is to improve lifestyle, given that the risk of severe clinical deterioration (20%) or major limb amputation (5%) over a 3- to 5-year period is low.[1,2] In most centers with extensive infrainguinal bypass experience, claudicants constitute only 15% to 30% of patients, with the majority of the remaining patients undergoing bypass for CLI. Although these data reflect practice patterns in tertiary referral centers, they may not reflect the realities of community-based practices.[3]

Critical Limb Ischemia

Patients with CLI generally require intervention. Such patients fall into Fontaine III and IV[4] and Rutherford 4 to 6 categories (see Chapter 103: Lower Extremity Arterial Disease: General Considerations).[5-7] The most recent European consensus document defines CLI as (1) persistent, recurring ischemic rest pain requiring opiate analgesia for at least 2 weeks and (2) ankle systolic pressure lower than 50 mm Hg or toe systolic pressure lower than 30 mm Hg, or (1) ulceration or gangrene of the foot or toes and ankle systolic pressure lower than 50 mm Hg or (2) toe systolic pressure lower than 30 mm Hg (or absent pedal pulses in diabetics).[8] Wolfe and Wyatt further subdivided patients meeting the standard definition of CLI into those with critical or with subcritical ischemia, based on subsequent amputation risk.[9] Subcritical ischemia is present in patients with rest pain and ankle pressure higher than 40 mm Hg. Critical ischemia is defined as rest pain and tissue loss or ankle pressure lower than 40 mm Hg. This distinction is based on a retrospective analysis of 20 publications analyzing 6118 patients. At 1 year, 27% of patients with subcritical ischemia achieved limb survival without revascularization, in contrast to only 5% in the group of patients with critical ischemia. In practice, these data indicate that certain extremely high-risk patients with subcritical ischemia might be managed medically (nonoperatively) but that virtually all patients with true CLI require either bypass or major limb amputation.

PREOPERATIVE ASSESSMENT

There is widespread recognition that patients requiring infrainguinal bypass frequently have medical co-morbidities, including diabetes mellitus, chronic obstructive pulmonary disease, and renal insufficiency; there is a particularly high prevalence of associated coronary artery disease (CAD). The incidence of perioperative myocardial infarction ranges from 2% to 6.5% following lower extremity arterial reconstruction; approximately 70% of both perioperative and late mortality in these patients is due to concomitant CAD.[10-13] It is clear that significant CAD is a nearly universal accompaniment of PAD. What remains controversial is determining which individuals are most likely to benefit from a detailed preoperative cardiac assessment and possible coronary intervention before undergoing infrainguinal bypass. Proposed algorithms have ranged from routine cardiac evaluation of all PAD patients to an almost nihilistic approach.[14]

Patients with CLI pose a more complex problem because there is a high anticipated amputation rate without lower extremity arterial reconstruction.[9] CLI patients have an even greater prevalence of CAD than claudicants, as well as a significantly reduced 5-year mortality, primarily due to associated CAD. However, because CLI patients also tend to be older and have a greater number of co-morbidities, cardiac intervention in such individuals has higher reported morbidity and mortality rates than in the general population of patients with isolated CAD targeted for intervention.[14] My approach in CLI patients is to assume that they all have significant CAD. Perioperative blood pressure control, antiangina regimens, and treatment for congestive heart failure (CHF) are optimized, and based on level I data,[15] perioperative beta blockade is employed if there are no contraindications.[16-18] I would recommend postponement of infrainguinal bypass in CLI patients to allow further cardiac evaluation only in the presence of frequent or unstable angina, recent myocardial infarction, poorly controlled CHF, or symptomatic or untreated arrhythmia. Even in these instances, the cardiac evaluation should be focused and expeditious. Invasive coronary intervention should be pursued only if the patient and anatomic characteristics are favorable, the benefit-to-risk ratio is high, and it can be performed without prolonged delay. In the absence of such cardiac instability, CLI patients are best treated with meticulous perioperative medical care and expeditious lower extremity reconstruction.[19,20] Prolonged delays before limb revascularization in CLI patients increase morbidity and amputation risk.[21] In patients requiring vascular reconstruction, the focus has turned sharply toward maximizing medical therapy rather than performing multiple, expensive, and sometimes ambiguous preoperative cardiac tests so that the patient can be "cleared for surgery." A large, well-designed prospective randomized trial failed to show a benefit of cardiac revascularization before vascular surgery in patients with stable cardiac symptoms.[22] (See Chapter 30: Preoperative Management for a detailed discussion of perioperative cardiac evaluation and treatment.)

PREOPERATIVE IMAGING

Infrainguinal bypass requires a careful assessment of the extent of arterial disease as well as a detailed anatomic characterization of the inflow and outflow arteries (see Chapter 103: Lower Extremity Arterial Disease: General Considerations). In most patients, standard arteriography is still the "gold standard." Computed tomographic angiography (CTA) has improved and is now the dominant preoperative imaging modality for aortic aneurysm disease; however, in the periphery, the small caliber of the infrainguinal artery and the presence of calcification in multiple vessels (associated with increasing age and diabetes) limit CTA's applicability, especially in CLI patients.[23] Magnetic resonance angiography (MRA)[24] is continually improving,[25-29] and particularly for patients with claudication, preoperative duplex imaging, also referred to as duplex arterial mapping (see Chapter 15: Vascular Laboratory: Arterial Duplex Scanning),[30,31] may provide sufficient anatomic information to proceed directly to the operating room without formal arteriography. In the latter circumstance, immediate pre-bypass arteriography in the operating room is a reasonable approach. For most patients, however, especially for those with CLI, I prefer to perform the initial diagnostic angiography at a separate sitting, for several reasons. One reason is that, for an increasing number of CLI patients, endoluminal techniques are a reasonable option.

Based on a careful preangiographic assessment, including the indications for intervention, anatomic considerations (based on duplex imaging), patient's functional status, co-morbidities, and availability of vein conduit (see Chapter 104: Lower Extremity Arterial Disease: Decision Making and Medical Treatment), I try to determine whether a given patient with TASC type C or D disease would be best served by endoluminal therapy or open bypass. If the former is the case, I vigorously pursue endoluminal treatment at the time of diagnostic arteriography. If open bypass is the plan, I focus on optimal visualization of potential target arteries and obtain multiple views, as required, to ascertain that no unexpected inflow disease is present that would require treatment before proceeding with infrainguinal bypass. Detailed high-quality diagnostic arteriograms can be obtained and reviewed carefully before proceeding with bypass. In some patients, selection of outflow arteries may be difficult, and this area of decision making can be improved if films are reviewed and discussed with colleagues. Confining the initial procedure to diagnostic or therapeutic angiography obviates time constraints and scheduling difficulties that arise in the operating room when trying to perform angiography and open reconstruction in one sitting. I reserve the latter approach for carefully selected patients whose arterial anatomy has already been fairly well delineated by preoperative MRA or duplex scanning. This confines the "one-stop approach" primarily to claudicants undergoing bypass for isolated, single-level femoropopliteal disease.

Figure 109-1 Detailed diagnostic arteriography with fixed imaging, proper timing, and appropriate catheter placement almost always identifies suitable target arteries. Each of the patients depicted had popliteal artery occlusion and extensive trifurcation and long-segment tibial disease, but diagnostic studies identified suitable target arteries in the foot. **A,** Completion arteriogram following inframalleolar posterior tibial bypass in a patient with diabetes and forefoot gangrene. Despite a small-caliber outflow vessel, the bypass remains patent, and the ischemic foot ulcers healed and have not recurred at 2 years. **B,** Completion arteriogram following bypass to a diseased dorsal pedal artery. Despite poor outflow and diseased arch and pedal vessels, the graft remains patent at 1 year. This patient with diabetes healed and ambulates with a transmetatarsal amputation.

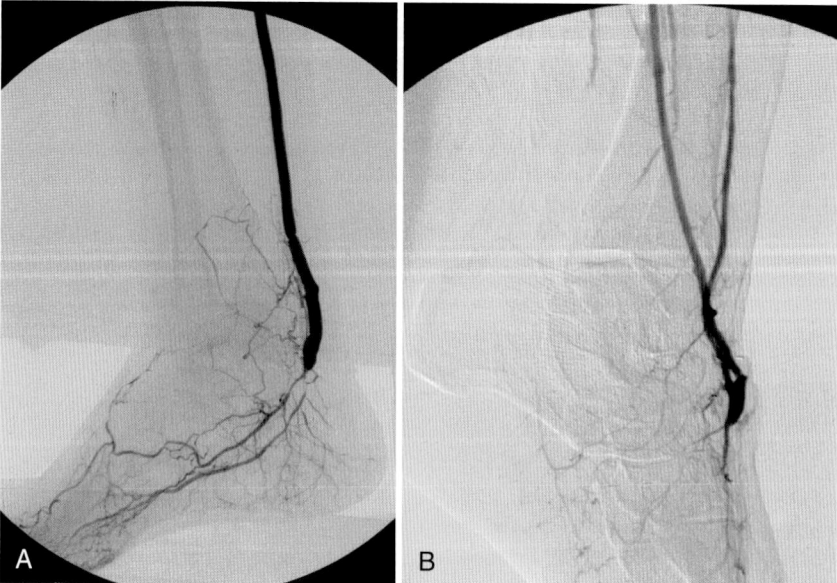

Defining Bypass Target Arteries

In nearly all patients in whom infrainguinal bypass is indicated, suitable target arteries can be identified (Fig. 109-1) if diagnostic angiography is properly performed.[32,33] Only a tiny fraction of individuals, usually those with multiple failed reconstructions, have no identifiable target artery.[34] Detailed runoff views are necessary, including magnification and lateral views of the foot. Such films can be obtained in nearly all patients with adjunctive techniques such as foot warming, local administration of intra-arterial vasodilators, and proper positioning of the diagnostic catheter. It is frequently helpful to advance the catheter selectively into the SFA or popliteal artery to obtain adequate views of the infrapopliteal and pedal circulations, especially in patients with diabetes mellitus. Intra-arterial runoff films with bolus injections performed while the diagnostic catheter is positioned in the aorta may fail to adequately define the runoff. If percutaneous access has been achieved from a contralateral, retrograde femoral approach, selective films can be obtained by advancing a wire and then an appropriate diagnostic catheter over the aortic bifurcation and selectively down the affected extremity. In selected patients with normal inflow based on physical examination and noninvasive studies, an ipsilateral antegrade approach may be more expeditious to identify suitable runoff vessels, with the additional advantage of requiring a reduced contrast load (Fig. 109-2). Such an approach is especially useful in diabetic patients with renal insufficiency and noninvasive studies that suggest isolated infrapopliteal disease.

Despite optimal angiographic techniques, there may be a small number of patients in whom no suitable target can be identified. Selective exploration of dorsal pedal or distal posterior tibial arteries with flow detectable by Doppler or duplex imaging may identify a graftable recipient artery. Pomposelli and associates reported a surprisingly high

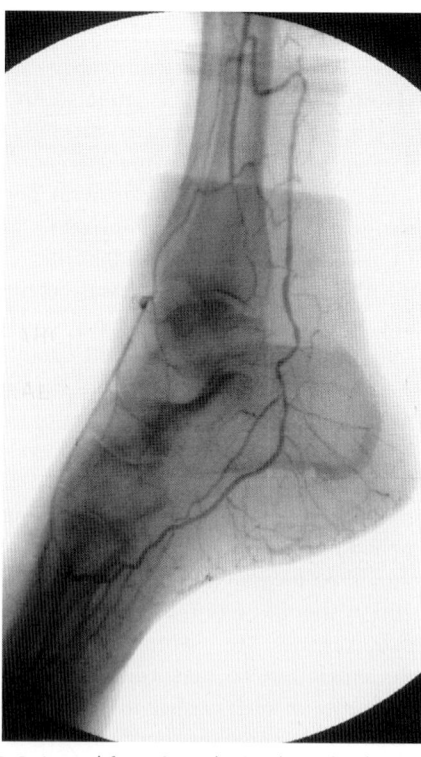

Figure 109-2 Lateral foot view obtained via distal selective superficial femoral arterial catheter injection identifies excellent collaterals from the distal peroneal artery to both the dorsal pedal and posterior tibial circulations.

success rate under these circumstances,[34] although I believe that this situation is relatively uncommon if diagnostic angiography has been pursued to its fullest advantage. In short, there are few patients who are truly unreconstructable from an anatomic standpoint owing to the lack of a suitable outflow target vessel.

Autogenous Vein Assessment

Since Kunlin's first description of the successful use of autogenous vein to bypass femoropopliteal arteriosclerosis obliterans,[35,36] there is near universal agreement that autogenous vein is the best conduit for infrainguinal bypass at all levels.[37,38] The great saphenous vein (GSV) is the most readily available and durable conduit. Assessment of vein availability and quality is critical and should be carried out before embarking on the operation.[39-41] I routinely perform duplex mapping of the GSV in all patients before surgery; if the ipsilateral GSV is absent, unsuitable, or of insufficient length to perform the anticipated bypass, I also scan the ipsilateral small saphenous vein, the contralateral great and small saphenous veins, and the upper extremity veins, if necessary, to locate a suitable vein and to identify any extenuating circumstances that might arise during the conduct of the operation. Patients are scanned with a light tourniquet in place with the limb dependent, as described by Blebea and colleagues.[42] I prefer to use veins that are soft, compressible, and at least 3 mm in diameter. Calcified or sclerotic veins are rejected. Soft, compressible veins between 2 and 3 mm in diameter are worthy of exploration, but if they do not distend appropriately, the operation should be modified either by harvesting a better-quality vein (based on preoperative duplex studies) or by shortening the length of the proposed bypass, if possible, by selecting alternative inflow or outflow sites. The type and quality of the bypass conduit are the most important determinants of infrainguinal bypass success; efforts to maximize conduit quality will be rewarded.

Vein harvesting can be performed through long continuous incisions, through skip incisions, or endoscopically. Endoscopic vein harvest has become common in cardiac surgery. Although there are a few enthusiasts, it has not been widely adopted by vascular surgeons for leg bypass, likely owing to equipment costs, learning curve issues, and concerns about damaging vein segments when a long conduit is needed. There are no convincing data to support any specific harvesting technique.[43-47] Regardless of the harvesting technique, poor-quality or marginal vein should be rejected. The search for high-quality vein is worth the time and effort, even if vein splicing or bypass shortening is required. Every effort should be made to perform all infrainguinal bypasses with vein conduit (an all-autogenous policy). Long-term results should not be sacrificed for the sake of expediency at the initial operation. Saphenous vein performs well in the reversed,[48-52] nonreversed,[53] and in situ[54-62] configurations; the technique chosen is dictated primarily by conduit availability, anatomic considerations, and surgeon preference and experience.

OPERATIVE PLANNING

Operative planning for infrainguinal bypass involves the most complex decision making a vascular surgeon is called on to provide. More than any other operation, infrainguinal bypass taxes the surgeon's ingenuity and requires him or her to anticipate and carefully consider numerous alternatives and potential complications both in the preoperative evaluation and during the conduct of the reconstruction itself. Foremost, the major anatomic lesions and their hemodynamic significance must be identified.[63-65]

Concomitant Inflow Disease

Adequate inflow should be ensured before commencing with infrainguinal bypass. Selected inflow lesions can be treated either percutaneously in advance, at the time of the preoperative diagnostic angiogram, or at the same operative sitting if need be. Iliac artery lesions of hemodynamic significance should be addressed in nearly all claudicants before proceeding with infrainguinal bypass. For patients with CLI, an iliac lesion with a resting gradient of less than 5 to 10 mm Hg may be acceptable if the pulse and Doppler waveform at the selected inflow site (e.g., femoral artery) are normal. In patients with claudication or CLI presenting with rest pain alone in the absence of tissue loss, an isolated iliac angioplasty without concomitant infrainguinal bypass may suffice if the iliac lesion is of sufficient hemodynamic importance. In such patients with tandem lesions, the profunda-popliteal collateral index may be helpful in predicting whether an inflow procedure alone will be sufficient to alleviate the patient's symptoms.[63] An index greater than 0.25 indicates a large pressure gradient across the knee joint and suggests that inflow disease correction and profundaplasty alone are unlikely to be adequate.[66-68]

Proximal Anastomotic Site

Before operation, the surgeon must define the inflow source, which need not be the CFA. There is abundant evidence that originating shorter bypasses from the deep femoral, superficial femoral, popliteal, or, in rare cases, one of the tibial arteries results in patency rates equivalent to those achieved when the CFA serves as the bypass origin. Short bypasses are frequently useful in patients with diabetes mellitus and primary infrapopliteal arterial occlusive disease, as well as in individuals with limited available vein conduit who present with failure of a previous reconstruction. Based on hemodynamic data and anatomic imaging, the surgeon should commence the operation with the optimal inflow site in mind. However, if unanticipated arterial disease is identified or vein quality and length are worse than anticipated once the operation is under way, the surgeon should already have alternative bypass origins in mind that can be used to shorten the length of the bypass without compromising hemodynamics. If there is uncertainty about the appropriateness of the inflow site at exploration, its hemodynamic suitability should be assessed by direct intra-arterial pressure measurements that can be compared with the transduced radial artery pressure. A resting gradient exceeding 10 mm Hg is significant, as is a drop in pressure exceeding 15% following the administration of intra-arterial papaverine.[64,65,69] If a significant gradient is identified at the selected inflow site, a more proximal inflow site above the culprit lesion should be selected, or the responsible lesion should be addressed by local endarterectomy or angioplasty. This problem occasionally arises with iliac or common femoral lesions whose hemodynamic significance was not appreciated at the time of preoperative arteriography, particularly lesions consisting primarily of posterior plaque that may have been masked if appropriate oblique projections were not obtained.

Associated Femoral Endarterectomy

Whenever the CFA is used as the site of origin for bypass, significant occlusive disease involving the origin and proximal deep femoral artery should usually be addressed at the time of the infrainguinal bypass. The endarterectomy often begins in the CFA. Following the division of veins that cross the anterior surface of the deep femoral artery, the femoral arteriotomy is carried out beyond the posterior tongue of disease that extends a variable distance down the deep femoral artery, usually at least to its first or second portion. Tacking sutures may or may not be needed at the distal endpoint. The arteriotomy can be closed with a vein patch or a segment of endarterectomized SFA. This patch can then be opened longitudinally to serve as the origin for the infrainguinal bypass (modified Linton's patch technique; Fig. 109-3). Alternatively, if the vein caliber is good (>4 mm), a longer venotomy can be made in the vein conduit, which then serves simultaneously as a profundaplasty patch and the bypass origin. The latter technique should not be used if the arterial wall is markedly thickened or if the caliber of either the native donor artery or the vein graft artery is small, to avoid compromising the origin of the vein graft at the heel of the anastomosis. Incorporation of a venous side branch as part of the anastomotic heel is another useful technique when the donor

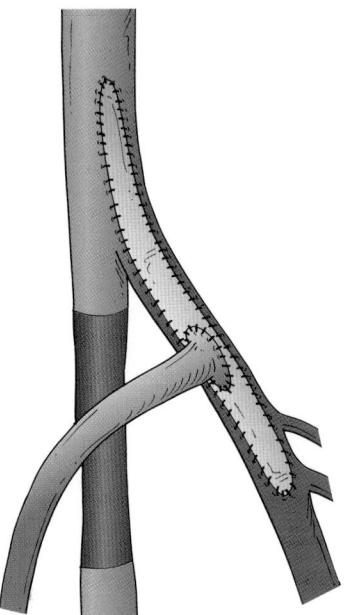

Figure 109-3 Linton's vein patch technique following endarterectomy of the distal common and proximal deep femoral arteries, with anastomosis of the reversed vein graft to the patch.

arterial wall is thick or there is a caliber mismatch between the donor artery and the vein bypass conduit (Fig. 109-4). Correction of significant deep femoral disease at the time of infrainguinal bypass is clinically important; should the bypass ever fail, adequate deep femoral artery perfusion may prevent the development of severe, recurrent limb ischemia.

Distal Anastomotic Site

Although inflow artery selection is generally straightforward, outflow site selection frequently requires greater judgment. The general principle of infrainguinal reconstruction is to bypass all hemodynamically significant disease and to insert the bypass into the most proximal limb artery that has at least one continuous runoff artery to the foot. Thus, if the popliteal artery reconstitutes distal to an SFA occlusion, and at least one tibial or peroneal artery is continuous to the foot, the popliteal artery would be selected as the outflow site. It is possible, however, and sometimes desirable to bypass to an isolated or so-called blind popliteal segment.

Isolated Popliteal Target

An isolated popliteal artery is defined as a patent popliteal artery segment at least 5 cm long but with only geniculate collaterals and no major distal tibial or peroneal runoff artery in direct continuity with the foot. Such bypasses function surprisingly well and are especially useful in patients with limited vein availability.[70-75] They may also be more useful in patients with claudication or rest pain than in those with frank tissue necrosis, for whom anything less than providing pulsatile flow directly to the foot may be insufficient. In the presence of tissue loss, I prefer bypass to an artery in direct continuity with the foot. Five-year assisted primary or secondary patency rates of 50% to 74% have been reported for such blind-segment popliteal bypasses.[73] Successful bypasses to isolated tibial artery segments have also been reported.[71]

Tibial, Peroneal, and Pedal Targets

Although most claudicants require only femoropopliteal bypass, a high proportion of patients with CLI require tibial or pedal bypass. In general, the most proximal segment of tibial or peroneal artery that is continuous with the foot should be chosen as the outflow site. Thus, a patent anterior tibial or posterior tibial artery in direct continuity with the foot and pedal arch would be chosen over the peroneal artery as an outflow site if suitable vein length is available. There is still some controversy over whether one should choose the proximal or midperoneal artery or a patent pedal artery for patients with tissue loss.[76] Most authors have found no adverse effects on graft patency or limb salvage for peroneal bypasses compared with tibial or pedal bypasses,[77-79] but Pomposelli and others have made a strong case for pedal bypass,[34] particularly in diabetic patients with

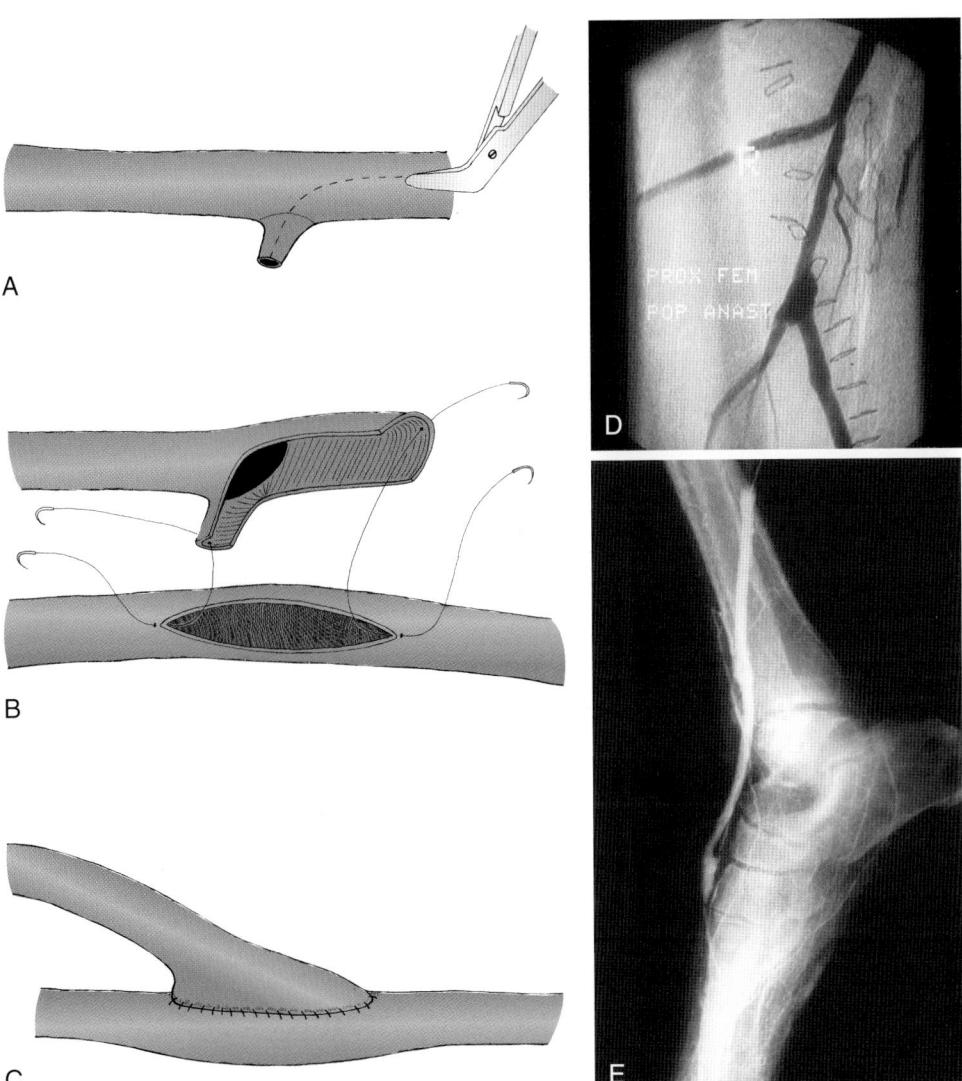

Figure 109-4 The venotomy through the reversed vein is extended through a suitable side branch (**A**) and anastomosed to the inflow artery (**B** and **C**) to avoid anastomotic stenosis at the graft heel.[35,300] This technique can be used at either the proximal anastomosis (**D**) or the distal anastomosis (**E**) and is useful when the vein caliber is small or the arterial wall is thickened.

tissue loss.[80] They emphasize the importance of restoring a pedal pulse and maximizing forefoot reperfusion. The pedal arteries are also more superficial and more easily exposed than the anatomically disadvantaged, deeply located peroneal artery. If the bypass must originate in the groin and the proximal or midperoneal artery is of good quality on arteriography and has abundant collaterals with the foot (see Fig. 109-2), I generally perform a shorter bypass to the peroneal artery, especially if vein conduit length is a limiting factor. If the peroneal artery is diseased or does not appear to collateralize well with the foot, I preferentially bypass to the foot or ankle and splice a vein if required to obtain sufficient length. I prefer dorsal pedal or paramalleolar posterior tibial–plantar artery insertion sites for short bypasses originating from the popliteal artery in diabetic patients with tissue loss.[81] Shortening the bypass in such patients allows one to optimize vein conduit quality, and the choice of an inframalleolar target artery maximizes forefoot perfusion.

OPERATIVE EXPOSURES

Standard Anterior Approach to the Common Femoral and Profunda Femoris Arteries

A thorough knowledge of anatomy and facility with multiple surgical exposures are critical to the success of infrainguinal bypass.[82] The standard approach to the CFA and the profunda femoris artery (PFA) is provided by a vertical incision overlying the CFA. This anterior approach allows complete exposure and mobilization of the CFA and its bifurcation; more proximal exposure can be obtained by division of the recurrent portion of the inguinal ligament or the entire ligament (Peter Martin incision). Distal extension allows exposure of the PFA. Division of the lateral femoral circumflex vein offers access to the proximal PFA; careful progressive division of numerous crossing veins allows extensive exposure of the PFA. In selected patients, alternative exposures have been described.

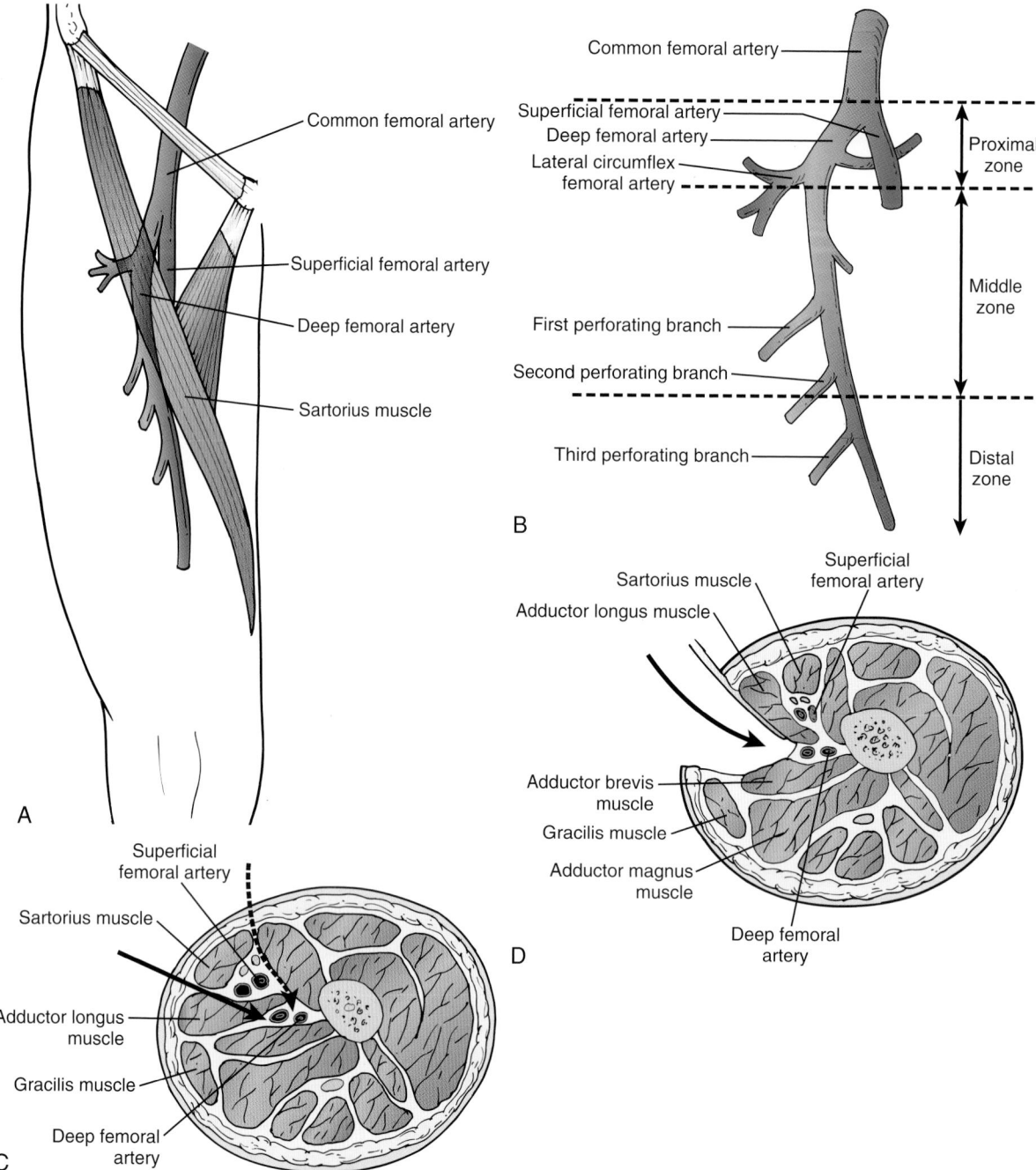

Figure 109-5 Alternative approaches to the distal deep femoral artery (DFA)[85] are useful for reoperative femorodistal bypass and when it is desirable to shorten the bypass because of limited length of vein conduit.[86] **A,** Location of the DFA. Note the surface landmarks used to identify its course. **B,** The DFA can be divided into three zones: proximal, middle, and distal. **C,** Transverse section of the thigh (viewed from above) shows the plane of dissection when the anteromedial approach (*solid arrow*) is used. Alternatively, the DFA can be approached through an even more anterior route (*dashed arrow*) by making an incision along the lateral border of the sartorius and retracting this muscle and the superficial femoral neurovascular bundle medially to reach the distal DFA. **D,** Posterior approach to the distal DFA. Note the fascial plane and structures separating the DFA from superficial femoral vascular structures and isolating it from the subsartorial canal.

Alternative Approaches to the Profunda Femoris Artery

If previous infection or scarring from multiple previous reconstructions makes standard exposure difficult, and if there are no significant occlusive lesions in the CFA or proximal PFA, the mid or distal PFA can be approached laterally, anteromedially, or posteromedially (Fig. 109-5).[71,83-86] The lateral approach is the most useful for infrainguinal bypass; the incision is placed in the upper thigh lateral to the sartorius muscle. The sartorius and SFA are retracted medially. The raphe between the adductor longus and vastus medialis is incised to expose the PFA. This approach is useful when vein conduit length is limited or femoral triangle scarring is prohibitive. The surgeon must be certain that there are no hemodynamically significant lesions proximal to the PFA if this approach is used. With these caveats in mind, use of the PFA as an origin for distal bypass does not compromise long-term patency[85,86]; similarly, the SFA[87] and popliteal arteries[85-88] can be used as an inflow source in carefully selected patients without compromising graft patency.

Exposures of the Popliteal and Tibioperoneal Arteries

The standard exposures of the above-popliteal and below-knee arteries are through medial leg incisions, usually made by deepening the saphenectomy incision. Lateral approaches to these vessels are occasionally useful and are well described elsewhere.[88] The posterior tibial and proximal to midperoneal arteries are usually approached medially. The distal third of the peroneal artery is most expeditiously exposed by means of

a lateral leg incision directly over the distal fibula. A short segment of fibula is carefully removed to expose the distal peroneal artery immediately beneath it.

Posterior exposures of the popliteal, posterior tibial, and peroneal arteries are sometimes useful (Fig. 109-6).[89,90] Diabetic patients frequently have relatively normal inflow to the popliteal trifurcation. If the inflow site is the below-knee popliteal artery and the most appropriate target artery is the distal posterior tibial or distal peroneal artery, and if the lesser saphenous vein is of good quality based on duplex imaging, the entire operation can be conducted with the patient in a prone position through a posterior approach. These approaches have been well described by Ouriel[90] and should be considered not only in selected reoperative situations (e.g., failed bypass via a medial approach) but also if conduit length is limited and ipsilateral GSV is unavailable. Commitment to an all-autogenous bypass approach requires ingenuity and familiarity with numerous anatomic exposures and techniques to allow shortening of the bypass or to permit operation in a virgin field that is unscarred by previous operations. When

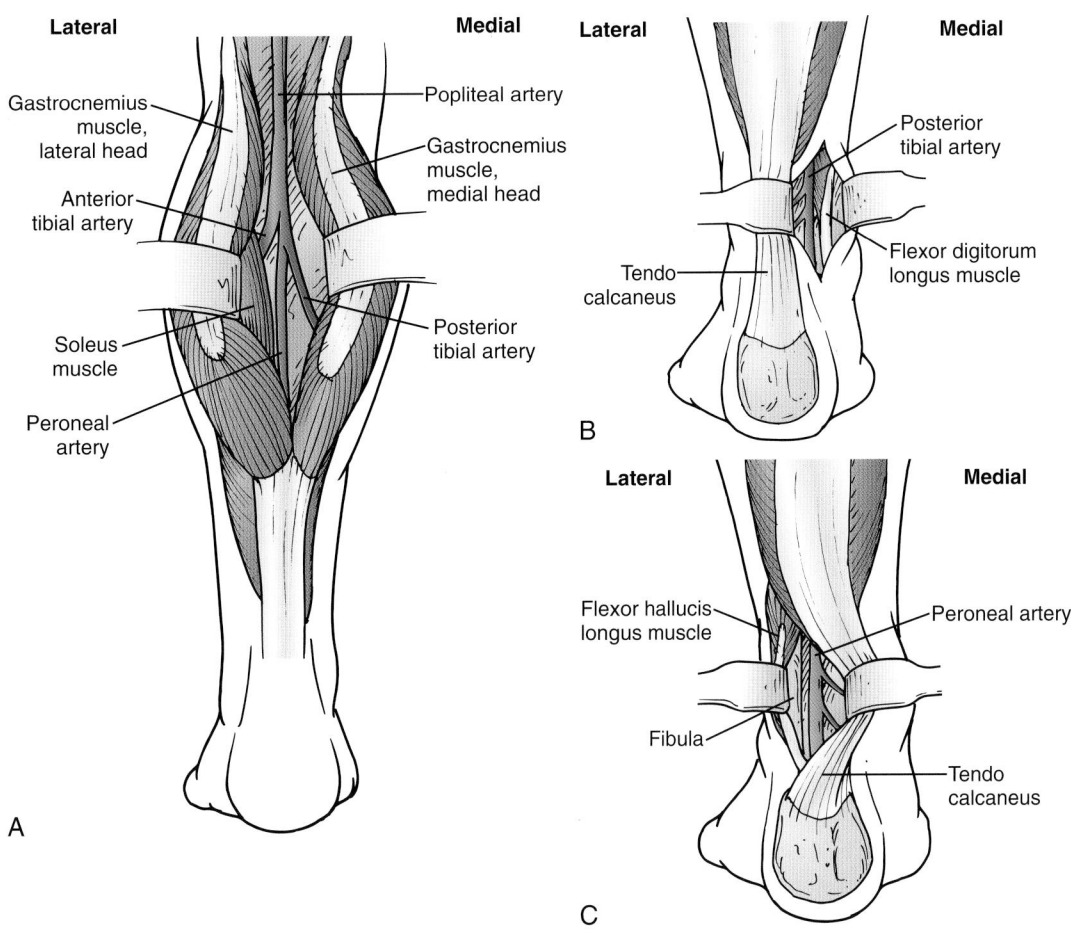

Figure 109-6 Posterior exposures.[301] **A,** Exposure of the popliteal and proximal crural arteries through a posterior approach. The two heads of the gastrocnemius muscle are separated, and the soleus muscle is lysed from its tibial origin. **B,** Exposure of the posterior tibial artery through a posterior approach. The tendo calcaneus is retracted laterally. The flexor digitorum longus muscle is reflected medially in the lower portion of the calf because the artery lies posterior to the lateral border of this muscle near the level of the malleoli. **C,** Exposure of the peroneal artery through a posterior approach. The tendo calcaneus is retracted medially, and the flexor hallucis longus muscle is reflected laterally to expose the artery in the groove next to the fibula.

using such distal origin bypass grafts, a pneumatic tourniquet instead of vascular Silastic loops or clamps is occasionally useful in the presence of severe distal arterial calcification.[91] A thorough working knowledge of alternative exposures and the occasional use of the pneumatic tourniquet are of great benefit when performing re-operative bypass.

■ CHOICE OF CONDUIT

Autogenous conduit options for infrainguinal bypass include ipsilateral and contralateral GSV,[92] small saphenous vein,[93,94] superficial femoral vein,[95] arm (basilic and cephalic) vein,[96-101] endarterectomized segments of the SFA,[102] cryopreserved vein,[103-105] and radial artery.[106,107] Prosthetic options include Dacron, heparin-bonded Dacron (HBD), human umbilical vein (HUV), polytetrafluoroethylene (PTFE) with and without a distal cuff, and, most recently, expanded PTFE (ePTFE) covalently bonded with heparin. In my group's reported 10-year experience, we performed 93% of infrainguinal bypasses with all-autogenous conduits.[108]

Autogenous Grafts

The preferred conduit is the GSV, as it outperforms all other conduit choices. If the ipsilateral GSV is absent, I do not hesitate to harvest the contralateral GSV and see no merit in saving this vein for possible use later.[92] Numerous reports suggest that the contralateral GSV is subsequently needed in no more than 20% to 25% of patients. I therefore advocate using it when necessary and performing a more difficult alternative vein reconstruction at a later time in those relatively few patients who require it. Exceptions occur whenever the contralateral limb is already ischemic, as manifested by severe claudication, rest pain, or ischemic ulceration. If the contralateral limb is asymptomatic and the ankle-brachial index (ABI) exceeds 0.6, I have experienced no significant wound healing complications from harvesting the GSV from the groin to the midcalf level. This approach usually allows the bypass to be performed with one segment of GSV and obviates the harvesting of arm vein and vein splicing. Other groups prefer to harvest arm vein if the ipsilateral GSV is unavailable and to save the contralateral GSV for later use.[96,109]

Alternative veins are used when the GSV is unavailable or of insufficient length.[110] Duplex mapping is useful in identifying suitable vein sources. The small saphenous vein is suitable if the proposed bypass is relatively short. It is possible to perform a common femoral–to–above-knee popliteal bypass or a PFA–to–below-knee popliteal bypass with one complete segment of lower saphenous vein harvested from the ankle to the knee. If a longer bypass with spliced vein is necessary, I prefer to use arm vein because it is less awkward to harvest. LoGerfo and colleagues[111] and Holzenbein and coworkers[100] described novel techniques of harvesting the upper arm basilic, median cubital, and cephalic veins in continuity with valve lysis of the basilic segment and use of the cephalic segment in a reversed configuration to provide a relatively long, unspliced autogenous conduit. The femoropopliteal

deep vein is occasionally useful for shorter bypasses but is difficult to harvest; arm vein is therefore generally preferred. Treiman and associates reported the use of the radial artery as a bypass conduit in selected patients requiring short infrageniculate bypasses, with good early results.[107] Cryopreserved vein grafts are expensive and have not performed well in clinical practice[103,104]; they may serve a niche role when revascularization is required following the removal of an infected bypass graft and autogenous vein is unavailable to create a new bypass through clean tissue planes.[104]

Prosthetic Grafts

PTFE is the most commonly used prosthetic conduit for infrainguinal bypass, although recent reports suggest that in the above-knee position, it is not superior to Dacron.[112-114] A prospective randomized trial from the United Kingdom reported by Devine and colleagues suggested that HBD was superior to PTFE for above-knee popliteal bypasses.[115] The 3-year primary patency for HBD was 55%, compared with 42% for PTFE ($P < .044$). Both of these patency rates are inferior to those of GSV, however, and the early apparent advantage of HBD over PTFE disappeared with longer follow-up.[116]

Vein Cuffs

For bypasses that insert below the knee, the addition of a vein cuff confers a significant patency advantage (52% patency at 2 years for PTFE with vein cuff versus 29% for PTFE with no cuff) and also improves limb salvage (84% versus 62%; $P < .03$).[117] My own experience and that of others suggests that a distal vein cuff or collar results in improved 2- to 3-year patency for infrageniculate bypass when PTFE is required.[118-122] Nevertheless, the results are still inferior to those of vein bypasses, even when using alternative veins; these data emphasize the validity of the all-autogenous policy. If vein is truly limited, however, PTFE is an acceptable choice, and available data suggest that distal anastomotic modification with autogenous tissue is a worthwhile adjunct. The only prospective randomized clinical trial used a Miller cuff (Fig. 109-7).[117] A distal Taylor patch (Fig. 109-8)[118,120] and the St. Mary's boot (Fig. 109-9)[122] may yield equivalent results.

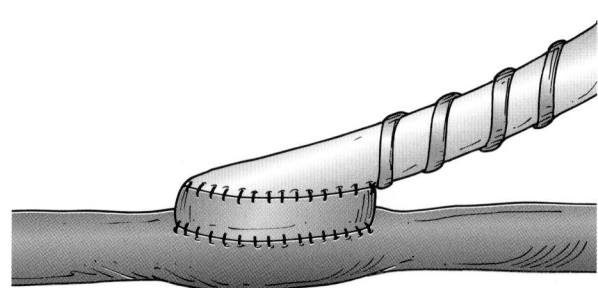

Figure 109-7 The Miller cuff technique[119,302] improved the patency of below-knee popliteal and tibial polytetrafluoroethylene bypass grafts when used as a distal anastomotic adjunct in a controlled randomized clinical trial.[117]

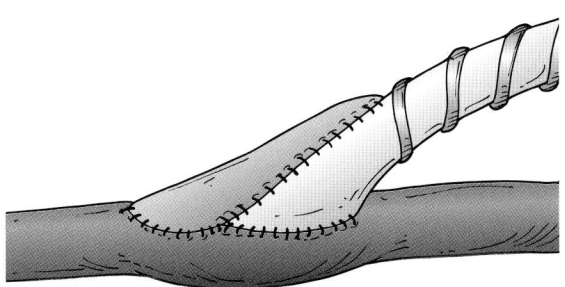

Figure 109-8 The Taylor patch technique can improve the patency of infrageniculate polytetrafluoroethylene bypass grafts.[118,120]

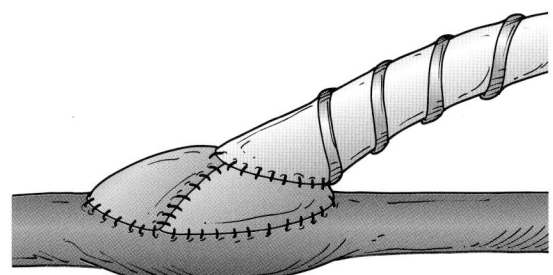

Figure 109-9 The St. Mary's boot or prosthetic venous collar technique[122] combines the attributes of the Taylor patch and the Miller cuff.

Human Umbilical Vein and Adjunctive Arteriovenous Fistula

HUV is less commonly employed than PTFE, primarily because it is thicker and more cumbersome to handle and because of concerns about subsequent aneurysmal degeneration.[123] Dardik and associates reported excellent results using HUV with an adjunctive distal arteriovenous fistula to promote increased graft flow velocity[124]; there are no prospective trials comparing this technique to alternative prosthetic conduits such as PTFE. A single prospective trial did not demonstrate any benefit of the addition of an arteriovenous fistula to femoroinfrapopliteal bypass with vein cuff.[125]

Heparin-Bonded PTFE

The most recent addition to the inventory of prosthetic infrainguinal bypass conduits is ePTFE, to which heparin has been covalently bonded. The commercially available product was originally called Carmedia BioActive Surface (CBAS).[126] Preclinical studies suggest that biologically active heparin has been successfully covalently bonded to ePTFE without causing systemic anticoagulative effects.[127] The drug is biologically active, at least in baboons and dogs, for up to 12 weeks.[128] In animal models of thromboresistance (short 3- and 4-mm grafts), CBAS appears to prevent early ePTFE graft thrombosis; this effect may persist up to 180 days, although not as strikingly. It also appears to reduce early platelet and fibrin deposition in animal models.

There is no proof, however, that these experimental findings will translate into improved prosthetic graft patency in humans. The five published reports of CBAS for peripheral infrainguinal bypass suffer from major flaws, including lack of randomization, lack of control groups, small numbers of patients, selection bias, large numbers of patients with relatively prosthetic-friendly above-knee popliteal insertion sites, lack of intermediate follow-up (beyond 2 years), and flawed or unreliable life-tables.[126,129-132] In two of these five series, anastomotic adjuncts such as patches were used in addition to CBAS grafts, further confounding interpretation. In addition, aggressive combination antiplatelet therapy (oral and low-molecular-weight heparin) was used by nearly all the authors; this combination is not routinely used in North America.

If one assumes that there is no patient overlap between the two studies from the same center (an assumption that may well be false),[129,132] the entire published human experience with CBAS infrainguinal grafts consists of 356 grafts with the following insertion site distribution: 142 (41%) above-knee popliteal, 115 (33.5%) below-knee popliteal, 75 (21.8%) femorocrural or tibial, and 24 indeterminate (one study does not specify target arteries[133]). The estimated number of patients available with documented follow-up in all five human clinical CBAS studies combined is as follows: 95 above-knee popliteal, 45 below-knee popliteal, and 25 femorocrural at 1 year; and 48 above-knee popliteal, 16 below-knee popliteal, and 9 femorocrural at 2 years. The data and follow-up length are thus insufficient to support assertions of improved patency conferred by covalently bonded heparin grafts. Long-term studies of this intriguing bioactive graft are needed to determine whether covalent heparin bonding confers any significant patency benefit. Heparin-induced thrombocytopenia has also been reported with their use.

Graft Comparison

Table 109-1 summarizes the available level I data comparing conduit types with outcome.[114-120,125,134-138] Vein is superior to all prosthetic materials, even in the above-knee position.[138,139,140] The randomized clinical trials comparing HUV with PTFE have been inconclusive.[136,137,141] The addition of rings to PTFE conferred no benefit in the single prospective randomized clinical trial conducted.[142] Thus, the most prudent recommendation is that autogenous vein be used whenever possible for infrainguinal bypass. This dictum holds true not only for primary infrainguinal bypasses but also for reoperations, in which vein conduits outperform all other options.[143,144] For long bypasses, ipsilateral GSV, contralateral GSV, and spliced vein are employed in decreasing order of preference. If only 5 to 15 cm of extra length is required and a more distal origin site is not feasible, eversion endarterectomy of a proximal segment of the SFA with anastomosis to the available vein conduit is a useful technique that avoids the harvesting and splicing of additional vein (Fig. 109-10).[102] For shorter bypasses, arm vein or lower saphenous vein is effective, with the latter being especially useful when a posterior approach is applicable.

If vein is truly unavailable, PTFE, HUV, or Dacron is a reasonable option for above-knee bypass. The initially

Table 109-1 Patency of Above-Knee Popliteal Bypass and Below-Knee Popliteal or Infrapopliteal Bypass Grafts

Graft Type and Study	Patency (%)					P Value
	1-Yr	2-Yr	3-Yr	4-Yr	5-Yr	
Above-Knee Popliteal Bypass: Dacron versus PTFE						
Devine and McCollum, 2004[116] (n = 209)						.055
Heparin-bonded Dacron	71		54	46		
PTFE	62		44	35		
Post et al., 2001[113] (n = 194)						NS
Dacron			64			
PTFE			61			
Green et al., 2000[112] (n = 240)						NS
Dacron					43	
PTFE					45	
Robinson et al., 1999[114] (n = 108)						NS
Dacron	70	56	47			
PTFE	72	52	52			
Above-Knee Popliteal Bypass: HUV versus PTFE						
McCollum et al., 1991[137] (n = 191)						NS (.27)
HUV	68	63	57			
PTFE	61	56	48			
Aalders and van Vroonhoven, 1992[136] (n = 96)						NS
HUV	90	67*			71.4†	
PTFE	80	63			38.7	
Eickhoff et al., 1987[141] (n = 105)						.001
HUV (below knee)	74			42		
PTFE	53			22		
PTFE: Ringed versus Nonringed						
Gupta and Lee, 1991[142] (n = 122; above- and below-knee popliteal bypass)						NS
Ringed			74			
Nonringed			68			
PTFE: Vein Cuff versus No Cuff						
Stonebridge et al., 1997[117] (n = 261)						
Above-knee popliteal						NS
Cuff	80	72				
No cuff	84	70				
Below-knee popliteal						.03
Cuff	80	52				
No cuff	65	29				
Above-Knee Popliteal Bypass: Vein versus Prosthetic (PTFE or HUV)						
Klinkert et al., 2003[138] (n = 151)						.035
Vein					76	
PTFE					52	
Johnson et al., 2000[140] (n = 752)						.01
Vein		81			73	
HUV		70			53	
PTFE		69			39	
Tilanus et al., 1985[298] (n = 49)						<.001
Vein					70	
PTFE					37	
Veith et al., 1986[299] (n = 845)						
Above-knee popliteal (n = 176)						>.25
Vein				61		
PTFE				38		
Below-knee popliteal (n = 153)						<.05
Vein				76		
PTFE				54		
Infrapopliteal (n = 204)						<.001
Vein				49		
PTFE				12		

*Patency determined at 18 months.
†Patency determined at 6 years.
HUV, human umbilical vein; NS, not significant; PTFE, polytetrafluoroethylene.

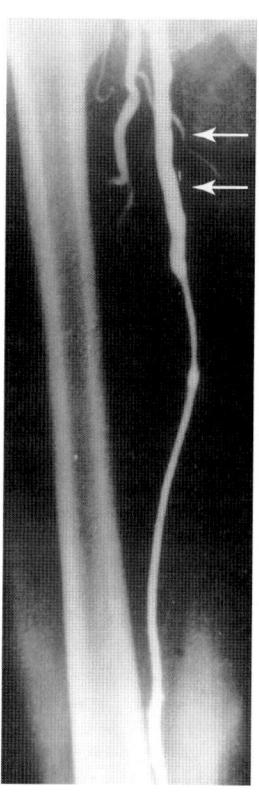

Figure 109-10 When vein length is limited, an eversion endarterectomy of a proximal superficial femoral artery segment (*arrows*) can be performed.[102] The everted arterial segment is anastomosed to the available vein graft to create an all-autogenous conduit of sufficient length to perform the required bypass.

favorable results with HBD were not confirmed during subsequent follow-up,[115,116] so there appears to be no advantage to HBD conduit for above-knee bypass. A recently published prospective randomized trial of HUV versus HBD showed no difference in patency in the above-knee popliteal position,[145] and published trials of PTFE versus Dacron have shown no clear difference.[112-114,116] For infrageniculate insertion sites, PTFE with distal anastomotic modification (cuff, boot, or patch) is recommended if vein is unavailable. There is inadequate evidence to state a preference in terms of standard ePTFE versus heparin-bonded or carbon-coated PTFE. The single prospective randomized trial of standard PTFE versus carbon-impregnated PTFE for infrageniculate bypass showed approximately 30% primary patency, with no difference between groups at 3 years.[146]

BYPASS TECHNIQUE

Reversed, nonreversed, and in situ conduits appear to work equally well. The choice is primarily one of surgeon preference. Arm veins pose special challenges. Regardless of which type of conduit is used, meticulous technique and gentle handling of the vein are critical.

Reversed Vein Bypass

Harvest of the GSV begins with a groin incison two fingerbreadths lateral to the pubic tubercle. Preoperative duplex vein mapping and drawing a line with indelible ink directly over the vein conduit are helpful in following the course of the vein and avoiding the creation of skin flaps. The saphenofemoral junction at the fossa ovalis should be identified to ensure that the GSV and not an anterior or large posteromedial branch is being exposed. Once the main trunk is identified, the incision is extended distally, directly over the vein, with a No. 10 blade or Cooley scissors. I frequently leave short skin bridges, especially in the thigh and about the knee level, to avoid the creation of long flaps. If exposure or branch ligation is difficult, or if the course of the main vein is unclear, the skin directly over the vein is divided. The periadventitial tissue, not the vein wall itself, is grasped gently to avoid damage to the conduit. Side branches are meticulously ligated and divided with 3-0 or 4-0 silk; leaving a short stump is preferable to placing a ligature too close to the main trunk and compromising the lumen. When first exposed, the vein should be soft and blue. Sclerotic segments are whitish and rubbery. Vein spasm can turn a blue vein white and should be treated with local papaverine irrigation.

Sufficient length of vein should be harvested to perform the proposed bypass. If adequate vein of good quality is not available, alternative inflow or outflow arteries should be considered to shorten the bypass; otherwise, alternative vein must be harvested from another site and spliced on a back table. Vein quality is extremely important, and segments less than 3 mm should not be used. Once an adequate length of vein is identified, it is ligated proximally and distally and prepared on the back table by a senior surgeon while the rest of the team exposes the inflow and outflow arteries.

The vein is cannulated with a 3-mm olive tip or Marx tip needle and gently distended with cooled autologous blood (50 to 60 mL) to which 1000 units of heparin and 60 mg of papaverine have been added. The vein should flow readily, should distend smoothly, and should be free of fibrotic, nondistensible segments, strictures at branch ligature sites, and bleeding from missed branches. Missed or small avulsed branches are repaired with longitudinally oriented 6-0 or 7-0 Prolene sutures on a BV-1 or BV-175 needle. Overly forceful distention of the conduit should be avoided because it damages the endothelium. The entire length of the conduit is inspected to ensure that there are no sclerotic areas, no areas of persistent spasm, and no bleeding branches. Once preparation is complete, the distal end of the vein is ligated with 3-0 silk, leaving the suture ends long; the prepared conduit is stored in chilled blood until the graft is ready to be tunneled. Proper intraoperative planning should result in minimal vein storage time. Many believe that autologous blood, rather than saline, better preserves graft endothelium.[147]

Proper graft tunneling of reversed grafts is important. For primary leg bypasses with GSV, I prefer to tunnel the graft in a deep anatomic plane to avoid kinking and graft exposure should wound complications ensue. For above-knee popliteal bypasses, a subsartorial plane is frequently easier than a true anatomic tunnel. A large-caliber hollow-bore metal tunneler with a removable obturator is used. For below-knee popliteal and proximal–to–midposterior tibial or peroneal bypasses, I generally prefer an anatomic tunnel between the two heads of the gastrocnemius for initial bypasses. It is often wise to tunnel reoperative bypasses subcutaneously; this approach avoids scarring and makes graft surveillance and revision easier, which is advantageous because the alternative vein conduits often used in these circumstances are at higher risk for the development of graft stenosis. Bypasses to the anterior tibial artery can be tunneled through the interosseous membrane (anatomic) or a lateral subcutaneous plane.

Arm Vein Harvest and Vein Splicing

If leg vein length is inadequate or unavailable, or if additional conduit is required, arm vein should be used. Arm veins, especially the basilic vein, are more fragile and demanding to harvest. Branches should be carefully identified and ligated a short distance away from their junctions with the main trunk to avoid troublesome bleeding from an injury at the crotch between the branch and the parent vein. Large branches are double-ligated. The initial irrigation and distention of the vein are performed with heparinized saline and papaverine because defects in thinner-walled arm veins are more difficult to visualize and repair if blood is used as the initial irrigant. Once major leaks have been controlled, the vein graft is prepared and stored in chilled blood as mentioned earlier. It is worth considering that arm veins frequently harbor abnormal segments containing intrinsic lesions such as webs, synechiae, and sclerotic valves. Angioscopy of such high-risk conduits may be a useful adjunct (see later under "Angioscopy").

In Situ Vein Bypass

In situ bypass can be used successfully in many patients with intact ipsilateral GSVs. Proponents suggest that the vein-artery size match is frequently optimized by this technique.[148] This technique requires the use of a radial cutting blade (Mills valvulotome)[56] or fixed-diameter circumferential blades such as the Hall[57] or Lemaitre valvulotomes to accomplish valve lysis.[60,149] The proximal segment of GSV is initially mobilized in the groin as it would be for reversed vein bypass, described earlier. The distal GSV is then mobilized in the region of the projected distal arterial anastomosis. The vein may be exposed by an open technique along its entire length, via skip incisions, or endoscopically. After systemic heparinization, the vein is transected below a Satinsky clamp placed at the saphenofemoral junction, and the stump is closed with running 5-0 Prolene suture. The most proximal valve is excised under direct vision with Potts scissors, and the vein is spatulated and sewn end to side to the selected arterial anastomotic site, usually the CFA. Arterial flow is allowed into the vein conduit; if the conduit is of large caliber, a circumferential valvulotome can be inserted from distal to proximal to lyse the valves. Many surgeons prefer to more carefully control valve lysis by progressive serial valvulotomy via large side branches, progressing from proximal to distal. The Mills valvulotome is introduced via side branches; the leaflets are usually just distal to branches and are oriented parallel to the skin. Under arterial pres-

sure, the valve sinuses distend, and the valve leaflets are displaced toward the center of the lumen, where they can be safely engaged by the valvulotome and cut by sharp retraction on the valvulotome under direct visualization. The final valves are lysed from the distal end of the vein. The quality of the vein and the success of lysis are then assessed; flow should be highly pulsatile from the end of the conduit before performing the distal anastomosis.

After completion of the anastomoses, the quality of pulsation and flow is assessed by palpation and hand-held Doppler interrogation. The entire graft should be evaluated from proximal to distal; it can be manually compressed or occluded distal to the Doppler probe. The presence of continuous outflow despite distal graft compression indicates an arteriovenous fistula; these branches should be ligated. With either the reversed or the in situ technique, careful handling of the vein is important. The assurance of adequate valve lysis and the detection of major arteriovenous fistulae can be challenging; the type of completion study used depends on the type, source, and quality of the conduit and surgeon preference.

■ INTRAOPERATIVE COMPLETION STUDIES

Insufficient or inadequate arterial exposure; inappropriate inflow or target artery selection (Fig. 109-11); intrinsic conduit defects; technical defects associated with clamp injury, local endarterectomy, anastomosis creation (Fig. 109-12), and valve lysis; graft tunneling errors (Fig. 109-13); and coagulation or platelet aggregation abnormalities can all complicate infrainguinal bypass. The surgeon should strive to avoid these complications but must be prepared to recognize and correct them should they arise. Ignorance is not bliss, and the best opportunity to correct a problem is at the initial operation. Failing to address a significant defect and hoping for the best compromises patient outcome and increases stress on the operating surgeon. "Take-backs" to the operating room for hemorrhage or graft thrombosis are inevitable, but their frequency can be markedly reduced by meticulous technique, prudent decision making, and routine completion studies to ensure a technically optimal result.

There are four options for completion assessment, which can be used alone or in combination: (1) distal pulse palpation and Doppler flow assessment, with and without manual compression of the graft[150,151]; (2) completion arteriography[152-154]; (3) intraoperative duplex scanning, with and without papaverine administration[155,156]; and (4) angioscopy.[157-169]

Doppler Flow Assessment

Doppler flow assessment should always be performed. Restoration of a palpable distal pulse or Doppler flow that clearly diminishes with manual occlusion of the bypass graft documents graft patency. These techniques are only sufficiently sensitive to detect major conduit, technical, or outflow prob-

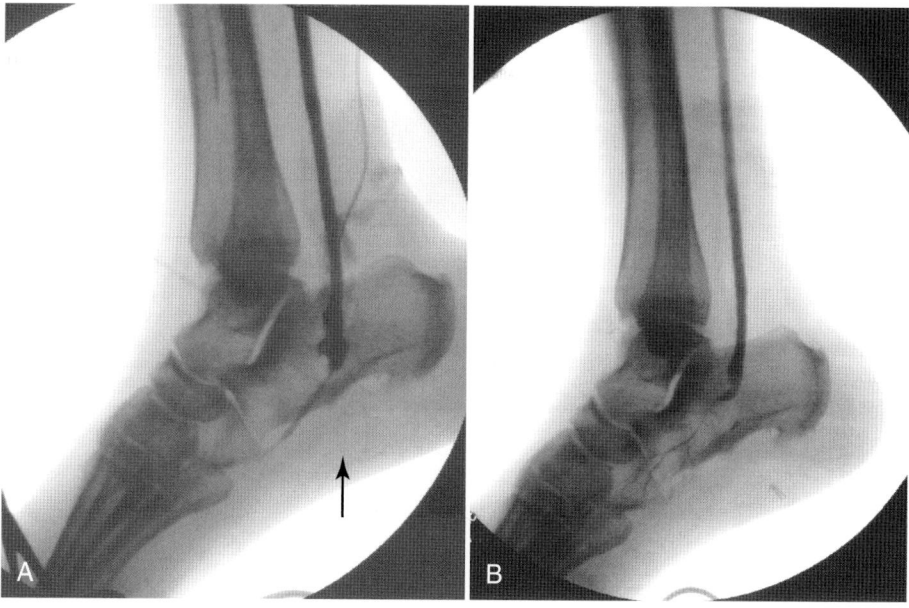

Figure 109-11 A, Completion arteriography demonstrates poor runoff, with minimal branching of the target plantar artery (*arrow*). The initial exposure was inadequate, leading to incorrect selection of the target artery (lateral plantar). **B,** The anastomosis was relocated to the medial plantar artery, and the graft remains patent 2 years postoperatively.

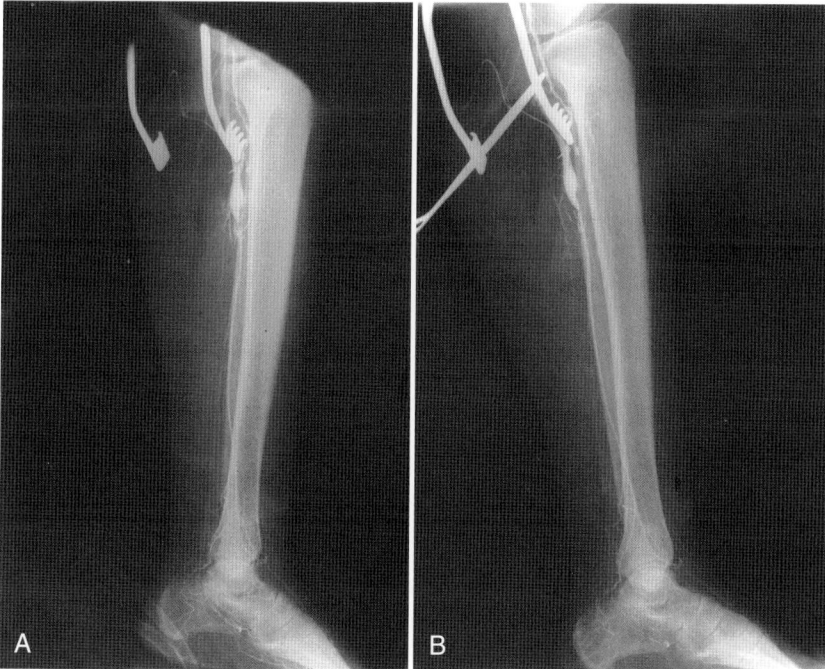

Figure 109-12 A, Completion arteriography identifies a significant distal anastomotic defect, despite a good graft pulse and distal continuous wave Doppler signal. **B,** The anastomosis was re-explored, the defect was corrected, and the graft is patent at 3 years.

lems, however. Therefore, other, more complex techniques should also be employed.

Arteriography

For reversed vein conduits, arteriography is the simplest and most effective completion study. With improved intraoperative imaging capabilities, it has become relatively easy to rapidly evaluate the conduit, tunnel, anastomoses, and outflow for significant graft-threatening lesions with minimal contrast material and little additional time (see Fig. 109-13). Renwick and coworkers identified defects requiring correction in 27%

of infrainguinal bypasses using intraoperative angiography, despite a normal appearance by visual inspection and external pulse palpation.[153] The 2-week primary patency was 100%, compared with 72% in a control group without completion arteriograms. Mills and associates prospectively evaluated 214 consecutive infrainguinal bypass grafts with routine completion angiography and identified significant lesions requiring revision in 8% of grafts, with a higher incidence in tibial than popliteal reconstructions.[152] The 30-day primary patencies were 99% for femoropopliteal bypasses and 93% for femorodistal grafts. Angiography may not be sufficiently sensitive to detect incomplete valve lysis during the performance of in situ or nonreversed grafts.[164,166]

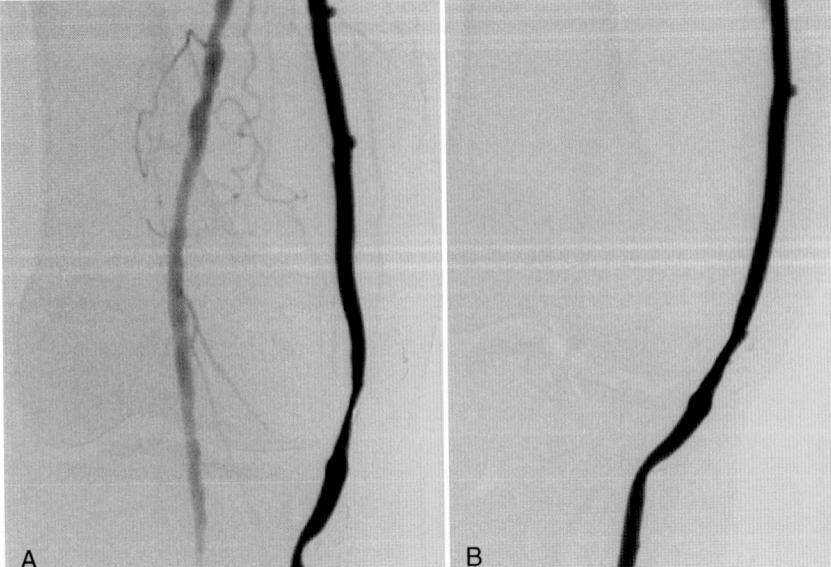

Figure 109-13 A, Routine completion arteriography identifies an unsuspected site of graft compression in the tunnel, despite a good distal graft pulse and continuous wave Doppler signal. **B,** The site was explored, the compression was released, and the graft is patent at 2 years.

Duplex Ultrasound

Bandyk,[155] Johnson,[156] and their colleagues have long championed intraoperative duplex scanning following such reconstructions and report significant abnormalities requiring correction in 12% of cases. Lesions associated with focal peak systolic velocities exceeding 250 cm/sec are repaired. In low-flow grafts without identifiable technical defects, if target artery relocation or graft extension is not possible, consideration is given to either performing an adjunctive arteriovenous fistula to augment graft flow velocity or administering postoperative anticoagulation. The short-term patency of infrainguinal bypasses with normal intraoperative duplex scanning is superb. Intraoperative graft duplex scanning requires the availability of a machine and a technician, however, and most surgeons are less familiar with this technique and find it more cumbersome to use. These issues have prevented its widespread application, although I have found it useful in difficult "redo" cases, particularly when using alternative, spliced, or valve-lysed vein segments.[170]

Angioscopy

Angioscopy has been employed to evaluate the conduit by many clinical investigators,[157-169] who have used it to evaluate harvested arm vein[159] or as an adjunct to valve lysis to permit in situ bypass with minimal skin incisions.[171-173] Marcaccio and associates analyzed the use of intraoperative angioscopy in a series of 113 arm vein bypasses and identified significant intraluminal disease in 62.8% of cases; previous thrombosis with recanalization (54%) was the most commonly encountered lesion, followed by complex weblike lesions at valve sites or possibly associated with previous venipuncture.[165] Angioscopy was used to correct 95.8% of vein abnormalities judged to be significant and allowed an "upgrade" of the conduit quality. The 1-month patency rate was 95.5% in grafts judged to be normal initially or following repair, compared with only 70% in conduits judged to be of inferior quality even after attempted repair. Wilson and colleagues reported a similar yield of prognostically important information with intraoperative angioscopic evaluation of conduits.[158] Angioscopy thus appears to most useful for assessing arm vein conduits or ensuring the adequacy of valve lysis for in situ conduits. Wound and vein harvest incisional complications can compromise outcome and prolong hospital stay.[174-178] Several groups have reported the adjunctive use of angioscopy to both assist in the performance of valve lysis and allow in situ bypass to be performed with minimal skin incisions[162,171-173,179-186]; whether these techniques improve outcome is uncertain.

Some objective assessment of the bypass, its anastomoses, and the outflow is an important component of infrainguinal bypass. I still recommend completion arteriography but recognize that duplex scanning and angioscopy are important adjuncts, especially in higher risk situations and when using nonreversed or in situ conduits in which complete valve lysis is critical. It seems even more important to perform routine completion studies in an era when the volume of open bypass procedures has fallen at most centers owing to a paradigm shift toward endovascular therapy.

RESULTS

Outcomes must be reported according to the Society for Vascular Surgery reporting standards.[5-7,187] Graft patency, limb salvage, and mortality are objective endpoints. Somewhat subjective endpoints are functional outcome and quality of life.

Objective Endpoints

The outcomes of infrainguinal bypass procedures have traditionally been reported solely in terms of graft patency, limb salvage, and patient survival rates. Several factors affect outcome when considered in these terms. Conduit type is the major determinant of long-term graft patency, with vein outperforming prostheses for all varieties of infrainguinal bypass. For vein conduits, vein quality[188-190] and caliber[190-192] are the most critical determinants of success. Vein grafts less than 3 to 3.5 mm in diameter are inferior whether used in situ or reversed.[191,193,194] GSV is superior to alternative vein sources.[110,193] Reduced graft patency has been attributed to high outflow resistance or poor runoff,[190,195,196] although poor runoff is somewhat difficult to define, and autogenous vein grafts frequently remain patent in the presence of rather striking outflow disease (Fig. 109-14). Other factors such as patient age and diabetes do not appear to adversely impact graft patency, although diabetic patients exhibit prolonged wound healing times.[196] Most investigators agree that the presence of end-stage renal failure is associated with reduced graft patency and increased limb loss and mortality.[223,197-205] Anesthetic type has not been conclusively shown to influence graft patency or perioperative mortality.[206,207]

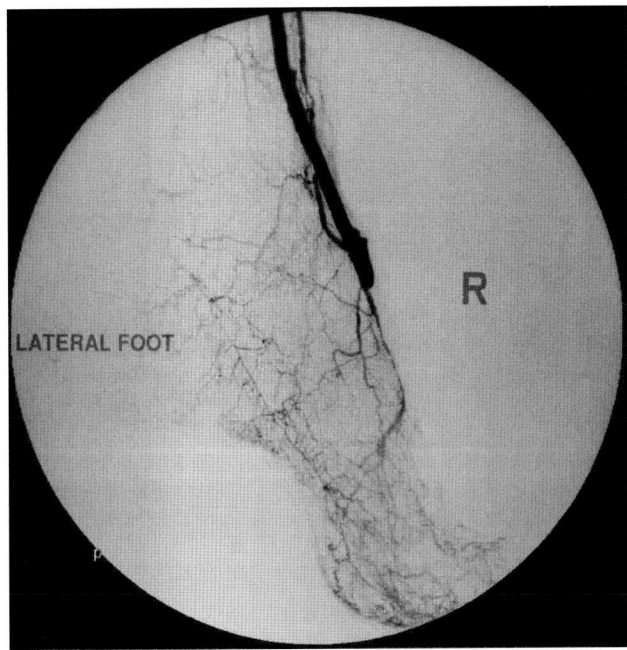

Figure 109-14 Distal view of completion arteriogram following popliteal artery–to–dorsal pedal artery reversed vein bypass in an 82-year-old diabetic man with chronic renal disease and a functioning renal transplant. Despite significant disease of the distal dorsal pedal artery, the patient's toe amputation healed and the graft has remained patent, with normal graft flow velocities, for more than 6 years.

Graft Patency

Patency Definitions. Patency may be primary, assisted primary (most applicable to vein grafts), or secondary. A graft with *primary patency* has been continuously patent without any actions being performed to maintain graft patency, except for treatment of more proximal or distal disease not involving the graft or its anastomoses. Dilatations or minor revisions performed for stenoses or other structural defects before occlusion occurs do not constitute exceptions because they are intended to prevent eventual graft failure.[5-7,187] A graft with *assisted primary patency* required an intervention (either percutaneous or open surgical) to maintain patency but never occluded. A graft with *secondary patency* thrombosed but was successfully thrombectomized. Primary patency thus reflects the durability of the initial reconstruction, assisted primary patency reflects the impact of graft surveillance and timely re-intervention, and secondary patency reflects the persistence of the surgeon in restoring graft patency following failure. The most meaningful endpoints are thus primary and assisted primary patency.

Comparison of Graft Types. Randomized prospective trials demonstrate equivalence between in situ and reversed vein conduits (Table 109-2).[208-215] The use of these techniques is thus dictated by operative considerations and surgeon preference and experience. Vein is superior to all prostheses, even in the above-knee popliteal position. Expected patency data, based on a previously published review by Dalman[216] and several recently published meta-analyses,[136,217-223] are summarized in Tables 109-3 to 109-6 and Figures 109-15 and 109-16.

Table 109-2 Patency of Reversed Vein and In Situ Bypass Grafts

Series and Graft Type	Patency (%)		
	RVG	In Situ	P Value
Watelet et al., 1987[213]: AK/BK popliteal (n = 100 grafts)*	88	71	NS
Harris et al., 1993[210]: AK/BK popliteal (n = 215 grafts)*	77	68	NS
Veterans Administration Cooperative Study Group 1988[208] (n = 461 grafts)†			
BK popliteal	75	78	NS
Infrapopliteal	67	76	NS
Wengerter et al., 1991[216] (n = 125 grafts)‡			
Overall	67	69	NS
<3-mm veins	37	61	NS
Watelet et al., 1997[214] (n = 91 grafts)§	70.2	64.8	NS

*Values at 36 months.
†Values at 24 months.
‡Values at 30 months.
§Ten-year results.
AK, above knee; BK, below knee; NS, not significant; RVG, reversed vein graft.

Table 109-3 Patency of Above-Knee Femoropopliteal Grafts

Graft Type	Primary Patency (%)*					
	1-Mo	*6-Mo*	*1-Yr*	*2-Yr*	*3-Yr*	*4-Yr*
Reversed saphenous vein	99	91	84	82	73	69
Arm vein	99	—	82	65	60	60
Human umbilical vein	95	90	82	82	70	70
Polytetrafluoroethylene	—	89	79	74	66	60

*All series published since 1981.

Table 109-4 Patency of Below-Knee Femoropopliteal Grafts

Graft and Patency Type	Patency (%)*					
	1-Mo	*6-Mo*	*1-Yr*	*2-Yr*	*3-Yr*	*4-Yr*
Primary Patency						
Reversed saphenous vein	98	90	84	79	78	77
In situ vein bypass	95	87	80	76	73	68
Secondary Patency						
In situ vein bypass	97	96	96	89	86	81
Arm vein	97	—	83	83	73	70
Human umbilical vein	88	82	77	70	61	60
Polytetrafluoroethylene	96	80	68	61	44	40
Limb Salvage						
Reversed saphenous vein	100	92	90	88	86	75
In situ vein bypass	97	96	94	84	83	—

*All series published since 1981.

Table 109-5 Patency of Infrapopliteal Grafts

Graft and Patency Type	Patency (%)*					
	1-Mo	*6-Mo*	*1-Yr*	*2-Yr*	*3-Yr*	*4-Yr*
Primary Patency						
Reversed saphenous vein	92	81	77	70	66	62
In situ vein bypass	94	84	82	76	74	68
Secondary Patency						
Reversed saphenous vein	93	89	84	80	78	76
In situ vein bypass	95	90	89	87	84	81
Arm vein	94	—	73	62	58	—
Human umbilical vein	80	65	52	46	40	37
Polytetrafluoroethylene	89	58	46	32	—	21
Limb Salvage						
Reversed saphenous vein	95	88	85	83	82	82
In situ vein bypass	96	—	91	88	83	83
Polytetrafluoroethylene	—	76	68	60	56	48

*All series published since 1981.

Table 109-6 Patency of Ankle and Below-Ankle Grafts

Graft and Patency Type	Patency (%)*				
	1-Mo	*6-Mo*	*1-Yr*	*2-Yr*	*3-Yr*
Primary Patency					
Reversed saphenous vein	95	85	81	—	—
Secondary Patency					
Reversed saphenous vein	96	90	85	81	76
In situ vein bypass	93	93	92	82	72
Foot salvage	99	94	93	87	84

*All series published since 1981.

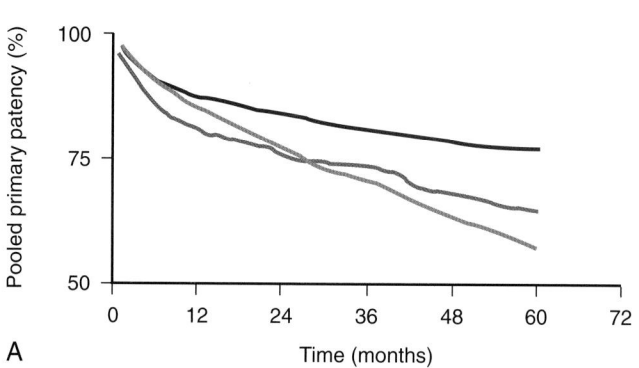

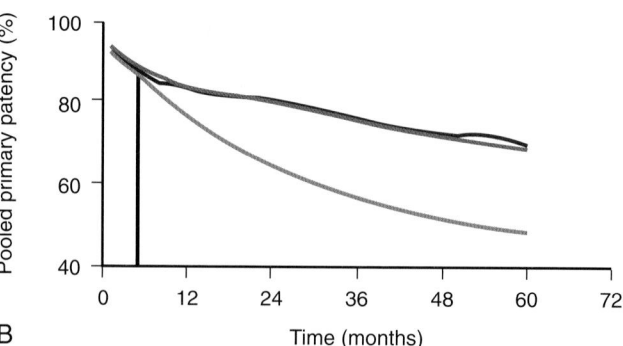

Figure 109-15 A, Meta-analysis of primary patency in claudicants for above-knee femoropopliteal polytetrafluoroethylene (PTFE) bypass grafts (*green line*), above-knee femoropopliteal saphenous vein bypass grafts (*red line*), and below-knee saphenous vein bypass grafts (*blue line*). **B,** Meta-analysis of primary patency in patients with critical ischemia for above-knee femoropopliteal PTFE bypass grafts (*green line*), above-knee femoropopliteal saphenous vein bypass grafts (*red line*), and below-knee saphenous vein bypass grafts (*blue line*). The *vertical line* indicates when above-knee saphenous vein grafts surpassed PTFE grafts.[134]

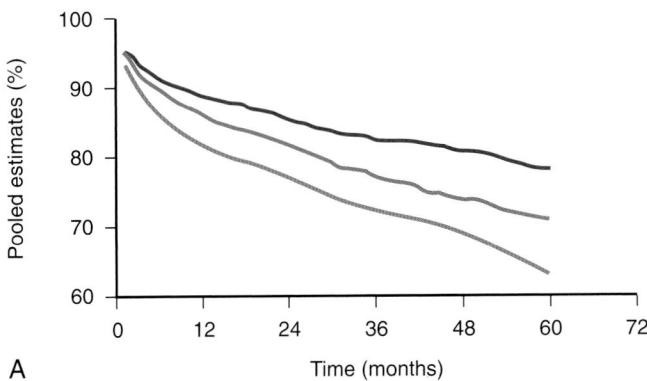

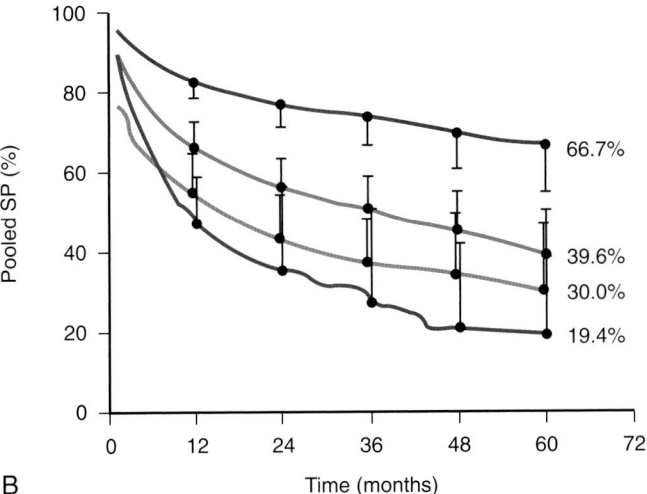

Figure 109-16 Patency of infrageniculate bypass grafts. **A,** Random effects meta-analysis of popliteodistal bypass grafts for primary patency (*green line*), secondary patency (*blue line*), and foot preservation (*red line*).[222] **B,** Meta-analysis survival curve of secondary patency (SP) for alternative autologous vein (*red line*), polytetrafluoroethylene (*blue line*), umbilical cord vein (*green line*), and cryopreserved vein (*purple line*). Bars are half the amplitude of 95% confidence intervals.[221]

Subjective Endpoints

Functional Outcome

While graft patency and limb salvage are objective and important endpoints, numerous investigators have recognized that functional outcomes are equally important. Nicoloff and coworkers emphasized that an ideal outcome—defined by the expectations of a patent graft, healed wound, no need for reoperation, independent living status, and continued ambulation—was extremely difficult to achieve in patients with CLI.[224] Only a small fraction of patients in their report (14.3%) met these basic criteria for success. Golledge and others from South Australia, using similar criteria, showed that only 22% of patients had an ideal outcome.[225] Abou-Zamzam and colleagues identified preoperative independence and ambulation as the best predictors of postoperative independence and continued ambulation.[226] These data emphasize the severity of underlying co-morbidities in CLI patients and the difficulties encountered in obtaining functional limb salvage.

Goshima and coworkers from the University of Arizona analyzed a consecutive series of 318 patients undergoing infrainguinal bypass, 72% for CLI.[227] Three nontraditional outcome measures were used to explore outcomes and define the clinical realities of treating patients with CLI: index limb reoperation rate within 3 months of bypass, hospital readmission rate within 6 months, and wound healing time. Perioperative mortality was less than 1%, mean length of initial hospital stay was 9 days, 30-day graft patency was 97%, and 3-month limb salvage was 97%. Five-year limb salvage in a similar group of patients from the same center was 91%, and the costs of bypass combined with graft surveillance and revision for 5 years were equal to or less than those for patients undergoing major limb amputation.[228] However, 49% of patients required at least one reoperation within 3 months, and 50% required readmission to the hospital within 6 months. The cumulative length of stay for all readmissions was 11 days. More than half of CLI patients required more than 3 months of postoperative care to achieve wound healing. The presence of preoperative tissue loss increased the odds of reoperation by 3.1-fold (95% confidence interval [CI] 1.9 to 6.8), whereas ischemic tissue loss, renal failure, and diabetes were independently associated by multivariate analysis with the need for readmission. Diabetes mellitus was the sole independent risk factor for prolonged wound healing (odds ratio 3.4; 95% CI 2.3 to 6.2).

Further studies using such functional or patient-related outcomes are needed to place the role of infrainguinal bypass in perspective,[222,229-236] particularly to allow comparisons with less invasive techniques such as subintimal angioplasty or even primary amputation in selected high-risk patients with CLI. Although it is generally agreed that nearly all patients with CLI are best treated with surgical revascularization, it is clear that both economic and functional outcome issues mandate the consideration of alternative therapies, at least for certain subsets of patients with CLI, such as individuals confined to chronic care facilities, those who are minimally ambulatory, and patients with extensive tissue loss and infection who are receiving chronic renal replacement therapy.[223,226,233,236-239] This issue is addressed in depth in Chapter 104 (Lower Extremity Arterial Disease: Decision Making and Medical Treatment).

Quality of Life

A substantial amount of new data, derived primarily from two large prospective trials (PREVENT III [Prevention of Recurrent Venous Thromboembolism] and BASIL [Bypass versus Angioplasty in Severe Ischemia of the Leg]),[178,193,204,229,230,240-246] is beginning to put the role of successful bypass in the proper perspective. It also lends support to long-standing impressions regarding the effectiveness of leg bypass in relieving ischemic symptoms and improving quality of life (QoL) in properly selected patients.[229-231,246-251] Patients with true CLI have a markedly reduced QoL compared with a normal control population,[231,246] and their QoL is markedly improved by successful bypass.[246,249,250] It is also becoming evident, especially in CLI patients, that ongoing graft patency, at least for the first 1 to 2 years, is critical to the maintenance of this QoL improvement.[245,246,252,253] Tissue loss at presentation and graft-related events or failure of percutaneous transluminal angioplasty (PTA) during the first 1 to 2 years after the index revascularization are associated with reduced QoL and increased resource utilization. Thus, although the early BASIL results showed no difference in outcomes between bypass and PTA for CLI,[252] the presented but as yet unpublished intermediate follow-up analysis demonstrates that bypass is more effective than PTA in all but the most unfit patients. The bypass-first group had a better amputation-free survival (relative risk [RR] 0.85) and a lower all-cause mortality than the angioplasty-first group (RR 0.65; $P < .009$), likely due to the high failure rate of PTA and the more frequent need for re-intervention to maintain patency (data presented to the Vascular Society of Great Britain, Manchester, November 2007, and to the Veith annual meeting, New York City, November 2008). For patients with severe ischemia, particularly diabetics and those with tissue loss, ongoing vascular patency is important for maintaining QoL and preventing amputation.[227,245] These important findings may eventually lead to a gentle swing of the therapeutic pendulum away from endovascular therapy and back toward open bypass, at least for relatively fit CLI patients with TASC type C or D disease, available vein conduit, and an estimated life expectancy of more than 2 years.[253,254]

POSTOPERATIVE MANAGEMENT

Following bypass, patients should generally be maintained on their preoperative medical regimens for the control of angina, arrhythmia, CHF, and hypertension. Patients with a recent history of CHF are at high risk for prolonged hospital stay and readmission.[204,225,227] Care should be taken to avoid volume overloading in these patients, and they may require supplemental diuresis. Perioperative beta blockade should be continued in the absence of contraindications; in moderate- and high-risk patients undergoing vascular surgery, beta blockade with targeted heart rate control reduces cardiac complications and improves mortality.[16-18]

Antiplatelet Therapy

Most patients with PAD are already receiving antiplatelet therapy, usually aspirin (81 or 325 mg daily). Aspirin has well-recognized cardiac and cerebral protective effects and may also improve early graft patency.[255-265] Clopidogrel may also be used,[266] but it is more expensive and may have an increased risk of complications compared with aspirin alone. Most vascular surgeons consider antiplatelet therapy essential for patients undergoing infrainguinal bypass.

Anticoagulation

There are insufficient data on which to base a recommendation concerning anticoagulation following lower extremity bypass. A single long-term, randomized, prospective trial of 130 patients by Kretschmer and colleagues from Vienna demonstrated improved vein graft patency and limb salvage rates and improved patient survival in those randomized to receive phenprocoumon.[267] An important clinical report, the Dutch Bypass Oral Anticoagulants or Aspirin (BOA) trial, summarized a study of 2690 lower extremity bypass patients randomized to anticoagulation versus antiplatelet therapy (aspirin).[268-270] Although overall differences were not significant, subgroup analysis suggested that oral anticoagulation improved vein graft patency compared with aspirin, whereas aspirin improved prosthetic graft patency compared with anticoagulation. If these data can be confirmed, it would likely alter the typical practice in North America, where surgeons tend to treat vein graft patients with aspirin and to anticoagulate those with prosthetic grafts. The BOA trial, however, noted that anticoagulated patients had nearly double the major bleeding risk of patients on antiplatelet therapy, suggesting that anticoagulation should be used selectively in subgroups at greatest risk.

Such a selective approach has been recommended by the University of Florida group, based on a small randomized study of patients with high-risk vein grafts.[271] High-risk grafts were defined on the basis of poor arterial runoff, suboptimal vein conduit, and reoperative cases. Patency (74%) and limb salvage (81%) rates at 3 years in the high-risk group randomized to warfarin and aspirin were significantly higher than in the aspirin-only group (51% and 31%, respectively), although again, bleeding was much more common in the group receiving warfarin.

Although this seems to be a logical approach, a Veterans Affairs cooperative trial reached a different conclusion based on 665 patients with infrainguinal bypasses who were randomized to aspirin and warfarin versus aspirin alone.[272] Vein graft patency was not increased by the addition of warfarin to aspirin; in contrast, prosthetic graft patency was significantly improved by anticoagulation, but at the expense of double the risk of hemorrhagic events. These data all suggest a potential role for postoperative anticoagulation that requires larger trials with higher statistical power to permit an evidence-based recommendation. Until then, most surgeons will continue to routinely employ antiplatelet therapy (aspirin 81 to 325 mg daily) and add anticoagulation in selected groups at highest risk (e.g., prosthetic infrageniculate grafts, poor outflow, reoperative cases, poor or alternative vein conduit).

Wound Care

All patients with CLI are at risk for pressure ulcers not only in the affected limb but also in the contralateral limb and the sacrum. Unremitting nursing care is essential to prevent these complications. Considerable wound care is also required to achieve healing of ischemic foot lesions and forefoot amputations. Foot infection should have been controlled before revascularization. Basic science wound studies suggest that débridement and formal toe and forefoot amputations for areas of tissue ulceration or gangrene should be delayed 4 to 10 days following bypass to maximize tissue reperfusion and allow the clear demarcation of marginal areas (see Chapter 112: Diabetic Foot Ulcers; Chapter 113: Podiatry Care; Chapter 114: Lower Extremity Amputation: General Considerations; and Chapter 115: Lower Extremity Amputation: Techniques and Results).

COMPLICATIONS

The major early postoperative complications of infrainguinal bypass are wound problems, bleeding, graft occlusion, graft infection, and death (see Table 104-2). The results of the PREVENT III trial from 83 enrolling centers likely reflect realistic complication rates in clinical practice.[242] The authors of this study reported the following early complication rates in a prospective trial of more than 1400 infrainguinal vein grafts in patients with CLI: death (2.7%), myocardial infarction (4.7%), major amputation (1.8%), graft occlusion (5.2%), major wound complications (4.8%), and graft hemorrhage (0.4%). Late complications include persistent lymphedema, graft infection, graft aneurysm, and graft stenosis.

Early Graft Occlusion

With experienced judgment and intraoperative attention to detail, early graft occlusion should be an uncommon event. Should a graft fail in the early postoperative period, the most important principle is to identify and correct the underlying cause.[273] If no cause can be identified, the prognosis for long-term patency is poor. The outcome is much more favorable if the cause can be ascertained and addressed. The most common correctable culprits are anastomotic, local endarterectomy, or clamp defects; valve defects; poor conduit quality; or inadequate outflow. When the patient is returned to the operating room, one can usually begin by exploring the distal anastomosis first. If the graft hood is pulsatile, an arteriogram is performed. If not, the hood is opened and gentle distal thrombectomy and graft thrombectomy are performed with balloon catheters of appropriate caliber. If the graft is a reversed vein, both proximal and distal anastomoses usually require exploration. An uninflated balloon catheter is passed from proximal to distal; a second catheter can be tied to the first one and drawn uninflated proximally. The tie is cut, the second catheter is inflated, and the graft is then thrombectomized from proximal to distal. Once the thrombus has been evacuated, heparinized saline is forcibly irrigated through the graft to flush any residual thrombotic debris out the distal graftotomy. Both anastomoses can then be carefully inspected; if a distal anastomotic defect is identified, the graftotomy can be extended down the outflow artery and closed with a patch. If no defects are identified, the graft incisions are closed, and thorough arteriography of the entire graft and the outflow is performed. Significant conduit or anastomotic lesions should

be corrected. If unsuspected or previously unappreciated outflow disease is identified, the graft should be extended beyond the lesion or to an alternative outflow artery if available. If a marginal vein conduit was used at the initial procedure and no focal defect is identified at re-exploration, one should consider replacing the conduit; this decision is difficult and may require the harvesting of additional vein or, if none is available, converting to a prosthetic conduit if outflow is sufficient.

Late Graft Occlusion

Late graft occlusion should be treated only if the patient's symptoms are severe enough to warrant intervention. When vein conduit is limited, I attempt thrombolysis, mechanical thrombectomy, or both and treat the underlying lesion responsible for graft failure. The results of this approach are generally poor, however. My preference for late graft occlusions is to perform a new bypass with autogenous vein, which provides superior results and durability.[144] If vein is unavailable and thrombolysis is contraindicated or fails, a "redo" bypass with PTFE and a vein patch or cuff is the best option. The optimal therapy for graft occlusion is to prevent its occurrence by identifying graft-threatening stenosis before the onset of graft occlusion through routine postoperative duplex graft surveillance.

GRAFT SURVEILLANCE

Vein graft surveillance is critical to the long-term outcome of infrainguinal bypass. It has been well documented for more than 3 decades that nearly one third of autogenous vein grafts develop lesions that threaten graft patency.[274] Most such lesions, especially in the first 1 to 2 years following graft implantation, are intrinsic to the graft itself and result from intimal hyperplasia.[275-277] Later, inflow and outflow lesions may develop and reduce graft flow, thus threatening ongoing graft patency. All these lesions can be readily identified, graded for severity, and monitored for progression by means of a simple program of ABI determination and duplex graft surveillance.[108,212,228,278-289] I obtain the first study within 4 weeks of surgery, either before hospital discharge or at the first postoperative visit.[279] Serial studies are performed every 3 months for 1 year, every 6 months for 2 additional years, and annually thereafter. Grafts with focal lesions associated with a peak systolic velocity greater than 300 cm/second or a velocity ratio greater than 3.5 to 4.0 undergo prophylactic repair to prevent graft stenosis.[287,288] Grafts that develop low-flow velocities over time (peak systolic velocity <45 cm/sec throughout the graft) or a drop in ABI exceeding 0.15 in the absence of detectable graft lesions undergo arteriography to search for inflow, outflow, or missed graft lesions. Abundant clinical data from multiple investigators and a single prospective randomized trial by Lundell and associates[290] suggest that vein graft surveillance improves long-term vein graft patency by approximately 15%. Although one trial questioned the benefit of vein graft surveillance,[244] that surveillance protocol was flawed, the endpoints were inappropriate, and the follow-up was too short to detect a difference.[284] Cost-benefit analyses both in Europe[289] and in the United States[228] confirm that vein graft surveillance is cost-effective. Graft occlusion is a morbid and costly event,[228,245] and its prevention is worthwhile. Graft surveillance of prosthetic grafts has not been shown to be beneficial.[291,292]

■ TREATMENT OF GRAFT AND ANASTOMOTIC STENOSES

Graft stenoses are solitary and focal in approximately 80% of cases. Multiple focal synchronous or metachronous lesions are identified in 15% to 20% of grafts; diffuse long-segment graft narrowing, presumably due to myointimal hyperplasia, is uncommon (3% to 5% of cases).[276] If recurrent limb ischemia requires treatment in the latter circumstance, graft replacement is the treatment of choice.

There are multiple options for the treatment of focal graft lesions; selection of the optimal therapy depends primarily on the length of the lesion, the timing of its occurrence (early [<3 to 6 months] versus late [>3 to 6 months]), and patient co-morbidities. Focal lesions that develop after the sixth post-operative month respond fairly well to PTA,[293,294] and recent data suggest that use of a cutting balloon is superior to standard balloon angioplasty.[295,296] If a graft stenosis is treated by PTA, it should be closely followed by duplex ultrasound because the recurrence rate is generally higher than after open repair. Stent placement in infrainguinal vein grafts should be avoided.

If open repair is chosen, there are several options, depending primarily on the characteristics and location of the lesion. Circumferentially fibrotic midgraft lesions are best treated with excision and segmental interposition vein grafts. Less extensive lesions are amenable to vein patch angioplasty. There are no data demonstrating the superiority of patch versus interposition grafting,[283] but circumferentially fibrotic, napkin ring–like lesions are better treated with replacement. Focal, less fibrotic lesions, particularly related to valves, can be treated with valve excision and vein patch through a longitudinal graftotomy that extends proximal and distal to the site of the lesion. An intraoperative completion angiogram or duplex scan should be performed to document resolution of the lesion.

Focal juxta-anastomotic lesions often develop in the vein graft itself, immediately adjacent to the arterial anastomosis.[276] These lesions can be treated by either patch angioplasty or short interposition grafts (Fig. 109-17). Another option that eliminates the need to harvest additional vein conduit is proximal anastomotic translocation.[297] This procedure involves resecting the lesion and oversewing the graft stump near its origin. If the vein graft below the stenosis is of good caliber, the graft can be transposed to an alternative inflow artery. For example, if the original anastomosis was to the CFA, and if the PFA is large and its origin is free of disease, the PFA can be exposed, and the graft can be mobilized below the proximal stenosis and swung over or transposed to reorigi-

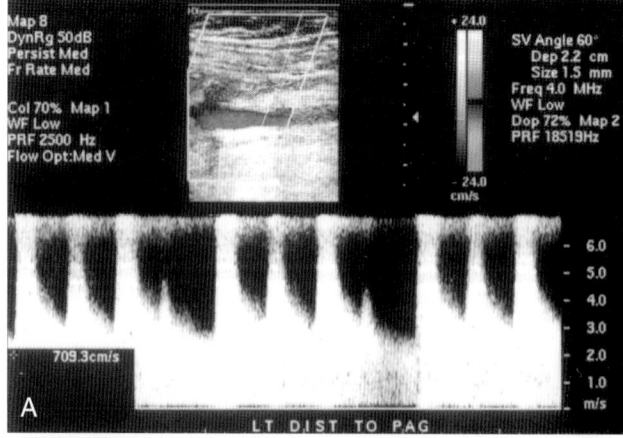

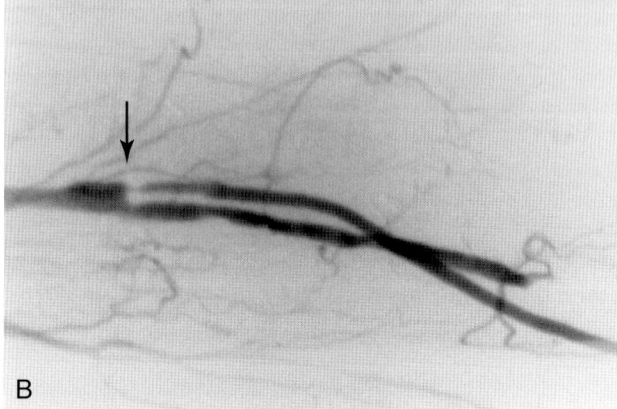

Figure 109-17 Duplex surveillance identified a critical vein graft stenosis in the proximal aspect of a femoropopliteal vein graft. **A,** Marked spectral broadening and pronounced elevation of both the peak systolic and end-diastolic velocities is diagnostic of a high-grade vein graft stenosis. **B,** A focal, severe proximal graft stenosis (*arrow*) was confirmed by arteriography and treated with a short interposition vein graft harvested from the upper extremity.

nate from the PFA. Distal juxta-anastomotic stenoses can usually be vein patched, but if the outflow artery has also developed progressive occlusive disease, a better option is a jump graft to a more distal target artery if one is available. These procedures have been described in detail elsewhere.[297]

Acknowledgments

The illustrations were drawn by Joseph L. Mills, Jr.

SELECTED KEY REFERENCES

Conte MS, Bandyk DF, Clowes AW, Moneta GL, Seely L, Lorenz TJ, Namini H, Hamdan AD, Roddy SP, Belkin M, Berceli SA, DeMasi RJ, Samson RH, Berman SS, PREVENT III Investigators. Results of PREVENT III: a multicenter, randomized trial of edifoligide for the prevention of vein graft failure in lower extremity bypass surgery. *J Vasc Surg.* 2006;43:742-751.
  Landmark study of a novel molecular therapy for the prevention of vein graft failure in patients undergoing infrainguinal revascularization for CLI. Despite a well-conceived trial design, an impeccably executed study, and high-quality surgical results at multiple centers, the proposed molecular therapy was found to result in no significant improvement in any of the primary endpoints.

Edwards JM, Taylor LM, Porter JM. Treatment of failed lower extremity bypass with new autogenous vein bypass. *J Vasc Surg.* 1990;11: 132-145.

This study argues strongly for the performance of a new vein bypass as the most definitive and durable therapy after failure of a previously placed graft.

Faries PL, Arora S, Pomposelli FB Jr, Pulling MC, Smakowski P, Rohan DI, Gibbons GW, Akbari CM, Campbell DR, LoGerfo FW. The use of arm vein in lower-extremity revascularizations: results of 520 procedures performed in eight years. *J Vasc Surg.* 2000;31:50-59.

This Boston group has long championed an all-autogenous approach. Their study shows that autogenous arm vein can be used successfully in a wide variety of lower extremity revascularization procedures and achieves excellent patency and limb salvage rates, generally much higher than those reported for prosthetic or cryopreserved grafts.

Mills JL, Fujitani RM, Taylor SM. The characteristics and anatomic distribution of lesions that cause reverse vein graft failure: a five-year prospective study. *J Vasc Surg.* 1993;17:195-206.

Postoperative duplex surveillance was prospectively performed over a 66-month period in 227 patients after infrainguinal vein graft placement to determine the causes of graft failure. The authors found that a significant portion of these failures occurred during the intermediate postoperative period (3 to 18 months), usually as a result of focal intrinsic vein graft lesions that are readily detectable by duplex. They concluded that duplex vein graft surveillance is warranted by the 21% incidence of potentially remediable graft failure.

Stonebridge PA, Prescott RJ, Ruckley CV. Randomized trial comparing infrainguinal polytetrafluoroethylene bypass grafting with and without vein interposition cuff at the distal anastomosis. The Joint Vascular Research Group. *J Vasc Surg.* 1997;26:543-550.

This study was undertaken to determine whether an interposition vein cuff improved the short- and medium-term patency and limb salvage rates of femoral above-knee and below-knee popliteal artery PTFE bypass procedures. The authors found that there was no improvement in patency rate with the use of a distal anastomosis interposition vein cuff in above-knee PTFE grafts, but there was a statistically significant advantage when PTFE grafts were anastomosed to the popliteal artery below the knee. Vein cuffs or patches seem to be beneficial in those relatively uncommon patients requiring infrageniculate bypass in whom autogenous vein is not available.

Szilagyi DE, Elliot J, Hageman JH, Smith RF, Dall'olmo CA. Biologic fate of autogenous vein implants as arterial substitutes: clinical, angiographic, and histo-pathological observations in femoro-popliteal operations for atherosclerosis. *Ann Surg.* 1973;178:232-246.

Infrainguinal vein grafts implanted in 377 patients over a 10-year period were studied by serial arteriography to determine their natural history. This study set an early standard for long-term follow-up and demonstrated its importance in patients undergoing such procedures.

Watelet J, Soury P, Menard JF, Plissonnier D, Peillon C, Lestrat JP, Testart J. Femoropopliteal bypass: in situ or reversed vein grafts? Ten-year results of a randomized prospective study. *Ann Vasc Surg.* 1997;11:510-519.

Long-term studies with good follow-up provide the best information about treating patients with chronic diseases. For example, this study reported the results of 100 femoropopliteal bypass procedures performed in 91 patients over 5 years who were randomly divided into two statistically comparable groups: 50 in situ vein grafts and 50 reversed vein grafts. One conclusion: small veins do not work as well, even when used in situ.

REFERENCES

The reference list can be found on the companion Expert Consult Web site at *www.expertconsult.com.*

CHAPTER 110

Infrainguinal Disease: Endovascular Treatment

Mikel Sadek and Peter L. Faries

Endovascular treatment (ET) is increasingly the first option for treating infrainguinal peripheral arterial disease (PAD). Percutaneous transluminal angioplasty (PTA) with adjunctive stenting is a well-validated and increasingly used technology, and it is the technique most frequently employed for infrainguinal ET. An alternative to transluminal angioplasty is subintimal angioplasty (SIA), also referred to as percutaneous intentional extraluminal revascularization. SIA is used to cross occluded vascular lesions, and recanalization is performed by intentionally exiting the vascular lumen, entering the subintimal plane, and then reentering the vascular lumen distal to the lesion. The diseased arterial segment is subsequently balloon-dilated in the subintimal plane to achieve revascularization.[1] Stenting is an adjunctive procedure used either routinely or selectively for the treatment of complex lesions or persistent stenosis or to correct intraprocedural complications.

Early experiences with PTA of lower extremity lesions were characterized by poor immediate and long-term outcomes.[2,3] Factors contributing to these poor outcomes included the presence of long-segment disease, compromised distal outflow, and the presence of chronic occlusion. ET of infrainguinal PAD has since gained acceptance owing to reported improvements in outcome and diminished rates of morbidity and mortality compared with standard surgical bypass.[4-6] Novel technologies and refinements of previous technologies are enabling ET for increasingly complex vascular pathology. Patients with multiple co-morbidities or those lacking adequate autogenous conduits may derive particular benefit from an endovascular approach, because the utility of standard bypass is more limited in these cases.[7]

This chapter focuses on the measures of success for infrainguinal ET, the factors that influence procedural outcome, and the results from recent clinical trials that demonstrate the safety and efficacy of infrainguinal ET. For additional information on preoperative testing, planning, and specific endovascular techniques, refer to Chapter 85 (Technique: Endovascular Therapeutic), Chapter 103 (Lower Extremity Arterial Disease: General Considerations), and Chapter 104 (Lower Extremity Arterial Disease: Decision Making and Medical Treatment).

ENDOVASCULAR PLANNING

Most studies demonstrate that infrainguinal ET can be carried out with limited periprocedural risk.[8,9] Nevertheless, the deci-

sion to proceed with infrainguinal ET rather than an open surgical approach requires a thorough risk-to-benefit analysis based on the information acquired from the history, physical examination, noninvasive imaging, and diagnostic angiography. Salient features of the history and physical examination when planning an intervention include (1) indication (claudication versus critical limb ischemia [CLI]), (2) disease location and severity, (3) extent of disability and lifestyle limitations, (3) medical co-morbidities and anesthetic risk, (4) prior lower extremity reconstructions or interventions, and (5) prospects for long-term functional status and survival. For detailed discussions of duplex ultrasonography, computed tomographic angiography (CTA), magnetic resonance angiography (MRA), and digital subtraction angiography, refer to Chapter 103 (Lower Extremity Arterial Disease: General Considerations). Additional variables that may influence the decision-making process include the expertise of the treating physician, the consequences of ET failure, and the long-term costs of care.

GUIDELINES FOR TREATMENT

Guidelines for infrainguinal ET have evolved with the accumulation of experience and data. In 1994, the American Heart Association (AHA) Task Force compiled a list of recommendations for the use of PTA in the infrarenal vasculature.[10] The anatomic criteria were divided into four categories of increasing severity, based on the premise that milder disease should be managed with PTA and more complex disease should be managed with surgical revascularization. The AHA Task Force criteria were formulated in general terms and relied on a body of evidence collected before the routine use of stenting. Improvements in reporting standards, longer postintervention follow-up, advances in technique, and the more prevalent use of adjunctive technologies such as stenting have contributed to improved outcomes and consequently to refinements in the guidelines for ET of infrainguinal PAD.[11,12] The revised Trans-Atlantic Inter-Society Consensus (TASC) guidelines are the most recent to be devised.[12] These guidelines distinguish the treatment of femoropopliteal and infrapopliteal disease.

Femoropopliteal

The new TASC femoropopliteal criteria reflect the fact that increasingly complex disease can be managed using endovascular techniques (Table 110-1). TASC type A lesions are

Table 110-1 Trans-Atlantic Inter-Society Consensus Classification of Femoropopliteal Disease

Type	Lesion Characteristics
A	Single stenosis ≤10 cm Single occlusion ≤5 cm
B	Multiple stenoses or occlusions, each ≤5 cm Single stenosis or occlusion ≤15 cm not involving infrageniculate popliteal artery Single or multiple lesions in the absence of continuous tibial vessels to improve inflow for tibial bypass Heavily calcified occlusion ≤5 cm Single popliteal stenosis
C	Multiple stenoses or occlusions totaling >15 cm with or without heavy calcification Recurrent stenoses or occlusions that need treatment after two endovascular interventions
D	Chronic occlusion of common or superficial femoral artery >20 cm or involving popliteal artery Chronic occlusion of popliteal artery and proximal trifurcation vessels

Table 110-2 Categories of Chronic Limb Ischemia

Grade	Category	Clinical Description	Objective Criteria
0	0	Asymptomatic disease	Normal treadmill or reactive hyperemia test
	1	Mild claudication	Completes treadmill exercise*; AP after exercise >50 mm Hg but at least 20 mm Hg lower than resting value
I	2	Claudication between categories 1 and 3	Between categories 1 and 3
	3	Moderate claudication	Cannot complete standard treadmill exercise*; AP after exercise <50 mm Hg
II†	4	Severe claudication	Resting AP <40 mm Hg; ankle or metatarsal PVR flat or barely pulsatile; TP <30 mm Hg
III†	5	Ischemic rest pain	Resting AP <60 mm Hg; ankle or metatarsal PVR flat or barely pulsatile; TP <40 mm Hg
	6	Minor tissue loss‡ Major tissue loss§	Same as 5

*Five minutes at 2 miles per hour on a 12% incline.
†Grades II and III correspond to critical limb ischemia.
‡Nonhealing ulcer or focal gangrene with diffuse pedal ischemia.
§Extending above transmetatarsal level, or foot no longer salvageable.
AP, ankle pressure; PVR, pulse volume recording; TP, toe pressure.

suitable candidates for ET; TASC type D lesions necessitate surgery, owing to ET's prohibitive failure rate; and TASC types B and C lesions can be treated using either endovascular or surgical revascularization, depending on the clinical scenario. There is some evidence that in patients with high-grade disease (e.g., TASC type C or D) who are facing imminent limb loss but are not candidates for surgical reconstruction, endovascular reconstruction may be beneficial.[13-17] For a detailed description of the TASC classification system, see Chapter 104 (Lower Extremity Arterial Disease: Decision Making and Medical Treatment).

Infrapopliteal

Consensus regarding the effectiveness of ET for infrapopliteal arterial occlusive disease is limited. This is reflected by the TASC guidelines, which do not delineate specific anatomic criteria for infrapopliteal ET.[12] These guidelines state that infrapopliteal angioplasty and stenting should be reserved for limb salvage therapy; there is insufficient evidence to recommend their use for the treatment of intermittent claudication. The only specific recommendation is that in a patient with CLI and medical co-morbidities who is being treated for infrapopliteal occlusion, ET may be attempted if in-line flow to the foot can be re-established. The TASC guidelines also mention that failed angioplasty usually does not preclude subsequent bypass. Therefore, as is the case with femoropopliteal disease, if a patient is at high risk for surgical bypass and is facing imminent limb loss, PTA may be considered to avoid amputation.[18,19]

RESULTS

Reporting Standards

The revised Society for Vascular Surgery Lower Extremity Ischemia Reporting Standards (also known as the Rutherford guidelines) emphasize the need for uniform and objective criteria for evaluating the success of interventions for infrainguinal PAD.[20] These guidelines recommend the use of specific clinical criteria or stages, as well as vascular laboratory data, to evaluate outcomes. With respect to chronic limb ischemia, affected limbs are categorized according to the following spectrum of symptoms: asymptomatic disease, mild claudication, moderate claudication, severe claudication, ischemic rest pain, minor tissue loss, and major tissue loss (Table 110-2). Additional clinical and noninvasive hemodynamic criteria are used to quantitate changes in preprocedure and postprocedure clinical status (see Table 103-3 in Chapter 103: Lower Extremity Arterial Disease: General Considerations).[20] Although the revised Rutherford guidelines remain the standard for reporting on lower extremity PAD, they have been applied more consistently to reports of surgery than to those of ET. Consequently, it may be useful to update and re-enforce the use of standardized criteria for reporting the outcomes of lower extremity PAD treated endovascularly.[21]

Definitions of Successful Intervention

The complexity of infrainguinal ET has resulted in the creation of multiple definitions of success. The measures of success reported most commonly in the literature include clinical response with regard to symptom resolution and limb salvage, technical success, primary patency, assisted primary patency, secondary patency, and target lesion revascularization. Depending on the study design and the intent of the investigators, significant variability exists in the use of these outcomes.

Clinical Response

The literature is characterized by significant heterogeneity in the reporting of clinical status for patients with infrainguinal PAD treated with ET. The clinical variables that are evaluated most commonly and exhibit the greatest clinical relevance are resolution of symptoms, limb salvage, and patient survival.

Resolution of symptoms and limb salvage have been defined using various combinations of the following clinical criteria: sustained absence of symptoms or improvement by at least one (claudication) or two (tissue loss) categories according to the Rutherford classification; freedom from claudication among claudicants; 50% improvement in claudication distance; complete resolution of rest pain; relief of rest pain without the use of analgesics; resolution of claudication or rest pain and healing of ulcers with no or only minor amputations at 6 weeks; healing of ulcers; total ulcer healing; healing of minor amputations required for gangrene; freedom from areas of gangrene; absence of any requirement for revascularization; freedom from minor amputations; absence of amputation; standing and walking without a prosthesis; freedom from amputations proximal to the forefoot or ankle; and freedom from any clinical deterioration. The most appropriate measure of clinical response according to the revised Rutherford guidelines combines clinical and noninvasive imaging data—for example, an increase of at least 1 point on the Rutherford scale concomitant with an ankle-brachial index (ABI) improvement of 0.15 or greater.[20]

Technical Success

The majority of studies have used angiographic criteria to define the technical success of infrainguinal ET. Technical success is most often defined as the presence of antegrade flow through the treated lesion at the termination of the procedure.[22-24] Certain studies have added further refinements and other requirements, such as the presence of less than 25% to 30% residual stenosis by angiography at the termination of the procedure, flow to the pedal arch, and vascular laboratory studies demonstrating a duplex-derived peak systolic velocity ratio of 1.5 or less at the treatment site or an ABI improvement of 0.15 or greater.[25-28] One study specifically defined technical success as good flow on angiography at the termination of the procedure and good flow on duplex ultrasonography before hospital discharge.[29] Conversely, technical failure has been defined as failure to revascularize the target vascular lesion.[30]

Hemodynamic Success

In addition to the concepts of clinical response and technical success, hemodynamic success is used to document the degree to which the procedure has improved limb blood flow. Hemodynamic success is defined as an increase in ABI of 0.10 to 0.15 or greater. Conversely, an ABI increase of less than 0.10 to 0.15 or a decrease in ABI is considered a hemodynamic failure.[20] Another reported definition of hemodynamic success is the absence of an ABI decrease greater than 0.15 from the maximum early postprocedural level, or the demonstration of biphasic or triphasic waveforms with a peak systolic velocity less than 200 cm/sec or a peak systolic velocity ratio less than 2 at the site of the intervention.[31] Using angiographic criteria, hemodynamic success has also been defined as the absence of occlusion or less than 30% to 50% residual stenosis in the treated vessel.[32,33] According to the Rutherford guidelines, hemodynamic success must be accompanied by an improvement in clinical response to be designated a clinical success.[20]

Primary Patency

The definition of primary patency has been variably interpreted in different studies. For arterial grafts, the definition of patency is clear, but in most cases of ET, the artery was patent before treatment, so most investigators have included recurrent stenosis as well as thrombosis in the definition of patency after ET. Primary patency is most frequently defined as the duration of follow-up in which there is an absence of occlusion or significant restenosis within the treated segment. For the definition of primary patency, the degree of allowable restenosis varies between 30% and 50%, depending on the cited literature.[34-36] Other reported measures of primary patency have used data from noninvasive vascular studies to define significant recurrent stenosis: velocity ratio greater than 2 or ABI decrease greater than 0.15 results in loss of primary patency.[23,26,37] Primary patency is typically reported in the context of a Kaplan-Meier life-table analysis.

Assisted Primary Patency

The definition of assisted primary patency is simply primary patency (as defined earlier) requiring the assistance of a subsequent interventional procedure to maintain patency or treat a significant recurrent stenosis. Typically, re-intervention in nonoccluded but restenotic arteries carries the same or lower risks of morbidity and mortality as those associated with primary ET.[38] In addition, lower rates of primary patency have been observed for infrainguinal PAD compared with more proximal arterial vasculature disease. Therefore, in conjunction with aggressive postprocedural monitoring, preocclusion re-intervention may be required to prolong the duration of clinical patency in the cohort of patients undergoing infrainguinal ET. Assisted primary patency is reported with Kaplan-Meier life-table analysis.

Secondary Patency

The definition of secondary patency differs from that of assisted primary patency in that it refers to patency that has been restored after occlusion of the treated arterial segment. Salvage of an occlusive lesion is currently achieved with safety and efficacy levels that approach those reported for re-intervention of a preocclusive lesion. Therefore, outcomes reported in terms of secondary patency are frequently similar to those using assisted primary patency. Secondary patency is also reported with Kaplan-Meier life-table analysis.

Target Lesion Revascularization

The concept of target lesion revascularization (TLR) was first applied to the percutaneous treatment of coronary artery disease to accurately identify the need to re-intervene in a previously treated atherosclerotic lesion.[39,40] TLR is typically defined as a re-intervention performed on a restenosis at or within 5 mm of the lesion treated during the index procedure. In contrast, target vessel revascularization is defined as any repeat intervention, whether endovascular or open, that occurs in the same vessel treated during the index procedure. The concept of TLR is used to assess the safety and efficacy of percutaneous treatment, and the information it provides differs from that obtained from evaluating patency. TLR may, however, overestimate the benefit of an intervention because patients may elect not to undergo repeat intervention if their symptoms are mild, such as claudication. Thus, significant restenosis could occur at the site of ET for claudication, causing a return of symptoms but no TLR. For this reason, most regard TLR as a less accurate reporting method than the patency measures described earlier.

Determinants of Outcome

The primary determinants of outcome for patients undergoing infrainguinal ET include lesion characteristics, pattern of vascular disease, patient demographics and co-morbid diseases, clinical situation, and intraprocedural factors (Box 110-1). The majority of data can be gathered preoperatively during the history and physical examination and through the use of noninvasive testing. At the time of intervention, additional information with regard to lesion-specific characteristics may be obtained.

Lesion Characteristics

Location. ET of proximal, larger caliber arteries results in improved immediate and long-term outcomes compared with the treatment of distal, smaller caliber arteries. Improved long-term patency has been reported for aortic and iliac artery lesions compared with infrainguinal lesions.[41,42] For infrainguinal disease, preliminary results suggest a trend toward improved outcomes following the treatment of femoropopliteal lesions compared with infrapopliteal lesions.[43,44] This trend is reflected in the revised TASC criteria, which delin-

---

> **Box 110-1 Determinants of Outcome of Endovascular Treatment**
>
> **LESION CHARACTERISTICS**
> - Lesion location
> - Stenosis versus occlusion
> - Lesion length
> - Multiple same-segment stenoses
>
> **PATTERN OF VASCULAR DISEASE**
> - Multilevel disease
> - Runoff status
>
> **PATIENT DEMOGRAPHICS**
> - Gender
> - Co-morbidities (e.g., diabetes)
>
> **CLINICAL SITUATION**
> - Indication for intervention
> - Recurrent stenosis
>
> **INTRAPROCEDURAL FACTORS**
> - Dissection or residual stenosis
> - Initial hemodynamic response

---

eate a broad range of indications for ET of femoropopliteal lesions but continue to restrict infrapopliteal ET to limb salvage therapy.[12]

Stenosis versus Occlusion. Historically, ET of stenotic lesions yields better immediate and long-term outcomes than does the treatment of occluded lesions.[45-47] However, more recent data indicate an improvement in the technical success rates associated with the treatment of occluded lesions.[1] Long-term outcomes with regard to symptom resolution, limb salvage, and clinical patency continue to be superior for stenoses compared with occlusions. This may be a reflection of the increased overall disease burden that accompanies occlusive lesions.[8,46] Accordingly, the TASC criteria characterize occlusion as an anatomic factor that adversely affects outcome following ET.[12]

Length. The results of ET of infrainguinal PAD are affected by lesion length. The length of the treated lesion is inversely correlated with successful outcome in terms of technical success, symptom resolution, limb salvage, and clinical patency.[45,47,48] Early experience demonstrated that treated lesions shorter than 2 cm exhibited significantly greater patency than longer lesions. Five-year patency rates were approximately 75% for lesions less than 2 cm, versus 50% for longer lesions.[48,49] Consequently, some investigators suggested that a long lesion should be considered a relative indication for stent placement. Outcomes following SIA, however, seemed to show a limited dependency on lesion length and more dependency on the presence of normal vessel above and below the lesion.[25] These considerations are likewise reflected in the revised TASC criteria, which diminish the emphasis on lesion length as a deleterious factor.[12]

Multiple Same-Segment Stenoses. ET of multiple same-segment or multifocal stenoses results in worse outcomes compared with focal stenoses or lesions. The rationale is that multiple same-segment lesions represent multiple potential sites for immediate or long-term failure. Initially, 3-year patency rates of 20% following the treatment of long, multifocal stenoses were reported, compared with 68% following the treatment of focal stenoses.[50] More recently, using a hybrid approach consisting of surgery and percutaneous techniques for the treatment of multifocal stenoses, 2-year primary and assisted primary patency rates were 79% and 86%, respectively.[51]

Pattern of Vascular Disease

Multilevel Disease. Factors influencing the outcome of ET of multilevel disease are likely similar to those affecting multiple same-segment lesions. In multilevel disease, each lesion has its own failure rate and has the potential to impact the entire reconstruction. The outcome of multilevel disease is thought to be more favorable following surgery compared with ET.[12,52] In addition, patients with multilevel disease are frequently older, have multiple risk factors for atherosclerosis, and have lower baseline ABIs, putting them at increased risk for perioperative complications and long-term failure.[53-55]

Runoff Status. Similar to the effect of outflow vessel quality on the success of open bypass, the success of infrainguinal ET correlates directly with improved runoff status. In patients treated for femoropopliteal stenoses, the 5-year clinical success rate was 53% in patients with good runoff, compared with 31% in patients with poor runoff, in a representative study.[46] The same study demonstrated that in patients treated for occlusions, the 5-year clinical success rate was 36% in patients with good runoff and 16% in patients with poor runoff. More recent data from a report evaluating 324 infrainguinal interventions confirmed the deleterious effect of poor runoff.[38] One-year primary patency rates were significantly diminished in patients with impaired tibial runoff (fewer than three vessels) compared with patients having normal tibial runoff (three vessels)—52% versus 83%.

Patient Demographics

Gender. Female gender is frequently cited as a factor that negatively influences the outcome of open or endovascular reconstruction. However, conflicting evidence exists concerning the patency and clinical success rates of infrainguinal intervention in women compared with men.[30,56] One potential reason for these outcome differences is that the treated vessels, as well as the inflow and outflow vessels, are typically smaller in women. Even though female gender has been reported to be an independent risk factor for failure of lower extremity vascular reconstruction, these differences may be accounted for by the increased incidence of associated adverse factors in women, including CLI, diabetes, and infrapopliteal disease.[57]

Co-morbidities. Outcomes of infrainguinal ET are worse in patients with diabetes, and the incidence of infrapopliteal disease is high in this patient subgroup. The interaction of these closely linked risk factors may explain the increased failure rates following ET.[58] After controlling for lesion location, however, the reported results are more variable. In some studies, diabetes does not independently predict poor outcome.[59-61] Other reports suggest that type 1 and type 2 diabetes mellitus and hypertension are independent risk factors for progression to CLI following infrainguinal ET for claudication.[44,62,63] End-stage renal disease may also decrease the success rate for endovascular infrainguinal therapy. A significant increase in SIA failure has been observed in patients with renal failure.[64] In addition, diabetes and renal failure are found more commonly in patients presenting with CLI, which may also explain the diminished patency rates observed in these patient cohorts.[65]

Clinical Situation

Indication for Intervention. The indication for intervention represents one of the strongest predictors of immediate and long-term outcome for patients undergoing infrainguinal ET. With respect to lesion characteristics, multilevel disease, and co-morbidities, patients with CLI present with more complex disease than those with claudication. Several studies have demonstrated that patients with claudication demonstrate better outcomes than those with CLI when evaluating symptom resolution, limb salvage, and overall patency.[10,46,48]

Recurrent Stenosis. Historically, the results of dilatation of recurrent infrainguinal stenoses were poor. Consequently, surgical reconstruction was recommended for recurrent stenoses. One study that characterized the early treatment experience of recurrent stenoses demonstrated that the 1-, 2-, and 3-year clinical success rates were 41%, 20%, and 11%, respectively, for ET, compared with 84%, 72%, and 72%, respectively, for surgical reconstruction.[66] Owing to improved techniques and devices, there is a trend to apply ET more aggressively for recurrent stenoses.[67] Definitive recommendations for the treatment of restenotic lesions have not been made because the data are insufficient to assess effectiveness.

Intraprocedural Factors

Dissection or Residual Stenosis. In addition to preprocedural factors that might affect the outcome of infrainguinal ET, intraprocedural factors may play a role. Flow-limiting dissections and residual stenoses of 30% or greater occur with an estimated combined frequency of 10% with ET.[10,68] Traditionally, intraprocedural dissection or residual stenosis was a significant prognostic indicator of poor immediate and long-term outcome. With the advent of stent placement to prevent acute occlusion, early failure rates have improved significantly.[69]

Initial Hemodynamic Response. Gauging immediate postprocedural anatomic success can be accomplished using digital subtraction angiography; however, ABI is also a significant prognostic indicator. An improvement in postprocedure ABI correlates with superior immediate and long-term outcome.[20]

Treatment Outcomes

Femoropopliteal: Angioplasty (Fig. 110-1)

Before the routine use of stenting, data for conventional femoropopliteal PTA revealed initial technical success rates of 80% to 95%. However, long-term patency rates were significantly worse compared with those of patients treated for isolated aortoiliac disease. Reported primary patency rates were 47% to 63% (1 year), 38% to 51% (3 year), and 26% to 45% (5 year).[45-47,70,71] A meta-analysis evaluated the long-term outcomes for femoropopliteal PTA from 19 studies conducted between 1993 and 2000.[9] The study included 923 balloon dilatations and illustrated the significant impact of occlusive lesions and CLI on long-term outcome: 3-year patency rates

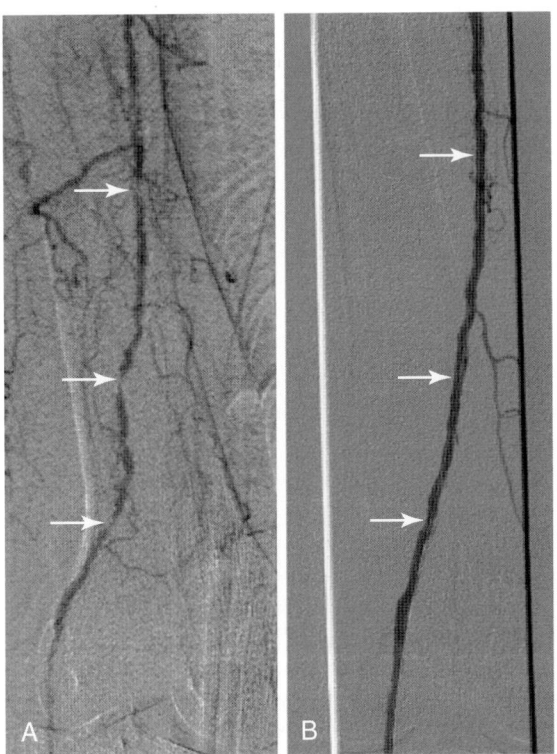

Figure 110-1 A 102-year-old woman with progressive cyanosis and early gangrene of the right great toe associated with ulceration. **A,** Arteriography demonstrates diffuse infrainguinal disease, including multiple same-segment stenoses and occlusions of the superficial femoral artery (*arrows*). **B,** Recanalization of the stenoses and occlusions was performed using a glide wire. After angioplasty of the superficial femoral artery using a 4-mm angioplasty balloon, angiography demonstrates resolution of the underlying stenoses and occlusions (*arrows*), with no evidence of significant residual stenosis or flow limitation. For this reason, no stents were placed.

were 61% for stenoses in claudicants, 48% for occlusions in claudicants, 43% for stenoses in patients with CLI, and 30% for occlusions in patients with CLI (Fig. 110-2).

SIA is a newer technique used to treat complex lesions and longer occlusions. The treatment of femoropopliteal artery occlusions using SIA was evaluated in 200 consecutive patients.[72] Technical success was achieved in 80% of the patients treated and was not affected significantly by lesion length. In addition, hemodynamic and clinical patencies at 3 years were 46% and 48%, respectively. A recent systematic review evaluated studies from 1966 through May 2007 focusing specifically on infrainguinal SIA.[8] A meta-analysis could not be performed because of the significant heterogeneity among the studies. The data incorporated 23 cohort studies and 1549 patients. Technical success ranged from 80% to 90%. One-year clinical success was achieved in 50% to 70% of patients, with limb salvage occurring in 80% to 90% of patients; primary patency approximated 50% in most series.

Although the use of angioplasty for complex femoropopliteal disease results in compromised durability, some evidence suggests that the transiently improved arterial circulation might confer a limb salvage benefit to patients who cannot undergo surgery due to prohibitive risk.[15] An early retrospective evaluation of 97 treated limbs in 86 patients exhibiting end-stage occlusive disease in whom vascular reconstruction was not feasible demonstrated a technical success rate of 90%, 1-year primary patency of 43%, and overall limb salvage of 76%.[73] A more recent study evaluating 50 patients with severe femoropopliteal disease demonstrated a technical success rate of 78% and a limb salvage rate of 42% at 2 years.[13]

Femoropopliteal: Angioplasty versus Bypass

The "gold standard" for comparing alternative therapies is the randomized controlled trial. Recruitment and randomization are inherently challenging in such trials when the treatments exhibit marked differences. One of the initial trials of surgical revascularization versus PTA randomized 255 patients.[74] Kaplan-Meier life-table analysis demonstrated no statistically significant difference in outcomes at 4 years. Nevertheless, patients treated with surgical revascularization demonstrated a trend toward improved primary patency but higher annual mortality rates, and patients treated with PTA exhibited a trend toward improved limb salvage. The Bypass versus Angioplasty in Severe Ischemia of the Leg (BASIL) trial was a multicenter randomized controlled trial that assigned 452 patients to a surgery-first or angioplasty-first approach.[75] The primary endpoint was amputation-free survival, and at 6 months' follow-up, there was no significant difference in amputation-free survival between the two groups (Fig. 110-3). Health-related quality of life, as measured by the EuroQol 5-D and Short Form 36, did not differ significantly between the two groups. The minimally invasive nature of PTA, improvements in technology, and growing operator experience have increased the aggressiveness with which complex infrainguinal lesions are approached using ET.[12]

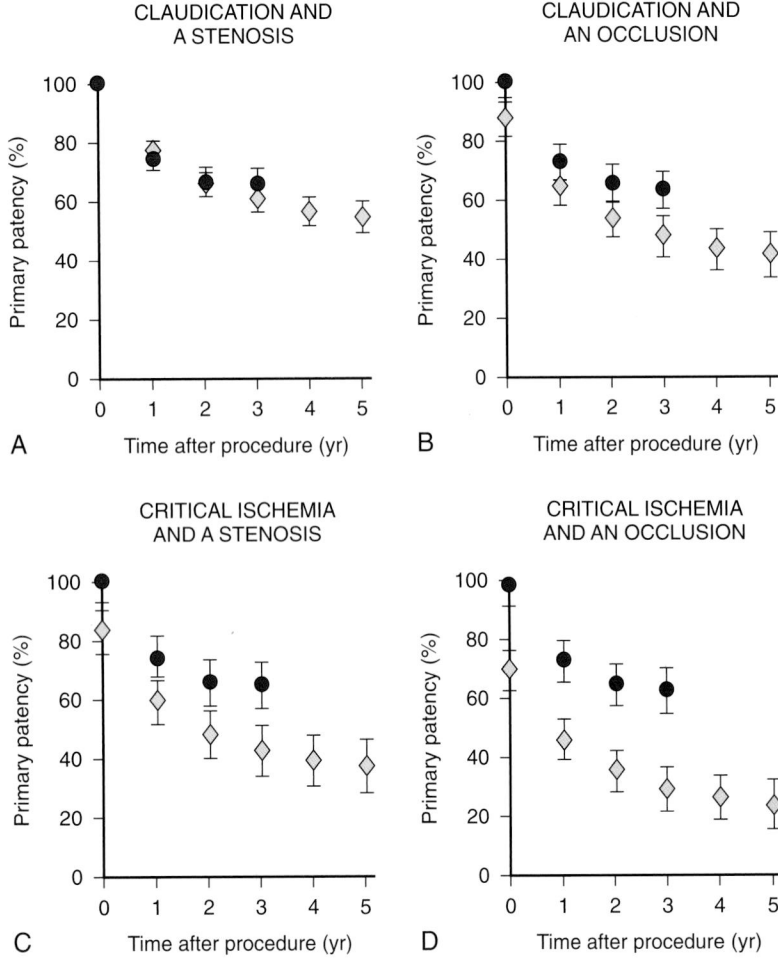

Figure 110-2 Cumulative primary patency rates and 95% confidence intervals (error bars) for femoro-popliteal balloon dilatation (diamonds) and femoro-popliteal stent implantation (circles), depending on lesion type (stenosis versus occlusion) and clinical indication (claudication versus critical ischemia). **A,** Graph shows that the estimates for primary patency following percutaneous transluminal angioplasty and stent placement are similar in patients with claudication and femoropopliteal stenosis. **B–D,** Graphs show that the estimates for primary patency following percutaneous transluminal angioplasty and stent placement are different in patients with critical ischemia and femoropopliteal occlusion. *(From Muradin GS, Bosch JL, Stijnen T, Hunink MG. Balloon dilation and stent implantation for treatment of femoropopliteal arterial disease: meta-analysis. Radiology. 2001; 221:137-145.)*

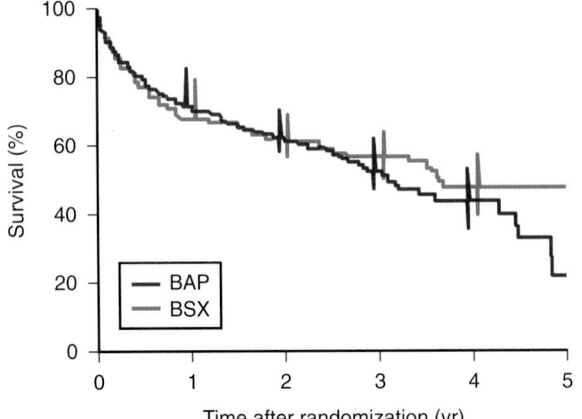

Figure 110-3 Amputation-free survival after bypass surgery (BSX) and balloon angioplasty (BAP). Bars show 95% confidence intervals for survival after 1, 2, 3, and 4 years of follow-up, which were calculated from the cumulative hazards. *(From Adam DJ, Beard JD, Cleveland T, et al. Bypass versus angioplasty in severe ischaemia of the leg (BASIL): multicentre, randomised controlled trial. Lancet. 2005; 366:1925-1934.)*

Femoropopliteal: Angioplasty versus Stenting

With the application of ET to lesions of increasing complexity, stent placement has become integral to the management of infrainguinal disease (Fig. 110-4). Several trials have been published since the routine incorporation of stenting for infrainguinal PAD. Although the results have been inconsistent, stenting appears to be useful as a salvage procedure for suboptimal angioplasty. The initial experience from retrospective cohort studies demonstrated 1-year primary patency rates ranging from 49% to 81%.[76-80] A meta-analysis evaluating 19 studies from 1993 to 2000, which included 473 stent placements, demonstrated 3-year patency rates ranging from 63% to 66%.[9] Unlike the data for PTA, long-term patency following stent placement does not correlate with clinical indication or lesion type. Consequently, PTA and stenting appear to generate more favorable outcomes than PTA alone for severe femoropopliteal disease.

More recently, a number of randomized controlled trials were designed to compare PTA alone with PTA and stenting. The following reports describe the results using balloon-expandable stents. Vroegindeweij and coworkers randomized 51 patients to undergo either PTA or PTA with stenting.[81]

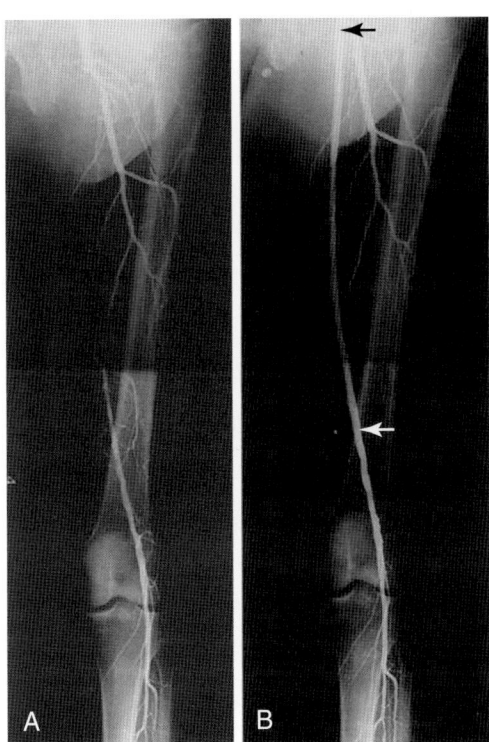

Figure 110-4 A, Arteriogram showing a 24-cm-long segmental occlusion of the superficial femoral artery. **B,** Angiographic results after angioplasty and stent placement. The stented segment is 31 cm long (*arrows*). *(From Conroy RM, Gordon IL, Tobias JM, et al. Angioplasty and stent placement in chronic occlusion of the superficial femoral artery: technique and results.* J Vasc Interv Radiol. *2000;11:1009-1020.)*

One-year clinical success, hemodynamic success, and primary patency did not differ significantly between the two groups. Grimm and colleagues randomized 30 patients to undergo either PTA alone or PTA with stenting.[82] At 39 months' follow-up, there were no significant differences in primary or secondary patency rates between the two groups. Cejna and associates randomized 154 limbs to undergo either PTA alone or PTA with stenting.[83] Although the rate of technical success was higher in patients undergoing PTA with stenting (99%, versus 84% with PTA alone), clinical success, hemodynamic success, primary patency, and secondary patency did not differ significantly between the two groups at 1 and 2 years after intervention. Becquemin and coauthors randomized 227 patients with persistent disabling claudication or CLI to undergo either routine or selective stent placement using a balloon-expandable Palmaz stent.[84] The primary endpoint evaluated was greater than 50% stenosis at 1-year follow-up, which did not differ significantly between the two groups. In addition, freedom from new vascular events and overall survival were not significantly different. These studies all indicate that the routine use of balloon-expandable stents for the treatment of femoropopliteal disease is not justified.

The lack of long-term efficacy associated with balloon-expandable stents for the treatment of femoropopliteal disease resulted in the pursuit of alternative stenting technologies, including the use of self-expanding nitinol stents. Conroy and

associates evaluated the results of treating 61 arteries in 48 men with chronic femoropopliteal occlusions, primarily using the Wallstent (Boston Scientific, Natick, MA).[85] The patients exhibited primary and secondary patency rates of 25% and 38%, respectively, at 4 years' follow-up. Lugmayr and colleagues evaluated the treatment of 54 extremities in 44 patients with short, complex stenoses and occlusions that were treated using the Symphony stent (Boston Scientific).[86] Technical success was achieved in 100% of patients. Three-year primary and secondary patency rates were 76% and 87%, respectively. Three retrospective studies were performed to evaluate the SMART stent (Cordis, Miami Lakes, FL); they demonstrated 2-year primary patency rates of 60% to 84%.[87-89]

Schillinger and coworkers performed a randomized controlled trial of 154 patients with severe claudication or CLI due to superficial femoral artery (SFA) disease who underwent either angioplasty with optional stenting or angioplasty with routine stenting.[90] The mean length of the treated segments did not differ significantly between the two study groups. Thirty-two percent of patients in the optional stenting group underwent stent placement, most commonly owing to inadequate results following angioplasty. One-year restenosis rates differed significantly; they were 63% in the optional stenting group and 37% in the routine stenting group (Fig. 110-5). In addition, patients treated with routine stenting were able to walk a greater distance before the recurrence of symptoms at 6 and 12 months compared with those treated with optional stenting.

Using current technology, stent placement appears to be strongly indicated as an adjunct to suboptimal angioplasty for the treatment of post-PTA dissection and residual stenosis. Newer technologies, including drug-eluting stents and covered stents, are discussed later.

Infrapopliteal: Angioplasty

Data on infrapopliteal PTA are limited (Fig. 110-6). There is no level I evidence for the treatment of patients with claudication or CLI due to infrapopliteal disease.[7] Ingle and colleagues performed a retrospective review of 67 patients with CLI treated with infrapopliteal angioplasty.[91] The technical success rate was 86%, and Kaplan-Meier life-table analysis demonstrated a 3-year limb salvage rate of 94% and freedom from CLI in 84%. Krankenberg and associates evaluated 78 patients with intermittent claudication as an indication for infrapopliteal angioplasty.[92] Procedural success occurred in 89% of patients; there were six complications, all of which were managed conservatively. Clinically, patients exhibited significant improvement in walking distance and ABI. Markose and Bolia performed a retrospective review of 46 patients with CLI treated using infrapopliteal angioplasty. The study demonstrated a technical success rate of 80% and a 2-year limb salvage rate of 87%.[1] Vraux and Bertoncello performed a retrospective review of 50 limbs in 46 patients treated with SIA for occluded tibial vessels.[24] Technical success was achieved in 82%, and technical failure did not preclude surgery when appropriate. One-year primary, secondary, and

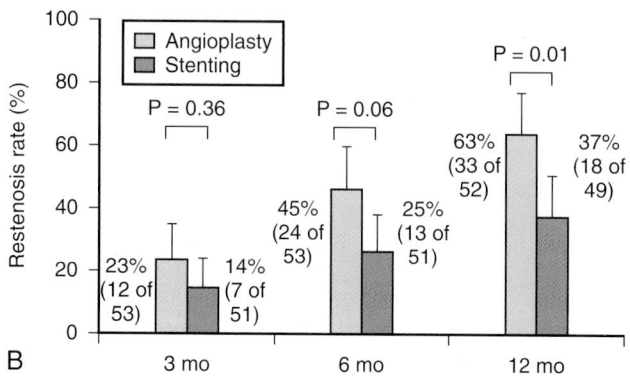

A

B

Figure 110-5 Rates of restenosis (defined as stenosis >50%). **A,** Rates of restenosis determined by angiography at 6 months, analyzed according to the intention-to-treat principle and according to the treatment actually received. Stenting demonstrated significantly diminished rates of restenosis compared with angioplasty when evaluated using angiography. **B,** Rates of restenosis in the same patients determined by duplex ultrasonography at 3, 6, and 12 months, analyzed according to the intention-to-treat principle. Error bars indicate 95% confidence intervals. At 6 and 12 months, stenting demonstrated significantly diminished rates of restenosis compared with angioplasty when evaluated using duplex ultrasonography. *(From Schillinger M, Sabeti S, Loewe C, et al. Balloon angioplasty versus implantation of nitinol stents in the superficial femoral artery. N Engl J Med. 2006;354:1879-1888.)*

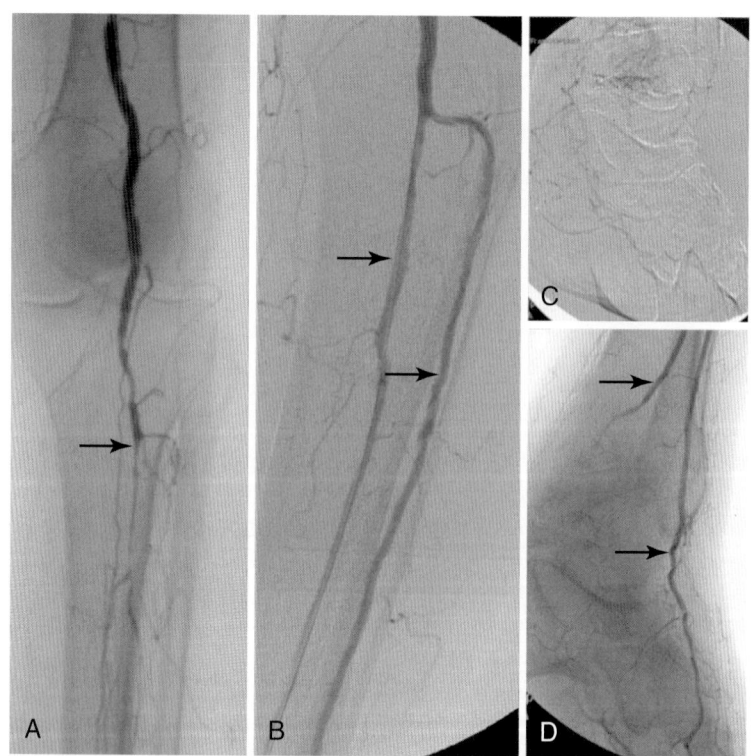

Figure 110-6 A 64-year-old diabetic woman with prior right femoropopliteal bypass who presented with gangrene of the left second and third toes and nonpalpable pedal pulses. **A,** Arteriography demonstrates occlusion of the tibial arteries (*arrow*). **B,** Recanalization and subintimal angioplasty of the tibial arteries was performed, with resolution of the occlusive lesions. There is no evidence of significant residual stenosis or flow limitation (*arrows*). **C,** Preintervention arteriography demonstrates no reconstitution in the pedal vasculature. **D,** Postintervention arteriography demonstrates reconstitution of the pedal vasculature (*arrows*). On follow-up examination, the patient had a palpable dorsal pedal pulse, healing of her toe amputation sites at 3 months, and no evidence of restenosis at 12 months.

clinical patency rates were 46%, 55%, and 63%, respectively. The 2-year limb salvage rate was 87%.

Infrapopliteal: Angioplasty and Stenting

Data on the use of bare metal and drug-eluting stents for the treatment of infrapopliteal PAD are also limited (Fig. 110-7). Feiring and colleagues evaluated stent-supported angioplasty as the treatment for 82 patients with CLI or lifestyle-limiting claudication.[93] The study reported a technical success rate

of 94%, a significant improvement in ABI, and a 96% limb salvage rate in patients treated for CLI. Clair and coworkers performed a retrospective review of 23 vessels in 19 patients who underwent infrainguinal angioplasty for limb-threatening ischemia.[18] Technical success was achieved in 22 of the treated vessels, and 16 patients demonstrated improved wound healing or relief of rest pain. The study did not demonstrate the long-term efficacy of infrapopliteal intervention; however, it did suggest that it should be considered in selected high-risk patients who may not be anatomically or physiologically suited for open bypass.

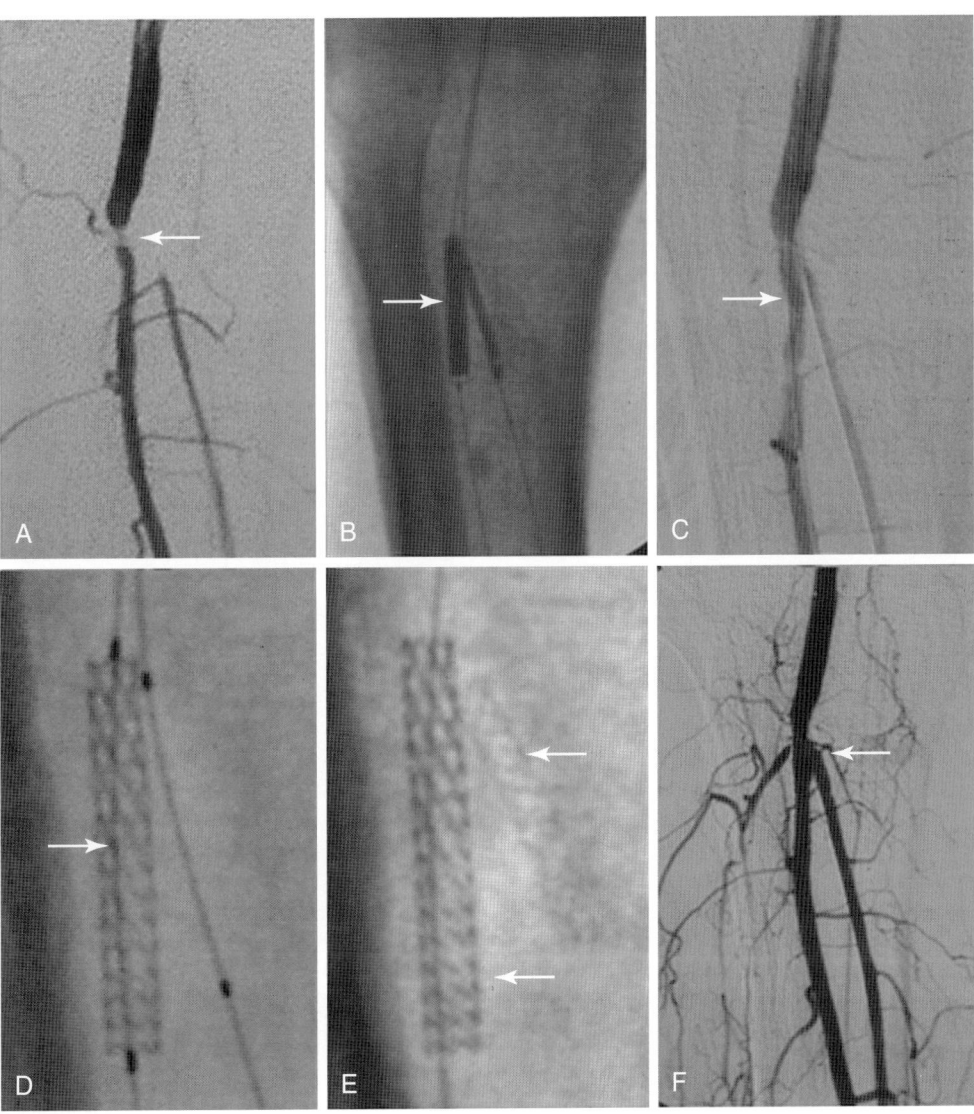

Figure 110-7 A 78-year-old man with multiple co-morbidities, a right fifth toe ulcer present for 6 weeks, and an inadequate great saphenous vein conduit. **A,** Arteriography demonstrates a bifurcation lesion of the tibioperoneal trunk (*arrow*). **B,** Recanalization was performed using an antegrade approach with two 0.014-inch wires. The lesion was treated using the kissing balloon technique (*arrow*). **C,** A flow-limiting dissection was noted following balloon angioplasty (*arrow*). **D** and **E,** The bifurcation lesion was subsequently treated by sequential stent deployment (kissing stents) with balloon protection (*arrows*). **F,** Completion arteriography demonstrates resolution of the bifurcation lesion (*arrow*), with no evidence of residual stenosis or flow limitation.

Bosiers and colleagues performed a retrospective review of 681 below-knee percutaneous interventions in 443 patients with CLI.[94] The distribution of disease severity according to Rutherford criteria was as follows: category 4 (n = 355), category 5 (n = 82), and category 6 (n = 6). Patients were treated with angioplasty alone, angioplasty and stenting, or laser atherectomy using the excimer laser (Spectranetics Corporation, Colorado Springs, CO). The overall primary patency rates for laser atherectomy at 6 months and 1 year were 85.2% and 74.2%, respectively (Fig. 110-8). The overall limb salvage rates for laser atherectomy at 6 months and 1 year were 97.0% and 96.6%, respectively (Fig. 110-9). Subset analyses did not demonstrate statistically significant differences between angioplasty alone and angioplasty with stenting: the 1-year primary patency rate was 68.6% for angioplasty alone, versus 75.5% for angioplasty with stenting; limb salvage was 96.7% for angioplasty alone and 98.6% for angioplasty with stenting. These results compare favorably to historical surgical controls, but further study is required to determine the role of angioplasty alone or angioplasty with stenting in the treatment of infrapopliteal PAD. It is striking that 80% of patients in this series had ischemic rest pain rather than tissue loss as the indication for intervention; this differs markedly from most open bypass series and suggests differing patient selection criteria.

COMPLICATIONS

The decision to proceed with ET as opposed to surgical revascularization in the infrainguinal arteries must be based on a careful risk-to-benefit analysis. ET is frequently chosen because of lower rates of morbidity and mortality in the perioperative period. The AHA Task Force guidelines on PTA were created after reviewing 12 series with 3784 patients undergoing ET for lower extremity PAD.[10] The complications were categorized according to location: puncture site, angioplasty site, distal vessel, and systemic (Table 110-3). Complications associated with the puncture site, angioplasty site, and distal vessel occurred in 10% of patients, and systemic complications occurred in 1% of patients. In a more

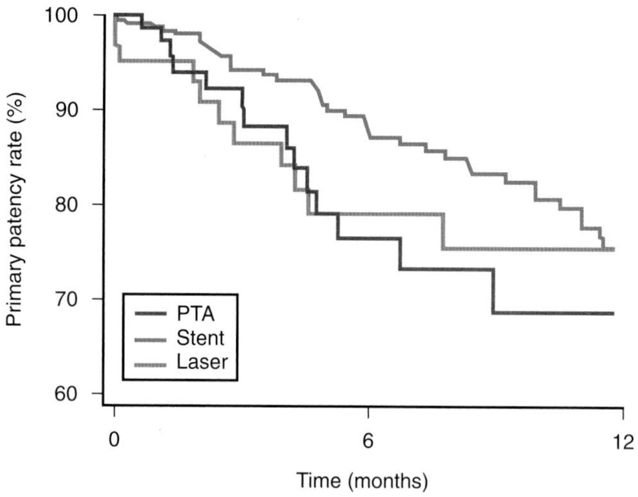

Figure 110-8 Primary patency of interventions performed using percutaneous transluminal angioplasty (PTA) alone, PTA with stenting (Stent), and laser-based intervention strategies (Laser). *(From Bosiers M, Hart JP, Deloose K, et al. Endovascular therapy as the primary approach for limb salvage in patients with critical limb ischemia: experience with 443 infrapopliteal procedures. Vascular. 2006;14:63-69.)*

Figure 110-9 Limb salvage rates of interventions performed using percutaneous transluminal angioplasty (PTA) alone, PTA with stenting (Stent), and laser-based intervention strategies (Laser). *(From Bosiers M, Hart JP, Deloose K, et al. Endovascular therapy as the primary approach for limb salvage in patients with critical limb ischemia: experience with 443 infrapopliteal procedures. Vascular. 2006;14:63-69.)*

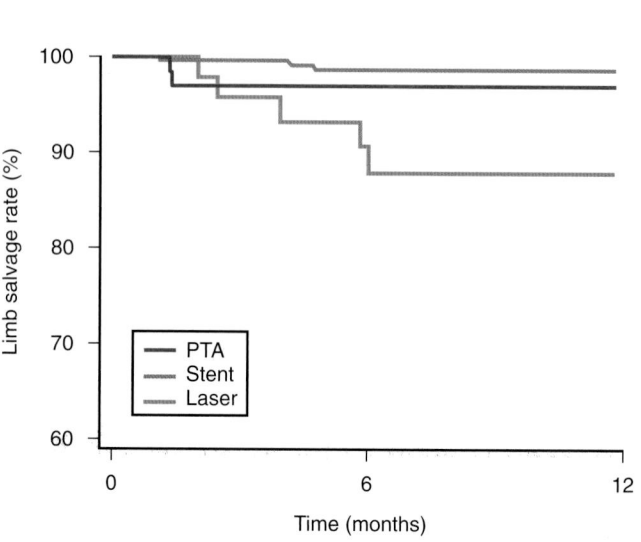

Table 110-3 Complications of Angioplasty

Complication	Percentage
Puncture site	4.0 (total)
Bleeding	3.4
False aneurysm	0.5
Arteriovenous fistula	0.1
Angioplasty site	3.5 (total)
Thrombus	3.2
Rupture	0.3
Distal vessel	2.7 (total)
Dissection	0.4
Embolization	2.2
Systemic	0.4 (total)
Renal failure	0.2
Myocardial infarction (fatal)	0.2
Consequences	
Surgical repair	2.0
Limb loss	0.2
Mortality	0.2

From Pentecost MJ, Criqui MH, Dorros G, et al. Guidelines for peripheral percutaneous transluminal angioplasty of the abdominal aorta and lower extremity vessels. A statement for health professionals from a special writing group of the Councils on Cardiovascular Radiology, Arteriosclerosis, Cardio-Thoracic and Vascular Surgery, Clinical Cardiology, and Epidemiology and Prevention, the American Heart Association. *Circulation.* 1994;89:511-531.

recent systematic review of 23 cohort studies that included 1549 patients, the most frequently reported complications were groin hematoma, arterial perforation, and distal embolization.[8] The overall complication rates averaged between 8% and 17% for patients presenting with claudication or CLI. Complication rates did not differ significantly when the studies were divided into those that evaluated the treatment of femoropopliteal vessels (7% to 20%) and those that evaluated the treatment of infrapopliteal vessels (8% to 16%).

Acute Failure

The most commonly reported cause of acute (<30 days) failure of ET for infrainguinal PAD is technical failure. Technical failures frequently result from post-PTA flow-limiting dissections and residual stenoses. Other mechanisms of acute failure include acute thrombosis and distal embolization, which may result in tissue loss despite successful revascularization. An early report evaluating 318 iliac artery and femoropopliteal artery angioplasty procedures demonstrated an acute failure rate of 17%.[95] Nevertheless, patients did not fare worse after the procedure compared with before it. Subsequent reports also demonstrated that technical failure had a minimal effect on the ability to perform subsequent arterial bypass.[91]

Advances in endovascular techniques and device technology, coupled with improved learning curves, may diminish acute failure rates in patients treated for infrainguinal PAD.[96] Stenting has played a prominent role in diminishing acute failure rates by allowing the salvage of post-PTA flow-limiting dissections and residual stenoses. However, the

increasingly complex disease being approached using ET has resulted in additional acute failures. Reported technical success rates continue to range between 80% and 90%.[8,96] Routine periprocedural antiplatelet therapy is essential to optimize technical success, maintain patency, and mitigate cardiovascular complications.[97]

Late Failure

The most common cause of late (>30 days) failure in patients treated with ET is recurrent stenosis. Recurrent stenosis results from an exaggerated response to intervention, causing flow-limiting stenosis or occlusion. The pathophysiologic cause of restenotic lesions is intimal hyperplasia, which results from the migration of vascular smooth muscle cells from the vessel wall media to the intima. Once in the intima, the vascular smooth muscle cells proliferate, produce extracellular matrix proteins, and contribute to the development of restenosis.[98] Progressive atherosclerosis is another significant cause of late failure, particularly more than 1 year post procedure.[99]

Failed angioplasty is usually easier to manage than failed bypass surgery. Patients tend to present with recurrent, subacute ischemic symptoms rather than acute limb-threatening ischemia. Therefore, most re-interventions for late failure can be performed electively. Recurrent stenoses or occlusions can be managed using endovascular procedures with safety and efficacy profiles comparable to those of the index cases.[61,100,101] Many investigators recommend the use of angioplasty with stenting when treating recurrent infrainguinal lesions.[61,101,102]

■ PERIPROCEDURAL MANAGEMENT
Clinical

The periprocedural management of patients undergoing infrainguinal ET parallels that for other endovascular procedures. Patients require bed rest for 4 to 6 hours after the angiographic sheath has been removed to prevent hemorrhage, pseudoaneurysm, and hematoma formation at the puncture site. In addition, patients with tissue loss require appropriate wound care. Late failure of infrainguinal ET is not uniformly accompanied by the recurrence of ischemic ulceration or gangrene. In these cases, once wound healing has been achieved, the augmented level of arterial perfusion may no longer be necessary to preserve the intact integument.

Medical

Periprocedural medical treatment for infrainguinal PTA and stent placement is strongly recommended owing to the increased risk of thrombosis at the site of intervention. Postprocedural medication regimens are intended to maintain patency as well as mitigate the cardiovascular risk factors that are frequently present in patients with PAD. The rationale for the use of antiplatelet agents and anticoagulants has largely been extrapolated from the literature on coronary angioplasty and stenting. Unfractionated heparin is typically administered at the onset of the procedure to achieve an activated clotting time of 250 seconds or greater. Before performing PTA and stenting, antiplatelet therapy is typically initiated, consisting of aspirin, clopidogrel, or both. The regimen is generally continued for 30 days but may be continued indefinitely, barring any contraindications.[97] For more detailed information on medical treatment, see Chapter 104 (Lower Extremity Arterial Disease: Decision Making and Medical Treatment).

FOLLOW-UP

Surveillance

The majority of published reports have used a combination of clinical follow-up and noninvasive imaging to monitor patients after the intervention. A typical postoperative regimen consists of performing a clinical examination, measuring the ABI, and obtaining pulse volume recording and duplex studies at 1, 3, 6, 9, and 12 months and then yearly thereafter, assuming the treated lesion is stable. Evidence of failure includes worsening of symptoms, as measured by the Rutherford scale, and noninvasive imaging demonstrating greater than 30% to 50% restenosis.[20] The proposed utility of performing such frequent follow-up is to prevent occlusion by instituting timely intervention for restenosis.[38]

Most restenoses are detectable by duplex surveillance and ABI measurements. If more detailed anatomic information is required before re-intervention, CTA or MRA can be used. The major limitations of CTA include radiation exposure, artifacts from excessive calcification, and the risk of contrast-induced nephropathy associated with iodinated contrast material.[103] Stenting may also result in significant artifacts. MRA has become a prominent imaging technique for the diagnosis and planning of endovascular interventions in patients with PAD. The accuracy of MRA exceeds 93%.[104] Stents may produce artifacts or signal loss, so MRA has limited utility in imaging previously stented arterial segments. In contrast to CTA, calcium does not produce significant artifacts with MRA. MRA must be employed with caution, however, and it is contraindicated in patients with pacemakers, defibrillators, spinal cord stimulators, intracerebral shunts, and cochlear implants. In addition, the use of a gadolinium contrast agent, once thought to be safe in patients with renal insufficiency, has now been associated with nephrogenic systemic fibrosis, a rare but potentially fatal complication.[105]

Long-term Management

Long-term management following infrainguinal ET requires careful monitoring and concomitant treatment of modifiable atherosclerotic risk factors. These modifiable risk factors are similar to those affecting the majority of patients with PAD: tobacco use, obesity, hyperlipidemia, hypertension, diabetes, inflammation, and antiplatelet therapy. Aggressive attempts at smoking cessation, reduction to an ideal body weight with diet and exercise, and the control of hypercholesterolemia with pharmacologic therapy are essential to mitigate cardiovascular risk and may confer some benefit with respect to PAD symptoms. In addition, aggressive control of hypertension has a demonstrated survival benefit in patients with PAD.[106,107]

All symptomatic PAD patients should be prescribed low-dose aspirin to reduce cardiovascular morbidity and mortality.[97] Clopidogrel may also be considered as monotherapy. A recent trial comparing dual therapy consisting of clopidogrel and aspirin with aspirin alone did not demonstrate any benefit of dual therapy with regard to myocardial infarction, stroke, or vascular death.[108,109] Chapter 104 (Lower Extremity Arterial Disease: Decision Making and Medical Treatment) addresses these important considerations in depth.

SPECIAL CONSIDERATIONS

Anatomic

Common Femoral Artery

Common femoral artery (CFA) plaque is generally bulky and eccentric and may involve the bifurcation. In addition, it is frequently continuous with disease in the iliac artery or the SFA. If an endovascular approach is attempted, angioplasty alone is preferred to angioplasty with stenting because the CFA resides in a region of high mobility, which may result in stent fracture or compromise. In addition, stent placement prohibits percutaneous access through the treated site and reduces open surgical options at this easily accessible site. A retrospective analysis of 18 patients with CFA disease who were treated using PTA demonstrated 1- and 3-year primary patency rates of 59% and 37%, respectively.[26] More recently, an analysis was conducted on 33 limbs in 27 patients undergoing CFA angioplasty and stenting. Technical success was achieved in 100% of patients, and 30-month and 3-year primary patency rates were 86% and 83%, resepectively.[110] In general, surgical repair of the CFA is more commonly recommended because surgical exposure and repair of the artery are straightforward and associated with low morbidity and high patency rates. In addition, surgical repair may be combined with proximal or distal endovascular interventions as deemed necessary.[111-113]

Profunda Femoris Artery

Disease of the profunda femoris artery (PFA) may not respond favorably to PTA because it usually presents as an orifice lesion, at the femoral bifurcation, or as diffuse disease. In addition, there are few clinical situations in which temporary improvement in PFA perfusion assists with limb salvage. Older series demonstrated a reasonable technical success rate for PFA angioplasty; however, long-term follow-up was lacking.[114,115] More recently, the safety and efficacy of percutaneous profundaplasty were demonstrated in a case series evaluating balloon angioplasty as the treatment for 31 patients with severe limb ischemia.[116] Procedural success was achieved in 91% of patients, and freedom from revascularization was achieved in 88% of patients with an average follow-up of 34 months. Nevertheless, because of the consistently good results achieved with surgical repair, that is still the modality most commonly recommended for the treatment of PFA disease.[117]

Adjunctive Techniques and Special Devices

A number of adjunctive techniques and special devices have been developed to treat more complex lesions (Fig. 110-10; see also Chapter 85: Technique: Endovascular Therapeutic).

Lesion-Crossing Techniques

Controlled Blunt Microdissection. A number of new crossing techniques have been devised to improve the technical success rates associated with the treatment of increasingly complex lesions. Controlled blunt microdissection is a technique with specific utility for chronic, heavily calcified occlusions. The catheter (CMD, Cordis, Warren, NJ) uses a set of articulating jaws to create a passage in either the true lumen or the subintimal plane, and the passage is subsequently dilated and stented. An evaluation of 36 patients with 44 chronic, symptomatic infrainguinal occlusions demonstrated angiographic success in 91% of the treated lesions.[118] One patient exhibited in-stent thrombosis, which responded well to intra-arterial thrombolysis. Long-term data are not available.

Crosser Catheter. The Crosser catheter (FlowCardia Inc., Sunnyvale, CA) for the treatment of chronic occlusions is similar in design to the CMD. To create a passage through an occluded lumen, the head of the catheter mechanically vibrates at 20 kHz, resulting in a stroke depth of approximately 20 μm. Technical success rates of 63% to 76% have been reported in the coronary tree. The ongoing Peripheral Approach to Recanalization in Occluded Totals (PATRIOT) trial is designed to evaluate the safety and efficacy of the Crosser catheter in the treatment of femoropopliteal disease.

Reentry Devices. Two devices have been used to facilitate true lumen reentry. The Outback LTD reentry catheter (Cordis) has been used with SIA, and after entry into the subintimal space, the catheter can be oriented toward the true lumen by appropriately aligning its distal radiographic markers. In an evaluation of 100 consecutive endovascular occlusions in which the distal true lumen could not be reentered initially and the Outback LTD catheter was subsequently used, there was a 95% technical success rate for reentering the true lumen and completing the intervention.[119] The Outback LTD reentry catheter was recalled by the Food and Drug Administration in August 2008 owing to a mechanical dysfunction that prevented cannula retraction. The Pioneer catheter (Medtronic Vascular Inc., Minneapolis,

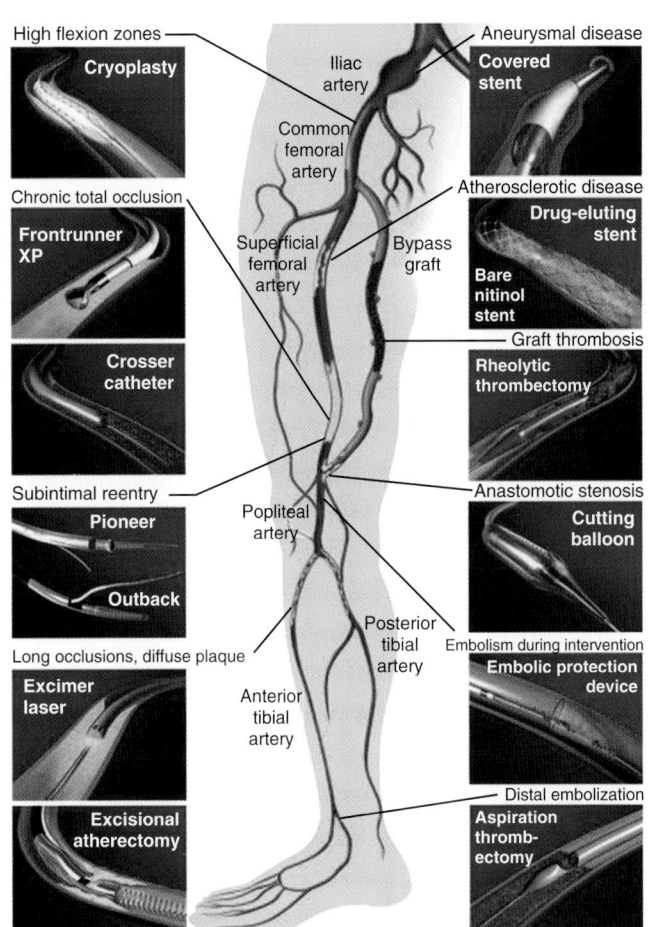

Figure 110-10 Overview of new technologies for lower extremity revascularization. *(From Rogers JH, Laird JR. Overview of new technologies for lower extremity revascularization.* Circulation. *2007;116:2072-2085.)*

MN) uses a nitinol reentry needle in combination with intravascular ultrasound to assist with reentry into the true lumen. The safety and efficacy of the device have been demonstrated preliminarily.[120]

Drug-Eluting Stents

Drug-eluting stents are designed to limit the proliferative process of neointimal hyperplasia. For example, sirolimus-eluting stents have been shown to inhibit neointimal hyperplasia in the coronary vasculature.[121] The Sirolimus Coated Cordis SMART Nitinol Self-Expandable Stent for the Treatment of SFA Disease (SIROCCO) I trial randomized 36 patients with SFA disease to treatment with either sirolimus-eluting or bare metal stents. Intimal hyperplasia was assessed using quantitative angiography. Although the drug-eluting cohort demonstrated improved patency at 1 year, the study failed to achieve the primary endpoint, which was improved mean in-stent restenosis at 2 years (23% in the sirolimus group versus 31% in the control group; not significant).[122]

The SIROCCO II trial was a randomized study that evaluated the use of slow-eluting sirolimus stents (n = 29) versus bare metal stents (n = 28) in patients presenting with chronic limb ischemia due to SFA occlusions or stenoses.[123] Using quantitative angiography, SIROCCO II failed to demonstrate a difference in the primary endpoint of improved mean in-stent restenosis. In another study comparing sirolimus-eluting stents (n = 29) with bare metal stents (n = 29) in patients who underwent suboptimal SIA, sirolimus-eluting stents demonstrated increased primary patency, significantly decreased in-stent restenosis, and fewer target lesion re-interventions at 6 months.[124] Clinically, there were no reported differences in mortality, minor amputation, or limb salvage rates. Another drug-eluting stent currently under investigation is the Zilver PTX Stent Platform (Cook Medical, Bloomington, IN), which uses paclitaxel.[125]

Stent-Grafts

Stent-grafts attempt to duplicate the prosthetic femoropopliteal bypass using endovascular techniques. The Viabahn stent-graft (W. L. Gore & Associates Inc., Flagstaff, AZ) comprises a self-expanding nitinol stent bonded to a graft made of expanded polytetrafluoroethylene (PTFE). A randomized controlled trial comparing the Viabahn stent-graft to open femoral above-knee PTFE bypass in 100 patients with SFA occlusive disease demonstrated that 1-year primary and secondary patency rates did not differ significantly between the two groups.[126] The Viabahn versus Bare Nitinol Stent Trial (VIBRANT) is currently enrolling patients and will help clarify the potential contribution of stent-grafts to the treatment of infrainguinal PAD.

Debulking Devices

Debulking devices consist of excisional atherectomy, rotational atherectomy, and excimer laser devices (Fig. 110-11). The SilverHawk Plaque Excision System (SilverHawk, Redwood City, CA) is the prototype excisional atherectomy device. It uses a high-speed cutting blade that excises a strip of plaque that is subsequently stored in a nosecone. In a study of 131 lesions in 84 patients presenting with Rutherford category 2 to 5 ischemia treated using the SilverHawk device,

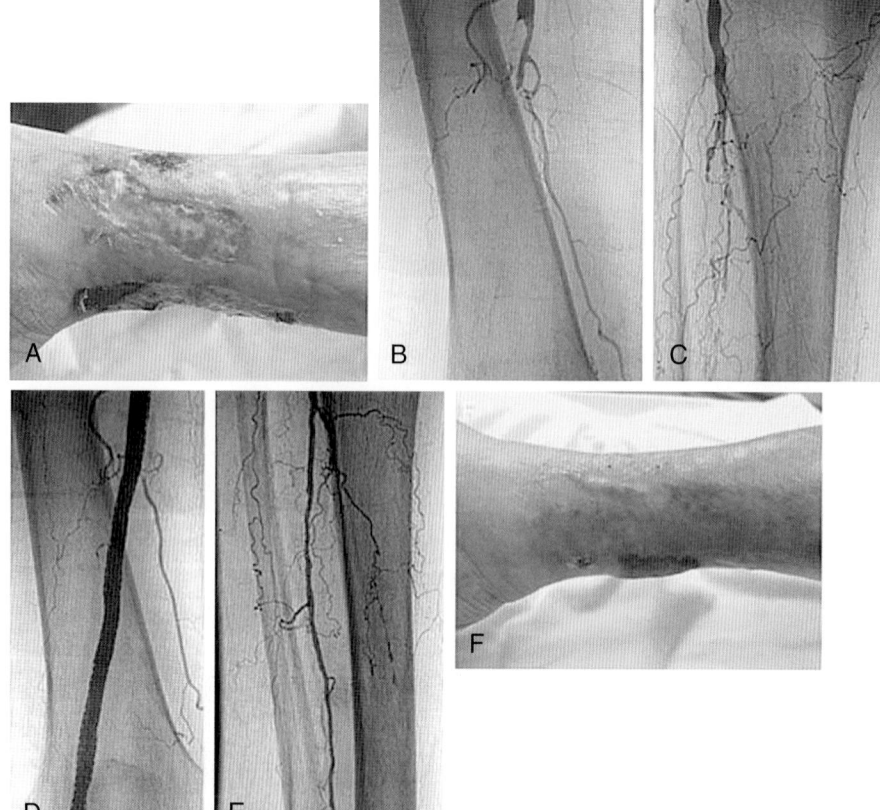

Figure 110-11 Treatment of multilevel disease with plaque excision. A 91-year-old woman with intractable pain, ischemic ulceration (**A**), and an ankle-brachial index of 0.16 underwent angiography, which demonstrated occlusions of the proximal superficial femoral artery (**B**) and all tibioperoneal arteries (**C**). Following treatment with plaque excision and stenting in the superficial femoral artery (**D**) and plaque excision alone in the peroneal artery (**E**), the patient exhibited sustained wound healing at 6 months' follow-up (**F**). *(From Kandzari DE, Kiesz RS, Allie D, et al. Procedural and clinical outcomes with catheter-based plaque excision in critical limb ischemia. J Endovasc Ther. 2006;13:12-22.)*

technical success was achieved in 86% of cases undergoing atherectomy alone and in 100% of cases using additional adjunctive modalities.[127] In addition, primary and secondary patency rates were improved in patients who were treated for de novo lesions compared with those treated for restenoses. In another evaluation of 76 limbs in 69 patients presenting with Rutherford category 5 and 6 ischemia, the procedural success rate was 99%, and the 6-month limb salvage rate was 87%.[128] With regard to rotational atherectomy devices, published results are pending for interventions using the Pathway Medical PV (Pathway Medical Technologies, Redmond, WA) and the Orbital Atherectomy System (Cardiovascular Systems, St. Paul, MN).

The excimer laser (ClirPath, Colorado Springs, CO) uses a 308-nm ultraviolet wavelength and functions by ablating tissue on contact, without causing a rise in temperature in the surrounding tissue. In a study evaluating use of the excimer laser for 411 consecutive procedures in 318 patients with long SFA occlusions, technical success was 90.5%, and 1-year secondary patency was 70.5%.[129] In the Laser Angioplasty for Critical Limb Ischemia (LACI) trial, 423 lesions were treated in 145 patients who were poor candidates for surgical revascularization; the reported 6-month limb salvage rate was 93%.[130]

Cryoplasty

Cryoplasty is a technique that combines balloon angioplasty with cold therapy, which is hypothesized to modify plaque

behavior, reduce elastic recoil, and induce smooth muscle cell apoptosis.[131] Liquid nitrous oxide is the cooling agent. The PolarCath system (Boston Scientific, Natick, MA) for cryoplasty was evaluated in a prospective multicenter registry that included 102 patients. Procedural success was observed in 94% of patients. At 9 months, primary, assisted primary, and secondary patencies were 70%, 94%, and 98%, respectively.[132] A prospective multicenter trial of cryoplasty was conducted on 111 limbs in 106 CLI patients with infrapopliteal lesions. Reported procedural success was 97%, and the 1-year limb salvage rate was 85%.[133]

Embolic Protection Devices

Embolic protection devices were first used in the carotid and coronary circulations, and their use in the lower extremities is being evaluated. However, that entails a unique set of obstacles: a greater atheroembolic burden, marked variation in the diameter of infrainguinal vessels, problems with delivery owing to longer disease segments, and problems with filter retrieval. Currently, the most likely use for embolic protection devices when performing infrainguinal ET is for patients with poor runoff and those undergoing thrombolytic therapy who are at high risk for embolization (Fig. 110-12).[134-136]

Cutting Balloon

The cutting balloon (Boston Scientific, Natick, MA) is equipped with four microsurgical blades that are bonded lon-

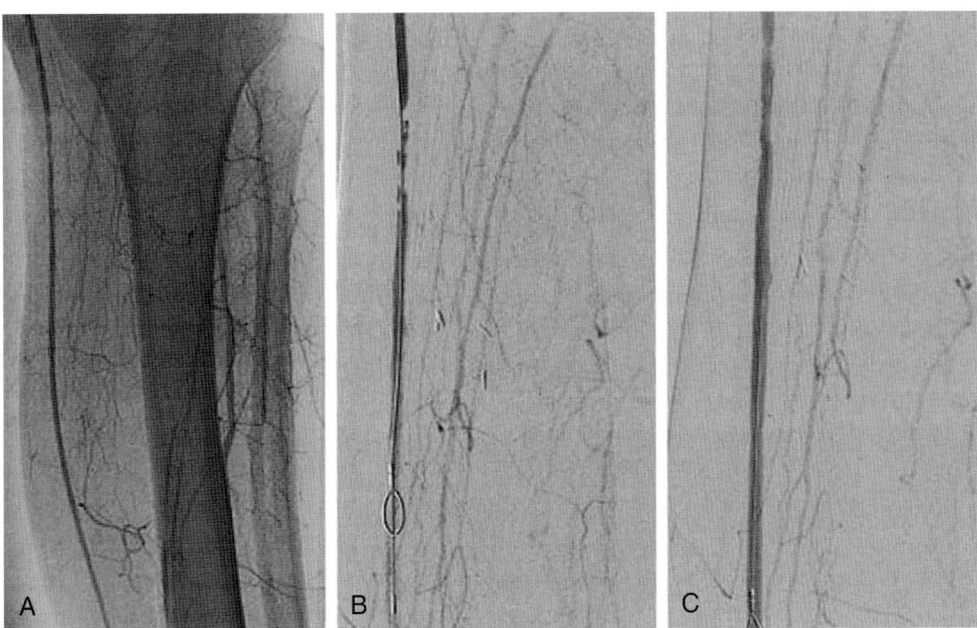

Figure 110-12 A, High-grade stenosis of midfemoral–posterior tibial saphenous bypass graft. **B,** With the EPI FilterWire distal to the lesion, angioplasty with a 3-mm balloon catheter is performed. **C,** Immediately after angioplasty, there is good flow through the lesion. *(From Wholey MH, Toursarkissian B, Postoak D, et al. Early experience in the application of distal protection devices in treatment of peripheral vascular disease of the lower extremities.* Catheter Cardiovasc Interv. *2005;64:227-235.)*

gitudinally to a balloon. The proposed mechanism of action is controlled (and thus less) disruption of the vessel wall, resulting in more controlled dilatation at lower balloon inflation pressures. In a comparison of conventional balloon angioplasty and cutting balloon angioplasty in 36 patients with failing infrainguinal bypass grafts, initial success was better for the cutting balloon cohort, but 1-year primary patency did not differ between the two groups.[137] A retrospective review evaluating the use of cutting balloon angioplasty in 93 infrapopliteal lesions in 73 patients demonstrated a procedural success rate of 100% and a 1-year limb salvage rate of 90%.[138] Twenty percent of the patients required stenting as a salvage procedure for dissection or residual stenosis.

■ FUTURE DIRECTIONS

ET for infrainguinal PAD continues to evolve. Progress can be attributed to refinements of existing technologies, development of new techniques and devices, and increasing practitioner experience with a broad array of devices and techniques. Despite this rapid evolution, the durability of infrainguinal ET continues to be suboptimal, emphasizing the need not only for further technical improvements but also for more detailed knowledge about the basic processes of intimal hyperplasia and atherosclerosis. Randomized controlled trials are needed to determine the best strategies for treating various lesion subtypes and comparing alternative modes of therapy. In addition, all trials need to strictly adhere to reporting standards so that therapies can be accurately assessed and compared.

SELECTED KEY REFERENCES

Adam DJ, Beard JD, Cleveland T, Bell J, Bradbury AW, Forbes JF, Fowkes FG, Gillepsie I, Ruckley CV, Raab G, Storkey H; BASIL trial participants. Bypass versus angioplasty in severe ischaemia of the leg (BASIL): multicentre, randomised controlled trial. *Lancet.* 2005; 366:1925-1934.
Multicenter randomized controlled trial comparing surgical bypass to lower extremity angioplasty.

Bosiers M, Hart JP, Deloose K, Verbist J, Peeters P. Endovascular therapy as the primary approach for limb salvage in patients with critical limb ischemia: experience with 443 infrapopliteal procedures. *Vascular.* 2006;14:63-69.
Large retrospective review of 443 infrapopliteal endovascular procedures.

Met R, Van Lienden KP, Koelemay MJ, Bipat S, Legemate DA, Reekers JA. Subintimal angioplasty for peripheral arterial occlusive disease: a systematic review. *Cardiovasc Intervent Radiol.* 2008;31:687-697.
Systematic review of SIA for the treatment of infrainguinal PAD.

Muradin GS, Bosch JL, Stijnen T, Hunink MG. Balloon dilation and stent implantation for treatment of femoropopliteal arterial disease: meta-analysis. *Radiology.* 2001;221:137-145.
Recent meta-analysis evaluating the use of ET for femoropopliteal PAD.

Norgren L, Hiatt WR, Dormandy JA, Nehler MR, Harris KA, Fowkes FG; TASC II Working Group. Inter-society consensus for the management of peripheral arterial disease (TASC II). *J Vasc Surg.* 2007;45S:S5-S67.
Primary consensus guidelines describing the current management of PAD.

Rutherford RB, Baker JD, Ernst C, Johnston KW, Porter JM, Ahn S, Jones DN. Recommended standards for reports dealing with lower extremity ischemia: revised version. *J Vasc Surg.* 1997;26: 517-538.
Primary guidelines describing the reporting standards for lower extremity PAD.

Schillinger M, Sabeti S, Loewe C, Dick P, Amighi J, Mlekusch W, Schlager O, Cejna M, Lammer J, Minar E. Balloon angioplasty versus implantation of nitinol stents in the superficial femoral artery. *N Engl J Med.* 2006;354:1879-1888.
First randomized controlled trial to demonstrate the superiority of self-expanding nitinol stents compared with angioplasty alone in the treatment of superficial femoral artery occlusive disease.

REFERENCES

The reference list can be found on the companion Expert Consult Web site at *www.expertconsult.com.*

CHAPTER 111

Nonatheromatous Popliteal Artery Disease

Thomas L. Forbes

Based in part on a chapter in the previous edition by Lewis J. Levien, MB BCh, PhD, FCSSA.

The vast majority of patients experiencing lower extremity ischemic symptoms have atherosclerotic occlusive disease. However, in the absence of significant atherosclerotic risk factors, especially in younger and more active individuals, nonatheromatous causes must be considered. Adventitial cystic disease of the popliteal artery and popliteal artery entrapment syndrome are by far the most common of these rare pathologies; more unusual causes, including fibromuscular dysplasia of the iliac arteries, also exist. Similar to the more common atherosclerosis, the symptoms associated with non-atheromatous causes of popliteal artery occlusive disease range from claudication of varying severity to critical limb ischemia (CLI). Given the younger population affected and their rarity, these conditions are often not diagnosed in a timely fashion, resulting in prolonged disability or occasionally progression to CLI.[1]

EMBRYOLOGY

The embryologic origins of the arterial system are more completely described in Chapter 2 (Embryology), but it is important to review some of the key features to understand the anatomy associated with pathologies affecting the popliteal artery (Fig. 111-1).

The lower extremity arterial system arises from two arteries—the axial and external iliac arteries—both of which originate from the umbilical artery. The femoral artery originates from the external iliac artery and progresses distally in the anterior compartment, while the axial artery elongates distally in the posterior compartment. At this stage of development, around 42 days of intrauterine life, the axial artery is divided into three segments, depending on its relationship to

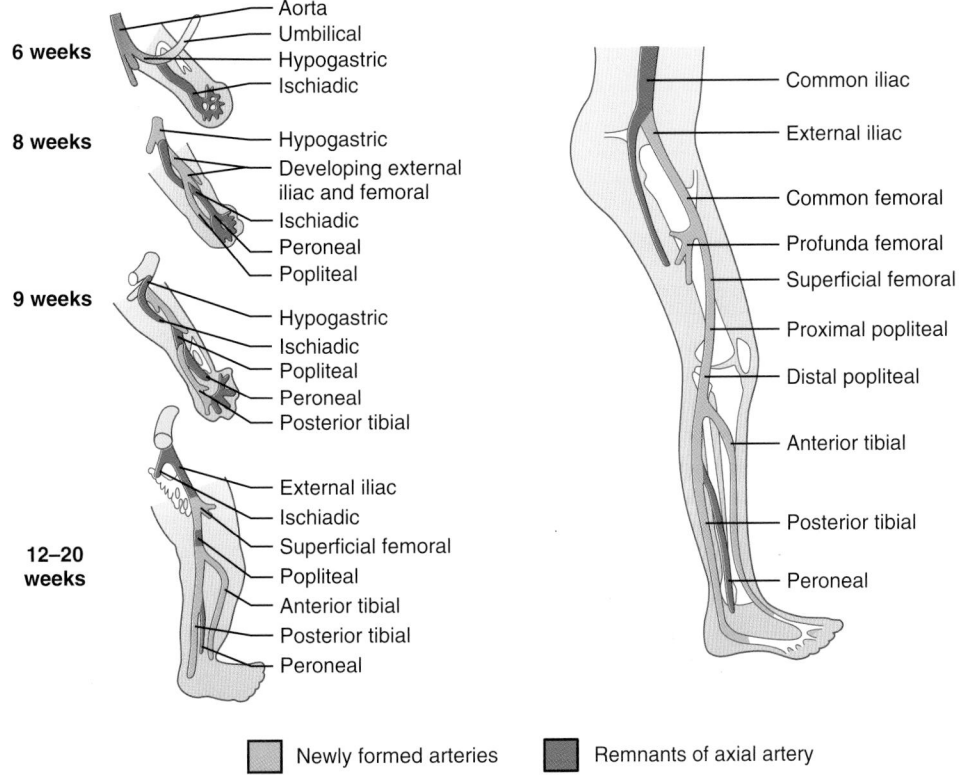

Figure 111-1 Embryologic derivation of the popliteal and other lower limb arteries. Remnants of the axial artery and arteries that develop with later differentiation are indicated. *(From Levien LJ, Benn C. Adventitial cystic disease: a unifying hypothesis. J Vasc Surg. 1998;28:193-205.)*

the popliteus muscle (proximal, deep, and distal); a bridging artery, the ramus communicans superius, joins the femoral artery and the proximal segment of the axial artery through the adductor hiatus. During the next week of development, the proximal component of the axial artery gives rise to a branch that runs superficial to the popliteus muscle and joins with the distal segment of the axial artery; the deep segment of the axial artery involutes. The fully developed popliteal artery results from the fusion of several arterial elements.[2]

Initially, both heads of the gastrocnemius muscle originate from the proximal tibia. With development, these migrate craniad along the femur to different extents. The final position of the medial head of the gastrocnemius muscle is more proximal to that of the lateral head and immediately caudal to the adductor hiatus, with the popliteal artery lying immediately lateral.[2] These dynamic processes of muscle and arterial development create the potential for anatomic variations that can result in nonatheromatous popliteal artery abnormalities.

■ ADVENTITIAL CYSTIC DISEASE

Epidemiology

Adventitial cystic disease was first reported in the medical literature in 1947 with the description of a case involving the external iliac artery.[3] Since then there have been approximately 400 cases reported in the world literature, with the popliteal artery most commonly affected (85% of cases).[4] In the vast majority of cases, popliteal artery involvement is unilateral; there has been only one published report of bilateral lesions.[5] The next most common arteries involved are the external iliac and femoral arteries,[6] but involvement has been noted in most of the arteries lying adjacent to joint spaces (Fig. 111-2).[7] Additionally, although it is primarily and most commonly a disorder of the arterial system, there have been isolated reports of adventitial cystic disease involving the iliofemoral and saphenous veins.[8]

Adventitial cystic disease affects predominantly males, with a male-female ratio of 5:1. The typical age at diagnosis is the mid-30s. Some investigators have reported a slightly older age at diagnosis in women, who are often in their 50s.[9] It must be remembered, however, that the diagnosis is often delayed, given the relatively young age of these patients and the absence of atherosclerotic risk factors. As a result, there is uncertainty regarding the age at which the pathologic abnormality would be apparent in an asymptomatic person. This disease has been observed primarily in western Europe, Australia, Japan, and elsewhere in Asia. Fewer cases have been reported in North America, with the majority occurring on the East Coast.[10,11] The prevalence of adventitial cystic disease has been variously reported as 1 in 1200 patients with claudication, regardless of age, and 1 in 1000 diagnostic angiograms.[11] These reports include predominantly symptomatic patients, so the incidence of adventitial cystic disease in the general asymptomatic population is still unknown.

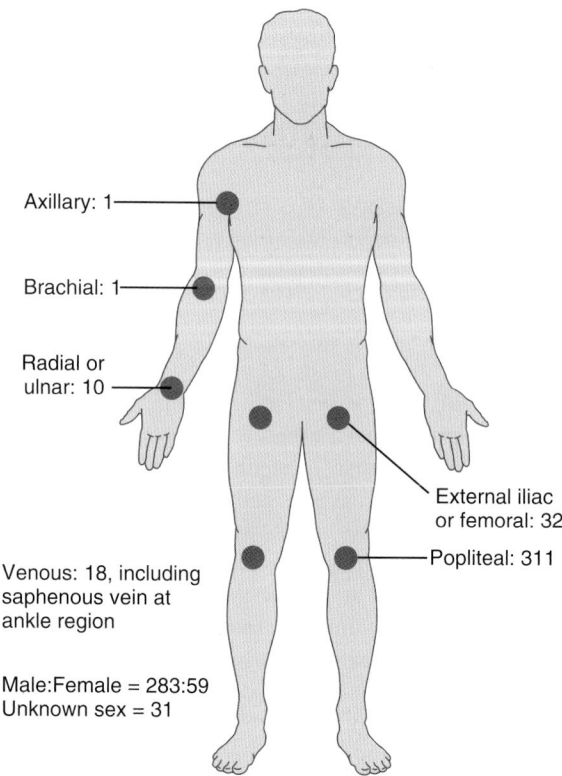

Figure 111-2 Anatomic location and sex in 375 published cases of adventitial cystic disease.

Pathogenesis

Etiology

The precise cause of adventitial cystic disease remains unclear and somewhat controversial, but there has been some recent clarification. Previously, four predominant theories of etiology and pathogenesis had been described by numerous authors: the repetitive trauma, ganglion, systemic disorder, and developmental theories.[9,11] Although convincing data to support the validity of the first three theories are scarce, they are briefly discussed in the following paragraphs.

Repetitive Trauma Theory. Proponents of this theory suggest that repeated flexion and extension of the knee joint lead to chronic injury of the popliteal artery characterized by cystic degeneration.[7,9,12] It is thought that this repetitive distraction movement of the popliteal artery causes intramural hemorrhage between the adventitia and media, which causes cyst formation when combined with adventitial enzymatic activity. An extension of this theory suggests that subjecting the knee joint (not the popliteal artery) to this repetitive movement and stress leads to joint degeneration and changes in the surrounding connective tissue. Consequently, these connective tissue cells secrete a substance containing hydroxyproline that results in adventitial cyst formation.[12]

Although the repetitive trauma theory is somewhat attractive, given its simplicity and relative intuitiveness, there are few scientific data to support it. Repetitive trauma as a causative factor does not explain cases occurring in arteries that are not subjected to such stress or in younger patients who have not been subjected to the same duration of this stimulus as have older patients. If this theory were correct, we would expect more cases of adventitial cystic disease in more active individuals or athletes, and there would be a positive correlation between age and incidence of the disease. Neither is the case.

Ganglion Theory.
Proponents of this theory of pathogenesis have been prompted by the similar content of simple ganglions and popliteal artery cysts.[7,9,13] Specifically, both types of cystic structures contain high levels of hyaluronic acid. Additionally, some support is offered by periodic case reports of synovial cystic structures and Baker's cysts directly involving adjacent vascular structures.[14] Presumably, in the case of the popliteal artery, these synovial cysts enlarge and track along arterial branches, where they implant in the adventitia of the popliteal artery itself.[4] Support for this theory would include evidence of histologic similarities between the lining and chemical content of the cystic fluid in the synovium and that of popliteal artery cysts. Decades ago, several researchers failed to find any such similarities, resulting in this theory's falling into disfavor.[15] Specifically, fluid from these cysts has a much higher hyaluronic acid content than from synovial cysts.[16]

Systemic Disorder Theory.
The third theory of pathogenesis for adventitial cystic disease, also lacking much supporting evidence, is that of a systemic disorder—specifically, the existence of a systemic mucinous or myxomatous degenerative condition. This was first postulated in 1967,[17] but since then, there has been little epidemiologic or pathologic supporting evidence, and this systemic condition has never been discovered. In addition, reports of bilateral disease are exceedingly rare,[5] as are cases of synchronous or metachronous cysts in different vascular locations. These presentations and distributions would be expected to be more common with an underlying systemic cystic disorder.

Developmental Theory.
At this time, the developmental theory of pathogenesis enjoys the greatest degree of acceptance and has the most convincing body of evidence. Also known as the cellular inclusion theory, it proposes that adventitial cystic disease occurs when mesenchymal mucin-secreting cells are implanted in the adventitia of the vessel during development. Levien and Benn highlighted the embryologic development of these arteries in support of this proposal.[7] They recognized that these nonaxial arteries form from vascular plexuses between 15 and 22 weeks of embryologic development adjacent to developing joints. During this time, mesenchymal cell rests forming these joints can be incorporated into closely adjacent vessels and may be responsible for subsequent cyst formation when these mesenchymal cells start to secrete mucoid material.

Connections between the knee joint capsule and an adjacent popliteal artery adventitial cyst have periodically been identified by preoperative imaging and intraoperatively.[3,4,9,17-20]

On the one hand, the presence of such a connection could lend support to the ganglion theory of development, with the connection representing a direct communication between the joint capsule and the arterial adventitial layer through which synovial cysts can migrate.[4,19,20] On the other hand, proponents of the developmental theory claim that these communications represent a residuum of the embryologic process, when mesenchymal cells of the adjacent joint are included in the adventitia of the nearby developing artery.[4,7] As mentioned previously, the biochemical analysis of these adventitial cysts does not support the ganglion theory because these cysts have a greater hyaluronic acid concentration than synovial cysts.[16]

All four theories of development have been proposed as rational explanations for adventitial cystic disease at one time or another. However, the prevailing opinion and, more important, the current body of evidence largely support the developmental theory as the most rational explanation. In the absence of convincing supporting evidence, the other three theories can be viewed in the appropriate historical context.

Pathology

Popliteal artery adventitial cysts are filled with a gelatinous mucoid material. Microscopic examination reveals a simple cuboid cell lining in the adventitial layer, with a notable absence of any coexisting microscopic features of atherosclerotic disease (Fig. 111-3). Grossly, the popliteal artery may appear enlarged and sausage-like, with adhesions to adjacent structures (Fig. 111-4). The cyst is usually unilocular but can be multilocular. Cyst contents are usually clear or yellow but can be dark red following hemorrhage. At the time of operation, these cysts are apparent following incision of the adventitial layer.

Clinical Presentation

Arterial

The typical patient with adventitial cystic disease of the popliteal artery is male, is in his mid-30s, and complains of the fairly sudden onset of short-distance calf claudication.[11] The duration of symptoms is generally relatively short (weeks to a few months), and except in unusual cases, these symptoms are unilateral.[5] The differential diagnosis includes popliteal artery entrapment syndrome (discussed later in this chapter) and premature atherosclerosis. Given the focality of these cysts, the young age of patients, and the otherwise normal status of inflow and outflow vessels, progression to CLI is exceedingly unusual with adventitial cystic disease, although the severity of claudication can progress and become disabling. It appears that the cysts have been present and slowly enlarging for extended periods before patients enter the symptomatic phase. These enlarging cysts lead to progressive compression of the arterial lumen and can result in a "functional" occlusion of the artery without necessarily causing complete thrombosis. In fact, in cases of apparent arterial occlusion without

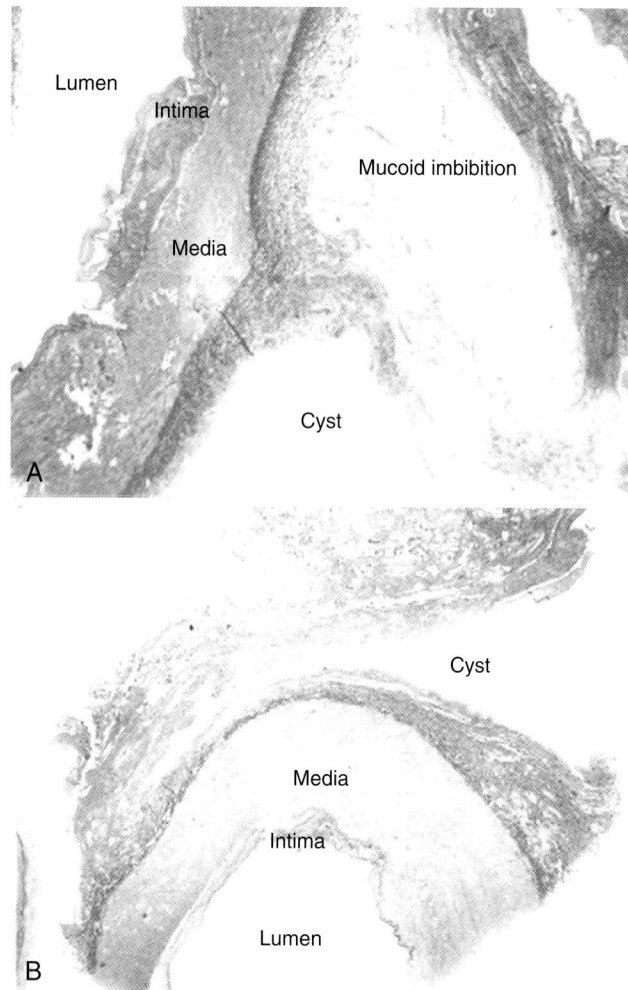

Figure 111-3 A and **B,** Specimen stained with elastica van Gieson showing mucoid-filled cysts between the adventitia and media of the popliteal artery. *(From Tsilimparis N, Hanack U, Yousefi S, et al. Cystic adventitial disease of the popliteal artery: an argument for the developmental theory. J Vasc Surg. 2007;45: 1249-1252.)*

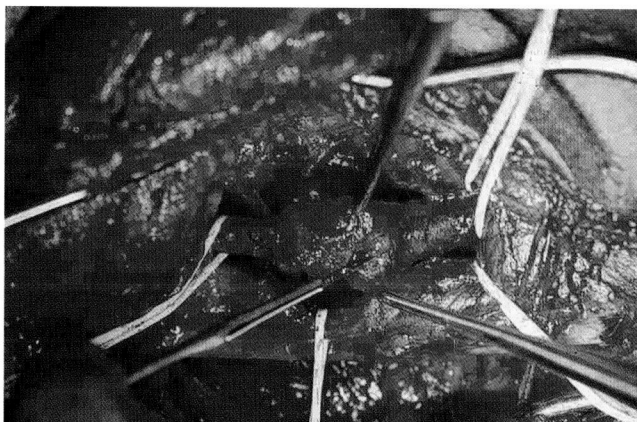

Figure 111-4 Appearance of popliteal artery affected by adventitial cystic disease. Exposure is through a posterior approach. The artery is often adherent to other structures and appears enlarged.

Venous

Rare and unusual cases of lower extremity venous involvement with adventitial cystic disease have been reported sporadically.[8] As with arterial involvement, these venous cysts occur predominantly in males; they most commonly involve the iliofemoral venous segments, with only occasional instances of popliteal or saphenous vein involvement. The most common presentation of this rare condition is similar to that of deep venous thrombosis. Typically, a young, healthy male presents with painless swelling of the lower extremity. Venous adventitial cystic disease should be considered when there is evidence of extrinsic compression on venous duplex imaging or a filling defect on venography. The optimal method of management of venous adventitial cystic disease is not well defined, but most authors advocate operative exploration involving a venotomy with evacuation of the cyst contents, followed by cyst wall excision in the hope of minimizing the risk of recurrence.

Diagnostic Evaluation

Noninvasive studies are consistent with an isolated arterial lesion. Ankle-brachial indices are unaffected at rest and drop following exercise. This pattern should raise the suspicion of an arterial cause of the patient's symptoms and prompt further investigation.

As with all other arterial pathologies, we have seen a steady progression of diagnostic modalities from standard angiography and Doppler ultrasound technologies to cross-sectional imaging with computed tomography (CT) and magnetic resonance imaging (MRI). Although all these methods have advantages and disadvantages with regard to adventitial cystic disease, current recommendations advocate the use of duplex scanning followed by CT or MRI as the best diagnostic modality for this pathology.[11]

Noninvasive Testing

Doppler ultrasound should be considered the first diagnostic tool for this disorder.[22,23] It is noninvasive and inexpensive

thrombosis, evacuation of cyst contents can restore arterial patency, supporting the pathophysiology of extrinsic luminal compression with a normal intimal layer. Of course, prolonged compression of a compromised lumen can lead to popliteal artery thrombosis and a fixed occlusion. There have been anecdotal reports of spontaneous cyst resolution,[21] but this appears to be extremely rare and should not be considered a feature of this disorder.

Approximately two thirds of patients present with popliteal artery stenosis rather than occlusion. On physical examination, this may be demonstrated by normal or diminished pedal pulses and by an audible bruit in the popliteal fossa. Pedal pulses that are present at rest may disappear with flexion of the knee (Ishikawa's sign), representing a functional stenosis that proceeds to occlusion with this physical manipulation. This is in contradistinction to popliteal artery entrapment, in which case pedal pulses disappear with gastrocnemius muscle contraction caused by active plantar flexion or passive dorsiflexion of the foot.[11]

and, in the appropriate hands, can yield important information. The number of cysts and their dimensions can be easily evaluated; their presence, along with elevated Doppler velocities through the affected segment, can be considered diagnostic for adventitial cystic disease. The boundary between the cyst and the arterial lumen is depicted by a fine bright line that pulsates. Ultrasound can also differentiate these cysts from popliteal artery aneurysms by the absence of flow signals in the cysts themselves. Following intervention, Doppler ultrasound is a useful postoperative surveillance tool to rule out cyst recurrence and residual or recurrent stenosis.

Angiography

Angiography has been the traditional diagnostic modality for adventitial cystic disease as well as most other arteriopathies. Complete popliteal artery occlusion is demonstrated in up to one third of cases, and the remaining studies demonstrate an eccentric compression of the popliteal artery lumen known as the "scimitar" sign (Figs. 111-5 and 111-6).[23] Caution is warranted, however, because stenosis can be missed on anteroposterior views and may be evident only with lateral projections. In the absence of arterial thrombosis, this eccentric stenosis in the absence of post-stenotic dilatation is a specific diagnostic sign of adventitial cystic disease. However, the diagnostic capability of conventional angiography is limited in the case of arterial occlusion. In this situation, angiography provides little accurate information regarding arterial wall pathology and the surrounding soft tissue.[11] In a young individual, angiography does not necessarily differentiate between adventitial cystic disease and popliteal artery entrapment syndrome in cases of popliteal artery occlusion.

Computed Tomography and Magnetic Resonance Imaging

CT is being used more extensively in cases of popliteal artery disease (Fig. 111-7). Its main contribution to the evaluation of adventitial cystic disease is to differentiate this pathology from popliteal entrapment syndrome and aneurysmal formation, especially in cases of popliteal artery occlusion or thrombosis. CT is superior to angiography in this regard, especially

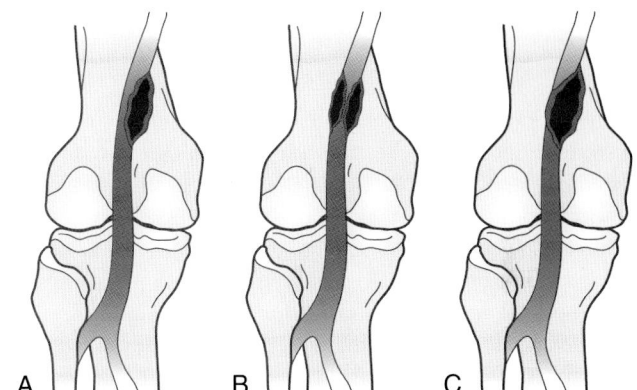

Figure 111-5 Adventitial cysts can occur in variable locations on the popliteal artery. The expanding cyst may indent the artery, resulting in the "scimitar" sign (**A**); encircle the artery, resulting in the "hourglass" sign (**B**); or completely occlude the vessel (**C**).

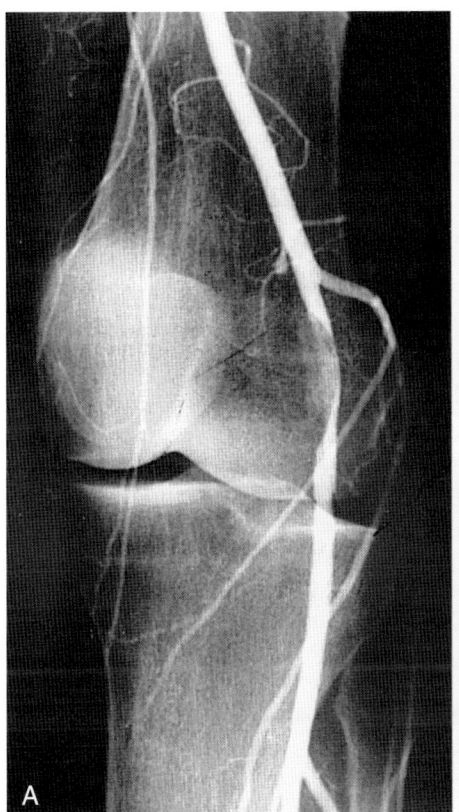
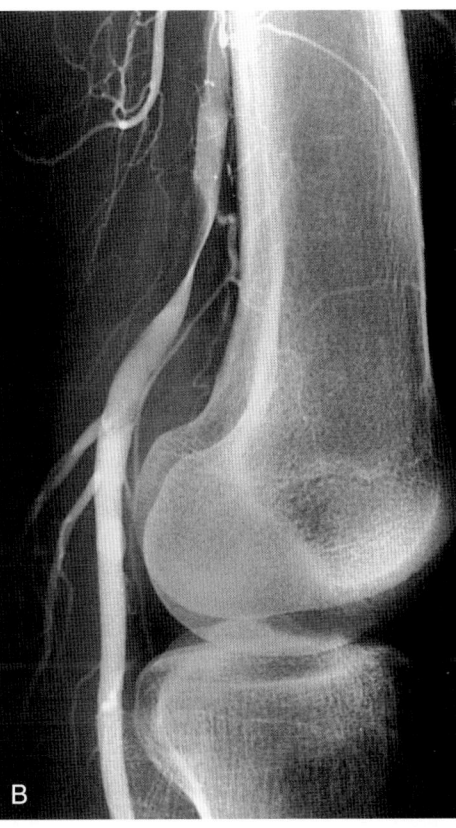

Figure 111-6 A, Femoral angiogram shows compression of the right popliteal artery by an adventitial cyst. **B,** Lateral view of another patient shows anterior compression of the popliteal artery above the knee.

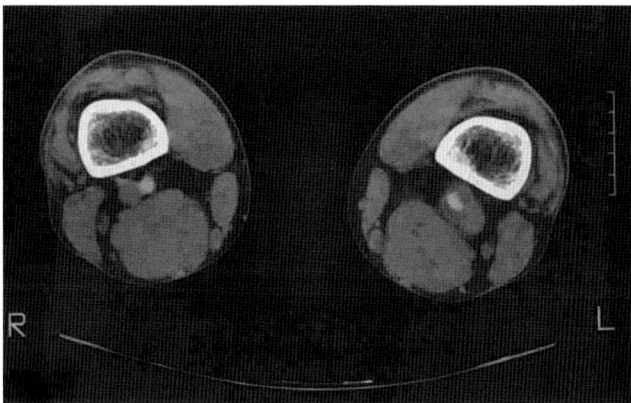

Figure 111-7 CT of popliteal fossa displays adventitial cystic disease of the left popliteal artery. The contralateral artery is unaffected.

Table 111-1 Management Options for Adventitial Cystic Disease of the Popliteal Artery, from Highest to Lowest Risk of Recurrence

Treatment	Risk of Recurrence (%)
Nonresectional (Stenosed Artery)	
Transluminal angioplasty	≈100
Imaging-guided cyst aspiration	0-33
Operative cyst evacuation and excision	6-33
Resectional (Thrombosed Artery)	
Arterial resection and reconstruction	0-6

in the case of arterial occlusion; CT has the ability to demonstrate the nature of the cysts and their relationship to surrounding structures.[24] It can also exclude the muscular abnormalities apparent in popliteal artery entrapment syndrome.

In the past decade, MRI has supplanted other techniques as the optimal diagnostic modality for adventitial cystic disease in the view of some investigators.[25] Obvious advantages of MRI over CT include the avoidance of ionizing radiation and intravascular contrast agents. MRI clearly depicts the extent of cystic involvement, and many authors consider it essential during the planning of surgical intervention. The typical finding on MRI is an "hourglass" deformity in the popliteal artery. Technically, some authors recommend formatting MRI to include T2-weighted and gradient-echo sequences for suspected cases of adventitial cystic disease.[11]

Despite these strongly held beliefs, there is little convincing evidence to support the use of MRI over CT. However, few investigators would argue against the use of a cross-sectional imaging modality for the diagnosis of adventitial cystic disease and subsequent treatment planning. The additional information on cyst extent and anatomy provided by these techniques compared with conventional angiography can be invaluable, especially in cases of complete arterial occlusion. Doppler ultrasound remains useful as an initial diagnostic test and as an instrument of postoperative surveillance.

Treatment

The literature pertaining to treatment strategies for popliteal adventitial cystic disease ranges from anecdotal reports to descriptions of small series. Given the rarity of this arteriopathy, no individual center has accumulated the critical mass of patients required to offer clear guidelines about its treatment and management. Treatment recommendations are based on an evaluation of cumulative experience as opposed to randomized controlled studies. In addition, information on recurrence rates is rare. Because most case descriptions are anecdotal, so are descriptions of recurrence. Therefore, data

on recurrence risks are best described as greater or less risk versus other treatment options, as opposed to citing of specific percentages.

Generally, management options for adventitial cystic disease can be divided into resectional and nonresectional procedures (Table 111-1).[4,11] Resection, with subsequent arterial reconstruction, is more commonly used in cases of complete popliteal artery occlusion secondary to thrombosis or in the presence of extensive degeneration of the arterial wall. In the majority of instances when nonocclusive stenoses are encountered, nonresectional methods are recommended.

Nonresectional Methods

Nonresectional methods of treatment previously described in the literature include the following:

- Percutaneous transluminal angioplasty
- CT- or ultrasound-guided percutaneous cyst aspiration
- Cyst evacuation with or without cyst excision

These treatment methods are listed in order of increasing chance of initial success and decreasing recurrence rate. Angioplasty has been discarded as a treatment option by most investigators. Its ineffectiveness is based on the normal intimal layer of these arteries and the compliant arterial segment, which can cause recoil and restenosis as early as 24 hours following balloon dilatation.[26] Preservation of the secretory lining of the adventitial cysts following angioplasty almost universally leads to disease recurrence.

Cyst Aspiration. Promising short-term outcomes have been achieved with CT- or ultrasound-guided cyst aspiration. The technique is well described, including the precise positioning of the needle tip to avoid the popliteal vein and tibial and peroneal nerves.[11,27] Although the technique is relatively simple and minimally invasive, treatment failures following percutaneous cyst aspiration are not unusual in cases of multiple loculations and highly viscous cyst fluid. This can result in incomplete cyst evacuation and recurrence in up to a third of patients.[11] Imaging-guided cyst aspiration has a place in the management of this arteriopathy, but given the risk of incomplete evacuation and recurrence, it should be limited to those patients who refuse operative intervention and agree to close imaging surveillance and probable re-intervention.

Cyst Excision or Cyst Evacuation. Operative exposure of the involved popliteal artery is best achieved via a posterior approach with the patient prone, using an S-shaped incision. This approach is described under "Types I to V, Normal Popliteal Artery." In the case of a stenosed popliteal artery, incision into the cyst and evacuation of its contents are usually sufficient to restore arterial patency. Recurrence rates following this form of treatment may be as high as 10%,[11] however, causing some authors to recommend cyst excision and evacuation to limit the chance of recurrence.

Resectional Methods

In instances of popliteal artery thrombosis or extensive arterial degeneration, a resectional treatment option is preferred. The affected popliteal artery is explored through a posterior approach, and the extent of arterial resection is determined by the length of arterial involvement on preoperative cross-sectional imaging and intraoperative findings. Arterial reconstruction is performed with an autogenous venous conduit of the surgeon's choice. Through a posterior approach with the patient prone, the small saphenous vein is available if it is of adequate caliber. If not, an alternative vein must be harvested. Although recurrence of adventitial cystic disease after such resective therapy is unusual, there have been reports of recurrence after vein graft interposition following arterial resection.[28] Presumably this was due to incomplete resection of the involved artery at the original operation.

Recurrence

Recurrence of adventitial cystic disease has been described following all methods of therapy, although it is less likely with resection of the cyst or the involved artery. Choice of therapy is determined by the luminal status of the popliteal artery. In nonoccluded arteries, nonresectional methods, including imaging-guided cyst aspiration, or operative cyst evacuation and excision offer good short-term outcomes. The operative approach is most definitive and has the lowest chance of recurrence. In instances of popliteal artery thrombosis, resection is advocated, with excision of the involved artery and reconstruction with an autogenous conduit. Given the recurrence risk with all these therapies, indefinite and periodic postoperative surveillance with ultrasound is necessary.

■ POPLITEAL ARTERY ENTRAPMENT SYNDROME

Epidemiology

Similar to adventitial cystic disease, popliteal artery entrapment syndrome should be considered a possible diagnosis in any young individual with exertional calf discomfort. As an anatomic variant, entrapment of the popliteal artery has been recognized for more than 100 years, but it was not until 40 years ago that the term *popliteal artery entrapment syndrome* was used to describe the clinical entity.[2,29] The true incidence of this syndrome is difficult to determine, but it is apparently more common than initially thought. The corresponding anatomic abnormalities were observed in 3.5% of individuals in a postmortem study,[30] and it is estimated that up to 60% of young individuals with claudication symptoms suffer from popliteal artery entrapment syndrome.[31] This makes it more common than adventitial cystic disease. Those affected tend to be quite active, giving this syndrome the moniker the "jogging disease."

The vast majority (up to 80%) of reported cases have occurred in men, with over half affected before reaching 30 years of age.[32,33] Cases of popliteal artery entrapment syndrome in women older than 50 years have been reported but are unusual.[34] Of course, the anatomic variant is present since its embryologic origin in utero, but it appears that at least several decades are necessary for the development of symptoms. Popliteal artery entrapment syndrome has been described as being simultaneously symptomatic in both lower extremities in approximately 30% of cases.[35] Interestingly, upon investigation, patients with unilateral symptoms were found to have bilateral anatomic abnormalities two thirds of the time.[35] Rare instances of bilateral popliteal artery occlusion secondary to popliteal artery entrapment have been reported.[36]

Pathogenesis

Etiology

The anatomy observed in the different types of popliteal artery entrapment is best understood by considering the embryologic development of the various structures of the popliteal fossa (see "Embryology"). Similar to the development of the lower extremity arterial system, the in utero development of the gastrocnemius muscle is a dynamic process with the potential for the occurrence of several anatomic abnormalities. Specifically, the medial head of the gastrocnemius muscle arises from the posterior fibula and lateral tibia, and during subsequent medial limb bud rotation and knee extension, it migrates across the popliteal fossa to its final attachment on the posterior aspect of the medial femoral condyle.[35] As described previously, the popliteal artery forms superficial to the popliteus muscle at about the same time as this medial migration of the medial head of the gastrocnemius muscle across the popliteal fossa (Fig. 111-8).

Classification

With an appreciation of the embryologic development of the popliteal fossa, a classification system based on this developmental anatomy was developed. The basis of this system was the Heidelberg classification, which originally described three types (I to III) of popliteal artery entrapment syndromes (Fig. 111-9).[37] At present, the classification system describing popliteal artery entrapment syndrome consists of six variants, types I to VI.

Type I. In type I entrapment syndrome, the popliteal artery completes its development before migration of the medial

Figure 111-8 Migration of the medial head of the gastrocnemius muscle through the popliteal fossa during formation of the popliteal artery. **A,** The medial head of the gastrocnemius muscle begins to migrate from the region of the fibula. At this stage, the axial distal popliteal artery lies deep to the popliteus muscle. **B,** The distal portion of the popliteal artery involutes as the medial head of the gastrocnemius muscle passes from lateral to medial. The proximal popliteal artery is derived from fusion with the developing femoral plexus, whereas the midportion of the popliteal artery is formed from the persistent axial artery remnant. **C,** A new or nonaxial distal popliteal artery now forms superficial to the popliteus muscle, after the medial head has migrated through the popliteal fossa. **D,** Normal definitive popliteal anatomy. *(From Levien LJ, Veller MG. Popliteal artery entrapment syndrome: more common than previously recognised. J Vasc Surg. 1999;30: 587-598.)*

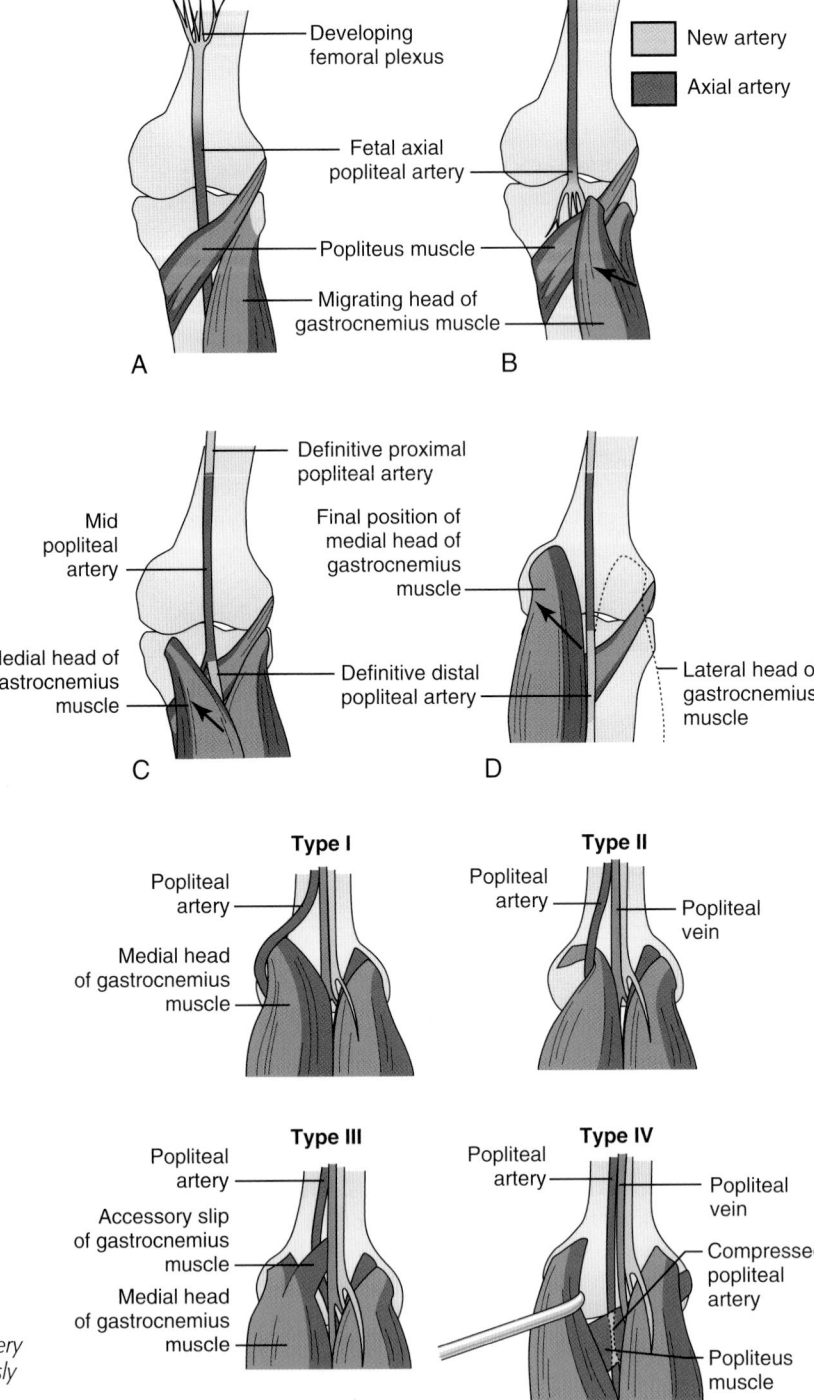

Figure 111-9 Types of popliteal artery entrapment syndromes. *(From Levien LJ, Veller MG. Popliteal artery entrapment syndrome: more common than previously recognised. J Vasc Surg. 1999;30:587-598.)*

head of the gastrocnemius muscle, which then pushes the artery medially during migration. This results in the popliteal artery's lying medial to a normally situated gastrocnemius muscle and is associated with an anatomic and radiologic medial deviation of the artery.[35]

Type II. With type II popliteal entrapment, the artery is displaced medially, but the medial head of the gastrocnemius muscle has a variable attachment on the lateral aspect of the medial femoral condyle or intercondylar area. In this case, the artery forms prematurely and partially arrests the migration

of the gastrocnemius muscle, resulting in the artery's being positioned medial to an abnormally attached muscle. In contrast to the normal position of gastrocnemius muscle insertion in type I entrapment, type II is defined by an abnormal femoral insertion site.

Type III. Type III entrapment is a result of an abnormal muscle slip or fibrous band that arises from either the medial or lateral femoral condyle.[35] Type III entrapment occurs when embryologic remnants of the gastrocnemius muscle remain posterior to the popliteal artery or when the artery develops within this muscle mass. Occasionally a double origin of the gastrocnemius muscle can surround and compress the popliteal artery.

In summary, types I to III represent the same anatomic variant, the degree of which depends on the temporal relationship between popliteal artery development and migration of the medial head of the gastrocnemius muscle.

Type IV. The mechanism resulting in type IV entrapment is fundamentally different from that causing types I to III. Type IV entrapment occurs with persistence of the axial artery as the mature distal popliteal artery. This artery remains in its embryologic position, deep to the popliteus muscle or fibrous bands.[35]

Type V. The mechanism causing type V entrapment can be that of any of the previously mentioned types; however, in addition, both the popliteal artery and popliteal vein are involved or entrapped. This subtype has been estimated to occur in approximately 10% to 15% of popliteal entrapment cases.[2,33]

Type VI. An additional type of entrapment—previously known as "functional" entrapment, or type F—is now commonly referred to as type VI entrapment. This occurs in otherwise healthy individuals who describe the typical symptoms of entrapment and show appropriate compression of the artery with stress maneuvers in the absence of an explanatory anatomic abnormality.[35] The anatomic abnormality in type VI entrapment has been difficult to determine, but it has been proposed that an especially lateral attachment of the medial head of the gastrocnemius muscle to the posterior aspect of the medial femoral condyle predisposes to this condition. Close to half of these asymptomatic individuals show reduction or complete occlusion of popliteal artery flow with such stressor mechanisms as plantar flexion or dorsiflexion against resistance.[38] Hypertrophy of this muscle following regular exercise is thought to result in compression of the posteromedial aspect of the popliteal artery. When subjected to MRI examination, individuals with functional entrapment and popliteal artery occlusion with stressor maneuvers tend to have a more extensive midline position of the medial head of the gastrocnemius muscle. When compared with normal controls, patients with functional entrapment have more of this muscle attached toward the supracondylar femoral midline, around the lateral border of the medial femoral condyle, and within the intercondylar fossa.[39] This more midline position of the muscle is likely a variation of normal embryologic development that predisposes to functional entrapment with strenuous activities or exercise that results in gastrocnemius muscle hypertrophy.

Pathology

A classification of the progression of histologic changes in popliteal artery entrapment syndrome has been described.[40] These histologic changes are the result of continuing arterial compression causing the progression from fibrosis of the various arterial layers to complete occlusion or thrombosis (Fig. 111-10). In this pathologic classification scheme, the fibrosis is confined to the adventitia in stage 1; it extends into the media in stage 2, which may result in post-stenotic dilatation or aneurysm formation. In stage 3, the artery may become

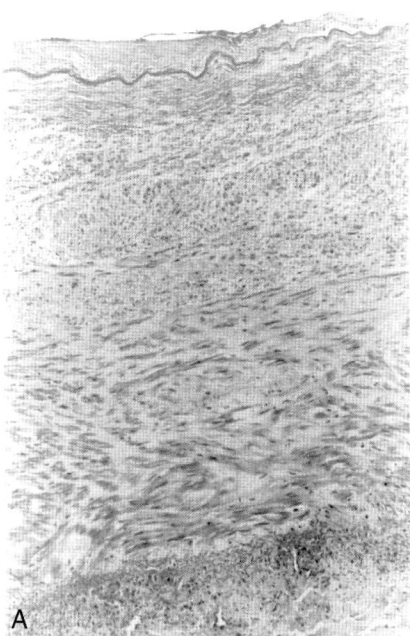
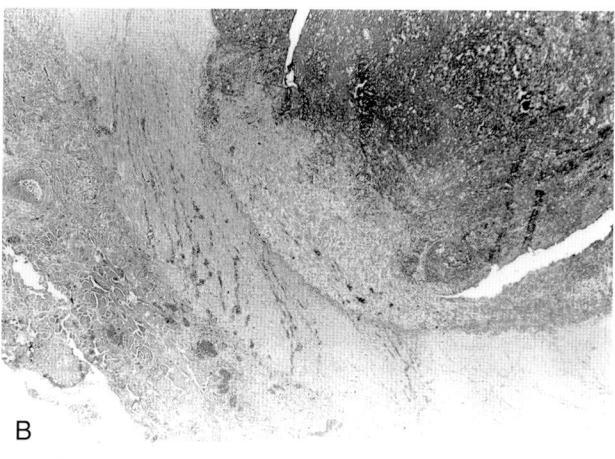

Figure 111-10 Histologic appearance of a popliteal artery shows stage 2 disease with significant degeneration of the media (**A**) and stage 3 disease with extensive destruction of the media and hyperplasia of the intima complicated by thrombosis (**B**).

thrombogenic, independent of the compression, as the fibrosis extends into the intimal layer.[33] The degree of arterial damage does not appear to be directly related to the duration of compression or popliteal entrapment.[1] The major clinical significance of these findings is the potential thrombogenicity of a chronically entrapped popliteal artery that might not be corrected with any surgical intervention short of arterial replacement.

Clinical Presentation

The most common presentation of an individual with popliteal artery entrapment syndrome is that of a young, healthy man who participates in sports and has symptoms of claudication. However, a range in the severity of associated symptoms has been described, and a grading scale describing these symptoms was recently proposed following a forum specifically convened to discuss popliteal artery entrapment syndrome[2]:

- *Class 0:* Asymptomatic
- *Class 1:* Pain, paresthesia, and cold feet after physical training (e.g., jogging, heavy work)
- *Class 2:* Claudication while walking (>100 m)
- *Class 3:* Claudication while walking (<100 m)
- *Class 4:* Rest pain
- *Class 5:* Necrosis

In a large series of patients, 46% of patients had class 1 symptoms, 35% class 2, 14% class 3, and 2% class 5.[2] None had class 4.

The vast majority (70% to 90%) of patients with symptomatic popliteal artery entrapment present with intermittent calf claudication. This classically resolves with rest. In some cases, the claudication symptoms may be atypical and paradoxical, in that they worsen with standing or walking but improve with more vigorous exercise, or they may occur immediately after the onset of walking rather than after walking a longer distance. Patients occasionally describe symptoms of coldness, blanching, and numbness. All types of entrapment (except type VI) can involve the tibial nerves and result in certain degrees of paresthesia. The minority of patients (10%) present with signs and symptoms of chronic CLI, and even fewer present with acute limb ischemia. Venous entrapment (type V) is suggested by calf cramping or symptoms more typical of a compartment syndrome, including swelling and a feeling of fullness.[33]

Typically, pedal pulses are palpable and normal at rest in these individuals, as long as compression of the popliteal artery has not progressed to occlusion. These pulses disappear with passive dorsiflexion or active plantar flexion of the foot. These maneuvers tense the gastrocnemius muscle against the entrapped artery, temporarily occluding the patent lumen. They should also be performed on the contralateral asymptomatic limb. If left untreated, chronic entrapment causes progressive fibrosis of the popliteal artery, resulting in a thrombogenic intimal surface and eventual arterial thrombosis and occlusion.[35] Occlusion of the artery can be heralded by the sudden onset of more severe calf claudication with absent pedal pulses. This can occur after an episode of strenuous exercise and should result in a high degree of suspicion for popliteal artery entrapment syndrome when it occurs in a young adult with no manifestations of or risk factors for atherosclerosis.

Post-stenotic dilatation or aneurysmal degeneration of the popliteal artery can occasionally occur and be a source of distal emboli, as can thrombus formation in a normal-caliber entrapped artery.[40]

Diagnostic Evaluation

Once the diagnosis of popliteal artery entrapment syndrome has been entertained in the context of an appropriate history and physical examination, several noninvasive diagnostic tests can be performed to confirm this suspicion. The specific diagnostic and imaging protocol varies greatly among centers. Generally, the most common initial tests are distal pressure measurement and duplex scanning, combined with dynamic provocative maneuvers that cause gastrocnemius muscle contraction—namely, active plantar flexion and passive dorsiflexion of the ankle with the knee in full extension.[41]

Noninvasive Testing

Segmental pressures are taken with the Doppler probe placed on the posterior tibial artery during calf muscle contraction and relaxation. Readings are repeated several times, and care should be taken to avoid moving the probe during muscle contractions. Similarly, duplex studies are performed with visualization of the popliteal artery during calf muscle contraction and relaxation. The duplex interrogation must be repeated several times because the popliteal artery can be pushed deeper into the popliteal fossa during muscle contraction, negatively affecting visualization and volume recordings. Although a positive duplex test with provocative maneuvers should prompt further investigation, it should not form the only basis for operative intervention. Very high (72%) false-positive rates have been reported, resulting in an overestimation of popliteal artery compression.[33]

Angiography

Although cross-sectional imaging techniques have gained ground, angiography remains the mainstay of investigation at many centers. However, angiography without provocative maneuvers can have low sensitivity in cases of arterial occlusion or a patent artery that is minimally displaced.

Generally, the diagnosis of popliteal artery entrapment syndrome should be considered when at least two of the following angiographic features are apparent[1]:

- Medial deviation of the proximal popliteal artery
- Focal occlusion of the mid–popliteal artery
- Post-stenotic dilatation of the distal popliteal artery

Medial deviation of the artery is most often apparent in types I, II, and III popliteal artery entrapment, but it may be a subtle finding and is subject to variation in observers' interpretation. Focal occlusion of the mid–popliteal artery in young patients without risk factors for or evidence of atherosclerotic disease is due to either adventitial cystic disease of the popliteal artery or popliteal artery entrapment syndrome in most cases. Post-stenotic dilatation of the distal popliteal artery is apparent in an estimated 12% of angiograms of patients with popliteal artery entrapment.[1] Angiography has the additional advantage of delineating tibial artery anatomy following emboli from a post-stenotic dilatation of an entrapped popliteal artery or a thrombogenic entrapped artery.

Several angiographic views should be obtained both in the neutral position and during provocative maneuvers such as passive dorsiflexion and active plantar flexion of the foot with the knee in full extension. These views increase the sensitivity of angiography in cases of popliteal artery entrapment syndrome because compression or occlusion is often not apparent in the neutral position without active contraction of the gastrocnemius muscle (Fig. 111-11). This contrasts with adventitial cystic disease of the popliteal artery; in that case, although stressor maneuvers (i.e., knee flexion) can cause complete arterial occlusion, the arterial stenosis or compression from adventitial cysts is readily apparent at rest or in the neutral position (previously described as the "scimitar" sign).

Computed Tomography and Magnetic Resonance Imaging

Less invasive imaging alternatives such as CT and MRI can be particularly useful in cases of popliteal artery entrapment syndrome when the artery is occluded. They can illustrate the particular anatomic relationships between the artery and muscle in the popliteal fossa and identify anomalous muscular insertions (Fig. 111-12). Although these claims are subjective and not backed up by extensive evidence, some investigators claim that MRI is superior to CT in this regard and should be the diagnostic test of choice in young patients suffering from intermittent claudication.[33]

Treatment

In most cases of symptomatic popliteal artery entrapment syndrome, surgical intervention is indicated and should be offered. This is especially true for types I to V entrapment; the decision may be less clear in type VI entrapment, depending on the severity of symptoms. Generally, intervention during an earlier clinical stage results in a more limited operation—namely, myotomy alone rather than arterial reconstruction. This statement is based on knowledge of the natural history of entrapment, which is one of progressive arterial fibrosis and damage and eventual thrombosis and occlusion. As a result, most authors advocate surgical correction of types I to V popliteal artery entrapment to avoid the risk of later significant arterial degeneration.[1]

The basic principles of intervention include release of arterial entrapment, restoration of normal anatomy, and restoration of arterial flow.[33] These goals are best achieved with operative procedures because endoluminal therapies do not deal with muscular entrapment. There have been reports of small numbers of patients with occluded popliteal arteries undergoing endoluminal interventions and thrombolysis followed by myotomy several weeks later. These patients were

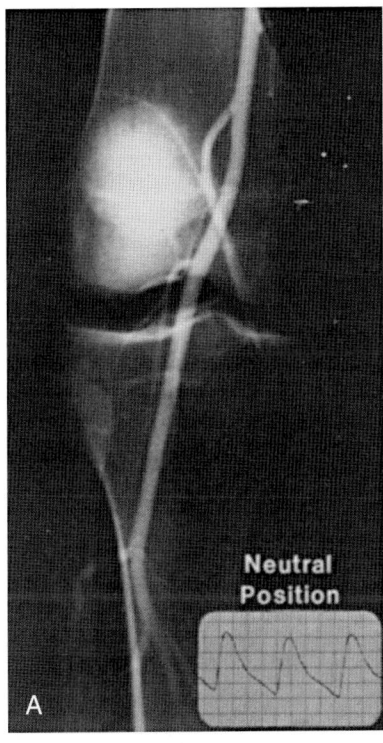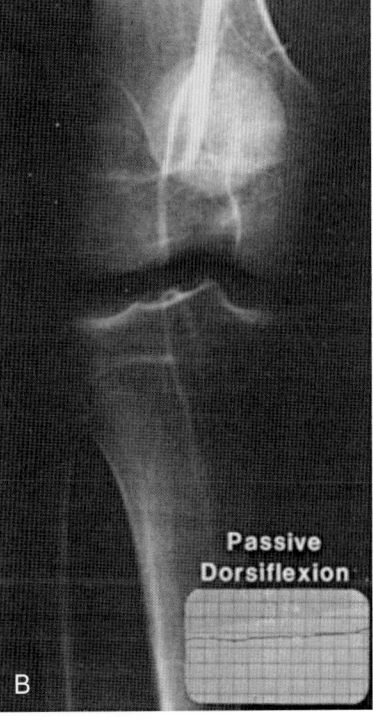

Figure 111-11 A, Angiogram reveals a normal course of the popliteal artery with a normal ankle pulse volume recording (*inset*) when the foot is in the neutral position. **B,** With passive dorsiflexion of the foot, the popliteal artery becomes occluded, and the ankle pulse volume recording becomes flat (*inset*).

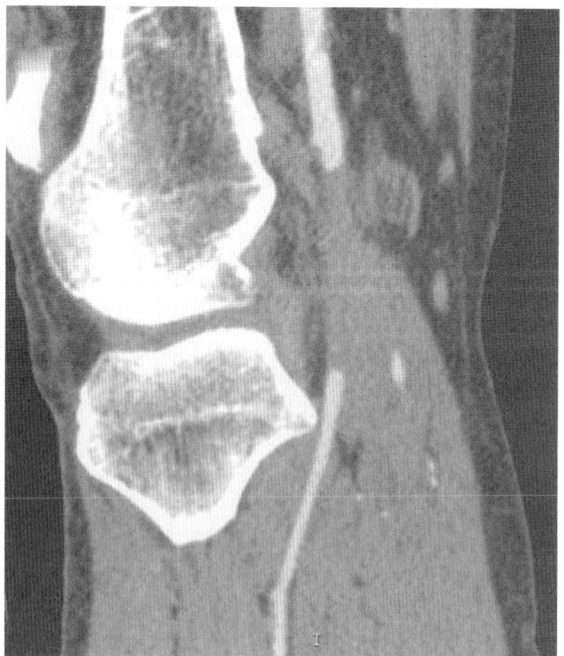

Figure 111-12 Computed tomographic angiography reveals popliteal artery occlusion due to popliteal artery entrapment syndrome.

Table 111-2 Management Options for Popliteal Artery Entrapment Syndromes

Status of Artery	Entrapment Type	Operation	Surgical Approach
Normal	I and II	Myotomy	Medial
	III and IV	Myotomy	Posterior
	V	Myotomy	Medial or posterior
	VI	Myotomy if symptomatic	Medial or posterior
Abnormal (occluded, stenosed, or post-stenotic dilatation or aneurysm)	I to VI	Decompression and arterial resection and replacement or exclusion and bypass	Medial or posterior

anticoagulated for various periods.[42] Anticoagulation and the preservation of a potentially thrombogenic popliteal artery are suboptimal treatment options in this young, healthy, active patient population.

The specific approach for an individual patient is dictated by the anatomy, the clinical presentation, and the status of the popliteal artery (Table 111-2). These different scenarios are discussed in the following sections.

Types I to V, Normal Popliteal Artery

These symptomatic patients have normally patent popliteal arteries at rest but display evidence of occlusion during non-invasive investigations and angiography with provocative

maneuvers, as previously described. Preoperative investigations often indicate whether the entrapped artery is suffering from damage or fibrosis, but it is often not until operative exposure and palpation of the artery that the degree and extent of fibrosis are apparent. In the absence of arterial fibrosis and in the presence of a normal-appearing artery, therapy limited to musculotendinous release is sufficient to restore normal anatomy.[33] In one large series, three quarters of limbs were treated in this manner with myotomy of the medial head of the gastrocnemius muscle, abnormal muscle slips, or tendinous bands. When followed for up to 10 years, patients treated in such a manner were able to return to their prior sports activities, did not require any further interventions, and maintained patency of their popliteal arteries.[35]

Musculotendinous release can be performed through either a posterior or a medial approach. Posterior exposure of the entrapped popliteal artery is performed with the patient in the prone position through an S- or Z-shaped incision (Fig. 111-13). Proponents of this approach highlight the operative flexibility it offers the surgeon, the wider degree of inspection possible, the greater ease of identifying and addressing the specific anatomic abnormality, and an adequate exposure to complete an arterial reconstruction if necessary.[33,43] Following incision, flaps are raised to expose the deep fascia, which is incised longitudinally, avoiding injury to the median cutaneous sural nerve. Sacrifice of the lesser saphenous vein can facilitate exposure. As the vessels are approached, the tibial nerve is encountered and mobilized. The popliteal vein is identified passing between the heads of the gastrocnemius muscle deep in the popliteal fossa. The popliteal artery, which is not in its normal position, is identified higher in the popliteal space and followed distally. The artery's abnormal course can be medial to the medial head of the gastrocnemius muscle or entrapped by anomalous muscular structures or tendinous tissue.[1,43]

Through this posterior exposure, the medial head of the gastrocnemius muscle or the entrapping musculotendinous bands are completely divided. It most cases, it is not necessary to reattach the muscle because the medial head of the gastrocnemius muscle can be divided with no adverse functional sequelae, even in these young, active patients.[44] In entrapment types III and IV, it is usually not necessary to divide the tendon of the medial head of the gastrocnemius muscle; mobilization of the muscular portion of the medial head off the posterior aspect of the femoral condyles usually suffices to relieve compression of the artery.[1]

With this scenario, the medial operative approach is most suited for popliteal artery entrapment types I and II and is less appropriate for types III and IV, where it may be more difficult to delineate the arterial and muscular anatomy. Entrapment types III and IV may best be explored via the posterior approach. Type V entrapment can be explored through either route, depending on the underlying muscular abnormality. The medial approach seems to result in a quicker return to normal athletic activities in these active patients and less incision-related morbidity.[35] Similar to the posterior approach, the medial head of the gastrocnemius muscle is divided when

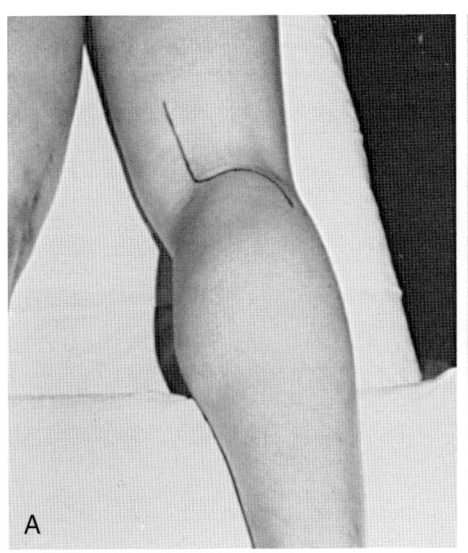 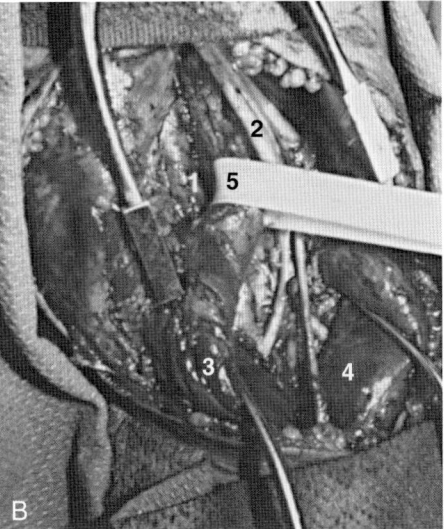

Figure 111-13 A, An S-shaped incision in the popliteal fossa is used for the posterior approach. **B,** Anatomic structures identified through the posterior incision are the popliteal artery (1), tibial nerve (2), medial head of the gastrocnemius muscle (3), lateral head of the gastrocnemius muscle (4), and a Penrose drain (5) wrapped around the accessory slip of the gastrocnemius muscle, which caused arterial compression.

approached from its medial aspect, permitting complete arterial decompression.

Types I to V, Abnormal Popliteal Artery

Arterial bypass or replacement is indicated in cases of complete thrombosis, arterial wall degeneration from the chronic entrapment, thrombus formation on the intimal surface, fibrotic narrowing of the artery, and post-stenotic dilatation or aneurysm formation.[1] When the popliteal artery shows evidence of chronic damage, even if the extent is only minimal fibrosis, it should be replaced or bypassed in its entirety. Allowing continued flow through the native artery leaves a residual intimal surface with unpredictable thrombogenic potential in a young, active individual and provides a setup for symptom recurrence due to arterial thrombosis.

Early reports of this syndrome described numerous instances of thromboendarterectomy with or without vein patch angioplasty. This approach produced inferior results, with a higher incidence of arterial thrombosis and reocclusion compared with arterial replacement with an autogenous conduit.[33] Once a popliteal artery is occluded or thrombosed, it should be considered beyond repair and be replaced.

This arterial reconstruction can be performed through a posterior or a medial approach. The posterior approach permits use of the lesser small vein as the venous conduit, but it is less useful in cases requiring a more distal reconstruction. There are several advantages to the medial approach, including the ease of harvesting the more proximal great saphenous vein if a conduit of larger caliber is required. Additionally, it is much easier to expose the more distal popliteal artery, or tibial arteries, through a medial exposure if a more distal revascularization is required.[1] This may be the case with extensive post-stenotic dilatation or with tibial artery occlusion secondary to thromboemboli from the entrapped popliteal artery.

In these cases, the entrapment is first relieved by dividing the muscle or tendinous segment causing the arterial compression. Resection of the thrombosed artery and a short interposition venous graft are then performed. Alternatively, a short venous bypass graft can be performed, with exclusion of the occluded artery to prevent distal thromboemboli. If post-stenotic dilatation or aneurysm formation has occurred, arterial resection and venous replacement are performed; alternatively, ligation and exclusion of the affected arterial segment are performed, followed by bypass of the excluded segment with autogenous vein.[1]

Type VI, Symptomatic

It is widely recognized that type VI functional entrapment due to hypertrophy of the medial head of the gastrocnemius muscle can lead to progressive popliteal artery damage, fibrosis, and eventual thrombosis. Most authors support an aggressive approach to surgical intervention when faced with symptomatic patients with functional entrapment.

In these cases, surgical decompression can occur through either a medial or a posterior approach. Transection of the muscular portion of the medial head of the gastrocnemius muscle, with preservation of the tendon, is sufficient to relieve symptoms.[33,34] To ensure adequate decompression, one must take care to completely transect the muscular fibers from the posterior aspect of the lateral femoral condyle and the intercondylar area.[1]

Type VI, Asymptomatic

As mentioned previously, up to half the normal, asymptomatic population may exhibit signs of popliteal artery compression with provocative measures such as active plantar flexion and passive dorsiflexion of the foot. This can be demonstrated by the loss of pedal pulses with these maneuvers or by angiographic investigation. When these individuals are truly asymptomatic, there is little evidence to support prophylactic operative intervention. These asymptomatic individuals are best followed.[33]

Similarly, although bilateral popliteal artery entrapment is common, often only one extremity is symptomatic (43% of cases).[32] These asymptomatic contralateral extremies should be investigated, but surgical exploration is seldom recommended in the absence of symptoms or positive investigations.[32]

SELECTED KEY REFERENCES

di Marzo L, Cavallaro A. Popliteal vascular entrapment. *World J Surg.* 2005;29:S43-S45.
Short paper summarizing the findings and recommendations of the 1998 Popliteal Vascular Entrapment Forum.

Dix FP, McDonald M, Obomighie J, Chalmers N, Thompson D, Benbow EW, Smyth JV. Cystic adventitial disease of the femoral vein presenting as deep vein thrombosis: a case report and review of the literature. *J Vasc Surg.* 2006;44:871-874.
Excellent description of the rare venous involvement in this disorder.

Henry MF, Wilkins DC, Lambert AW. Popliteal artery entrapment syndrome. *Curr Treat Options Cardiovasc Med.* 2004;6:113-120.
Practical summary of the treatment options and recommendations for popliteal artery entrapment syndrome, as well as a succinct description of the important embryologic development.

Levien LJ, Veller MG. Popliteal artery entrapment syndrome: more common than previously recognized. *J Vasc Surg.* 1999;30:587-598.
One of the largest clinical series of popliteal artery entrapment syndrome, encompassing 48 patients treated over a 10-year period.

Tsilimparis N, Hanack U, Yousefi S, Alevizakos P, Ruckert RI. Cystic adventitial disease of the popliteal artery: an argument for the developmental theory. *J Vasc Surg.* 2007;45:1249-1252.
Excellent discussion of the theories of the etiology of this syndrome, with a strong defense of and argument for a unifying developmental theory.

Tsolakis IA, Walvatne CS, Caldwell MD. Cystic adventitial disease of the popliteal artery: diagnosis and treatment. *Eur J Vasc Endovasc Surg.* 1998;15:188-194.
One of the largest published reviews, encompassing a 41-year experience with 264 cases.

REFERENCES

The reference list can be found on the companion Expert Consult Web site at *www.expertconsult.com.*

CHAPTER 112

Diabetic Foot Ulcers

George Andros and Lawrence A. Lavery

Diabetes is the most common underlying cause of foot ulcers, infections, ischemia, and amputations in the United States and Europe. Despite advances in vascular surgery, wound care, and medical management of diabetes, the statistics have not improved for lower extremity complications in the United States. The incidence of ulceration and amputation has declined in Sweden and the Netherlands and appears to be leveling off in Germany and Great Britain.[1,2] Diabetic foot ulceration (DFU) is important because 85% of all diabetic lower extremity amputations, both major and minor, are preceded by an ulcer.[3] Ulceration and its management strategies, which include intensive foot and wound care, treatment of infection, débridement, revascularization, and amputation, remain the number one reason for the hospitalization of diabetic patients, as has been the case for many years.

EPIDEMIOLOGY

Diabetes and diabetic foot complications are epidemic. Changes in the ethnic and cultural composition of the American population have likely contributed to the growing prevalence of diabetes in the United States. There are several reasons to anticipate an increase in the incidence of ulceration and amputation, including the increasing incidence of diabetes not only in the United States but worldwide, an aging population of baby boomers, an increasingly obese population, and the lack of a national plan for recognizing amputation risks and promoting education and ulcer prevention.

Likelihood of Amputation

Lower extremity amputation may best exemplify the impact of diabetes because it is a measure of end-stage disease and treatment failure. Overall, patients with diabetes are 15 to 30 times more likely to have an amputation than are patients without diabetes.[2,4,5] There are 90,000 amputations performed on individuals with diabetes in the United States annually. Seventy percent to 80% of all nontraumatic amputations occur in those with diabetes. After a major limb loss, 50% of contralateral limbs develop a serious lesion. After the initial index amputation, 9% to 17% of patients experience a second amputation within the same year,[1] and 25% to 68% of amputees have their contralateral extremity amputated within 5 years.[6,7]

Diabetes-related foot complications and amputations are disproportionately more common in men and in minorities.

The incidence of lower extremity amputation is 50 to 60 per 10,000 persons with diabetes per year in non-Hispanic whites. These rates are 150% higher in Hispanics and 170% to 240% higher in African Americans in the United States.[2] In non-Hispanic whites, 56% of amputations occur in patients with diabetes, whereas 75% of amputations in African Americans and 86% of amputations in Hispanics are due to diabetes.[5,8] Across all race and ethnic groups, the incidence of diabetes-related amputation is more than twice as high in men compared with women. The level of amputation is similar across race and ethnic groups: about 50% of amputations involve the foot, and 50% are below or above the knee. With respect to major limb amputation, the ratio of below-knee to above-knee amputations reported in the literature is highly variable. The recently updated Trans-Atlantic Inter-Society Consensus document (TASC II) reported a ratio of 1:1,[9] while other reports estimate the ratio to range from 1.7 to 5:1.[2,5,10] The reported ratios are likely a reflection of patient mix as well as referral and practice patterns.

Incidence of Foot Ulcers

Up to 25% of patients with diabetes will suffer from a foot ulcer during their lifetime.[3] Ulceration is a pivotal factor in the causal pathway to infection and amputation. Approximately 50% of diabetic foot ulcers become infected, and 20% of these require amputation.[3] The incidence of DFU ranges from 2.0% to 6.8% per year in the general diabetic population.[6,8,11] In more than 85% of lower extremity amputations, a wound is a critical aspect of the causal pathway.[8,12-14] It is uncommon for an adult with diabetes to develop a limb infection without a wound as a precipitating factor. Hematogenous soft tissue and bone infections are distinctly unusual. Lavery and coworkers evaluated a cohort of 1666 patients over 2.5 years and reported that 151 patients (9%) developed 199 foot infections.[13] Osteomyelitis was the diagnosis in 20% of these infections. Foot wounds preceded all but one soft tissue infection, and every case of osteomyelitis was preceded by ulceration.

Ulcer Recurrence

After healing, ulcer recidivism is very high. Once a person with diabetes develops a foot ulcer, the risk of recurrent foot ulcer, infection, and amputation is significant. Additional comorbidities confer markedly increased risk. For example, the presence of sensory neuropathy or peripheral arterial disease

(PAD), in addition to diabetes, increases the risk of these adverse outcomes more than 50-fold.[14-16]

ETIOLOGY

The etiology of DFU is complex, and an ulcer is rarely the result of a single factor. DFUs are caused by a combination of (1) autonomic, motor, and sensory neuropathy; (2) abnormal foot mechanics, leading to increased pressure and shear; (3) structural foot deformities coupled with limited joint mobility, which amplify the effects of neuropathy; (4) PAD; (5) trauma; and (6) poorly fitting shoes.[6,17,18] Heel ulcers, for example, commonly have two essential components: gravitational (decubitus) pressure transmitted to the heel, and ischemia.[19] In general, foot ulcers are the cumulative result of repetitive trauma that literally wears a hole in the skin.

The development of foot ulcers is often a matter of poor biomechanics.[13,17,18] Ulcer prevention requires attention to this pivotal and often misunderstood component of pedal energy transfer. Shear and stress develop on the sole of the foot at the site of high pressures resulting from structural foot deformity and limited joint mobility. Structural deformities such as claw toes, hallux valgus, dislocated metatarsophalangeal joints, and limited motion of the ankle and first metatarsophalangeal joint are regularly associated with foot ulcers. Dorsiflexion of the ankle joint should be 10 degrees from neutral, and dorsiflexion of the first metatarsophalangeal joint should be about 50 degrees from neutral. A combination of clawing of the toes and dislocation of the metatarsophalangeal joints causes retrograde buckling and dislocation. These forces cause the toes to be dislocated dorsally and the metatarsal head to be pushed in a plantar direction. In such cases, the metatarsal head is actually pushed through the bottom of the foot. Ulcers on the great toe often develop because of arthritis or limited motion of the first metatarsophalangeal joint. At toe-off in gait, the reduced motion causes more pressure and shear forces under the first metatarsal head or at the interphalangeal joint of the great toe. Ulcers on the tips of claw toes usually arise because of constant pressure and weight bearing. Bony prominences in the midfoot and unilateral flatfoot often result from Charcot's neuro-osteoarthropathy, neuropathic fracture, or a tear of the posterior tibialis tendon; these areas may ultimately become sites of ulceration. Classically, ulcers on the metatarsal heads (the "ball" of the foot) occur at sites of high pressure and shear forces that are exposed to repetitive injury (normal walking). In the presence of sensory neuropathy, a normally painful insult to soft tissues is not recognized until an ulcer develops and is detected fortuitously by inspection or malodor rather than pain. Ulcers on the dorsum or sides of the foot are usually due to ill-fitting shoes.

The importance of bony deformities that expose the overlying skin to trauma cannot be overemphasized. Because diabetics with neuropathy lack normal sensation, they may select shoes that are too small. In addition, progressive bunion and hammertoe deformities may require patients to purchase ill-fitting shoes that are wider and deeper than needed in the past. Because of neuropathy, patients may sustain penetrating injuries such as lacerations and puncture wounds that are not recognized owing to the loss of protective sensation.

CLINICAL PRESENTATION

DFUs can develop on any part of the feet, ankles, or toes. Yet despite their common occurrence, DFUs are often missed and must be actively sought. Claudication and rest pain occur less often in diabetics with neuroischemic ulceration than in nondiabetics with purely ischemic lesions; ulcers overlying the medial and lateral malleoli and metatarsophalangeal joints may cause pain despite neuropathy and the absence of infection because of penetration to the bone. When a patient presents with pain, drainage, malodor, or local or systemic signs of infection, medical attention is necessarily focused on the foot. However, because symptoms may be sparse owing to neuropathy, any physician who examines a diabetic patient is obliged to screen for DFUs. The essential elements of a screening examination include a history of foot wounds, amputations, or lower extremity bypass surgery or angioplasty; inspection of all surfaces of the foot for ulcers or preulcerative lesions; and an evaluation for neuropathy, PAD, structural foot deformities, and mobility of the ankle and metatarsophalangeal joints. Screening to identify risk factors in the diabetic foot can be capably performed by a nurse or trained technician.[12,14,17,19] The patient must remove shoes and socks for the examination; all surfaces of the foot and ankle, including the spaces between all the toes, the soles, and the heels, must be inspected for fissuring, cracks, blisters or bullae, calluses, and ulcers. The shoes should also be inspected for sites of wear or pressure and palpated for foreign bodies and irregularities such as extruding nails. Once an ulcer has been discovered, the process of understanding its cause begins. Details of the vascular examination are presented under "Clinical Evaluation."

Ischemia

The belief that the angiopathy caused by long-standing diabetes exists on a microvascular level and is therefore not amenable to enhancement has been conclusively disproved.[20-22] Microvascular basement membrane changes at the capillary level are well known in diabetes, especially in the kidney. However, the clinically important arterial changes in the lower extremity occur at the macrovascular level.

Anatomy of Occlusive Disease

Characteristically, diabetic occlusive lesions spare the arteries above the knee but involve the infrapopliteal arteries with calcific single or multiple stenoses and occlusions. In more than 90% of patients, one or more of the large arteries at the ankle and in the foot are spared (Fig. 112-1). In most cases the peroneal artery in the calf remains patent and is the last of the three crural arteries to occlude. It provides pedal cir-

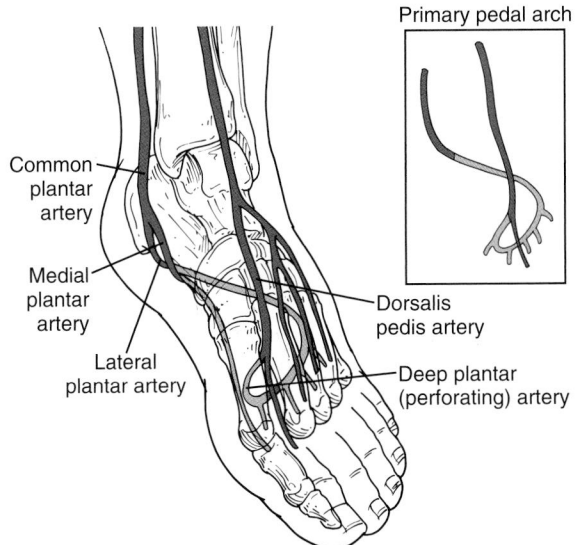

Figure 112-1 Pedal arterial anatomy. Because the deep plantar artery is nearly always occluded in advanced diabetic arterial disease, there is rarely a continuous connection between the dorsal forefoot and the plantar hindfoot circulations. The lighter portion of the primary pedal arch is the plantar arch.

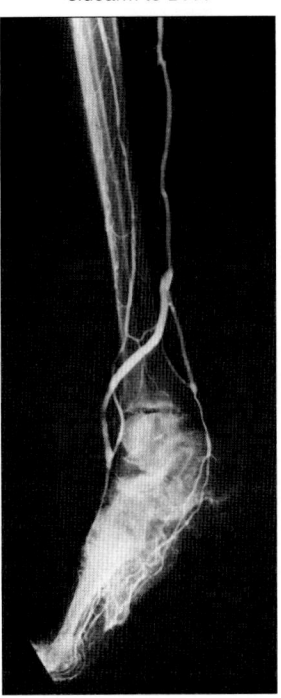

Figure 112-2 If forefoot and hindfoot ulcerations occur in the absence of a patent primary pedal arch, healing may be enhanced by creating a bifurcated bypass when both the anterior and posterior tibial arteries are patent. DPA, dorsal pedal artery; PTA, posterior tibial artery.

culation through its terminal branches, the anterior and posterior perforating arteries, to collaterals of the dorsal pedal and posterior tibial and plantar arteries. The primary pedal arch is almost always incomplete, but in most cases at least a segment of the plantar arch retains patency, if not continuity with the anterior and posterior circulation. Consequently, bypass to a single tibial or peroneal artery usually provides good blood flow to the foot. Infrequently only a single infrapopliteal artery segment remains patent, without direct communication to the foot arteries. In this situation, bypass to the "isolated segment" is the only revascularization option but has a reasonable success rate.[23-25] Reports that heel ulcers are slow to heal after bypass to the dorsal pedal artery[26] and its collateral runoff suggest that the pedal circulation, somewhat analogously to the coronary circulation, is compartmentalized.[23,27] If the ulcer is in the hindfoot, bypass to the posterior pedal–plantar artery axis is preferred. Forefoot and toe ulcers should preferentially receive dorsal pedal bypasses if possible. Midfoot, plantar, and combined toe and heel ulcers can be treated with bifurcated grafts to both the dorsal pedal and posterior tibial branches if these arterial targets are available (Fig. 112-2).

Clinical Evaluation

Clinical symptoms are often not helpful in the diagnosis of ischemia in patients with diabetes. DFUs are seldom foreshadowed by claudication, a common symptom of PAD in atherosclerotic patients without diabetes. Either the patient has infrapopliteal arterial occlusions, which do not usually cause claudication, or the patient walks too little or too slowly to experience calf pain. The aortoiliofemoral segment seldom develops occlusive lesions in diabetic patients, so buttock and thigh symptoms are rare; impotence, an occasional occur-

rence in aortoiliac occlusive disease, develops in diabetics by other pathogenetic mechanisms. The superficial femoral and popliteal arteries are more often affected in patients with diabetes than is the aortoiliac segment, so when claudication is present, it is usually experienced in the calf. Diabetic patients with foot ulcers and gangrene are often found to have a strong popliteal pulse and absent pedal pulses. This finding is due to a highly prevalent pattern of predominantly tibial artery occlusive disease in diabetics; moreover, it portends a high likelihood that the patient is a suitable candidate for revascularization, because the peroneal artery or the inframalleolar pedal arteries are usually spared. These general observations underscore the importance of the physical examination in the initial vascular assessment.

The increasing incidence of diabetic vascular disease has led to the emergence of new patterns of diabetic arteriopathy. These lesions include exophytic and "coral reef" plaques and stenoses involving the iliofemoral segment (Fig. 112-3). Arterial calcification, first noted by West[28] to be a hallmark of diabetic arteriopathy in the tibial arteries, is now recognized as widespread throughout the arterial system. This frequently results in noncompressible arteries in major arterial segments. Clinical signs such as absent foot pulses, pallor with elevation, dependent rubor, atrophic integument, and absent hair growth are common manifestations of PAD in diabetics.

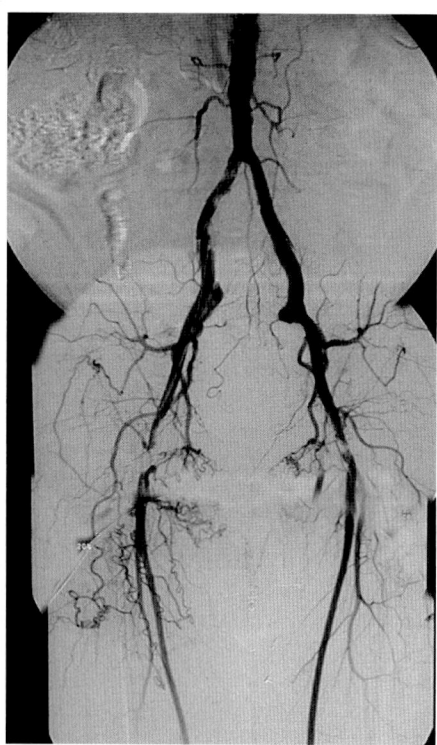

Figure 112-3 Calcific iliofemoral arterial occlusions are occurring more frequently and are often associated with "coral reef" exophytic plaques.

Noninvasive Testing

The ankle-brachial index (ABI) is a reference standard for the diagnosis of PAD. In persons without diabetes, the sensitivity and specificity of ABI measurements are 97% and 100%, respectively, compared to angiographically determined disease. However, because of medial calcification in those with diabetes, noninvasive arterial pressure measurements in the legs are falsely elevated owing to noncompressibility in up to 40% of patients. The presence of a spuriously high ABI (>1.3) requires additional testing such as toe systolic pressure, toe-brachial index, skin perfusion pressure, or duplex ultrasound to assess perfusion to the foot.[29-34] Toe pressures are usually accurate in diabetic patients because the digital arteries are seldom calcified, although in rare cases even these vessels can be noncompressible (see Chapter 14: Vascular Laboratory: Arterial Physiologic Assessment).[35,36]

Predicting Wound Healing

Numerous methods of assessment, including ABI, transcutaneous oxygen pressure (tcPo2), toe pressure, duplex ultrasound, and skin perfusion pressure, have been used to predict wound healing and select amputation level. None of these tests, either singly or collectively, is completely accurate in the prediction of ulcer healing. Confounding factors such as co-morbidities, wound severity, and infection are not included in the analysis. A variety of cut-points have been used for each of these tests in different study populations and often with different clinical endpoints, making the interpretation of data

difficult. For instance, Kalani and coworkers evaluated tcPo2 and toe pressures in 50 DFUs during a 12-month period.[31] Transcutaneous oxygen measurements on the dorsum of the foot greater than 25 mm Hg demonstrated sensitivity, specificity, and positive predictive values of 85%, 92%, and 79%, respectively, for healing; the corresponding values for toe pressures greater than 30 mm Hg were 15%, 97%, and 67%. Likewise, Apelqvist and coworkers evaluated 314 consecutive patients with DFUs.[35] Not one patient healed primarily with an ankle pressure less than 40 mm Hg, but no upper limit that prevented amputation could be identified. Primary healing was achieved in 85% of patients with a toe pressure greater than 45 mm Hg, and only 36% of patients healed without amputation with a toe pressure less than 45 mm Hg. The relative risk of major amputation is 2.6 times higher in patients with tcPo2 less than 20 mm Hg, 2.5 times higher in those with toe pressure less than 20 mm Hg, and 5.8 times higher in those with ankle pressure less than 50 mm Hg.[29]

Doppler skin perfusion pressure has shown promise in predicting wound and amputation healing potential. The technique is not widely used, but several studies indicate good positive and negative predictive values for determining wound healing when used alone or in combination with toe pressure. Adera and colleagues used skin perfusion pressure, tcPo2, and toe pressure to evaluate 52 patients with peripheral vascular disease and wounds.[37] Skin perfusion pressure less than 30 mm Hg had a negative predictive value of 90% and a positive predictive value of 75%. For major amputation, the negative and positive predictive values were 100% and 83%, respectively; for minor amputations, they were 75% and 67%. Yamada and associates evaluated 211 patients with ischemic wounds and reported a sensitivity and specificity of 72% and 88%, respectively, to predict healing when the skin perfusion pressure was greater than 40 mm Hg.[32] The accuracy of predicting healing was improved when skin perfusion pressure was combined with a toe pressure greater than 30 mm Hg.

Arterial Imaging

Three techniques of arterial imaging are currently in widespread use. Magnetic resonance angiography (MRA) and computed tomographic angiography (CTA) have become more effective for stratifying the severity of diabetic PAD, for decision making, and for selecting appropriate revascularization procedures (see Chapter 21: Computed Tomography and Chapter 22: Magnetic Resonance Imaging) Although MRA and CTA share the advantage of being noninvasive, the nephrogenic fibrosis syndrome associated with gadolinium administration in patients with azotemia has raised concerns about MRA. Likewise, the need to administer iodinated contrast material in diabetic patients, who often have impaired renal function, may limit CTA's broader use. As a consequence, many clinicians select contrast digital subtraction arteriography as their first option. By using selective catheterization techniques, highly detailed images of the arterial anatomy can be obtained with low volumes of iso-osmolar contrast material. In addition, the use of carbon dioxide gas as the "contrast" agent has several advantages: it is not nephrotoxic, is inexpensive, and is painless on injection (see Chapter 18: Arteriography). By combining selective catheterization with carbon dioxide and the judicious use of non-ionic iso-osmolar contrast in a "hybrid" arteriographic technique, high-quality images, including multiple views of the foot, can be obtained with almost no risk of renal impairment. Comprehensive detailed arterial images are essential for categorizing the anatomic severity of diabetic PAD and for planning the appropriate revascularization strategy. In most cases, if an endoluminal intervention is to be performed, it can be done concomitantly with the diagnostic or "strategic" arteriogram.

Diabetic Neuropathy

By the time diabetes is first diagnosed, 13% of patients have reliable evidence of diabetic peripheral neuropathy (DPN). After 10 years, DPN is present in at least 50% of patients. This complication, together with retinopathy, nephropathy, and diabetic arteriopathy, is due to the prolonged effects of hyperglycemia. Current evidence suggests that the progression of these diverse complications in patients with both type 1 and type 2 diabetes can be retarded by precise glycemic control (see Chapter 27: Atherosclerotic Risk Factors: Diabetes). Neuropathy is one of the most common risk factors for foot ulcers and lower extremity amputation. Even though testing criteria have been established and the tools and tests are inexpensive, noninvasive, and easy to use, neuropathy is often not evaluated.

Components

There are three components of diabetic neuropathy: sensory, motor, and autonomic. The combined effect of this triad is a foot that cannot respond to pain and is biomechanically impaired, with increased foot pressures, limited joint mobility, and poorly hydrated skin that cannot appropriately respond to injury.

Sensory Neuropathy. The damage from sensory neuropathy affects the large myelinated alpha fibers. Its distribution is usually symmetric in a stocking-and-glove pattern; as a result, patients are unable to perceive injury to their feet because the primary protective or warning systems are defective. This fundamental pathophysiologic impairment is referred to as the loss of protective sensation. Affected patients sustain repetitive, unrecognized injuries to their feet that culminate in full-thickness ulcerations. An ulcer in an insensate foot is usually painless. However, neuropathy can have a wide range of severities and symptoms. Loss of protective sensation does not necessarily mean complete absence of sensation or pain. So-called painful-painless ulcers may develop because of ischemia or deep sepsis; these require prompt attention and intervention. This scenario can also represent damage to both large myelinated nerves and small unmyelinated nerves, so the patient may have burning symptoms because of small-fiber damage and deep, gnawing pain and numbness because of large-fiber neuropathy.

Motor Neuropathy. Motor neuropathy often occurs later in the course of DPN and contributes to intrinsic muscle wasting of the feet and hands. Short, weak flexors and extensors that are overpowered by long, stronger flexors and extensors in the foot contribute to structural foot deformities such as claw toes, dislocated metatarsophalangeal joints, and ankle equinus (Fig. 112-4). Motor neuropathy changes the biomechanics of the foot and directly contributes to increased shear and pressure under the ball of the foot, the most common site

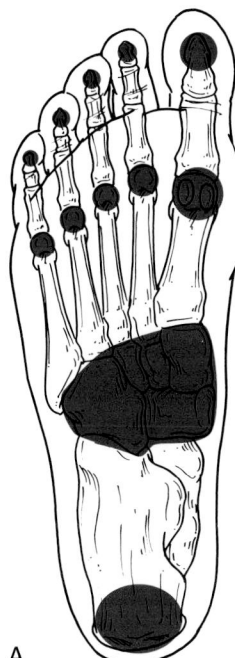
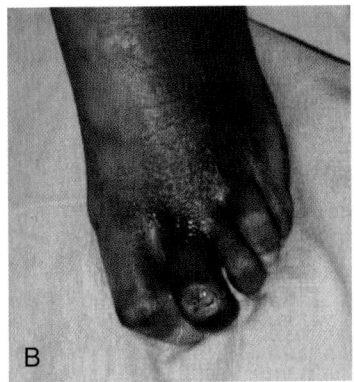
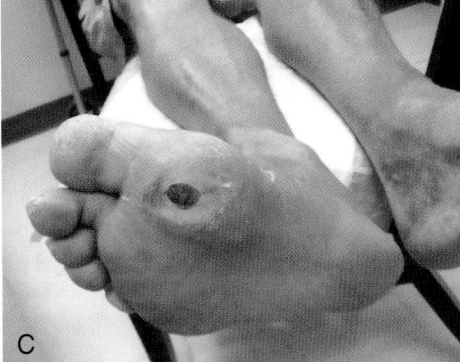
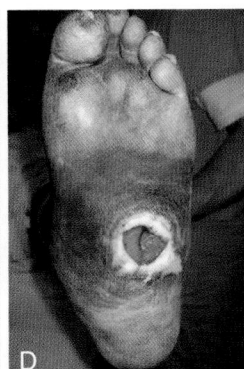

Figure 112-4 Diabetic foot deformity due to motor neuropathy produces pressure points at specific bony prominences (**A**), which the patient often cannot feel because of sensory neuropathy and loss of protective sensation. Ulceration frequently develops at these sites of increased pressure or shear: hammertoes or claw toes (**B**), metatarsal head mal perforans ulcer (**C**), and midfoot collapse, or Charcot's foot (**D**).

of neuropathic foot ulcers. Severe motor neuropathy contributes to the development of the "intrinsic minus" foot, or the appearance of a high arch structure because of muscle wasting and weakness.

Autonomic Neuropathy. Autonomic neuropathy (sympathetic dysfunction) causes shunting of blood and loss of sweat and oil gland function. The result is dry skin that cracks and fissures; often, this first manifests as skin breakdown on the heel. The intrinsic "autosympathectomy" caused by autonomic neuropathy explains why surgical sympathectomy fails to improve skin blood flow or to benefit the ulcerated diabetic foot.

Diagnostic Tests

There are several methods to identify sensory neuropathy, including history, vibration perception testing, and pressure assessment. These simple noninvasive investigations have good sensitivity and specificity for identifying persons with loss of protective sensation and can be performed by nurses or technicians in a few minutes. Armstrong and coworkers reported that a simple history of neuropathy symptoms such as numbness, tingling, burning, or the sensation of insects crawling on the feet can help identify patients at risk for foot ulcers.[38]

Patients sometimes mistake the symptoms of DPN for those of PAD. In addition to reporting numbness, tingling, burning, and formication, they may complain that their feet are cold even though they have strong peripheral pulses, the integument is warm to touch, and there are no other signs of ischemia. Additional complaints may include various other sensations: a feeling of thick feet, the sensation that mud is caked on the bottom of the feet, or the feeling of walking in "cement shoes."

Monofilament Testing. Semmes-Weinstein monofilament testing is one of the most common methods used in the United States to screen for sensory neuropathy.[6,19,38] The 10-g monofilament measures pressure sensation and is inexpensive and easy to use. The test apparatus consists of a nylon monofilament attached to a handle; it is designed to provide 10 g of force when it is buckled perpendicular to the test surface of the skin. It is important to explain to the patient that this is not a needle, and a nurse or technician should demonstrate that the monofilament bends on the patient's hand or arm (Fig. 112-5).

The monofilament is pushed perpendicular to the skin with enough pressure to bend the filament, forming a semicircle on the patient's hand; it is held for approximately 1 second and then removed. Approximately 10 sites on each foot will be tested, and the patient is instructed to say "yes" every time he or she feels pressure or thinks he or she feels pressure. The nurse or technician may need to prompt the patient by asking, "Do you feel this?" The test is performed with the patient's eyes closed. Sites to be tested include the first, third, and fifth digits; first, third, and fifth metatarsal

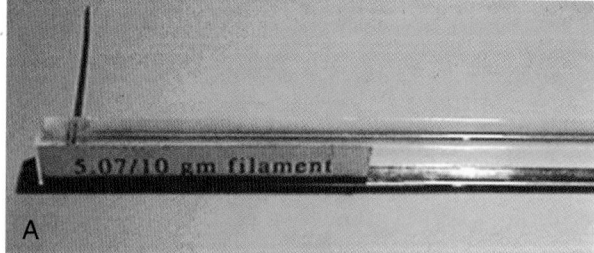
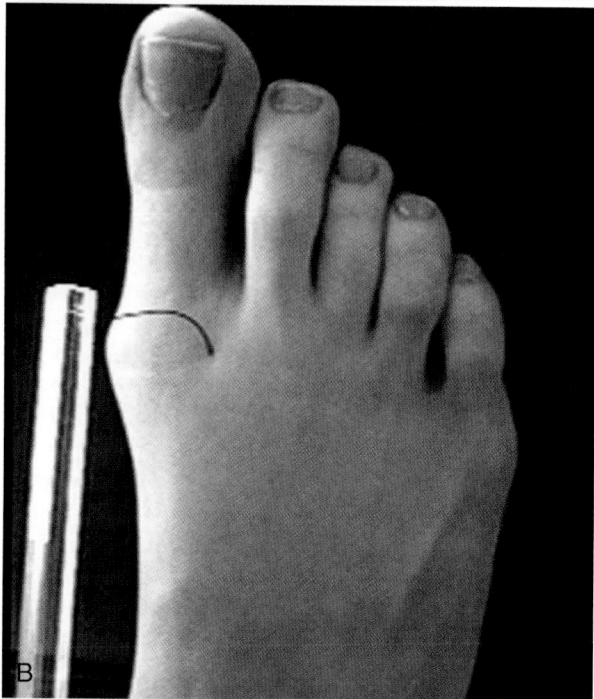

Figure 112-5 A and **B,** Testing for sensory neuropathy with Semmes-Weinstein monofilament is performed in both feet in 3 to 10 sites, depending on the individual protocol.

heads; base of the fifth metatarsal; heel; arch; and dorsum of the foot.[38] Any site at which the patient does not accurately identify the presence of pressure is scored as an abnormal response and is associated with neuropathy with loss of protective sensation.

Vibration Testing. Vibration perception testing, also an A myelinated fiber sensory modality, can be evaluated with a 128-Hz tuning fork or a vibration perception threshold (VPT) testing device. The tuning fork is struck and placed on a bony prominence, such as the great toe or metatarsal head, and the patient is instructed to signify when the vibration stops. The examiner then makes a subjective judgment of whether the level of vibration perception is abnormal. The VPT tester (Diabetica Solutions, San Antonio, TX) is designed to measure vibration sensation on a semiquantitative scale from 0 to 100. The instrument consists of a handpiece with a testing probe on the end, a motor, a rheostat, and a voltmeter. It is applied perpendicular to the distal tip of the erect hallux and is held gently so the weight of the probe is the only applied force. The rheostat is slowly increased until the subject senses the vibration and informs the examiner. Before starting the test, the nurse or technician demonstrates the process on the patient's hand. The level of perceived vibration is read in volts. Vibration sensation less than 25 volts has been associated with an increased risk of foot ulceration.[38]

DIABETIC FOOT RISK ASSESSMENT

Several classification systems have been developed to assess foot risk in patients with diabetes (discussed in more detail under "Ulcer Classification"). This issue is clinically complex, and a number of factors must be considered, including nutrition, glucose control, co-morbidities, wound characteristics (e.g., location, size, depth), neuropathy, peripheral vascular disease, and infection. Three essential factors, however, comprise the short list; wound depth, infection, and PAD. These factors are predictive of healing, amputation, and final amputation level. It is important to remember that in many cases the wound needs to be surgically débrided of callus and necrotic tissue for appropriate evaluation. Wounds that initially appear gangrenous and fetid may be less virulent after they have been cleaned and débrided. Foot wounds should be explored with a sterile metal probe to assess the anatomic depth of the wound (probe to bone).

FOOT INFECTION

Diagnosis

Soft tissue and bone infections in persons with diabetes are often challenging and difficult to diagnose. Consensus documents by the Infectious Diseases Society of America (IDSA) and the International Working Group on the Diabetic Foot (IWGDF) have been published to help direct the assessment, classification, and treatment of infection.[39,40] The diagnosis of infection is based on the presence of two or more local signs of inflammation (erythema, swelling, local warmth, local pain, purulent drainage).[41,42] However, the clinical signs and symptoms of infection are blunted in persons with diabetes by sensory neuropathy, lack of pain, vascular disease, and impaired cellular immunity. Infection of the diabetic foot is one of the major reasons for amputation and hospitalization.[6,13] The diagnosis of infection may rely on subtle signs and a high index of suspicion. Despite abscess and extensive tissue necrosis, patients with diabetes do not have a normal systemic or local inflammatory response. Importantly, they often do not feel ill or appear to be unwell. They are often afebrile, with only minimal or mild local signs of redness and swelling. There may be a subtle history of malaise or "flulike" symptoms.

Superficial swabs of the wound bed are unreliable in the diagnosis of infection because wounds are colonized by a variety of microorganisms that fail to reflect the true bacterial pathogen when a clinical infection is present. The widespread and indiscriminate use of antibiotics is not warranted, especially because it has demonstrably increased the prevalence of antibiotic-resistant infection.[6,17,41]

Osteomyelitis

The diagnosis of osteomyelitis is challenging; clinical assessment alone often provides insufficient evidence. The reported sensitivity of clinical examination to diagnose bone infection ranges from 0% to 54%. Ancillary testing is needed to improve diagnostic accuracy. The "gold standard" is bone biopsy. However, the use of extensive testing needs to be combined with clinical acumen and common sense. In clinic and hospital settings, bone scans and magnetic resonance imaging (MRI) are often ordered before plain radiographs have been obtained. Percutaneous bone biopsy is inexpensive and more accurate in both establishing a definitive diagnosis and identifying bacterial pathogens.

Probe to Bone. The "probe-to-bone" test has been widely adopted to diagnose bone infections in the foot.[43] Palpation with a sterile metallic probe can increase the accuracy of diagnosing osteomyelitis. The technique is simple and inexpensive. However, the positive and negative predictive values and sensitivity and specificity of this test are controversial and are dependent on the clinical setting. A landmark study by Grayson and coworkers used this technique in a group of 76 patients admitted to the hospital for limb-threatening infections.[43] As might be expected, there was a high prevalence of bone infection (66%) that was proved by bone biopsy, surgical exploration, or radiologic studies. The authors reported a very high positive predictive value (89%) and low negative predictive value (56%), with a sensitivity of 66% and a specificity of 85% if the bone was palpable with a sterile probe. Lavery and associates[44] and Shone and colleagues[45] reported data on two groups treated as outpatients with a much lower prevalence of osteomyelitis (20%). In both studies the positive predictive value was much lower than in Grayson's study (57% and 53%) and the negative predictive value was higher (97% and 85%). This indicates that a positive probe-to-bone test improves the pretest probability only slightly, but a negative test most likely rules out a bone infection.

Imaging Studies. Changes in plain film radiographs may lag several weeks behind the clinical course. In the setting of acute osteomyelitis, typical findings include soft tissue swelling, periosteal reaction, irregularity of the bony cortex, and demineralization. Chronic osteomyelitis is characterized radiographically by thick sclerotic bone and interspersed radiolucencies, periosteal elevation, and sinuses. Positive plain radiographs are associated with a wide range of sensitivities (28% to 93%) and specificities (50% to 92%). Radionuclide tests have a sensitivity of 45% to 100% and a specificity of 0% to 100%. More recent studies have shown a sensitivity of 77% to 100% and a specificity of 82% to 100% for technetium 99m leukocyte labeling techniques. MRI is highly sensitive (75% to 100%) for diagnosing bone infection, with a specificity ranging from 75% to 89%. The reliability of both radiographs and bone scans is diminished in the presence of arterial disease or Charcot's arthropathy or after recent surgery or trauma.[24,46]

Bacteriology

The type and variety of bacterial pathogens in diabetic foot infections depend on host immunity, mechanism of injury, wound depth, and severity of infection. The most common pathogens in mild to moderate infections are *Staphylococcus aureus* and *Streptococcus* species. Puncture wounds that result from penetrating injuries through footwear are usually associated with a high prevalence of *Pseudomonas* infection in patients without diabetes.[47] However, most puncture-related infections in persons with diabetes are due to *Staphylococcus* and *Streptococcus* species.[48] Limb-threatening infections classically present with mixed bacterial flora of gram-positive and gram-negative aerobic and anaerobic pathogens.[42]

Wound Cultures

The IDSA has produced a useful classification system for diabetic foot infections that addresses obtaining cultures as well as guidelines for treatment (Table 112-1). Ulcers that are not infected should not be cultured or treated with antibiot-

Table 112-1 Infectious Diseases Society of America's Diabetic Foot Infection Classification

Infection Severity	Treatment Recommendations
Uninfected Ulcer	No antibiotics recommended
Mild Infection	
Involves skin and subcutaneous tissue ≤2 cm of erythema surrounds ulcer Minimal necrosis	Gram-positive coverage with cephalexin, clindamycin, or trimethoprim-sulfamethoxazole 7-14 days of antibiotic therapy
Moderate Infection	
Penetrates to tendon, bone, or joint >2 cm of erythema surrounds ulcer Deep abscess or local gangrene	Broad-spectrum coverage Hospital admission for incision and drainage or if oral therapies have failed Amoxicillin-clavulanate, levofloxacin Piperacillin-tazobactam, ampicillin-sulbactam Fluoroquinolone with clindamycin MRSA coverage if history of MRSA, risk factors, or positive culture: trimethoprim-sulfamethoxazole, ertapenem, linezolid, or vancomycin 2-4 wk of antibiotic therapy
Severe Infection	
Systemic response to infection Fever, leukocytosis Metabolic complications	Broad-spectrum antibiotics Requires hospitalization 2-4 wk of antibiotic therapy for soft tissue infection 4-6 wk of antibiotic therapy for bone infection

MRSA, methicillin-resistant *Staphylococcus aureus*.
Modified from Armstrong DG, Lavery LA, eds. *Clinical Care of the Diabetic Foot.* Alexandria, VA: American Diabetes Association Press; 2005.

ics.[6,17] Superficial wound swabs should not be used for culture and sensitivity because these often provide cultures that are representative of superficial colonization. Community-acquired mild to moderate infections usually respond to empirical therapy, so cultures are not required.[41,44] Deep-tissue aerobic and anaerobic cultures are required in several scenarios: if the infection is not responding to empirical therapy; if the wound is deep; or if there is extensive tissue necrosis, a fetid odor, or crepitus. Ideally, tissue specimens for cultures are obtained from the débrided base of the wound.

Antibiotics

Initial empirical therapy for mild infections should be directed primarily against gram-positive pathogens and consists of oral outpatient administration of agents such as cephalosporins (cephalexin, cefadroxil), amoxicillin-clavulanate, levofloxacin, trimethoprim-sulfamethoxazole, or clindamycin.[42] More severe infections require hospitalization and initial treatment with empirical broad-spectrum antibiotics to cover gram-positive and gram-negative bacteria; appropriate antimicrobials include piperacillin-tazobactam, carbapenems (ertapenem, imipenem), or fluoroquinolones (levofloxacin, ciprofloxacin).[42] Once cultures and sensitivities are available, the antibiotic spectrum can be narrowed. The increasing incidence of methicillin-resistant *Staphylococcus aureus* (MRSA) has made empirical antibiotic selection more difficult. Empirical coverage for MRSA should be reserved for patients with known risk factors for MRSA or previous positive cultures. In addition to vancomycin, several newer antibiotics are available to treat MRSA, such as daptomycin, linezolid, and tigecycline.

Ulcer Classification
IWGDF Classification

The most widely accepted risk classification for DFUs is based on consensus recommendations from the IWGDF (Table 112-2).[39] This system was adapted from the Insensitive Foot Classification developed at the Carville Hansen Disease Center. Foot complications and clinical outcomes increase dramatically with the risk profile of the population. In separate studies, Peters and Lavery[15] and Mayfield and colleagues[16] used the IWGDF's risk classification to demonstrate that the frequency of foot complications increases as risk criteria increase. Lavery and coworkers stratified a subpopulation with PAD and demonstrated a significant increase in the incidence of foot ulceration, reulceration, infection, amputation, and hospitalization compared with patients with neuropathy and foot deformity but without previous foot pathology or PAD.[14]

Meggitt-Wagner System

One of the most frequently referenced DFU classification systems was initially described by Meggitt[49] in 1976 and subsequently popularized by Wagner[50] in 1981. The Meggitt-

Table 112-2 Diabetic Foot Risk Classifications

Classification	Risk Group				
	0	**1**	**2**	**3**	**4**
International Working Group on the Diabetic Foot[39]	No neuropathy No PAD	Peripheral neuropathy No deformity or PAD	Peripheral neuropathy and deformity or PAD	History of ulcer or amputation	—
Modified International Working Group on the Diabetic Foot[15]	No neuropathy No PAD	Peripheral neuropathy No deformity or PAD	2A: Peripheral neuropathy and deformity 2B: PAD	3A: History of ulcer 3B: History of amputation	—
Lavery-Peters[14]	—	No neuropathy No PAD	Neuropathy ± deformity No PAD	PAD ± neuropathy	History of ulcer or amputation

PAD, peripheral arterial disease.

Table 112-3 Meggitt-Wagner Classification of Diabetic Foot Ulcers

Grade	Description
0	Preulcerative lesion
1	Superficial ulcer
2	Ulcer extending deep to tendon, bone, or joint
3	Deep ulcer with abscess or osteomyelitis
4	Forefoot gangrene
5	Whole-foot gangrene

Table 112-4 University of Texas Wound Classification System

Class	Wound Depth			
	0	**1**	**2**	**3**
A	Preulcerative lesion or healed ulcer site	Superficial wound; no tendon, capsule, or bone involvement	Wound extends to tendon or capsule	Wound extends to bone or joint
B	+ Infection − PAD	+ Infection − PAD	+ Infection − PAD	+ Infection − PAD
C	− Infection + PAD	− Infection + PAD	− Infection + PAD	− Infection + PAD
D	+ Infection + PAD	+ Infection + PAD	+ Infection + PAD	+ Infection + PAD

PAD, peripheral arterial disease.

Wagner system uses six wound grades that consider factors related to depth, infection, and peripheral vascular disease (Table 112-3). Infection is included in only one of the six ulcer grades.[50] Moreover, PAD is included in only the last two grades based on the end-stage finding of gangrene. This system does not allow the classification of superficial wounds that are infected or wounds of different depths affected by PAD. The only criteria for PAD are forefoot gangrene and whole-foot gangrene. The Meggit-Wagner classification system lacks more subtle, clinically relevant, and objective measure of PAD.

PEDIS System

The PEDIS (perfusion, extent, depth, infection, and sensation) ulcer classification system was developed by an international consensus panel for research purposes.[40] Although it provides guidelines for reporting standards, the PEDIS system has not found widespread implementation or validation.

University of Texas System

The University of Texas ulcer classification system was developed and validated to provide a more consistent evaluation of depth, infection, and PAD (Table 112-4).[51] The rationale for including depth is based on the observation that wounds involving deep structures, such as tendons or joint capsules, are more likely to develop cellulitis, abscess, and osteomyelitis. Wounds that probe to bone are associated with a higher risk of bone infection. In addition, deeper wounds are associ-

ated with prolonged healing, soft tissue infection, and amputation. The rationale for including infection and PAD is that these are two of the factors that most often lead to amputation, poor wound healing, and hospitalization.

The University of Texas system uses a 4-by-4 matrix (classes A to D, wound depths 0 to 3) to provide a consistent and systematic evaluation of these three factors. The frequency and level of amputation increase in deeper wounds and in the presence of infection and PAD.[51] For example, patients with wounds that penetrate to bone with infection and PAD (grade 3D) were 90 times more likely to require amputation than those with superficial wounds without infection or PAD.[51] A methodical consideration of depth, infection, and vascular disease should allow physicians, nurses, and podiatrists to more accurately quantify wound severity and predict clinical outcomes.

Treatment

Débridement and Drainage

The best "antibiotic" is often surgical débridement, as reflected in the surgical adage: "Don't let the sun set on undrained pus." When there is abscess or necrotic tissue, removing the nidus of infection is imperative. The choice between aggressive surgical débridement with limited digit or ray amputation (and the prospect of limb salvage) and pre-emptive above-ankle amputation hinges on the ability to remove nonviable tissue and eliminate limb-threatening infection. These options should be weighed in the context of a long-term strategy to retain a functional extremity. Initial incision and drainage should decompress the infection and facilitate drainage from all affected anatomic spaces. Wounds are left open, and drains are placed. Often a second débridement in the operating room is scheduled within 48 to 72 hours to remove remaining nonviable tissue. When there is extensive soft tissue damage and all or a portion of the foot is not viable, amputation at the most functional level should be considered. In patients with a truly unsalvageable foot due to extensive gas or invasive infection with extensive pedal tissue necrosis, a two-stage approach—initial rapid guillotine amputation at the ankle level, followed by below-knee amputation and closure after the elimination of sepsis (generally 5 to 7 days)—is prudent.

Infection tends to follow the path of least resistance in the diabetic foot. Infection can travel up the foot along tendon sheaths and tissue planes and may not be clinically obvious by external inspection alone; detailed knowledge of potential pathways of extension is therefore important for the surgeon who explores a diabetic foot infection. The sole has four layers of muscles that are often involved in deep plantar space infections. The evaluation of foot ulcers and infections should include insertion of a sterile probe to identify tunneling and tracks that penetrate to tendon sheaths or extend along fascial planes in the foot. Plantar space infections often have erythema extending from the ulcer toward the medial arch, with tenderness on palpation of the arch or along the flexor tendons. However, in patients with severe neuropathy, even deep infection may be asymptomatic, and the patient's poor inflammatory response may mask the clinical signs of infection. Deep plantar space infections are more likely to have a mixed bacterial flora that includes anaerobes. They are therefore more likely to have a fetid smell. In some cases soft tissue emphysema can be appreciated with plain film radiographs.

Exploration and débridement of infection may require a step-by-step exploration of the plantar compartments of the foot, with a layered approach to dissection. The incision for plantar space infections begins at the ulcer site and extends along the course of the long flexor tendons in the direction of the porta pedis at the medial arch and proximally along the tarsal tunnel if necessary. Each fascial plane or muscle layer should be adequately evaluated and explored if abscess or necrotic tissue is identified.

The first fascial layer in the foot involves the space from the skin to the plantar fascia. The plantar fascia attaches to the tuberosity on the plantar aspect of the calcaneus and extends distally to the toes. The second layer also originates from the calcaneal tuberosity and consists of three intrinsic foot muscles: abductor hallucis, flexor digitorum brevis, and abductor digiti minimi brevis. These muscles are just deep to the plantar fascia. The flexor digitorum brevis provides tendons to the lateral four toes. The abductor digiti minimi brevis inserts into the lateral side of the base of the proximal phalanx of the fifth toe, and the abductor hallucis inserts into the medial side of the proximal phalanx of the great toe. The third fascial space involves the flexor hallucis longus, flexor digitorum longus, quadratus plantae, and lumbricals. The flexor hallucis longus originates from the posterior aspect of the fibula, and the flexor digitorum longus originates from the posterior tibia. They both enter the foot through the tarsal tunnel along the medial arch and insert into the distal phalanx of the toes. The fourth plantar space includes the flexor hallucis brevis, adductor hallucis, and flexor digiti minimi. The deepest layer involves the interossei, peroneal longus, and tibialis posterior.

The spaces in the foot can be further divided into medial, central, and lateral compartments based on the medial and lateral intermuscular septa of the plantar fascia. Ulcers under the great toe or first metatarsal communicate with the medial compartment. Ulcers of the middle three rays communicate with the central compartment, and fifth toe and metatarsal ulcers communicate with the lateral compartment.

Arterial Revascularization

After the initial control of sepsis, the vascular status is assessed as previously described. Before any formal amputation—either minor or major—is contemplated, arterial imaging is essential, and contrast angiography is preferred.[20-23,52] Without it, a salvageable limb may be amputated because remediable arterial obstructions have been overlooked and left untreated. A course of regular wound débridement, ultimate control of gangrene or sepsis, negative-pressure wound therapy, skin grafting, or definitive amputation can succeed only if the foot has adequate arterial perfusion. What might have been sufficient circulation for an intact, uninfected foot may be inadequate once ulceration, sepsis, and gangrene develop. Healing cannot occur unless the circulation is optimized by either open or endoluminal therapy. Likewise, débridement of an ischemic, ulcerated foot will only exacerbate gangrene until the circulatory insufficiency has been rectified. How much augmentation of blood flow is required is usually proportional to the extent of gangrene and sepsis.

Once acute or infected ulceration is superimposed on chronic ischemia, therapy is initially, and appropriately, directed toward drainage and débridement, antibiotics, and offloading. This approach addresses the acute problem but ignores the fact that healing and limitation of amputation can occur only when the underlying chronic ischemia is treated. Therefore, underlying ischemia should be evaluated and addressed by open or endovascular means as soon as the infection has been controlled. Fortunately, the majority of arterial lesions accompanying DFUs (>95%) are amenable to revascularization. In general, in the presence of major tissue necrosis with recent infection, it is usually necessary to restore a pedal pulse if healing is to occur. These salutary circumstances should be borne in mind before one rejects open or endoluminal therapy in favor of proceeding directly and irretrievably to amputation.

Digital Amputation

Foot-sparing amputations include isolated toe, toe-metatarsal, transmetatarsal, Lisfranc's, Chopart's, and Syme's amputations. The goal is to select an amputation level with adequate soft tissue coverage to provide a durable and usable extremity. An amputation that requires no prosthesis is the optimal goal. Osteomyelitis, focal gangrene, or extensive soft tissue infection often necessitates amputation of a single toe. A common approach is to place two converging, elliptical incisions ("fish mouth") over the base of the toe, with a linear incision extending over the metatarsophalangeal joint or the proximal interphalangeal joint on the dorsum of the foot, depending on the amount of viable tissue. The joint is disarticulated, and the toe is removed. If necessary, the head of the metatarsal can be resected to allow subsequent soft tissue closure. (See Chapter 115: Amputation: Techniques and Results.)

Midfoot Amputation

When there is extensive soft tissue infection of the forefoot or when multiple toes are not viable, a transmetatarsal amputation can prove durable and highly functional. The plantar incision is made at the toe sulcus and extended medially and laterally just proximal to the first and fifth metatarsal heads. The dorsal incision is then placed over the metatarsal necks, and the metatarsals are resected at this level following the normal metatarsal parabola. The first metatarsal should be resected shorter than the second. The third, fourth, and fifth metatarsals should be cut sequentially shorter than the adjacent metatarsal bone. A good-quality plantar fat pad is essential for a durable residual limb. If there is extensive soft tissue infection or a thin, atrophied fat pad under the resected metatarsal bones, the risk of reulceration is high. Importantly, if there is ankle equinus, a percutaneous lengthening of the Achilles tendon to allow 5 to 10 degrees of dorsiflexion can reduce forefoot pressures and reduce the risk of reinjury. Whenever possible, primary closure of a clean amputation is preferred because it provides the best chance of healing. (See Chapter 115: Amputation: Techniques and Results.)

■ CHARCOT'S ARTHROPATHY

Charcot's arthropathy or neuroarthropathy is a fracture and dislocation process of the foot and ankle that occurs in patients with sensory and autonomic neuropathy. Fracture is often associated with unrecognized injury or minor trauma that might otherwise appear innocuous.[6,17] Patients with Charcot's arthropathy classically present with a painless, hot, swollen foot. Others may present with what initially seems to be a unilateral flatfoot deformity, with the arch of the foot "suddenly" collapsing. Patients generally have excellent arterial pulses and severe sensory neuropathy. We and others have noted anecdotally that diabetic patients with sensory neuropa-

thy and ischemia sometimes develop Charcot's arthropathy following the restoration of foot perfusion by pedal bypass.

Diagnosis

Charcot's arthropathy is often misdiagnosed as infection unless the treating physician has a high index of suspicion. The differential diagnosis includes infection, osteomyelitis, deep venous thrombosis, posterior tibialis tendon dysfunction, and even bone tumor. Imaging studies can be misleading, especially early. Plain film radiographs often show periosteal elevation, multiple fractures, and, in some cases, osteopenia that can be misinterpreted as osteomyelitis by an inexperienced radiologist or surgeon. Many patients are treated for osteomyelitis even though they have never had a wound (injury). Bone scans and MRI are usually not reliable to differentiate bone infection, trauma, fracture, and postsurgical inflammation. The surgeon should have a clear diagnosis of bone infection versus Charcot's fracture before planning an amputation, especially in the absence of a wound. A bone biopsy is the "gold standard" to diagnose bone infection. A Jamshidi needle used under fluoroscopy permits the surgeon to obtain a bone specimen for a definitive diagnosis; it also minimizes the ambiguity associated with imaging techniques, which may be expensive.

Radiographic Appearance

The midfoot is the most common site of Charcot's fracture. The result is often a convex arch, with the head of the talus and navicular bones or the cuboid projecting from the bottom of the foot; in advanced cases these midfoot bones may be destroyed, with the weight of the extremity borne by the malleoli. Ulcers often occur at these sites because of the abnormal pressure and shear forces created by the collapse of the arch (Fig. 112-6). Failure of these wounds to heal is usually not due to ischemia. Rather, it is a combination of neuropathy, bony abnormality, pressure, shear, and repetitive local trauma.

Treatment

The treatment for Charcot's arthropathy is cast immobilization with a total-contact cast.[53] This method of therapy allows

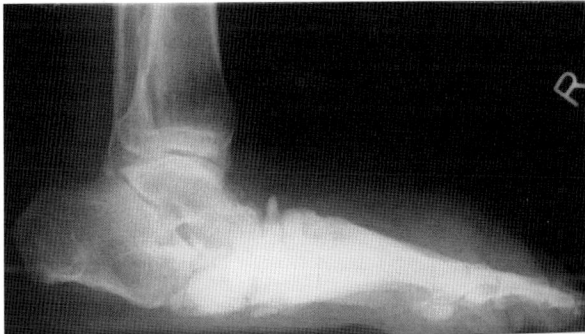

Figure 112-6 Radiographic appearance of midfoot collapse that produces rocker-bottom foot.

patients to continue to ambulate while preventing progressive deformity. Charcot's fractures in diabetics may take two to three times longer to heal than fractures at the same site in persons without diabetes. Casts must be checked and changed weekly to evaluate the fit, assess the ulcer, and perform débridement when required. Serial plain radiographs should be obtained during the acute phase. A total-contact cast is generally required for 3 to 6 months to reach a state of quiescence for acute Charcot's arthropathy. Metal braces and ankle-foot orthoses have also been used but are less effective than casts.[53]

Reduction of stress is indicated to decrease weight bearing on the affected extremity. Although total non–weight bearing is ideal, patients are often noncompliant. Partial weight bearing with assistive devices (e.g., crutches, walkers) is acceptable and does not seem to compromise healing time (see Chapter 113: Podiatry Care). However, some patients are physically unable to remain non–weight bearing with crutches, so walkers or wheelchairs may be preferred to reduce pressure on the fractured extremity. Full weight bearing in the acute phase tends to lengthen total time in the cast.

Management after cast removal is focused on lifelong protection of the involved extremity. Patient education and specialized, regular foot care are integral. Following cast removal, a protective foot brace or accommodative footwear should be prescribed, such as a modified ankle-foot orthosis, a Charcot-restraint orthotic walker, or a double metal upright ankle-foot orthosis. Custom footwear includes extra-deep shoes with rigid soles and a plastic or metal shank. If ulcers are present, a rocker-bottom sole can be used, with the addition of Plastazote inserts for those with insensate feet. Continued use of custom footwear in the postacute phase is essential for foot protection and support. Ongoing vigilance by the patient and foot care specialist is mandatory to prevent recurrence.

Surgical procedures are uncommonly performed but are based on the location of the disease and on the surgeon's preferences and experience with Charcot's arthropathy. They include osteotomy, exostosectomy of a bony prominence, arthrodesis, screw and plate fixation, open reduction and internal fixation, major arch reconstructive surgery, Achilles tendon lengthening with fusion, autologous bone grafting, and, rarely, major amputation. Healing times are frequently prolonged after surgery; total-contact casts and pressure reduction remain the cornerstones of therapy.[53,54]

■ ULCER PREVENTION

Management of DFUs, from their diagnosis to the prescription of proper footwear and offloading, can be a time-consuming and arduous undertaking. Ulcer prevention is equally challenging but rewarding not only for patients, their families, and their doctors but also for all members of the community who bear the cost of these potentially devastating lesions. A more comprehensive presentation of DFU prevention and methods of offloading is found in Chapter 113 (Podiatry Care).

SELECTED KEY REFERENCES

Andros G, Harris RW, Dulawa LB, Oblath, RW, Salles-Cunha SX. The need for arteriography in diabetic patients with gangrene and palpable pedal pulses. *Arch Surg.* 1984;119:1260-1263.
These authors recognized that clinically acceptable pedal pulses may hide inadequate foot perfusion and recommended that patients with DFUs have contrast arteriography to diagnose occult arterial occlusive disease that could be revascularized and prevent unnecessary amputations.

Armstrong DG, Lavery LA, Harkless LB. Validation of a diabetic wound classification system: the contribution of depth, infection and ischemia to risk of amputation. *Diabetes Care.* 1998;21:855-859.
The first validated and clinically practical DFU classification system (the so-called University of Texas system) that addressed the multifactorial nature of wound severity.

Grayson ML, Gibbons GW, Balogh K, Levin E, Karchmer AW. Probing to bone in infected pedal ulcers. A clinical sign of underlying osteomyelitis in diabetic patients. *JAMA.* 1995;273:721-723.
Using the simple technique of exploring the depths of DFUs with a small metallic probe, these authors investigated the possible presence of osteomyelitis, an important determinant of limb salvageability.

Lavery LA, Armstrong DG, Murdoch DP, Peters EJ, Lipsky BA. Validation of the Infectious Diseases Society of America's diabetic foot infection classification system. *Clin Infect Dis.* 2007;44:562-565.
Reports studies that validated the IDSA's system of classifying diabetic foot infections and stratifying infection severity based on clinical findings.

LoGerfo FW, Coffman JD. Current concepts. Vascular and microvascular disease of the foot in diabetes. Implications for foot care. *N Engl J Med.* 1984;311:1615-1618.
Addresses several important facts regarding diabetic vascular disease: (1) occlusive lesions of the infrapopliteal vessels are the most important sites of blood flow restriction; (2) the pedal arteries are usually soft enough to serve as the distal outflow site for distal bypasses; and (3) small-vessel disease in the distal foot, toes, and arteriolar level and beyond does not preclude wound healing if the larger arteries of the calf are successfully bypassed.

Wagner FW Jr. The dysvascular foot: a system for diagnosis and treatment. *Foot Ankle.* 1981;2:64-122.
Disseminates the concept that it is important to stratify the severity of ulceration based on size, depth, and clinical presentation.

REFERENCES

The reference list can be found on the companion Expert Consult Web site at *www.expertconsult.com.*

CHAPTER 113

Podiatry Care

Lee C. Rogers and David G. Armstrong

A podiatrist is a doctor who practices medicine and surgery of the human foot and ankle. The scope of practice for podiatrists varies by state and country, and in some cases it includes treatment of the entire lower extremity. The surgical expertise of each podiatrist varies depending primarily on his or her postdoctoral residency or fellowship training. A podiatrist can complete a history and physical examination, order laboratory work or imaging, and deal with a broad range of medical conditions and their treatment.

■ THE SPECIALTY OF PODIATRY

The history of podiatry is rich. The mention of foot specialists dates back to the Egyptians circa 1500 BC. Both Napoleon and Abraham Lincoln relied on the services of foot specialists. New York was the first state to license podiatrists in 1895. The *Journal of the American Podiatric Medical Association* was first published in 1907. One of the profession's early advocates, William M. Scholl, graduated from Illinois Medical College (now Loyola University) with an MD in 1904. His grandfather was a shoemaker in Germany, and Scholl was appalled by the lack of foot care in the United States. He invented several foot care products, resulting in the creation of a global company that was worth $77 million in 1968, the year of Scholl's death.

Training

A candidate for podiatric medical school must first complete 4 years of undergraduate training. There are nine colleges of podiatric medicine in the United States, located in New York, Philadelphia, Miami, Cleveland, Chicago, Des Moines, Phoenix, Oakland, and Los Angeles. Most of them require candidates to sit for the Medical College Admission Test (MCAT) to be considered for admission. Podiatric medical school consists of a 4-year program and includes coursework in the basic sciences and clinical training. Graduates receive the Doctor of Podiatric Medicine (DPM.) degree. All states require graduates to complete a residency in order to practice. Podiatric residencies last 3 years and are accredited by the Council on Podiatric Medical Education. Some podiatrists complete additional fellowship training in diabetic limb salvage, trauma and reconstruction, pediatrics, infectious disease, or research.

Scope of Practice

The podiatrist and the vascular surgeon often share patients. Podiatrists are trained to perform a clinical peripheral vascular examination and often order and interpret noninvasive vascular studies. They rely on the vascular surgeon when an elective surgical candidate has marginal or poor peripheral flow, which is a frequent occurrence in the care of the diabetic foot. Figure 113-1 illustrates the philosophy of cross-referral. The sigmoid curve represents the probability of healing based on toe pressures. When a patient is referred to a multidisciplinary team, the vascular team treats wounds that are profoundly ischemic, with the goal of improving flow and pushing the wound up the curve. Conversely, when flow is adequate, the podiatry team manages wound healing, offloading, reconstruction, and prevention. Patients falling in the middle of the curve are frequently managed simultaneously by combined efforts.

■ DIABETIC FOOT ULCERS

Epidemiology

Up to 25% of patients with diabetes have a foot ulcer during their lifetime.[1] Approximately 50% of such ulcers become

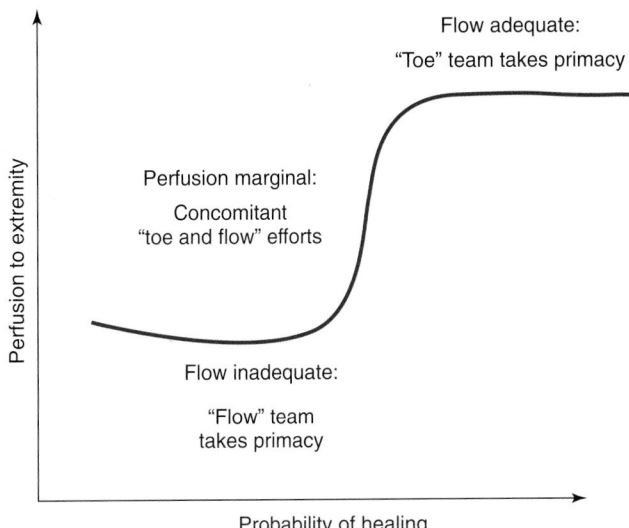

Figure 113-1 Team approach to diabetic foot care, based on adequacy of flow.

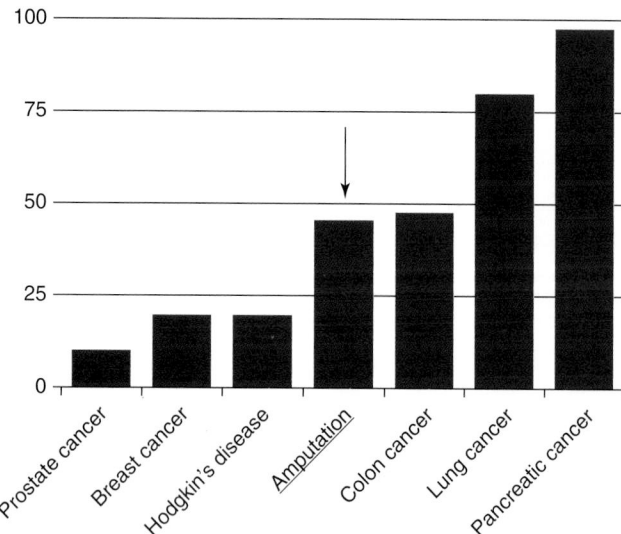

Figure 113-2 Five-year relative mortality rate for major lower extremity amputation compared with that for various cancers.

infected, and in 20% of these cases, amputation is required.[2] There are 81,000 major amputations performed on individuals with diabetes in the United States annually. About 60% of all nontraumatic amputations occur in those with diabetes.[3] After a major limb loss, the contralateral limb develops a serious lesion in 50% of cases.[4] The 5-year adjusted mortality rate after a major limb amputation is 46%.[5] This is higher than the mortality rate for many forms of cancer (Fig. 113-2). The cost of treating diabetic foot ulcers (DFUs) and performing amputations was nearly $30 billion in the United States in 2007.[6] This is discussed in detail in Chapter 112 (Diabetic Foot Ulcers).

Etiology

The etiology of DFUs is well understood. The factors leading to DFUs are peripheral neuropathy, foot deformity, and trauma.[7] Neuropathy is the key component of all DFUs. A patient with a loss of protective sensation does not have the "gift of pain," as the late orthopedic surgeon and medical missionary Paul Wilson Brand wrote.[8] Pain warns of impending tissue damage. In a sensate individual, when an area of the foot becomes tender, the gait is subconsciously altered to place less pressure on that area. Without this feedback loop, the tender area continues to receive pressure until tissue damage is irreversible. Trauma can be either high-pressure acute, such as a puncture wound, or repetitive low to moderate pressure. In an individual with peripheral sensory neuropathy, unopposed repetitive cycles of low to moderate stress first cause a callus, followed by a bulla and then a hematoma, until the skin envelope ulcerates. Foot abnormalities associated with DFUs can be visible or mechanical. Visible deformities include bunions, hammered or clawed digits, Charcot's foot, or cavus foot. Mechanical deformities cannot be identified by superficial visual inspection and require an examination of joint motion.

Normal gait is divided into swing, contact, midstance, and propulsive phases. Peak pressure and the line of progression follow an orderly path from the heel, through the lateral aspect of the midfoot, coursing medially through the forefoot, and eventually the push-off of the hallux. This allows a remarkable amount of force to be dissipated over a relatively large unit area. Diabetes, limited joint mobility, and aging alter this normal process and, in the presence of peripheral neuropathy, set the stage for the development of DFUs.

Limited joint mobility is as important as deformity in predicting ulceration.[9,10] If the extent of ankle motion does not exceed 10 degrees of dorsiflexion, the abnormality is termed equinus (named after horses, which walk on their toes). In patients with diabetes, the tendons, including the Achilles tendon, become glycosylated and less elastic.[10] A less elastic Achilles tendon plantar flexes (or resists dorsiflexion) and concentrates plantar pressures under the forefoot. A neuropathic patient with ankle equinus has a risk ratio of 2.3 for developing a forefoot ulcer.[11] The most common location for a DFU is under the hallux.[12] Limited dorsiflexion at the first metatarsophalangeal joint (hallux limitus) increases plantar pressure under the distal hallux during toe-off. The hallux should normally be able to dorsiflex more than 45 degrees. Degenerative joint disease at this location is also common in nondiabetic people, but the presence of pain prevents ulceration and causes them to seek treatment. Hallux limitus in the presence of neuropathy has an associated risk ratio of 4.6 for ulceration.[11]

Prevention

To prevent DFUs, one must address the causative factors: neuropathy and trauma.

Neuropathy

Neuropathy can be reduced or delayed by precise glucose control. Both the Diabetes Control and Complications Trial[13] (type 1 diabetes) and the United Kingdom Prospective Diabetes Study[14] (type 2 diabetes) showed a reduction or delay in the onset of peripheral neuropathy when glucose was precisely controlled. However, there is no high-quality evidence that any treatment can *reverse* diabetic neuropathy. Some have proposed that it can be reversed by means of peripheral nerve decompression. Proponents of this approach generally cite trials that are poorly designed or use unaccepted diagnostic methods to demonstrate the restoration of sensation.[15] Recently, the American Academy of Neurology published a position statement cautioning against the use of invasive procedures that lack sound evidence and are based on misconceptions regarding the pathophysiology of diabetic neuropathy.[16] Other methods have not proved effective. A double-blinded randomized controlled trial showed that monochromatic infrared light had no effect on peripheral sensory neuropathy.[17] Both alpha lipoic acid and aldose reductase inhibitors have been evaluated in well-designed trials for sensory neuropathy, with mixed results.[18,19] Additional trials are needed to determine whether the potential benefit of these treatments can translate into a restoration of sensation significant enough to reduce the incidence of DFUs. There have been single trials investigating B vitamins, magnesium, zinc, methylcobalamin, and vitamin E, but no consensus has been reached on their effectiveness.

Pressure Reduction

In individuals who already have sensory neuropathy, the focus should be on reducing areas of high plantar pressure and preventing trauma. Pressure reduction can include internal (surgical) and external (bracing and shoeing) approaches. Surgical reduction of pressure to heal or prevent DFUs is reviewed later in this chapter.

External pressure offloading consists of the use of custom and noncustom devices and shoes. Abundant evidence proves that custom insoles and footwear reduce plantar pressure in diabetics with neuropathy.[20,21] Translating these data into clinical practice has been difficult, however. Custom-molded diabetic shoes reduced the rate of DFUs by 53% in one trial.[22] Another study showed little effect, but the control group in that study also received shoes (noncustom).[23] Shoes can prevent trauma, but proper patient education is required to ensure compliance. Shoes should be worn at all times, including during ambulation at home.

Injection of silicone as a tissue filler to reduce pressure under bony prominences has been used, with clinical success.[24] Our group is studying the injection of poly-L-lactic acid (Sculptra) to reduce pressure in areas of preulceration. The effect is determined by dynamic computerized peak plantar pressure and ultrasonic tissue thickness measurements (unpublished data).

The home measurement of skin temperature has the most robust data of any prevention strategy. An increase in temperature is one of the cardinal signs of inflammation. Tissue inflammation increases the local temperature before dermal breakdown and can warn a patient of impending ulceration. Three randomized controlled trials have shown a reduction in the incidence of DFUs by 73% through the use of routine foot temperature monitoring.[25-28] However, at the time of this writing, the thermometers cost $150, require a prescription, and are not reimbursable by insurance.

Team Approach

Another effective means of DFU prevention is the formation of a multidisciplinary diabetic foot care team. A large population-based observational study reported a 69% reduction in the diabetes-related amputation rate over 5 years after the implementation of better-organized foot care.[29] Another study found that a multidisciplinary team consisting of physicians, podiatrists, and nurses led to a 51% reduction in ulceration in a high-risk population (previous ulcer history) over a 2-year period.[30]

Natural History

Foot ulceration is the main risk factor for limb loss in diabetic patients.[31] The natural history of diabetes-related lower extremity amputation can be described as a staircase (Fig. 113-3). The first step is the diagnosis of diabetes, followed by the onset of neuropathy. If an ulcer occurs, it may be complicated by peripheral arterial disease, which slows healing. The coup de grace is often an ascending infection leading to the urgent need for amputation. There are interventions to prevent each advancing "step" and, ultimately, prevent a major amputation. It is imperative that the ulcerated diabetic foot be free from infection and receive adequate blood flow in order to heal in a timely fashion. If one can heal a DFU or at least prevent it from becoming infected, most amputations can be avoided. This topic is discussed in Chapter 112 (Diabetic Foot Ulcers).

Diagnosis

First and most urgently, the wound must be inspected for signs of infection and, if present, managed appropriately. The diagnosis of diabetic foot infection is based primarily on the clinical presentation. Signs of infection include purulence, erythema, edema, and malodor. Because persons with diabetes may have a blunted immune response, laboratory testing should not be relied on to establish the diagnosis of infection; leukocytosis is present in only 46% of diabetic patients with moderate to severe foot infections.[32]

The Infectious Diseases Society of America (IDSA) has produced guidelines for the diagnosis and classification of diabetic foot infection, based on clinical signs and symptoms (Table 113-1). The IDSA divides infections into four categories: uninfected, mild, moderate, and severe.[33] This classification system has recently been validated and is a good clinical predictor of the outcome of diabetic foot infection.[34]

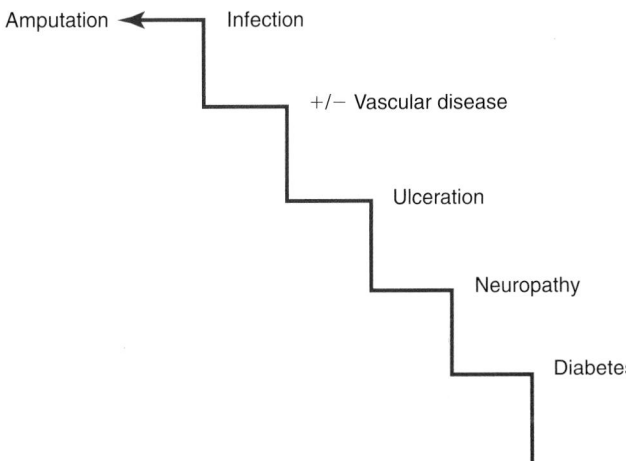

Figure 113-3 Common natural history of major lower extremity amputation. Each step in this "stairway to amputation" is a target for intervention to prevent the escalation to amputation.

Table 113-1 Classification of Diabetic Foot Infection

Clinical Presentation	IDSA Infection Severity	Threatened Limb Class
Wound without purulence or inflammation	Uninfected	N/A
Presence of >2 manifestations of inflammation, cellulitis <2 cm surrounding ulcer, no systemic symptoms	Mild infection	Non–limb threatening
Infection with >2 cm of surrounding cellulitis; any infection with the presence of gangrene, abscess, deep involvement, or gas in the tissue; no systemic signs or symptoms	Moderate infection	Limb threatening
Infection as above with the presence of systemic signs or symptoms	Severe infection	Life and limb threatening

IDSA, Infectious Diseases Society of America; N/A, not applicable.

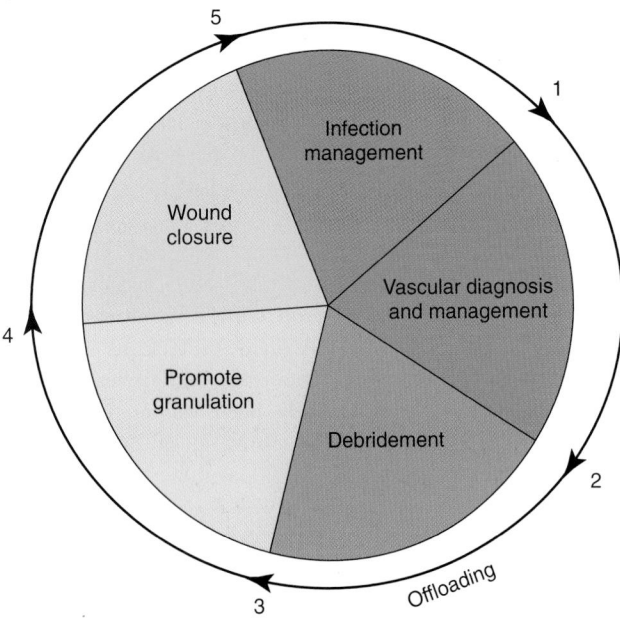

Figure 113-4 Diabetic foot ulcers should be treated in an orderly fashion according to this pie algorithm. Each piece of the pie should be considered, beginning with "infection management." "Offloading" is important throughout the life cycle of the wound and encircles the algorithm.

Treatment

An overview of the treatment of DFUs is presented in Figure 113-4.

Mechanical Offloading

Effective pressure reduction is the cornerstone of treatment for DFUs. Repetitive trauma and pressure on the wound bed are two of the primary reasons for ulcer persistence.[35] Excessive plantar pressure and shear forces prevent the formation

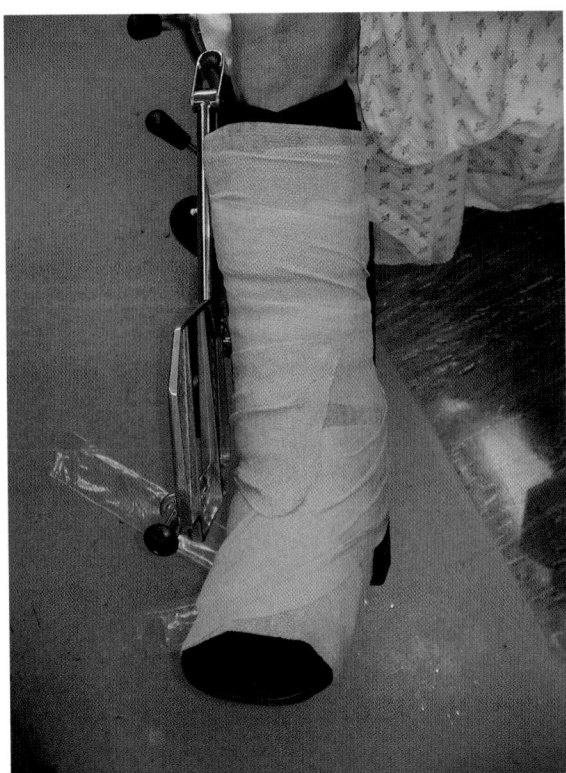

Figure 113-5 The instant total-contact cast is a removable cast-walker rendered irremovable by a cohesive bandage or fiberglass.

of adequate granulation tissue. The total-contact cast (TCC) has been the "gold standard" for offloading the ulcerated foot. However, it is time-consuming to apply and must be applied by those with experience because it can cause ulcers if used improperly. This has led some to investigate the use of non-custom off-the-shelf devices. In the laboratory, removable cast-walkers (RCWs) offload the plantar foot as well as the TCC does, and they do so better than postoperative shoes and half shoes.[36] In clinical practice, however, TCCs are better at healing ulcers. This can be explained by the nature of RCWs—that is, they are removable. Armstrong and colleagues hid pedometers inside RCWs and also gave patients pedometers to wear on their hips.[37] Subjects were instructed to use the RCWs at all times while ambulating. The investigators found a significant discordance between the hip and RCW pedometers, indicating that the patients were not compliant with instructions to wear their offloading devices at all times and suggested that improved outcomes would be achieved with a nonremovable device. The instant TCC is a removable walking cast-boot rendered irremovable by applying a layer of cohesive bandage, plaster, or fiberglass (Fig. 113-5). The instant TCC is an effective, easy-to-use offloading device that ensures patient compliance.[38]

Surgical Offloading

Surgical offloading involves either an exostosectomy to remove a plantar prominence or joint reconstruction to lower

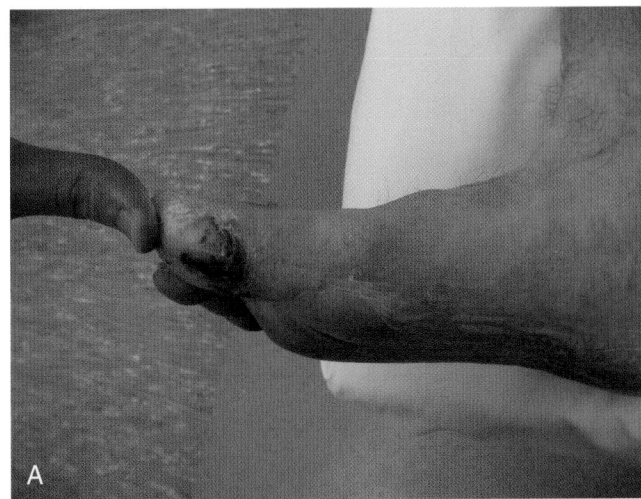

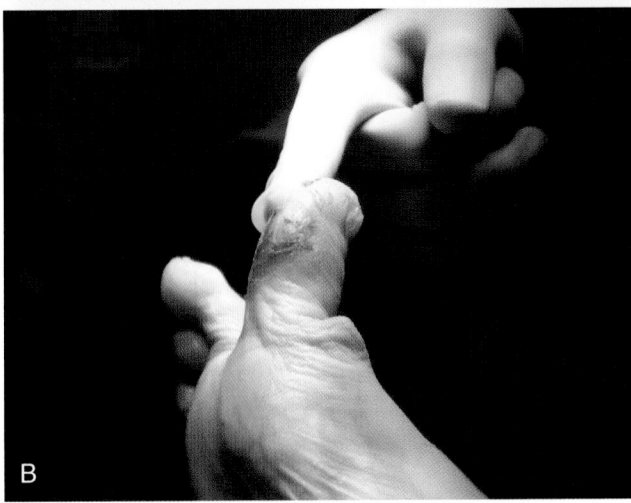

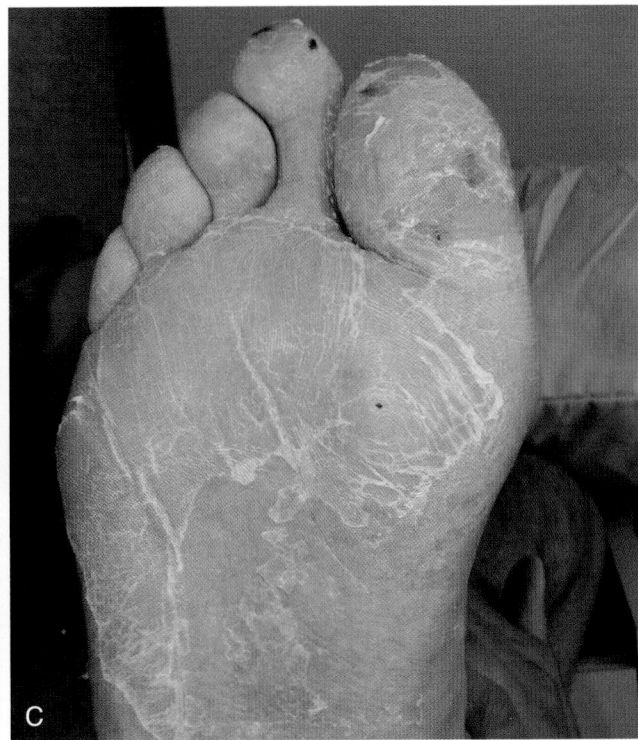

Figure 113-6 A, Preoperative view of limited mobility of the hallux (hallux limitus) with a distal hallux ulcer. **B,** Intraoperative view illustrating an improvement in dorsiflexion after resection of the base of the proximal phalanx. **C,** Hallux ulcer healed within 3 weeks of surgery.

peak plantar pressure distal to the joint. Plantar hallux ulcers in the presence of hallux limitus respond well to a base resection of the hallux proximal phalanx (Keller arthroplasty; Fig. 113-6). This operation improves dorsiflexion and reduces plantar pressure on the distal hallux during toe-off.[39] Plantar forefoot ulcers can heal faster when a tendo Achillis lengthening (TAL) is performed.[40] The standard TAL is accomplished through three stab incisions, posing minimal surgical risk (Fig. 113-7). Although this "lengthening" might be considered more of a "weakening" of the posterior muscle group, it results in muscle tendon balancing and reduces forefoot pressures. This relatively short-lived pressure reduction can lead to ulcer healing and prevent recurrence (Fig. 113-8).[41] Possible complications of this procedure include Achilles tendon rupture, calcaneal gait (increased weight-bearing time on the calcaneus), and heel ulcer.

In a foot that demonstrates both equinus and varus—that is, the foot is inverted and pressure is placed on the plantar or lateral fifth metatarsal area—an additional tendon procedure might be of benefit. The tibialis anterior tendon transfer is performed through three anterior incisions. The tendon is

transected from its normal insertion on the medial cuneiform and transposed laterally into the lateral cuneiform or cuboid; it is usually secured with a bone anchor. This eliminates the forces that pull up on the medial midfoot, transferring pressure laterally. The new function of the tibialis anterior is a more central dorsiflexion action.

With a single plantar metatarsal ulcer and no equinus, one might consider a metatarsal head resection. This procedure is commonly performed when osteomyelitis is present in the metatarsal head from a chronic tracking ulcer. The incision is made dorsally over the metatarsophalangeal joint, and the head is removed by osteotomizing the neck of the metatarsal. Occasionally, when there are multiple foci of pressure or ulcerations under plantar metatarsal heads, a panmetatarsal head resection is indicated, which can significantly reduce plantar forefoot pressures (Fig. 113-9). The heads of metatarsals 1 through 5 are removed through multiple dorsal longitudinal incisions or through one plantar transverse incision in the sulcus, distal to the metatarsal heads. Some surgeons prefer to perform a fusion of the first metatarsophalangeal joint instead of resecting it.

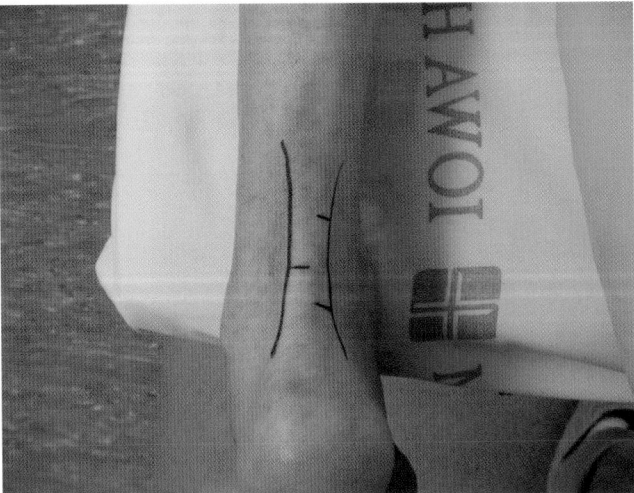

Figure 113-7 Triple-hemisection approach to Achilles tendon lengthening. The linear markings connote the outline of the left Achilles tendon medially and laterally. Two transverse stab incisions are made medially and one is made laterally, all 1 cm apart, transecting slightly more than 50% of the tendon substance. The foot is then forcibly dorsiflexed to create a sliding effect of the tendon.

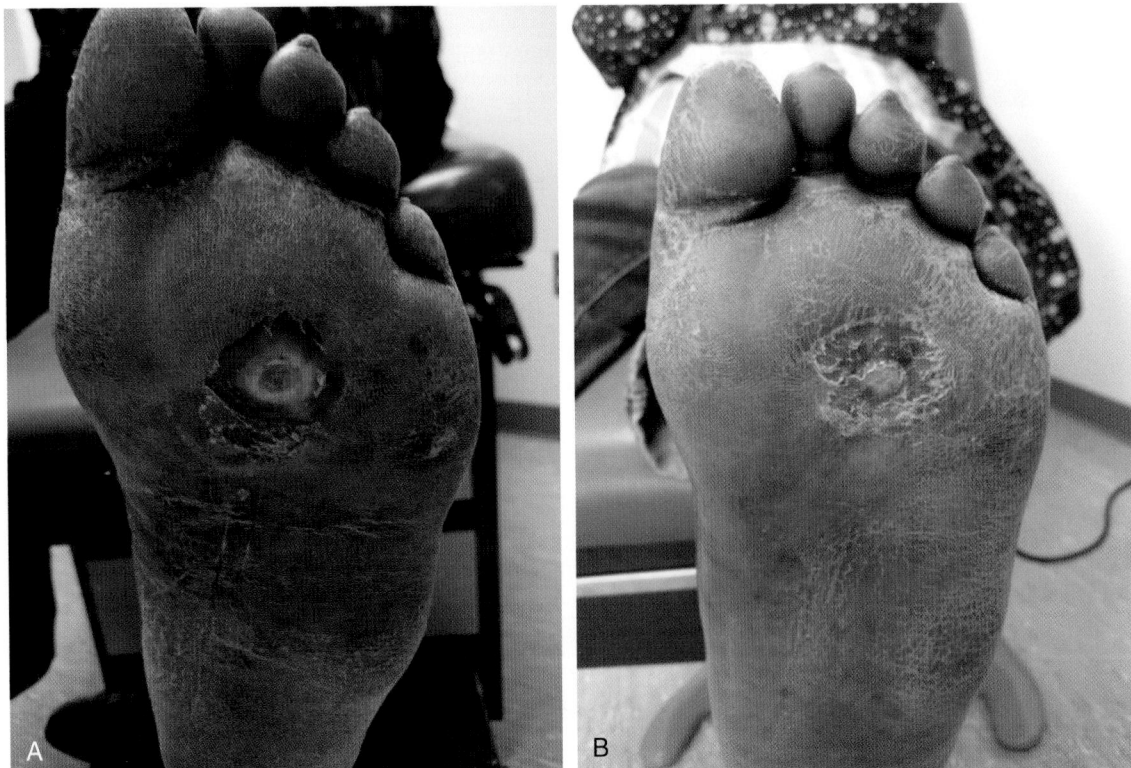

Figure 113-8 A, Preoperative view of a plantar forefoot ulcer in the presence of Achilles contracture (equinus). **B,** Three weeks postoperatively, the plantar ulcer has healed.

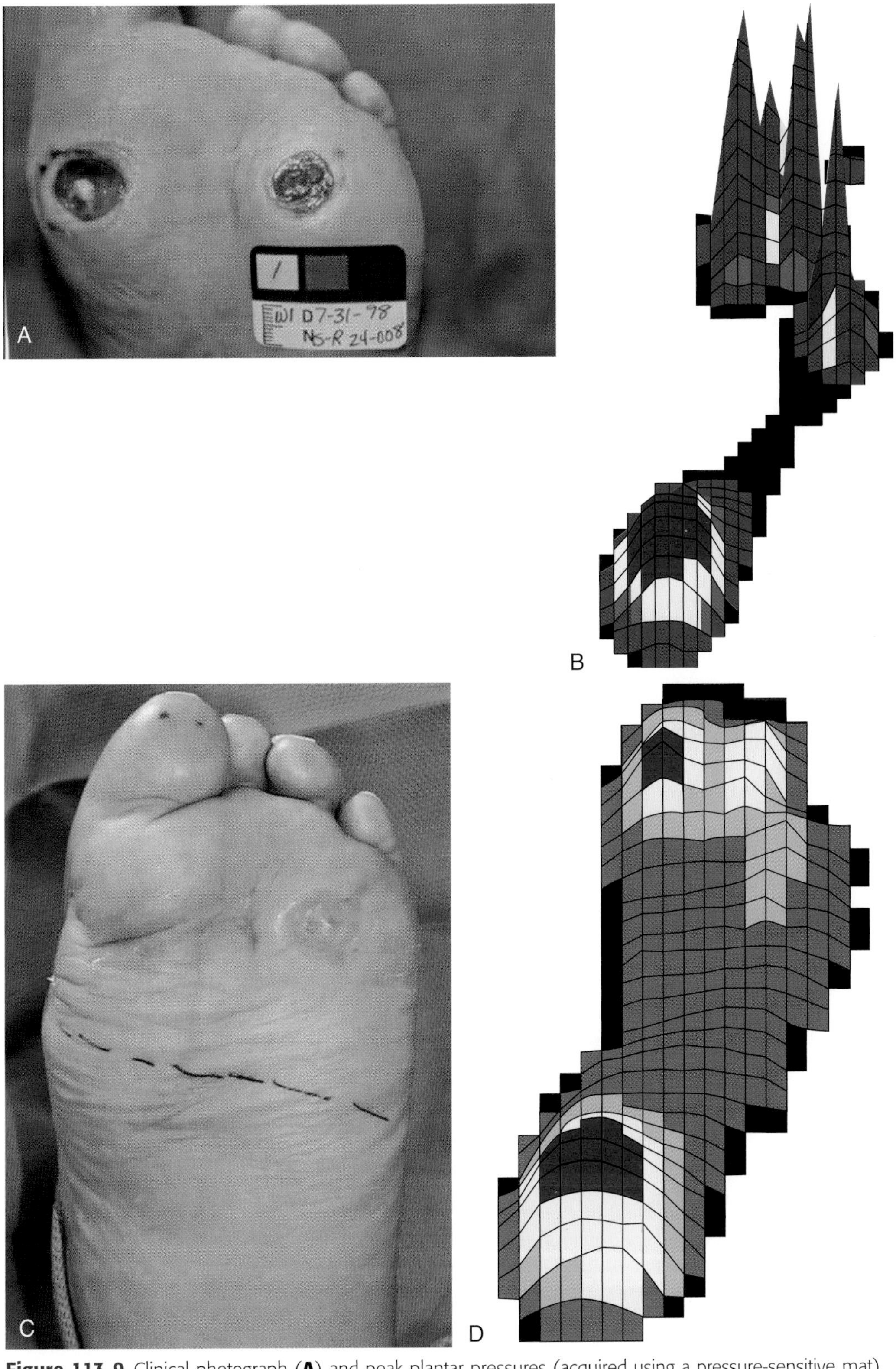

Figure 113-9 Clinical photograph (**A**) and peak plantar pressures (acquired using a pressure-sensitive mat) (**B**) of a foot with ulcers under metatarsal heads 1 and 5. After panmetatarsal head resection, the ulcers have healed (**C**), and the peak plantar pressures have been reduced (**D**). *Red color* connotes the zones of highest pressure, and the magnitude of this pressure is depicted by the height of the peaks.

Results of Diabetic Foot Surgery

In persons with normal baseline circulation (or in those who have been revascularized), there has been increased interest in performing reconstructive diabetic foot surgery. However, this approach has led to an ill-defined mélange of indications and contraindications. To address this confusion, Armstrong and Frykberg proposed classifying nonvascular diabetic foot surgery into four categories, based on indications and perceived risk: elective, prophylactic, curative, and emergency. This system, which focuses on historical variables such as neuropathy, presence of ulceration, and limb-threatening infection,[42] was validated in a study we reported in 2006.[43] Designed as a cohort model, the study involved abstracting medical records from 180 patients with diabetes requiring foot surgery and assigning them equally to the four classes. There was a strong and significant trend toward increasing postoperative infection, ulceration, reulceration, and amputation with higher surgical class (Fig. 113-10).[43]

Class I: Elective

Elective diabetic foot surgery is performed on a sensate (non-neuropathic) patient to reduce pain or improve function.[42] Assuming good metabolic control, these patients are at no greater risk for the development of complications than corresponding patients without diabetes.[43]

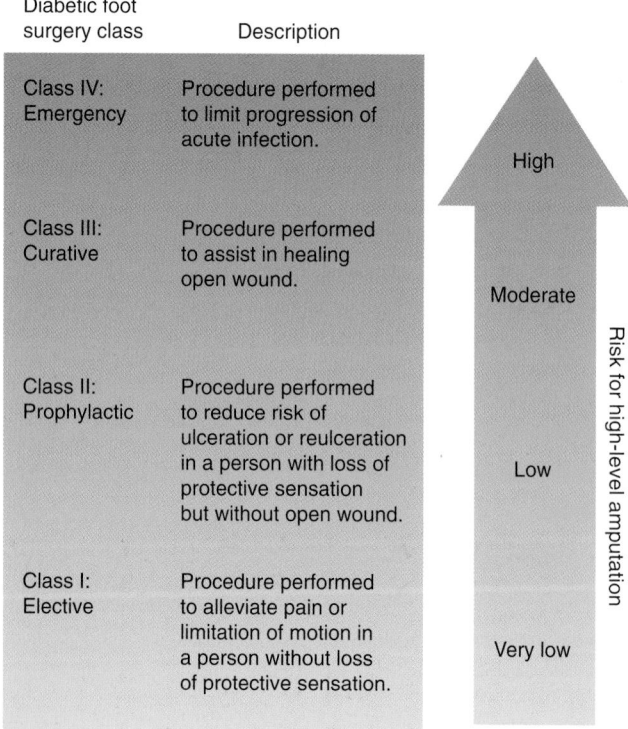

Figure 113-10 Armstrong-Frykberg classification of diabetic foot surgery. Risk of amputation increases as a function of complications and the indications for performing the given procedure.

Class II: Prophylactic

Prophylactic surgery is performed to alleviate deformity in a person with neuropathy but without an open ulcer. The goal of prophylactic surgery is to reduce plantar vertical and shear stress. Armstrong and coworkers compared postoperative complications in people with and without diabetes undergoing a single hammertoe correction (arthroplasty).[44] After a follow-up period of 3 years, there were no complications in either the neuropathic diabetic patients with no history of ulceration or the nondiabetic subjects. However, those with a history of ulceration were more likely to experience a postoperative infection (14.3%). Long-term outcomes after these procedures were uniformly good, with 96.3% of patients remaining ulcer free for a mean of 3 years. In a later work, we reported a postoperative infection rate of 6.7% following class II surgery.[43]

At least 4 in 10 people with Charcot's neuro-osteoarthropathy develop an ulcer, and their risk ratio for ulceration is up to 36-fold higher than normal.[11] Those presenting with an unstable foot secondary to this condition can often achieve bony fusion and limb salvage with surgical reconstruction; however, most people with Charcot's neuro-osteoarthropathy do not require surgical intervention.[45]

Limited joint mobility in the foot is essentially equivalent to overt deformity.[9] A common example is hallux limitus, in which limited first metatarsophalangeal joint dorsiflexion increases pressure at the distal hallux during ambulation, specifically during toe-off. This can lead to the formation of calluses and blistering under the great toe and the subsequent development of a wound. This is a clear indication for prophylactic surgery to increase motion and thereby reduce pressure.

Class III: Curative

Curative diabetic foot surgery is designed to heal the wound and reduce the risk of reulceration.[42] Rosenblum and colleagues reported their experience with hallux interphalangeal joint arthroplasty in 45 feet for chronic neuropathic ulcers of the great toe.[46] Overall, 41 feet (91%) healed and had no evidence of recurrence in the follow-up period. The authors reported an 11% postoperative complication rate and a 4% infection rate.

Ankle equinus (<10 degrees of dorsiflexion at the ankle joint) increases plantar forefoot pressures and may increase the risk of ulceration.[47] TAL has been shown to reduce plantar forefoot pressures by a mean 27% and is beneficial in preventing ulceration.[48] Lin and associates suggested there was more rapid healing of previously recalcitrant plantar wounds with a TAL procedure, as well as a lower rate of recurrence.[49] Mueller and coworkers, in a randomized controlled trial, similarly reported a trend toward lower ulcer recurrence when performing TAL.[41]

Class IV: Emergency

Emergency surgery connotes procedures performed to reduce the risk of proximal spread of acute infection. Patients who may require revascularization must be evaluated by a vascular surgeon in the immediate perioperative period. However, drainage or damage-control débridement of a limb- or life-threatening infection should not necessarily be delayed if the time to obtain consultation will be prolonged.[42] These procedures often include partial or whole-foot amputation.

■ CHARCOT'S ARTHROPATHY

The Charcot foot ulcer can be particularly troublesome to offload and deserves special mention. Charcot's arthropathy or neuroarthropathy is a fracture and dislocation process of the foot and ankle that occurs in patients with sensory and autonomic neuropathy. Fracture is often associated with unrecognized injury or minor trauma that might otherwise appear innocuous.[50,51] Charcot arthropathy patients classically present with a painless, hot, swollen foot. Others may present with what initially seems to be a unilateral flatfoot deformity, with the arch of the foot "suddenly" collapsing. Patients generally have excellent arterial pulses and severe sensory neuropathy. Diabetic patients with sensory neuropathy and ischemia have been reported to develop Charcot's arthropathy following in situ pedal bypass, after perfusion to the foot has been restored. Certain cases require surgical reconstruction and arthrodesis. In some cases, a simple exostosectomy can reduce pressure enough to heal an ulcer[52]; many others require complete foot reconstruction (Fig. 113-11).[53]

Charcot's arthropathy is often misdiagnosed as an infectious process unless the treating physician has a high index of suspicion. The differential diagnosis includes infection, osteomyelitis, deep venous thrombosis, posterior tibialis tendon dysfunction, and even bone tumor. Imaging studies can be misleading, especially early in the course of the disease. Plain film radiographs often show periosteal elevation, multiple fractures, and, in some instances, osteopenia that may be misinterpreted as osteomyelitis by an inexperienced radiologist or surgeon. Many patients are treated for osteomyelitis even though they have never had a wound (injury). Bone scanning and magnetic resonance imaging are usually not reliable for differentiating bone infection, trauma, fracture, and postsurgical inflammation. The surgeon should have a clear diagnosis of bone infection before planning an amputation, especially in the absence of a wound. A bone biopsy is the "gold standard" to diagnose bone infection. A Jamshidi needle used under fluoroscopy permits the surgeon to obtain a bone specimen for a definitive diagnosis, and it minimizes the ambiguity associated with more expensive imaging techniques.

The midfoot is the most common site of Charcot's fracture. The result is often a convex arch, with the head of the talus and navicular bones or the cuboid projecting from the bottom of the foot; in some cases, the talus bone may be

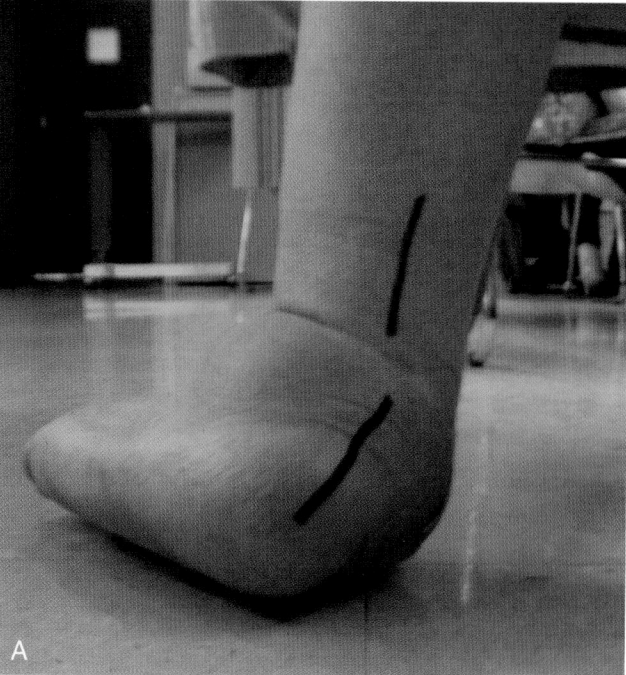

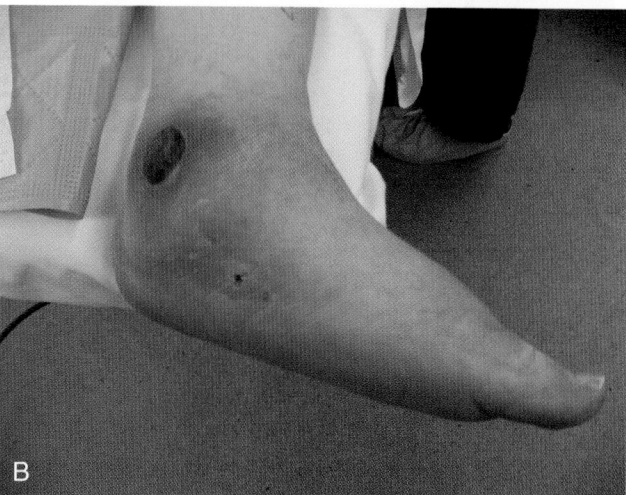

Figure 113-11 Charcot ankle joint with dislocation and ankle valgus (**A**), causing the patient to bear weight on the medial malleolus, which subsequently ulcerated (**B**).

destroyed, with the weight of the extremity borne by the malleolus, which easily ulcerates (Fig. 113-12). Ulcers often occur because of abnormal pressure and shear forces created by the collapse of the arch. When these wounds fail to heal it is usually not due to ischemia but rather to a combination of neuropathy, bony abnormality, pressure, shear, and repetitive local trauma. The treatment for both ulcers and active Charcot arthropathy is cast immobilization. Charcot's fractures may take two to three times longer to heal than fractures at the same site in persons without diabetes.

Techniques to Expedite Healing

Wound care has become exceedingly complex. However, by adhering to important basic principles of wound inspection, ongoing reassessment, débridement, and the promotion of

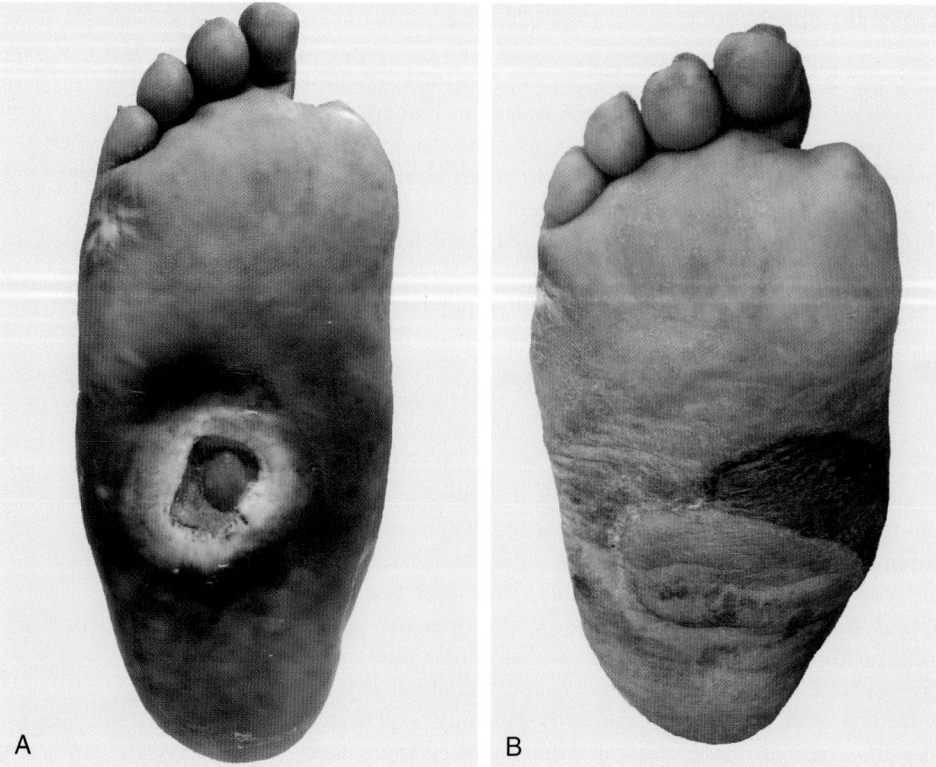

Figure 113-12 A, Plantar diabetic foot ulcer under a Charcot foot deformity. **B,** Healing of the ulcer 12 weeks after a midfoot reconstruction, medial plantar artery flap, and split-thickness skin grafting.

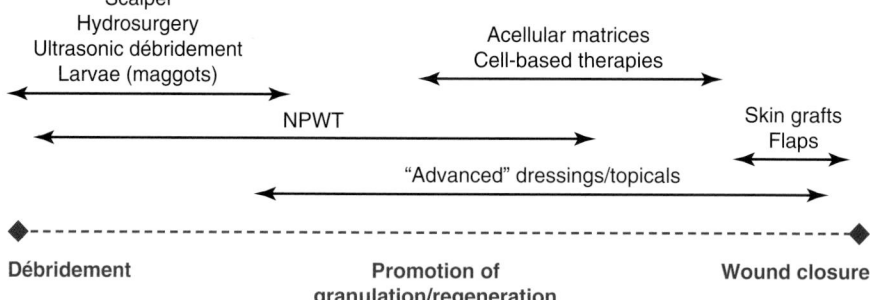

Figure 113-13 This "wound management spectrum" shows how modalities cross boundaries slightly, creating effects in multiple categories. NPWT, negative-pressure wound therapy.

tissue substructure and granulation tissue, and by applying a variety of closure techniques, healing can be achieved in most patients and accelerated in many.

Once infection, vascular insufficiency, and pressure have been addressed, a purely neuropathic wound should heal in a timely fashion if the following recommendations are followed. DFUs respond to débridement, promotion of granulation tissue, and closure. The modalities to achieve each of these treatment goals are displayed in Figure 113-13.

Débridement

Débridement removes devitalized tissue, bioburden, and senescent cells and promotes healing through bleeding. By débriding a wound, one converts a chronic, slowly healing wound to a healthier, more acute state.[54] When débriding a wound, it is important to remove all necrotic and nonviable tissue. The surgeon should not be concerned about the defect caused by the initial débridement because removing this tissue

is important to attain closure. Most wounds require serial débridements. Cardinal and coworkers found that DFUs that were débrided at each visit had a significantly greater chance of healing in 12 weeks than did ulcers débrided less often.[55]

There are five methods of wound débridement: mechanical, autolytic, enzymatic, surgical, and biosurgical. Mechanical débridement has fallen out of favor as a primary method, but it consists of applying wet gauze dressings, allowing them to dry, and then removing the dry gauze, thereby "ripping" off the surface layer (wet-to-dry dressing). Autolytic débridement is achieved by covering the wound with an occlusive dressing and allowing the wound's proteolytic enzymes to lyse the fibrotic or necrotic tissue. This is rarely recommended, owing to the risk of infection and the availability of better methods. Enzymatic débridement uses a cream such as collagenase to remove devitalized tissue.

Surgical débridement is the most common and effective method.[55] It can be simply using a scalpel or using a newer modality such as a hydroscalpel (Versajet, Smith & Nephew,

Memphis, TN), which allows for a precise depth of débridement.[56] The Versajet uses a handpiece that creates a Venturi effect and a stream of saline with a force up to 15,000 pounds per square inch. It is typically performed in an operating room setting. Another recent development for wound débridement involves ultrasound. The SonicOne (Misonix, Farmingdale, NY) is a new device that combines ultrasound with an adjustable irrigation system to adequately débride a wound.

Maggot (larval) débridement therapy (Medical Maggots, Monarch Labs, Irvine, CA) has gained recent attention and might be considered a new category of débridement—biosurgical.[57] Though it is certainly not a new treatment, our understanding of these "biosurgeons" has grown, and the use of maggot débridement has increased in the United States. Maggots arrive in a sterile vial containing 250 to 500 larvae. They are placed inside a fibrotic wound and covered with a mesh dressing for 3 days. The species *Phaenicia sericata* (green blowfly) is unique in that it consumes only fibrotic or necrotic tissue and will not digest living granulation tissue (Fig. 113-14). Occasionally, multiple applications are required. These are the only living organisms to be approved as a medical device by the Food and Drug Administration (FDA). The use of medical maggots has been shown to increase the number of "antibiotic-free days" during débridement,[58] and they are also effective against methicillin-resistant *Staphylococcus aureus* (MRSA).[59]

Promotion of Granulation Tissue/Regeneration

Once a wound has been thoroughly débrided, granulation tissue is necessary before wound closure. This process, also called wound bed preparation, starts by achieving an appropriate moisture balance in the wound. The principle of keeping wounds moist without maceration has been demonstrated to accelerate epithelialization.[60] Multiple dressing types and topical therapies exist (Fig. 113-15), and there is little evidence that any one dressing is more effective than another. Most practitioners use multiple dressing types throughout the life of the wound to adapt to the changing wound environment.

Negative-Pressure Wound Therapy

Few advances in wound healing have been as groundbreaking as negative-pressure wound therapy (NPWT). The Wound VAC (Kinetic Concepts Inc., San Antonio, TX) is the only NPWT device with any evidence to support its use. The VAC uses a piece of foam in contact with the wound bed, covered by an occlusive dressing, and placed under negative pressure (usually –125 mm Hg). The VAC produces high-quality granular tissue that has a characteristic rough appearance. It is essentially a wound simplification device, converting complicated (deep) wounds to simple (shallow) ones (Fig. 113-16). The VAC device can decrease the depth and area of large diabetic foot wounds, speeding closure.[61] In a recent randomized controlled trial evaluating its use after partial

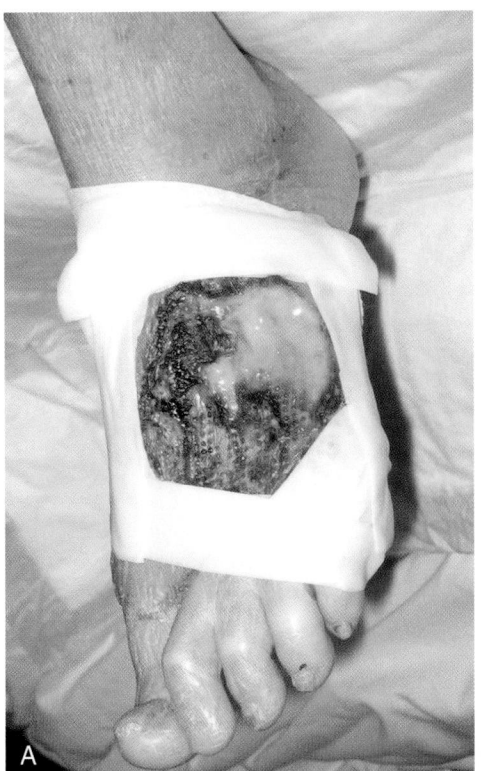

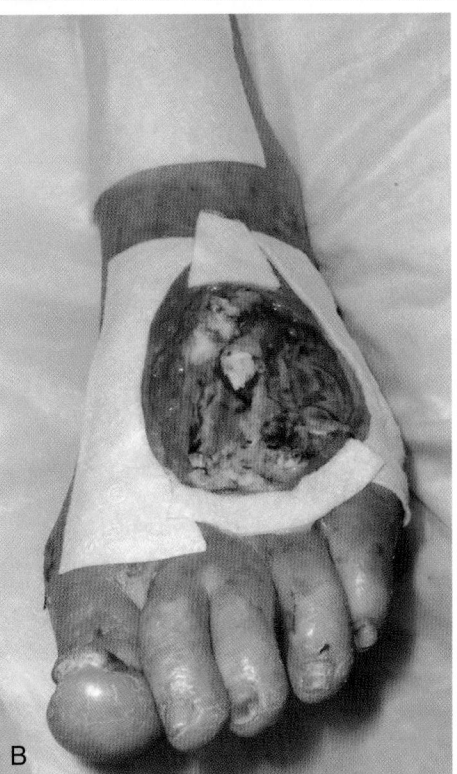

Figure 113-14 Extensively fibrotic and necrotic dorsal foot wound before (**A**) and after (**B**) one application of maggots for débridement.

diabetic foot amputations, the VAC was found to be more effective than the standard of care, and it limited the number of secondary amputations.[62] Because DFUs are so costly, the rapid response provided by the Wound VAC lowers the cost of care delivered to those with chronic wounds.[63] Occasion-

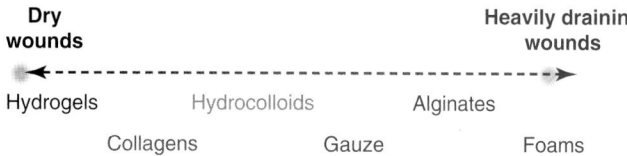

Figure 113-15 Dressings can be used to attain proper moisture balance in a wound. These dressings are categorized based on their effects on wound moisture.

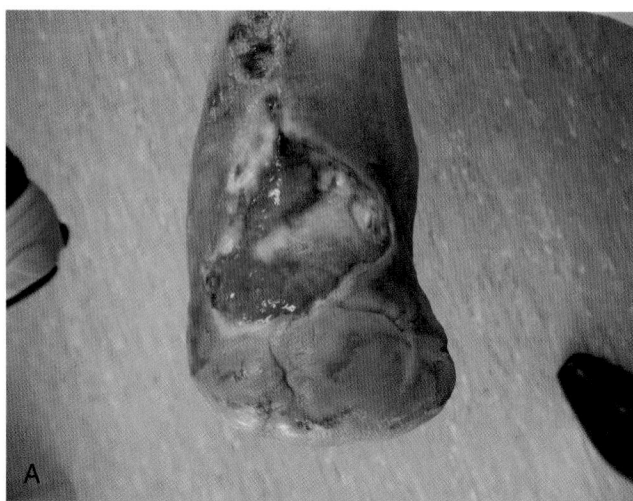

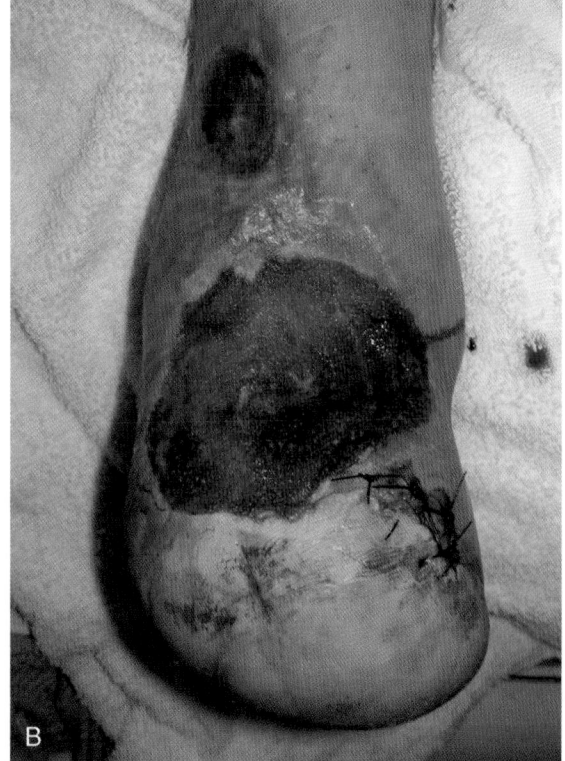

Figure 113-16 A, Wound with fibrotic tissue in the base, before débridement. **B,** After proper débridement and promotion of granulation tissue with the Wound VAC, the wound bed is prepared for closure.

ally, in shallow DFUs, it is difficult to keep the VAC foam from shearing. To prevent this, one can reduce the thickness of the foam or bridge the track pad to the dorsal foot. Once a wound becomes shallow and covered in granulation tissue, it is time to consider discontinuing the VAC and progressing to wound closure.

Growth Factors

Growth factor therapy has been theorized to speed the healing of chronic ulcers.[64] Recombinant human platelet-derived growth factor (PDGF) is available in the United States by prescription. Original trials reported a 32% decrease in the time to complete closure when combined with good wound care.[65] PDGF therapy is expensive, and it should be used only by those with experience in wound care. It has no effect on fibrotic or necrotic tissue and should be applied only to a thoroughly débrided wound. Aggressive, serial débridements improve outcomes.[66]

Stem Cells

Chronic diabetic ulcers exhibit cells that are phenotypically senescent, incapable of not only mitosis but also apoptosis. These cells may be unresponsive to growth factor application. Débridement of the superficial layer of the wound bed and margins aids in removing these cells. Bone marrow contributes to dermal wound healing by the mobilization and peripheral circulation of progenitor cells.[67] Direct application of autologous marrow-derived stem cells topically or by periwound injection may speed this process, resulting in robust granular tissue that will accept a skin graft or substitute.[68] Others have harvested and expanded marrow-derived stem cells in culture and reapplied them to chronic ulcers with success.[69-71]

Wound Closure

After preparing a vascularized wound bed, wound closure should be performed as rapidly as possible to avoid complications. Wound closure can be obtained by split-thickness skin graft, plastic surgical flaps, or bioengineered tissue.

Skin Grafts

Split-thickness skin grafting is a viable, minimally invasive, and cost-effective method to cover large granular defects.[72] Split-thickness grafts perform best on non–weight-bearing surfaces of the foot, including the dorsal, medial, lateral, and arch areas. Although meshed grafting can reduce the rate of seroma and hematoma formation, some have shown that unmeshed grafts perform equally well.[73] Another method to improve the adherence and survival of meshed split-thickness skin grafts is the use of NPWT as a bolster dressing,[74] which reduces seroma and hematoma formation and shear forces. A nonadherent interface must be interposed between the foam and the graft. The negative pressure can be used continuously for 4 to 5 days after grafting; then it is discontinued, and standard dressings are applied. Because split-thickness grafts are not suitable for weight-bearing surfaces, some have recommended donor glabrous skin grafts in these locations.[75]

Tissue Flaps

Large soft tissue defects and wounds with exposed deep structures such as bone require more aggressive measures to obtain closure. Multiple types of soft tissue flaps can be used to manage these defects. The flaps should be based on current vascular flow and not assumed anatomic flow, because patients with diabetes may have segmental or regional arterial occlusions. With fasciocutaneous flaps, the fascia and superficial tissue are rotated into place to cover a defect. One of the more common fasciocutaneous flaps performed in the diabetic foot is a medial plantar artery flap, which can be rotated laterally to cover a subcuboid ulcer or proximally to cover a plantar calcaneal defect. The toe fillet flap can be used to cover submetatarsal head ulcers, but it requires sacrifice of a digit.[76] For plantar central metatarsal head ulcerations, the attached toe can be filleted with a central plantar incision, the nail removed, and the skin advanced in a plantar direction to cover the ulcer site. In rare cases, the hallux may be sacrificed; however, this can have a deleterious impact on gait and plantar pressure afterward. In these cases, the incision is made laterally between the dorsal and plantar digital neurovascular bundles; the flap is then lifted from the bone and can be advanced laterally (Fig. 113-17). Muscle flaps are used to cover exposed bone, such as the extensor digitorum brevis flap or the abductor hallucis (and digiti minimi) flap. The exposed muscle can be covered with a split-thickness skin graft. Free flaps involve the autotransplantation of a vascularized myocutaneous area to the recipient site and microvascular reanastomosis.[77]

Bioengineered Tissue

In shallow wounds without exposed deep structures, bioengineered tissues such as Apligraf and Dermagraft are useful

adjuncts and are sometimes termed "living skin equivalents." Apligraf (Organogenesis, Canton, MA) is a living dermal bilayer consisting of a dermis and epidermis. Apligraf has been studied extensively and is approved by the FDA for use in DFUs and venous leg ulcers. It has a shelf life of approxi-

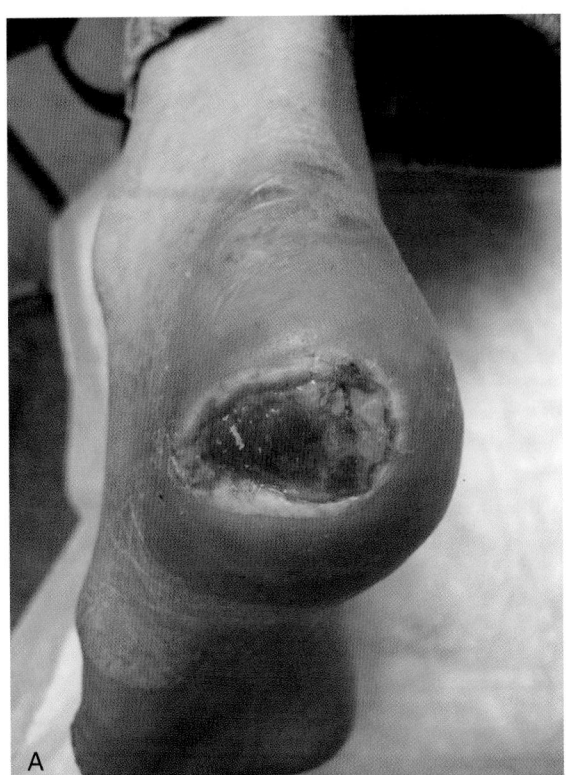

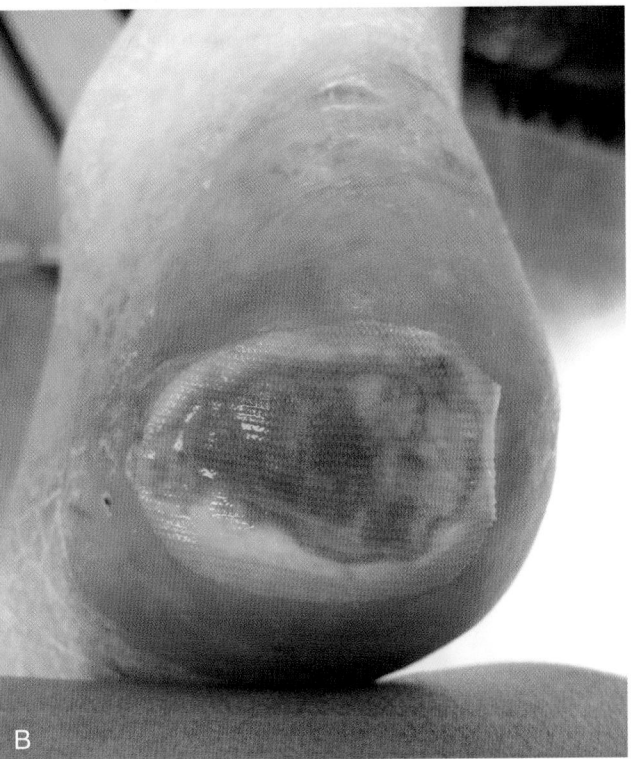

Figure 113-18 Heel ulcer before (**A**) and after (**B**) application of Dermagraft bioengineered skin substitute. It is secured in place with a dressing.

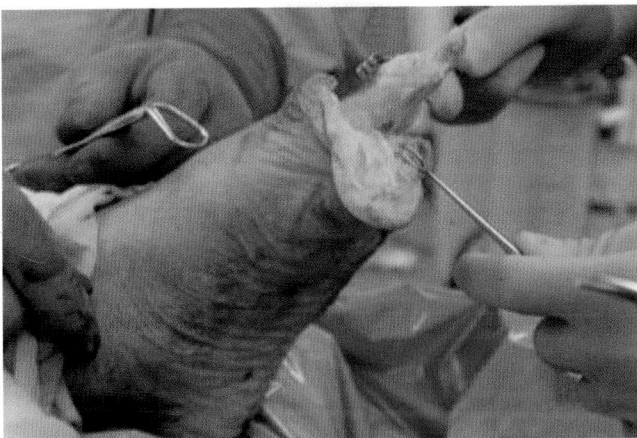

Figure 113-17 Toe fillet flap of the hallux is lifted from the underlying bone. The incision is made laterally, and the soft tissue is lifted full thickness from the periosteum to ensure that the digital arteries are captured in the flap.

mately 10 days. It must be secured to the wound with sutures or another type of anchor. In a large multicenter trial, weekly applications (up to five) resulted in a 63% healing rate, compared with 38% among controls at 12 weeks.[78] Dermagraft (Advanced BioHealing, Inc., La Jolla, CA) is a single layer consisting of living fibroblasts on an absorbable mesh that is FDA approved for DFUs. It is cryopreserved and has a shelf life of 90 days. After thawing, it is applied to the ulcer and secured with a dressing (Fig. 113-18). It is applied weekly for up to 8 weeks.[79] In a randomized controlled trial, Dermagraft resulted in a 30% healing rate over 12 weeks, compared with 18% in the control group. Dermagraft was also associated with a lower rate of ulcer-related adverse events.[80]

GraftJacket (Wright Medical Technology, Inc., Arlington, TN) is an acellular dermal matrix made from irradiated cadaveric skin. Although it was reported to be beneficial for ulcer healing in one published trial,[81] the authors found that its best use was to cover exposed deep tissue, such as tendon and bone. It can be meshed and sutured into place over fenestrated bone, and with the application of NPWT, it leads to granular tissue formation. When used to close ulcers, our experience indicates that it replaces "like with like" tissue, such that plantar weight-bearing skin is regenerated if used in those areas.

TREATMENT SELECTION

Determining whether to perform a split-thickness skin graft or use bioengineered tissue depends on the location of the wound and the suitability of the host. Generally, split-thickness skin grafting works best on wounds without pressure or shearing forces, such as dorsal, medial, lateral, or ankle wounds. In our experience, plantar foot and heel wounds do not fare well with skin grafts, and we prefer a bioengineered tissue. A recent prospective case-control study comparing split-thickness skin grafting with standard wound care found an obvious difference in healing times.[82] Mean healing time in the skin graft group was 28 ± 5 days, versus 122 ± 7 days in the control group ($P < .05$). Interestingly, split-thickness skin grafts were used on plantar heel and foot wounds, without an increase in failure rates. The 5-day postoperative healing rate was found to be a good predictor of complete healing of the skin graft. The mean healing time for split-thickness skin grafts was less than that for a skin equivalent.[78]

SELECTED KEY REFERENCES

Armstrong DG, Lavery LA. Negative pressure wound therapy after partial diabetic foot amputation: a multicentre, randomised controlled trial. *Lancet.* 2005;366:1704-1710.
Randomized controlled trial evaluating use of the Wound VAC in diabetic patients undergoing partial foot amputation. It resulted in faster granulation tissue formation and a reduction in secondary amputations.

Attinger CE, Janis JE, Steinberg J, Schwartz J, Al-Attar A, Couch K. Clinical approach to wounds: debridement and wound bed preparation including the use of dressings and wound-healing adjuvants. *Plast Reconstr Surg.* 2006;117(7 Suppl):72S-109S.
Review of débridement for cutaneous wounds from the surgeon's perspective.

Lipsky BA, Berendt AR, Deery HG, Embil JM, Joseph WS, Karchmer AW, LeFrock JL, Lew DP, Mader JT, Norden C, Tan JS, Infectious Diseases Society of America. Diagnosis and treatment of diabetic foot infections. *Clin Infect Dis.* 2004;39:885-910.
Complete review of diabetic foot infections and treatment guidelines from opinion leaders in the United States and Europe.

Reiber GE, Vileikyte L, Boyko EJ, del Aguila M, Smith DG, Lavery LA, Boulton AJ. Causal pathways for incident lower-extremity ulcers in patients with diabetes from two settings. *Diabetes Care.* 1999;22: 157-162.
Pivotal article illustrating the triad of DFU causes: peripheral neuropathy, foot deformity, minor trauma.

Singh N, Armstrong DG, Lipsky BA. Preventing foot ulcers in patients with diabetes. *JAMA.* 2005;293:217-228.
Thorough review of the current strategies to prevent foot ulcers in patients with diabetes. Also includes new lifetime foot ulcer incidence data, indicating that 25% of those with diabetes are affected.

Steed DL, Donohoe D, Webster MW, Lindsley L. Effect of extensive debridement and treatment on the healing of diabetic foot ulcers. Diabetic Ulcer Study Group. *J Am Coll Surg.* 1996;183:61-64.
Study confirming the additive effect of serial débridement in combination with advanced therapies.

Wrobel JS, Connolly JE. Making the diagnosis of osteomyelitis. The role of prevalence. *J Am Podiatr Med Assoc.* 1998;88:337-343.
Article debunking the probe-to-bone concept. In the clinic setting, the prevalence of osteomyelitis makes the probe-to-bone test no more sensitive than a coin flip.

REFERENCES

The reference list can be found on the companion Expert Consult Web site at *www.expertconsult.com*.

CHAPTER 114

Lower Extremity Amputation: General Considerations

Wayne W. Zhang and Ahmed M. Abou-Zamzam, Jr.

Major lower extremity amputations continue to be part of all vascular practices, despite the general approach of aggressively attempting to salvage limbs. Though often viewed as a failure of treatment, major amputation should be considered an important, definitive treatment option. The convergence of several important factors, such as the aging of the population and the epidemic of diabetes and peripheral arterial disease (PAD), suggests that amputations will be an increasingly important issue facing patients and surgeons.

The goal of amputation is to remove all infected, gangrenous, and ischemic tissue and provide the patient with the longest functional limb. Avoidance of repeated amputations and nonhealing operative sites is crucial for the patient's optimal recovery and best functional rehabilitation or palliation.

EPIDEMIOLOGY

In the United States, approximately 60,000 major amputations (above the ankle) are performed annually.[1-3] In 2003, 115,749 amputations of all types were performed in the United States, which included 55,574 major amputations.[1] Diabetes and PAD remain the major risk factors for lower extremity amputation worldwide.[4] Studies show that 25% to 90% of all amputations are associated with diabetes.[2,4] Patients with diabetes have a 10-fold greater risk of amputation than those without diabetes.[3] This association is due to the presence of neuropathy and infection, as well as the markedly increased prevalence of PAD in this patient population.

Variation in Amputation Rates

There is significant regional variation in the performance of amputation around the world, which suggests that factors other than strict medical issues may affect amputation rates.[4-6] A study from the United Kingdom cited significant regional variation in amputation rates and stressed the need for consensus guidelines.[5] The Global Lower Extremity Amputation Study Group reported that the highest amputation rate (for a first major amputation) was 44 per 100,000 population per year among Navajo men, and the lowest rate was 2.8 per 100,000 per year in Madrid, Spain.[4] Physician experience plays a key role in the selection of amputation as a treatment. In the treatment of critical limb ischemia, surgeon caseload and hospital volume have been shown to affect amputation rates, with low volumes being associated with higher amputation rates.[7]

A study of a Medicare claims database demonstrated that the supply of vascular specialists influences the rate of amputation. A 0.30 increase in the number of vascular surgeons per 10,000 Medicare beneficiaries led to a 1.6% reduction in amputations.[8] The distribution of vascular surgeons and interventional radiologists in the United States is strongly correlated not only with regional medical needs but also with local climate, education, crime, and transportation. This observation suggests that policies to increase the supply of vascular specialists in underserved areas may reduce regional disparities in amputation rates.[8] Patient and health care provider education has also been demonstrated to reduce amputation rates.[9] Earlier identification of patients at risk leads to more timely referral, treatment, and intervention.

Effect of Ethnicity and Economic and Social Status

A complex interaction exists between race or ethnicity and amputation rates. In certain groups, such as the Native American Navajo population, amputation rates appear to be related to the high incidence of diabetes.[4] However, African Americans are more likely than Caucasians to undergo amputation as opposed to revascularization, even when controlling for the presence of diabetes.[10-12] These differences have been attributed to variations in access to health care, treatment of comorbidities, and possible physician and patient factors. Insurance status also has an effect on amputation rates. Patients without insurance coverage have higher rates of amputation than those with access to health insurance.[12] Data from the National Inpatient Sample documented that 34% of the 691,833 patients presenting with lower extremity ischemia from 1998 to 2002 underwent amputation. The primary amputation rates were significantly higher among patients who were nonwhite, low income, and without commercial insurance.[13] Similar results showed that African American patients were 1.7 times more likely to have both primary and repeat amputation than white or other patients.[14]

Effect of Revascularization Rates

Trends in the interplay between revascularization and amputation rates are complicated. Over a 10-year period, the Mayo Clinic reported a 50% reduction in amputation rates that corresponded to increased rates of lower extremity revascularization by both surgical and endovascular techniques.[15] A Finnish study also demonstrated that an increase in revascularization rates correlated with a decrease in major amputation rates in elderly patients.[16] A recent U.S. study of two national (Nationwide Inpatient Sample and National Hospital Discharge Survey) and four state databases demonstrated that both the number of lower extremity revascularizations and the number of major amputations have declined, despite a substantial increase in lower extremity endovascular interventions. From 1998 to 2003, the volume of major amputations decreased 16% regionally (New York, California, New Jersey, and Florida) and 15% nationally. However, minor amputations increased 4% regionally and 3% nationally.[1] It has been speculated that the improved limb salvage rates are partially due to earlier endovascular interventions in less critical lesions and to procedures in high-risk patients who are not candidates for open bypass. Other possible contributing factors to lower rates of amputation include improved medical management, risk factor modification, and wound care methods used in these patients.

High-risk patients treated with endovascular intervention have superior rates of limb salvage and maintenance of ambulation compared with patients undergoing primary amputation. However, these patients have no better functional benefit than those treated with primary amputation after 1 year.[17] The medium-term results of the Bypass versus Angioplasty in Severe Ischemia of the Leg (BASIL) trial indicate that the outcomes of bypass surgery–first and balloon angioplasty–first strategies are similar in terms of amputation-free survival.[18]

The ideal balance of endovascular and open surgical reconstructions has yet to be determined for lower extremity ischemia. Nationwide Inpatient Sample data suggest that lower extremity revascularizations have reached a plateau of around 140,000; similarly, major amputation may have settled near 60,000 annually.[1] The total number of revascularizations may be higher because same-day endovascular procedures might not be included in the Nationwide Inpatient Sample database. The Trans-Atlantic Inter-Society Consensus (TASC) II Working Group documented that the incidence of major amputations varies from 12 to 50 per 100,000 population per year.[19] With the aging of the population, future trends in these areas will have a great effect on health care expenditures.

■ INDICATIONS FOR AMPUTATION

Indications for amputation have traditionally been divided into acute ischemia, chronic ischemia, foot infection, severe traumatic injury, and lower extremity skeletal or soft tissue malignancies. The last two indications are beyond the scope of this chapter and are not discussed. In the presence of acute ischemia, major amputation is undertaken for irreversible ischemia, for severe ischemia with no revascularization options, or following unsuccessful attempts at revascularization. Amputation for chronic ischemia may be performed owing to failure of revascularization, lack of suitable conduit

or target arteries, severe patient co-morbidities or poor functional status, or extensive gangrene or infection such that foot salvage is not possible. Pedal sepsis without ischemia constitutes another major subgroup of patients undergoing amputation; this presentation is extremely common in patients with diabetes and associated neuropathy. Because the underlying indications for amputation frequently overlap, it can be difficult to compare indications for and outcomes of amputations reported in the literature.

Impact of Diabetes

The presence of PAD and diabetes, either alone or in combination, contributes to the majority of major nontraumatic lower extremity amputations. Many general classifications, however, overemphasize the role of diabetes and understate the role of concomitant ischemia. Malone reported the indications for amputation as follows: complications of diabetes (60% to 80%), infection without diabetes (15% to 25%), ischemia without infection (5% to 10%), chronic osteomyelitis (3% to 5%), trauma (2% to 5%), and miscellaneous (5% to 10%).[20] These general classifications have a certain degree of overlap and mask the true interaction between ischemia and diabetes. This simplistic breakdown does not provide any insight into the true influence of ischemia or the full potential of revascularization to reduce amputation rates. Also, ischemia may occur in an acute or chronic setting, and because no revascularization is entirely successful, amputation may ultimately follow revascularization.

Impact of Tissue Loss and Anatomy

In a 2003 report, our group sought to more clearly categorize the indications for major amputation to explain why amputations continue to be performed despite aggressive revascularization programs.[21] When identifying the indications for amputation, it must be recognized that with chronic ischemia, limb loss may ultimately occur despite revascularization. Also, patients may present initially with acutely ischemic limbs that are beyond any hope of salvage. The influence of gangrene and pedal sepsis must also be considered, because they have a significant impact on the options for limb salvage. Last, patient co-morbidities and ambulatory status influence the decision for amputation.

The TASC II Working Group reported that the rate of primary amputation in chronic critical leg ischemia is approximately 25%. Unreconstructable vascular disease is the most common indication for secondary amputations, which account for nearly 60% of patients.[19] To more clearly delineate the reasons for major amputation in an academic vascular practice, a series of 131 consecutive major lower extremity amputations were reviewed, and the indications for amputation clearly classified (Table 114-1). In this setting, more than 50% of patients who underwent amputation had prior attempts at limb salvage via revascularization or had no anatomically feasible revascularization options. This group of patients had exhausted the armamentarium of vascular

Table 114-1 Indications for Major Amputation by Vascular Surgeons

Indication for Major Amputation	Percentage of Cases (N = 131)
Critical limb ischemia with failed revascularization	39
Extensive pedal gangrene	15
Unreconstructable arterial anatomy	11
Overwhelming pedal sepsis	9
Excessive surgical risk	9
Nonviable, acutely ischemic foot	8
Nonambulatory status	8

From Abou-Zamzam AM Jr, Teruya TH, Killeen JD, Ballard JL. Major lower extremity amputation in an academic vascular center. *Ann Vasc Surg* 2003; 17:86-90.

surgery. Seventeen percent of patients were not considered candidates for aggressive attempts at limb salvage owing to a preexisting nonambulatory status (8%) or the presence of excessive surgical risk (9%). Additionally, 32% of patients had nonsalvageable limbs at presentation due to extensive pedal gangrene, pedal sepsis, or a nonviable foot that dictated primary amputation.

Similar findings were reported by Nehler and colleagues in a series of 172 major amputations.[22] The indication for amputation was critical ischemia in 87% and complications of diabetic neuropathy without significant ischemia in 13%. Forty-six patients (30%) had prior bypass failures or amputations despite patent reconstructions, and 10 (6%) had no revascularization options; therefore, 36% had exhausted the resources of revascularization. Eighty-five patients (55%) underwent primary amputation because of severe co-morbidities, poor functional status, extensive necrosis, or a combination of these factors. In another series of 125 major amputations, 38% of procedures were performed following failed revascularizations.[23]

Impact of Delay in Presentation

The significant role of delay in patient presentation cannot be overstated. The mean time to vascular surgery consultation was 73 days for pedal tissue loss and 27 days for ischemic rest pain in the report by Nehler and colleagues.[22] This delay likely accounts for the large percentage of primary amputations in their series and underscores the need for patient and physician education. Indeed, in a report by Bailey and cowork-ers, only 24% of patients with critical limb ischemia were perceived as needing "urgent" vascular consultation, with a mean 8-week duration of symptoms before vascular evaluation.[24] This suggests that delayed patient presentation involves not just patient factors but also physician factors.

■ PRIMARY AMPUTATION VERSUS REVASCULARIZATION

The most important aspect of determining the need for amputation is the initial decision whether to attempt limb

salvage or proceed with major amputation. Despite wide-spread discussion of great triumphs in revascularization, there is a growing awareness that primary amputation may be the best approach in specific patient subsets. As stated earlier, more than 140,000 lower extremity revascularizations are performed annually in the United States. In recent years, open revascularizations have been partially replaced by endovascular procedures, yet nearly 60,000 major amputations are still being performed each year.[1] This implies that the ratio of amputation to revascularization may be close to 1:2 nationally. Many specialty centers may have a much lower ratio owing to the filtering effect of referring physicians. Many patients perceived as not being candidates for revascularization are treated locally with amputation and are never referred to these high-volume centers specializing in revascularization.

The ratio of major primary amputation to revascularization differs among facilities and may vary because of surgeon experience and practice protocols. A prospective study in an academic vascular surgery practice demonstrated that 43% of the 224 patients presenting with limb-threatening ischemia were treated by primary amputation, and 57% were treated with revascularization.[25] Diabetes mellitus, end-stage renal disease, tissue loss, and poor functional status were all predictors of treatment with amputation as opposed to revascularization.

Groups Benefiting from Primary Amputation

The perceived improved outcomes following revascularization compared with amputation have driven the belief that revascularization is always the better option. However, an examination of the data demonstrates that functional outcomes following amputation may not be markedly different from those following revascularization for specific patient subgroups. A recent report by Taylor and associates analyzed 553 patients who underwent 627 primary major limb amputations.[26] In patients younger than 60 years, functional outcomes following below-knee amputation were similar to those of patients undergoing successful revascularization. Such information lends credence to the observation that primary amputation should be considered not a failure of therapy but a viable, important treatment option.[22,26,27]

The recent trend in percutaneous revascularization has raised the question of how to treat patients who are considered "unfit" for open surgical revascularization. Taylor and coworkers recently reported an analysis of 314 patients treated for critical limb ischemia who were unsuitable for open revascularization owing to medical, functional, or mental co-morbidities.[17] Patients were treated with either percutaneous transluminal angioplasty (PTA) or major amputation. The 131 patients treated with PTA had higher rates of maintenance of ambulation and independent living compared with the 183 patients treated with amputation. However, the PTA group had a higher mortality rate, and the advantages in ambulation and independent living lasted only 12 months and 3 months, respectively. Therefore, despite hopes to the contrary, in patients with critical limb ischemia who are unfit for open revascularization, PTA is no better than primary amputation.

Indeed, in those with extensive foot lesions, severe co-morbidities, or very unfavorable anatomy, primary amputation is often the best treatment option.[22,26,27] Because of delayed referral, many patients ultimately requiring amputation present to the vascular surgeon with extensive pedal necrosis, which makes salvage unlikely, regardless of arterial targets for revascularization. End-stage renal disease presents a particularly difficult challenge, and the presence of advanced heel gangrene in this group of patients may best be treated with primary amputation.[28,29] An attempt at limb salvage that ultimately ends with major amputation despite "successful" revascularization is a scenario seen in all vascular practices. These multiple operations have additive morbidities that can diminish the likelihood of eventual prosthetic use and successful rehabilitation.

A very reasoned approach to patients presenting with critical limb ischemia is necessary. A thoughtful strategy considering the patient's co-morbidities, the status of the foot, and the complexity of the required revascularization has been outlined by Nehler and colleagues.[27] In a good-risk patient with minimal pedal tissue loss, an aggressive attempt at revascularization, with use of alternative vein conduits, may be appropriate. However, when the patient's overall health status is poor or the foot lesions are extensive, primary amputation must be considered.

■ PREOPERATIVE EVALUATION

The preoperative evaluation of a patient undergoing major amputation should be rational and expeditious, and it should strive to reduce perioperative complications and mortality. Preoperative regional and systemic evaluation is critical. Regional evaluation should include the duration and severity of limb ischemia, extent of tissue loss, presence of wound infection, and anatomic considerations for revascularization. Preoperative medical co-morbidities, ambulatory ability, mental status, and life expectancy should also be evaluated systematically.

A standard evaluation with a thorough history and physical examination should be performed in all patients. Acute congestive heart failure, unstable angina, or concurrent myocardial infarction must be addressed. A thorough cardiac evaluation is not necessary in the absence of active cardiac symptoms, evidence of congestive heart failure on history or physical examination, or acute issues on the electrocardiogram.[30,31] It is important to recognize, however, that most patients presenting for amputation have had limited activity and may not manifest overt cardiac disease owing to the lack of physiologic stress, so even minor cardiac symptoms should be concerning.

Reducing Risk

Perioperative treatment with beta blockade has been beneficial in the general vascular surgery population,[32-34] but these important studies included few patients undergoing major amputation. However, owing to the shared risk factors, the positive impact of beta blockers can likely be extrapolated from critical limb ischemia patients to the amputation population. The management of associated hypertension, diabetes, and renal failure should be optimized. The timing of hemodialysis in relation to operation is important in managing fluids and electrolytes in the perioperative period. An aggressive approach to normalize glucose levels is essential to ensure proper wound healing.

The incidence of venous thromboembolism in the perioperative period is high. Yeager and coworkers documented that the perioperative rate of deep venous thrombosis (DVT) was 11% following major amputation.[35] Interestingly, more than half the thromboses were present preoperatively. Furthermore, 17% of all amputation-related deaths are caused by pulmonary emboli.[2] These statistics underscore the infirm nature of these patients and the importance of surveillance and prophylaxis for venous thromboembolism. There are limited prospective comparisons of DVT prophylaxis regimens in the amputation population. Prophylaxis with either subcutaneous unfractionated heparin or low-molecular-weight heparin appears to be safe and effective.[36]

Managing Infection

Special consideration should be given to patients presenting with extensive pedal infection necessitating amputation. Aggressive control of infection, with surgical extirpation of the source and adjunctive intravenous antibiotics, is the mainstay of treatment. The two-stage approach of guillotine amputation followed by formal amputation several days later has a lower complication rate than single-stage amputation.[37] Guillotine amputation is a rapid procedure, but an additional operation to treat the amputation stump is necessary.

Another option in patients who are moribund is a physiologic cryoamputation, which can be performed safely at the bedside.[38,39] The materials needed to perform cryoamputation are dry ice, a large plastic bag, an umbilical tape to use as a tourniquet, towels, blankets, adhesive tape, and a heating pad. After parenteral analgesics are administered, an umbilical tape is tied around the affected extremity just proximal to the diseased area. A large plastic bag is placed over the distal leg and filled with dry ice, circumferentially covering the leg. The dry ice bag is wrapped with blankets and secured with adhesive tape. A heating pad covered with a protective towel is placed around the proximal extremity adjacent to the frost line. The opposite leg should be covered with numerous blankets to avoid collateral injury. The frost line and the frozen limb should be checked periodically by the nursing staff, and dry ice added as needed. This bedside procedure alleviates any time pressures for amputation, controls infection, and allows optimal treatment of associated conditions. If necessary, a cryoamputation can be maintained for several weeks. When the patient's status improves, he or she may be taken to the operating room for a one-stage amputation.

Addressing Associated Heart Disease

The evaluation of any potential amputee depends on the urgency of the intervention. In patients with acute ischemia, embolic disease directs the focus of the investigation toward embolic sources—most often cardiac. Any arrhythmias or recent myocardial infarction with ventricular thrombus must be investigated and addressed. Echocardiography and anticoagulation are key aspects of perioperative management. Preoperatively, however, the focus is on stabilizing an unstable patient. The nonviable limb should be amputated in a timely manner, with most diagnostic testing taking place in the postoperative period.

Patients with acute ischemia related to thrombosis of chronically diseased arteries have the same risk factors as patients presenting with chronic ischemia. In these patients, the role of extensive perioperative cardiac evaluation is unclear. Indeed, most reports of preoperative cardiac evaluation have excluded patients undergoing amputation, focusing instead on those undergoing aneurysm repair or lower extremity revascularization.[30,40-42] Comparable perioperative mortality rates regardless of extensive preoperative cardiac evaluation call the practice of preoperative "cardiac clearance" into question.[43] Guidelines issued in 2007 by the American College of Cardiology and the American Heart Association clarified that the purpose of preoperative cardiac evaluation is not to give medical clearance but rather to evaluate the patient's current medical status and cardiac risks over the entire perioperative period. These guidelines recommend that no test be performed unless it is likely to influence the patient's treatment.[32]

Planning Rehabilitation

Throughout the perioperative evaluation, it is important to involve rehabilitation medicine specialists, physical therapists, nurses, and prosthetists in the care of these patients. Centers with dedicated multispecialty teams have much more successful rehabilitation outcomes.[44] Addressing the patient's concerns regarding postoperative recovery, the timing of prosthetic use, and ultimate functional goals is best done in the preoperative period.

▪ AMPUTATION LEVEL SELECTION

The goals of amputation are (1) to eliminate all infected, necrotic, and painful tissue; (2) to have a wound that heals successfully; and (3) to have an appropriate remnant stump that can accommodate a prosthesis. The length of the preserved limb has important implications for rehabilitation. Prosthetic use following major amputation puts an increased

energy demand on the patient. Unilateral below-knee amputees require a 10% to 40% increase in energy expenditure for ambulation, and above-knee amputees require 50% to 70% more energy to ambulate.[2] This differential may explain why the successful rehabilitation rate is much lower following above-knee amputation (AKA) than below-knee amputation (BKA). Prosthetic use is reportedly 50% to 100% following BKA but only 10% to 30% following AKA.[22,44-46] Interestingly, the true rate of ambulation is significantly lower than that of prosthetic use, and it shows a steady attrition in the 5 years following amputation.[22,45] Partial foot or toe amputations are minor procedures that preserve the majority of the extremity and allow ambulation without the need for bulky prostheses. Most minor amputations, including toe and ray amputations, lead to minimal increases in energy expenditure and require simple orthotic inserts.

Failure of an amputation to heal is multifactorial. Much emphasis has been placed on assessing blood flow at the level of the amputation to predict wound healing. However, failure may be caused not just by ischemia but also by infection, hematoma, or trauma. This explains why no single test can predict with 100% accuracy the ability of an amputation to heal or, conversely, its inability to heal. Most tests are better at predicting wound healing than failure to heal. Thus, using any single test may lead to unnecessarily proximal amputation.

The importance of optimizing level selection is underlined by the need to revise BKAs to AKAs in 15% to 25% of patients.[2,21,22,47] This revision rate is frequently accompanied by a perioperative mortality rate of greater than 5%.[2] Such events also lead to increased patient anxiety and fear of repeated, more proximal amputations.

Objective Testing and Clinical Judgment

The drive to maximize limb length in amputees and to minimize the need for revisions has led to a search for the optimal modality for selecting an amputation level. Physical findings (pulses, skin quality, extent of foot ischemia or infection, skin temperature), noninvasive hemodynamic tests (segmental arterial pressures, Doppler waveforms, toe pressures), invasive anatomic tests (angiographic scoring systems), and physiologic tests (skin blood flow, skin perfusion pressure, muscle perfusion, transcutaneous oxygen measurements) have all been extensively investigated.

Pulse Palpation and Physical Findings

Physical examination is the essential first step in determining the level of amputation. The extent of gangrene and infection dictates the maximal length attainable. In this evaluation, the presence of dependent rubor should be considered analogous to gangrene because this tissue is ischemic. The presence of pulses should be accurately assessed. The presence of a palpable pulse immediately proximal to a proposed amputation level predicts successful healing in nearly 100% of patients undergoing either major or minor amputation.[48,49] However, the absence of a pulse does not necessarily lead to failure of wound healing; therefore, sole reliance on the presence of a pulse leads to unnecessarily proximal amputations.

Using "clinical judgment," which incorporates physical findings and consideration of the patient's overall status, yields wound healing rates of 80% in BKAs and 90% in AKAs. Wagner and colleagues found that objective data may supplement clinical judgment but not replace it; more distal amputations were achieved with clinical judgment than with sole reliance on objective examinations.[50] Experience is important; therefore, the determination of amputation level should not be relegated to junior surgeons or trainees.

Skin Temperature Measurements

The subjective interpretation of skin temperature as a guide for amputation is not reliable. However, several investigators have demonstrated that objective, direct skin temperature measurement may predict amputation healing with an accuracy of 80% to 90%.[2,50,51] In a study comparing several noninvasive techniques, direct skin temperature measurement at the level of amputation with a threshold of 90°F demonstrated the best accuracy.[50] Special attention must be paid to room temperature, and comparison with a normal contralateral extremity can be helpful.

Ankle and Toe Pressure Measurements

The use of noninvasive hemodynamic tests has been extensively evaluated. Frequently employed tests are segmental arterial pressures, Doppler waveforms, and toe pressures. Absolute ankle pressures greater than 60 mm Hg can predict the healing of BKAs with an accuracy of 50% to 90%. Calf pressures and thigh pressures have shown similar reliability.[2] However, Wagner and colleagues found that Doppler-derived pressures at the thigh, popliteal, calf, and ankle levels are less reliable than clinical judgment in predicting the healing of BKAs.[50] This inaccuracy may be due in part to the high prevalence of diabetes in this population, making measured pressures less reliable because of medial calcinosis.

The ankle-brachial index (ABI) should always be obtained, regardless of the presence of a palpable pulse. Marston and colleagues reported on the role of ABI in predicting the need for amputation in a cohort of high-risk patients with critical limb ischemia treated with meticulous wound care but without revascularization. In patients with an ABI less than 0.5, 28% and 34% of limbs required amputation at 6 and 12 months, respectively, versus 10% and 15% of limbs in patients with an ABI greater than 0.5 (P = .01).[52]

The use of toe pressures has been advocated as being predictive of forefoot amputation healing. Vitti and associates demonstrated universal failure of minor amputations in patients with diabetes and toe pressures less than 38 mm Hg.[53] However, there was no similar threshold value in patients without diabetes, limiting the usefulness of this parameter.

Arteriography

Invasive testing with arteriography has been investigated as a means of determining amputation level, but the correlation between arteriographic findings and healing potential has been poor. Dwars and coworkers found that angiographic scores did not correlate with amputation healing.[49] In fact, in their report, angiographic patency tended to be greater in limbs with failed or delayed healing than in limbs with successful healing.

Radioisotope Scans, Scintigraphy, and Skin Perfusion Pressure

All physiologic tests attempt to predict wound healing based on tissue perfusion or oxygen delivery at the proposed level of amputation. One technique of measuring skin blood flow involves injecting an intradermal isotope (xenon 133 or iodine 125) and then calculating blood flow by measuring the isotope washout rate using nuclear medicine scanning devices.[20,54] Malone and associates initially reported excellent results with xenon 133 clearance, with an accuracy of 92% to 97%.[55] However, in a follow-up report, this same group found that the overlap in values between patients with healed and failed amputations made this test too unreliable.[54]

Sarikaya and coworkers used technetium (Tc) 99m sestamibi scintigraphy to predict the healing of extremity amputation based on deep tissue perfusion.[56] Perfusion to the ischemic limb was evaluated preoperatively based on the Tc 99m sestamibi uptake pattern. Nonviable tissue in the extremity was suggested by a clear-cut edge of perfused muscle. The most distal level of amputation was determined above the nonviable tissue. In their 25 patients, the proposed level of amputation based on physical examination and Doppler study was changed to a lower level after Tc 99m sestamibi scintigraphy in 65% of cases, and all amputation wounds healed.

Skin perfusion pressure is another physiologic test to determine amputation level. This test involves a scintigraphic technique in which intracutaneous iodine 123 is injected at different amputation levels. External pressure is applied, and by measuring the washout of isotope, the skin perfusion pressure is determined. A level less than 20 mm Hg was predictive of wound failure in 89% of amputations, and a reading greater than 20 mm Hg predicted healing in 99%.[49] Skin perfusion pressure can also be measured by laser Doppler velocimetry, thus avoiding the need for isotopes and markedly simplifying the test.

Skin fluorescence employs a Wood's or ultraviolet light following the intravenous injection of fluorescein dye. A qualitative determination of regional blood flow is used to determine the level of amputation. Success rates in predicting healing have ranged from 86% to 100%.[20] Owing to the wide availability of these tools and no requirement for radioisotope, this technique is more accessible than scintigraphic techniques. However, the fluorescein technique may be more affected by the presence of inflammation and cellulitis than are scintigraphic techniques.

Table 114-2 Prediction of Wound Healing by Noninvasive Vascular Studies[63]

Study	Threshold (mm Hg)	Wound Healing (%)		Sensitivity (%)	Specificity (%)
		Below Threshold	*Above Threshold*		
SPP	40	10	69	72	88
tcPo$_2$	30	14	63	60	87
TBP	30	12	67	63	90
ABP	80	11	45	74	70

ABP, ankle blood pressure; SPP, skin perfusion pressure; TBP, toe blood pressure; tcPo$_2$, transcutaneous oxygen pressure.

Transcutaneous Oxygen Measurements

Transcutaneous oxygen measurement is a completely noninvasive method that is widely used to select an amputation level. A small sensor is placed on the skin in the area of interest. By heating the sensor and skin to 44°C, local skin hyperemia results in decreased flow resistance and arteriolarization of capillary blood. The partial pressure of oxygen measured transcutaneously (tcPo$_2$) approximates the true arterial oxygen pressure in the area of interest.[57] The sensors can be placed anywhere on the body, and readings are given in millimeters of mercury (mm Hg). Absolute readings can be recorded, or readings in areas of interest can be indexed to a reference site (often the chest). The probes are small and atraumatic, and multiple sites can be tested simultaneously, depending on the machine. Readings in the supine position are more predictive than measurements in the dependent position or during supplemental oxygen breathing.[58] The values recorded are reliable and show an acceptable day-to-day variability in repeat measurements.[59]

Transcutaneous oxygen levels have an accuracy of 87% to 100% in predicting wound healing.[2,48,54,60] Malone and coworkers reported no amputation failures in patients with tcPo$_2$ greater than 20 mm Hg and universal failure when tcPo$_2$ was less than 20 mm Hg.[54] Unfortunately, other investigators have not confirmed any consistent absolute tcPo$_2$ threshold.[2,48,50] Some authors have reported a useful tcPo$_2$ threshold of 30 mm Hg, while others have reported 16 mm Hg as a cutoff value. In general, tcPo$_2$ readings greater than 40 mm Hg are associated with healing and readings less than 20 mm Hg are associated with failure.[57,61] The lack of a consistent minimal level is likely due to the fact that nutrient blood flow may be present even in the setting of tcPo$_2$ readings of 0 mm Hg. The tcPo$_2$ may be artificially low in the setting of infection, inflammation, or edema, and repeat measurements are advised once such processes have resolved. Incidentally, in addition to modest utility in predicting wound healing, tcPo$_2$ has accuracy in predicting outcome following revascularization. Increases in tcPo$_2$ of greater than 30 mm Hg following revascularization are predictive of a successful clinical outcome.[60]

In direct comparisons with segmental pressures and skin blood flow, tcPo$_2$ has been the most accurate predictor of wound healing.[54] This applies not only to major amputation but also to forefoot amputation.[20,62] Transcutaneous oxygen measurements are also more accurate than fluorescein dye injections.[28,42] In addition, tcPo$_2$ has several advantages over other tests in terms of ease of measurement, reproducibility, and simple instrumentation that can be readily introduced into any vascular laboratory.

Yamada and colleagues studied 211 patients with 403 ischemic limbs using skin perfusion pressure, toe pressure, ankle pressure, and tcPo$_2$.[63] The correlations between these methods demonstrate that the combination of skin perfusion pressure and toe pressure can accurately predict wound healing. However, the combination of skin perfusion pressure and tcPo$_2$ did not result in a more accurate prediction. A meaningful approach to the accurate determination of amputation level must therefore include a combination of physical findings, clinical judgment, and objective testing.[48-50,54,57]

Technique Selection

Whether skin temperature, skin blood flow or perfusion, or transcutaneous oxygen measurements are used depends on local experience and availability. Measurement of tcPo$_2$ is easily incorporated into a noninvasive vascular laboratory, requires minimal equipment and training, and is reliable and reproducible. For these reasons, our preferred objective test is tcPo$_2$, with a threshold value of 30 mm Hg. However, strict utilization of a single objective method, rather than taking all available clinical data into account, leads to unnecessarily proximal amputations and denies patients the best opportunity for successful rehabilitation. The various methods of predicting wound healing and their accuracies are shown in Table 114-2.[63]

REHABILITATION CONSIDERATIONS

In 2005, 1.6 million people in the United States were living with the loss of a limb. Thirty-eight percent of them had amputations secondary to vascular disease. It is projected that the number of people living with the loss of a limb will more than double by the year 2050 to 3.6 million.[64] Rehabilitation is crucial for maximizing the functional outcome of these patients. The significant physical and psychological changes following major amputation make rehabilitation a complex process. Integrated rehabilitation requires an interdisciplinary team that incorporates members from surgery, internal and family medicine, psychiatry, physical therapy, occupational therapy, prosthetics, social services, nursing, nutrition, and recreational therapy.

Table 114-3 Energy Expenditure and Ambulation Rate at Various Amputation Levels

Amputation Level	Energy Expenditure above Normal (%)	Ambulation Rate (%)
Below-knee amputation		80
Long stump	10	
Short stump	40	
Knee disarticulation	71.5	31 (prosthesis fitting rate)
Above-knee amputation	63	38–50
Hip disarticulation	82	0–10 (vascular patients)

From Tang PCY, Ravji K, Key JJ, et al. Let them walk! Current prosthesis options for leg and foot amputees. *J Am Coll Surg* 206:548, 2008.

As mentioned earlier in this chapter, greater energy expenditure is required for ambulation in patients with higher levels of amputation. Energy expenditure and ambulatory rates at various amputation levels are shown in Table 114-3.[65] Many studies have shown that BKA patients have a significantly greater chance to achieve ambulation than AKA patients. In general, the goal is the preservation of maximal limb length at which a healed stump wound can be achieved.

Preoperative evaluation and amputation level selection should always include postoperative rehabilitation considerations. Preoperative ambulatory ability, co-morbidities, age, and mental status affect rehabilitation potential. Patients with limited preoperative ambulatory function, age older than 70 years, dementia, end-stage renal disease, and advanced coronary artery disease perform poorly following amputation.[26]

A comprehensive treatment plan should be developed at the beginning of rehabilitation and updated frequently based on the patient's condition. A dedicated team approach clearly improves the ultimate outcome for amputees.[44,62] One report documented that successful rehabilitation following major amputation increased from 69% before the institution of a coordinated team approach to 100% after the development of such a team.[44]

Medical assessment and treatment should be targeted to optimize the patient's overall condition. Addressing co-morbidities increases the patient's ability to participate in the rehabilitation process. Pain management is essential to ensure that amputees can actively participate in intensive rehabilitation and prosthetic training. Assessment and modification of health risk factors can improve long-term functional outcome. All patients should be encouraged to exercise daily to improve their performance of activities of daily living.

Amputation Wound Dressings

A soft gauze dressing with a mild compression wrap is the most widely used dressing following lower extremity amputation. Patients remain nonambulatory until the fitting of a permanent prosthesis 4 to 6 weeks after surgery. There are concerns that this type of dressing may delay effective physical therapy and rehabilitation. An alternative technique known as

immediate postoperative prosthesis (IPOP) placement, proposed by Berlemont in the 1950s, has been documented to improve primary healing rates and rehabilitation rates.[65] IPOP, which must be applied at the initial operation, combines a rigid postoperative dressing with a temporary prosthesis and has been advocated for the early rehabilitation of nonischemic amputees. Concerns from surgeons include lack of familiarity with the prosthesis, fear of placing a hard cast on a potentially compromised remnant limb, and the inability to inspect the wound frequently.[66]

Moore reported that with the use of IPOP and xenon clearance to select the amputation level, postamputation healing rates increased from 75% to 100%.[67] In unilateral amputees who were ambulatory before surgery, a 100% prosthetic rehabilitation rate was achieved when IPOP was placed. More recent studies support the contention that IPOP facilitates postoperative recovery, wound healing, rehabilitation, and independent ambulation.[68,69] In addition, new custom-made removable IPOP dressings allow surgeons to inspect stump wounds more easily.[66] In addition, rigid postoperative dressings are now available without an attached prosthesis; these protect the stump, minimize edema, and lead to earlier prosthetic fitting and training.[70]

Prosthesis Selection and Training

Prosthetic training plays an important role in rehabilitation. An appropriate durable prosthesis should be prescribed based on the individual's situation. Advanced prosthetic technology provides amputees with more choices. New functional designs and ultralight materials help amputees live independently. Various lower extremity prostheses are commercially available for patients following AKA and BKA (Figs. 114-1 and 114-2).[65]

The advantages and disadvantages of different types of prostheses and the indications for their use depend on the individual patient and should be fully explored by the experienced prosthetist.[65] For example, microprocessor-controlled above-knee prostheses are now typical of the high-technology products (see Fig. 114-1B). These "intelligent" prostheses can change the orifice size, based on different walking speeds, to allow the appropriate shin swing time. The shin includes numerous sensors to accumulate biomechanical data, such as vertical loading amplitude and sagittal knee movement, to determine the direction and angular acceleration of the artificial knee joint. A software analysis system can optimize prosthetic characteristics through a process of data sampling and calculations up to 60 times in a 1.2-second gait cycle.[65] A patient wearing one of these prostheses can easily step up and sit on an examination table (see Fig. 114-1C).

Different types of prostheses are available to meet the needs of amputees with different amputation levels, physical conditioning, and exercise demands.[65] In general, persons of smaller stature with a slow to moderate cadence are better suited to smaller, simpler, and lighter hydraulic swing-control prostheses. Taller, more active ambulators benefit from larger, more powerful hydraulic swing-control prostheses.[71]

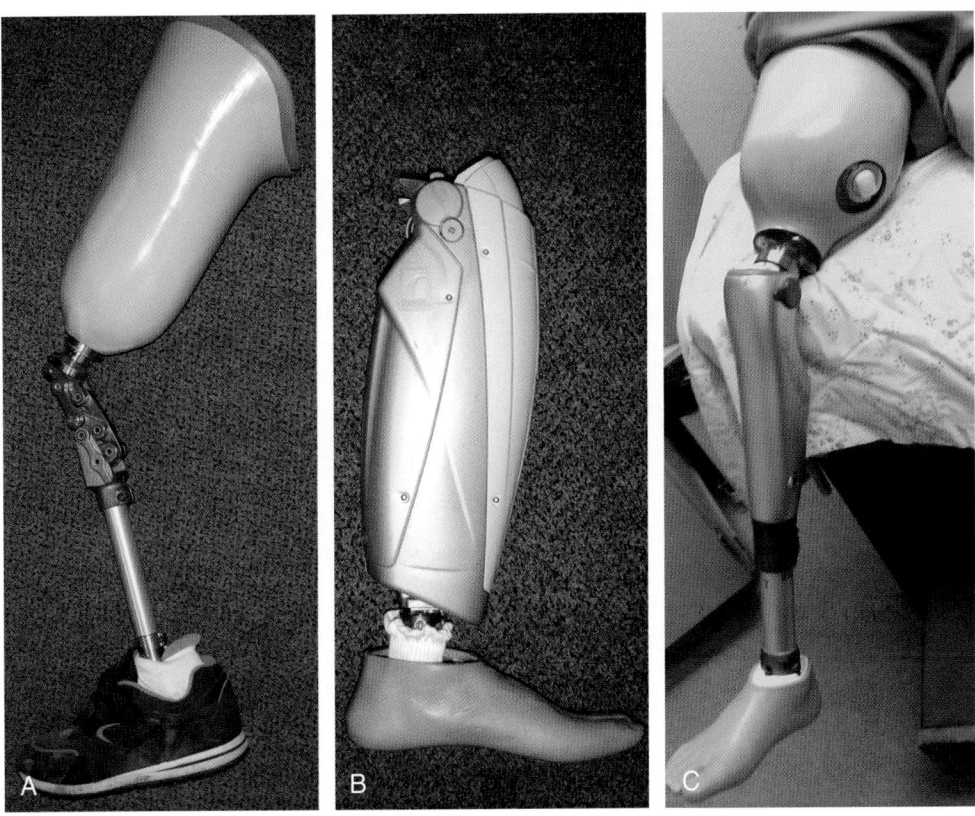

Figure 114-1 Above-knee prostheses. **A,** Standard mechanical knee with swing control. **B,** "Intelligent" transfemoral microprocessor-controlled prosthesis. **C,** Patient with "intelligent" above-knee prosthesis seated on an examination table.

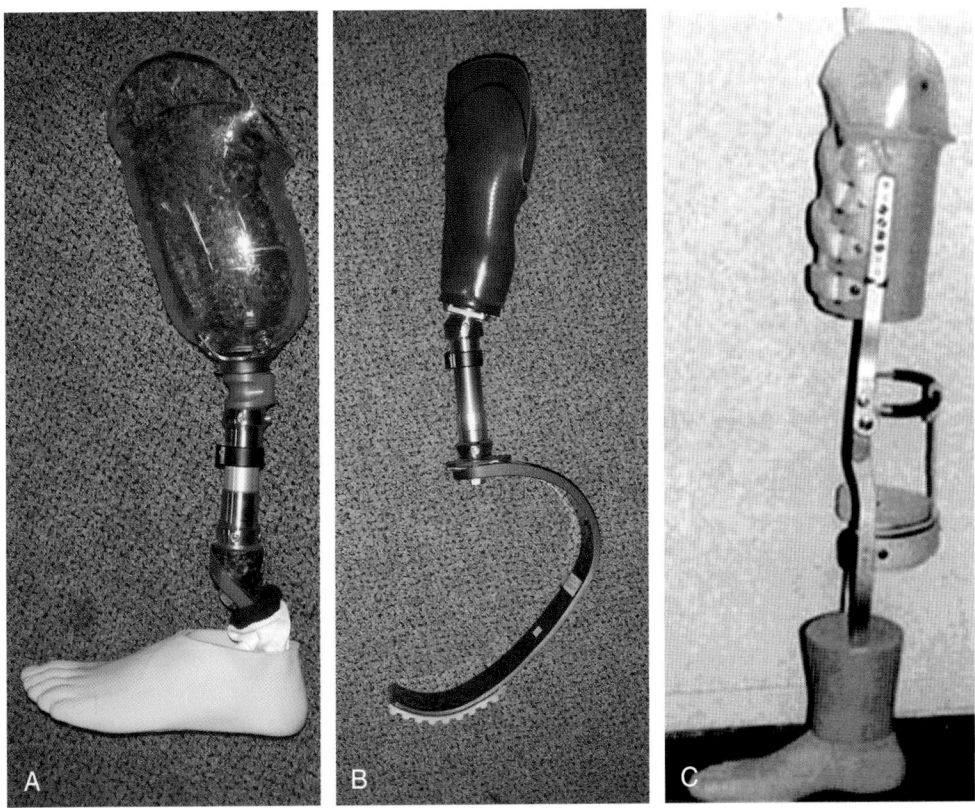

Figure 114-2 Below-knee prostheses. **A,** Standard prosthesis with solid ankle and cushioned heel foot. **B,** Dynamic, energy-conserving athletic prosthesis. **C,** Below-knee prosthesis for patients with wound difficulties.

Below-knee prostheses are generally much more lightweight than above-knee prostheses. The below-knee prostheses vary and include standard passive ankle designs, energy-conserving ankles, and open-type sockets that can accommodate slowly healing stumps (see Fig. 114-2).

Reasonable goals must be set for each patient. Many patients may not walk independently, but many wear prostheses, and the large majority return to their home environments. Although all patients may be offered the eventual fitting of a prosthesis, only a fraction will actively walk with their prostheses. In a recent series of major amputations, 29% of patients were able to walk outside the home with a prosthesis, 42% used a prosthetic limb, and 92% of patients were able to return to community living.[22]

FUNCTIONAL OUTCOME

Results of lower extremity amputation are discussed in detail in Chapter 115 (Amputation: Techniques and Results). However, the assessment of functional performance following major amputation is a complex issue that influences decision making, so it is also addressed here. The most important factors that influence functional outcome are age, preoperative functional status, co-morbidities, mental status, amputation level, stump healing status, unilateral versus bilateral amputation, and postoperative rehabilitation.

Impact of Amputation Level and Co-morbidities

Among amputees with healed stumps, 80% of those with BKAs can achieve ambulation, compared with only 38% to 50% of patients with AKAs.[72,73] Taylor and coworkers documented that patients older than 70 years had a 3-fold greater chance of not wearing a prosthesis, a 3.1-fold greater chance of death, a 2.3-fold greater chance of being nonambulatory, and a 4-fold greater chance of losing functional independence at 1 year compared with patients younger than 50 years.[26] Patients aged 70 years or older and those with limited preoperative ambulatory ability, dementia, end-stage renal disease, and advanced coronary artery disease all had a significantly higher chance of experiencing death, nonambulatory status, and loss of functional independence and never using a prosthesis. AKA patients who were not ambulatory preoperatively had a 10-fold greater chance of not wearing a prosthesis and twice the chance of death at 1 year. Amputees with dementia were 2.4 times less likely to wear a prosthesis. Patients with advanced co-morbidities, including coronary artery disease, end-stage renal disease, and severe chronic obstructive pulmonary disease, also had a greater chance of not ambulating following amputation.[26]

Through-knee amputation is not commonly performed because of poor soft tissue coverage and a higher risk of wound complications. However, in the patients with adequate residual skin and subcutaneous tissue, through-knee amputation is an option. Through-knee amputees are able to achieve higher normal and maximal walking speeds with lower relative energy expenditure than above-knee amputees. In elderly patients or those with significant co-morbidities preventing them from postoperative ambulation, through-knee amputation allows earlier weight bearing with a lower risk of wound complications compared with BKA.[65]

Minor amputations, such as digital, ray, transmetatarsal, and midfoot amputations, are considered limb salvage procedures. Patients with digital or ray amputation may walk with little additional energy expenditure. Partial foot amputation requires less ambulation energy than more proximal amputation. Pinzur and associates demonstrated that energy demands after midfoot, Syme's, below-knee, through-knee, and above-knee amputations are directly related to the level of amputation.[74]

Impact of Age

Patients younger than 60 years with well-controlled co-morbidities who were ambulating preoperatively can anticipate an ambulatory rate of 70%, a survival rate of 80% at 1 year, and an independent living rate of 90% following major amputation.[26] A Canadian study showed that although older patients had more co-morbidities at admission, they benefited as much as younger people from an intensive rehabilitation program with a comparable length of stay.[75] However, younger amputees continued to improve after 3 months, whereas older patients tended to plateau. In selected patients who developed stump wound complications but had good perceived healing potential, a "redo" BKA yielded better functional outcomes than conversion to an AKA.[76] Integrative and vocational rehabilitation combined with newly designed prostheses allow high-level amputation patients to achieve independent lifestyles. Interdisciplinary management should be employed in the care of all amputees. Pre- and postoperative optimization of a patient's medical condition, intensive rehabilitation, wound care, pain management, and proper prosthesis fitting all significantly improve the patient's ultimate functional outcome.

Fate of the Contralateral Limb after Amputation

Following a major amputation, many patients worry about the fate of their remaining limb. Patients surviving more than 3 years after the first amputation have a significant chance of needing a contralateral amputation.[77] Fifteen percent to 35% of amputees with diabetes lose their remaining leg within 5 years.[78] The presence of renal failure is a particularly poor prognostic indicator of second limb amputation.[21] These facts underscore the need for diligence in protecting and surveying the remaining limb. Continued efforts focused on patient education and preventive foot care are essential. Periodic evaluation and management of PAD in the contralateral limb after unilateral amputation is important for the long-term functional outcome of these patients.

Depression after Amputation

As in other areas of vascular surgery, the successful completion of the operation is only the beginning of the patient's recovery. Although the surgeon may initially focus on the surgical wounds, other considerations are unique to the recovery of an amputee. Depression is common following major amputation, especially in younger amputees.[79] The loss of a limb has been compared to the loss of a spouse in terms of magnitude. Although the feeling of bereavement abates over the first year, many amputees experience a continued sense of loss extending beyond 1 year.[80] In the recovery period, although positive outcomes should be stressed, clinical screening and appropriate medical therapy for depression should be considered. Amputees with significant depression may become malnourished owing to loss of appetite; malnutrition may delay healing, contribute to the development of pressure ulcers, and seriously affect the patient's overall recovery.

Successful rehabilitation can decrease the severity and incidence of depression following amputation.[81] Social discomfort, the appearance of the prosthesis, and individual coping skills should be addressed to aid in the recovery process.[82-84] The psychological impact of the loss of independence may be minimized by aggressive, focused rehabilitation that openly addresses the concerns of the amputee. Dealing with these issues requires the participation of psychologists, nurses, and geriatric and rehabilitation specialists.

SELECTED KEY REFERENCES

Abou-Zamzam AM Jr, Gomez NR, Molkara A, Banta JE, Teruya TH, Killeen JD, Bianchi C. A prospective analysis of critical limb ischemia: factors leading to major primary amputation versus revascularization. *Ann Vasc Surg.* 2007;21:458.
Prospective look at patients presenting with limb-threatening ischemia and the factors that lead to amputation versus revascularization.

Nehler MR, Hiatt WR, Taylor LM Jr. Is revascularization and limb salvage always the best treatment for critical limb ischemia? *J Vasc Surg.* 2003;37:704.
Excellent discussion of the issues involved in deciding on revascularization versus primary amputation, including a clear decision algorithm.

Norgren L, Hiatt WR, Dormandy JA, Nehler MR, Harris KA, Fowkes FG, TASC II Working Group. Inter-society consensus for the management of peripheral arterial disease (TASC II). *J Vasc Surg.* 2007;45S:S5.
Excellent review of the current data and approach to PAD.

Nowygrod R, Egorova N, Greco G, Anderson P, Gelijns A, Moskowitz A, McKinsey J, Morrissey N, Kent KD. Trends, complications, and mortality in peripheral vascular surgery. *J Vasc Surg.* 2006;43:205.
Article covering the trends in amputation and revascularization, with a good framework for discussing the current role of amputation in the United States.

Tang PCY, Ravji K, Key JJ, Mahler DB, Blume PA, Sumpio B. Let them walk! Current prosthesis options for leg and foot amputees. *J Am Coll Surg.* 2008;206:548.
Succinct review of prostheses available for amputees.

Taylor SM, Kalbaugh CA, Blackhurst DW, Hamontree SE, Cull DL, Messich HS, Robertson RT, Langan EM 3rd, York JW, Carsten CG 3rd, Snyder BA, Jackson MR, Youkey JR. Preoperative clinical factors predict postoperative functional outcomes after major lower limb amputation: an analysis of 553 consecutive patients. *J Vasc Surg.* 2005;42:227.
Review of the clinical factors predictive of functional outcome in a large cohort of patients treated with major amputation.

Yamada T, Ohta T, Ishibashi H, Sugimoto I, Iwata H, Takahashi M, Kawanishi J. Clinical reliability and utility of skin perfusion pressure measurement in ischemic limbs—comparison with other noninvasive diagnostic methods. *J Vasc Surg.* 2008;47:318.
Excellent outline and comparison of the various methods of determining amputation level in ischemic limbs.

REFERENCES

The reference list can be found on the companion Expert Consult Web site at *www.expertconsult.com.*

CHAPTER 115

Lower Extremity Amputation: Techniques and Results

John F. Eidt and Venkat R. Kalapatapu

Based in part on chapters in the previous edition by Kenneth R. Woodburn, MD, FRCSG (Gen.);
C. Vaughan Ruckley, MB ChM, FRCSE; and Richard A. Yeager, MD.

Amputation of a damaged limb is one of the oldest and, argu-ably, most effective surgical procedures. A properly performed amputation holds the promise of pain relief for patients with advanced ischemia, control of infection in the setting of extremity sepsis, and cure of malignancy confined to the limb. Unfortunately, vascular surgeons often regard amputation as the terminal battle in the war against atherosclerosis and an admission of personal failure. As such, amputation is too fre-quently relegated to the least experienced member of the surgical team to perform at the end of the day with insufficient guidance. This chapter emphasizes the therapeutic value of a well-done amputation and describes the technical details essential to successful amputation surgery.

As one of the oldest surgical procedures, amputation has been refined over many centuries.[1] Progress in amputation surgery was hindered by early surgeons' inability to manage the critical triad of infection, hemorrhage, and pain. Before antisepsis was introduced by British surgeon Joseph Lister in 1867, more than half of all amputees died from infection. Before the introduction of general anesthesia, surgical speed was the only way to limit pain and hemorrhage. A variety of novel amputation devices was developed by 16th-century French and German barber-surgeons to achieve rapid removal of the offending limb. The introduction of vessel ligatures by Ambrose Paré in 1529 put an end to the barbaric use of mass cauterization with scalding oil. Another technical landmark was the introduction of the hemostatic tourniquet by another French surgeon, Morell, who is said to have first used the technique successfully in the battle of Besançon in 1674.[1]

GENERAL PRINCIPLES

Regardless of the level of amputation, a number of general principles apply (Box 115-1). The surgeon must be satisfied that there is sufficient arterial perfusion to sustain healing. In addition, it is important to ensure the structural integrity of the bony architecture of the residual limb. For example, in some patients with diabetes and Charcot's degenerative osteo-arthropathy of the foot, formal transtibial amputation may be superior to complex foot salvage procedures. Meticulous attention to detail and gentle handling of soft tissues are vital in creating a well-healed and functional amputation stump. The use of skin hooks or fine-toothed forceps to retract the skin is preferable to the use of crushing instruments such as DeBakey-type forceps. Some surgeons condemn the use of any grasping instruments and rely on gentle finger traction

Box 115-1 General Principles of Amputation Surgery

- Assess arterial perfusion and bone architecture
- Handle all tissue with atraumatic technique
- Excise all nonviable and infected tissue
- Apply tourniquet to minimize blood loss
- Eliminate all sharp bone edges and fragments
- Minimize number of cuts across muscle
- Transect nerves sharply and allow to retract
- Minimize use of electrocautery
- Close wounds under no tension
- Perform myodesis or myoplasty to stabilize antagonistic muscle groups
- Use drains to reduce dead space
- Provide prophylaxis for deep venous thrombosis
- Administer prophylactic antibiotics
- Avoid weight bearing until adequate wound healing
- Use protective soft and rigid dressings
- Avoid excessive cosmetic tailoring of wounds
- Isolate infected or gangrenous tissue

alone. Hemostasis is best obtained with fine suture ligatures, and the use of electrocautery should be minimized. The knife blade should be maintained perpendicular to the skin surface to avoid a bevel, and the skin should not be separated from the underlying fascia to prevent ischemia. In planning the amputation, the surgeon should avoid placing surgical scars on weight-bearing surfaces. If possible, the skin should be separated from the cut surface of bone by a myofascial layer to prevent the formation of adherent scar, which may be a source of pain. Skin flaps should be approximated without tension. Although the maintenance of limb length is generally desirable, removal of all nonviable and infected tissue is a higher priority. Excessively redundant soft tissue interferes with proper prosthetic fit and should be avoided. An amputa-tion site has a remarkable capacity for remodeling, so com-pulsive trimming of small dog-ears and other minor cosmetic irregularities is usually best avoided. The use of a hemostatic tourniquet is beneficial in reducing blood loss.[2] Antagonistic muscle groups should be stabilized to prevent muscle atrophy and skeletal misalignment.[3] The term *myoplasty* is used to describe the suture fixation of antagonistic muscle groups to each other; with *myodesis*, the musculotendinous unit is sutured directly to bone. Sharp bone edges should be contoured, and bony prominences should be beveled. Nerves should be sharply transected proximal to weight-bearing surfaces to avoid painful neuroma. Excessive periosteal stripping is generally contraindicated because it can result in the formation of ring sequestra or bony overgrowth. Drains may be used and are usually removed after 1 to 2 days.

Postoperatively, surgeons should be mindful that accidental injury to the recent amputation is a frequent cause of failure; this may be preventable by the liberal use of both rigid and soft protective dressings. In most cases, weight bearing should be completely avoided until the wounds are well healed. All amputation patients should receive appropriate prophylaxis against deep venous thrombosis (DVT). We prefer low-molecular-weight heparin administered subcutaneously until ambulation is initiated.[4] All patients receive perioperative intravenous prophylactic antibiotics appropriate for skin flora.[5]

When approaching an infected limb, several unique factors must be considered. Mechanical barriers, such as impervious plastic sleeves or iodinated adhesive skin drapes, should be used to isolate infected areas. Open "drainage" or guillotine amputation should be considered in most cases of gross infection.[6-10] Delayed primary closure after the septic process is controlled (two-stage approach) may preserve limb length. Antibiotic coverage should be based on Gram stain and culture results.

■ AMPUTATION TYPES

Toe and Ray Amputation

Anatomy

There are two phalanges in the first toe and three in each of the remaining four toes (Fig. 115-1). The interphalangeal and metatarsophalangeal joints are hinge joints. Each has an articular capsule and medial and lateral collateral ligaments. The plantar surface of the articular capsule is strengthened to form a fibrous plate, the plantar ligament, which limits toe extension. The flexor hallucis longus and flexor digitorum longus tendons insert on the distal phalanges. The flexor hallucis brevis inserts on the proximal phalanx of the first toe. There are typically two sesamoid bones contained within the flexor hallucis brevis tendon that articulate with the plantar surface of the first metatarsal head.

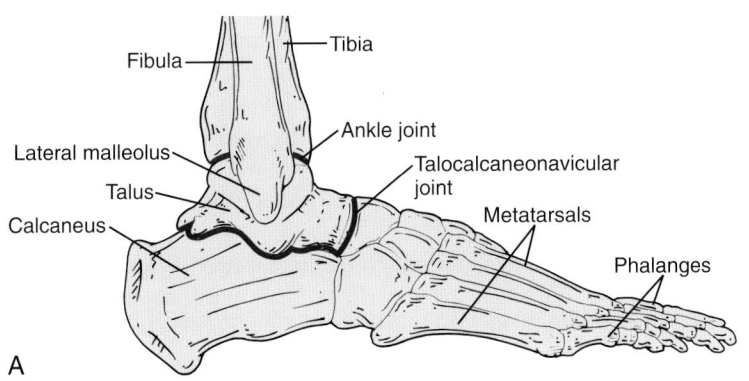

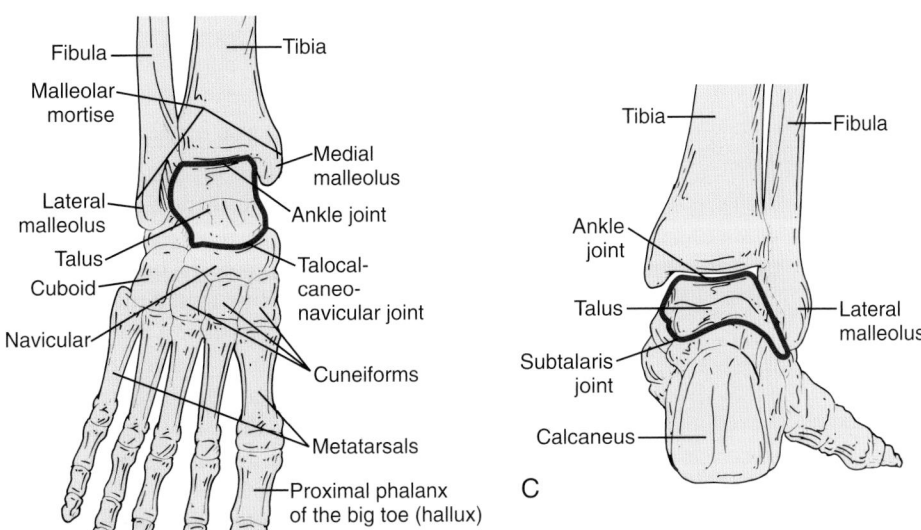

Figure 115-1 Bone anatomy of the foot.

Technique: Toe Amputation

Toe amputation is appropriate for wounds limited to the middle and distal toe and not involving the skin over the metatarsal head. More proximal wounds typically necessitate ray amputation. Ankle or digital nerve block is preferred for most toe amputations, but spinal, epidural, or general anesthesia may be chosen. Care should be taken to avoid direct puncture of the pedal arteries or excessive infiltration of anesthetic in the dysvascular foot because of the risk of exacerbating ischemia. Some surgeons avoid the use of ankle and digital blocks in the setting of local foot sepsis for fear of spreading cellulitis. The foot and toes should be scrubbed vigorously with an antiseptic soap. Iodine-impregnated adhesive drapes are impractical on the toes, but a surgical glove may be useful to isolate a necrotic or septic area.

Partial or complete amputation of the toe can be performed. Almost any incision that results in tension-free coverage of the transected bone can be chosen; however the simplest technique for complete amputation of the toe is based on the racket incision, so named because its shape is similar to that of a tennis racket (Fig. 115-2). For amputation of the first and fifth toes, we prefer to orient the handle of the racket on the medial or lateral surface of the respective metatarsal head. For the second, third, and fourth toes, the handle of the racket is oriented longitudinally along the dorsal surface of the digit. For partial amputation of the toe, a transverse or vertical fish-mouth skin incision may be used.

The flexor and extensor tendons are divided at the level of the skin incision and allowed to retract. The bone is divided at the appropriate level. If disarticulation is desired, a No. 15 knife blade is inserted into the joint, and the joint capsule is incised sharply to avoid injury to surrounding soft tissue. Because the articular cartilage is poorly vascularized, we prefer to excise the cartilage with a rongeur. We also gently shape the exposed bone to eliminate any bony projections that might lead to wound or skin problems. The wound is irrigated vigorously, and careful hemostasis is obtained. Excessive use of electrocautery is avoided. The skin is closed without tension in one layer using nonabsorbable monofilament suture. Weight bearing is completely prohibited until adequate healing is observed.

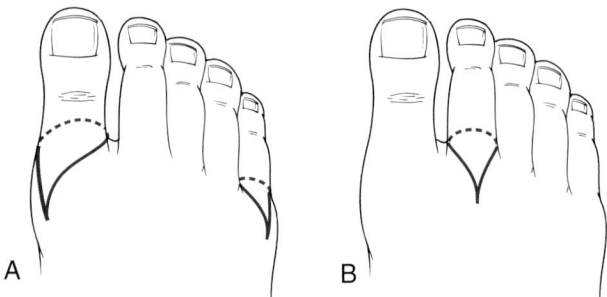

Figure 115-2 A, Racket incision for first and fifth toe amputation. **B,** Racket incision for second, third, or fourth toe amputation.

Technique: Ray Amputation

Ray amputation involves amputation of the toe along with all or part of the corresponding metatarsal head. Although a single isolated ray amputation sometimes proves durable, multiple ray amputations narrow the foot excessively and create biomechanical instability. This increases the amount of weight that must be borne by the remaining metatarsal heads and can lead to new areas of increased pressure, callus formation, and ulceration. Ray amputation may be useful in the treatment of blue toe syndrome caused by microatheroembolism involving the entire toe if there is insufficient skin to cover the exposed metatarsal head. Ray amputation may also be useful in the treatment of malperforans ulcers in the neuropathic diabetic foot, especially in the setting of osteomyelitis of the metatarsal head. Because a hallux valgus deformity commonly develops following isolated second toe amputation, complete second ray amputation may be preferable because it reduces the angle between the first and third metatarsals.

In a typical ray amputation, we modify the racket incision by extending the handle of the racket to provide sufficient exposure of the shaft of the metatarsal (Fig. 115-3). The extensor tendons are divided and allowed to retract, and the shaft of the metatarsal is transected with a power saw. The distal segment of metatarsal is engaged with a bone hook, and distal traction is applied while the remaining plantar soft tissue attachments are divided. Care is taken to stay close to the bone to avoid injury to adjacent digital arteries and nerves. Sesamoid bones are excised, and the flexor tendons are transected under tension to facilitate retraction.

In comparison to the lateral four rays, the first metatarsal and great toe contribute disproportionately to the mechanics of normal ambulation. In a normal stride, the foot contacts the ground on the posterolateral aspect of the heel. The weight is transferred progressively along the lateral plantar surface of the foot and then across the metatarsal heads from lateral to medial. Finally, the foot lifts off primarily from the first metatarsal head and the great toe. Although near-normal foot mechanics can be achieved after amputation of one of the lateral four rays, amputation of the great toe and first metatarsal head markedly alters normal ambulation and may result in destructive forces within the architecture of the foot. Recurrent ulceration following first ray amputation has been reported in up to 60% of patients.[11] Some orthopedic surgeons recommend formal transmetatarsal amputation of all five rays rather than isolated first ray amputation.[12] The contrarian viewpoint holds that transmetatarsal amputation may require revision or reamputation in 20% to 40% of patients and that above-ankle amputation is necessary in one of five patients.[13,14] Thus, there is a lack of consensus in the literature, and the final decision between first ray amputation and complete transmetatarsal amputation should be individualized, based on patient and surgeon preferences.

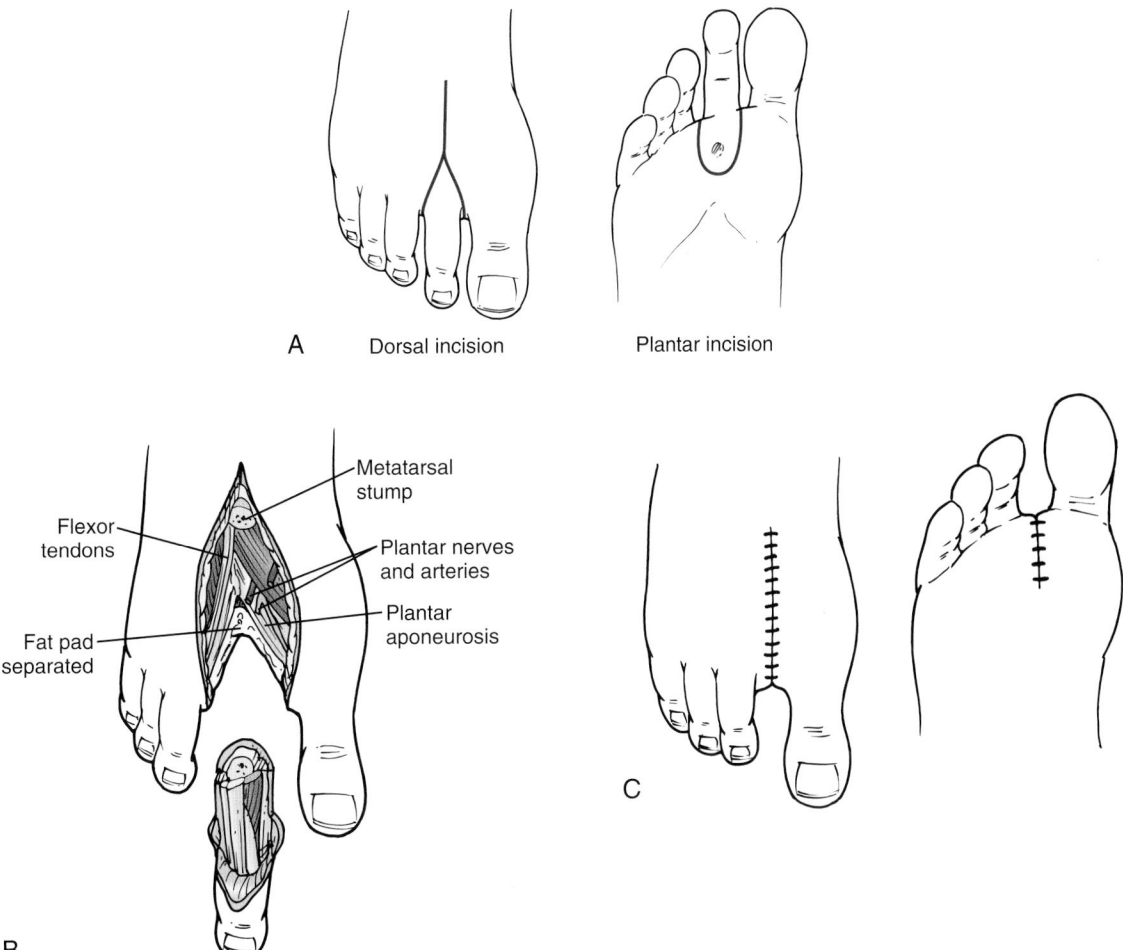

Figure 115-3 **A,** Ray amputation incision. Note the plantar extension to include a malperforans ulcer. **B,** Transection of the metatarsal shaft. **C,** Closure with nonabsorbable suture under no tension.

Postoperative Considerations

No weight bearing is allowed until the wound is thoroughly healed. We usually use a simple bulky soft dressing to protect the wound. A rocker-bottom shoe with a metatarsal bar that unloads pressure from the toes may be effective in selected patients. Approximately 25% of toe amputations fail to heal and require additional amputation at a higher level.[15] Of these higher amputations, approximately 40% are at the transtibial level.[16] With the use of appropriate orthoses and foot care, many patients achieve durable ambulation following toe or ray amputation.

Transmetatarsal Amputation

Anatomy

The metatarsal heads are stabilized by a series of segmental deep transverse metatarsal ligaments that connect the plantar ligaments of the adjacent metatarsophalangeal joints (see Fig. 115-1). Proximally, the metatarsals articulate with the three cuneiforms—medial, intermediate, and lateral—and the cuboid bone. These bones are connected by the dorsal and plantar tarsometatarsal and the interosseous cuneometatarsal ligaments. The tarsometatarsal, or Lisfranc's, joint connects the midfoot to the forefoot.

Technique

Transmetatarsal amputation (TMA) is appropriate for wounds involving the entire forefoot. TMA may be preferable to isolated first ray amputation in selected patients because TMA has better healing rates and, owing to improved foot mechanics, better rehabilitation rates. TMA also offers the benefits of full limb length, normal shoe wear, and near-normal ambulation. A one-stage TMA should generally not be undertaken in the setting of severe forefoot infection. In this situation, a guillotine débriding amputation should be considered, followed by formal wound closure after control of sepsis. A partial-thickness skin graft may be an effective method to salvage an open TMA wound if it is restricted to non–weight-bearing surfaces. TMA is contraindicated if there is excessive bone deformity in the midfoot and hindfoot, which would not be structurally sound.

The entire lower leg and foot are prepared and draped. A pneumatic tourniquet is placed on the lower leg. A latex bandage is used to exsanguinate the foot before tourniquet inflation, unless there is significant forefoot sepsis. The incision extends from a point just medial to the first metatarsal head transversely across the dorsum of the foot at the level of the distal metatarsal shaft and ends on the lateral side of the fifth metatarsal head (Fig. 115-4).[17] The incision then extends at right angles onto the plantar surface of the foot, creating a plantar flap that extends up to the base of the toes. The extensor tendons and sheaths are divided at, or slightly proximal to, the level of the dorsal skin incision to expose the metatarsal shafts. The periosteum is divided just proximal to the metatarsal heads, and the metatarsals are transected using a sharp power saw. We prefer to divide the metatarsals in a gentle curve from medial to lateral, with each successive shaft being 3 to 5 mm shorter than the previous one. Some surgeons advocate transecting the metatarsal shaft with a 30- to 45-degree plantar-oriented bevel to facilitate lift-off during ambulation. Following transection of the bone, the distal metatarsal fragments can be grasped with a bone clamp or bone hook and retracted distally while the plantar myofascial attachments to the meta-

tarsal heads are sequentially divided. The flexor tendons and sheaths are poorly vascularized and should be excised individually, along with other fibrocartilaginous structures on the plantar flap, taking care not to incise too deeply. The tourniquet is deflated, and bleeding is controlled with fine suture ligatures. Use of electrocautery is minimized. The wound is irrigated, and the plantar flap may be trimmed to fit if necessary. The wound is closed in two layers with interrupted absorbable sutures in the fascia. The skin is closed loosely with interrupted nonabsorbable monofilament sutures or staples.

Postoperative Considerations

A posterior plaster splint that maintains the foot at 90 degrees is applied. Weight bearing is prohibited until adequate healing is observed, usually after 3 to 4 weeks. TMA is a relatively durable procedure following initial healing. Primary healing can be expected in 50% to 75% of patients following TMA.[18-21] Revision to a higher level is necessary in approximately 25% to 40% of TMAs.[15] A vacuum dressing may be

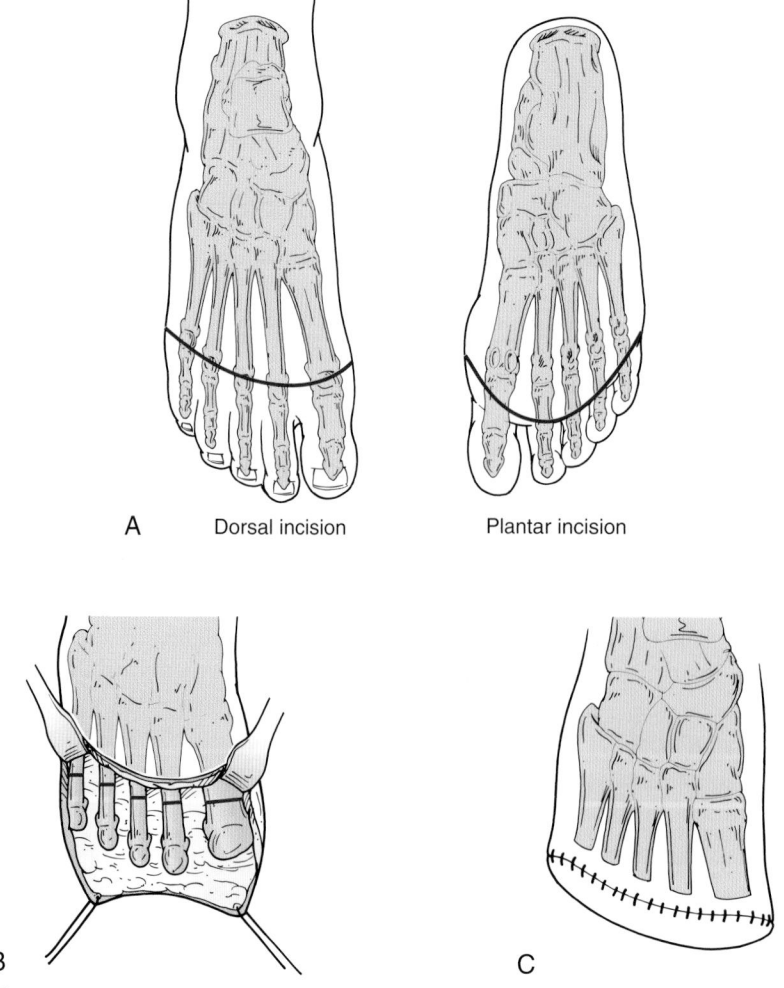

A   Dorsal incision   Plantar incision

B   C

Figure 115-4 Technique of transmetatarsal amputation. **A,** Dorsal and plantar incisions, with disarticulation of the metatarsophalangeal joints. **B,** Level of bone transection. **C,** Closure with monofilament suture.

effective in avoiding more proximal amputation.[22] With appropriate orthoses, patients can be expected to ambulate with an almost imperceptible gait alteration following complete healing.

Midfoot and Hindfoot Amputation

Three proximal foot amputations may be appropriate in vascular surgery patients (Fig. 115-5): Lisfranc's tarsometatarsal disarticulation, Chopart's midfoot amputation, and Syme's amputation.[23,24] Two other hindfoot amputations that are rarely employed are the Boyd's and Pirogoff's amputations.[17,23,25,26] These hindfoot amputations are performed primarily in children to preserve length and growth centers.

The use of midfoot and hindfoot amputations in diabetic patients remains controversial. Many surgeons recommend formal transtibial (below-knee) amputation if TMA cannot be performed or has failed. Others suggest that increased limb salvage rates can be achieved with the use of unconventional foot amputations.[25,27] Recently, it has been shown that the preservation of leg length may give diabetics a survival advantage. Stone and coworkers reported that diabetics undergoing proximal foot amputations had better function and survival than those undergoing below-knee amputations (BKAs).[26] These findings were not observed in dialysis-dependent diabetics, however.

Anatomy

The tibia and the fibula articulate with the talus via the talocrural joint. The ligaments that join these bones are the deltoid, anterior and posterior talofibular, and calcaneofibular ligaments. The talus articulates with the calcaneus at the subtalar joint. The medial and lateral talocalcaneal ligaments and the cervical ligament support this joint. The talocalcaneonavicular joint is a multiaxial joint supported by the talonavicular and plantar calcaneonavicular ligaments. Supination (inversion) at this joint is produced by the tibialis anterior and posterior. Pronation (eversion) is produced by the peroneus longus and brevis. A heavy fibrofatty heel pad is firmly adherent to the calcaneus and skin and provides protection during heel strike (see Fig. 115-1).

Because the strong ankle extensor attachments are divided in the performance of midfoot and hindfoot amputation, the Achilles tendon exerts unopposed plantar flexor forces on the residual foot. The Achilles tendon may require division or lengthening to prevent the development of an equinus deformity.

Lisfranc's and Chopart's Amputations

Lisfranc's. Lisfranc first described this amputation in 1815. The incision results in a long plantar flap (see Fig. 115-5; Fig. 115-6). Tendons and synovial sheaths are divided at the level of the skin incision. The first, third, fourth, and fifth tarsometatarsal joints are disarticulated. The second metatarsal is divided 1 to 2 cm distal to the medial cuneiform.[29] To reduce the risk of the patient's developing equinovarus deformity, Sanders has recommended a modification of the Lisfranc amputation that preserves the base of the fifth metatarsal and the insertion of the peroneus brevis.[25] The Achilles tendon is released by either transection or Z-plasty.[28,30] The plantar fascia on the flap is approximated to the dorsal periosteum with absorbable sutures. The skin is approximated with interrupted monofilament sutures or staples.

Chopart's. Chopart described this amputation in 1814. It involves a long plantar flap similar to that used in the Lisfranc amputation (see Figs. 115-5 and 115-6). This amputation is performed through the talocalcaneonavicular joint and the calcaneocuboid joint. To prevent equinovarus deformity resulting from unopposed plantar flexion, an Achilles tenectomy is recommended. The extensor hallucis longus and the tibialis anterior tendons may be reattached to the talar neck. The extensor digitorum longus may be reattached to the calcaneus.[29] The wound is irrigated and closed in layers.

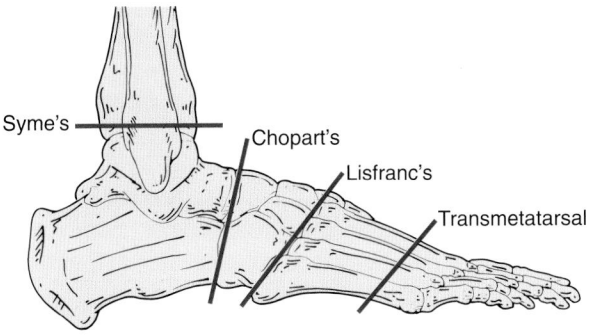

Figure 115-5 Levels of foot amputation.

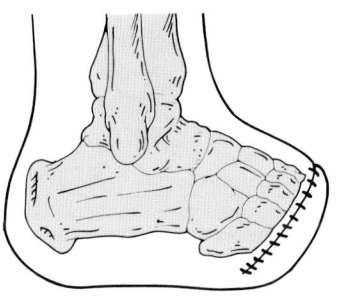
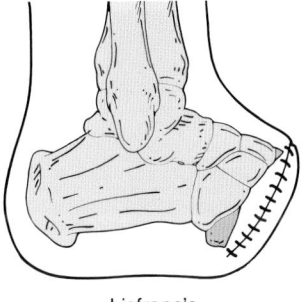
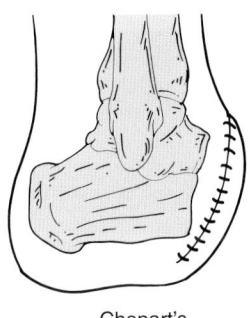

Figure 115-6 Diagram of completed transmetatarsal, Lisfranc's, and Chopart's amputations.

Postoperative Considerations. Because the Lisfranc and Chopart amputations result in a dramatic alteration in normal foot biomechanics, their durability may be limited. A short-leg plaster cast is used over the sterile dressings. The cast must be molded to ensure that the talus is slightly dorsiflexed in relation to the tibia and that the calcaneal tuberosity is parallel to the long axis of the tibia. The cast is changed weekly to check wound healing. Weight bearing is allowed after 6 weeks. Patients with a Lisfranc amputation need little more than a shoe filler with an ankle lace-up shoe. Patients with a Chopart amputation need a custom-fitted ankle-foot orthosis with a filler to hold the shoe adequately.

Syme's Amputation

Syme first described this amputation in 1843. The anterior incision extends across the ankle just distal to the tip of each malleolus (see Fig. 115-5; Fig. 115-7). The posterior incision extends from the malleoli vertically down and across the sole of the foot. The extensor tendons are divided at the level of

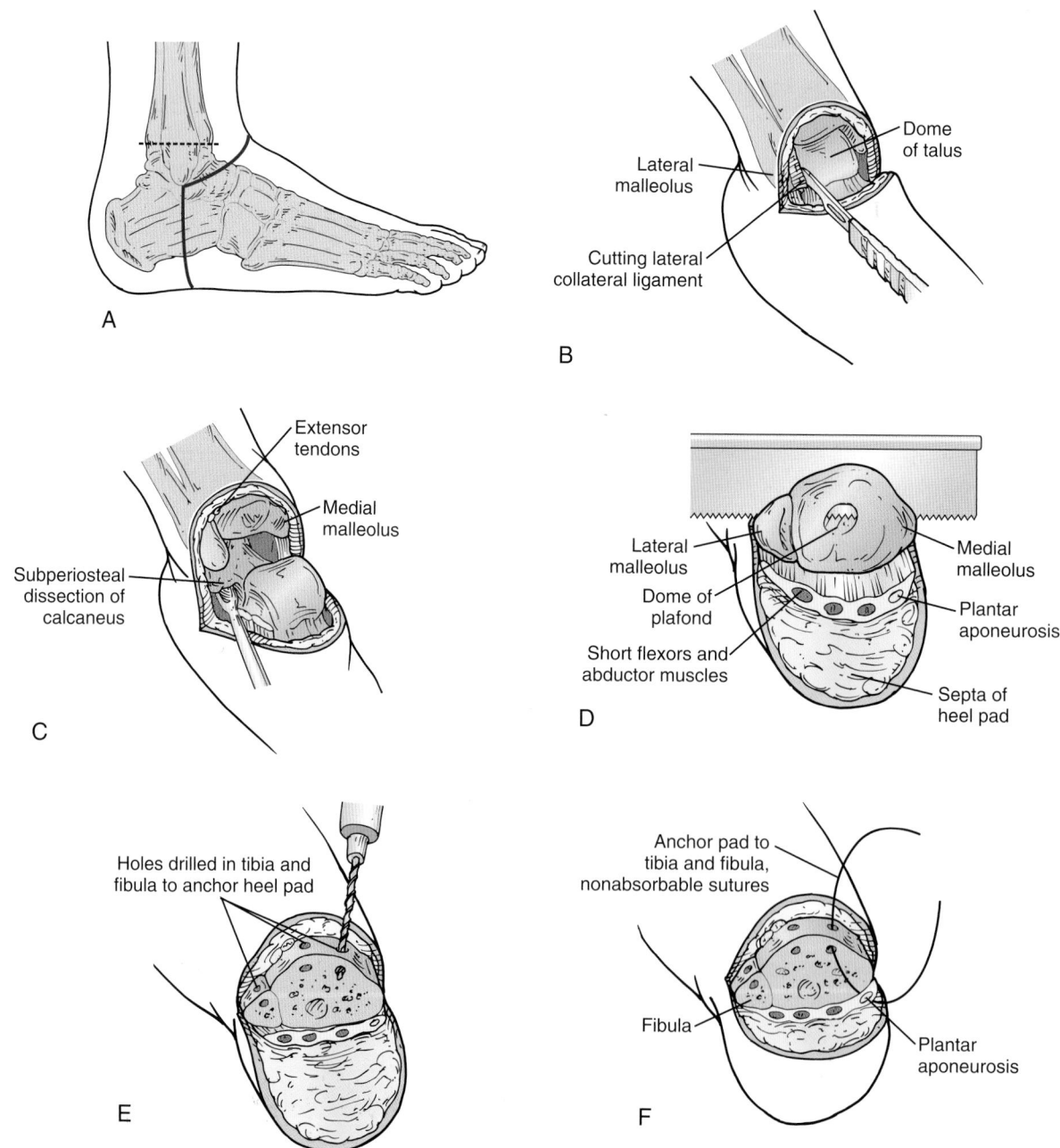

Figure 115-7 Syme's amputation. **A,** Skin incision and bone transection level. **B,** Exposure of the ankle and division of the ligaments. **C,** Soft tissue dissection from the calcaneus. **D,** Division of the tibia and fibula. **E,** Holes drilled in the anterior aspect of the tibia and fibula. **F,** Fascia lining the heel pad sutured to the bone.

the skin incision. The dorsalis pedis artery is ligated and divided. The ankle joint capsule is incised while plantar flexing the foot. The medial and lateral ankle ligaments are divided. The tendons of the posterior tibialis and flexor hallucis longus are transected, taking care to avoid injury to the posterior tibial artery. The heel fat pad is carefully dissected by staying close to the calcaneus to avoid buttonholing. The ankle joint is disarticulated, and the specimen is passed off the table. In a one-stage amputation, the malleoli are divided with a saw at the level of the articular surface of the tibia, and the width is reduced by vertical bone excision. Holes are drilled in the medial, anterior, and lateral parts of the distal tibia and fibula to secure the heel pad directly under the tibia. In a two-stage Syme amputation, the wound is closed by suturing the heel flap to the dorsal fascia. Six weeks later, the malleoli are removed through separate vertical incisions. (The reader is referred to references 31 and 32 for a detailed description of midfoot amputations.)

Postoperative Considerations.

The chief advantage of the Syme amputation is the preservation of limb length, which may obviate the need for a prosthesis during brief periods of weight bearing, such as during transfer from bed to wheelchair. The disadvantages include the slight leg-length discrepancy, which may lead to biomechanical side effects in more proximal or contralateral joints. Further, the prosthesis is typically bulky at the ankle and less cosmetically appealing than a conventional below-knee prosthesis, which can be designed with a near-normal ankle profile. In addition, because it is an end weight-bearing stump, the heel fat pad may be unstable and can migrate medially, exposing the distal tibia to excessive force. Thus, the Syme amputation has its greatest utility in young, healthy trauma patients with extensive forefoot injuries who are highly motivated to avoid transtibial amputation. We consider the presence of diabetic neuropathy a specific contraindication to Syme's amputation because of the inability to protect the stump from injuries such as scalding and pressure.

Transtibial (Below-Knee) Amputation

Anatomy

There are four muscle compartments in the leg (Fig. 115-8). The anterior compartment contains the tibialis anterior, extensor hallucis longus, and extensor digitorum longus muscles and the deep peroneal nerve. The lateral compartment contains the peroneus longus and brevis muscles and the superficial peroneal nerve. The posterior compartment is subdivided into superficial and deep parts. The superficial posterior group consists of the gastrocnemius and soleus muscles. The deep posterior compartment contains the tibialis posterior, flexor digitorum longus, and flexor hallucis longus muscles. The tibial nerve is adjacent to the posterior tibial artery. The tibia and fibula are connected distally by a fibrous inferior tibiofibular joint that is sacrificed in conventional BKA. The skin of the leg is supplied by fasciocutaneous per-

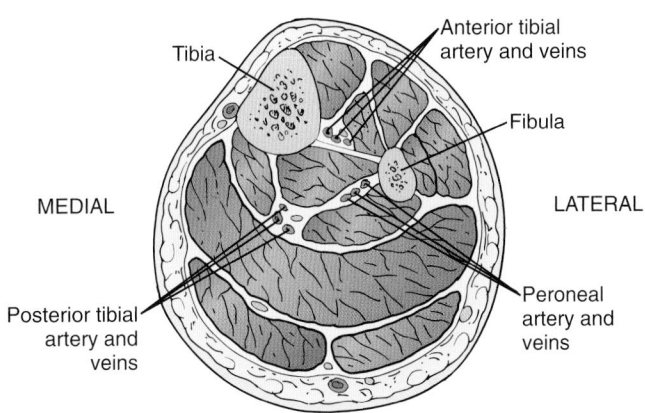

Figure 115-8 Anatomy of the leg at the level of transtibial amputation.

forating arteries that arise from the posterior tibial, anterior tibial, sural, saphenous, and peroneal arteries (Fig. 115-9). Of note, the sural artery arises from the popliteal artery proximal to the tibial trifurcation and supplies the gastrocnemius muscle and the posterior skin. The saphenous artery accompanies the saphenous vein and nerve below the knee and supplies the skin of the anteromedial leg, along with perforating branches of the posterior tibial artery.[33] To preserve adequate blood supply to the skin via these fasciocutaneous perforators, the skin and subcutaneous tissues should not be separated from the underlying fascia.

Technique

Five types of flaps are used in transtibial amputation techniques (see Fig. 115-9).

Posterior Flap.

The most common technique employs a long posterior flap as described by Burgess.[34-36] Optimally, the tibia should be divided 10 to 12 cm (three or four fingerbreadths) distal to the tibial tuberosity; however, we have observed functional stumps with as little as 5 cm of residual tibia (Fig. 115-10). The anterior incision extends from one half to two thirds of the leg's circumference. A thicker posterior flap results in more prominent dog-ears but may be better vascularized. The length of the posterior flap is approximately one third the circumference of the leg and should be gently curved to reduce dog-ears. After venous exsanguination and application of a pneumatic thigh-high tourniquet, the skin and fascia are incised together, beginning with the transverse component and then extending to complete the posterior flap. The anterior and lateral compartment muscles are divided. The periosteum of the tibia is incised circumferentially, and the tibia is divided using a power saw perpendicular to the long axis of the bone. The anterior lip of the tibia is beveled to eliminate sharp edges that may protrude through thin skin. The fibula is divided with a saw no more than 1 to 2 cm proximal to the tibia. Excessive resection of the fibula results in a conical stump that is difficult to fit with a prosthesis. The posterior flap is completed by dividing the residual

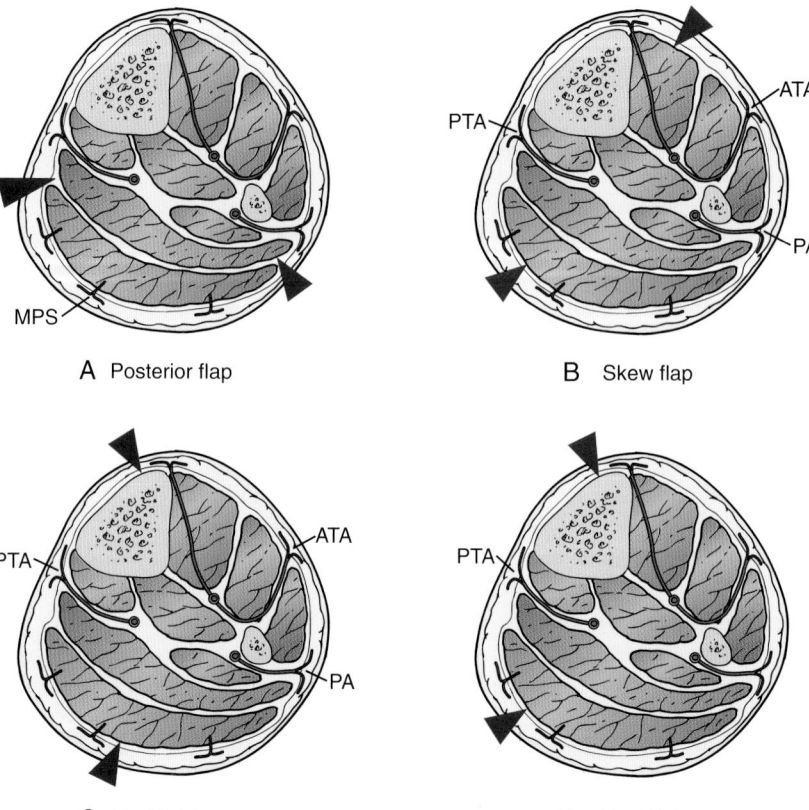

Figure 115-9 Blood supply to the skin at the level of transtibial amputation. Note the location of skin incisions (*red arrowheads*). **A,** Posterior flap. **B,** Skew flap. **C,** Sagittal flap. **D,** Medial flap. ATA, anterior tibial artery; MPS, musculocutaneous perforators from the sural artery; PA, peroneal artery; PTA, posterior tibial artery.

posterior compartment musculature at a plane just deep to the tibia and fibula with a long amputation knife. Major vascular bundles are suture ligated. The tourniquet is released, and complete hemostasis is obtained. The tibial and peroneal nerves are sharply divided and allowed to retract to avoid the formation of a neuroma. If necessary, the posterior flap can be trimmed, but excessive attempts to eliminate dog-ears should be avoided because the stump will remodel with time. Some surgeons prefer to advance the posterior flap 3 to 4 cm proximal to the tibial osteotomy.[37] If the posterior flap is too bulky to allow tension-free closure, the soleus muscle can be excised at the level of the tibial osteotomy, taking care to preserve the gastrocnemius muscle and fascia. The sural nerve is identified in the subcutaneous tissue in the middle of the posterior flap and divided 5 or 6 cm proximal to the skin edge to prevent neuroma formation. The wound is irrigated to remove bone dust. The deep fascia is approximated with interrupted absorbable sutures, taking care to completely cover the tibia without tension. The skin is closed with staples or monofilament suture.

Sagittal Flap.

If creation of a long posterior flap is not possible, sagittal or skew flaps may be used. In the sagittal flap technique described by Persson, equal-length medial and lateral myocutaneous flaps are developed (see Fig. 115-9).[38] A myoplasty is performed to cover the tibia by suturing the anterior and lateral compartment muscles to the medial component of the gastrocnemius and soleus. In a randomized comparison of sagittal versus posterior flaps, there was no significant difference in outcome.[39]

Skew Flap.

In the skew technique, equal anteromedial and posterolateral fasciocutaneous flaps are created (see Fig. 115-9; Fig. 115-11). The posterior muscle flap is identical to the conventional long posterior flap based on the gastrocnemius muscle.[40] The skew technique may be of particular benefit when there is inadequate skin to create a conventional long posterior flap.

Fish-Mouth Flap.

Before the development of the long posterior flap, the creation of equal anterior and posterior flaps was the most common transtibial amputation technique. The chief disadvantage was the anterior flap's vulnerability to ischemia. This so-called fish-mouth incision has no advantages over alternative techniques and is rarely indicated.

Medial Flap.

A medially based flap technique was described by Jain and colleagues and may be appropriate in selected patients (see Fig. 115-9; Fig. 115-12).[41] Based on thermographic imaging, a long medial flap and a shorter lateral flap are designed. The reported results have been satisfactory, but there is little to recommend this flap over the more common long posterior technique. A Cochrane review published in 2004 concluded that there was insufficient evidence to establish the superiority of one transtibial amputation technique over the others.[42]

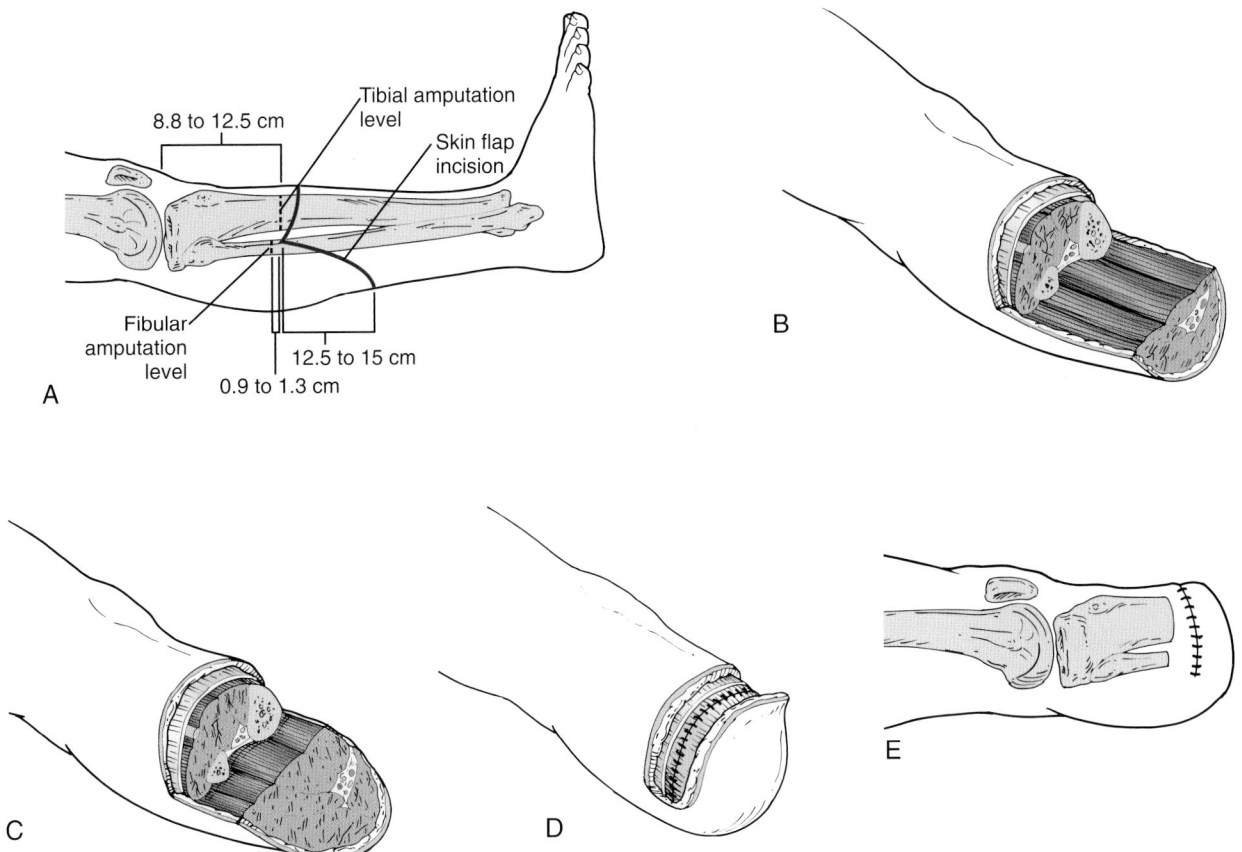

Figure 115-10 Transtibial amputation. **A,** Marking the skin incisions. **B,** Fashioning the flaps after bone transection. **C,** The soleus muscle is tailored to create a proper flap. **D,** The posterior deep fascia is sutured to the anterior deep fascia and periosteum. **E,** Closure of skin flaps.

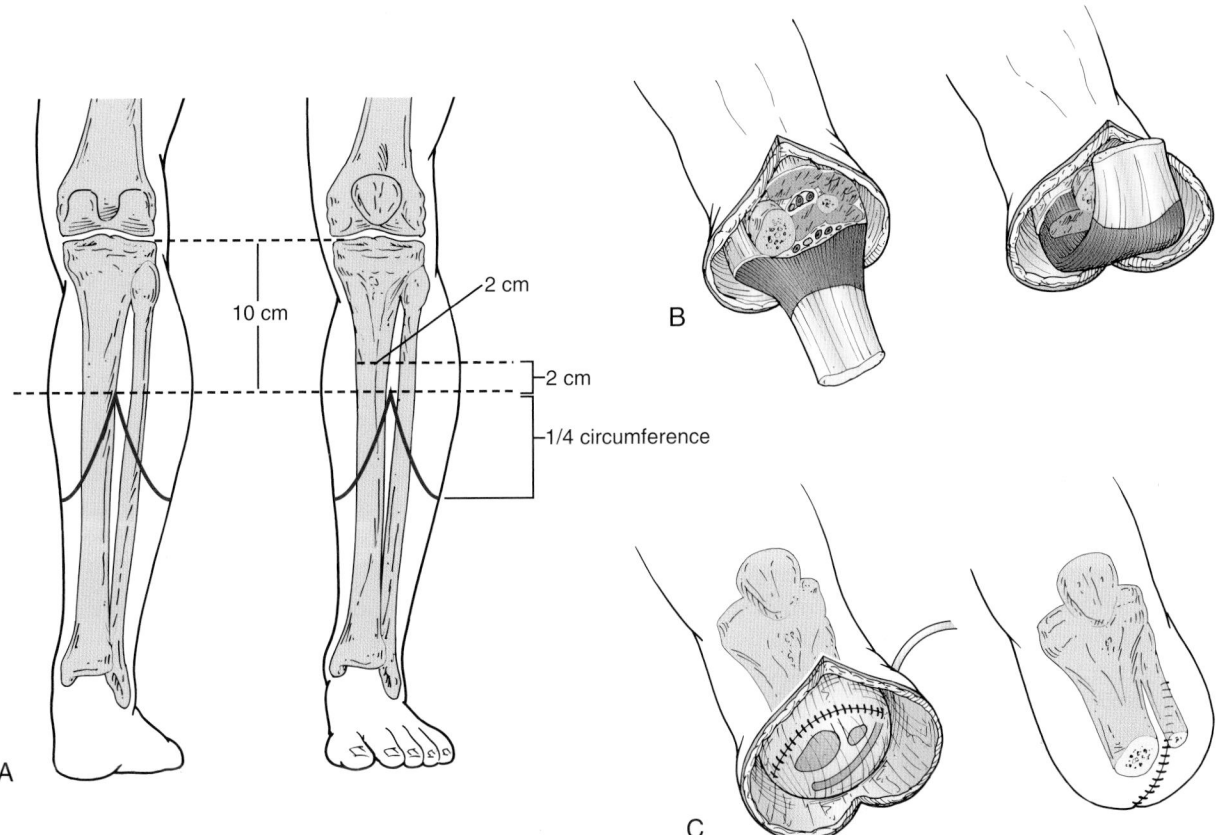

Figure 115-11 Skew flap. **A,** The incisions result in equal anteromedial and posterolateral skin flaps. The tibia is transected 10 to 12 cm distal to the joint line. **B,** The gastrocnemius muscle flap covers the tibia. **C,** The skin is closed with nonabsorbable sutures.

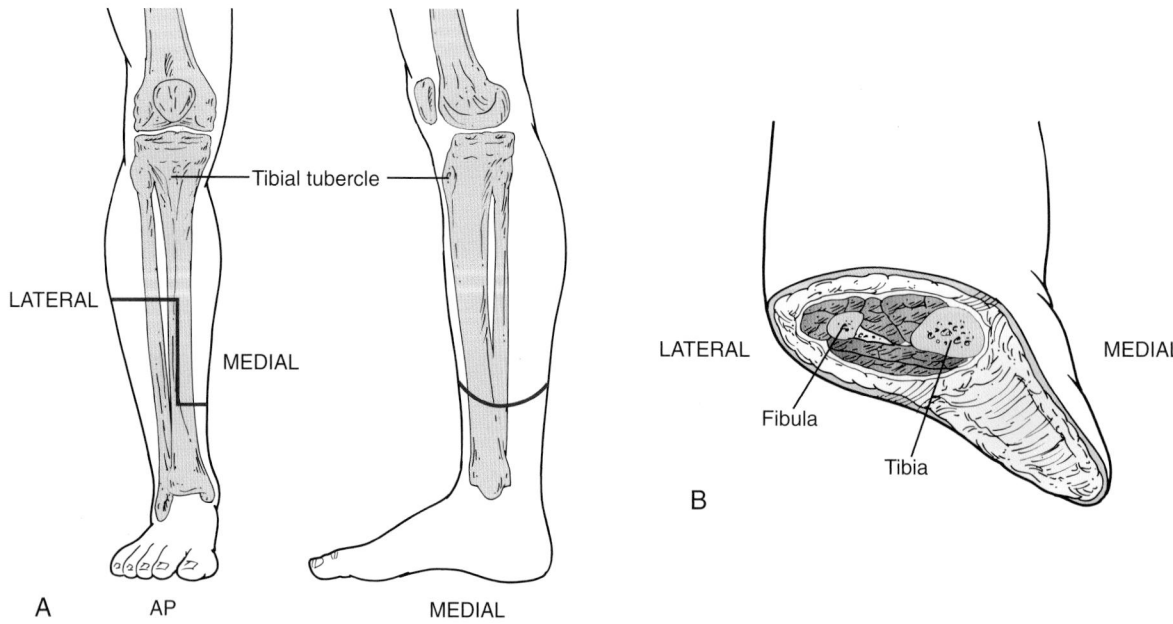

Figure 115-12 A, Skin incision for a medially based flap. **B,** View of the flap after transection. AP, anteroposterior.

Guillotine Amputation.
In the setting of severe sepsis involving the foot, some surgeons prefer to perform an initial débriding amputation to arrest the ascending infection, followed by a formal BKA at a later date. The advantage of the so-called guillotine amputation is the complete, rapid removal of the septic source. Disadvantages include the need for a second procedure and additional anesthetic, inevitable prolongation of hospitalization, increased cost, and danger of damage to the posterior flap, necessitating above-knee amputation (AKA). In two small trials, the two-stage amputation was associated with a lower overall reinfection rate.[6,7]

Cryoamputation.
In selected patients with infected gangrene, severe ischemia, or myonecrosis and with severe medical co-morbidities precluding safe anesthesia, cryoamputation has been used. The technique involves the use of dry ice to "hard-freeze" the extremity. This results in a physiologic amputation such that organic acids and other toxic byproducts are effectively quarantined in the frozen limb. Proponents of this technique report improved mortality in comparison to emergency amputation in a frail, elderly population.[43-45] Complications associated with cryoamputation include migration of the frost line above the intended level and a substantial need for revision.[46] In summary, physiologic cryoamputation controls local infection, avoids emergency surgery, and allows for medical stabilization before surgery.[45,46] Modern surgical and anesthetic techniques make cryoamputation predominantly of historical interest.

Postoperative Considerations

Following transtibial amputation, a rigid dressing is used to prevent postoperative knee contracture. We prefer a simple knee immobilizer with Velcro straps because it is widely avail-

able and can be easily removed to examine the wound. A foam cylinder can be cut to shape and inserted into the end of the knee immobilizer to provide additional protection to the stump. After adequate wound healing, an elastic stump "shrinker" should be applied to reduce edema. Ambulation is undertaken gradually under the direction of a multidisciplinary rehabilitation team.

Approximately 20% to 30% of wounds fail to heal primarily following transtibial amputation. Of these, about 50% can be salvaged at the same level. Amputation at a higher level is necessary in 10% to 20%.[16,47] Complete healing of a transtibial amputation may be protracted. Nehler and associates reported that at 100 days after surgery, only 55% of transtibial amputations were completely healed.[47]

Through-Knee Amputation

Anatomy

The femur articulates with the tibia via the knee joint, and the fibula articulates with the tibia via the superior tibiofibular joint. The stability of the knee joint depends on the anterior and posterior cruciate ligaments and the medial and lateral collateral ligaments. The patellar ligament is the central portion of the common tendon of the quadriceps femoris, which inserts on the tuberosity of the tibia.

Technique

Through-knee amputation has been recommended as an alternative to transfemoral amputation in selected patients because it results in a longer lever arm and uses a simple end weight-bearing prosthesis as opposed to ischial weight bearing with an AKA prosthesis. It is technically more demanding

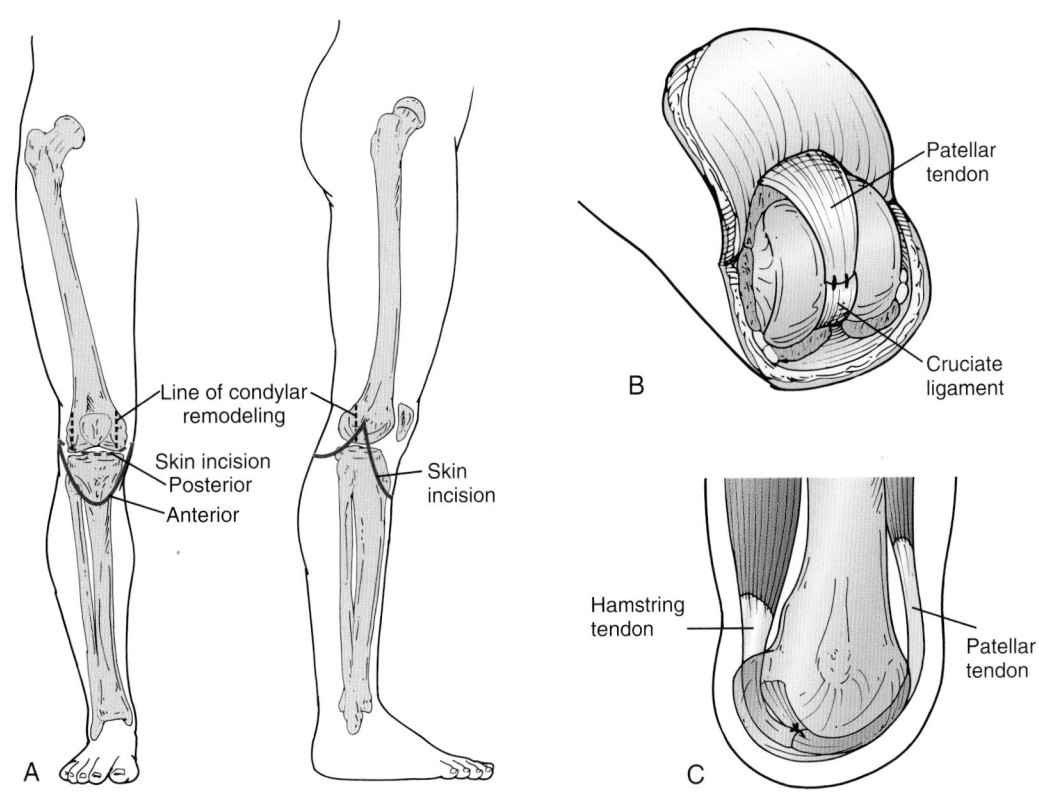

Figure 115-13 A, Fish-mouth incision for through-knee amputation. **B** and **C,** The patellar tendon is sutured directly to the residual cruciate ligament and the hamstring tendon, seen from anterior (**B**) and lateral (**C**) aspects.

than a transfemoral amputation. Wound problems leading to higher-level amputation are more common than after transfemoral amputation. The superiority of the functional outcome has led some authors to recommend through-knee amputation rather than transtibial amputation in selected patients with acceptable rehabilitation potential.[48] We reserve this technique for younger patients with above-average rehabilitation potential who are not candidates for transtibial amputation. Data supporting the use of through-knee amputation in nonambulatory patients are inconclusive.

The technique described here is the modified Gritti-Stokes amputation (Fig. 115-13).[29] A sterile tourniquet is applied above the knee after venous exsanguination. Equal anterior and posterior flaps are marked, although sagittal flaps may be used. The apex of the anterior flap is between the distal patella and the tibial tuberosity. The skin is incised, and the medial and lateral collateral ligaments are divided. The patellar tendon is divided at its insertion into the tibia. The joint capsule is incised. The cruciate ligaments are divided. The popliteal artery and vein are identified, ligated, and divided. The popliteus muscle and gastrocnemius muscles are divided. The remaining attachments of the hamstring are divided, and the knee is disarticulated. The distal femur is divided at the level of the adductor tubercle, just distal to the insertion of the adductor magnus, at an anteroposterior angle of 10 degrees. The transected end of the patellar tendon is sutured to the cruciate ligaments and the hamstring tendons. The wound is irrigated with sterile saline and closed in layers with interrupted absorbable sutures. The Mazet modification of the through-knee amputation involves removing the posterior, medial, and lateral projections of the femoral condyles. The patellar tendon and hamstrings are sutured to one another in the intercondylar notch under slight tension using nonabsorbable sutures.[49]

Postoperative Considerations

Nonunion or migration of the patella may occur in 3% of patients. This can be prevented by stable three-point transfemoral fixation. Reamputation at a higher level occurs in 10% to 15% of patients after through-knee amputation.[50] A soft dressing is appropriate. Care is taken to avoid any tight circumferential bandage that acts like a tourniquet.

Transfemoral (Above-Knee) Amputation
Anatomy

The muscles of the thigh are divided into three groups: the anterior group consists of the sartorius, quadriceps femoris, and tensor fasciae latae; the medial group includes the gracilis, pectineus, and adductor longus, brevis, and magnus; and the posterior group consists of the biceps femoris, semitendinosus, and semimembranosus. The adductor muscles insert into the posterolateral femur along a narrow ridge called the linea aspera.

Technique

A hemostatic tourniquet may be used if the femur is sufficiently long. In most patients, the femur can be divided at the junction between the middle and distal thirds (Fig. 115-14). Almost any incision that results in sufficient soft tissue coverage can be used. A transversely oriented fish-mouth incision with equal anterior and posterior flaps is commonly used, but sagittal flaps are equally effective. Some surgeons prefer a simple circular incision that is progressively deepened as the bone is approached. The superficial femoral artery and vein are divided and suture ligated. The femur is transected proximal to the skin incision, and the specimen is passed off the table. The edges of the transected femur are shaped with a rasp if desired. The sciatic nerve is divided sharply and allowed to retract. The wound is irrigated. It is important to flex the patient's hip before wound closure. If there is any tension, the femur should be shortened.

Owing to the release of the strong posteromedial adductor muscles, the unopposed hip flexors cause abduction and flexion of the proximal femur. To avoid this dysfunctional and unsightly complication, stabilization of the adductors is strongly recommended. Myopexy is performed by sewing the muscles of the posterior and medial compartment to the periosteum anterolateral to the femur. Some orthopedic surgeons recommend direct myoplasty of the adductor muscles using nonabsorbable suture through holes drilled in the anterolateral femur. After either myoplasty or myopexy, the deep fascia is approximated with absorbable suture. The skin is closed using either staples or interrupted monofilament sutures.

Postoperative Considerations

Preventing fecal and urine wound contamination is challenging after above-knee amputation. Care must be taken to avoid constrictive, circumferential dressings that impair blood flow. A simple and effective dressing consists of Vaseline gauze or nonadherent gauze on the suture line covered with a protective sheet of adhesive Ioban.

The energy required for ambulation with an AKA is approximately 50% higher than after a BKA. Less than 10% of elderly vascular amputees can be expected to ambulate effectively after transfemoral amputation.[51]

Hip Disarticulation
Anatomy

The hip joint is a multiaxial ball-and-socket joint. The ligamentous structures of the joint are the fibrous capsule, acetabular labrum, ligament of the head of the femur, and iliofemoral, ischiofemoral, pubofemoral, and transverse acetabular ligaments. The muscles that surround the hip joint are divided into three groups—anterior, posterior, and inferior. The anterior group, lateral to medial, includes the rectus femoris, iliopsoas, and pectineus. Anterior to this group are the sartorius and tensor fasciae latae. The posterior group consists of the piriformis, obturator internus, quadratus femoris, and obturator externus.

Technique

An anterior racket incision or a long posterior flap incision can be used (Fig. 115-15).[52] The anterior racket incision starts 1 inch medial to the anterior superior iliac spine, extends toward the pubic tubercle, and continues posteriorly, distal to the ischial tuberosity and just distal to the gluteal crease. The incision is then turned back anteriorly, medial to the greater trochanter and the anterior inferior iliac spine, and joins the starting point. The incision for the long posterior flap starts about 1 inch parallel to the inguinal ligament anteriorly and extends posteriorly to create the posterior flap. The length of the posterior flap is one and a half times the anteroposterior diameter at the level of the hip joint. After the skin incision, the femoral vessels are ligated. The sartorius is divided at its origin, and the iliopsoas is divided at its insertion. Next the pectineus muscle is divided at its origin from the pubis. The gracilis muscle and all three adductors are divided at their origins. The obturator neurovascular bundle is divided. The obturator externus muscle is divided from its insertion to the lesser trochanter. The hamstrings (semimembranosus, semitendinosus, and biceps femoris) are divided at the ischial tuberosity. Next, the tensor fasciae latae, gluteus maximus, and rectus femoris are divided. Finally, the muscles attached to the greater trochanter are divided. The ligamentum teres

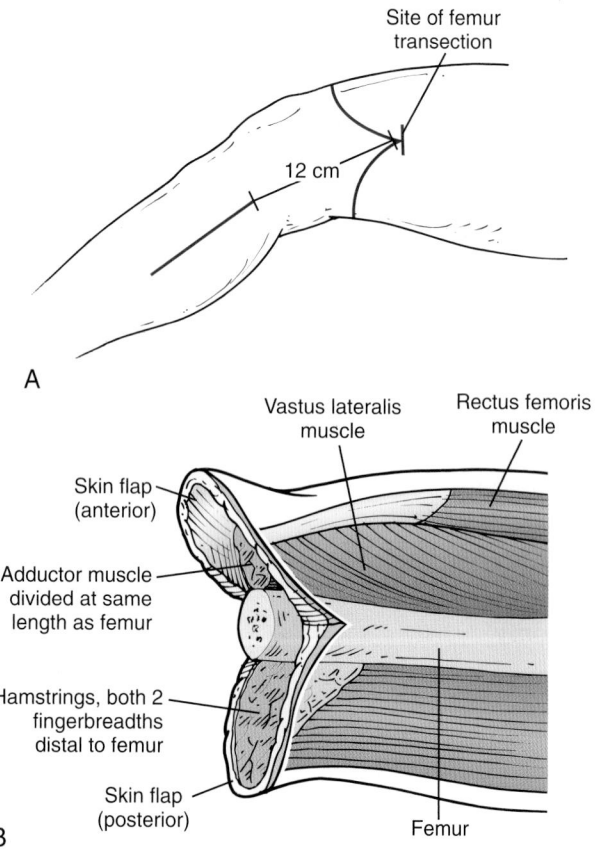

Figure 115-14 A, Fish-mouth incision for long transfemoral amputation. **B,** Cutaway view of transfemoral amputation.

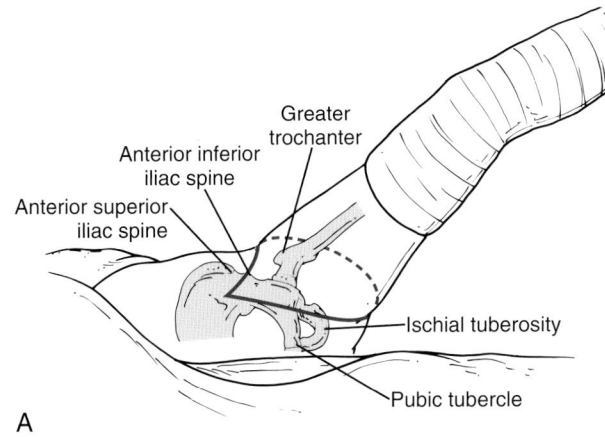

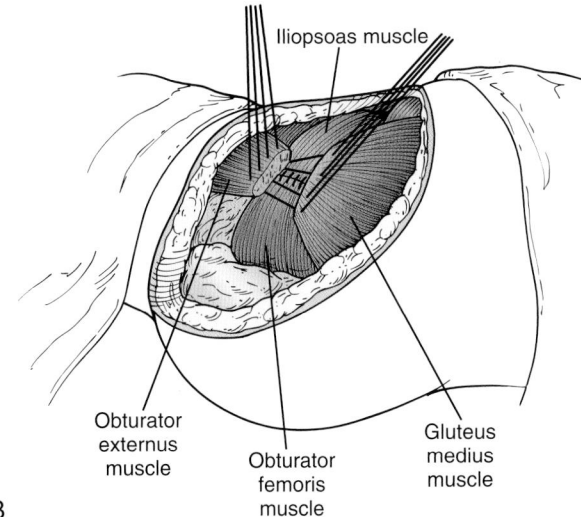

Figure 115-15 A, Racket incision for hip disarticulation. **B,** Two-layer myoplasty over the acetabulum.

is divided, and the capsule of the hip joint is incised. The sciatic nerve is transected, which retracts posterior to the piriformis muscle. The specimen is passed off the table. Myoplasty is then performed by joining two groups of muscles over the acetabulum. First, the posterior quadratus femoris is sutured to the anterior iliopsoas. Second, the lateral gluteus medius is sutured to the medial obturator externus. The gluteal fascia is then approximated to the inguinal ligament. The skin is closed loosely with staples.

Postoperative Considerations

Drains and a Foley catheter are left in place for a few days. Wound soilage from stool and urine should be prevented. The skin over the sacrum and posterior hip should be inspected daily. Attention to prophylaxis against venous thromboembolism is particularly important in this group of patients.

■ PRINCIPLES OF POSTOPERATIVE CARE

Postoperative care of amputation patients requires multidisciplinary cooperation. Anesthesiology, rehabilitation medi-

cine, physical therapy, and psychiatry services may all contribute to the patient's recovery. Pain management and psychological support are critical to successful amputation surgery. The surgeon carries the responsibility of ensuring that the other members of the rehabilitation team are committed to the patient's successful recovery.

The ideal postoperative dressings share the following characteristics: they protect the wound from contamination and trauma, allow easy access for wound examination, prevent contractures, and minimize edema without restricting arterial inflow. A wide variety of soft, semirigid, and rigid removable dressings has been developed, but there is no consensus regarding the optimal method of stump treatment.[53,54]

In an effort to reduce the time to ambulation with a prosthesis, the strategy of applying an immediate postoperative prosthesis (IPOP) was developed.[55] In our experience, wound healing is the rate-limiting step in rehabilitation after amputation for vascular disease, and we have not found immediate plaster dressings to be beneficial. Advocates of IPOP report that more patients are able to achieve effective prosthetic ambulation at an earlier time in comparison to conventional rehabilitation.[55,56] The primary drawbacks are that successful IPOP requires the commitment of a skillful multidisciplinary team, which is not universally available, and that the rigid prosthesis limits access to the wound for examination.[54,57,58] The reader is directed to an excellent discussion of postoperative prosthetic options in Chapter 114 (Lower Extremity Amputation: General Considerations).

■ OUTCOMES
Operative Mortality

Historically, operative mortality following lower extremity amputation was as high as 30% to 40%.[59-61] The excessive mortality associated with amputation was frequently invoked as justification for complex conventional or endovascular limb salvage procedures even in frail, nonambulatory patients with significant co-morbidities. Contemporary surgical publications indicate an improvement in overall operative mortality following amputation. For major lower extremity amputation, the currently reported 30-day operative mortality ranges from 4% to 9%.[62-64] Operative mortality for minor amputations at the ankle and below is approximately 2% to 4%.[16,19,20,47]

The majority of lower extremity amputations are performed for ischemia and diabetes. Trauma and malignancy account for the remainder.[65,66] The most common causes of death following amputation are cardiac (46%), sepsis (16%), and pneumonia (11%).[67]

Several recent reports have identified predictors of operative mortality after amputation for vascular indications. There is an association between the level of amputation and operative mortality, a finding that presumably reflects the severity of systemic cardiovascular disease rather than the magnitude of the procedure.[68] Operative mortality for transfemoral amputation ranges from 11.1% to 17.5%; for transtibial amputation, it ranges from 3.6% to 9.4% (Table 115-1).[47,64,68-72]

Table 115-1 Thirty-Day Mortality, 1-Year Survival, and Reamputation Rates

Series	Year	Number of Patients	30-Day Mortality (%)		1-Year Survival (%)		Reamputation Rate	
			BKA	AKA	BKA	AKA	BKA to AKA (%)	Contralateral Major Amputation (%)
Kazmers[a]	2000	8696	9.4	16.1				
Feinglass et al.[70]	2001	4061	6.3	13.3	77	59		
Mayfield et al.[74]	2001	5180	7.0	11.1				
Abou-Zamzam et al.[63]	2003	131					19.6	10.7 (at 3 yr)
Nehler et al.[47]	2003	172					19	
Cruz et al.[81]	2003	296	12	17			12	17 (at 7 yr)
Aulivola et al.[67]	2004	959	5.7	16.5	74.5	50.6	9.4	19.8 (at 11 yr)
Sandnes et al.[68]	2004	6919	6.1	13.5	80.4	64.6		
Subramaniam[b]	2005	954	4.2	17.5	78.2	62.1		
Ploeg et al.[64]	2005	122	5.2	17.8			14.3	
Dillingham et al.[16]	2005	3565			64.5	49.6	9.4	9.4 (at 1 yr)
Stone et al.[26]	2007	508	3.6	13.6			11.5	21 (at 5 yr)

AKA, above-knee amputation; BKA, below-knee amputation.
[a]Kajmers A, Perkins A, Jacobs L. Major lower extremity amputation in Veterans Affairs Medical Centers. *Ann Vasc Surg.* 2000;14:216-222.
[b]Subramaniam B, Pomposelli F, Talmar D, et al. Perioperative and long-term morbidity and mortality after above-knee and below-knee amputations in diabetics and nondiabetics. *Anesth Analg.* 2005;100:1241-1247.

For example, in 954 major lower extremity amputations at Beth Israel Deaconess Boston, the overall 30-day mortality was 8.6%; the mortality was 16.5% for AKA and 5.7% for BKA.[67] Sandnes and coworkers reported that 30-day operative mortality for transtibial amputation in Washington State has remained remarkably stable over a 14-year period (Fig. 115-16).[68] During the most recent 5-year period, the 30-day mortality for BKA was 6.1%, versus 13.5% for AKA.[68] In a large study by the Department of Veterans Affairs, the 30-day mortality for BKA was 6.3%, compared with 13.3% for AKA.[70]

In addition to level of amputation, a variety of markers of systemic illness have been shown to be related to operative mortality. Malnutrition, as evidenced by decreased serum albumin, was shown to predict operative mortality in the Department of Veterans Affairs National Surgical Quality Improvement Program database.[70] Several recent reports identified diabetes as a risk factor for perioperative death. Schofield and colleagues reported that diabetes conferred a 55% increased risk of mortality after lower extremity amputation when compared to nondiabetic subjects.[73] Dillingham and associates reported that although diabetes did not result in elevated operative risk, diabetic amputees were more likely to be severely disabled, experience their initial amputation at a younger age, progress to higher level amputations, and die at a younger age than their nondiabetic counterparts.[16] Increased age is associated with increased operative mortality, as is advanced cardiac, pulmonary, and renal disease.[74] A Finnish study reported that age older than 65 years and amputation above the knee (or higher) were associated with elevated operative mortality.[75] Guillotine amputation for sepsis was associated with a 30-day mortality rate of 14.3%, compared with 7.8% in those undergoing elective amputation.[67] There is no consistent evidence that either race or gender is independently associated with operative mortality.[68] In summary, severe cardiac, pulmonary, and renal disease; level of amputation; advanced age; malnutrition; and diabetes appear to be significant predictors of perioperative death.

Long-term Survival

It is estimated that the prevalence of major lower extremity amputation due to vascular disease in the United States was approximately 500,000 in 2005.[76] The entry of baby boomers into the geriatric age group is expected to increase this number by 50% in the next 15 years.[76] Long-term survival in amputees is significantly less than in age-matched controls. In a representative report by a group from Denver, the overall survival after major lower extremity amputation was 78% at 1 year and 55% at 3 years.[47] As previously found for 30-day mortality, the level of amputation is also associated with long-term mortality (see Table 115-1). The approximate 1-year survival is 65% to 80% after BKA and 50% after AKA (Fig. 115-17).[16,64,67,68,73] Based on Medicare data from 1997 to 1998, Dillingham and associates reported 1-year survival of 65% for BKA and 50% for AKA.[16] Aulivola and colleagues reported 1-year survival of 74.5% after BKA and 50.6% after AKA.[67] Based on 21,000 amputations over 20 years, Ebskov reported that the 1-year median survival time was only 1.0 year for transfemoral amputation and 2.4 years for transtibial.[77] Increased long-term mortality is also associated with diabetes and renal failure.[67,77] In a British study of 390 patients who underwent lower extremity amputation, the median time to death was 27.2 months in diabetics and 46.7 months in nondiabetics.[73] In patients on dialysis, Aulivola and colleagues reported 1-year survival of only 51.9% following major lower extremity amputation; in contrast, 75.4% of patients with normal renal function were alive at 1 year. In addition, nondialysis patients with preoperative creatinine levels greater than 2 mg/dL (176.8 μmol/L) had similar survival rates to their dialysis-dependent counterparts, with 55.9% alive at 1 year.[67] Patients presenting with critical limb ischemia have a

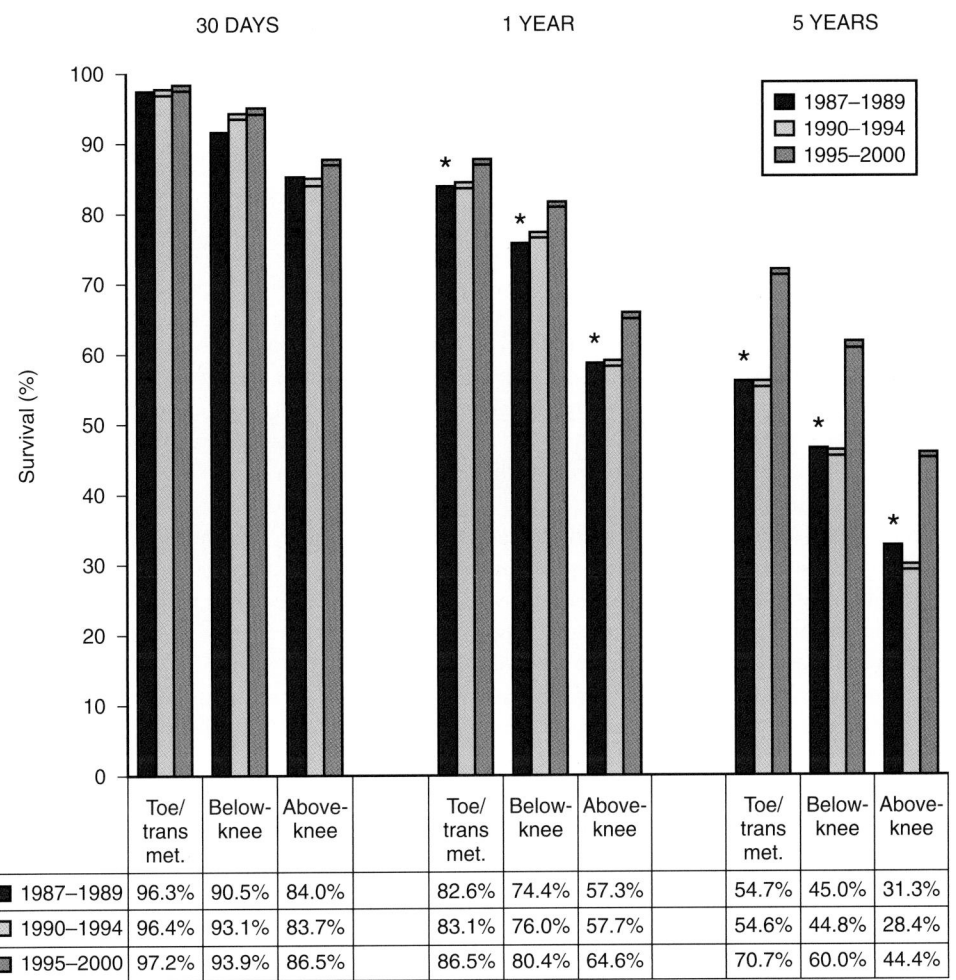

	30 DAYS				1 YEAR				5 YEARS		
	Toe/ trans met.	Below-knee	Above-knee		Toe/ trans met.	Below-knee	Above-knee		Toe/ trans met.	Below-knee	Above-knee
■ 1987–1989	96.3%	90.5%	84.0%		82.6%	74.4%	57.3%		54.7%	45.0%	31.3%
□ 1990–1994	96.4%	93.1%	83.7%		83.1%	76.0%	57.7%		54.6%	44.8%	28.4%
▨ 1995–2000	97.2%	93.9%	86.5%		86.5%	80.4%	64.6%		70.7%	60.0%	44.4%

Figure 115-16 Bar graph showing survival at 30 days, 1 year, and 5 years following foot (toe/transmetatarsal), below-knee, and above-knee amputations during three periods (1987–1989, 1990–1994, and 1995–2000). (*P < .001 when post-1995 is compared with pre-1995.) *(From Sandnes DK, Sobel M, Flum DR. Survival after lower-extremity amputation. J Am Coll Surg. 2004;199:394-402.)*

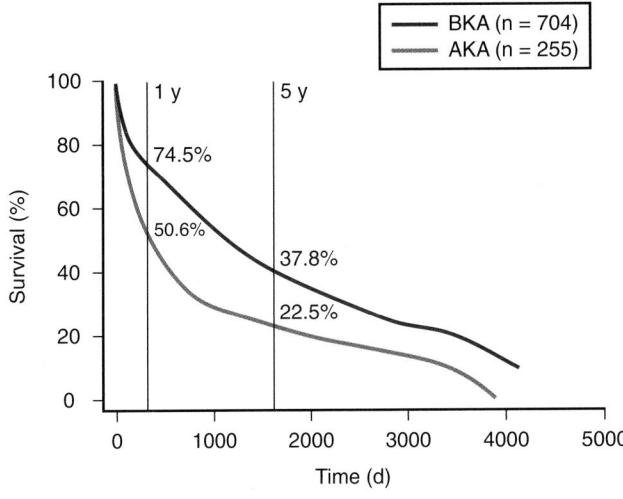

Figure 115-17 Long-term survival following below-knee amputation (BKA) and above-knee amputation (AKA). *(From Aulivola B, Hile CN, Hamdan AD, et al. Major lower extremity amputation: outcome of a modern series. Arch Surg. 2004;139:395-399.)*

higher mortality than patients presenting with either infection or trauma as the indication for amputation. Long-term survival has not clearly been shown to be related to gender, race, history of hypertension, or previous revascularization procedures. There is evidence that long-term survival following major lower extremity amputation has improved in recent years.[62,68]

Functional Outcome

Once healing has been achieved following toe, ray, and transmetatarsal amputations, near-normal ambulation with conventional footwear is likely. Shoe fillers and simple orthoses are usually sufficient to allow ambulation for the majority of patients.[11,13,17-20]

Following transtibial amputation for vascular disease, bipedal ambulation with a prosthesis is uncommon. The reported outcome of rehabilitation varies widely, depending on the definition of success. Two recent reports from well-known academic centers indicate that only about 25% of major lower extremity amputees ambulate with a prosthesis outside the home.[47,78] These patients were unable to use a prosthesis for a variety of reasons, including mental illness, cardiopulmonary insufficiency, inadequate balance, and stump problems.[47,79] Taylor and coworkers identified significant preoperative factors independently associated with not wearing a prosthesis. In order of greatest to least risk, they were nonambulatory status before amputation (odds ratio [OR] 9.5), AKA (OR 4.4), age older than 60 years (OR 2.7), homebound but ambulatory status (OR 3.0), dementia (OR 2.4), end-stage renal disease (OR 2.3), and coronary artery disease (OR 2.0).[80] Older transfemoral amputees rarely (<10%) ambulate successfully with a prosthesis.[47,78,81] Dialysis-dependent renal failure is a strong predictor of nonambulatory status.

Despite the fact that few vascular amputees ambulate with a prosthesis outside the home, most maintain their preoperative living status. Thus, most patients who were living independently before major amputation remain independent postoperatively. Highly motivated patients—as evidenced by a commitment to a strict rehabilitation program, including smoking cessation and weight loss—are more likely to achieve long-term success.[82] In addition, patients with financial resources that allow participation in a well-organized rehabilitation program are more likely to be successful. Taylor and coworkers identified the following statistically significant preoperative factors that were independently associated with a failure to maintain an independent living status (in decreasing order of influence): age 70 years or older (hazard ratio [HR] 4.0), age 60 to 69 years (HR 2.7), level of amputation (HR 1.8), homebound ambulatory status (HR 1.6), and dementia (HR 1.6).[80] Thus, elderly transtibial amputees with dementia are unlikely to maintain an independent living status.

Reamputation

Following an initial toe amputation, approximately 50% of patients eventually undergo additional ipsilateral or contralateral amputations. Following foot or ankle amputation, nearly 35% of patients progress to a higher level amputation within 1 year.[16] The rate of revision following major proximal amputations remains disturbingly high, despite the availability of a variety of methods for selecting the appropriate amputation level. Wound problems develop in 20% to 30% of patients following transtibial amputation.[47,67,81] About half of these amputations are salvaged at the transtibial level. Additionally, reamputation at the transfemoral level has been reported in 9.4% to 19.6% of transtibial amputees.[16,47,63,64,67,81] It has also been reported that 9.4% to 17% of transtibial amputees undergo contralateral major amputation within as little as 12 months.[16,63,67,81,83] Not surprisingly, the risk of ipsilateral reamputation at a higher level is inversely related to the level of the index amputation. Diabetic patients are almost twice as likely to have reamputation as nondiabetics.[15,73] The 1-, 3-, and 5-year ipsilateral reamputation rate for patients who are diabetic are as follows: for toe amputees, 22.8%, 39.6%, and 52.3%, respectively; for ray amputees, 28.7%, 41.2%, and 50%, respectively; for midfoot amputees, 18.8%, 33.3%, and 42.9%, respectively; and for major amputees, 4.7%, 11.8%, and 13.3%, respectively.

Complications

Local

Bleeding. Reoperation for postoperative bleeding is reported in 3% to 9% of major lower extremity amputations.[47,62] Postoperative hematomas may be underreported and may be an undetected cause of amputation failure. Patients on anticoagulants, including DVT prophylaxis, are at a higher risk for hematoma formation.

Infection. Wound infection following major lower extremity amputation has been reported in 13% to 40% of patients.[5,7,84] An increased risk of wound infection is associated with diabetes, preoperative wound infection, malnutrition, malignancy, advanced age, lack of insurance, wound hematoma, and prior prosthetic bypass grafts. Complete removal of synthetic graft material at the time of amputation can decrease the rate of stump infection.[85]

The role of antibiotics in amputation surgery is three-pronged: (1) prophylaxis in a patient without infection, (2) treatment of postamputation wound infection, and (3) perioperative treatment of extremity sepsis. In general, prophylactic broad-spectrum antibiotics should be administered perioperatively to all amputees to reduce the incidence of wound infection. Surveys of the bacteriology of amputation wound infections confirm a wide spectrum of aerobic and anaerobic species.[84] Anaerobic coverage should be considered for diabetics. A recent report from the United Kingdom demonstrated a reduction in amputation wound infection from 22.5% to 5% following a prophylactic 5-day course of broad-spectrum antibiotics in comparison to the standard three-dose regimen.[5] Not surprisingly, the incidence of *Clostridium difficile* colon infection was higher in patients receiving the 5-day course of antibiotics (7.5% versus 0%).

Following elective amputation, the wound should be examined for signs of infection, including erythema, excessive warmth, and foul drainage, especially in a patient with unexplained fever or excessive stump pain. Superficial infections can initially be treated with broad-spectrum antibiotics and removal of skin sutures. Deeper infections necessitate more aggressive drainage and débridement. Vacuum dressings are particularly effective in this setting.[22]

In a patient with active extremity sepsis before amputation, treatment should be based on fundamental surgical principles: abscess drainage, débridement of all nonviable tissue, and avoidance of complete wound closure. Broad-spectrum antibiotics are selected in accordance with the local antibiogram. Antibiotic coverage should be promptly adjusted in response to wound culture and sensitivities. Débriding amputation at the toe, forefoot, or ankle level may allow the surgeon to control the septic process before definitive amputation in 5 to 7 days.

Contracture.
Flexion contractures at the hip and knee joint develop in 3% to 5% of major lower extremity amputations. A fixed flexion contracture at the knee that exceeds 15 degrees prohibits effective prosthetic ambulation. Contractures are more common in older patients, especially those with dementia and prior ipsilateral stroke. Failure to provide adequate postoperative analgesia may also result in flexion contracture. Once a significant contracture develops, it may be impossible to correct with physical therapy or surgery.[86] Prevention of contracture is thus an essential component of a successful rehabilitation program. A rigid, removable dressing should be applied to prevent knee contractures. Hip flexion contracture can sometimes be retarded by placing the patient prone for brief periods. An aggressive postoperative knee exercise program should be undertaken as soon as permitted by pain tolerance and wound healing.

Systemic

Cardiac.
Myocardial infarction is the most common cause of death following lower extremity amputation. In a study of 154 patients undergoing 172 major amputations, 10 of 16 (62.5%) perioperative deaths were due to cardiac disease.[47] Another report of 959 amputations reported a cardiac complication rate of 10.2%.[67] Complications included arrhythmias (2.6%), congestive heart failure (4.2%), and myocardial infarction (3.4%). Cardiac complications continue to be a significant cause of long-term mortality in these patients. Use of beta blockers may decrease the rate of perioperative myocardial infarction and should be considered standard care unless specifically contraindicated.

Pulmonary.
The incidence of pulmonary complications, including atelectasis and pneumonia, is approximately 5% after major lower extremity amputation.[67] Identification of patients at risk and appropriate pre- and postoperative pulmonary care may decrease the rate of these complications. DVT prophylaxis should be administered to all amputees in accordance with their individual risk for bleeding.

Venous Thromboembolism.
Without prophylaxis, DVT has been reported in up to 50% of patients following major lower extremity amputation.[4,87-89] Prophylaxis with low-molecular-weight heparin can reduce the incidence of DVT to approximately 10%.[4] All patients should receive some form of DVT prophylaxis following lower extremity amputation. A sequential compression stocking on the contralateral leg may be beneficial.

Renal Failure.
The incidence of new-onset renal failure after major lower extremity amputation is between 0.6% and 2.6%.[47,67] Renal failure is associated with increased operative and long-term mortality.

Stroke.
Postoperative stroke has been reported to occur in 0.28% to 1.4% of patients following major amputation.[47,62] The reported incidence of perioperative stroke-related mortality after major lower extremity amputation is 7.3%.[90]

Psychiatric.
Post-traumatic stress disorder is common (20% to 22%) after amputations for combat or accidental injuries; for vascular amputations, the incidence is less than 5%. Depression following amputation can result from an adjustment reaction to the surgery and to sudden disability. Risk factors for major depressive disorder include young age at the time of amputation, pain, neurotic personality, lifestyle, and poor coping skills.[91,92]

Pain.
Chronic pain is reported by up to 95% of amputees.[93] The diagnosis of phantom pain, best described as a painful sensation in the missing limb, should be made only after other causes of stump pain have been eliminated, including ischemia, infection, neuroma, and pressure-related wounds. Chronic ischemic stump pain may be difficult to detect by physical examination alone but is confirmed by a transcutaneous oxygen tension less than 20 mm Hg. Chronic infection, particularly related to residual prosthetic graft material, may be a cause of pain. Neuroma can develop at the site of transection of virtually any peripheral nerve. The pain is usually well localized to the site of injury and can be transiently or permanently blocked with anesthetic injection. Pressure points that develop over bone spurs or pathologic bone formation should be eliminated. In addition, depression appears to complicate the treatment of pain in many amputees.[93]

True phantom pain is a complex, poorly understood pain syndrome that is sometimes described as a burning, aching, or electrical pain in the amputated limb. The incidence of phantom pain widely varies in the literature from 5% to 85%, depending on the diagnostic criteria.[94,95] Inadequate control of both pre- and postoperative pain may increase the risk of chronic amputation pain.[96] Preemptive epidural anesthesia has been used to reduce the incidence and severity of phantom pain.[97] Gabapentin has not been consistently effective in the treatment of phantom pain.[98] Multimodality pain management is the cornerstone of a successful amputation rehabilitation program.[98]

SELECTED KEY REFERENCES

Aulivola B, Hile CN, Hamdan AD, Sheahan MG, Veraldi JR, Skillman JJ, Campbell DR, Scovell SD, LoGerfo FW, Pomposelli FB Jr. Major lower extremity amputation: outcome of a modern series. *Arch Surg*. 2004;139:395-399.
Comprehensive, contemporary report of outcomes after major lower extremity amputation.

Barnes R, Cox B. *Amputations: An Illustrated Manual*. Philadelphia: Hanley & Belfus; 2000.
Beautifully illustrated atlas of commonly performed lower extremity amputations.

Early JS. Transmetatarsal and midfoot amputations. *Clin Orthop Rel Res*. 1999;361:85-90.
Excellent reference for midfoot amputation techniques.

Faber DC, Fielding P. Gritti-Stokes (through-knee) amputation: should it be reintroduced? *South Med J*. 2001;94:997-1001.
Good review of through-knee amputation.

Moore WS, Malone, JM. *Lower Extremity Amputation*. Philadelphia: WB Saunders; 1989.
Still a valuable resource for descriptions of hip disarticulation and other major amputations.

Nawijn SE, van der Linde H, Emmelot CH, Hofstad CJ. Stump management after trans-tibial amputation: a systematic review. *Prosthet Orthot Int.* 2005;29:13-26.
Review of the literature on rehabilitation after transtibial amputation.

Nehler MR, Coll JR, Hiatt WR, Regensteiner JG, Schnickel GT, Klenke WA, Strecker PK, Anderson MW, Jones DN, Whitehill TA, Moskowitz S, Krupski WC. Functional outcome in a contemporary series of major lower extremity amputations. *J Vasc Surg.* 2003;38:7-14.
Review of functional outcome after lower extremity amputation.

Richardson D. Amputations of the foot. In: Canale S, Beaty J, eds. *Campbell's Operative Orthopedics*. Philadelphia: Elsevier; 2008:595-596.

The standard of care for orthopedic surgery for many years. The description of amputation techniques is very well done.

Robinson KP. Amputations in vascular patients. In: Bell PRF, ed. *Surgical Management of Vascular Disease*. London: WB Saunders; 1992: 609-635.
Detailed description of the skew flap technique for transtibial amputation.

Tang PCY, Ravji K, Key JJ, Mahler DB, Blume PA, Sumpio B. Let them walk! Current prosthesis options for leg and foot amputees. *J Am Coll Surg.* 2008;206:548-560.
Very nice review of prosthetic options after lower extremity amputation.

REFERENCES

The reference list can be found on the companion Expert Consult Web site at *www.expertconsult.com*.

Upper Extremity Arterial Disease | *Section* **16**

Louis M. Messina

CHAPTER 116

Upper Extremity Arterial Disease: General Considerations

James M. Edwards

A large number of diseases can affect the arterial circulation in the upper extremity, unlike in the lower extremity, where atherosclerosis is responsible for the vast majority of vascular disease. The reason for this disparity is unknown and has been the subject of only cursory research. Upper extremity arterial reconstruction is much less common than lower extremity arterial reconstruction in most vascular surgical practices and accounts for less than 5% of patients with limb ischemia.[1] This chapter provides an overview of upper extremity arterial diseases. Subsequent chapters will review in detail the diagnosis, natural history, and treatment of specific diseases that affect the upper extremity circulation. These disease processes span from the common, Raynaud's disease and atherosclerosis, to the uncommon, occupation-induced diseases and trauma.

EPIDEMIOLOGY

Although upper extremity arterial diseases can be subdivided in a number of different ways, the two most important ways are by anatomic location and etiology. Location is categorized as affecting small or large arteries; etiology is categorized as either vasospasm or occlusive disease.[1] Small-artery and large-artery diseases have widely differing causes, pathophysiologies, and treatments, although the initial clinical findings may be similar. Even though patients with vasospasm or occlusive disease may have the same clinical manifestations, differentiation of these two disease states has obvious important clinical implications.

Because the causes of upper extremity arterial disease are many but the incidence of these diseases is low, the discussion of epidemiology is complex. The one exception is Raynaud's syndrome. As many as 20% to 30% of people who live in cold climates will complain of cold-induced finger discomfort.[2] Fortunately, finger ischemia does not develop in the vast majority of these patients because they have primary Raynaud's syndrome, caused by cold-induced vasospasm. Only a minority of patients have secondary Raynaud's syndrome, caused by a significant associated disease process such as scleroderma that is responsible for the development of severe ischemia because of digital artery occlusion.[3] However, scleroderma, with a 3:1 female-male ratio, is present in approximately 50,000 patients, with an incidence of about 10 cases per million population in the United States.[4]

Significant arterial disease involving the upper extremity affects just a small proportion of the population. The age distribution of patients is broad, with conditions such as autoimmune disease being seen in both the young and old and atherosclerosis occurring primarily in elderly patients with diabetes or renal failure (or both). Box 116-1 lists the possible causes of significant hand and finger ischemia, and Table 116-1 details which portion of the arterial system that they affect. Three disease processes from this table—vasculitis, thromboangiitis obliterans, and Takayasu's disease—are discussed in Chapter 76 (Vasculitis and Other Arteriopathies), Chapter 77 (Thromboangiitis Obliterans), and Chapter 78 (Takayasu's Disease).

PATHOGENESIS

Occlusive disease can affect both large and small arteries or a combination of both. The most frequent cause of occlusive disease of large arteries is atherosclerosis, which is most common in the subclavian artery but may extend more distally into the forearm, especially in diabetic patients. An inflammatory obliterative process caused by autoimmune diseases can also cause occlusion of large arteries. In addition, occlusion secondary to an inflammatory arteritis can result in small-artery occlusion and can have a vasospastic component (see Chapter 76: Vasculitis and Other Arteriopathies; Chapter 77: Thromboangiitis Obliterans; and Chapter 78: Takayasu's Disease). A similar pattern of large- and small-artery disease occurs in arterial thoracic outlet syndrome, where stenosis of the subclavian artery can be accompanied by emboli that cause digital ischemia (see Chapter 124: Thoracic Outlet Syndrome: Arterial). Finally, upper extremity arterial aneurysm, though rare, can embolize or thrombose and cause ischemia.

Raynaud's syndrome has a unique pathogenesis and is more common in the upper than the lower extremity (see Chapter 119: Raynaud's Syndrome). Patients with Raynaud's syndrome most commonly have symptoms of cold-induced pain, numbness, and color changes in the fingers. Because the first large group of patients with finger ischemia was described by Maurice Raynaud in 1888, the eponym Raynaud's has been used to describe this group of patients.[5] Patients with digital artery ischemia caused by primary Raynaud's syndrome have decreased blood flow because of vasospasm (transient occlusion of the digital arteries as a result of exposure to cold or other stresses), whereas patients with Raynaud's syndrome secondary to underlying connective tissue disease may progress to a more severe occlusive lesion that continuously

Box 116-1 Causes of Severe Hand Ischemia

ARTERIAL VASOSPASM

- Ergotism
- Idiopathic vasospastic Raynaud's syndrome
- Vinyl chloride exposure

ARTERIAL OBSTRUCTION

Large-Artery Causes

- Atherosclerosis
- Thoracic outlet compression
- Arteritis
  Takayasu's
  Giant cell
- Fibromuscular disease

Small-Artery Causes

- Connective tissue diseases
  Scleroderma
  Rheumatoid arthritis
  Sjögren's syndrome
  Systemic lupus erythematosus
- Myeloproliferative disorders
  Thrombocytosis
  Leukemia
  Polycythemia
- Buerger's disease
- Hypersensitivity angiitis
- Cold injury
- Henoch-Schönlein purpura
- Cytotoxic drugs
- Hypercoagulable states
- Arterial drug injection

PROXIMAL LARGE-ARTERY SOURCES OF EMBOLISM TO DISTAL SMALL ARTERIES

- Ulcerated or stenotic atherosclerotic plaque
  Aortic arch
  Innominate artery
  Subclavian artery
- Aneurysms
  Innominate artery
  Subclavian artery
  Axillary or brachial artery
  Ulnar artery

From Landry GL, Moneta GL, Taylor LM. Severe hand ischemia. In: Pearce WH, Matsumura JS, Yao JST, eds. *Trends in Vascular Surgery 2003*. Chicago: Precept Press; 2004:280.

obstructs blood flow into the digit. The differences in digital blood flow between vasospasm and obstruction with and without cooling are demonstrated diagrammatically in Figure 116-1.

ETIOLOGIES AND RISK FACTORS

Etiologies

The diseases leading to the most severe upper extremity arterial ischemia are autoimmune or connective tissue diseases such as scleroderma, rheumatoid arthritis, systemic lupus, and others.[6] Autoimmune diseases are surprisingly common, and most patients with autoimmune disease have secondary Raynaud's syndrome (see Chapter 119: Raynaud's Syndrome). Scleroderma is the most common associated disease in the majority of reports detailing causes of upper extremity arterial ischemia from tertiary referral centers. Risk factors for autoimmune disease in the general population are not well understood.

Thromboangiitis Obliterans

Patients with Buerger's disease (thromboangiitis obliterans) have segmental thrombotic occlusions of the small and medium-sized arteries of the extremities.[7,8] These lesions have the usual features of atherosclerosis but characteristically also have an inflammatory process of the artery that can encase the adjacent vein and nerve (see Chapter 77: Thromboangiitis Obliterans). Even though the lower extremities are more frequently involved, approximately 50% of patients also have upper extremity involvement with resulting digital ischemia. Tobacco smoking is the major risk factor for the development of Buerger's disease, although it has also been reported after prolonged marijuana use.[9]

Vibration Injury

Finger and hand ischemia secondary to small-artery disease caused by the long-term use of vibrating tools was first described in the early 1900s.[10,11] The initial group of patients consisted of stonecutters, but since that time similar groups in various occupations have been described, including

Table 116-1 Arterial Diseases and Artery Affected

	Subclavian	Axillary	Brachial	Forearm	Hand
Atherosclerosis	•				
Giant cell arteritis	•				
Takayasu's disease	•	•			
Fibromuscular dysplasia		•			•
Embolic		•	•		•
Connective tissue disease				•	•
Diabetes mellitus				•	•
Repetitive trauma					•
Hypercoagulation					•
Cryoglobulins					•
Pressors/polyvinyl chloride					•

WARM   COLD

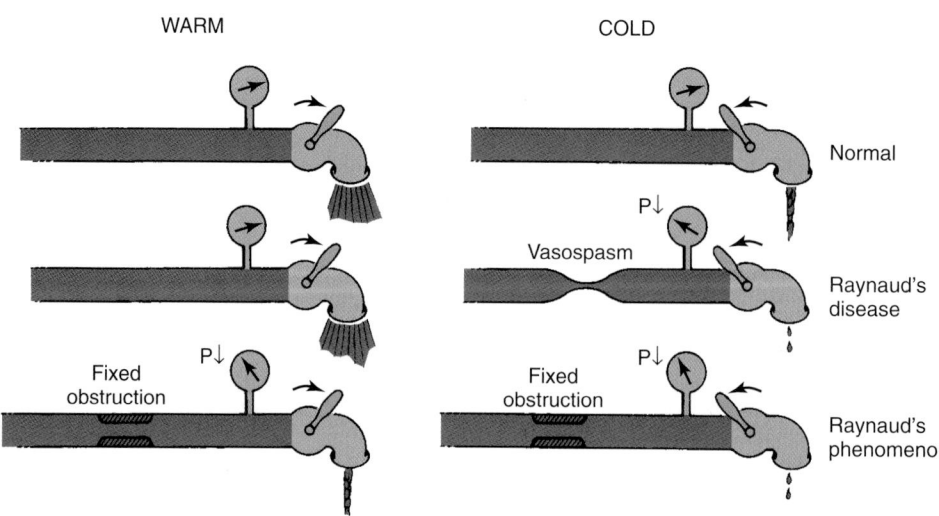

Figure 116-1 Effect of exposure to cold on normal fingers, fingers with primary Raynaud's disease, and fingers with Raynaud's phenomenon secondary to fixed arterial obstruction and vasospasm. Faucets represent arteriolar sphincters. When a faucet handle is turned to the right, the arterioles are dilated; when it is turned to the left, the arterioles are constricted. Gauges represent digital arterial pressure, with increasing pressure indicated by clockwise rotation of the handle. Digital blood flow is represented by the output of the faucets.

welders/grinders in shipyards, timber fellers, and most recently, windshield replacement technicians in the auto glass industry.[12] This condition has been termed hand-arm vibration syndrome (HAVS) or vibration-induced white finger (see Chapter 120: Occupational Vascular Problems). Patients with HAVS will first have Raynaud's syndrome, but in the late stage, usually after decades of using vibrating tools, digital artery occlusive disease is seen.[13,14] Not all vibrating tools appear to cause HAVS, however, and certain frequencies are now well substantiated in the occupational health literature to be associated with HAVS. HAVS appears to be a cumulative trauma injury in that there is a long latent period before workers become symptomatic. The theory is that the initial period of exposure causes little damage, subsequent use causes additive damage, but it is only after the damage has built up to a certain level that workers begin noting Raynaud's symptoms. Exposure of workers to these harmful frequencies—and consequently the development of HAVS—is now limited by occupational health agencies. The rules allow use of low-power tools for longer periods than tools that impart more energy to the worker's hands. These rules are meant to limit damage to workers so that they never cross the threshold to symptoms during their working lifetime.

Risk Factors

Risk factors for large-artery occlusive disease of the upper extremity are similar to those for arterial disease elsewhere in the body. Tobacco is the most significant risk factor, with hyperlipidemia, hypertension, diabetes, male gender, and age also being important (see Chapter 4: Atherosclerosis; Chapter 25: Atherosclerotic Risk Factors: General Considerations; Chapter 26: Atherosclerotic Risk Factors: Smoking; Chapter 27: Atherosclerotic Risk Factors: Diabetes; Chapter 28: Atherosclerotic Risk Factors: Hyperlipidemia; and Chapter 29: Atherosclerotic Risk Factors: Hypertension). Atherosclerosis may cause upper extremity ischemia through a variety of

mechanisms. The most common is occlusive disease, with involvement of the origin of the subclavian artery being a common finding in patients with significant atherosclerosis. Aneurysms of the upper extremity arteries are rare but can occur in the subclavian or axillary arteries. Patients with diabetes or renal failure, or both, particularly those undergoing dialysis, may have accelerated atherosclerosis and not infrequently have involvement of both large and small arteries of the upper extremity that can lead to significant hand ischemia.[15]

There are a number of less commonly seen causes of upper extremity arterial ischemia, including trauma, iatrogenic injury, fibromuscular dysplasia of the forearm and hand arteries, frostbite, and malignancy.[16-19] Furthermore, small aneurysms of branches of the axillary artery may develop from repetitive injury in athletes and result in distal embolization (see Chapter 120: Occupational Vascular Problems).

■ CLINICAL FINDINGS

Acute Ischemia

As with the lower extremities, patients may have acute or chronic symptoms of ischemia. Only 10% to 20% of patients with acute limb ischemia will have their upper extremity affected. This small group of patients is more likely to be female and to be older than those with lower extremity ischemia.[20] Patients with severe ischemia will have symptoms that include pain, paresthesias, and paralysis. Physical examination reveals a diminution or absence of brachial, radial, or ulnar pulses; pallor of the extremity; dependent rubor; and reduced temperature. Because of the rich collateral network in the upper extremity, acute occlusion of upper extremity arteries rarely results in tissue loss, although if it is left uncorrected patients will often have significant symptoms. It has been estimated that interruption of the axillary artery results in limb loss in less than 10% of cases and that interruption of the brachial artery distal to the deep brachial artery branch results in finger gangrene in less than 5% of cases. Surgical correction of acute upper extremity ischemia is described in Chapter 117 (Upper Extremity: Revascularization).

Chronic Ischemia

Patients with chronic upper extremity ischemia may complain only of a subjective change in sensation, hand temperature, and muscle pain with use. However, patients may also have digital and hand pain that may be associated with ulcers or gangrene of the digits. Findings on physical examination may be normal at rest, but typically the hand and digits are cool and the brachial and wrist pulses are reduced or absent. Chronic upper extremity ischemia may be seen in conjunction with dialysis access, and in the early stages the patient may complain only of ischemic pain while on dialysis.[15] In this situation a noticeable increase in wrist pulses or Doppler signals, or both, may be noted with fistula compression. Management of dialysis access steal is detailed in Chapter 75 (Hemodialysis Access: Nonthrombotic Complications).

◼ DIAGNOSTIC EVALUATION

Clinical Evaluation

Evaluation of patients with upper extremity ischemia begins with a detailed history and physical examination. The history should specifically focus on signs and symptoms of connective tissue disease such as dry eyes, dry mouth, and arthritis. Other pertinent historical details that should be sought are a history of trauma, even remote trauma, as well as an occupational history to determine whether the patient has used vibrating tools or been exposed to toxin.

Patients with complaints of digital artery ischemia should be examined in a warm room and during cold weather should be allowed to rewarm before being examined. A complete arterial examination, including bilateral brachial pressure, palpation of pulses, and Doppler insonation of the forearm arteries at the wrist and palmar arch, may provide valuable information about the level of arterial occlusion. Auscultation of the supraclavicular and infraclavicular fossae may lead to the detection of subclavian artery stenosis. The hands should be examined carefully and temperature, capillary refill, and ulcers or other lesions noted. The fingers should be examined for clubbing, sclerodactyly, and telangiectasia and the nail beds for splinter hemorrhages. Clubbing is associated with chronic pulmonary disease, and patients with clubbing and cold fingers may have low arterial oxygen levels as the basis of their complaints. Telangiectasia and sclerodactyly are commonly seen with advanced scleroderma but may occur with other connective tissue diseases. Splinter hemorrhages in the nail beds are seen with emboli. A complete upper extremity neurologic examination, including muscle mass, muscle strength, and sensation, may give important information regarding external compression of the neurovascular bundle, as well as advanced HAVS.

Vascular Laboratory Evaluation

Basic vascular laboratory testing consists of segmental pressure measurements of the upper extremity and finger pressure measurements and waveforms. These tests will detect the presence of arterial occlusive disease. Small-artery disease is defined as disease of the arteries within the hand. Typically, the arterial examination is normal to the level of the wrist, and finger pressure is reduced. With large-artery occlusive disease, arterial pressure is reduced at the wrist with no further reduction at the finger level. Cold sensitivity may be measured by a variety of testing methods, the simplest of which is recovery of finger temperature after immersion in ice water. In the presence of a classic history of cold-induced color changes, testing for cold sensitivity is not required for clinical diagnosis. A schematic approach outlining the evaluation process is shown in Figure 116-2. The noninvasive vascular laboratory tests listed typically provide the information needed to diagnose and treat patients with upper extremity arterial disease because most patients do not require invasive intervention. However, in a few patients, particularly those with significant

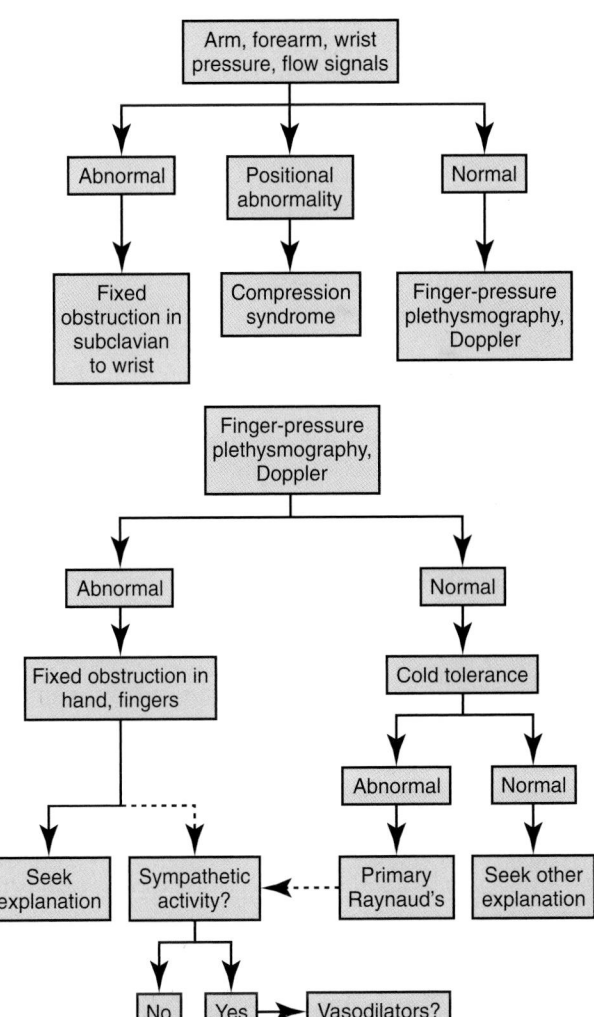

Figure 116-2 Approach to the noninvasive diagnosis of upper extremity ischemia. *(From Sumner DS. Noninvasive assessment of upper extremity and hand ischemia.* J Vasc Surg. *1986;3:560.)*

unilateral digital ischemia, a cause is not obvious, and further and more invasive evaluation is needed.

Other Imaging

If embolic disease is suspected, both duplex examination of the upper extremity arteries and transthoracic or transesophageal echocardiography are recommended. If these tests do not reveal a peripheral or cardiac source of emboli, the aortic arch and intrathoracic upper extremity arteries should be imaged. The arch and its branches are imaged well by arteriography, which also allows detailed digital artery views to be obtained. Both magnetic resonance arteriography (MRA) and computed tomographic arteriography (CTA) now provide excellent resolution, may give additional details through three-dimensional reconstructions, and are less invasive than catheter-based arteriography,[21] but if a patient has evidence of small-artery disease and either CTA or MRA is normal, catheter arteriography is indicated. At times the large-artery defect may be subtle, as can occur in arterial thoracic outlet disease. When unilateral hand or arm ischemia develops in an athlete, multiple views of the subclavian and axillary arteries should be obtained to detect small aneurysms in major arteries or their smaller branch vessels (see Chapter 120: Occupational Vascular Problems).

Arteriography, whether intra-arterial arteriography, CTA, or MRA, should be performed in both upper extremities because it is common to find bilateral arterial digital occlusion even when only one extremity is symptomatic, which is an indication of a systemic vascular disease. Thus, a patient with diffuse occlusion of all the fingers of both hands and high-titer antinuclear antibodies would not undergo further testing because the diagnosis of an underlying autoimmune disease is likely and an inflammatory arteritis is inferred. However, a patient with an acute onset of ischemia in two fingers and normal screening blood test results would have upper extremity arterial duplex ultrasonography, echocardiography, and bilateral arteriography recommended if the initial noninvasive vascular laboratory tests and blood tests did not provide a source for the ischemia.

Blood Tests

The basic blood tests needed to screen for underlying autoimmune disease include the erythrocyte sedimentation rate, C-reactive protein, antiphospholipid antibodies, antinuclear antibody titer, and rheumatoid factor. If these tests are negative, the likelihood of an underlying autoimmune disease is low. If positive, referral to a rheumatologist is indicated both for further delineation of the disease process and for treatment.

■ SELECTION OF TREATMENT

Patients who have normal results on physical examination, screening vascular laboratory tests, and blood work but a posi-

tive test for or a history of vasospasm with exposure to cold can safely be diagnosed as having primary Raynaud's syndrome and be reassured that they have a benign condition.[22] They are no more likely than the general population to have an autoimmune disease diagnosed in the future. In this group of patients symptoms wax and wane over time, depending on factors such as stress and climate, but progression to digit-threatening ischemia is extremely rare. Avoidance of cold is the mainstay of therapy in this group, with medical therapy added for the most severe cases (see Chapter 119: Raynaud's Syndrome).

Patients with occlusive disease and a negative test for autoimmune conditions may have large-artery disease, typically atherosclerosis, or small-artery disease from processes such as embolic events, industrial exposure, or hypersensitivity angiitis. This group has an intermediate risk for progression that is dependent on the natural history of the underlying cause of the obstruction.[22] Medical therapy is not particularly helpful in this group because no medications have clearly been demonstrated to increase resting blood flow distal to an occlusion.

Patients with both arterial obstruction and an underlying disease have the worst prognosis and the highest risk for ulceration and tissue loss. These patients are likely to progress slowly over time. Interestingly, if ulceration is not present at the initial consultation, it is unlikely to develop in the future, and those with ulceration have only a 50% chance of further ulceration developing.[22]

There are few surgical options for small-artery occlusive disease. Thoracic sympathectomy is not generally beneficial in improving blood flow and aiding healing of ischemic lesions (discussed in Chapter 121: Thoracic Sympathectomy). Sympathectomy is now often performed via a thoracoscopic approach, but there is little evidence that performing sympathectomy by this approach is as effective as performing it by a transcervical approach or thoracotomy.[23] Because the limited ability of thoracic sympathectomy to provide long-term relief may be due to collateral nerve pathways, periarterial digital sympathectomy performed in the common digital arteries in the hands has been suggested as a superior alternative, and a number of small series claim long-lasting benefit from such a procedure.[24,25]

Subclavian artery occlusion, subclavian artery aneurysm, thoracic outlet syndrome with arterial damage or occlusion, fibromuscular disease, and upper extremity arterial trauma with symptoms are best treated by revascularization. In the past this has been accomplished by open bypass, but over the last decade interventional techniques such as angioplasty with stenting and endovascular grafting have been used in some cases with good results. Revascularization options for large-artery occlusive disease are discussed in Chapter 117 (Upper Extremity Arterial Disease: Revascularization). If revascularization is unsuccessful or if the injury or subsequent ischemia leads to a nonviable extremity, amputation may be necessary. Upper extremity amputation is rare, and the options are discussed in Chapter 118 (Upper Extremity Arterial Disease: Amputation).

MEDICAL MANAGEMENT

Long-acting vasodilators work reasonably well in patients with primary Raynaud's syndrome, and about 50% of patients note improvement of symptoms and tolerance of medication. However, these drugs typically do not lead to symptomatic improvement in patients with occlusive Raynaud's syndrome. The two medications that have been shown to be beneficial in randomized double-blinded controlled trials are extended-release nifedipine at a dose of 30 mg daily and losartan, 50 mg twice daily.[26,27] Both medications reduce the severity and frequency of cold-induced symptoms in about 75% of patients, although some patients have significant side effects that cause them to discontinue the medications. Most of my patients do not take these medications year-round. Rather, they take them either from late fall to late spring or when they know that they will be facing significant cold exposure, such as during a ski vacation.

An exhaustive list of other medications that have been tried for symptomatic obstructive upper extremity ischemia is detailed in Chapter 119 (Raynaud's Syndrome). The mainstay of medical management for patients with atherosclerotic causes consists of control of risk factors, as discussed in Section 3 (Atherosclerotic Risk Factors).

SELECTED KEY REFERENCES

Brotzu G, Susanna F, Roberto M, Palmina P. Beta-blockers: a new therapeutic approach to Raynaud's disease. *Microvasc Res.* 1987;33:283-288.

This paper was one of the first reports that detailed how directed pharmacologic intervention in the microvascular control system could be used to treat Raynaud's syndrome. Although beta blockers are not currently used to treat Raynaud's syndrome, this paper was the first to attempt therapy based on a specific defect that had been identified in the microcirculation in patients.

Cherniack M, Brammer AJ, Lundstrom R, Meyer JD, Morse TF, Neely G, Nilsson T, Peterson D, Toppila E, Warren N. The Hand-Arm Vibration International Consortium (HAVIC): prospective studies on the relationship between power tool exposure and health effects. *J Occup Environ Med.* 2007;49:289-301.

This report summarizes current knowledge about the relationship between upper extremity ischemia and exposure to vibration.

Cooke JM, Marshall JM. Mechanisms of Raynaud's disease. *Vasc Med.* 2005;10:293-307.

This is an excellent summary of current knowledge about the pathophysiologic mechanisms of Raynaud's disease.

Edwards JM, Porter JM. Associated diseases with Raynaud's syndrome. *Vasc Med Rev.* 1990;1:51-58.

This paper gives an exhaustive summary of diseases that are associated with Raynaud's syndrome.

Landry GJ, Edwards JM, Taylor LM Jr, Porter JM. Long-term outcome of prospectively analyzed patients with Raynaud's syndrome. *J Vasc Surg.* 1996;23:76-86.

This report summarizes long-term clinical outcomes in a group of Raynaud's patients monitored for many years. This is one of the largest patient groups and provides important information on long-term clinical outcomes.

Walcher J, Strecker R, Goldacker S, Winterer J, Langer M, Bley TA. High resolution 3 tesla contrast-enhanced MR angiography of the hands in Raynaud's disease. *Clin Rheumatol.* 2007;26:587-589.

This report details what hopefully will be widely available in the near future in terms of minimally invasive detailed upper extremity arteriography.

REFERENCES

The reference list can be found on the companion Expert Consult Web site at *www.expertconsult.com.*

CHAPTER 117

Upper Extremity Arterial Disease: Revascularization

Sean P. Roddy and R. Clement Darling III

Upper extremity arterial occlusive disease is responsible for less than 5% of all cases of limb ischemia.[1] Even in high-volume centers, arm reconstructions account for only 3% of elective limb revascularizations. Palmar and digital artery occlusive disease is the most common cause of upper extremity ischemia, whereas large-vessel disease, including arteries proximal to the wrist, account for less than 10% of cases of upper extremity arterial occlusive disease. This chapter deals with revascularization for both acute and chronic ischemia involving the intrinsic arteries of the upper extremities, including the axillary, brachial, radial, ulnar, and palmar arteries. Raynaud's syndrome (see Chapter 119: Raynaud's Syndrome), thoracic outlet obstruction (see Chapter 124: Thoracic Outlet Syndrome: Arterial), and occlusive disease of the great vessels (see Chapter 100: Brachiocephalic Artery Disease: Surgical Treatment) are described elsewhere. Because the volume of these procedures is small, it is difficult to draw evidence-based conclusions on the optimal approach for patients with upper extremity ischemia. What is known is that patients with diabetes mellitus and chronic renal failure make up a significant proportion of those with digital gangrene. Treatment presents a challenge that often involves difficult reconstruction, meticulous wound care, and patience.

■ CLINICAL FINDINGS

Patients may have either acute or chronic ischemic symptoms, as discussed in detail in Chapter 116 (Upper Extremity Arterial Disease: General Considerations).

Acute Arm Ischemia

Arms with acute ischemia account for only a fifth of all acutely threatened limbs. Women are affected twice as often as men, and patients are significantly older than those with acute symptoms in the lower extremity.[2] Because most reports of acute arm ischemia generally involve those who required surgery, the denominator is difficult to calculate. Between 9% and 30% of patients seen by vascular surgeons with upper extremity arterial occlusive disease are managed conservatively because of significant co-morbid conditions or minimal symptomatology. Postoperative mortality rates for brachial embolectomy are as high as 12%.[3] However, after successful brachial embolectomy, 95% of patients will remain free of symptoms.[4] Patients managed conservatively are probably underreported in the literature. In the few reported series,

assessment of symptoms and disability tends to be inconsistent. However, in a series of 95 patients described by Baird and Lajos in 1964 with arm ischemia managed without surgery, 32% were left with permanent disability in the arm.[5] In 1977, Savelyev and coauthors reported that 75% of patients managed conservatively had a poor functional outcome.[6] More recently, in 1985 Galbraith and associates confirmed that 50% of their conservatively managed patients had persistent exercise-induced forearm pain (a claudication equivalent).[7] Therefore, although conservative management is appropriate for some patients with acute ischemia, for those with a reasonable life expectancy, all efforts should be made to restore blood flow.

Chronic Arm Ischemia

Whereas chronic leg ischemia is usually due to atherosclerosis, the causes of chronic arm ischemia are more diverse. Although atherosclerosis is still one etiology, consideration must be given to other pathologies such as thoracic outlet syndrome, iatrogenic injury after arm catheterization, and rarer causes such as Takayasu's or giant cell arteritis and radiation-induced injury. Hand and finger ischemia has been reported with increasing frequency in patients with end-stage renal disease.[8,9] The etiologic backgrounds of this disease process are multiple and include thrombosis, accelerated atherosclerosis, and diffuse arterial calcification. The origin of this condition may well involve atherosclerosis, but there is a well-described association with calciphylaxis.[10] Manifestations range from digital pain at rest and ulceration to gangrene. Initial assessment is by noninvasive studies such as pulse volume recordings or duplex ultrasound, followed by magnetic resonance or computed tomographic angiography. Confirmation of these findings can be obtained by aortic arch and arm catheter angiography. Occlusive lesions will be located in the axillary, brachial, or forearm arteries. Each requires separate treatment strategies.

Another clinical situation of hand ischemia encountered in patients with end-stage renal disease is that associated with an ipsilateral upper extremity arteriovenous fistula. The onset of hand ischemia is a devastating complication of upper extremity hemodialysis access. Arteriovenous shunts are almost always associated with some degree of reduced arterial flow to the distal circulation. Untreated, this may produce pain, ulceration, and gangrene in a previously viable extremity. Although prevention of this complication remains paramount,

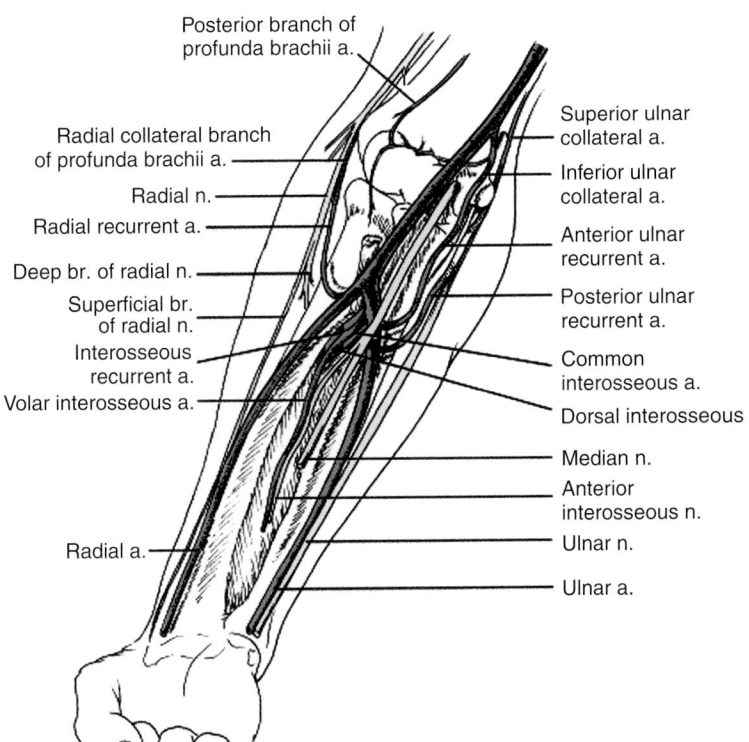

Figure 117-1 Forearm nerve and vessel anatomy. The brachial artery typically bifurcates just below the elbow. *(From Valentine RJ, Wind CG.* Anatomic Exposures in Vascular Surgery. *2nd ed. Philadelphia, PA: Lippincott Williams & Wilkins; 2003.)*

several techniques are available to manage this problem once diagnosed. Chapter 75 (Hemodialysis Access: Nonthrombotic Complications) describes the diagnosis and management of steal-associated ischemia and critical upper extremity ischemia caused by infrabrachial disease in renal failure patients.

REVASCULARIZATION

Endovascular Treatment

Endovascular therapies for the treatment of arterial occlusive disease have increased in popularity over the last decade with the improvement in catheter, balloon, and stent technology. The majority of lower extremity revascularizations in large vascular surgery practices are now done percutaneously. However, the upper extremity has not shared the same paradigm shift, possibly because of the infrequency of interventions or the causes of the arterial disease. Most institutional reviews that describe treatment of occlusions in the axillary, brachial, radial, and ulnar arteries still involve surgical bypass or embolectomy.[11,12] There are scattered reports of emergency placement of covered stents in the axillary artery in trauma patients.[13] There are also reports of small series of patients treated by axillary artery angioplasty for radiation-induced occlusion, by brachial artery atherectomy, and by radial artery stenting for digital gangrene, but their numbers are low and follow-up is minimal.[14-16] Therefore, dissection and exposure of the arterial anatomy for revascularization will

be described at the most common levels of intervention (Fig. 117-1).

Surgical Treatment

Arterial Exposure

Axillary Artery. The patient is placed supine and the arm is draped circumferentially. The axillary artery is exposed with a transverse incision 2 cm below the middle third of the clavicle (Fig. 117-2). The underlying pectoralis major muscle is divided, when possible, in the decussation between the sternal and clavicular portions. Despite the descriptions found in most operative texts, this point is not always readily apparent. Division of the pectoralis major exposes the clavipectoral fascia, which is divided. The axillary artery is located cephalic to the vein. It is dissected carefully to avoid injury to the surrounding cords of the brachial plexus. The second part of the axillary artery can be exposed by dividing the pectoralis minor muscle. If needed, the distal third of the axillary artery may also be exposed. An oblique incision is made along the lateral margin of the pectoralis major muscle with the arm abducted 90 degrees relative to the thorax. Once the subcutaneous tissue is divided, the axillary sheath is located near the posterior and inferior border of the coracobrachialis. Careful dissection avoids injury to the medial and lateral cords of the brachial plexus medially and the median and ulnar nerves laterally.

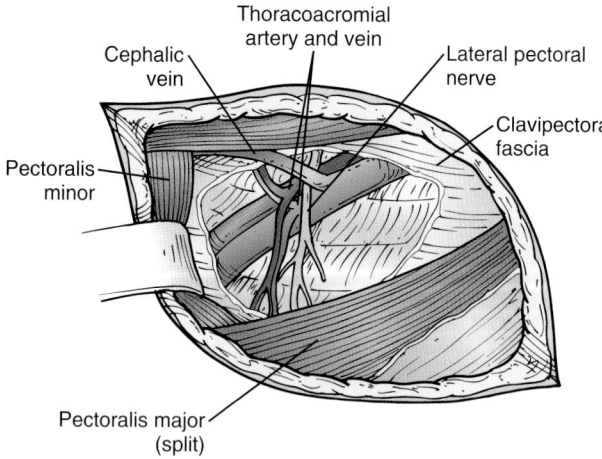

Figure 117-2 Exposure of the first portion of the axillary artery. The clavipectoral fascia is opened to expose the axillary sheath. The pectoral nerves and vessels, as well as the cephalic vein, are seen in the operative field.

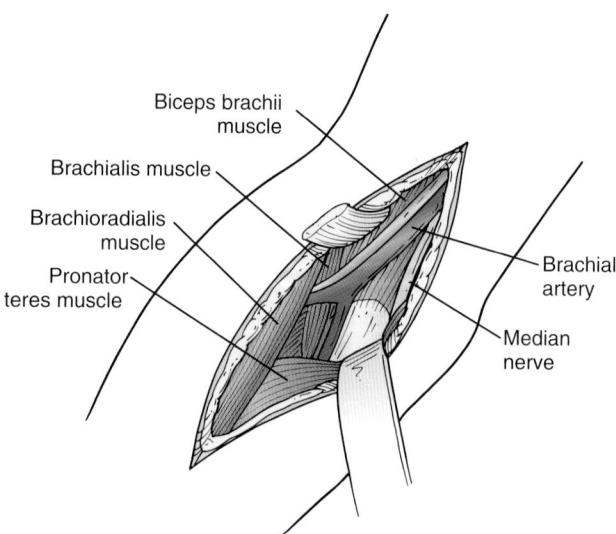

Figure 117-3 Exposure of the brachial artery at the elbow. The bifurcation of the brachial artery can be exposed by retracting the pronator teres and flexor muscle mass. The radial artery can be followed the length of the incision, but the larger ulnar artery dives between the heads of the flexor digitorum superficialis.

Brachial Artery. The mid or distal brachial artery is exposed through a medial incision over the bicipital groove. This allows access to the proximal or middle third of the brachial artery. The basilic vein and cutaneous branches of the median nerve are located within the subcutaneous tissue and should be avoided during dissection. Traction or transection of the median antebrachial cutaneous nerve may lead to hyperesthesia or anesthesia along the medial dorsal surface of the forearm. This occasionally occurs after dialysis access (e.g., basilic vein transposition) and can be debilitating for the patient. In some cases it can even preclude use of a patent and mature fistula. The brachial sheath is then incised longitudinally. The median nerve is the most superficial structure encountered. The nerve is gently mobilized and retracted to allow access to the brachial artery. Crossing vein branches should be divided to minimize the risk of injury to the posteriorly located ulnar nerve.

The distal third of the brachial artery and its bifurcation, in contrast, are exposed in the antecubital fossa (Fig. 117-3). A lazy S–shaped incision is recommended to expose the origins of the ulnar and radial arteries. Sometimes a vertical incision is used. However, there is a legitimate concern about contracture of the elbow with vertical incisions. The skin and subcutaneous tissues are divided. Care is taken to preserve the superficial veins, especially the median antecubital vein, because it may be required for autogenous patch angioplasty closure. The bicipital fascia is incised and the brachial artery is seen coursing between the biceps tendon laterally and the median nerve medially. Dissection is continued distally until the ulnar and radial arteries are encountered. The radial artery is really a continuation of the brachial artery. The ulnar artery, on the other hand, comes off the brachial artery medially and, within 2 to 3 cm, dives beneath the pronator and epitrochlear muscles.

Radial Artery. The course of the radial artery in the forearm follows an oblique line from the brachial artery pulse medial

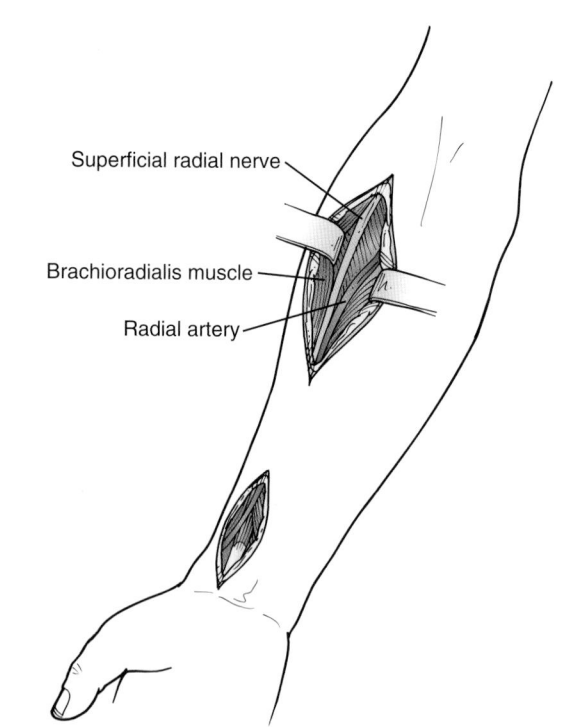

Figure 117-4 The radial artery in the midforearm can easily be exposed beneath the brachioradialis.

to the biceps tendon to the styloid process of the radius. In the midforearm, the radial artery is medial to the brachioradialis and lateral to the flexor carpi radialis. A lateral longitudinal incision is made. The muscles are separated to reveal the radial artery as needed (Fig. 117-4).

At the wrist the radial artery is exposed by a longitudinal incision between the tendons of the flexor carpi radialis and the brachioradialis muscles. This is the traditional site of the radial artery pulse in normal subjects. The artery is superficial and exposure is relatively straightforward. The superficial branch of the radial nerve is often located near the lateral aspect of the artery. Injury can result in troublesome paresthesias along the lateral aspect of the thumb.

Ulnar Artery. The ulnar artery extends from the medial epicondyle of the humerus to the pisiform bone. In the midforearm, the ulnar artery lies beneath the deep fascia between the bellies of the flexor digitorum laterally and the flexor carpi ulnaris medially (Fig. 117-5). The ulnar nerve joins the artery on its lateral aspect for its distal two thirds. It may be injured if not carefully identified and preserved.

At the wrist, the ulnar artery is lateral to the flexor carpi ulnaris (it is the most medial tendon palpable at the wrist). For exposure, this tendon is identified and a vertical skin incision is made lateral to it. The ulnar artery is relatively deeper than the radial artery at the wrist but just as easily exposed. The palmar cutaneous branches of the ulnar nerve are superficial to the artery here and should be preserved.

Interosseous Artery. The interosseous arteries of the forearm are naturally the smallest and most deeply situated of the forearm vessels. They are the embryologic analogue to the peroneal artery in the lower extremity, an artery of supply to the distal extremity musculature. The initial few millimeters of the common interosseous artery can be accessed by following the ulnar artery down from the bra-

chial artery, dividing some of the fibers of the superficial flexor digitorum, and looking for the large branch going lateral and deep from the ulnar artery.

The common interosseous bifurcates into an anterior (or volar) interosseous and a posterior (or dorsal) interosseous just proximal to the forearm interosseous membrane. Exposure of the length of the anterior interosseous artery is best done through the same incision used to expose the midportion of the ulnar artery and then to separate the flexor carpi ulnaris from the superficial flexor digitorum. After an incision long enough to release the fascia is made, the superficial flexor digitorum is elevated along with the median nerve and dissection is carried along the volar surface of the flexor digitorum profundus. Next, the flexor pollicis longus is elevated toward the radius to expose the anterior interosseous neurovascular bundle; some fibers of the flexor pollicis longus may partially cover the anterior interosseous artery and need to be divided. The posterior interosseous artery is best approached through a dorsal forearm skin incision along the medial aspect of the radius. This artery is usually smaller and less often used for revascularization.

Palmar Arteries. Exposure of the palmar arteries is not routinely performed in many vascular surgery centers. The blood supply of the hand is nourished by the superficial and deep palmar arches. The superficial palmar arch is supplied by a branch of the radial artery and the ulnar artery. The deep palmar arch is supplied by the radial artery itself and a deep branch of the ulnar artery. Exposure of the radial artery, ulnar artery, and superficial palmar arch is relatively straightforward, and these vessels match the distal tibial or pedal vessels in the leg in size. The deep palmar arch is much more difficult to expose and deeply located and thus is relatively inaccessible.

Exposure of the distal radial artery can be performed as described earlier. Alternatively, exposure can be accomplished by making a vertical incision over the anatomic snuff-box (the snuff-box lies between the extensor pollicis longus tendon posteriorly and the tendons of the extensor pollicis brevis and abductor pollicis longus anteriorly). After deepening of the incision through subcutaneous tissue, the radial artery can be exposed in the floor of the snuff-box (Fig. 117-6). Because there are no significant nerves at this level, it is often chosen as a site for hemodialysis access.

Exposure of the deep palmar arch, by contrast, is considerably more taxing and disabling. It runs across the palm at a level with the proximal border of the outstretched thumb. An incision is made along the medial border of the thenar eminence. Extensive dissection of the superficial and deep flexor tendons of the hand, as well as division of the oblique head of adductor pollicis, is required to gain access to its origin.

Distal ulnar artery and superficial palmar arch exposure is best accomplished via a curved incision along the lateral border of the hypothenar eminence (Fig. 117-7). The aponeurotic layer is divided and the artery is then exposed in the upper part of the palm at the origin of the superficial palmar arch. No major nerves pass in the vicinity, and a reasonable

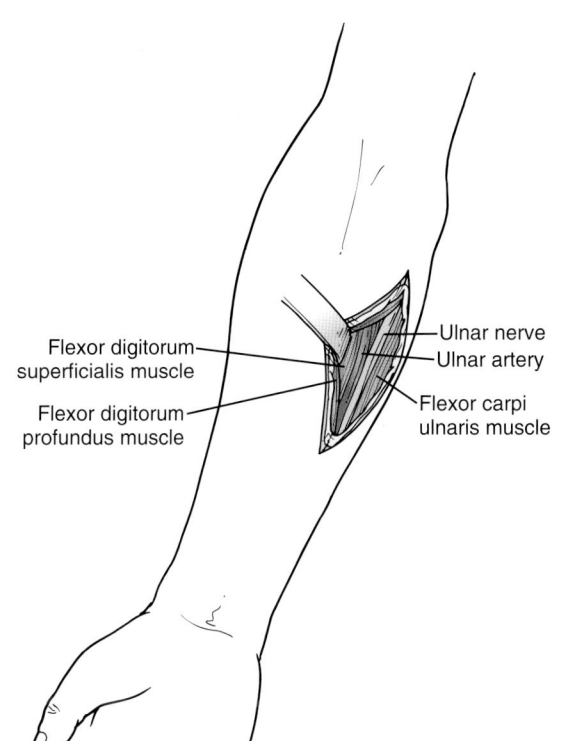

Figure 117-5 Exposure of the forearm ulnar artery. The ulnar artery in the midforearm is reached between the flexor carpi ulnaris and flexor digitorum superficialis.

Flexor digitorum superficialis muscle
Flexor digitorum profundus muscle
Ulnar nerve
Ulnar artery
Flexor carpi ulnaris muscle

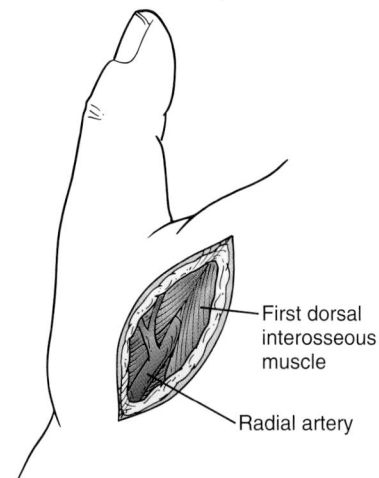

Figure 117-6 The segment of radial artery beyond the extensor pollicis longus tendon is exposed.

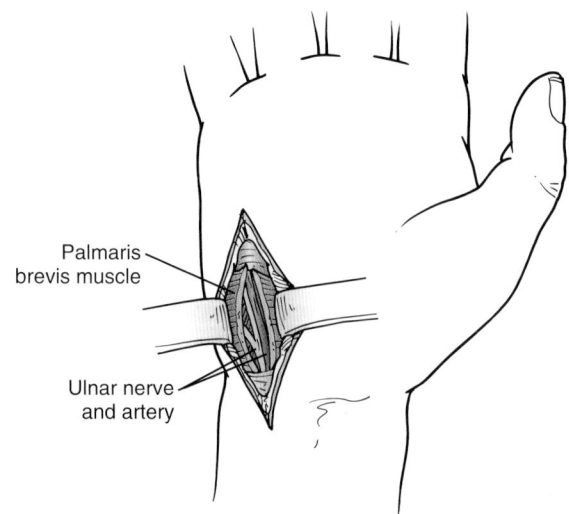

Figure 117-7 The ulnar artery and nerve beyond the tunnel of Guyon are exposed beneath the palmaris brevis muscle and hypothenar fascia.

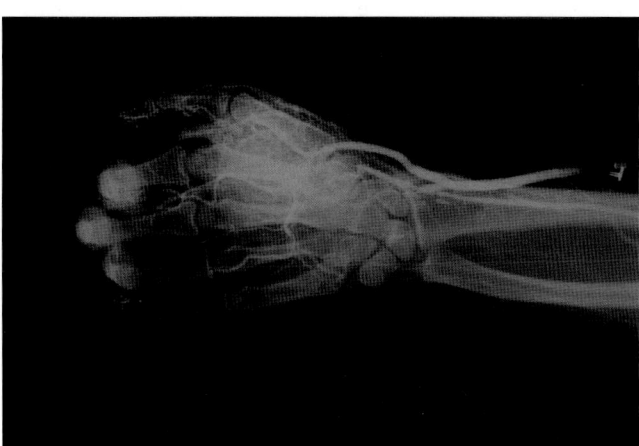

Figure 117-8 Palmar artery bypass completion arteriogram.

length of artery can usually be exposed for an arterial anastomosis. Alternatively, the superficial palmar arch can be exposed in the palm by making an incision along one of the larger vertical or oblique skin creases.

Bypass Conduit and Tunneling

Autogenous vein is the conduit of choice for upper extremity reconstructions. The great saphenous vein is preferable, although use of in situ cephalic vein has been described.[17] The more joints that the bypass crosses, the lower the patency rate.[18] After systemic heparinization, the venous conduit is excised and its side branches ligated with fine polypropylene suture or silk ties. The vein is distended with a solution of dextran, heparin, and papaverine (500-mL bag of dextran 40 + 120 mg papaverine + 1000 units heparin). The excised conduit may be used in either reversed or orthograde (nonreversed) orientation, depending on the taper of the conduit. If orthograde orientation is used, the proximal anastomosis is performed, the conduit is distended, and the valves are rendered incompetent by passage of a retrograde Mills valvulotome. Prosthetic reconstructions in this setting have lower patency rates than do venous bypasses and should be avoided.[11] Management of infection in prosthetic grafts can also be challenging.

Bypasses originating from the axillary artery are preferably tunneled anatomically along the axis of the axillary and brachial arteries because they are then less prone to movement or distortion. They may also be positioned anteriorly in the subcutaneous plane. However, superficial bypasses are more prone to distraction injuries from forcible abduction of the shoulder. Therefore, redundancy is paramount to avoid harming the conduit. As another alternative, there is at least one case report of a retrohumeral approach for tunneling an axillary-based reconstruction.[19]

Bypasses based on brachial artery inflow are most often tunneled in the subcutaneous plane. This facilitates physical examination for appropriate evaluation of bypass patency,

ensures surveillance of the bypass with duplex if readily available, and avoids manipulation of the rich forearm nerve network. Alternatively, if good-quality basilic or cephalic veins are present, an in situ bypass may be performed.

In the case of distal radial artery reconstructions, the graft is tunneled over the anatomic snuff-box onto the dorsum of the hand, between the thumb and index finger, to join the deep palmar arch (Fig. 117-8) or even a digital vessel in the absence of a complete arch (Fig. 117-9). In the case of ulnar artery reconstruction, the course of the vein graft is more direct and it passes superficial to the flexor retinaculum at the wrist to join the superficial palmar arch.

Transbrachial Embolectomy

The majority of arm emboli are cardiac in origin (75%). The most common site for emboli is the brachial artery (60%), followed by the axillary artery (26%). In situ thrombosis accounts for only 5% of episodes of arm ischemia.[20] Usually, there is an underlying embolic source such as atrial

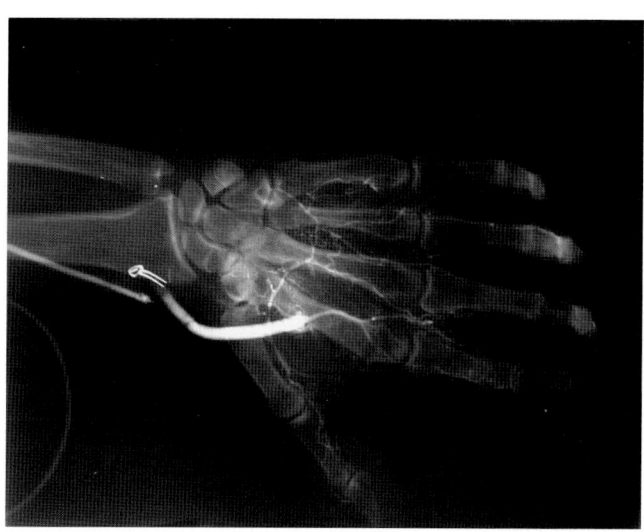

Figure 117-9 Digital artery bypass completion arteriogram.

fibrillation. The majority of brachial embolectomies are performed under local anesthesia with monitored anesthesia care.

When an embolectomy is planned, several considerations are essential. If preoperative imaging (usually duplex ultrasound) has demonstrated occlusion of the distal brachial artery, it is important to expose the origins of both forearm arteries because the embolectomy catheter must be passed down each artery. If the catheter is passed blindly down the brachial artery, it will most likely travel down the radial artery. This will probably re-establish flow to the hand in the majority of patients. However, it may fail to restore adequate flow if the ulnar is the dominant arterial blood supply or if the catheter passes down the common interosseous artery, which does not provide any direct flow to the hand. We usually make a vertical arteriotomy in the brachial artery. Clot, frequently encountered at the bifurcation, can readily be removed. The brachial artery may be pulseless, indicative of an embolus lodged more proximally. However, one concern with proximal passage of an embolectomy catheter is dislodgment of debris that may embolize the vertebral artery near the origin of the subclavian artery. If there is any concern, contrast-enhanced angiography is warranted to define the anatomy. Once inflow is established, a size 2 or 3 embolectomy catheter is passed distally down each forearm vessel. The arteriotomy can be closed primarily with running fine polypropylene suture if the artery is sufficiently large. If there is any doubt, the artery should be closed with a vein patch. Usually, a segment of vein can be harvested from the antecubital fossa.

After closure, an intraoperative continuous wave Doppler probe should be applied to each artery to ensure the presence of adequate flow. Completion angiography is at the discretion of the surgeon but should be performed if the hand still appears ischemic, especially if extensive thrombus has been extracted from forearm arteries. Occasionally, embolization may have been a chronic process and resulted in distal arterial occlusion that cannot be completely resolved with embolectomy, but arteriography can be used to detect residual fresh thromboembolic material. If there is any suspicion of an inflow lesion, intraoperative arteriography can be performed by either the femoral or brachial route to diagnose and treat such lesions.

Postoperative Management and Follow-up

Postoperatively, surveillance with pulse volume recordings or Doppler segmental pressure measurements can be used to document the adequacy of the bypass. Duplex ultrasonography is used to determine the patency of the reconstruction and allow early detection of stenoses during surveillance of the venous conduit. Anticoagulation is essential after embolectomy. Recurrent embolization occurs in a third of patients after successful embolectomy if systemic anticoagulation is not instituted. Even in patients placed on warfarin in Edinburgh after embolectomy, 11% sustained a further embolus if they had ongoing atrial fibrillation.[2]

Complications

Major complications that may occur after upper extremity arterial surgery include brachial plexus and median or ulnar nerve injury. Such injury is usually a result of traction and should be avoided by careful dissection during operative exposure. The use of electrocautery should be minimized to lessen the chance of direct thermal injury to the underlying nerves at all levels.

As with any arterial bypass, graft thrombosis can also occur. Some series found female smokers and patients with longer bypasses crossing multiple joints to have the lowest patency.[11,20] An inflow lesion in the subclavian artery can also cause acute arm ischemia (e.g., ulcerated plaque, thrombosed subclavian artery aneurysm, or arterial thoracic outlet syndrome). In such situations, even a technically perfect brachial embolectomy will fail to restore normal hand perfusion. Moreover, if the arteries are relatively free of atherosclerotic disease, embolectomy of the distal radial and ulnar vessels may result in arterial spasm. This problem is more commonly seen in women and children. However, it is a diagnosis of exclusion, and the first priority must be removal of retained embolic debris. If spasm is identified, topical or intra-arterial vasodilators such as papaverine, warm saline irrigation, and time should relieve the constriction and result in an adequately perfused hand.

■ ALTERNATIVE THERAPY

Sympathectomy has been used with isolated reports of success,[21,22] but the experience in most centers has been less than optimal (see Chapter 121: Thoracic Sympathectomy). Thrombolysis of acutely occluded axillary or brachial arteries has been described with reasonable outcomes.[23] However, in one large series, success was reported in just over half of the limbs treated, and 8 of 55 patients required surgical thrombectomy.[24]

There have also been reports of excellent outcomes of acute arm ischemia with the use of rotational thrombectomy devices such as the Straub Rotarex system (Straub Medical, Wangs, Switzerland) or the Omnisonics OmniWave device (OmniSonics Medical Technologies, Inc., Wilmington, MA).[25] However, experience is limited to case reports, with no large published series.

TRAUMA

Upper extremity trauma is relatively frequent and can be iatrogenic or noniatrogenic (see Chapter 153: Vascular Trauma: Thoracic and Chapter 155: Vascular Trauma: Extremity).

Iatrogenic Trauma

Brachial Artery

Brachial artery pseudoaneurysm or occlusion related to cardiac catheterization is one of the most common indications for arterial surgery in the upper extremity.[26] The presence of a pseudoaneurysm may be suggested by a mass at the puncture site, evidence of distal occlusion or embolization, or neurologic complications related to compression within the sheath, usually in the nature of paresthesias. The diagnosis can generally be made with duplex ultrasonography (Fig. 117-10), and direct repair with evacuation of the hematoma compressing the median nerve can be performed under local anesthesia. Occlusion of the brachial artery as a result of catheter insertion often requires more extensive reconstruction that usually involves a segmental bypass with either saphenous vein or cephalic vein from the ipsilateral arm. If recognized promptly, any propagated thrombus that may be present either proximal or distal to the puncture site can be extracted with a balloon embolectomy catheter. Delayed recognition of this problem will often necessitate a longer-segment interposition graft with autogenous vein.

Radial Artery

The radial artery is the second most common site of upper extremity iatrogenic arterial injury as a result of catheterization. Partial or complete occlusion of the radial artery after cannulation for monitoring purposes was apparent in 25% of 1699 patients undergoing cardiovascular surgery in a series by Slogoff and colleagues. None of these patients had hand ischemia.[27] Fortunately, with the usually good collateral filling across the palm from the ulnar artery, although the involved hand may be clinically pale, with depressed Doppler or pulse volume waveforms, usually the fingers remain viable with intact neurologic function. Unless there is some obvious evidence of severe cyanosis demarcation, neuropathy, or sensorimotor deficit, we would generally recommend a period of observation after removal of the arterial catheter. Heparinization is desirable but not mandatory. Many of these cases will improve with conservative treatment. In the few cases in which the hand either acutely or subacutely appears to be severely ischemic, repair with a short autogenous bypass of the radial artery above and below the puncture site is usually sufficient to effect improvement. Radial and ulnar artery vascular access for cardiac catheterization using up to 6 Fr sheath systems is increasing. Occlusion rates have been reported to be approximately 5% in either vessel,[28] and the overwhelming majority are asymptomatic.

Noniatrogenic Trauma

Trauma related to blunt injury or penetrating trauma is unfortunately a common source of upper extremity problems.[29]

Penetrating Trauma

Penetrating trauma is generally evident on evaluation in the emergency department. Repair of the injury is not usually

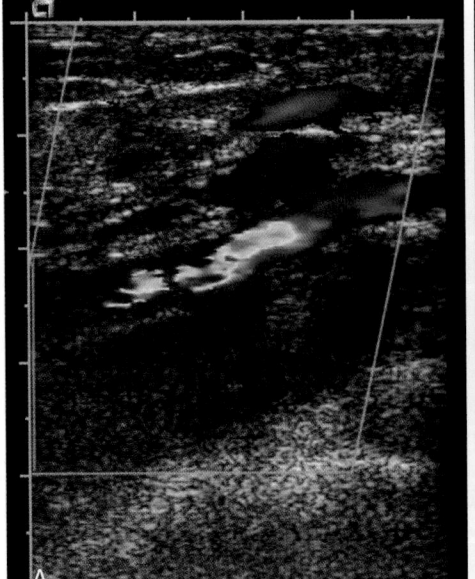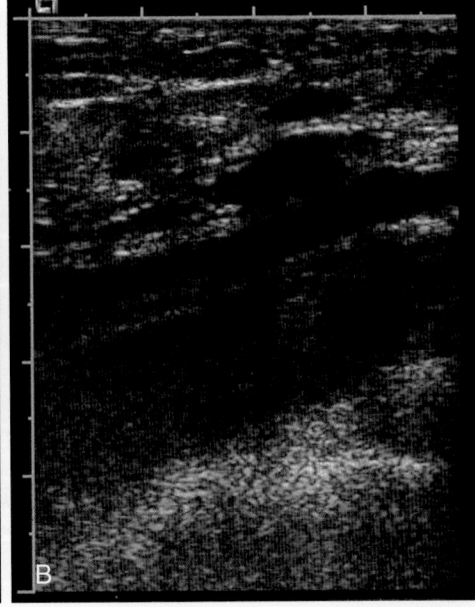

Figure 117-10 Brachial artery pseudoaneurysm after cardiac catheterization as seen through color duplex (**A**) and B-mode (**B**) ultrasound imaging.

complex, but obtaining proximal arterial control can be challenging. Injury to the subclavian arteries may require anterior thoracotomy or a trapdoor-type incision, or both (see Chapter 153: Vascular Trauma: Thoracic). Injury to the axillary arteries is often best managed by prior exposure of the subclavian artery from a supraclavicular approach. Proximal control of the brachial arteries can usually be managed with a more proximal medial upper arm incision. Radial and ulnar artery injuries can often be managed with relatively local control, although exposure of the brachial artery at the elbow is always an option. Alternatively, application of a tourniquet may allow direct wound exploration. Patients with isolated radial or ulnar artery injuries and clinical evidence of satisfactory hand perfusion in all five digits can be managed by ligation of the affected artery. However, it is often not much more difficult to simply repair the involved artery with local vein. Whether to ligate or bypass an isolated forearm arterial injury in a pink viable hand is still debated.

Delayed Recognition

Delayed recognition of arterial injury related to penetrating trauma may occasionally result in pseudoaneurysm formation, and sometimes arteriovenous fistulae are also formed by this kind of injury. Consequently, there should be a relatively low threshold for obtaining arterial imaging for any penetrating trauma that may produce an arterial injury. Many forearm injuries related to broken glass may produce an occult radial or ulnar artery injury that is not identified at the initial inspection but may result in further hemorrhage and even the development of compartment syndrome days later. Given the potential difficulty with follow-up of these patients, imaging at the time of initial evaluation is recommended to avoid delayed recognition of these injuries.

Blunt Trauma

Management of blunt trauma producing arterial injury is somewhat more complicated because of the difficulty in diagnosing and localizing the injury. The force of an impact strong enough to injure the artery may result in associated neurologic compromise and long-bone fracture. Frequently, these patients benefit from preoperative arteriography. Ongoing hemorrhage is not generally the problem, and exposure can be directed at the injured site. However, it is also more likely that there will be associated extensive venous injury and the development of venous hypertension after reconstruction of the arterial lesion. In these cases, either direct repair of the vein or a short autogenous bypass of the injured venous segment is useful to decompress the venous hypertension in the affected arm and thereby decrease the swelling and continued hemorrhage from the wound, although this remains controversial.[30]

Pediatric Supracondylar Fractures

One area of controversy is the treatment of type III supracondylar fractures of the humerus in children who lack a palpable radial pulse after the injury. Long-term ischemia from arterial occlusion in a child may lead to Volkmann's contracture, which results in permanent flexion and a clawlike deformity of the hand and fingers. The brachial artery may be pinched, avulsed, or thrombosed as it wraps around the fracture site. Orthopedic reduction is the accepted first treatment, with neurovascular re-evaluation after stabilization. If the pulse returns, no further treatment is necessary besides observation. If it does not and the hand appears white, pale, and ischemic, operative exploration is preferred. Debate exists in the literature regarding the optimal treatment when the pulse is not palpable but the hand is pink and viable. Some describe a conservative approach with serial examination.[31] Others favor aggressive operative reconstruction whenever possible,[32] either direct arterial repair with patch angioplasty or bypass using the great saphenous vein around the area of injury. Care must be taken with arterial manipulation in children to avoid spasm whenever possible. Fortunately, the incidence of this type of upper extremity ischemia is low.

TAKAYASU'S ARTERITIS AND GIANT CELL ARTERITIS

Takayasu's arteritis and giant cell arteritis frequently involve the subclavian and axillary arteries.[33] Takayasu's arteritis typically occurs in a young woman in the second or third decade and is associated with an acute or subacute illness with fever, malaise, arthralgias, abdominal pain, weight loss, and myalgias (see Chapter 78: Takayasu's Disease). Giant cell arteritis differs in that it is more frequently seen in women in the fifth decade or later (see Chapter 76: Vasculitis and Other Arteriopathies). Constitutional symptoms are similar, with frequent involvement of the ophthalmic and posterior ciliary arteries.

Treatment of both these diseases often requires corticosteroid therapy and, in some cases, other immunosuppressive drugs. Giant cell arteritis typically responds well to corticosteroids, whereas Takayasu's arteritis more frequently requires the addition of other agents such as cyclophosphamide. Frequently, treatment is maintained for several weeks until the erythrocyte sedimentation rate has normalized and the patient's constitutional symptoms have improved. Maintenance therapy over years is useful to prevent relapse.

Arterial reconstruction in these patients is more successful after the acute illness has been treated, and therefore operations should be delayed if at all possible.[34] Surgery during the time of acute inflammation is much more likely to result in acute occlusion of the bypass and should be avoided. Treatment of distal subclavian or axillary artery disease (or both) can be performed with either an endovascular treatment such as balloon angioplasty or a prosthetic or saphenous vein graft, depending on the relative size of the artery and the available conduit.[14] Involvement of the aortic arch and arch vessels with type I Takayasu's arteritis may require either direct aortic reconstruction through a median sternotomy or extra-anatomic revascularization such as femoroaxillary artery prosthetic bypass in some cases.

SELECTED KEY REFERENCES

Babu SC, Piccorelli GO, Shah PM, Stein JH, Clauss RH. Incidence and results of arterial complications among 16,350 patients undergoing cardiac catheterization. *J Vasc Surg.* 1989;10:113-116.
Review of adverse outcomes after arterial catheterization in an extensive patient population.

Chang BB, Roddy SP, Darling RC 3rd, Maharaj D, Paty PS, Kreienberg PB, Ozsvath KJ, Mehta M, Shah DM. Upper extremity bypass grafting for limb salvage in end-stage renal failure. *J Vasc Surg.* 2003;38:1313-1315.
A series that describes the technique, conduit, and results in patients with chronic renal insufficiency who underwent upper extremity bypass.

Myers SI, Harward TR, Maher DP, Melissinos EG, Lowry PA. Complex upper extremity vascular trauma in an urban population. *J Vasc Surg.* 1990;12:305-309.
Review of the interventions for complex upper extremity trauma with arterial injury.

Nehler MR, Dalman RL, Harris EJ, Taylor LM Jr, Porter JM. Upper extremity arterial bypass distal to the wrist. *J Vasc Surg.* 1992;16:633-640; discussion 640-642.
A series that describes the feasibility of revascularization to the distal part of the arm.

Roddy SP, Darling RC 3rd, Chang BB, Kreienberg PB, Paty PS, Lloyd WE, Shah DM. Brachial artery reconstruction for occlusive disease: a 12-year experience. *J Vasc Surg.* 2001;33:802-805.
This is a large series of brachial artery reconstructions that demonstrates the infrequency of the operation but also that the interventions can result in limb salvage.

REFERENCES

The reference list can be found on the companion Expert Consult Web site at *www.expertconsult.com.*

CHAPTER 118

Upper Extremity Arterial Disease: Amputation

Niten N. Singh and W. Darrin Clouse

Based in part on a chapter in the previous edition by Joyesh K. Raj, MD, and Michael J. V. Gordon, MD.

Upper extremity amputation remains infrequent in today's vascular surgery practice. Loss of a portion of the arm and hand is usually a devastating and life-altering event. Although surgical therapies may be aimed either at initial salvage attempts or, with reconstructive principles in mind, at maximizing function after amputation, such efforts are only the beginning of a life full of challenges for these individuals. Rehabilitative, social, financial, and psychological considerations are important and may be different from those with lower extremity loss.

■ EPIDEMIOLOGY

In 2005, there were some 1.6 million amputees living in the United States, with upper extremity amputees accounting for 541,000 of them, and it is anticipated that these numbers will more than double over the next 4 decades.[1] Approximately 185,000 patients undergo amputation each year in the United States, and it is estimated that anywhere from 10% to 25% of these amputations involve the arm and hand.[1,2] It seems that this relative proportion remains constant as the overall number of amputations performed increases. Most amputations in the upper extremity (93%) involve minor amputation at the wrist or within the digits.

Etiology

The majority of upper extremities requiring amputation are the result of trauma (80% to 90%).[1,2] It is not surprising, then, that upper extremity amputees are generally younger (20 to 40 years old on average) and predominantly male. Other etiologies do contribute, however. Vascular disease and tumors are the next most common indications and represent 7% and 0.6% of upper extremity amputations, respectively.[1,2] Even less frequent causes include infections, congenital anomalies, and iatrogenic reasons, such as complications related to catheterization, vasopressors, and vascular access. Thus, the general indications for amputation of portions of an arm or hand include tissue destruction, vascular compromise, and tumor. This overall distribution is in contradistinction to that of lower extremity amputation, where vascular disease is the inciting etiology in near 80%.[1,2]

Ischemia as the cause of upper extremity amputation usually results from trauma. Atherosclerosis is distinctly less common in the arteries of the arm and is a rare form of peripheral arterial disease.[3] Even in more chronic scenarios, the most frequent reason for upper extremity revascularization is traumatic injury.[4,5] Emboli from more proximal atherosclerotic or cardiac origins are much more common than chronic occlusive disease.[6] Occupational arterial trauma is relevant to the arm, and several are well described (see Chapter 120: Occupational Vascular Problems). Such trauma may include vibration-induced white finger, hypothenar hammer syndrome, and athletic-associated conditions such as quadrilateral space syndrome and arterial thoracic outlet compression resulting in subclavian aneurysm. Arterial trauma or embolization related to drug use has clearly been illustrated. Apart from atherosclerosis, a variety of less common arterial disorders leading to extremity arterial insufficiency may affect the arm, including vasospastic disorders (e.g., Raynaud's disease), small-vessel diseases (e.g., Buerger's disease), and radiation-induced arteritis.

Trauma and Military Injuries

Recent experiences from Operation Iraqi Freedom (OIF) and the Global War on Terrorism (GWOT) have provided some new insight into traumatic vascular injury of the upper extremity and upper extremity amputation. Such insight is mostly due to the significance of extremity injury during this conflict and war in general. Many of the principles of amputation were developed during the American Civil War and persist today. Stansbury and colleagues characterized the amputations that occurred in 8000 U.S. troops after injuries to extremities during the first 5 years of GWOT.[7] They found that 7.4% of major limb injuries required amputation. This is not unique, however, because a purported need for amputation occurred in more than 8% of extremities during the Vietnam War. In both wars, some 18% of amputees required multiple limb amputations.

Interestingly, the experience in the upper extremity is somewhat different from that in the lower one. With nearly 3400 major upper extremity injuries recorded, the arm amputation rate was 3.1%. This figure is in contrast to a rate of 8.5% in almost 4000 major lower extremity injuries, even though the incidence of neurovascular injury was similar in the two groups at approximately 15%. The authors surmised that this disparity could be related to several factors. Nearly 90% of extremity injuries were due to explosive mechanisms, which are most common at ground level such that the legs may sustain more significant destruction. Furthermore, the increased infection and nonunion rates cited in the lower extremities may have played a role. Finally, the surgical push for arm salvage because of limited functional prosthetic options for the upper extremity may have created a higher threshold for amputation.

Nevertheless, the experience in Iraq clearly depicts the seriousness of arterial injury in the upper extremity during OIF.[8,9] At the 332nd EMDG (Expeditionary Medical Support Group) Air Force Theater Hospital in Balad, Iraq, almost 10% of patients with upper extremity arterial injury who underwent arm salvage treatment ultimately lost the limb in the early period. Yet if those sustaining upper extremity arterial trauma are able to be successfully revascularized, the prospect of limb salvage into the later phases of treatment and rehabilitation is excellent.[10] This reaffirms a small body of literature indicating that in those with significant neurovascular, bony, and soft tissue upper extremity injury, aggressive limb salvage attempts are often successful.[11-20] Moreover, even though disability after upper limb salvage is usual, intensive therapy can lead to improvement over the longer term. Thus, unless absolutely clear from a destructive or systemic indication, early amputation should be avoided. The extreme views on this topic are seen in communications by those espousing limb reimplantation techniques.[21,22] Furthermore, the visibility of upper extremity amputation in our GWOT troops has led to an appreciation by society and produced an environment whereby prosthetic technologies, broadened therapeutic applications, and rehabilitative principles have been advanced for those missing a segment of an arm or hand.

Nontraumatic Disease

When nontraumatic vascular compromise in the upper extremity is the pathologic pathway leading to a limb-threatening process, treatment should be directed at correction of the underlying condition. This may be relatively simple and systemic, such as cessation of smoking in those with Buerger's disease; operatively straightforward, as with thromboembolectomy; or more complex and infrequent, such as sympathectomy for vasospastic diseases and bypasses, with or without thrombolytic therapy, for occlusive disease. Should the process affecting the upper extremity be focal, the surgical principles of treating limb-threatening conditions apply so that the best possible function can be provided for the patient. Unfortunately, some diseases involving the arm and hand are more diffuse, lead to regional pain syndrome, are difficult to treat, and have less clearly described therapeutic outcomes. All of this may proceed to a final pathway that simply requires some form of amputation. If such is the case, the principle of conservatism and conservation of parts is critical because aggressive surgical procedures may both aggravate the ischemic process and impede eventual function.

■ GENERAL OPERATIVE CONSIDERATIONS

Initial Management

As stated earlier, the majority of amputations are secondary to trauma and are usually managed in staged fashion to pre-serve as much of the arm as possible. This principle dates back to the care of battlefield injuries during World War II.[23] As opposed to the lower extremity, which requires only adequate soft tissue coverage in anticipation of a functional prosthesis, an upper extremity amputation must be both functional and cosmetically acceptable. With this in mind, definitive decisions on the level and length of amputation should not be made in the acute setting. Sequential stepwise débridement and later definitive closure are the keys to successful technical and functional results. One of the advancements over recent years is wound care and wound bed preparation before closure. The use of negative pressure therapy to promote granulation and assist in flap and graft coverage has become a mainstay in treatment. This technology is used even in the modern battlefield scenario, with multiple débridements and placement of these devices early after injury.[24] Although the basic techniques of surgery and débridement have not changed, emotional and functional rehabilitation has improved dramatically. Advancements in prosthesis design and functionality have allowed these patients to return to meaningful positions in today's society. Factors that play major roles in individualizing the surgical strategy for upper extremity amputation include etiology, age, handedness, occupation, associated injuries and physiologic state, accessibility to state-of-the-art occupational and physical therapies, and cultural settings.

Arterial Assessment

For both traumatic and nontraumatic indications, the level of upper extremity amputation required fundamentally depends on adequate arterial perfusion. The use of physical examination in conjunction with noninvasive studies such as duplex ultrasound, segmental pressure measurement, pulse volume recording, infrared photoplethysmography, laser Doppler techniques, transcutaneous oxygen tension ($tcPo_2$) measurement, and occasionally even arteriography before amputation can ensure that no ischemic component of the injury will prevent healing. Each evaluation technique has benefits and shortcomings. As described in Chapter 116 (Upper Extremity Arterial Disease: General Considerations) and Chapter 117 (Upper Extremity Arterial Disease: Revascularization), use of noninvasive tests can be invaluable in facilitating success. This is no less true in amputation, and though rare when compared with lower extremity evaluation, low pressure, poor arterial waveforms, and low $tcPo_2$ along the extremity must be recognized and management altered appropriately.

Guidance suggesting the appropriate blood flow for healing at specific levels has largely been described for lower extremity amputation (see Chapter 114: Lower Extremity Amputation: General Considerations). Within the context of tissue perfusion, however, these same principles can be applied to the upper extremity. Generally, healing will occur at the hand level when digital pressure is 40 mm Hg or higher and wrist Doppler pressure is above 60 mm Hg. For hand-level procedures, healing is unlikely to occur when digital pressure is less than 20 mm Hg. At the forearm and arm levels, healing will almost always take place when wrist or brachial pressure is at least 60 mm Hg or when tcPo$_2$ is 40 mm Hg or greater. Healing is less predictable when tcPo$_2$ is between 20 and 40 mm Hg and wrist or brachial Doppler pressure is less than 50 mm Hg. Pulse volume recordings may provide evidence of collateralization and suggest a higher likelihood of success, yet they remain nonspecific when blunted. Once a level for amputation is chosen, simple ligation of blood vessels during the procedure is usually sufficient as long as tissue coverage of these structures can be obtained.

Preservation of Length

Although preservation of length is a fundamental principle of amputation surgery, length does not always correlate directly with function, depending on the type of prosthetic application contemplated. However, in general it is important to retain and salvage as much residual stump as possible to maximize the ultimate functional outcome. To this end, several reconstructive techniques have been described to salvage stump length,[25-30] including plastic and orthopedic surgery techniques such as bone and free tissue transfer. These techniques have been applied selectively and may be helpful in certain instances, particularly elective planned procedures when the cause is tumor resection or isolated traumatic injury and the procedures may need to be performed in staged fashion. Length-preservation techniques have a limited role when the underlying pathology involves vascular insufficiency because of concern for viability and perfusion of the grafted tissue. Moreover, selective reimplantation methods and even hand transplantation have been suggested in an attempt to maintain viable, functional tissue and length for the upper extremity.[21,22,31] In fact, in select scenarios, such as clean traumatic severing without much tissue loss or associated trauma, these methods must be given initial consideration. However, in most acute trauma settings this decision cannot be made, and minimizing loss of length should be the goal. One concept that should be considered is that longer length may result in poorer healing whereas shorter length results in decreased function. Thus, acute amputation should be performed at a level at which healing is likely and function maximized. Also, if at all possible the elbow joint should be retained to facilitate later prosthetic function.

Soft Tissue Coverage

Historically, maintenance of length depended on local soft tissue coverage; if soft tissue coverage was not adequate, one merely shortened the extremity until closure could be achieved. As mentioned earlier, skin grafts, free flaps, and composite tissue transfer have dramatically changed this approach. Skin grafts are applicable when the underlying soft tissue bed is acceptable, but one must be sensitive to the ultimate functional needs of the amputation site; in some cases, skin grafts may not be durable enough to tolerate therapy and the use of prostheses. Local flaps (see under

"Fingertip Amputation") abound, but their applicability is limited because of the anatomy at more proximal amputation sites. Pedicled flaps (regional or distal) have a long, productive history in hand surgery; however, they have been increasingly replaced by free tissue transfers. This change is based on (1) better matching of the tissue transferred (in terms of thickness and ultimate functional performance), (2) avoidance of additional surgery (whether for division or thinning of the flap), and (3) lack of the joint limitations that result from the immobility that is typically necessary with pedicled flaps. Free tissue transfer is increasingly being accomplished at sites proximal to the hand to achieve more satisfactory results.

Nerves

Prevention of neuroma is the most difficult problem in upper extremity amputation. As in all of medicine, the existence of many methods of treatment usually indicates that none of them is exceptionally good. Such is the case with prevention of neuroma. Distal ligation, proximal ligation, coagulation, chemical ablation of the end, simple division, traction and division, nerve repair to other divided nerves, and immediate burial of the transected nerve end have all been attempted with varying degrees of success. The desire to eliminate painful focal sensation must be balanced against the secondary loss of sensibility induced by many of these techniques. A divided nerve always attempts to regenerate and, in so doing, produces a neuroma of variable clinical significance. Thus, in reality the goal is not to prevent the formation of a neuroma altogether but to prevent the patient from experiencing the pain or dysesthesias from the neuroma that will predictably develop. In general, locating the divided, free nerve end as far from external stimuli as possible and placing it in a healthy, nonscarred bed of tissue are the best preventive measures. In addition, early postoperative therapy (desensitization or sensory re-education) is an extremely important determinant of the patient's ability to tolerate the dysesthesias that result from an amputation. Targeted reinnervation by way of nerve transfer techniques has also been described as a means of improving residual muscle function and sensory aspects of the stump and thus prosthetic utility.[32] Such procedures can be performed in either a planned elective or staged scenario.

Bone and Cartilage

Whatever length is ultimately chosen for the amputation, the bony prominences must be optimally contoured. Lack of attention to bony prominences or irregularities in bony contour leads to aesthetic abnormalities and difficulty fitting prostheses. Inadequate débridement of traumatized tissue and displaced bony fragments, improper initial contouring of bone, or failure to identify bone-producing periosteum, which must also be contoured, is the source of such difficulties. Visual identification of the periosteum is easiest during initial management of the injury, and achievement of a natural bone contour is greatly assisted by palpating the end of the bone through the skin before closure. This is even more important in amputations through joints, where natural anatomic flares of the bone produce aesthetically unnatural contours and interfere with prosthetic fitting.

Tendons

The hand represents a very delicate balance between extensor and flexor forces. It is extremely difficult to duplicate the balance of these forces through myodesic methods (i.e., suturing of tendons or muscles to bones) or myoplastic techniques (i.e., suturing of tendons or muscles to tendons or muscles of the opposite functional group; for example, suturing an extensor tendon directly to a flexor tendon over a bony amputation site). In general, then, such techniques are not used distally in the fingers and hand because they often add to the functional deficit. However, they do have value proximally, where the balance is not as critical and re-education and adaptation are easier.

■ SPECIFIC AMPUTATIONS
Fingertip Amputation

Distal finger amputations are extremely common. The most frequent mechanism causing such injuries is a crushing blow, such as from a closing door. Although many people arrive at the emergency department with the tip of the finger available for reattachment, the injury is usually too distal for microsurgical reattachment. Many surgeons have attempted composite reattachment (i.e., reattachment without specific revascularization) with generally poor results. At present, such composite grafts are not indicated except in young children (<2 years), in whom there is an increased chance of graft survival.[33] Most composite grafts fail because (1) the amount of tissue is generally more than can survive the ischemia until new circulation develops and (2) the zone of injury is greater than the area of amputation (i.e., the tip is usually damaged and thus is not capable of surviving as a composite graft).

Technique

If the proximal portion of the distal phalanx is not severely injured such that the insertions of the flexor digitorum profundus and extensor tendons are intact, preservation of that portion of bone is indicated for functional length. If these areas are damaged beyond repair, disarticulation through the distal interphalangeal joint is indicated. The flexor digitorum profundus tendon should never be sutured over the tip or to the extensor tendon because this can weaken grip in the hand (the quadriga effect).[34] The bone of the distal phalanx should be of adequate length to support the nail bed and nail growth.[35] Generally, these amputations occur through a portion of the nail bed. If enough proximal nail bed (≈50%) is present to provide a functional nail, the bed should be repaired under optical magnification with absorbable 6-0 or 7-0 suture.

The distal phalanx is usually rongeured back so that the end of the bone is not exposed. The digital nerves are identified, distracted distally, and divided so they will be at least 1 cm from the fingertip stump to avoid neuroma formation in this location. If the final cutaneous defect is then less than 1 cm², simply allowing the wound to close by secondary intention is acceptable. Other wound closure techniques have been attempted, including every conceivable type of local or regional flap. However, given the fact that flap closures are frequently insensate and do not reduce healing time, ultimate functional recovery appears to be better after secondary healing because the resulting scar contracture diminishes the size of the sensory defect.

Skin Grafts

If the cutaneous defect is greater than 1 cm², the amount of time needed for closure and the ultimate functional result may not warrant healing by secondary intention. If there is no exposed bone, a skin graft is possible. The temptation is to use the amputated part as a donor source for the skin graft. This practice should be avoided because the amputated portion has been traumatized and the overall success of such skin grafts is disappointing. However, one advantage of these grafts is that they may serve as temporary biologic dressings even if they do not survive.

Nontraumatized skin graft donor sites that may be considered are

- The ulnar border of the palm (within the operative field and a good color match)
- The forearm (the medial portion of the forearm or the elbow crease, although hypertrophic scarring can lead to some cosmetic deformity)
- The groin (a well-hidden donor area, although the color match is not good and some unwanted hair may also be transferred)

Local Flap Closure

As mentioned previously, many alternative flaps are often useful for cutaneous defects of the fingertip; some of the more common local flaps include

- The Kutler flap,[36] a lateral V-Y flap for closure of a central tip defect
- The Atasoy flap,[37] a palmar V-Y flap
- The palmar flap,[38] based on both digital neurovascular bundles in which the entire soft tissue coverage of the digit above the tendon sheath is elevated and advanced to cover the tip of the finger
- Radius- or ulna-based local flaps, which preserve cutaneous innervation on the appropriate digital nerve,[39] with skin grafting of the donor site as necessary

In addition to these local flaps, numerous regional flaps can be used, such as dorsal skin cross-finger flaps, palmar skin cross-finger flaps, and thenar flaps. Although it is sometimes necessary to use these regional pedicled flaps, they carry significant additional morbidity by creating joint stiffness because of the obligatory period of immobility needed for attachment of the flap. Even in young people who have had good physical therapy, long-term problems can result.

Digit-Level Amputations

Midfinger Amputation

Amputations that leave more than half the proximal phalanx may be functional for the patient. These amputations represent variations of fingertip amputations. First, the bone is rongeured back a short distance to allow soft tissue coverage. Tendons that have been separated from their bony insertions by the amputation are placed on traction, divided, and allowed to retract into the palm. Digital nerves are a potentially more difficult problem. It is preferable to divide them under mild traction and allow them to retract beneath healthy vascularized tissue. Excessive traction may denervate the new tip of the digit. If traction is not applied, however, the cut nerve remains adjacent to the amputation site, which can lead to postinjury trauma and produce significant pain. The associated soft tissue defect is managed in the same manner as a fingertip amputation.

Proximal Phalanx

Amputation proximal to the midportion of the proximal phalanx is not typically a functional amputation. If enough digit remains, it may be possible for patients to wear a cosmetic prosthesis that may allow some functional restoration; however, most patients find the remaining digit a nuisance (Fig. 118-1). The effects of proximal digital amputation vary with the finger involved. For example, an index finger, which is second in importance to the thumb, when amputated proximally can become a hindrance to function of the hand. Because the patient uses the middle finger for activities such as writing, the index finger stump becomes an obstacle. With middle or ring finger amputations, each time the person reaches into his or her pocket or purse for a small object, the object falls through the opening left in the hand by the remaining short digit. The small fingers play a role in gripping objects, and if the finger becomes immobile, it may become caught on objects. Because of these issues, patients frequently choose to undergo secondary ray amputation. Regardless of the certainty of this denouement, ray amputation should not be offered to the patient at the time of initial wound closure. Elective resection of the remaining portion of the digit is a decision that each patient should arrive at by experience.

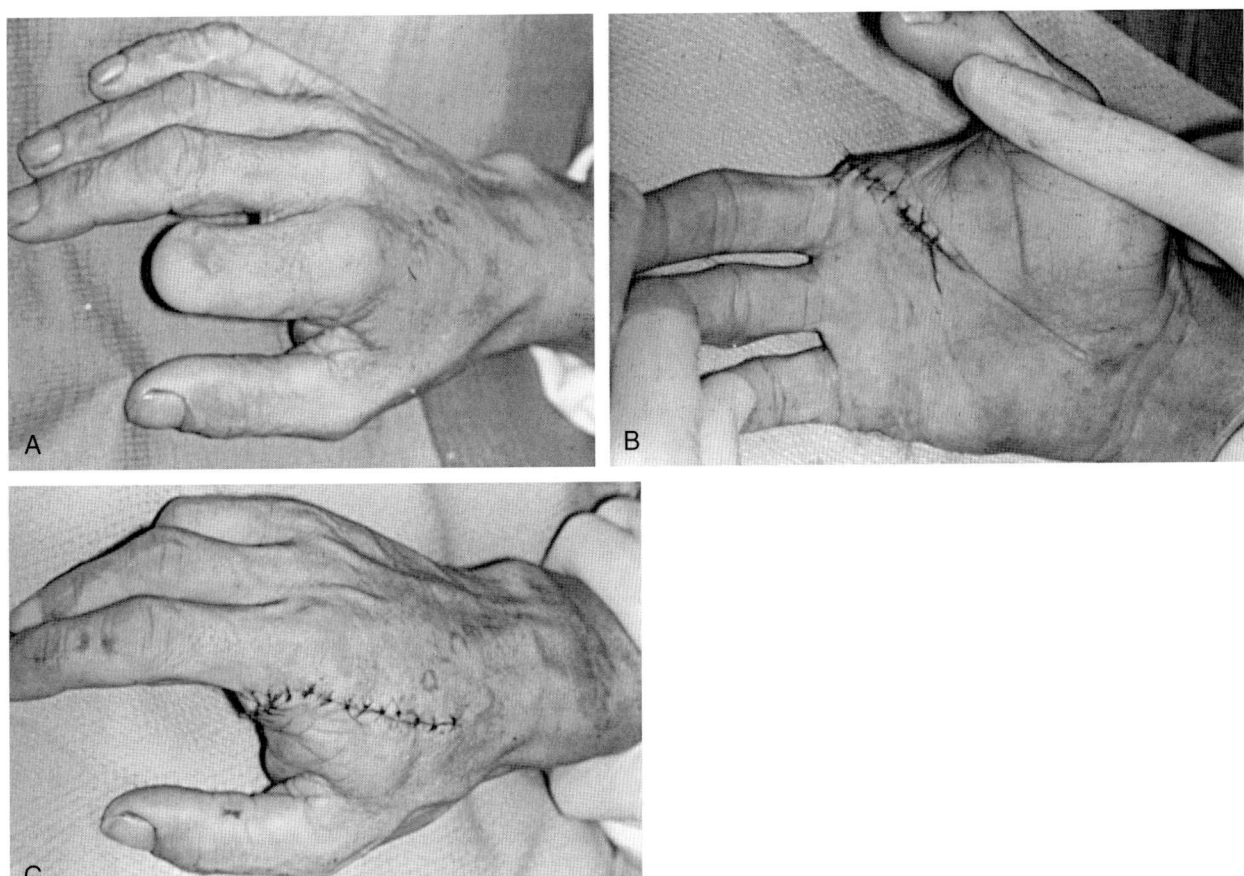

Figure 118-1 A, Loss of the index finger at the proximal interphalangeal joint. The patient does not effectively use the index remnant but instead bypasses it to use his long digit. He requested elective ray resection because he thought that the remnant was in the way and unsightly. **B** and **C,** Successful ray amputation is shown with a more natural hand contour.

Ray Amputation

Ray amputation, which includes removal of the injured finger to the metacarpal base, often provides a far more cosmetically acceptable hand, especially with an index ray amputation. This technique usually involves a dorsal longitudinal incision over the index metacarpal along with a palmar skin incision over the proximal phalangeal level. Alternatively, a circumferential racket incision may be used. Minimal digital nerve neurolysis should be done to prevent pain. Attention to myodesic and myoplastic techniques is critical because improper attachment of the remaining muscle and tendons to the lumbrical and interosseous muscle or nearby periosteum can downgrade intrinsic hand function significantly. In addition, care should be taken when performing a fifth ray amputation because the extensor carpi ulnaris inserts at the base and wrist function can therefore be affected.

In most cases, the appearance of a three-fingered hand with normal border contours is so natural that it goes unnoticed. Nevertheless, the operation is not without its own set of risks. First, the procedure narrows the palm by 20% to 25%, which reduces the hand's ability to stabilize objects. Second, the operation is a more extensive procedure that produces more proximal postoperative pain, edema, and stiffness than caused by the original injury to the digit. However, in the final analysis, ray amputation is very functional and cosmetically appealing, and there are few dissatisfied patients.

Thumb Amputation

Because it accounts for 40% of the function of the hand, the thumb deserves special attention in any amputation involving the hand. Clearly, the major emphasis is on reattachment of the thumb. However, the desire for reattachment has led some surgeons to attempt reimplantation in circumstances that would otherwise be considered contraindications (e.g., severe avulsion injuries). The standard of care is now to attempt reimplantation of the thumb if possible, and encouraging results have been achieved even after avulsion injuries.[40] Nonreimplantable amputations at the level of the interphalangeal joint are functional, and most patients do not request or require additional reconstruction. These stumps still provide the opposition function for the fingers. Revision of thumb amputations proximally to allow closure should not be performed as in the other fingers, and thought should be given to rotational, advancement, and free flaps.[41] More proximal thumb amputations can be reconstructed by pollicization (using a remaining finger, usually the index finger, and myodesic techniques to create a thumb), osteoplasty, bone-lengthening techniques, or toe-to-thumb transfer (great toe, second toe, or toe wraparound).

Hand-Wrist Amputations

Whatever tissue can be preserved during hand amputation should be salvaged. A hand with a short palm may seem dysfunctional, but as an assist hand it may be preferable to a prosthesis. A transcarpal amputation allows supination and pronation of the forearm, as well as flexion and extension of the wrist. A prosthesis can be fitted for this type of amputation as well. Wrist disarticulation is preferred to more proximal forearm amputation because it has the same advantages of a transcarpal amputation except that wrist flexion and extension are lost. Wrist disarticulation is performed by creating a long palmar and short dorsal flap; ligating the radial and ulnar arteries proximal to the wrist; identifying the median, radial, and ulnar nerves and distracting and dividing them; dividing all tendons; disarticulating the joint; and resecting the tips of the radial and ulnar styloid processes. The resultant smooth contour can easily be fitted for a prosthesis.

The radial, ulnar, and median nerves can present difficulties during hand-wrist amputation. The ulnar and median nerves are frequently avulsed at a more proximal level with these traumatic amputations; if they are apparent in the wound, they can be severed with mild traction and allowed to retract. Retraction of the ends usually positions the nerves away from contact with a prosthesis. The sensory branch of the radial nerve, however, is quite superficial throughout its course in the forearm (covered only by the brachioradialis muscle). Neuromas from this nerve are not uncommon, and division of the nerve in the proximal part of the forearm may be considered at the time of the initial amputation. Sensibility of the forearm skin is not directly determined by these nerves but instead is controlled by the brachial cutaneous nerves, and improper management of the brachial cutaneous nerves can cause difficulties similar to those that occur with the superficial branch of the radial nerve. However, it is preferable not to divide these nerves far proximally because sensibility of the forearm skin will be sacrificed.

Forearm Amputations

The optimal level for a forearm amputation is the junction of the middle and distal third of the forearm. The issue with the distal third of the forearm is the relative paucity of padding in this area because of the thin skin and subcutaneous tissue. This factor can be more evident in patients with ischemia because this area is notably prone to skin breakdown. So important is the elbow that the use of free-flap soft tissue coverage to preserve length or even distraction osteogenesis (Ilizarov technique[27]) is a viable consideration in the case of very short below-elbow amputations. With the exception of these very special cases, however, heroic efforts at preserving length are not usually indicated.

Heeding these caveats, the surgeon can trim the bony tissues adequately to permit soft tissue closure. The technique is as follows: creation of equal anterior and posterior skin flaps; ligation of the radial and ulnar arteries; distraction and division of the medial, radial, and ulnar arteries; transection of the muscle bellies; division of the radius and ulna; and closure of the deep fascia followed by the skin (Fig. 118-2). Reconstruction of the amputation is generally accomplished by means of a fitted prosthesis. As described by Tubiana, however, bilateral upper extremity amputations can be func-

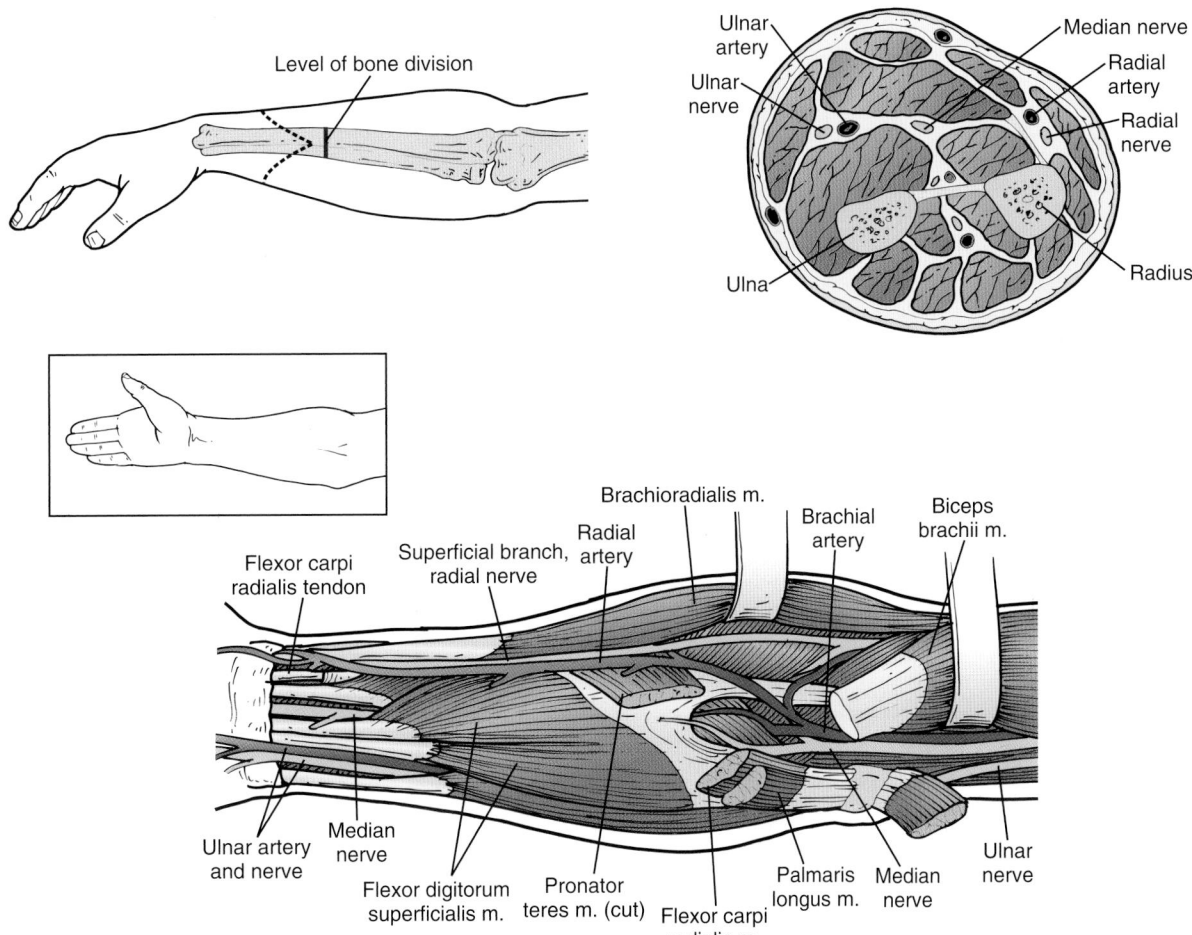

Figure 118-2 Forearm amputation is relatively straightforward: division of soft tissue at the junction of the distal third and proximal two thirds of the forearm and several centimeters distal to the level of bony division. Proper muscle coverage is achieved with myofascial closure. *(Adapted with permission from Maxwell MC. Amputations in trauma. In: Thal ER, Weigelt JA, Carrico CJ, eds.* Operative Trauma Management: An Atlas. *2nd ed. New York, NY: McGraw-Hill; 2002:449.)*

tionally improved with the Krukenberg procedure, in which a sensate pincer is created between the radius and ulna (Fig. 118-3).[42] The pincer is motorized by the pronator teres muscle, and this procedure allows preservation of proprioception and stereognosis. Although the cosmetic result is far from desirable, the functional improvement is great, and the procedure should be given serious consideration in the rare instances of bilateral injuries, in blind individuals, or when prosthetic reconstruction is not practical.[43]

Elbow Disarticulation

If the elbow joint is not salvageable, elbow disarticulation is preferred over distal humeral transection. In addition to maintaining length, humeral rotation can be transmitted to the elbow, and the broad flare of the condyles makes for a good prosthetic fit. When compared with the forearm, which has two bones with a functional noncircular cross-section and thin soft tissue coverage that allows transmission of rotational forces (pronation and supination), the upper part of the arm has a single bone with a relatively circular cross-section and less rotational stability because of its thicker soft tissue. The

amputation technique is similar to that described earlier in that anterior and posterior skin flaps are created; the brachial artery is ligated; the median, ulnar and radial nerves are distracted and divided; the joint capsule is opened and the forearm removed; and a muscle flap (brachialis or triceps) is then used to cover the humerus (Fig. 118-4). As noted, there has been an emphasis on retaining all of the humerus if possible. In so doing, however, the upper part of the arm may appear longer than the normal (unamputated) arm when fitted with an internal elbow joint prosthesis. It is possible to use an external elbow joint option, but these joints are substantially less durable. Another approach to this problem involves construction of an artificial asymmetry by means of angulation osteotomy in which bone is resected yet epicondylar stability is retained.[44] This method has gained popularity in Europe but is not routinely practiced in the United States because of the obvious cosmetic deformity in the proximal remaining stump.

Upper Arm Amputations

Surgical considerations for above-elbow amputations are essentially the same as those for forearm amputations with

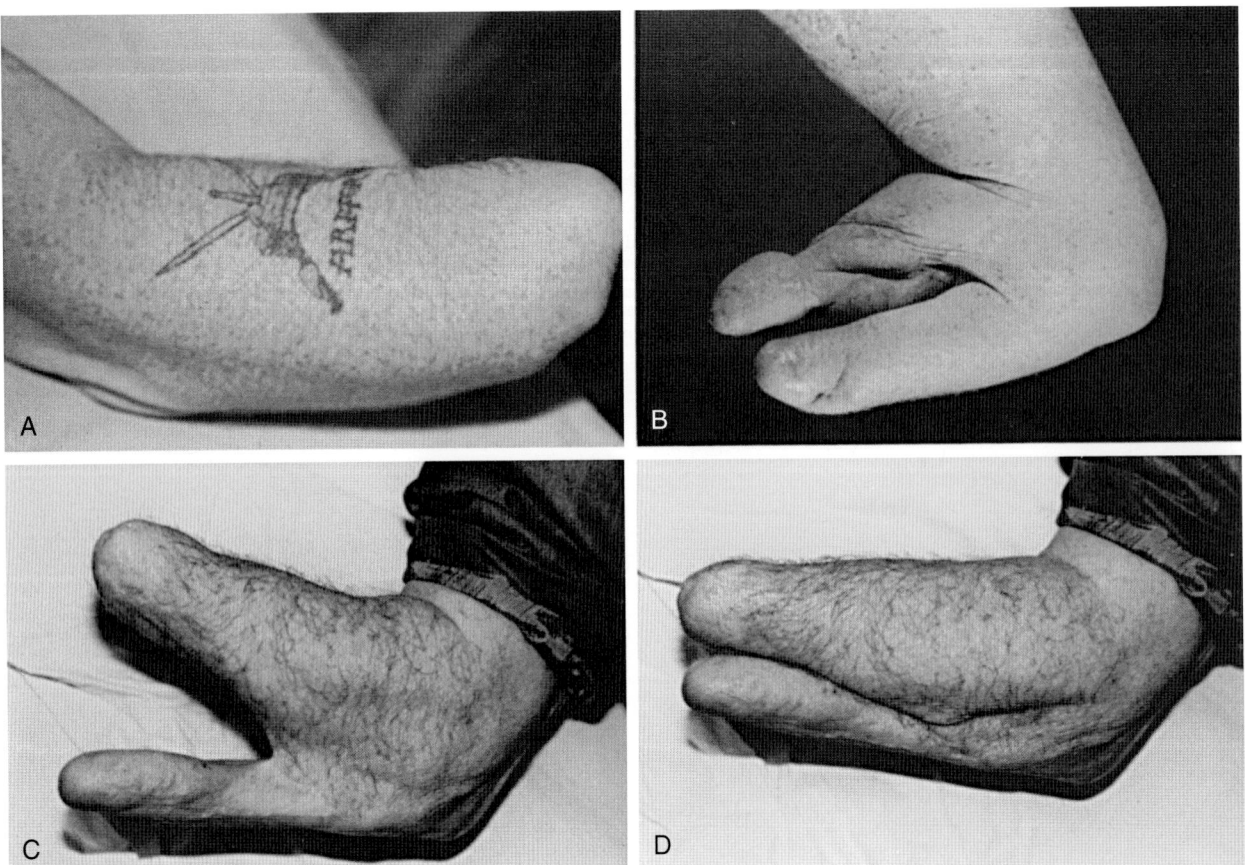

Figure 118-3 Classically, in a double-arm or blind amputee, the Krukenberg procedure has been performed. By separating the ulna and radius, proprioception and a simple pincer grasp mechanism have been maintained.

respect to the treatment of bone, muscles, tendons, nerves, and skin. A transcondylar amputation functions essentially the same as an elbow disarticulation. More proximal amputations must include an elbow lock mechanism to stabilize the musculature and future prosthetic joint in full extension or flexion and a turntable mechanism that will serve as humeral rotation. Taking into account the location of the elbow lock, which extends 4 cm from the distal amputation site, the transhumeral amputation should be made 4 cm proximal to the elbow (see Fig. 118-4).[45]

Reimplantation remains a viable option, and Wood and Cooney have reported that reimplantation should be considered even with high amputations.[22] A multidisciplinary approach is required and involves early arterial and venous shunting followed by bony fixation, definitive vascular repair with attention to maximizing venous outflow, and finally nerve and soft tissue reconstruction. Functional recovery of the hand may not occur, yet it may be possible to convert an obvious above-elbow amputation to a below-elbow amputation, which is far more functional. The shorter the remaining stump, the more difficult the prosthetic fit and the less functional the prosthesis will be. As a result, several new techniques have been developed to facilitate this type of reconstruction. The use of free flaps can provide additional soft tissue and bone length for a short upper arm amputation. Functional restoration of the glenohumeral joint may be

accomplished with a free fibular transfer. The proximal humerus can be replaced with the fibula and its proximal joint with reattachment of the muscular insertions.[25,26] Particularly in patients with malignant tumors, limbs that would otherwise have to be sacrificed can now be salvaged. Fibular flaps can also be used in conjunction with soft tissue coverage from a latissimus dorsi flap (pedicled or free) to provide acceptable upper arm length for fitting a prosthesis.

One final technique used to achieve adequate bony length is distraction osteogenesis, as mentioned previously.[27-29] Although this technique was developed in the 1960s by Ilizarov, it did not become widely recognized and used worldwide until the 1990s. The scattered reports of this method of treatment have been encouraging. As indicated previously, every effort should be made to avoid high amputations. Even when the amputation will be a functional shoulder disarticulation (amputation proximal to the insertions of the deltoid and pectoralis major), maximal proximal length of the humerus should be sought for either prosthetic fitting or potential reconstruction by these complex plastic and orthopedic techniques.

Shoulder Disarticulation and Forequarter Amputations

Shoulder disarticulation and forequarter, or scapulothoracic, amputation are the most complex and difficult procedures

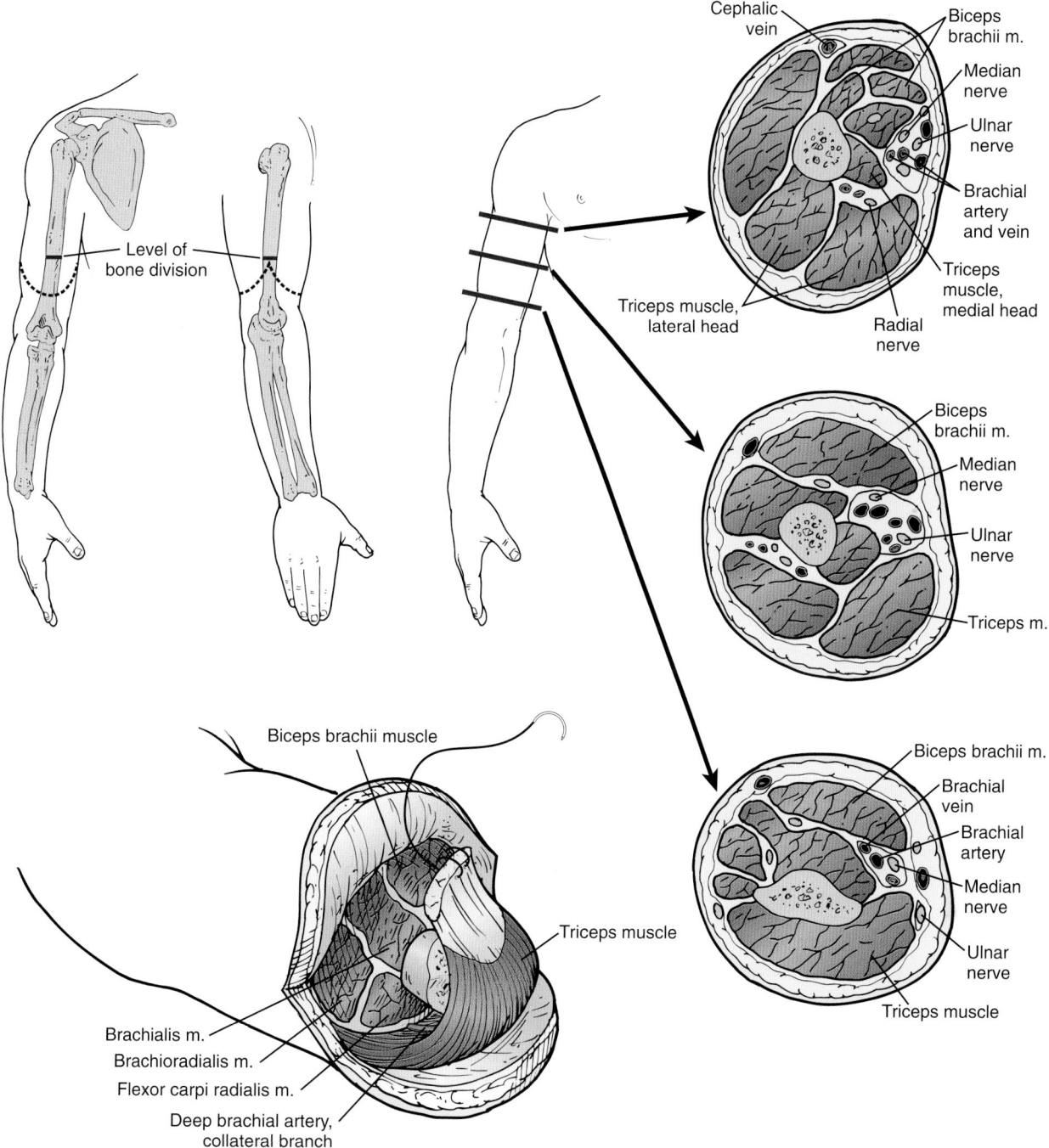

Figure 118-4 Upper arm amputation can be performed at several levels. The initial operation should be focused on maintaining as much humeral length as possible and the epicondyles, if salvageable. *(Adapted with permission from Maxwell MC. Amputations in trauma. In: Thal ER, Weigelt JA, Carrico CJ, eds.* Operative Trauma Management: An Atlas. *2nd ed. New York, NY: McGraw-Hill; 2002:451.)*

from a prosthetic and functional standpoint. Considerations are (1) loss of potential motor units as drivers of the prosthetic device and (2) difficulty fitting the prosthesis to contours. The shoulder disarticulation (after rounding off any bony prominences that may cause wear) leaves a contour adequate to provide a snug fit for the prosthesis (Fig. 118-5). In addition, scapular function is retained and can be used (with some difficulty) as a motor unit for the prosthetic device. A forequarter amputation (which is done almost exclusively for malignant

processes), however, offers little hope for functional restoration of the limb, and prosthetic application is challenging.[46]

The surgical techniques for these amputations are well described in the literature. The shoulder disarticulation may be modified by retention of the humeral head to assist in contouring or may be a true disarticulation with complete removal of the humerus. Regardless, the deltoid and pectoral muscles along with their overlying myofasciocutaneous tissue provide the flap coverage. Occasionally, if the deltoid is not

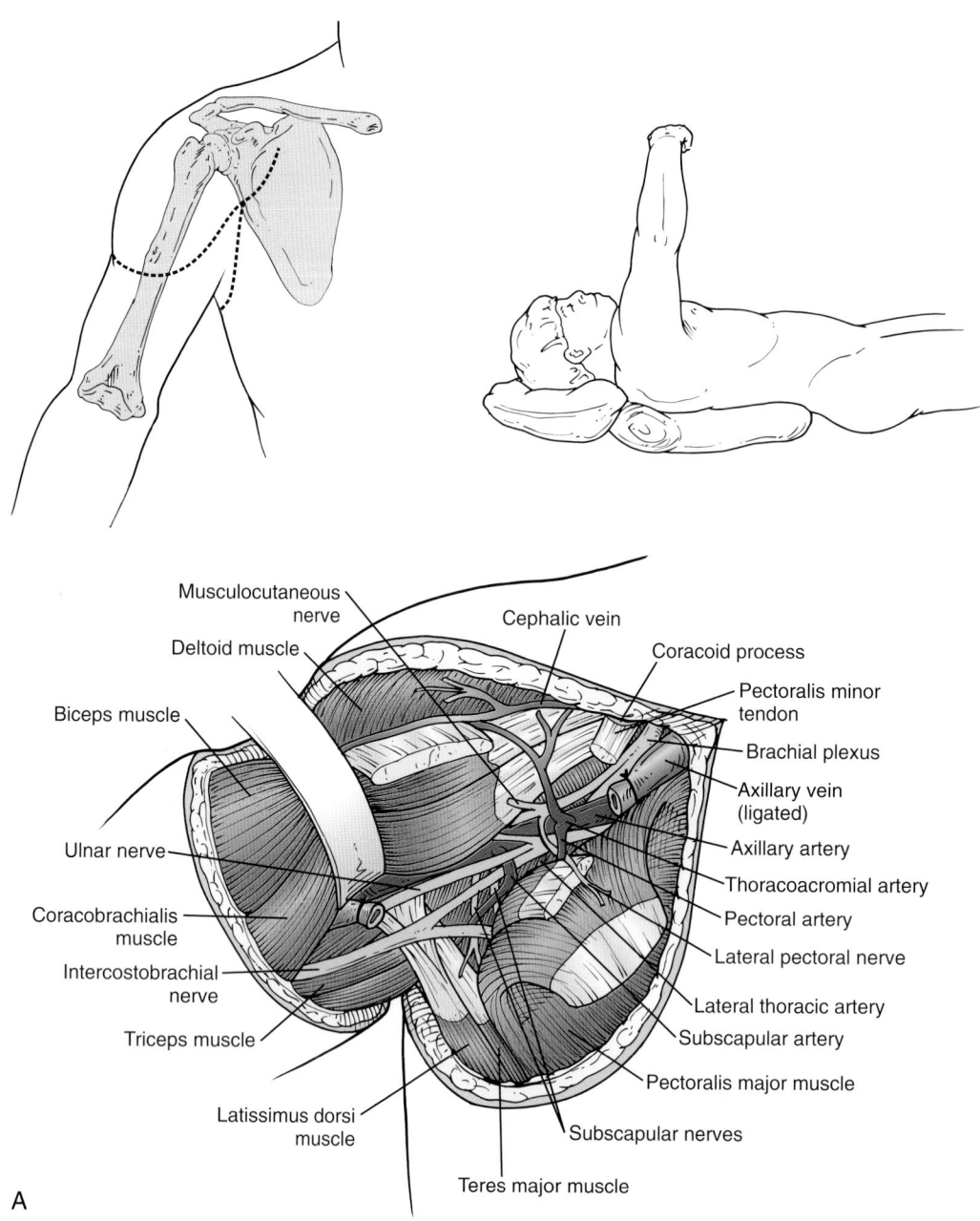

Figure 118-5 Shoulder disarticulation as classically described. **A,** Skin incision and initial anterior approach with division of the anterior attachments, brachial plexus, and subclavian vessels.

available, an inferior axillary fasciocutaneous flap may be necessary. The latissimus dorsi and pectoralis major are reattached to either the glenoid capsule or the humeral head remnant. The tendinous components of the rotator cuff are also attached to the glenoid capsule. In a modified technique their insertions are undisturbed, which reduces movement and thus pain in the joint area. It also stabilizes the muscles for future myoelectric control points.

There are two approaches to forequarter amputation. The anterior approach, described by Berger,[47] and the posterior approach, described by Littlewood,[48] differ only in exposure of the vascular structures hidden behind the clavicle. Both approaches are well accepted. Any available remaining myo-

fascial components are used to provide closure. The same principles that were described previously apply: removing the bony prominences, treating the nerves and muscles, and providing adequate soft tissue coverage.

POSTOPERATIVE MANAGEMENT AND COMPLICATIONS

Wound Treatment

Aside from the standard surgical principles of postoperative wound care and post-traumatic injury care, the principles of postoperative management after upper extremity amputation

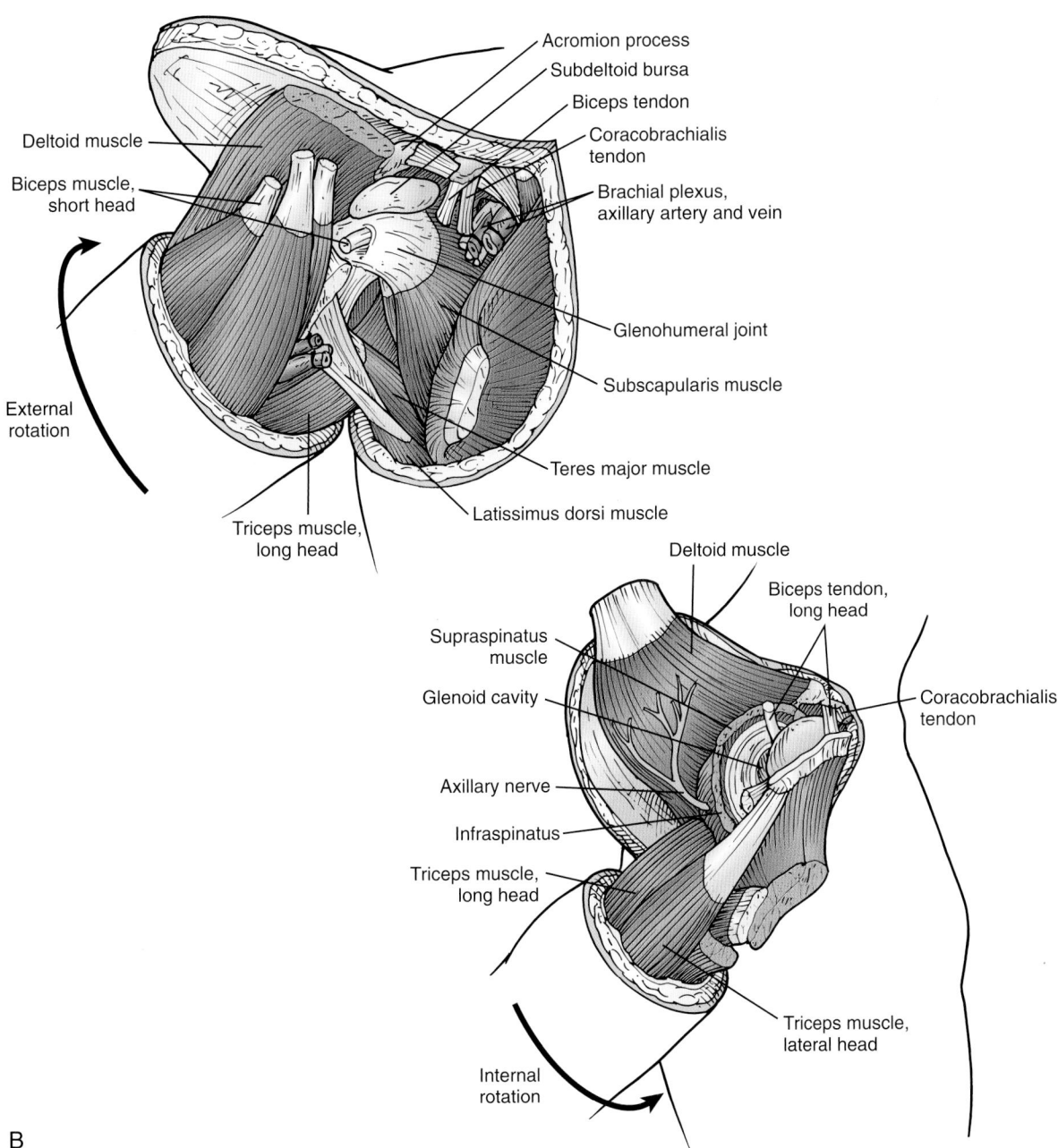

Acromion process
Subdeltoid bursa
Biceps tendon
Coracobrachialis tendon
Brachial plexus, axillary artery and vein
Glenohumeral joint
Subscapularis muscle
Teres major muscle
Latissimus dorsi muscle

Deltoid muscle
Biceps muscle, short head
External rotation
Triceps muscle, long head

Deltoid muscle
Biceps tendon, long head
Supraspinatus muscle
Glenoid cavity
Coracobrachialis tendon
Axillary nerve
Infraspinatus
Triceps muscle, long head
Triceps muscle, lateral head
Internal rotation

B

Figure 118-5, cont'd B, Completion of all anterior and posterior attachment transections.

Continued

are supportive. There should be a low threshold for the use of drains in areas of potential space because hematoma and seroma formation is not uncommon and might not only delay rehabilitation and prosthetic placement but also place tissue viability at risk and increase the potential for infection. Drain removal as soon as possible is encouraged to reduce infection risk. Early physical activity and rehabilitation are encouraged. Compressive dressings are used immediately. Full range-of-motion exercises of the elbow and shoulder should be started immediately when these structures are preserved. Local amputation site concerns revolve around infection, wound healing, and the viability of specialized reconstructive methods, such as free flaps if used. Infection is rare and, even when trauma is the indication for amputation, should gener-

ally occur in less than 5% of cases. Failure of complex tissue transfers, if performed, occurs in 3% to 8% of upper extremity reconstructions early and becomes even rarer in later evaluation.[49]

Poor wound healing and the concerns of flap ischemia and stump necrosis, which are well appreciated in lower extremity amputation, occur infrequently in upper extremity amputation but must be recognized if they occur. Potential systemic complications of upper extremity amputation are related to septic events, associated traumatic injuries, or systemic consequences of either a global vascular process or organ system co-morbidity. As with treatment of any ischemic injury, should upper extremity amputation be performed subsequent to attempts at limb salvage and revascularization or after significant crush

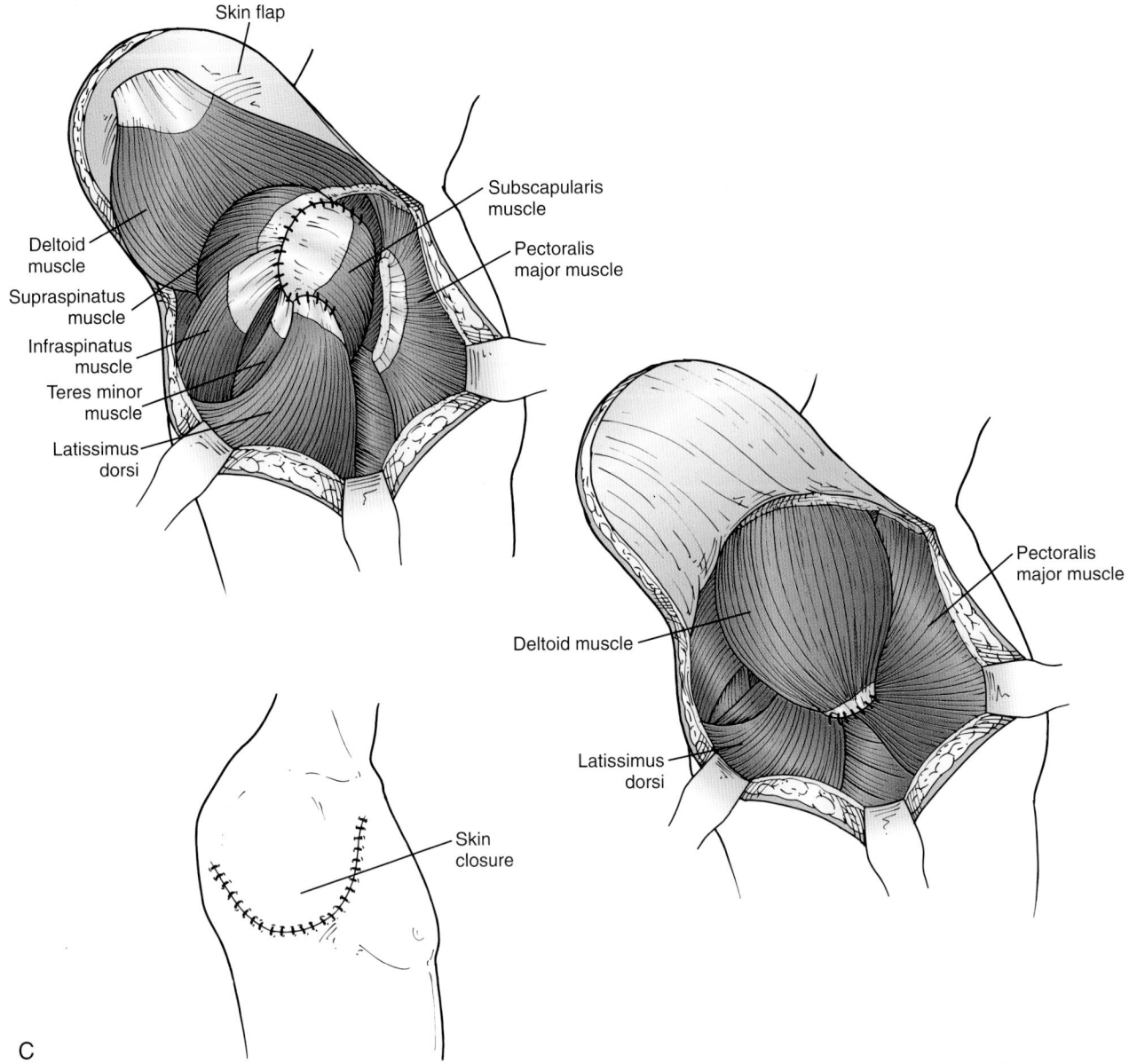

Figure 118-5, cont'd C, Sequential closure over the glenoid of the scapularis muscle, other rotator cuff components, latissimus dorsi muscle, pectoral muscle, and deltoid muscle. *(Adapted with permission from Maxwell MC. Amputations in trauma. In: Thal ER, Weigelt JA, Carrico CJ, eds.* Operative Trauma Management: An Atlas. *2nd ed. New York, NY: McGraw-Hill; 2002:453-457.)*

injury, one should be attuned to the potential for significant rhabdomyolysis and myoglobinuria. The threat of this problem is usually less than in the lower extremity because of smaller muscle mass, shorter arm length, and thus attainment of collateral flow, yet it remains a possibility, and proper hydration and urine alkalinization should be instituted, if necessary.

Phantom Pain

Phantom sensations occur over time in the majority of patients undergoing upper extremity amputation. Long-term phantom pain, in varying degrees, occurs in 40% to 80% of patients.[50,51] In an evaluation of upper extremity amputees from the Iran-Iraq War over an average of 17.5 years, phantom pain occurred in 32%.[52] Treatment methods for phantom pain are numerous and usually multidimensional but can be generally categorized as pharmacologic, surgical, psychological, and neurostimulatory. Newer evaluations of motor cortical changes and alterations in hemispheric function after upper extremity amputation may in the near future lead to novel therapeutic methods to treat postamputation pain syndromes.[53] It has been suggested that loss of the dominant hand is an independent predictor for the development of more significant phantom limb pain.[54]

Psychosocial Rehabilitation

When compared with lower extremity amputees, those losing part of the arm or the hand suffer from a higher rate of psychological disorders such as depression, anxiety, and post-traumatic stress disorder. Although overall this area is relatively poorly studied, it appears that some 30% to 40% of upper extremity amputees will require psychological care afterward.[55] This is specifically related to the complex impact that the upper extremity and its components have on daily function. The effect that hand function has on both the patient's quality of life and his or her psychological well-being is recognized. It is therefore understandable that loss of hand function, not to mention the physical aspects of the hand and arm, directly leads to a grieving process and possibly longer term psychological disorders.

Physical Rehabilitation

Rehabilitation for those with upper extremity amputation is complex and onerous, and to date, the technology and functionality of upper extremity prosthetics have lagged behind those of the lower extremity because of the intricate movements and fine sensorimotor function in the native arm and hand. Replicating these attributes has been difficult. The rehabilitative principles used for upper extremity amputees are not unique. They encompass residual limb soft tissue shrinkage and shaping, desensitization, maximization of range of motion, skin health and mobility, muscle strength, augmentation of self-reliance and daily activities, and finally, exploration of prosthetic options.[56] These key features are focused on issues that provide a reduction in postamputation pain and maximize the potential for meaningful prosthetic use.

Prostheses

Prostheses used in the upper extremity fall into three categories: purely aesthetic, body powered, and myoelectrically powered.[57,58]

Aesthetic prostheses are simply that. They usually consist of silicone and are made to produce a lifelike appearance so that the amputee can have a relatively normal body habitus (Fig. 118-6). They have very minimal function.

Body-powered prostheses are simple mechanical devices that are controlled by residual body motion and function

(Fig. 118-7). They are, in general, the most durable of prostheses and are used for most significant physical activity by amputees. Indeed, young upper extremity amputees use these types of prostheses for swimming, rock climbing, and performing most athletic activities.

Myoelectrically controlled prostheses use electrodes to convert the electrical stimulation of residual muscle groups

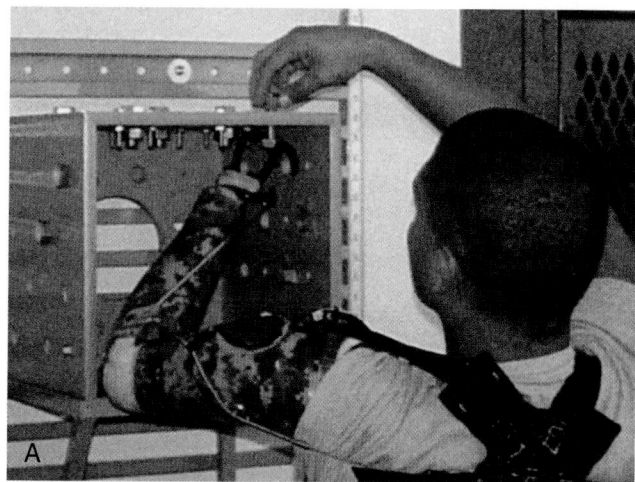

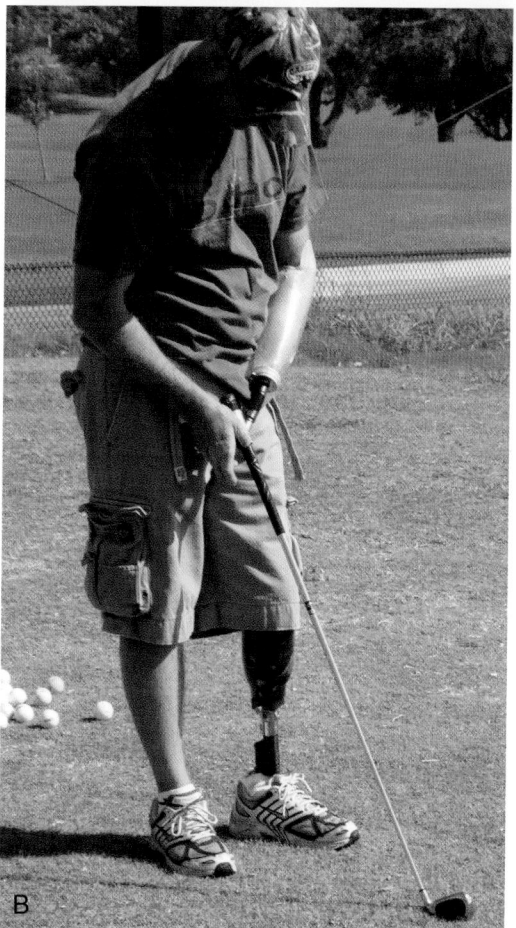

Figure 118-7 A, Body-powered left arm prosthesis in a young soldier after transhumeral amputation. Note the pincer terminal device, cable powered by proximal movements at the shoulder girdle harness. **B,** Forearm sleeve body-powered golf prosthesis with a terminal device for the club handle.

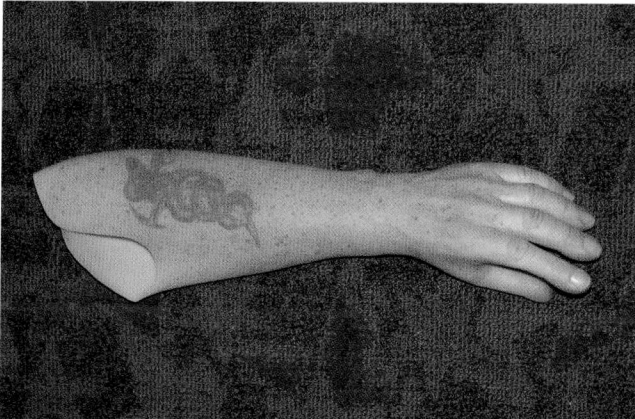

Figure 118-6 Aesthetic forearm and hand silicone prosthesis.

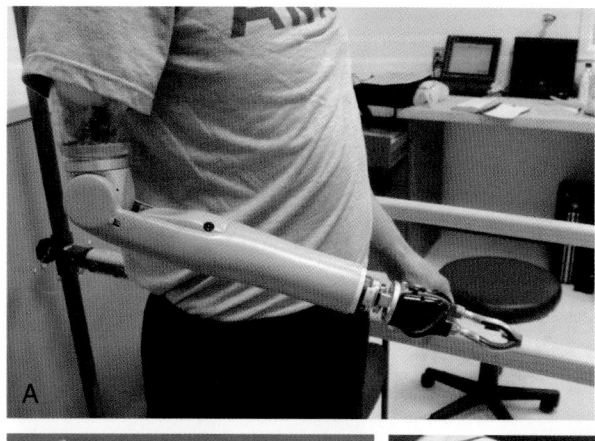
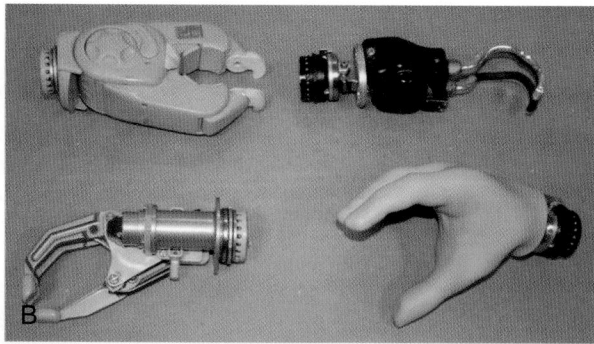
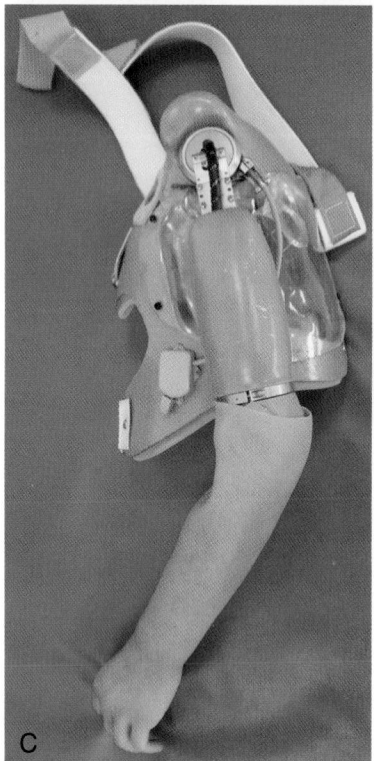
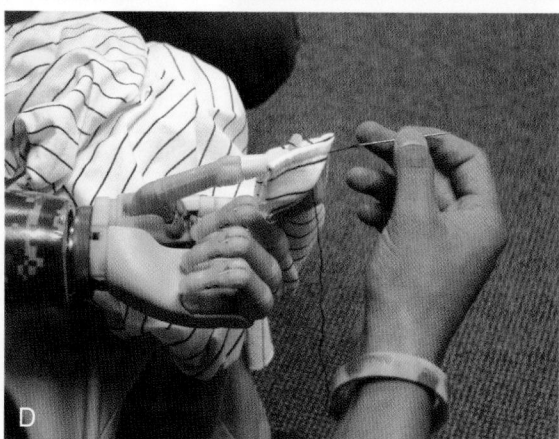

Figure 118-8 A, Contemporary myoelectric arm prosthesis with a classic pincer terminal device. **B,** Various detachable terminal devices used on myoelectric upper extremity prostheses for differing needs. **C,** Shoulder girdle–mounted myoelectric arm prosthesis with a silicone aesthetic cover. **D,** The i-LIMB hand (Hangar Orthopedic Group, Inc., Bethesda, MD) is a new hand prosthesis with myoelectric control that is able to simulate nearly normal hand motion.

into current used to power the prosthesis. This has made movements such as wrist rotation and finger movement a reality, and many terminal devices may be attached to the prosthesis to allow various functions (Fig. 118-8). Although they permit greater degrees of freedom, these prostheses are much more complex, more expensive, and less durable for hard physical activity. Progress in myoelectric technologies continues at a rapid pace. In addition, the Defense Advanced Research Projects Agency, in affiliation with Johns Hopkins University, is now developing and testing an upper extremity prosthesis that is myoelectrically controlled with nearly all the degrees of freedom of a human arm (Fig. 118-9).[59] The residual muscles are surgically reinnervated, with or without splitting, for maintenance of cortical functioning to enable muscle contraction and thus application of the myoelectric prosthesis. This technique, targeted reinnervation, has recently been applied clinically and is currently undergoing investigation at

several sites.[32,60] Another complex, contemporary method of neural control of biomechanical upper extremity prostheses involves the placement of electrodes directly on the cerebral cortex.[61] As this technique continues to undergo study and improvement, integration of direct cortical signaling into mechanical endpoints is proving to be intricate. It is likely that in the near future a prosthetic mechanical arm controlled by the patient's own neurologic processes and with almost normal function may be an everyday reality.

LONG-TERM OUTCOMES

There are few reports of late outcomes after upper extremity amputation. Meaningful comparative information is difficult to obtain because of differing causes, levels of amputation, and amputee age, in addition to many other variables. The rate of late stump revision remains poorly defined for similar reasons,

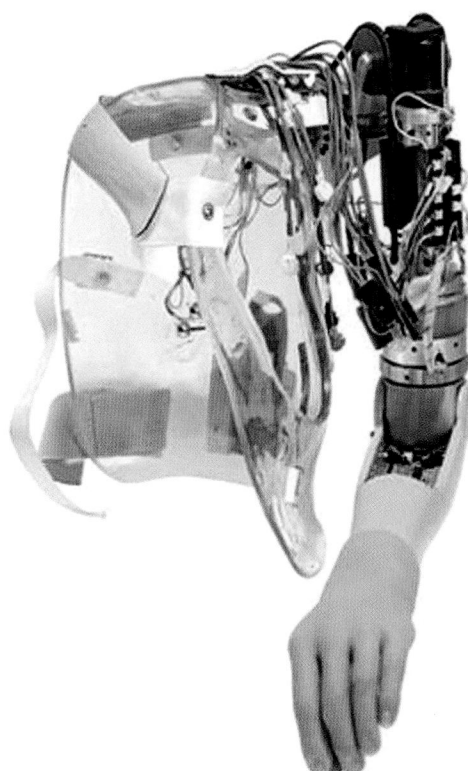

Figure 118-9 Complex myoelectric upper extremity prosthesis developed at Johns Hopkins in conjunction with the Defense Advanced Research Project Agency. Note the color-coded electrodes, which are placed on certain muscle groups for myoelectric control or on various aspects of muscles after targeted reinnervation surgery to allow areas of each muscle to independently transmit current.

but late revision is not uncommon and is influenced by both disease and either prosthesis-induced or prosthetic technology–specific concerns. Such concerns may include late skin and musculoskeletal changes and complications necessitating revision, such as ulcers, stump necrosis, dermatitis, infection, or disease recurrence in the stump, as with malignancy and vasculitis. In addition, revision of the bony and soft tissue stump components to allow fitting and use of more modern prostheses may be chosen.

In general, attitudes toward prosthesis use in proximal upper extremity amputees are poor, and currently, as many as 40% would rather not use their prosthesis.[62] Even those with hand-based amputations can find return to activities of daily living and job performance challenging.[63] Return to employment has a positive effect on prosthesis use.[64] However, the patient's education level appears to play an important role in postamputation employment. Weed and colleagues found that more than 70% of those with at least some college education were employed after amputation whereas only 23% of those with a high-school or less education were employed.[65] The potential for these long-term physical, socioeconomic, and psychological problems again re-enforces the need for upper extremity amputees to have access to a multidisciplinary

institution regardless of whether they choose to seek contemporary rehabilitation and prosthetic options.

SELECTED KEY REFERENCES

Calandruccio JH. Amputations of the hand. In: Canale ST, Beaty JH, eds. *Campbell's Operative Orthopedics.* St. Louis, MO: Mosby Elsevier; 2008:660-674.
This reference chapter contains the latest insight into hand-based amputation. Similar to the chapter by Cleveland, it provides technical outlines and decision making for all aspects of hand amputation. The procedural summaries and graphics are clear, concise, and overall superb.

Chung KJ. *Hand and Upper Extremity Reconstruction with DVD: A Volume in the Procedures in Reconstructive Surgery Series.* St. Louis, MO: Saunders Elsevier; 2008.
This volume highlights the plastic and reconstructive surgery aspects of the hand and upper extremity. It will provide a resource, including operative video, describing the newest techniques and options surrounding both hand and upper extremity conservation and loss.

Cleveland KJ. Amputations of the upper extremity. In: Canale ST, Beaty JH, eds. *Campbell's Operative Orthopedics.* St. Louis, MO: Mosby Elsevier; 2008:625-638.
This definitive reference provides a state-of-the-art technical description of upper extremity amputation and the factors involved in operative decision making at each level. It includes excellent step-by-step summaries and graphics/pictures.

Meier RH, Atkins DJ. *Functional Outcome of Adults and Children with Upper Extremity Amputation.* New York, NY: Demos Medical Publishing; 2004.
This source provides comprehensive state-of-the-art information on reconstructive methods, rehabilitation, prosthetic options, and long-term care concerns in those undergoing upper extremity amputation.

O'Shaughnessy KD, Dumanian GA, Lipschutz RD, Miller LA, Stubblefield K, Kuiken TA. Targeted reinnervation to improve prosthesis control in transhumeral amputees. *J Bone Joint Surg Am.* 2008;90: 393-400.
This communication provides a glimpse of the future by describing the state-of-the-art surgical techniques developed to provide the most complex neuromuscular biomechanical control of upper extremity prosthetics to date.

Smith DG, Michael JW, Bowker JH. *Atlas of Amputations and Limb Deficiencies: Surgical, Prosthetic, and Rehabilitation Principles.* Rosemont, IL: American Academy of Orthopedic Surgeons; 2004.
This reference provides the basic principles of surgical techniques and the global aspects of postamputation care by the level of amputation required.

Stansbury LG, Lalliss SJ, Branstetter JG, Bagg MR, Holcomb JB. Amputations in U.S. military personnel in the current conflicts in Afghanistan and Iraq. *J Trauma.* 2008;22:43-46.
This manuscript provides a description of the incidence, cause, and outcomes of extremity injury and amputation during the Global War on Terrorism.

Ziegler-Graham K, MacKenzie EJ, Ephraim PL, Travison TG, Brookmeyer R. Estimating the prevalence of limb loss in the United States: 2005 to 2050. *Arch Phys Med Rehabil.* 2008;89:422-429.
This article provides the most current epidemiologic estimates of amputation in the United States, as well as projections for amputee care in the future.

REFERENCES

The reference list can be found on the companion Expert Consult Web site at *www.expertconsult.com.*

CHAPTER 119

Raynaud's Syndrome

Gregory J. Landry

Based in part on a chapter in the previous edition by Roger F. J. Shepherd, MB BCh.

Raynaud's syndrome (RS) is defined as episodic pallor or cyanosis of the fingers caused by vasoconstriction of small digital arteries or arterioles occurring in response to cold or emotional stress. Digits are generally normal between attacks. Although this term typically applies to the fingers, the toes can also be affected. RS may occur as an isolated clinical entity or in association with one or more of a variety of systemic disease processes.

The hallmark of RS is the change in skin temperature and color brought on by exposure to cold. A typical vasospastic attack is characterized by the sudden onset of pallor of part or all of one or more digits. Cyanosis follows as static blood in the capillaries becomes desaturated. The attack subsides with the return of arterial inflow, and postischemic vasodilatation results in hyperemia and rubor of the skin (Figs. 119-1 and 119-2).

■ TERMINOLOGY

Historical Perspective

In 1862, Maurice Raynaud, a French physician, titled his thesis for the Academy of Medicine "On Local Asphyxia and Symmetrical Gangrene of the Extremities."[1] In this paper he described 25 patients with intermittent digital ischemia and recognized the relationship of local cold and emotional stress in the causation of these episodes. He attributed the attacks of digital ischemia to excessive sympathetic activity producing vasoconstriction of the digital arteries. He also described the classic tricolor skin changes of digital pallor, cyanosis, and rubor that are now associated with his name. These patients with intermittent vasospastic episodes of digital ischemia were hence diagnosed as having "Raynaud's disease."

Raynaud's original series included a mixture of patients; some did have a primary vasospastic disease, but others with gangrene of the fingers probably had significant arterial obstruction. In 1901, Hutchinson recognized that there can be multiple causes of Raynaud's observations and coined the term "Raynaud's phenomenon" to indicate the presence of an underlying abnormality causing this disorder.

Current Perspective

In clinical practice, use of the term *Raynaud's disease* or *Raynaud's phenomenon* has not been intuitive. These terms are commonly misunderstood and are often mistakenly interchanged; as a result, they have lost much of their original

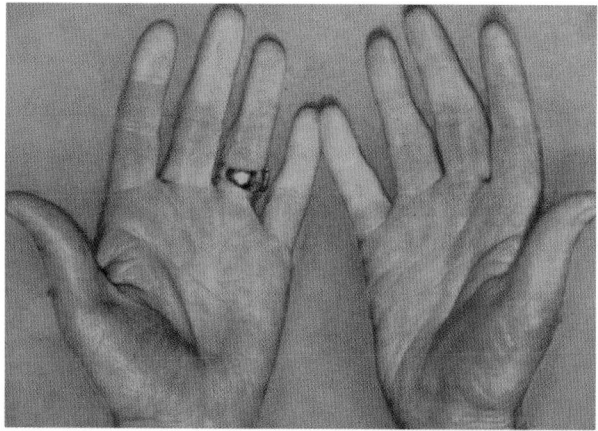

Figure 119-1 Palmar view of the hands of a patient with a typical example of Raynaud's syndrome. Note that attacks of digital vasospasm cause well-demarcated pallor affecting one or more fingers brought on by exposure to cold or emotional stress.

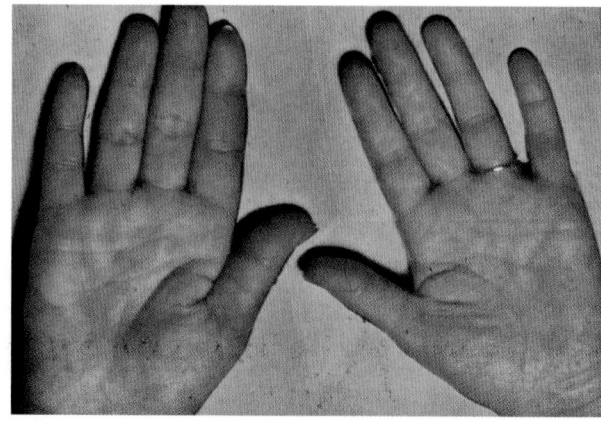

Figure 119-2 Palmar view of the hands of a patient with Raynaud's syndrome demonstrating both pallor and cyanosis in multiple fingers.

meaning. Review of the Raynaud's literature is complicated by the lack of a standard accepted diagnostic classification. For this reason many have advocated replacing the old terms "Raynaud's disease" and "Raynaud's phenomenon" with *Raynaud's syndrome*.[2]

RS can be subdivided into two groups: (1) primary RS, in which patients have idiopathic vasospasm, and (2) secondary RS, in which patients have an underlying disease causing symptomatic episodes. It has also been helpful to classify patients with Raynaud's syndrome as having either vasospastic or obstructive disease. This has important clinical utility because it underscores the different pathologic mechanisms, treatment options, and outcomes of these two groups.

EPIDEMIOLOGY

Prevalence

RS is a common disorder. Its prevalence in the general population varies greatly with climate and ethnic origin. A number of epidemiologic studies investigating disease prevalence have been performed, primarily in populations in colder climates. Overall estimates of disease prevalence in the general population range from 3.3% to 22.0%, with a prevalence of 0.5% to 8.3% in men and 2.5% to 21% in women.[3-20] White women consistently have been noted to have a higher prevalence of RS than men. In African American[16] and Asian[8] populations, the gender prevalence is equal.

Incidence

Longitudinal population-based studies have been carried out to determine the annual incidence of RS in the general population. In a 14-year study in a community in southern France, the annual incidence of new cases of primary RS was 0.25% with a declining incidence with age.[21] Of patients in whom RS was initially diagnosed, remission of symptoms was observed in 33%, thus suggesting that primary RS is a transient phenomenon in many people. Similar findings were noted in an epidemiologic analysis of the Framingham Offspring Study cohort. Over a 7-year period, the incidence of new-onset RS was 2.2% in women and 1.5% in men. Remission of Raynaud's symptoms occurred in 64% of those with primary RS at the beginning of the study period.[22] In subjects with persistent disease, there was no limitation in activities because of RS. These studies were the first to report significant disease remission in patients with primary RS. No predictive factors for remission have been identified, but it is thought to be due to a general decrease in vascular reactivity with age.

PATHOGENESIS

Normal Arterial Flow to the Hand

Circulation in the hand is complex with frequent anatomic variants. The deep and superficial arches supply the metacar-

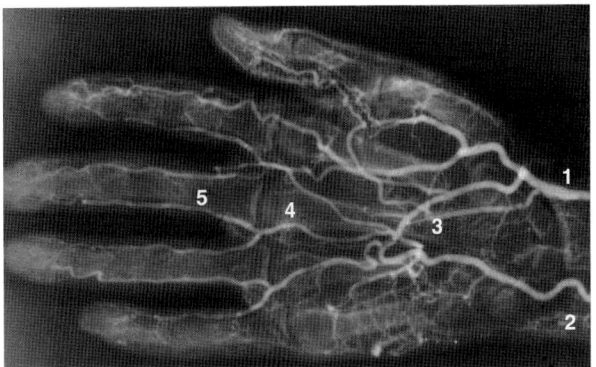

Figure 119-3 Normal hand arterial anatomy. 1, Radial artery; 2, ulnar artery; 3, deep palmar arch; 4, common digital (metacarpal) artery; 5, proper digital artery.

pal arteries and in turn the proper digital arteries (Fig. 119-3). In most patients, branches of both the deep and superficial arches provide blood flow to all five fingers, and the two palmar arches provide important collateral flow between the radial and ulnar system.[23] The superficial arch is incomplete in 21.5% of people.[24] Severe digital ischemia can occur with occlusion of the radial or ulnar artery and an incomplete superficial arch.

The metacarpal arteries in the palm originate from the superficial arch and provide blood flow to the digits. At the web space the common digital (metacarpal) arteries branch to supply the proper digital arteries that run the length of each finger. In at least 86% of extremities, all five digits are supplied by arteries from both the deep and superficial arches.[23] Each finger has two digital arteries, which is important in preventing critical ischemia if one digital artery becomes occluded. The end of the finger is highly vascular with a dense network of blood vessels in the pulp space of the fingers.

Regulation of Blood Flow in the Digits

Blood flow in the digits is highly variable and can range from less than 1 mL/min per 100 mL of tissue to 180 mL/min.[25] Blood flow to the skin of the digits has two functions, nutritional and thermoregulatory. Only a very small proportion of digital blood flow (<10%) is needed to provide nutrients and oxygen to the tissues.[26] Approximately 80% to 90% of blood flow through the digits is controlled by thermoregulatory mechanisms and serves an important role in controlling body temperature.[27] Blood vessels that are superficially located in the skin dilate to radiate excess heat to the environment, and this reduces body core temperature. In response to cold, these arteries constrict to decrease blood flow and conserve body heat. One hand can lose 800 calories of heat per minute, which causes a fall in esophageal temperature of 0.6°C in 9 minutes.[28]

Changes in digital blood flow occur as a result of changes in ambient temperature, and this is effected in part by the central nervous system with input from the cerebral cortex, hypothalamus, and medullary vasomotor centers. The hypothalamus changes body temperature by altering sympathetic outflow to the digital vessels via the medulla, spinal cord, sympathetic ganglion, and local nerves. The sympathetic nerves innervate vascular smooth muscle in the digital arteries and regulate vessel diameter and blood flow. Activation of the sympathetic nerves on vascular smooth muscle causes vasoconstriction, and decreased sympathetic activity allows vasodilatation.

The fingers and the palms contain many arteriovenous (AV) anastomoses, and blood can return to the venous circulation before reaching the distal small capillaries. Studies by Coffman and others have shown that reflex sympathetic vasoconstriction produced by total-body cooling causes a marked decrease in total digital blood flow; however, capillary blood flow is not affected.[27,29] This is due to constriction of AV shunts while maintaining nutritional blood flow to the fingers. During vasodilatation, 80% to 90% of finger blood flow is shunted through AV anastomoses. In warm environments, digital blood flow is increased by shunting more blood through these AV fistulae. The AV shunts are also under the control of the sympathetic nervous system.[30] In response to cold exposure or body cooling, increased sympathetic tone causes the digital AV shunts to close; hence, less blood flows through the digits and core body temperature is maintained.

Maximum vasoconstriction in response to cold occurs at 10°C to 20°C. At lower temperatures, cold-induced vasodilatation results in slight reopening of arteries to allow a trickle of blood into the digits. In 1930, Lewis measured blood flow in the finger with a thermoelectric junction and found during immersion in cold water that vasoconstriction occurred initially followed by alternating periods of vasodilatation.[31] With cold exposure, there is a regular rhythmic fluctuation in finger flow caused by periods of vasoconstriction and vasodilatation in the fingers every 30 seconds to 2 minutes.[32] Other investigators have found similar rhythmic fluctuations in finger flow with a frequency of 5 to 10 per minute.[33] These alternating periods of vasoconstriction and dilatation have been called the hunting response.[34] This cold-induced vasodilatation, which protects the fingers from freezing in a cold environment, is impaired in those with secondary RS because of the presence of occlusive arterial disease.

Mechanisms of Primary Vasospasm

Historical Perspective

The exact cause of the vasospastic attacks in primary RS is unknown. There is no demonstrable structural abnormality of the digital arteries. Whether primary RS represents an exaggeration of the normal thermoregulatory mechanisms causing constriction of digital vessels in response to cooling or is due to a specific local or systemic fault remains an area of controversy.

Raynaud in 1862 speculated that sympathetic nervous system hyperactivity was the sole cause of vasospasm.[1] This position was disproved by Lewis in 1929, who demonstrated that blockade of digital nerve conduction did not prevent vasospasm. Lewis proposed the theory of a "local vascular

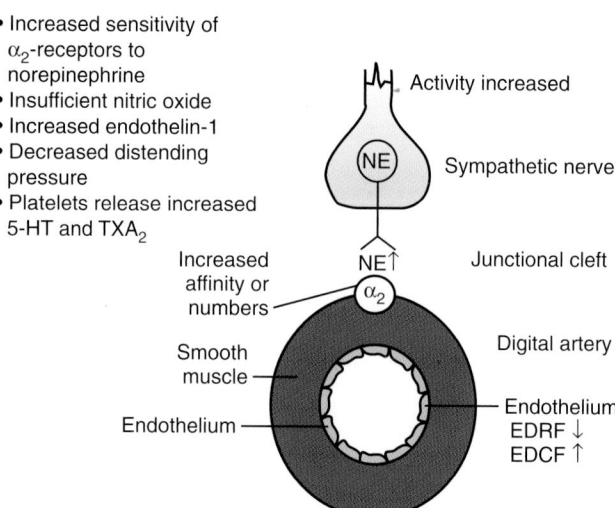

PRIMARY RAYNAUD'S DISEASE: POTENTIAL MECHANISMS

- Increased sensitivity of α₂-receptors to norepinephrine
- Insufficient nitric oxide
- Increased endothelin-1
- Decreased distending pressure
- Platelets release increased 5-HT and TXA₂

Figure 119-4 There are many potential causes of vasospastic attacks in primary Raynaud's syndrome. Norepinephrine (NE) released from the sympathetic nerve ending acts on the postjunctional α2-receptor located on vascular smooth muscle. Local cooling enhances the response of the α2-receptor, thereby causing increased arterial contraction. Endothelial dysfunction may lead to insufficient nitric oxide or increased endothelin-1, which changes the balance toward arterial constriction. Activated platelets release thromboxane A₂ (TXA₂) and serotonin (5-hydroxytryptamine [5-HT], which may aggravate arterial vasospasm. A decrease in intraluminal distending pressure may decrease the "critical closing pressure" threshold and result in a vasospastic attack. EDCF, endothelium-derived contracting factor; EDRF, endothelium-derived relaxing factor.

fault" in the digital arteries causing increased sensitivity of the blood vessel to cold.[35] He also found that cooling of the proximal part of the finger but keeping the distal portion warm would still cause distal vasospasm. He concluded that this must be due to local factors causing constriction of the more proximal digital artery by cold. Over the past 80 years, the exact nature of the "local vascular fault" has not been fully elucidated; however, recent research has greatly increased our understanding of what is likely to be a multifactorial problem involving a combination of vascular, neural, and humoral factors (Fig. 119-4).[36]

Vascular Abnormalities

Impaired Vasodilatation. Vascular endothelial cells synthesize a number of vasodilating and vasoconstricting substances.[37-40] Endothelial-derived relaxing factors include nitric oxide (NO), prostacyclin, adenosine triphosphate (ATP), and bradykinin. NO is a potent vasodilator synthesized from the amino acid L-arginine by the activity of the enzyme NO synthase. NO diffuses from the endothelium into smooth muscle, where it activates guanylate cyclase to increase intracellular cyclic guanosine monophosphate (cGMP), which leads to vascular relaxation.

A deficiency of one or more of these factors could potentially increase the responsiveness of digital arteries to vasoconstrictive influences and increase the likelihood of vasospasm. This has most extensively been studied in patients with RS secondary to scleroderma, in whom a reduction in mRNA for NO synthase has been demonstrated.[41] Decreased levels of asymmetric dimethylarginine, an inhibitor of endothelial NO synthase, have also been demonstrated in patients with secondary RS.[42] The role of NO in primary RS is less clear.

A number of studies have suggested endothelial dysfunction as an important cause of RS. In one study, patients underwent a series of sequential infusions with acetylcholine, prostacyclin, glyceryl trinitrate, and L-arginine. Patients with a history of RS had a greater digital artery vasodilator response to intra-arterial glyceryl trinitrate (an endothelium-independent vasodilator) than to acetylcholine (an endothelium-dependent vasodilator), whereas in control patients, the difference in response was less pronounced.[43]

Increased Vasoconstriction. The endothelial cell also produces factors that cause vessel contraction, such as endothelin-1 (ET-1), which is a potent vasoconstrictor, as well as a promoter of fibroblast and smooth muscle proliferation. Other endothelium-derived contracting factors include angiotensin II, thromboxane A_2, and superoxide anion, an oxygen-derived free radical. Patients with primary RS have been found to have increased circulating and intraplatelet serotonin.[44] The thromboxane A_2 and serotonin produced by platelets can induce vasospasm.

Normally, endothelial cells continually form and release enough NO to keep vascular smooth muscle relaxed. If the endothelium is damaged, NO production is decreased and vasoconstrictor substances such as endothelin may predominate.[45] Increased levels of ET-1 would potentiate arterial contraction by other agents such as norepinephrine and serotinin.[46] Plasma ET-1 levels become elevated in response to the cold pressor test, which may suggest an association between the rise in ET-1 levels and cold-induced vasoconstriction.[47] Whole-body cooling also increases ET-1 levels in women with primary RS.[48] A threefold rise in ET-1 concentration has been reported in subjects with primary RS.[49]

Angiotensin is another endogenous peptide with vasoconstrictive effects that has been implicated in the mechanism of vasospasm. Despite the frequent use of angiotensin-converting enzyme (ACE) inhibitors in patients with RS, the mechanism of involvement of angiotensin in RS is unknown. Increased circulating levels of angiotensin II have recently been noted in patients with scleroderma.[50] Activation of the renin-angiotensin system, however, has not been demonstrated in patients with primary RS.[51]

Neural Factors

Adrenergic Factors.
In recent years, the focus of RS pathophysiology has been on alterations in peripheral adrenoceptor activity. Early studies with the sympathetic blocking

drug reserpine demonstrated increased digital blood flow in patients with RS.[29] Laboratory studies showed a marked reduction in cold-induced digital arterial vasospasm after the intra-arterial administration of reserpine.[52] This suggested that patients with RS may possess abnormal adrenergic receptors that become increasingly sensitive to stimulation after exposure to cold.

Characterization of α_1- and α_2-adrenoceptors has led to an improved understanding of the mechanisms of RS. α_1-Adrenoceptors are located postsynaptically and, when stimulated, produce vasoconstriction. α_2-Adrenoceptors are located both presynaptically and postsynaptically. Whereas stimulation of presynaptic α_2-receptors inhibits norepinephrine release and has a vasodilatory effect, stimulation of postsynaptic α_2-receptors induces vasoconstriction. Sympathetic nerves can respond to cold and emotional stress by releasing neurotransmitters such as norepinephrine, which acts on the postsynaptic α_2-receptor and causes vascular smooth muscle contraction. Cold also causes increased affinity of the α_2-receptor for norepinephrine, which results in enhanced smooth muscle contraction in the cold.[53,54]

Experimentally, the relative roles of α_1- and α_2-receptors in regulating digital blood flow was evaluated by plethysmography during the intra-arterial infusion of saline or adrenergic antagonists.[55] In normal controls, infusion of the selective α_1-antagonist prazosin resulted in a significantly greater increase in digital arterial flow than did infusion of the α_2-antagonist yohimbine. In contrast, in patients with RS, the vasodilatory effect of yohimbine was equal to that of prazosin. This demonstrated that although α_1-receptors are the dominant determinant of digital arterial flow in controls, in patients with RS, α_2-receptors also play a prominent role.

The mechanism of α_2-mediated vasoconstriction in RS is not completely understood. An elevation in the number of α_2-receptor sites and α_2-receptor hypersensitivity in patients with RS have been proposed as potential mechanisms. Alternatively, alterations in the number of receptors exposed at any one time may occur in patients with RS. It has recently been demonstrated that with cooling, the α_2-receptors redistribute from the interior of the vascular smooth muscle cells to the membrane, where they can be activated by norepinephrine to induce vasoconstriction. This cold-induced redistribution of receptors appears to be under the control of Rho kinase, a guanosine triphosphate–binding protein known to be involved in cell motility and contraction.[56,57]

Neurally Mediated Impairment in Vasodilatation.
Nerves supplying blood vessels produce a number of vasodilatory substances. Calcitonin gene–related peptide (CGRP) is a vasodilator released by sensory afferent fibers. Immunohistochemical studies have shown a reduction in the number of CGRP-immunoreactive nerve fibers in biopsies of finger skin from patients with both primary RS and RS secondary to scleroderma.[58] Intravenous infusion of CGRP has been shown to improve blood flow in patients with severe secondary RS.[59]

Sympathetic nerves also release substance P, a vasodilator, as well as neuropeptide Y and ATP, which are vasoconstrictor agents.[60] The vasoconstrictor effect of ATP is also augmented in response to cold. Though not as well studied as CGRP, altered concentrations of these agents have been demonstrated in patients with RS.

The parasympathetic nerves release acetylcholine and vasoactive intestinal peptide, both of which are vasodilators. Acetylcholine acts in an endothelial-dependent fashion, and vasoactive intestinal peptide is endothelial independent. With endothelial damage, as in atherosclerosis or small-vessel fibrosis in scleroderma, acetylcholine-induced vasodilatation is impaired.

Centrally Mediated Mechanisms.
Though typically induced by cold, emotional stress is recognized as a potential trigger of vasospasm, which implies that there is a central neural component to the mechanism of RS. The nature of this neural component is not well defined and is difficult to demonstrate. Digital cutaneous vasoconstriction is prolonged in RS patients subjected to stressors when compared with controls, and this appears to be associated with a rise in serum ET-1 levels. Thus, the centrally mediated neural mechanisms appear to be superimposed on locally released ET-1. Overall, however, the centrally mediated mechanisms appear less prominent than the peripherally mediated neural mechanisms.[36]

Humoral Factors

Many circulating humoral factors have been implicated in the pathogenesis of RS, particularly in secondary and vibration-induced forms. Whether these factors are the cause or the effect of vasospasm is unclear, but several associations have clearly been shown.

Platelet Activation.
Activation of platelets has been demonstrated in patients with RS. Elevated circulating levels of activated platelet products such as thromboxane and β-thromboglobulin have been induced by cooling of subjects with RS. Serotonin (5-hydroxytryptamine) is another product of platelet activation that has been detected at increased levels in the plasma and platelets of patients with RS.[44] However, serotonin has not been identified at increased levels in venous samples taken during episodes of vasospasm.[61] Ketanserin, a serotonin receptor antagonist, has been shown to accelerate digital rewarming after episodes of vasospasm.[62] Paradoxically, the selective serotonin reuptake inhibitor fluoxetine, which raises plasma levels of serotonin, has also been shown to decrease the frequency and severity of vasospastic attacks.[63] Thus, the role of serotonin in the pathogenesis of RS remains to be defined.

Fibrinolysis.
Abnormalities of fibrinolysis have primarily been implicated in secondary RS. Elevated levels of tissue plasminogen activator inhibitor have been shown in patients with scleroderma.[64] An impairment in thrombolysis is thought to predispose to fibrin deposition and vascular obstruction.[36]

Blood Rheology.
Abnormalities in red blood cell deformability and viscosity have also been described in RS. Reduced red blood cell deformability has been demonstrated in secondary but not primary RS and may reflect free radical damage to the erythrocyte membrane.[65] Blood viscosity increases with cold exposure but appears to do so to a greater degree in patients with primary RS than in normal controls.[66]

Hormonal Factors

RS is more frequent in women than men and, in women, is more frequent and severe between menarche and menopause. In postmenopausal women, the prevalence of RS is increased significantly in women receiving hormone replacement therapy.[67] This has led to interest in the potential relationship between hormonal factors and RS. Investigators have demonstrated tonically elevated sympathetic tone in the cutaneous circulation in women in comparison to men.[68] How this translates to an increase in RS in women is unclear, but adrenergic effects have been implied. In human cell culture and in mouse models, estrogen has been demonstrated to increase the expression of α_2-adrenoceptors.[69] The role of estrogen in the pathogenesis of RS remains an area of ongoing research.

Genetic Factors

Approximately one quarter of patients with primary RS have a family history of RS in a first-degree relative.[70] The recognized familial clustering of RS cases has led investigators to search for a genetic cause. From an epidemiologic standpoint, however, it has been difficult to differentiate genetic factors from shared environmental causes. The strongest evidence to date of the importance of genetic factors has been provided by twin studies that control for shared environmental causes such that differences in the prevalence of RS between monozygotic and dizygotic twins can be explained only by genetic differences. In the largest study to date, Cherkas and associates demonstrated a doubling of risk for RS in monozygotic twin pairs versus dizygotic twins.[71] Although a number of chromosomal regions have been evaluated in genomic studies, no significant differences in allelic frequency have been detected between patients with RS and normal controls.

■ RISK FACTORS
Gender

RS predominantly affects young women, but it can affect both sexes and occur in any age group, including children. Older studies have noted that RS affects women four times more often than men. More recent surveys indicate that men are commonly affected, with a male-female ratio closer to 1:1.6.[72]

Age

The usual age at onset of primary RS ranges from 11 to 45 years. A study of 474 patients with RS by Allen and Brown reported an average age of 31 years.[73] Nigrovic and colleagues recently reported a series of 123 cases of RS in children younger than 19 years. The mean age at the time of diagnosis was 13 years.[74] As with adults, the majority (70%) of the children had primary RS. Older patients with RS are more likely to have a contributing underlying arterial disease.

Smoking

Even though smoking has been shown to impair vasodilatation and decrease cutaneous circulation,[75] the link between smoking and primary vasospastic RS is less clear. Most epidemiologic studies have shown no association between smoking and primary RS in women. In a study of the Framingham Heart Study Offspring Cohort, no association was found between smoking and RS in women; however, there was a significant association in men, particularly in those with other cardiovascular risk factors, with an odds ratio of 2.6.[76] The reason for gender differences in smoking effects is unclear.

Alcohol

As with smoking, the effect of alcohol consumption on RS remains to be clarified. The effects of mild, moderate, and heavy alcohol consumption and red wine consumption were evaluated in the Framingham Heart Study Offspring Cohort study.[76] In a multivariate logistic regression model, heavy alcohol consumption was a significant risk factor for RS in women (odds ratio, 1.69) but not in men. Moderate alcohol consumption was protective in men (odds ratio, 0.51) but did not reach statistical significance in women. Red wine consumption had a protective effect in both men and women, thus adding to the growing body of literature demonstrating the cardiovascular protective effects of red wine consumption.[77]

Occupational Exposure

Occupational arterial disease manifested as RS can result from the use of vibratory tools or from repetitive pounding on the palm of the hand. Traumatic ulnar artery occlusion, or hypothenar hammer syndrome, is common in carpenters and mechanics but can occur in any occupation in which instruments or hand tools are used.[78]

Vibration-induced RS was first recognized in 1918 by Hamilton,[79] and it has been estimated that as many as 1.2 million American workers involved in a variety of occupations using vibrating tools are now at risk.[59] Terms that have been used to describe RS caused by chronic vibration include *hand-arm vibration syndrome* and *vibration-induced white finger*. The risk for vibration-induced RS is proportional to the duration of exposure.[80] In a study of workers who used compressed air drills to clean castings, 4% had RS by 2 years, 48% by 3 years, and 55% by 10 years.[81] McLafferty and colleagues examined 16 automobile glass workers who used a pneumatic air knife for removal of automobile windshields. The mean onset of

RS was 3 years, and workers had used the vibrating knife for an average of 2450 hours. None of the workers improved after they stopped using the air knife, and a third worsened.[82]

Chronic vibration appears to cause structural damage to the arterial wall with hypertrophy of the intima and media. Vibration is believed to cause sympathetic overactivity, endothelial damage, and smooth muscle hypertrophy leading to vibration-induced vasospasm.[83,84] In addition, formation of microthrombi can lead to fixed digital ischemia and fingertip necrosis. The prognosis may be poor because of the development of digital artery obstruction after prolonged exposure to vibration. It is unknown whether vibration-induced RS is reversible in the earlier stages. Early symptoms may include tingling and numbness from peripheral nerve damage. Preventive measures, including wearing gloves, providing a cushioned surface on handles, and avoiding prolonged exposure, may minimize the damage[85] (see Chapter 120: Occupational Vascular Problems).

Drugs and Medications

Beta Blockers

β-Adrenoreceptor blocking drugs are well-established medications for arterial hypertension and cardiac disease. Beta blockers, however, can cause arterial vasospasm through inhibition of β_2-mediated arterial vasodilatation. The incidence of RS in hypertensive patients taking beta blockers was 40% in a Scandinavian study in which patients responded to a questionnaire.[86] It is doubtful that all symptoms were drug related because half of these patients had symptoms before starting antihypertensive therapy and 18% of those taking diuretics also complained of RS. Approximately 5% of patients treated with beta-blocker medications for hypertension require discontinuation of the medication or dose reduction because of RS.[87]

Vasospasm occurs with both selective and nonselective beta blockers. Drugs with combined α- and β-adrenoceptor blocking activity such as labetalol would be expected to cause less symptomatic vasospasm.[88] However, in a double-blinded crossover trial of propranolol and labetalol, no differences in finger temperature or symptoms were found.[89]

Despite these concerns, most patients with RS do tolerate beta blockers, and many studies show no adverse effects on digital blood flow. In a double-blinded crossover trial in 16 patients with RS, Coffman and Rasmussen compared the hemodynamic effects of 80 mg/day of propranolol versus 100 mg/day of metoprolol with placebo.[90] There was no significant difference from placebo in finger systolic pressure or fingertip capillary flow measured in a warm or cold environment. In addition, there was no significant change in the number of vasospastic attacks in patients treated with a beta blocker. Another study also found no adverse effects of intravenous beta blockers on finger skin temperature and laser Doppler blood flow when compared with placebo.[91] Both of these studies would indicate that the use of beta blockers is not contraindicated in most patients with RS.

Chemotherapy Agents

A number of case reports suggest an increased incidence of RS in chemotherapy patients.[92] Vinblastine and bleomycin are used for the treatment of testicular cancer and lymphoma and can induce RS in 2.6% of patients undergoing chemotherapy.[93] Cisplatin, carboplatin, and gemcitabine have been associated with the development of ischemic ulcers in patients with scleroderma and should be used with caution in these patients.[94] Interferon alfa is used for the treatment of leukemia and melanoma, and rare cases of RS with digital ulceration have been reported after several months of therapy.[95]

Other Drugs and Toxins

The ergot preparations used for migraine headaches are a well-known cause of severe extremity vasospasm and ischemia with absent pulses.[96] Amphetamine and cocaine abuse can also cause arterial vasoconstriction.[97,98] Other drugs that have been reported to be associated with RS have included oral contraceptives and cyclosporine. Bromocriptine, an ergot derivative and dopamine agonist used to treat Parkinson's disease, may cause mild RS, but discontinuation of the medication is not usually required.[99]

Endocrine Disorders

Endocrine diseases that have been associated with RS include hypothyroidism, Graves' disease, Addison's disease, and Cushing's disease. These are all unusual causes of vasospasm.

Increased Blood Viscosity

Blood flow varies indirectly with blood viscosity, and any abnormality that increases blood viscosity results in decreased blood flow. Disorders that affect blood viscosity include cryoglobulinemia, paraproteinemia in myeloma, and polycythemia. Cold-induced precipitation of proteins increases the viscosity of blood. Cryoglobulins occur with malignancies such as lymphomas and some viral infections and can cause skin necrosis and gangrene of the fingers, toes, and ears. Hepatitis C in particular is associated with secondary cryoglobulinemia.[100] Treatment of cryoglobulinemia is plasmapheresis to remove the cryoglobulin, steroids, and chemotherapy to treat the underlying malignancy (Fig. 119-5).[101]

Malignancy

A wide range of cancers have been associated with secondary RS. Digital ischemia is an uncommon but well-recognized paraneoplastic manifestation of malignancy. The most common malignancies associated with RS are adenocarcinoma of the lung, stomach, colon, pancreas, ovaries, testes, and kidney; hematologic malignancies, including myeloma and leukemia; lymphomas; melanoma; and astrocytomas.[102-105] Possible mechanisms of arterial disease caused by malignancy

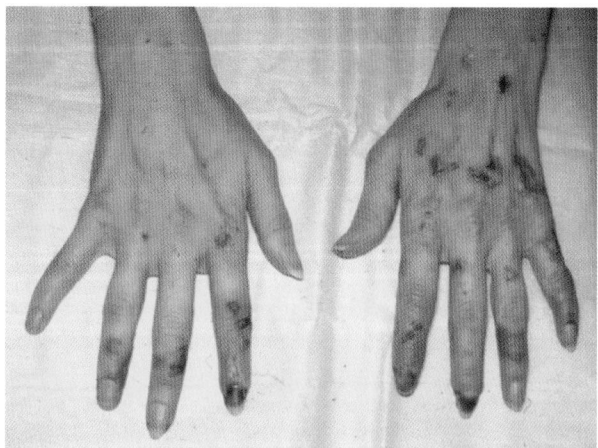

Figure 119-5 Cryoglobulinemia type 1 associated with low-grade lymphoma in a 70-year-old woman. Cryoglobulins cause small-vessel occlusive arterial disease with cutaneous necrosis involving the extremities. Digital ischemia improved with plasmapheresis, chemotherapy, and prednisone.

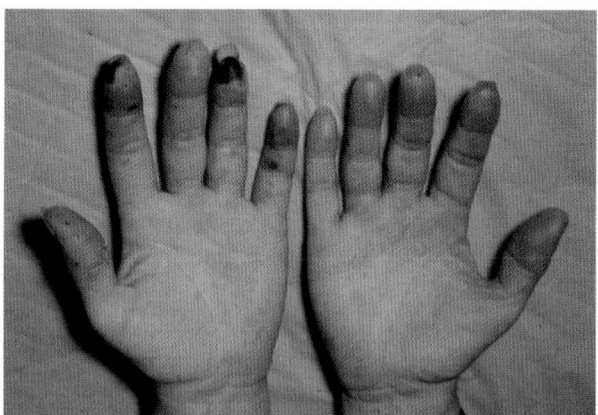

Figure 119-6 Paraneoplastic vasculitis with gangrene of several digits in a patient in whom small cell lung cancer was recently diagnosed. The digital ischemia improved with chemotherapy.

may include coagulopathy, cryoglobulinemia, or small-vessel vasculitis (Fig. 119-6).

Treatment of the cancer may result in remission of the Raynaud symptoms and digital ischemia.[106] RS associated with malignancy has a sudden onset at an older age with severe symptoms and asymmetric digital involvement. Many patients (80%) progress to digital infarction and gangrene.[102]

■ CLINICAL FINDINGS

The clinical manifestations are the basis for the diagnosis of RS. Coffman suggested the following criteria for the diagnosis of RS: "Episodic attacks of well demarcated blanching or cyanosis of one or more digits brought on by cold exposure or emotion."[99] "Episodic" means that the attacks are reversible as opposed to persistent ischemia. A well-demarcated change occurs with local vasospasm, and this avoids the problem of overdiagnosis in normal individuals who simply have pale fingers.

All three color changes do not have to be present to make the diagnosis of RS. Gifford and Heins reported in 1957 that 65% of 133 patients had classic white to blue to red changes; however, many patients describe only episodic pallor or cyanosis of the fingers.[107] A study of 78 patients by Maricq and associates found that white (38%) or blue (44%) was the most common color change reported by patients.[72] Maricq and Weinrich used color charts to assist patients with description of their symptoms.[108] Rarely does the patient have a spontaneous episode of vasospasm at the physician's office, and it is surprisingly difficult to provoke a typical vasospastic episode in the vascular laboratory.

Although the clinical findings may be variable, the typical patient describes attacks of pallor involving part or all of one or many fingers brought on by exposure to cold with full and rapid recovery on rewarming of the digits. The episodes are self-limited and may last from less than a minute to generally not more than 10 to 20 minutes. Local warming of the hands is usually successful in terminating attacks. Pallor may involve part of the digit or the entire finger. Vasospastic attacks most commonly involve the fingers but can affect both the fingers and toes in up to a third of patients (Fig. 119-7). For reasons that have never been clarified, the thumbs are frequently spared. This was demonstrated in a recent study in which the frequency and severity of vasospastic episodes were equal in the second through fifth digits and significantly greater than in the thumb in both primary and secondary RS.[109]

Attacks may occur several times a day to several times a week. Episodes of vasospasm are more common in the cooler winter months, and some patients have few or no attacks during the summer. Unusual manifestations include vasospasm of the nose, ear, and nipple.[110] Other vascular beds prone to vasospasm include the coronary and cerebral vessels. Patients with Prinzmetal's angina are more likely to have RS and migraine headaches, thus suggesting a common factor causing generalized vasospasm.[111]

Pain is not usually a feature during the pallor or cyanotic phase of primary RS. The absence of pain and lack of tissue damage during arterial vasospasm may be because during cooling of the fingers, as well as vasoconstriction, there is also cold-induced intermittent vasodilatation, and this allows just enough blood flow to protect the fingers from severe ischemia or freezing. Minor finger discomfort, but not pain, may occur during the hyperemic recovery phase.

In contrast, patients with underlying occlusive disease have little or no reserve and cannot increase digital blood flow, with the result that ischemic damage can occur during exposure to cold. These patients with secondary RS are more likely to complain of digital pain on rewarming of cold fingers because the blood flow cannot increase to match the increased metabolic activity of the finger.

ASSOCIATED DISEASES

Disorders Associated with Secondary Raynaud's Syndrome

Secondary causes of RS all have one thing in common: they cause some degree of fixed vascular obstruction to blood flow, which decreases the threshold for cold-induced vasospasm. When the artery is narrowed because of preexisting large- or small-vessel disease, there is a lower "critical closing pressure," and a relatively normal vasoconstrictor response to cold or other stimuli will result in temporary closure of the vessel. Any disease that narrows the vessel lumen of the digital arteries or increases blood viscosity may cause RS. RS is common in connective tissue diseases (CTDs) such as scleroderma, where intimal hyperplasia, thrombosis, and fibrosis result in luminal narrowing of the digital arteries, but this process may also involve the more proximal arteries of the hand and forearm. The abnormal plasma proteins in myeloma and other hematologic cancers cause hyperviscosity and decreased blood flow.

The list of secondary causes of RS is extensive (Box 119-1). In a large series of 1039 patients with RS referred to the Oregon Health Sciences University from 1970 to 1995, more than half had primary vasospasm with no identifiable disease.[112] In those with associated abnormalities, the most common underlying disorder was CTD, which accounted for 27% of cases of RS. Scleroderma was the most likely CTD, followed by undifferentiated and mixed CTD. Atherosclerosis was less common, followed by "hypersensitivity angiitis," Buerger's disease, cancer, and vibration-induced white finger. In clinical practice, differentiation between primary and secondary RS has always been challenging. Table 119-1 outlines the clinical features differentiating primary from secondary RS.

Connective Tissue Disease

Systemic Sclerosis

RS occurs in more than 90% of patients with systemic sclerosis and can be the initial symptom in a third of patients.[56]

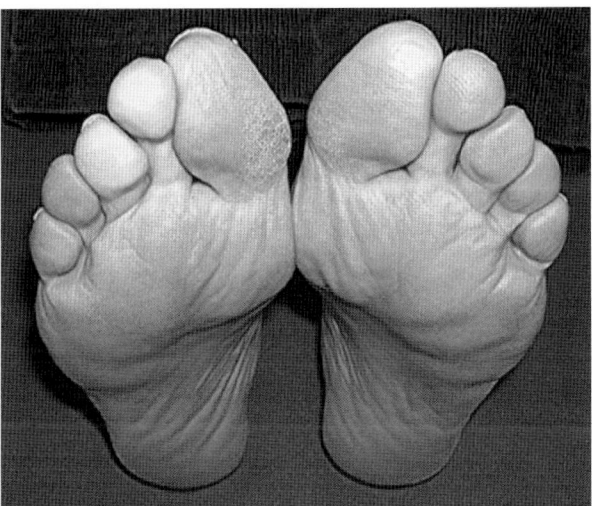

Figure 119-7 Digital vasospasm can affect the toes as well as the fingers.

Box 119-1 Conditions Associated with Secondary Raynaud's Syndrome

CONNECTIVE TISSUE DISEASES
- Progressive systemic sclerosis (scleroderma)
- Systemic lupus erythematosus
- Rheumatoid arthritis
- Sjögren's syndrome
- Mixed connective tissue disease
- Overlap connective tissue disease
- Dermatomyositis and polymyositis
- Vasculitis (small, medium-sized vessels)

OCCLUSIVE ARTERIAL DISEASE
- Atherosclerosis
- Thromboangiitis obliterans (Buerger's disease)
- Giant cell arteritis
- Arterial emboli (cardiac and peripheral)
- Thoracic outlet syndrome

OCCUPATIONAL ARTERIAL DISEASE
- Hypothenar hammer syndrome
- Vibration induced

DRUG-INDUCED VASOSPASM
- β-Adrenergic blocking drugs
- Vasopressors
- Ergot
- Cocaine
- Amphetamines
- Vinblastine/bleomycin

MYELOPROLIFERATIVE AND HEMATOLOGIC DISEASE
- Polycythemia rubra vera
- Thrombocytosis
- Cold agglutinins
- Cryoglobulinemia
- Paraproteinemia

MALIGNANCY
- Multiple myeloma
- Leukemia
- Adenocarcinoma
- Astrocytoma

INFECTION
- Hepatitis B and C antigenemia
- Parvovirus
- Purpura fulminans

Table 119-1 Clinical Features Distinguishing Primary from Secondary Raynaud's Syndrome

Type	Gender	Other Features
Primary	Usually female	Age <45 years Vasospasm of multiple or all digits Normal vascular examination No skin abnormalities at room temperature Normal laboratory studies
Secondary	Male or female	Any age Single or multiple digits involved Abnormal pulse examination Vascular laboratory abnormalities Positive serologic abnormalities

Systemic sclerosis is the most common CTD associated with RS.[26,113,114] Systemic sclerosis is also called scleroderma, which is derived from the words "skleros" (hard) and "derma" (skin). This rare multisystem disease of unknown etiology affects an estimated 40,000 to 165,000 people in the United States with an incidence of 20 to 75 cases per 100,000.[115]

Scleroderma is characterized by fibrosis of the skin and internal organs and causes widespread small-vessel vasculopathy and fibrosis. Small arteries, arterioles, and capillaries are affected by obliterative and proliferative structural changes in the vessel wall that cause tissue ischemia.

The pathogenesis of arterial disease is probably initiated by proliferation of smooth muscle cells in the blood vessel intima causing luminal narrowing. Activated platelets release platelet-derived growth factors and thromboxane A_2, which can induce vasoconstriction and stimulate the growth of endothelial cells and fibroblasts. Fibrin is deposited within and around vessels and causes vessel obstruction.[115]

The most characteristic feature of scleroderma is tightening or thickening of the skin, initially noted as puffiness of the fingers and hands. In advanced scleroderma, the skin becomes tight and shiny. Joint contracture leads to a clawhand deformity. Ulcers typically form at the fingertips and over joints. These ulcers may be refractory to therapy, are slow to heal, and cause significant ischemic digital pain (Figs. 119-8 to 119-10).

Systemic sclerosis is divided into two subsets, depending on the degree of skin involvement: limited scleroderma and

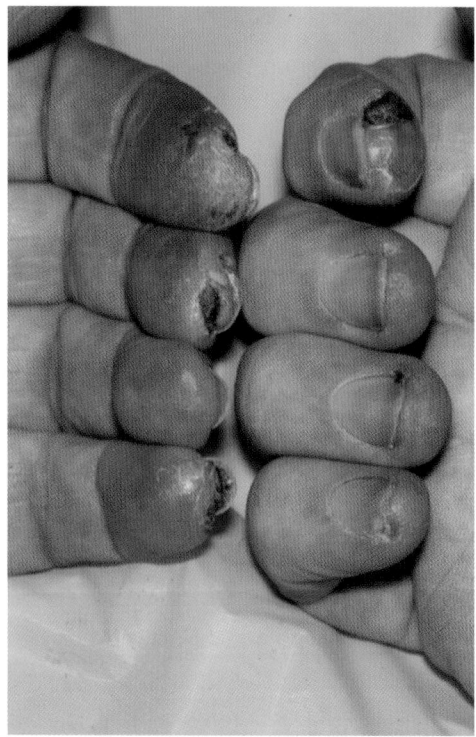

Figure 119-8 Raynaud's syndrome secondary to limited systemic sclerosis in a young male patient. Cyanotic discoloration is apparent on the left second and third fingers. The diagnosis of scleroderma can be made by physical examination. There is resorption with healed ulcerations of several fingertips.

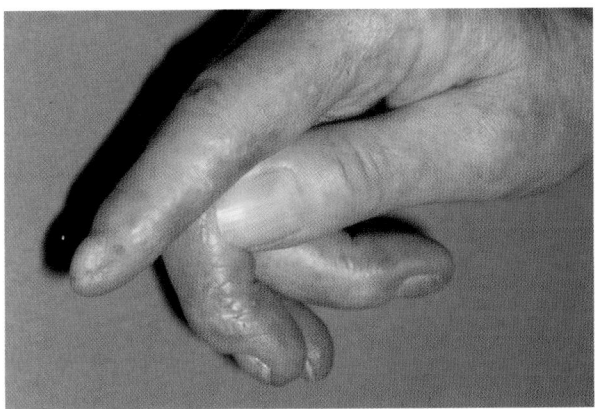

Figure 119-9 Systemic sclerosis. Note the tight, shiny, fibrotic skin encasing the fingers.

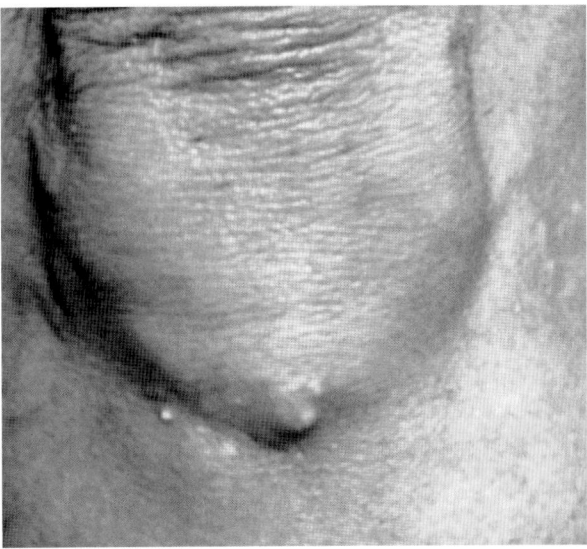

Figure 119-11 Calcinosis manifested as multiple areas of subcutaneous calcification in a patient with scleroderma.

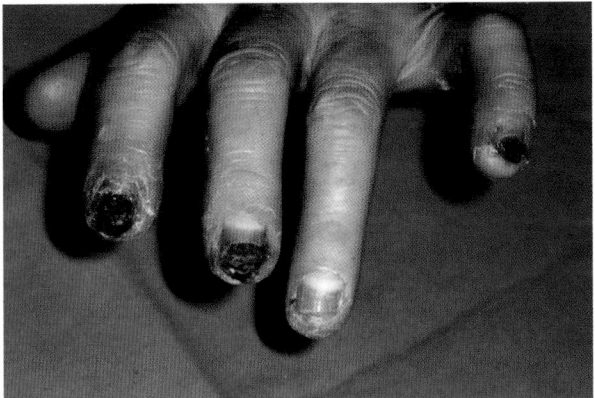

Figure 119-10 Advanced scleroderma with flexion contracture of the fingers and ulceration of multiple fingertips. Even with the best wound care, these ulcers can be difficult to heal.

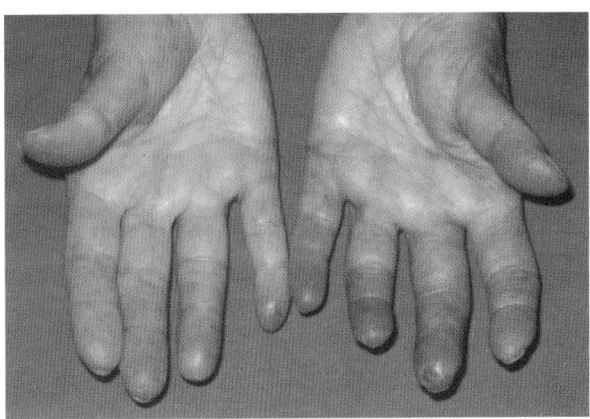

Figure 119-12 CREST syndrome (calcinosis, Raynaud's syndrome, esophageal dysmotility, sclerodactyly, telangiectasia). A pathognomonic finding in systemic sclerosis is sclerodactyly and telangiectasia of the fingers.

diffuse systemic scleroderma.[116] Limited scleroderma is by definition limited to the distal ends of the limbs without truncal involvement. Patients with limited scleroderma may have features of the CREST syndrome: calcinosis, RS, esophageal dysmotility, sclerodactyly, and telangiectasia. Calcinosis refers to subcutaneous calcification found in the fingers, forearms, and pressure points (Fig. 119-11). These calcium deposits may cause local tenderness and can ulcerate and exude a white, hard material. Telangiectases are prominent on the fingers and hands, as well as on the face and mucous membranes. The finding of multiple small telangiectases is pathognomonic for scleroderma (Fig. 119-12). Esophageal dysmotility leads to dysphagia, regurgitation, and aspiration. Despite these complications, limited scleroderma is thought of as the more benign disease with a long, often stable course and a low incidence of heart, lung, or kidney complications. RS may be present for a number of years before other signs of scleroderma become evident.

Diffuse systemic sclerosis causes skin thickening of the proximal parts of limbs and the trunk. It is often rapidly progressive with a short interval between the onset of RS and severe multiorgan disease. The diffuse form has a much worse prognosis, with a 10-year survival rate of 40% to 60% versus greater than 70% in those with the limited form of

scleroderma. Scleroderma renal involvement results in severe hypertension and renal failure. ACE inhibitors may decrease intraglomerular pressure and should be considered for all patients with scleroderma renal disease. Dyspnea, hypoxia, and resulting pulmonary hypertension occur in scleroderma lung disease. Digital involvement is disabling, but death results from the cardiac and pulmonary complications of scleroderma. Once hypoxia or right heart failure develops, mean survival is less than 2 years.[114]

Mixed and Undifferentiated Connective Tissue Disease

Mixed CTD is an overlap syndrome with features of at least two CTDs: usually, scleroderma and systemic lupus erythematosus with elevated antinuclear antibody. Eighty-four percent of patients with mixed CTD have RS.[117] Undifferentiated CTD is a term used to describe CTD that lacks the characteristics of any distinct CTD. Undifferentiated CTD may have a mixture of clinical findings, including polyarthritis, RS, lupus-type symptoms, sicca syndrome, and photosensitivity. RS is present in approximately 50% of patients with undifferentiated CTD, but in contrast to other forms of RS secondary to CTD, it tends to follow a benign course.[118]

Systemic Lupus Erythematosus

Lupus can affect all age groups but most frequently occurs in young women. Arthralgias, rash, pericarditis, pleuritis, and glomerulonephritis are some of the frequent features, usually with a positive antinuclear antibody. RS is a frequent manifestation of systemic lupus erythematosus and occurs in 20% to 50% of affected patients.[119]

Small-Vessel Vasculitis

Rheumatoid arthritis and Sjögren's syndrome can be complicated by digital ischemia secondary to small-vessel vasculitis and obliterative fibrosis, sometimes with skin necrosis or digital gangrene. RS occurs in approximately 13% of patients with Sjögren's syndrome and 17% of those with rheumatoid arthritis.[120] Other small-vessel vasculitides include Wegener's granulomatosis, microscopic polyarteritis nodosum, and cutaneous livedo vasculitis.

Arterial Occlusive Disease

Arterial occlusive disease of the upper extremity can result from atherosclerosis, a variety of systemic disorders, emboli from the heart or more proximal arteries, and local trauma causing arterial thrombosis.[121] Occlusive arterial disease at any level causes decreased transluminal distending pressure in the distal artery and can precipitate RS.

Thromboangiitis obliterans (Buerger's disease) is a non-atherosclerotic inflammatory disorder that involves the distal small and medium-sized arteries in the fingers and toes and progresses proximally.[122] Although Buerger's disease can be manifested as distal extremity vasospasm, it often causes chronic ischemia with very painful fingertip ulcerations and necrosis. Typically, Buerger's disease occurs in male smokers younger than 45 years. In up to half of patients a migratory superficial thrombophlebitis develops. Arteriography can be diagnostic of vascular obstruction by demonstrating chronic vessel thrombosis and inflammatory changes with alternating segmental occlusion and arterial dilatation, often with the pathognomonic finding of corkscrew collaterals. The proximal arteries are normal with no evidence of atherosclerosis. The only way to prevent progression of thromboangiitis obliterans is absolute cessation of all tobacco products (Fig. 119-13) (see Chapter 77: Thromboangiitis Obliterans).[123]

Erythromelalgia

Erythromelalgia is a rare syndrome characterized by recurrent episodes of burning pain, erythema, and heat usually

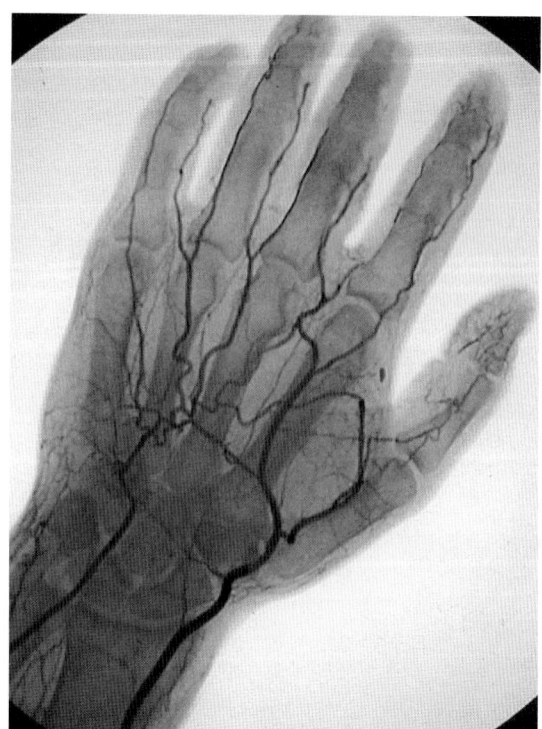

Figure 119-13 A young male patient with thromboangiitis obliterans and digital vasospastic attacks. An upper extremity angiogram documents occlusive arterial disease involving several digits. Angiographic findings in thromboangiitis obliterans may show palmar and digital artery occlusions and irregularity, sometimes with corkscrew collaterals. The angiographic findings, however, are often not specific for Buerger's disease and can be seen with vasculitis and repetitive hand trauma.

involving the lower extremities, although the upper extremities may also be involved. Episodes may begin with an itching sensation before progressing to burning and pain, and affected individuals often go to great lengths to keep the affected extremities cool. Although the spectrum of symptoms is the opposite of RS, the two conditions occasionally coexist, and both represent abnormalities in vasoreactivity.[124] As with RS, the pathophysiology of erythromelalgia is poorly understood.

Associated conditions include thrombocythemia, polycythemia rubra vera, CTDs, diabetes, hypertension, and certain malignancies. Treatment with aspirin is most effective in patients with associated myeloproliferative disorders. Calcium channel blockers may be effective but might paradoxically exacerbate the symptoms.[125]

■ DIAGNOSIS

Although many tests have been found useful for the diagnosis of RS, no consensus exists on the optimal battery of clinical and diagnostic tests. A suggested list of criteria for the diagnosis of primary RS and differentiation of primary from secondary RS is as follows: (1) vasospastic attacks precipitated by cold or emotional stress, (2) symmetric attacks involving both hands, (3) absence of tissue necrosis or gangrene, (4) no history or physical findings suggestive of a secondary cause, (5) normal nail fold capillaries, (6) normal erythrocyte sedimentation rate, and (7) negative serologic findings, particularly a negative test for antinuclear antibodies.[126,127]

History

The diagnosis of RS is made on the basis of historical features. Historical information should be sought regarding symptoms of CTDs, including arthralgia, dysphagia, skin tightening, xerophthalmia, and xerostomia. Symptoms of large-vessel occlusive disease, exposure to trauma or frostbite, a drug history, and a history of malignancy should also be sought.

Physical Examination

The diagnosis of RS is primarily made by the history, and physical examination in patients with suspected RS is often normal. Nonetheless, determination of primary or secondary disease is aided by a focused physical examination. The vascular examination should determine the presence of large-, medium-, or small-vessel occlusive disease and should detect signs of a CTD.

The skin of the hands and fingers should be inspected for ulceration or hyperkeratotic areas on the fingertips suggestive of healed ulcers. The hand and fingers should be examined for evidence of skin thinning, tightening, sclerodactyly, or telangiectases, all of which may suggest associated autoimmune disease. Splinter hemorrhages under the nails may be a normal finding in manual workers with hand trauma but is also a sensitive indicator of distal atheroemboli (Fig. 119-14).

Pulse examination should include palpation of the subclavian, brachial, radial, and ulnar arteries. Palpation above the clavicle can determine the presence of a cervical rib or aneurysm of the subclavian artery, or both. A palpable thrill indicates high-grade arterial stenosis. Auscultation over large arteries for a bruit, in particular over the sternoclavicular joint and above the clavicle, may identify an arterial stenosis.

A palpable radial or ulnar pulse at the wrist does not mean that the arteries are patent into the hand. The most common site of blockage of the ulnar artery is at the hypothenar eminence where it crosses the hook of the hamate. The Allen test should be performed in every patient with suspected RS to detect the presence of radial or ulnar artery occlusion and to test for completeness of the ulnar arch.

Vascular Laboratory Evaluation

The noninvasive vascular laboratory is an important adjunct to the office-based clinical assessment of patients with RS.[128] It provides objectivity to the clinical evaluation and assists in decision making for medical and surgical treatment. Vascular laboratory testing can assist in differentiating between fixed arterial obstruction and pure vasospasm and can provide assessment of the location and severity of the circulatory impairment.

The diagnosis of RS should not be made on the basis of any laboratory test,[99] and the vascular laboratory should not take the place of a good history and physical examination.[23] Even though attacks of RS are classically brought on by exposure to cold, it is surprisingly difficult to reproduce an attack of vasospasm in the vascular laboratory, even with digital cooling. Quantitative evaluation of vasospasm has also been difficult,[129] and symptoms do not always correlate with finger skin blood flow measurements.[130]

The most useful noninvasive laboratory tests for RS include room-temperature evaluation of arm, hand, and digital arterial perfusion, supplemented by measurement of digital temperature, systolic blood pressure, and laser Doppler flow of the fingers before and after local digital cooling.

Segmental Pressure Measurements

To evaluate for large-vessel occlusive arterial disease, segmental blood pressure measurements in the upper extremity can be obtained. Pneumatic cuffs are placed on the brachial, upper elbow, and wrist levels, and systolic blood pressure is measured. A pressure differential exceeding 10 mm Hg between levels may be significant and indicative of proximal occlusive arterial disease. The wrist-brachial ratio can be calculated, but there may be a wide range of normal values (as low as 0.8) because of variation in cuff size and arm diameter.[129]

Finger Systolic Blood Pressure

Finger systolic pressure is measured by applying small digital cuffs to the proximal part of the finger. The cuff is inflated above systolic blood pressure to occlude the digital artery. As the cuff is slowly deflated, the pulse returns to the distal part of the finger, and systolic blood pressure can be assessed by pulse-volume recording, strain-gauge plethysmography, or photoplethysmography.[131,132] Decreased systolic pressure

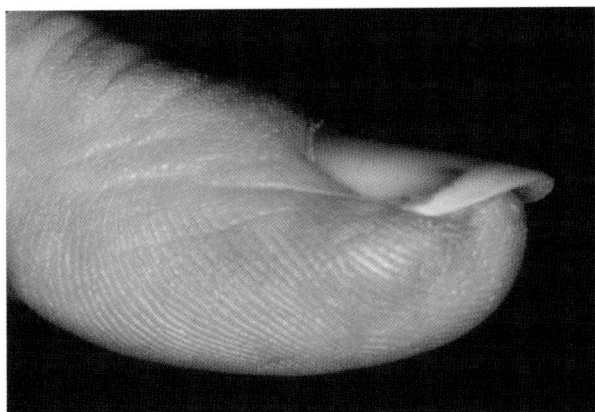

Figure 119-14 Splinter hemorrhages under the nails may be a normal finding with local trauma but can also be an important indicator of distal atheroembolism, as seen in this patient. Note the splinter hemorrhages under the nail and subtle skin mottling consistent with microembolization.

usually indicates fixed arterial occlusive disease in that finger; however, the range of normal digital pressure is variable and is influenced by temperature.

The normal finger-brachial index may range from 0.8 to 1.3. The fingers are especially temperature sensitive, and cool fingers can result in falsely low indices. When the fingers are very cold, digital indices may be unobtainable until the fingers have warmed. Conversely, when the fingers are warm, finger systolic blood pressure may be lower than arm pressure by 10 mm Hg. Noncompressible vessels (similar to those in the lower extremity) can result in supranormal digital pressure.

A difference of more than 15 mm Hg between fingers or an absolute finger systolic blood pressure of less than 70 mm Hg may indicate occlusive disease.[129] Because the digits have dual arteries, early disease with occlusion of one of the digital arteries cannot be detected by finger pressure measurement if the contralateral artery is open.

Evaluation of digital plethysmographic waveforms is also useful, particularly for identifying obstructive RS. Patients with obstructive RS have blunted waveforms, whereas patients with vasospastic RS have either normal waveforms or a "peaked pulse." The peaked pulse pattern, first described by Sumner and Strandness, appears to reflect increased vasospastic arterial resistance.[133]

Cold Challenge Testing

A number of tests have been designed to measure patients' response to a cold challenge. Although this would intuitively seem to be the ideal way to diagnose RS, the optimal method of digital and systemic cooling and measurement of the cold response remains elusive. The first vascular laboratory test used widely for the objective diagnosis of RS was the measurement of recovery in fingertip temperature after digital exposure to ice water.[134] There are many variations of the cold immersion test with various immersion times and temperatures. A standard protocol is to record baseline digital temperatures with a temperature probe at the end of the finger pulp. The hands are then immersed in cold water at 4°C for 20 seconds. The hands are dried, and digital skin temperature is recorded for each finger as the hands and fingers gradually warm to ambient room temperature. The length of time that it takes for the hands to rewarm to baseline is noted by recording finger temperatures or laser Doppler flux at 5-minute intervals until recovery of preimmersion temperatures. A delay in rewarming suggests a tendency for vasospasm. Patients with RS typically take more than 10 minutes and sometimes 30 minutes or longer to return to resting finger temperature as opposed to less than 10 minutes for normal subjects. However, although the ice water immersion test is 100% specific, it is only 50% sensitive and therefore is neither sufficiently accurate nor reproducible for routine clinical use.[135,136]

The digital blood pressure response to 5 minutes of digital occlusive hypothermia as described by Nielsen and Lassen has proved to be a more accurate method of diagnosing RS in the vascular laboratory. This method uses a double-inlet plastic cuff for local digital cooling. A cuff that can be sequentially cooled is placed on the proximal phalanx of the test finger, with a cuff maintained at room temperature placed on the proximal phalanx of a reference finger. The test is repeated at several temperatures, and the result is expressed as the percent drop in finger systolic pressure with cooling.[137,138] In an evaluation of this test at the Oregon Health Sciences University, this test was found to be 87% specific and 90% sensitive for an overall accuracy of 92%.[139]

Duplex Ultrasound

The role of duplex scanning has traditionally been limited in the diagnosis of RS, with its utility typically being restricted to the evaluation of proximal upper extremity arterial obstruction or aneurysmal disease. The use of color-flow Doppler to assess the digital arteries after cold exposure has been reported.[140] Recently, however, power Doppler has emerged as a means of evaluating the digital arteries for the diagnosis of RS. Lee and colleagues compared power Doppler with a 10-MHz scan head focused at 5 mm with nail fold capillaroscopy for the diagnosis of primary and secondary RS.[141] The investigators were able to correctly diagnose RS in all cases and were able to correctly classify patients as having primary or secondary RS in 89% of cases.

Fingertip Thermography

Skin surface temperature can be used as an indirect index of capillary blood flow in the skin. At temperatures lower than 30°C, blood flow is proportional to skin surface temperature. At temperatures higher than 30°C, larger increases in flow may not be appreciated because of the minimal increase in skin temperature. Patients with vasospasm have increased vascular tone leading to decreased blood flow and decreased surface skin temperature.

Measurement of skin temperature can be combined with cold challenge testing. Foerster and colleagues recently described a dual sensor device in which the measured fingertip is placed in a thermal chamber that can be set to different temperatures. The chamber is equipped with both digital thermography and infrared plethysmography to record recovery of both temperature and pressure after a cold challenge. Using a cutoff of 6 minutes to achieve 63% of the precooling skin temperature, the authors reported a sensitivity of 74% and a specificity and positive predictive value of 95% in diagnosing RS.[142,143]

Laser Doppler

Laser Doppler Flux. Laser Doppler is a noninvasive test that measures microvascular skin perfusion in the fingers. A laser Doppler probe transmits a low-powered helium-neon light via a quartz glass fiberoptic system. The light is scattered by both static and moving tissue. Most moving structures are red blood cells. Laser light scattered by moving red blood cells undergoes a shift in frequency according to the Doppler

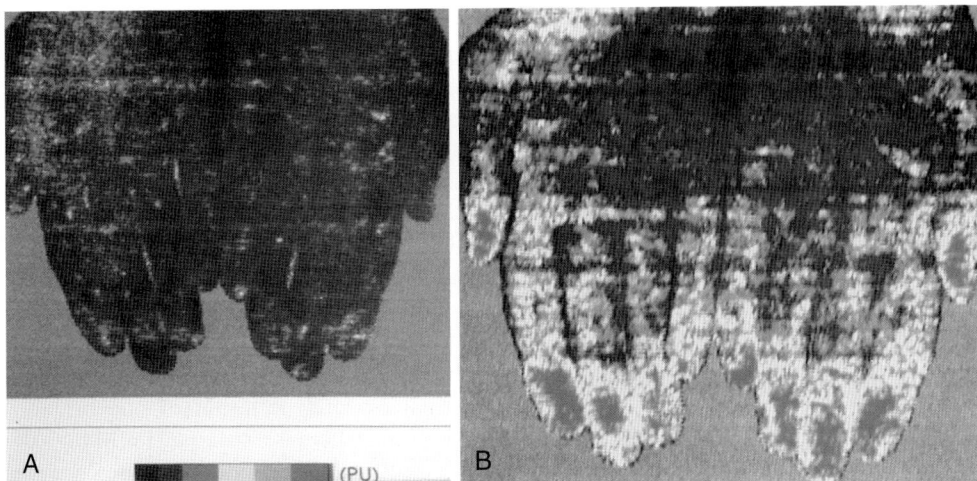

Figure 119-15 Scanning laser Doppler imaging shows low laser Doppler flow as a result of vasospasm (**A**). After warming the hands (**B**), a marked increase in digital blood flow is seen. On examination, the fingers were cool, with resting digital temperatures of 28° C. Physical examination was normal, and there was no evidence of occlusive arterial disease. Blood tests, including a complete blood count, sedimentation rate, cryoglobulin, antinuclear antibody, and extractable nuclear antigens, all were negative. Primary Raynaud's syndrome was diagnosed and the patient was treated with a long-acting nifedipine medication.

effect. The scattered light is detected by a photodetector in the probe and produces an output signal proportional to the flux (number and velocity) of red blood cells in the volume of tissue illuminated.

Baseline measurements are highly variable and affected by emotion, sympathetic tone, and environmental temperature. Cold stress testing can be combined with laser Doppler by cooling the fingers with a laser Doppler probe.[144] When finger temperatures are decreased, vasoconstriction results in decreased skin blood flow and reduced laser Doppler flux. With slow rewarming there is an increase in laser Doppler flux. The normal response to cooling is a decrease in skin temperature and a symmetric decrease in laser Doppler flow.[145,146] Several studies have demonstrated the ability to combine laser Doppler flow with cold challenge testing to establish the diagnosis of RS.[144,147] A wireless laser Doppler device has also been combined with cold provocation and an arm-raising test to diagnose and evaluate the response to therapy in patients with systemic sclerosis.[148]

Laser Doppler Imaging (Scanning Laser Doppler).

Laser Doppler flowmetry allows measurement of skin perfusion at a single point. To account for the heterogeneity in digital arterial flow, a new technique of laser Doppler imaging has been developed.[149] This technique allows measurement of blood flow over an area rather than a single point and also is noncontact, thereby obviating the potential effect of direct skin pressure on digital arterial flow. Because the Doppler probe does not come in contact with the patient, scanning laser Doppler can be used to assess blood flow at the base of ulcers or other wounds and is able to scan the entire hand.

Laser Doppler imaging can be combined with a thermal challenge to assess recovery of skin perfusion for the diagnosis

of RS. A number of small pilot studies have demonstrated the effectiveness of laser Doppler imaging in diagnosing RS,[150] differentiating primary from secondary RS,[151] and evaluating response to vasodilator therapy.[152] Unfortunately, the great deal of variability limits interpretation, and scanning laser Doppler has not found the same applicability as single-digit Doppler probes (Fig. 119-15).

Current research focuses on comparing thermography, which measures changes in skin surface temperature, and laser Doppler imaging, which measures microcirculatory flow, in their ability to diagnose RS. Interestingly, most studies show that the two modalities do not have a strong correlation.[153] It is thought that laser Doppler imaging is more sensitive to changes in blood flow and therefore more likely to show inhomogeneities than is the dampened temperature response.[154] Thus, the two technologies are not interchangeable but, rather, provide complementary information.

Imaging Studies
Magnetic Resonance Angiography

Magnetic resonance angiography is excellent for imaging the upper extremity arteries and can provide accurate imaging of the hand and wrist vessels. Its resolution is not as good as that of contrast-enhanced angiography, which remains the "gold standard" for arterial imaging (Fig. 119-16).[155]

Contrast-Enhanced Angiography

Contrast-enhanced angiography remains the best imaging modality when a detailed examination is necessary to look for the cause of digital ischemia, such as microembolism from an

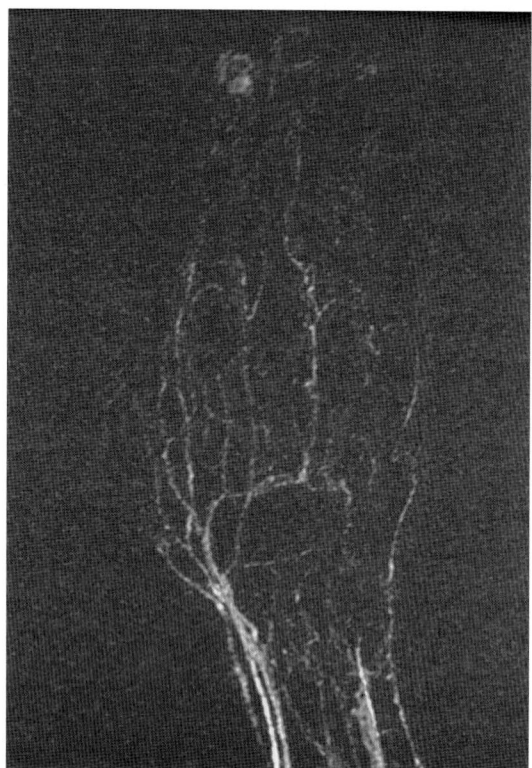

Figure 119-16 Magnetic resonance angiography of the hand shows distal ulnar artery occlusion, an incomplete deep palmar arch, and severe disease of digital arteries with only faintly visualized arteries to the index, middle, and ring fingers. This patient had a 3-year history of Raynaud's symptoms and recent onset of ischemic pain involving the right index finger. Digital ischemia was refractory to vasodilator medication, and the patient was treated with an upper extremity pneumatic pump to improve arterial perfusion to the fingers.

ulcerated plaque, thrombus in an ulnar artery, the tapered narrowing of vasculitis, or the corkscrew collaterals of thromboangiitis obliterans. As an invasive test, angiography is reserved for patients with severe disease or those who may be candidates for intervention with thrombolytic agents, angioplasty, or surgical revascularization.

Angiography is not generally indicated in most patients with CTD but may be helpful when searching for another cause of hand ischemia such as atheroembolism or arterial thrombosis. Angiography in patients with CTD shows distal occlusive arterial disease in the hand and fingers. The digital arteries are the most severely involved and demonstrate segmental or total occlusion of one or both digital arteries. Sometimes there is a striking lack of digital vessels and a lack of new or collateral vessels. In more severe cases, the common digital and palmar arch vessels are affected. Distal ulnar artery involvement can occur in up to 50% of patients, but usually the radial artery is spared.[156] A nonspecific vasculitic appearance with alternating occlusive disease and arterial dilatation can be seen in many conditions, including Buerger's disease, trauma, small-vessel vasculitis, and CTDs. All can have similar angiographic findings (Fig. 119-17).

Nail Fold Capillary Microscopy

The superficial capillaries in the nail fold can be visualized by applying a drop of immersion oil over the cuticle of the finger to make it translucent and imaging with a low-powered microscope or an ophthalmoscope at 40 diopters. Although all fingers are evaluated, assessment is typically most accurate in the fourth and fifth fingers because of greater skin

Figure 119-17 Bilateral upper extremity arteriogram of the left (**A**) and right (**B**) hands in a patient with mixed connective tissue disease. There were features of scleroderma and CREST syndrome with strongly positive antinuclear antibody. The patient had an ischemic right index fingertip that did not respond to topical nitroglycerin (see also Fig. 119-12).

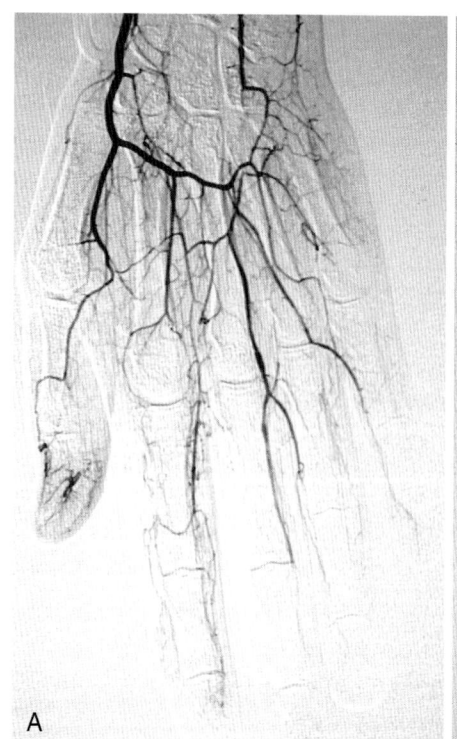
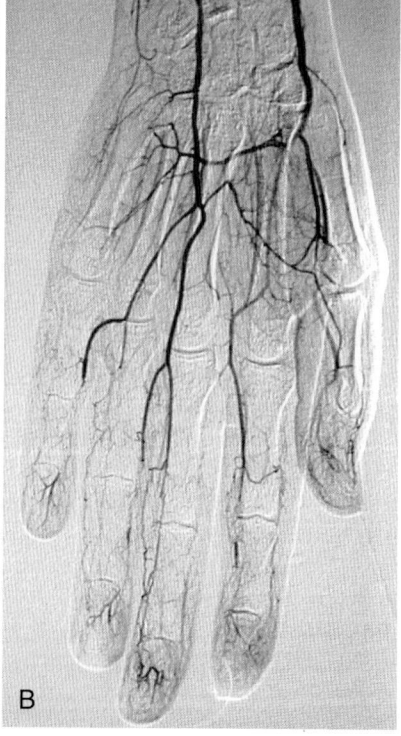

transparency at these levels.[157] Normal capillaries are seen as regularly spaced hairpin loops encompassing a venous limb and an arterial limb. The arterial limb has a narrower diameter with more rapid flow, and the venous limb has a larger diameter with slower capillary flow.[23]

Abnormal capillaries are seen in scleroderma and mixed CTD as enlarged, tortuous, and deformed or as loop dropout causing avascular areas.[158,159] Furthermore, the presence of abnormal nail folds in patients without CTD is a strong predictor of the subsequent development of CTD. With a mean follow-up of 6.5 years, Meli and colleagues demonstrated that 80% of patients with abnormal nail fold findings at the time of initial diagnosis of RS eventually developed CTD, primarily scleroderma, CREST, and mixed CTD. Thus, there may be significant prognostic utility in the use of nail fold capillaroscopy in the early phases of RS.[160]

Serologic Testing

Serologic studies may help confirm the diagnosis of CTD and are also useful in screening for occult underlying CTD. Useful screening tests include antinuclear antibody and rheumatoid factor. Antinuclear antibodies are present in 95% of patients with systemic sclerosis.[115] They are not specific for scleroderma and can be present in a number of other CTDs—in particular, lupus erythematosus. A positive antinuclear antibody raises suspicion but on its own does not make the diagnosis of a CTD. Several autoantibodies are specific for systemic sclerosis, including topoisomerase 1, centromere, scl-70, RNA polymerase 1, and U3 RNP. Anticentromere antibody is associated with limited CREST syndrome. As opposed to vasculitis, the erythrocyte sedimentation rate is usually normal in CTD.

Rheumatoid factor is an antibody directed against the Fc region of IgG and has been used as a diagnostic marker for rheumatoid arthritis.[161] More specific but less frequently used diagnostic markers include antiperinuclear factor, antikeratin antibodies, and anti–cyclic citrullinated peptide antibody.

■ SELECTION OF TREATMENT

Natural History

Knowledge of the natural history of RS is important in patient counseling and treatment recommendations. The natural history differs greatly between primary vasospastic and secondary obstructive causes.

Primary Vasospastic Raynaud's Syndrome

Primary vasospastic RS is a benign disorder. Several natural history studies have demonstrated a low incidence of finger ulcers or tissue loss in the presence of vasospasm. In a longitudinal study from Oregon, digital ulcers occurred in 5% of patients in whom vasospastic RS was initially diagnosed when observed for more than 10 years.[112] Others have demonstrated regression of disease with time, as previously noted.[21,22]

Secondary Obstructive Raynaud's Syndrome

Patients with obstructive RS follow a more virulent course. In patients monitored for more than 10 years, over half experienced digital ulcerations and 20% to 25% required digital or phalangeal amputations.[112]

Risk for Development of Connective Tissue Disease

The onset of RS may precede the clinical onset of CTD by up to several years. A number of studies have looked at the future risk for development of CTD in patients in whom primary RS was initially diagnosed. The rate of conversion to a CTD in patients with initially primary RS ranges from approximately 5% to 19% in the medical literature. Patients with apparent primary RS should be told that the risk for development of a CTD is low but that follow-up evaluation is recommended.

Some patients at the time of their evaluation are found to have subtle abnormalities by history, examination, or blood tests that may be suspicious for but not diagnostic of CTD (such as a low positive antinuclear antibody or abnormal nail fold microscopy). These patients are at higher risk for the future development of a CTD. In a 12-year retrospective study, Ziegler and coauthors reported that the rate of progression to CTD in 147 patients with primary RS was 14.1%, 9.2% in "pure" primary RS but 30.3% in patients with initial positive antinuclear antibodies or finger skin thickening. Higher age at the time of diagnosis was also a significant predictor of conversion to a CTD.[162] Hirschl and colleagues, in a 10-year prospective surveillance study of 307 patients with primary RS, reported a 1% annual incidence of conversion to secondary RS. A number of factors were predictive of conversion, including older age at onset, a shorter duration of symptoms, abnormal findings on the thoracic outlet test, and an initial antinuclear antibody titer greater than 1:320.[163]

Approach to Treatment

The approach to therapy for RS should be individualized according to the patient's symptoms, the frequency of vasospastic attacks, the underlying disease, and the risk for development of ischemic ulceration, gangrene, or digital loss. For most patients with primary RS there is no cure; however, a number of simple measures can be effective in reducing the frequency and duration of attacks. Preventive measures consisting of education and reassurance and avoidance of exposure to cold constitute the basis of therapy for most patients.

Management principles can be considered in three groups: nonpharmacologic behavioral therapy, pharmacologic treatment, and interventional-surgical procedures. Potential therapies in the future could be specifically targeted to one of the many underlying abnormalities responsible for RS, including the endothelium, autonomic nervous system, or specific neurohumoral and hematologic factors.

MEDICAL TREATMENT

Nonpharmacologic Therapy

Preventive Measures

Most patients with primary RS have only mild symptoms that do not require the use of vasodilatory medications. These patients are best managed with a conservative program that stresses the concepts of heat conservation and avoidance of factors that cause arterial vasoconstriction. Education and reassurance are the mainstay of therapy. Patients with primary RS should be reassured that they have a benign disorder with little risk of progression, finger ulcers, or digital loss. Patients should be educated about the nature and prognosis of primary RS, in particular emphasizing that the underlying arterial circulation is normal and that episodes of pallor and cyanosis are an exaggeration of the normal response of the finger arteries to cold exposure and emotional stress.

Simple measures to maintain warmth and avoid cold are effective. Protection from cold involves the use of mittens to keep the fingers warm in cold weather. Chemical or electrical hand warmers can be obtained at sporting goods stores.[164] In a recent randomized trial, ceramic-impregnated gloves that absorb ambient infrared light to generate heat resulted in significantly improved hand function and visual analogue pain scores when compared with a placebo group wearing cotton gloves.[165] Additionally, the concept of whole-body warmth should be stressed. Situations likely to cause vasospasm should be avoided or minimized. In severe cases, patients may elect to spend more time in warmer climates. Avoiding agents that cause vasoconstriction, such as nicotine and vasoconstricting medications, is also an important aspect of therapy.[166]

Behavioral Therapies and Maneuvers

Temperature Biofeedback. Temperature biofeedback is a type of mind/body therapy whereby patients are taught methods of self-regulation of skin temperature.[167] Control of autonomic functions such as temperature control can be learned. Temperature sensors are placed on the patient's skin, and instructions are given on raising skin temperature. Significant time must be invested—it may take 12 sessions of biofeedback training lasting 45 minutes each to learn the techniques of relaxation and meditation.[168] The primary goal is to teach methods of avoiding RS attacks; however, with training, individuals can learn to reverse the existing vasospasm. Vasodilatation is thought to occur through a non-neural β-adrenergic mechanism, as well as a reduction in α-sympathetic activity.[168]

Temperature biofeedback has been studied in randomized trials with variable results. Randomized controlled trials from three independent investigators demonstrated significant improvements in the frequency and severity of vasospastic attacks in the group of patients receiving biofeedback,[169-171] but these trials were small, with fewer than 30 patients in each. In one large (N = 313) randomized multicenter trial, biofeedback was no better than a control group treated with nifedipine. In fact, nifedipine-treated patients had 56% fewer RS attacks than did the biofeedback group.[172] Although the results of this study dampened overall enthusiasm for the use of biofeedback to treat RS, a significant criticism of this trial was the fact that only 35% of the subjects in the biofeedback group were able to successfully learn hand-warming techniques. There is a learning curve with biofeedback, and the results may depend on the training. Behavioral therapy can help some patients, but not all can learn temperature control techniques.

Pharmacologic Therapy

Pharmacologic therapy is indicated for patients with severe symptoms whose activities of daily life are affected and who do not respond to simple conservative measures. Most patients with mild or moderate symptoms respond well to conservative measures and do not need vasodilator medications. Some patients have symptoms and require medications only during the cold winter months and not during the warmer summer months.

The goal of pharmacologic therapy is to decrease the frequency and intensity of vasospastic episodes rather than cure the underlying cause. The potential side effects and adverse consequences of medications should be balanced against the expected benefit. Vasodilator medications are more effective in patients with primary RS. Individuals with secondary RS often have fixed obstructive arterial disease, and vasodilators are less effective or at times have no benefit at all.

A number of medications are routinely used for RS (Table 119-2); however, no currently available drugs are specifically approved by the U.S. Food and Drug Administration for the treatment of RS. Choosing the one best medication has been difficult because of the lack of large prospective, randomized, double-blinded studies comparing the efficacy of different medications in RS. There is a significant placebo effect in published clinical trials ranging from 20% to 40%,[26] a fact that needs to be taken into consideration when interpreting the results of uncontrolled trials. Most clinical trials rely on the patient's self-assessment of the frequency and severity of RS, and laboratory confirmation of benefit has been difficult to discern.

Calcium Channel Blockers

Calcium channel blockers are the most commonly prescribed and extensively researched medications for vasospasm associated with RS. These drugs share a common mode of action and inhibit the influx of extracellular calcium ions into the smooth muscle cell by blocking specific ion channels in the cell membrane. The contractile process of the smooth muscle in the arterial wall is dependent on extracellular calcium, and a reduction in calcium influx causes vascular smooth muscle relaxation and arterial dilatation. Because they do not act on a receptor, they are considered direct-acting vasodilator drugs. The three main classes of calcium channel blockers differ in their mode of action on the slow calcium channels

Table 119-2 Drugs Used for the Treatment of Raynaud's Syndrome

Class	Drugs	Comments
Calcium channel blockers (dihydropyridine)	Nifedipine, nicardipine, felodipine	First-line therapy, best effect in vasospastic RS
α₁-Adrenergic blockers (nonselective)	Phenoxybenzamine, phentolamine	Limited applicability because of side effects (orthostatic hypotension, tachycardia)
α₁-Adrenergic blockers (selective)	Terazosin, doxazosin, prazosin	Second-line therapy, may cause hypotension
Angiotensin II receptor blockers	Losartan	Second-line therapy
Angiotensin-converting enzyme inhibitors	Captopril	Variable results in clinical trials
Serotonin reuptake inhibitors	Fluoxetine	Second-line therapy
Topical nitrates	2% Nitroglycerin	May provide symptom relief but limited by side effects
Phosphodiesterase 5 inhibitors	Sildenafil, vardenafil, tadalafil	May be beneficial in ulcer healing in patients with secondary RS, not studied in primary RS
Endothelin inhibitors	Bosentan	Used for pulmonary hypertension, not yet approved to treat RS
Prostaglandin analogues	Iloprost	Intravenous medication used primarily in Europe, not available in the United States

and vary in their selectivity for vascular or cardiac tissue. The three classes are dihydropyridines, phenylalkylamines such as verapamil, and benzothiazepines such as diltiazem.

Dihydropyridines such as nifedipine are the most potent in relaxing vascular smooth muscle and are better vasodilators than diltiazem or verapamil. However, as a consequence of this vasodilatory property, dihydropyridines are also more likely than other calcium channel blockers to cause the adverse effects of flushing and peripheral edema, which may require discontinuation of the medication. An unusual erythromelalgia-like syndrome can result from dihydropyridine medications.[125] Diltiazem is less potent and consequently has fewer adverse effects.[173] Verapamil has more cardiac than peripheral vascular selectivity and is not a good peripheral vasodilator.

Dihydropyridine calcium channel blockers are the best studied of all calcium channel blockers and have been shown in multiple studies to be effective therapy for RS. There are more than 10 drugs in this class that share similar properties. Nifedipine has been and continues to be the gold standard, but most of the newer dihydropyridines (including amlodipine, nicardipine, felodipine, isradipine, and nisoldipine) all appear to be efficacious. Long-acting or sustained-release preparations of calcium channel blockers are preferred.

Other dihydropyridines have also been used for RS. Felodipine was found to be equally efficacious as nifedipine in a double-blinded, crossover trial of 16 patients.[174] Nisoldipine reduced the number but not the severity of attacks in 19 patients with primary RS in a European controlled, double-blinded trial of 19 patients.[175] Isradipine has also been studied in RS with documented benefit.

Nifedipine. Nifedipine is considered by many to be the drug of first choice if pharmacologic treatment of symptoms is required. A 66% reduction in frequency of attacks has been reported in a recent multicenter randomized controlled trial of 313 patients with primary RS treated with a sustained-release form of nifedipine versus placebo.[172] Of note, adverse side effects necessitating discontinuation of nifedipine occurred in 15% of patients. A recent meta-analysis of 12 randomized controlled trials demonstrated an overall 33% reduction in severity of attacks as graded on a visual analogue scale, with an average of 2.8 to 5.0 fewer attacks per week in patients treated with nifedipine, and similar findings were reported in five additional studies with other dihydropyridine calcium channel blockers.[176] In patients with secondary RS, beneficial effects have also been demonstrated, though to a lesser degree than in those treated for primary RS.[177]

Laboratory studies have been inconsistent in documenting improved blood flow or less susceptibility to vasospastic attacks with nifedipine therapy. In some studies, nifedipine has been shown to improve the temperature recovery time after cold immersion of the hands and fingers.[145] In other studies using cold provocation, nifedipine-treated patients were found to have less of a decrease in finger systolic pressure in the cooled finger than were subjects given placebo.[178] Similar findings were reported in a recent study of 158 patients with primary RS who were randomized to sustained-release nifedipine. The digital blood pressure response to local finger cooling from 30° C to 10° C was measured. Patients treated with nifedipine had a higher relative mean digital systolic blood pressure during finger cooling than did those treated with placebo.[179]

Amlodipine. Amlodipine is similar to nifedipine but has a longer half-life. In a 3-week Italian trial, amlodipine, 10 mg once daily, was found to reduce the frequency of vasospastic attacks by 25% (from a baseline of 11.4 attacks to 8.6 attacks per week). Amlodipine has a theoretical advantage of fewer adverse effects because of its long half-life of more than 24 hours; however, adverse reaction in this study were common and included ankle edema in 55%, flushing in 10%, and headache in 20%.[180]

Nicardipine. In most studies, nicardipine has been shown to be effective in the treatment of vasospasm and can be administered by the oral or intravenous route. Only a few studies have been able to document improvement based on any laboratory test. Oral slow-release nicardipine (20 mg two times daily) was better than placebo in a randomized, double-blinded, crossover, placebo-controlled trial. The number of

RS episodes decreased and the severity of discomfort and hand disability scores improved in 21 patients (18 women and 3 men) with RS who had no underlying disease. Two discontinued the trial because of headache. The time to peak flow after postischemic reactive hyperemia was significantly reduced after nicardipine.[181]

Some investigators have found nicardipine to be of no benefit in either primary or secondary RS. No statistically significant differences in the number, duration, or severity of vasospastic attacks were found between nicardipine and placebo in a double-blinded, placebo-controlled, crossover study of oral nicardipine (30 mg three times a day) in 25 patients (16 with primary and 9 with secondary RS). Microcirculatory assessment by finger skin temperature and laser Doppler flux measured during a finger cooling test also showed no differences in nicardipine- and placebo-treated patients.[182]

Intravenous nicardipine has been shown to raise resting skin temperature in those with primary RS and improve recovery after cold-induced vasospasm, but again these effects were not seen in patients with secondary RS.[183]

α₁-Adrenergic Blockers

There are two major types of α₁-blockers. Nonselective α₁-blockers include phenoxybenzamine and phentolamine, which today are primarily used to control hypertensive emergencies in patients with pheochromocytoma and are rarely used for any other purposes because of the high incidence of adverse side effects, including orthostatic hypotension and reflex tachycardia.

Selective α₁-adrenergic receptor blocking agents include prazosin and the longer-acting terazosin (Hytrin) and doxazosin (Cardura). When the sympathetic nerve is stimulated, norepinephrine is released from the nerve terminal and crosses the synapse to act on the α₁-receptor located on vascular smooth muscle. Drugs such as prazosin cause competitive inhibition of the postsynaptic α₁-receptor, thus blocking the vasoconstrictor action of norepinephrine. At the same time, the presynaptic α₂-receptor located on the nerve terminal remains intact. The norepinephrine released feeds back on the α₂-receptor to limit further release of catecholamines and prevent the tachycardia seen with nonselective α₁-blockers.

Prazosin is a selective α₁-adrenergic antagonist that significantly reduces the number of attacks in both primary and secondary RS.[184] Side effects are less frequent but can include postural hypotension (first-dose phenomenon), which usually resolves within several days as tolerance develops.[185] In a double-blinded, placebo-controlled, crossover study of 24 patients, prazosin was reported to be superior to placebo in the treatment of RS. Subjective benefit with a significant reduction in the number and duration of attacks was noted in two thirds of patients treated with prazosin (1 mg three times a day) versus placebo, with improvement in finger blood flow assessed during a finger cooling test. Complete relief was observed in only two patients (8%).[186] Long-acting forms of

prazosin include doxazosin and terazosin, which allow once-daily dosing. These drugs have also been shown to be effective therapy for RS by decreasing the number, intensity, and duration of attacks.[187]

The selective α₂C-adrenergic blocking agent OPC-28326 was recently assessed in a single-center, double-blinded, placebo-controlled, randomized trial in patients with RS secondary to scleroderma.[188] This agent's selectivity for the α₂C-receptor has the theoretical advantage of causing less systemic hypotension and therefore has greater tolerability. Study endpoints were recovery of skin temperature and plethysmographic digital blood flow after cold challenge. Patients treated with 40 mg of OPC-28326 experienced significant improvement in skin temperature recovery when compared with placebo. There was no difference in recovery of digital blood flow. Side effects were more common than with placebo, but none were serious or sustained.

Nitrates

Nitrates have been used for the treatment of RS as oral, topical, or intravenous preparations but in general are not first-line therapy. All forms are limited by side effects, particularly headaches and hypotension. Topical nitrates in the form of 2% nitroglycerin ointment (¼ to ½ inch) or as a transdermal patch can be applied locally to an ischemic finger and have been shown to be effective in the treatment of RS in randomized controlled trials.[189,190] In cases of digital ulceration, drug-induced vasodilatation of normal proximal vessels can cause a steal phenomenon by dilating the proximal arteries at the expense of distal finger blood flow and thereby resulting in worsening ischemia (Fig. 119-18).

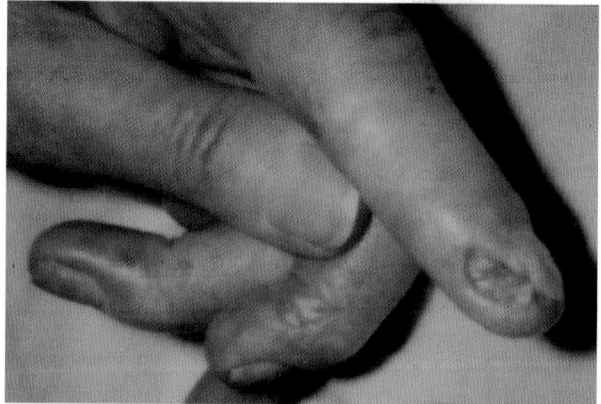

Figure 119-18 This patient was evaluated for acute ischemia of the fingertip. She was found to have positive antinuclear antibody and anticentromere antibody. An angiogram showed severe digital artery occlusive disease consistent with a connective tissue disease. Topical nitroglycerin ointment often fails to improve blood flow in the setting of critical ischemia as a result of severe underlying fixed small-vessel occlusive disease. The patient was treated with multiple agents, including oral, topical, and intravenous vasodilators; antiplatelet therapy; doxazosin; and nifedipine.

Renin-Angiotensin System Mediators

Mediators of the renin-angiotensin system, such as ACE inhibitors and angiotensin II receptor blockers, are indirect vasodilators that can mitigate the effects of angiotensin II, a potent vasoconstrictor. This has led to the hypothesis that these drugs may be of benefit in both primary and secondary RS.[191]

Angiotensin-Converting Enzyme Inhibitors.
Captopril has been the most extensively used of the ACE inhibitors for the treatment of RS. Doses range from 25 to 75 mg daily in divided doses. In an initial single-armed observational study, patients with both primary and secondary RS reported significant decreases in both the frequency and severity of RS attacks after 3 months of therapy.[192] In a subsequent randomized, controlled, crossover trial of 15 subjects with primary RS, captopril caused a significant increase in cutaneous blood flow measured with both laser Doppler flowmetry and photoplethysmography, but no change in the frequency or severity of RS attacks was noted.[193] Likewise, enalapril has not been shown to improve the frequency or severity of RS attacks in randomized controlled trials.[194] The long-acting ACE inhibitor quinapril also had no effect on the occurrence of digital ulcers or the frequency or severity of RS attacks in a randomized placebo-controlled trial.[195] Thus, the role of ACE inhibitors in the treatment of RS remains to be clarified, although captopril seems to have more promise than enalapril. In addition to its vasodilatory properties, ACE inhibitors also have antifibrotic properties, and their use should be considered in all patients with systemic sclerosis and hypertension to prevent scleroderma renal crisis.

Angiotensin II Receptor Blockers.
Losartan is an angiotensin II receptor type 1 antagonist. In a recent randomized controlled study, losartan, 50 mg daily, was found to be more effective than nifedipine, 40 mg daily, in reducing the frequency and severity of vasospastic episodes in patients with primary RS and those with RS secondary to systemic sclerosis after 12 weeks of therapy.[196] No significant differences in laser Doppler flow after cold challenge were seen between the two groups. Significantly fewer adverse effects were noted in the losartan group than in those taking nifedipine (39% versus 12%, $P = .005$). Though losartan is promising, larger trials with longer follow-up are required to more clearly define the role of losartan in the treatment of RS.

Serotonin Reuptake Inhibitors

Fluoxetine is a selective serotonin reuptake inhibitor. A significant reduction in attack frequency and severity was found in both primary and secondary RS treated with fluoxetine, 20 mg daily, but not in those treated with nifedipine, 40 mg daily, in a crossover trial. Laboratory testing showed improvement in recovery after a cold challenge test, with the greatest improvement seen in women with primary RS.[197] Clonazepam, a benzodiazepine with serotonergic effects, has been

shown to promote digital ulcer healing in patients with scleroderma.[198]

Phosphodiesterase Inhibitors

The phosphodiesterase type 5 (PDE5) inhibitors sildenafil, tadalafil, and vardenafil have recently garnered considerable interest in the treatment of secondary RS. These medications are selective inhibitors of cGMP-specific PDE5, which increases cGMP and thereby results in enhanced cGMP-dependent microvascular and macrovascular dilatation.[199] Thus, in addition to their use in the treatment of erectile dysfunction, the PDE5 inhibitors have been investigated for use in nonerectile indications such as pulmonary hypertension and RS.[200]

Of the available PDE5 inhibitors, the strongest evidence for use in RS lies with sildenafil. A placebo-controlled, double-blinded, crossover trial comparing 4 weeks of therapy with sildenafil, 50 mg twice daily, versus placebo was performed in 16 subjects with secondary RS not responsive to standard vasodilator therapy.[201] Significant improvements in RS symptoms, as measured by the Raynaud's Condition Score, and in capillary blood flow, as measured by laser Doppler, were detected with sildenafil therapy, regardless of the order of treatment. The frequency of RS attacks was reduced by 33% and the duration of attacks by 44% with sildenafil therapy versus placebo. Beneficial effects on ulcer healing were also observed, and only two patients had side effects requiring cessation of sildenafil therapy. Thus, despite being a small study, the data made a strong argument for the effectiveness of sildenafil in the treatment of secondary RS. In contrast, to date no studies have demonstrated the effectiveness of sildenafil in treating primary RS.[202]

In case series and small open-label pilot studies, beneficial effects on the frequency and severity of RS have also been demonstrated with the longer half-life agents vardenafil[203] and tadalafil.[204] More clinical trials with larger patient enrollment will be required to more fully define the role of PDE5 inhibitors in the treatment of RS.

An additional phosphodiesterase inhibitor that has been investigated as a potential treatment of RS is the PDE III inhibitor cilostazol. In a recent randomized, double-blinded trial, 40 patients with RS (19 primary, 21 secondary) were randomized to 6 weeks of cilostazol therapy versus placebo.[205] Arterial flow was measured by brachial artery vasoreactivity and laser Doppler flow, in addition to measuring patient symptoms with standardized questionnaires. Patients treated with cilostazol demonstrated improvements in brachial artery diameter but no change in microvascular flow or symptoms. Thus, cilostazol does not appear to have a role in the treatment of RS.

Endothelin Inhibitors

Endothelin is a potent vasoconstrictor and also causes cell proliferation. Bosentan is an endothelin receptor antagonist that has been shown in case series to have numerous beneficial effects in patients with secondary RS, including improvement in pain and disease activity, prevention and healing of digital ulcers, and improved peripheral thermoregulation. Bosentan is currently used to treat idiopathic pulmonary hypertension and pulmonary hypertension associated with scleroderma. It is not currently approved for the treatment of RS.[206,207]

Prostaglandins and Analogues

Prostaglandins are vasodilators that have been used for patients with critical digital ischemia secondary to fixed occlusive disease.

Epoprostenol.
Epoprostenol is a naturally occurring prostaglandin with potent vasodilatory and antiplatelet actions that can be given through a peripheral line as a continuous intravenous infusion. Epoprostenol (Flolan) is now available in the United States and has been approved for the treatment of primary pulmonary hypertension and pulmonary hypertension associated with scleroderma. For patients with pulmonary hypertension, it is administered as a continuous ambulatory infusion through an indwelling catheter via a small infusion pump. Major side effects are flushing, headache, nausea, vomiting, and hypotension.

Patients with severe RS and digital ischemia have been treated with epoprostenol administered as a continuous intravenous infusion (0.5 to 2 ng/kg/min) for 1 to 3 days. In one double-blinded, placebo-controlled study, 12 patients with severe RS received intravenous epoprostenol. A significant increase in fingertip skin temperature and laser Doppler flow was documented before and after a finger cooling test, but improved blood flow was not sustained and the beneficial effects were gone after 1 week.[208]

Iloprost.
Iloprost is a prostacyclin analogue that has been reported to reduce the severity, frequency, and duration of RS attacks and promote healing of ischemic ulcers.[209] Iloprost is investigational in the United States. In addition to its vasoactive properties, iloprost is thought to have antioxidant properties. Scleroderma patients treated with iloprost were found to have elevated levels of native antioxidants (catalase and superoxide dismutase) and decreased levels of malondialdehyde, a product of free radical release and lipid peroxidation, when compared controls.[210] In systemic sclerosis, complete healing of ulcers was observed 10 weeks after treatment in six of seven patients receiving an intravenous infusion of iloprost (0.5 to 2 ng/kg/min) administered as a 6-hour infusion over 5 consecutive days, as opposed to no healing of ulcers in those treated with saline placebo. In this study, improvement was sustained over the 9-week follow-up period.[211]

Intravenous iloprost was more effective than oral nifedipine in a 12-month prospective, single-blinded trial. Forty-six patients with systemic sclerosis were randomized to receive intravenous iloprost (at a rate of up to 2 ng/kg/min) over a period of 8 hours for 5 consecutive days and then once every 6 weeks. Raynaud's severity score was decreased and skin thickening was reduced. The study was limited by the adverse effects of headache, nausea, and vomiting during iloprost infusion.[212]

Another smaller study also found benefit of iloprost in patients with systemic sclerosis and RS. Over the 16-week study, 12 patients with systemic sclerosis were treated with iloprost administered by intravenous infusion on 3 consecutive days for 8 hours or randomized to nifedipine orally. Both agents produced reductions in the mean number, duration, and severity of attacks of RS. Hand temperature and blood flow increased with iloprost but not with nifedipine; however, healing of digital ulcers occurred in both groups.[213] Other prostaglandin analogues, such as alprostadil, have also been demonstrated to be effective in the symptomatic treatment of RS secondary to CTDs.[214]

Most studies have failed to show any significant improvement in RS or digital ischemia with oral formulations of iloprost. A multicenter trial of 143 patients with RS secondary to systemic sclerosis who were randomized to oral iloprost or placebo found no significant difference in the number or duration of attacks.[215] Another trial of 103 patients with scleroderma and RS showed only minimal benefit with oral iloprost, but adverse side effects required discontinuation of the medication in a number of patients.[216]

Antiplatelet Therapy

There is no evidence that antiplatelet therapy is of benefit in primary RS, but therapy with aspirin or clopidogrel should be considered for most patients with RS secondary to atherosclerosis.

Anticoagulation

Anticoagulation with intravenous or subcutaneous heparin may prevent further thrombosis in acute ischemia. Chronic anticoagulation is not generally indicated for most patients with small-vessel occlusive disease because the underlying process is an obliterative and not a thrombotic vasculopathy.

Alternative Therapies

Fish Oil.
Fish oil may decrease thromboxane A_2 production, increase prostacyclin synthesis, and reduce plasma viscosity; however, ingestion of a large number of fish oil capsules is required daily. One controlled trial failed to demonstrate any benefit in patients with secondary RS.[217]

Arginine.
L-Arginine is a substrate for NO synthesis and has a theoretical benefit of improving endothelial dysfunction in patients with both primary and secondary RS, but relatively few studies have been able to show any benefit. In one study, brachial artery infusion of either L-arginine or sodium nitroprusside (a direct donor of NO) decreased vasospastic attacks in 15 patients with scleroderma. Attacks were induced by

holding a beaker of ice water for 2 minutes and reducing the room temperature to 4° C. Attacks were fewer in hands infused with L-arginine.[218]

In another study of 20 patients with primary RS, there was no improvement in endothelium-dependent vasodilatation in a double-blinded, crossover trial of oral L-arginine (8 g daily for 28 days).[219] Patients with systemic sclerosis have reduced vasodilatation in response to acetylcholine and nitroglycerin because of fixed occlusive disease. Another study by Khan and Belch found that administration of L-arginine did not improve vasodilatation.[220]

Ginkgo biloba. Extracts of *Ginkgo biloba* have been used in Chinese medicine since at least the 14th century for a variety of conditions, including cognitive disorders, memory disturbances, dementia, and circulatory disorders. Seredrine, a high-potency extract of *Ginkgo biloba*, was evaluated in a randomized, placebo-controlled trial in patients with primary RS.[221] Patients randomized to the treatment group experienced fewer attacks per day than those given placebo after a 10-week treatment course, with a 56% drop in event rates versus 27% in the placebo group. In contrast, there were no differences in the duration and severity of attacks, nor were any differences in hemorheologic endpoints observed. This was, however, a small pilot study with only limited statistical power.

Acupuncture. Acupuncture may be of benefit in some patients. In a small, randomized trial, acupuncture was found to be effective in reducing the frequency and severity of attacks in patients with primary RS. The mechanism of action is believed to be stimulation of sensory nerves causing release of vasodilators such as substance P and CGRP.[222,223]

Laser Therapy. Laser therapy has been investigated as a potential treatment of a variety of vascular and rheumatologic disorders, including RS. Although most reports of efficacy are anecdotal, a recent randomized controlled trial evaluated low-level laser therapy with a diode laser versus sham therapy.[224] Forty-eight subjects underwent treatment consisting of five sessions per week for 3 weeks. The frequency and intensity of attacks were significantly reduced in the laser-treated group in comparison to sham therapy. It is hypothesized that laser therapy alters membrane permeability, thereby influencing postsynaptic α-adrenergic receptors, although the exact mechanism of action remains to be determined.

Nerve Stimulation. Transcutaneous nerve stimulation has also been used in some patients to induce vasodilatation with varying results.[225] Spinal cord stimulators are occasionally indicated for the treatment of various intractable pain syndromes of the upper extremities. There are several case reports of the use of spinal cord stimulators for the treatment of severe RS.[226,227] A spinal cord stimulator may reduce pain and promote ulcer healing in severe cases of secondary RS with trophic lesions.

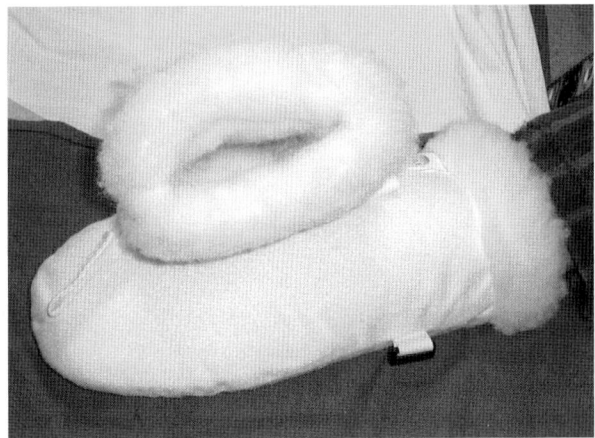

Figure 119-19 A vascular mitten protects and maintains warmth of the hands. Patients with critical hand and finger ischemia can have further compromise in distal perfusion as a result of cool ambient room temperature causing vasoconstriction. A vascular mitten keeps the hands at body temperature and maximizes distal finger blood flow by avoiding cold-induced vasoconstriction.

Management of Critical Digital Ischemia

In most cases, digital ulcers can be managed conservatively, which includes keeping the extremity at body temperature with the use of a vascular mitten, providing local therapy for digital ulcers with wound care products to prevent infection, and protecting the finger from trauma (Fig. 119-19). Local débridement of dead tissue or removal of the fingernail is sometimes necessary, but local amputation of the end of a digit may be necessary in 10% to 20% of patients. Whenever possible, amputation should be avoided because the amputation site may take longer to heal (if ever) than the original ulcer, and this can result in further skin necrosis at the amputation stump and necessitate a more proximal amputation.

Intermittent pneumatic compression is an established therapy for atherosclerotic limb ischemia after all surgical and medical options have been exhausted. Currently, several pumps are on the market, similar to the venous pumps used for thromboembolic prophylaxis but with more rapid and higher compression cycles. An increase in digital laser Doppler flow during the pump phase may indicate improved distal perfusion during pneumatic pumping of the upper extremity (Fig. 119-20).

■ SURGICAL THERAPY

Sympathectomy

Cervicothoracic Sympathectomy

Cervicothoracic sympathectomy was previously used as a surgical treatment of RS but is less frequently performed now.[228] Cervicothoracic sympathectomy is rarely if ever indicated for those with primary RS but may be effective in some patients who have critical ischemia of the digits, in particular to alleviate pain. The benefit may be short-lived.

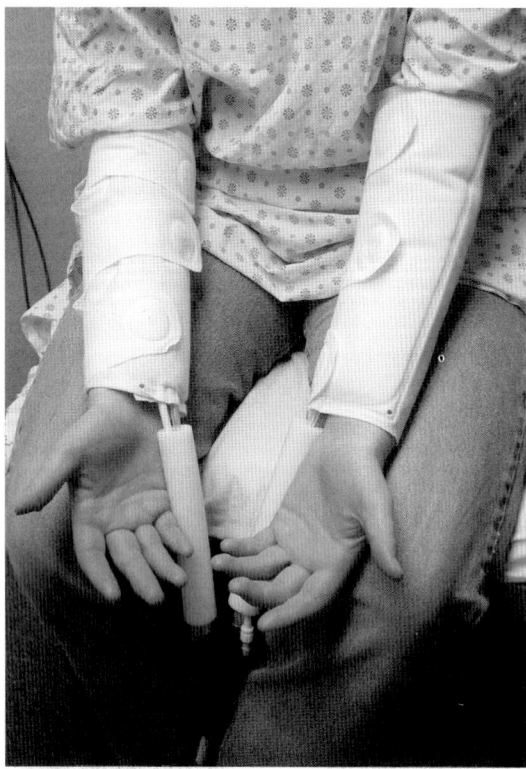

Figure 119-20 Pneumatic pumping of both upper extremities in a patient with digital ischemia secondary to scleroderma.

Thoracoscopic Sympathectomy

Currently, thoracoscopic sympathectomy has supplanted open cervicothoracic sympathectomy as the technique of choice because it limits complications such as pneumothorax, phrenic nerve injury, and Horner's syndrome. The frequency of Horner's syndrome is directly related to the level of transection. Therefore, most thoracic sympathectomies performed by any technique now exclude excision of the T1 sympathetic ganglia (see Chapter 121: Thoracic Sympathectomy). Initial improvement is followed by a high relapse rate because of regeneration of nerve fibers, hypersensitivity to catecholamines, or progression of underlying disease.

In a recent retrospective study, Thune and colleagues reported immediate relief of symptoms in 83% of patients but a 60% recurrence rate at a median follow-up of 40 months.[229] Forty-three percent of patients reported that they regretted undergoing the operation, which led the authors to conclude that sympathectomy should be reserved for patients with only the most severe cases of RS.

In contrast, Maga and coworkers reported significant improvement at 5 years in basal capillary flow rates and digital symptoms in 25 patients undergoing thoracoscopic sympathectomy for primary RS refractory to medical therapy.[230] These patients also had concomitant hyperhidrosis, which may indicate that this subset of patients with both conditions may get durable symptomatic relief. Likewise, Matsumoto and associates reported 28 patients with refractory RS or digital ulcers who underwent endoscopic thoracic sympathectomy.[231] Although initial relief was achieved in 93%, symptoms recurred in 82%. However, all ulcers healed without

recurrence, and at a median follow-up of 5 years, 89% reported overall improvement in symptoms in comparison to their preoperative state.

Lumbar Sympathectomy

In contrast to thoracic sympathectomy, excellent results have been achieved with lumbar sympathectomy, with long-term symptomatic relief noted in more than 90% of patients undergoing this procedure.[232] Lumbar sympathectomy remains a viable option in the rare patient with severely symptomatic lower extremity vasospasm. It is amenable to minimally invasive laparoscopic techniques.[233]

Digital Arterial Sympathectomy

Adventitial stripping of hand and digital arteries has been successful in healing ulcers and improving ischemic pain.[234,235] The results are anecdotal with no controlled trials comparing digital arterial sympathectomy with other less invasive treatment modalities. Therefore, its use in general is discouraged and should be considered only in refractory cases at risk for tissue loss.

Other Treatments

Percutaneous sympathetic blockade with a variety of agents, including mepivacaine and bupivacaine,[236] has also been shown to be an effective treatment of refractory RS. A 2-week infusion of mepivacaine through a thoracic sympathetic catheter placed in the T2 vertebral segment was shown to facilitate ulcer healing in refractory secondary RS.[237] Recently, a chemical sympathectomy produced by injecting botulinum toxin adjacent to the digital arteries has been proposed.[238] In a small study of 11 patients with refractory secondary RS, significant pain relief with a decreased frequency of vasospastic episodes was achieved in all patients with a mean follow-up of 9.6 months. Healing of digital ulcers was promoted, and only three patients reported side effects of hand weakness after the injections.

SELECTED KEY REFERENCES

Carpentier PH, Satger B, Poensin D, Maricq HR. Incidence and natural history of Raynaud phenomenon: a long-term follow-up (14 years) of a random sample from the general population. *J Vasc Surg.* 2006;44:1023.

This excellent epidemiologic study examines the incidence of new-onset Raynaud's syndrome in the general population. It is also one of the first studies to demonstrate disease regression over time in patients with primary vasospastic Raynaud's syndrome, with 33% of patients experiencing resolution of symptoms.

Cherkas LF, Williams FM, Carter L, Howell K, Black CM, Spector TD, MacGregor AJ. Heritability of Raynaud's phenomenon and vascular responsiveness to cold: a study of adult female twins. *Arthritis Rheum.* 2007;57:524.

This is one of the first studies to demonstrate a genetic component of Raynaud's syndrome, with a doubling of risk in first-degree relatives of affected individuals. These findings suggest that patients with Raynaud's syndrome may have as yet undefined susceptibility genes that may be amenable to targeted therapy.

Comparison of sustained-release nifedipine and temperature biofeedback for treatment of primary Raynaud phenomenon: results from a randomized clinical trial with 1-year follow-up. *Arch Intern Med.* 2000;160:1101.

This randomized trial did not demonstrate the effectiveness of temperature biofeedback but does provide level 1 evidence demonstrating the effectiveness of nifedipine over placebo.

Fries R, Shariat K, von Wilmowsky H, Böhm M. Sildenafil in the treatment of Raynaud's phenomenon resistant to vasodilatory therapy. *Circulation.* 2005;112:2980.

This randomized, controlled crossover trial provides strong evidence in support of sildenafil as a promising new therapy for the treatment of secondary Raynaud's syndrome. It is, however, a small trial that needs to be confirmed in a larger study population.

Herrick AL. Pathogenesis of Raynaud's phenomenon. *Rheumatology.* 2005;44:587.

This article summarizes the current understanding of the pathogenesis of Raynaud's syndrome and examines the interplay of both vascular and neural components. Implications for novel therapeutic options are also discussed.

Landry GJ, Edwards JM, McLafferty RB, Taylor LM Jr, Porter JM. Long-term outcome of Raynaud's syndrome in a prospectively analyzed patient cohort. *J Vasc Surg.* 1996;23:76.

This is one of the largest studies to date of a prospectively evaluated patient cohort with both primary and secondary Raynaud's syndrome. It provides useful prognostic information on the development of connective tissue diseases and the long-term risk for digital ulcerations or the need for digital amputations.

Matsumoto Y, Ueyama T, Endo M, Sasaki H, Kasashima F, Abe Y, Kosugi I. Endoscopic thoracic sympathectomy for Raynaud's phenomenon. *J Vasc Surg.* 2002;36:57.

This case series confirmed the high rate of symptomatic recurrence of Raynaud's symptoms after sympathectomy but does demonstrate the potential important role of sympathectomy in facilitating digital ulcer healing.

Suter LG, Murabito JM, Felson DT, Fraenkel L. Smoking, alcohol consumption, and Raynaud's phenomenon in middle age. *Am J Med.* 2007;120:264.

This large epidemiologic study clarified the role of smoking and alcohol consumption in the pathogenesis of vasospastic Raynaud's syndrome and also highlighted gender-specific differences in risk factors.

Thompson AE, Pope JE. Calcium channel blockers for primary Raynaud's phenomenon: a meta-analysis. *Rheumatology.* 2005;44;145.

This excellent meta-analysis summarizes current evidence in support of the use of calcium channel blockers for the treatment of Raynaud's syndrome.

Wigley FM, Korn JH, Csuka ME, Medsger TA Jr, Rothfield NF, Ellman M, Martin R, Collier DH, Weinstein A, Furst DE, Jimenez SA, Mayes MD, Merkel PA, Gruber B, Kaufman L, Varga J, Bell P, Kern J, Marrott P, White B, Simms RW, Phillips AC, Seibold JR. Oral iloprost treatment in patients with Raynaud's phenomenon secondary to systemic sclerosis: a multicenter, placebo-controlled, double-blind study. *Arthritis Rheum.* 1998;41:670.

Although intravenous iloprost has been shown to be an effective treatment of Raynaud's syndrome, it is not practical to use on an extended basis. The search continues for an effective oral preparation. Unfortunately, in this and other randomized, controlled trials, oral iloprost performed no better than placebo.

REFERENCES

The reference list can be found on the companion Expert Consult Web site at *www.expertconsult.com.*

CHAPTER 120

Occupational Vascular Problems

Mark K. Eskandari

Upper extremity work-related injuries are a major societal problem in regard to disability, cost, and loss of workdays. Occupational injuries affecting the shoulders, arms, and hands have been recognized for nearly 300 years and are generally categorized into injuries caused by accidents at work and injuries resulting from long-standing repetitive tasks.[1] Injuries in the latter category are due to small but additive amounts of tissue damage sustained from repetitive motions; they are known collectively as *cumulative trauma disorders*. According to data released by the U.S. Bureau of Labor Statistics, cumulative trauma disorders account for more than 50% of all occupational illnesses in the United States today.[2] Although most of these injuries affect the musculoskeletal system, injuries to arteries and veins are known to occur.[3] Work-related vascular injuries develop because of excessive or exaggerated job-related physical activity involving the shoulders, arms, or hands. Arterial occupational trauma includes vibration-induced white finger syndrome, hypothenar hammer syndrome, acro-osteolysis, electrical burns, extreme thermal exposure, and athletic injuries.

MANUAL LABOR INJURIES

Injury to arteries in the upper extremity is relatively common given the extensive use of the arms in manual labor.

Vibration-Induced White Finger

The first cases of this type of injury were reported in Rome in 1911 by Loriga.[4] Cottingham in 1918 noted blanching and numbness of the hands after using pneumatic drills,[5] and subsequent reports by Taylor and Pelmear[6] and Ashe and associates[7] firmly established vibration-induced white finger as a discrete clinical entity associated with hand ischemia. According to Taylor and Pelmear, the disease can be divided into five categories, as shown in Table 120-1[6]; this classification has been accepted as a standard by workers in this field. It is particularly useful in determining workers' compensation.

Clinical Findings and Risk Factors

The term *vibration-induced white finger* was favored by the Industrial Injuries Advisory Council in 1970 to describe symptoms similar to those of Raynaud's phenomenon— numbness, paresthesias, stiffness, coldness, and blanching of

Table 120-1 Stages of Vibration-Induced White Finger

Stage	Condition of Digits	Work and Social Interference
0	Vibration exposure but no signs or symptoms	No complaints
0T	Intermittent tingling	No interference with activities
0N	Intermittent numbness	No interference with activities
1	Blanching of 1 or more fingertips, with or without tingling and numbness	No interference with activities
2	Blanching of 1 or more fingers with numbness, usually in winter	Slight interference with home and social activities; no interference with work
3	Extensive blanching; frequent episodes in summer and winter	Definite interference at work, at home, and with social activities; restriction of hobbies
4	Same as stage 3: extensive blanching, most fingers involved, frequent episodes in summer and winter	Same as stage 3, but occupation changed to avoid further vibration exposure because of the severity of signs and symptoms

Updated from Taylor W, Pelmear PL, eds. *Vibration White Finger in Industry.* New York, NY: Academic Press; 1975.

one or more digits—that were caused by exposure to vibration.[8] Other investigators have used the terms *Raynaud's of occupational origin* or *traumatic vasospastic disease*. Regardless of the designation, the common initial symptoms are those of Raynaud's phenomenon secondary to prolonged use of vibrating mechanical tools.

In the early stages, vibration injury may be manifested as slight tingling and numbness. Later, the tips of one or more fingers exposed to vibration experience attacks of blanching, usually precipitated by cold. With continued exposure to vibration, the affected area increases in size, and the blanching extends to the entire finger exposed to vibration. Attacks of white finger typically last about 1 hour and terminate with reactive hyperemia (red flush) and often considerable pain. Prolonged exposure to vibration may induce bluish black cyanosis in the affected fingers. Only about 1% of cases progress to ulceration or gangrene.[9] Hand-held tools (e.g., pneumatic hammers and drills, grinders, and chain saws) are associated with vibration-induced white finger. Such injury potential is not restricted to a few types of tools but applies to a variety of situations in which workers' hands are subjected to signifi-

Box 120-1 Tools Associated with Vibration-Induced White Finger

- Pneumatic tools
- Riveting tools
- Caulking tools
- Drilling tools
- Clinching and flanging tools
- Rotary bur tools
- Pneumatic hammers
- Chain saws
- Grinders
- Pedestal tools
- Hand-held tools
- Chipping hammers
- Concrete vibrothickener
- Concrete-leveling vibrotables

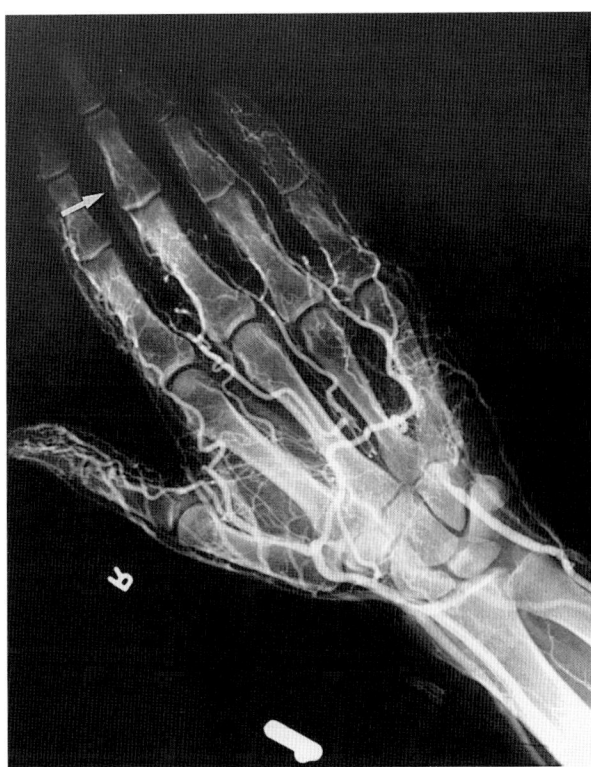

Figure 120-1 Arteriogram of the hand in a vibratory tool worker. Occlusion of the digital arteries (*arrow*) is apparent.

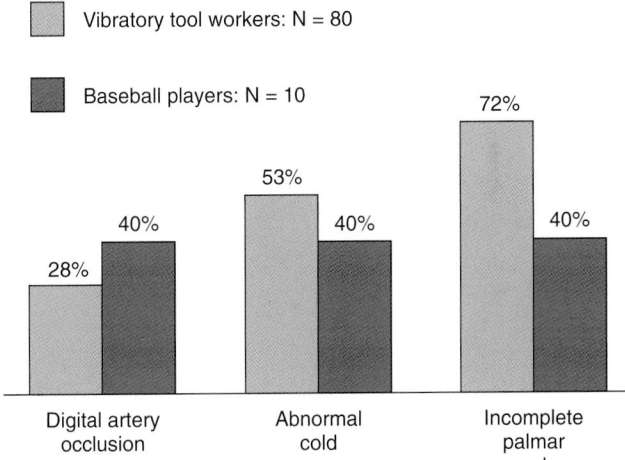

Figure 120-2 Incidence of digital artery occlusion, abnormal cold response, and incomplete palmar arch by Doppler examination in vibratory tool workers and baseball players. *(From Bartel P, Blackburn D, Peterson L, et al. The value of non-invasive tests in occupational trauma of the hands and fingers. Bruit. 1984;8:15.)*

cant vibration exposure.[8] Box 120-1 lists the types of tools that commonly cause vibration-induced white finger.

The exact mechanism of injury is unknown. Repetitive trauma from vibration of the tool is the main cause of the problem. The frequency of the vibration and the intensity of the trauma that it produces affect the extent of damage to the endothelium.[10] Local platelet adhesion seems to be an important factor in arterial occlusion. It has been shown that sympathetic hyperactivity, in combination with local factors such as vibration-induced hyperresponsiveness of the digital vessels to cold, may be responsible for the finger-blanching attacks.[11]

Diagnosis

The diagnosis is made from a history of using vibrating tools and from the classic Raynaud symptoms. For a vasospastic condition, the most promising single objective test is cold provocation and recording of the time until digital temperature recovers (see Chapter 14: Vascular Laboratory: Arterial Physiologic Assessment). Digital artery occlusion is best detected by recording the systolic pressure of the affected fingers with transcutaneous Doppler ultrasound[12-14] or duplex scanning.[15] In advanced disease, arteriography is helpful. Barker and Hines first documented arterial occlusion by brachial arteriography in a group of workers who complained of hand blanching and attacks of numbness.[16] Other authors have reported on the use of arteriography in investigating this injury.[17-19]

Arteriographic changes in vibration tool injury are confined largely to the hands. Multiple segmental occlusions of the digits and sometimes a corkscrew configuration are seen.[19] The intensity of the symptoms and the extent of the digital artery occlusion depend on the magnitude of the vibration, the frequency of the vibration, and lifetime exposure.[20] In advanced cases, occlusion of digital arteries is common. Of 80 workers (chippers) with vibration-induced white finger investigated at the Blood Flow Laboratory at Northwestern Uni-

versity, 25 (31%) exhibited a significant reduction in systolic pressure in one or more digits.[21] In 6 of the 25 workers, arteriography showed digital artery occlusion (Fig. 120-1). Incompleteness of the palmar arch was seen not only in the symptomatic hand but also in the contralateral, asymptomatic one. Symptoms of Raynaud's syndrome were present in 73 of 80 workers (91%). Abnormal cold response was observed in 53% of the workers (Fig. 120-2).

Treatment

Treatment of vibration-induced white finger consists of relief of Raynaud's symptoms. Surgical treatment, such as cervical sympathectomy or digital sympathectomy, is rarely indicated or needed. The most important step is to discontinue the use of vibrating tools by changing jobs or rotating on and off that particular task. In most instances, prevention is more effective than cure. Factory standards should conform to standards suggested by the American Conference of Governmental Industrial Hygienists in 1984,[22] and perhaps more operations should be automated to eliminate human exposure to vibratory insults. In advanced cases, a calcium channel blocker such as nifedipine (30 to 80 mg daily) may be useful. Calcium antagonists inhibit the response of arterial smooth muscle to norepinephrine and have been reported to be effective.[23] Intravenous infusion of a prostanoid (prostaglandin E_1, prostacyclin, or iloprost) is usually reserved for patients with digital gangrene.[24]

Hypothenar Hammer Syndrome

The predisposing factor in the development of hypothenar hammer syndrome is repetitive use of the palm of the hand in activities that involve pushing, pounding, or twisting. The anatomic site of the ulnar artery in the area of the hypothenar eminence makes it vulnerable. The terminal branches of the ulnar artery (deep palmar branch and superficial arch) arise in a groove named Guyon's tunnel, which is bounded medially by the pisiform and the hook of the hamate and dorsally by the transverse carpal ligament. Over a distance of 2 cm, the ulnar artery lies superficially in the palm and is covered only by skin, subcutaneous tissue, and the palmaris brevis muscle (Fig. 120-3). When this area is repeatedly traumatized, ulnar or digital arterial spasm, aneurysms, occlusion, or a combination of these lesions can result. Embolization from an aneurysm may cause multiple digital artery occlusions distally. The type of arterial abnormality observed often depends on the nature of the vessel damage.

Clinical Findings and Risk Factors

Intimal damage often results in thrombotic occlusion, whereas injury to the media causes palmar aneurysms (Fig. 120-4).[25] This type of occupational injury has been called the hypothenar hammer syndrome.[26] In 1934, Von Rosen provided the first descriptive report of this condition,[27] and subsequently it was recognized as an occupational disease.[28]

Table 120-2 lists the types of workers in whom this syndrome developed in reported series.[29] Among 79 workers who habitually used their hands as a hammer, Little and Ferguson found that 11 (14%) showed evidence of ulnar artery occlusion in one or both hands.[30] The traditional dogma regarding

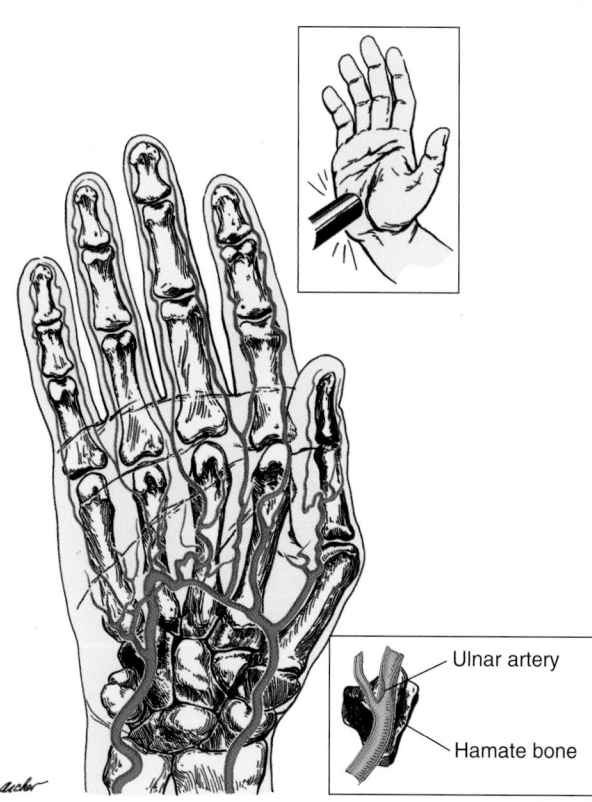

Figure 120-3 Mechanism of ulnar artery injury (*upper inset*) in a patient with hypothenar hammer syndrome. The terminal branch of the ulnar artery is vulnerable to injury because of its close proximity to the hamate bone (*lower inset*).

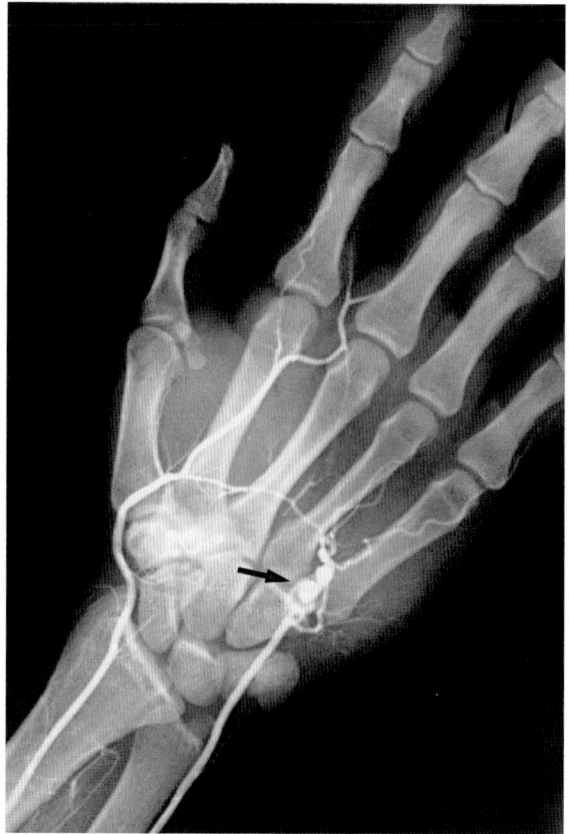

Figure 120-4 Arteriogram of the hand of a carpenter. Note the aneurysm of the ulnar artery (*arrow*) caused by repetitive trauma from using the hand as a hammer.

Table 120-2 Occupations of 33 Patients with Hypothenar Hammer Syndrome

Occupation	Number of Patients
Mechanic/automobile repair	15
Lathe operator	3
Fitter and turner	2
Tire braider	2
Carpenter	2
Engineer	2
Machinist	2
Painter	1
Butcher	1
Gardener	1
Tool and die worker	1
Bus conductor	1

Modified from Pineda CJ, Weisman MH, Bookstein JJ, et al. Hypothenar hammer syndrome: form of reversible Raynaud's phenomenon. *Am J Med* 1985;79:561. With permission of Excerpta Medica, Inc.

the etiology of hypothenar hammer syndrome has been challenged by Ferris and colleagues.[31] These investigators reviewed the arteriographic and histologic findings of 21 patients treated for hypothenar hammer syndrome. Similar radiographic findings of "corkscrew" elongation of the ulnar artery in the dominant and nondominant hands were identified in 12 of 13 patients with bilateral angiograms. Additionally, in patients undergoing surgical resection and bypass grafting of symptomatic aneurysms, the histologic findings were consistent with fibromuscular dysplasia with superimposed trauma. Based on this evidence, they proposed that the etiology of hypothenar hammer syndrome depends on the presence of underlying ulnar artery fibromuscular dysplasia in the presence of repetitive palmar trauma.

Clinically, patients report symptoms of Raynaud's syndrome. In the series of patients described by Conn and colleagues, the ring finger was most often involved.[26] The traditional triphasic color changes (white-blue-red) and thumb involvement are uncommon.[29] Physical examination may disclose a prominent callus over the hypothenar eminence, coldness or mottling of the involved fingertip, and atrophic ulceration. A positive Allen test result, which indicates ulnar artery occlusion, is common. Occasionally, an aneurysm is observed as a pulsatile mass in the hypothenar eminence.

Diagnosis

The diagnosis is suggested by a history of repetitive trauma to the dominant hand and physical finding of a pulsatile mass in the palm. B-mode ultrasound scanning is particularly useful in confirming the presence of an ulnar artery aneurysm. Traditional arteriography is helpful in diagnosis of hypothenar hammer syndrome and in planning treatment. Arteriography defines the type of vascular lesion (spasm, aneurysm, occlusion), shows its site and extent, and identifies the presence of significant collateral vessels. Frequently, these patients have an incomplete superficial palmar arch, even in the asympto-

matic hand. More recently, high-resolution contrast-enhanced magnetic resonance angiography has been used as a noninvasive modality in place of standard angiography.[32,33]

Treatment

Treatment of ulnar artery occlusion is often supportive, and surgical intervention is seldom needed or possible.[34] Catheter-directed intra-arterial thrombolytic therapy may be beneficial if patients are seen within several weeks of the onset of ischemic symptoms. Occasionally, an ulnar aneurysm is uncovered by thrombolysis. Aneurysms of the ulnar artery should be resected to eliminate the source of emboli and can be treated by resection with end-to-end anastomosis or by an interposed vein graft. Satisfactory long-term results have been reported with this approach.[35]

Occupational Acro-osteolysis

Occupational acro-osteolysis was first described by Wilson and colleagues in workers exposed to polyvinyl chloride.[36] Many of these workers have ischemic symptoms in the hand with resorption of the distal phalangeal tufts, similar to that seen with scleroderma. The dominant initial symptoms are those of Raynaud's syndrome. Few reports of angiography in this syndrome have been published to document damage to the digital arteries.[37-39] Findings include multiple arterial stenoses and occlusions of the digital arteries, along with nonspecific hypervascularity adjacent to the areas of bony resorption. The reason for the hypervascularity is not clear, but it may be related to stasis of contrast medium in digital pulp arteries secondary to shortening and retraction of the fingers. Some of these digits were clubbed, a finding that has also been associated with hypervascularity in the fingertips. Treatment is supportive.

Electrical Burns

Electrical burns inflict tissue destruction in relation to the voltage applied. Currents of less than 1000 V cause injuries limited to the immediate underlying skin and soft tissue. High voltage (>1000 V) usually causes extensive damage as the current travels from the point of entry to the point of exit. No tissue is immune to the devastating effects of high-voltage injury, and arterial injury may occur. The upper extremity, especially the hand, is more often involved than other parts of the body because of its grasping function. The arterial injury is often manifested by arterial necrosis with thrombus or bleeding, and occasionally gangrene of the digits develops.

Bookstein described the angiographic changes in the upper extremity after electrical injury, including extensive occlusion of the ulnar and digital arteries and thrombosis of the radial artery.[37] Arterial spasm may also be present. Later on, damage to the media may cause aneurysm formation. Figure 120-5 shows a brachial artery aneurysm in a patient who had sustained electrical burns 9 months earlier. Treatment depends

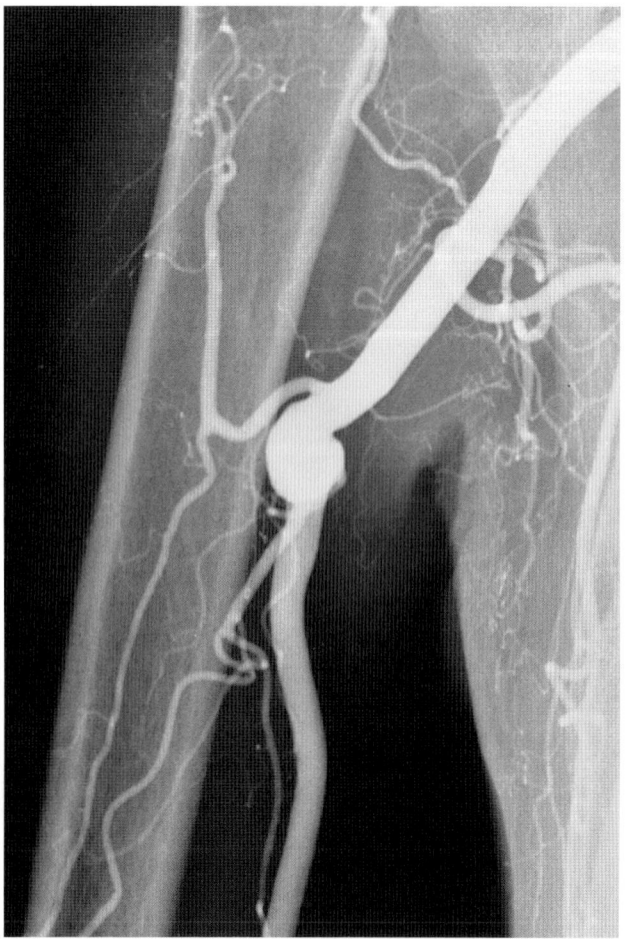

Figure 120-5 Aneurysm of the brachial artery in an electrician who had sustained a high-voltage electrical burn 9 months previously.

on the associated soft tissue and bone injuries.[40] Occlusion of a major artery documented by arteriography requires bypass grafting, and good results have been reported.[41]

Extreme Thermal Injuries

Vasomotor disturbances in the hands of individuals exposed to extreme chronic thermal trauma are typically manifested as Raynaud's syndrome. Workers at highest risk for thermal injuries are those in a profession in which their hands are subjected to chronic exposure to cold, such as slaughterhouses, canning factories, and fisheries.[42,43] Epidemiologic studies examining this dilemma are limited. The action of alternating ice-cold and hot exposure, use of plastic gloves in cold exposure, and long-term exposure to cold seem to be identifiable risk factors. Treatment is supportive.

ATHLETIC INJURIES

Athletes, particularly professionals who engage in strenuous or exaggerated hand or shoulder activity, may be susceptible to hand or upper extremity ischemia as a result of arterial injury. Hand ischemia is often manifested as Raynaud's

syndrome, symptoms of sudden arterial occlusion, or embolization to the digits. Three types of arterial injury are common: hand ischemia, quadrilateral space syndrome, and thoracic outlet compression of the subclavian-axillary artery. The exact incidences are unknown; however, vascular injury has been reported in professional and competitive participants in baseball, karate, volleyball, handball, Frisbee, and lacrosse and in weightlifters and butterfly swimmers.[21,29,44-48]

Hand Ischemia

Repetitive trauma is the principal cause of hand ischemia in athletes.

Clinical Findings and Risk Factors

The mechanisms of ischemia fall into two main categories: (1) direct digital artery injury or (2) embolization from a source more proximal in the upper extremity. Nearly all hand activity involved in any sport can cause blunt force injury to the arteries.[49] Though infrequent, hand ischemia secondary to direct digital arterial trauma is encountered more often in handball players, baseball catchers, and practitioners of karate. Among baseball players, hand ischemia is more common in pitchers, catchers, and first-basemen because of frequent contact with the baseball. Figure 120-6 illustrates occlusion of the palmar

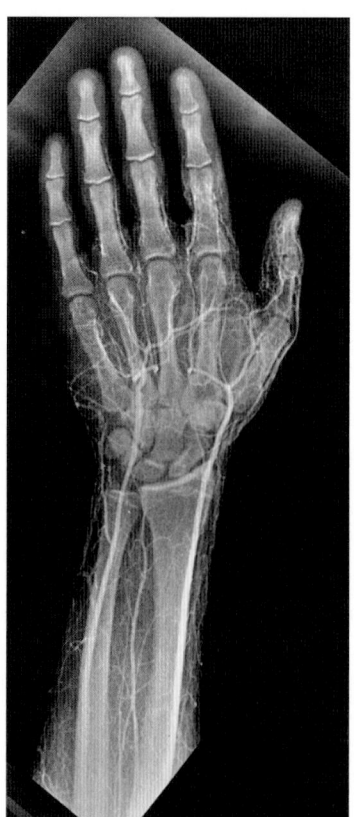

Figure 120-6 Occlusion of the palmar arch in a Frisbee player. Because of the injury, there is poor filling of contrast media in the second, third, fourth, and fifth fingers.

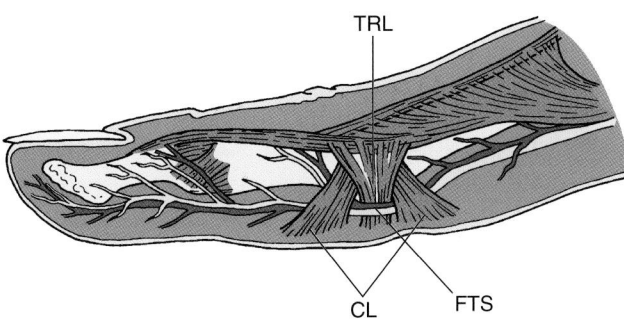

Figure 120-7 With the proximal interphalangeal joint in hyperextension, Cleland's ligaments may compress and occlude the vascular supply to the fingertip. CL, Cleland's ligaments; FTS, flexor tendon sheath; TRL, transverse retinacular ligament.

arch in a Frisbee player; ischemia of all fingers occurred suddenly after he caught the Frisbee. It has been suggested that handball players with more than 200 hours of accumulated playing time are at greater risk for symptomatic alterations in perfusion.[50,51]

Professional baseball players, particularly catchers, are predisposed to the development of chronic hand ischemia. Many catchers have symptoms of Raynaud's syndrome, especially in the off-season when they engage in outdoor activity in cool autumn or winter weather. Lowrey reported decreased digital perfusion to the index finger of the glove hand in 13 of 22 baseball catchers examined by Doppler flow detection and the Allen test.[52] Of 10 professional catchers studied in the author's laboratory, 40% had evidence of digital artery occlusion.[52] In view of the speed of the baseball and the impact of the force on the hands, perhaps arterial injury in professional baseball catchers occurs more often than would be expected.

Another form of hand ischemia occasionally observed in baseball pitchers is compression of the digital artery by Cleland's ligament. These ligamentous structures are found on the palmar surface of the digits and span from the phalanx to the subcutaneous tissue (Fig. 120-7). The proposed mechanism is compression of the digital vessels with hyperextension of the proximal interphalangeal joints.

Treatment

Treatment of hand ischemia depends on the clinical findings. With acute injury, a conservative approach involving intravenous infusion of dextran and pain control is in order. Surgical intervention is rarely needed; however, attempts at digital sympathectomy or release of Cleland's ligaments have met with some short-term success.[53] Preventing injury is important and can be accomplished by the use of gloves with padding and other protective devices.[52]

Quadrilateral Space Syndrome

Quadrilateral space syndrome was first described in 1983 by Cahill and Palmer, who reported on the diagnosis and surgical treatment of 18 patients with this entity.[54] The quadrilateral space is defined as the area bordered by the teres minor supe-

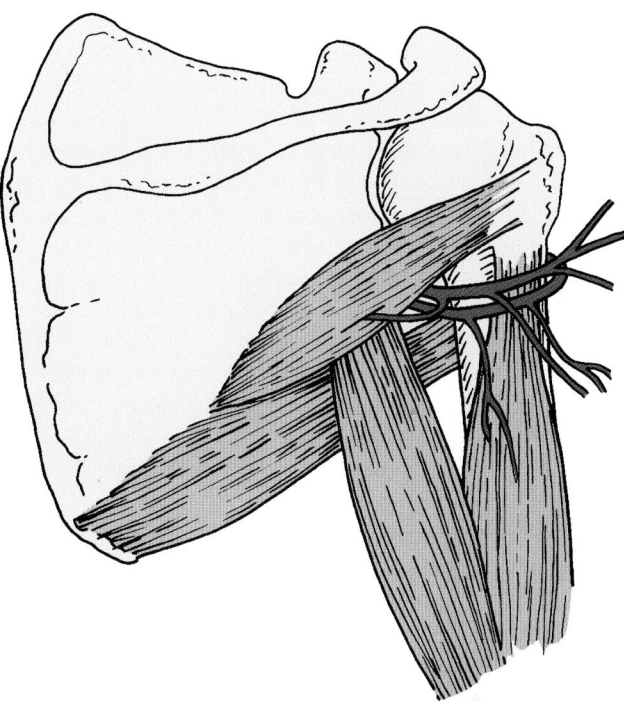

Figure 120-8 The posterior humeral circumflex artery and axillary nerve traverse the interval of the quadrilateral space.

riorly, the humeral shaft laterally, the teres major inferiorly, and the long head of the triceps muscle medially (Fig. 120-8).[55] Found within this space are the posterior humeral circumflex artery and the axillary nerve. Compression of the posterior humeral circumflex artery within this space has been shown to occur with the arm in the "cocked" position (abduction and external rotation). Chronic compression and trauma to this artery in throwing athletes, particularly pitchers, can lead to aneurysmal dilatation or occlusion. Aneurysms in this location are prone to distal embolization in the hand. Surgical treatment of aneurysms in this location involves ligation of the posterior humeral circumflex artery.[56] The anterior and posterior humeral circumflex arteries provide blood supply to the humeral head, and at least one of the two vessels must be preserved or repaired to prevent avascular necrosis.

Thoracic Outlet Compression

Athletes who engage in overextended shoulder motion, such as baseball pitchers, butterfly swimmers, weightlifters, and oarsmen, are potential candidates for thoracic outlet compression. Injuries to the subclavian artery or vein have been reported in these athletes.

Clinical Findings and Risk Factors

In professional baseball pitchers, the injury is most likely due to the violent throwing motion. The act of pitching has five phases: (1) wind-up, (2) cocking, (3) acceleration, (4) release and deceleration, and (5) follow-through. Most injuries occur during the acceleration and deceleration phases.[57] It has been estimated that a fastball creates 600 inch-lb of forward momentum at release of the ball. It is understandable that soft tissue injury may occur because of the force absorbed by the shoulder and the elbow.[58]

Symptoms are more common in pitchers whose throwing motion is overhand rather than sidearm. Symptoms are pain in the region of the elbow associated with easy fatigue and loss of pitch velocity after several innings. Raynaud's syndrome has also been observed in these pitchers. Making the diagnosis is often difficult, and a complete evaluation by an orthopedic surgeon to rule out musculoskeletal abnormalities is mandatory. Duplex scanning and transcutaneous Doppler flow detection with the athlete in the pitching position help detect compression of the subclavian or axillary artery. Finally, a definitive diagnosis is established by arteriography with positional exposure (Figs. 120-9 and 120-10).

Arterial injury to the pitching arm affects the subclavian artery,[45] the axillary artery,[44] and the humeral circumflex arteries.[54] Compression on the subclavian or axillary artery is often due to hypertrophy of the anterior scalene or the pectoralis minor muscle; however, arterial injury can occur at the costoclavicular space, humeral head, or quadrilateral space. In 1964, Tullos and colleagues were the first to report an axillary artery thrombus secondary to compression of the pectoralis minor in a major league pitcher.[44] In 1978, Strukel and Garrick reported on three competitive baseball pitchers with thoracic outlet compression.[59] Until Fields' report on athletic injury in the thoracic outlet,[60] the injury had received little attention. The report by Fields and associates on a major league pitcher who suffered a catastrophic stroke resulting from subclavian artery thrombosis with proximal clot propagation is of great interest.[45] The humeral head and the pectoralis minor muscle and other shoulder muscles have been shown to be hypertrophied in pitchers; these structures are more prone to cause local trauma to the nearby vessels in this group of athletic individuals.[61,62]

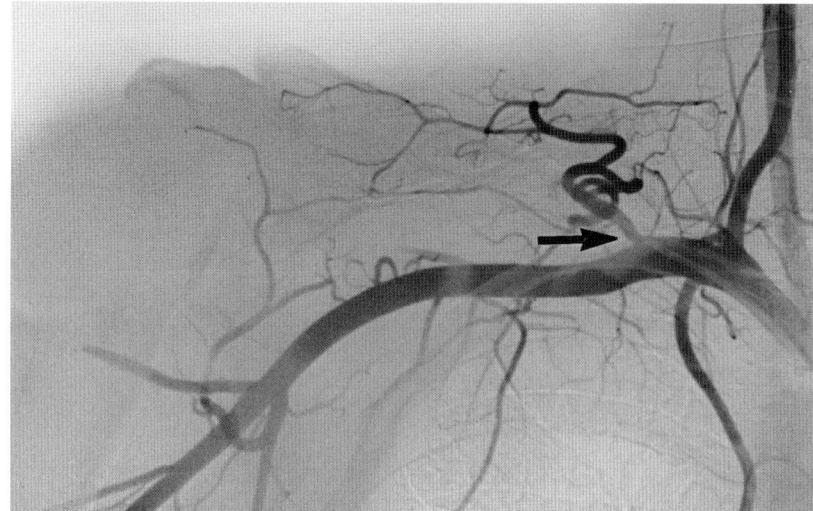

Figure 120-9 Arteriogram of the right subclavian artery (*arrow*) in a professional baseball pitcher. No injury is seen when the arm is placed in neutral position.

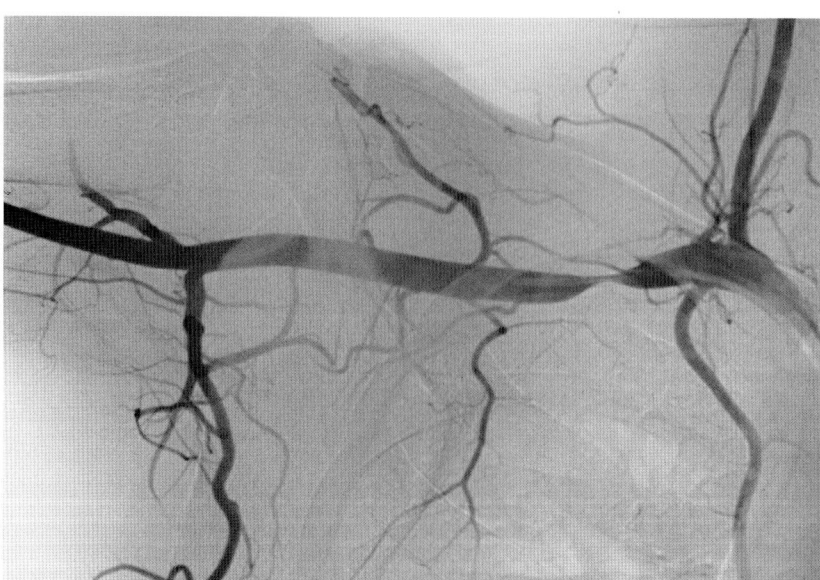

Figure 120-10 In the same patient shown in Figure 120-9, there is compression of the subclavian artery when the arm is placed in the pitching position (hyperabduction).

It is now recognized that aneurysm formation in the anterior and, more commonly, the posterior circumflex arteries as a result of repetitive athletic activity is responsible for severe hand ischemia secondary to distal embolization.[63] Tethering of the axillary artery between the chest and the loop of circumflex arteries around the humeral neck can produce a traction injury resulting in intimal damage with subsequent thrombosis or aneurysm formation. Distal embolization occurs because of retrograde extrusion of clot from the side branch aneurysm with persistent excessive activity of the upper extremity. Such injury has been observed in baseball pitchers and volleyball players (Fig. 120-11).[61,64,65] Reekers and coworkers believe that the downward pull of the humeral head during the "smash" in volleyball is a mechanism of axillary artery trauma akin to pitching.[65] In both instances, the circumflex artery is not the only one affected; aneurysm formation in the suprascapular and subscapular arteries has also been reported.[66] Additionally, direct trauma from the head of the humerus can cause compression on the axillary artery with similar sequelae.[61,64,67]

In addition to arterial injury, thrombosis of the subclavian-axillary vein, so-called effort thrombosis or Paget-Schroetter syndrome, has been reported in baseball pitchers,[68] weightlifters,[69] and competitive swimmers.[70] The presumed mechanism of injury is similar to that of the arterial system, and treatment options are similar.

Treatment

Treatment depends on the extent of injury. Compression only is best treated by division of the offending muscle and tendon. Occlusion of a major artery requires bypass grafting together with decompression of the thoracic outlet. Traditional reconstruction is advocated; however, some authors have reported on the successful use of an extra-anatomic bypass over the pectoralis muscle after arterial injury in pitchers.[71] Aneurysms of the circumflex artery and thrombosis in the axillary artery are best treated via a transaxillary approach with resection of the aneurysm, vein grafting, or both, if indicated.[67] Management of acute venous thrombosis is controversial and varies from anticoagulation alone to decompressive surgery to venoplasty and stenting.[72-75] In athletes, some form of decompression is needed to return to competitive activity. To return a professional athlete to full activity, close consultation with a trainer or sports medicine specialist and carefully supervised rehabilitation are necessary.

SELECTED KEY REFERENCES

Ferris BL, Taylor LM Jr, Oyama K, McLafferty RB, Edwards JM, Moneta GL, Porter JM. Hypothenar hammer syndrome: proposed etiology. *J Vasc Surg*. 2000;31:104.
This report nicely describes the anatomy and pathophysiology of hypothenar hammer syndrome. It also suggests that an underlying arterial problem (i.e., fibromuscular dysplasia) may be a predisposing condition.

McLelland D, Paxinos A. The anatomy of the quadrilateral space with reference to quadrilateral space syndrome. *J Shoulder Elbow Surg*. 2008;17:162.
A great reference and illustration of the quadrilateral space and the associated syndrome.

Nasu Y, Kurozawa Y, Fujiwara Y, Honma H, Yanai T, Kido K, Ikeda T. Multicenter study on finger systolic blood pressure test for diagnosis of vibration-induced white finger. *Int Arch Occup Environ Health*. 2008;81:639.
This contemporary multicenter study demonstrates the sensitivity and specificity of using noninvasive systolic blood pressure measurements to make the diagnosis of vibration-induced white finger. Included are the techniques of performing this testing.

REFERENCES

The reference list can be found on the companion Expert Consult Web site at *www.expertconsult.com*.

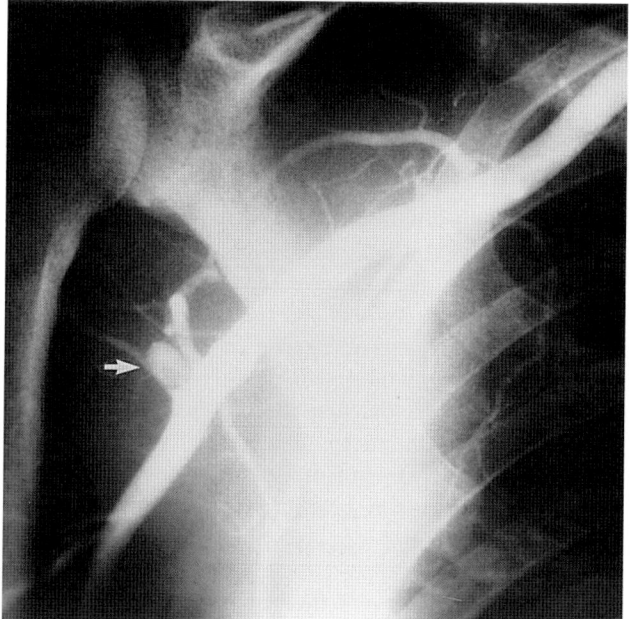

Figure 120-11 Artery of a major league baseball pitcher. Note the aneurysm of the posterior humeral circumflex artery (*arrow*).

CHAPTER 121

Thoracic Sympathectomy

Nelson Wolosker and Paulo Kauffman

The first studies on the anatomy of the autonomic nervous system are attributed to Galen in the second century AD, but it was only in the last decade of the 19th century that effects resulting from blockade of the preganglionic and postganglionic neurons were described by Langley.[1] The first sympathectomy is attributed to Alexander in 1889, who tried to treat an epileptic patient with this surgical procedure.[2] He was followed by Jonnesco, who in 1896 performed sympathectomy on a large number of epileptic patients.[3] In 1899, Jaboulay resected the lower cervical chain in a patient with exophthalmos and goiter.[4] Because of lack of success in the operative treatment of these conditions, as well as many others with no effective medical or surgical alternatives (migraine, renal pain, poliomyelitis, etc.), interest in intervention on the sympathetic nervous system waned for a time.

The first successful clinical application of sympathectomy occurred in patients with angina pectoris. The knowledge that afferent visceral fibers could transmit sensory impulses through the sympathetic chain to the central nervous system led Jonnesco in 1916 to successfully perform cervicodorsal sympathectomy for angina pectoris with the aim of pain suppression.[5] The first to use cervical sympathectomy to treat a patient with hyperhidrosis (HH) was Kotzareff in 1920.[6] In 1924, Hunter tried to use sympathectomy to reduce muscle tonus in patients with spastic paralysis.[7] Although this intervention did not show any beneficial effect on this condition, he observed a significant increase in circulation in denervated limbs.[6] This led to its use in treating Raynaud's disease and other types of vasospastic disease. In 1924, Diez reported 100% success in treating 150 cases of thromboangiitis obliterans (TAO) in the upper limbs.[8]

There was a technical evolution in open surgery involving different surgical approaches to resect the sympathetic ganglia: supraclavicular (cervical),[9] axillary transthoracic,[10] dorsal (posterior),[11] dorsal midline,[12] and anterior transthoracic.[13] By the end of the 1930s, the main indications for cervicodorsal sympathectomy had started to be delineated: HH, TAO, and vasospastic conditions.

Using the development of thoracoscopy introduced by Jacobaeus in 1910,[14] Hughes in 1942 performed the first thoracoscopic sympathectomy.[15] Kux in 1953 was the first to publish a large experience with this method.[16] However, despite the good results, for unknown reasons this technique did not achieve international acceptance for practically 30 years. In the 1980s, the endoscopic technique was used to perform sympathetic denervation in the upper limbs by a few groups of surgeons.[17]

In the 1990s, advances in optical systems and instruments for thoracoscopic surgery made it possible to use video-assisted thoracoscopy to perform sympathectomy.[18] The low morbidity, good cosmetic results, decrease in incidence of Horner's syndrome, and short hospital stay stimulated patients with HH to request their physicians to use video-assisted thoracic sympathectomy (VATS). Because these patients are young and healthy and VATS is an elective procedure, there have been positive outcomes, and this type of surgery is increasingly being performed. Over the last 10 years, thousands of operations have been reported in hundreds of articles, which has led to technical improvements and better results.

■ ANATOMY

Sympathetic Ganglia

The motor sympathetic route is formed by three neurons (Fig. 121-1). The cell body of the first neuron is located in the sudomotor and vasomotor centers. Its axon projects along the dorsal longitudinal and spinovestibular fascicles to the cell body of the second neuron (preganglionic neuron), which is located in the intermediolateral nucleus of the spinal gray matter, between the first thoracic and second lumbar vertebrae. Its axon (the preganglionic fiber) exits the medulla through the ventral root of the spinal nerves and, through the white communicating branch, projects to the paravertebral ganglion, where it forms a synapse with the cell body of the third neuron, the postganglionic neuron. Its axon (the postganglionic fiber) leaves the sympathetic chain through the gray communicating branch into the spinal nerve and is distributed peripherally. The ganglia are also interconnected longitudinally by axons from preganglionic neurons that run rostrally or caudad to the neighboring ganglia of the chains.

As in the somatic nervous system, the axon of the preganglionic neuron exits from the segment in which its soma is located. There is one sympathetic paravertebral ganglion for each spinal segment, and the sympathetic fiber that originates from the ganglion innervates the area of the spinal nerve corresponding to that segment. Thus, for example, the T2 ganglion supplies sympathetic innervation for structures of the D2 dermatome.

Sympathetic Innervation of the Upper Limbs

The preganglionic fibers responsible for innervation of the upper limbs originate from the second to eighth medullary segments, most of them below the fourth segment. The fibers enter the paravertebral sympathetic chain through the white communicating branches of the corresponding ganglia and have an ascending pathway in which a synapse is formed with cells located in the second thoracic ganglion, the stellate ganglion, and probably the middle cervical ganglion.

It is of surgical interest that no preganglionic fibers enter the sympathetic chain above the first thoracic ganglion and that the latter participates in innervation of the limb in only 10% of cases.

Palmar and axillary sweating, or sudoresis, diminishes after T3 or T4 ablation, and ischemia diminishes after ablation of T1 to T3.

Sympathetic Innervation of the Ocular Structures

The sympathetic preganglionic fibers controlling the smooth muscles of the eye are rostral from the anterior roots of T1 and T2. The fibers enter the sympathetic chain by the corresponding ganglia but do not form synapses. The synapses are subsequently formed when they ascend to the superior cervical ganglion. The postganglionic fibers, through the carotid plexus, head toward the ocular-pupillary apparatus. Consequently, resection of the stellate ganglion causes the Claude Bernard–Horner syndrome (enophthalmos, myosis, and ptosis).

Sympathetic Innervation of the Cephalic Segment

Sympathetic innervation of the head and neck originates from the medullary segments T1 to T5. The preganglionic fibers ascend the sympathetic chain and form synapses with the first thoracic ganglion and the inferior cervical ganglion. Most of the postganglionic fibers responsible for innervation of the face originate from T2, which implies that craniofacial sweating diminishes after T2 ablation.

Sympathetic Innervation of the Heart

Sympathetic innervation of the heart is supplied higher from the three cardiac nerves (superior, medium, and inferior) arising from the three cervical ganglia and also from the thoracic cardiac nerves arising from the first six or seven thoracic paravertebral ganglia. Most fibers converge at the cardiac plexuses. These nerves are more abundant in the fourth and fifth thoracic segments than at higher levels.

◼ PHYSIOLOGY

The sympathetic chain supplies the smooth muscles of blood vessels through adrenergic fibers and the sweat glands through

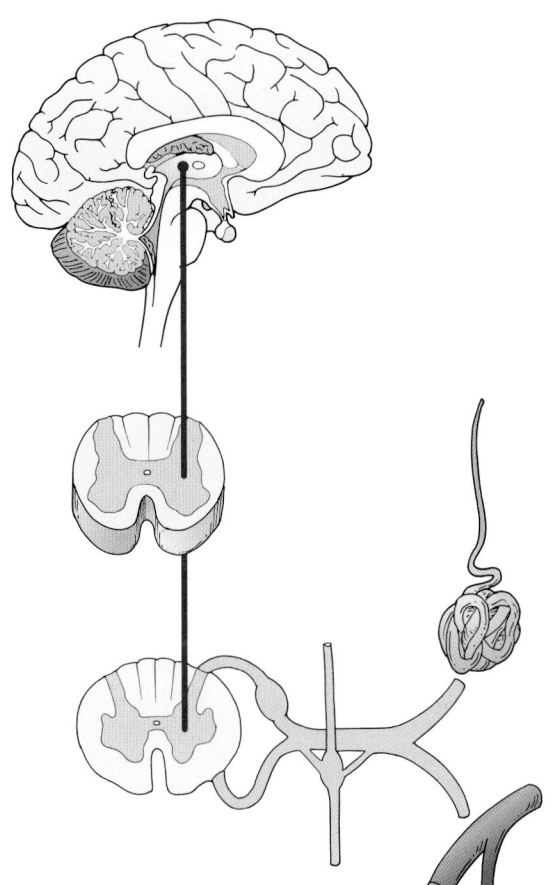

Figure 121-1 The motor sympathetic route. The cell body of the first neuron is located in the sudomotor and vasomotor centers, the second neuron (preganglionic neuron) is located in the intermediolateral nucleus of the spinal gray matter, and the third neurons are located in the paravertebral ganglia.

In the neck there are normally three ganglia in the sympathetic chain. The superior cervical ganglion results from fusion of the first four sympathetic cervical ganglia; it is located at the level of the transverse process of the second and third cervical vertebrae and supplies the head and neck. The middle cervical ganglion is located at the level of the sixth cervical vertebra. The inferior cervical ganglion is generally fused with the first thoracic ganglion (T1) to form the cervicothoracic ganglion (stellate ganglion), which is located anterior to the head of the first rib and covered by the pleura.

In the thoracic region, the ganglia of the sympathetic chain are positioned anterior to the transverse processes of the thoracic vertebrae and are covered by the parietal pleura. They are fewer in number than the spinal thoracic nerves because of fusion of the first thoracic ganglion with the inferior cervical ganglion, fusion of the last thoracic ganglion with the first lumbar ganglion, and fusion of the thoracic ganglia with each other. The greater and lesser splanchnic nerves are formed by preganglionic fibers originating from the 5th to the 12th thoracic medullary segments. They cross the corresponding sympathetic ganglia without forming synapses with them and innervate the medulla of the adrenal glands.

cholinergic fibers. In the vascular system, which is different from other systems, there is no antagonistic innervation between the sympathetic and parasympathetic fibers. Control of vasomotor tonus depends only on the sympathetic vasoconstrictor fibers; thus, vasoconstriction results from an increase in sympathetic activity and vasodilatation from a decrease in sympathetic activity.

The autonomic nervous system has a considerable influence on vessels, with greater development of the smooth muscle layer of the vessel wall in relation to its caliber. Hence, arterioles are most affected by sympathetic activity. Consequently, the autonomic nervous system has a great influence on skin circulation and is of little importance in the great vessels and muscular arteries.

Autocrine sweat glands are innervated by the nonmyelinic C fibers of the sympathetic nerves, and acetylcholine is the chemical mediator. Local or systemic administration of cholinergic agents induces sweating, whereas the use of atropine blocks sweating. Although sweating in the palmar and plantar regions may result from emotional stimuli, and abundant sweating is observed under clinical conditions in which catecholamines are released by the adrenal glands, administration of adrenergic agents through any route does not produce stimulation of the sweat glands.[15] Blocking preganglionic fibers does not stop sweating caused by stimulation of the postganglionic fibers, nor does the local administration of cholinergic agents. However, if the postganglionic fibers are cut, such secretion will no longer occur through local stimulation by any pharmacologic agent. This is an exception to Cannon's law ("When one unit in a series of efferent neurons is destroyed, increased irritability to chemical agents is developed in the structure that has been isolated and the effect is greater in the part that is directly denervated"). Heating of the skin may cause sweating in this situation through an unknown mechanism.

Different neural centers control the various types of apocrine sweat glands in a reflex manner. Thus, emotional sweating is controlled by a cortical center, thermal sweating by a hypothalamic center, gustatory sweating by medullary nuclei, and spinal sweating by cells of the intermediate-lateral region of the spinal cord.

The nerve centers and pathways that control emotion-induced sweating are not fully known, although it seems that they are located in the frontal lobes. Emotion-induced stimuli can increase sweating, especially in the palmar and plantar regions.

Under baseline conditions, few impulses pass to the sweat glands, and nonsensory sweating (perspiration) is always present, partly because of the activity of the glands and partly because of loss of water through the epidermis.

■ INDICATIONS FOR CERVICODORSAL SYMPATHECTOMY

The current indications for cervicodorsal sympathectomy are limited to essential HH and selected cases of critical ischemia of the hand, complex regional pain syndrome (CRPS),[19] long QT syndrome refractory to clinical treatment,[20] and Raynaud's syndrome.[21]

Idiopathic Hyperhidrosis

Essential or idiopathic HH is the production of excessive quantities of sweat beyond what is required for the organism's thermoregulatory needs. The causal mechanism is not exactly known, but it is accepted that it is a result of stimulation of the sympathetic nervous system at the central level rather than being due to exercise or heat.[22]

HH is most typically limited to the palms, soles, or axillae in a symmetric manner. It may also affect the craniofacial segment. HH may arise during childhood, but it is more intense during adolescence, a transitional period of life in which the great psychological stress associated with hormonal and sexual maturation triggers or worsens conditions that are associated with a *psychosomatic component*, such as HH. This condition may persist into adulthood, but it decreases in intensity in some patients.[22] HH affects approximately 3% of the population, and in 13% to 57% of patients it can be associated with a family history of HH.[23] Climate is not an etiologic factor, but hot weather exacerbates sweating.[24]

Palmar HH generally takes on greater clinical significance than plantar or axillary HH because it creates significant problems within the educational, social, professional, and affective spheres that can worsen any emotional issues that such patients may already have. These individuals moisten everything that they touch, which makes writing, reading, and school activities difficult. From a social and affective point of view, these patients withdraw from the world by avoiding handshakes, parties, dances, and dating. They tend to be almost constantly holding a cloth so that they can dry their hands.[25]

Professionally, palmar HH may incapacitate such individuals from working in various activities. Thus, industrial workers with this condition who handle metals have been labeled "rust makers" because of the corrosive action of their sweat.[26] Other activities may become dangerous under these circumstances, such as situations in which patients handle electrical and electronic equipment.

Plantar HH is frequently associated with palmar or axillary HH and is worsened by the use of closed shoes, which hinder evaporation and favor skin maceration. The constant dampness provides conditions for fungal or bacterial infection, thereby causing a bad smell, not only on the feet but also from socks and shoes.[27]

Axillary HH tends to appear at puberty with the increased production of sexual hormones. This causes social embarrassment to patients because the sweat runs down the body and dampens and damages their clothes. These patients avoid wearing colored clothes and sometimes use rolls of paper or even sanitary pads in their axillae. The symptoms of axillary HH are disabling both professionally and socially for almost all patients who seek surgical treatment.[28] Likewise, craniofacial HH and facial rubor may cause social phobia.[29]

Nonsurgical treatment may be attempted in cases of moderate HH. However, it requires constant adherence by the patient because its results are temporary or have little effect. In cases of severe HH, only surgical treatment will provide results that are more consistent and long lasting.[30]

Ischemia of the Hand

Selected patients with hand ischemia, particularly those with TAO and distal arterial obstructions, ulcers in the fingers, or ischemic pain, may benefit from sympathectomy.[31]

TAO, also known as Buerger's disease, is an obliterative disease characterized by inflammatory changes in the small and medium-sized arteries and veins (see Chapter 77: Thromboangiitis Obliterans). The lower limbs are more frequently affected, but the upper limbs can also be compromised. TAO usually occurs in young men (between 20 and 40 years of age) who smoke cigarettes. The cause is unknown, but it has not been documented in nonsmokers, thus implicating cigarette smoking as a primary etiologic factor.[32] Occlusions start in the distal vessels of the extremities, progress proximally, and culminate in distal gangrene. Frequently, sympathetic overactivity is observed (coldness, excessive sweating, and cyanosis), probably caused by persistent and severe pain.[33]

Clinical treatment consists of the patient's giving up smoking and avoiding vasoconstriction from exposure to cold or drugs, together with supportive care directed toward controlling pain with the use of analgesics. Bypass grafts are seldom helpful because TAO rarely affects large vessels.

For selected cases of critical ischemia of the hands, cervicodorsal sympathectomy has been used to improve cutaneous vasodilatation, control ischemic rest and vasomotor phenomena, and assist in healing of the skin if patients do not respond to conservative management.[34] However, there is no randomized comparison with other treatments, and because the disease can be improved by smoking cessation, it is difficult to judge the benefit of sympathectomy in published studies.

Complex Regional Pain Syndrome

CRPS, also known as causalgia, reflex sympathetic dystrophy, post-traumatic pain syndrome, shoulder-hand syndrome, and Sudeck's atrophy, is a term that has been used since 1994. It describes a regional pain condition that often occurs after injury, is disproportionate to the inciting event, and is associated with signs of vasomotor dysfunction and sudomotor activity. It often results in impairment of motor function.[35] CRPS is categorized into two subtypes, type I (formerly reflex sympathetic dystrophy) and type II (formerly causalgia) (see Chapter 161: Complex Regional Pain Syndrome).

When CRPS is left untreated, hyperalgesia, allodynia, signs of vasomotor dysfunction, and edema can be seen initially. After 3 to 6 months there is increased pain, and sensory dysfunction and motor or trophic changes (or both) develop (dystrophic stage). Finally, the pain decreases but there are still sensory disturbances (atrophic stage).[36,37]

Treatment includes physical therapy (indispensable), psychotherapy, pharmacologic therapy, and surgical therapy. The key to success is starting treatment in the early stages of the disease process.[38] Pharmacologic therapy includes anti-inflammatory agents, corticosteroids, anticonvulsants, antidepressants, sympatholytic drugs, and other drugs used to treat any type of neuropathic pain. Opioid analgesics are helpful occasionally, but their use remains controversial.

Sympathetic blockade with local anesthetic has been used to control pain in selected patients. If it is effective, this technique can be repeated, together with physical therapy to recover functionality of the limb.[39] Peridural or intrathecal infusions of anesthetic drugs can be used in selected patients who do not respond to conservative treatment. Because of proximity to receptor sites, the therapeutic effect of intrathecal drug application lasts longer and the rate of systemic side effects is reduced. However, there are catheter-related technical problems such as catheter dislocation, obstruction, kinking, and disconnection or rupture, as well as drug-related side effects.[40]

Spinal cord stimulation is efficacious in CRPS type I (level B recommendation) that is resistant to medication or other treatments. High-frequency transcutaneous electrical nerve stimulation and repetitive transcranial magnetic stimulation are noninvasive and suitable as preliminary or add-on therapies and provide satisfactory pain relief to many patients, including those resistant to medication or other therapies.[41]

Chemical sympathectomy with phenol or alcohol seems to have at best a temporary effect limited to cutaneous allodynia. Because studies reported in the literature have only a few patients and poorly defined outcomes, well-designed studies on the effectiveness of the procedure are needed.[42]

Sympathectomy can be used in selected patients who do not respond to nonsurgical treatment or in those who have good but transient benefit from pharmacologic sympathetic blockade (see Chapter 161: Complex Regional Pain Syndrome).

Long QT Syndrome

Long QT syndrome is an idiopathic congenital disorder characterized by a lengthened QT interval on electrocardiograms and associated with a high incidence of severe tachyarrhythmia, syncope, and sudden death. The young age of most of these patients and the high morbidity and mortality in untreated individuals have led to a search for effective therapies.

There is no clinical or radiologic evidence of heart disease. Severe episodes typically occur during intense physical exercise or emotional crises, which has led to the supposition that the sympathetic nervous system plays an active part in the genesis of the problem. The mortality rate in untreated patients reaches as high as 78%. Beta blockers are effective in preventing such crises in 75% to 80% of cases.[43]

Sympathectomy is only potentially indicated in patients who even with appropriate clinical treatment continue to have syncopal crises (about 20% to 25% of patients).

Raynaud's Syndrome

Raynaud's disease and phenomenon are characterized by episodic spasm of arterioles, usually in the digits, which demonstrate intermittent pallor or cyanosis, and are precipitated by exposure to cold, emotional upset, or drugs. Raynaud's disease, most common in young women, is idiopathic. Raynaud's phenomenon is secondary to other conditions such as connective tissue disorders, blood diseases, neurologic disorders, obstructive arterial diseases, trauma, drug intoxication (ergot), dysproteinemias, and primary pulmonary hypertension (see Chapter 119: Raynaud's Syndrome).

During the crisis patients may complain of pain, hypothermia, numbness, and paresthesias in the affected fingers. When these episodes are frequent and intense, they may cause obstruction of arteries in the fingers and palms that subsequently results in ischemic lesions in the fingers, which are very painful and resistant to healing.

Treatment of Raynaud's syndrome is essentially clinical. Sympathectomy has been used in rare patients who despite adequate clinical treatment continue to have severe symptoms or trophic lesions that heal with difficulty. However, it is difficult to judge the benefit of such sympathectomy because randomized trials have not been performed and the natural history is variable.

■ SURGICAL TECHNIQUE

Open Surgery

Until the 1990s and before VATS, open surgery was the "gold standard" for cervicodorsal sympathectomy. Several approaches are available for open surgery, each with its own advantages and disadvantages. There are three main accesses, the paravertebral, transthoracic, and supraclavicular routes. Nowadays, the open technique is indicated only when VATS cannot be accomplished because of technical reasons or an associated open operation is being performed.

The paravertebral route, mainly used by neurosurgeons, offers wide exposure of the sympathetic chain; however, it involves extensive dissection and sectioning of several muscular bunches and requires a long period for recovery.[44]

The transthoracic axillary approach has the advantages of superior exposure, easier access to the sympathetic chain for wide incisions, lower risk for Horner's syndrome, and good cosmetic results. The main complication is postsympathetic neuralgia, which lasts long and extends the recovery time.[45]

The supraclavicular approach requires extrapleural access and thus allows the operation to be accomplished bilaterally in a single operation. The resulting scar becomes practically invisible in a short period, convalescence is fast with little pain, the hospital stay is short, and surgical complication rates are low. The disadvantage is that the stellate ganglion is the point of reference for identifying the sympathetic chain and simple manipulation can result in Horner's syndrome, although in most cases it is transitory.[46]

Video-Assisted Thoracic Sympathectomy

At present, VATS is considered the gold standard for cervicothoracic sympathectomy. Several approaches (two ports, three ports, four ports, lateral, dorsal, etc.) are available, each with its own advantages and disadvantages.[47] An easy and practical technique (two ports) is described in the following paragraphs.

Instrumentation

The basic equipment includes a 15-degree angled thoracoscope, a video camera with monitor and DVD recorder, a light source, video endoscopic instruments, electrocautery (harmonic or not), and a nerve hook and vascular clips.

Anesthesia

The patient usually undergoes double-lumen endotracheal general anesthesia, which makes it possible to stop the patient's ventilation and consequently collapse the lung on the side that will undergo surgery. When necessary, bronchoscopy is used to verify tube positioning. Selective intubation is used in patients undergoing resection of the fourth ganglion of the thoracic sympathetic chain. When thermoablation is performed on the second or third ganglion, a simple lumen tube may be used in conjunction with adequate control over lung ventilation.

Long-acting anesthetic agents are avoided to allow immediate extubation at the end of the procedure.

Positioning

The patient is placed in a dorsal decubitus, semi-seated position with the trunk raised approximately 45 degrees. Two small pads are placed under the shoulders to create a space between the axillae and the surgical table and to bring the shoulders forward, thereby avoiding distention of the brachial plexus when the arms are positioned in 90 degrees of abduction on the arm rests. Another pad under the knees and a securing strap at the hip level allow the legs to be positioned comfortably and impede patient movement on the surgical table when it is rotated laterally to bring the sites for surgery forward (right or left) (Fig. 121-2).

Technique

In cases of HH, which represents more than 95% of cases and in which only thermoablation of the third or fourth sympathetic ganglia is performed, two mini-incisions about 1 cm in length are made. The first of the incisions is made on the anterior axillary line at the level of the fourth or fifth intercostal space to introduce a video camera. The second incision at the second or third intercostal space on the medial axillary line is used to introduce the surgical instruments—electric or ultrasonic bistoury, scissors, dissecting forceps, retractable hook, and aspirator—into the pleural cavity (Fig. 121-3). In

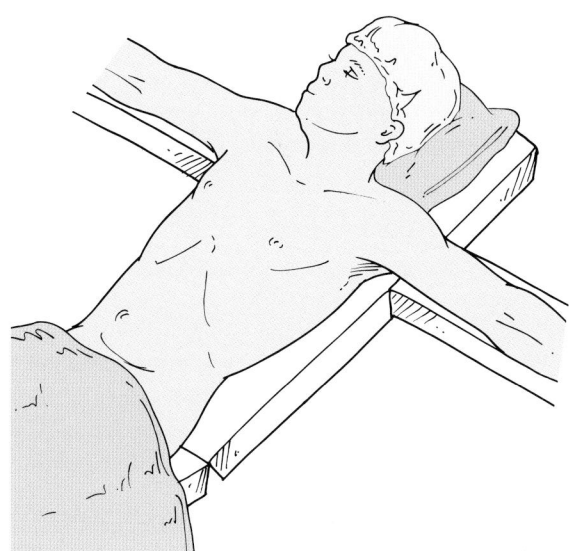

Figure 121-2 Patient in a dorsal decubitus, semi-seated position. The trunk is raised approximately 45 degrees and both arms are abducted.

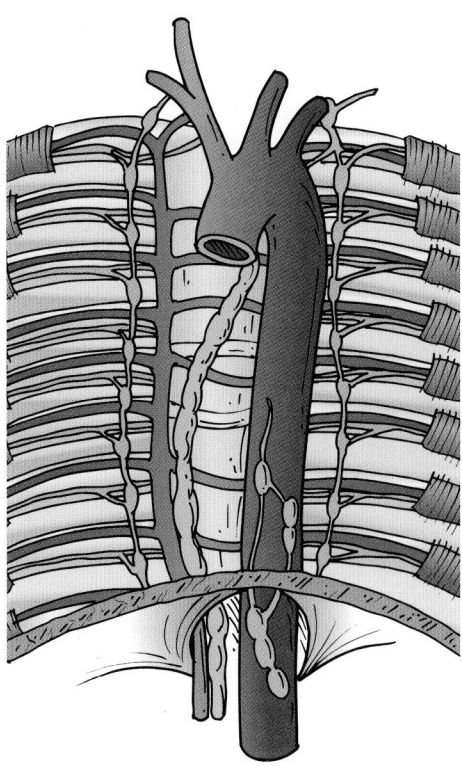

Figure 121-4 Sympathetic chain coursing above the heads of the costal arches. The stellate ganglion is located anterior to the head of the first rib, the T2 ganglion is between the second and third ribs, the T3 ganglion is between the third and fourth ribs, and the T4 ganglion is between the fourth and fifth ribs.

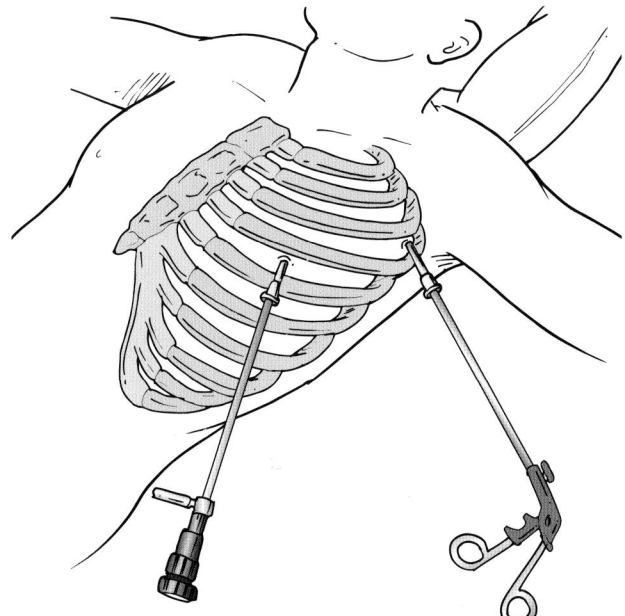

Figure 121-3 Port placement: one in the fourth or fifth intercostal space on the anterior axillary line, and one in the medial axillary line in the second or third intercostal space.

cases in which the stellate ganglion has to be resected, to facilitate the dissection, a third mini-incision is made a little anteriorly in the posterior axillary line, a few millimeters lateral to the hemiclavicular line.

Trocars 5.5 mm in diameter are introduced into all the incisions to keep the pathway open and protect the structures of the thoracic wall. Carbon dioxide insufflation into the pleural cavity has been used in some centers to improve surgical access. However, this procedure is not free of risk, and it may cause cardiovascular problems, even when used at low pressure.[48] To avoid these complications, we have preferred

using open pneumothorax, which has proved to be sufficiently satisfactory.

Once the video camera has been installed into the pleural space, the other instruments are always introduced under direct view to provide greater safety for the patient. The sympathetic chain is identified through the parietal pleura as a whitish, longitudinal, multinodular cord that forms a slight prominence in the lateroposterior region of the thoracic vertebrae, above the heads of the costal arches (Fig. 121-4). In elderly patients or in individuals with a greater degree of fatty tissue, the sympathetic chain sometimes becomes difficult to distinguish. In such cases, the chain is identified by touch with the endosurgical instruments (Fig. 121-5). The parietal pleura is sectioned above the chain and is also dissected by blunt separation. The communicating branches are coagulated and sectioned to the extent desired (Fig. 121-6). The chain is then sectioned above the costal arches, and the segment isolated is cauterized (Fig. 121-7). Application of vascular clips to the main sympathetic trunk instead of thermoablation is an alternative.

After achieving hemostasis, a 14 or 16 Fr aspiration probe is placed through the upper trocar and connected to a negative pressure aspirator. The anesthetist is then asked to ventilate the collapsed lung until complete expansion has been achieved. This can be verified by direct viewing on the video monitor. The video camera and the aspirating probe are then

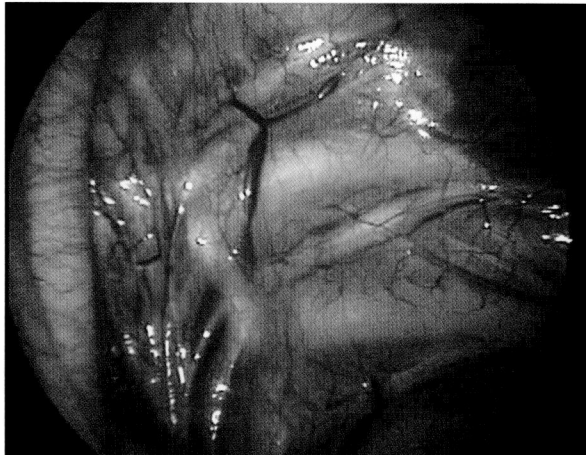

Figure 121-5 Thoracoscopic normal anatomy of the sympathetic chain.

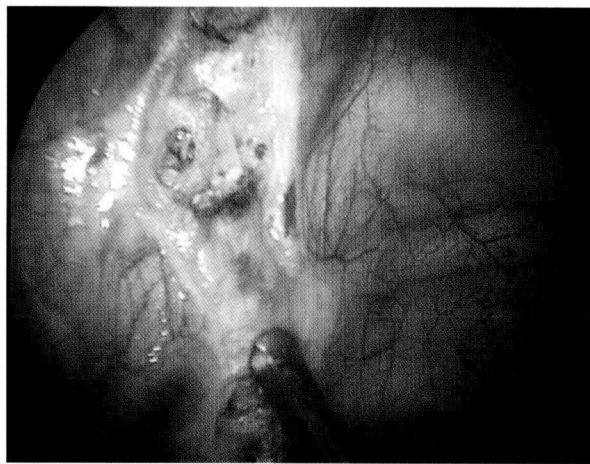

Figure 121-6 Sympathetic chain sectioned above and below the ganglia.

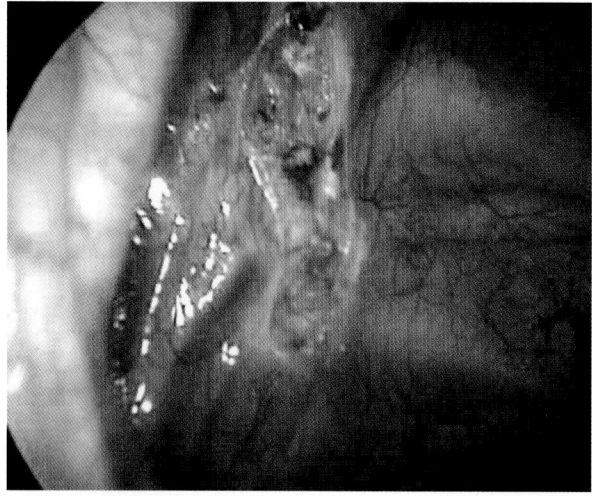

Figure 121-7 Sympathetic chain cauterized.

removed, and the corresponding incision is sutured. Occlusive bandages are left on the surgical incisions for 24 hours.

In the postanesthesia recovery room, chest radiography is requested to observe the expandability of the lung and check for the possible presence of residual pneumothorax.

Technical Difficulties

Pleural adhesions are found fairly frequently during endoscopic operations (3% to 5%). When they are weak, it is easy to release them; however, firm and extensive pleural adhesions caused by previous pleuropulmonary diseases, which are found in a few patients, may make it impossible to perform VATS. In these cases, open surgery is the best option. Unfortunately, such adhesions cannot be diagnosed preoperatively by routine chest radiography.[49]

The presence of an azygos lobe is an infrequent anatomic variation that makes it difficult or sometimes impossible to carry out VATS.[50] Preoperative chest radiography may identify this anomaly.

Technical Alternatives

Alternatives to ganglia resection in cases of HH are the application of vascular clips to the main sympathetic trunk and transection of the main sympathetic trunk (sympathectomy). In both techniques, transmission of sympathetic impulses from the lower sympathetic ganglia through the stellate ganglia to the limbs is interrupted.

Sympathectomy and thoracoscopic clipping are acceptable methods. The early results are comparable to sympathectomy, but the long-term results are unknown. Sympathectomy is a good alternative when the anatomy is not appropriate for sympathectomy (large veins over the sympathetic chain).[51] Clipping the trunk has the potential benefit of unclipping (reverse operation) in case of intolerable compensatory HH.[52,53] Large-scale prospective studies with long-term follow-up are needed in both techniques.

Contraindications

Contraindications to VATS are lung infections that evolve with pleural effusion and require puncture or drainage, lung diseases that cause dense pleural adhesions such as tuberculosis, previous thoracic surgery, thoracic radiotherapy, sinus bradycardia, and clinical conditions in which endotracheal anesthesia is contraindicated.[54] Obesity has also been considered a contraindication to VATS; even though overweight patients have a high degree of satisfaction with the operation, it may be difficult to identify the sympathetic chain when it is covered by a greater layer of adipose tissue. In addition, such patients have a higher risk for severe compensatory HH.[55]

Complications (Box 121-1)

Pneumothorax. The most common perioperative complication is pneumothorax. Most patients (75%) have some

Box 121-1 Complications Associated with Thoracoscopic Sympathectomy

COMMON
- Compensatory sweating (70% to 100%)
- Segmental atelectasis (1% to 5%)
- Pneumothorax (1% to 5%)
- Subcutaneous emphysema (1% to 2%)

RARE (<1% OF CASES)
- Horner's syndrome
- Hemothorax
- Pleural effusions
- Injury to the vagus nerve
- Injury to the phrenic nerve
- Injury to the subclavian artery and vein

residual gas in the thorax at the end of surgery; however, thoracic drainage is necessary in only a small number of these patients (0.4% to 2.3%).[56] Tension pneumothorax after surgery is rare. It results from direct injury to the lung at the time of trocar insertion or from tearing of an apical adhesion when the lung is depressed.

Apical bullae may occasionally be found, and they may rupture during anesthesia when high pulmonary insufflation pressure is used at completion of the surgical procedure. This complication can be prevented by careful reinsufflation at the end of the operation. It is important to carry out chest radiography during the immediate postoperative period to rule out the possibility of significant pneumothorax because in this situation pleural drainage has to be performed, usually for 24 hours.[57] Subcutaneous emphysema around the trocar insertion site confined to thoracic wall may occur in 2% to 7% of patients.[58] Treatment is conservative if not associated with pneumothorax.

Hemorrhage. Significant intraoperative hemorrhage is rare and mostly originates from intercostal vein disruption during dissection of the sympathetic chain. It may also occur at the trocar insertion site. Laceration of the subclavian artery and intercostal artery pseudoaneurysm requiring thoracotomy have been reported.[59]

Chylothorax. Chylothorax is an extremely rare complication resulting from laceration of the accessory thoracic duct.[60]

Cardiac. Transitory bradycardia during sympathectomy occurs in another 1.2% of patients,[61] but recovery takes place after a few minutes of clinical observation. Extensive thoracic sympathectomy may have a beta-blocker effect leading to a moderate decrease in heart rate at rest and during maximum exercise.[62] Intraoperative cardiac arrest was reported in only two patients during the surgical procedure, but they were both successfully resuscitated.[63] Caution is necessary in patients with already present or previous bradycardia. There are no reports in the literature of deaths caused by VATS.

Neurologic. Severe postoperative pain is a common event. Most patients report acute pain, especially when breathing in deeply, for some hours after the operation, but a significant number complain of pain of lower intensity that is more constant in the dorsal region, which may occasionally require analgesics for weeks.[64]

Paresis and paresthesia in the upper limbs occurred in 2.9% of patients as a result of tension on the brachial plexus caused by their position on the surgical table.[65] In most patients these manifestations regressed within 3 days to 3 weeks. Some authors have reported neuralgia in the medial region of the arm, which usually disappears after 6 weeks.[66]

Horner's syndrome is a side effect from complete sympathetic denervation of the upper limb when the stellate, T2, and T3 ganglia are resected.[50] However, in cases of HH, in which only T3 or T4 is manipulated nowadays, this complication is considered rare. It results from direct or indirect injury to the stellate ganglion, from transmission of heat when performing T2 thermoablation with an electric bistoury, or from excessive traction on the sympathetic chain during dissection or thermoablation.

Causes of Failure

Incomplete Denervation. Late activation of the intermediate ganglia (microscopic aggregates of ganglion cells distributed in the communicating branches or even in the anterior roots of the cervical and brachial spinal nerves) could explain failure of sympathetic denervation of the upper limbs.[13]

Regeneration. There is no evidence of regeneration of the sympathetic ganglion cells. However, if only the axis cylinder is sectioned, regeneration of new fibers from the ganglion cell may occur. This may have a negligible effect in operations in which the paravertebral ganglia are removed.[46]

Functional Reorganization (Collateral Nerve Sprouting). Degenerated fibers produce humoral substances that stimulate close intact nerves to establish connections with denervated ganglion cells.[67] Hence, cutting only the preganglionic fibers responsible for innervation of the upper limbs (the fibers that pass by the stellate ganglion on their pathway to the superior cervical ganglion) would give rise to favorable conditions in the stellate ganglion for sprouting.[68] Furthermore, there may be a functional connection between these branches and the ganglion cells present in the spinal nerves, which would explain the return of sympathetic activity in the limb.

TARGET GANGLIA

The extent of thermoablation, resection, or interruption of the sympathetic chain is a very important subject (Table 121-1). With improvements in surgical techniques for treating HH, therapeutic success has been achieved even when sympathectomy is performed at levels distant from the stellate

Table 121-1 Denervation Levels for Different Indications

Disease	Denervation Level
Palmar hyperhidrosis	T4 or T3
Axillary hyperhidrosis	T4
Craniofacial hyperhidrosis	T2
Facial rubor	T2
Complex regional pain syndrome	Stellate ganglion, T2, and T3
Vascular disease	Stellate ganglion, T2, and T3
Raynaud's syndrome	Stellate ganglion, T2, and T3
Long QT syndrome	Left side, from the stellate ganglion to T4 or T5

ganglion (T3 and T4 ganglia). This has corresponded to a significant reduction in the complications that were most feared before the advent of VATS: Horner's syndrome and compensatory HH.

Palmar Hyperhidrosis

In cases of palmar HH, physicians initially used to resect the T2 and T3 ganglia with good results (anhidrosis); however, it was a difficult procedure associated with a high incidence of Horner's syndrome and severe compensatory HH.[69] Subsequently, based on the principle that interruption of the transmission of sympathetic impulses from the lower sympathetic ganglia through the stellate ganglia resolves HH, thermoablation of T2 accelerated this procedure and gave similar results.[70] However, intervention on the T2 ganglion resulted in a high rate of compensatory HH (>75% of cases) because a very extensive area is denervated, including the cephalic, cervical, and upper limb segments. This collateral effect has been responsible for dissatisfaction in 4% of patients.[71] To minimize this problem, thermoablation of T2 was initially replaced by thermoablation of T3 and currently T4, which has led to similar results of palmar anhidrosis but considerably decreased compensatory HH.[72] This is probably due to preservation of sympathetic tonus in the cephalic segment.

Patients who undergo T3 ablation usually have totally dry hands and need to use skin moisturizers, whereas patients who undergo T4 ablation have continued low levels of sweating (not HH but a little greater than normal physiologic levels), which is considered to be a therapeutic success.[73]

Other alternatives are sympathicotomy[74] (without the removal of ganglia) and blockade by endoscopic clipping,[75] a technique that can eventually be reversed by removal of the clips.[76]

Axillary Hyperhidrosis

Resection of the second to fourth ganglia of the thoracic sympathetic chain was the first step in treating axillary HH.[77] It was replaced by thermoablation of T3 and T4[78] and currently by single T4 thermoablation,[79] which results in excellent therapeutic success (anhidrosis), less severe compensatory HH, and a higher rate of satisfaction.

Other alternatives are sympathicotomy[80] and blockade by endoscopic clipping.[57,72]

Craniofacial Hyperhidrosis or Facial Rubor

Sympathetic denervation of the face and head can be obtained by thermoablation of the T2 ganglion.[81] Sympathetic blockade of T3 with clips is an alternative for these patients.[82]

Complex Regional Pain Syndrome, Vascular Disease, and Raynaud's Syndrome

Sympathetic denervation of the upper limb needs to be as complete as possible if sympathectomy is used for these conditions; hence, the stellate ganglion, T2, and T3 should be included.[50,65]

To avoid incomplete denervation of the limb, the communicating branches of T1 and Kuntz's nerve have to be ablated as well.[83] This approach is always associated with the presence of Horner's syndrome.

Long QT Syndrome

Sympathectomy is performed only on the left side, from the stellate ganglion to T4 or T5.[84]

RESULTS

Hyperhidrosis

The results of VATS in patients with HH have been uniformly very good. The immediate postoperative period is uneventful in almost 95% of patients, which permits these individuals to be discharged on the following or the same day.

The success rate in abolition of HH (i.e., anhidrosis) is very high and ranges from 96% to 100% for palmar HH,[85,86] 63% to 100% for axillary HH,[87,88] and 87% to 100% for craniofacial HH.[89]

In addition to traditional outcome data (anhidrosis and subjective satisfaction), quality of life analyses are also being used in the evaluation of patients with HH. The objective satisfaction rate combines the overall result with the adverse effects, thus resulting in lower rates of "overall satisfaction" of around 85%.[90]

Though nonspecific for treating the plantar HH that is usually associated with palmar or axillary HH, VATS was shown to immediately reduce plantar sweating in more than 80% of patients; however, there is a reduction to smaller degrees of improvement (60%) over a 1-year period after surgery.[91] There is no convincing anatomic-physiologic explanation for this improvement. Perhaps correction of palmar HH by the intervention leads to greater emotional equilibrium, thereby lowering sympathetic nervous stimuli to the feet.

Recurrence of palmar or axillary HH has been reported in 1% to 13% of operated patients[67] and in 2% of patients with craniofacial HH.[87] The main cause of the recurrence is technical failure. Reoperation is usually successful. Weak adhesions are found in these situations, but they do not cause significant difficulties for the procedure.

Transitory occurrence of sweating of variable intensity in the denervated segment during the first postoperative week (third to fifth postoperative days) is observed in 13% of cases. It lasts for a maximum of 36 hours and is caused by the release of neurotransmitter at the end of the sympathetic postganglionic fibers as they degenerate.[92]

One adverse effect from sympathectomy is gustatory sweating. It is unrelated to the level of sympathetic chain blockade, its incidence is variable (ranging from 6% to 32%), and it is probably related to eating habits in different regions. In most cases it is of light to moderate intensity and does not interfere with quality of life.[93]

Compensatory HH consists of an increase in the severity of sweating in locations that were previously normal. This is the most frequent and most feared side effect of thoracic sympathectomy. Reported rates of compensatory HH are higher than 75%, and when severe, it is considered the main cause of patient dissatisfaction.[94] It occurs mainly on the abdomen, back, and thighs, and it becomes more uncomfortable on hot days, during physical exercise, and in hot work environments.[95] It may diminish over time, or the patient may learn to live with it. Compensatory HH may also affect the feet, although this is infrequent.[27]

Compensatory HH has a high correlation with the level and extent of resection.[96] The higher the interruption or resection of the sympathetic chain, the more the afferent fibers responsible for inhibition of sweating would be harmed, thereby causing a considerable increase in the quantity and intensity of compensatory HH. By performing thermoablation of only the T4 ganglia for palmar or axillary HH, there is a significant decrease in the quantity and intensity of compensatory HH,[62] which leads to an improvement in quality of life. Another risk factor for compensatory HH is a high body mass index.

The rate of compensatory HH and its severity are tolerated better by children, and their postoperative satisfaction is higher than that of adolescents and adults. Therefore, VATS is indicated in children as early as possible.[97]

Because of the importance of compensatory HH, it is necessary to alert all patients with HH to this risk before they choose sympathetic denervation or an alternative technique.

Vascular Diseases

Sympathectomy is seldom used at present to treat vascular insufficiency because of the availability of bypass and interventional procedures. When used, it is performed for digital and palmar obstructions associated with necrotic lesions of the fingers.[98] In selected patients, sympathectomy has been reported to decrease pain and assist in clinical treatment.[99,100]

Complex Regional Pain Syndrome

VATS is highly effective in reversing symptoms when performed early in the evolution of CRPS, at which time it has a success rate of 80% to 90%. However, sympathectomy is ineffective if delayed until joint contracture or nerve atrophy has occurred.[101]

Long QT Syndrome

Favorable results from left thoracic sympathectomy in high-risk patients (preventing complications) have been demonstrated in the literature since the 1970s. VATS is associated with a significant reduction in the incidence of aborted cardiac arrest and syncope in high-risk patients with long QT syndrome when compared with pre-left cardiac sympathetic denervation events, but changes in the QT interval after sympathectomy are variable and the clinical results cannot be fully predicted.[102] In a group of high-risk patients undergoing left cardiac sympathetic denervation, 46% remained asymptomatic; syncope occurred in 31%, aborted cardiac arrest in 16%, and sudden death in 7%.[44]

Raynaud's Syndrome

The results of sympathetic denervation in cases of Raynaud's syndrome (disease and phenomenon) in the upper limbs are transitory.[103] Vasospastic episodes reappear within a short time, and dissatisfaction with the procedure is observed in almost 50% of patients, especially because of the appearance of compensatory HH in more than 60% of cases.[104] This has led most authors to no longer recommend cervicothoracic sympathectomy for such patients.[105]

SELECTED KEY REFERENCES

de Campos JR, Kauffman P, Werebe Ede C, Andrade Filho LO, Kusniek S, Wolosker N, Jatene FB. Quality of life, before and after thoracic sympathectomy: report on 378 operated patients. *Ann Thorac Surg.* 2003;76:886.
The authors analyzed the results and complications of thoracic sympathectomy and proposed a questionnaire to assess the quality of life of patients.

Krasna MJ. Thoracoscopic sympathectomy: a standardized approach to therapy for hyperhidrosis. *Ann Thorac Surg.* 2008;85:S764.
This article presents a complete review of existing approaches and techniques, as well as the author's summary and preferences for thoracoscopic sympathectomy.

Kwong KF, Hobbs JL, Cooper LB, Burrows W, Gamliel Z, Krasna MJ. Stratified analysis of clinical outcomes in thoracoscopic sympathicotomy for hyperhidrosis. *Ann Thorac Surg.* 2008;85:390, discussion 393.
The authors identified clinical variables associated with successful surgical treatment of hyperhidrosis and facial blushing in a group of 608 patients who underwent thoracoscopic sympathicotomy.

Libson S, Kirshtein B, Mizrahi S, Lantsberg L. Evaluation of compensatory sweating after bilateral thoracoscopic sympathectomy for palmar hyperhidrosis. *Surg Laparosc Endosc Percutan Tech.* 2007;17:511.
The authors evaluated the compensatory sweating after bilateral thoracoscopic sympathectomy for palmar hyperhidrosis.

Lin CC, Wu HH. Endoscopic T4-sympathetic block by clamping (ESB4) in treatment of hyperhidrosis palmaris et axillaries: experiences of 165 cases. *Ann Chir Gynaecol.* 2001;90:167.
This article was the first to study T4 sympathetic blockade in patients with palmar and/or axillary hyperhidrosis by clamping (ESB4) in the treatment of 165 patients.

Lin TS, Wang NP, Huang LC. Pitfalls and complication avoidance associated with transthoracic endoscopic sympathectomy for primary hyperhidrosis (analysis of 2200 cases). *Int J Surg Invest.* 2001;2:377.
The authors present their experience (2200 patients who underwent thoracic sympathectomy) in treating palmar and axillary hyperhidrosis and discuss methods for resolving potential problems during and after transthoracic endoscopic sympathectomy.

Munia MA, Wolosker N, Kauffman P, de Campos JR, Puech-Leão P. A randomized trial of T3-T4 versus T4 sympathectomy for isolated axillary hyperhidrosis. *J Vasc Surg.* 2007;45:130.
The authors compared the initial results of sympathectomy using two distinct levels for treating axillary sudoresis—T3-T4 versus T4—in a prospective and randomized manner.

Strutton DR, Kowalski JW, Glaser DA, Stang PE. US prevalence of hyperhidrosis and impact on individuals with axillary hyperhidrosis: results from a national survey. *J Am Acad Dermatol.* 2004;51:241.
This is the first article estimating the prevalence of hyperhidrosis in the U.S. population and assessing the impact of sweating on those affected by axillary hyperhidrosis.

Wolosker N, Yazbek G, Ishy A, de Campos JR, Kauffman P, Puech-Leão P. Is sympathectomy at T4 level better than at T3 level for treating palmarpalmar hyperhidrosis? *J Laparoendosc Adv Surg Tech A.* 2008; 18:102.
The authors compared the results of VATS at the T4 denervation level with those from VATS at the T3 level for the treatment of palmar hyperhydrosis in a prospective manner.

Yoon DH, Ha Y, Park YG, Chang JW. Thoracoscopic limited T-3 sympathicotomy for primary hyperhidrosis: prevention for compensatory hyperhidrosis. *J Neurosurg.* 2003;99(1 Suppl):39.
The authors evaluate the role of limited thoracoscopic T3 sympathicotomy for primary hyperhidrosis.

REFERENCES

The reference list can be found on the companion Expert Consult Web site at *www.expertconsult.com.*

CHAPTER 122

Thoracic Outlet Syndrome: General Considerations

Richard J. Sanders

The history of thoracic outlet syndrome (TOS) began more than 250 years ago. It is summarized in Box 122-1 and can be read in full discussion in the Appendix (see the Expert Consult Web site).

DEFINITION AND CLASSIFICATION

TOS is a constellation of upper extremity symptoms and signs resulting from compression of the neurovascular bundle in thoracic outlet area. The three components of the bundle in the thoracic outlet area are the brachial plexus, subclavian vein, and subclavian artery. Thus, there are three types of TOS, depending on which structure is compressed: neurogenic (nTOS), venous (vTOS), and arterial (aTOS). Their distinct symptoms and signs are described in Table 122-1.

Box 122-1 History of Thoracic Outlet Syndrome

PERIOD I: CERVICAL RIB: 1740-1927
- Anatomic description: 1740, Hunauld[1]; 1869, Gruber[2]
- Embryology: 1912, Todd[3]; 1913, Jones[4]
- First surgical resection: 1861, Coote[5]
- Physiology of subclavian aneurysms: 1916, Halsted[6]

PERIOD II: CERVICAL RIB SYNDROME WITHOUT A CERVICAL RIB: 1907-1956
- Anomalous first rib: 1907, Keen[7]
- Initial first rib resection: 1910, Murphy[8]
- Congenital bands and ligaments: 1920, Law[9]
- Scalene anticus syndrome: 1927, Adson and Coffey[10]; 1938, Naffziger and Grant[11]
- Costoclavicular syndrome: 1939, Eden[12]
- Middle scalene muscle as a cause of symptoms: 1929, Stiles[13]
- Pectoralis minor syndrome (hyperabduction syndrome): 1945, Wright[14]

PERIOD III: MODERN ERA OF THORACIC OUTLET SYNDROME: 1956 TO PRESENT
- Name, thoracic outlet syndrome: 1956, Peet et al.[15]; 1958, Rob and Standeven[16]
- Three approaches for first rib resection:
  - 1962: Posterior—Clagett[17]
  - 1966: Transaxillary—Roos[18]
  - 1968: Infraclavicular—Gol et al.[19]
- Histochemical microscopy demonstrating scalene muscle pathology:
  - 1986: Machleder et al.[20]
  - 1990: Sanders et al.[21]

EPIDEMIOLOGY

Age and Gender

Most patients are 20 to 50 years of age. Less than 5% are teenagers, whereas 10% are older than 50 years. Seldom is any form of TOS seen in patients older than 65.

Seventy percent are female. There is no explanation for the female preponderance, but perhaps it is related to the observation that 70% of cervical ribs also occur in females.

Prevalence

TOS is uncommon, but its true incidence is unknown because many people with upper extremity pain and paresthesia have TOS that has escaped diagnosis by health care providers who may have failed to recognize it.

Incidence

We have found nTOS to be by far the most common form, accounting for more than 95% of all TOS patients. vTOS occurs in 2% to 3%, whereas aTOS is the least common, being seen in less than 1% of patients. The incidence of each type may vary depending on geography and the referral base.

PATHOGENESIS

Etiology

The most common cause of nTOS is neck trauma that involves a hyperextension neck injury. Whiplash in a motor vehicle accident is the most common injury. Other frequent causes are repetitive stress injuries in the workplace and falls on slippery floors or icy walkways.

vTOS is most often the result of developmental anomalies of the costoclavicular space and repetitive arm activities such as throwing, swimming, or working with the arms overhead for long periods.

aTOS is usually associated with a cervical or anomalous first rib or, rarely, an anomalous insertion of the anterior scalene muscle. Symptoms and signs are the result of arterial emboli arising from subclavian artery aneurysms or stenosis that resulted from the abnormal rib.

Table 122-1 Comparison of the Three Types of Thoracic Outlet Syndrome

	Neurogenic	Venous	Arterial
Incidence	95%+	3%	1%
Etiology	Neck trauma (auto accident with whiplash), RSI at work, falls on the floor or ice	Repetitive overhead shoulder movements and/or coagulopathy	Cervical rib or anomalous first rib; rarely, congenital band
Predisposing factors	Cervical rib, congenital band, scalene triangle muscle variations	Congenital narrowing of the costoclavicular space by the costoclavicular ligament or the subclavian tendon compressing the subclavian vein	Cervical rib or anomalous first rib eliminating space under the artery
Pathology	Scalene muscle fibrosis; occasionally, anomalous 1st rib or cervical rib	Subclavian vein stenosis with or without thrombosis	Subclavian artery stenosis, thrombosis or aneurysm formation with mural thrombus and emboli
Symptoms	Extremity pain, paresthesia, weakness plus neck pain and occipital headache, Raynaud's phenomenon, chest pain for pectoralis minor syndrome	Swelling of the whole arm, cyanosis, pain	Pain, paresthesia, pallor, coldness; digital ischemia; arm claudication; seldom are there neck or shoulder symptoms
Physical examination	Positive response to provocative maneuvers; tenderness over the scalenes, pectoralis minor	Arm swelling, cyanosis, pain	Those with arterial occlusion: decreased pulses at rest, perhaps color changes and ischemic fingertips, distal emboli
Diagnostic tests	EMG/NCV, MAC measurement,[22] scalene muscle block; MRI to rule out other conditions; pectoralis minor block	Venogram (best), duplex scan	Neck radiograph, duplex scan, arteriogram, digital pressures and waveforms, arteriography
Nonsurgical treatment	Physical therapy	Fibrinolysis, anticoagulants	None; surgery is the only Rx
Surgical treatment	Scalenectomy with or without rib resection or transaxillary 1st rib resection (see Chapter 123: Thoracic Outlet Syndrome: Neurogenic), pectoralis minor tenotomy	1st rib resection and subclavian vein venolysis plus postoperative PTA if necessary or endovenectomy with vein patch. See Chapter 125 (Thoracic Outlet Syndrome: Venous)	Embolectomy, thrombectomy, artery/aneurysm resection, grafting. See Chapter 124 (Thoracic Outlet Syndrome: Arterial)

EMG, electromyography; NCV, nerve conduction velocity; MAC, medial antebrachial cutaneous nerve; MRI, magnetic resonance imaging; PTA, percutaneous transluminal angioplasty; RSI, repetitive strain injury; Rx, treatment.

Predisposing Factors

These syndromes result from a combination of developmental anomalies in the thoracic outlet and physical activities and life events that predispose individuals to become symptomatic. In nTOS, predisposing factors include scalene muscle anomalies, narrow scalene triangles, congenital ligaments or bands, roots of the plexus arising high near the apex of the scalene triangle, and cervical ribs. A common initiating event is neck trauma, which causes symptoms in patients with developmental anomalies of the thoracic outlet. All patients with cervical ribs are predisposed to the development of some form of TOS, most commonly nTOS. In such patients, neck trauma may precipitate symptoms, but in some patients with no history of trauma, the rib and arm activities of daily living can cause nTOS.

In vTOS, the predisposition is the relationship of the subclavian vein to the subclavius tendon and costoclavicular ligament and dimensions of the costoclavicular space. In most patients with vTOS, the subclavian vein lies tightly against the costoclavicular ligament, and the subclavius tendon is compressing the top of the vein within a narrowed costoclavicular space. With the vein in this compressed position, repetitive arm movements can easily traumatize the vein and produce fibrosis, stenosis, and eventually thrombosis.

In aTOS, a cervical or anomalous first rib, developmental anomalies of the anterior scalene muscle, and activities of daily living are the cause of symptoms.

Pathology

The common pathologic findings in most patients with nTOS are (1) developmental anomalies of the thoracic outlet and fibrosis of the scalene muscle and (2) conversion of muscle fibers from fast twitch to slow twitch[20,21] (see Chapter 123: Thoracic Outlet Syndrome: Neurogenic). The fact that transaxillary first rib resection for the treatment of nTOS has become popular since its introduction by Roos in 1966 has led some to believe that the first rib is the underlying cause of the pathology.[18] This is not universally believed to be true. Many think that in nTOS the attachments to the first rib are the more likely cause. Support for this theory is that the results of anterior and middle scalenectomy without first rib resection are similar to those of scalenectomy with first rib resection.[23]

However, although the first rib is not the underlying pathology, its removal avoids the complication of having the lower trunk of the brachial plexus become fixed to the rib by scar tissue in patients in whom the lower trunk is touching the first rib. It is for this reason that the first rib is selectively

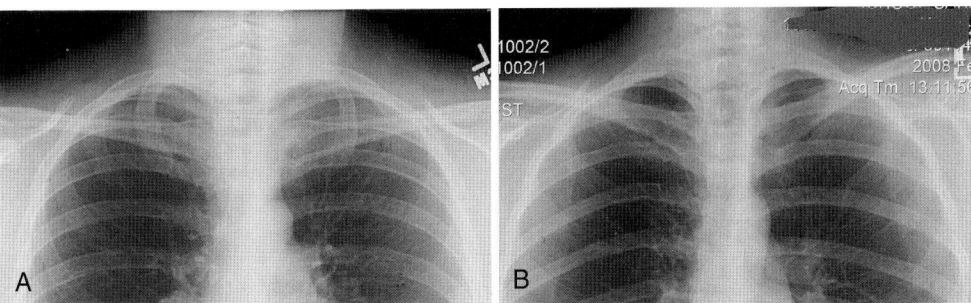

Figure 122-1 A, Fairly vertical first rib that is resting against the lower trunk of the brachial plexus and is usually excised. **B,** Curved first rib that lies free of the lower trunk and is not usually removed.

removed after scalenectomy when the lower trunk is seen to be touching the first rib. We have found that the shape of the first rib on chest radiography usually predicts who will require first rib resection and who will not (Fig. 122-1).

The pathology of vTOS is a focal area of scarred subclavian intima that has narrowed the lumen to just a few millimeters. Thrombus is the final event that occludes the vein and precipitates acute symptoms of upper extremity deep venous thrombosis.

In aTOS the most common pathology is subclavian artery stenosis accompanied by post-stenotic dilatation that gives the appearance of an aneurysm. Thrombus forms within the dilated portion of the artery just distal to the stenosis, as mural thrombus does in an aneurysm. The disease process is usually asymptomatic until emboli are dislodged.

Pathophysiology

Although the pathophysiology of nTOS may vary depending on the specific predisposing and causative factors, it is usually associated with an underlying narrowed scalene triangle. These patients are asymptomatic until neck trauma stretches and tears some of the anterior and middle scalene muscle fibers. This mechanism explains the neck pain that usually appears within the first 24 hours of a neck injury. Over the next few days, swelling of the muscles from bleeding or inflammation (or both) results in compression against the nerve roots of the brachial plexus. This compression then causes upper extremity pain and paresthesia, the onset of which is usually delayed a few days or weeks after the initial trauma. As the muscle injury heals and the swelling subsides, scar tissue replaces the blood that collected within the muscle, which accounts in part for the muscle fibrosis. The extremity symptoms persist because the scarred muscle compresses the nerves, as the swollen muscle had. Persistent neck pain results from the scarred scalenes, and occipital headaches may occur as referred pain from scalene muscle spasm.

Data supporting the scalene muscles as the site of pathology include (1) histologic studies of the scalene muscles that show an average of three times more scar tissue in the scalene muscles of nTOS patients than in control patients (see Chapter 123: Thoracic Outlet Syndrome: Neurogenic), (2) the strong correlation between positive responses to scalene muscle blockade and positive responses to surgery,

and (3) the fact that the rate of improvement after surgery for nTOS is the same as that for scalenectomy with or without first rib resection.

The pathophysiology of vTOS begins with subclavian vein thrombosis. The symptoms of swelling and pain result from venous hypertension. Symptoms improve as a result of collateral formation and eventual recanalization of the vein in many patients.

In aTOS, the pathophysiology is based on the effects of arterial compression by an anomalous first rib, cervical rib, or anterior scalene muscle. Subclavian artery stenosis produces fluid hemodynamics that results in post-stenotic dilatation or aneurysm formation, mural thrombus, and distal embolization.

ANATOMY

Three Spaces

Three separate spaces are present in the thoracic outlet area: the scalene triangle, the costoclavicular space, and the pectoralis minor (PM) space (Fig. 122-2A). The scalene triangle (Fig. 122-2B) is the most common site of brachial plexus compression. When present, cervical ribs (Fig. 122-3) and anomalous first ribs (Fig. 122-4) also compress the plexus in this location. The costoclavicular space, between the first rib and clavicle (Fig. 122-2C), is traversed by all three structures and is the site of subclavian vein compression. The PM space is actually outside the thoracic outlet area, but compression of the upper extremity neurovascular bundle can occur in this space between the PM muscle and ribs of the chest wall. Although this might better be termed axillary compression syndrome, it is appropriate to consider the PM space as an extension of the thoracic outlet area because compression here is common and the axillary and the thoracic outlet neurovascular bundles contain the same elements (Fig. 122-5).

Frequency

The space most frequently involved in TOS is the scalene triangle (see Fig. 122-2B). Only since 2004 has it been postulated that a very close second may be the PM space. Between 2004 and 2007, the PM space was involved in more than 75% of our TOS patients (unpublished data).

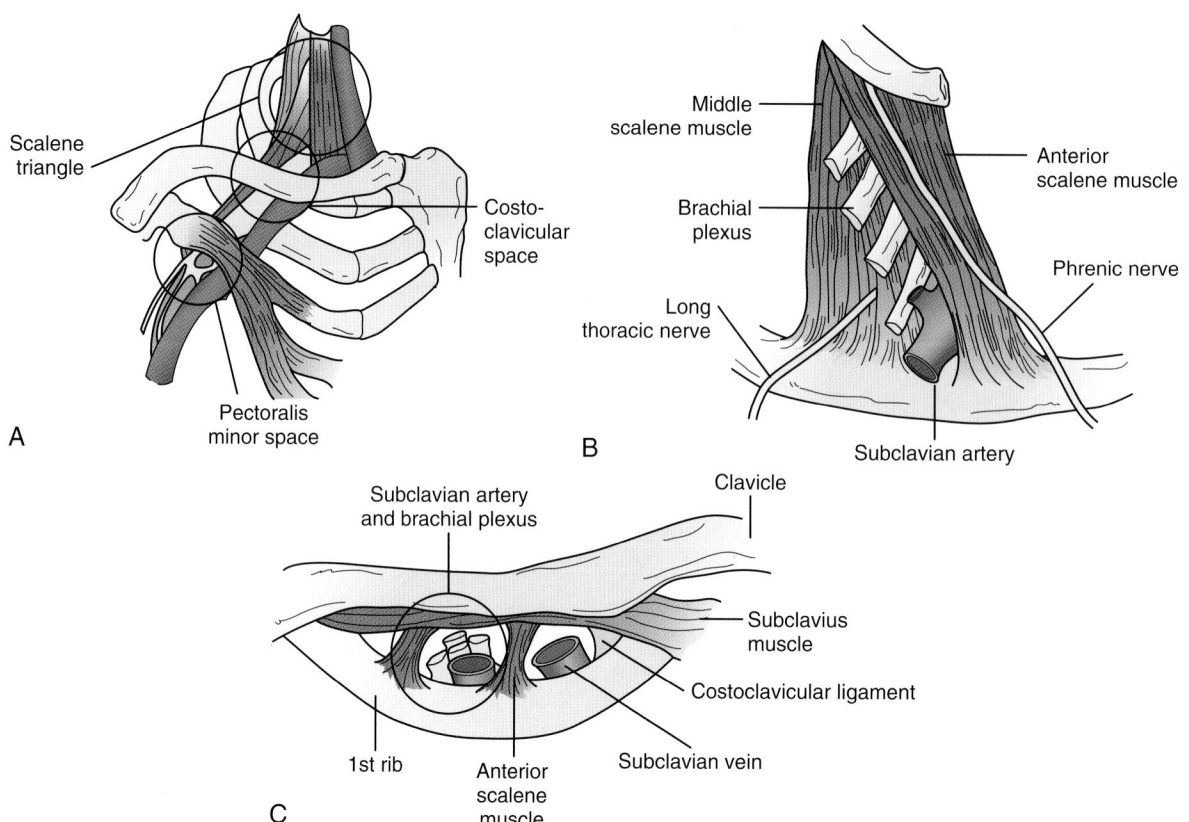

Figure 122-2 A, Anatomy of the thoracic outlet area with the three major spaces. **B,** Scalene triangle with the phrenic and long thoracic nerves located in the most common positions. **C,** Costoclavicular space revealing the subclavian vein being separated by the anterior scalene muscle from the subclavian artery and brachial plexus. *(A, from Sanders RJ, Haug CE. Thoracic Outlet Syndrome: A Common Sequela of Neck Injuries. Philadelphia, PA: JB Lippincott; 1991:34. B, from Sanders RJ, Haug CE. Thoracic Outlet Syndrome: A Common Sequela of Neck Injuries. Philadelphia, PA: JB Lippincott; 1991:46. C, from Sanders RJ, Haug CE. Thoracic Outlet Syndrome: A Common Sequela of Neck Injuries. Philadelphia, PA: JB Lippincott; 1991:39.)*

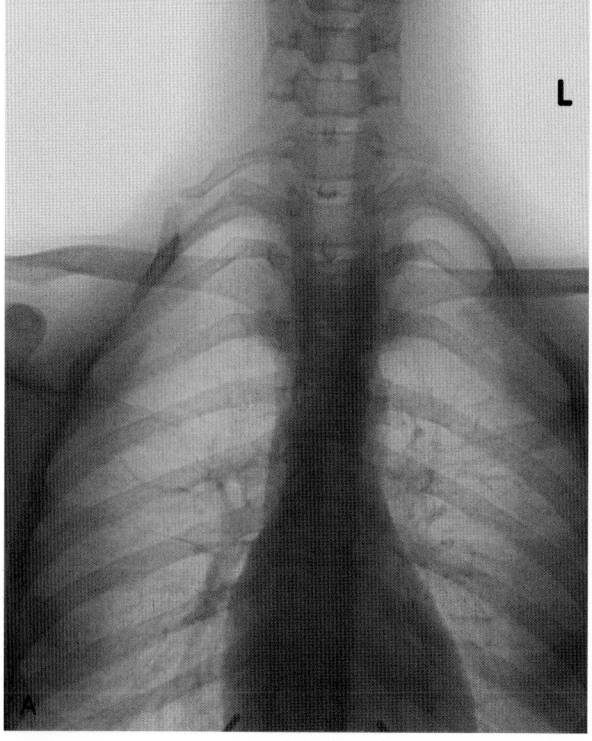

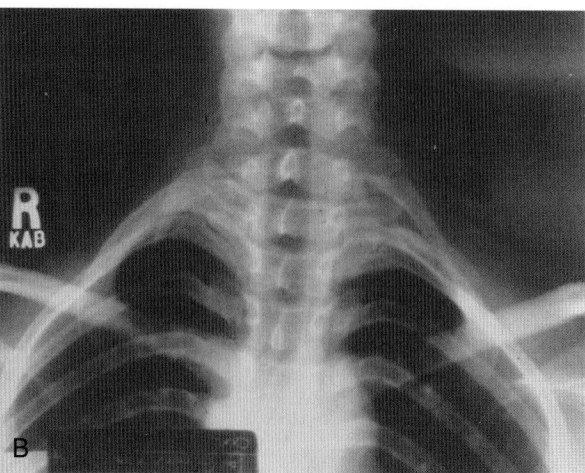

Figure 122-3 A, Right complete cervical rib with a true joint between the cervical rib and a small process arising from the top of the first rib. **B,** Bilateral cervical ribs, incomplete on the right and complete on the left. *(B, from Sanders RJ, Haug CE. Thoracic Outlet Syndrome: A Common Sequela of Neck Injuries. Philadelphia, PA: JB Lippincott; 1991:43.)*

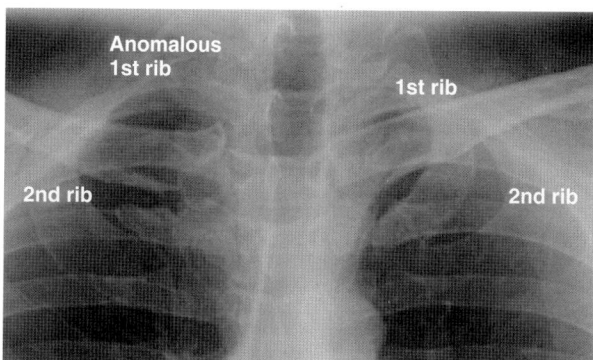

Figure 122-4 Anomalous right first rib. That this is an anomalous first rib and not a cervical rib is demonstrated by comparing the normal first rib on the patient's left with the abnormal rib on the patient's right. Note the symmetry of the two second ribs. An anomalous right first rib and normal left first rib arise from the symmetric transverse processes of T1.

Nerves

In addition to the brachial plexus, the phrenic and long thoracic nerves are seen during supraclavicular dissections. Very close to the area but rarely seen are the dorsal scapular nerve and cervical sympathetic chain.

Brachial Plexus

The brachial plexus arises from nerve roots C5 to T1. In the scalene triangle area the five nerve roots become three trunks. The anterior and posterior divisions and cords of the plexus are usually formed proximal to the PM space, so it is the branches of the plexus that lie under the PM muscle, along with the axillary artery and vein.

Phrenic Nerve

Arising primarily from C4, the phrenic nerve usually receives branches from C3 and C5. It is single in 87% and double or triple in 13% of individuals. A double phrenic nerve usually results from the C5 branch to the phrenic nerve's failing to fuse with the C4 branch in the neck. It may fuse below the clavicle or in the mediastinum. The phrenic descends 84% of the time from the lateral to the medial side of the anterior scalene muscle. In the other 16% the phrenic nerve remains on the lateral side.[24] Each phrenic nerve accounts for 20% of the breathing capacity. In neck dissections, a helpful landmark is that the nerve lies just below the transverse cervical artery.

Long Thoracic Nerve

The long thoracic nerve arises primarily from C6 and usually receives contributions from C5 and C7. The C5 and C6 branches run through the muscle belly of the middle scalene muscle, where they can usually be observed to join. The C7 branch arises from the posterior aspect of the nerve root and often descends below the middle scalene before joining the other two branches.

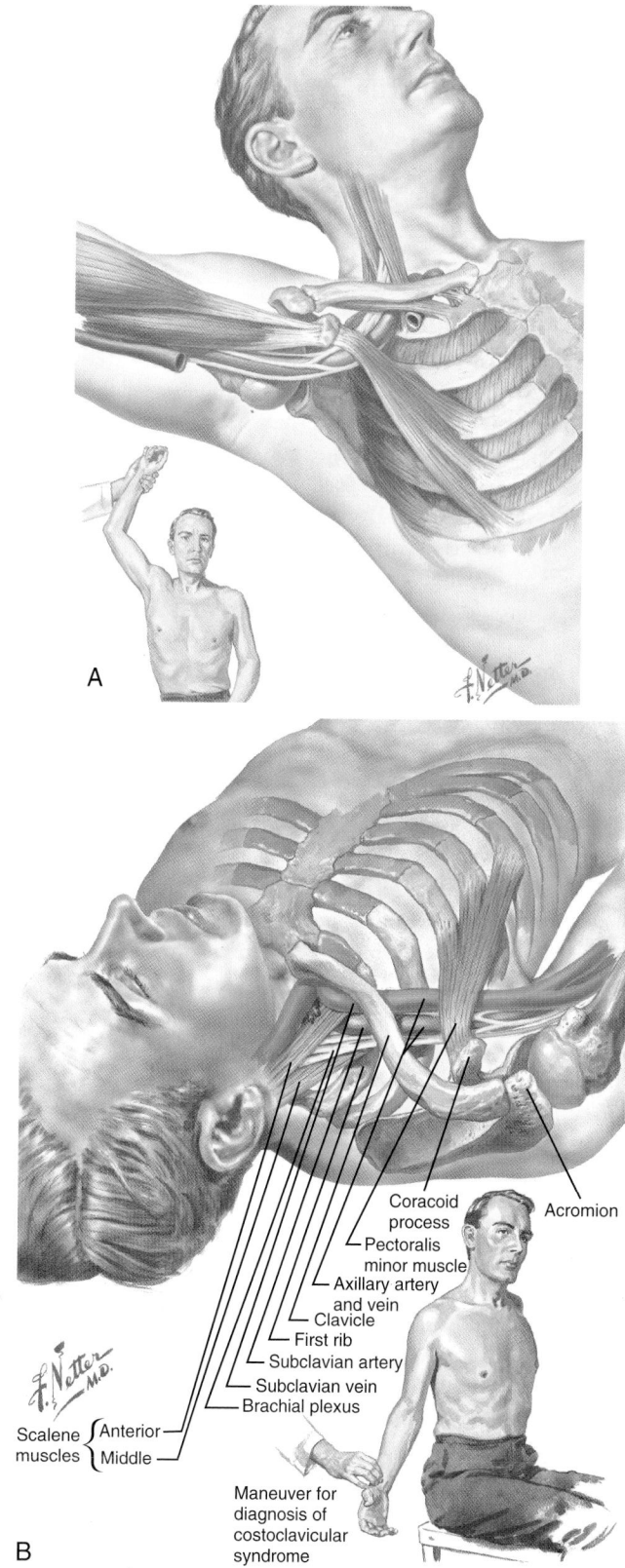

Figure 122-5 A and **B,** Two views of the thoracic outlet area demonstrating the pectoralis minor space in the foreground. The axillary artery and vein are continuations of the subclavian artery and vein. At the axillary level the brachial plexus has already formed its cords, so it is the branches that are seen under the pectoralis minor. *(From Lord JW Jr, Rosati LM. Thoracic outlet syndromes. Ciba Symp. 1971;23:1-13.)*

Dorsal Scapular Nerve

The dorsal scapular nerve, the first branch of C5, courses through the cephalic portion of the middle scalene muscle and then descends lateral to the muscle. However, it may course very close to the area of dissection in supraclavicular approaches to thoracic outlet decompression.

Cervical Sympathetic Chain

Though not usually in the operative field of supraclavicular procedures, the cervical sympathetic chain lies over the transverse processes of the cervical vertebrae and is therefore very close to the origin of the anterior and middle scalene muscles. As a result, when cautery is used to excise the scalene muscles at their transverse process origins, the current may reach and damage the cervical sympathetic chain. This is the probable explanation for the occasional case of Horner's syndrome observed after supraclavicular scalenectomy. Since we have stopped excising scalene muscles all the way to bone, we no longer are seeing Horner's syndrome. Use of bipolar cautery can reduce the incidence of this complication but does not totally eliminate it.

Scalene Muscle Variations and Anomalies

A significant number of anatomic variations in scalene muscles have been observed both in the normal population and in patients with nTOS. They are too common to be called anomalies. These variations might be regarded as factors predisposing to TOS but are not regarded as causes.

Splitting of the Anterior Scalene around C5 and C6.
Such splitting was noted in 45% of cadavers and in only 21% of nTOS patients.[24]

Scalene Minimus Muscle.
This muscle arises from the transverse processes of the lower cervical vertebrae, runs in front of C8 and T1 and behind the subclavian artery, and inserts on the first rib or Sibson's fascia. Its incidence is 25% to 55%.[25]

Interdigitating Muscle Fibers.
Such fibers commonly run between the anterior and middle scalene muscles. They were noted in 75% of nTOS patients and in only 40% of cadavers.

Scalene Triangle Width.
The width of the scalene triangle varies from very narrow to quite wide, with the distance between the two scalene muscles at their insertion on the first rib ranging from 0.3 to 2.0 cm. The nerve roots emerge lower in a wide triangle than in a narrow triangle (Fig. 122-6). Observations during surgery have revealed that most nTOS patients have the narrower type of triangle.[24]

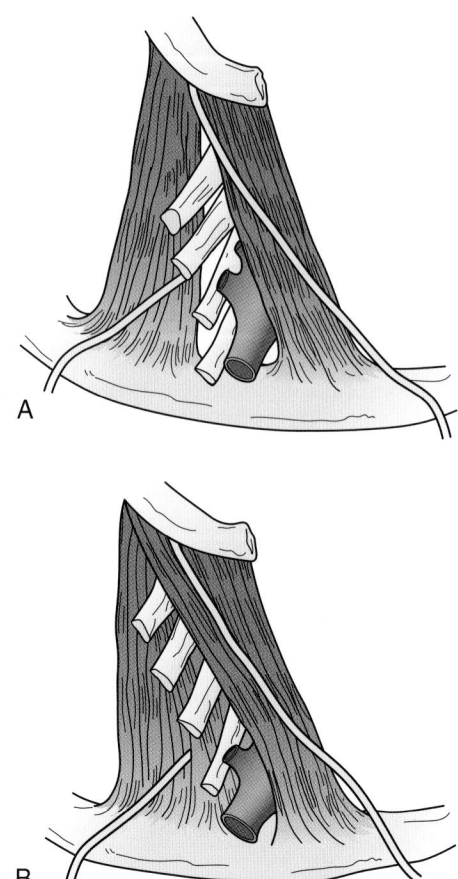

Figure 122-6 Scalene triangle variations. **A,** The usual relationships found in cadavers. The triangle is wider and the nerves emerge lower in the triangle than in most patients with neurogenic thoracic outlet syndrome. There is minimal contact between nerve and muscle. **B,** A narrow triangle in which the nerves emerge high and are touching the muscles as they emerge. Contact between nerve and muscle is stronger than in **A.** *(From Sanders RJ, Roos DB. The surgical anatomy of the scalene triangle. Contemp Surg. 1989;35:11-16.)*

Congenital Bands and Ligaments.
These structures are frequently observed in the normal population, with an incidence as high as 63%.[26] Although bands have been observed in almost every area of the scalene triangle and have been nicely classified,[27] their role is as a predisposing factor rather than a direct cause.

Relationship of the Subclavian Vein to the Phrenic Nerve.
The phrenic nerve usually runs posterior to the subclavian vein. However, in 5% to 7% of individuals the phrenic nerve runs anterior to the vein and in this position can be a rare cause of subclavian vein obstruction[28] (Fig. 122-7). A case of this is seen in Figure 122-8. This patient was treated by dividing the subclavian vein, letting the nerve fall behind the vein, and anastomosing the vein anterior to the nerve.

Relationship of the Subclavian Vein and Costoclavicular Ligament.
The subclavian vein lies on top of the first rib just before it is joined by the jugular vein. It is touched medially by the costoclavicular ligament and superiorly by the

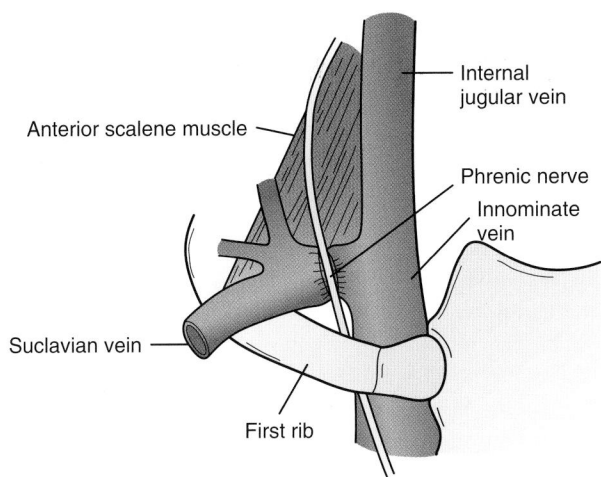

Figure 122-7 Prevenous phrenic nerve lying anterior to the subclavian vein and compressing it. This occurs in 5% to 7% of cases. *(From Sanders RJ, Haug CE. Thoracic Outlet Syndrome: A Common Sequela of Neck Injuries. Philadelphia, PA: JB Lippincott; 1991:241.)*

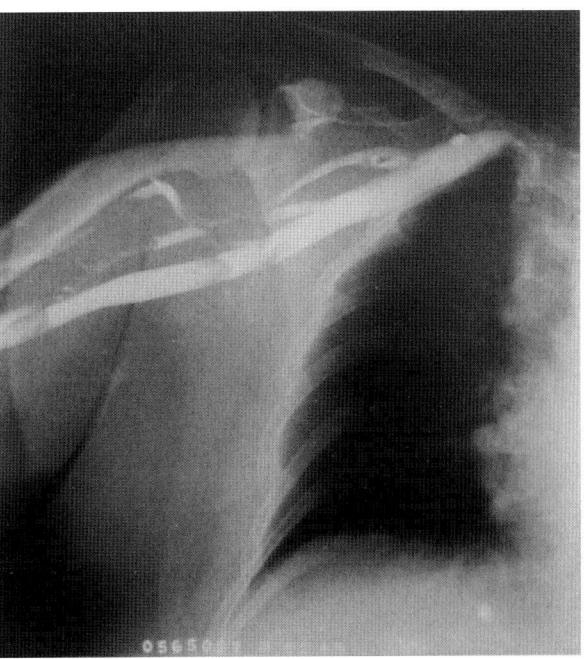

Figure 122-8 Nonthrombotic obstruction of the subclavian vein by a phrenic nerve lying anterior to the vein rather than in the usual posterior position. *(From Sanders RJ, Haug CE. Thoracic Outlet Syndrome: A Common Sequela of Neck Injuries. Philadelphia, PA: JB Lippincott; 1991:237.)*

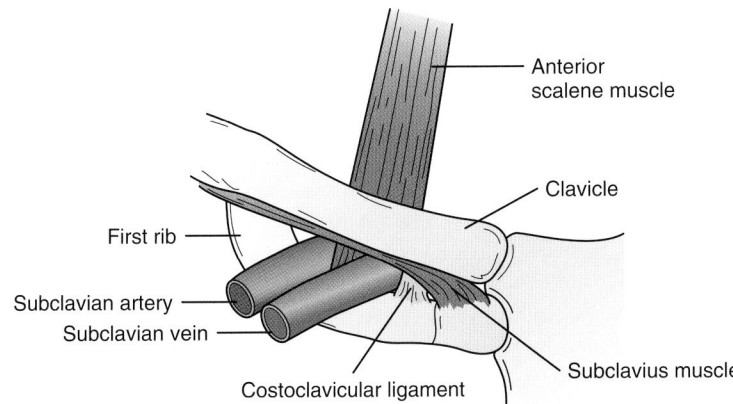

Figure 122-9 Anatomy of the subclavian vein and ligaments. The subclavian vein is in close contact with the costoclavicular ligament, subclavius tendon, and anterior scalene muscle because it lies on the first rib. *(From Sanders RJ, Haug CE. Thoracic Outlet Syndrome: A Common Sequela of Neck Injuries. Philadelphia, PA: JB Lippincott; 1991:236.)*

subclavius tendon. A variation in the position of the vein is its position a little more medially on the first rib so that it is partially compressed by the costoclavicular ligament. Variations in the thickness of the subclavius tendon can also result in compression of the vein from above. These variations in position between the three structures predispose to the development of subclavian vein obstruction. Obstruction is then caused by excessive overhead use of the upper extremity, which results in the vein's being repeatedly pushed against the ligament or tendon (or both) and the first rib (Fig. 122-9).

Cervical Ribs and Anomalous First Ribs

Incidence

Anomalous or rudimentary first ribs are often overlooked on routine chest radiographs. The first report was a 1939 study

of 5000 chest radiographs. This study found the incidence of anomalous first ribs and cervical ribs to be 0.76% and 0.74%, respectively. Anomalous ribs occurred equally in women and men. In contrast, the female-male ratio of cervical ribs was found to be 7:3.[29] No one has yet provided an explanation for this difference.

Both ribs are narrower and lie higher than a normal first rib. The only difference between the two is that a cervical rib arises from the transverse process of C7, whereas an anomalous first rib arises from the transverse process of T1 (see Fig. 122-4). It is more than of academic interest to note the distinction between anomalous and cervical ribs. It is common to excise the first rib with the cervical rib. However, if the rib is an anomalous first rib, the second rib below it should not usually be removed. An exception is if the anomalous first rib is so fused to the second rib that the second rib is significantly thinned and deformed when removing the anomalous first rib; in that case, excision of the second rib is justified.

Complete versus Incomplete Cervical Ribs

About 30% of cervical ribs are complete ribs fused to the first rib by a true joint or a fibrous attachment. The other 70% are incomplete cervical ribs with no direct attachment to the first rib. However, most of these incomplete ribs have a tight fascial band extending from the tip of the cervical rib to the first rib.[27] The cervical rib and attached band lie within the middle scalene muscle, thereby narrowing the space within the scalene triangle through which the nerve roots of the plexus must pass. Thus, an incomplete cervical rib with its band can act like a complete rib.

Significance

Cervical and anomalous first ribs can push against the subclavian artery and cause stenosis with or without post-stenotic aneurysm formation, or more often they will push against the lower trunk of the brachial plexus and cause a neuropathy. However, most cervical and anomalous first ribs remain asymptomatic throughout life. When symptoms do develop, they are usually neurogenic. In a recent review of 47 nTOS operations involving abnormal ribs, 15% were anomalous first ribs and 85% were cervical ribs. Spontaneous onset of symptoms occurred in 50% of patients with complete cervical ribs versus only 20% with incomplete ribs. Neck trauma preceded the onset of symptoms in the other 80% with incomplete ribs and in the 50% with complete ribs.[30]

Association with Arterial and Neurogenic Thoracic Outlet Syndrome

Cervical ribs or anomalous first ribs are almost always seen in patients with aTOS. On the other hand, symptomatic cervical ribs are more likely to produce symptoms of nTOS than aTOS. Over a 28-year period during which more than 1000 nTOS operations were performed, there were 39 cervical ribs and 7 anomalous first ribs, for an incidence of about 4%. Among the same group of 1000-plus TOS patients, there were only 9 with aTOS—5 with complete cervical ribs and 4 with anomalous first ribs—for an incidence of less than 1%.[30]

Objective Findings

Ulnar neuropathy on electrodiagnostic studies and hand atrophy occur in only a small minority of patients with cervical ribs and nTOS symptoms. Both were present in only 3 of 39 patients (8%) in one study[30] and were noted in 8 of 45 patients (18%) in another.[31] Improvement in symptoms and signs after surgery is the same in patients with cervical ribs as in those without. In the few patients with cervical ribs and hand atrophy, the neurologic deficit persisted after surgery in more than half.[31]

■ MISSED DIAGNOSIS
Timing of Diagnosis

A diagnosis of nTOS is seldom made in the emergency department immediately after an injury, and seldom can it be made in the first few weeks. Although symptoms of pain in the head, neck, and shoulder girdle often develop within a few days of a neck injury, pain in the arms and paresthesia in the hands may be delayed several days or weeks and occasionally even months. Most often the initial symptoms will be due to cervical spine strain. Therefore, a diagnosis of nTOS should be deferred for at least a few weeks from the onset of symptoms. Furthermore, it is not critical to make this diagnosis early. The initial treatment of nTOS is the same as for cervical strain, namely, rest, gentle stretching exercises, anti-inflammatory drugs, muscle relaxants, and analgesics. If the symptoms have not subsided after a few months, physical examination should be reliable enough to make a diagnosis.

Failure to Recognize Abnormal Ribs on Radiographs

Subclavian artery thrombosis is easily recognized by the presence of an ischemic hand and an arteriogram demonstrating axillosubclavian artery obstruction. However, sometimes overlooked is an anomalous first rib or a cervical rib that elevated the subclavian artery and was the original cause of the problem. Subclavian artery obstruction seldom develops in young people. When it does occur, it is unlikely to be due to arteriosclerotic occlusive disease and more likely to be an abnormal rib or an inflammatory condition such as Takayasu's arteritis. It is important to determine the cause preoperatively and excise an offending rib at the time of arterial reconstruction. There have been cases in which vein grafts and prosthetic grafts have been compressed and occluded by an unremoved abnormal rib.

In patients with nTOS it is important to obtain and correctly read neck radiographs to detect cervical and anomalous first ribs. Patients with abnormal ribs in whom symptoms of pain and paresthesia develop should be given a short trial of nonsurgical therapy, but if there is no response in 2 to 3 months, additional conservative therapy is unlikely to succeed.

Incomplete History

Obtaining a history of some type of neck trauma preceding the onset of symptoms is helpful in considering a diagnosis of nTOS. The absence of such a history should make the examiner look hard for other diagnoses. Although nTOS can occur spontaneously, more than 80% of patients have a history of some type of neck trauma, the most common being whiplash injuries from motor vehicle accidents, falls on slippery surfaces or down stairs, and repetitive stress injury from hours on keyboards, assembly lines, or various other occupations.

Specific Symptoms

When asked about their symptoms, many patients will mention pain in the arm and numbness in the hand but fail to describe additional symptoms. It is important that the examiner not accept the initial symptoms as the complete list. The patient should be asked specifically about occipital headache and pain over the trapezius, neck, chest, and shoulder girdle. A patient who has symptoms confined to the forearm and hand is more likely to have carpal or cubital tunnel syndrome and not nTOS. On the other hand, a patient who has pain in the neck and shoulder girdle plus occipital headache may well have nTOS or compression in more than one area, a double-crush syndrome.[32]

Incomplete Physical Examination

The standard neurologic examination often fails to detect nTOS. In addition to tenderness over the scalene muscles and reduced sensation to very light touch in the fingers, an examination for nTOS should include elicitation of symptoms by a variety of provocative maneuvers. The Adson test is the best known of these maneuvers but is now largely considered to be in the category of historical interest (see "Inaccurate Provocative Tests").[10] In addition, there are several other provocative maneuvers, including neck rotation, head tilt, 90-degree abduction in external rotation, and the elevated arm stress test position. For standardization of the 90-degree abduction in external rotation position, the arms should be elevated in the same plane as the trunk, neither too far forward nor too far backward (Fig. 122-10). The most effective provocative test is the upper limb tension test of Elvey[33,34] (Fig. 122-11). This test is comparable to straight-leg raising in the lower extremity and is worth incorporating into every examination for upper extremity symptoms. A positive response indicates compression of either the cervical nerve roots or brachial plexus at the level of the spine, thoracic outlet, or PM

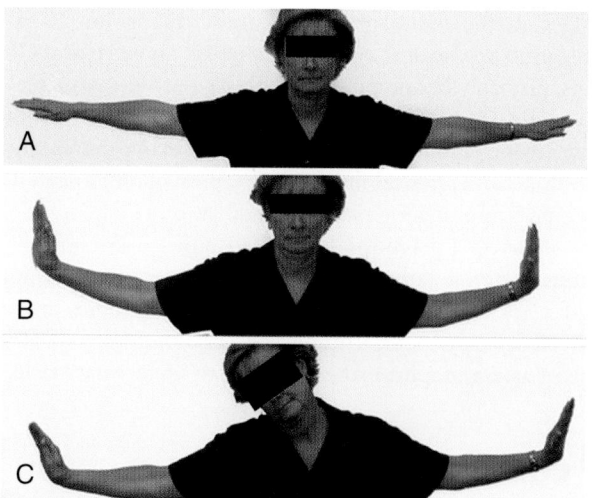

Figure 122-11 Upper limb tension test, modified from Elvey. Each maneuver progressively stretches the brachial plexus. **A,** Arms abducted to 90 degrees with the elbows extended. **B,** Wrists dorsiflexed. **C,** Head tilted ear to shoulder. *(From Sanders RJ, Hammond SL, Rao NM. Diagnosis of thoracic outlet syndrome. J Vasc Surg. 2007;46:601-604.)*

space. A negative response is usually adequate to rule out the diagnosis of nTOS.

Inaccurate Provocative Tests

Provocative positions such as the Adson maneuver and its modifications are intended to put stress on the neurovascular bundle. In Adson's original description of his test, he noted "A decrease or obliteration of the radial pulse or blood pressure is a pathognomonic sign of scalenus anticus syndrome (this is one of the syndromes included in TOS)."[10,35] However, in 1947, the same year of Adson's last report, Gage and Parnell noted that 50% of normal individuals had a positive Adson test.[36] Subsequently, others have demonstrated similar high rates of positive Adson tests in healthy volunteers.[27,37-41]

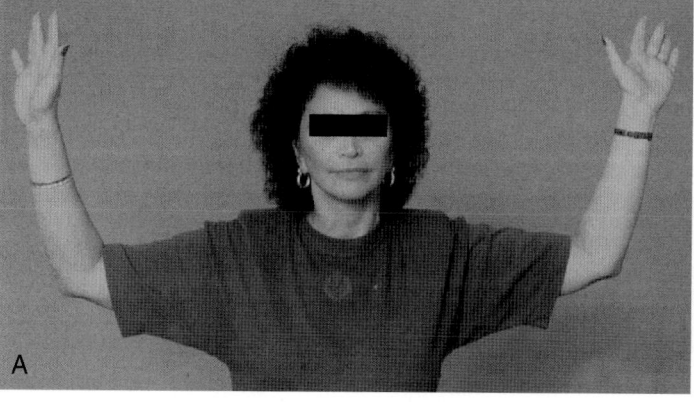
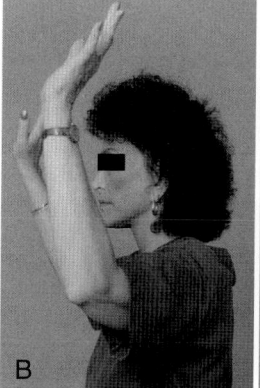
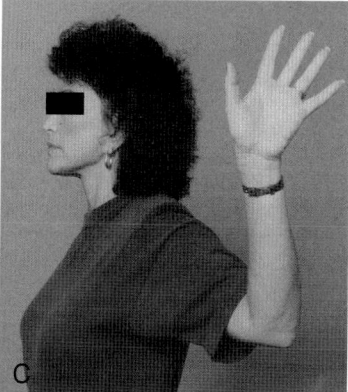

Figure 122-10 Ninety-degree abduction in external rotation. The patient is asked to hold this position for 3 minutes. Most patients with neurogenic thoracic outlet syndrome will note reproduction of their symptoms of pain, paresthesia, and weakness within 60 seconds. **A,** Correct position with the elbows in the same plane as the shoulders. **B,** The arms are too far forward with too much shoulder adduction. **C,** The arms are too far back because of too much shoulder abduction. *(From Sanders RJ, Haug CE. Thoracic Outlet Syndrome: A Common Sequela of Neck Injuries. Philadelphia, PA: JB Lippincott; 1991:81.)*

Despite the abundant evidence indicating its unreliability, the Adson test is still currently popular among many clinicians, probably because it is the only *objective* test available on physical examination. This is unfortunate because it has led to an erroneous diagnosis of vTOS or aTOS in patients whose symptoms and physical findings are typical of nTOS and who have no symptoms or physical findings of aTOS or vTOS. The erroneous diagnosis has led to unnecessary studies to confirm arterial pathology, such as pulse volume recordings, duplex scans, and even arteriography. Such studies are not indicated, waste medical resources, waste money, and in the case of arteriography, expose patients to unnecessary risks.

■ CONTROVERSIES

Objective versus Subjective Diagnostic Criteria

Questions have been raised regarding the diagnostic criteria for nTOS. No one disputes the existence of aTOS and vTOS because these conditions can be detected by objective methods. However, most patients with nTOS lack objective findings, which means that diagnoses must be made by subjective criteria alone. Objective criteria for nTOS, specifically ulnar neuropathy on electromyographic studies and atrophy of the thenar eminence, are usually found only in patients with cervical or anomalous first ribs. By one classification, patients with objective criteria have "true" nTOS, whereas those lacking objective changes are labeled "disputed" nTOS.[42] This classification was created by its author to discourage surgery for nTOS because such surgery has resulted in a number of nerve injuries, some causing severe disability.

Even though all physicians would like to have objective criteria to establish a diagnosis, most nTOS patients lack such criteria. The history, physical examination, and response to a scalene muscle block may be the best criteria available. Although at the present time there appears to be promise in measuring the responses of the medial antebrachial cutaneous (MAC) nerve, more studies are needed for confirmation before accepting its validity.[22,43] Until objective testing is available, subjective criteria must be used. It should be noted that the results of surgery in patients with objective criteria are no better than those in patients without such criteria.[30]

Not a Diagnosis of Exclusion

Because most nTOS patients lack objective diagnostic criteria, it is important that the diagnosis of nTOS be made on the basis of several positive findings on physical examination. A patient with just arm pain or hand paresthesia who has few positive physical findings should not be labeled as having nTOS simply because no other diagnosis can be found.

■ FUTURE DEVELOPMENTS

TOS continues to be a challenge. In the past 50 years many new innovations in this area have added to our understanding of the diagnostic criteria, pathology, conservative treatment,

and surgical management of the three types of TOS. In the future we expect to see more progress in this field. Currently, studies are ongoing in three areas that hold promise. A new objective electrodiagnostic test has recently been reported; a film containing hyaluronidase to reduce scar formation and thereby compression of the nerve roots may reduce recurrence and make reoperations less difficult; and new attention is being focused on pectoralis minor syndrome (PMS), which is in the area of the thoracic outlet but has received too little attention. The following sections will update these three new areas.

New Diagnostic Study for Neurogenic Thoracic Outlet Syndrome

The MAC nerve is the lowest branch of the inferior trunk of the brachial plexus and appears to be more sensitive to compression than other branches of the plexus are. In 2004, abnormal MAC measurements of amplitude were recorded in 16 patients with clinical signs of nTOS and normal electromyography/nerve conduction velocity studies.[22] In all patients, the amplitude of the symptomatic arm was lower than that of the asymptomatic arm of the same patient.

Another study of the MAC test was performed between 2004 and 2006 in 41 patients operated on for clinical signs of nTOS.[43] Although Seror's study measured only amplitude,[22] the later study found that latency was a little more helpful than amplitude. Four diagnostic criteria were established and their normal ranges determined from measurements in 19 volunteers. In this electromyography laboratory, the diagnostic criteria established were a latency of 2.4 msec or less, difference in latency between the symptomatic and asymptomatic sides of at least 0.2 msec, amplitude of less than 10 µV, and amplitude ratio between the asymptomatic and symptomatic sides of 2.0 or greater. Using these four criteria, 40 of the 41 patients had at least one abnormal reading, and 56% had at least three of the four criteria in the abnormal range.[43] In applying these criteria it is important that each electrodiagnostic laboratory establish its own diagnostic criteria in healthy volunteers because precise technique and equipment may vary. For example, in our laboratory, orthodromic determinations were obtained by stimulating distally from the antecubital fossa and measuring over the volar forearm at 12 cm, a modification of the Seror protocol.[22,43] MAC nerve determinations could prove to be a better objective test than is currently available to support the diagnosis of nTOS.

Antiadhesion Material
Seprafilm

Studies of methods to prevent postsurgical adhesions began appearing in 1996 and 1997.[44,45] The material initially tried was composed of hyaluronic acid and methylcellulose and was called Seprafilm. It is totally absorbed in body tissues in 3 to 4 weeks and has significantly reduced adhesions after abdominal and pelvic surgery.[46-49] Based on these early studies, antiadhesive materials have been tried in other areas for the same purpose. In animal studies it has reduced peridural fibrosis at laminectomy sites[50] and prevented adhesions after tenolysis.[51,52]

Because postoperative scarring is the most common cause of recurrent nTOS, Seprafilm was used in an attempt to reduce adherence of scar tissue to the nerves of the plexus in 249 patients over a 3-year period.[53] Unfortunately, the failure rate was unchanged, perhaps because of the short life of Seprafilm. Its only advantage seemed to be that during reoperations the plexus was a little easier to find. The nerve roots were still fairly compressed by layers of scar tissue in the 10 patients who underwent reoperations.

SurgiWrap

Another material, SurgiWrap,[54] was suggested to us by Dr. James Avery of San Francisco. SurgiWrap is a polylactic acid film, is easier to handle than Seprafilm, and is not absorbed for several months. It has been used for the past 3 years in more than 175 patients undergoing supraclavicular scalenectomy for nTOS, with or without first rib resection. The early results are better than those of Seprafilm. Final evaluation has not yet been made, but to date there have been only eight reoperations for recurrence. At each of the reoperations, once the nerve roots were identified, the layers of scar close to the epineurium could be separated from the nerve root fairly easily without entering the nerve sheath. This was not true with Seprafilm (personal communication).

▪ PECTORALIS MINOR SYNDROME

Little attention has been paid to PMS since it was initially described in 1945 and called "hyperabduction syndrome"[14] or "subcoracoid compression." Over the next 60 years only three articles were written on the subject, the last being in 1984.[55-57] In 2004, the addition of pectoralis minor tenotomy (PMT) to operations performed for recurrent nTOS was described in 13 patients,[58] and it was Dr. George Thomas of Seattle who suggested that we begin looking for PMS. By 2007, PMS was recognized in more than 75% of our patients who had symptoms and signs of nTOS.

Separately, seven patients have been seen with nonthrombotic axillary vein obstruction secondary to PM compression. Their symptoms were the same as those with axillary-subclavian vein thrombosis, but less severe. They were all relieved of symptoms by PMT.[59] In addition, axillary artery compression by the PM muscle has been noted in a few isolated patients. These patients have also been treated by PMT plus appropriate arterial repair.[60,61]

Etiology

Based on patients' histories, neurogenic PMS is associated with trauma or excessive exercise of the shoulder girdle. The common denominator appears to be activities that can hyperabduct the shoulder and thereby stretch the PM muscle, which is attached to the coracoid process of the scapula.

Pathology

The pathology is believed to be a tight PM muscle that compresses branches of the brachial plexus, the axillary artery, and the axillary vein.

Symptoms

Because most patients with PMS also have nTOS, some of the symptoms are similar to those seen in nTOS patients: pain in the neck, trapezius, shoulder, and upper extremity; paresthesia in the hand; and weakness. In addition, the particular symptoms suggesting PMS are pain in the anterior portion of the chest and axilla. Patients with PMS alone have fewer and milder symptoms in the head and neck areas than do nTOS patients.

Physical Examination

Positive findings include tenderness near the PM insertion, located 2 to 3 cm below the coracoid process, and tenderness in the axilla. Moreover, most patients with PMS also have some of the positive physical findings of nTOS in the extremity, but they often do not have positive findings in the neck and do not demonstrate duplication of symptoms with neck rotation and head tilt. If patients do have these physical findings, they are mild.

Diagnostic Testing

PM muscle block is the most helpful diagnostic test. It is performed by injecting 4 mL of 1% lidocaine into the PM muscle near its insertion into the coracoid process. It is not necessary to inject it right at the coracoids; 1 to 2 cm near it will suffice. A 1½-inch, No. 22 needle is introduced 2 to 3 cm below the clavicle with the needle aimed 45 degrees cephalad. Aspiration is important because it is easy to enter one of the axillary vessels. If this occurs, the needle is backed out a few millimeters and redirected a little more superficially. The 4 mL is injected over a wide area while keeping the needle moving and injecting only as it is partially withdrawn. A good result is noted within a few minutes by improvement in symptoms at rest, as well as reduced findings on repeat physical examination. Note that the 45-degree cephalad angle is important to avoid entering an interspace and producing pneumothorax.

Cause of Recurrent Symptoms after Surgery for Neurogenic Thoracic Outlet Syndrome

Patients with recurrent symptoms after thoracic outlet decompression operations are frequently found to have chest pain and tenderness over the PM tendon. PMS is often a part of the recurrence and may have been present and overlooked at the time of the first TOS operation. If these patients have a good response to PM muscle blockade, they may be candidates for PMT alone. Patients responding well to this test can undergo a very low-risk procedure and thereby be spared reoperations in scarred areas.

Treatment

Choice of Surgery: Pectoralis Minor Tenotomy Alone or with Thoracic Outlet Decompression

Because symptoms of the two conditions are similar, it is difficult to differentiate between nTOS and PMS, and the two frequently coexist. Even in patients who experienced excellent improvement with PMT alone, a preoperative diagnosis of both conditions had often been made.

Responses to PM muscle block and scalene muscle block have been used to help determine which condition to treat first or whether both areas require decompression simultaneously. Patients who note excellent relief of symptoms at rest and improvement of most physical findings after PM blockade are offered PMT alone. Patients who show only partial improvement after a PM block are then given a scalene block. If there is further improvement in symptoms at rest and on repeat physical examination, decompression of both areas is recommended. If there is a poor response to the PM block and a good response to the scalene block, just thoracic outlet decompression is offered.

Conservative Treatment

Initial treatment is reduction or cessation of repetitive upper extremity activities, correction of posture, and stretching exercises of the PM muscle by holding the shoulders in a military position (hyperabducted) or by stretching into the corner of a wall or into an open doorway. If successful, no further treatment is needed.

Surgical Treatment

If conservative measures fail, surgical PMT is indicated for partially disabling symptoms.

Technique. In the past, PMT has been performed through an infraclavicular incision. However, we have changed the incision to a 5- to 7-cm transaxillary incision about 1 cm above the bottom of the axillary hairline. The procedure is performed under local anesthesia (1% lidocaine and 0.2% ropivacaine) with heavy sedation provided by an anesthesiologist. After dividing the subcutaneous fat, blunt dissection identifies the PM muscle, which is followed deep until it is found inserting into the coracoid process. In some patients the pectoralis major and minor are fused. The coracoid process is the place to find the plane between the two muscles. Once found, the PM is isolated and divided at the coracoid process with a cautery. The end of the muscle is elevated and 2 to 3 cm of muscle excised to prevent the muscle end from attaching to the nerves of the plexus. Care is taken to not excise too much muscle for fear of injuring the pectoral nerve. The axillary neurovascular bundle is explored and any bands or ligaments of clavipectoral fascia are divided. One patient

Table 122-2 Results of Pectoralis Minor Tenotomy (PMT) as the Only Operation*

| Operation | Number of Operations | Results (%) | | |
		Good/ Excellent	Fair	Failed
Primary PMT in patients with PMS as the only diagnosis	50	86	6	8
Primary PMT in patients with combined PMS and TOS	49	37	14	49[†]
PMT for recurrent nTOS	70	74	11	15
Total	**169**			

*Follow-up time: 3 months to 2 years. Operations were performed over a period of 3 years, 2005 to 2007.
[†]Thirteen of 24 patients recorded as failures subsequently underwent scalenectomy, some with and some without first rib resection. Twelve of the 13 have had good improvement at a follow-up of 3 to 18 months.
nTOS, neurogenic thoracic outlet syndrome; PMS, pectoralis minor syndrome; PMT, pectoralis minor tenotomy; TOS, thoracic outlet syndrome.

was encountered with a Langer arch bilaterally.[62] The wound is closed and the patient discharged the same day.

Results. Between 2005 and 2007, 276 PM operations were performed. The procedures fell into five groups: PMT alone (carried out in 169 patients), PMT as the primary operation for patients with PMS alone (50 patients), PMT as the primary operation for patients with combined PMS and nTOS (49 patients), and PMT performed as the only procedure for recurrent TOS (70 patients). In addition, PMT was added as an additional procedure to accompany 80 primary TOS operations and 26 recurrent TOS operations (unpublished data).

The results with 2-month to 2-year follow-up revealed a success rate of 92% in patients with PMS alone but only 51% in those with combined PMS and nTOS. Patients with recurrent nTOS and PMS who received only PMT had a failure rate of just 15% (Table 122-2). Because follow-up times are short, longer times will be needed to determine the durability of this procedure. However, in patients with PMS alone, all failures but one were seen in the first 3 months.

Combined operations, PMT plus thoracic outlet decompression, were performed both as a primary operation and for recurrent TOS. These patients had some improvement from the PM block and significantly more improvement from the scalene block. The results to date (Table 122-3) are better than those in the past for the same operations without PM decompression.

Significance

The importance of recognizing PMS is seen in the impact that it has had on our TOS operations. In 2004, the first 100 operations performed for TOS were all TOS decompression. In 2007, of the first 100 operations performed, 46 were for TOS and 54 were for PMS. In addition, 33 of the 46 operations for TOS were accompanied by PMT. Thus, more than half of the patients seen initially for TOS were treated with the PMT procedure.

Table 122-3 Results of Pectoralis Minor Tenotomy Combined with Decompression of Thoracic Outlet Syndrome*

Operation	Number of Operations	Results (%)		
		Good/ Excellent	*Fair*	*Failed*
Primary TOS operation + PMT	80	75	12	13
Neurolysis for recurrent NTOS + PMT	26	77	12	11
Total	106			

*Follow-up time: 3 months to 2 years. Operations were over a period of 3 years, 2005 to 2007.
nTOS, neurogenic thoracic outlet syndrome; PMT, pectoralis minor tenotomy

The only group with a poor success rate was the combined PMS and nTOS group. These patients were offered the simple PMT procedure because they experienced good relief of symptoms after the PM block. Half the group succeeded in avoiding the larger TOS operation; among patients in whom PM decompression failed, none were made worse. To date, 13 of the 24 patients who failed have undergone thoracic outlet decompression, with relief in 12. Three more are awaiting surgery.

Broader Application of Pectoralis Minor Tenotomy

Because it has been shown that PMT causes no impairment of shoulder function,[63] it has been added to the initial approach in all transaxillary first rib resections, whether for nTOS or vTOS. Exposure is improved and retraction made easier by dividing rather than retracting the PM tendon. The subclavian vein can then be followed proximally until the first rib is identified. This technique helps avoid accidental removal of the second rib.

SELECTED KEY REFERENCES

Cormier JM, Amrane M, Ward A, Laurian C, Gigou F. Arterial complications of the thoracic outlet syndrome: fifty-five operative cases. *J Vasc Surg.* 1989;9:778-787.
Though 20 years old, this is still an excellent, comprehensive description of the strategy and results of managing arterial TOS.

Gage M, Parnell H. Scalenus anticus syndrome. *Am J Surg.* 1947; 73:252-268.
The uselessness of the Adson test was noted in 1947 because 50% of normal volunteers lost their pulses with this maneuver.

Machanic BI, Sanders RJ. Medial antebrachial cutaneous nerve measurements to diagnose neurogenic thoracic outlet syndrome. *Ann Vasc Surg.* 2008;22:248-254.
Description of an electrodiagnostic test that appears to be the first good objective test for neurogenic TOS and has fairly good specificity and sensitivity.

Melby SJ, Vedantham S, Narra VR, Paletta GA Jr, Khoo-Summers L, Driskill M, Thompson RW. Comprehensive surgical management of the competitive athlete with effort thrombosis of the subclavian vein. *J Vasc Surg.* 2008;47:809-821.
Good summary of the current management of subclavian vein thrombosis.

Molina JE, Hunter DW, Dietz CA. Paget-Schroetter syndrome treated with thrombolytics and immediate surgery. *J Vasc Surg.* 2007;45: 328-334.
Good summary of one current strategy for treating subclavian vein thrombosis.

Roos DB. New concepts of thoracic outlet syndrome that explain etiology, symptoms, diagnosis, and treatment. *Vasc Surg.* 1979;13: 313-321.
Classic description of transaxillary first rib resection by its originator.

Sanders RJ, Jackson CGR, Banchero N, Pearce WH. Scalene muscle abnormalities in traumatic thoracic outlet syndrome. *Am J Surg.* 1990;159:231-236.
Objective evidence of scalene muscle pathology in neurogenic TOS.

Sanders RJ, Hammond SH. Management of cervical ribs and anomalous first ribs causing neurogenic thoracic outlet syndrome. *J Vasc Surg.* 2002;36:51-56.
Largest report to date of the management of cervical ribs and the results of treatment.

Sanders RJ, Pearce WH. The treatment of thoracic outlet syndrome: a comparison of different operations. *J Vasc Surg.* 1989;10:626-634.
Though 20 years old, it is still the only report comparing transaxillary first rib resection, scalenectomy alone, and combined scalenectomy and first rib resection by the same surgeons.

REFERENCES

The reference list can be found on the companion Expert Consult Web site at *www.expertconsult.com*.

CHAPTER 123

Thoracic Outlet Syndrome: Neurogenic

Robert W. Thompson and Matt Driskill

An increasing body of experience demonstrates that excellent outcomes can be achieved by a comprehensive, multidisciplinary approach to neurogenic thoracic outlet syndrome (nTOS), including a prominent role for surgical treatment in well-selected patients.[1-3] Nonetheless, uncertainties in diagnosis and disappointing results of treatment have led some authorities to question the need for surgical management of nTOS and even to challenge whether the condition actually exists.[4-6] The purpose of this chapter is to review current understanding of the diagnosis, optimal management, and surgical techniques for nTOS. Because the vascular (arterial and venous) forms of thoracic outlet syndrome (TOS) give rise to distinct clinical syndromes and require variations in management, these conditions are covered in Chapter 124 (Thoracic Outlet Syndrome: Arterial) and Chapter 125 (Thoracic Outlet Syndrome: Venous).

ANATOMY

As shown in Figure 123-1, the anatomy of the thoracic outlet region is composed of several bony and soft tissue structures, as well as the nerves and blood vessels that pass through this area. The anatomy of the thoracic outlet is described in detail in Chapter 122 (Thoracic Outlet Syndrome: General Considerations). There are a number of important variations in these structures that may be associated with nTOS, including changes extending from gross anatomy to the microscopic structure of the scalene muscles.

Nerves in the Thoracic Outlet

The space formed by the scalene triangle is traversed by the five nerve roots arising from spinal levels C5 through T1 that make up the *brachial plexus*. Although each of these nerves can be identified as individual structures on entering the scalene triangle, they begin to fuse into the initial trunks of the brachial plexus within this space and as they pass over the first rib. The three trunks of the brachial plexus include the *upper trunk* (formed by fusion of the C5 and C6 nerve roots), the *middle trunk* (composed of the C7 nerve root), and the *lower trunk* (formed by fusion of the C8 and T1 nerve roots). Further merging and branching of these trunks outside the thoracic outlet forms the divisions, cords, and terminal nerves of the brachial plexus.

Additional nerves of surgical importance pass through the thoracic outlet, including the phrenic nerve, the long thoracic nerve, and the cervical sympathetic chain. The *phrenic nerve*

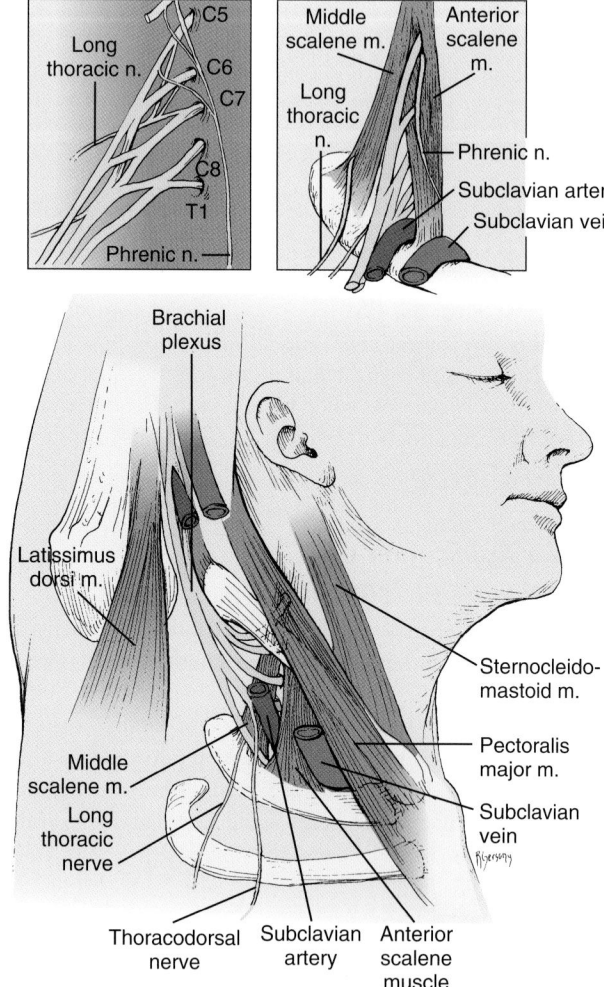

Figure 123-1 Anatomy of the thoracic outlet. The surgical anatomy of the thoracic outlet is centered on spinal nerve roots C5 through T1, which interdigitate to form the brachial plexus as they cross under the clavicle and over the first rib. The long thoracic and phrenic nerves also arise within the thoracic outlet region. The brachial plexus nerve roots pass through the scalene triangle, bordered by the anterior and middle scalene muscles on each side and the first rib at the base. The subclavian artery also courses through the scalene triangle in direct relation to the brachial plexus nerve roots. The subclavian vein crosses over the first rib immediately in front of the anterior scalene muscle before joining with the internal jugular vein to form the innominate vein. Symptoms of neurogenic thoracic outlet syndrome are often exacerbated by arm elevation, where greater strain is placed on the neurovascular structures passing through the scalene triangle. *(Redrawn from Thompson RW, Petrinec D. Surgical treatment of thoracic outlet compression syndromes. I. Diagnostic considerations and transaxillary first rib resection. Ann Vasc Surg. 1997;11: 315-323.)*

forms from the C4 nerve root at the lateral border of the anterior scalene muscle, where it also receives contributions from the C3 and C5 nerve roots. It passes lateral to medial as it descends along the anterior surface of the scalene muscle and then behind the subclavian vein into the mediastinum, where it subsequently innervates the diaphragm. Unilateral phrenic nerve palsy is thereby characterized by paralysis of the ipsilateral hemidiaphragm. The *long thoracic nerve* arises as three branches from the C5, C6, and C7 nerve roots. It passes through the belly of the middle scalene muscle, where its three components typically fuse to form a single nerve. It then descends to supply the serratus anterior muscle. Dysfunction of the long thoracic nerve results in the defect described as a "winged scapula." The *cervicodorsal sympathetic chain* consists of a series of interconnected ganglia passing between the neck and the upper part of the chest; it lies along the posterior inner aspect of the ribs. At the level of the first rib, fusion of several ganglia results in formation of the large stellate ganglion, which supplies part of the face and upper extremity. Interruption of the sympathetic chain is occasionally indicated in some patients with nTOS in whom the neurogenic symptoms have become amplified by concomitant reflex sympathetic dystrophy. Horner's syndrome occurs when the sympathetic fibers passing through the upper half of the stellate ganglion are interrupted, which results in ptosis, ipsilateral pupillary constriction, and vasodilatation with absence of facial sweating.

Musculofascial Variations

The conventional description of scalene triangle anatomy probably occurs in no more than a third of individuals, with variations in the soft tissue structure of this region being very common.[7,8] Because many of these variations occur too frequently to be termed true anomalies, it is unclear whether they add significantly to the potential for anatomic compression of neurovascular structures or they simply represent anatomic variants with little relationship to symptoms. For example, the posterior aspect of the anterior scalene muscle is frequently firm and tendinous and can potentially exert pressure on adjacent nerve roots. It may also give origin to fascial bands that extend from the posterior surface of the muscle to the thickened extrapleural fascia over the dome of the pleura (Sibson's fascia) or that circumscribe the subclavian artery. The most common muscular variation in this region is the *scalene minimus muscle*, a structure that originates within the plane of the middle scalene muscle. This muscle passes between various nerve roots of the brachial plexus and inserts on the first rib in conjunction with the anterior scalene muscle; thus, it may contribute to nerve root compression when present. Additional soft tissue variations include fascial bands that pass across or between individual nerve roots and subsequently attach to either the first rib or the extrapleural fascia. During operations for TOS it is particularly common to encounter a dense fascial band crossing over the origin of the T1 nerve root where it passes from underneath the first rib to contribute to the brachial plexus. Although the surgical

Table 123-1 Classification of Congenital Bands and Ligaments within the Scalene Triangle

Type	Description
1	Extends from the anterior tip of an incomplete cervical rib to the middle of the first thoracic rib; inserts just posterior to the scalene tubercle on the upper rib surface
2	Arises from an elongated C7 transverse process in the absence of a cervical rib and attaches to the first rib just behind the scalene tubercle; associated with extension of the transverse process of C7 beyond the transverse process of T1 on anteroposterior spine radiographs
3	Both originates and inserts on the first rib; starts posteriorly near the neck of the rib and inserts anteriorly just behind the scalene tubercle
4	Originates from a transverse process along with the middle scalene muscle and runs on the anterior edge of the middle scalene muscle to insert on the first rib; the lower nerve roots of the brachial plexus lie against this band
5	Scalene minimus muscle arises with the lower fibers of the anterior scalene muscle, runs parallel to this muscle but passes deep to it to cross behind the subclavian artery and in front of or between the nerve roots, and inserts on the first rib; any fibers passing anterior to or between the plexus but posterior to the artery
6	Scalene minimus muscle inserting onto Sibson's fascia over the cupula of the pleura instead of onto the first rib; labeled separately to distinguish its point of insertion
7	Fibrous cord running on the anterior surface of the anterior scalene muscle down to the first rib and attaching to the costochondral junction or sternum; lies immediately behind the subclavian vein, where it may be a cause of partial venous obstruction
8	Arises from the middle scalene muscle and runs under the subclavian artery and vein to attach to the costochondral junction
9	Web of muscle and fascia filling the inside posterior curve of the first rib and compressing the origin of the T1 nerve root

Adapted from Roos DB. Congenital anomalies associated with thoracic outlet syndrome. *Am J Surg*. 1976;132:771-778.

significance of these structures is not entirely clear, a spectrum of other muscular and fascial variations in this region has been described and classified by several investigators (Table 123-1), and in recent years, it has become possible to detect many of these anatomic variations with magnetic resonance imaging (MRI) techniques.[9,10]

Bony Anomalies

Cervical ribs occur in approximately 0.45% to 1.5% of the population and in up to 5% of patients with TOS. They arise in the plane of the middle scalene muscle and typically attach to the midlateral portion of the first rib; the anomalous rib may join the first rib as an immobile bony fusion or as a fully developed joint (Fig. 123-2A).[11] *Incomplete cervical ribs* may also occur and arise as a bony or cartilaginous extension from the C7 cervical vertebrae without extension to join the first rib; in some cases they are attached to the first rib only by a band of cartilage or tendinous tissue (Fig. 123-2B). *Rudimentary first ribs* are not as frequently recognized as cervical rib anomalies, and their actual incidence is unknown. These structures consist of a first rib that tends to lie higher in the neck than normal and often inserts into the second rib rather

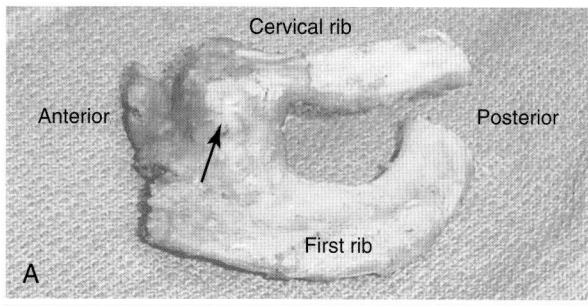

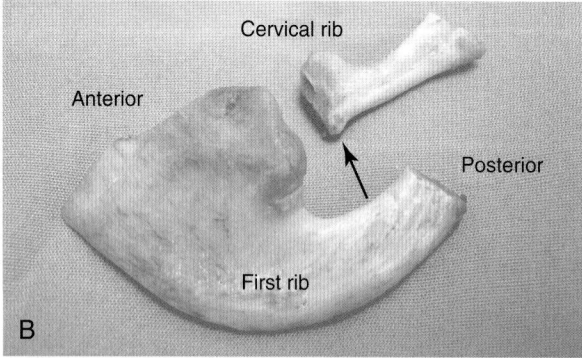

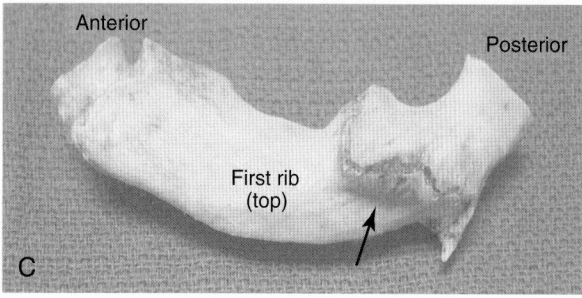

Figure 123-2 Operating room photographs depicting first rib anomalies associated with neurogenic thoracic outlet syndrome. **A,** Resected specimen of a cervical rib and attached first rib exhibiting a fully developed joint (*arrow*). **B,** Resected specimen of a cervical rib and accompanying first rib with attachment through a fibrous connection and a large exostosis on the first rib (*arrow*). **C,** Resected specimen of a first rib that contained thickened callus associated with a healed fracture site from previous trauma (*arrow*).

than the sternum. *Previous trauma* may also result in abnormalities of the first rib, such as fractures with the formation of thickened callus at the site of bony healing (Fig. 123-2C).

Histopathology

Microscopic studies of scalene muscles from patients with nTOS have consistently revealed two major abnormalities: (1) predominance of type I muscle fibers and (2) endomysial fibrosis (Fig. 123-3).[12,13] Although the anterior scalene muscle normally has an equal distribution of type I ("slow-twitch") and type II ("fast-twitch") muscle fibers, in patients with nTOS, up to 78% of the scalene muscle fibers are type I, with type II fibers exhibiting atrophy and pleomorphism. Alongside these changes there is marked thickening of the connective tissue matrix that surrounds individual muscle fibers and a twofold increase in connective tissue content in comparison to normal scalene muscles; additionally, in some cases there are mitochondrial abnormalities resembling those seen in muscular dystrophy. Because biopsy of unaffected muscles in patients with nTOS fails to reveal similar abnormalities, these changes do not represent a general myopathy but only a local abnormality. These findings are therefore thought to reflect the histopathologic changes occurring after long-standing muscle injury, sustained muscle spasm, and abnormal tissue remodeling, most likely resulting from previous trauma to the scalene muscles. These observations are therefore consistent with the frequent history of neck trauma in patients with nTOS.

■ ETIOLOGY
Predisposing Anatomic Factors

Current concepts indicate that nTOS is caused by a combination of predisposing anatomic factors and previous neck trauma. Indeed, the normal anatomy of the thoracic outlet

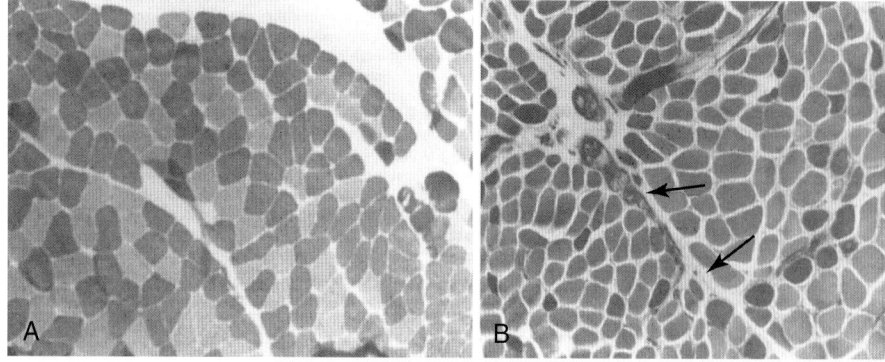

Figure 123-3 Scalene muscle histopathology showing changes consistently observed in neurogenic thoracic outlet syndrome (nTOS). Sections of the anterior scalene muscle were stained with myosin ATPase (pH 9.4) to visualize the fiber types, with type I fibers staining lightly and type II fibers staining dark (original magnification ×100). **A,** Normal muscle has an equal distribution of type I and type II fibers. **B,** Muscle from a patient with nTOS exhibits predominance of type I fibers, atrophy of type II fibers, and a significant increase in the connective tissue matrix between fibers (*arrows*). (*Redrawn from Sanders RJ. Thoracic Outlet Syndrome: A Common Sequela of Neck Injuries. Philadelphia, PA: JB Lippincott; 1991.*)

serves as a predisposing factor for the development of nTOS because the neurovascular structures that traverse this region are prone to compression even during the course of regular daily activity. Activities involving sustained or repeated elevation of the arm or vigorous turning of the neck may place additional tension on the scalene muscles, thereby potentiating any positional compression of the underlying nerve roots. This anatomic predisposition may be further increased by congenital structural variants such as scalene muscle variations, abnormal tendinous bands, or cervical rib anomalies. However, because many individuals harbor such variations in the absence of neurogenic symptoms, anatomic factors are considered a predisposing factor for nTOS rather than a distinct and separate cause, and they appear only to lower the threshold for the development of symptoms after injury.

Neck Trauma

Most patients with nTOS describe some form of previous trauma to the head, neck, or upper extremity, followed by a variable interval before the onset of progressive upper extremity symptoms.[1] The interval between injury and the onset of symptoms may range from days and weeks to several years. This frequent delay in symptoms is thought to reflect the variable time frame for scalene muscle injury to result in sustained compression and irritation of the brachial plexus nerve roots and may therefore obscure the relationship between a specific injury and the development of nTOS. In some patients the inciting injury has been long forgotten, and a history of trauma may be overlooked if not specifically sought by the examining physician. Persistent use of the upper extremity in activities that promote brachial plexus compression may further exacerbate progression of symptoms over time and result in progressive disability, and many patients do not seek medical attention until the symptoms are well advanced. Thus, it is important to recognize that low-grade repetitive trauma can also contribute to this disorder.

Repetitive Strain Injury

Over the past several decades it has become increasingly evident that not all patients with nTOS have their condition brought on by a specific traumatic event. In many cases the injury may be the result of repetitive activities that inadvertently place strain on the scalene muscles over long periods, such as prolonged work at computer keyboards. TOS occurring in this circumstance is considered to be a form of repetitive strain injury. In these cases it is also likely that age-related changes in posture (e.g., slumping of the shoulders and stooping of the neck) superimposed on congenital variations of the scalene musculature may be significant factors leading to the development of extrinsic neural compression.

Pathophysiology

nTOS is thought to develop as a result of scalene muscle trauma, the pathophysiologic response to muscle injury, and

anatomic factors predisposing to compression of the brachial plexus nerve roots as they pass through the scalene triangle. Hyperextension injury of the anterior scalene muscle probably leads to acute and chronic inflammation and a reparative process that includes fibrosis and persistent muscle spasm. Chronic changes in the scalene musculature also include fibrotic contracture and stiffening, as well as histopathologic alterations reflecting persistent muscle injury. The resulting changes in the scalene muscles probably potentiate nerve root compression and irritation, which may be exacerbated by positional effects and lead to progression of symptoms over time. Intermittent exacerbation of neurogenic symptoms may occur as a result of additional scalene muscle injury that produces local inflammation and spasm, interspersed with periods in which symptoms are quiescent. Unfortunately, knowledge of the specific pathophysiologic mechanisms leading to nTOS is limited, and there remain many gaps in our understanding of this complicated disorder.

■ CLINICAL FINDINGS

The diagnosis of nTOS rests largely on recognition of clinical patterns, with diagnostic suspicion raised by a stereotypical history and a description of symptoms characteristic of the disorder. The provisional diagnosis of nTOS is supplemented by physical examination and may be supported by a limited number of diagnostic studies. In most cases such studies are of value primarily in the exclusion of other (more common) conditions within the differential diagnosis because no single diagnostic test has a sufficiently high degree of specificity to completely prove or exclude the diagnosis of nTOS.[14]

Symptoms
Demographics

nTOS most frequently occurs in individuals between 20 and 40 years of age, and approximately 70% of affected patients are women. nTOS may arise in individuals engaged in a variety of occupational or recreational activities, most often those involving repeated use of the arm or arms in elevated positions or after a spectrum of injuries to the head, neck, or upper extremity. nTOS may also develop in patients with no apparent predisposition (i.e., no anatomic variations or history of trauma). There are no medical conditions or known inherited patterns predisposing to nTOS.

Pain and Paresthesia

The primary symptoms of nTOS include pain, dysesthesia, numbness, and weakness. These symptoms usually occur throughout the affected hand or arm without any localization to a specific peripheral nerve distribution, and they often involve different areas of the entire upper extremity. Extension of symptoms from the hand to the shoulder, neck, and upper part of the back is not infrequent, and in many patients the symptoms in the neck or upper part of the back may be perceived as the most functionally disabling. Although most patients with nTOS have symptoms affecting just one upper extremity, bilateral symptoms are not uncommon; in such cases the dominant extremity is often more symptomatic at initial evaluation, but the opposite extremity may become involved over time, perhaps as a result of compensatory overuse. The lack of distribution of symptoms into patterns referable to a single peripheral nerve and the frequent extension of symptoms to the shoulder, neck, and back allow distinction of nTOS from nerve compression disorders affecting the ulnar nerve at the elbow (cubital compression syndrome), the median nerve at the wrist (carpal tunnel syndrome), or other related conditions. Different symptomatic manifestations of nTOS may be observed, depending on the brachial plexus nerve roots that are principally involved: upper plexus disorders (nerve roots C5, C6, C7) are dominated by symptoms in the distribution of the radial and musculocutaneous nerves, whereas lower plexus disorders (nerve roots C7, C8, T1) most commonly involve the median and ulnar nerves. In many cases, however, it is not possible to draw these distinctions because of a wider distribution of symptoms.

Positional Effects

Almost all patients affected by nTOS describe reproducible exacerbation of symptoms by activities that require elevation or sustained use of the arms or hands. These activities may include simply reaching for objects overhead, lifting, prolonged typing or work at computer consoles, driving a motor vehicle, speaking on the telephone, shaving, and combing or brushing the hair. Positional effects may also be brought on by lying supine, especially when the arms are positioned overhead, and can result in pain and difficulty sleeping at night.

Headache

Headaches are a common complaint associated with nTOS.[15] They most likely occur as a result of referred pain to the occiput because of secondary spasm within the trapezius and paraspinous muscles. Headaches associated with nTOS are therefore typically occipital, whereas frontal headaches are not specifically associated with nTOS. Although nTOS and migraine headaches are often seen together, there is currently no evidence for a specific link between these conditions.

Weakness and Muscle Atrophy

Prolonged, severe extrinsic compression of peripheral nerves can result in muscle weakness and atrophy, but such findings are actually rare in patients with nTOS, probably because of the intermittent nature of nerve compression in nTOS, which produces pain and other neural symptoms but prevents permanent motor nerve dysfunction. Most commonly, hand or arm pain with use of the affected extremity may lead to the perception of weakness and cause the patient to avoid use of the arm or positions that exacerbate symptoms; this distinction should be sought during evaluation to help identify other

conditions that may be responsible for the symptoms of muscle weakness. The presence of authentic muscle weakness may therefore indicate particularly severe and long-standing compression of the brachial plexus nerve roots as a result of either nTOS or another condition.

Disability

The majority of individuals with positional complaints related to nTOS are affected to only a mild and tolerable degree. These symptoms are usually due to transient irritation of the brachial plexus with certain positions of the arm or during certain activities, and to some extent such symptoms are frequent in the normal population. There is little risk of progressive injury in these situations, and no specific intervention is warranted.

There remains a smaller subset of patients with clinically significant nTOS, however, who exhibit progressively disabling symptoms that effectively prevent them from working or carrying out simple daily activities. These patients often describe progressive disability and a long history of consultations with different physicians and partial or ineffective treatments. Such patients may have been prevented from working for a long time before consultation or may have attempted to persist in work-related activities despite ongoing neurogenic symptoms. Part of the initial assessment of a patient with nTOS is therefore concerned with assessing the extent of the patient's disability and expectations for the potential to continue or return to work. It is particularly helpful in this regard to obtain a detailed description from the patient of activities that exacerbate the symptoms associated with nTOS, as well as activities normally required in the workplace. Documentation of this assessment is often important if restrictions from work are necessary in the management of these patients and in guiding decisions about the role of surgical treatment.

Vascular Symptoms and Complex Regional Pain Syndrome

Vascular symptoms should be specifically sought in the history of patients with suspected TOS, particularly discoloration or coldness in the hands and fingers. It is important to note that ischemia is actually very unusual in such patients, whereas symptoms of vasomotor disturbance are not uncommon in those with long-standing or severe nTOS. Indeed, in some the symptoms of TOS may have progressed to resemble those of complex regional pain syndrome type I (CRPS-I; formerly known as reflex sympathetic dystrophy), with persistent vasospasm, disuse edema, and extreme hypersensitivity. The acuity of these symptoms often leads to avoidance and withdrawal from even light touch of the affected extremity. The diagnosis of CRPS-I can be supported by vascular laboratory studies revealing abnormal vasoconstrictive responses (cold pressor tests) or imaging studies of the hand microcirculation, but in most cases the diagnosis is made on clinical grounds. Identification of this condition in patients with nTOS is important because it may lead to an earlier recommendation for operative treatment and consideration of concomitant cervical sympathectomy.

When a history suggesting arterial insufficiency or thromboembolism exists, vascular laboratory studies and contrast-enhanced arteriographic imaging are necessary to exclude the presence of subclavian artery aneurysm or occlusive disease. Conversely, a history of arm swelling, cyanotic discoloration, and distended subcutaneous collaterals may indicate venous TOS secondary to obstruction of the subclavian vein, which requires contrast-enhanced venography for full evaluation. Identification of these conditions in patients with nTOS is vital because the coexistence of neurogenic and vascular forms of TOS will have an impact on the decisions and plans for surgical treatment.

Physical Examination

Physical examination is initially directed toward eliciting the degree of neurogenic disability and identifying particular factors that exacerbate painful hand and arm complaints. The range of motion of the upper extremity and lateral motion of the neck are assessed under both passive and active conditions. Pain and tenderness over the shoulder joint are evaluated as potentially being related to rotator cuff pathology, and tenderness over the trapezius muscle may indicate fibromyalgia. A thorough peripheral nerve examination is performed to exclude ulnar nerve entrapment or carpal tunnel syndrome, two conditions that may mimic the symptoms of nTOS. The base of the neck is examined to identify the extent of any local muscle spasm over the scalene triangle itself, as well as over the trapezius, pectoralis, and parascapular muscles, and to localize specific areas that reproduce the individual patient's symptom pattern on focal digital compression. The presence of "trigger points" is sought to identify specific sites where palpation re-creates the patient's typical symptoms of upper extremity pain and paresthesia. Localization of such trigger points over the scalene triangle serves to strongly re-enforce the diagnosis of nTOS.

Perhaps the most useful component of physical examination is the 3-minute elevated arm stress test ("EAST"), in which the patient is positioned with the arms elevated in a "surrender" position and asked to repetitively open and close the fists. Most patients with nTOS report a rapid onset of their typical upper extremity symptoms with EAST and are often unable to complete the exercise beyond 30 to 60 seconds. When there is no difficulty performing the 3-minute EAST, the diagnosis of nTOS is suspect and an alternative explanation for the symptoms should be sought more vigorously.

In some patients, compression of the neurovascular bundle as it passes underneath the pectoralis minor muscle tendon is a substantial factor contributing to nTOS. This situation is sometimes described as the "hyperabduction syndrome" or the "pectoralis minor syndrome" and is identified by localized tenderness and reproduction of the upper extremity neurologic symptoms on palpation over the pectoralis minor muscle. Given that pectoralis minor tenotomy may be an effective

primary or adjunctive treatment in such individuals, it is important during the initial physical examination to identify this increasingly recognized component of nTOS.

Vascular Examination

The Adson maneuver is commonly used to identify positional compression of the subclavian artery by detecting ablation of the radial pulse when the patient inspires deeply and turns the neck away from the affected extremity, with or without elevation of the arm. Although this maneuver does not specifically reveal nerve root compression, positive findings may be associated with nTOS. It is important to recognize that a positive Adson sign is also common in the asymptomatic general population. This maneuver may therefore serve to support but not prove the diagnosis of nTOS. It is equally important to recognize that negative findings of arterial compression do not exclude a diagnosis of nTOS. Most physicians experienced with TOS therefore find the Adson test to be of little specific value.

Patients with symptoms of nTOS may on occasion have vascular findings related to either arterial or venous TOS. It is important that these conditions be identified early in the evaluation because their presence may lead to specific tests and modified treatment recommendations. During physical examination, the surgeon should seek evidence of arterial compromise to the upper extremity, such as sympathetic overactivity with vasospasm, digital or hand ischemia, cutaneous ulceration or emboli, forearm claudication, or the pulsatile supraclavicular mass or bruit characteristic of a subclavian artery aneurysm. Comparison of blood pressure in each arm is also valuable to identify any evidence of arterial occlusion. Venous TOS, in contrast, may be associated with hand and arm edema, cyanosis, enlarged subcutaneous collateral veins, and early forearm fatigue in the absence of arterial compromise.

Diagnostic Tests

A wide variety of diagnostic tests and imaging studies are used for the evaluation of patients with nTOS, and most patients have had a number of such studies before consultation with the vascular surgeon. The results of specific diagnostic tests are negative or equivocal in most cases of nTOS, and no specific diagnostic test or imaging study can replace the clinical diagnosis of this condition. Thus, the principal value of the studies described in the following sections is to exclude other conditions, thereby helping strengthen the diagnosis of nTOS.

Radiography

Plain radiographs of the neck are helpful in determining whether an osseous cervical rib or an abnormally wide transverse process of the cervical vertebrae is present. Although each of these findings may solidify the diagnostic impression of TOS, neither of them is essential.

Cross-Sectional Imaging

The results of computed tomography, MRI, and other imaging examinations are usually negative in nTOS because the anatomic factors leading to intermittent or positional nerve compression are generally beyond the resolution of these studies. Even in situations in which an apparent imaging abnormality exists in the region of the scalene triangle, it is usually impossible to prove the functional importance of such abnormalities with respect to the patient's upper extremity complaints. Imaging studies are nonetheless important to exclude other conditions that could be responsible for the upper extremity symptoms, such as degenerative cervical disk or spine disease, shoulder joint pathology, or various forms of intracranial pathology.

In recent years, advances in MRI and data processing have led to higher resolution scans with three-dimensional reconstruction, along with the ability to detect localized abnormalities in nerve function (MR "neurography").[9,10,16,17] As this technique becomes used more frequently in patients with and without nTOS, there is reason to believe that it may provide an improved diagnostic tool to supplement clinical evaluation with an accurate "objective" test for this challenging problem.

Neurophysiologic Testing

Electromyography (EMG) and nerve conduction studies (NCS) are often used early in the evaluation of patients suspected of having nTOS, particularly when the symptoms are suggestive of a specific radiculopathy, a peripheral nerve syndrome, or a general myopathy. Positive results of neurophysiologic testing are therefore useful in that they point to specific conditions that must be evaluated further. Unfortunately, the results of conventional EMG/NCS are usually negative in nTOS because the nerve root compression occurs in an extremely proximal location and is intermittent and not typically associated with permanent changes in motor nerve function.[18] Negative results from these studies are nonetheless valuable in the diagnostic evaluation of some patients by helping exclude other conditions from further consideration. Positive EMG/NCS findings in patients with nTOS are a poor prognostic sign in the absence of an alternative explanation because they indicate an advanced stage of neural damage that may be unlikely to resolve despite adequate decompression. Recent evidence suggests that electrophysiologic testing of sensory nerve abnormalities may be more useful in the diagnosis of nTOS than conventional EMG/NCS. For example, Machanic and Sanders compared the response to medial antebrachial cutaneous nerve and C8 nerve root stimulation in 41 patients with a clinical diagnosis of nTOS and in 19 asymptomatic controls and reported that electrophysiologic testing had a high degree of sensitivity and specificity.[19]

Scalene Muscle Blocks

Injection of local anesthetic into the anterior scalene muscle may be used as an adjunct to the clinical diagnosis of nTOS, particularly in predicting the potential response to surgical decompression.[20] A successful scalene muscle block is indicated by relief of symptoms in the hand or arm, along with a reduction in local tenderness over the anterior scalene muscle. Injection of anesthetic to the level of the brachial plexus precludes accurate interpretation of this test because the temporary numbness and weakness in the arm will make assessment of pain relief unreliable. Although scalene muscle block is not necessary in patients with clear-cut symptoms in whom the diagnosis is not questioned, it is most useful in patients with an equivocal diagnosis of nTOS. Thus, Sanders and others have reported a strong correlation between relief of symptoms after scalene muscle block and success of surgical decompression.[20-22] A variation of scalene muscle block as a treatment of nTOS that has shown promising early results is the use of locally injected botulinum toxin.[23] However, side effects of botulinum toxin may occur early after treatment (e.g., dysphagia), the duration of beneficial effects with botulinum toxin is often limited to 3 to 6 months, and the effects of repeated treatment are diminished by the systemic immune response to the injected protein. Thus, in the absence of further studies, this approach cannot yet be generally recommended.

Angiography and Vascular Laboratory Studies

Vascular laboratory studies and angiography are not usually necessary in making the diagnosis of nTOS. However, patients with clinical features that suggest an arterial component of their disorder should undergo positional noninvasive vascular laboratory studies consisting of measurement of segmental arterial pressure, waveform analysis, and Duplex imaging, and contrast-enhanced arteriography may be necessary to completely exclude or prove the existence of a fixed arterial lesion. Similarly, patients in whom venous TOS is suspected should be studied by duplex ultrasound, and in those who have a negative duplex study but in whom the clinical findings remain suspicious for venous TOS, contrast-enhanced venography should be performed if not done previously in the context of an "effort thrombosis" event. In each case it is important to specifically alert the vascular radiologist of the need to perform positional maneuvers during radiologic examination and to consider bilateral studies if there is any suggestion of contralateral symptoms. Indeed, in patients with proven arterial or venous TOS, contrast-enhanced studies of the asymptomatic contralateral extremity are sometimes recommended.

Making the Diagnosis

Most patients suspected of having nTOS who consult a vascular surgeon have been referred to help resolve a diagnostic dilemma, especially when previous tests and consultations have resulted in uncertainty and a long list of conditions have already been considered in the diagnostic evaluation (Table 123-2). Although some of these entities can be distinguished by specific findings or tests, one is often left with a diagnosis

Table 123-2 Differential Diagnosis of Neurogenic Thoracic Outlet Syndrome

Condition	Differentiating Features
Carpal tunnel syndrome	Hand pain and paresthesias in the median nerve distribution, positive findings on nerve conduction studies
Ulnar nerve compression	Hand pain and paresthesias in the ulnar nerve distribution, positive findings on nerve conduction studies
Rotator cuff tendinitis	Localized pain and tenderness over the biceps tendon and shoulder pain on abduction; positive findings on MRI; relief from NSAIDs, local steroid injections, or arthroscopic surgery
Cervical spine strain/sprain	Post-traumatic neck pain and stiffness localized posteriorly along the cervical spine, paraspinal tenderness, relief with conservative measures over a period of weeks to months
Fibromyositis	Post-traumatic inflammation of the trapezius and parascapular muscles; tenderness, spasm, and palpable nodules over affected muscles; may coexist with TOS and persist after surgery
Cervical disk disease	Neck pain and stiffness, arm weakness, and paresthesias involving the thumb and index finger (C5-C6 disk); improvement in symptoms with arm elevation; positive findings on CT or MRI
Cervical arthritis	Neck pain and stiffness, arm or hand paresthesias infrequent, degenerative rather than post-traumatic, positive findings on spine radiographs
Brachial plexus injury	Caused by direct injury or stretch; arm pain and weakness, hand paresthesias; symptoms constant, not intermittent or positional; positive findings on neurophysiologic studies

CT, computed tomography; MRI, magnetic resonance imaging; NSAIDs, nonsteroidal anti-inflammatory drugs; TOS, thoracic outlet syndrome.

of exclusion. A surgeon recognizing nTOS should not be dissuaded by the impression that these problems are frequently associated with psychiatric overtones, dependency on pain medications, and ongoing litigation. Many patients with nTOS have suffered a progressively disabling condition at a relatively young age, without the satisfaction of diagnostic certainty or a reliable sense of prognosis. Careful evaluation can usually detect patients with strong clinical evidence of nTOS, as well as identify those most likely to respond to treatment.[24] The evaluating surgeon must therefore be willing to expend considerable time and energy to provide these patients with a thorough evaluation, detailed information, lengthy discussion, and ongoing support. The suspected nature of the condition is explained, the diagnostic and therapeutic uncertainties that surround nTOS are discussed, and an honest but reassuring outline of treatment expectations is presented. Surgeons making this effort are typically rewarded by grateful patients with renewed hope for long-awaited improvement.

■ CONSERVATIVE MANAGEMENT
Physical Therapy

Physical therapy serves as the initial treatment of almost all patients with nTOS.[25] It is important that the patient be referred to a therapist with experience, expertise, and interest in TOS because management of this condition is different from that of other disorders affecting the neck, shoulder, and upper extremity.[26] Many physical therapists do not have great experience with nTOS, and incorrect approaches to therapy can result in worsening of symptoms and premature failure of conservative management.[27]

Evaluation

The physical therapist treating a patient with nTOS outlines a specific plan for initial treatment over a 4- to 6-week period, to be followed by reassessment of progress. Initial assessment includes evaluation of posture, alignment, and movement patterns of the patient, with a specific focus on areas of impairment that may contribute to compression of the brachial plexus. Such areas include the slope of the shoulder girdle, the angle of the clavicle, the position of the scapula on the thorax, the position of the humerus in the glenoid, posturing of the head and neck, and alignment of the cervical and upper thoracic spine. The therapist also examines dynamic patterns, such as scapular mechanics and timing during upper extremity movements, as well as any changes in muscle length, strength, or recruitment that may put stress on the brachial plexus (Fig. 123-4).

Treatment

The therapist uses the results of individually based assessment to help educate patients on specific faults that may be contributing to their condition, instruct them in an exercise program, and possibly initiate the use of external devices, such as bracing or taping, to take stress off the anatomic compression sites.[28] The principal areas of anatomic compression addressed include the scalene triangle, the costoclavicular space, and the area between the pectoralis minor and the coracoid process. Additionally, scapular mechanics may be at a disadvantage in patients with nTOS and lead to additional stress with overhead motion. Treatment is focused on correcting the impairments in posture and movement that may be contributing to the physical stress and thereby causing or exacerbating symptoms.[29] Particularly in patients with nTOS, the therapist directs efforts to correct the faults in movement that contribute to compression, traction, and stress on the brachial plexus, including daily postures, work duties, and hobbies that may be contributing to the poor posture and disordered movement patterns. The initial goals of physical therapy are therefore to maintain and improve range of motion of the neck and affected upper extremity by using a combination of passive and assisted exercises.[30-32] In particular, exercises designed to relax and stretch the scalene muscle are used along with hydrotherapy, massage, and other techniques. These efforts may be accompanied by the use of nonsteroidal anti-inflammatory agents, muscle relaxants, and non-narcotic pain medications, as needed. Once initial improvement has been achieved, subsequent effort can be focused on

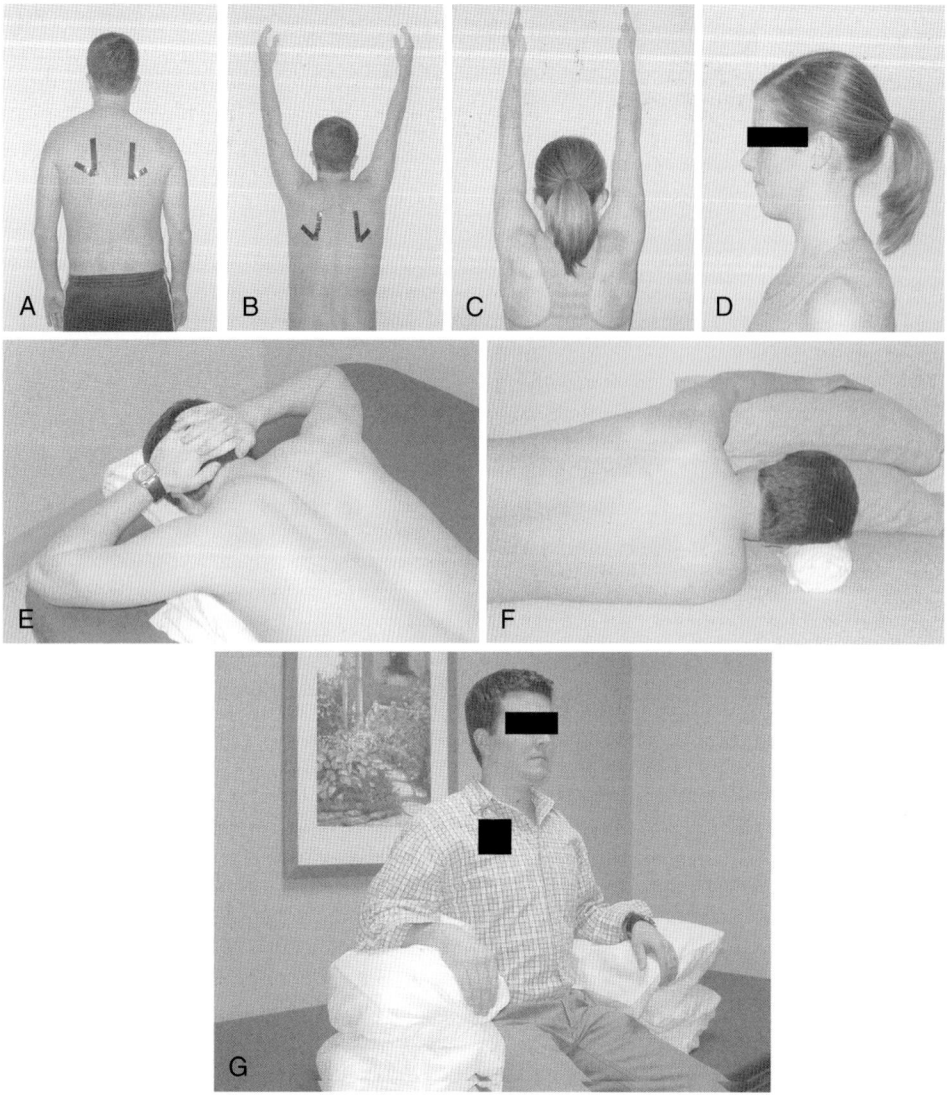

Figure 123-4 Physical therapy for neurogenic thoracic outlet syndrome. **A,** An example of postural assessment, including scapular depression with an increased slope of the right shoulder girdle. **B,** Implementing an exercise to improve a scapular depression fault. **C,** Upper trapezius muscle recruitment while standing facing a wall. **D,** Addressing cervical spine alignment. **E,** Strengthening the middle trapezius musculature. **F,** Exercises addressing overhead mechanics initiated in a gravity-lessened position. **G,** Sitting with the arms supported helps take weight off the shoulder girdle.

strengthening the muscles of posture and increasing achievable levels of activity.

Results

After the initial course of physical therapy, the physician reassesses the progress made and outlines plans for future treatment. Most patients with mild symptoms of nTOS or those in whom therapy has been started early after the onset of symptoms will exhibit significant improvement. Therapy is then continued in the expectation that continued benefits will preclude the need to consider surgical treatment. Although in our experience this outcome is achieved in only 20% to 30% of patients referred for management of nTOS,

the proportion of patients responding to conservative treatment is much higher in a more general population.[33] If progress with the initial course of conservative management has been unsatisfactory, the basis for the diagnosis of nTOS is reviewed and any further testing thought to be appropriate is carried out. When the patient has not responded sufficiently to conservative management and the physician is confident of the diagnosis of nTOS, surgical treatment is considered.[34] Even when this decision appears predictable at the time of the initial visit, helping to form an established relationship between the patient and physical therapist is a valuable first step in treatment because physical therapy and rehabilitation will remain an important part of patient care after surgery.

■ SURGICAL TREATMENT
Historical Background

The first operations for thoracic outlet compression were focused on the treatment of subclavian artery aneurysms in patients with a cervical rib, as described by Coote in 1861.[35] By the turn of the century, "cervical rib syndrome" was widely recognized, and in 1927 Adson and Coffey described the use of anterior scalenotomy for the treatment of this condition, including symptomatic patients without a cervical rib anomaly.[36] The term "thoracic outlet syndrome" was introduced by Peet and colleagues in 1956,[37] and in the 1960s several new operative approaches to TOS were described, including posterior thoracotomy (Clagett) and transaxillary first rib resection (Roos).[38,39] Although transaxillary first rib resection became popular and was used widely during the 1970s, disenchantment arose when the results were found to be no better than those of scalenectomy and when a national survey indicated a significant incidence of permanent nerve injuries after this operation.[22,40] It also became appreciated that symptomatic recurrences after transaxillary first rib resection often involved reattachment of the unresected scalene muscle to the remaining end of the first rib or adjacent tissues, which led to diminished enthusiasm for first rib resection and a re-emphasis on alternative operative approaches to include more complete scalene muscle resection.[41] Combined use of the supraclavicular and transaxillary approaches was reported in 1984 by Qvarfordt and coauthors,[42] followed by further description of the supraclavicular approach by Sanders and Raymer and by Reilly and Stoney.[43,44] During the past decade the supraclavicular approach appears to have become the most commonly used approach in current practice. Although a number of other operative techniques for thoracic outlet decompression have also been described, this section will focus on the transaxillary and supraclavicular approaches.

With regard to selection of the operative approach, it is now generally accepted that nTOS may arise from compression of the brachial plexus nerve roots at several different levels by different etiologic factors, not solely as a consequence of bony deformation by the first rib. Numerous soft tissue anomalies within the thoracic outlet have been described and classified, each of which can give rise to symptomatic neural compression. Significant factors playing a role in this process appear to include scalene muscle injury with spasm, scarring, and fibrotic inflammatory reactions surrounding the brachial plexus nerve roots, which may also be associated with pathologic changes in the scalene musculature. Current approaches to surgical treatment must take each of these potential contributing factors into account when selecting the optimal treatment for individual patients.

Transaxillary Approach

The primary advantages of transaxillary first rib resection include a relatively limited field of operative dissection, a cosmetically placed skin incision, and sufficient exposure to reliably accomplish resection of the anterolateral first rib. This approach also makes it possible to achieve at least partial resection of the anterior scalene muscle, as well as identification and removal of most anomalous ligaments and fibrous bands that may be associated with TOS. Disadvantages of the transaxillary approach include incomplete exposure of the structures composing the scalene triangle, difficulty achieving complete anterior and middle scalenectomy or brachial plexus neurolysis, and the necessity for first rib resection in all cases. This approach is also limited when vascular reconstruction is needed, and in such cases the addition of a separate incision or repositioning of the patient is required.

Under general anesthesia, the patient is positioned supine with the back of the table raised about 30 degrees. A small towel pack is placed behind the shoulder to elevate the affected side. The arm is prepared circumferentially and wrapped in a stockinette, and the sterile field includes the neck, upper part of the chest, and posterior aspect of the shoulder to the scapula. The arm is not placed on a table or crossbar; rather, it is held and positioned by a reliable, flexible, and sturdy assistant (Fig. 123-5).

A transverse skin incision is made at the lower border of the axillary hairline and extended from the anterior border of the latissimus dorsi to the lateral edge of the pectoralis major (see Fig. 123-5). This incision is carried through subcutaneous tissue directly to the chest wall, with blunt dissection used to establish a plane extending to the apex of the axilla. The long thoracic, thoracodorsal, and second intercostobrachial nerves are identified near the chest wall to avoid direct injury. Excessive elevation of the arm (unique to transaxillary exposure) is a potential mechanism of injury to the second inter-

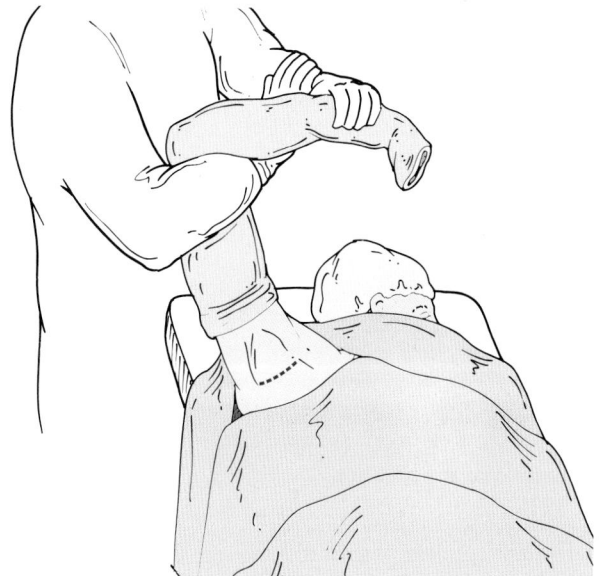

Figure 123-5 Positioning for transaxillary first rib resection. With the arm carefully elevated by a reliable assistant, the initial skin incision is made at the lower edge of the axillary hairline. (*Redrawn from Thompson RW, Petrinec D. Surgical treatment of thoracic outlet compression syndromes. I. Diagnostic considerations and transaxillary first rib resection. Ann Vasc Surg. 1997;11:315-323.*)

costobrachial cutaneous nerve that can result in postoperative pain and numbness along the medial aspect of the upper part of the arm. The first rib is typically palpable at the upper reaches of the areolar tissue plane along the chest wall. By using a Deaver retractor to gently lift the subcutaneous tissue and axillary contents away from the chest wall, the first rib is more clearly exposed in the upper aspect of the wound. It is necessary to carefully lift the arm to facilitate this exposure, both at this stage and throughout the remainder of the procedure, and the operating surgeon should use a fiberoptic headlight to properly illuminate the operative field.

The exposure obtained during the transaxillary approach is generally limited to the operating surgeon. It is therefore important that the surgeon be constantly aware of how the assistants are positioned and where the retractors are located with respect to the nerve roots and blood vessels. To avoid serious injury, the blades of the retractors must not apply excessive traction to the neurovascular structures visible above the first rib. In addition to the nerve roots of the brachial plexus, proper attention must be directed to avoiding traction on the long thoracic nerve, which exits the plane between the middle and posterior scalene muscles before coursing over the first rib to the serratus anterior muscle. Periodic inspection

of the retractors along with relief for the assistants is recommended and can be accomplished as a staged approach to the operation as described by Machleder.[46]

Once the first rib is sufficiently exposed, the subclavian vein and artery are identified along with the intervening anterior scalene muscle (Fig. 123-6A). These structures are carefully dissected such that the anterior scalene tendon can be encircled with a right-angle clamp just above its insertion onto the scalene tubercle of the first rib, which is typically palpable as a slight bony prominence. The anterior scalene muscle is exposed over several centimeters superior to the first rib, and while taking care to avoid the phrenic nerve, the muscle is divided with scissors at the highest level feasible. The importance of resecting a portion of the scalene muscle rather than simply dividing it at the level of the first rib itself has been underscored by analysis of the factors causing recurrent TOS.

The soft tissues attaching to the inferior and medial borders of the first rib are progressively divided with scissors, beginning with the attachments medial to the subclavian vein (the subclavius muscle tendon and the costosternal and costoclavicular ligaments). A periosteal elevator is used to scrape the inferior border of the rib, including underneath the rib

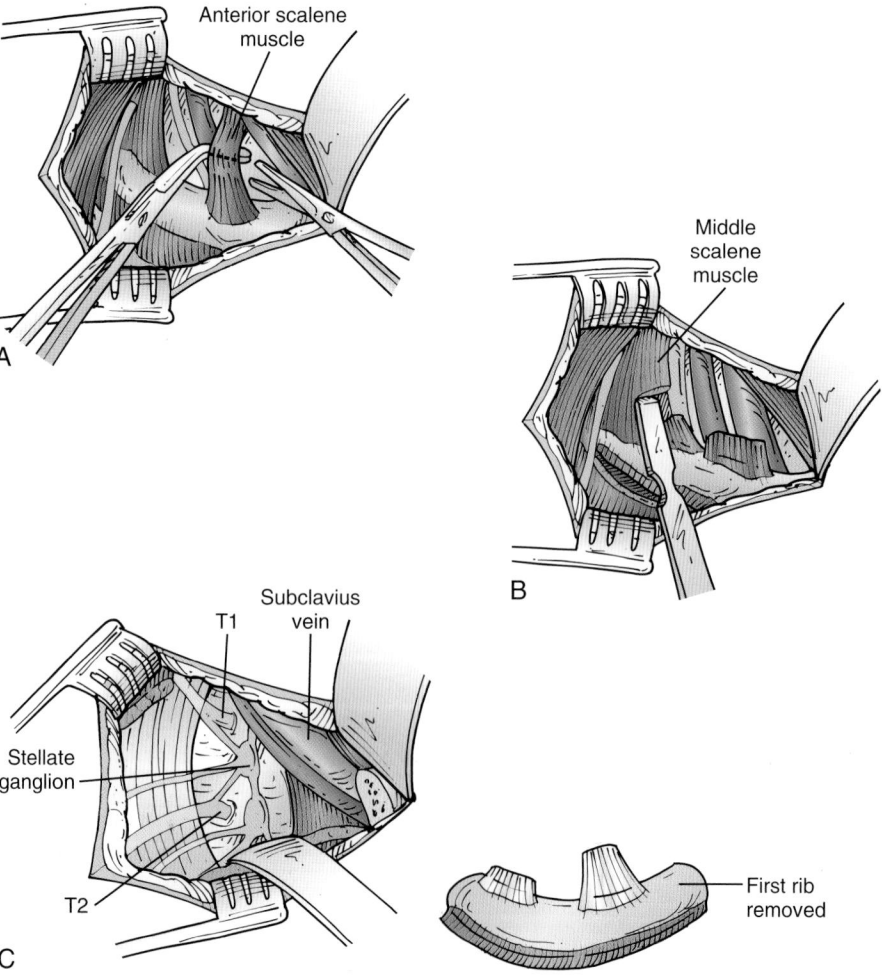

Figure 123-6 Transaxillary first rib resection. **A,** Transaxillary division of the anterior scalene muscle. The tendinous insertion of the anterior scalene muscle onto the first rib is elevated with a right-angle clamp and divided with scissors. **B,** Detachment of the middle scalene muscle. After the intercostal attachments to the first rib are divided, a periosteal elevator is used to detach the middle and posterior scalene muscles. Injury to the proximal portion of the long thoracic nerve is prevented by staying directly on the rib. **C,** Removal of the first rib. The anterior and posterior aspects of the first rib are divided, with the operative specimen including the resected portion of the anterior scalene muscle and the site of attachment of the middle scalene muscle. (*Redrawn from Thompson RW, Petrinec D. Surgical treatment of thoracic outlet compression syndromes. I. Diagnostic considerations and transaxillary first rib resection.* Ann Vasc Surg. *1997;11:315-323.*)

from the vantage point of the exposure used. The intercostal muscle is fully divided and the parietal pleura is pushed away from the deep aspect of the rib by blunt dissection. The middle scalene muscle is detached from the superior surface of the rib, posterior to the brachial plexus nerve roots (Fig. 123-6B). Although the proximal aspect of the long thoracic nerve is not directly visualized during this maneuver, injury to this nerve must be prevented to avoid postoperative serratus anterior muscle weakness. Such injury is best prevented by keeping the periosteal elevator directly on the rib during detachment of the scalene muscle and consequently avoiding any tendency to stray laterally where the long thoracic nerve can be easily injured. The long thoracic nerve is thereby gently pushed away from the rib indirectly as the middle scalene muscle is detached, which effectively protects it despite the lack of direct visualization. Once the posterior surface of the first rib is exposed and the T1 nerve root is in full view to protect it from injury, a bone-cutting instrument is carefully applied across the neck of the rib. The lateral portion of the divided rib is pulled downward and its anterior aspect is cut in similar fashion, just medial to the subclavian vein at the costochondral junction. The first rib is then fully detached and removed from the operative field (Fig. 123-6C). A bone rongeur is used to trim the remaining ends of the bone to a smooth surface well beyond the neurovascular structures. With an additional amount of extrapleural dissection, the same exposure can be used to perform adjunctive cervical sympathectomy for patients with nTOS complicated by CRPS.

Any additional soft tissue bands found to be crossing the brachial plexus nerve roots are sought and carefully divided, particularly those that may insert on Sibson's fascia, the thickened aspect of the apical pleural surface. After hemostasis is achieved, the wound is irrigated and the lung is inflated to detect any breaks in the pleural lining. If small air bubbles are observed during positive pressure ventilation or if the irrigation fluid appears to be lost into the pleural space, a small chest tube may be placed through a separate wound. The incisional wound is closed in two layers after placing a small closed suction drain in the operative field.

Supraclavicular Approach

The *supraclavicular approach* carries the advantage of wider exposure of all anatomic structures associated with thoracic outlet compression. It permits complete resection of the anterior and middle scalene muscles, as well as brachial plexus neurolysis with direct visualization of all five nerve roots. In many cases symptomatic relief of nTOS can be achieved by extended scalenectomy without the need for first rib resection, an option permitted by the supraclavicular approach. This approach also allows resection of cervical ribs, anomalous first ribs, or the normal first rib. A further advantage is that all forms of vascular reconstruction can also be accomplished through supraclavicular exposure; although removal of the anteromedial portion of the first rib and distal control of the vessels may require the addition of a second infracla-

vicular incision, this is performed without the need for repositioning the patient. The balance of advantages and disadvantages between the supraclavicular and the transaxillary approaches has now led many groups to prefer the supraclavicular approach to TOS, with some adopting a highly selective approach in which resection of the first rib is reserved solely for patients with vascular complications.[45]

Under general anesthesia, the patient is positioned supine with the head of the bed elevated 30 degrees. The hips and knees are flexed and the neck is extended and turned to the opposite side. The neck, upper part of the chest, and upper extremity are prepared into the field with the arm wrapped in a stockinette and then held comfortably across the abdomen. This allows arm movement through an extended range of motion during the operation, which may be necessary to assess any residual neurovascular compression after scalenectomy. A transverse skin incision is made two fingerbreadths above the clavicle, beginning at the lateral border of the sternocleidomastoid muscle (Fig. 123-7A). This incision is carried through the platysma muscle layer to expose the scalene fat pad. Several supraclavicular cutaneous nerves cross the operative field in this region. Although division of these sensory nerves results in postoperative numbness and dysesthesia below the clavicle, when necessary, division of these small cutaneous branches does not appear to produce significant problems.

The scalene fat pad is mobilized beginning at the lateral border of the internal jugular vein. As this tissue plane is entered, the fat pad is progressively dissected off the anterior surface of the anterior scalene muscle and reflected laterally (Fig. 123-7B). Within the investing fascia of the muscle the phrenic nerve is identified coursing in a lateral-to-medial direction. The inferior and superior attachments of the scalene fat pad are divided between ligatures to allow full exposure of the anterior scalene muscle. Lateral retraction of the scalene fat pad then permits exposure of the underlying roots of the brachial plexus.

The anterior scalene muscle is dissected while taking special effort to avoid excessive traction on the phrenic nerve (Fig. 123-8A). The C5 and C6 roots of the brachial plexus and the subclavian artery are observed at the lateral edge of the anterior scalene, and care is taken to avoid injury to these structures during mobilization of the anterior scalene muscle. The proximal subclavian artery must also be well visualized and protected at the medial edge of the scalene muscle. After circumferential mobilization of the anterior scalene muscle to its site of attachment to the first rib, a finger or right-angle clamp is passed behind the muscle, and the muscle tendon is sharply divided at its insertion (Fig. 123-8B). This is done under direct vision with curved scissors rather than the cautery. There may be additional slips of muscle or tendon that must be divided more posteriorly, including direct attachments of the muscle to the thickened pleural lining behind the rib itself.

Once the insertion of the anterior scalene muscle has been divided, the muscle is lifted superiorly to detach it from the additional structures underneath, including the pleural apex,

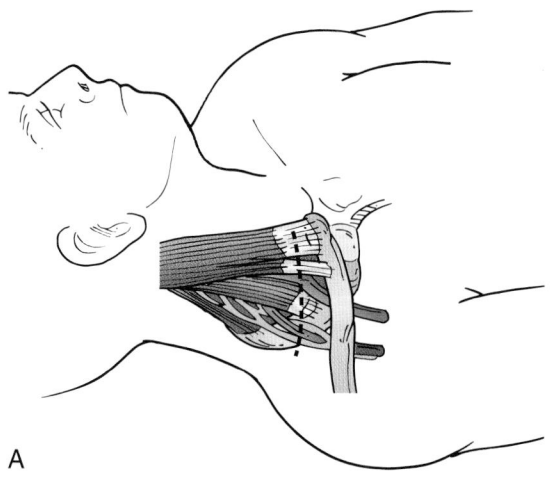

A

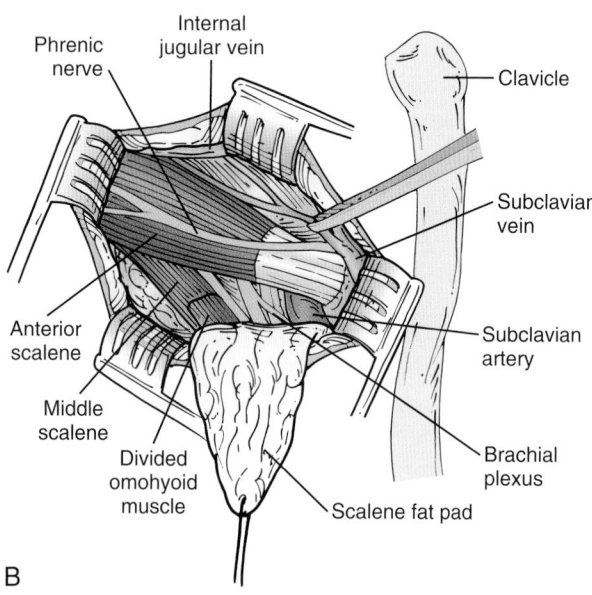

B

Figure 123-7 Positioning for supraclavicular thoracic outlet decompression. **A,** A transverse skin incision is made two fingerbreadths above the clavicle to obtain full exposure of the structures associated with the scalene triangle. **B,** The scalene fat pad is mobilized laterally to expose the underlying anterior scalene muscle, and the phrenic nerve is identified and protected. The omohyoid muscle is divided. The subclavian artery and the upper roots of the brachial plexus are identified behind the lateral edge of the anterior scalene muscle. (*Redrawn from Thompson RW, Petrinec D. Surgical treatment of thoracic outlet compression syndromes. I. Diagnostic considerations and transaxillary first rib resection. Ann Vasc Surg. 1997;11:315-323.*)

the subclavian artery, and the brachial plexus nerve roots (Fig. 123-8C). This dissection is carried superiorly to the level of the scalene muscle origin on the transverse process of the sixth cervical vertebra. Great care must be taken to avoid irretrievable neural injury while removing muscle fibers interdigitating with the proximal roots of the upper brachial plexus.

The entire anterior scalene is then removed and sent to the neuromuscular pathology laboratory.

After anterior scalenectomy and removal of any scalene minimus fibers, each of the nerve roots contributing to the brachial plexus is identified and meticulously dissected free of inflammatory scar tissue (Fig. 123-8D). Moderately dense fibrotic tissue encasing the nerve roots is not uncommon in patients with nTOS; because this scar tissue may contribute to nerve root compression, irritation, and neurogenic symptoms, failure to perform adequate neurolysis may be one cause of persistent symptoms. During the course of this dissection it is also important to ensure full mobility of the upper aspect of roots C5 and C6, which might remain entrapped by any residual scalene muscle or other fibrous tissue at the apex of the scalene triangle. Similarly, the origin of the T1 nerve root may be compressed by the posterior neck of the first rib. Relief from this source of nerve compression requires adequate visualization of the proximal first rib to achieve complete nerve root mobility. This aspect of the operation is not complete until each nerve root from C5 to T1 is completely dissected throughout its course in the operative field.

Osseous cervical ribs or their soft tissue counterparts occur within the same plane as the middle scalene muscle. Although the middle scalene muscle lies posterior to the roots of the brachial plexus, in some cases its insertion on the first rib may occur as far anteriorly as the scalene tubercle (the site of attachment of the anterior scalene muscle). The composition of the middle scalene muscle may also be firm and tendinous in this region, thereby serving as another potential source of nerve root compression and irritation. The attachment of the middle scalene muscle is divided from the first rib with a periosteal elevator or curved Mayo scissors and the dissection extended to a point posterior to the brachial plexus nerve roots (Fig. 123-8E). If a cervical rib is present in the plane of the middle scalene muscle, it may also be detached from the first rib at this time. It is important to note the separation between the middle scalene and posterior scalene muscles, as defined by the oblique course of the long thoracic nerve. Muscle tissue anterior to this nerve is detached along the plane delineated by the long thoracic nerve while leaving the nerve intact. To avoid motor dysfunction of apposition of the scapula to the chest wall, it is also important to recognize that the long thoracic nerve may be represented by two or three branches at this level rather than a single nerve as often described.

After resection of the anterior and middle scalene muscles and completion of a thorough brachial plexus neurolysis, an intraoperative decision is made regarding the potential role of the first rib in neurovascular compression. The surgeon's finger is placed alongside the subclavian artery and brachial plexus nerve roots while the arm is elevated through a normal range of motion at the shoulder to allow any residual compression to be readily detected during arm elevation. In many patients with nTOS there is little residual compression by the first rib after adequate scalenectomy, and in these cases retention of the first rib may be considered. In contrast, the first rib should be removed if there is any question that it might

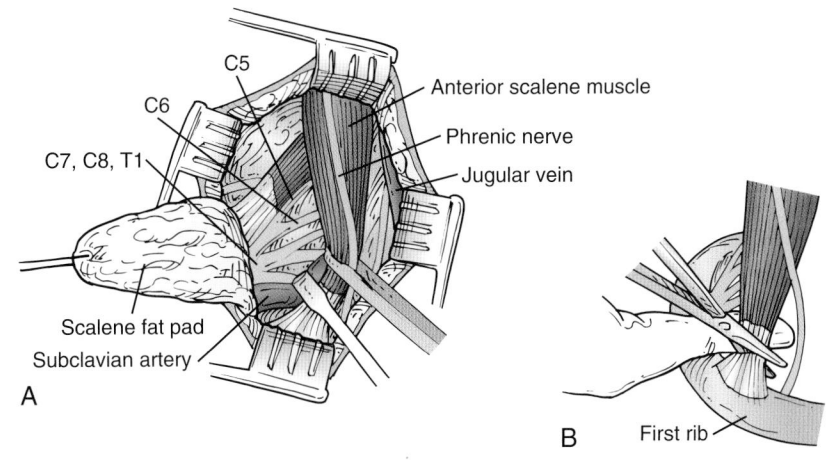

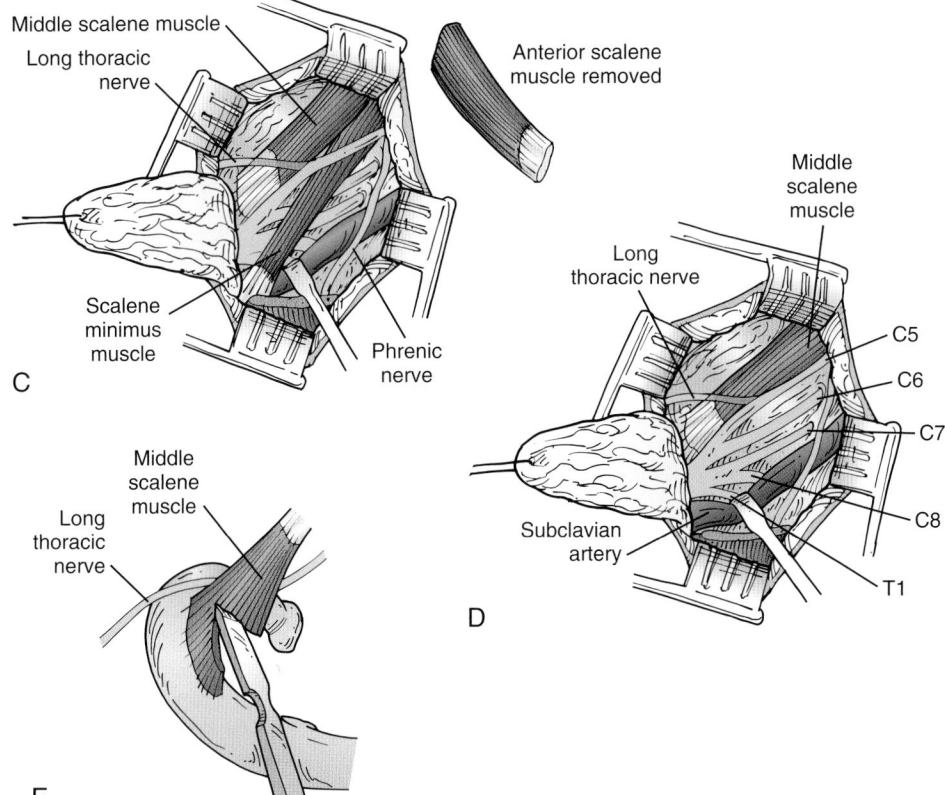

Figure 123-8 Supraclavicular scalenectomy and neurolysis. **A,** The anterior scalene muscle is circumferentially mobilized from the underlying subclavian artery and roots of the brachial plexus. **B,** The insertion of the anterior scalene muscle on the first rib is sharply divided with scissors, and the surgeon's finger protects the subclavian artery and roots of the brachial plexus. **C,** The anterior scalene muscle is reflected superiorly and dissected free of underlying structures to the level of its origin. Any muscle fibers passing between the upper nerve roots of the brachial plexus are also removed, including the scalene minimus muscle, if present. **D,** Complete dissection of the brachial plexus nerve roots from C5 to T1 is accomplished by resection of all perineural scar tissue. **E,** The middle scalene muscle is detached from the first rib with a periosteal elevator while taking care to protect the long thoracic nerve. All muscle tissue lying anterior to the long thoracic nerve is resected. *(Redrawn from Thompson RW. Treatment of thoracic outlet syndromes and cervical sympathectomy. In Lumley JSP, Hoballah JJ, eds. Springer Surgery Atlas Series: Vascular Surgery. London: Springer-Verlag; 2009:103-118.)*

contribute to residual neurovascular compression, as well as in all patients with arterial or venous TOS.

First rib resection is readily accomplished through the supraclavicular approach given the exposure already achieved at this stage of the operation (Fig. 123-9). Any remaining fibers of the middle scalene muscle are detached from their insertion on the top of the posterior first rib with a periosteal elevator. This dissection is always performed under direct vision to protect the C8 and T1 nerve roots. Using a fingertip covered with gauze, the pleural membrane is bluntly dissected away from the inferior aspect of the first rib. The intercostal muscle attachments to the first rib are divided with a perios-

teal elevator to relieve the posterior and lateral aspects of the first rib of all soft tissue attachments, and any remaining attachments are divided along the anterolateral aspect of the rib up to the scalene tubercle. The brachial plexus nerve roots are displaced anteriorly to expose the posterior neck of the rib. While the assistant protects the nerve roots with a fingertip, a rib cutter is inserted over the neck of the isolated first rib and applied. A Kerrison bone rongeur is used to resect additional amounts of bone as needed to ensure that the end of the rib will not impinge on the lower nerve roots and to create a smooth surface on the posterior stump of the first rib. The proximal portion of the rib is displaced inferiorly to open

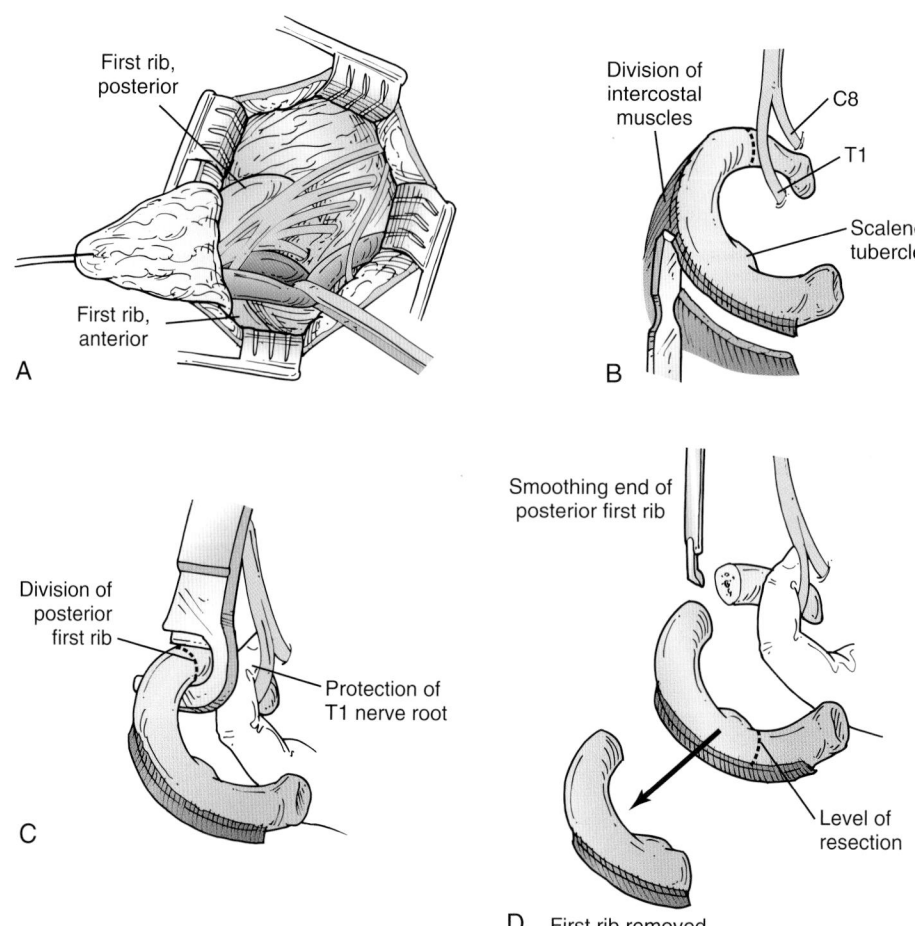

Figure 123-9 Supraclavicular first rib resection. **A,** The first rib is shown in relation to the brachial plexus roots and the subclavian artery. **B,** The intercostal attachments to the first rib are divided. **C,** After division of the anterior first rib just proximal to the level of the scalene tubercle, the brachial plexus is reflected anteriorly to visualize the posterior neck of the rib. The T1 nerve root is displaced by a finger while the neck of the rib is divided. The anterior rib is cut and the specimen is removed from the field. **D,** The remaining posterior edge of the rib is remodeled to a smooth surface with a Kerrison bone rongeur while ensuring that there is no residual impingement on the T1 nerve root. The anterior edge of the rib is similarly remodeled to a smooth surface (not shown). *(Redrawn from Thompson RW. Treatment of thoracic outlet syndromes and cervical sympathectomy. In Lumley JSP, Hoballah JJ, eds.* Springer Surgery Atlas Series: Vascular Surgery. *London: Springer-Verlag; 2009:103-118.)*

the anterior costoclavicular space, and a bone cutter is inserted at a level immediately medial to the scalene tubercle to divide the proximal rib. The first rib is then extracted from the operative field and discarded, and the proximal end of the rib is remodeled to a smooth surface with a bone rongeur.

On completion of the operation, several sheets of a bioresorbable hyaluronate membrane (Seprafilm, Genzyme Biosurgery, Cambridge, MA) are placed within the wound to limit the potential for postoperative scarring. One sheet is placed posterior to the brachial plexus nerve roots, a second is used to wrap the individual nerve roots, and a third is placed anteriorly, between the surface of the brachial plexus and the scalene fat pad. A closed-suction drain is placed in the supraclavicular field, and the scalene fat pad is reapproximated over the brachial plexus before wound closure.

Pectoralis Minor Tenotomy

When there is evidence on physical examination of brachial plexus nerve root irritation at the level of the subpectoral space ("hyperabduction syndrome"), pectoralis minor tenotomy may be added to either transaxillary or supraclavicular decompression to ensure thorough relief of the nerve compression. Pectoralis minor tenotomy may also be performed

as an isolated procedure when this site is the dominant location of nerve compression symptoms or when localized findings are present in patients who have previously undergone thoracic outlet decompression by other approaches (persistent or recurrent nTOS). As shown in Figure 123-10, a short vertical incision is made in the lateral infraclavicular space adjacent to the deltopectoral groove. The lateral edge of the pectoralis major muscle is gently retracted medially, and the underlying pectoralis minor muscle is encircled. The pectoralis minor tendon is then divided under direct vision, immediately inferior to its insertion on the coracoid process.

Cervical Sympathectomy

Patients with disabling nTOS may at times be seen with sympathetic overactivity resulting in painful vasospasm, delayed healing of digital skin lesions, and CRPS. In these situations the primary procedure performed for thoracic outlet decompression can be accompanied by cervical sympathectomy. This step adds little to the procedure itself and may be of substantial benefit with respect to alleviating vasospastic complaints or facilitating healing of digital lesions. The cervical sympathetic chain is first identified by palpation through the supraclavicular wound as a rubber band–like structure

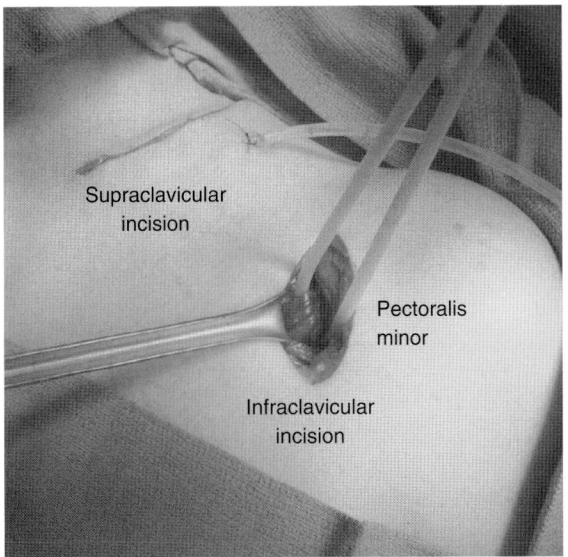

Figure 123-10 Pectoralis minor tenotomy. Operative view of the left lateral infraclavicular incision used to isolate the pectoralis minor muscle tendon, performed in conjunction with a supraclavicular thoracic outlet decompression procedure.

passing vertically over the neck of the first or second rib. The sympathetic chain is elevated with a vagotomy nerve hook and mobilized to the level of the third rib by sharply dividing its lateral rami. The stellate ganglion is also identified just above the level of the first rib. After placing metal clips at each end of the sympathetic chain it is divided sharply and removed; to reduce the incidence of Horner's syndrome, the proximal extent of sympathetic resection is marked by the lower half of the stellate ganglion.

Postoperative Management

An upright chest radiograph is performed in the recovery room after all thoracic outlet decompression procedures (Fig. 123-11), in part to detect residual pneumothorax or pleural fluid, which may be present in up to 10% of patients. These small air or fluid collections are carefully observed with the expectation of spontaneous resolution; although transthoracic aspiration may be necessary for a large or expanding pneumothorax, we have not found this necessary. Postoperative pain relief is provided by intravenous opioids until adequate control can be achieved with oral medications, and we

Section **16** **Upper Extremity Arterial Disease**

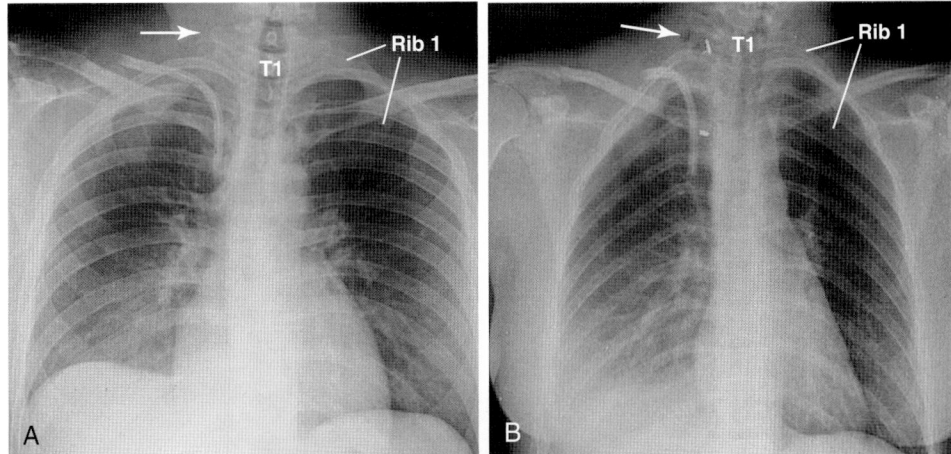

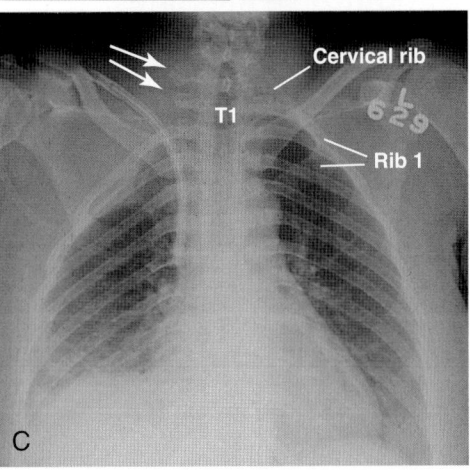

Figure 123-11 Postoperative chest radiographs **A,** Chest radiograph after right supraclavicular decompression. The closed-suction drain is seen extending from the neck into the pleural apex, and the posterior end of the resected first rib is indicated (*arrow*). **B,** Chest radiograph after right supraclavicular decompression with an adjunctive cervical sympathectomy for reflex sympathetic dystrophy. The posterior end of the resected first rib is indicated (*arrow*), with the extent of sympathetic chain resection demonstrated by the position of radiodense clips at the first and fourth thoracic levels. **C,** Chest radiograph after right supraclavicular decompression with resection of the cervical and first ribs. The posterior ends of the resected cervical and first ribs are indicated (*arrows*).

routinely prescribe oral narcotics, muscle relaxants, and non-steroidal anti-inflammatory agents for at least the first 2 weeks after surgery. The closed-suction drain is removed 3 days after surgery unless persistent lymphatic fluid is present, in which case the patient is discharged and the drain is removed in the outpatient office once the leak has subsided. Secondary procedures to control a persistent lymph leak are rarely necessary.

There are no strict restrictions with respect to use of the upper extremity after surgery, but patients are advised to avoid excessive reaching overhead or heavy lifting. Physical therapy is resumed as soon as feasible, usually on discharge from the hospital or in the first postoperative week. Patients are cautioned against activities that can result in muscle strain, spasm, and significant pain in the trapezius and other neck muscles, and a gradual return to use of the upper extremity is encouraged. The majority of patients resume fairly regular activity within several weeks after surgery and, in most cases, are permitted a cautious return to light-duty work by 4 to 6 weeks. Work restrictions are recommended to prevent heavy activity during the early stages of return to work, particularly to avoid excessive use of the upper extremity by lifting or repetitive activities that may contribute to postoperative complaints. It is important to recognize that patients with long-standing nTOS often have residual symptoms of dysesthesia, numbness, or other complaints that may not be eliminated by thoracic outlet decompression; although these symptoms may be tolerable, the surgeon must provide continuing support and reassurance during the period of recovery and rehabilitation. Physical therapy is continued as long as necessary to allow the patient to return to an optimal level of function, and patients are seen at least yearly to assess the long-term results of operative intervention.

SURGICAL COMPLICATIONS

Nerve Injuries

The most serious complications associated with thoracic outlet decompression are injuries to the brachial plexus nerve roots. Though infrequent, the rate of nerve injuries reported to occur after transaxillary first rib resection was one of the factors leading many to diminish their enthusiasm for this procedure in the 1980s.[22,40] Such injuries can occur through both direct and indirect mechanisms; limited exposure during the transaxillary approach can leave the upper nerve roots susceptible, and traction on the brachial plexus during retraction can also injure the nerve roots in a manner not recognized until after the operation. Although these factors are decreased in procedures done through the supraclavicular route given the improved exposure of the nerve roots, brachial plexus palsies can still occur as a result of retraction. In the absence of direct injury, however, these complications are temporary and will usually resolve within weeks to several months of the operation.

Phrenic nerve dysfunction is relatively common after supraclavicular thoracic outlet decompression and occurs in

approximately 10% of patients. This is again most often associated with retraction of the nerve for anterior scalenectomy and results in temporary diaphragmatic paralysis. This finding is often not perceived by the patient given adequate compensation by the contralateral diaphragm, and the diagnosis may require chest fluoroscopy. Although most patients with phrenic nerve palsy are asymptomatic and exhibit respiratory difficulty only with extremes of exertion, patients with underlying lung disease before surgery may have more significant symptoms. Even though these symptoms will typically resolve within weeks to months of surgery after recovery of phrenic nerve and diaphragmatic function, in some cases full recovery may take up to 10 months.

In patients with bilateral TOS requiring surgery on the contralateral side, it is essential to ensure that any degree of phrenic nerve paresis has completely resolved before the second operation. Although unilateral paralysis of the diaphragm is generally innocuous and asymptomatic in most patients, it is necessary to keep in mind that however carefully performed, contralateral surgery in this setting may result in a patient with complete diaphragmatic paralysis and severe ventilatory incapacity. We therefore routinely perform fluoroscopic visualization of diaphragmatic function to ensure complete return of innervation before planning any form of contralateral surgery.

Lymph Leakage

It is not uncommon to observe minor postoperative lymphatic fluid collections in the area of the wound or emanating from the closed-suction drain, at least within the first week after surgery. This may occur despite ligation of the thoracic duct on the left side and is usually due to leakage of lymph fluid from small tributaries subjected to higher fluid pressure than normal. In the majority of cases these lymph leaks will resolve spontaneously with time, generally within several weeks. Secondary surgical procedures for persistent lymph leak are only rarely necessary.

RESULTS OF SURGERY

Outcome Measures

Thoracic outlet decompression for the treatment of nTOS is intended to provide functional relief of preoperative upper extremity symptoms that have been refractory to conservative management. Assessment of results therefore depends on functional evaluation of symptoms and the patient's somewhat subjective perception of the degree of disability. Because this depends in large part on the extent of disability that existed before surgery, reported results may vary considerably in patients with differing degrees or duration of disabling symptoms before surgical treatment. Unfortunately, there are no well-defined classification schemes in common use with which to stratify patients undergoing surgical treatment.

Published reports on surgical treatment of nTOS also vary widely in how outcomes for different operations are defined.

Thus, a second difficulty in assessing the results of surgery remains the absence of well-established outcome measures or reporting standards for thoracic outlet decompression. Most authors classify results into four separate categories: (1) *excellent*, with complete relief of all symptoms; (2) *good*, with relief of major symptoms but some persistent symptoms; (3) *fair*, with partial relief but persistence of some major symptoms; and (4) *poor*, with no improvement. In general, patients who have results in the excellent, good, or fair categories will believe that the operation was worthwhile, whereas those in the poor category will think that the operation was a failure.

Another variable complicating the interpretation of outcomes of surgical treatment is the type of operation performed. As is evident from the earlier discussion, several different operations are currently in use for nTOS, each having its advantages and disadvantages. No single operation has been adopted by all those who perform surgery for nTOS, and the operations performed by some may have changed over time. Although each operative approach has its advocates and detractors, it has been difficult to demonstrate a significant difference in outcome between the different procedures in common use. Further complicating these assessments is the fact that some reports do not distinguish between patients undergoing surgery for nTOS versus those being treated for arterial or venous TOS, thus making it impossible to separate the results of treatment of nTOS alone.

It is recognized that the overall success of operations for nTOS can be considered only in the context of long-term outcomes. Most of these operations are performed in relatively young and active individuals, with the aim of improving function for many years. Because the degree of improvement obtained in the first few months after surgery may diminish with time, the durability of successful outcomes becomes another important measure of results. Unfortunately, many reports in the literature do not include follow-up or assessment of results beyond several months to a few years, which makes it difficult to assess differences that may exist among different operations over longer periods.

Finally, it is uncertain whether the results reported by those regularly performing operations for nTOS can be extended to those who perform thoracic outlet decompression only on an occasional basis because these are technically demanding operations not often performed by the majority of vascular surgeons. Thus, varying experience with different operations for TOS may also be a confounding factor in interpreting the results reported in various series.

Operative Results

Anterior Scalenotomy/Scalenectomy.
Anterior scalenotomy was initially described by Adson and widely applied until the 1960s. A summary of eight reports published between 1947 and 1987 in which the results were described in a total of 241 patients undergoing anterior scalenotomy indicated that the overall outcomes for this operation were good in 26% to 89% (mean, 58%), fair in 0% to 39% (mean, 9%), and poor in 7% to 60% (mean, 33%).[47-54]

Anterior scalenectomy was popularized by Adson as a means to avoid potential injury to the brachial plexus in patients with cervical ribs. In six reports of this procedure published up to 1989 and encompassing a total of 338 patients, there were good results in 26% to 89% (mean, 56%), fair in 0% to 39% (mean, 13%), and poor in 7% to 60% (mean, 31%).[55-60]

At present neither of these operations is performed frequently for nTOS, in part because the long-term results do not appear to be as good as those achieved with approaches involving resection of the first rib.

Transaxillary First Rib Resection.
Since its introduction by Roos in 1966, transaxillary first rib resection has been one of the most frequently performed operations for nTOS. By 1989, more than 3000 of these operations were reported in 21 separate publications. The largest of these series included 1315 patients, with a successful outcome in 92% and a failure rate of 8%. As summarized in Table 123-3, the overall rate of good outcomes for transaxillary first rib resection has ranged from 52% to 100% (mean, 80%), with fair outcomes in 0% to 25% (mean, 6%), and failure of surgery in 0% to 41% (mean, 15%).

Supraclavicular First Rib Resection with Anterior and Middle Scalenectomy.
This procedure has become one of the more commonly performed operations for nTOS over the

Table 123-3 Collected Results for Transaxillary First Rib Resection

Series	Year	Number of Operations	Outcomes (%)		
			Good	Fair	Poor
Sanders et al.[61]	1968	69	90	0	10
Roeder et al.[62]	1973	26	92	4	4
Hoofer and Burnett[63]	1973	135	100	0	0
Dale[64]	1975	49	94	0	6
Kremer and Ahlquist[65]	1975	48	86	0	14
McGough et al.[66]	1979	113	80	13	7
Youmans and Smiley[67]	1980	258	75	16	9
Roos[68]	1982	1315	92	0	8
Batt et al.[69]	1983	94	80	0	20
Sallstrom and Gjores[70]	1983	72	81	12	7
Heughan[71]	1984	44	75	0	25
Quarfordt et al.[42]	1984	97	79	0	21
Narakas et al.[53]	1986	43	77	0	23
Tagaki et al.[54]	1987	48	79	0	21
Davies and Messerschmidt[72]	1988	115	89	0	11
Selke and Kelly[73]	1988	460	79	14	7
Stanton et al.[74]	1988	87	85	4	11
Wood et al.[75]	1988	54	89	9	2
Cikrit et al.[60]	1989	30	63	0	37
Lindgren et al.[76]	1989	175	59	0	41
Lepantalo et al.[77]	1989	112	52	25	23
Jamieson and Chinnick[78]	1996	380	53	25	22
Totals		**3824**	**80**	**6**	**15**

Adapted from Sanders RJ. *Thoracic Outlet Syndrome: A Common Sequela of Neck Injuries.* Philadelphia, PA: JB Lippincott; 1991.

Table 123-4 Collected Results for Supraclavicular Scalenectomy/First Rib Resection

Series	Year	Number of Operations	Outcomes Reported (%)		
			Good	Fair	Poor
Graham and Lincoln[79]	1973	78	91	5	4
Thompson and Hernandez[80]	1979	15	87	0	13
Thomas et al.[81]	1983	128	83	13	4
Reilly and Stoney[44]	1988	39	59	33	8
Loh et al.[59]	1989	22	68	23	9
Hempel et al.[3]	1996	770	86	13	1
Axelrod et al.[82]	2001	170	65	17	18
Totals		**1222**	**77**	**15**	**8**

Adapted from Sanders RJ. *Thoracic Outlet Syndrome: A Common Sequela of Neck Injuries.* Philadelphia, PA: JB Lippincott; 1991.

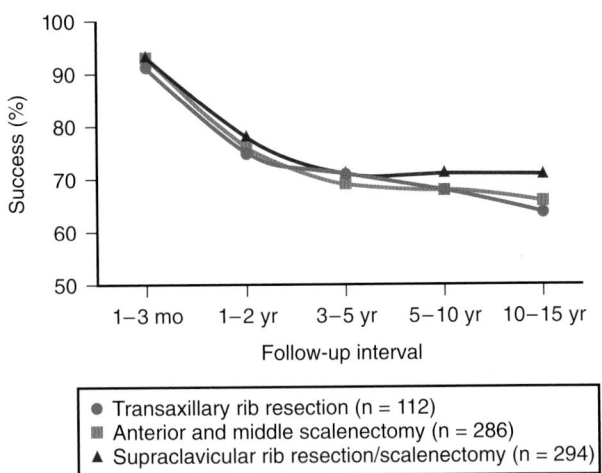

Figure 123-12 Long-term results of three operations for neurogenic thoracic outlet syndrome (nTOS). The outcomes of 692 patients undergoing a primary operation for nTOS are shown in life-table format, with follow-up intervals extending to 10 to 15 years. Data indicate the results for patients undergoing transaxillary first rib resection (n = 112), anterior and middle scalenectomy (n = 286), or supraclavicular scalenectomy with first rib resection (n = 249). There was no statistically significant difference between the three operations. *(Redrawn from Sanders RJ.* Thoracic Outlet Syndrome: A Common Sequela of Neck Injuries. *Philadelphia, PA: JB Lippincott; 1991.)*

past 2 decades. Table 123-4 summarizes the results of surgery from seven different publications that included a total of 1222 patients, the largest being the series reported by Hempel and colleagues (770 operations). Overall, the results for supraclavicular decompression were good in 59% to 91% (mean, 77%), fair in 0% to 33% (mean, 15%), and poor in 1% to 18% (mean, 8%).

Comparison of Surgical Approaches

The most comprehensive analysis of results for nTOS has been presented by Sanders, in which the life-table method was used to compare outcomes for different operative procedures.[1,22,83,84] In a comparison of patients undergoing transaxillary first rib resection (n = 112), anterior and middle scalenectomy (n = 286), or supraclavicular scalenectomy with first rib resection (n = 249), there was no difference in the initial success rate among these three procedures (91%, 93%, and 93%, respectively). As shown in Figure 123-12, the percentage of patients with successful outcomes also declined over time with all three procedures. Although the long-term success with supraclavicular scalenectomy and first rib resection appeared to be somewhat better at 10 to 15 years (71%) than the results with either anterior scalenectomy (66%) or transaxillary first rib resection (64%), there was no statistically significant difference among these operations. It must therefore be concluded that at the present time there is no demonstrable difference in either short- or long-term outcomes among these three operative approaches as applied to nTOS.

Predicting the Outcome of Surgery

Because patient selection for operative treatment remains an important variable in assessing outcomes for nTOS, attempts have been made to identify preexisting patient-specific factors that might influence surgical results. Franklin and associates examined injured workers in the state of Washington who had undergone an operation for nTOS between 1986 and 1991

and found that 60% of those with a work-related injury remained disabled 1 year after surgical treatment.[85] There appeared to be no differences in outcome based on the type of operation performed, the presence of any particular provocative test results, or the experience of the operating surgeon, but significant predictors of ongoing disability included the amount of work disability before surgery, longer intervals between injury and diagnosis of nTOS, and older age at the time of surgery. This study has frequently been cited to indicate poor outcomes for surgical treatment of nTOS in the presence of work-related injury and disability claims. However, the scope of its applicability is limited because it is a database study restricted to injured workers, and the results can be interpreted to suggest that better outcomes might be achieved with more accurate diagnosis of nTOS after work-related injury and earlier application of surgical treatment in this clinical setting.

Axelrod and coworkers also examined potential associations between preexisting psychological factors and socioeconomic characteristics and the long-term outcomes of patients undergoing surgery for nTOS.[82] Supraclavicular thoracic outlet decompression in 170 patients was considered successful in 65%, with 35% remaining on medications and 18% reporting ongoing disability. Multivariate logistic regression models revealed several independent risk factors significantly associated with persistent disability, including major depression, not being married, and having less than a high-school education. The authors suggest that further prospective studies are needed to address the potential impact of preoperative treatment of depression in patients undergoing operations for nTOS.

In evaluating the potential role of specific anatomic factors in outcomes of surgery, Sanders and Hammond reviewed their long-term operative results in 54 patients with nTOS associated with a cervical rib or anomalous first rib.[11] Although the overall success rate for surgery was 72%, the etiology of the symptoms was a significant variable in outcome, with failure in 42% of patients with symptoms after a work-related injury or repetitive stress, in 26% of patients with symptoms after an automobile collision, and in 18% of those with symptoms of a nonspecific cause. The failure rate was also substantially affected by the operation performed: 75% in those undergoing cervical rib resection without first rib resection in the work-related injury group (and 38% in the non–work-related group) versus 25% in those undergoing cervical rib resection along with resection of the first rib in the work-related group (and 20% in the non–work-related group). The authors concluded that (1) the presence of a cervical rib or anomalous first rib in patients with nTOS does not improve the success rate of surgery over that in patients without rib abnormalities; (2) neck trauma is the most common cause of nTOS, even in patients with abnormal ribs; (3) cervical and anomalous first ribs are predisposing factors rather than the cause of nTOS; and (4) surgery for nTOS in patients with cervical ribs should include both cervical rib and first rib resection.

Finally, in a recent study of 85 patients with nTOS treated by either surgery or botulinum toxin chemodenervation, Jordan and coauthors reported no differences between treatment-responsive and treatment-resistant patients with respect to work disability status or compensation claims, anomalous anatomy detected by ultrasonography, or alterations in subclavian artery flow detected by duplex sonography.[24] They did observe, however, that treatment-resistant patients had a higher frequency of sensory complaints extending beyond the lower trunk dermatomes (42% versus 10%), weakness extending beyond the lower trunk myotomes (19% versus 2%), a history of previous non-TOS surgery on the neck or upper limbs (50% versus 17%), co-morbid conditions of fibromyalgia or CRPS (81% versus 12%), and depression (35% versus 10%). Importantly, treatment-resistant patients also responded less frequently to scalene muscle test blocks than did treatment-responsive patients (38% versus 100%). This study thereby demonstrates the adverse effect of certain co-morbid conditions and diffuse upper extremity symptoms on surgical outcomes and highlights the clinical value of diagnostic scalene muscle blocks in the modern management of nTOS.

It can be concluded from the studies just cited that certain preexisting clinical features appear to be associated with diminished success of operative treatment of nTOS, particularly work-related injury, long-standing symptoms, major depression, diffuse upper extremity symptoms, and lack of a response to anterior scalene muscle blocks. The existence of such characteristics should not exclude individual patients from being considered for surgical treatment, and further studies are needed to evaluate potential interventions that might improve outcomes. Nonetheless, knowledge of these associations should be clearly communicated to patients con-

templating operative treatment of nTOS, and the potential influence of specific factors on the outcome of surgery should be discussed when appropriate.

Ongoing Symptoms

Patients with neurogenic symptoms after thoracic outlet decompression for nTOS are characterized as having either persistent or recurrent symptoms.

Persistent Symptoms. Persistent symptoms are those that were not relieved even for a short period by the initial operation. In most cases persistent symptoms are due to another condition and the diagnosis should be completely re-evaluated. If the symptoms cannot be attributed to another condition and they resist conservative management for at least several months, the possibility of persistent nTOS is then considered. If the initial operation consisted of transaxillary first rib resection, persistent symptoms may occur if there was inadequate relief of compression of the upper nerve roots because scalenectomy was not performed. In these cases, reoperative supraclavicular scalenectomy should be considered. Although it is unusual to observe persistent nTOS after supraclavicular scalenectomy, it may be considered if the procedure did not include first rib resection. In such cases it may be reasonable to consider a reoperation to remove the first rib by either the transaxillary or supraclavicular route.

Recurrent Symptoms. Recurrent symptoms of nTOS are considered to be present when the patient had good initial results from the operation but recurrent symptoms developed later. The majority of such recurrences take place within the first 2 years of the primary operation. The symptoms are often the same as those present before the initial operation, and the diagnosis is made in the same manner as described earlier. If reoperation is considered, the choice of procedure again depends on the type of operation performed initially. If a transaxillary first rib resection was performed, reoperation should be undertaken via a supraclavicular approach and should include scalenectomy, brachial plexus neurolysis, and resection of any remaining portion of the first rib. Experience with such operations shows that the stump of the anterior scalene muscle has often become attached to the extrapleural fascia or the brachial plexus nerve roots; it is also common to find a segment of the posterior rib still present because this portion cannot be resected easily through the transaxillary approach. If the initial operation was a supraclavicular scalenectomy, a repeat operation should include first rib resection. Because the cause of recurrent nTOS after supraclavicular scalenectomy and first rib resection is usually the formation of perineural adhesions, reoperation through the supraclavicular route may still be of value since it permits complete brachial plexus neurolysis to be achieved. Reoperations are associated with a higher risk for nerve and vascular injury than primary procedures are, so the decision to reoperate should not be taken lightly and the procedure should be performed by an individual with considerable experience in these operations.

SELECTED KEY REFERENCES

Axelrod DA, Proctor MC, Geisser ME, Roth RS, Greenfield LJ. Outcomes after surgery for thoracic outlet syndrome. *J Vasc Surg.* 2001;33:1220-1225.
This publication provides an excellent summary of current results of surgical treatment of nTOS.

Demondion X, Bacqueville E, Paul C, Duquesnoy B, Hachulla E, Cotten A. Thoracic outlet: assessment with MR imaging in asymptomatic and symptomatic populations. *Radiology.* 2003;227:461-468.
This publication depicts the use of novel MRI-based imaging techniques to identify patients with anatomic abnormalities associated with nTOS, an approach that may find broad application in the future.

Hempel GK, Shutze WP, Anderson JF, Bukhari HI. 770 consecutive supraclavicular first rib resections for thoracic outlet syndrome. *Ann Vasc Surg.* 1996;10:456-463.
This report summarizes an unusually large single-institution experience with supraclavicular operations for TOS, with excellent outcomes described.

Jordan SE, Ahn SS, Gelabert HA. Differentiation of thoracic outlet syndrome from treatment-resistant cervical brachial pain syndromes: development and utilization of a questionnaire, clinical examination and ultrasound evaluation. *Pain Physician.* 2007;10:441-452.
A recent study validating a comprehensive approach to identify patients with nTOS who are most likely to benefit from operative treatment.

Jordan SE, Machleder HI. Diagnosis of thoracic outlet syndrome using electrophysiologically guided anterior scalene blocks. *Ann Vasc Surg.* 1998;12:260-264.
A description of a useful and widely applicable technique for confirming the clinical diagnosis of nTOS.

Machanic BI, Sanders RJ. Medial antebrachial cutaneous nerve measurements to diagnose neurogenic thoracic outlet syndrome. *Ann Vasc Surg.* 2008;22:248-254.
This recent report describes improved use of an electrophysiologic test with a surprisingly high specificity for nTOS, which may be useful in both diagnosis and assessment of treatment.

Roos DB. Transaxillary approach for first rib resection to relieve thoracic outlet syndrome. *Ann Surg.* 1966;163:354-358.
A classic description of operative techniques for transaxillary first rib resection.

Roos DB. Congenital anomalies associated with thoracic outlet syndrome. *Am J Surg.* 1976;132:771-778.
The classic description of anatomic variations in the thoracic outlet that can be responsible for neurovascular compression syndromes.

Sanders RJ. *Thoracic Outlet Syndrome: A Common Sequela of Neck Injuries.* Philadelphia, PA: JB Lippincott; 1991.
This book provides perhaps the most comprehensive presentation available regarding all aspects of the etiology, diagnosis, treatment, and outcomes of TOS.

Sanders RJ, Raymer S. The supraclavicular approach to scalenectomy and first rib resection: description of technique. *J Vasc Surg.* 1985;2:751-756.
A classic description of operative techniques for supraclavicular thoracic outlet decompression.

REFERENCES

The reference list can be found on the companion Expert Consult Web site at *www.expertconsult.com.*

CHAPTER 124

Thoracic Outlet Syndrome: Arterial

Stephen T. Smith and R. James Valentine

Arterial complications from compression of the subclavian artery represent the least common type of thoracic outlet syndrome (TOS), but they are also the strongest indication for operative intervention. Arterial manifestations usually follow a progressive course characterized by extrinsic compression, post-stenotic dilatation, aneurysmal degeneration, and secondary embolization. Because arterial TOS is typically associated with anomalous osseous structures, this form of TOS has a more easily definable clinical picture. In fact, arterial TOS was probably the first form to be described.[1] The first reported resection of a bony abnormality causing a subclavian aneurysm was by Coote in 1861.[2] Compression of the subclavian artery and brachial plexus was first termed "Naffziger syndrome"[3] and evolved to the modern term of *thoracic outlet syndrome* after a 1956 publication by Peet and colleagues.[4]

PATHOPHYSIOLOGY

Arterial complications of TOS are associated with bony abnormalities in almost all cases. Cervical ribs that cause subclavian artery damage tend to be short, broad, and complete and usually articulate with the first rib as a pseudarthrosis.[5] This differs from the longer, thinner, and incomplete cervical ribs generally associated with neurogenic TOS. The cervical rib pushes the subclavian artery forward, where it is compressed between the first rib and the anterior scalene muscle. This compression causes injury to the inferior aspect of the third segment of the subclavian artery, which may lead to localized intimal damage or post-stenotic dilatation. Less common causes of arterial TOS include anomalous first ribs, fibrocartilaginous bands associated with the anterior scalene muscle,[6] and hypertrophic callus from healed clavicle fractures.[7] The post-stenotic dilatation associated with chronic arterial compression may progress to aneurysmal change, whereas localized intimal damage may lead to embolization or thrombosis. The relative frequencies of anatomic abnormalities are shown in Table 124-1.[6,8-10]

EPIDEMIOLOGY

The frequency of arterial TOS in the general population is undefined, but data abstracted from published series suggest that it is the least common form of symptomatic TOS. The largest single-institution experience of patients treated for all varieties of TOS was reported by Urshel and Kourlis.[11] Over

Table 124-1 Relative Frequencies of Anatomic Abnormalities Causing Arterial Thoracic Outlet Syndrome

Abnormality	Frequency (%)*
Cervical rib	63
Anomalous 1st rib	22
Fibrocartilaginous band	10
Clavicular fracture	4
Enlarged C7 transverse process	1

*Percentages represent a compendium of 93 reported patients from four large series.[6,8-10]

a period of 6 decades the authors performed primary neurovascular decompression on 5102 patients, including 4183 (82%) for neurogenic TOS, 625 (12%) for venous TOS, and 294 (6%) for arterial TOS. In another series of 200 consecutive transaxillary decompression procedures performed at a single referral center, Makhoul and Machleder reported that 160 (80%) had neurogenic symptoms, 33 (16.5%) had venous obstruction, and 7 (3.5%) had arterial obstruction.[12] Sanders and coauthors reported that less than 1% of their TOS patients had symptoms of arterial compression.[13]

Most patients with symptoms of arterial TOS are young, active adults. The mean age in most published series is 37 years, with a similar proportion of men and women reported.[8,9,14] The condition appears to be related to bony abnormalities or trauma in nearly every circumstance. No familial predisposition has been described.

CLINICAL FINDINGS

Patients with arterial TOS have a characteristic history and findings on physical examination, but diagnosis requires confirmation with objective testing.

Signs and Symptoms

The most common manifestation is hand ischemia as a result of microembolization. However, arterial TOS can be associated with less dramatic symptoms, and many cases go unrecognized because the condition tends to occur in young patients without atherosclerotic risk factors. Early in the disease process, patients may have mild symptoms of exertional arm pain or unilateral Raynaud's syndrome. Moderate to severe exertional pain may be associated with subclavian artery thrombosis. Occasionally, a subclavian artery aneurysm may be palpable in an asymptomatic patient. Though rare, cerebrovascular accidents from retrograde propagation of subclavian thrombus have been reported.[15-19]

Clinical Assessment

Clues to the diagnosis of arterial TOS include young age of the patient and the tendency for symptoms to be unilateral, which helps differentiate the condition from systemic pathologic states. The directed physical examination should consist of measurement of blood pressure in both upper extremities and auscultation for bruits in the supraclavicular fossa. A bruit may be elicited on shoulder abduction or the overhead arm position if it is not present in the relaxed position. Specific findings on physical examination include a palpable cervical rib or a pulsatile supraclavicular mass. Evidence of microembolization to the hand may also be present, including digital ischemia or splinter hemorrhages.

■ DIAGNOSTIC EVALUATION

Arterial TOS is a clinical diagnosis made by combining important elements from the history and physical examination. The following adjuncts may help support the diagnosis or suggest an alternative cause of the patient's symptoms.

Compression Maneuvers

Compression maneuvers have historically been used to aid in the diagnosis of TOC, but none is accurate. The Adson test, as originally described, "consists of having the patient take a long breath, elevate his chin and turn it to the affected side. This is done as the patient is seated upright, with his arms resting on his knees."[20] Ablation or reduction of the radial pulse with this maneuver is considered a positive test result. This finding has not proved accurate, however, because the incidence of false-positive results in normal, healthy volunteers ranges from 9% to 53%.[13,21-24] However, a negative test result may be helpful in ruling out the diagnosis and prompting evaluation for an alternative cause. Another compression maneuver is the abduction–external rotation test, also referred to as the elevated arm stress test popularized by Roos and Owens.[25] In this test the patient externally rotates and abducts the arms greater than 90 degrees. Development of hand pain or paresthesias within 60 seconds is considered a positive result. This test is used for the diagnosis of neurogenic TOS but is not helpful for arterial TOS[13] (see Chapter 123: Thoracic Outlet Syndrome: Neurogenic).

Noninvasive Vascular Laboratory Studies

Duplex Ultrasonography

Duplex ultrasound examination of the subclavian and axillary arteries may demonstrate aneurysmal changes or elevated flow velocities correlating with a compressive stenosis. The clavicle may interfere with complete ultrasound imaging of the subclavian artery, but significant ulcerations and intimal disruption may be visible. Compression maneuvers have been recommended during sonographic evaluation, with decreased subclavian diameter or changes in peak systolic velocity thought to be diagnostic of arterial TOS. One study evaluating multiple compression maneuvers and imaging locations found that arm abduction to 130 degrees while imaging in the costoclavicular space was the most discriminating technique.[26] However, as with the pulse-monitored compression maneuvers described earlier, there are a high number of false-positive results in normal, healthy volunteers. Studies have shown that compression maneuvers are associated with complete occlusion or significant stenosis of the subclavian artery in approximately 20% of normal subjects.[27,28] Therefore, positive ultrasound tests during compression maneuvers should be used only to confirm a suspected diagnosis of arterial TOS.

Pulse Volume/Segmental Pressure Recording

Pulse volume or Doppler segmental pressure recordings taken at multiple levels in the upper extremities can help localize the level of arterial obstruction if embolization has occurred as a result of arterial TOS. Reduced digital waveforms in the affected extremity and normal contralateral findings indicate arterial insufficiency consistent with stenosis or distal embolism. Digital waveforms can also be interpreted along with compression maneuvers, but these tests have a high number of false-positive results in normal subjects.

Radiographic Studies

Roentgenography

Chest radiographs, including cervical spine views, will often demonstrate the offending bony pathology. Cervical ribs, elongated transverse cervical processes, and large clavicle fracture calluses are easily seen (Fig. 124-1). Anomalous first ribs and fibrocartilaginous bands are not likely to be detected on plain radiographs.

Computed Tomography

Computed tomography with intravenous contrast-enhanced angiography (CTA) is a useful test to secure the diagnosis and aid surgical planning. CTA may identify the exact point of compression and the extent of arterial pathology that requires treatment. With the ability to manipulate these images in three dimensions, there is usually no need for catheter-based arteriography. In fact, CTA has replaced catheter-based angiography as the main radiographic test for diagnosing arterial TOS in some centers. CTA can also be used to evaluate the distal arterial circulation, but catheter-based angiography may still be necessary to visualize the small arteries of the distal end of the arm and hand. Because compression of the neurovascular structures in the thoracic outlet is common in normal,

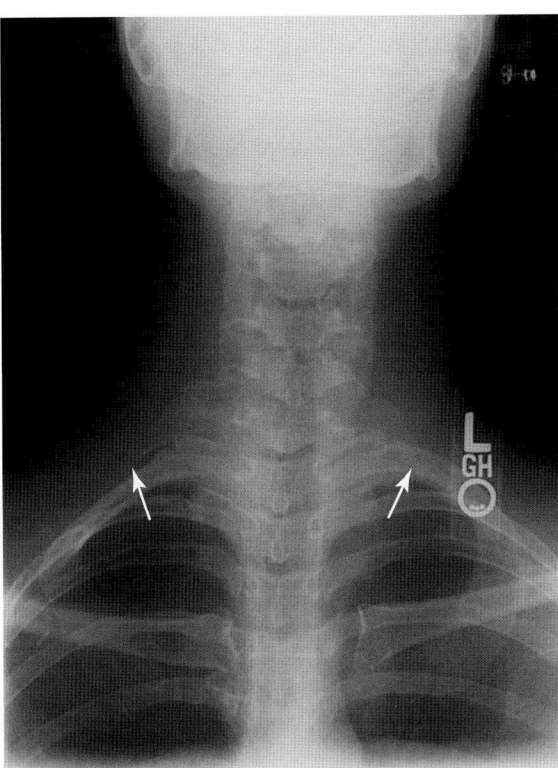

Figure 124-1 Chest radiograph demonstrating bilateral cervical ribs (*arrows*) in a patient with arterial thoracic outlet syndrome.

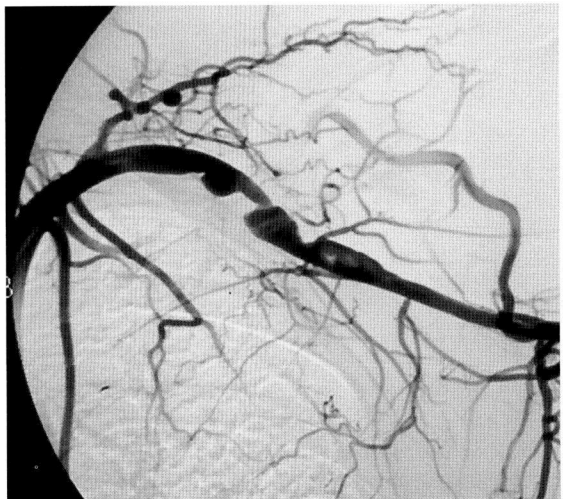

Figure 124-2 Left subclavian arteriogram demonstrating a subclavian aneurysm with thrombus.

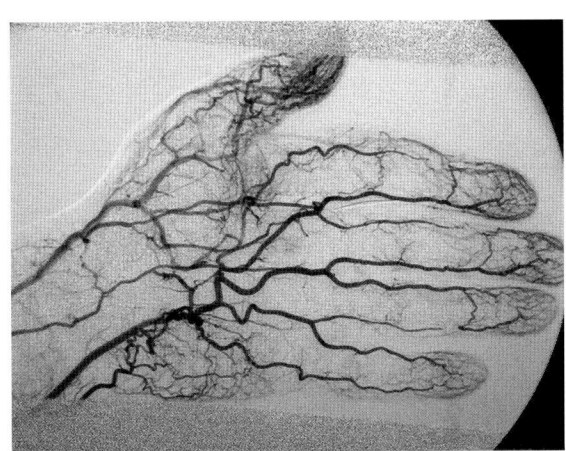

Figure 124-3 Hand arteriogram demonstrating distal embolization in the first, second, and third digits.

healthy subjects,[29] dynamic compression maneuvers should be used only to confirm the diagnosis in patients with suspected arterial TOS.

Magnetic Resonance Angiography

Although magnetic resonance angiography (MRA) may be an acceptable substitute for CTA or catheter-based angiography in some centers, the sensitivity of MRA for diagnosing arterial TOS appears to be low. Two reports of MRA in patients with arterial symptoms had a 37% and 42% incidence of false-negative findings.[26,30] Therefore, a negative MRA should not be used to rule out the diagnosis of clinically suspected arterial TOS.

Catheter-Based Angiography

Upper extremity arteriography represents the "gold standard" for evaluation of arterial TOS. This test is important in operative planning because it localizes the exact point of arterial compression, provides an assessment of the nature and extent of arterial damage, and permits evaluation of the distal circulation (Fig. 124-2). Additional views incorporating dynamic compression maneuvers may be useful to highlight compression points in symptomatic patients. To assist in operative planning, runoff images should be obtained to identify normal anatomic variants, as well as acquired abnormalities. As noted earlier, CTA for operative planning is gradually replacing catheter-based arteriography. However, arteriography with

magnified views remains the best method for demonstrating embolic occlusion of the small arteries of the hand and fingers (Fig. 124-3).

Laboratory Testing

No specific laboratory tests are necessary to diagnose arterial TOS. However, specific laboratory assays are important to exclude systemic causes of upper extremity ischemia such as vasculitis or connective tissue disorders. The specific tests appropriate for evaluation of vasculitis are discussed in Chapter 76 (Vasculitis and Other Arteriopathies), and those for connective tissue disorders are discussed in Chapter 119 (Raynaud's Syndrome).

DIFFERENTIAL DIAGNOSIS

Although arterial TOS has characteristic findings, other causes of upper extremity ischemia may be suspected from the history and physical examination (Box 124-1). A history of

---

Box 124-1 Differential Diagnosis of Arterial Thoracic Outlet Syndrome

- Embolization from other sources
  - Cardiac
  - Aortic arch
  - Hypothenar hammer syndrome
  - Acquired or congenital coagulopathies
- Vasculitis
  - Takayasu's arteritis
  - Giant cell arteritis
- Radiation-induced arteritis
- Connective tissue disorders
  - Marfan syndrome
  - Ehlers-Danlos syndrome type IV
  - Pseudoxanthoma elasticum
- Arterial dissection
- Atherosclerotic upper extremity disease
- Traumatic
  - Humeral head compression of the axillary artery
  - Circumflex humeral artery pseudoaneurysm (baseball pitchers)

---

cardiac pathology, particularly mitral valve stenosis or atrial fibrillation, supports a cardioembolic etiology. A family history of venous thromboembolic disease suggests an underlying hypercoagulable state, and further tests to exclude paradoxical embolus may be warranted. Risk factors for atherosclerosis, particularly heavy tobacco use, raise the possibility of atherosclerotic occlusive disease as the underlying etiology. Associated symptoms of polymyalgia rheumatica suggest the possibility of vasculitis, whereas symptoms of arthritis, dermatitis, and esophageal dysmotility warrant evaluation for connective tissue disease. Other possible causes include dissection, radiation injury, and trauma—all of which can be suspected from the history and evaluated with the imaging studies just discussed.

Screening

There is no role for screening of asymptomatic patients to diagnose arterial TOS. As noted previously, dynamic compression maneuvers are associated with a significant rate of false-positive results in asymptomatic patients; therefore, positive tests should be viewed with caution. On the other hand, it is reasonable to evaluate the opposite side in a patient with symptomatic arterial TOS. Although the incidence of bilateral arterial TOS is not known, the frequency of bilateral TOS of all types is reported to be 10% to 26%.[31,32] Treatment may be indicated for evidence of arterial dilatation or severe intimal degeneration, even in asymptomatic individuals. Patients with upper extremity occlusive or aneurysmal symptoms should be evaluated as discussed earlier under "Clinical Assessment."

■ TREATMENT

Medical Treatment

In contrast to neurogenic TOS, there is no role for conservative treatment of symptomatic patients with arterial TOS, although it may be appropriate for some asymptomatic patients. Even though the natural history is not well known, simple compression without evidence of arterial degeneration does not appear to carry a significant risk for complications in asymptomatic patients. Therefore, watchful waiting and the use of serial noninvasive tests such as duplex ultrasonography may be a reasonable approach. In addition, every attempt should be made to reduce compressive forces in the thoracic outlet. This is especially true for high-performance athletes engaged in repetitive overhead arm motion such as professional baseball pitchers and tennis players. Aggressive physical therapy and modification of arm motion have been recommended in these cases.[33]

The natural history of arterial abnormalities in asymptomatic patients with arterial TOS is not completely understood. However, some patients have profound hand ischemia as the first manifestation of arterial TOS. Therefore, it seems reasonable to treat patients, especially young, active individuals, with subclavian artery compression and documented arterial pathology such as arterial dilatation or severe intimal disruption before symptoms ensue. The role of anticoagulation in these circumstances is not known.

Principles of Surgical Treatment

The three main components of treatment include relieving the arterial compression, removing the source of embolus, and restoring the distal circulation. At a minimum, relieving the arterial compression involves resection of cervical ribs and any other identified anomalies causing impingement in the thoracic outlet. As discussed later, most authors also recommend routine division of the anterior scalene muscle and resection of the first rib to avoid recurrence. Removing the source of embolus involves resecting a subclavian aneurysm or repairing an arterial stenosis with intimal damage. The success of arterial reconstruction is usually related to the status of outflow in the limb. Restoring the distal circulation may involve any combination of thrombolysis, thromboembolectomy, or bypass.

The decision to repair an artery after thoracic outlet decompression should be individualized. Resolution of post-stenotic dilatation after decompression of the thoracic outlet has been described,[6,34,35] but it is not certain that all lesions will heal spontaneously. Likewise, it is not known whether associated intimal damage will resolve after decompression. At some point, post-stenotic dilatation progresses to the point of being considered an aneurysm. Symptomatic patients with subclavian artery aneurysms tend to have recurrent thromboembolic complications that may lead to digit or limb loss. Because of the numerous collaterals around the shoulder, the natural history of subclavian artery thrombosis is uncertain.

However, there is a reported risk for retrograde propagation with resultant stroke.[15-19] Furthermore, most patients will have significant arm fatigue with exercise.

Selection of Treatment

The appropriate treatment is dictated by the degree of arterial damage and the status of the distal circulation. Some definitions are important to consider here because they classically differ from other anatomic sites. Aneurysm of the subclavian artery associated with TOS is defined as an increase in diameter greater than two times the diameter of the adjacent segment of artery.[34,36] Post-stenotic dilatation associated with TOS is then defined as an increase in diameter of less than twice that of the adjacent segment.

Scher Classification

The Scher classification system for arterial TOS provides a guide to appropriate treatment and is summarized in Table 124-2.[36] Stage I describes compression of the subclavian artery with minor post-stenotic dilatation and no intimal disruption. Appropriate treatment consists of decompression of the thoracic outlet, including cervical or first rib resection (or both); division of the anterior scalene muscle; and resection of any anomalous fibrous pathology. As noted earlier, regression of post-stenotic dilatation after thoracic outlet decompression has been reported.[6,34,36] Scher stage II includes subclavian arteries with intimal damage, aneurysmal change, and mural thrombus. Appropriate treatment includes decompression of the thoracic outlet and reconstruction of the subclavian artery. Scher stage III includes patients with distal embolization. Treatment should include a combination of thrombolysis or thromboembolectomy, thoracic outlet decompression, and vascular reconstruction.

Surgical Treatment

Surgical treatment is indicated for all symptomatic patients with ischemia and for asymptomatic patients with aneurysmal degeneration or intimal damage. As noted previously, asymptomatic individuals with compression of the subclavian artery at the thoracic outlet do not require surgical intervention, but they should be monitored because their natural history is unknown. There are no specific contraindications to repair of arterial TOS; however, a few patients may be unfit for open surgery because of severe uncorrectable co-morbid conditions.

Relevant Anatomy

The most common offending osseous abnormality in arterial TOS is a cervical rib, which accounts for about two thirds of cases (see Table 124-1). As noted earlier, multiple other abnormalities may be encountered, including abnormal first ribs, fracture calluses, fibromuscular bands, and soft tissue defects.[5-7] Figure 124-4 demonstrates several of these abnormalities. Sanders and Haug have reported that up to 12% of patients with arterial TOS have fibrous bands without any definable osseous abnormality.[10]

Operative Planning and Strategy

The first principle of treatment is decompression of the thoracic outlet. This may involve resection of a cervical rib or fibrous bands or scalenectomy, but most experts agree that the first rib should usually be resected in addition to other associated pathology.[8] The first rib is a fixed structure that maintains tension in the thoracic outlet and, once released, allows the neurovascular bundle to relax and fall inferiorly. More importantly, it represents a common insertion for fibromuscular structures that cause vascular compression but are not recognized at the time of surgery.

There are two main approaches to thoracic outlet decompression: supraclavicular and transaxillary. Each has some advantages. Proponents of the transaxillary approach describe more complete visualization of the first rib for resection. However, this approach is not generally suitable for vascular reconstruction and is therefore more commonly used to treat neurogenic TOS (see Chapter 123: Thoracic Outlet Syndrome: Neurogenic).[37] The supraclavicular approach facilitates removal of cervical ribs. This exposure allows identification of the cause of compression, resection of the first rib, and subsequent vascular reconstruction. For this reason we favor supraclavicular exposure whenever arterial reconstruction is necessary. A large subclavian aneurysm or intimal damage that extends beneath the clavicle may require infraclavicular exposure in addition to the supraclavicular incision. This allows complete exposure of the subclavian and axillary arteries for vascular reconstruction. A single incision that affords both supraclavicular and infraclavicular exposure has been described.[38] Rarely, the subclavian artery has a focal abnormality that can be repaired by simple resection and

Table 124-2 Scher Staging Classification of Complications of Arterial Thoracic Outlet Syndrome

Stage	Arterial Complication	Treatment
0	Asymptomatic subclavian artery compression	No treatment indicated
I	Stenosis of the subclavian artery with minor post-stenotic dilation. No intimal disruption	Decompression of the thoracic outlet
II	Subclavian artery aneurysm with intimal damage and mural thrombus	Decompression of the thoracic outlet Subclavian artery reconstruction
III	Distal embolization from subclavian artery pathology	Thrombolysis or thromboembolectomy Decompression of the thoracic outlet Vascular reconstruction

Adapted from Scher LA, Veith FJ, Haimovici H, et al. Staging of arterial complications of cervical rib: guidelines for surgical management. *Surgery.* 1984;95:664-669.

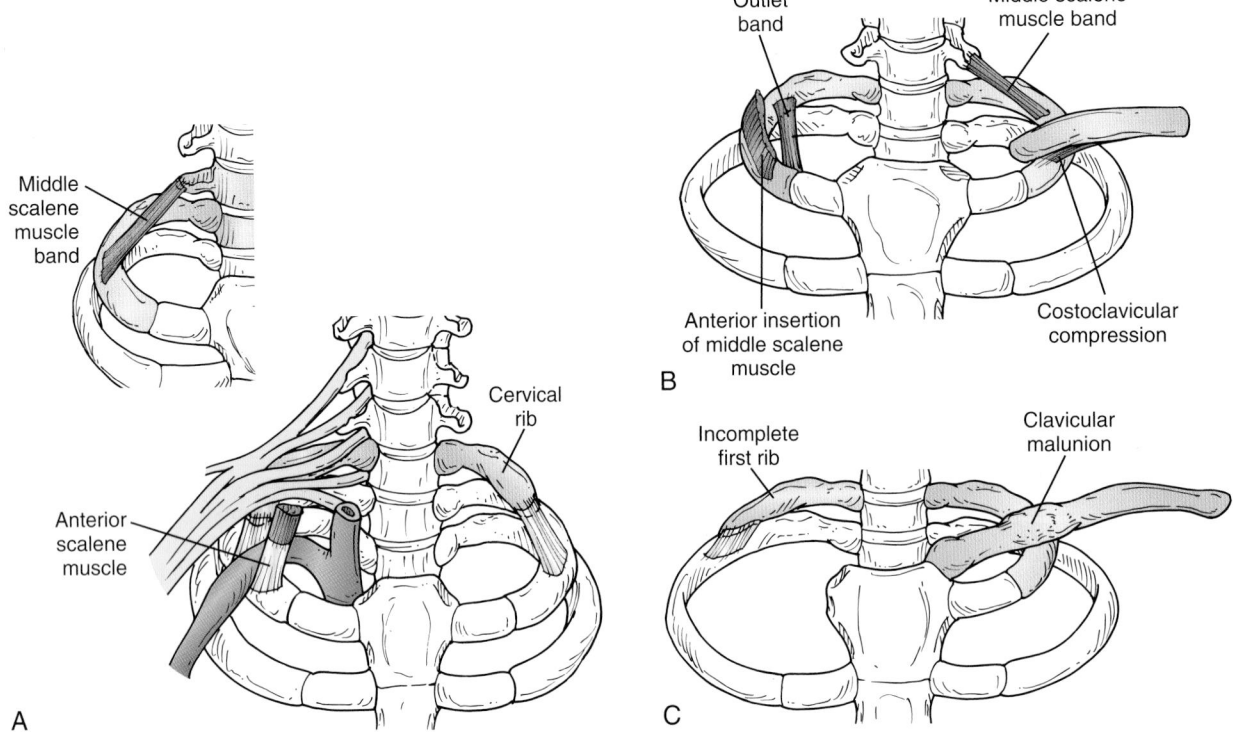

Figure 124-4 Pathologic conditions commonly associated with arterial thoracic outlet syndrome. **A,** Cervical ribs with associated fibrous bands and a middle scalene muscle band. **B,** Fascial bands and anomalous muscle insertions. **C,** Incomplete first rib and clavicular fracture callus. *(From Valentine RJ, Wind GG.* Anatomic Exposures in Vascular Surgery. *2nd ed. Philadelphia, PA: Lippincott Williams & Wilkins; 2003:124-125. By permission.)*

primary anastomosis. More commonly, a conduit is required for replacement of the subclavian artery. Although some consider the great saphenous vein to be the conduit of choice, reconstruction can be accomplished with femoral vein, ringed polytetrafluoroethylene, or Dacron. Ringed polytetrafluoroethylene or femoral vein may offer some advantage in longer bypasses because these grafts resist kinking as they traverse under the clavicle. The femoral vein conduit also appears to offer superior patency.[39]

Technique

The details of supraclavicular exposure are presented in Chapter 122 (Thoracic Outlet Syndrome: General Considerations) and elsewhere.[37,40] However, a few technical points are worth additional emphasis. After the scalene fat pad is mobilized, the phrenic nerve is mobilized off the surface of the anterior scalene before it is divided (Fig. 124-5A). The middle scalene is then divided off the first rib while taking care to avoid the long thoracic nerve (Fig. 124-5B). Attachments are freed via an extraperiosteal approach, and the first rib is divided just distal to the tubercle (Fig. 124-5C). The divided rib can then be used as a lever to assist with mobilization before dividing it anteriorly (Fig. 124-5D).

Endovascular Options

Although open surgical reconstruction is the standard approach to arterial complications of TOS, there have been reports of endovascular repair of the subclavian artery combined with surgical decompression of the thoracic outlet.[41,42] The importance of adjunctive decompression cannot be overemphasized because failure to decompress the thoracic outlet can lead to stent fracture or collapse, restenosis, and thrombosis.[43] Early reports of endovascular repair in highly selected patients are encouraging, but increased experience and longer-term outcome data are needed to determine the validity of this approach.

Distal Revascularization

Patients with Scher stage III have upper extremity ischemia as a result of distal embolization. The presence of any degree of motor deficit or a significant sensory deficit should be considered an indication for immediate surgery, including embolectomy. Brachial artery embolectomy does not always require a separate distal arm incision because large emboli can be extracted through the subclavian artery in some cases. Although embolectomy is usually sufficient, distal bypasses are sometimes necessary in patients with chronic embolization. Patients with milder ischemia may be appropriate for thrombolysis before surgical repair.[44] Thrombolysis may be particularly important in patients who have complete thrombosis of the forearm and hand vessels on arteriography. The role of catheter-directed thrombolysis is considered further in Chapter 158 (Acute Ischemia: Treatment). Sympathectomy does not have a significant role in the management of these patients, except in cases of ischemic causalgia.[14]

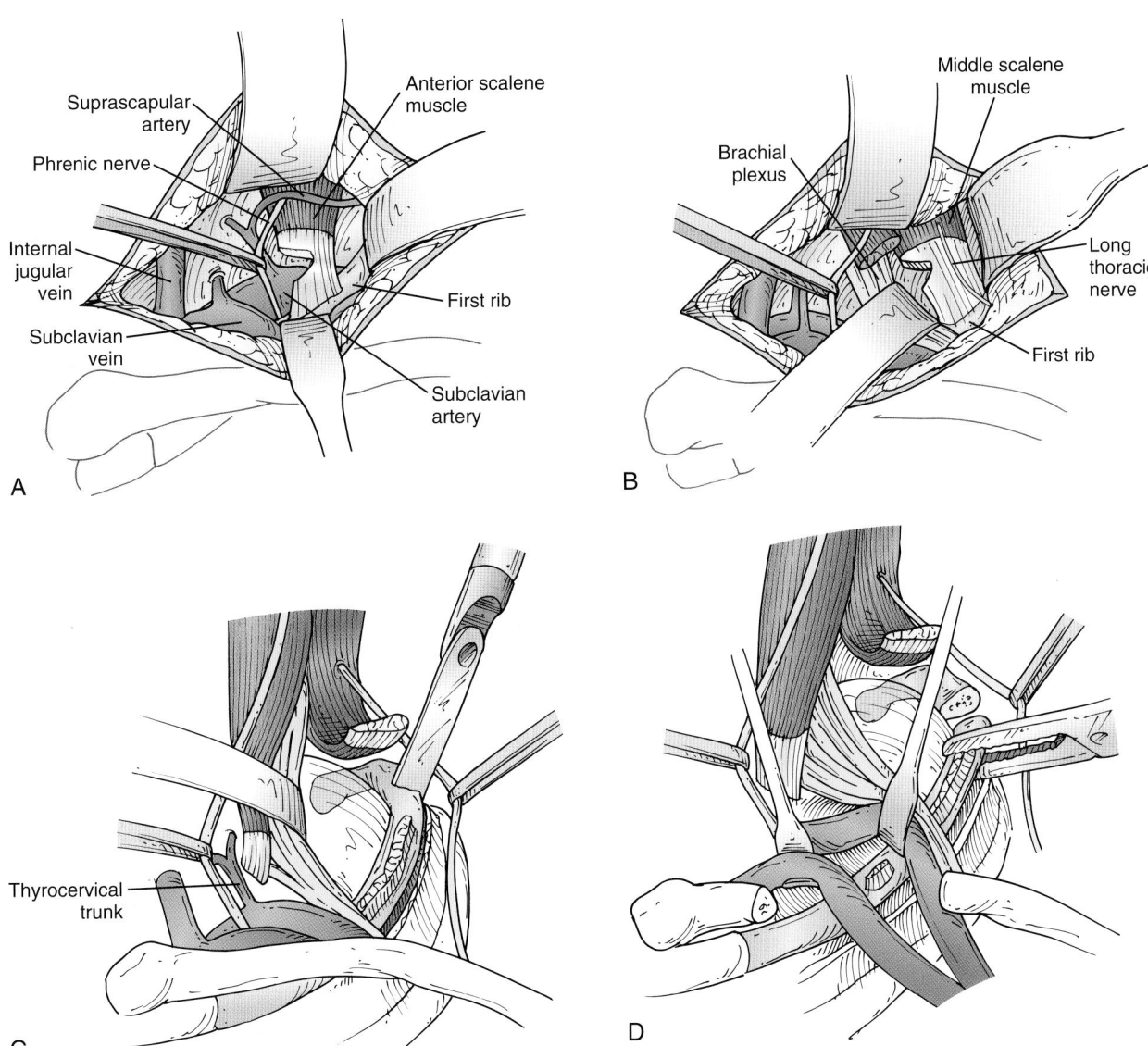

Figure 124-5 Operative view of the supraclavicular approach to thoracic outlet decompression. **A,** After mobilization of the scalene fat pad, the phrenic nerve should be identified and carefully elevated before the anterior scalene muscle is divided. **B,** The long thoracic nerve should be identified and protected during division of the middle scalene muscle. **C,** Attachments are freed via an extraperiosteal approach to prevent recurrent symptoms from reossification of the periosteal bed. **D,** Division of the first rib should be performed under direct vision to minimize the possibility of damage to the brachial plexus. After the first rib is divided just distal to the tubercle, the divided rib can be held as a lever to aid in clearing the overlying vessels. (*A, from Valentine RJ, Wind GG. Anatomic Exposures in Vascular Surgery. 2nd ed. Philadelphia, PA: Lippincott Williams & Wilkins; 2003:130. By permission. B, from Valentine RJ, Wind GG. Anatomic Exposures in Vascular Surgery. 2nd ed. Philadelphia, PA: Lippincott Williams & Wilkins; 2003:131. By permission. C, from Valentine RJ, Wind GG. Anatomic Exposures in Vascular Surgery. 2nd ed. Philadelphia, PA: Lippincott Williams & Wilkins; 2003:132. By permission. D, from Valentine RJ, Wind GG. Anatomic Exposures in Vascular Surgery. 2nd ed. Philadelphia, PA: Lippincott Williams & Wilkins; 2003:133. By permission.*)

Postoperative Management

In addition to supportive care, patients may benefit from physical therapy and range-of-motion exercises to shorten convalescence. Arterial repairs should be monitored with serial physical examination and noninvasive studies such as duplex ultrasound. Examination intervals vary from institution to institution, but the Oregon group has recommended examinations at 3 months postoperatively and every 6 months thereafter.[9]

Definition of Success and Determinants of Outcome

Successful outcome after treatment of arterial TOS is determined by relief of symptoms, avoidance of recurrence, patency of arterial bypasses, and limb salvage. Published series report complete relief of symptoms in more than 90% of patients.[6,8-10] Gelabert and Machleder have identified the following reasons for failed procedures: inaccurate diagnosis, failure to identify and correct the proximal embolizing lesion, and inadequate decompression.[14] Unlike neurogenic TOS, recurrence of arterial TOS is very rare in patients who have undergone complete thoracic outlet decompression and adequate arterial reconstruction. Bypass patency rates are reported in the range of 90% to 100%, depending on the status of the outflow vessels.[6,8,14] Limb salvage rates should approach 100% for Scher I and II lesions; distal embolization may result in finger amputation in Scher III patients, but arm amputation is distinctly uncommon.[14,22]

Results

Long-term results are related to the status of the distal vasculature. Limbs with compromised outflow secondary to embolization have a poorer prognosis. One of the largest series examined 55 cases of arterial TOS.[8] The early results showed no mortality and a low rate of morbidity (7%). The long-term results (mean follow-up, 5 years 8 months) of thoracic outlet decompression and vascular reconstruction were excellent, with 91% remaining asymptomatic and 9% experiencing exertional symptoms only. Of the four patients who were symptomatic at late follow-up, three originally had distal ischemia and required thromboembolectomy for brachial artery occlusions. There were no amputations in this series. In another series of 27 limbs with arterial TOS, Durham and colleagues reported 100% patency at a median of 38 months' follow-up in patients who underwent extensive saphenous vein reconstruction.[6] For Scher stage I lesions, decompression of the thoracic outlet alone is sufficient, with excellent results and the expectation that the post-stenotic dilatation will regress within a year.[6]

Complications

Operative mortality is negligible in these typically young patients. Morbidity is related to the closely related anatomic structures in the thoracic outlet and includes pneumothorax, hemothorax, chylous leak, brachial plexopathy, and vascular injury. Injury to the phrenic or long thoracic nerves is also possible. Rarely, injury to the cervical sympathetic chain may result in Horner's syndrome. The overall morbidity rate in published series ranges from 7% to 40%,[6,9,45] with pleural entry and transient brachial plexus injury being most frequent.

SELECTED KEY REFERENCES

Cormier JM, Amrane M, Ward A, Laurian C, Gigou F. Arterial complications of the thoracic outlet syndrome: fifty five operative cases. *J Vasc Surg.* 1989;9:778-787.
Largest published series of patients treated for arterial thoracic outlet syndrome and followed for a mean of more than 5 years.

Sanders RJ, Haug C. Review of arterial thoracic outlet syndrome with a report of five new instances. *Surg Gynecol Obstet.* 1991;173:415-425.
Comprehensive overview of the pathophysiology, clinical findings, and treatment options for arterial thoracic outlet syndrome.

Scher LA, Veith FJ, Haimovichi H, Samson RH, Ascer E, Gupta SK, Sprayregens S. Staging of arterial complications of cervical rib: guidelines for surgical management. *Surgery.* 1984;95:664-669.
Original article describing the modern classification of arterial thoracic outlet syndrome.

Thompson RW, Petrinec D, Toursarkissian B. Surgical treatment of thoracic outlet syndromes. II. Supraclavicular exploration and vascular reconstruction. *Ann Vasc Surg.* 1997;11:442-451.
Well-illustrated technical description of the surgical treatment of arterial thoracic outlet syndrome.

REFERENCES

The reference list can be found on the companion Expert Consult Web site at *www.expertconsult.com.*

CHAPTER 125

Thoracic Outlet Syndrome: Venous

Andres Schanzer and Louis M. Messina

Paget–von Schroetter syndrome was defined by Hughes in 1949 when he undertook a comprehensive review of the world's literature related to subclavian and axillary vein thrombosis.[1] In 1875, Paget had defined the syndrome of acute arm swelling and pain and thought that it was due to vasospasm.[2] However, in 1884, von Schroetter was the first to attribute these symptoms of acute upper extremity pain and swelling to subclavian and axillary vein thrombosis.[3]

Subsequent to this publication, primary subclavian-axillary vein thrombosis was most often identified in individuals who participated in activities that involve repetitive, vigorous exertion of the upper extremity. Primary subclavian-axillary vein thrombosis is common in young athletes and people employed in occupations that require repetitive activities with the arms elevated. Thus, in otherwise healthy individuals, subclavian venous compression occurs intermittently during strenuous activity, usually with the arm positioned in an elevated position. In such circumstances, the repetitive external compression of the vein occurs between the clavicle and the underlying subclavius muscle and fibers of the costocoracoid ligament from above and by the first rib and the anterior scalene muscle inserting on the tubercle of the first rib from below (see Chapter 122: Thoracic Outlet Syndrome: General Considerations). Such repetitive compression causes external vein wall compression, endothelial injury, and intermittent stasis. Eventually, perivenous fibrosis and endothelial injury lead to acute thrombosis.

PRIMARY SUBCLAVIAN-AXILLARY VEIN THROMBOSIS

Epidemiology

Primary upper extremity deep venous thrombosis (DVT) is a rare disorder that occurs in 2 per 100,000 individuals per year.[4] The annual incidence in the general population is 0.1%, and it increases with aging to as high as 1%.[5] It is estimated that upper extremity DVT accounts for approximately 2% to 4% of all cases of DVT.[5,6] Upper extremity DVT can be a relatively common occurrence in a hospital, with an estimated prevalence of 2 cases per 1000 hospital admissions.[7]

Etiology

Venous thoracic outlet syndrome (TOS) is a condition that ultimately results in thrombosis or severe narrowing of the subclavian-axillary vein secondary to chronic extrinsic mechanical compression. This clinical syndrome has been referred to as "effort thrombosis" because of its association with young, otherwise healthy individuals who engage in activities requiring repetitive arm and shoulder motion.[8-11] The venous pathology is a direct result of repetitive injury to the subclavian vein at the level of the costoclavicular space, the most medial aspect of the thoracic outlet (Fig. 125-1). The key anatomic structures contributing to compression of the subclavian vein and recurrent venous trauma are the first rib, the clavicle with its associated subclavius muscle and fibrous costocoracoid ligament, and the anterior scalene muscle and tubercle.[1,10,12,13] A cycle of alternating post-traumatic inflammation and quiescence leads to perivenous fibrosis, endothelial injury, stasis of blood flow, and thrombosis.[12]

Although venous TOS can occur in the absence of any identifiable anatomic abnormality,[14,15] a diverse array of anomalies associated with the thoracic outlet has been reported at the time of surgery, including abnormalities of the anterior scalene, subclavius, pectoralis minor, and scalenus minimus

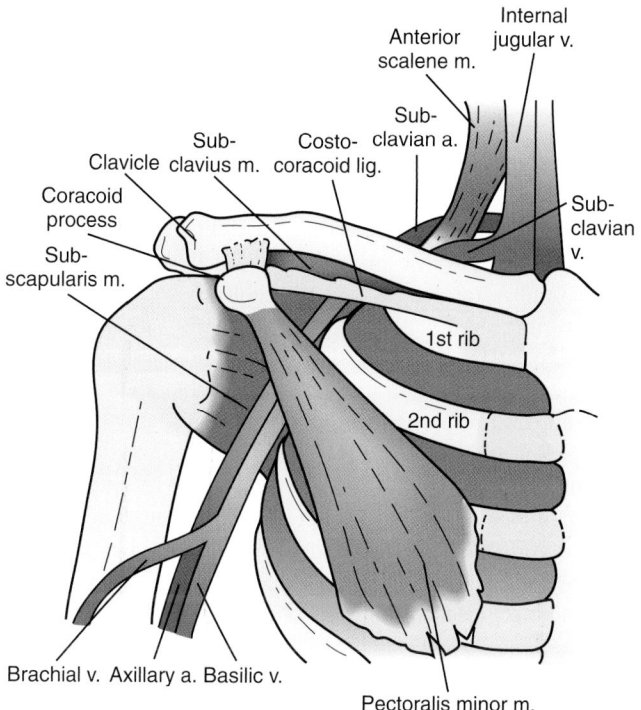

Figure 125-1 Anatomy of the thoracic outlet.

muscles; bony abnormalities of the clavicle and ribs; and ligamentous abnormalities of the costocoracoid ligament.[10,14-20] In many cases, compression of the subclavian-axillary vein may occur at the costoclavicular space without progression to thrombosis. This point is underscored by venographic studies evaluating the contralateral extremity in patients with confirmed subclavian-axillary vein thrombosis; although significant compression with provocative measures is visualized in 56% to 80% of contralateral limbs, the incidence of bilateral thrombosis is markedly less at 2% to 15%.[9,21-27]

Clinical Findings

Venous TOS usually develops in young, healthy patients with few, if any, co-morbid conditions. The mean age at diagnosis is 32 years, with the majority of patients affected between the second and fourth decades.[27] Traditionally, men have been reported to be affected more often than women; however, the largest series published to date (312 affected extremities) reported an equal gender ratio.[27] Individuals who perform strenuous or sustained upper extremity activities, whether athletic or occupational, are particularly prone to the development of subclavian-axillary vein thrombosis. The dominant arm is involved in the clear majority of cases.[26]

Upper extremity edema is the hallmark characteristic associated with subclavian-axillary vein thrombosis. The edema is often, though not always, accompanied by pain and cyanosis of the affected extremity. The edema usually involves the shoulder, arm, and hand and is characteristically nonpitting. Dilated superficial veins over the shoulder, neck, and anterior chest wall can often be visualized as collateral veins that accommodate to the increased venous hypertension (a pattern often referred to as "first rib bypass venous collaterals").[12] A minority of patients may also have symptoms of neurogenic TOS (see Chapter 123: Thoracic Outlet Syndrome: Neurogenic). This association may be due to the presence of multiple anomalies of the thoracic outlet anatomy and performance of repetitive upper extremity arm activities.

Most patients complain of some degree of pain, which is often described as "aching," "stabbing," or a feeling of "tightness" that worsens with exertion.[10] Extended use of the arm may cause an increase in arterial blood flow for which the limited collateral venous bed is unable to compensate; this leads to increased venous hypertension and subsequently to worsening symptoms of venous stasis and arm congestion. Depending on the timing of evaluation and treatment, the occlusion and resulting symptoms can be acute or chronic.

Urschel and Razzuk reported that of all patients with venous TOS in their 30-year experience (312 extremities), 93% complained of arm swelling, 77% demonstrated bluish discoloration, 66% had aching pain with exercise, and only 8% reported minimal symptoms.[27] Similarly, Swinton and coauthors reported in their series that 52% of patients were symptomatic, 39% were completely disabled, and only a small proportion, 9%, were asymptomatic.[28]

The two most severe potential complications of subclavian-axillary vein thrombosis are pulmonary embolism and upper extremity phlegmasia cerulea dolens (venous gangrene). Fortunately, both are reported to occur relatively infrequently. The reported incidence of pulmonary embolism secondary to subclavian-axillary vein thrombosis is less than 12%.[1,10,11,29-31] Furthermore, the small clot burden, as compared with iliofemoral DVT, may reduce the clinical impact of this entity. Venous gangrene is exceedingly rare and has been limited to case reports in patients with malignancy or an underlying hypercoagulable state.[32] There have been no published reports of venous gangrene occurring secondary to venous TOS.

Diagnostic Evaluation

The diagnosis of subclavian-axillary vein thrombosis requires recognition of the clinical signs and symptoms just presented, followed by definitive imaging studies.

Duplex Ultrasound. Duplex ultrasonography is the first step in confirming a clinical suspicion of venous TOS. Overlying structures such as the clavicle may make duplex interrogation of the vascular structures coursing through the thoracic outlet challenging. Therefore, duplex examinations relying on B-mode ultrasound alone have historically demonstrated low sensitivity (54%) and high specificity (100%) for the detection of subclavian-axillary vein thrombosis.[33] Recent technologic advances such as color-flow duplex, used in conjunction with indirect criteria suggesting the presence of an occlusion (evaluation for phasicity of flow with respiration and augmentation with compressive maneuvers), have led to markedly increased sensitivity (81% to 100%) while maintaining high specificity (82% to 100%).[23,34-38] See under "Secondary Subclavian-Axillary Vein Thrombosis" for a comprehensive review of the role of duplex scanning in this diagnosis, as well as an algorithm should the results of duplex scanning be equivocal.

Magnetic Resonance and Computed Tomographic Venography

Magnetic resonance venography (MRV) is another noninvasive imaging modality that has been used with increasing frequency for the diagnosis of venous TOS.[17,39-41] Although the sensitivity and specificity of MRV have been reported to be comparable to those of duplex ultrasound, we have not found this test to be necessary for patients with suspected venous TOS. The cost and time required for completion of the examination are substantial, and we have therefore continued to choose duplex ultrasound. With time and more accumulation of data, the role of MRV in patients with suspected subclavian-axillary vein thrombosis will be better defined.

Computed tomographic venography (CTV) shows high concordance with duplex ultrasound. When imaging of the extremity veins and pulmonary arteries is considered clinically indicated, CTV can be used to reliably diagnose DVT.

Venography

Venography remains the "gold standard" for the diagnosis of venous TOS and also plays a fundamental role in the current standard treatment of the condition. Invasive catheter-based imaging should be reserved for patients whose condition warrants an intervention. The patient is placed in the supine position, and the entire arm is circumferentially prepared into the field. The basilic vein is percutaneously punctured under ultrasound guidance. Cephalic vein access will often result in an incomplete diagnostic study because the cephalic vein often drains directly into the subclavian vein, thereby bypassing the axillary vein; thrombosis of this critical portion will therefore be missed. If thrombosis is visualized (Fig. 125-2), thrombolysis of the subclavian-axillary vein can be initiated with this approach. Once thrombolysis is successful or in patients found to have a patent but

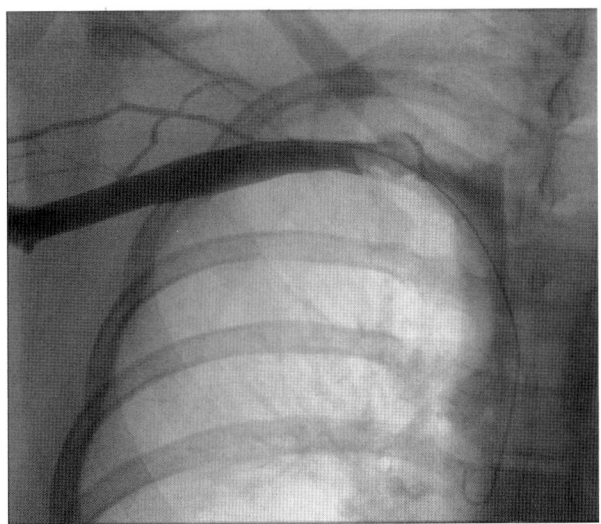

Figure 125-2 Venogram revealing an acute primary subclavian-axillary vein thrombosis.

severely narrowed subclavian-axillary vein, positional venography is performed. Positional venography involves a venogram of the subclavian-axillary vein segment performed in full adduction and then in 90 degrees of abduction with external rotation ("hand-on-head" position) (Fig. 125-3). These positional images are helpful to confirm the presence of extrinsic compression of the subclavian vein at the level of the thoracic outlet.

Evaluation of the collateral circulation is another important function of venography. The extent of collateralization provides information about the hemodynamic significance of the occlusion or stenosis and about the chronicity of the occlusion. Chronicity of the occlusion, in turn, plays a key role in dictating management and therefore has therapeutic implications. Accordingly, we classify patients into one of three categories based on their history and venographic findings: (1) acute subclavian-axillary vein thrombosis, (2) chronic or recurrent subclavian-axillary vein thrombosis, or (3) high-grade symptomatic subclavian-axillary vein stenosis.

Treatment

Anticoagulation Alone

Historically, treatment of acute primary subclavian-axillary vein thrombosis consisted of rest and elevation of the affected extremity, accompanied by a variable duration of systemic anticoagulation. Several retrospective reviews have demonstrated this approach to venous TOS to be associated with significant long-term morbidity and patient disability.[1,10,16,26,42] Hughes and colleagues reported on the conservative management of 320 patients with primary subclavian-axillary vein thrombosis, 40% of whom had persistent symptoms or limited recovery.[1] Likewise, in separate publications, Adams and DeWeese, Tilney and colleagues, and Urschel and Razzuk each reported high rates of residual functional impairment after treating patients with venous TOS in this manner (approximately 70%, 75%, and 74%, respectively).[10,26,27]

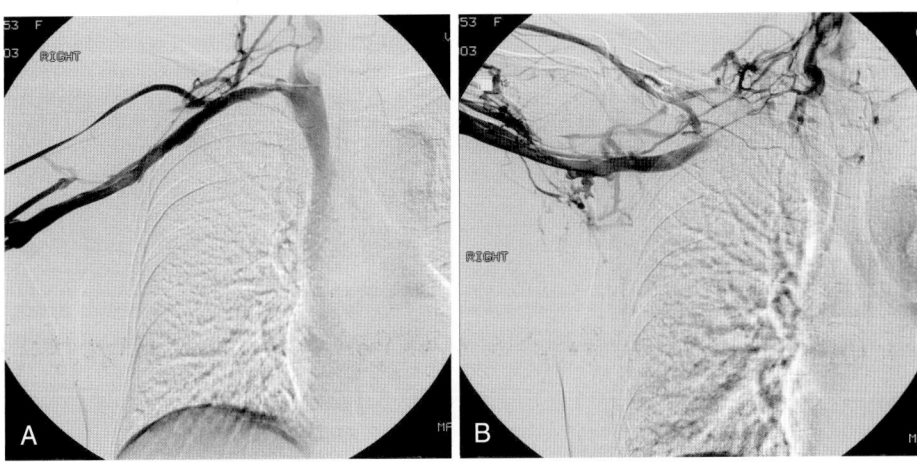

Figure 125-3 Venogram of the subclavian-axillary vein after successful thrombolysis with the extremity in full adduction (**A**) and in full abduction (**B**).

Thrombolytic Therapy

The early use of catheter-directed thrombolysis has emerged as the preferred initial management strategy in the modern treatment paradigm of venous TOS.[12,27,38,43-46] Because subclavian-axillary thrombus is much more localized than lower extremity DVT, this approach usually lyses the subclavian-axillary vein clot quickly to restore luminal patency. In 1981, Zimmerman and associates documented, in a small case series, the successful use of systemic urokinase in 82% of patients with acute primary subclavian-axillary thrombosis.[47] Since this initial series, many authors have demonstrated high rates of success in re-establishing patency with catheter-directed thrombolysis (Fig. 125-4).[38,43-46] Lee and colleagues reported their experience treating 64 patients with primary subclavian-axillary thrombosis. As the first step in their treatment algorithm, 54 patients with symptom onset within 7 days underwent attempted catheter-directed thrombolysis; 100% experienced successful restoration of luminal patency.[38] If thrombolysis is initiated within 14 days of the onset of symptoms, the results are generally reported to be excellent.[9,44] Treatment with thrombolysis in patients with greater than 14 days of symptoms is possible,[43,46] albeit with a decreased chance for successful re-establishment of luminal patency.

Thrombolysis Technique.
Although numerous thrombolytic agents and devices are available, the technical concepts for all are similar. Under ultrasound guidance, the ipsilateral basilic vein is accessed, and a wire is advanced centrally across the thrombosed vein into the superior vena cava (SVC) or right atrium. A catheter containing side holes for delivery of drug is then positioned across the thrombosed region. An infusion of thrombolytic agent is then commenced and continued for usually less than 48 hours, with intermittent reimaging to assess for progress. See Chapter 35 (Thrombolytic Agents) for a complete review of the pharmacology related to the available thrombolytic agents.

Alternatively, numerous mechanical thrombectomy devices that feature clot maceration and aspiration can be used at the initial procedure and during subsequent re-imaging.[48-50] The two devices commonly used by our group are the AngioJet (Possis, Minneapolis, MN) and the Trellis Peripheral Infusion System (Bacchus Vascular, Santa Clara, CA). These technologies, albeit at greater cost, allow more rapid clot dissolution than can be achieved with traditional thrombolysis infusion. The AngioJet functions by high-pressure injection of fluid through a distal catheter pore with simultaneous rapid aspiration through an adjacent pore. Secondary to the Bernoulli effect, an eddy current is created that results in low pressure and subsequent clot maceration and aspiration. In contrast, the Trellis system is a multilumen catheter with two compliant balloons at the distal end and infusion holes located between these balloons. An integrated wire is connected to a drive unit that oscillates the wire within the isolated region to macerate the clot and disperse the infused fluid (i.e., lytic agent). The isolated area between the occluding balloons can then be aspirated through the catheter lumen.

Post-thrombolysis Management.
At the conclusion of thrombolysis, patients can be divided into two major categories: (1) unsuccessful thrombolysis and (2) successful thrombolysis. Patients with unsuccessful thrombolysis, defined as persistent total occlusion of the subclavian-axillary vein, should receive warfarin anticoagulation and measures aimed at control of local symptoms, such as rest, compression, and elevation. Unsuccessful thrombolysis of acute subclavian vein thrombosis is rare and almost always seen in patients who have had repeated episodes of lysis, anticoagulation, and rethrombosis. Although we do not offer these patients surgical treatment, a limited number of authors, in small series, have recommended aggressive regimens that include thoracic outlet decompression with variable lengths of chronic anticoagulation. Using this strategy in a group of 42 patients, Urschel and Razzuk reported a 57% rate of recanalization and resolution of symptoms.[27] de Leon and colleagues reported 100% success in their small cases series of four patients who underwent thoracic outlet decompression and were then maintained on chronic anticoagulation until recanalization was documented.[51]

Patients in whom thrombolysis was successful, defined as those with re-establishment of subclavian-axillary vein patency, can be further subdivided, based on completion positional venography, according to the absence or presence of demonstrable extrinsic compression at the thoracic outlet.

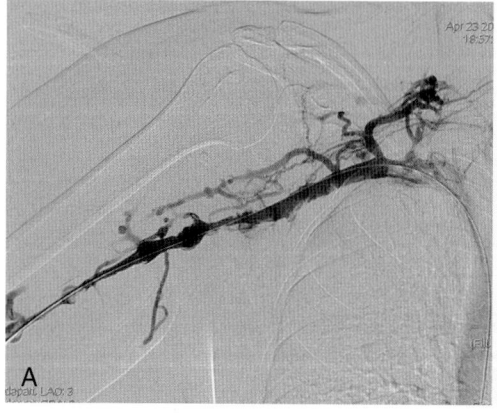
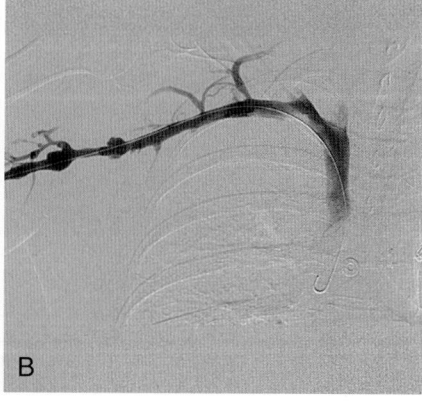

Figure 125-4 Venogram of the subclavian-axillary vein before (**A**) and after (**B**) thrombolysis.

Section **16** Upper Extremity Arterial Disease

Patients without extrinsic compression will not benefit from thoracic outlet decompression and should be treated with 3 to 6 months of systemic anticoagulation.[52]

In patients found to have venous TOS, no effort is made at the completion of successful thrombolysis to dilate a persistent subclavian vein stenosis. We favor immediate thoracic outlet decompression and intraoperative venography and subclavian vein angioplasty. At the other end of the spectrum, some recommend 3 to 6 months of systemic anticoagulation after successful thrombolysis.[18,53] Management of patients with extrinsic compression, or radiographically documented venous TOS, is discussed under "Surgical Decompression of the Thoracic Outlet."

Surgical Decompression of the Thoracic Outlet

Patients with persistent stenosis or signs of extrinsic compression on positional venography after thrombolysis remain at significant risk for recurrent thrombosis with anticoagulation alone.[46] In addition, if the underlying pathophysiology has not been addressed, adjunctive therapies such as balloon angioplasty or stent placement may provide satisfactory immediate results but lack sufficient durability to be used as definitive therapy.[38,43,54-56] Multiple reports have confirmed that the radial force associated with either a self-expanding or balloon-expandable stent is not adequate to compensate for the compressive force between the first rib and clavicle; stent deformation, fracture, and thrombosis in this setting are the norm rather than the exception (Fig. 125-5). Therefore, stents have no role in the treatment of venous TOS before surgical decompression.

Once subclavian-axillary vein patency has been restored and extrinsic compression has been demonstrated, first rib resection with external venolysis should be performed. Although some authors advocate deferring surgical decompression for 1 to 3 months after thrombolysis to allow healing of the venous endothelium and resolution of the acute inflammatory process,[18,53] most now agree that decompression

should take place during the same hospitalization as the thrombolysis to decrease the significant risk for reocclusion that may occur between thrombolysis and deferred surgery.[9,27,43,45,46,57,58] Immediate operative decompression, even as early as 4 hours after thrombolysis,[59] has been demonstrated to be safe and effective. This shift to immediate surgery has virtually eliminated the vein rethrombosis rate of 6% to 18% that has been reported to occur during the waiting period.[9,53,60]

Surgical Techniques

Paraclavicular Approach. The patient is placed on the operating room table in the semi-Fowler position. A small roll is placed transversely posteriorly just below the shoulders. The head is extended and rotated away from the operative site. The neck, chest, and affected extremity are prepared and draped sterilely. The arm, forearm, and hand are wrapped in a stockinette. During the procedure the arm is maintained in the adducted position, the elbow is flexed at 90 degrees, and the arm is fixed so that there is no tension on the brachial plexus throughout the procedure.

A transverse incision is made one fingerbreadth above the clavicle beginning at the lateral border of the sternocleidomastoid muscle and extended just beyond the external jugular vein. Extensive inferior and superior subplatysmal flaps are created. Portions of the clavicular head of the sternocleidomastoid muscle can be divided to provide exposure. The scalene fat pad is then mobilized on a lateral pedicle. This mobilization is initiated by taking down the medial attachments of the fat pad at the level of the internal jugular vein. Usually, the tissue is tied with 3-0 silk suture to prevent postoperative lymph leakage. The dissection is carried down to the junction of the internal jugular and subclavian vein and extended laterally to the insertion of the external jugular vein into the subclavian vein. Finally, the fat pad is mobilized superiorly until one encounters the cutaneous nerves of the chest and shoulder region. A self-retaining retractor (Omnitract, Minneapolis, MN) is put into position.

The medial and lateral borders of the anterior scalene muscle are mobilized, and the phrenic nerve is identified (Fig. 125-6A). The phrenic nerve is never directly grasped with an instrument. Rather, a generous length of fascia on either side of the nerve is incised and used to retract the phrenic nerve and expose the anterior surface of the anterior scalene muscle. Mobilization of the phrenic nerve is continued down to the thoracic inlet. The anterior scalene muscle is incised directly from its insertion on the tubercle of the first rib (Fig. 125-6B). It is then dissected posteriorly while hemostasis is maintained with a bipolar cautery. Frequently, a portion of the anterior scalene or a separate scalenus minimus will pass beneath the subclavian artery. The muscle is dissected proximally to the point of its attachments to the transverse processes of the cervical spine and then excised. The plane in the deep cervical fascia is developed laterally with a moistened sponge to expose the brachial plexus and the middle scalene muscle. After locating the long thoracic nerve, the middle scalene muscle is

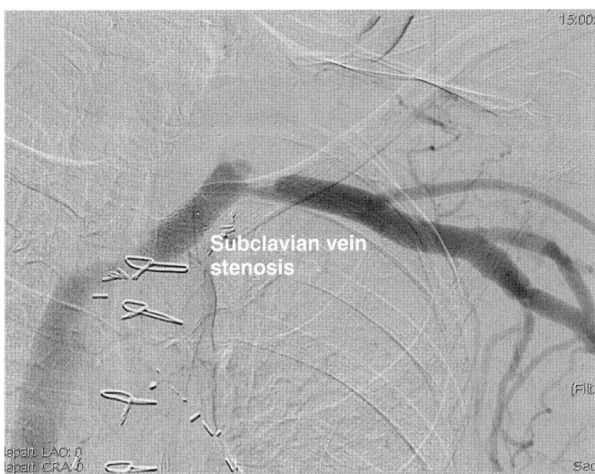

Figure 125-5 Deformed balloon-expandable stent 6 weeks after treatment of primary subclavian-axillary thrombosis.

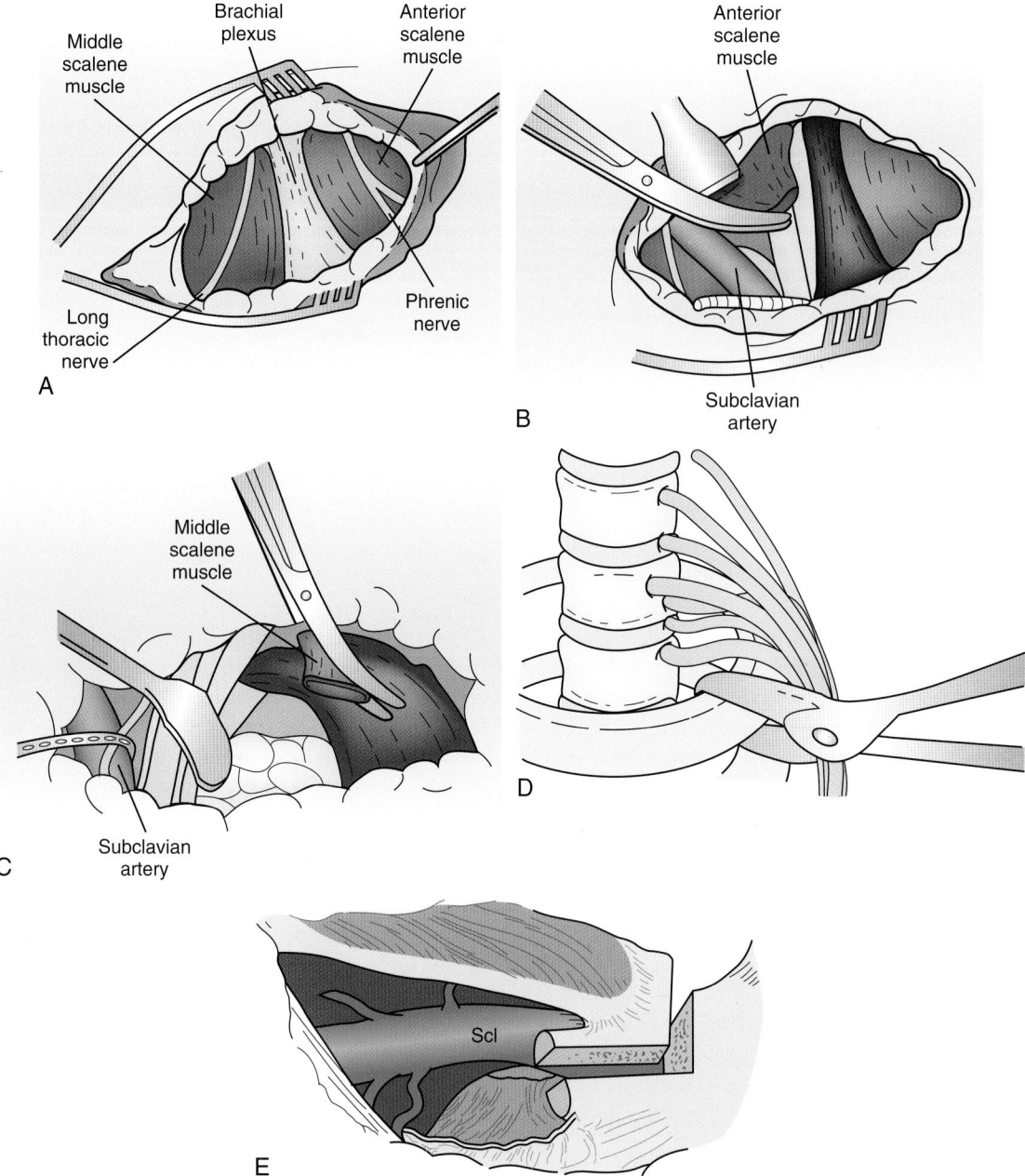

Figure 125-6 Paraclavicular approach. **A,** The brachial plexus is noted in its position between the anterior and middle scalene muscles. The phrenic nerve is seen coursing in a lateromedial direction across the anterior surface of the anterior scalene muscle. The supraclavicular nerves are being retracted. Also shown is the long thoracic nerve exiting from the posterior border of the middle scalene muscle. **B,** Division of the anterior scalene insertion from the first rib. The subclavian artery will be directly behind the anterior scalene muscle. **C,** The middle scalene muscle is divided from the first rib. **D,** The first rib is divided with a rib cutter. **E,** Transmanubrial extension of the subclavicular incision to the center of the sternum and vertically up to the sternal notch exposes the entire subclavian (Scl) and innominate veins without any need to remove or divide the clavicle. *(A–D, from Schneider DB, Azakie A, Messina LM, Stoney RJ. Management of vascular thoracic outlet syndrome. Chest Surg Clin North Am. 1999;6:781-803. E, from Molina JE, Hunter DW, Dietz CA. Paget-Schroetter syndrome treated with thrombolytics and immediate surgery. J Vasc Surg. 2007;45:328-334.)*

mobilized and then resected, with the long thoracic nerve used as the superior and lateral limits of this resection (Fig. 125-6C). The resection is carried down to the first rib. A periosteal elevator is used to dissect the attachments of the middle scalene muscle from the first rib. Often, some of the fibers of the middle scalene muscle extend to the second rib and are incised with Metzenbaum scissors. A plane is devel-

oped between the region of insertion of the anterior scalene and middle scalene muscles beneath the clavicle with a periosteal elevator. The intercostal fibers are incised similarly. The first rib is resected with a bone cutter or a Kerrison rongeur just distal to its articulation with the vertebra (Fig. 125-6D). Similarly, it is excised as medially as possible near its junction with the sternum. The subclavian vein is inspected and dissected circumferentially should any perivenous fibrosis be present.

It is critical that the first rib be resected at its junction with the sternum. To accomplish this, it is sometimes helpful to make a small counterincision just beneath the clavicle. The pectoralis major and minor fibers are separated and the rib identified. The remainder of the surface of the rib is then dissected with a periosteal elevator while taking care to note the location of the subclavian vein. This often requires resection of a portion of the subclavius muscle. After the rib is dissected thoroughly, it is resected up to the sternal junction (Fig. 125-6E). The scalene fat pad is reattached with interrupted 3-0 Vicryl suture. A Blake drain is placed routinely, and the platysma and skin are closed.

A lateral extension is added to the operating table, and the affected arm is abducted. The basilic vein is punctured and venography is performed in both the neutral and fully rotated positions with the hand over the head. Complete thoracic outlet decompression will reveal no compression of the vein with the arm rotated above the patient's head. Should residual stenosis be present, it can usually be dilated with balloon angioplasty. If this is not possible, the subclavian vein is opened, the residual chronic thrombus is removed, and a vein patch is placed. In our experience, more extensive replacement of the subclavian vein has not been necessary. Placement of stents after decompression should rarely be necessary.

Patients are not continued on anticoagulation postoperatively other than aspirin. They are usually able to be discharged on oral pain medication within 48 to 72 hours. When patients have had more than one cycle of thrombosis and thrombolysis or when concern persists that the vein remains prothrombotic, patients receive 3 to 6 months of postoperative anticoagulation.

Infraclavicular Approach. In Molina and colleagues' relatively large series of 114 patients who underwent treatment of venous TOS, all thoracic outlet decompressions were performed through an infraclavicular-only approach.[45] This approach is well described and involves partial resection of the anterior half of the first rib, removal of the subclavius tendon, and division of the anterior scalene tendon and part of the middle scalene muscle to the level of the subclavian artery. In this series, all patients underwent vein patch angioplasty of the subclavian vein with a segment of harvested great saphenous vein (Fig. 125-7A). Of note, in 12 patients found to have long stenoses (>2 cm), transmanubrial extension of the incision was performed. This consisted of extending the incision medially across the sternum to the midline and then angling 90 degrees up toward the sternal notch (Fig. 125-7B). These select patients were then managed with 6 weeks of postoperative arm immobilization. Angioplasty plus stent placement was used as an alternative strategy in seven patients with residual stenoses not amenable to local patch angioplasty. In this small group of patients, all stents were reported to remain patent on duplex follow-up (mean follow-up of 14 years). To date, this remains the largest published experience of central vein stenting after thoracic outlet decompression.

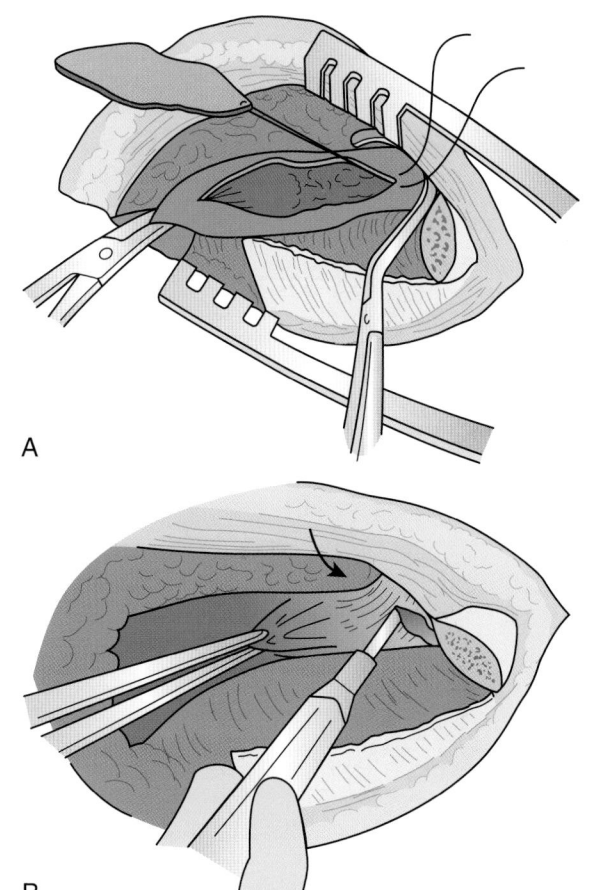

Figure 125-7 Infraclavicular approach. **A,** The saphenous vein patch is laid over the strictured segment of the vein. **B,** The key to success is complete mobilization of the subclavian vein by detaching it anteriorly from the sternum (*arrow*) until the vein is easily exposed in the operative field. This allows sufficient margin for placement of the medial clamp between the site of the stricture and normal innominate vein. (*A and B, from Molina JE, Hunter DW, Dietz CA. Paget-Schroetter syndrome treated with thrombolytics and immediate surgery. J Vasc Surg. 2007;45:328-334.*)

Transaxillary Approach. Several groups prefer and report excellent results with the use of a transaxillary surgical approach for first rib resection, scalenectomy, and venolysis (Fig. 125-8A).[27,53,61,62] For a scholarly description of the technical steps required for successful transaxillary first rib resection, we recommend the review on this topic by Urschel and Razzuk.[27] The key features include an incision below the axillary hairline between the pectoralis major and latissimus dorsi muscles. As the dissection is carried through the subcutaneous tissue cephalic to the first rib, attention is directed toward preservation of the intercostal brachial cutaneous nerve (exits between the first and second ribs). The anterior scalene muscle is divided and resected up into the neck. The first rib is dissected subperiosteally and separated from the adherent parietal pleura. The anterior portion of the rib is dissected off the subclavian vein, the costoclavicular ligament is divided, and the rib is transected at the sternal border. The posterior rib is dissected off the subclavian artery and brachial plexus,

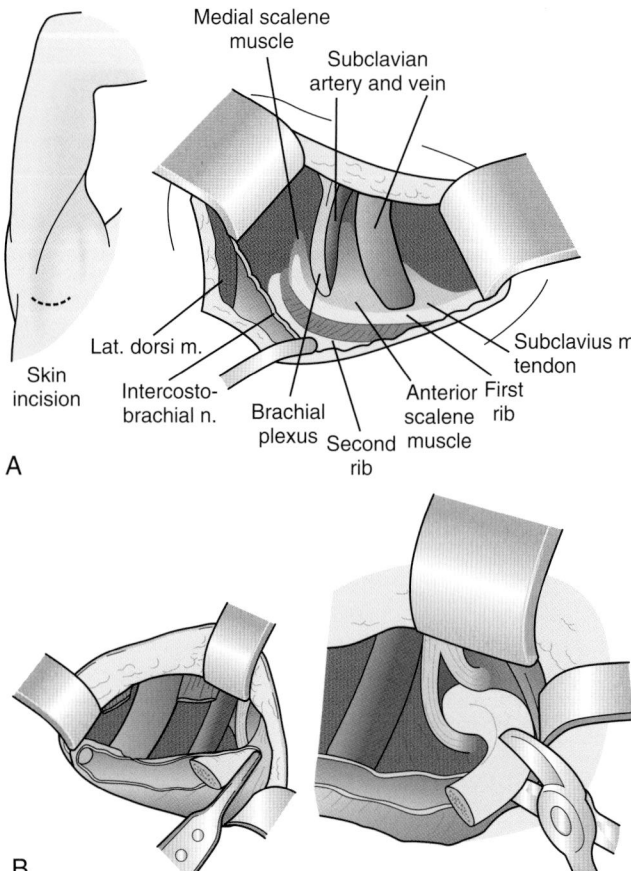

Figure 125-8 Transaxillary approach. **A,** View of the thoracic outlet from the transaxillary approach. **B,** The posterior part of the rib is dissected subperiosteally to the transverse process, where it is divided with rib shears. The rib may be resected posteriorly with an Urschel-Leskell re-enforced rongeur. Care is taken to avoid injury to the C8 and T1 nerve roots as the middle scalene muscle is dissected from the rib. *(A, from Machleder HI. Evaluation of a new treatment strategy for Paget-Schroetter syndrome: spontaneous thrombosis of the axillary-subclavian vein. J Vasc Surg. 1993;17:305-315. B, from Schneider DB, Azakie A, Messina LM, Stoney RJ. Management of vascular thoracic outlet syndrome. Chest Surg Clin North Am. 1999;6:781-803.)*

the middle scalene muscle is divided, and the rib is transected at the level of the transverse process of the vertebra (Fig. 125-8B). Complete venolysis is then carried out before closure of the wound.

Vein Treatment after First Rib Resection

The main controversy in the treatment of venous TOS continues to revolve around how best to manage the subclavian-axillary vein after surgical decompression of the thoracic outlet is completed. The presence of residual subclavian vein stenosis, even after relief of the extrinsic compression, is not uncommon.[46,53,63] Recommended strategies to deal with these intrinsic lesions have spanned a diverse spectrum ranging from completion venography and angioplasty with[63] or without[46] stenting to extensive venous reconstructions including thrombectomy, patching, or bypass.[38,43,45] No direct com-

parisons between these two strategies have been performed to date, but it is clear that extensive venous reconstructions are accompanied by a higher complication rate. This issue is underscored by the experience of Melby and colleagues, in which 44% of their 32 patients underwent direct subclavian-axillary vein reconstruction and 100% experienced resolution of their symptoms (no patency data reported).[43] However, 22% of their patients required secondary operations for complications. Furthermore, if closure of adjunctive radiocephalic fistulae is also included as a secondary procedure, the overall rate of secondary procedures increases to 53%. In this experience, no intraoperative venography was used to assess the status of the subclavian vein after decompression of the thoracic outlet. As a consequence, no attempts at intraoperative angioplasty of residual lesions were undertaken.

Our group has favored an endovascular approach after thoracic outlet decompression, as originally described by Messina and colleagues at the University of California, San Francisco.[46] This strategy is expeditious, safe, and effective. In this study, 25 patients routinely underwent completion venography, with angioplasty as necessary, at the time of thoracic outlet decompression. Their overall results demonstrated 100% technical success, 100% resolution of symptoms, and 1-year primary and secondary patency rates of 92% and 96%, respectively. No postoperative anticoagulation was used in these patients. Based on these excellent results with angioplasty alone, it is only when a residual fixed filling defect is seen on completion venography that our group performs extensive venous reconstruction (Fig. 125-9). In our experience this situation is definitely the exception rather than the norm. The essential point is that intraoperative venography can direct the surgeon to the most appropriate treatment of a residual stenosis.

Results

For the most part, reports on the treatment of venous TOS are limited to case series, often with relatively small sample sizes. Nonetheless, in aggregate, the overwhelming evidence suggests that in properly selected patients, restoration of subclavian-axillary vein patency and decompression of the thoracic outlet result in excellent and durable outcomes. Table 125-1 summarizes the results of multiple series that have used, albeit with varying techniques, strategies to achieve the goal of vein patency and decompression of the thoracic outlet in patients with venous TOS. Although subclavian vein occlusion after abduction can be documented in a high percentage of the contralateral limbs of these patients, the risk for thrombosis has proved to be very low and therefore prophylactic procedures are not recommended.

■ SECONDARY SUBCLAVIAN-AXILLARY VEIN THROMBOSIS

By the 1970s, secondary upper extremity DVT became increasingly associated with the use of central venous cathe-

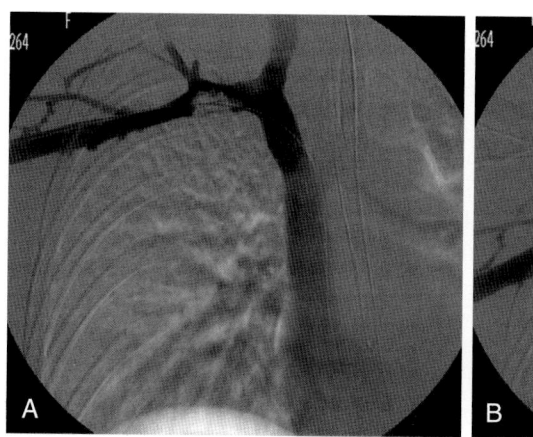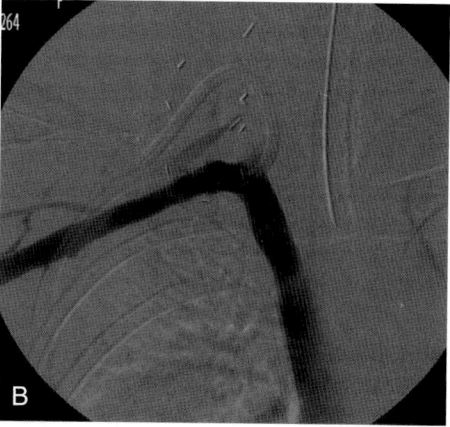

Figure 125-9 Venogram of the subclavian-axillary vein demonstrating (**A**) a fixed filling defect that was unresponsive to angioplasty after thrombolysis, paraclavicular first rib resection, circumferential venolysis, and scalenectomy and (**B**) patency with elimination of any residual stenosis after open thrombectomy and vein patch angioplasty.

Table 125-1 Results of Surgical Thoracic Outlet Decompression for Primary Subclavian-Axillary Thrombosis Published since 2000

		Results		
Series	Number of Patients	Clinical Success (%)	Secondary Patency (%)	Mean Follow-up (Mo)
Urschel and Razzuk[27]	277	95	NR	NR
Schneider et al.[46]	25	100	96 (1 yr)	10
Lee et al.[38]	29	93	97 (4 yr)	52
Doyle et al.[44]	34	100	92 (5 yr)	33
Molina et al.[45]	97	100	100 (5 yr)	62
Melby et al.[43]	32	100	NR	43

NR, not reported.

ters for chemotherapy, bone marrow transplantation, dialysis, and parenteral nutrition. Secondary upper extremity DVT can also be seen in patients with nephrotic syndrome, mediastinal tumors, malignancy, local surgery or trauma, and hypercoagulable states.

The most common causes of secondary subclavian vein thrombosis are catheter-induced thrombosis, cancer, and congestive heart failure. However the vast majority are secondary to various types of venous catheters such as pacemaker wires, tunneled catheters, peripherally inserted central catheters, and subcutaneous ports. Catheter-related subclavian-axillary venous thrombosis can be a serious disease resulting in pulmonary embolism and postphlebitic syndrome. In fact, catheter removal itself can be a cause of pulmonary embolism. As a catheter is removed, the fibrin sheath can break loose and embolize into the pulmonary circulation.[6]

Epidemiology

The reported overall incidence of catheter-related venous thrombosis has varied widely from 2% to 26% of all central venous catheters placed.[8,64] However, more recent studies suggest a much lower incidence of 5% or less.[11,37,65-67] In a recent prospective study of the risk factors for and incidence of catheter-related thrombosis in adult patients with cancer, 444 patients were studied for 76,713 patient-days of follow-up. The incidence of symptomatic catheter-related venous thrombosis was 4.3%, or 0.3 per 1000 catheter-days. Risk factors associated with a higher incidence of venous thrombosis were more than one attempt at insertion of the catheter, a history of a previous venous catheter use, and ovarian cancer.

In various studies, approximately 33% to 60% of patients with catheter-related venous thrombosis are asymptomatic The incidence of pulmonary embolism in patients with catheter-related thrombosis is between 15% and 25%, a not insubstantial figure.[68]

Pathogenesis
Etiology

Catheter-related central venous thrombosis is caused by a variety of factors. The vein wall can be damaged during catheter insertion, and the ongoing presence of the catheter can cause local stasis and inflammation of the endothelium. If, in addition, the patient has a hypercoagulable state such as cancer or sepsis, all of Virchow's triad is present: stasis, hypercoagulability, and intimal injury. The rate of thrombosis is not necessarily due to the duration of catheter placement.[66,69-71] In patients in whom upper extremity DVT develops as a result of implanted pacemaker wires, the presence of a low ejection fraction (<40%) has been shown to be associated with a higher incidence of venous thrombosis.[6]

Risk Factors

Cancer patients have up to an eightfold increased risk for venous thrombosis of the upper extremity.[5] In a recent population-based control study, it was also shown that immobilization of the arm, oral contraceptive use, a family history of venous thrombosis, and prothrombotic mutations increase the odds ratio from 2.0 to 3.1. Obese patients (body mass index >30 kg/m²) undergoing surgery have a 23-fold increase in upper extremity venous thrombosis over nonobese patients not undergoing surgery.

Natural History

The natural history of secondary upper limb DVT is poorly defined. With the use of sensitive methods, up to 50% of patients with lower extremity DVT will be found to have evidence of pulmonary embolism.[72] However, in the vast majority of these patients the pulmonary embolism produces few or no symptoms. There have been very few similar such studies examining the incidence of pulmonary embolism after upper limb DVT regardless of the etiology, primary or secondary. The incidence of pulmonary embolism in patients with upper limb DVT that is catheter related has varied from 0% to 50%. The average risk for pulmonary embolism after catheter-related subclavian-axillary vein thrombosis is approximately 20%. This risk for pulmonary embolism is higher after secondary than after primary upper limb venous thrombosis.

The incidence of post-thrombotic syndrome after secondary upper limb DVT has been difficult to characterize because of the diversity of causes, the frequency of serious concurrent illnesses such as cancer and its imposed early mortality, and lack of follow-up. In the largest such study, Hingorani and coworkers studied 170 patients with catheter-related upper limb thrombosis and found that persistent symptoms of pitting edema and pain developed in 7% after a mean follow-up of 13 months. Thus, from every standpoint—the risk for pulmonary embolism and the risk for chronic postphlebitic syndrome—catheter-related DVT should be treated aggressively.[29]

Clinical Findings

The clinical features of upper extremity DVT vary from asymptomatic to life-threatening massive pulmonary embolism. The most common initial signs are arm edema, shoulder and arm pain, heaviness of the extremity, and obvious dilated subcutaneous veins on the chest wall and arm. There may be increased erythema and limb temperature. Conditions that may mimic upper extremity DVT are lymphatic edema, external venous compression, and hematoma within muscle.[66] The signs and symptoms of upper extremity venous thrombosis are nonspecific and therefore can be misleading.

Diagnostic Evaluation

As indicated, the clinical diagnosis of upper extremity DVT is nonspecific.[66] Among symptomatic patients, a positive diagnosis is made in less than 50% of such patients. Thus, it is critical that an objective diagnostic algorithm be used appropriately to confirm or exclude the diagnosis of upper extremity DVT. The most commonly performed diagnostic studies are duplex ultrasonography, contrast-enhanced venography, MRV, and CTV.

Duplex Ultrasound

Duplex ultrasonography is the most frequently used diagnostic modality for the evaluation of patients suspected of having DVT of the upper limb. The study is noninvasive, does not require the use of a nephrotoxic contrast agent, and does not involve ionizing radiation. In addition, it can be performed at the bedside or in the emergency department should that be necessary. The use of diagnostic ultrasound in the upper extremity is different from that in the lower extremity. In the upper extremity there are areas in which compressibility of the targeted vein is not possible, such as the region of the axillary vein beneath the clavicle. In addition, it is not possible to compress the brachiocephalic vein or SVC. Acoustic shadowing can further obscure the duplex B-mode image. Nonetheless, for regions in which it is possible, compressibility of the vein is the main diagnostic criterion. In addition, the echogenicity of the suspected clot and examination of flow characteristics, including phasicity, pulsatility, and variation with the Valsalva maneuver, are critical, particularly in the regions in which compressibility cannot be completed. Finally, the color-flow filling of the vein adds an additional means of confirming the presence or absence of a clot.

The reported accuracy of duplex ultrasonography varies widely. However, one fundamental point concerning duplex ultrasonography is that its accuracy will always vary with the experience of the vascular laboratory in which it is performed. Thus, one cannot extrapolate the published results of sensitivity and specificity to every laboratory. Nonetheless, the overall sensitivity of duplex ultrasound has been recorded in the range of 78% to 100%, with a specificity of 82% to 100%.[37,68,72] It is notable that over the last 20 years there has been a significant improvement in the diagnostic accuracy of duplex ultrasound and the diagnosis of upper limb DVT.

Digital Subtraction, Magnetic Resonance, and Computed Tomographic Venography

Digital subtraction venography remains the gold standard. However, it is an invasive study that uses a potentially nephrotoxic agent and requires exposing the patient to ionizing radiation. In addition, in up to 20% of patients it may not be feasible because of the presence of a severe contrast allergy or inability to cannulate a vein in the edematous extremity. The primary role of digital venography is in a patient in whom the duplex ultrasound findings are equivocal. In such patients some other objective study should be undertaken to confirm or reject the diagnosis. One alternative is MRV. This study has gained popularity for use in the diagnosis of venous thrombosis in virtually any area of the body. Its merits are that it is a noninvasive study and can image all veins, including the central ones. MRV correlates well with contrast-enhanced venography.[68] It uses the breakdown of hemoglobin into methemoglobin, which yields a decreased T1 signal that gives rise to an increased signal ratio in heavily T1-rated sequences. Finally, CTV is reserved for patients in whom no other diagnostic study can be undertaken in a reasonable time frame and particularly in patients in whom external compression of a vein is thought to account for the patient's symptoms and signs. CTV also has value in that it can detect central vein thrombosis and the presence of pulmonary emboli.

Diagnostic Test Selection

A prospective randomized study was undertaken to compare the role of duplex color ultrasonography and digital contrast-enhanced venography for the diagnosis of upper limb venous thrombosis.[37] In this study the sensitivity and specificity of duplex ultrasonography were 82% (95% confidence interval, 70% to 93%) and 82% (95% confidence interval, 72% to 90%), respectively. Venous incompressibility correlated very well with the presence of thrombosis on digital venography. However, in only 50% of instances in which isolated flow abnormalities were noted on duplex ultrasonography was a thrombus found on digital venography. Thus, the diagnostic study of choice for all patients suspected of having upper limb DVT is duplex ultrasonography. Should the results of that study prove equivocal, the first noninvasive alternative would be MRV, followed by either digital contrast-enhanced venography or CTV.

Treatment

The goal of treatment of secondary upper extremity DVT is to prevent pulmonary embolism and to achieve recanalization of the vein. Most patients with secondary upper limb DVT improve after removal of the venous catheter and institution of anticoagulation therapy. If a catheter causes extensive axillary vein thrombosis resulting in marked edema, thrombolytic therapy may be considered. However, in the vast majority of patients, removal of the catheter plus systemic anticoagulation for a period of 3 months is indicated. Patients with secondary upper limb DVT who may have contraindications to systemic anticoagulation, such as concurrent gastrointestinal bleeding, recent neurosurgery, or the presence of pulmonary embolism despite anticoagulation, may be candidates for SVC filter placement. SVC filters are not used widely, but in small limited studies they have been shown to be effective in preventing recurrent pulmonary embolism. The long-term patency rates of the small number of SVC filters that have been placed have been reported to be very high.[73] Nonetheless, concerns persist about the risk of SVC filter migration or thrombosis resulting in SVC syndrome. Because fatal pulmonary embolism from upper extremity DVT has been documented to be very rare and evidence of the safety of filters is limited, clinical judgment must be used in recommending their deployment.[74]

Prophylaxis

A number of studies have been undertaken in patients who are known to have malignancies and have central venous cath-

eters to determine whether prophylactic warfarin or low-molecular-weight heparin will reduce the thrombosis rate.[75,76] Some of these trials have shown a decreased incidence of DVT and a low risk of bleeding. However, more recent trials have not found that prophylaxis with anticoagulants reduces the risk for symptomatic catheter-related upper limb DVT.[77-80] Young and colleagues recently completed a multicenter trial of prophylaxis with low-dose warfarin, dose-adjusted warfarin, or no prophylaxis and did not find any benefit of a reduction in symptomatic catheter-related upper limb DVT.[80] Thus, on the basis of these and other results, the American College of Chest Physicians consensus guidelines no longer recommends routine anticoagulant prophylaxis.[81]

Secondary upper extremity DVT is neither a rare nor a benign disease process. Catheter-related upper limb DVT requires prompt diagnosis and treatment. The key factors in reducing the incidence of catheter-related thrombosis are the skill and training of the individual inserting the catheter, a history of previous failed attempts at percutaneous catheter placement, and the presence of prothrombotic gene mutations, surgery, immobilization of arm, oral contraceptive use, and a family history.[5] With proper technique and careful surveillance, the incidence of catheter-related subclavian vein thrombosis can be minimized.

SELECTED KEY REFERENCES

Molina JE, Hunter DW, Dietz CA. Paget-Schroetter syndrome treated with thrombolytics and immediate surgery. *J Vasc Surg.* 2007;45: 328-334.
This study reports one of the largest series of patients to undergo treatment of venous thoracic outlet syndrome. The outcomes were excellent and the discussion emphasizes many key issues that are central to the management of this challenging syndrome.

Sajid MS, Ahmed N, Desai M, Baker D, Hamilton G. Upper limb deep vein thrombosis: a literature review to streamline the protocol for management. *Acta Haematol.* 2007;118:10-18.
Comprehensive review of key studies describing the etiology, diagnosis, and management of upper limb venous thrombosis.

Schneider DB, Dimuzio PJ, Martin ND, Gordon RL, Wilson MW, Laberge JM, Kerlan RK, Eichler CM, Messina LM. Combination treatment of venous thoracic outlet syndrome: open surgical decompression and intraoperative angioplasty. *J Vasc Surg.* 2004;40:599-603.
This study describes the first significant series of patients who underwent venothrombolysis, immediate surgical decompression of the thoracic outlet and intraoperative venography, and definitive treatment of residual stenosis. The outcomes indicate that in most patients it is unnecessary to delay surgical decompression, and the study emphasizes the importance of intraoperative venography to determine the optimal strategy for treating any residual stenosis.

Urschel HC Jr, Razzuk MA. Paget-Schroetter syndrome: what is the best management? *Ann Thorac Surg.* 2000;69:1663-1668; discussion 8-9.
This study provides a clear and detailed description of the transaxillary approach to thoracic outlet decompression.

REFERENCES

The reference list can be found on the companion Expert Consult Web site at *www.expertconsult.com.*

Arterial Aneurysms | *Section* **17**

Richard P. Cambria

CHAPTER 126

Arterial Aneurysms: General Considerations

Peter F. Lawrence and David Rigberg

An arterial aneurysm is one of the most common vascular diseases causing disability and death. It occurs in most arteries throughout the body and is particularly common in the elderly. Aneurysms have a variety of sizes, shapes, and locations; to help with classification and standardization for clinical decision making, the Ad Hoc Committee on Reporting Standards of the Society for Vascular Surgery defined an aneurysm as "a permanent localized (i.e., focal) dilation of an artery having at least a 50% increase in diameter compared to the expected normal diameter of the artery in question."[1] With this definition as the standard, it is important to know the normal diameter of each artery throughout the body so that clinicians will be able to determine when an artery becomes aneurysmal (Fig. 126-1; Table 126-1). These mea-

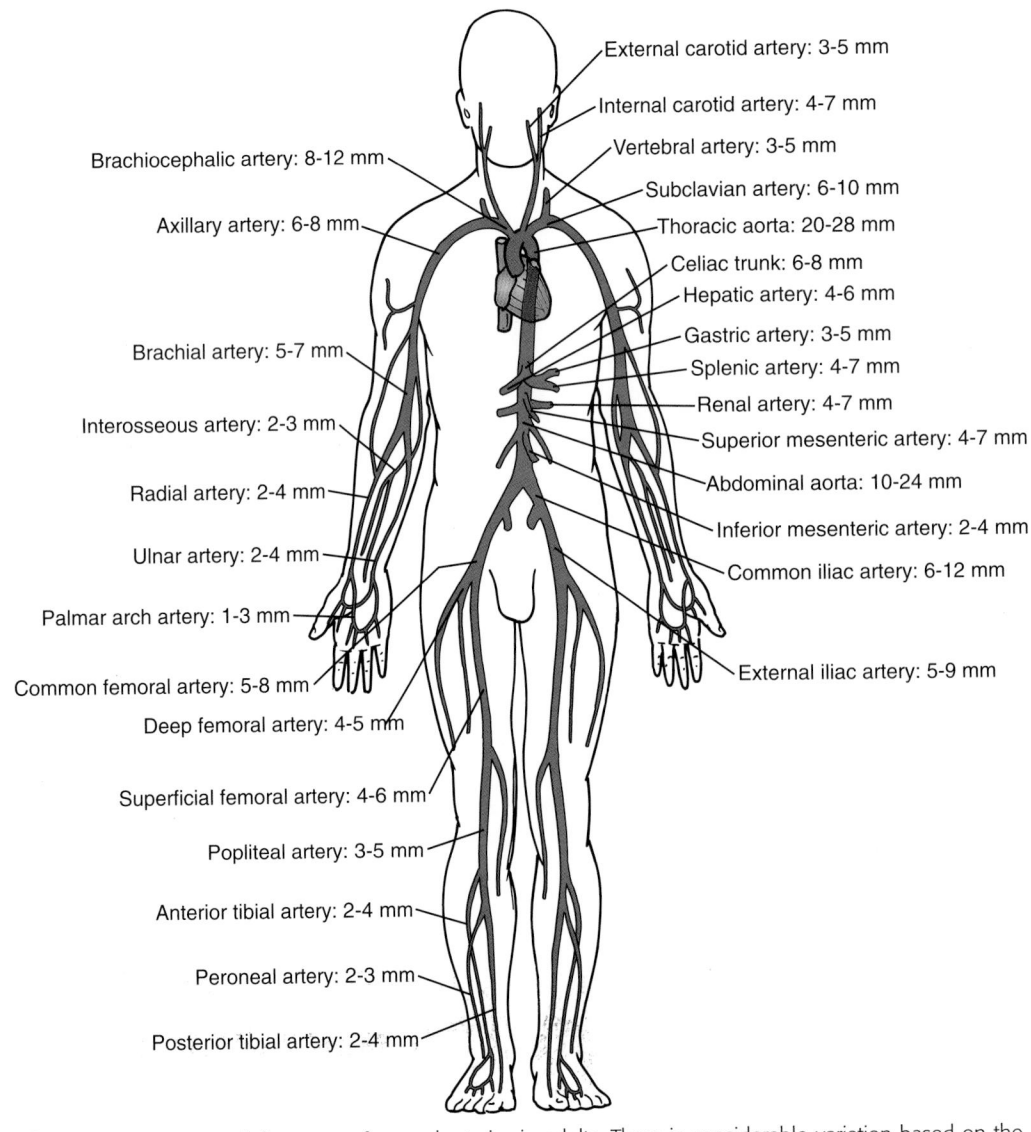

External carotid artery: 3-5 mm
Internal carotid artery: 4-7 mm
Vertebral artery: 3-5 mm
Subclavian artery: 6-10 mm
Thoracic aorta: 20-28 mm
Celiac trunk: 6-8 mm
Hepatic artery: 4-6 mm
Gastric artery: 3-5 mm
Splenic artery: 4-7 mm
Renal artery: 4-7 mm
Superior mesenteric artery: 4-7 mm
Abdominal aorta: 10-24 mm
Inferior mesenteric artery: 2-4 mm
Common iliac artery: 6-12 mm
External iliac artery: 5-9 mm

Brachiocephalic artery: 8-12 mm
Axillary artery: 6-8 mm
Brachial artery: 5-7 mm
Interosseous artery: 2-3 mm
Radial artery: 2-4 mm
Ulnar artery: 2-4 mm
Palmar arch artery: 1-3 mm
Common femoral artery: 5-8 mm
Deep femoral artery: 4-5 mm
Superficial femoral artery: 4-6 mm
Popliteal artery: 3-5 mm
Anterior tibial artery: 2-4 mm
Peroneal artery: 2-3 mm
Posterior tibial artery: 2-4 mm

Figure 126-1 Range of diameters of normal arteries in adults. There is considerable variation based on the gender and age of the individual.

Table 126-1 Normal Arterial Size Based on a Compilation of Studies Using Different Imaging Modalities

Vessel	Range of Reported Mean (cm)	Range of Reported Standard Deviation (cm)	Sex	Assessment Method
Thoracic aorta, root	3.50-3.72	0.38	Female	Computed tomography
	3.63-3.91	0.38	Male	Computed tomography
Thoracic aorta, ascending	2.86	—	Female, male	Chest radiography
Thoracic aorta, mid-descending	2.45-2.64	0.31	Female	Computed tomography
	2.39-2.98	0.31	Male	Computed tomography
Thoracic aorta, diaphragmatic	2.40-2.44	0.27-0.32	Female	Computed tomography
	2.43-2.69	0.27-0.40	Male	Computed tomography, intravenous arteriography
Abdominal aorta, supraceliac	2.10-2.31	0.27	Female	Computed tomography
	2.50-2.72	0.24-0.35	Male	Computed tomography
Abdominal aorta, suprarenal	1.86-1.88	0.09-0.21	Female	Computed tomography
	1.98-2.27	0.19-0.23	Male	Computed tomography
Abdominal aorta, infrarenal	1.66-2.16	0.22-0.32	Female	Computed tomography intravenous arteriography
	1.99-2.39	0.30-0.39	Male	Computed tomography intravenous arteriography
Abdominal aorta, infrarenal	1.19-1.87	0.09-0.34	Female	B-mode ultrasound, computed tomography, intravenous arteriography
	1.41-2.05	0.04-0.37	Male	B-mode ultrasound, computed tomography, intravenous arteriography
Celiac	0.53	0.03	Female, male	B-mode ultrasound
Superior mesenteric	0.63	0.04	Female, male	B-mode ultrasound
Iliac, common	0.97-1.02	0.15-0.19	Female	Computed tomography
	1.17-1.23	0.20	Male	Computed tomography
Iliac, internal	0.54	0.15	Female, male	Arteriography
Femoral, common	0.78-0.85	0.07-0.11	Female	Computed tomography, B-mode ultrasound
	0.78-1.12	0.09-0.30	Male	Computed tomography, B-mode ultrasound, M-mode ultrasound
Popliteal	0.90	20	Male	B-mode ultrasound
Tibial, posterior	0.30	0.01	Male	M-mode ultrasound
Carotid, common	0.77	0.08	Female	Arteriography
	0.63-0.84	0.10-0.14	Male	Arteriography, M-mode ultrasound
Carotid, bulb	0.92	0.10	Female	Arteriography
	0.99	0.10	Male	Arteriography
Carotid, internal	0.49	0.07	Female	Arteriography
	0.55	0.06	Male	Arteriography
Brachial	0.39	0.04	Female	M-mode ultrasound
	0.42-0.44	0.01-0.04	Male	M-mode ultrasound

Adapted by permission from Johnston KW, Rutherford RB, Tilson MD, et al, for the Subcommittee on Reporting Standards for Arterial Aneurysms, Ad Hoc Committee on Reporting Standards, Society for Vascular Surgery and North American Chapter, International Society for Cardiovascular Surgery. Suggested standards for reporting on arterial aneurysms. *J Vasc Surg.* 1991;13:452-458.

surements have been determined by various methods, including cadaveric studies, angiography, computed tomography, and ultrasonography. The size of the abdominal aorta and iliac arteries has been shown to be related to gender, age, and pulsatile expansion of the aorta during systole.[2]

HISTORICAL PERSPECTIVE

The earliest report of surgery for an aneurysm is from the 3rd century, and numerous surgeons reported performing ligation of feeder and runoff vessels from aneurysms in the 17th and 18th centuries. Matas, in 1888, performed the first definitive repair, endoaneurysmorrhaphy, by ligating the branches of a brachial artery aneurysm from inside the aneurysm sac.[3] However, it was not until suture repair of arteries became

feasible that aneurysms could be approached with preservation of blood flow. The first such operation was performed by Dubost in 1951 when he replaced an abdominal aortic aneurysm (AAA) with a thoracic aortic homograft harvested from a recently deceased 20-year-old. Dubost was inspired to pursue the treatment of cardiovascular diseases after Blalock and Bahnson performed a series of operations in Paris in 1947, and it is notable that he performed his procedure only 4 years later. This patient lived for 8 years postoperatively.[4] In 1954, Blakemore and Voorhees published their series of 17 aortic (and 1 popliteal) aneurysms repaired with Vinyon "N" cloth prostheses (with materials provided by the Union Carbide and Carbon Corporation).[5] This work launched the modern age of synthetic replacement of aneurysms. The following year, Cooley and DeBakey presented their work on repair of thoracic aneurysms with homografts.[6]

Section **17** Arterial Aneurysms

Open repair was refined over the next 4 decades, and by the dawn of the endovascular era, perioperative mortality for open repair of AAAs ranged from as low as 1.2% in single-institution series to 3.8% in studies looking at the general population. Parodi and coauthors reported the first repair of an aortic aneurysm with an aortic stent-graft in 1991; this was followed by the introduction of Food and Drug Administration–approved endografts.[7] There followed a rapid progression from a tube graft design to the currently used bifurcated systems. Recent data show that 73% of AAA repairs in the United States were done via an endovascular approach from 1998 to 2004, and this number is in all likelihood even higher now.[8] The introduction of thoracic endografts was also followed by their rapid diffusion into clinical practice. Newer techniques using fenestrated endografts allow continued perfusion of visceral branches arising from aneurysmal portions of the aorta such that even complex thoracoabdominal lesions can be approached through an all-endovascular approach. These procedures remain limited to a few specialized centers, but as the technology behind fenestrated grafts improves, these grafts may also see use on a much larger scale. Peripheral aneurysms have undergone a similar evolution from open repair with autogenous bypass to endovascular repair.

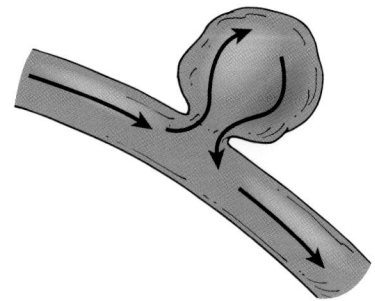

Figure 126-2 Schematic representation of a pseudoaneurysm. The expelled blood reenters the artery during the cardiac cycle so that the blood leaving the vessel returns as well. The "wall" of the pseudoaneurysm is composed of the surrounding tissue; these tissues can allow growth or even rupture if the blood escapes their confines.

ANEURYSM CLASSIFICATION

True versus False Aneurysms

The initial distinction that must be drawn when classifying aneurysms is between "true" and "false" lesions. *True aneurysms* involve all three layers of the arterial wall, regardless of the underlying pathology. *False aneurysms* (or "pseudoaneurysms") are differentiated from true aneurysms by the presence of blood flow outside the normal layers of the arterial wall. At its most basic level, a pseudoaneurysm is simply a hole in an artery that allows extravasation of blood into a contained space outside the artery; it remains pulsatile because of the "to-and-fro" motion of blood in the aneurysm sac. The wall of the false aneurysm is composed of the compressed, surrounding tissues, not the wall of the artery from which the lesion arises (Fig. 126-2). These aneurysms can be associated with needle sticks, infectious processes, or disruption of arterial anastomoses (see Chapter 43: Local Complications: Anastomotic Aneurysms) (Fig. 126-3).

Anatomic Categories

Aneurysms can be categorized according to their anatomic, pathologic, or etiologic characteristics. *Ectasia* refers to an intermediate stage of enlargement when an artery is less than 50% enlarged, whereas *arteriomegaly* refers to diffuse, continuous enlargement of multiple arterial segments dilated to greater than 50% of normal. *Aneurysmosis* is used by some authors to describe the combination of aneurysms with arteriomegaly.[9] *Fusiform aneurysms* are the most common anatomic type and occur when there is generalized enlargement of a limited segment of the vessel, with all layers of the artery

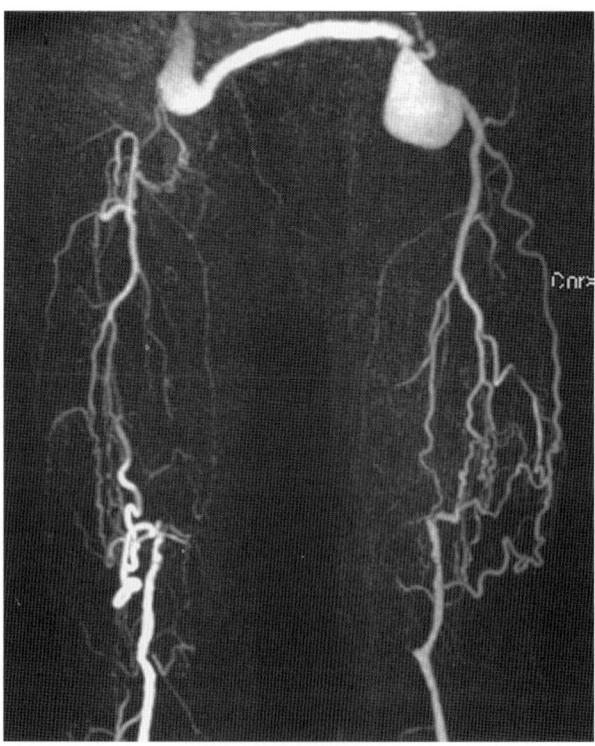

Figure 126-3 This magnetic resonance arteriogram demonstrates bilateral anastomotic pseudoaneurysms 10 years after right-to-left femorofemoral bypass grafting was performed. Femoral pseudoaneurysms can reach dramatic sizes and become symptomatic secondary to venous or neural compression.

involved. *Saccular aneurysms* occur when a focal weakness in a portion of the arterial wall results in an asymmetric bulge in the vessel (Fig. 126-4). Saccular morphology is common in aneurysms that develop distal to the left subclavian artery after chest trauma (Fig. 126-5). Although saccular lesions are frequently considered to be more prone to rupture, recent literature suggests that such is not the case; it is more likely that there are issues related to the cross-sectional asymmetry of aneurysms that confer a risk for rupture, but even this must be carefully controlled for so that it is not simply a reflection of tortuosity.[10,11]

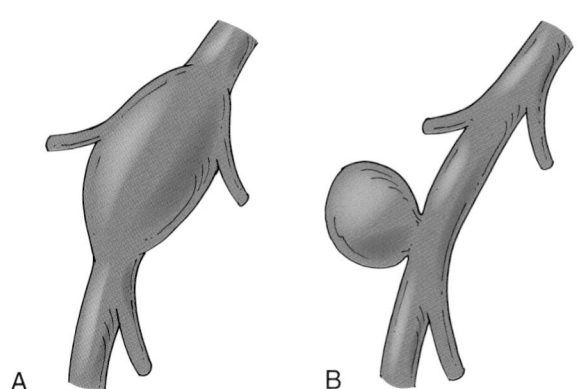

Figure 126-4 Schematic diagrams of fusiform (**A**) and saccular (**B**) aneurysms. The presence of a saccular lesion should prompt evaluation for a variety of causes, including post-traumatic pseudoaneurysm and infection.

Etiologic Categories

The underlying histopathology is useful to define an aneurysm as resulting from a degenerative/atherosclerosis etiology, an inflammatory process, arterial dissection with degeneration, trauma, infection, or a congenital etiology.

Degenerative

Most non-iatrogenic aneurysms encountered by vascular surgeons, particularly AAAs, are due to a complex, degenerative etiology (see Chapter 8: Arterial Aneurysms). They have often been incorrectly termed *atherosclerotic*, although these lesions are not typically associated with occlusive disease. Rather, these aneurysms involve a complex degenerative process, and even though the terms *atherosclerotic* and *degenerative* are frequently used interchangeably in this setting, the term *degenerative* is currently preferred. There is usually some degree of calcification and atherosclerotic pathology present in AAAs, and some data support atherosclerosis as a causative agent in the development of these lesions. For example, primates fed atherogenic diets are prone to the development of aneurysms.[12] However, there are also data that these atherosclerotic changes represent a secondary phenomenon. Experimental work has demonstrated the tendency of atheromatous plaque to develop in areas of reduced shear stress and turbulent flow; both these conditions are present at the level of the infrarenal aorta and within an aneurysm.[13] With regard to a degenerative process, the strongest evidence is provided by the role of metalloproteinases, a family of elastases recognized to be elevated in aneurysm specimens. Moreover, there are postulated to be reduced levels in the native antiproteolytic system, most notably tissue inhibitor of metalloproteinase-1,[14] in addition to a complex inflammatory process (see Chapter 8: Arterial Aneurysms).

Inflammatory

Inflammatory AAAs are characterized by a thick inflammatory wall with a fibrotic process in the retroperitoneum that may

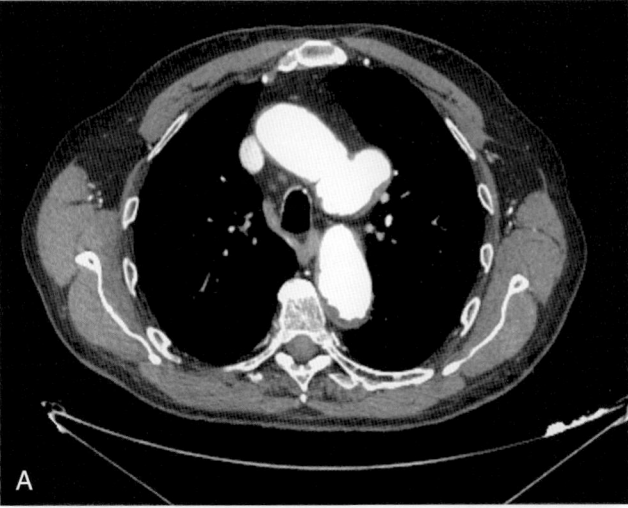

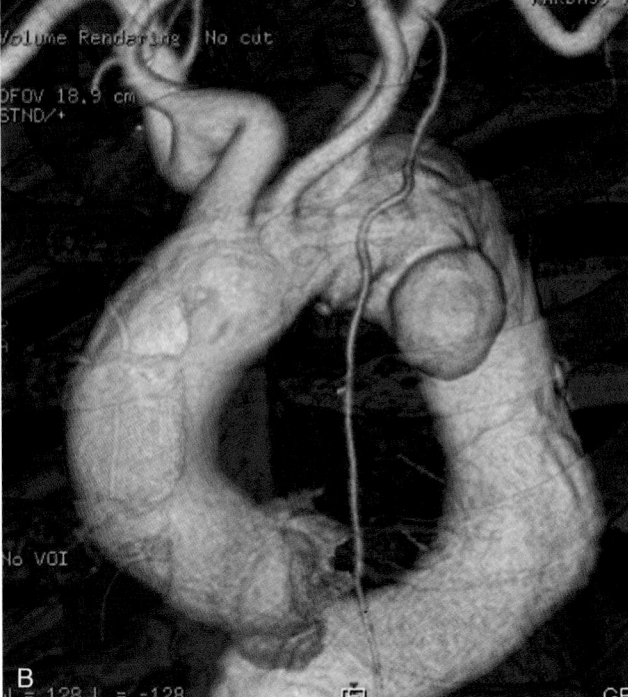

Figure 126-5 Axial slice (**A**) and three-dimensional computed tomographic reconstruction (**B**) of a saccular aneurysm arising from the aorta just distal to the origin of the left subclavian artery.

encase not only the aneurysm but also surrounding structures such as the ureters (Fig. 126-6). Current theories suggest that there is a spectrum of inflammation with all AAAs and that inflammatory aneurysms represent the extreme variant. On a molecular level, similar patterns of human leukocyte antigen (HLA) expression are seen with both inflammatory and non-inflammatory AAAs, thus lending further support to this theory.[15] Careful preoperative assessment is critical when approaching these lesions because of the high incidence of injury to adjacent structures.

Aneurysms can also be associated with a variety of rheumatologic inflammatory conditions such as Takayasu's arteritis and giant cell arteritis, polyarteritis nodosa, Behçet's

Section **17** Arterial Aneurysms

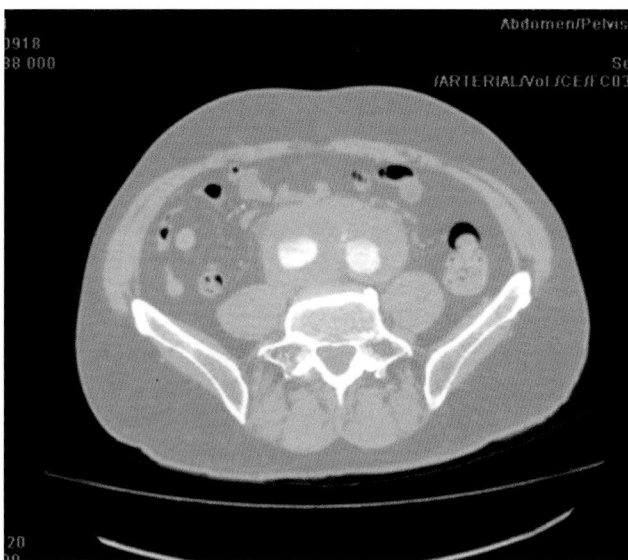

Figure 126-6 Computed tomographic scan demonstrating an inflammatory abdominal aortic aneurysm with extension to the common iliac arteries bilaterally. Note the thick inflammatory process involving the vessels, in this case extending all the way to the iliac artery bifurcations.

disease, and Cogan's syndrome. They can range from large aortic lesions to the multiple visceral aneurysms seen with polyarteritis nodosa (see Chapter 140: Aneurysms Caused by Connective Tissue Abnormalities).

Postdissection Aneurysms

Aneurysms may also develop after arterial dissection, particularly in the thoracic aorta, where up to 20% of aneurysms are related to previous dissections. The outer wall of the false lumen of a dissection can degenerate and eventually develop into a true aneurysm (see Chapter 135: Aortic Dissection). An underlying pathologic condition that can lead to the dissection itself is cystic medial necrosis. Histologically, the hyalin of the media is replaced by a disordered ground substance; the composition varies depending on the underlying pathology, which is usually either Marfan's syndrome or Ehlers-Danlos syndrome. Dissections can also lead to the development of aneurysms in other anatomic distributions, such at the skull base after internal carotid artery dissections.

Traumatic

Aneurysms that result from traumatic arterial disruption are by definition false aneurysms, as described earlier.

Developmental Anomalies

Aneurysms can also develop in the presence of anomalous arterial anatomy, although the underlying pathology in this situation has not been clearly defined. In more than 40% of

cases, aneurysms develop in persistent sciatic arteries (a fetal connection between the hypogastric artery and the popliteal artery), which may be secondary to repetitive trauma or even local connective tissue abnormalities.[16,17] This "degenerative" process can also occur in the presence of an aberrant right subclavian artery and an associated Kommerell diverticulum. These aneurysms develop at the origin of the aberrant subclavian vessel from the aortic arch (see Chapter 137: Upper Extremity Aneurysms).

Infectious

Infectious (or "mycotic") aneurysms can result from primary arterial infection or secondary infection of a preexisting aneurysm (see Chapter 139: Infected Aneurysms).[18] Aneurysms of the aortic arch and innominate artery were previously associated with syphilitic infection, but such infected aneurysms have become much less common. Infections related to human immunodeficiency virus can also lead to aneurysms, and they are often found in atypical locations.[19] *Candida* and other fungal organisms (true "mycotic" lesions) are likewise associated with aneurysm formation. Infection can also lead to disruption of anastomotic suture lines with the formation of pseudoaneurysms; this can occur in the presence or absence of synthetic graft material.

Congenital

Aneurysms in children are uncommon, tend to be congenital, and usually involve the aorta. They are associated with a variety of anomalies, such as tuberous sclerosis, aortic coarctation, and Marfan's syndrome. Case reports in the literature also describe congenital aneurysms in the subclavian, axillary, iliac, and brachial arteries, although they are exceedingly rare.[20,21]

Location Categories
Aorta

Aneurysms occur throughout the length of the aorta, starting at its ascending portion. Lesions in this location can be atherosclerotic aneurysms or can represent secondary dilatation after a type A aortic dissection. Isolated thoracic aneurysms were found in 0.9% of autopsies in Sweden[22] and represent 3% of repairs in the United States.[23] By far the most common type of aneurysm of the aorta is an atherosclerotic aneurysm affecting the infrarenal aorta. An estimated 2500 elective repairs per year are performed in the state of California alone, and our national data indicate more than 32,000 cases annually and a total of just over 105,000 patients receiving the diagnosis.[23,24] These aneurysms are classified as *infrarenal*, *juxtarenal*, or *suprarenal* with respect to their relationship to the renal artery ostia.

Thoracoabdominal aneurysms are less common than infrarenal AAAs and were noted in 0.03% of autopsies in a Swedish series.[22] Because operative morbidity and mortality can be considerable, it is not useful to estimate the incidence from the overall number of surgical repairs, but in 1994 there were approximately 100 thoracoabdominal repairs in California[25] and 362 cases in the United States.[23]

Iliac

Iliac aneurysms usually occur in the presence of AAAs. Of patients admitted to the hospital with a diagnosis of iliac aneurysm in 1994, only 11% had an iliac aneurysm in the absence of an AAA.[23] Autopsy data revealed an incidence of 0.03% for solitary iliac artery aneurysms, and in only one of the seven patients in this Swedish series did the lesion rupture.[26] These lesions usually involve the common iliac artery; it is unusual for internal iliac aneurysms to occur in the absence of common iliac disease, whereas external iliac aneurysms are exceedingly rare.[27]

Femoral

Common femoral artery aneurysms are most commonly pseudoaneurysms that occur after percutaneous arterial puncture, angiography, or aortobifemoral bypasses. The rate is highly dependent on the type of procedure performed and the size of the access catheter; approximately 0.05% to 4% of femoral punctures lead to this complication.[28] Degenerative aneurysms of the common femoral artery are rare, although this vessel can be involved with arteriomegaly. Superficial femoral and profunda femoris artery aneurysms are also unusual, as are aneurysms of the tibial and pedal vessels (see Chapter 136: Lower Extremity Aneurysms).

Popliteal

Popliteal aneurysms are the most common peripheral aneurysms, and their association with AAAs should lead an astute clinician to investigate for their presence. Data suggest that up to 10% of patients with AAAs have some combination of femoral or popliteal aneurysm, with the number being much higher in men and lower in women.[29] The presence of synchronous and metachronous bilateral popliteal artery aneurysms is also reported to occur in approximately 40% to 60% of patients.[23]

Visceral

The most common of the visceral artery aneurysms is renal, and they represent 0.3% of aneurysm repairs overall in our series versus 0.1% for the other visceral vessels.[23] Renal artery aneurysms are associated with fibromuscular dysplasia, arteritis, and dissections, although they are most commonly "degenerative." The splenic and mesenteric arteries are most commonly affected by aneurysm, followed by the hepatic and celiac vessels. Visceral aneurysms can also occur in association with diseases such as polyarteritis nodosa.

Cerebrovascular

Aneurysms of the intracranial circulation are relatively common, whereas those of the extracranial carotid arteries are very uncommon. Carotid aneurysms typically involve, in decreasing frequency, the internal, common, and external carotid arteries and are most commonly atherosclerotic or associated with fibromuscular dysplasia. The annual number of carotid aneurysm repairs in the United States is lower than 750.[23] Subclavian aneurysms are also unusual, with 305 cases reported in a single year.[23] True degenerative aneurysms at this site are rare; rather, they may occur as a result of the chronic trauma seen with thoracic outlet syndrome or as lesions secondary to infections. These lesions need to be differentiated from degenerative lesions associated with an aberrant right subclavian artery and Kommerell diverticulum of the aorta, as described earlier.

Upper Extremity

The only aneurysm commonly occurring in the upper extremity is an iatrogenic brachial pseudoaneurysm associated with cardiac catheterization or other procedures requiring arterial cannulation. False aneurysms of the axillary artery can result from trauma and can be manifested dramatically as a pulsatile axillary mass. Hypothenar hammer syndrome can lead to unusual aneurysms of the ulnar artery secondary to repetitive trauma to the vessel by the hamate bone.

■ REPAIR

Aneurysm repair data by location are summarized in Table 126-2.

Table 126-2 Relative Frequency of Aneurysm Repair in the United States Based on National Hospital Discharge Survey Data from 1994

Type of Aneurysm	Total Number Repaired	Total Aneurysm Repairs (%)
Abdominal aortic	32,389	62.3
Lower extremity	8112	15.6
Ruptured abdominal aortic	6623	12.7
Thoracic	1471	2.8
Neck	746	1.4
Isolated iliac	667	1.3
Ruptured thoracic	374	0.7
Thoracoabdominal	362	0.7
Upper extremity	296	0.6
Subclavian	257	0.5
Renal artery	133	0.3
Visceral	47	0.1
Splenic	36	0.1
Other	436	0.8

Reproduced by permission from Lawrence PF, Gazak C, Bhirangi L, et al. The epidemiology of surgically repaired aneurysms in the United States. *J Vasc Surg.* 1999;30:632-640.

MULTIPLE ANEURYSMS
Aortic

It has been recognized for some time that aneurysmal disease of the aorta is commonly a multifocal process. Some of the seminal work in this arena was reported by Crawford and Cohen and was based on their review of more than 1500 aortic aneurysm patients.[30] In this series, strong associations were noted between aneurysms of the thoracic aorta and the abdominal aorta. Of patients with AAAs, 12% also had thoracic aneurysms. More than 50% of patients with thoracic lesions had other aneurysms, the majority of which were AAAs. Further work in this arena was published by Gloviczki and coauthors[31]; they specifically addressed the question of managing these patients and reviewed their series of 102 patients undergoing repairs of multiple aneurysms (Fig. 126-7). In just over 50% of these patients the second aneurysm was recognized or present at the time of the initial repair. For the remaining patients, the mean time from initial repair to appearance of the second aneurysm was over 5 years (range, 68 days to almost 18 years). Their analysis indicated that patients with either aortic dissections or Marfan's syndrome were at particular risk for the development of multiple thoracic aneurysms, and they concluded that patients undergoing repair of aortic aneurysms need diligent evaluation for synchronous lesions and longitudinal follow-up for metachronous aneurysms.

Peripheral

The multicentric nature of aneurysms has also been noted in other circulatory beds. Stanley's group reported on their series of almost 90 popliteal aneurysms and noted that 44% of them were bilateral.[32] Patients with popliteal aneurysms were also found to have aneurysms of the abdominal aorta (62%), the iliac arteries (36%), and the femoral arteries (38%). The likelihood of peripheral aneurysms occurring in the presence of AAAs is much less, with a reported range of 1% to 10%. Rare lesions, such as profunda femoris aneurysms, are associated with multiple lesions as well. A recent Mayo Clinic series demonstrated that almost half the patients in its small series with these lesions had popliteal aneurysms and a third had aortoiliac aneurysms.[33]

Familial

Patients with aneurysms occasionally have a relative who has either the same type of aneurysm or a different aneurysmal lesion that develops in the patient's lifetime. Before the era of careful risk factor modification, it was assumed that these patients had risk factors in common with their relatives that were not adequately controlled. However, in some patients and families who have no risk factors or have undergone good risk factor modification, these aneurysms still develop, thus suggesting a genetic or metabolic etiology for some aneurysms. Some 15% of AAA patients will have a first-order relative also affected by the disease.[38]

Arteriomegaly

Arteriomegaly is associated with multiple aneurysms[34] and is an example of a condition with a possible metabolic or genetic basis for these lesions. Although the natural history of arteriomegaly is not firmly established, there are higher rates of limb loss in these patients than in those with isolated aneurysms, and there is also a strong familial predilection, with more than a third of patients with arteriomegaly having an affected first-degree relative.[35]

Abdominal Aorta

There is a familial predilection for AAAs, with the sibling of an AAA patient having eight times the risk for an AAA as the patient's spouse (see Chapter 127: Abdominal Aortic Aneurysms: Evaluation and Decision Making).[36] This is also true for aneurysms of the thoracic aorta.[37] These same familial relationships have not been found for peripheral aneurysms, but ultrasound screening examinations are currently recommended for first-degree relatives of patients with aortic aneurysms and arteriomegaly (but not peripheral aneurysms) because 7% of first-degree relatives of AAA probands have been shown to have aneurysms and 5.5% of first-degree rela-

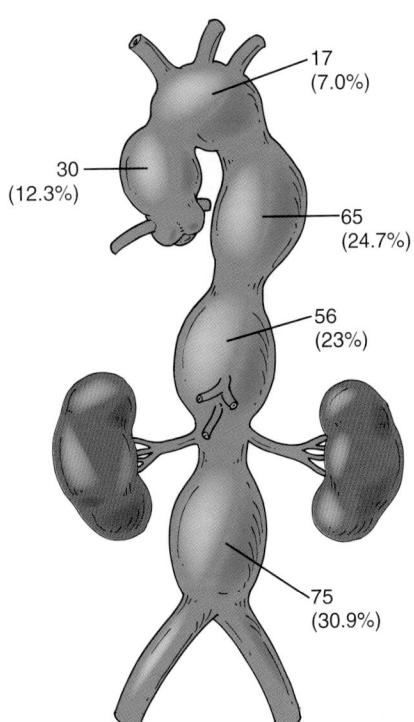

Figure 126-7 Graphic representation of the location and distribution of 243 aortic aneurysms in 102 patients. Individual patients had from two to four lesions, and almost 70% of patients had involvement of the infrarenal aorta. *(Reproduced by permission from Gloviczki P, Pairolero P, Welch T, et al. Multiple aortic aneurysms: the results of surgical management. J Vasc Surg. 1990;11:19-27.)*

17 (7.0%)

30 (12.3%)

65 (24.7%)

56 (23%)

75 (30.9%)

tives of arteriomegaly probands were found to have aneurysms. In women with aneurysms, the risk of their children having aneurysms is so high that the term *black widow syndrome* is applied; it refers to the increased risk of rupture in females with familial aortic aneurysm.[38]

SELECTED KEY REFERENCES

Blakemore AH, Voorhees AB. The use of tubes constructed from Vinyon "N" cloth in bridging arterial defects—experimental and clinical. *Ann Surg.* 1954;140:324-333.
Although this is an old reference, the original article is available online and is excellent first-hand reporting of the early use of prosthetics for repair of aneurysms in both the laboratory and clinical settings.

Johnston KW, Rutherford RB, Tilson MD, Shah DM, Hollier L, Stanley JC, for the Subcommittee on Reporting Standards for Arterial Aneurysms, Ad Hoc Committee on Reporting Standards, Society for Vascular Surgery and North American Chapter, International Society for Cardiovascular Surgery. Suggested standards for reporting on arterial aneurysms. *J Vasc Surg.* 1991;13:452-458.
This article summarizes the details on normal artery size, etiology, and location of aneurysms, as well as determination of the definition of arterial aneurysm.

Lawrence PF, Gazak C, Bhirangi L, Jones B, Bhirangi K, Oderich G, Treiman G. The epidemiology of surgically repaired aneurysms in the United States. *J Vasc Surg.* 1999;30:632-640.
This article gives an accounting of the distribution of aneurysm repair in the United States over the course of a year and is an excellent source for understanding the epidemiology of aneurysm repair.

Ogata T, MacKean GL, Cole CW, Arthur C, Andreou P, Tromp G, Kuivaniemi H. The lifetime prevalence of abdominal aortic aneurysms among siblings of aneurysm patients is eightfold higher than among siblings of spouses: an analysis of 187 aneurysm families in Nova Scotia, Canada. *J Vasc Surg.* 2005;42:891-897.
This paper presents data regarding the familial tendency of abdominal aortic aneurysms and demonstrates increased prevalence of these aneurysms in blood relatives.

Rigberg DA, McGory ML, Zingmond DS, Maggard MA, Agustin M, Lawrence PF, Ko CY. Thirty-day mortality statistics underestimate the risk of repair of thoracoabdominal aortic aneurysms: a statewide experience. *J Vasc Surg.* 2006;43:217-222; discussion 223.
A report on thoracoabdominal aneurysm mortality for the state of California that demonstrates the mortality associated with these lesions in the period after hospital discharge. It includes an invited discussion on the implications of the findings.

REFERENCES

The reference list can be found on the companion Expert Consult Web site at *www.expertconsult.com*.

Section **17** Arterial Aneurysms

CHAPTER 127

Abdominal Aortic Aneurysms: Evaluation and Decision Making

Mark F. Fillinger

Based in part on a chapter in the previous edition by Marc L. Schermerhorn, MD, and Jack L. Cronenwett, MD.

Surgical outcomes are closely linked to patient selection, which can be complex in the case of abdominal aortic aneurysm (AAA) repair. This is particularly true because of the availability of endovascular aneurysm repair (EVAR), which increases the complexity of decision making. In a patient with an AAA, the decision to operate is based on three primary factors: the risk of the aneurysm's rupturing, the risk associated with aneurysm repair, and the patient's life expectancy. There is a fourth factor, the patient's personal preference, but this can be heavily influenced by the information assimilated by the patient with regard to the other three primary factors. Such a basic framework for decision making makes the process appear overly simple. Unfortunately, it is not possible to accurately calculate rupture risk, procedure risk, and life expectancy for individual patients based on the literature and actuarial tables. Decades of work have not yielded complete knowledge of these factors, much less their interaction in a specific patient at a specific time. However, much information is available to guide clinical decision making, as discussed in this chapter.

■ BACKGROUND

Size Definitions

Aneurysms are defined as focal dilatations at least 50% larger than the expected normal arterial diameter.[1] A practical working definition of an AAA is a transverse diameter of 3 cm or greater and, for a common iliac aneurysm, a transverse diameter greater than 1.8 cm, based on average values for normal individuals. The normal aortic diameter gradually decreases from the thorax (28 mm in men) to the infrarenal location (20 mm in men).[2] At all levels, the normal aortic diameter is approximately 2 mm larger in men than in women and increases with age and increased body surface area.[2] A large ultrasound screening study by Lederle and colleagues found that increasing age, male gender, black race, and increasing height, weight, body mass index, and body surface area were all independently associated with increased infrarenal aortic diameter but that the effect of all these variables was small.[3] Because the average infrarenal aortic diameter was 2 cm in these patients, use of a 3-cm definition for an infrarenal AAA was recommended, without the need to consider a more complicated definition based on factors such as gender or body surface area. Although such definitions are useful for

large patient groups, in clinical practice with individual patients, it is more common to define an aneurysm as a 50% or greater enlargement over the diameter of the adjacent, nonaneurysmal artery.[1] This is particularly true for patients with unusually small arteries, in whom even a 2.5-cm local dilatation of the infrarenal aorta might be aneurysmal if the adjacent aorta were only 1.5 cm in diameter. Rather than being termed atherosclerotic, AAAs are more accurately referred to as degenerative or nonspecific in etiology (see Chapter 8: Arterial Aneurysms). Degenerative aneurysms account for more than 90% of all infrarenal AAAs.

Aneurysm Locations

Nearly all AAAs involve the infrarenal aorta, but only about 5% to 15% of AAAs undergoing surgical repair also involve the suprarenal aorta.[4,5] By definition, because suprarenal AAAs extend above the renal arteries, they require reimplantation of at least one renal artery during AAA repair. The term *juxtarenal* is used to describe AAAs that do not involve the renal arteries but because of proximity require clamping above the renal arteries to complete the proximal aortic anastomosis (see Chapter 128: Abdominal Aortic Aneurysms: Open Surgical Treatment). Although 25% of AAAs also involve the iliac arteries,[4] isolated iliac artery aneurysms are rare (<1% of aortoiliac aneurysm repairs).[6] Isolated aneurysms of the suprarenal aorta are extremely rare unless they have an associated thoracic or infrarenal component. Concomitant thoracic aneurysms have been found in 12% of patients with AAAs, but this is probably a high estimate based on a selected referral practice.[7] Nonetheless, in a population-based study, 5% of patients who underwent AAA repair subsequently died as a result of a thoracic aortic aneurysm.[8] Peripheral aneurysms of the femoral or popliteal artery are present in approximately 4% of patients with AAAs.[9]

■ EPIDEMIOLOGY

Impact of Rupture

In the United States, ruptured AAAs are the 15th leading cause of death overall and the 10th leading cause of death in men older than 55 years, a rate that has held steady for the past 2 decades.[10,11] In 1991, AAAs caused more than 8500 hospital deaths in the United States,[12] which underestimates their true number because 30% to 50% of all patients with ruptured AAAs die before they reach a hospital.[13] In addition, 30% to 40% of patients with ruptured AAAs die after reaching a hospital but without surgery.[13] When combined with an operative mortality rate of 40% to 50%,[14-17] this results in an overall mortality of 80% to 90% for AAA rupture.[13,15,18,19] This high mortality rate has not changed since the 1980s despite improvements in operative technique and perioperative management that have reduced elective surgical mortality to less than 5% in most series.[14] There is growing evidence that endovascular repair of ruptured aneurysms may lower the mortality rate significantly,[20] but rupture remains a high-mortality event because only a minority of patients survive to have an attempt at repair.

The effectiveness of elective AAA repair means that most deaths from AAAs are theoretically preventable. Elective AAA repair is one of the most frequent vascular surgery procedures, with a relatively constant volume of 40,000 operations performed annually in the United States since the 1990s.[12,21] Despite the frequency of elective repair, however, death from AAA rupture has remained relatively constant because many AAAs are undetected or untreated. In a review of ruptured AAAs that were easily palpable, more than 50% either were not detected or were not referred for treatment despite recent medical examination.[22] Ruptured aneurysms also impose a substantial financial burden on overall health care costs. One report from 1984 estimated that $50 million and 2000 lives could have been saved if AAAs had been repaired before they ruptured.[23] Another study showed that emergency operations for AAAs resulted in a mean financial loss to the hospital of $24,655 per patient.[24]

Incidence

AAAs primarily affect the population older than 50 years. They are two to six times more common in men than in women and are two to three times more common in white men than in black men.[12,25-27] Screening studies have provided information on incidence rates of AAA formation (the likelihood of an AAA developing). In the Huntingdon, United Kingdom, screening program for men older than 50, the incidence of new AAAs was 3.5 per 1000 person-years.[28] New AAAs were discovered in 2% of patients screened a second time at a mean of 5.5 years after an initial negative study. In a screening study of U.S. male veterans, Lederle and colleagues found new AAAs in 2.6% of patients 4 years after an initial normal aortic ultrasound study, for an incidence of 6.5 per 1000 person-years.[29] In men, AAAs begin to occur at about 50 years of age and reach a peak incidence near 80.[30-32] In women, AAA onset is delayed, beginning around age 60, with the incidence continuing to increase thereafter (Fig. 127-1).[30-32] Overall, the age-adjusted incidence of both asymptomatic and ruptured AAAs is twofold to sixfold higher in men than in women. A significant increase in the incidence of asymptomatic AAAs has been noted in the past 2 decades,[27,30,33] in part because of increased case finding as a result of

more frequent use of ultrasonography and other imaging modalities.

Incidence of Rupture

There also seems to have been a real increase in the incidence of aortic aneurysmal disease. The finding of a 2.4% per year increase in the age-adjusted incidence of death from AAA rupture from 1952 to 1988 supports this assumption[33] because this statistic is less influenced by more frequent abdominal imaging. An analysis of hospital deaths in the United States indicated that AAA rupture rates stabilized from 1979 to 1990, with 4 deaths per 100,000 in white men.[12] There is recent evidence that this rate may have started to decrease slightly in the United States, coincident with the commercial availability of endovascular AAA repair. Because the overall rate of AAA repair did not increase over this same period, this decrease in rupture rate is presumably due to the fact that EVAR enables elective repair in higher risk patients. The reported incidence of ruptured AAA varies from 1 to 21 per 100,000 person-years.[33] For patients older than 50 years, the incidence of AAA rupture is much higher because AAA increases dramatically with age (see Fig. 127-1).[13] A population-based study of ruptured AAAs by Choksy and associates in England noted an incidence of 76 per 100,000 person-years for men and 11 per 100,000 person-years for women older than 50 years, for a male-female ratio of 6.9:1.[34] The median age at rupture was 76 in men and 81 in women. The median AAA size at rupture was 8 cm, but 4.5% of the ruptured AAAs were smaller than 5 cm in diameter (measured at autopsy or surgery). The overall mortality associated with rupture was 78%, and three fourths of these deaths occurred outside the hospital.

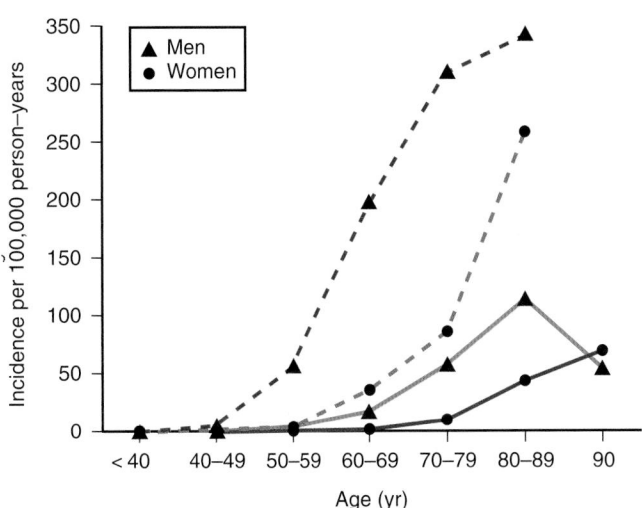

Figure 127-1 Incidence of clinically apparent and ruptured abdominal aortic aneurysms (AAAs) from population-based studies. *Dashed lines,* incidence of all AAAs; *solid lines,* incidence of ruptured AAAs.

Prevalence

Prevalence estimates for asymptomatic AAAs (likelihood of having an AAA) are more accurate than incidence estimates (likelihood of an AAA's developing) now that large ultrasound screening surveys have been performed. Ultrasound screening and autopsy series indicate that the prevalence of AAAs (≥3 cm) is 3% to 10% for patients older than 50 years in the Western world.[33] Necropsy studies from Sweden and the United States have shown increases in the detection of AAAs over the past several decades. In Sweden, the age-standardized prevalence of AAAs at necropsy increased by 4.7% per year for men and 3% per year for women between 1958 and 1986.[31] In Kansas City, the prevalence of necropsy-detected AAAs increased 1.5-fold for men and 2.5-fold for women between 1950-1959 and 1970-1984.[32] In a Veterans Affairs (VA) screening study of more than 73,000 patients 50 to 79 years old, the prevalence of AAAs 3 cm or greater was 4.6% and that of AAAs 4 cm or greater was 1.4%.[35]

Influence of Risk Factors

The prevalence of AAAs in a given population depends on the presence of risk factors associated with AAAs, including older age, male gender, white race, positive family history, smoking, hypertension, hypercholesterolemia, peripheral vascular occlusive disease, and coronary artery disease (CAD).[36] Although these risk factors are associated with increased AAA prevalence, they may not be independent predictors and may be markers rather than causes of AAA disease. Of these risk factors, age, gender, and smoking have the largest impact on AAA prevalence.[27,33,37] In the VA study, smoking was the risk factor most strongly associated with AAAs.[35] The relative risk of having an AAA 4 cm or greater (versus <3 cm) was fivefold higher in smokers than in nonsmokers, and the risk increased significantly with the number of years of smoking. The excess prevalence associated with smoking accounted for 75% of all AAAs that were 4 cm or greater in this study.[35] Other relatively important risk factors that increased AAA prevalence in this study were male gender (5.6-fold risk), age (1.7-fold risk per 7-year increase), white race (2-fold risk), and positive family history (2-fold risk); diabetes decreased the risk (0.5-fold risk). Less important independent risk factors for increased AAA prevalence were height, CAD, any atherosclerosis, high cholesterol level, and hypertension. Associations for AAAs 3 to 3.9 cm (most AAAs found) were similar but weaker.[35] Other investigators have confirmed the association of smoking, gender, and age with AAAs.[26,36,38-48] In a pooled study of more than 3 million subjects, the relative risk for aortic aneurysm–related events in current smokers was generally 3 to 6, as opposed to 1 to 2 for CAD or cerebrovascular disease and 5 to 12 for chronic obstructive pulmonary disease (COPD).[49] Among smokers, AAA prevalence in one study was increased not only by the number of cigarettes smoked and increasing depth of inhalation but also by elevated mean arterial or diastolic blood pressure.[42] In another study of male smokers, AAA prevalence increased with increasing age, years

Table 127-1 Independent Risk Factors for Detecting an Unknown 4-cm-Diameter or Larger Abdominal Aortic Aneurysm during Ultrasound Screening

Risk Factor	Odds Ratio*	95% CI
Increased Risk		
Smoking history	5.1	4.1-6.2
Family history of AAA	1.9	1.6-2.3
Older age (per 7-yr interval)	1.7	1.6-1.8
Coronary artery disease	1.5	1.4-1.7
High cholesterol	1.4	1.3-1.6
COPD	1.2	1.1-1.4
Height (per 7-cm interval)	1.2	1.1-1.3
Decreased Risk		
Abdominal imaging within 5 yr	0.8	0.7-0.9
Deep venous thrombosis	0.7	0.5-0.8
Diabetes mellitus	0.5	0.5-0.6
Black race	0.5	0.4-0.7
Female gender	0.2	0.1-0.5

*Odds ratio indicates relative risk in comparison to patients without that risk factor.
AAA, abdominal aortic aneurysm; CI, confidence interval; COPD, chronic obstructive pulmonary disease.
From Lederle FA, Johnson GR, Wilson SE, et al: The aneurysm detection and management study screening program: validation cohort and final results. Aneurysm Detection and Management Veterans Affairs Cooperative Study Investigators. *Arch Intern Med.* 2000;160:1425.

of smoking, systolic and diastolic blood pressure, and cholesterol.[50] Although there is less agreement that hypertension increases AAA prevalence, it does increase rupture risk in patients with established AAAs.[36,39,41-43,51,52] Larger screening studies using multivariate analysis that included patients whose hypertension had been controlled with medications have found hypertension to be an independent predictor for the development of AAAs.[35,39,43] An analysis of patients enrolled in screening studies in the United Kingdom showed that after adjustment for other risk factors, use of calcium channel blockers was associated with an increased risk for AAAs (odds ratio, 2.6; 95% confidence interval [CI], 1.5 to 4.3). Use of beta blockers showed a trend toward protection, but this did not reach statistical significance (odds ratio, 0.6; 95% CI, 0.4 to 1.1).[53] Although statins may have an effect on the rate of aneurysm expansion, there is no evidence regarding prevalence. Medication use and aneurysms will be discussed in more detail later in this chapter. The estimated impact of various risk factors on AAA prevalence is summarized in Table 127-1.

Familial Clustering

Familial clustering of patients with AAAs has been well described in the literature. Of patients undergoing AAA repair, 15% to 25% have a first-degree relative with a clinically apparent AAA as compared with only 2% to 3% of age-matched control patients without AAAs.[54-61] Conversely, 7% of siblings of patients with AAAs have a clinically apparent AAA.[62] This prevalence increases if ultrasound screening of relatives is performed. Webster and coworkers showed that ultrasound screening of siblings of a patient with an AAA yielded AAAs 3 cm or larger in 25% of the male and 7% of the female siblings older than 55 years.[58] The likelihood that relatives will have an AAA increases if the proband (patient with the AAA) is a woman. If the proband is a man, 7% of relatives have a clinically apparent AAA, but if the proband is a woman, 12% of these relatives have an AAA.[62] It is estimated that first-degree relatives of a patient with an AAA have a 12-fold increased risk for aneurysm development themselves.[56] Brothers of a patient with an AAA have an 18-fold increased risk for the development of an AAA—highest in the 50- to 60-year-old range.[57] Analysis of patients with familial aneurysms indicates that on average these patients are 5 to 7 years younger and are more frequently women.[55,57] In the surgical series by Darling and associates of patients undergoing AAA repair, women accounted for 35% of the patients with a positive family history of AAAs but for only 14% of the patients without familial AAAs.[55] Although AAAs are much less common in women than in men, women with AAAs are more likely to have affected relatives. For a given patient with an AAA (male or female), however, brothers are still at least twice as likely as sisters to have an AAA.

CLINICAL FINDINGS AND DIAGNOSIS

Although AAAs are primarily a disease of the elderly, they can develop in patients younger than 50 years. As reported by Muluk and coworkers, AAAs in younger patients are more often symptomatic, familial, and on average 1 cm larger at initial evaluation than in older patients.[63] This finding may relate to fewer incidental abdominal imaging studies performed in younger patients such that AAAs escape detection until they are larger or symptomatic. Younger patients tend to have more proximally located AAAs, with 46% being juxtarenal or higher as opposed to 18% at this level in older patients. Smoking is nearly universal in young patients with AAAs, whereas only 23% have a defined etiology such as Marfan's syndrome.[63]

Nonruptured Abdominal Aortic Aneurysms

Most nonruptured AAAs are asymptomatic and discovered during abdominal imaging for an unrelated condition. Occasionally, patients may feel a "pulse" in their abdomen or palpate a pulsatile mass. Rarely, large AAAs cause symptoms from local compression, such as early satiety, nausea, or vomiting from duodenal compression; urinary symptoms secondary to hydronephrosis from ureteral compression; or venous thrombosis from iliocaval venous compression. Posterior erosion of AAAs into adjacent vertebrae can lead to back pain. Even without bony involvement, AAAs can cause chronic back pain or abdominal pain that is vague and ill defined. Acute ischemic symptoms can result from distal embolization of the thrombotic debris contained within an AAA. Ischemic symptoms appear to be more common with smaller AAAs, especially if the intraluminal thrombus is irregular or fissured.[64] Acute thrombosis of an AAA occurs rarely but causes

catastrophic ischemia. Atheroembolism is much more common than acute AAA thrombosis, but both combined occur in less than 2% to 5% of patients with AAAs.[64] Nonetheless, an aortic aneurysm source for distal atheroemboli must always be considered, especially in patients without overt atherosclerotic occlusive disease. Such symptoms are nearly always an indication for AAA repair.

Ruptured Abdominal Aortic Aneurysms

Most AAAs that become symptomatic do so because of rupture or acute expansion. Ruptured AAAs are discussed in detail in Chapter 130 (Abdominal Aortic Aneurysms: Ruptured). In a review of stable but symptomatic patients with a suspected ruptured AAA, computed tomography (CT) showed a ruptured aneurysm in 30%, a nonruptured AAA in 50%, and other pathology to explain the symptoms in 20% of patients.[65] This is valuable information because patients with symptomatic but nonruptured aneurysms (termed acutely expanding) have a substantially higher operative mortality rate than do those undergoing elective AAA repair (average of 23%).[66,67] This higher mortality probably results from a combination of factors, including suboptimal preoperative evaluation, case planning, and management of co-morbid disease, as well as less experienced emergency surgical and anesthesia teams. Emergency repair is less likely to be endovascular, with the attendant differences in mortality rates (discussed later under "Operative Risk" under the heading "Factors Affecting Clinical Decision Making"). Because acute expansion is considered an immediate precursor of rupture, however, such patients must undergo expeditious AAA repair.

Physical Examination

Although most clinically significant AAAs are potentially palpable during routine physical examination, the sensitivity of this technique depends on AAA size, obesity of the patient, skill of the examiner, and focus of the examination.[68] With physical examination alone, the diagnosis is made in 29% of AAAs 3 to 3.9 cm, 50% of AAAs 4 to 4.9 cm, and 75% of AAAs 5 cm or larger.[69] Although a focused physical examination detected 50% of 3.5- to 6-cm-diameter AAAs, they had all been missed on a recent, nonfocused examination.[68] Conversely, AAAs may be falsely suspected in thin patients with a prominent but normal-sized aorta or in patients with a mass overlying the aorta that transmits a prominent pulse. Patients with hypertension, a wide pulse pressure, or a tortuous aorta can also have prominent aortic pulsation that may be mistaken for an AAA. The positive predictive value of physical examination for identifying AAAs greater than 3.5 cm in diameter is only 15%.[70] The accuracy of physical examination in measuring the size of a known AAA is also poor, with the size usually being overestimated because of intervening intestine and abdominal wall tissue. As a result of these factors, most AAAs are detected by incidental abdominal imaging studies performed for other reasons. In a review of 243 patients who underwent elective AAA repair, Chervu and colleagues found that 38% were initially detected by physical examination whereas 62% were detected by incidental radiologic studies, even though 43% of them were palpable on subsequent examination.[71] Of these clinically significant AAAs, 23% were not palpable even when the diagnosis was known, and in obese patients, two thirds were not palpable. These findings emphasize the fact that many significant AAA are missed on physical examination and that ultrasound screening has a potential role in high-risk patients, as discussed later.

Imaging

Ultrasound

Several imaging modalities are available to confirm the diagnosis of AAA. Abdominal B-mode ultrasonography is the least expensive, least invasive, and most frequently used examination, particularly for initial confirmation of a suspected AAA and follow-up of small AAAs. Measurements of diameter with ultrasound have an interobserver variability of approximately 5 mm in 84% of studies and are more accurate in the anteroposterior than in the lateral dimension.[72] Visualization of the suprarenal aorta and iliac arteries may be obscured by bowel gas or be difficult in obese patients. Ultrasonography cannot accurately determine the presence of rupture[73] and often cannot accurately determine the upper extent of an AAA.[74] When compared with CT, ultrasound typically underestimates the diameter of AAAs by 2 to 4 mm in the anteroposterior direction.[72,75-77] In general, ultrasound is used to diagnose and monitor AAAs until the aneurysm approaches a size at which repair may be considered, whereupon more advanced imaging is used for preoperative evaluation.

Computed Tomography

CT is more expensive than ultrasound and involves exposure to radiation and intravenous contrast material, but it provides more accurate measurement of diameter, with 91% of studies showing less than 5-mm interobserver variability.[72] Accuracy can be increased by using standardized techniques, electronic calipers, and magnification.[75] Intraobserver variability under these conditions is within 2 mm in 90% of cases.[75] Ultrasonography and CT can overestimate AAA diameter if an oblique rather than a perpendicular section is obtained in a tortuous aneurysm. This results in an elliptical rather than a circular cross-section, and unless the aneurysm cross-section is truly asymmetric, the larger diameter of the ellipse overestimates the true AAA diameter (see Chapter 21: Computed Tomography). CT scanning is largely used in the preoperative assessment of patients with AAAs (see under "Aneurysm Evaluation" under the heading "Individual Patient Decision Making"), but it is also particularly useful for excluding AAA rupture in a stable but symptomatic patient.

■ SCREENING

Because asymptomatic AAAs are often not discovered until they rupture, the potential benefit of ultrasound screening

programs is apparent. Though only recently reimbursed by Medicare with the "welcome to Medicare" physical examination, screening programs have been in place for years in other countries.[52,78-86] Screening is generally considered appropriate when a disease has a long latency period, when the disease can be detected by the screening study at an early stage, when intervention at an early stage would improve outcome relative to intervention at a later stage, and when the screening study is inexpensive, is accurate, has minimal risk, causes little or no pain, and is cost-effective. An important caveat is that steps should be taken to ensure a high attendance rate for screening to avoid the "healthy volunteer effect." People who are most likely to attend screening tend to be more health conscious and may benefit less than people who refuse. This effect is particularly important for a disease associated with smoking and uncontrolled hypertension. Targeted ultrasound screening for AAAs is recommended to focus effort on people most at risk (e.g., older age, male gender, smoking history, positive family history). In the absence of effective medical therapy, it seems reasonable to withhold screening from people who would not be offered intervention if the disease were discovered (patients unfit for even EVAR).

Prospective Trials

Two nonrandomized studies and four randomized controlled trials have been completed that address these issues and are summarized in a review by Lederle.[87]

Nonrandomized Trials

In the Gloucestershire Aneurysm Screening Programme, all men aged 65 to 73 were offered ultrasound screening.[81] No prescreening evaluation of potential fitness for AAA repair by a general practitioner was made. The attendance rate was 84%. AAAs larger than 4 cm were detected in 2.2% of the volunteers scanned, and during subsequent follow-up there was a 66% reduction in overall AAA-related mortality (including deaths resulting from elective repair and rupture), which was statistically significant. In the Huntingdon, United Kingdom, trial, general practitioners reviewed their lists of male patients older than 50 years.[88] They excluded those considered unfit for potential AAA repair. The remaining patients were invited for ultrasound screening and had an attendance rate of 74%. A significant (49%) reduction in future ruptured AAAs was noted in patients who were invited. Even though only 74% to 84% of patients were screened in these two studies, detection of small AAAs and subsequent management reduced rupture risk by half in the entire group of patients invited for AAA screening.

Randomized Trials

The first randomized trial of AAA screening enrolled 6058 unselected 65- to 80-year-old men in Chichester, United Kingdom, 74% of whom attended screening.[89] AAAs (≥3 cm) were detected in 7.6%. AAA-related death was subsequently reduced by 41% at 5 years and 21% at 10 years, but this difference was not significant.[82] The investigators also enrolled 9342 unselected 65- to 80-year-old women, 65% of whom attended screening.[83] The prevalence of AAA in women was just 1.3%. Women did not seem to benefit from screening because there was no difference in elective AAA repair, ruptured AAA, or AAA-related mortality at 5 or 10 years in women offered screening. The average age of women with a ruptured AAA was 6 years older than men. For both men and women it is important to note that the comparison was between those *offered* screening and those who were not offered screening. The Chichester group noted that a substantial number of ruptured AAAs occurred in patients invited for screening who refused screening, did not adhere to follow-up, refused surgery, or were considered unfit for surgery after AAA was diagnosed. This study highlights the importance of preselecting only individuals who may benefit from screening.

In the second randomized trial of AAA screening, all 12,658 65- to 73-year-old men in Viborg County, Denmark, were randomized.[84] The attendance rate was 76%. AAA (≥3 cm) was diagnosed in 4%. In-hospital AAA-related mortality was reduced by 68% in men invited for screening ($P <$ .01). Outpatient deaths were not recorded, however. Additionally, studies reporting simply a reduction in AAA-related deaths fail to account for the timing of death. Patients who die as a result of elective surgery for screening-detected AAAs tend to die sooner than patients who die as a result of rupture of an undiagnosed AAA, thus resulting in a greater loss of life-years per death in the screened group.

The Multicentre Aneurysm Screening Study (MASS) was a well-designed, carefully conducted, and thoughtfully analyzed randomized trial that involved 70,495 men aged 65 to 74 years and excluded 4% who were considered unfit for possible surgical repair.[85] Of the 33,839 patients randomized to ultrasound screening (versus no screening), 80% accepted and were scanned. The aorta was not visualized in 1.2%, and AAAs larger than 3 cm were detected in 5%. The 33,961 control patients were not contacted. After a mean follow-up of 4 years, there were 113 AAA-related deaths in controls and 65 in the invited group. To account for the timing of death, the investigators calculated the rate of AAA-related death per 1000 person-years of follow-up. It was 0.85 in the control group and 0.49 in the invited group, with a hazard ratio of 0.58 (95% CI, 0.42 to 0.78; P = .0002). The incidence of nonfatal ruptured AAAs was similarly reduced in the invited group (hazard ratio, 0.59; 95% CI, 0.45 to 0.77; P = .00006). Although there were more deaths as a result of elective AAA repair in the screened group (15 versus 9), this was more than offset by the reduction in deaths from ruptured AAAs (37 versus 91). AAA-related death was similar in the two groups over the first year, but after 1 year the curves continued to separate over the remainder of the trial period, thus suggesting that the benefit may still increase over time. AAA-related death accounted for only 3% of all deaths in control patients and 2% of deaths in patients invited for screening. It is not likely that any single trial would be large enough to show a

significant reduction in all-cause mortality. The 32% reduction in AAA-related mortality rate was significant, however.

A meta-analysis by Bohm and colleagues in which the long-term results from all the major screening studies were analyzed was large enough (with more than 125,000 patients) to demonstrate not only a 44% reduction in the AAA-related mortality rate but also a small but statistically significant reduction in overall mortality in the long-term (7- to 15-year) results.[90]

Quality of Life

Quality of life was also assessed carefully in the MASS trial.[85] At all times and in all groups, anxiety, depression, and health status measures were within the age- and gender-matched population norms. Patients who screened positive for AAA had slightly lower scores, however, on some physical and mental health scales and self-rated health immediately after screening. Patients undergoing surgery versus surveillance had lower scores in mental health at 3 months, but the scores were similar by 12 months. Self-rated health at 3 and 12 months was also better in those who underwent surgery versus surveillance and was similar to ratings by patients screening negative. These results are comparable to those of previous studies and indicate that AAA screening does not have a negative impact on quality of life.[67,91-94]

Cost-Effectiveness

In a parallel publication, the MASS group showed that screening men aged 65 to 74 for AAA is cost-effective with an incremental cost-effectiveness ratio of $30,000 per life-year saved when analyzed after only 4 years (the duration of the trial) and a projected cost-effectiveness ratio of $8500 per life-year saved after 10 years.[95] After adjusting for the quality of life changes described earlier, the cost-effectiveness ratio at 4 years is increased slightly to about $38,000 per quality-adjusted life-year saved, which it is well within the range of other widely accepted practices, from coronary artery bypass to dialysis.

Recommendations

All randomized trials have shown at least a trend toward reduced AAA-related mortality with ultrasound screening. This benefit was shown best in the largest trial, which in addition to large numbers also had a high attendance rate. If the attendance rate is low, it becomes more likely that patients at greatest risk will not undergo screening and the overall benefit may be reduced or lost. Targeting patients at greatest risk for AAA is likely to increase the benefit. Screening seems reasonable for men older than 60 years who would be candidates for at least endovascular repair. Screening may be beneficial for women if they have other risk factors for AAA such as a smoking history or a family history of AAA. Because familial AAAs tend to occur at a younger age, screening in patients with a family history should be performed earlier, such as at 50 to 55 years.

In 2005, the U.S. Preventive Services Task Force (USPSTF) updated recommendations relative to AAA screening.[96,97] These articles provide an update of the 1996 USPSTF recommendations on the topic based on several important studies, including those already described. The USPSTF recommended screening for AAAs with ultrasonography in males 65 to 75 years of age who have ever smoked (not solely current smokers). Because "ever smoked" is defined as lifetime consumption of at least 100 cigarettes, this encompasses 69% of men aged 65 to 75 in the United States. This is a "grade B" recommendation ("at least fair evidence … improves important health outcomes and concludes that benefits outweigh harms") that upgraded the recommendation in the previous review, which could recommend neither for or against screening ("grade C"). The USPSTF recommendation for women was against screening, but it failed to take into account specific risk factors that may make screening cost-effective in selected groups.[98,99] The Society for Vascular Surgery and the Society for Vascular Medicine and Biology recommended more comprehensive screening that reflects the concerns noted earlier and yet would still be cost-effective relative to other common screening tests.[99] Currently it appears that women with a family history of aneurysm will be covered, but the final result is not yet clear.

If an initial screening study is negative, there is little additional value for future repeat ultrasound scans.[28,29,100,101] In all studies, additional small AAAs were detected in 2% to 4% at 4 to 12 years of follow-up, but almost all were less than 4 cm and none were considered likely to require repair during the life of the patient. It is unlikely that repeat screening would be helpful for most patients. Repeat screening may be reasonable, however, in patients with a positive family history who undergo an initial scan at a young age.

■ FACTORS AFFECTING CLINICAL DECISION MAKING

The choice between observation and prophylactic surgical repair of an AAA for an individual patient at any given time should take into account (1) the risk for AAA rupture under observation, (2) the operative risk associated with repair, (3) the patient's life expectancy, and (4) the personal preferences of the patient.[102,103]

Aneurysm Rupture Risk

Estimates of the risk for AAA rupture are imprecise because large numbers of patients with AAAs have not been observed without intervention. Even in the recent randomized trials, a high percentage of patients in the "observation" groups undergo repair, thus underestimating rupture risk. Studies conducted before the widespread application of surgical repair documented the likelihood of large AAAs to rupture, although many of these AAAs were both large and symptomatic, thus

Table 127-2 Range of Potential Rupture Rates for a Given Size of Abdominal Aortic Aneurysm

AAA Diameter (cm)	Rupture Risk (%/yr)
<4	0
4-5	0.5-5
5-6	3-15
6-7	10-20
7-8	20-40
>8	30-50

From Brewster DC, Cronenwett JL, Hallett JW Jr, et al. Guidelines for the treatment of abdominal aortic aneurysms. Report of a subcommittee of the Joint Council of the American Association for Vascular Surgery and Society for Vascular Surgery. *J Vasc Surg.* 2003;37:1106-1117.

overestimating rupture risk.[104,105] Even autopsy studies[106,107] may underestimate the diameter at rupture because the aneurysm is no longer pressurized at autopsy, and rupture risk may be overestimated because there is no way of knowing how many patients with asymptomatic aneurysms did not undergo autopsy. Varying populations, referral patterns, surgical intervention rates, imaging methods, and definitions of how to measure diameter lend further variability to the data, as evidenced by the wide range of potential rupture risk in the literature for a given aneurysm size (Table 127-2). Data are insufficient to develop an accurate prediction rule for AAA rupture in individual patients, which makes surgical decision making difficult. Knowledge of the available natural history data can assist in making these decisions, however.

Aneurysm Diameter

For the past 5 decades the primary determinant of rupture risk has been the maximum aneurysm diameter, based on a pivotal study reported by Szilagyi and colleagues in 1966.[108] These authors compared the outcomes of small-diameter and large-diameter aneurysms and found that patients with larger aneurysms (>6 cm) were much more likely to die of a ruptured aneurysm. Foster and coworkers confirmed these results in 1969 by reporting rupture in 16% of AAAs less than 6 cm in diameter versus rupture in 51% of AAAs greater than 6 cm in patients managed nonoperatively.[109] In these series AAA diameter was determined by physical examination and abdominal radiography, both of which are now known to overestimate actual diameter, such that the actual size for their definition of a 6-cm AAA was closer to 5 cm. Early autopsy studies also demonstrated that larger AAAs are more prone to rupture.[106] One series found that rupture had occurred in 5% of AAAs 5 cm or less in diameter, in 39% of AAAs 5 to 7 cm in diameter, and in 65% of AAAs 7 cm or greater in diameter.[107] These studies firmly established the effect of size on AAA rupture and provided a sound basis for recommending elective repair for large AAAs because even these early studies showed a marked improvement in survival after operative repair.[108,109]

Defining Rupture Risk. In a Minnesota population-based study of 176 patients with AAAs selected for nonoperative management, the estimated annual rupture risk was zero for AAAs less than 4 cm, 1% per year for AAAs 4.0 to 4.9 cm, but 11% per year for AAAs 5.0 to 5.9 cm.[110] These rates also probably underestimate rupture risk, however, because 45% of AAAs underwent elective repair during follow-up, presumably those at greatest risk for rupture within any size category.[110] In another study of 114 patients with small AAAs initially selected for nonoperative management, Limet and associates observed rupture in 12% during a 2-year follow-up despite elective repair in 38% because of rapid expansion.[111] This yielded an annual rupture rate of zero for AAAs less than 4 cm in diameter, 5.4% per year for AAAs 4 to 5 cm in diameter, and 16% per year for AAAs larger than 5 cm in diameter. Because this was a referral-based study, it probably overestimated rupture risk for the entire population but may accurately portray the group of patients referred for surgical consultation.

In another referral-based study of 300 patients with AAAs initially managed nonoperatively, however, the observed annual rupture risk during a 4-year follow-up was only 0.25% per year for AAAs smaller than 4 cm, 0.5% per year for AAAs 4 to 4.9 cm, and 4.3% per year for AAAs larger than 5 cm in diameter, even though only 8% of the patients underwent elective repair.[112]

Data from the United Kingdom Small Aneurysm Trial (UKSAT; see under "U.K. Small Aneurysm Trial") provide the most recent estimates of AAA rupture risk in patients randomized to nonoperative management. The annual rupture risk was 0.3% for AAAs 3.9 cm or smaller, 1.5% for AAAs 4.0 to 4.9 cm, and 6.5% for AAAs 5.0 to 5.9 cm.[113] These numbers do not accurately represent the rupture risk for women, who made up only 17% of the trial and had a 4.5-fold higher risk for rupture than men did. It is also likely that these numbers underestimate the actual annual rupture risk for small AAAs because some underwent repair for rapid expansion or the development of symptoms.

Despite differences in precise estimates, all the aforementioned studies show that rupture risk increases substantially with AAA diameter between 5 and 6 cm.

Large Diameters. A study of patients with aneurysms larger than 5.5 cm by Conway and coworkers indicated that more than 50% will ultimately rupture when surgery is deferred because of high operative risk.[114] In this high-risk group, the median time to rupture was only 19 months for patients with 5.5- to 5.9-cm AAAs and just 9 months for patients with AAAs larger than 7 cm.[114] Even in patients under close surveillance, the aneurysm rupture rate is substantial when larger than 5.5 cm and rises exponentially with size. Lederle and colleagues reported on 198 predominantly male veterans with AAAs 5.5 cm or larger who were unfit for or refused surgery.[115] The 1-year rupture risk was 9% for AAAs 5.5 to 5.9 cm, 10% for AAAs 6 to 6.9 cm, and 33% for AAAs 7 cm or larger based on the initial diameter. The subgroup of patients with an initial AAA diameter of 6.5 to 6.9 cm had an annual rupture risk of 19%.[115,116]

Method of Measurement. Most aneurysms have an elliptical cross-section on axial CT imaging, and large studies have suggested that rupture risk is more closely associated with the minor axis.[117,118] This makes sense with regard to three-dimensional reconstructions of CT imaging data, which demonstrate that the elliptical axial cross-section in most aneurysms is more commonly due to tortuosity than to a truly asymmetric shape.[117] For aneurysms with a truly asymmetric shape, the larger "diameter" in the elliptical cross-section appears to be a more appropriate estimate of rupture risk.[117] Despite these issues, many studies fail to precisely report how maximum aneurysm diameter was determined, and many centers still use the "major axis" diameter to estimate rupture risk for all aortic aneurysms. Thus, even though maximum aneurysm diameter remains the "gold standard" for estimating rupture risk, it is far from ideal.

Aneurysm Wall Stress

From a biomechanical perspective, AAA rupture occurs when the forces within an AAA exceed the wall's "bursting strength." Laplace's law indicates that the wall tension of a symmetric shape such as a cylinder or sphere is directly proportional to its radius and intraluminal pressure and inversely proportional to wall thickness. Actual AAAs are not ideal symmetric shapes and have walls of variable thickness and strength. Over the years, multiple authors have suggested that mathematical modeling of aneurysm asymmetry may prove superior to simple maximum diameter.[119-124] The application of engineering principles to the analysis of actual aneurysms has only recently been possible. At this point, multiple studies have demonstrated that finite element analysis of AAA wall stress with three-dimensional CT reconstructions is better than diameter for estimating rupture risk.[125-127]

Finite Element Analysis. In 2002, in the first report using finite element analysis on a large cohort of AAA patients with and without rupture, Fillinger and colleagues reported that finite element analysis of AAA wall stress with three-dimensional CT reconstructions is better than diameter for differentiating AAAs at or near the time of rupture.[125] Aneurysm wall stress also predicted the location of rupture, a finding that has been reproduced in small aneurysms (Fig. 127-2).[128] Moreover, they found that calculated indices previously suggested to better predict rupture risk (e.g., ratio of maximum AAA diameter to normal infrarenal diameter) were not helpful.[125] The lack of utility for calculated indices was later confirmed in a much larger cohort of 259 AAAs, including 122 with documented rupture.[117]

In 2003, Fillinger and coauthors reported on the first large series of finite element analysis in patients with AAAs under observation; they evaluated aneurysms that had elective repair deferred because of co-morbid conditions or were thought to be at low risk for rupture.[127] In this study of 105 patients, wall stress was superior to AAA diameter for predicting rupture risk in patients under observation (Fig. 127-3). Equally important, the study indicated that aneurysm wall stress is elevated

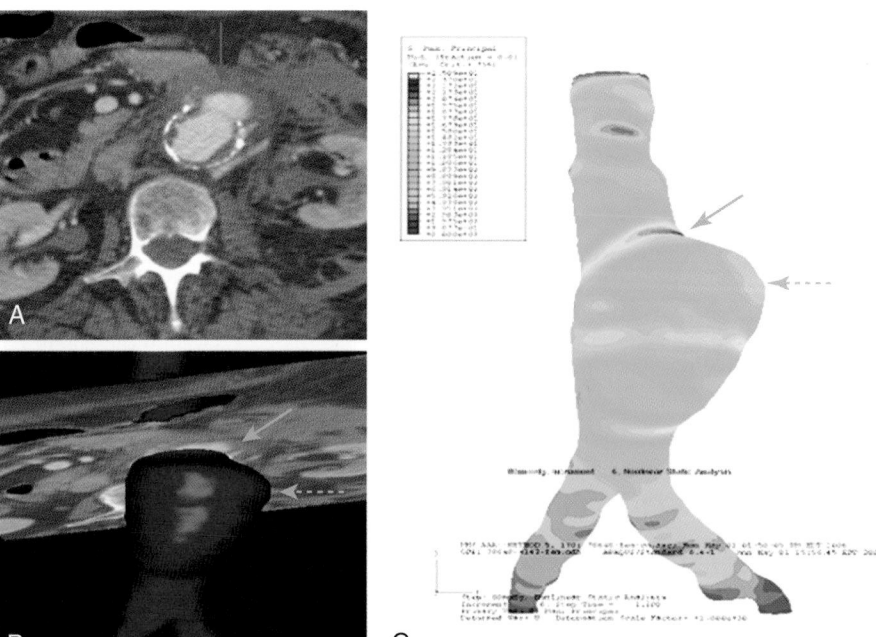

Figure 127-2 Wall stress analysis of a small abdominal aortic aneurysm (AAA) (≤5-cm maximum diameter). **A,** AAA rupture noted on CT. **B,** Three-dimensional model of the aneurysm with the CT slice merged for context. Note that the native aneurysm wall boundaries, and not the hematoma, were modeled for the stress analysis. **C,** Maximal wall stress is demonstrated in *red* at the location of the actual rupture. As is typical, the location of maximum stress and rupture (*solid arrow in B and C*) is not at the cross-section with the maximum diameter (*dashed arrow in B and C*). (*Modified from Truijers M, Pol JA, Schultzekool LJ, et al. Wall stress analysis in small asymptomatic, symptomatic and ruptured abdominal aortic aneurysms.* Eur J Vasc Endovasc Surg. *2007;33:401-407.*)

well in advance of the time of rupture, thereby allowing sufficient time to repair the aneurysm before a catastrophic outcome.[127] Using multivariate analysis with proportional hazards modeling, it was determined that peak wall stress was the greatest predictor of rupture (hazard ratio, 25), followed by gender (hazard ratio, 3), and that after accounting for wall stress and gender, diameter did not predict rupture. Thus, it appears that wall stress can be a useful clinical tool with the potential to replace the diameter method in use for the past 4 decades. At this point the strength of the data and the size of the patient cohorts already rival or exceed that of the data initially used to determine the clinical use of aneurysm diameter to estimate rupture risk in the 1960s. The method has also been validated in more than one institution and in multiple countries.[126,128,129] The technique of using aneurysm wall stress to predict rupture risk remains to be validated in a large multicenter cohort using a standardized, broadly applicable technique, although one such study is currently under way.[117] There is also reason to believe that refining the computer modeling to include wall strength along the lines of Vorp's group will improve estimates of rupture risk even further.[130] Until multicenter validation studies of finite element methods are completed, however, the gold standard will continue to be based on diameter.

Aneurysm Shape

Clinical opinion also holds that shape is important and that eccentric or saccular aneurysms present a greater risk for rupture than do more diffuse fusiform aneurysms. The utility of clinical impression appears to be variable, however. Vorp and associates used computer modeling to show that wall stress is substantially increased by an asymmetric bulge in

AAAs.[124] The influence of asymmetry was nearly as important as diameter over the clinically relevant range tested. The large-scale asymmetric bulges modeled in the referenced study are not the same as a symmetric saccular aneurysm, however, and saccularity alone does not appear to enhance rupture risk.[117,118] In contradistinction to a symmetric saccular aneurysm, localized outpouchings or "blebs" ranging from 5 to 30 mm are commonly observed on AAAs intraoperatively or on CT scans.[131] These areas of focal wall outpouching are associated with thinning of the tunica media elastin and have been suggested to increase rupture risk, although this is not firmly established.[132] Calcification within the wall may increase wall stress focally but may not be useful as a clinical tool.[133-135] The effect of intraluminal thrombus on rupture risk is also debated, with studies suggesting that thicker thrombus may increase the risk for rupture, decrease the risk for rupture, or have no effect.[117,134,136-140] The practical impact of these variables on AAA rupture risk (alone or in the context of finite element analysis) requires further study.

Other Risk Factors

Although maximum aneurysm diameter is a good predictor of rupture risk in summary data involving large numbers of patients, some aneurysms rupture at an unusually small size.[106,141,142] In some series, 10% to 24% of the ruptured aneurysms were 5 cm or less in maximum diameter, including a study of consecutive patients with imaging before rupture.[113,142] At least one population-based study has reported extremely low rupture rates for smaller aneurysms,[143] but nearly half of the AAAs underwent repair during follow-up. Even in prospective studies with frequent observation and timely surgical intervention for symptoms, rapid expansion,

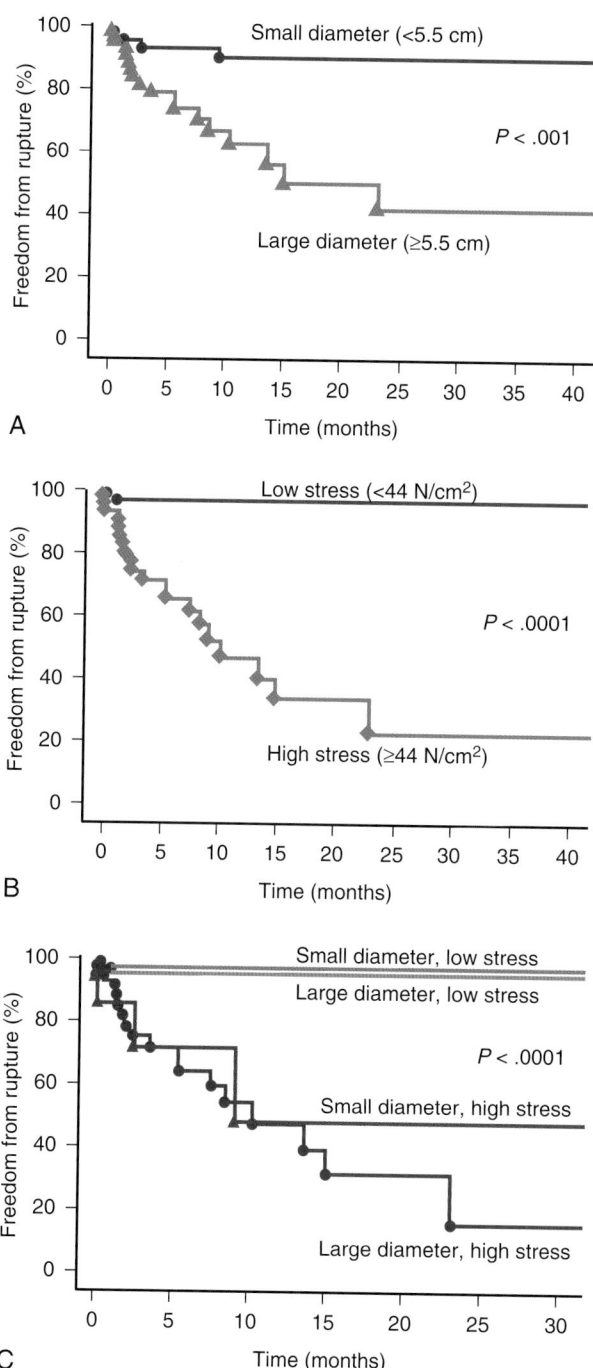

Figure 127-3 Life-table comparison of rupture risk in subsets with small- and large-diameter AAA stratified by low and high wall stress. **A,** Larger diameter was a highly significant predictor for a higher rate of rupture, as shown for aneurysms larger than 5.5 cm. **B,** High stress was also a highly significant predictor for a higher rate of rupture. **C,** Subgroups were analyzed for combinations of small and large diameter and low and high wall stress by using the same thresholds as in the other life-tables. Low-stress aneurysms had a low rupture rate whether they were small or large diameter, and high stress aneurysms had a high rupture rate regardless of diameter. *(From Fillinger MF, Marra SP, Raghavan ML, Kennedy FE. Prediction of rupture risk in abdominal aortic aneurysm during observation: wall stress versus diameter. J Vasc Surg. 2003;37: 724-732.)*

or expansion to 5.5 cm, the rupture rate was as high as 2% per year, depending on gender and aneurysm size.[113,144,145]

The simple observation that not all AAAs rupture at a specific diameter suggests that other patient- and aneurysm-specific variables influence rupture. Several studies have used multivariate analysis to examine the predictive value of various clinical parameters on AAA rupture risk. The UKSAT monitored 2257 patients over the 7-year period of the trial, including 1090 randomized patients and an additional 1167 patients who were ineligible for randomization.[113] There were 103 documented ruptures. Predictors of rupture using proportional hazards modeling (adjusted hazard ratio in parentheses) were female gender (3.0), initial AAA diameter (2.9/cm), smoking status (never smokers, 0.65; former smokers, 0.59— both versus current smokers), mean blood pressure (1.02/mm Hg), and forced expiratory volume in 1 second (FEV_1) (0.62/L). The mean diameter for ruptures was 1 cm lower for women (5 cm) than for men (6 cm). Data from Fillinger and colleagues in which CT scan measurements of 122 ruptured AAAs were evaluated indicate that the average size of ruptured aneurysms in women is 5 mm smaller than in men.[117] The UKSAT was the first to show that smoking status predicts rupture independently of chronic pulmonary disease.[113] These data suggest that smoking has a two-tiered effect in that FEV_1, probably a measure of the duration and quantity of smoking, is related to rupture but also that AAAs in current smokers are more likely to rupture than are AAAs in former smokers, even after adjusting for FEV_1. The UKSAT analysis is reenforced by other independent work. In an early study, Cronenwett and associates determined that larger initial AAA diameter, hypertension, and COPD were independent predictors of rupture.[141] By comparing patients with ruptured and intact AAAs at autopsy, Sterpetti and colleagues also concluded that larger initial AAA size, hypertension, and bronchiectasis were independently associated with AAA rupture.[107] Patients with ruptured AAAs more frequently had hypertension (54% versus 28%), emphysema (67% versus 42%), and bronchiectasis (29% versus 15%). In a review of 75 patients with AAAs managed nonoperatively, Foster and coworkers noted that death from rupture occurred in 72% of patients with diastolic hypertension but in only 30% of the entire group.[109] Among 156 patients with AAAs managed nonoperatively, Szilagyi and colleagues found that hypertension (>150 mm Hg) was present in 67% of those who experienced rupture but in only 23% of those without rupture.[146] More recently, work by Fillinger and associates has demonstrated an independent effect of current smoking on rupture risk even when shape is accounted for.[117] With current techniques, female gender may even be an independent risk factor when using finite element analysis for wall stress.[127] Thus, multiple reports implicate hypertension, COPD, female gender, and current smoking status as important risk factors for AAA rupture independent of AAA size, and some of these factors may be independent of shape and wall stress as well.

Family History. Although a positive family history of AAA is known to increase the prevalence of AAAs in other first-degree relatives, it also seems that familial AAAs have a higher risk for rupture. Darling and colleagues reported that the frequency of ruptured AAAs increased with the number of first-degree relatives who have AAAs: 15% with two first-degree relatives, 29% with three first-degree relatives, and 36% with four or more first-degree relatives.[55] Rupture was more likely in women with familial aneurysms (30%) than in men with familial AAAs (17%). Verloes and associates found that the rupture rate was 32% in patients with familial AAAs versus 9% in patients with sporadic aneurysms and that familial AAAs ruptured 10 years earlier (65 versus 75 years old).[57] These observations suggest that patients with a strong family history of AAA may have an individually higher risk for rupture, especially if they are female. These studies did not consider other potentially confounding factors, however, such as AAA size, which might have been different in the familial group. Further epidemiologic research is required to determine whether a positive family history is an independent risk factor for AAA rupture in addition to a risk factor for increased AAA prevalence.

Expansion Rate. Although rapid AAA expansion is presumed to increase rupture risk, it is difficult to separate this effect from the influence of expansion rate on absolute diameter, which alone could increase rupture risk. Numerous studies have established that aneurysms expand more rapidly as they get larger.[111,147-150] Limet and colleagues[111] calculated the median expansion rate of small AAAs to be $e^{0.106t}$, where t = years. For a 1-year interval, this formula predicts an 11% increase in diameter per year, nearly identical to the 10% per year calculation reported by Cronenwett and colleagues in 1990.[147] Two studies have reported that the expansion rate was larger in ruptured than in intact AAAs but that these ruptured AAAs were also larger.[111,151] Other studies have found that absolute AAA diameter rather than expansion rate predicted rupture.[143,141] Studies of patients with thoracoabdominal aneurysms indicate that both initial diameter and the subsequent expansion rate are independent predictors of rupture.[152] One study with seven ruptures in 39 patients examined with serial three-dimensional CT scans found expansion rate to be a predictor of rupture.[152]

Determinants of AAA expansion rate in a patient population can be studied in a more robust fashion. The UKSAT showed that current smoking is predictive of more rapid expansion whereas former smoking is not.[153] In addition to these factors, hypertension and pulse pressure have been identified as independent predictors of a more rapid expansion rate.[147,149,151,154] Finally, two studies have shown that increased thrombus content within an AAA and the extent of the aneurysm wall in contact with thrombus are associated with more rapid expansion.[117,140,155] Santilli and colleagues pointed out that the median expansion rate is lower than the mean and may be more appropriate given the skewed nature of the data.[154] The median expansion rate may be more useful for predicting expansion for an individual patient and should be reported in future studies. Though far from being proven, rapid AAA expansion is frequently regarded as a risk factor

for rupture and often is used as a criterion for elective repair of small AAAs. Furthermore, calculating predicted AAA expansion is useful to inform patients about when a currently small AAA will probably reach the threshold size for elective repair in the future.

Operative Risk

Operative mortality is the most widely reported of all aneurysm-related statistics in the literature. A review by Blankensteijn and coworkers found that population-based studies reported mortality rates as high as 8% after open AAA repair (prospective) and as a whole are significantly higher than single-center reports, which averaged 3.8%.[156] A review by Hallin and colleagues found a weighted operative mortality for elective open AAA repair of 5%,[17] consistent with the UKSAT figure of 5.6%,[157] U.S. hospital discharge data (5.6% in a review of 360,000 repairs),[158] and the Canadian Aneurysm Study (4.8%).[159] EVAR has substantially improved these mortality rates, as discussed later under "Operative Risk" under the heading "Factors Affecting Clinical Decision Making."

Prediction Algorithms for Open Repair

A meta-analysis by Steyerberg and associates found six independent risk factors for operative mortality (in order of importance): creatinine greater than 1.8 mg/dL (159 μmol/L), congestive heart failure, electrocardiographically detected ischemia, pulmonary dysfunction, older age, and female gender.[160] They created a prediction rule that took into account a surgeon's specific operative mortality (Table 127-3). Despite the logic and elegance of this model, it has not been validated in other trials, including the UKSAT, where the Steyerberg prediction rule did not work as well as expected.[157] The Glasgow Aneurysm Score is a more recent prediction algorithm for operative mortality after open repair that likewise shows promise, but it also has an accuracy rate in the 75% range, which means that it will fail in a substantial number of patients.[161-163] Multiple scoring systems have been developed, but none are better than the 75% to 80% range.[161] Consistent themes in the studies by Steyerberg and colleagues, Hallin and associates, the Canadian Aneurysm Study, L'Italien, and the UKSAT suggest that cardiac disease (congestive heart failure, ischemia on electrocardiography), pulmonary disease, and renal insufficiency are all strong predictors of operative mortality, with lesser effects of age and gender if adjusted for other co-morbid factors. Coronary bypass within 5 years and negative cardiac stress testing appear to have a protective effect.[164] Nesi and coworkers performed a retrospective evaluation of the Eagle score, Glasgow Aneurysm Score, Leiden score, modified Leiden score, and Vanzetto score in a consecutive series of 286 patients.[161] For the Glasgow Aneurysm Score, Leiden score, modified Leiden score, and Vanzetto score, receiver operating characteristics curve analysis for prediction of in-hospital mortality showed an area under the curve of 0.749 (P = .01), 0.777 (P = .008), 0.788 (P = .006), and 0.794 (p = .005), respectively (i.e., 75% to 80% predictive ability).

Table 127-3 Predicting Operative Mortality after Elective Open Abdominal Aortic Aneurysm Repair: Steyerberg Prediction Model*

SURGEON-SPECIFIC AVERAGE OPERATIVE MORTALITY

	Mortality (%)					
	3	**4**	**5**	**6**	**8**	**12**
Score	−5	−2	0	+2	+5	+10

INDIVIDUAL PATIENT RISK FACTORS

	Age			Gender		Cardiac Co-morbidity			Renal Co-morbidity	Pulmonary Co-morbidity
	60	**70**	**80**	**Male**	**Female**	**MI**	**CHF**	**ECG Ischemia**	**Creatinine >1.8 mg/dL (159.1 µmol/L)**	**COPD, Dyspnea**
Score	−4	0	+4	+4	0	+3	+8	+8	+12	+7

ESTIMATED INDIVIDUAL SURGICAL MORTALITY, TOTAL SCORE

	Mortality (%)									
	1	**2**	**3**	**5**	**8**	**12**	**19**	**28**	**39**	**51**
Total score	−5	0	5	10	15	20	25	30	35	40

*Based on the total score from the sum of scores for each risk factor, including the surgeon-specific average mortality for elective abdominal aortic aneurysm repair and estimated patient-specific mortality.
CHF, congestive heart failure; COPD, chronic obstructive pulmonary disease; ECG, electrocardiogram; MI, myocardial infarction.
From Steyerberg EW, Kievit J, de Mol Van Otterloo JC, et al: Perioperative mortality of elective abdominal aortic aneurysm surgery: a clinical prediction rule based on literature and individual patient data. *Arch Intern Med.* 1995;155:1998.

Table 127-4 Variables for Models of Operative Mortality after Open Repair of Abdominal Aortic Aneurysm

Preoperative Risk Factor	Eagle Score	Glasgow Aneurysm Score	Leiden Score	Modified Leiden Score	Vanzetto Score
Age	1 if >70 yr	Years	0 if 70 yr; 1 every 2.5 yr (60 = −4; 80 = +4)	0 if 70 yr; 1 every 2.5 yr (60 = −4; 80 = +4)	1 if >70 yr
Female gender			4	4	
Myocardial infarction			3	3	1
Angina pectoris	1				1
Myocardial disease		7			
Q waves on ECG	1				1
ST/T changes on ECG			8*		1†
Ventricular ectopy	1				
Hypertension with LVH					1
Congestive heart failure			8	8	1
Diabetes mellitus	1				1
Cerebrovascular disease		10			
Renal disease		14‡	12§	12¶	
Pulmonary disease			7	7	
Center-specific average surgical mortality			0 if 5% (3% = −5; 4% = −2; 6% = 2; 8% = 5; 12% = 10)		

*If ST-segment depression is >2 mm from baseline.
†If ST-segment depression is ≥1 mm from baseline.
‡If history of chronic and acute renal failure and/or urea >56 mg/dL (20 mmol/L) and/or creatinine >1.7 mg/dL (150 µmol/L).
§If creatinine >1.8 mg/dL (160 µmol/L).
¶If creatinine >2.0 mg/dl (180 µmol/L).
Cerebrovascular disease, all grades of stroke, including transient ischemic attack; COPD, chronic obstructive pulmonary disease; ECG, electrocardiogram; LVH, left ventricular hypertrophy; myocardial disease, documented myocardial infarction and/or ongoing angina pectoris; pulmonary disease, COPD, emphysema, dyspnea, or previous pulmonary surgery.
From Nesi F, Leo E, Biancari F, et al. Preoperative risk stratification in patients undergoing elective infrarenal aortic aneurysm surgery: evaluation of five risk scoring methods. *Eur J Vasc Endovasc Surg.* 2004;28:52-58.

The Eagle risk score was less accurate in predicting in-hospital mortality. The factors included in the various risk models for open repair are shown in Table 127-4. Operative details such as suprarenal versus infrarenal aortic cross-clamping for open repair are also important (see Chapter 128: Abdominal Aortic Aneurysms: Open Surgical Treatment).

Impact of Volume and Specialty

Substantial variation in operative mortality after open AAA repair has been demonstrated among institutions. The *Dartmouth Atlas of Vascular Healthcare* demonstrated that surgeon volume is important, with operative mortality rates of 4% when a surgeon performed more than 10 AAA repairs per year

Table 127-5 Receiver Operating Curve Analyses Performed for Risk-Scoring Systems of Mortality and Morbidity after Elective Endovascular Aneurysm Repair

Scoring System			Mortality		Morbidity	
	AUC	95% CI	P Value	AUC	95% CI	P Value
GAS	0.678	0.48-0.87	0.046	0.637	0.51-0.76	0.330
V-POSSUM	0.663	0.51-0.81	0.067	0.624	0.51-0.74	0.550
m-CPI	0.629	0.45-0.81	0.148	0.549	0.42-0.68	0.451
CPI	0.646	0.49-0.81	0.100	0.542	0.41-0.67	0.509

AUC, area under the curve (a perfect accuracy of 100% corresponds to an AUC of 1.0); CI, confidence interval; CPI, Customised Probability Index; GAS, Glasgow Aneurysm Score; m-CPI, modified-Customised Probability Index; V-POSSUM, Vascular Physiology and Operative Severity Score for the enumeration of Mortality and Morbidity.
From Bohm N, Wales L, Dunckley M, et al. Objective risk-scoring systems for repair of abdominal aortic aneurysms: Applicability in endovascular repair? *Eur J Vasc Endovasc Surg.* 2008;36:172-177.

versus 8% for surgeons performing fewer than 4 AAAs per year.[158] Surgical specialty was also found to have an impact, with the lowest mortality rates achieved by vascular surgeons (4.4%), followed by cardiac surgeons (5.4%) and general surgeons (7.3%). Dimick and colleagues also found that hospital volume played a role, with 30-day mortality rates of 3% in hospitals performing more than 35 AAA repairs per year and 5.5% in hospitals performing fewer than 35 AAA repairs per year.[165] Because there is an association between surgeon volume and hospital volume and specialty, Dimick and associates used multivariate analysis to account for this and found that surgeon volume, hospital volume, and surgical specialty were independently associated with operative mortality rates in elective open AAA repair.[165]

Impact of Endovascular Repair

EVAR has had a significant impact on the operative mortality of AAA repair. With very large studies now reported, including large statewide and nationwide studies and randomized trial data, the mortality rate for EVAR is consistently lower than that for open AAA repair. New York State data indicated that in-hospital mortality in 2001 was 3.55% for open repair and 1.14% for EVAR ($P = .0018$), and in 2002 these rates were 4.21% versus 0.8% ($P < .0001$), respectively, despite a higher frequency of co-morbid conditions in the EVAR patients.[166] In a 2001 U.S. National Inpatient Sample of more than 7000 patients, EVAR demonstrated benefits in morbidity (18% versus 29%; $P = .0001$), mortality (1.3% versus 3.8%; $P = .0001$), median length of stay (2 versus 7 days; $P = .0001$), and rate of discharge to an institutional facility versus home (6% versus 14%; $P = .0001$).[167] Multivariate analysis indicated that only open AAA repair and age older than 80 years were strong independent predictors ($P = .0001$ for all) for mortality or discharge to an institutional facility.[167] More recently, Dillavou and coworkers found similar results from a 5% U.S. national Medicare sample over a 3-year period, including a significantly lower mortality rate for EVAR (odds ratio for 30-day mortality, 0.34; 95% CI, 0.22 to 0.50; $P < .001$).[168] Similar results have also been found in analysis of prospectively collected data such as the National Surgical Quality Improvement Program database.[169]

Table 127-6 Variables for Models of Operative Mortality after Endovascular Aneurysm Repair

Scoring System	Formula
Glasgow Aneurysm Score (GAS)	Age + if CAD +7; if CVD, +10; if RF, +14
Modified-Customised Probability Index (M-CPI)	If CAD, +13; if CCF, +14; if BP, +7; if COPD, +7; if RF, +16; if beta blocker −15; if statin −10
Customised Probability Index (CPI)	If CAD, +13; if CCF, +14; if CVD, +10; if BP, +7; if COPD, +7; if RF, +16; if beta blocker, −15; if statin, −10

BP, treated hypertension; CAD, coronary artery disease (myocardial infarction, revascularization, angina, severe valve disease [m-CPI only], or arrhythmia [m-CPI only]); CCF, uncontrolled congestive cardiac failure; COPD, chronic obstructive pulmonary disease (<60% forced expiratory volume in 1 second [m-CPI only]); CVD, cerebrovascular disease (stroke, transient ischemic attack); RF, renal failure (creatinine >2.04 mg/dL [180 μmol/L]).
From Bohm N, Wales L, Dunckley M, et al. Objective risk-scoring systems for repair of abdominal aortic aneurysms: applicability in endovascular repair? *Eur J Vasc Endovasc Surg.* 2008;36:172-177.

Prediction Algorithms for Endovascular Aneurysm Repair

As with open repair, creating an index of mortality or morbidity risk for specific patients undergoing EVAR is difficult despite good population-based statistics. Table 127-5 displays the predictive capability of various scoring systems relative to morbidity and mortality after EVAR. Most of the scoring systems are not even statistically significant, and those that are have modest accuracy. The difficulty in creating an index is in part due to the lower morbidity and mortality rates with EVAR, which creates few "outcomes" unless the number of patients is large. As can be seen from Table 127-6, the variables used in models for EVAR are similar to those for open repair and include age, cardiac disease, renal insufficiency, and cerebrovascular disease. At least one study has demonstrated that the Glasgow Aneurysm Score has reasonable accuracy in estimating operative risk for both open and endovascular repair in a population of patients who are candidates for both procedures.[170]

Other Measures of Operative Risk

Factors other than mortality are also important in assessing operative risk and comparing EVAR and open AAA repair.

Functional Outcome. Shorter hospital stay after EVAR has been well documented.[167-169,171-173] Less frequently reported is disposition at discharge. Patients undergoing open repair are threefold to fivefold more likely than patients undergoing EVAR to be discharged to a facility other than home.[167,168,173,174] The patients undergoing EVAR in the referenced studies were older and had more co-morbid conditions, but this may have been offset somewhat by patients undergoing suprarenal aortic cross-clamping in the open repair group that were not coded for exclusion. Nonetheless, the speed of recovery after EVAR versus open AAA repair is an important factor. A retrospective study of functional status after open AAA repair by Williamson and coworkers suggested that up to a third of patients believe that they never fully recovered from open repair, and 18% would not undergo the procedure again even knowing the risk for rupture.[175] Despite the shorter hospital stay and recovery time and better quality of life in the very short term,[176] quality of life at 12 months appears to be similar for open repair and EVAR in the average patient.[171]

Subsequent Interventions. On the other hand, differences in the rate of secondary intervention after EVAR versus open repair have been documented thoroughly, with multiple studies demonstrating that the rate of secondary intervention for the aneurysm is significantly higher for EVAR, at approximately twofold to threefold, especially in earlier studies.[171,172,177] Conversion to open repair and rupture are lower in more recent studies, but secondary interventions, mostly endovascular, are still common.[172,173,177]

More recently, however, another pertinent issue has been raised with regard to nonvascular hospital admissions and procedures for patients undergoing open repair. Schermerhorn and colleagues studied perioperative rates of death and complications, long-term survival, rupture, and re-interventions after open AAA repair versus EVAR in propensity score–matched cohorts of Medicare beneficiaries undergoing repair during 2001 to 2004.[173] Perioperative mortality was lower after endovascular repair than after open repair (1.2% versus 4.8%; $P < .001$), and the reduction in mortality increased with age (2.1% difference for those 67 to 69 years old versus 8.5% for those 85 years or older; $P < .001$). Late survival was similar in the two cohorts, although the survival curves did not converge until after 3 years. By 4 years, rupture rates were low but rupture was more likely in the EVAR cohort than in the open repair cohort (1.8% versus 0.5%; $P < .001$), as was re-intervention related to the AAA (9.0% versus 1.7%; $P < .001$), although most re-interventions were minor. The principal new finding was that within 4 years of the operation, surgery for laparotomy-related complications was more likely in patients who had undergone open repair (9.7% versus 4.1% in those who had undergone EVAR; $P < .001$), as was hospitalization without surgery for bowel obstruction or abdominal wall hernia (14.2% versus 8.1%; $P < .001$). Thus, the more frequent late re-interventions related to EVAR are counterbalanced by an increase in laparotomy-related re-interventions and hospitalizations after open surgery.

Endovascular versus Open Aneurysm Repair

Despite significant differences in population-based data regarding operative risk, the results might not be indicative of the true differences in open repair and EVAR because of nonrandom samples and selection bias. Ultimately, these questions were at least partially answered by randomized clinical trials, primarily EVAR-1 and the Dutch Randomized Endovascular Aneurysm Management (DREAM).[171,178] These trials randomized patients with AAAs larger than 5.5 cm to EVAR or open repair. Both trials showed lower 30-day mortality for EVAR but similar all-cause mortality at later time points. The larger of these two studies was EVAR-1, which had a 30-day mortality of 1.6% for EVAR and 4.6% for open repair ($P = .007$).[171] There was a higher rate of secondary intervention in the EVAR group but a persistent, significant reduction in aneurysm-related death at 4 years. As already mentioned, all-cause mortality was similar in the two groups by 2 years in both studies,[171,172] which highlights the importance of best medical management of associated (primarily cardiovascular) disease in patients with AAAs to optimize life expectancy.

Life Expectancy

Clinical decision making for AAA requires knowledge regarding life expectancy, but determining this for an individual patient is not a simple proposition. One of the difficulties in estimating life expectancy is that it is not a simple linear function. A typical 60-year-old surviving AAA repair has a 13-year life expectancy, but a 70-year-old surviving AAA repair has a 10-year life expectancy, and an 80-year-old has a 6-year life expectancy (Table 127-7).[179,180] Patients who survive elective

Table 127-7 Life Expectancy in Years for Patients Surviving Abdominal Aortic Aneurysm Repair by Age, Gender, and Race

Age (yr)	Total	Male		Female	
		White	*Black*	*White*	*Black*
60	13	12	11	14	13
65	11	11	10	12	11
70	10	9	8	10	10
75	8	8	7	9	8
80	6	6	6	7	6
≥85	5	4	4	5	5

Data from Schermerhorn M. Should usual criteria for intervention in abdominal aortic aneurysms be "downsized," considering reported risk reduction with endovascular repair? *Ann N Y Acad Sci.* 2006;1085:47-58; and Schermerhorn ML, Finlayson SR, Fillinger MF, et al. Life expectancy after endovascular versus open abdominal aortic aneurysm repair: results of a decision analysis model on the basis of data from EUROSTAR. *J Vasc Surg.* 2002;36:1112-1120.

AAA repair have a reduced life expectancy when compared with the age- and gender-matched population.[181-183] These values are not as good as those of the age-matched general population because of the associated co-morbid diseases typical of aneurysm patients. Therein lies the second major problem with determining life expectancy—aneurysm patients have a relatively high incidence of CAD, pulmonary disease (COPD), hypertension, renal insufficiency, hyperlipidemia, cerebrovascular disease, and cancer. One extensive review of 32 articles by Norman and colleagues found that the mean 5-year survival rate after AAA repair was 70% as opposed to 80% for the general population.[86] The UKSAT participants found (after adjustment for age, gender, and AAA diameter, but not cardiac disease) that both FEV_1 and current smoking status (plasma cotinine) predicted late death.[184] Although it is not possible to precisely calculate life expectancy for individual patients, estimates can be made with this information.

Patient Preferences

When decision making is borderline because of comparable rupture and operative risk, patient preferences are very important. Some patients have great fear of surgery, whereas others may have great fear of their AAA, often based on anecdotal experiences of friends and family. It is important to discuss these issues openly with patients. In addition, it is important to assess a patient's quality of life before deciding to attempt to prolong life with AAA repair. Although this is simple in concept, it is sometimes difficult in debilitated elderly patients or those with mental deterioration. In such cases, discussion with the extended family and primary care provider may provide helpful insight.

Randomized Clinical Trials

Two randomized trials have provided substantial information to assist the clinical decision-making process.

U.K. Small Aneurysm Trial

The UKSAT was the first randomized trial to compare early surgery with surveillance for AAAs 4 to 5.5 cm, and it enrolled 1090 patients aged 60 to 76.[185] Patients undergoing surveillance were monitored by repeat ultrasound every 6 months for AAAs 4 to 4.9 cm and every 3 months for AAAs 5 to 5.5 cm. If AAA diameter exceeded 5.5 cm, the expansion rate was more than 1 cm per year, the AAA became tender, or repair of an iliac or thoracic aneurysm was needed, elective surgical repair was recommended. At the initial report in 1998 after a mean 4.6 years of follow-up, there was no difference in survival between the two groups (Fig. 127-4). Survival was initially worse in the early-surgery group because of operative mortality, which was unexpectedly high at 5.8%. After 3 years, patients who had undergone early surgery had better late survival, but the difference was not significant. More than 60% of patients randomized to surveillance eventually under-

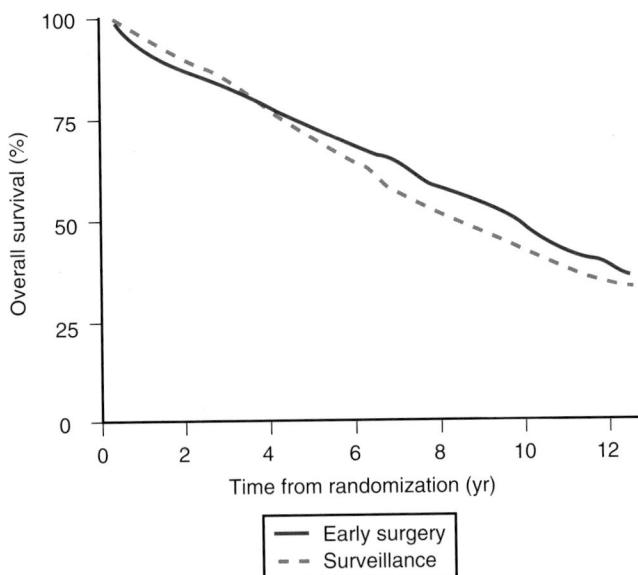

Figure 127-4 Survival of early surgery and surveillance groups in the U.K. Small Aneurysm Trial. *(From Powell JT, Brown LC, Forbes JF, al. Final 12-year follow-up of surgery versus surveillance in the UK Small Aneurysm Trial.* Br J Surg. *2007;94:702-708.)*

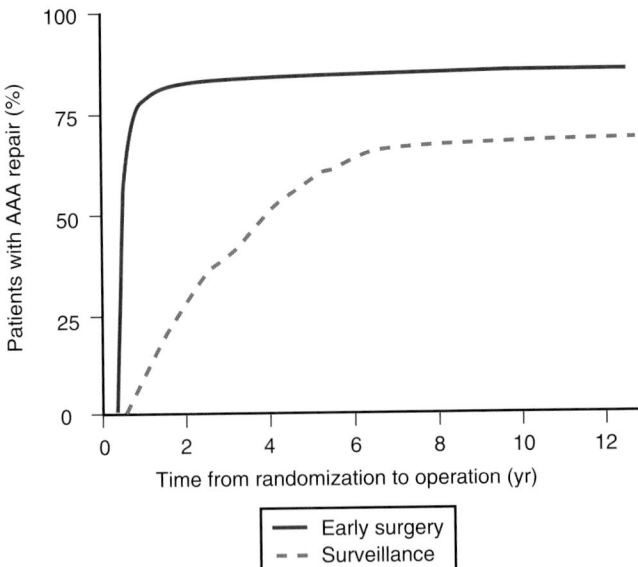

Figure 127-5 Proportion of patients undergoing abdominal aortic aneurysm repair in the early surgery and surveillance groups in the U.K. Small Aneurysm Trial. *(From Powell JT, Brown LC, Forbes JF, et al. Final 12-year follow-up of surgery versus surveillance in the UK Small Aneurysm Trial.* Br J Surg. *2007;94:702-708.)*

went surgery at a median of 2.9 years (Fig. 127-5). Rupture risk in patients undergoing careful surveillance was 1% per year. Operative mortality was 5.8% in the early-surgery group and 7.2% in the surveillance group, which included more emergency and urgent repairs than in the early-surgery group. The operative mortality was more than twice the rate used in power calculations for design of the trial, thus causing some to question the generalizability of these results.

Aneurysm Detection and Management Study

The Aneurysm Detection and Management (ADAM) study conducted at U.S. VA hospitals was published in 2002.[145] In this trial, 1163 veterans (99% male) age 50 to 79 years with AAAs 4 to 5.4 cm were randomized to early surgery versus surveillance. Surveillance entailed ultrasound or CT every 6 months with elective surgery for expansion to 5.5 cm, expansion of 0.7 cm in 6 months or greater than 1 cm in 1 year, or development of symptoms attributable to the AAA. Patients with severe heart or lung disease were excluded, as were patients who were not thought to be likely to comply with surveillance. As in UKSAT, there was no survival difference after a mean follow-up of 4.9 years. Similarly, more than 60% of patients in the surveillance arm underwent repair. Initial AAA diameter predicted subsequent surgical repair in the surveillance group: 27% of patients with AAAs initially 4 to 4.4 cm underwent repair during follow-up as compared with 53% of patients with AAAs 4.5 to 4.9 cm and 81% of patients with AAAs 5 to 5.4 cm. Operative mortality was 2.7% in the early-surgery group and 2.1% in the surveillance group. The ADAM study confirmed the results of the UKSAT by showing a lack of benefit of early surgery for AAAs 4 to 5.5 cm even if operative mortality is low and compliance with surveillance is high because most patients ultimately require surgery as their AAA expands.

Long-term Results

In 2002, the UKSAT participants published the results of long-term follow-up.[186] At 8 years there was a small survival advantage in the early-surgery group (7.2% improved survival; $P = .03$). The proportion of deaths caused by rupture of an unrepaired AAA was low (6%), however. The early-surgery group had a higher rate of smoking cessation, which may have contributed to a reduction in overall mortality. An additional 12% of surveillance patients underwent surgical repair during extended follow-up, thus bringing the total to 74%. Fatal rupture occurred in only 5% of men but in 14% of women, such that risk of rupture was approximately three times higher for women. This finding prompted the UKSAT participants to recommend a lower diameter threshold for elective AAA repair in women. A separate analysis of the UKSAT showed that a strategy of early surgery for small AAAs is more costly but associated with small gains in health-related quality of life at the latter analysis.[187] When followed even longer, mortality rates became similar once again because mortality from comorbid diseases dominated later in the lives of these elderly patients.

Decision-Making Summary

Randomized trials indicate that in general it is safe to wait for AAA diameter to reach 5.5 cm before performing surgery in selected men who would be compliant with surveillance, even if their operative mortality is predicted to be low. Compliance in these carefully monitored trials of selected patients was

high, however. In another VA population, Valentine and associates reported that 32 of 101 patients undergoing AAA surveillance were not compliant despite several appointment reminders and that 3 or 4 of these 32 patients experienced rupture.[188] Additionally, the increased rupture risk for women seen in UKSAT suggests that a smaller threshold is appropriate for women. It appears that the average size at rupture is 5 mm smaller for women than for men based on a study of more than 120 ruptured aneurysms,[117] and ruptures in UKSAT were mostly in 5- to 5.5-cm AAAs, thus suggesting that 5 cm may be an appropriate threshold for good-risk female patients.[189] Risk factors other than gender may influence the decision, as discussed earlier. Finally, waiting for the aneurysm to reach the 5- or 5.5-cm threshold is appropriate when the AAA is nontender and not expanding more rapidly than the established thresholds. Overall, the UKSAT and ADAM studies highlight the need to individualize treatment based on a careful assessment of individual patient characteristics (rupture risk, operative risk, life expectancy, and patient preferences).

◼ INDIVIDUAL PATIENT DECISION MAKING

Patient Evaluation

A careful history, physical examination, and basic laboratory data are the most important factors for estimating perioperative risk and subsequent life expectancy. These factors not only may influence the decision to perform elective AAA repair but may also focus preoperative management to reduce modifiable risk. Assessment of daily activity level, stamina, and stability of health is important in this regard and can be translated into metabolic equivalents to help assess cardiac and pulmonary risk.[190]

Coronary Artery Disease

Because CAD is the largest single cause of early and late mortality after AAA repair, its assessment is critical (see Chapter 30: Preoperative Management and Chapter 38: Systemic Complications: Cardiac). It is well established that patients with AAAs have a high prevalence of CAD. In a classic study of routine preoperative coronary arteriography, Hertzer and coauthors reported that only 6% of patients with AAAs had normal arteries, 29% had mild to moderate CAD, 29% had advanced compensated CAD, 31% had severe correctable CAD, and 5% had severe uncorrectable CAD.[191] Furthermore, this study established that clinical prediction of the severity of CAD is imperfect because 18% of patients without clinically apparent CAD had severe correctable CAD on arteriography as compared with 44% of patients whose CAD was clinically apparent. This pivotal study has led to intense effort to identify risk factors and algorithms that would more accurately predict the presence of severe CAD and justify its correction before AAA repair or lead to avoiding

AAA repair. A number of clinical parameters, such as angina, history of myocardial infarction, Q wave on the electrocardiogram, ventricular arrhythmia, congestive heart failure, diabetes, and increasing age, have been reported to increase the risk for postoperative cardiac events.[192] Various combinations of these risk factors have been used to generate prediction algorithms, as discussed earlier. In general, these algorithms identify low-risk, high-risk, or intermediate-risk patients. For high-risk patients, such as those with unstable angina, more sophisticated cardiac evaluation is required, whereas low-risk patients may undergo elective AAA repair without further testing. For intermediate-risk patients, who represent the vast majority with AAAs, decision making is more difficult and is discussed in detail in Chapter 38 (Systemic Complications: Cardiac).

Other Risk Factor Evaluation

COPD is an independent predictor of operative mortality with open AAA repair[157,159] and should be assessed by pulmonary function studies with or without room air–arterial blood gas measurement in patients who have apparent pulmonary disease (see Chapter 39: Systemic Complications: Respiratory). In some cases, preoperative treatment with bronchodilators and pulmonary toilet can reduce operative risk.[193] In more extreme cases, pulmonary risk may reduce life expectancy substantially, and in these cases, formal pulmonary consultation may be helpful to estimate survival. Serum creatinine, as an estimate of the glomerular filtration rate, is one of the most important predictors of operative mortality,[159] and renal dysfunction should figure prominently in clinical decision making (see Chapter 40: Systemic Complications: Renal). The impact of other diseases, such as malignancy, on expected survival should also be considered carefully. Obviously, some of the aforementioned risk factors may be more important for open AAA repair than for EVAR in terms of perioperative mortality. These risk factors are also important for calculation of life expectancy, however, and thus must be considered to some degree no matter which type of repair is being considered.

Aneurysm Evaluation

Preoperative assessment of AAAs focuses primarily on determining whether a patient is an anatomic candidate for EVAR (see Chapter 129: Abdominal Aortic Aneurysms: Endovascular Treatment) or the optimal approach for open repair (see Chapter 128: Abdominal Aortic Aneurysms: Open Surgical Treatment). This is done with sophisticated preoperative imaging.

Computed Tomography

CT precisely defines the proximal and distal extent of an AAA, more accurately images the iliac arteries, and provides other important information for operative planning. This is particularly true with modern multidetector spiral CT with thin slices in the region of interest (see Chapter 21: Computed Tomography). Spiral CT allows not only accurate size measurements but also accurate definition of the relationship of an AAA to the visceral and renal arteries with computed tomographic angiography (CTA). Accordingly, CTA yields important information regarding the nature (open versus endovascular), extent, and complexity of surgery. Recent studies also indicate that incidental findings are present in the majority of CT scans, with 19% being clinically significant (e.g., tumor, horseshoe kidney, venous anomalies).[194] For juxtarenal or suprarenal aneurysms, CTA can define the most appropriate location for suprarenal cross-clamping. CTA with associated three-dimensional reconstruction has largely supplanted catheter angiography in the pretreatment assessment of AAA patients.[195] For these reasons, CTA has become the primary imaging modality in preoperative planning for AAA repair.

Magnetic Resonance Imaging

Magnetic resonance imaging (see Chapter 22: Magnetic Resonance Imaging) also provides a great deal more information than ultrasound does but has numerous issues (including cost, claustrophobia, problems detecting calcification) that have prevented it from being a standard imaging study for AAAs. Magnetic resonance angiography (MRA) is comparable to CTA in many respects with regard to accuracy of AAA measurement and evaluation, and it avoids radiation exposure (see Chapter 22: Magnetic Resonance Imaging). Despite the lack of ionizing radiation, MRA has not been the favored preoperative imaging technique, however, because when compared with CTA, it visualizes calcified plaque poorly, typically has half the spatial resolution, is more expensive, is technically more difficult to standardize, and is less well tolerated by claustrophobic patients. Historically, MRA was used in patients with renal failure, but recent studies have shown the risk of potentially fatal nephrogenic sclerosing fibrosis in patients with renal insufficiency who receive gadolinium contrast.[196,197] MRA with gadolinium is still useful when intravenous contrast administration is contraindicated because of allergic reaction, and flow-induced contrast can be used as well. In centers with sufficient experience using this technique, MRA has also been shown to be accurate in determining the presence of occlusive disease in intra-abdominal arteries (see Chapter 22: Magnetic Resonance Imaging). Improvements in the spatial resolution of spiral CTA, combined with its more rapid, less expensive technique, have largely relegated MRA to a secondary role in the evaluation of AAAs.

Arteriography

Historically, conventional arteriography was nearly always used for the preoperative evaluation of AAAs and adjacent arteries. In contemporary practice, however, catheter angiography is primarily used only to perform interventions such as renal artery stenting or rarely in patients with anomalies such as a horseshoe or pelvic kidney, where selective injections might be used to determine the renal mass supplied by specific arteries. In patients with associated iliac disease, conventional arteriography is often not necessary in the era of CTA because the disease will be bypassed with open repair or stented with EVAR. Preoperative stenting of iliac stenoses to allow EVAR is typically not advantageous because the stent may interfere with large delivery systems. Occasionally, preoperative stenting of occlusive iliac disease may be useful when the intent is to perform AAA reconstruction with an open tube graft, but in presence of severe occlusive iliac disease, aortofemoral reconstruction is more durable. The development of EVAR initially renewed the need for arteriography for precise preoperative device measurement, but three-dimensional reconstruction from CTA has become the standard in most centers (see Chapter 129: Abdominal Aortic Aneurysms: Endovascular Treatment).[195]

Decision Making

Once the critical factors have been assessed, it is necessary to "operationalize" the concept that intervention for an AAA is appropriate when the cumulative risk for rupture exceeds the risk associated with repair within the context of patient life expectancy. For a young, healthy patient with a large aneurysm, the recommendation for intervention is a relatively easy decision. In healthy patients with aneurysms smaller than 5.5 cm in diameter and in high-surgical-risk patients with large aneurysms, however, the decision may not be simple.

Rupture Risk

Large clinical trials have demonstrated the relative safety of observation of AAAs with a maximum diameter of less than 5.5 cm, as discussed earlier.[144,145,185,198] In an effort to prevent rupture, however, these studies required frequent observation, including ultrasound or CT every 6 months, with surgical intervention for symptoms, rapid expansion, or growth to 5.5 cm. This resulted in a surgical intervention rate of greater than 60% in the "observation" group within several years for both of the major trials. Even with a high rate of intervention in a patient population willing to undergo frequent and reliable surveillance, the rupture rate may still be greater than 2% per year in some patient populations, primarily women.[113,144] Although observation is appealing in older, high-risk patients, in some studies aneurysms larger than 5.5 cm will rupture in more than 50% of patients when surgery is deferred because of high operative risk,[114] and many rupture within the first year of observation.[114,115] These issues illustrate the importance of the ability to predict AAA rupture risk. It appears that finite element analysis of maximum aneurysm wall stress will be a better predictor than diameter, but this has yet to be applied to large patient cohorts in a multicenter study using a standardized, broadly applicable technique. Pending availability of a better technique and more

definitive studies, the gold standard for most will continue to be 5.5-cm diameter, with the recommendation for repair modified by factors such as gender, current smoking, aneurysm anatomy, procedure risk, and the patient's life expectancy.[113,117,199,200] Despite all of this, current data suggest that aneurysm diameter as a criterion will be inadequate in 10% to 25% of patients by failing to repair an aneurysm soon enough or recommending a repair that may not be needed.[113-115,125,127,141,142,185]

Operative Risk

Operative mortality data favor EVAR, thus making it the procedure of choice in high-risk patients in particular, and based on EVAR-1, it appears that the aneurysm-related mortality benefit persists to at least 4 years.[171] A decision analysis study by Schermerhorn and associates used EuroSTAR (European Collaborators on Stent/Graft Techniques for aortic Aneurysm Repair) registry data to calculate quality-adjusted life expectancy and found that the relative benefits of EVAR versus open repair were most dependent on the operative mortality rate.[180] Other factors were also potentially important, but the difference between open repair and EVAR was small across the plausible range of most of these variables. This suggests that the key factor is the operative mortality rate, which is statistically in favor of EVAR based on randomized clinical trials. Thus, with modern-generation endografts, the best short-term and intermediate-term outcomes will be generated by EVAR in most patients. By the same token, however, mathematical models also demonstrate that EVAR should not substantially alter the diameter threshold in the majority of patients.[201]

High-Risk Patients

Regardless of whether we determine that the patient is best treated by EVAR or open repair, a number of algorithms discussed previously exist to estimate perioperative and long-term survival, but none of them are more accurate than 75% to 80%.[157,160-163] EVAR-2 demonstrated that we cannot simply assume benefit even in the context of a relatively noninvasive procedure and a patient with a large aneurysm. EVAR-2 also suggested, however, that efforts focused on improving a patient's overall health can lower operative risk beyond expectations at the initial evaluation (see Chapter 129: Abdominal Aortic Aneurysms: Endovascular Treatment). Other studies evaluating "high-risk" patients demonstrate that we cannot simply ignore patients in this category because many will have acceptable operative mortality rates and life expectancy.[202-204] The sometimes conflicting message in all of these studies demonstrates that the definition of "high risk" is nebulous and that there is not yet a clear algorithm that adequately quantifies life expectancy or operative risk in an individual patient. Moreover, more quantitative data are needed on quality of life, discharge home versus an institutional facility, laparotomy-related morbidity, and other factors that are critical to these elderly patients.

Table 127-8 Method of Portraying Risk Factors in a Unified Fashion for Patient-Specific Education

	Low	Medium	High
Diameter	<5 cm	5-6 cm	>6 cm
Gender	—	Male	Female
Wall stress	Low (<30 N/cm^2)	Medium (30-40 N/cm^2)	High (>40 N/cm^2)
Smoking	—	Never, former	Current
Pulmonary/COPD	None, mild	Moderate	Severe, steroids
Expansion rate	<0.3 cm/yr	0.3-0.6 cm/yr	>0.6 cm/yr
Family history	None	One	Multiple
Hypertension	None	Controlled	Uncontrolled
Statin use	On statin	Not on statin	

Risks are portrayed as "average," "lower than average," or "higher than average" for an example patient, depending on the presence or absence of a particular risk factor. They can also be displayed as calculated fields based on quantitative data from the literature or risk models when available.
COPD, chronic obstructive pulmonary disease.

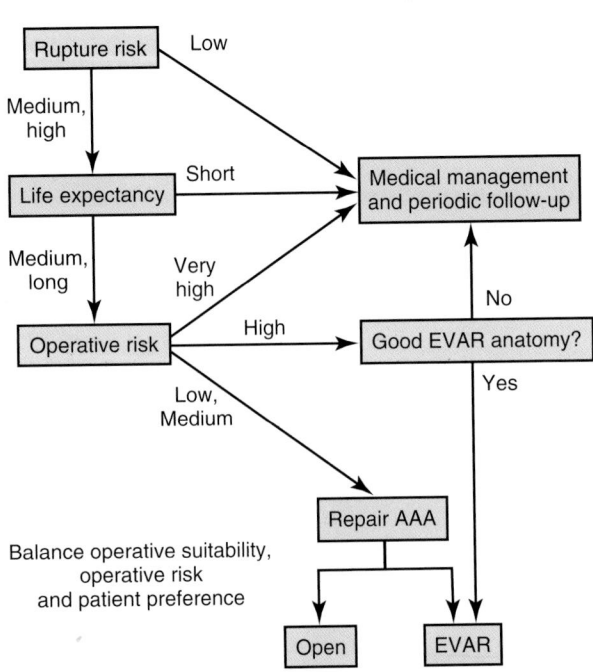

Figure 127-6 Basic decision-making algorithm. AAA, abdominal aortic aneurysm; EVAR, endovascular aneurysm repair.

Making the Decision

Although substantial data have been published to assist in clinical decision making, it remains an imprecise science when applied to individual patients. Estimates of rupture risk described earlier vary considerably and depend on multiple risk factors. At best, it is usually possible to estimate rupture risk only as low, average, or high, depending on the predominance of these risk factors (Table 127-8). Similarly, operative risk can be estimated, somewhat more precisely, by using the various algorithms discussed earlier to provide a stratification based on low, average, or high operative risk. Finally, life expectancy can be estimated on the basis of age and other co-morbid conditions (see Table 127-7). The basic decision-making algorithm is described in Figure 127-6. Though simplified, this decision model provides a framework in which to consider the key variables affecting the decision for EVAR versus open repair versus medical management (for details on comparison of open versus EVAR see Chapter 129: Abdominal Aortic Aneurysms: Endovascular Treatment).

Quantifiable metrics aside, nothing is likely to completely substitute for clinical experience. Somehow, experienced surgeons are able to sift through a massive amount of information and properly select patients who are appropriate for surgery with reasonable perioperative and long-term mortality rates.[202-204] This remains an opportunity and a challenge for vascular surgeons.

◼ MEDICAL MANAGEMENT OF ABDOMINAL AORTIC ANEURYSMS

Most aneurysms detected in screening studies are smaller than the standard thresholds for repair. Medical management in these patients should focus on reducing the risk of associated cardiovascular disease and decreasing the expansion rate of the AAA if possible. It has been suggested that the number of aneurysm repairs and ruptures could be cut nearly in half if

the rate of expansion in small aneurysms could be cut in half.[205] This estimate is based primarily on preventing aneurysms from reaching the threshold for rupture during the typical elderly aneurysm patient's lifetime. Medical management to reduce cardiovascular complications in this group is important but not widely practiced. For example, in the UKSAT and ADAM trials, cardiovascular events were the leading cause of death in the surveillance and surgery arms, but less than 20% of patients were receiving beta blockers during long-term follow-up.[145,186,206]

Smoking Cessation

The best evidence in terms of the potential effect of modifiable risk factors for expansion and rupture is for smoking. In a systematic review of eligible studies that included more than 3 million subjects, Lederle and colleagues determined that the relative risk for aortic aneurysm–related events in current smokers was generally 3 to 6, as compared with 1 to 2 for CAD or cerebrovascular disease and 5 to 12 for COPD. Pooled estimates indicated that in men the association of ever smoking with aortic aneurysm is 2.5 times greater than the association of ever smoking with CAD and 3.5 times greater than the association of ever smoking with cerebrovascular disease.[49] In a review of more than 100,000 health maintenance organization patients with a median 13 years of follow-up, other less important factors associated with aneurysm development (not expansion rate) were hypertension, high cholesterol, CAD, and claudication.[207] In terms of aneurysm expansion rate, however, the UKSAT multivariate analysis determined that only smoking was linked to increased aneurysm expansion rates (mean increase, 0.4 mm/yr); that peripheral arterial disease and diabetes were linked to a significantly slower expansion rate; and that age, gender, hypertension, and serum cholesterol level had no significant association with an altered expansion rate.[208] Thus, in terms of aneurysm development and expansion, tobacco use is the single most important modifiable risk factor.

Exercise Therapy

In terms of other modifiable risk factors, there is evidence to suggest that exercise therapy may be beneficial in patients with small aneurysms. Computational flow modeling studies of the aorta suggest that the decreased flow from prolonged sedentary conditions may promote aneurysmal degeneration.[209] Patients with traumatic above-knee amputation and spinal cord injury have an increased risk for AAA independent of other risk factors, including tobacco use.[209,210] Studies have been initiated to determine whether prospective intervention with supervised exercise will have an impact on the aneurysm expansion rate, but no results are yet available with regard to this intriguing potentially modifiable risk factor.

Medications

Beta Blockers

Beta blockade has been postulated to decrease the rate of AAA expansion, and this effect has been demonstrated in animal models.[211-215] Subsequent retrospective analyses in humans seemed to corroborate this finding.[44,216-218] However, two subsequent randomized trials failed to show any reduction in growth rate with beta blockade.[219,220] Furthermore, the randomized trial from Toronto showed that patients taking beta blockers had a worse quality of life and did not tolerate the medication well.[219] Even when the study analyzed only patients who tolerated the medication, there was no effect of propranolol on AAA expansion rate. Beta blockers do have a significant effect on perioperative and long-term mortality rates, however, and this effect appears to be independent of statin therapy, whether looking at heart rate effects or beta blocker use alone.[221,222]

Angiotensin-Converting Enzyme Inhibitors

Evidence is mixed with regard to angiotensin-converting enzyme inhibitors (ACEIs). Hackam and associates analyzed a large administrative database of more than 15,000 patients from Ontario, Canada, and found that ACEI use was less frequent in patients with ruptured aneurysms.[223] A case-control study and a post hoc analysis of UKSAT found no relationship between ACEI use and aneurysm expansion rates, however.[208,224] These potentially confounding results may be related to the patient populations because the ruptured aneurysm patients of the Canadian study had primarily previously undetected large aneurysms that had not been repaired, whereas the aneurysms in the latter two studies were primarily small aneurysms under close observation.

Doxycycline

Doxycycline, 150 to 200 mg daily, has been shown to slow the rate of AAA expansion in two small randomized prospective trials, whereas roxithromycin, 30 mg daily, was shown to reduce the expansion rate in a similar trial.[225-228] These antibiotics have activity against *Chlamydia pneumoniae*, which has been shown to be present in many AAAs.[229,230] Vammen and colleagues showed that antibodies to *Chlamydia* predicted expansion in small AAAs and suggested that antibody-positive patients may benefit from anti-*Chlamydia* treatment.[231] The medication's effect may not be related to its antibiotic properties, however. In the roxithromycin study there was no correlation between *Chlamydia* titers and the ability to inhibit aneurysm expansion. Doxycycline has been shown to suppress expression of matrix metalloproteinase (MMP) in human AAAs and to reduce aneurysm formation in animal models.[232-234] Baxter and coworkers demonstrated that clinically useful doses of 100 mg orally twice a day reduce plasma MMP-9 levels significantly.[225] In the randomized study by Mosorin and colleagues, a 3-month regimen of 150 mg daily resulted in half the expansion rate at 18 months when compared with the placebo group (32 patients total).[227] The reasonably low incidence of side effects has stimulated some clinicians to prescribe doxycycline for patients with small AAAs under surveillance or large aneurysms in patients unfit for repair, but issues of nausea, light sensitivity, and the duration of treatment needed for a benefit have prevented these medications from being widely adopted.

Statins

Recently, at least three studies have suggested that 3-hydroxy-3-methylglutaryl coenzyme A reductase inhibitors (statins) are associated with reduced aneurysm expansion rates.[224,235,236] As mentioned previously, there is no clear association between cholesterol and aneurysm expansion rates even though there is an association between cholesterol and the presence of aneurysm.[49,207] Similar to doxycycline, statins have been shown to decrease MMP-9 within the aneurysm wall,[237,238] thus suggesting a mechanism unrelated to cholesterol levels. Despite this potentially exciting association, however, there are no randomized prospective studies related to statins and aneurysms, and there are notable potentially confounding factors. As previously noted, diabetes and peripheral vascular occlusive disease were associated with significantly slower aneurysm expansion rates by multivariate analysis in the UKSAT.[208] Because these patients are more likely to be placed on a regimen of statins, the retrospective studies cannot definitively account for this. A recent retrospective study found no significant difference in the aneurysm expansion rate with statins in 132 patients, although there was a difference in aneurysm repair and rupture rates.[239] Thus, there is mounting evidence for the potential of medical therapy, but more investigation is warranted for definitive clinical guidelines. However, because many patients with AAAs may warrant statin therapy for secondary atherosclerosis prevention, this potential benefit on AAA expansion rate is a welcome observation. Cardiovascular events are the leading cause of death in AAA patients undergoing surveillance, and multiple studies have demonstrated that statins independently reduce death from cardiovascular causes and death from any cause in aneurysm patients.[221,222]

SELECTED KEY REFERENCES

Baas AF, Janssen KJ, Prinssen M, Buskens E, Blankensteijn JD. The Glasgow Aneurysm Score as a tool to predict 30-day and 2-year mortality in the patients from the Dutch Randomized Endovascular Aneurysm Management trial. *J Vasc Surg.* 2008;47:277-281.
First study to compare mortality prediction for both open and endovascular repair in patients who were candidates for both procedures. The large number of patients and the fact that they were randomized between the two procedures may provide the best insight to date regarding prediction indices that could be useful in preoperative counseling, although they are still far from ideal.

Baxter BT, Terrin MC, Dalman RL. Medical management of small abdominal aortic aneurysms. *Circulation.* 2008;117:1883-1889.
Comprehensive and up-to-date review of state-of-the-art medical management of small AAAs.

Blankensteijn JD, de Jong SE, Prinssen M, van der Ham AC, Buth J, van Sterkenburg SM, Verhagen HJ, Buskens E, Grobbee DE. Two-year outcomes after conventional or endovascular repair of abdominal aortic aneurysms. *N Engl J Med.* 2005;352:2398-2405.
Key randomized trial of EVAR versus open AAA repair. See Rutherford reference for context.

Brewster DC, Cronenwett JL, Hallett JW Jr, Johnston KW, Krupski WC, Matsumura JS. Guidelines for the treatment of abdominal aortic aneurysms. Report of a subcommittee of the Joint Council of the American Association for Vascular Surgery and Society for Vascular Surgery. *J Vasc Surg.* 2003;37:1106-1117.
Key reference outlining in a brief summary fashion all the key aspects for the treatment of AAAs.

Endovascular aneurysm repair versus open repair in patients with abdominal aortic aneurysm (EVAR trial 1): randomised controlled trial. *Lancet.* 2005;365:2179-2186.
Key randomized trial of EVAR versus open AAA repair. See Rutherford reference for context.

Endovascular aneurysm repair and outcome in patients unfit for open repair of abdominal aortic aneurysm (EVAR trial 2): randomised controlled trial. *Lancet.* 2005;365:2187-2192.
Key randomized trial of EVAR versus open AAA repair. See Rutherford reference for context.

Lederle FA, Johnson GR, Wilson SE, Ballard DJ, Jordan WD Jr, Blebea J, Littooy FN, Freischlag JA, Bandyk D, Rapp JH, Salam AA. Rupture rate of large abdominal aortic aneurysms in patients refusing or unfit for elective repair. *JAMA.* 2002;287:2968-2972.
The largest study to date of patients with "large" (>5.5 cm) aneurysms who refused or were unfit for elective repair. A high percentage had autopsy studies performed and most did not undergo surgery, thus demonstrating the natural history of these patients in a controlled environment.

Lederle FA, Wilson SE, Johnson GR, Reinke DB, Littooy FN, Acher CW, Ballard DJ, Messina LM, Gordon IL, Chute EP, Krupski WC, Busuttil SJ, Barone GW, Sparks S, Graham LM, Rapp JH, Makaroun MS, Moneta GL, Cambria RA, Makhoul RG, Eton D, Ansel HJ, Freischlag JA, Bandyk D. Immediate repair compared with surveillance of small abdominal aortic aneurysms. *N Engl J Med.* 2002;346:1437-1444.
Classic U.S. randomized trial comparing open AAA repair and surveillance with selected repair; similar results (mostly in men) were demonstrated despite a lower mortality rate for open repair in this study.

Lindholt JS, Norman P. Screening for abdominal aortic aneurysm reduces overall mortality in men. A meta-analysis of the mid- and long-term effects of screening for abdominal aortic aneurysms. *Eur J Vasc Endovasc Surg.* 2008;36:167-171.
Largest accumulation of AAA screening study results yet published (>125,000 patients) and includes long-term follow-up from the screening studies; a significant reduction in aneurysm-related and all-cause long-term mortality was demonstrated.

Powell JT, Brown LC, Forbes JF, Fowkes FG, Greenhalgh RM, Ruckley CV, Thompson SG. Final 12-year follow-up of surgery versus surveillance in the UK Small Aneurysm Trial. *Br J Surg.* 2007;94:702-708.
Update of long-term follow-up on the classic randomized trial comparing open AAA repair and surveillance with selected repair.

Rutherford RB. Randomized EVAR trials and advent of level I evidence: a paradigm shift in management of large abdominal aortic aneurysms? *Semin Vasc Surg.* 2006;19:69-74.
These four articles on randomized trials of EVAR versus open AAA repair go together, with a nice synopsis of the implications.

Schermerhorn ML, O'Malley AJ, Jhaveri A, Cotterill P, Pomposelli F, Landon BE. Endovascular vs. open repair of abdominal aortic aneurysms in the Medicare population. *N Engl J Med.* 2008;358:464-474.
Largest comparison of "matched" open and endovascular AAA repair cases to date, with more than 22,000 patients in each group. This is the first study to quantify the secondary procedures and hospitalizations related to the open abdominal incision (bowel obstruction and hernia repair), not just aorta-related interventions. It also captures the rate of discharge to skilled nursing facilities.

REFERENCES

The reference list can be found on the companion Expert Consult Web site at *www.expertconsult.com.*

Abdominal Aortic Aneurysms: Open Surgical Treatment

Brian G. Rubin and Gregorio A. Sicard

Open repair of abdominal aortic aneurysms (AAAs) is a central component of vascular surgery with a rich history (see Chapter 126: Arterial Aneurysms: General Considerations). With progressive refinement in operative techniques and perioperative care, centers of excellence now report 30-day perioperative mortality rates of 0% to 5% after elective infrarenal AAA repair.[1-4] In 1997, before the widespread adoption of endovascular aneurysm repair (EVAR), an estimated 37,000 patients in the United States underwent open surgical repair of an intact AAA.[5]

Rapid adoption of EVAR, however, has transformed the landscape of AAA treatment and significantly influenced the mix of patients considered for open repair.[6] Initially proposed for the treatment of patients considered to be at excessively high risk for open aneurysm surgery, EVAR has steadily increased as the primary therapy for elective AAA treatment in the United States.[7-9] Data from the Nationwide Inpatient Sample for 2003 indicated that 43% of nonruptured AAAs were treated by EVAR, less than a decade after the commercial availability of endografts in the United States. Recent series report that more than 60% of infrarenal AAAs are now treated with an endovascular approach,[10,11] and this percentage is expected to increase as endovascular experience becomes even more widespread and endograft technology continues to progress. Because EVAR is routinely used to treat infrarenal aneurysms in patients with straightforward arterial anatomy, the population of patients now treated by open surgical repair contains a greater percentage of those with complex aortic pathology, including juxtarenal and suprarenal aneurysms.[10,12-16] An important consequence of increasing EVAR use is the potential reduction in the total number or change in the type of open aortic aneurysm repairs as compared with the case mix before the endovascular era.[14,16,17]

TERMINOLOGY

AAAs can involve any segment of the intra-abdominal aorta from the supraceliac segment to the aortic bifurcation, with isolated infrarenal involvement being the most common. By definition, infrarenal aneurysms involve the aorta distal to the main renal arteries and have sufficient distance between the proximal extent of the aneurysm and the lowest main renal artery to permit clamp placement and construction of the proximal anastomosis below the clamp.[18] Although isolated aneurysms of the infrarenal aortic segment are the most common variant, approximately 25% involve the common iliac arteries as well.[19] The term *juxtarenal* or *pararenal* is used to describe aneurysms that have no normal aorta between the upper extent of the aneurysm and the renal arteries,[19] thereby requiring suprarenal (or higher) clamp placement to perform the proximal infrarenal anastomosis. AAAs that extend above at least one main renal artery but end below the celiac axis are classified as *suprarenal* and require revascularization of at least one renal artery. Suprarenal aneurysms account for approximately 5% of all AAAs,[19] although their reported frequency is increased in referral centers specializing in complex aortic reconstruction. Finally, extension of the aneurysm proximally to include the visceral aortic segment is considered a *total abdominal* aneurysm, also referred to as a type IV thoracoabdominal aneurysm according to Crawford and colleagues' classification.[20]

INDICATIONS

If not already performed, after the diagnosis of an AAA an imaging study is obtained to identify the location and size of the aneurysm (see Chapter 127: Abdominal Aortic Aneurysms: Evaluation and Decision Making). Patients considered for open AAA repair include those who opt for open surgical treatment (instead of EVAR) or whose anatomy precludes treatment with EVAR. Typically, the threshold for infrarenal AAA repair is 5.5 cm in maximum aortic diameter.[21,22] Because of a strong predominance of aortic aneurysms in men, trial data include few women. Therefore, an exact diameter threshold for intervention in women has not been clearly delineated, but it has been suggested that a smaller diameter may be appropriate (e.g., 5.0 cm).[23] For aneurysms requiring proximal clamp placement above the level of the renal arteries, the increased operative risk may warrant delaying elective surgery until a larger aortic diameter has been attained, with its associated greater risk for aneurysm rupture if left untreated. Specific guidelines on aortic diameters warranting intervention for the treatment of aneurysms above the infrarenal level have not been clearly outlined. However, because procedural risk increases with more proximal extension of the aneurysm or clamp location, the diameter at which surgical repair is recommended is typically slightly larger (0.5 cm) than that for aneurysms in an infrarenal location. These general guidelines serve only as starting points, and decision making must be individualized to reflect the unique risk-benefit analysis undertaken for each patient. General guidelines for AAA evaluation and treatment of aneurysms, as well as decisions regarding treatment with EVAR versus open repair, are discussed in Chapter 127 (Abdominal Aortic Aneurysms: Evaluation and Decision Making).

PATIENT ASSESSMENT

Because open AAA repair is a high-risk procedure, careful patient assessment is critical to obtain good results. A general strategy for preoperative assessment and management is addressed in Chapter 30 (Preoperative Management). In contrast to EVAR, open AAA repair requires aortic clamping, which causes increased peripheral arterial resistance and cardiac stress and alterations in renal arterial perfusion. Open repair is routinely performed with the patient under general anesthesia with or without epidural anesthetic supplementation. Because the physiologic repercussions of open AAA surgery differ significantly from those of EVAR, an evaluation of cardiac, pulmonary, renal, and coagulation status is standard before open repair (see Chapter 38: Systemic Complications: Cardiac; Chapter 39: Systemic Complications: Respiratory; and Chapter 40: Systemic Complications: Renal). An initial critical judgment is whether the patient's current quality of life is adequate to justify elective surgery aimed at increasing longevity. This decision is difficult in patients with deteriorating mental status or debilitating diseases, and consultation with family members is often essential. In patients considered to be at prohibitive risk for open AAA repair, EVAR is often recommended; however, its benefit in this patient subset remains controversial.[24,25] Risk stratification is a critical component in counseling patients about treatment options and is essential for identifying appropriate patients who will benefit from open AAA repair.

Risk Prediction

Open AAA repair is perhaps the most carefully studied vascular operation in terms of predictors of operative risk. Retrospective outcomes analysis in the Canadian Aneurysm Study identified electrocardiographic evidence of ischemia, chronic obstructive pulmonary disease, and elevated creatinine (>1.6 mg/dL [141 μmol/L]) as important predictors of increased mortality.[26] Operative mortality ranged from 1.9% when none of these risk factors were present to 50% when all three existed. Age older than 80 years also adversely influenced mortality.[26] A meta-analysis by Steyerberg and associates identified these same predictors plus congestive heart failure and female sex as independent risk factors for perioperative mortality.[27] Of these six factors, creatinine elevated to greater than 1.8 mg/dL (159 μmol/L) (odds ratio, 3.3) and congestive heart failure (odds ratio, 2.3) most strongly correlated with perioperative death. Perhaps surprisingly, application of this predictive model failed to adequately risk-stratify the majority of patients when applied in the U.K. Small Aneurysm Trial (UKSAT).[28] A more recent series of 790 patients at 11 New England hospitals identified age older than 70 years, history of chronic obstructive pulmonary disease, serum creatinine higher than 1.8 mg/dL (159 μmol/L), and supra-

Table 128-1 Number of Risk Factors and Predicted Mortality 1 Year after Open Repair of Abdominal Aortic Aneurysm

Number of Risk Factors	1-Year Mortality (%)
0	1
1	2-5
2	9-22
3	27-37
4	58

See text for details of risk factors.
Adapted from Beck AW, Goodney PP, Nolan BW. Predicting one year mortality after elective AAA repair. *J Vasc Surg.* 2009;4:838-843, discussion 843-844.

renal clamp placement as strong, additive predictors of mortality at 30 days and 1 year after open aneurysm repair (Table 128-1).[29]

PREOPERATIVE PLANNING

Computed Tomography

Computed tomography (CT) readily identifies important findings, including venous anomalies such as a duplicated vena cava or retroaortic left renal vein and renal abnormalities such as a horseshoe or pelvic kidney, and is the optimal imaging method for planning of open AAA repair. CT is also a sensitive technique to identify inflammatory aortic aneurysms. CT angiography (CTA) with three-dimensional reconstruction allows accurate measurements of luminal diameter orthogonal to the long axis of the aneurysm, thereby facilitating precise and reproducible measurements of aneurysm size and comparisons with previous studies. CTA is both a powerful tool for planning EVAR and beneficial in patients treated by open surgical repair (Fig. 128-1).[30] Information about wall characteristics such as circumferential or heavy calcification, intense periaortic inflammation, and the location and extent of intraluminal thrombus or plaque is important to note for determination of optimal clamp placement, specifically with the goal of avoiding potentially devastating atheroembolism (Fig. 128-2).[31] Superb spatial resolution allows the surgeon to resolve areas of severe angulation with three-dimensional reconstructions[32] (Fig. 128-3) and to identify the location and distances between renal and visceral vessels, as well as the presence of coexistent occlusive disease in the aortoiliac, renal, and splanchnic vessels (Fig. 128-4).[33] It cannot be stressed enough, however, that the three-dimensional reconstructed images must be correlated with their corresponding axial data slices, or important information can be overlooked. Finally, several CT findings have been reported to be predictive of "impending rupture" of the aneurysm. In patients with CT findings that include a crescent sign, discontinuous aortic calcification, aortic bulges or blebs, aortic draping, and aortic wall irregularity, Boules and coauthors reported that rupture occurred in 2 of 29 nonoperated patients within 72 hours (6.9%).[34] Twelve patients never underwent surgery by 1 year, with no additional ruptures occurring.

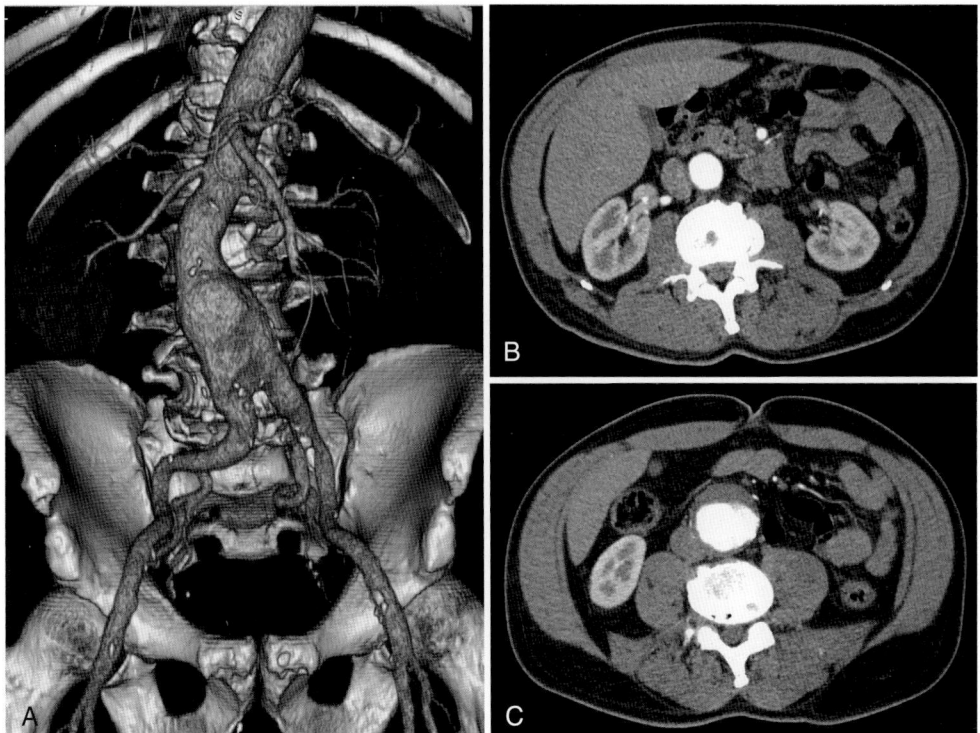

Figure 128-1 A, Three-dimensional reconstruction of contrast material filling the flow lumen demonstrates the overall geometry of an infrarenal aortic aneurysm, as well as patency of the visceral and renal arteries and iliac and femoral vessels bilaterally. **B,** Absence of significant calcification or thrombus in the infrarenal aortic neck. **C,** Thrombus within the aneurysm sac.

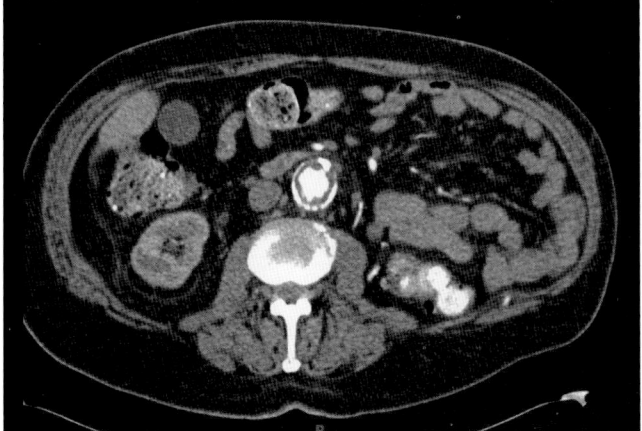

Figure 128-2 The neck of this patient's aneurysm contains both heavy circumferential calcification and circumferential thrombus. Clamp placement in this region should be avoided.

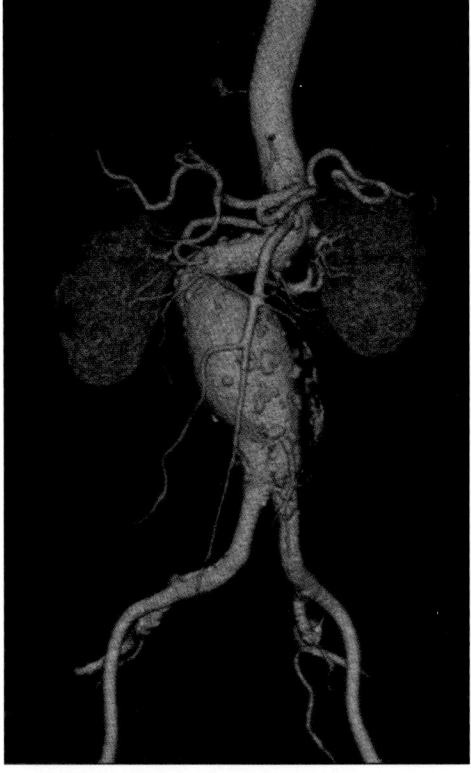

Figure 128-3 Three-dimensional reconstructed images of this patient's aorta demonstrate an infrarenal aneurysm with severe tortuosity in the neck.

A more extended discussion of CT techniques can be found in Chapter 21 (Computed Tomography).

Magnetic Resonance Angiography

Magnetic resonance angiography (MRA) is comparable to CT for measurement of aneurysm diameter and for preoperative planning (Fig. 128-5).[35-37] MRA has also been shown to be

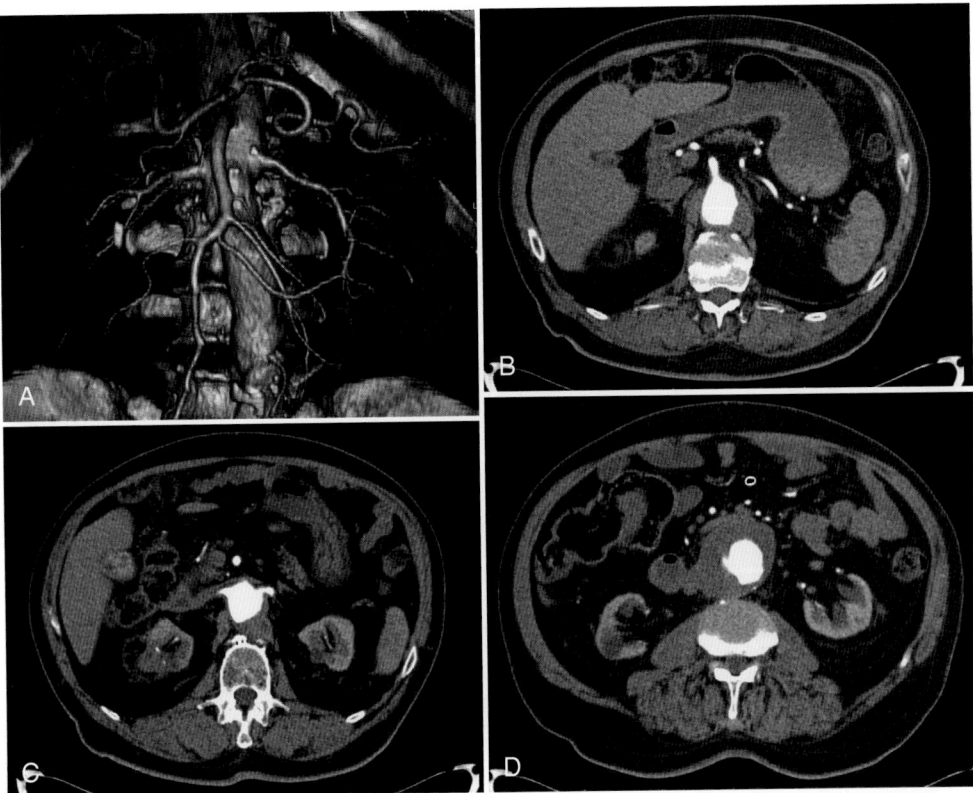

Figure 128-4 A, The three-dimensional reconstructed image alone fails to demonstrate the extent of aneurysm involvement, but correlation with individual slices of the CT scan shows that the aneurysmal degeneration involves the aorta at the level of the superior mesenteric artery (**B**), renal arteries (**C**), and infrarenal segments (**D**).

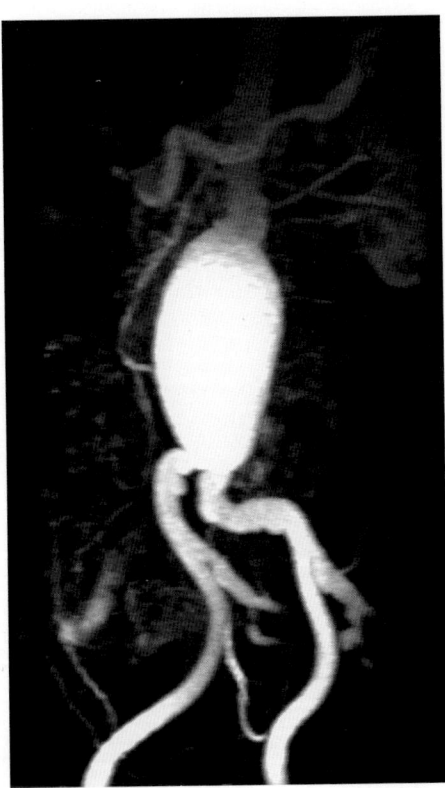

Figure 128-5 MRA is also suitable as an imaging modality for preoperative evaluation of the aorta and associated vessels.

accurate in determining the presence of occlusive disease in intra-abdominal arteries[38-40] and may be superior to CTA in detecting the extent of aortic involvement in inflammatory aneurysms.[41] MRA is discussed in detail in Chapter 22 (Magnetic Resonance Imaging).

Angiography

Angiography of the abdominal aorta and branch vessels is rarely necessary for planning open aortic reconstruction given the advances in cross-sectional imaging. However, in selected patients, conventional angiography may play a role, particularly in settings in which the initial diagnostic procedure is performed at the same time as an intervention (see also Chapter 18: Arteriography; Chapter 84: Technique: Endovascular Diagnostic; and Chapter 85: Technique: Endovascular Therapeutic). For example, percutaneous angioplasty and stent placement might be used to treat severe stenosis in a mesenteric or renal vessel and allow the surgeon to avoid more proximal clamp placement or additional revascularization procedures, thereby reducing the extent or complexity of the aortic operation. This strategy should generally be avoided with aneurysms that extend above the level of the renal arteries because clamp placement can crush or dislodge stents placed in the renal or visceral ostia.

■ SELECTION OF SURGICAL APPROACH

There are two potential surgical approaches for open surgical repair of an aortic aneurysm, transabdominal (TA) (transperitoneal) and retroperitoneal (RP). Other surgical techniques, such as laparoscopic aneurysm repair (see Chapter 107: Aortoiliac Disease: Laparoscopic Reconstruction)[42-45] and TA repair via a minilaparotomy incision, have been advocated but have not been widely adopted.[46-49] In many patients, either the TA or RP options are feasible, and in that setting the decision should be guided by the operating surgeon's preference. For some patients, however, there are relative advantages to selecting one approach over another, and the vascular surgeon must be comfortable with both techniques. The goal is to obtain adequate exposure of the aorta proximal and distal to the aneurysmal aortic segment. For both approaches, extension of the incision into the thorax is possible and frequently necessary, particularly for the treatment of aneurysms with greater proximal extent. A detailed description of each of these surgical techniques is covered later in this chapter.

Transabdominal Approach

The TA approach is widely used, in part because of every surgeon's familiarity with this incision and the rapidity of aortic exposure. It is the optimal approach in patients with previous RP surgery and is routinely used in patients with ruptured aortic aneurysms (see Chapter 130: Abdominal Aortic Aneurysms: Ruptured). Additionally, a TA approach is recommended for patients requiring exposure of (1) the mid or distal portions of the visceral vessels or right renal artery, (2) the right internal or external iliac arteries, (3) coexistent intra-abdominal pathology, or (4) a left-sided vena cava. Juxtarenal exposure can be challenging from a TA approach; mobilization or division of the left renal vein is possible but is associated with increased risk for renal dysfunction[50,51] or bleeding and should be avoided whenever possible. Rather, division of its adrenal, gonadal, and lumbar branches permits wide mobilization of the left renal vein.

Retroperitoneal Approach

The RP approach is typically performed through a left flank incision; however, a right RP approach is also possible.[52] RP exposure is preferred in patients with multiple previous intraperitoneal procedures or infections because of the adhesions generated by these processes, as well as in patients with abdominal wall stomas, ectopic kidneys, or inflammatory aneurysms.[53] A left RP approach provides more proximal aortic access than does a right RP approach because the latter is limited by the liver and its associated veins. The left RP approach, with or without mobilization of the left kidney anteriorly, facilitates juxtarenal and suprarenal aortic exposure and is also helpful in patients requiring transaortic endarterectomy of the celiac artery, superior mesenteric artery (SMA), or renal artery. We have also found the left RP approach to

be helpful in facilitating aortic exposure in obese patients because the abdominal pannus falls toward the patient's right side and away from the surgical field.[52,54]

Choice of Approach

Reported advantages of the RP approach include a more rapid return of bowel function,[55] fewer gastrointestinal complications,[52] reduced intraoperative crystalloid or blood requirements,[55] reduced postoperative pulmonary complications,[55] decreased length of intensive care unit and total hospital stay,[52,55,56] improved patient satisfaction,[55] expedited return to full function,[55] and decreased global cost.[52-55] Contradictory reports, however, challenge the validity of these studies and refute these purported benefits[57] or suggest that global improvements in perioperative care rather than use of the RP approach account for the reductions in morbidity.[54] Finally, with the use of visceral rotation maneuvers, a TA incision can still allow extensive exposure of RP structures, including the juxtarenal and suprarenal aortic segments.

Influence of Renal Anatomy

The presence of renal anomalies identified on preoperative imaging studies can influence selection of the surgical approach as well. During the fourth through ninth weeks of normal human embryologic development, the kidneys migrate from the pelvis into the abdomen and take their blood supply from vessels closest to them during their ascent. Ectopic kidneys may remain in the pelvis (pelvic kidney). If both kidneys are involved, the limited space in the pelvic cavity may result in the formation of a single renal mass (pancake kidney) without a surgical cleavage plane. In addition, an ectopic kidney may cross the midline and fuse with the contralateral renal parenchyma outside the pelvis, typically forming the inferior component of a single renal mass (cross-fused ectopia), although the ureters cross the midline to enter the bladder. Finally, the most common fusion anomaly, known as a horseshoe kidney, occurs when the fused portion of the renal mass is unable to ascend above the level of the inferior mesenteric artery (IMA). These congenital renal lesions are associated with anomalous renal blood supply, with multiple arteries typically arising from the mid and distal portions of the abdominal aorta and the proximal common iliac arteries (Fig. 128-6). In addition, the ureters course anteriorly and accordingly are more liable to injury. Favorable outcomes have been reported with both the RP and TA approaches, although most commonly an RP approach is favored for aortic reconstruction in these patients.[58-67] However, careful preoperative evaluation of each patient's unique anatomy should result in individualized decision making.

■ INTRAOPERATIVE MANAGEMENT

Intraoperative management of patients undergoing abdominal aortic surgery is a dynamic, complex, and challenging undertaking. The intraoperative course is remarkable for

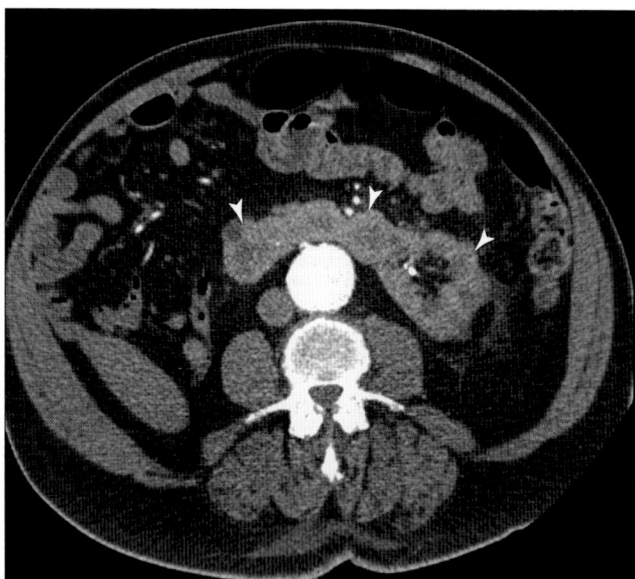

Figure 128-6 CT scan demonstrating a single fused renal parenchymal mass (*arrowheads*) located over an aneurysmal section of the aorta just above the level of the aortic bifurcation. This patient's horseshoe kidney received its arterial supply from six vessels arising at multiple levels ranging from above the superior mesenteric artery to the common iliac arteries bilaterally.

(1) hemodynamic and metabolic demands related to aortic cross-clamping and unclamping and (2) the consequences of organ ischemia during clamp placement. Replacement of blood loss, often by autotransfusion, and maintenance of normothermia are critical. See Chapter 31 (Intraoperative Management) for detailed discussion of anesthetic management considerations for patients undergoing major vascular surgery. Aspects unique to open AAA repair are discussed in the following sections.

Hemodynamic Changes during Aortic Surgery

The hemodynamic derangements subsequent to aortic cross-clamping and unclamping are profound and multifactorial.[68] Some important determinants include the level of aortic clamping and baseline cardiac function (including the possible presence of coronary artery disease or reduced ejection fraction). Equally as important are specific aspects of anesthetic management, such the choice of medications and their effects on the myocardium and vascular tone and maintenance of appropriate intravascular volume status.

Aortic Clamping

Aortic clamping initiates a series of complex metabolic and humoral responses that include the renin-angiotensin system and the sympathetic nervous system. Alterations in systemic physiologic processes, such as the production of metabolic acids, generation of oxygen free radicals, shifts in prostaglandin production, neutrophil and complement activation, and

possibly the release of myocardial depressant factors, have all been cited as additional important responses to aortic clamping.[68,69] The anesthesia team must therefore be aware of each patient's unique initial cardiac physiology, as well as the planned (and actual) level of aortic clamping, and meet changes in myocardial demand during the procedure by monitoring and normalizing preload, afterload, coronary blood flow, and contractility.

Aortic Clamp Level. The level of aortic clamp placement is the principal factor influencing cardiac function during aortic surgery.[70] Although the majority of abdominal aortic surgery is performed with a clamp placed below the level of the renal arteries, more proximal clamping results in hemodynamic changes of greater magnitude. Regardless of clamp location, aortic occlusion results in proximal arterial hypertension secondary to increased systemic vascular resistance. Arterial pressure typically increases after infrarenal clamping, with correspondingly greater increases associated with more proximal clamp placement. Aortic clamping results in redistribution of blood from organs distal to the aortic clamp toward the central venous circulation and organs proximal to the clamp. After infrarenal clamping, the splanchnic vasculature serves as a venous reservoir, which causes modest changes in preload, filling pressure, and cardiac output. With more proximal aortic clamping, particularly supraceliac clamping and reduced perfusion into the splanchnic venous system, blood volume shifts toward the heart, with marked increases in cardiac preload. Therefore, at least with infrarenal aortic cross-clamping, cardiac function is generally maintained in patients with normal preoperative myocardial function and coronary arterial anatomy. However, in patients with significant baseline cardiac impairment, decompensation can occur and result in myocardial ischemia, heart failure secondary to ventricular dysfunction, or both. One study reported a 30% incidence of myocardial ischemia in a group of patients with coronary artery disease after infrarenal aortic clamp placement.[71]

Aortic Declamping

Unclamping of the aorta is also associated with abrupt hemodynamic alterations, with hypotension initially being due to a sudden decrease in systemic vascular resistance. Other important contributory factors include central hypovolemia caused by vascular engorgement in distal, reperfused tissues and the release of previously sequestered vasodilatory metabolites back into the systemic circulation. Accordingly, management of resuscitation, electrolytes, and pressors is critically important during this step (see Chapter 31: Intraoperative Management).

Renal and Splanchnic Ischemia

Clamping the aorta in an infrarenal location typically produces minimal effect on renal and splanchnic blood flow, whereas suprarenal and supraceliac clamping can markedly alter perfusion. Although it is desirable to place the proximal clamp as distal on the aorta as possible to permit successful aneurysm repair, careful evaluation of clamp location is essential to avoid chronic thrombus or cholesterol embolization to the lower extremities, kidneys, or splanchnic arteries. Embolization after aortic clamp placement in hostile neck anatomy is associated with significant morbidity and mortality.[72]

Renal Dysfunction

Most commonly, the cause of renal failure associated with aortic surgery is acute tubular necrosis.[73] The incidence of renal dysfunction in patients undergoing elective AAA repair varies widely, depending on the magnitude of the surgery performed and the duration of renal ischemia. Renal insufficiency is more frequent after suprarenal than after infrarenal cross-clamping, with suprarenal clamp times longer than 30 minutes being associated with increased risk for postoperative renal failure.[74] Although clamp times of up to 50 minutes appear to be tolerated and associated with transient azotemia,[75] avoidance of intravascular volume depletion and intraoperative hypotension is essential.[73] Perhaps surprisingly, even infrarenal clamp placement reduces renal blood flow by up to 40%. Infrarenal aortic cross-clamping decreases renal cortical blood flow, increases renal vasculature resistance, and reduces the glomerular filtration rate.[76]

Renal Protection Agents. A number of renal protective agents have been proposed, including mannitol,[77] dopamine,[77] furosemide, fenoldopam,[78,79] and N-acetylcysteine.[80] Mannitol and furosemide are frequently used despite the absence of any clinically demonstrable benefit in humans undergoing elective aortic surgery.[69] The selective dopamine receptor agonist fenoldopam has vasodilatory and natriuretic effects, with demonstrated benefit in patients undergoing aortic clamping.[78,79] Some authors have suggested reserving fenoldopam for patients with preoperative renal dysfunction.[69]

Renal Cold Perfusion. For patients requiring suprarenal clamp placement, renal perfusion with cold (5° C) hyperosmolar crystalloid solution has been reported to be an effective renal protection strategy. The proposed mechanism is a decrement in oxygen consumption of roughly 7% for each degree drop in temperature,[73] with reduced metabolic demands during clamp-induced parenchymal ischemia resulting in less accumulated damage by the time of organ reperfusion. Cold perfusion with a reduction in renal temperature has been reported to improve outcomes in patients undergoing suprarenal clamping for suprarenal, supra-SMA, supraceliac, and thoracoabdominal aneurysm operations[20,81-84] and appears to be superior to near-normothermic perfusion of whole blood.[85,86]

Splanchnic Ischemia

An additional potential problem associated with supraceliac clamping is the development of coagulopathy. Ischemia of the hepatic and mesenteric circulation is an important contributor to intraoperative and postoperative coagulopathy.[87-90] Although the increased extent of surgical dissection, enlarged prosthetic surface area, and greater number of anastomoses all increase the risk for consumptive coagulopathy during procedures requiring supraceliac cross-clamping,[91] other potential explanations have been advanced to explain this common clinical occurrence, including disseminated intravascular coagulation,[87] altered heparin pharmacodynamics,[92] and perhaps, enhanced primary fibrinolysis.[93,94]

Finally, although the potential for lower extremity and colon ischemia must be considered during any aortic procedure, the consequences of inadequate perfusion are not typically manifested during conduct of the initial aortic surgery. Obviously, the adequacy of perfusion of the legs and colon should be evaluated and deemed sufficient before leaving the operating room at the time of the initial surgery.

■ SURGICAL TECHNIQUE
Midline Transabdominal Repair
Exposure

For TA exposure the patient should be placed in a supine position and prepared and draped from the nipples to the knees. Multiple incisions have been described (Fig. 128-7);

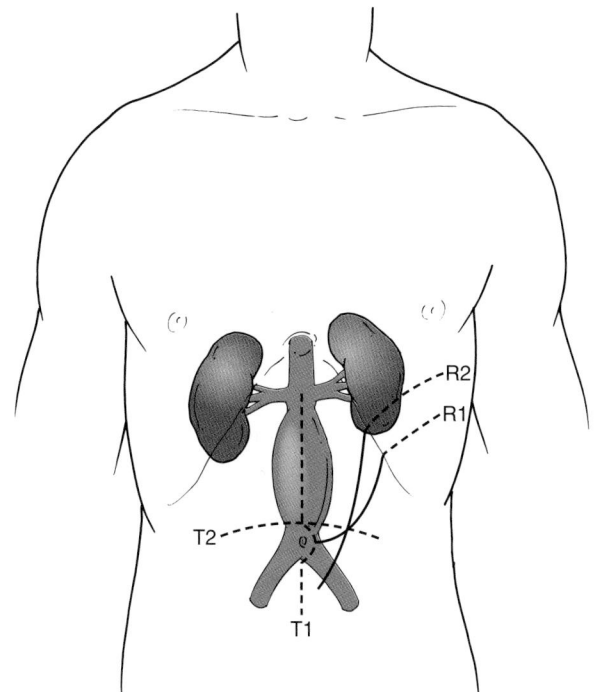

Figure 128-7 Surgical incisions for repair of abdominal aortic aneurysms, including a standard vertical laparotomy incision for the transperitoneal approach (T1) and retroperitoneal incisions for an infrarenal (R1) aneurysm alone or with iliac involvement (R2). For juxtarenal or more proximal aortic exposure, the incisions can be extended into the desired intercostal space. A transverse laparotomy incision has occasionally been used for transperitoneal exposure (T2).

Section **17** Arterial Aneurysms

however, a midline incision is most frequently used for a TA approach. The midline incision should extend from the xiphoid to the symphysis pubis to provide maximal exposure. Such exposure permits full exploration of the abdominal contents to rule out any intra-abdominal pathology that might not have been detected by preoperative CT scanning.

Once the intra-abdominal contents are inspected, the greater omentum and transverse colon are elevated superiorly. The small bowel is then mobilized to the right side of the abdomen to expose the retroperitoneum. The aorta is exposed by incising the posterior peritoneum starting just below the bifurcation of the aorta inferiorly and extending superiorly to the level of the ligament of Treitz just to the right of the inferior mesenteric vein. If necessary, the inferior mesenteric vein can be divided to allow retraction of the pancreas. Superior dissection of the posterior peritoneum exposes the left renal vein crossing over the neck of the aneurysm (Fig. 128-8). The left renal vein may be retroaortic, which should be identified on the preoperative CT scan. If the aneurysm extends to the level of the renal arteries and will require suprarenal clamping just below the SMA, the left renal vein should be mobilized to the level of its confluence with the inferior vena cava (IVC). Typically, broad mobilization of the left renal vein by division of its branches provides adequate exposure (Fig. 128-9). If the left renal vein must be divided, it should be done close to the junction of the vena cava (Fig. 128-10). This is rarely necessary because the use of other surgical approaches can obviate the need for renal vein ligation to obtain adequate exposure, and renal vein ligation is not without risk. If needed, however, ligation of the left adrenal and left gonadal veins must then be avoided because they provide important renal venous collaterals. In some situations, use of an Omni self-retaining retractor (Omni-Tract Surgical, St. Paul, MN) allows placement of a renal vein retractor under the left renal vein to improve exposure of the juxtarenal aorta and provide the necessary space for clamping.

Aortic Reconstruction

Most infrarenal AAA repairs can be performed with the use of a tube graft, which requires exposure of only the first 2 cm of the common iliac arteries. Circumferential mobilization of the common iliac arteries should be avoided to prevent venous injury. Similarly, identification of the ureters as they cross the iliac arteries should be accomplished. Before cross-clamping, systemic heparinization is initiated. Once proximal and distal control is achieved, the aneurysm is entered. The thrombus

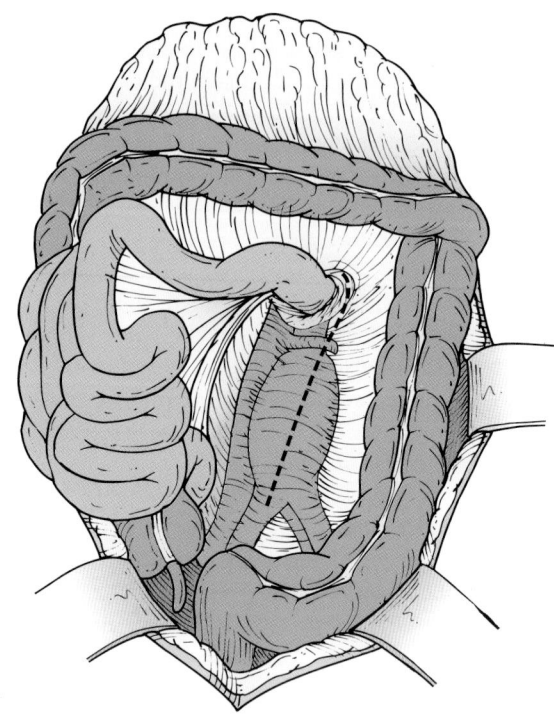

Figure 128-8 Standard inframesocolic aortic exposure. Via a transperitoneal approach, the posterior peritoneum overlying the aorta is incised from the level of the aortic bifurcation to the right of the inferior mesenteric vein up to the level of the left renal vein.

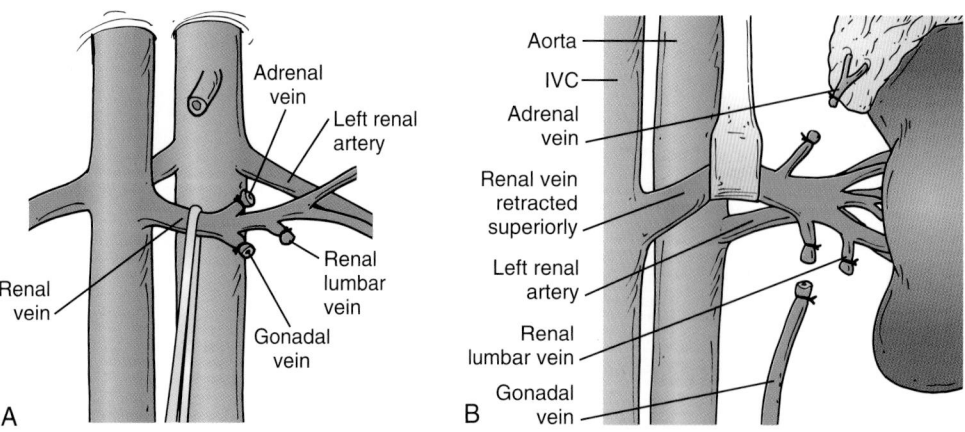

Figure 128-9 From a transperitoneal approach, additional exposure of the juxtarenal aorta can be achieved by ligation of the gonadal, adrenal, and lumbar branches of the renal vein. The renal vein can then be extensively mobilized and retracted inferiorly (**A**) or superiorly (**B**). IVC, inferior vena cava.

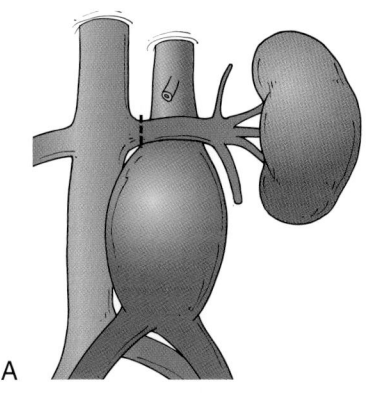

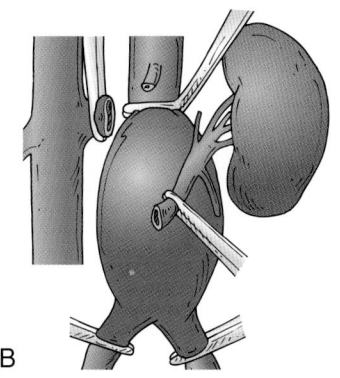

Figure 128-10 A and **B,** In rare cases requiring division of the left renal vein, it should be done close to the inferior vena cava with care taken to preserve all major venous collaterals of the left renal vein.

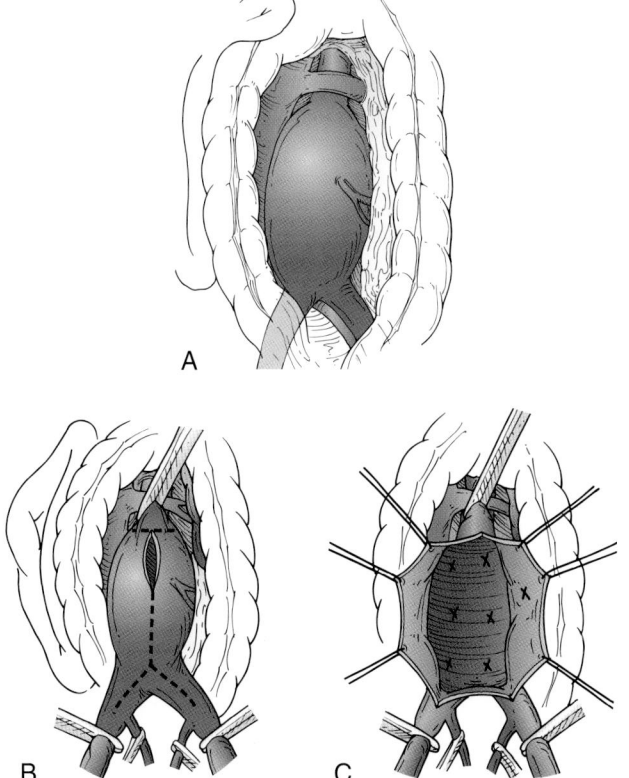

Figure 128-11 After identifying important vascular structures, including the left renal vein and inferior mesenteric artery (**A**), clamps are placed proximally and distally and the sac of the aneurysm is opened with a T-shaped proximal incision on the sac (**B**). The thrombus is evacuated, and backbleeding lumbar arteries, as well as the inferior mesenteric artery, are oversewn from within the sac (**C**).

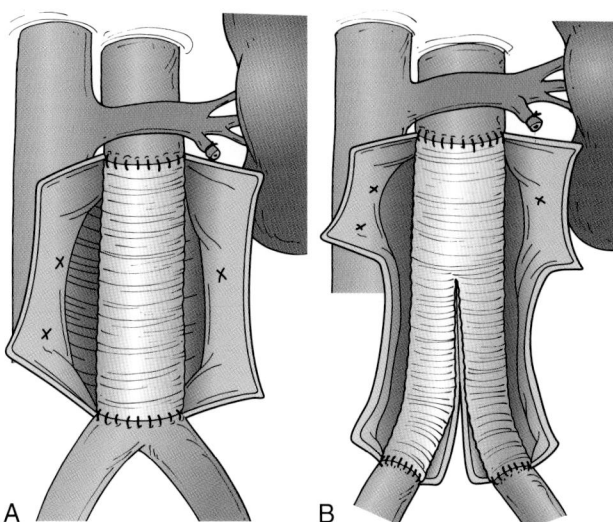

Figure 128-12 A, Endoaneurysmorrhaphy with a tube graft configuration. **B,** Endoaneurysmorrhaphy with a bifurcated graft configuration and distal anastomoses to the common iliac arteries.

ene suture (Fig. 128-12A). In cases in which the common iliac arteries are dilated (≥2 cm), the anastomosis can be performed to the distal common iliac artery, which requires mobilization of the internal and external iliac arteries (Fig. 128-12B). Identification of the ureters is important, and they should be retracted to avoid injury. If the anastomosis is performed in the common iliac artery, every attempt to preserve at least one internal iliac artery should be made. Before releasing the clamps, backbleeding and forward bleeding are allowed. Communication with the anesthesiologist before releasing the clamps is important to avoid large shifts in blood pressure.

Closure

After ascertaining hemostasis, the aneurysmal sac is closed over the graft with running absorbable suture. Closure of the posterior peritoneum with absorbable suture is performed to avoid contact of the bowel with the graft (Fig. 128-13). The abdominal wall is then closed with either interrupted or running nonabsorbable suture.

is evacuated, and any bleeding lumbar arteries are suture ligated from within the aneurysmal sac. The IMA is inspected for backbleeding if patent and can usually be ligated (see "Inferior Mesenteric Artery Management"). Either suture ligation from within the sac or external ligation of the IMA close to the AAA wall is performed (Fig. 128-11). An end-to-end anastomosis between the prosthetic graft and the aorta is performed proximally and distally with running polypropyl-

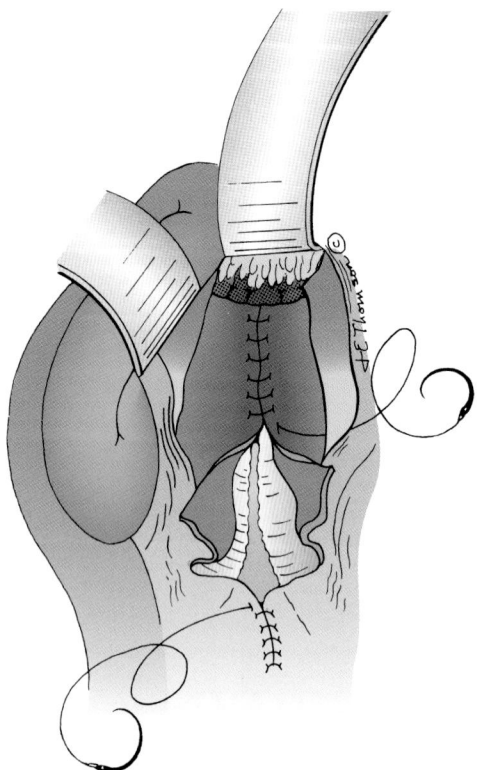

Figure 128-13 To protect the prosthetic graft from erosion into bowel and from exposure to contamination from intraperitoneal processes, the abdominal aortic aneurysm sac is closed over the graft, followed by careful reclosure of the posterior peritoneum.

Suprarenal Exposure

Anterior Supraceliac Clamping. The supraceliac aorta is exposed by dividing the gastrohepatic ligament, typically a thin layer, using electrocautery to expose the aortic crus of the diaphragm. Occasionally, the left lobe of the liver is enlarged, and its attachments to the retroperitoneum and diaphragm must be divided so that it can be mobilized anteriorly or to the right to facilitate aortic exposure. A nasogastric tube in place is easily palpated and allows the surgeon to identify the adjacent esophagus and avoid accidental injury. The aortic pulsation is also easily palpated, and the overlying fibers of the crus are divided with electrocautery during elective surgery so that several inches of proximal abdominal aorta can be exposed without difficulty. Care should be taken when encircling the aorta at this level so that any posterior lumbar branches are not avulsed. Continued exposure distally along the anterior aortic surface will eventually allow one to reach the celiac axis. Care must also be taken to not injure other important anterior structures that lie immediately inferior and anterior to the area of aortic exposure, such as the pancreas. During open repair of ruptured aortic aneurysms, the identical process is repeated but in more rapid fashion, often with blunt techniques of finger fracture to divide the gastrohepatic ligament and diaphragmatic fibers and maintenance of manual compression on the supraceliac aorta until clamp placement can be performed. (See Chapter 130: Abdominal Aortic Aneurysms: Ruptured.)

Medial Visceral Rotation. In patients in whom a TA exposure has been selected in whom the distance between the renal artery and the SMA is so small that a clamp will not be able to be placed above the renal arteries to treat a juxtarenal aneurysm, the surgeon will need to be familiar with medial visceral rotation maneuvers to expose the suprarenal aorta. Although the right medial visceral rotation maneuver can provide more proximal exposure (i.e., mobilizing the entire right colon in continuity with the duodenum and shifting the orientation of the SMA and root of the mesentery), in the case of aneurysm surgery, the preferred method is the left medial visceral rotation maneuver (Fig. 128-14). In this situation, the

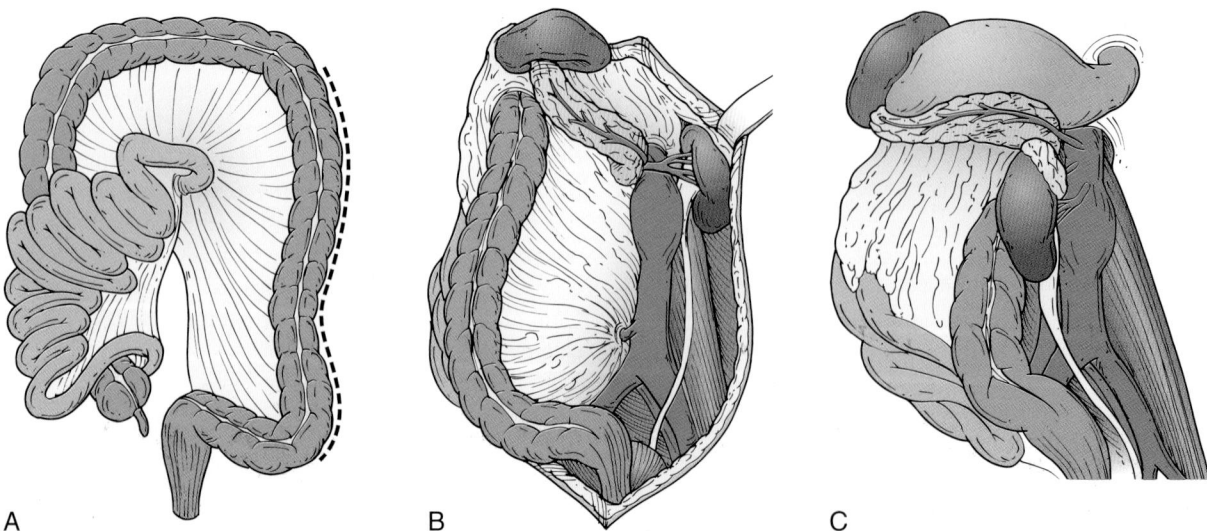

A   B   C

Figure 128-14 In a left medial visceral rotation performed via a transperitoneal approach, the left colon (**A**), spleen, and pancreas are mobilized laterally to medially until the suprarenal aorta is exposed. The left kidney can either be kept in the renal fossa or be mobilized medially (**B**). Division of the left crus of the diaphragm provides additional proximal exposure of the suprarenal aorta (**C**).

left colon, splenic flexure, spleen, and pancreas are mobilized laterally to medially until the suprarenal aorta is exposed. Depending on the extension and the location where the anastomosis will be performed, the left kidney can be either kept in the renal fossa or mobilized medially. If the kidney is brought up medially, the large lumbar vein that normally drains into the posterior wall of the left renal vein should be ligated. Division of the left crus of the diaphragm will provide exposure of the suprarenal aorta to the supraceliac aorta. Such exposure permits surgeons to select the location of the clamp from just above the renal arteries all the way up to the supraceliac aorta. If medial visceral rotation is indicated, this exposure allows placement of a suprarenal anastomosis. If suprarenal aortic dilatation is present, the beveled prosthetic graft should be sutured to include the celiac axis, SMA, and right renal artery, with as much aneurysmal aorta excluded as possible. In these cases, the left renal artery should be reimplanted into the graft or a limb presutured to the graft and then anastomosed to the left renal artery in end-to-end fashion. Topical (surface) cooling of the left kidney can be performed with ice or gentle irrigation of a cold heparinized solution (10 U/mL). For relatively brief periods of renal artery ischemia, ice is preferred because it tends to cause less systemic hypothermia with its attendant complications. Once the proximal anastomosis and reimplantation of the left renal artery have been carried out, the distal anastomosis is performed, either end to end to the aortic bifurcation or end to end to both distal common iliac arteries as needed. Use of a self-retaining retractor is important to avoid intermittent excessive retraction of the pancreas or spleen (or both) and injury to these organs. Left medial visceral rotation can likewise be used in patients with juxtarenal aneurysms and mesenteric and renal artery occlusive disease, in which case the aneurysm repair will be accompanied by transaortic endarterectomy of the visceral and renal vessels. When endarterectomy of the visceral and renal vessels is performed, careful dissection with a dural elevator and gentle outward traction should proceed until the atherosclerotic lesions are removed. Once the visceral vessels have been revascularized, use of intraoperative ultrasound to verify the lack of a flap in the renal or mesenteric vessels is required to avoid perioperative thrombosis of these vessels.

Retroperitoneal or Thoracoretroperitoneal Repair

Exposure

The patient is placed in a partial right lateral decubitus position with the left side of the torso rotated approximately 45 degrees. The patient is positioned on a beanbag to maintain this posture, and the table is flexed slightly with the kidney rest elevated.

The most common incision for RP repair of an infrarenal aneurysm is a curvilinear incision that extends to the 12th rib from the area of the umbilicus (Fig. 128-15). If an aortic tube graft is being considered, stopping the incision just medial to the left lateral border of the left rectus muscle is adequate. If

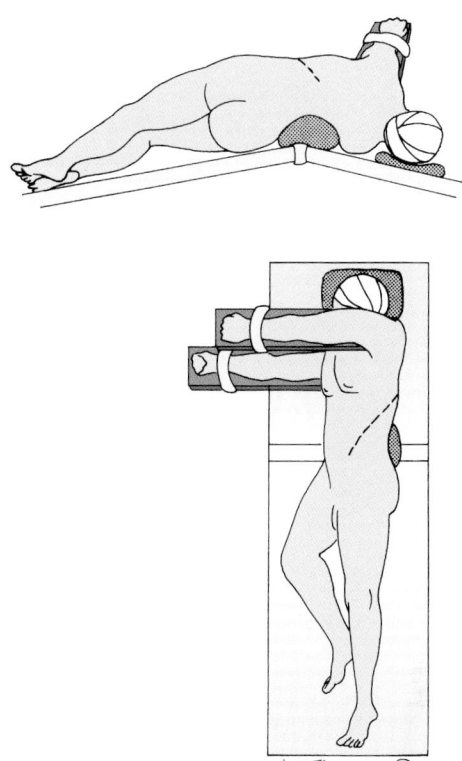

Figure 128-15 Positioning and incision for retroperitoneal exposure of the infrarenal aorta.

an aortobiiliac graft needs to be performed, the incision should be extended to approximately 2 to 3 cm below the umbilicus. In most patients, mobilization of the right common iliac artery can be carried out, not uncommonly to the level of the bifurcation of the right common iliac arteries. If the patient has a very large aneurysm in both the infrarenal aorta and the proximal right common iliac artery, intraluminal control of the distal iliac artery with a balloon occlusion catheter may be necessary, and many surgeons prefer to use this routinely for right iliac control. After the incision is extended to the 12th rib, part of the rib may need to be resected for maximal posterior exposure.

A common location to enter the retroperitoneum is at the junction of the lateral abdominal wall muscles and the posterior rectus sheath. After division of the anterior rectus sheath and muscle, the external oblique muscles are divided with electrocautery. The junction of the posterior rectus sheath and lateral abdominal wall muscle is incised until the peritoneum is identified. Blunt dissection of the peritoneum medially and cephalically provides excellent mobilization of the retroperitoneum. The lateral abdominal wall muscles are divided with electrocautery to either the tip of the 12th rib or past the tip of the 12th rib with partial removal of this rib. Further mobilization medially allows division of the posterior rectus sheath to fully expose the left retroperitoneum. The left ureter should be identified immediately and circled with a vessel loop to include the periureteral vascular plexus. This becomes an important technical factor to avoid devascularization of the ureter and resultant fibrosis. The ureter is

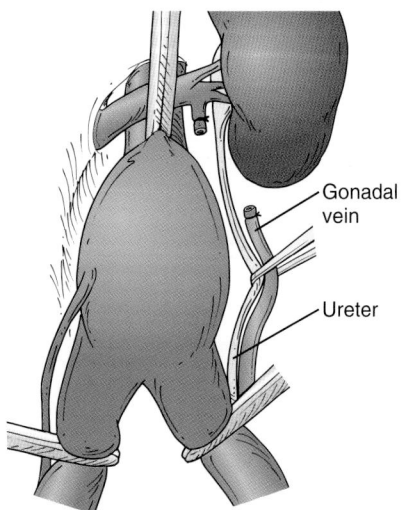

Figure 128-16 The gonadal vein can be traced up to its junction with the left renal vein and then ligated and divided to improve retroperitoneal exposure. The left ureter and its accompanying blood supply are encircled with a vessel loop.

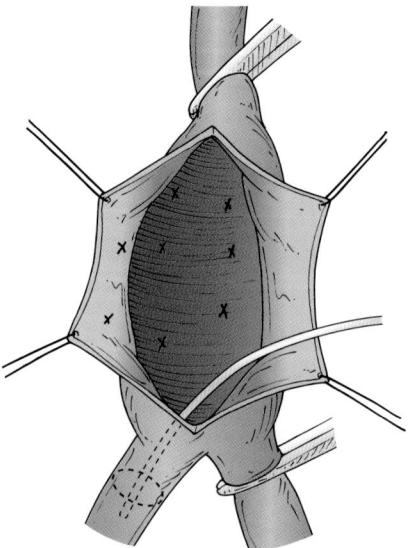

Figure 128-17 The right iliac artery can be controlled after the aneurysm sac has been entered by placement of a balloon occlusion catheter. This can be done to minimize dissection of the right common iliac artery, as well as to provide distal control when that vessel is heavily calcified and clamp placement is undesirable.

mobilized down to the left of the left common iliac artery inferiorly and superiorly to the renal pelvis. This maneuver, along with incising the lumbodorsal fascia overlying the left kidney, allows excellent visualization of the left gonadal vein, which is then dissected superiorly to its confluence in the left renal vein. Ligation of the junction of the gonadal vein with the left renal vein provides the exposure that is needed to appropriately isolate the infrarenal neck (Fig. 128-16). Superior mobilization of the left renal vein facilitates exposure of the aortic neck up to the level of the left renal artery. An alternative approach is to mobilize the left kidney anteriorly and medially, a maneuver that is required for adequate exposure of suprarenal aortic pathology and a commonly selected option when approaching infrarenal aortic aneurysms.

Once appropriate exposure and mobilization of the neck are achieved, attention is directed to the level of the bifurcation of the aorta. Close attention to the location of the pudendal nerves is important to avoid postoperative sexual dysfunction. The right common iliac artery can be exposed by further mobilization superior to the pudendal nerves or by ligation of the IMA flush with the aortic aneurysm. The left common iliac artery is easily visualized. If an anastomosis to the bifurcation of the left common iliac artery needs to be performed, mobilization of the external and internal iliac arteries is usually fairly simple to carry out.

Arterial Reconstruction

After placement of self-retaining retractors, the remainder of the procedure is carried out in a similar manner as described previously. The specific details of the type of self-retaining retractor used and placement of retracting blades vary according to surgeon preference and body habitus of the patient, but optimal performance is an essential aspect of aortic surgery. If balloon control of the right common iliac artery is necessary

after clamping the left common iliac and infrarenal aortic neck, the sac is opened primarily in the distal aorta to allow balloon cannulation of the right common iliac artery without excessive mobilization of intraluminal clot and potential embolization into the right common iliac artery (Fig. 128-17). After completion of the proximal and distal anastomoses, because the peritoneum was not entered, the only closure of RP contents involves the aneurysm sac if preferred by the surgeon, although this is not required. Because the duodenum is still attached to the anterior wall of the aorta, reperitonealization is not required.

Suprarenal Repair

If the aneurysm extends to above the renal arteries in a suprarenal location, the incision should be carried out in the 11th, 10th, or 9th intercostal space, depending on the aortic anatomy of the patient. Any exposure above the 11th intercostal space will usually enter the pleural space and require placement of a chest tube if the visceral pleura is violated. If the incision is kept between the 11th and 12th ribs, the pleural space can usually be avoided. RP exposure in this particular situation requires positioning the patient in a more right lateral decubitus position to allow wider posterior exposure.

Once the RP space is entered, the inferior surface of the diaphragm needs to be mobilized medially to expose Gerota's fascia. Mobilization of the peritoneum from the inferior surface of the diaphragm is continued until the left crus of the diaphragm is fully visualized. If suprarenal extension of the aneurysm has occurred, the left kidney should be mobilized superiorly and medially to expose the retroperitoneum up to the level of the diaphragm. The left crus of the diaphragm is divided for exposure up to 4 to 6 cm above the celiac axis

(Fig. 128-18). The large lumbar vein that drains into the posterior wall of the left renal vein should be ligated early to avoid avulsion.

After the location for the proximal aortic cross-clamp is identified, the dissection is carried out in a similar fashion inferiorly, but in this case the ureter is not mobilized laterally but maintained attached to the posterior peritoneum and retracted to the right. Placement of the appropriate self-retaining retractors will then provide the necessary exposure. Depending on the anatomy of the juxtarenal and suprarenal aorta, an incision is made for resection of the aneurysm and possible reimplantation of the left renal artery. If the aneurysm extends to the suprarenal location, the cross-clamp is usually applied above the celiac axis and the prosthetic graft is beveled, usually to include the right renal artery, SMA, and celiac axis. The left renal artery is reimplanted into the graft or bypassed with a sidearm from the graft. If a bypass to the left renal artery is needed, a side limb can be sutured to the main body of the prosthetic graft before cross-clamping the aorta to limit ischemia time in the left kidney (Fig. 128-19). The left kidney can be cooled externally with topical

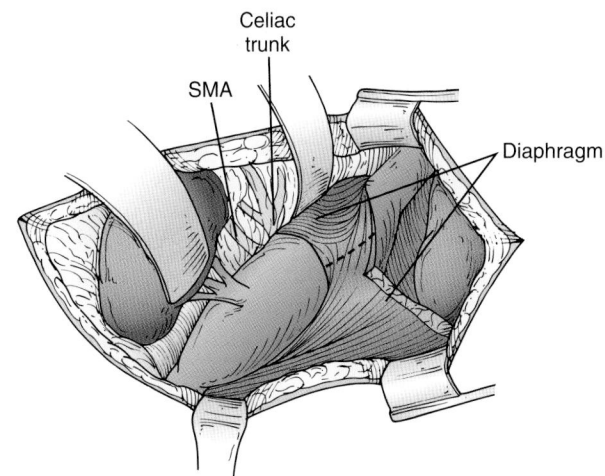

Figure 128-18 After the retroperitoneal space is entered, the inferior surface of the diaphragm is mobilized medially until the left crus of the diaphragm is fully visualized. The left kidney can be mobilized superiorly and medially to expose the retroperitoneum up to the level of the diaphragm. The left crus of the diaphragm is divided for exposure above the celiac axis. SMA, superior mesenteric artery.

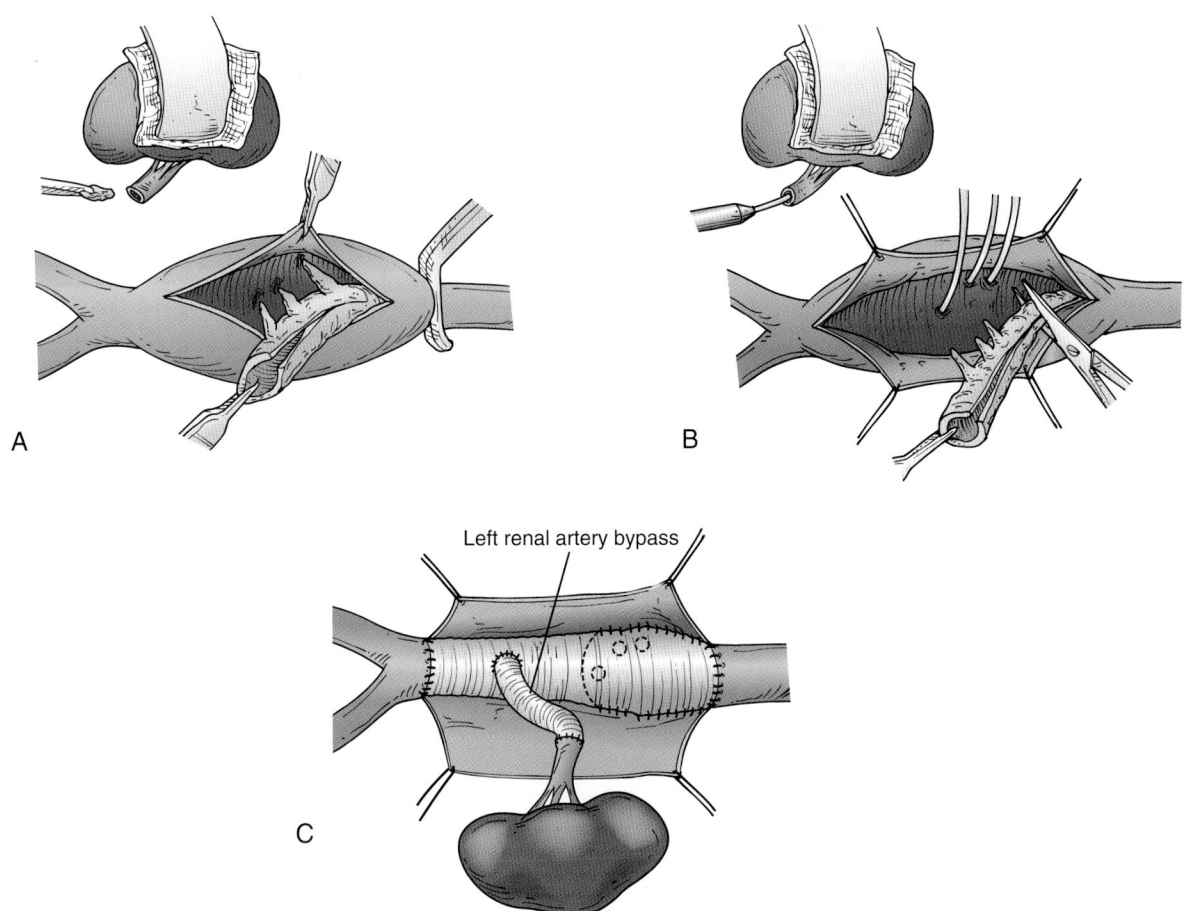

Figure 128-19 If necessary, endarterectomy of atherosclerotic occlusive disease involving the origin of the visceral vessels can be performed, and the left renal artery perfused with renal preservation solution. (**A** and **B**). In most instances, a beveled proximal anastomosis that includes an aortic inclusion patch encompassing the orifices of the celiac axis, superior mesenteric artery, and right renal artery is performed, whereas the left renal artery is typically reimplanted or bypassed separately off the aortic graft (**C**).

ice in gauze and held in place with a self-retraining retractor; alternatively, renal preservation solution at 5°C can be instilled into the left renal artery.

After revascularization of the right renal artery, SMA, and celiac axis, the left renal artery is revascularized to limit ischemia time in the left kidney. The distal anastomosis is then performed in accordance with the anatomy of the bifurcation of the aorta. If endarterectomy of the visceral and renal vessels is indicated, the same maneuver as described in the previous section, with medial visceral rotation, should be carried out to verify the patency of all the endarterectomized vessels.

Inferior Mesenteric Artery Management

Because of the morbidity and mortality associated with postoperative colonic ischemia, careful intraoperative assessment and prevention are essential. The safety of IMA ligation is contingent on other collateral pathways' providing adequate blood supply. Patients at risk include those with underlying celiac/SMA occlusive lesions, patients with previous bowel resection, patients with significant pelvic occlusive disease, and patients with hypotension in the perioperative period. Identification of a large meandering mesenteric or marginal artery indicates significant mesenteric occlusive disease, and careful preoperative assessment of the pathway of arterial blood supply to the bowel is essential. Intraoperatively, adequacy of the collateral colonic circulation is confirmed by assessing backbleeding of the IMA. The presence of backbleeding along with a normal-appearing colon would indicate that it is safe to ligate the IMA. Although Ernst and colleagues have suggested that the stump pressure index be used when considering reimplantation of patent IMAs,[95] this practice has not been widely embraced. Routine IMA reimplantation does not prevent postoperative colonic ischemia[96-99] but may be advantageous in patients in whom colonic perfusion is borderline.

◼ POSTOPERATIVE MANAGEMENT

Postoperative care is critical to avoid complications after AAA repair (see Chapter 32: Postoperative Management). A significant reduction in risk after aortic surgery is associated with a pattern of daily care by an intensive care unit physician[100] and a high nurse-to-patient ratio.[101] Mortality risk after open AAA repair has been extensively modeled, with outcomes after elective surgery correlating best with predictions using the Acute Physiology and Chronic Health Evaluation (APACHE) AAA model.[102] This model includes four independent predictive factors: age, acute physiology score (APACHE II), emergency surgery, and chronic health dysfunction (coronary artery disease, congestive heart failure, or chronic renal failure).[103]

Cardiac Complications

Myocardial ischemia as indicated by postoperative troponin-I levels should be checked as an important indicator of both immediate and delayed myocardial infarction (see Chapter 38: Systemic Complications: Cardiac).[104] Beta blockade should be continued in the postoperative period because this strategy has been documented to improve outcomes, particularly in patients at highest risk for cardiac complications.[105,106] Moreover, discontinuation of beta blockade in the postoperative period has been shown to increase cardiovascular mortality (29% versus 0% in patients in whom beta blockers are continued) and increase risk for myocardial infarction nearly 18-fold.[107]

Bleeding

Patients remain at an increased risk for bleeding in the immediate postoperative period. Even though the problem may occasionally be secondary to coagulopathy, the possibility of new or unrecognized hemorrhage requiring surgical control must be strongly considered. Although some fluid equilibration and redistribution can influence postoperative hemoglobin levels, platelet counts, and parameters of coagulation, the need for continuing transfusions should warn the surgical team of new or continued bleeding in the surgical field and prompt possible immediate re-exploration in the operating room. Attention to hemostasis before closing the incision, judicious monitoring in the intensive care unit, and early reoperation in the case of suspected bleeding remain important tools for dealing with bleeding after open aneurysm surgery.

There are two common culprit locations for significant postoperative hemorrhage. The first is unrecognized backbleeding from the lumbar or intercostal arteries. These vessels may not be actively bleeding when the aneurysm sac is initially inspected while the proximal clamp is still in place. After declamping and restoration of distal perfusion, however, previously hemostatic vessels may bleed. Careful inspection of the posterior aspect of the aneurysm sac at the conclusion of the procedure is essential to avoid this complication. The second common site of postoperative bleeding is from inadvertent splenic injury, often related to retractor placement. In this case we recommend careful, gentle initial retractor blade placement protected by a laparotomy pad. Despite attempts to protect the spleen from direct trauma, adhesions between intra-abdominal structures and the splenic capsule may be preexistent, and retraction on these other structures, such as bowel, can result in an indirect form of splenic trauma. From an RP approach, splenic hemorrhage is unlikely to be identified unless it results in hemodynamic instability during the initial procedure. Should hemorrhage out of proportion to the degree of blood loss in the surgical field develop in a patient undergoing RP surgery, opening the peritoneum to inspect the abdominal cavity for bleeding is recommended.

Venous Thrombosis

Deep venous thrombosis (DVT) and the associated risk for pulmonary embolism (PE) remain some of the most common preventable complications after surgery. In a series of patients undergoing open AAA repair who were not given preoperative DVT prophylaxis and studied postoperatively for 5 days with bilateral lower extremity venography, the incidence of DVT was 18%.[108] The majority of thrombi were located in the calf, with only 4% of patients having more proximal DVT. No clinically significant PEs ensued. Although DVT prophylaxis is routinely used in conjunction with major surgical procedures, its benefit in patients undergoing open AAA repair remains unclear, perhaps because these patients receive substantial intraoperative heparin routinely during these procedures. A review of the Cochrane Peripheral Vascular Diseases Group registry and the Cochrane Central Register of Controlled Trials revealed only two trials, both of which failed to demonstrate a benefit of postoperative anticoagulant therapy, with or without the addition of mechanical devices to augment venous return, in terms of DVT, PE, or mortality.[109] Despite the lack of strong supporting studies, many surgeons continue to use prophylactic anticoagulant therapy, mechanical devices, and early ambulation in an attempt to reduce the risk for perioperative DVT and PE. However, the most recent evidence-based guidelines from the American College of Chest Physicians, based on the results of four randomized trials of thromboprophylaxis after arterial surgery, suggested that clinicians not routinely use specific thromboprophylaxis other than early and frequent ambulation for patients undergoing vascular surgery procedures who do not have additional thromboembolic risk factors.[110] For patients undergoing major vascular surgery who have additional thromboembolic risk factors, prophylaxis with unfractionated or low-molecular-weight heparin or fondaparinux was recommended.

OUTCOMES

Early Survival

Early mortality rates after elective open surgical repair vary considerably in the literature. As pointed out by Blankensteijn and coauthors, part of the difference in outcomes stems from the type of study reported (e.g., population-based reports versus individual hospital-based series) and whether the data are collected prospectively or retrospectively.[111] Centers of excellence report 30-day mortality rates of 1% to 5%,[2-4,52,112,113] with individual physicians also reporting personal series with equally outstanding results.[113] The Brigham and Women's Hospital reported a 4.7% mortality rate in 128 high-risk patients and a 0% mortality rate in 444 average-risk patients.[112] A recent review of 30 published reports from centers of excellence identified a 3.2% mortality rate in 9291 patients with a "clear trend towards recent improvement."[114] These outcomes should not be extrapolated to other institutions or surgeons, however. Higher mortality rates ranging from 3.5% to 8.4% have been reported in population-based series (Table 128-2),[115-127] with one review of 64 studies documenting an average 5.5% mortality rate.[128] It should be noted that many surgical series report hospital or operative mortality rather than 30-day outcomes.

Table 128-2 Early Mortality in Population-Based Reports of Repair of Nonruptured Infrarenal Aneurysms

Series	Number of Patients	Mortality (%)	Data Source
Johnston and Scobie[115]	666	4.8	Canadian Society of Vascular Surgery
Lawrence et al.[116]	32,389	8.4	National Hospital Discharge Survey (U.S.)
Dimick et al.[117]	7980	3.8	National Inpatient Sample (U.S.)
Rigberg et al.[118]	9778	3.8	California Statewide
Heller et al.[119]	358,521	5.6	National Hospital Discharge Survey (U.S.)
Galland[120]	2680	4.8	British Joint Vascular Research Group
Bradbury et al.[121]	270	6.2	Royal Edinburgh Infirmary database
Bayly et al.[122]	671	6.3	Vascular Anaesthesiology Society of Great Britain and Ireland
Kazmers et al.[123]	3687	4.86	Veterans Affairs Medical Centers (U.S.)
Huber et al.[124]	16,450	4.2	National Inpatient Sample (U.S.)
Dardik[125]	2335	3.5	Maryland Health Service Cost Review
Akkersdijk et al.[126]	1289	6.8	Dutch National Medical Registration
Schermerhorn et al.[127]	22,830	4.8	Medicare beneficiaries (U.S.)

Determinants of Early Survival

Most series suggest a direct relationship between mortality and the number of preexisting co-morbid conditions, older patient age, female gender,[117,129,130] black race, and the surgeon's lack of specialty training in vascular surgery[131] and an inverse relationship with hospital and physician case volume.[132-134] Steyerberg and coworkers developed a clinical prediction rule based on data from their own institutional experience, as well as from a literature review.[27] They determined that congestive heart failure and cardiac ischemia on the electrocardiogram followed by renal impairment, a history of myocardial infarction, pulmonary impairment, and female gender predicted risk, in decreasing order. Cardiac, renal, and pulmonary co-morbidity were the most important risk factors for mortality in the clinical prediction rule. Finally, recent, prospective randomized trials have compared open surgery with EVAR (the EVAR-1[135] and Dutch Randomized Endovascular Aneurysm Management[136] [DREAM] trials) and open surgery with continued surveillance for small-diameter (4.0 to 5.4 cm) aneurysms (the UKSAT[21] and Aneurysm Detection and Management[137] [ADAM] trials). Mortality in the surgically treated patient study arms ranged from 2% (ADAM) to 4.7% (EVAR-1) to 5.8% (UKSAT, DREAM) across these series.

Section **17** Arterial Aneurysms

Table 128-3 Early Mortality Associated with Nonruptured Juxtarenal and Suprarenal Aneurysm Repair

Series	Number of Patients	Mortality (%)	Aneurysm Extent
Qvarfordt et al.[138]	77	1.3	Juxtarenal and suprarenal
Crawford et al.[139]	101	7	Juxtarenal
Poulias et al.[140]	38	5.2	Juxtarenal
Nypaver et al.[141]	53	3.5	Juxtarenal and suprarenal
Allen et al.[82]	65	1.5	Juxtarenal and suprarenal
Faggioli et al.[142]	50	7.1	Juxtarenal and suprarenal
Martin et al.[143]	57	1.8	Suprarenal
Chiesa et al.[144]	115	4.2	Juxtarenal and suprarenal
West et al.[12]	247	2.5	Juxtarenal and suprarenal
Sarac et al.[13]	138	5.1	Juxtarenal and suprarenal
Jean-Claude et al.[145]	180	5.8	Juxtarenal and suprarenal
Knott et al.[146]	126	0.8	Juxtarenal

Effect of Suprarenal Clamping

Perhaps surprisingly, early survival after open surgical repair requiring cross-clamping above the level of the renal arteries does not differ significantly in some series from the results cited earlier. This may reflect biases toward more careful patient selection or referral to specialized centers. Early mortality rates range from 0.8% to 7.1% (Table 128-3).[12,13,82,138-146] Differentiation between outcomes of juxtarenal versus suprarenal aneurysm repair is made difficult by the variability in aneurysm nomenclature among reports and the tendency to describe outcomes with both types of aneurysm configuration in a single report. It is worth noting that these excellent outcomes for more complex AAAs are inferior to outcomes of infrarenal repairs from these same centers.[26] Therefore, these results should not be generalized across all institutions and surgeons, where the results would be expected to be inferior. A recent regional experience found suprarenal clamping to be associated with higher 30-day and 1-year mortality after open elective infrarenal AAA repair.

Late Survival

As expected, age is the strongest predictor of life expectancy, which ranges from 18 years for a 60-year-old man to 5 years for an 85-year-old.[23] Survival in patients with AAA is lower than that in sex- and age-matched populations without AAA. In a report from 28 medical centers on 794 patients who survived elective AAA repair, survival rates were 94% at 1 year, 90% at 2 years, 84% at 3 years, 78% at 4 years, and 67% at 5 years.[147] Essentially every subsequent study has confirmed Crawford and colleagues' report that cardiac disease and cancer,[1] followed by stroke,[148] pulmonary disease, and renal failure,[4] are, in decreasing order, the principal causes of death in AAA patients. In Batt and associates' series, AAA repair was associated with a reduction in 5-year survival rates from 91% to 72% versus matched controls[149]; Johnston reported that 6-year survival rates decreased from 79.2% to 60.2%.[148] Several other centers have reported large series with similar outcomes.[1,150-153] Both Zöllner and coworkers[154] and Hallett and colleagues[152] identified reduced survival in patients with small aneurysms, many unoperated, and determined that the diminished survival in aneurysm patients was not due to aneurysm-related mortality.

Determinants of Late Survival

The principal factors determining long-term survival after identification or initially successful repair of AAAs are not aneurysm related. As would be anticipated, predictors of diminished long-term survival include age at the time of surgery, abnormal renal function, and the presence of cardiovascular disease.[1,147,148] Generally speaking, none of these factors are directly influenced by AAA repair. It is therefore not surprising that in extremely high-risk cohorts, in whom multiple negative prognostic factors often coexist, AAA repair may have no impact on survival.[24]

Although several of these reports included both infrarenal aneurysms and more complex AAAs, other reports have focused solely on long-term outcomes after repair of juxtarenal and suprarenal aneurysms. Martin and coauthors' report on 57 patients treated by suprarenal AAA repair at the Cleveland Clinic included 49 patients undergoing elective surgery, as well as 108 patients with Crawford types III and IV aneurysms.[143] Kaplan-Meier survival estimates for the entire series were 71% at 3 years and 50% at 10 years, with cause of death in long-term follow-up again being due to cardiovascular, pulmonary, and renal causes. Crawford and colleagues had previously reported 64% 3-year and 60% 5-year survival rates in patients undergoing thoracoabdominal repair, with late rupture of another aneurysm accounting for 12% of the deaths.[20] Both reports suggest that malignant disease is a less common cause of death and that cardiovascular disease is more common as a late cause of death than is infrarenal aneurysm.

Functional Outcome

Open AAA repair results in a significant early decrease in functional capability. Williamson and coauthors reported that 11% of previously ambulatory patients required transfer on discharge to a skilled nursing facility with an average length of stay of 3.7 months.[155] Of all patients treated, at 2 years' follow-up, 64% of the patients remained ambulatory, 22% required assistance, and 14% were nonambulatory. A third of the patients reported a decrease in functional activities such as shopping, driving, or traveling in comparison to their preoperative status. Two thirds of patients reported complete recovery by 3.9 months; however, the remainder thought that they had not fully recovered by 34 months. Eighteen percent of patients said that they would not undergo AAA repair again because of the recovery process. Arko and associates reported that after open AAA repair, 26% of patients required skilled nursing facility care on discharge and had an average recovery time of 99 days.[156] After 6 months, 75% of the patients were fully recovered, with activity levels decreased in 23%.

Prinssen and coauthors reported that open surgical repair compares favorably with EVAR as determined by Short Form (36) Health Survey (SF-36) and Euro-QoL-5D questionnaires at five time points in the first postoperative year.[157] In the early postoperative period there was a small yet significant advantage for EVAR. However, at 6 months and beyond, patients reported higher quality of life scores after open repair than after EVAR.

It remains uncertain, however, to what extent aneurysm surgery contributes to declining functional outcomes. Advancing age and co-morbid conditions also contribute to reductions in quality of life. ADAM trial data suggest that any difference in quality of life between open and EVAR treatment groups is small based on SF-36 health status questionnaires for the physical and mental subscales, with all showing a substantial decline in follow-up regardless of treatment group. The UKSAT used a similar questionnaire and found that for the surveillance subgroup, physical functioning, role functioning, social functioning, and body pain scores decreased in the initial 12 months after randomization. For patients randomized to early AAA repair, only physical functioning decreased, but health perception scores improved significantly.

Metachronous Aneurysms

A report from the Mayo Clinic identified 1112 patients who underwent AAA repair between 1970 and 1976. As expected, the most frequent cause of late death was coronary artery disease (46%).[158] Vascular lesions ultimately occurred in 94 patients and resulted in 8.4% of all late deaths. Forty-nine true, 14 anastomotic, and 5 dissecting aneurysms were detected in 5.4% of patients at a mean of 5.2 years after the initial aneurysm surgery. After a mean follow-up of 7.2 years in a contemporary group of 152 patients undergoing AAA repair, a Massachusetts General Hospital study found new aneurysms outside the surgically repaired aortic segment in nearly a quarter of the patients, thus underscoring the importance of continued surveillance directed toward the detection of other aneurysms.[159]

■ POSTOPERATIVE COMPLICATIONS

Early Complications

Many of the complications that occur early after AAA repair are common after any major surgical procedure. Because of the increased prevalence of preexisting atherosclerotic arterial disease and underlying pulmonary dysfunction in patients with AAA, the frequency of early postoperative complications, including myocardial infarction, acute pulmonary decompensation resulting in pneumonia or reintubation, and renal dysfunction, is also elevated. The cause of these problems and

potential interventions to reduce their severity or rates of occurrence are discussed in Section 6 (Complications). Three problems specifically related to conduct of the aortic procedure are addressed further in the following sections.

Colon Ischemia

A feared complication after aortic surgery is colon ischemia. Though uncommon after elective aortic operations, the mortality associated with AAA repair complicated by colon ischemia remains high (40% to 65%),[159] so vigilance and early recognition are essential. Colonic ischemia is much more common (7% to 27% clinically, up to 60% endoscopically) after repair of a ruptured AAA than after elective aneurysm surgery (0.6% to 3%).[96,98,160-164]

Clinical Findings. A high index of suspicion is essential inasmuch as pain is an unreliable marker because of incisional discomfort and the use of narcotic analgesia. Findings potentially suggestive of ischemic colitis include persistent acidosis and shock, increased immature white blood cells, elevated lactate levels, fluid sequestration,[165] or bloody bowel movements. Early identification is essential because progression to full-thickness necrosis is associated with mortality rates of 80% to 100%.[166] A network of collaterals from the SMA, IMA, internal iliac artery, and profunda femoris artery supply the sigmoid colon (Fig. 128-20). Bast and coworkers demonstrated that IMA stump pressure decreased from 61% to 58% of systemic pressure with transient clamping of the internal iliac arteries after AAA repair,[167] thus re-enforcing the notion of multiple robust collateral pathways for colon perfusion.

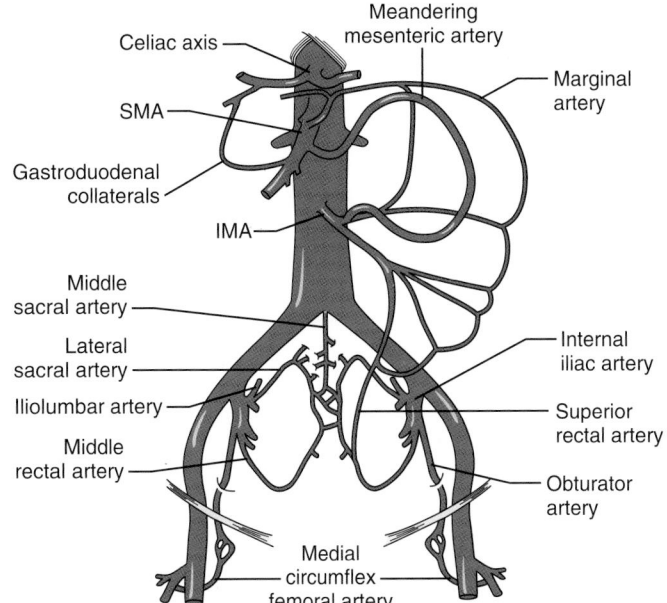

Figure 128-20 Multiple arterial pathways provide collateral blood supply to the sigmoid colon should the inferior mesenteric artery (IMA) be occluded or ligated at its origin during the conduct of open abdominal aortic aneurysm repair. SMA, superior mesenteric artery.

Aneurysm repair can compromise sigmoid blood flow by ligation of a patent IMA or internal iliac artery, embolization of debris into these arteries, prolonged hypotension, or injury to important collateral branches. Bowel infarction is infrequent because of the extensive collateral arterial pathways.

Evaluation and Treatment.

Systemic signs of infection or the occurrence of bloody rectal discharge should prompt urgent evaluation with a flexible sigmoidoscope.[98] The classic finding of bloody diarrhea in the early postoperative period occurs in only about 30% of cases,[162] with a significant proportion of patients exhibiting no symptoms at all.[167] Flexible sigmoidoscopy has been found to be a reliable determinant of colonic ischemia after ruptured AAA repair[168] and is important in guiding subsequent treatment. Patients with nonconfluent ischemia limited to the mucosa can be safely monitored by serial endoscopic examinations, whereas those with full-thickness ischemia should be treated by colonic resection after operative confirmation of the endoscopic findings.

Boley and colleagues described three forms of ischemic colitis. The mildest, most common form results in ischemia limited to the colonic mucosa and submucosa. Patients may have symptoms of abdominal pain, ileus, distention, or bloody diarrhea, but the disease resolves with adequate resuscitation and bowel rest alone. A more moderate form involves ischemia of the muscularis and may eventually result in ischemic stricture formation. The most severe form of colonic ischemia involves transmural ischemia and colonic infarction and fortunately is least common. Should it occur, however, bowel resection with fecal diversion, creation of an ostomy, and washout of the abdomen is required, ideally before perforation and abdominal soilage or sepsis occur, and is associated with risk for infection of the newly placed prosthetic graft.[169,170] In all forms of colonic ischemia, broad-spectrum antibiotic therapy is routinely initiated as well. Clinically insignificant colonic ischemia occurs at greater frequency than is often appreciated. Routine endoscopic surveillance studies have reported an incidence of 4.5% to 11.4% in patients after elective AAA repair,[170,171] whereas biopsy of the mucosa has identified ischemic changes in 30% of patients after aortic surgery, with half the patients having no macroscopically apparent ischemic changes.[172]

Lower Extremity Ischemia

At the conclusion of AAA repair, the peripheral pulses or Doppler signals are evaluated and compared with the preoperative status before leaving the operating room. Although some diminution in peripheral pulses will occasionally occur because of hypothermia or proximal redistribution secondary to ischemia/reperfusion, a reduced pulse requires either careful monitoring to ensure return of adequate perfusion within a few hours or additional surgery to treat new sites of thrombosis or embolization before leaving the operating room.

Arterial thrombosis can occur as a result of limited perfusion during periods of proximal clamping. It can be mini-mized by adequate anticoagulation during clamping and vigorous antegrade and retrograde flushing before completion of each anastomosis. Embolization of atheroemboli or macroscopic debris also occurs. Atheroembolization can usually be avoided by judicious clamp placement in nondiseased arterial segments. CT scanning helps select appropriate sites for clamp placement, and intraoperative palpation confirms the absence of disease. Macroembolization most commonly results when preexistent aortoiliac thrombus or plaque is inadequately removed from iliac outflow vessels. Direct inspection of the iliac arterial lumen with removal of macroscopic debris and vigorous flushing typically suffices to prevent this complication.

Spinal Cord Ischemia

Spinal cord ischemia can result in a range of clinical manifestations from mild transient paraparesis to permanent flaccid paralysis. Spinal cord ischemia is a rare complication after infrarenal aortic surgery.[173-181] Spinal cord ischemia after infrarenal abdominal aortic surgery appears to be an unpredictable and unpreventable event. Fortunately, even in patients with a more proximal extent of their AAAs, the risk remains quite small. Risk for paraplegia is directly related to the proximal extent of the aneurysm and the potential loss of previously patent internal iliac arteries.[143] A complex interplay of anatomic and surgical factors is responsible for maintaining or disrupting blood supply to the spinal cord. Some of these factors include the level and duration of aortic cross-clamping, interruption of the spinal cord blood supply via the artery of Adamkiewicz (greater medullary artery), the presence of intraoperative or postoperative episodes of hypotension, atheromatous embolization, and the absence of other adequate collateral vessels (radiculomedullary arteries other than the greater medullary artery, anterior spinal artery, or internal iliac arteries).[182] Although many of these factors are not under control of the operating surgeon, occlusion or division of these vessels combined with periods of severe hypotension can lead to spinal cord ischemia.[183] A discussion of the techniques of spinal cord protection can be found in Chapter 132 (Thoracic and Thoracoabdominal Aneurysms: Open Surgical Treatment).

Late Complications

Incisional Hernia or Bulge

While the molecular basis underlying AAA development is currently being unraveled, the propensity toward reduced tissue integrity in AAA patients is unmistakable. The finding of diastasis rectus is common on examination, and inguinal and other abdominal wall hernias occur with greater frequency in AAA patients than in patients with aortoiliac occlusive disease. It is not surprising, then, that after open AAA repair, incisional problems occur with increased frequency. Most series report a threefold to fivefold increase in postoperative incisional hernia in AAA patients when compared with cohorts with occlusive disease: greater than 10% (AAA patients) versus approximately 3% (aortoiliac occlusive disease).[184-187] Although careful surgical technique is always essential, this predilection for incisional hernia in aneurysm patients does not appear to be under the control of the operating surgeon. One common complaint related to the RP approach is the development of a flank bulge. Imaging studies typically reveal marked asymmetry with significant attenuation and muscular atrophy of the flank wall. Understanding the cause of this problem was aided by work from Gardner and associates, who noted that a bulge developed in 11% of patients after left RP incisions: in 19% of patients with incisions into the 11th intercostal space versus 3% of patients with incisions that avoided extension into the intercostal space.[188] Matsen and colleagues prospectively evaluated 50 patients and identified a 56% incidence 1 year after aortic reconstruction.[189] In 43% of these patients the bulge was deemed mild (<1-inch protrusion), and in 54% it was moderate (protrusion of 1 of 2 inches). Increased body mass index (>23) and incision length (>15 cm) correlated with bulge occurrence. Ballard and coworkers also reported a strong correlation between body mass index and risk for an RP incisional bulge, which occurred in 8% of patients whose incision extended from the tip of the 12th rib and spared the rectus muscles.[190] Treatment of incisional hernia typically involves wound reclosure with mesh re-enforcement. We have treated most symptomatic patients with RP bulges with a supportive binder and reserved flank wall reconstruction with mesh re-enforcement for the few patients with disabling symptoms or large defects.

Anastomotic Aneurysm and Other Graft-Related Complications

Anastomotic disruption can result in pseudoaneurysm formation and typically occurs as a result of continued arterial degeneration. Szilagyi and coauthors reported that anastomotic pseudoaneurysm occurred in 0.2% of aortic anastomoses, 1.2% of iliac anastomoses, and 3% of femoral anastomosis after 3 years.[174] Using yearly sonograms for surveillance of both patients with AAA and those with aortic occlusive disease treated surgically, Edwards and colleagues reported an incidence of aortic pseudoaneurysms of just 1% after 8 years but 20% after 15 years, with the average time to detection of a pseudoaneurysm being 12 years.[191] Hallett and coworkers reported anastomotic pseudoaneurysms in 4% of patients after 10 years.[192] In a subset of 94 of the original 680 patients from the Canadian Aneurysm Study willing to undergo a CT scan 8 to 9 years after AAA repair, proximal pseudoaneurysms were detected in 10% of patients.[193] Because these studies may include patients with anastomoses constructed with suture materials such as silk, with grafts fabrics no longer in use, or without the current emphasis on creation of anastomoses to completely normal aortic tissue, it is unclear whether contemporary open AAA repair patients remain at similar risk. Hertzer and associates reported on 1047 patients who survived their operations and remained available for follow-up study and commented on "the exemplary success of open infrarenal AAA repair."[4] The Cleveland Clinic practice was to

obtain a contrast-enhanced CT scan of the descending thoracic aorta and the visceral aortic segment every 3 to 5 years to rule out the possibility of new proximal aneurysms. At an average follow-up of 57 months, only four late graft complications (0.4%) were identified. Two graft infections, one graft limb occlusion, and one femoral pseudoaneurysm occurred and required operative treatment. Despite their low incidence, aortic pseudoaneurysms progressively enlarge and present a risk for rupture, so follow-up imaging studies may be appropriate to detect late asymptomatic pseudoaneurysms. It has been our practice to encourage surveillance imaging every 5 years after AAA repair to detect both anastomotic aneurysms and new sites of aneurysm formation in the thoracic and abdominal aorta.

In an update on the original Mayo Clinic report on graft-related complications, Hallett and coauthors reported on 307 patients who had undergone previous AAA repair between 1957 and 1990.[192] All patients were asked to undergo new aortic imaging studies. With follow-up as long as 36 years after the original procedure (mean of 5.8 years), 9.4% of patients had a graft-related complication identified, including 6.8% occurring in late follow-up. The lesions identified included anastomotic pseudoaneurysm (3.0%), graft thrombosis (2.0%), graft-enteric erosion/fistula (1.6%), graft infection (1.3%), anastomotic hemorrhage (1.3%), colon ischemia (0.7%), and atheroembolism (0.3%). The Canadian Aneurysm Study report on 680 patients with 6-year follow-up identified only three graft-related deaths (1.5%) in 205 cases.[148] A smaller study of 521 patients from Munich, Germany, undergoing elective AAA surgery found 1 patient who died of graft-related causes (0.2%) at 10 years of follow-up.[194] Other international series include reports from Japan, with no deaths from graft-related complications after AAA repair,[195] and from Finland, where 1.9% of late deaths were attributable to graft-related complications.[196] The Finnish series also reported late graft-related complications in 32 patients (15.4%), including proximal para-anastomotic pseudoaneurysms (2.9%) and distal pseudoaneurysms (8.7%); in 3.4% of patients the problem was bilateral or recurrent. Graft limb occlusion occurred in 5.3% of patients.

The most contemporary report consists of 152 patients operated on at the Massachusetts General Hospital between 1994 and 1998.[159] Surveillance imaging (CT and magnetic resonance imaging [MRI]) was obtained at a mean follow-up of 87 months. Late graft-related complications were identified in 2% of patients (mean follow-up, 7.2 years), including seven anastomotic pseudoaneurysms, four graft limb occlusions, and two graft infections.

◼ SPECIAL CONSIDERATIONS

Inflammatory Abdominal Aortic Aneurysms

Inflammatory AAAs are characterized by perianeurysmal fibrosis and inflammation, which results in marked thickening of the aneurysm wall that typically involves the anterior and lateral aspects most extensively. The inflammatory response results in adhesions to adjacent structures, specifically the duodenum and left renal vein anteriorly and the ureters.[197-199] Although hypervascularity and inflammatory changes of a mild form generally surround any aortic aneurysm,[166] this degree of intense inflammation is clinically identified in only approximately 5% of AAAs.[200] The etiology is unclear, although proposed causes include exacerbation of the standard perianeurysmal inflammatory response, chronic subacute rupture, or a variant form of RP fibrosis. Interestingly, treatment of the aneurysm often resolves the periaortic inflammation,[201,202] thus suggesting that the aortic pathology may be the cause of rather than a response to the inflammatory process. Resolution of the periaortic inflammation occurs after EVAR,[203] as well as after open aneurysm repair. The indications for repair of an inflammatory aneurysm are identical to those for noninflammatory aneurysms because the thickened aortic wall does not appear to protect against the risk for aortic rupture.

Diagnosis

Patients with inflammatory AAAs are nearly always symptomatic (93%),[202] with abdominal, back, or flank pain pain[197] and tenderness on aneurysm palpation.[198] Systemic complaints such as a febrile illness or weight loss are common. An elevated sedimentation rate is also routinely present.[202,204] The thick periaortic inflammatory process is readily identified as an enhancing rim surrounding the aorta with the standard techniques of contrast-enhanced CTA and MRA routinely obtained before any open aortic surgery.[41]

Surgical Treatment

Intraoperatively, from a transperitoneal approach, the anterior surface of the aortic wall has a characteristic pearly white appearance, with the duodenum (up 90% of cases) and left renal vein (50%) densely adherent to the aortic wall.[41,205] Attempts to dissect these structures free from the inflammatory mass can result in damage to the bowel wall with resultant contamination or bleeding. The inflammation can also involve the ureters (25%),[205,206] which can result in ureteral obstruction, draw them into unexpected portions of the surgical field, and make recognition of them difficult. These changes enhance the likelihood of ureteral injury during the course of aortic surgery. For these reasons, preoperative recognition of an inflammatory aneurysm is essential because alterations in approach can reduce some of the risk of injury to adjacent organ.[204]

Ureter Management. We consider placement of ureteral stents in all patients undergoing open repair of an inflammatory aneurysm, even those without ureteral obstruction, both to aid in identification of the ureter and to recognize ureteral injury promptly should it occur. An RP approach is considered standard management because it allows the surgeon to avoid injuring adherent structures and facilitates suprarenal

clamp placement in approximately 40% of patients in whom the inflammatory process makes infrarenal clamping unsafe.[207] Even in the setting of ureteral obstruction, ureterolysis is to be eschewed. Instead, ureteral obstruction is managed with an indwelling ureteral stent, which can be left in place until the inflammatory process resolves after AAA repair. Ureterolysis in patients with obstructive uropathy has not been demonstrated to result in improvement in renal function when compared with stent placement alone.[206,208]

Results

Elective operative mortality for inflammatory AAA repair is similar to that for noninflammatory aneurysms, although the risk for operative complications is increased.[199,202,204,207] The inflammatory changes resolve completely after AAA repair in most (53%) patients, but 47% have persistent inflammation, with involvement of the ureters in 32%.[202] Although prednisone treatment of inflammatory AAAs can reduce the fibrotic reaction,[209] its use should be reserved for the small percentage of patients after aneurysm repair who continue to manifest significant obstructive problems related to the persistent inflammatory condition.

Infected Abdominal Aortic Aneurysms

Primary infection of the abdominal aorta is an uncommon clinical entity that has been reported in only 0.65% of more than 6000 aneurysm repairs over a 30-year experience from the Henry Ford Hospital.[210] An infected AAA can result from a secondary infection of an established aneurysm.[211,212] Alternatively, aneurysmal degeneration can occur as a result of infection of a previously nonaneurysmal aortic segment. Most often, this occurs in the setting of underlying aortic wall abnormalities, such as severe atherosclerosis or calcification, which appears to facilitate localization and growth of infectious agents in nonaneurysmal but diseased portions of the aortic wall.[213] Potential causes of aneurysm infection can be contiguous spread of local infection, septic embolization from a distant site, or bacteremia. The microbiology of infected aortic aneurysms continues to change; it has evolved from syphilis and streptococcal species in the past to a predominance of staphylococcal and *Salmonella* infections today.[212-218] In the contemporary era with widespread antibiotic use and a growing number of immunocompromised patients, essentially any bacterial or fungal infection can lead to an infected aneurysm. Chapter 139 (Infected Aneurysms) provides greater detail on the topic of infected aneurysms.

Diagnosis and Treatment

The clinical entity of an infected aortic aneurysm must be differentiated from the finding of a positive culture of the aortic wall or thrombus obtained from asymptomatic patients during routine aortic surgery. In a series of 500 patients, Farkas and coauthors reported positive culture results in 185 patients (37%).[219] After an average follow-up interval of 35 months, in only a single patients did an aortic graft infection develop (6 years later) from a different organism than was cultured at the time of the original aneurysm repair.

The majority of patients (93%) with an infected aortic aneurysm are symptomatic,[212] but the initial clinical findings of an aortic infection are nonspecific, so the diagnosis is often delayed. Fever (76%),[212,213] abdominal or back pain (66%),[213] elevated sedimentation rate (86%),[212] bacteremia, and a pulsatile abdominal mass or aneurysm on imaging studies should suggest an infected AAA. A high index of suspicion is required, and an aneurysm can arise rapidly in a previously nonaneurysmal aortic segment.[220,221] Even in the absence of other clinical findings supportive of the diagnosis, a noncalcified, saccular aneurysm in an otherwise normal-appearing aorta should at least prompt consideration of a primary infected AAA, particularly if its location is atypical. Surgical options are discussed in Chapter 139 (Infected Aneurysms).

Venous Anomalies

Venous anomalies are uncommon but important anatomic variants. Their reported incidence varies depending on the means of detection and ranges from 1.5% (35 patients) in a series of 2427 aneurysm patients treated at the Mayo Clinic[222] to as high as 10% in radiologic series. Circumaortic left renal veins, also referred to as persistent renal venous collars, occur most commonly, followed in decreasing frequency by a retroaortic left renal vein and duplicated IVC. Accessory left renal veins and a preaortic IVC or iliac venous confluence are extremely rare. Their importance lies in their recognition preoperatively because failure to do so can result in torrential hemorrhage and even death. Eight of 35 patients in a series from the Mayo Clinic had significant venous hemorrhage because of injury to the anomalous vein, with 7 of these patients not having a preoperative diagnosis of the anomaly. In patients with circumaortic left renal veins, intraoperative recognition is difficult because the anterior component of the left renal vein is frequently stretched tightly across the aneurysm neck and dissection behind the aorta for clamp positioning is often done blindly after digital dissection of the tissues. With retroaortic left renal veins, absence of the typical landmark of the left renal vein overlying the planned proximal clamp zone should alert the operator to this anomaly.

Even after recognition it is important to note that two types of aberrant anatomy have been described and occur with roughly equal frequency. In one type, the retroaortic vein enters the IVC in an orthotopic position, whereas in the second type the vein runs more caudal and joins the IVC and gonadal and ascending lumbar veins, typically at the L4-L5 level.

Surgical techniques for addressing each of these venous anomalies must be individualized to each patient's aberrant anatomy and include alteration of aortic or iliac artery clamp position, retraction of the vein, or ligation and division of the anomalous vein.[223-226] Finally, it must be emphasized that careful review of the preoperative CT scan will delineate virtually all these venous anomalies.

Management of Concomitant Intra-abdominal Pathology

Identification of a second significant pathologic condition in association with an aortic aneurysm, such as cholelithiasis or pulmonary, gastrointestinal, or renal neoplasms, is frequent. Overall guidelines are to treat the most life-threatening process first and avoid simultaneous operations that increase the risk for prosthetic graft infection. Prioritization is determined by the urgency of addressing each of the identified conditions. For example, a nearly obstructing colorectal malignancy deserves to be addressed before elective surgery for a 5.5-cm infrarenal aneurysm. In addition, characterization of the secondary lesion may also have an impact on decision making regarding aneurysm repair. Identification and resection of a lung mass found to be an aggressive malignancy may ultimately result in a decision to avoid any surgical therapy for the aneurysm given the patient's abbreviated life expectancy. Alternatively, the findings may sway treatment options in favor of EVAR[227] to shorten the recovery period between surgeries or to avoid intra-abdominal surgery and make a subsequent intraperitoneal procedure more challenging.[228] In patients in whom treatment of the secondary procedure can be staged without increased risk, aneurysm repair should take priority. Simultaneous prosthetic graft placement and gastrointestinal tract operations should be avoided. The presence of cholelithiasis is associated with a low risk for progression to acute cholecystitis in the immediate perioperative period,[229] although subsequent cholecystectomy is often required.[230]

With the availability of laparoscopic surgery and other minimally invasive therapies such as cryoablation for conditions including renal lesions, treatment of the nonaortic problem can frequently precede open aneurysm repair with only a brief hiatus between the two procedures. Clean procedures such as renal resection[227,228] or oophorectomy can be performed simultaneously with open AAA repair, ideally after closure of the aneurysm sac and retroperitoneum over the prosthetic graft. Rupture of aortic aneurysms has been reported to occur after unrelated surgical procedures,[231] most commonly in patients with larger aortic aneurysms.[232] In these patients, AAA repair should be considered soon after the preceding operation, potentially during the same hospitalization. Occasionally, an unsuspected intra-abdominal problem is discovered during aneurysm repair. Typically, the AAA reconstruction should proceed. Exceptions to this rule, however, would be findings associated with an increased risk for prosthetic graft infection such an abscess or metastatic disease. In these settings, aneurysm repair should be abandoned. Fortunately, this is uncommon in the contemporary era of high-resolution preoperative imaging studies.

■ ISOLATED ILIAC ARTERY ANEURYSMS

Isolated iliac aneurysms, referring to iliac aneurysms without involvement of the abdominal aorta, constitute 0.6% to 2.0% of abdominal aortoiliac aneurysms.[233,234] Aneurysmal degeneration typically involves the common iliac (70% to 90%) or internal iliac (10% to 30%) arteries or both together[235,236]; external iliac artery involvement is rare. Bilateral common iliac artery aneurysms are identified approximately 50% of the time.[237]

Clinical Findings

Although their location makes detection by physical examination challenging, larger iliac aneurysms may sometimes be identified during abdominal, rectal, or pelvic examination.[236] Even though older reports suggest that iliac aneurysms are frequently symptomatic,[234] today they are often identified incidentally during abdominal imaging studies performed for other reasons. As a result, an increasing number of smaller, asymptomatic iliac aneurysms are now routinely being detected.[238] Larger aneurysms may have vague findings, typically caused by compression of adjacent pelvic structures. In symptomatic patients, the diagnosis is frequently delayed until the aneurysm is large and imaging studies finally reveal the cause of the complaint.[236] Local compression or erosive problems that affect adjacent pelvic structures can lead to ureteral obstruction, hematuria, iliac vein thrombosis, bowel obstruction, or neurologic deficit.[239]

Natural History

Before the era of widespread use of CT and MRI, larger isolated iliac aneurysms were more often initially found to have ruptured,[240] with a high resultant mortality rate.[236] Several reports have helped to more clearly define the natural history of isolated iliac aneurysms. Kasirajan and coauthors reported that none of the iliac aneurysms between 2.0 and 2.5 cm expanded in follow-up averaging 57 months but that a significant risk for rupture existed in patients with iliac aneurysms larger than 5.0 cm.[241] The authors suggested that surgical treatment was appropriate for aneurysms larger than 3 cm. Santilli and colleagues identified 189 patients with 323 iliac aneurysms in a report from a large U.S. Veterans Affairs hospital.[238] Symptoms occurred in just six patients (3.1%), including two ruptures, all with aneurysms larger than 4.0 cm. Smaller aneurysms (<3.0 cm) expanded more slowly than larger (3 to 5 cm) ones (11 versus 26 mm/yr). The authors concluded that (1) iliac aneurysms smaller than 3.0 cm could be monitored by annual ultrasound surveillance, (2) aneurysms 3.0 to 3.5 cm could be monitored with imaging every 6 months, and (3) aneurysms larger than 3.5 cm in good-risk patients should be considered for repair. Sandhu and Pipinos analyzed reports on patients with 473 isolated iliac aneurysms treated by open repair between the years 1985 and 2001. Sixty-three percent of patients were symptomatic, including 31% with rupture.[242] For emergency open surgery, mortality averaged 28%, whereas for elective operations it averaged 5%. Although not all anatomic variants can be treated with an endovascular approach, most contemporary series suggest endoluminal therapy as the preferred treatment route, with excellent initial outcomes being reported. Chapter 129

(Abdominal Aortic Aneurysms: Endovascular Treatment) addresses endoluminal treatment of aortoiliac aneurysms in depth.

Surgical Treatment

The approach to open surgical repair is determined by the presence of aortic dilatation or a contralateral iliac artery aneurysm. When the abdominal aorta is normal and iliac involvement is unilateral, simple interposition graft placement via either a TA or an RP approach ipsilateral to the side of the aneurysm is a reasonable option. However, if iliac involvement is bilateral, a TA approach is preferred. In the presence of early aneurysmal degeneration (ectasia) of the aorta, replacement of both the aorta and the aneurysmal iliac arteries is suggested because continued aortic expansion is likely. If aneurysmal degeneration involves the common iliac artery to its bifurcation, creation of the distal anastomosis to encompass the orifices of both the internal and external iliac arteries can be difficult, and preservation of flow into at least one internal iliac artery is considered essential. In AAA patients with an occluded IMA, colon perfusion is further decreased by occlusion of the internal iliac arteries,[243] although experience with EVAR suggests that bilateral internal iliac artery occlusion can be tolerated in many patients.[244] Because of collateral flow across the pelvis between the internal iliac artery branches, proximal ligation of an internal iliac aneurysm without distal ligation, endovascular occlusion, or endoaneurysmorrhaphy may result in persistent aneurysm expansion or rupture.[245] In the absence of contralateral internal iliac artery aneurysm or occlusion, internal iliac artery aneurysms are typically addressed endoluminally with embolization of outflow branches, filling of the aneurysm sac with coils, and exclusion from inflow with a covered stent. Open surgical treatment of internal iliac artery aneurysms with ligation of distal branches located deep in the pelvis can be challenging.

SELECTED KEY REFERENCES

Chaikof EL, Brewster DC, Dalman RL, Makaroun MS, Ellis KA, Sicard GA, Timaran CH, Upchurch GR. The care of patients with an abdominal aortic aneurysm: The Society for Vascular Surgery Practice Guidelines. *J Vasc Surg.* 2009;50:25-495.
SVS guidelines for decision-making for elective repair of abdominal aortic aneurysms including AAA size as well as assessment of factors that influence rupture risk, operative mortality, and life expectancy.

Conrad MF, Crawford RS, Pedraza JD, Brewster DC, Lamuraglia GM, Corey M, Abbara S, Cambria RP. Long-term durability of open abdominal aortic aneurysm repair. *J Vasc Surg.* 2007;46:669-675.
Open repair is a safe and durable option for the management of abdominal aortic aneurysms, with the freedom from graft-related reintervention superior to EVAR.

Johnston KW. Multicenter prospective study of nonruptured abdominal aortic aneurysm. Part II. Variables predicting morbidity and mortality. *J Vasc Surg.* 1989;9:437-447.
This article details the perioperative complications and their associated variables for patients undergoing open AAA repair.

Johnston KW. Nonruptured abdominal aortic aneurysm: six-year follow-up results from the multicenter prospective Canadian aneurysm study. Canadian Society for Vascular Surgery Aneurysm Study Group. *J Vasc Surg*. 1994;20:163-170.
Long-term outcomes after open AAA repair identified rare aneurysm-related deaths, with an increased risk of heart-related and stroke mortality.

Johnston KW, Rutherford RB, Tilson MD, Shah DM, Hollier L, Stanley JC. Suggested standards for reporting on arterial aneurysms. Subcommittee on Reporting Standards for Arterial Aneurysms, Ad Hoc Committee on Reporting Standards, Society for Vascular Surgery and North American Chapter, International Society for Cardiovascular Surgery. *J Vasc Surg*. 1991;13:452-458.
This article defines and classifies arterial aneurysms and recommends standards for describing the causes, manifestations, treatment, and outcome criteria.

Knott AW, Kalra M, Duncan AA, Reed NR, Bower TC, Hoskin TL, Oderich GS, Gloviczki P. Open repair of juxtarenal aortic aneurysms (JAA) remains a safe option in the era of fenestrated endografts. *J Vasc Surg*. 2008;47:695-701.
Report from the Mayo Clinic on outcomes of patients undergoing juxtarenal AAA repair.

Lederle FA, Johnson GR, Wilson SE, Chute EP, Hye RJ, Makaroun MS, Barone GW, Bandyk D, Moneta GL, Makhoul RG. The aneurysm detection and management study screening program: validation cohort and final results. Aneurysm Detection and Management Veterans Affairs Cooperative Study Investigators. *Arch Intern Med*. 2000;160:1425-1430.
US Veterans Administration trial of ultrasound surveillance and delayed surgery versus early operation for 4.0-5.5 cm aortic aneurysms.

Schermerhorn ML, O'Malley AJ, Jhaveri A, Cotterill P, Pomposelli F, Landon BE. Endovascular vs. open repair of abdominal aortic aneurysms in the Medicare population. *N Engl J Med*. 2008;358:464-474.
Report of US Medicare population outcomes comparing patients treated by open versus endovascular repair.

Sicard GA, Reilly JM, Rubin BG, Thompson RW, Allen BT, Flye MW, Schechtman KB, Young-Beyer P, Weiss C, Anderson CB. Transabdominal versus retroperitoneal incision for abdominal aortic surgery: report of a prospective randomized trial. *J Vasc Surg*. 1995;21:174-181; discussion 181-183.
Single institution report suggesting potential advantages of a retroperitoneal approach to AAA repair.

Young EL, Holt PJ, Poloniecki JD, Loftus IM, Thompson MM. Meta-analysis and systematic review of the relationship between surgeon annual caseload and mortality for elective open abdominal aortic aneurysm repairs. *J Vasc Surg*. 2007;46:1287-1294.
Meta-analysis of six series including more than 115,000 patients demonstrating improved outcomes for surgeons performing higher volumes of open AAA repair.

REFERENCES

The reference list can be found on the companion Expert Consult Web site at *www.expertconsult.com*.

Section 17 Arterial Aneurysms

Abdominal Aortic Aneurysms: Endovascular Treatment

Timothy A. M. Chuter and Darren Schneider

The field of endovascular aneurysm repair (EVAR) is a relatively new addition to the vascular surgery armamentarium. The necessary techniques and technology are still evolving, and papers on the subject are just snapshots of a moving object. The accumulated literature on EVAR offers little basis for sweeping conclusions regarding the field as a whole or even the current state of the art. Only a few studies provide level 1 evidence, and most published data relate only to specific devices and specific anatomy.

DEVICE AND TECHNIQUE DEVELOPMENT

EVAR did not enter the collective surgical consciousness until 1990, when Parodi and colleagues presented a small clinical series.[1] The importance of Parodi's presentation and subsequent paper on the subject cannot be overstated. Had vascular surgeons not heeded this wake-up call and started to acquire endovascular skills, it is possible that they would have been spectators, not participants, in the endovascular revolution.

Yet the idea of EVAR was far from new, even in 1990. No invention arises in a vacuum. There is almost always some "prior art" in the form of related ideas and devices, and most inventions depend on other enabling technologies. In the case of EVAR, the prior art included a variety of endovascular grafts, stents, and other graft attachment devices, whereas the enabling technology included arterial catheters, sheaths, guide wires, and fluoroscopic imaging.

Landmarks

Key landmarks in the development of EVAR are shown in Table 129-1.[2-10] This listing omits commercial devices that are no longer available and investigational devices that have yet to achieve widespread application, not that these unlisted devices are unimportant. One might argue that the failings of obsolete devices had more impact on the development of the field than did the purported advantages of those that remain in clinical use. The listed chronology relates to the year of first presentation or publication. The dates of conception and application are often difficult to establish to everyone's satisfaction, especially when these details determine intellectual property rights.

The results of endovascular repair of abdominal aortic aneurysms (AAAs) have improved steadily over the past 15 years[11] as the lessons of clinical experience were incorporated into system design.[11-22] Unfortunately, preclinical testing failed to identify many important failure modes because the rigors of the endovascular environment were poorly understood and there were few data relating the physical properties of a stent-graft to its long-term performance. As one might

Table 129-1 Key Events in the Development of Endovascular Aneurysm Repair

Event	Year	Description
New devices (experimental)	1951	Aneurysm wiring and electrocoagulation of the aneurysm sac[2]
	1969	Stent for arterial stenosis[3]
	1984	Stent for endoluminal repair of a pseudoaneurysm[4]
	1986	Stent-graft implantation under direct visual control[5]
	1987	Stent-graft implantation under fluoroscopic control[6]
	1988	Percutaneous stent-graft for aneurysm repair[7]
	1990	Balloon-expandable stent-graft[8]
	1991	Bifurcated aortobiiliac stent-graft[9]
New devices (clinical)	1986	Self-expanding aortoaortic stent-graft[10]
	1990	Balloon-expandable aortoaortic stent-graft[1]
	1993	Unibody bifurcated aortobiiliac stent graft[15]
	1994	Modular bifurcated aortobiiliac stent graft[16]
	1997	Unibody branched stent-graft[38]
	1999	Fenestrated stent-graft[40]
	2000	Modular multibranched stent-graft[41]
Regulatory approval (Europe)	1996	AneuRx bifurcated aortobiiliac stent-graft
	1997	Excluder bifurcated aortobiiliac stent-graft
	1998	Talent bifurcated aortobiiliac stent-graft
	1999	Zenith bifurcated aortobiiliac stent-graft
	2001	Aorfix bifurcated aortobiiliac stent-graft
	2005	Anaconda bifurcated aortobiiliac stent-graft
Regulatory approval (United States)	1999	AneuRx bifurcated aortobiiliac stent-graft
	2002	Excluder bifurcated aortobiiliac stent-graft
	2003	Zenith bifurcated aortobiiliac stent-graft
	2004	New fabric for AneuRx
	2004	New fabric for Excluder
Randomized studies (start date)	1999	EVAR-1, EVAR-2, and DREAM
	2001	OVER

DREAM, Dutch Randomized Endovascular Aneurysm Management; OVER, Open versus Endovascular Repair.

expect, the iterative cycle of device design, clinical trial, observed failure, and redesign resolved short-term problems more quickly than long-term problems.

Bifurcated Devices

The first major advance was the realization that one could not eliminate AAA perfusion, pressurization, dilatation, and risk of rupture without attaching both ends of the graft securely to nondilated arteries above and below the aneurysm.[1,17,18] This requirement proved to be something of a limitation for the original aortoaortic designs because most AAAs extend all the way to the aortic bifurcation.[19] No single design change expanded the application of EVAR more than the development of bifurcated aortoiliac stent-grafts.[15-17,20] At present, most bifurcated stent-grafts have a modular design, although unibody designs seem to be staging a minor comeback.[22]

Delivery Systems

Other advances in the short-term safety and applicability of EVAR resulted from improvements in the methods of stent-graft delivery. First- and second-generation delivery systems were bulky, blunt ended, and stiff.[14] The development of narrow, tapered, over-the-wire delivery systems greatly reduced the rate of iliac artery trauma and permitted endovascular treatment in an increasing number of women, who often have small iliofemoral access arteries.

Improved Efficacy

Subsequent design changes have eliminated late failure modes, thereby improving the long-term efficacy and durability of EVAR. Important lessons of the early experience included the following observations: any potential for movement between the apex of a stent and the fabric of the graft will lead to graft erosion,[23-25] short intercomponent overlaps lead to disconnection,[25] friction alone is not enough to prevent migration,[26,27] and porous fabrics allow aneurysm pressurization and dilatation (endotension), even in the absence of persistent aneurysm perfusion (endoleak).[28,29]

Improved Applicability

Improvements in safety, durability, and efficacy have generally been matched by improvements in applicability.[12,30-34] First-generation designs performed well within a narrow range of anatomic requirements, whereas modern designs have been shown to perform well in most cases of AAA. Refinements in endovascular technique have further expanded the scope of EVAR, but there are limits. Some patients cannot be treated with standard infrarenal devices because their aneurysms encroach on the origins of vital branches to the abdominal and pelvic viscera. These patients require surgical bypass to affected branches or complex stent-grafts containing holes (fenestrations) or branches.[35-43]

Fenestrated and Branched Grafts

The most important advance in fenestrated technique involved the use of a bridging catheter to guide the placement of small fenestrations over the renal artery orifices, followed by the insertion of a bridging stent to maintain close apposition and alignment.[35,36]

The first branched stent-grafts had a unibody design, with all their branches sewn in place before insertion.[37-39] Ingenious as they were, the irreducible complexity of the unibody approach prevented widespread application. Modular branched stent-grafts, which are assembled in situ from multiple components, are simpler and more versatile.[40-43] Their branches, which consist of covered stents, are inserted one by one to connect a series of fenestrations or short cuffs on the main graft with the corresponding visceral artery lumina.

ENDOVASCULAR ABDOMINAL AORTIC ANEURYSM REPAIR

Anatomic Substrate

Nobody would argue that stent-mediated graft attachment is as secure or as hemostatic as a suture-mediated surgical anastomosis, especially in the absence of a long zone of overlap between the proximal end of the stent-graft and a segment of nondilated infrarenal aorta (the neck). Indeed, an adequate neck is one of the few absolute requirements for successful EVAR. Difficult access and compromised distal implantation sites may cause problems, but these are almost always surmountable by using a wide variety of relatively low-impact maneuvers (see Chapter 86: Technique: Endovascular Aneurysm Repair). Treatment of a proximal type I endoleak, on the other hand, escalates rapidly up the scale of invasiveness to the level of complex endovascular reconstruction with fenestrations and branches or to laparotomy with aortic cross-clamping or visceral bypass. These issues should be considered when the aortic neck is less than ideal[27,44-47] and the potential patient is too high risk to tolerate open conversion.

Definition of Success

In surgical aneurysm repair, the open aneurysm imposes an absolute intolerance for leakage that does not apply in EVAR. There can be no anastomotic leaks or patent lumbar arteries by the end of an open surgical repair. No such limitations apply in the case of EVAR. The aneurysm is intact and leakage into the intact aneurysm (endoleak) is usually without immediate consequences. However, even though endoleaks may not affect the safety of repair, they do affect efficacy.

The efficacy of EVAR depends on the following chain of events: an endoluminal graft connects the nondilated arteries proximal to an aneurysm to the nondilated arteries distal to the aneurysm, thereby excluding the aneurysm's walls from the arterial circulation, reducing the pressure within its sac,[48-50] and preventing dilatation[51,52] and rupture. In the years

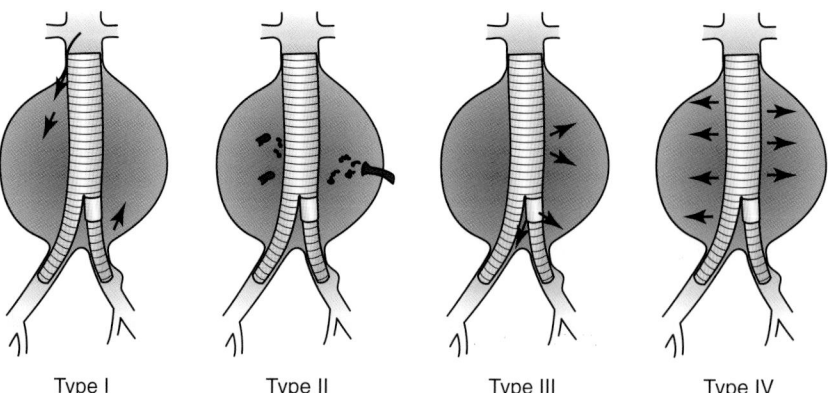

Figure 129-1 A type I endoleak (periprosthetic) occurs at the proximal or distal attachment zones (or at both). A type II endoleak is caused by retrograde flow from patent lumbar or inferior mesenteric arteries. A type III endoleak arises from a defect in the graft fabric, an inadequate seal, or disconnection of modular graft components. A type IV endoleak is due to graft fabric porosity, which often results in a generalized mild blush of contrast material within the aneurysm sac. (*From White GH, May J, Waugh RC, et al. Type III and type IV endoleak: toward a complete definition of blood flow in the sac after endoluminal AAA repair. J Endovasc Surg. 1998;5:305-309.*)

since stent-grafts were first used to treat aneurysms, each link of this chain has been examined and all the underlying assumptions found to be correct.

If this chain of causality is to remain intact, the first requirement is an absence of blood flow in the aneurysm sac. In the presence of an endoleak, one can assume that the aneurysm is still exposed to some arterial pressure and still at risk for dilatation and rupture.[50,51,53,54] Endoleaks have been categorized (Fig. 129-1) and subcategorized according to the location of the inflow.[55-57]

Types I and III Endoleak

A type I endoleak reaches the aneurysm around the end of the stent-graft, and a type III endoleak reaches the aneurysm through a defect in the wall of the stent-graft. Both these direct forms of endoleak are associated with high sac pressure,[51] aneurysm dilatation,[51] and aneurysm rupture.[58,59] Both may be considered indications of failed repair, hence their inclusion among the exclusion criteria for technical success.[57]

Type II Endoleak

Type II endoleak reaches the aneurysm by retrograde flow through lumbar or inferior mesenteric branches. The effects of this less direct form of endoleakage on sac pressure,[51] sac diameter,[51] and risk for rupture represent an intermediate state of partial treatment. EVAR may still be considered a technical and clinical success as long as a type II endoleak is not associated with aneurysm dilatation, aneurysm rupture, or re-intervention.

Type IV and V Endoleak

Type IV endoleak is a variant of type III endoleak characterized by diffuse leakage through the walls of the stent-graft

that resolves within a month of stent-graft insertion. The term *endotension* (also known as type V endoleak), originally coined to describe aneurysm pressurization leading to aneurysm dilatation,[60] was subsequently used to describe aneurysm pressurization in the absence of endoleak[61] and is now applied to cases of aneurysm dilatation in the absence of endoleak.[57] As if that were not confusing enough, there is a big overlap between endotension and type IV endoleak. Both are caused by a leaky stent-graft, and endotension eventually develops in many patients with type IV endoleak.[28,29,62]

Outcomes

Technical Success. Technical success is a short-term indication of satisfactory stent-graft insertion and function. In addition to the absence of direct (type I or III) endoleak, qualifiers for technical success include successful insertion and deployment of the stent-graft and the absence of significant twisting, kinks, or obstruction (>30% luminal stenosis or a pressure gradient >10 mm Hg) by intraoperative measurements.[57]

Clinical Success. Clinical success is an indication of ongoing stent-graft function. The criteria for clinical success include all the elements of technical success and exclude the following complications of EVAR or re-intervention for complications of EVAR: aneurysm-related death, aneurysm expansion (>5% volume, or >5-mm diameter), aneurysm rupture, surgical conversion, graft infection, graft migration, or failure of device integrity.[57]

Procedural Success. Procedural success is a term used mainly in industry-sponsored studies to describe the short-term outcome of stent-graft implantation. All that is required for procedural success is a live patient and a patent stent-graft in the intended position.

Many studies use aneurysm-related death as a primary endpoint.[63-68] This is a more precise endpoint than all-cause mortality because it allows the effects of aneurysm repair to be dissected from the effects of serious co-morbid conditions, which are prevalent among the elderly patients who have aortic aneurysms.

COMPARISON OF ENDOVASCULAR AND OPEN ANEURYSM SURGERY

Endovascular techniques and devices substitute transfemoral access to the aneurysm for direct transabdominal or retroperitoneal exposure and stent-mediated attachment for sutured anastomosis, thereby eliminating laparotomy, retroperitoneal dissection, and aortic cross-clamping, all of which are potential sources of physiologic stress, morbidity, and mortality. This difference changes the risk-benefit analysis entirely and accounts for the emergence of EVAR as an alternative to open surgery, even though the latter remains more effective, more durable, and less subject to anatomic constraints. Surgical repair is preferred for patients who have the physiologic reserve to tolerate laparotomy and aortic cross-clamping, whereas EVAR is preferred for patients who have a route of transfemoral access to the aneurysm and non-dilated arteries above and below the aneurysm for secure hemostatic stent-graft implantation. These preferences are even apparent in industry-sponsored, prospective comparisons of surgery and EVAR.[26,69-73] For example, pooled data in the Lifeline Registry showed that the surgical patients were younger (70 versus 73 years) and less likely to have coronary artery disease (59% versus 83%) or congestive heart failure (6% versus 10.5%) than the endovascular patients. Detailed anatomic data were not part of the Lifeline Registry. However, in the individual investigational device exemption studies, the surgical patients tended to have worse anatomy for EVAR with larger aortic aneurysms, shorter necks, and more iliac aneurysms.[22,26,69-73]

Difficulty of Comparison

The following factors complicate the comparison of EVAR and open surgical repair.

1. Both are prophylactic operations intended to prevent an event, aneurysm rupture, that occurs infrequently and unpredictably, depending on aneurysm size. Most of the mortality and morbidity of repair, by whatever method, occurs shortly after treatment, and the short-term results give a reliable indication of *safety*. A change in risk or aneurysm rupture becomes apparent only months or years after the intervention, and long-term results are required to assess *efficacy*.

2. Unless patients are randomized to one treatment or the other, there are likely to be significant differences between EVAR and surgical groups in both anatomy and physiology. Some patients are too high risk to undergo open repair and others lack the anatomic substrate for EVAR.

3. EVAR and surgery produce different complications. Many of the complications of EVAR, such as endoleak and migration, have no correlate in open surgical experience. Broadly defined complications, such as re-intervention, range widely in severity. For example, re-exploration of the abdomen for bleeding has a far greater impact than coil embolization of an inferior mesenteric artery for a type II endoleak.

4. Perioperative death is an infrequent occurrence in normal-risk patients, whatever method of repair.

5. The results of EVAR are dependent on the device, especially in the long term. It is difficult to interpret the findings of studies containing an unspecified mix of devices.

6. The results of EVAR are improving. Even the best studies are out of date as soon as they no longer describe the results obtained with current devices and current techniques.

7. It is becoming increasingly difficult to define a study population for whom a state of clinical equipoise between EVAR and surgery still exists. Given a choice, most patients will discount the long-term risks and opt for the least invasive alternative.

Physiologic Differences

Because of the less invasive nature of EVAR, it is hardly surprising that physiologic parameters show less derangement after EVAR than after open surgical repair. EVAR has less effect on pulmonary function,[74] cardiac function,[75,76] renal function, intestinal perfusion,[77] and catecholamine levels.[75,78] The sole exception is a poorly understood systemic inflammatory response to EVAR that is associated with low-grade fever and elevated levels of cytokines, including interleukin-6, C-reactive protein, and tumor necrosis factor.[79,80] In the early days of EVAR there were isolated reports of a severe response with sepsis and death, but these were probably related to some characteristic of the fabric component of the Stentor stent-graft because no occurrences of this type have been reported since the fabric was changed in 1996. The inflammatory response may be a more prominent feature of the postoperative course after EVAR, but it probably occurs to an equal extent after open surgery.[80] The most notable change is a rise in interleukin-6, possibly caused by disruption of mural thrombus. Although this response appears to be associated with clinical effects such as malaise, anorexia, and renal impairment, there is as yet no real understanding of its cause and no basis for recommendations regarding its prevention or treatment.

Mortality and Morbidity: Short-term Differences

Much of the early literature consisted of case series from individual centers without surgical controls. Many of these studies contained mixtures of low- and high-risk patients in urgent and elective circumstances. These studies consistently showed that EVAR results in fewer complications, more rapid recovery, shorter intensive care unit stay, and shorter hospital stay than is the case with open repair.[69,73,81-86] In general, women fare less well than men,[87-90] large aneurysms are more difficult to treat than small aneurysms,[91-93] and experienced operators get better results than inexperienced operators.[94-96] They were a poor basis for conclusions regarding the relative mortality rates of EVAR and open surgery and no basis for the unbridled enthusiasm that found expression in the concluding statements of many papers throughout the late 1990s. Industry-sponsored studies were larger but no better controlled, and their conclusions generally mirrored their stated objectives, which were to *prove* the safety and efficacy of one device or another.[26,69-73] These data provide a more complete picture when pooled by meta-analysis or accumulated in large registries.

Registries

The EuroSTAR (European Collaborators on Stent/Graft Techniques for Aortic Aneurysm Repair) registry[58,59,97] includes a wide range of endovascular devices that have been inserted in several European countries over a long period (1996 to 2005). The size and heterogeneity of the EuroSTAR database have made it a rich source of information on the effects of such variables as investigator experience, aneurysm size, aneurysm extent (with and without iliac aneurysms), patient gender, anesthesia type, and endoleak type. By 2005, when the registry closed, more than 10,000 patients had been enrolled. Of these, roughly 20% had been treated with devices that were subsequently removed from the market. When it became apparent that obsolete devices produced far worse results,[13] these cases were purged from the aggregated database. The vast majority of the EuroSTAR experience was obtained with AneuRx, Excluder, Talent, and Zenith stent-grafts, and perhaps the most important findings of the EuroSTAR study relate to device-specific differences in rates of long-term complications, such as migration, stent fracture, and limb occlusion (Table 129-2).[97] As a voluntary registry, EuroSTAR was subject to the potential for selective reporting. A requirement for preoperative enrollment was introduced in the latter part of the study to counter the risk that poor outcomes would be underreported.

The Lifeline Registry largely consists of pooled data from industry-sponsored comparisons of open and endovas-cular repair conducted in the United States from 1999 onward.[26,70-73,98] Unlike EuroSTAR, the Lifeline Registry includes data on surgical controls, and unlike EuroSTAR, in which the most common device was Zenith, the Lifeline Registry contains no Zenith cases. In addition, the only device-specific findings presented in publications of Lifeline data relate to the now-defunct Ancure device. More than half the aneurysms in the Lifeline Registry were smaller than 5.5 cm in diameter, which is important because aneurysm size is known to affect rates of technical success, re-intervention, and aneurysm rupture. Nevertheless, the 30-day mortality of EVAR in the Lifeline study (1.7%)[98] was almost identical to the rates in the EVAR-1 (1.6%)[64] and Dutch Randomized Endovascular Aneurysm Management (DREAM, 1.5%[65]) studies. On the other hand, the mortality rate for the open surgical arm in the Lifeline Registry (1.2%) was much lower than it was in EVAR-1 (4.6%), DREAM (4.8%), and other large trials of open repair, such as the U.K. Small Aneurysm Trial (5.8%)[99] and the Canadian aneurysm study (4.7%).[100] The only large multicenter with such a low perioperative mortality rate was the Veterans Affairs (VA) small aneurysm study,[101] where perhaps the low rates are explained by the more favorable anatomy found in small aneurysms. Alternatively, the Lifeline results may reflect the more favorable physiology of cases selected for surgical repair. The EVAR arm may have purged the open surgical arm of high-risk cases by offering an alternative means of treatment. If so, one of the underappreciated benefits of EVAR may be an improvement in the results of open repair.

Meta-analysis

A large segment of the available data on EVAR, consisting of 161 papers and 278,862 patients, was examined in a recent meta-analysis.[11] The relatively high overall mortality rate (3.3%) in the combined series[11] reflects the influence of poor early results. These authors used a technique of meta-regression to weight the effects of different studies over time and assess temporal changes in outcome. The data show striking heterogeneity, some of which is attributable to the effects of changing technique and device design. Meta-regression plots of both mortality rate (Fig. 129-2) and endoleak rate (Fig. 129-3) show steady improvement between 1992 and 2002. Based on the regression line, the perioperative mortality rate was estimated to have fallen to approximately 1.4% in 2002, which is very close to the rates seen in the Lifeline, EVAR-1, and DREAM studies (see earlier).

Clearly, the observed linear decline in mortality and endoleak rates cannot continue indefinitely. The line has to stabilize as further improvements in device design and insertion technique produce a diminishing return. Nevertheless, one would expect the current results of EVAR to be somewhat better than the results achieved in the EVAR-1 study,[64] which started in 1999, the DREAM study,[65] which started in 2000, and the EuroSTAR registry, which started in 1996. The field has changed substantially in the past decade, although

Table 129-2 Annual Incidence of Complications by Stent-Graft Type (per 1000 Patients)

	AneuRx	Ancure	Excluder	Talent	Zenith
Type I or II endoleak	52	86	50	66	41
Migration	43	5	11	24	7
Graft occlusion	19	33	11	23	35
Rupture	4	0	1	5	2

From Van Marrewijk CJ, Leurs LJ, Vallabhaneni SR, et al. Risk-adjusted outcome analysis of endovascular abdominal aortic aneurysm repair. *J Endovasc Ther.* 2005;12:417-429.

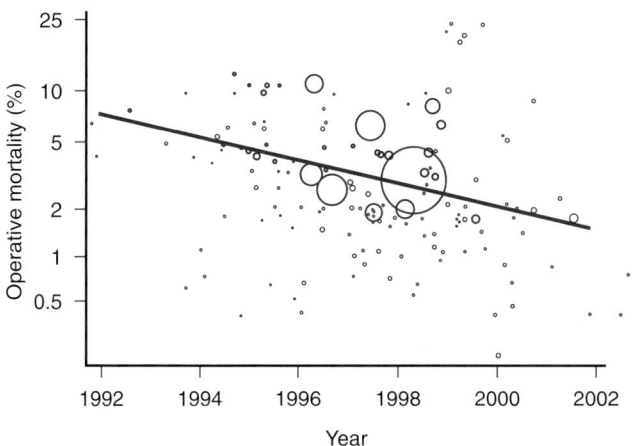

Figure 129-2 Mortality rate over time. *Circles* represent individual studies; the size of the circle is proportional to the inverse of the variance of the mortality of the estimate for that study and indicates the relative influence of that study in the meta-analysis. *(From Franks SC, Sutton AJ, Bown MJ, Sayers RD. Systematic review and meta-analysis of 12 years of endovascular abdominal aortic aneurysm repair. Eur J Vasc Endovasc Surg. 2007;33:154-171.)*

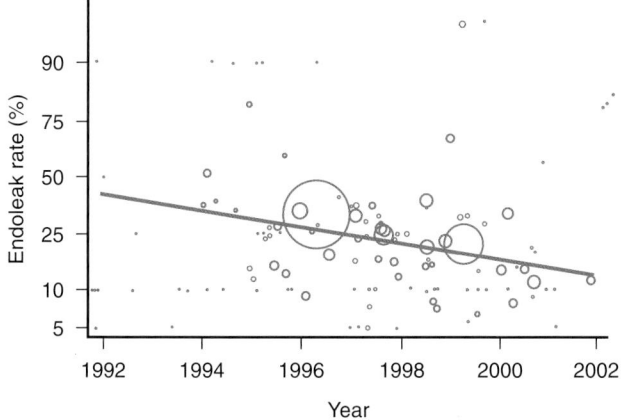

Figure 129-3 Endoleak rate over time. *Circles* represent individual studies; the size of the circle is proportional to the inverse of the variance of the mortality of the estimate for that study and indicates the relative influence of that study in the meta-analysis. *(From Franks SC, Sutton AJ, Bown MJ, Sayers RD. Systematic review and meta-analysis of 12 years of endovascular abdominal aortic aneurysm repair. Eur J Vasc Endovasc Surg. 2007;33:154-171.)*

most of these changes were directed at late failure modes, which have more of an effect on long-term results.

Randomized Trials

Two large randomized trials, EVAR-1 in the United Kingdom[64] and DREAM in the Netherlands,[65] have yielded the only level 1 evidence for comparisons between open and endovascular repair of AAA. Two other studies of this type, the Open versus Endovascular Repair (OVER) trial in the United States, and the Anévrisme de l'aorte abdominale: Chirurgie versus Endoprothèse (ACE) trial in France, are under way.

Patients with large aneurysms (>5.5 cm for EVAR-1, >5.0 cm for DREAM) were randomized to open or endovas-

cular repair, starting in 1999. The EVAR-1 study enrolled 1082 patients, 1017 of whom complied with their assigned therapy. The much smaller DREAM study enrolled 351 patients, 345 of whom complied with their assigned therapy. More than half the repairs were performed with Zenith stent-grafts (51% in EVAR-1, 57% in DREAM). The primary endpoint of both studies was overall mortality. Secondary endpoints included aneurysm-related mortality, perioperative morbidity, quality of life, and cost-effectiveness.

Both studies showed a striking difference in perioperative mortality rates between EVAR and surgery (1.7% versus 4.7% in EVAR-1, 1.2% versus 4.6% in DREAM), although the difference failed to reach statistical significance in the underpowered DREAM study. In the DREAM study, the combined rate of perioperative mortality and severe complications was 4.7% after EVAR and 9.8% after open surgery, mainly as a result of a higher rate of pulmonary complications. When compared with surgery, EVAR was associated with less blood loss, shorter operations, and shorter stays in the intensive care unit and hospital.

Mortality and Morbidity: Long-term Differences

Substantial data are available on the long-term behavior of first- and second-generation aortic stent-grafts.[12,17,26,62,102,103] Lacking are data on the long-term behavior of *current* stent-grafts. Long-term results inevitably reflect the performance of devices that were implanted long ago. Many of the early stent-grafts are no longer available, and many have been changed in important ways. Midterm results show a particularly striking difference between current stent-grafts and obsolete stent-grafts in rates of migration, re-intervention, conversion, and rupture.[12,13,74] Even some of the currently marketed stent-grafts, such as the AneuRx, Talent, and Excluder, are current in name only because they have changed in fundamental ways (see Table 129-1) to correct problems with long-term device performance.[2-10] It will be a while before we can be sure that these changes are effective and do not produce unexpected consequences, such as an increased migration rate. The Zenith stent-graft is a notable exception. The basic design has changed very little since 1998, and the long-term performance of the 1998 version is probably a sound predictor of the current design.[102] In addition, some of the most complete long-term follow-up data come from studies with a preponderance of Zenith stent-grafts (EVAR-1, DREAM, EuroSTAR). The Euro-STAR study is a particularly rich source of information on long-term stent-graft performance and other factors that influence the long-term outcome of EVAR (see "Complications of Endovascular Aneurysm Repair"), but it lacks a surgical control arm.[58,97] The EVAR-1[64] and DREAM[65] studies, on the other hand, have randomized surgical controls and are the most valid basis we have for comparison of long-term mortality rates, complication rates, cost, and patient well-being between EVAR and open surgery.

Randomized Trials

Life-table analysis (Fig. 129-4) of data from EVAR-1 shows that the initial 3% absolute survival advantage for EVAR persists to 4 years only in terms of aneurysm-related mortality (4% for EVAR versus 7% for surgery).[64] The difference in overall mortality is lost within 2 years of repair because of a higher death rate from cardiovascular causes in the EVAR group. The DREAM study showed a similar phenomenon, with 2-year survival rates of 89.7% for EVAR and 89.6% for surgery.[65] This excess mortality in the EVAR group is not explained by a higher rate of complications and re-interventions. EVAR is associated with a higher rate of complications and re-interventions (Fig. 129-5), but most are not life-threatening. The vast majority of complications after EVAR consisted of type II endoleaks, and the majority of re-interventions were performed to treat endoleaks, not lethal conditions such as graft infection or aneurysm rupture. It has been suggested that the stress of open surgical repair could have precipitated the death of patients who would otherwise have died within the next 2 years, as they did in the EVAR group, thereby causing the EVAR mortality rate to catch up. Indices of patient well-being showed a small advantage in favor of EVAR, but only for the first 3 months after repair. The total cost of treatment and 4-years of follow-up was significantly higher for EVAR than for open surgery.

Population-Based Results

As a rule, the best clinical outcomes are reported by academic centers with a high level of expertise and little interest in publishing unfavorable results. Even controlled, prospective, multicenter studies show the beneficial effects of rigorous patient and investigator selection. Thus, for an accurate picture of real-world experience one needs to examine a large, well-defined, but unselected population. Statewide and nationwide audits fill this role well, although procedure-specific information may be sparse because the study is usually based on administrative claims. Studies of this kind have confirmed the short-term advantages of EVAR over open AAA repair.[104,105] Only one study, an analysis of Medicare data from 2001 to 2004, has examined long-term results.[106] One can assume that most of the repairs in this study were performed with AneuRx stent-grafts because little else was available until 2003 and the transition to other devices was a slow process. The most notable finding of this study was the high rate of serious complications, such as ventral hernia (14.2%) and small bowel obstruction (9.7%), many years after open surgical repair. Endovascular AAA repair fared relatively well by comparison. As in the aforementioned randomized studies, the survival curves showed an early advantage for EVAR, followed by progressive convergence. The time to convergence reflected the magnitude of the perioperative survival advantage, which was a function of patient age. The overall perioperative mortality rate was

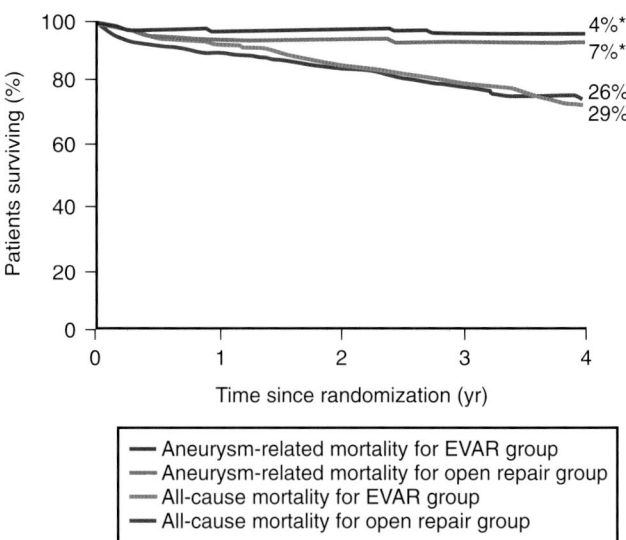

Figure 129-4 Kaplan-Meier curve of all-cause and aneurysm-related mortality. Mortality is derived from 4-year point estimates. EVAR, endovascular aneurysm repair. *(From Greenhalgh RM, Brown LC, Kwong GP, et al, for the EVAR trial participants. Comparison of endovascular aneurysm repair with open repair in patients with abdominal aortic aneurysm [EVAR trial 1], 30-day operative mortality results: randomized controlled trial. Lancet. 2004;364:843-848.)*

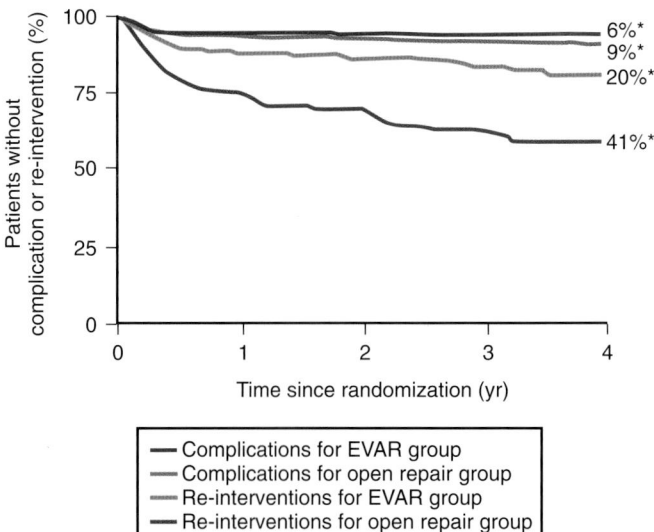

Figure 129-5 Kaplan-Meier curve of postoperative complications and re-interventions derived from 4-year point estimates for patients with complications or re-interventions. EVAR, endovascular aneurysm repair. *(From EVAR Trial Participants. Comparison of endovascular aneurysm repair with open repair in patients with abdominal aortic aneurysm [EVAR trial 1], 30-day operative mortality results: randomized controlled trial. Lancet. 364:843-848.)*

1.2% for EVAR and 4.8% for propensity score–matched surgical controls. Some of the "catch-up" mortality in the EVAR group is attributable to high rates of aneurysm rupture (1.8%) and major intervention (1.6%), which were not matched by similar complications in the surgical group.

These late failures of EVAR are consistent with the known failure modes of the AneuRx stent-graft, which was in widespread use throughout the United States at the time of the study.[26,97]

ENDOVASCULAR ANEURYSM REPAIR VERSUS MEDICAL MANAGEMENT

There is no doubt that EVAR is safer than open surgical repair, but the safest short-term option will always be no repair at all, especially in patients considered unfit for open surgery. These patients fare relatively poorly after EVAR, as demonstrated by various subset analyses of the EuroSTAR data[68] and the findings of the EVAR-2 study.[66]

EVAR-2 was a much smaller trial than EVAR-1. Starting in 1999 a total of 338 patients, all considered unfit for open repair, were randomized to EVAR (n = 166) or best medical therapy (n = 172). The perioperative mortality rate of EVAR was 9% (n = 15), but this was inflated by nine cases (5.4%) of aneurysm rupture while awaiting treatment. The aneurysm rupture rate during medical management was 9% per year, but this was artificially reduced by 20% as a result of "medically managed" patients undergoing aneurysm repair because either their health improved or their AAA became more worrisome to their surgeon. Interestingly, patients in the medical arm who crossed over to EVAR or even open surgery did extremely well. One can hypothesize that their ability to withstand surgery benefited from the delay and that surgeons made good selection of patients for surgery. Given AAA rupture in the EVAR group before surgery and crossover to surgery in the medical group, it is not surprising that an intention-to-treat analysis showed no difference in overall survival or aneurysm-related survival at 4 years, with high mortality rates from co-morbid conditions in both arms of the study.

Flawed as it is, the EVAR-2 study currently provides the only level 1 evidence regarding the relative mortality rates of endovascular versus no treatment in patients with large aneurysms. However, there are other studies of EVAR in high-risk patients[67,68,107,108] and studies of large aneurysms in patients considered unfit for surgery.[109] For example, quality assurance data from the VA study showed a perioperative mortality rate of 3.4% in such patients, whereas a subset analysis of data from five industry-sponsored Food and Drug Administration trials showed a perioperative mortality rate of 2.9%. Both studies had open surgical controls, which suggests that the "high-risk" patients in these studies were less ill than patients in the EVAR-2 study who were "unfit for open repair." The annual rupture rate in the VA large aneurysm study (9.4%) was almost identical to that seen in EVAR-2, but only for aneurysms smaller than 6 cm and just for the first year of follow-up. As one would expect, the rupture rate was an exponential function of aneurysm diameter. Aneurysms larger than 8 cm had a rupture rate of 26% within 6 months, and aneu-

rysms larger than 6.5 cm had a high likelihood of exceeding 8 cm by the next follow-up.

COMPARISONS OF DIFFERENT STENT-GRAFTS

Few complications in EVAR are entirely attributable to faulty technique; most can be traced to faulty stent-graft performance or at least failure to match device performance to patient anatomy. Indeed, specific complications represent specific failure modes and specific features of stent-graft design. Most of what we know about this subject comes from painful clinical experience, not preclinical testing. Yet very little of the published literature provides a sound basis for direct comparisons among different types or makes of stent-graft. Short-term data are of no use because most of the short-term problems were eliminated in the first few iterations of stent-graft evolution.[12,21,24] When it comes to comparisons of currently available stent-grafts, small studies or studies that require stratification into multiple small groups are also of limited value because the most significant endpoints often occur infrequently.

The EuroSTAR database is unique in having large numbers and long follow-up of the most widely used stent-grafts, AneuRx, Talent, Zenith, and Exluder,[68] together with a willingness to publish comparative data (see Table 125-2). The AneuRx and Talent stent-grafts had the highest rates of migration, endoleak (types I and III), and conversion. The Zenith stent-graft had the highest rates of limb occlusion and aneurysm shrinkage, whereas the Excluder stent-graft had the lowest. The Zenith stent-graft was also notable for having the lowest rate of migration.

The Lifeline Registry, on the other hand, cannot be used for device comparisons.[98] It lacks data on Zenith stent-grafts, and the only device-specific information relates to Ancure, a now-defunct stent-graft. It is possible to glean the necessary information from the corresponding industry-sponsored studies,[26,70-73] but differences in study design, follow-up, and definition complicate comparisons. For example, studies that rely on duplex ultrasonography for follow-up tend to underreport migration,[26] and some studies have a 5-mm threshold for migration,[71] whereas others have a 10-mm threshold.[26,72,73]

A few individual centers have reported comparisons of long-term stent-graft performance, but even relatively large studies of this type lack power once the overall experience is divided according to device type. As a result, striking differences often fail to reach statistical significance. A recent comparison of Zenith, Excluder, and AneuRx is a case in point.[108] All but 1 of the 10 cases of migration occurred with AneuRx repairs, yet "there was no difference between devices on actuarial analysis." Only the compound endpoint, graft-related adverse events, showed significant differences, with rates of 29% for Zenith, 35% for Excluder, and 43% for AneuRx.

COMPLICATIONS OF ENDOVASCULAR ANEURYSM REPAIR

Most of the complications of EVAR have no open surgical counterparts, especially in the long term. Many studies have demonstrated higher rates of late complication and re-intervention in EVAR patients, but until recently, the nonvascular complications of abdominal surgery, such as hernia and small bowel obstruction, have been overlooked.[106]

Endoleak

Endoleaks are categorized according to the route of flow into the space between the wall of the stent-graft and the wall of the aneurysm, as described earlier.[56,57,61] This naming scheme is valuable because the type of endoleak gives a good indication of the probable cause, prognosis, and treatment.[110-115]

Endoleak Detection

Contrast-enhanced computed tomography (CT) is and will probably remain the "gold standard" for detection of endoleaks, if only because most of what we know about the prognosis of endoleak is derived from CT-based follow-up. The sensitivity and specificity of CT are technique dependent. Low-resolution studies lack the localizing information needed to designate the endoleak type. A complete CT study acquires data in multiple phases. Arterial-phase images show types I and III endoleaks, delayed (2 to 3 minutes) images show type II endoleaks, and non–contrast-enhanced images show mural calcium, which might otherwise be misidentified as contrast-enhanced blood (endoleak). Three-dimensional reconstruction may help define the full extent of the endoleak cavity and the proximity to potential sources as a basis for diagnosis of the type of endoleak. There is no role for oral contrast agents.

Contrast-enhanced CT exposes the patient to two injurious agents, intravenous contrast material and radiation. The effects of serial contrast injections are illustrated by the postoperative changes in calculated glomerular filtration rate in a subset of the Zenith investigational device exemption study.[116] In every case, a progressive decline in renal function over the first 12 months, when the patients underwent five contrast-enhanced studies, was followed by improvement over the subsequent 12 months, when the patients underwent only one contrast-enhanced CT scan. The radiation exposure of a single CT scan is relatively low. However, multidetector arrays increase the dosage, and the cumulative dose of annual multidetector CT scans is a cause for concern.[117]

Alternative imaging modalities include magnetic resonance imaging (MRI)[118,119] and duplex ultrasound.[120-123] MRI is expensive and cannot be used to image ferromagnetic stent-grafts, such as the Zenith.[124] Moreover, gadolinium contrast is contraindicated in patients with renal failure. Duplex ultrasound is relatively inexpensive and innocuous. Papers on the potential role of duplex have focused on the sensitivity and specificity of the technique, with or without ultrasound con-

trast, for the detection of endoleak.[120-123] Most show acceptable sensitivity, although the accuracy of ultrasound varies with the experience of the technician and patient-related variables such as bowel gas and obesity. One relatively large study showed a sensitivity of 67%, with a large number of endoleaks seen on CT that were not apparent on ultrasound.[122] However, most of them were of the relatively benign type II. Ultrasound correctly identified all type I endoleaks. The same study showed a specificity of 91%. These false positives may be real endoleaks, but their significance is difficult to assess given that most of what we know about the behavior of endoleaks is based on the findings of CT-based follow-up.

Variations in the sensitivity of CT scanning for the detection of endoleak may help explain why large numbers of endoleaks seem to appear and disappear from one study to the next, why the number of type II endoleaks varies widely among studies, and why duplex ultrasound may demonstrate endoleaks not seen on CT. The diagnostic sensitivity of CT depends on contrast timing. Early acquisitions (arterial phase) show types I and III endoleaks, but not type II endoleaks, which are better seen on delayed views. An endoleak may still be present in the absence of a visible endoleak cavity, as evidenced by the common finding of contrast opacification of two adjacent lumbar arteries. The most likely type of endoleak to be missed is type II, but one has to be careful to not miss a type I or III endoleak. If three-dimensional reconstruction of high-resolution contrast-enhanced CT fails to settle the issue, there is a role for catheter angiography with a high frame rate, multiple obliquities, and a long acquisition time.

Type I Endoleak

Most type I endoleaks are identified and treated at the time of stent-graft implantation, as discussed in Chapter 86 (Technique: Endovascular Aneurysm Repair), and a persistent type I endoleak should be a rare finding on postoperative imaging. As always, treatment depends on the cause. Inaccurate (low) stent-graft placement leaves a gap between the proximal margin of the graft and the renal arteries, which can be bridged with a short aortic cuff. More often, the problem lies in patient selection, with a neck that is too short, too wide, or too angulated for hemostatic stent-graft implantation. Balloon dilatation will force even the stiffest stent-graft and most angulated necks into alignment, but only temporarily. More durable realignment can be achieved with a giant Palmaz stent bridging the proximal stent-graft and the suprarenal aorta.[125] Failing that, the seal zone has to be extended proximally into the pararenal aorta, and the technique has to make provision for flow to one or both renal arteries.

If endovascular maneuvers fail to improve the seal, one is faced with a variety of unpalatable choices: conventional open surgical repair, banding the neck with soft (nylon) umbilical tape or a segment of Dacron graft material,[126] coil embolization of the perigraft space, or leaving the endoleak untreated. There is no role for observation in the management of a type I endoleak because of the high likelihood of AAA rupture.[112]

The late appearance of a type I endoleak on follow-up studies indicates a loss of sealing at one of the implantation sites that is usually caused by downward migration of the proximal end of the stent-graft (see later under "Migration"). Type I endoleak can also occur as a result of neck dilatation, but in our experience this is rare (see later under "Neck Dilatation").

Type II Endoleak

In our experience, some form of type II endoleak is almost always apparent on the later images of high-resolution completion angiograms, but most resolve with the restoration of normal coagulation at the end of the operation. Postoperative CT scans show signs of type II endoleak in 10% to 20% of cases.[110-115] This range may represent variation in the timing of postoperative studies, variation in diagnostic sensitivity and diagnostic accuracy, or a real device-dependent variation in the incidence of type II endoleak. Although type II endoleak is not generally regarded as a failure of stent-graft performance, it is possible that differences in stent-graft compliance might influence the occurrence or persistence of a type II endoleak. Movement of the graft wall through the phases of the cardiac cycle might change the volume of the perigraft space and pump blood in and out of patent lumbar and inferior mesenteric branches.

Significance.
When compared with direct endoleaks (types I and III), type II endoleaks are relatively benign. As many as 80% of type II endoleaks resolve spontaneously within 6 months of stent-graft implantation,[12] and those that persist are unlikely to cause aneurysm pressurization,[113] dilatation, or rupture. A better understanding of the natural history of type II endoleak has led to a reduction in the rate of intervention. Indeed, high rates of re-intervention for type II endoleak can no longer be construed as evidence of a relationship between type II endoleak and poor outcome, but only evidence that surgeons once believed that type II endoleaks were a strong indication for re-intervention. These days, the usual indications for treatment of a type II endoleak are uncertainty of the diagnosis, aneurysm enlargement, and endoleak persistence.

Although no treatment is indicated for an uncomplicated type II endoleak, it is important to not miss the more dangerous types I and III that may also be present. CT-based endoleak designation is often based solely on the proximity of the endoleak cavity to probable sources of inflow. In cases of doubt, it may be possible to identify the source of flow by following the path of contrast material on catheter angiograms.

In general, mean sac pressure is high in the presence of a direct (type I or III) endoleak, low in the absence of an endoleak, and somewhere in between with a type II endoleak.[51] However, the range is wide, and some type II endoleaks are associated with high sac pressure, aneurysm dilatation, and a persistent risk for aneurysm rupture. There are many well-documented cases of aneurysm rupture in the absence of any

cause but an isolated type II endoleak, yet the risk is relatively low, especially if the aneurysm is small. Multivariate analysis of EuroSTAR data[59] showed no association between type II endoleak and risk for aneurysm rupture. If anything, type II endoleak had a protective effect. However, it is possible that the pressurizing effects of type II endoleaks were obscured by high rates of more malignant processes, such as migration and structural degradation (see later), because at the time of this analysis the EuroSTAR database included many highly unstable stent-grafts. If so, the apparent protective effect of type II endoleak may have been the result of close follow-up with early diagnosis and correction of otherwise catastrophic complications.

Persistent Endoleak.
Persistent type II endoleaks are usually associated with a large endoleak cavity,[127] continuous flow between inflow and outflow arteries,[128] numerous large lumbar and inferior mesenteric arteries,[129] and systemic hypertension.[130] None of these factors exerts a strong enough influence to warrant early treatment. Aneurysm dilatation remains the primary indication for intervention.[12,110-113] However, one cannot necessarily assume that a type II endoleak is the only process causing the aneurysm to dilate or that treating the endoleak will cause the aneurysm to shrink. Aneurysm dilatation often complicated repair with early versions of the Excluder and AneuRx stent-grafts (see "Endotension"). Under these circumstances, the presence of a type II endoleak presents a difficult diagnostic dilemma: what to treat, the stent-graft or the endoleak. In most such cases the best strategy is to treat the stent-graft first (see "Endotension") because it is the more likely cause of aneurysm dilatation based on the relative frequencies of pure endotension- and pure endoleak-induced aneurysm dilatation.

Treatment.
Options for treatment of a type II endoleak include conversion to open surgery, suture ligation of the feeding arteries (with the aneurysm open or intact), laparoscopic ligation or clipping of the feeding arteries, coil embolization of the feeding arteries, coil embolization of the endoleak cavity, and polymer embolization of the endoleak cavity. The transcatheter therapies can be accomplished through transarterial (usually transfemoral) or through translumbar access. Given the benign nature of type II endoleak, open surgical correction should be reserved for patients with large aneurysms and rapid dilatation after failed attempts at transcatheter therapy. Transcatheter treatment of a type II endoleak can easily become an exercise in futility. The endoleak behaves like an arteriovenous malformation, and coil occlusion of one branch artery supplying the type II endoleak inevitably leads to hypertrophy of another with persisting endoleak. The occlusive agent has to be injected directly into the endoleak cavity to have a durable effect. This can be difficult to achieve when the only transarterial route to the aneurysm is through a tiny ascending iliolumbar collateral. Transarterial embolization is more likely to succeed when the endoleak cavity is fed through a patent inferior mesenteric artery. It is usually possible to pass a microcatheter

through the middle colic branch of the superior mesenteric artery, around the colonic arcade, and through the left colic artery to the inferior mesenteric artery.[114] If transarterial access fails, translumbar access is an option.[115]

Type III Endoleak

In type III endoleak, blood reaches the aneurysm sac through gaps in the wall of the stent-graft at sites of component separation or graft erosion. Both forms of type III endoleak are rare,[12,131] both tend to occur long after stent-graft insertion,[12] and both depend on design features that have changed over the years,[25] which makes it difficult to estimate current rates of type III endoleak. Furthermore, if they are mentioned at all, type III endoleaks are usually bundled with type I endoleaks under the heading "direct" or "graft-related" endoleak.[59,92,132] Only modular stent-grafts are at risk for component separation, but all stent-grafts are at risk for "graft failure."[25,133-135] Published rates of type III endoleak range from 0% to 1.5%.[12,22]

Graft Separation.
Intercomponent separation is caused by the same hemodynamic forces that cause migration. With every pulse, flow and pressure slowly move the middle of the stent-graft away from the original line of insertion toward the outer curve of the aneurysm.[136] Unless the intercomponent connection is secure, the resulting tension eventually pulls the components apart (Fig. 129-6). In any given case, the risk of component separation depends on the anatomy of the aorta and the design of the stent-graft. Separation is more likely to occur if the limb is long and flexible, the intercomponent overlap is short, the aorta is angulated, the pressure in the aneurysm is low (high transmural pressure), and the aneurysm is large. In practice, there is not much one can do with high-risk anatomy other than implant a stent-graft with short stiff limbs and a long intercomponent overlap.

Fabric Erosion.
Fabric erosion is caused by the repetitive micromotion of graft fabric against a part of a stent, usually its apex (Fig. 129-7). The incidence can be greatly reduced by attaching the graft securely to the apex of the stent. The Vanguard experience illustrates this point in that most instances of fabric erosion followed breakage of the polypropylene sutures that previously held the stent and graft in close apposition.[23-25] Sutured attachment has the potential effect of inducing fiber separation and thereby causing small holes, which may transmit pressure (endotension) or flow (endoleak).

Significance.
The presence of a type III endoleak is one of the strongest predictors of rupture.[58] One of the primary goals of follow-up is diagnosis of component separation so that prompt re-intervention can be undertaken. All current stent-grafts have a continuous exoskeleton of radiopaque stents. Impending component separation is easy to identify on serial radiographs (see Fig. 129-6), whereas axial CT will give very little indication of a problem until complete loss of an inter-component seal causes a type III endoleak. CT scans are not

much better at identifying type III endoleak through a site of fabric erosion. Catheter angiograms can help localize the problem. Some authors have suggested that the diagnostic sensitivity for this form of type III endoleak is increased by occluding the graft with a balloon before injection of contrast agent into the suspect area.

Treatment.
The goal of treatment is to re-establish the continuity of the stent-graft by inserting an additional component to bridge the gap or cover the hole. It can be difficult to gain wire access through two components that no longer share the same longitudinal axis. In such cases, a guide wire is inserted through one component and snared through the other. We prefer a multilooped snare to a gooseneck snare and a 6 Fr angled sheath to a straight unvalved snare catheter. If localized fabric erosion is seen in the body of the graft or the midportion of the limb, a simple cylindrical extension may be all that one needs to patch the hole. Otherwise, it is safer to cover the entire graft (see the next section).

Endotension

Although the term *endotension* implies a state of aneurysm pressurization, the diagnosis usually signifies nothing more than aneurysm dilatation in the absence of a discernible endoleak. In that regard, the alternative term for endotension (type V endoleak) is somewhat confusing. Yet it is useful to think of endotension as a form fruste of endoleak, a kind of endoleak that is difficult to see, because regardless of whether there is an endoleak, the same causes of aneurysm dilatation make up the list of potential targets for intervention.

Causes.
Excluding an aneurysm from arterial flow does not guarantee exclusion from arterial pressure. Pressure may be transmitted through the thrombus lining of a porous stent-graft or through the thrombus lining of a large or irregular implantation site. Graft porosity on a macroscopic level appears to have been the explanation for the high rate of aneurysm dilatation after repair with the AneuRx stent-graft.[133] At a mean of 3 years after implantation, 12% of aneurysms had increased in diameter, 36% had decreased in diameter, and the rest remained within 5 mm of their original diameter. The explanation for the lack of shrinkage in a high proportion of cases is to be found in the findings of an analysis of explanted AneuRx stent-grafts,[137] which showed a mean of two holes per device, each with a mean area of 0.5 mm². These findings led to a change in the graft fabric in 2004, which appears to have been successful in producing lower rates of dilatation and higher rates of shrinkage, although long-term data are lacking.

The original Excluder stent-graft also was porous, but on a microscopic level. Within 3 years of repair, roughly 25% of patients experienced aneurysm dilatation, equally divided between cases of type II endoleak and endotension. MRI showed perigraft flush in these cases.[138] Open surgical repair usually reveals a mass of gelatinous material around the stent-graft.[139] The substitution of low-porosity

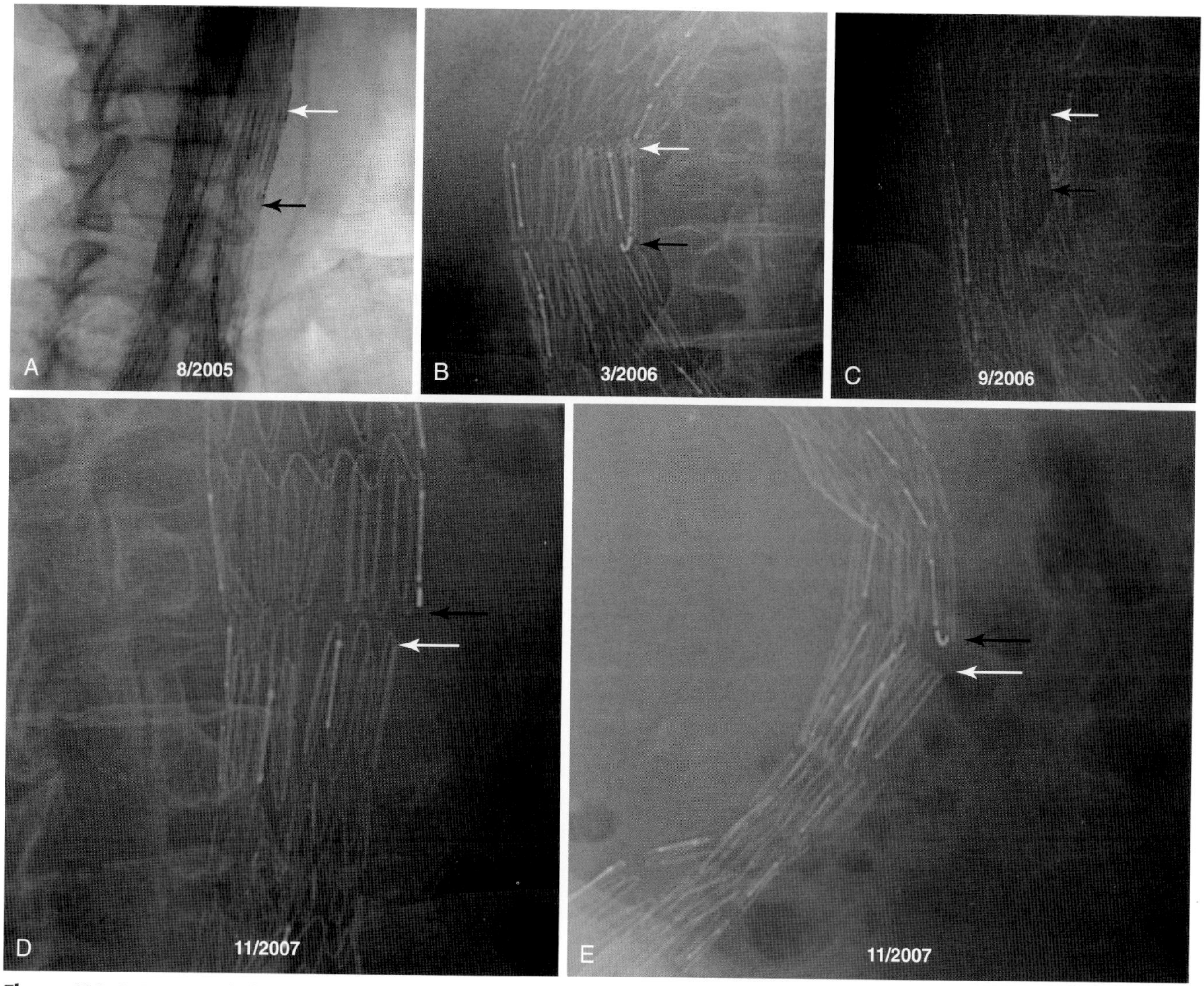

Figure 129-6 A–D, Serial plain radiographs of a Zenith stent-graft showing gradual separation of the components. **E,** A lateral view shows how much the stent-graft bowed forward into the large empty aneurysm. The *white arrow* indicates the top of the limb, and the *black arrow* indicates the bottom of the gate.

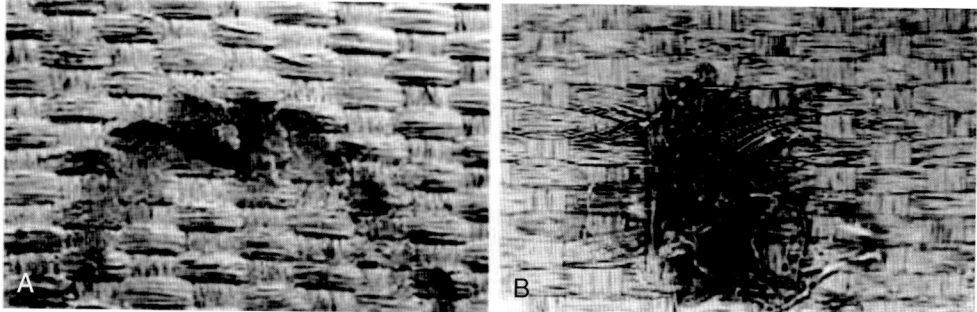

Figure 129-7 Two representative samples from in vitro simulation testing of the Vanguard stent-graft under various conditions of angulation and compression. **A,** Flattening of polyethylene fibers can be seen after repeated cycles of compression against a flat stent wire without the erosion that produces a hole. **B,** Fabric erosion that resulted in a hole after similar repeated compression cycles against the apex of an angled "zigzag" stent. *(From Beebe HG, Cronenwett JL, Katzen BT, et al. Results of an aortic endograft trial: impact of device failure beyond 12 months. J Vasc Surg. 2001;33:55-63.)*

polytetrafluoroethylene fabric appears to have reduced the rate, at least in the medium term.[140] One year after implantation of a low-permeability stent-graft in 48 patients, the sole case of aneurysm enlargement was associated with a type II endoleak.[29]

Diagnosis. The diagnosis of endotension rests on the finding of elevated sac pressure, aneurysm dilatation, or both. Until recently, the only way to measure sac pressure was through a catheter during re-intervention for endoleak. Consequently, most clinical decisions were based on changes in the diameter of the aneurysm sac. With the advent of implantable pressure sensors,[49,50,141] there is the potential to measure sac pressure noninvasively during routine follow-up, although issues related to the accuracy[52,55] and predictive value[142] of the technique have yet to be resolved.

Treatment. If the distal implantation site is suspect, the solution is to extend the stent-graft to a less diseased segment, generally the external iliac artery. Proximal extension, on the other hand, is limited by the proximity of the existing stent-graft to the renal arteries and the state of any remaining infrarenal aorta. In the absence of a nondilated infrarenal implantation site, open conversion may be the only way to protect against rupture.

If the stent-graft itself is suspect, the solution is to insert another of a less porous type.[143] In most cases the short body of the original AneuRx or Excluder stent-graft precludes implantation of another bifurcated stent-graft. There are two alternatives: implantation of a uniiliac Renu stent-graft together with contralateral limb occlusion and femorofemoral bypass, or implantation of three separate components, one cuff and two limbs (Fig. 129-8). The latter is less definitive but easier to accomplish through percutaneous access and just as effective based on the limited published experience.[143]

Migration

Hemodynamic forces tend to pull both ends of the stent-graft into the aneurysm. The graft limbs migrate toward the head and the trunk toward the feet. Nevertheless, the term *stent-graft migration* generally refers to unstable proximal attachment that results in caudad migration of the stent-graft. The forces on the stent-graft increase with the degree of angulation, the diameter of the trunk, and the pressure gradient across the walls of the stent-graft. Other things being equal, large-diameter, acutely angulated stent-grafts are the most likely to migrate.[44]

Proximal Fixation

Migration rates also vary with the type of proximal attachment. Based on the findings of simple pullout tests[144] and the relative migration rates of different devices,[97] it appears that barb-mediated attachment confers the greatest stability. A comparison of two devices, the AneuRx and the Ancure (see Table 125-2), both of which lack suprarenal stents, shows a higher incidence of migration with the *unbarbed* AneuRx than with *barbed* EVT/Ancure. A comparison of two devices, the Talent and the Zenith, both of which have suprarenal stents, shows a higher incidence of migration with the *unbarbed* Talent than with *barbed* Zenith. A similar set of comparisons shows that the suprarenal stent also contributes to a reduced incidence of migration. Neither the stiffness (column strength) of the stent-graft nor its incorporation into the wall of the aorta seems to play much of a role in stabilizing stent-graft position.[145] The result is a sixfold difference in migration rates between the AneuRx and Zenith stent-grafts.[97] Kaplan-Meier analysis of data from the AneuRx clinical trial showed migration in 19% of subjects at 3 years,[26,27] although individual centers have reported much higher rates.[146] The AneuRx stent-graft was implanted in large numbers of patients, mainly because until 2003 it was the only device approved for sale in the United States. This has left a vast reservoir of at-risk patients who need close follow-up and prompt treatment to prevent secondary type I endoleak and rupture.

Detection and Prevalence

Migration is a slow process, and the prevalence of significant migration increases steadily with the time from implantation.

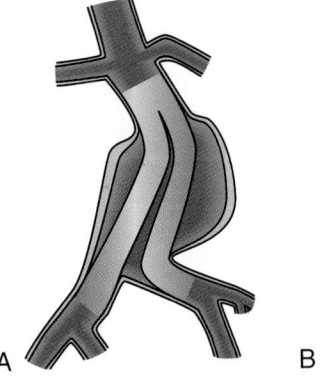 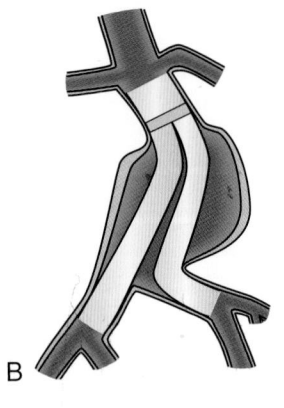 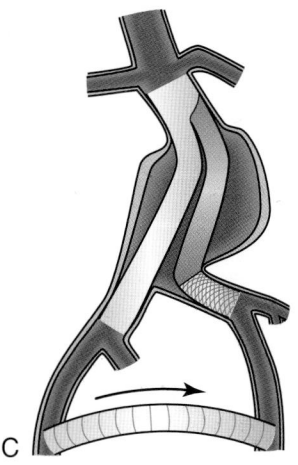

Figure 129-8 Relining of a leaky bifurcated stent graft (**A**) may be accomplished with multiple stent-graft components (**B**) or a single uniiliac stent-graft with a contralateral occluder and a femorofemoral bypass (**C**).

A   B   C

At any point in follow-up, the prevalence of migration depends on the characteristics of the device, the sensitivity of follow-up imaging, and the threshold distance for the diagnosis. There is often a long interval between the first signs of migration and the development of a type I endoleak. However, small changes in the shape or position of the stent-graft may be difficult to detect on routine imaging. The slice thickness of axial CT imposes a margin of error on localization of the renal arteries and the top of the stent-graft. There is no way to detect 5-mm migration on 5-mm-thick slices. Besides, it can be difficult, in the presence of an uncovered suprarenal stent, to identify the top of the graft. If CT scans are to be used for the diagnosis of migration, contrast enhancement and fine slices are mandatory, and three-dimensional reconstruction is helpful.

Plain radiographs are sensitive to changes in stent-graft shape,[147,148] but not stent-graft position, because the frame of reference (the spine) occupies a different plane, which results in parallax errors. Direct comparisons of serial plain radiographs in multiple views will seldom miss significant migration. It is a mistake to attribute bowing of the stent-graft to changes in the shape of the aneurysm. Aneurysms may change shape after EVAR, but they rarely shorten. Any redundancy indicates true lengthening of the stent-graft, as in the old Vanguard device; apparent lengthening of the stent-graft, as in component separation; or migration of the ends, proximal or distal.

Treatment

Options for treatment depend on the state of the neck. If the primary stent-graft has fallen out of a long straight neck, the addition of a proximal cuff will re-establish continuity and eliminate the endoleak. In our 'experience, short unbarbed cuffs fail to provide a durable remedy because the cuff is no more stable than the original stent-graft. The cuff can migrate out of the neck, or the primary stent-graft can migrate off the cuff. The Renu stent-graft (Cook Medical) was designed with the migrating AneuRx stent-graft in mind. It has a barbed uncovered stent for secure proximal attachment and two alternative configurations: straight aortoaortic and tapered aortoiliac. The tapered version allows more secure attachment to the primary stent-graft. It directs blood into one limb of the stent-graft, which requires a femorofemoral bypass for contralateral lower extremity perfusion. There is no need to insert a contralateral common iliac occluder because the contralateral limb of the original AneuRx stent-graft will serve this function. Standard bifurcated Zenith stent-grafts are too long to fit above the bifurcation of the original stent-graft, no matter how far it has fallen into the aneurysm.

Graft Limb Occlusion

Stent-grafts vary in their ability to tolerate compression or angulation.[97,149-151] Annualized occlusion rates of various stent-grafts in the EuroSTAR database are shown in Table 129-2. Unsupported limbs are more likely to occlude than fully stented limbs.[151,152] However, the stents themselves can reduce a graft's capacity for differential shortening and convert a bend into a kink. Optimal kink resistance is achieved by using short stents that are well spaced along the length of the limb. The original Zenith stent-graft, with an uninterrupted chain of long stainless steel Z-stents, had a high rate of limb thrombosis.[149]

Prevention

Implantation of a flexible self-expanding stent is a simple, safe, and effective remedy for kinking or compression.[149] The efficacy of adjunctive stenting is illustrated by the limb occlusion rates after EVAR with the unsupported Ancure stent-graft,[151] which were 13.4% for unstented limbs and zero for stented limbs. Similar findings have been reported after EVAR with Zenith stent-grafts.[149] Limb thrombosis occurred in 5.2% of patients (2.7% of limbs), all in the unstented group. No limb occlusions occurred in the presence of adjunctive bare-metal stents. In both studies, the additional stents were inserted to treat luminal compromise at the time of insertion in cases that would otherwise have been considered high risk for limb occlusion. In both series the majority of limb occlusions occurred within a month of stent-graft implantation, presumably in the absence of worrisome findings on completion angiography. Prophylactic stent implantation may therefore be warranted, even in the absence of overt kinking, when the limb crosses a narrow angulated segment of the common iliac artery or terminates in the external iliac artery.[149,152]

Treatment

There are endovascular and open alternatives for treatment of graft limb occlusion. Endovascular techniques involve thrombolysis or thrombectomy, followed by stent implantation to correct the underlying kinking or compression of the limb. Open surgical options include extra-anatomic bypass from the axillary artery or the contralateral femoral artery and conversion to surgical aneurysm repair. Both are effective in the short term, but endovascular techniques appear to yield a more durable result.[152]

Renal Artery Occlusion

Stent-grafts do not usually migrate proximally after implantation. A renal artery that is found to be covered on follow-up was most likely covered at the initial operation.[102] Partial renal artery occlusion can be difficult to identify on intraoperative angiograms and early postoperative CT scans. The wall of the stent-graft is too thin to create a filling defect in the renal profile, and even when the stent-graft covers much of the renal orifice, the renal artery lumen often fills with contrast-enhanced blood in the brief interval between angiographic images. One has to pay close attention to the position of radiopaque markers at the proximal edge of the graft and not be lulled into a false sense of security by the appearance of renal artery patency or even the location of markers, which may be as much as 2 mm from the proximal margin of the graft fabric.[102] Filling defects appear within the renal arteries only when thrombus starts to accumulate on the downstream side of the graft.

When suprarenal stents were first introduced, there was concern that they would induce hyperplasia and narrow the renal orifices, but to date no studies have shown this. Although most studies are relatively small and their negative findings may represent type II errors,[153,154] a recent meta-analysis with a large pooled data set found no significant difference (P = .39) in the time to renal impairment between those with suprarenal stents (37 months) and those without (45 months).[155]

Neck Dilatation

The pararenal and paravisceral segments of the aorta seem to be more resistant to dilatation than the infrarenal aorta. Nevertheless, serial studies of neck diameter after open surgical and endovascular AAA repair show that this area is far from stable.[46,156,157] The inevitability of neck dilatation used to be a favorite theme of "endoskeptics" worldwide, but their dire prophesies have not been borne out by clinical experience. The explanation for this outcome lies in the mechanical properties of self-expanding and balloon-expandable stent-grafts.

Etiology

Self-expanding stent-grafts are relatively compliant until they reach full expansion, at which point they become noncompliant. The partially expanded stent-graft transmits pressure to the surrounding aorta, which dilates and allows the self-expanding stent-graft to dilate as well. Once the stent-graft reaches its fully expanded diameter, it ceases to transmit the

aortic pressure wave to the wall of the surrounding aorta. Thus, an oversized, bottle-shaped stent-graft becomes a fully expanded, can-shaped stent-graft, whereupon dilatation ceases (Fig. 129-9).

The ratio between the diameter of the stent-graft within the neck and the diameter within the aneurysm sac is an indicator of the degree of residual oversizing. The process of neck dilatation can be followed by plotting this ratio against the duration of follow-up. In our experience with Zenith stent-grafts, the ratio increases in a linear fashion as the neck dilates and then plateaus as the stent-graft reaches its fully expanded state (unpublished data). At this point, which occurs 2 to 5 years after stent-graft implantation, further neck dilatation would no longer be matched by further stent-graft dilatation, and the resulting mismatch could cause loss of wall contact with a type I endoleak and migration. However, this is not what happens. Long-term follow-up of more than 325 Zenith cases, for example, showed no instances of secondary type I endoleak.[102]

Balloon-expandable stent-grafts are different. They have very low compliance from the time of implantation and never transmit the aortic pressure wave to the wall of the surrounding aorta, hence the lack of neck dilatation.[158,159]

Prevention

The protective effect of the noncompliant stent-graft depends on close contact with the aorta. Any channel between them will transmit arterial pressure to the aortic wall, even if that channel is filled with thrombus, and cause neck dilatation and secondary type I endoleak. Little can be done to correct this process once it has begun other than substituting suprarenal fenestrated repair for standard infrarenal repair. Indeed, many in Europe and Australia, where fenestrated stent-grafts are widely available, now prefer primary fenestrated stent-graft implantation to implantation

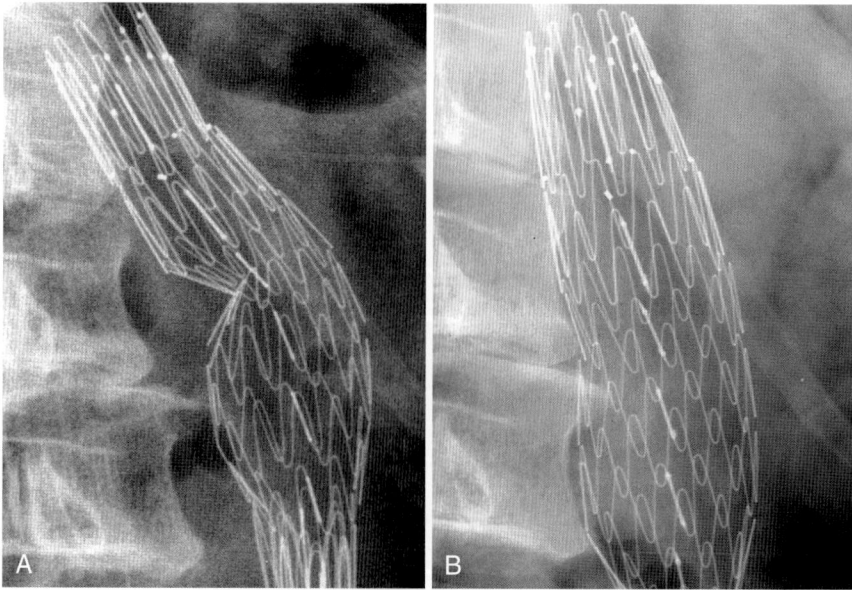

Figure 129-9 Abdominal radiographs 1 week (**A**) and 4 years (**B**) after implantation of a Zenith stent-graft. Note the effect of neck dilatation on stent-graft profile.

of a very large (36 mm) stent-graft in an already dilated neck. When fenestrated stent-grafts are not available, the best option may be to avoid EVAR when the proximal neck characteristics suggest future progression to a pararenal aneurysm.[160,161]

Stent-Graft Infection

Unlike a graft implanted during open surgery, an endovascular graft has less risk of direct contamination from the patient's skin or the surgeon's gloves. However, it may be at greater risk for hematogenous seeding because unlike an open surgical graft, it never becomes incorporated into surrounding tissue. There is also a risk of contamination during catheter-based re-intervention, which used to be a common occurrence when stent-grafts were less stable and type II endoleaks were treated more aggressively. The net effect is an infection rate after EVAR of 0.43%,[162] which approximates the lower end of the range for surgical grafts.

Pelvic Ischemia

Buttock claudication is the most common but by no means the most severe manifestation of pelvic ischemia after internal iliac artery occlusion during EVAR. Others complications include buttock necrosis, colon necrosis, spinal ischemia, lumbosacral plexus ischemia, and erectile dysfunction. The reported rates of each complication vary. Buttock claudication occurs at a rate of 16% to 50%.[163,164] An analysis of pooled data from 20 published studies showed a rate of buttock claudication of 29% after unilateral and 32% after bilateral internal iliac artery occlusion.[165] The same review reported erectile dysfunction rates of 15% and 17% after unilateral and bilateral internal iliac artery occlusion, respectively. The other listed complications are rare. The most feared complication, ischemic colitis, occurs in less than 2% of elective EVAR cases.[166]

The aforementioned manifestations of pelvic ischemia secondary to internal iliac artery occlusion usually occur when the common iliac artery is too wide for stent-graft implantation and the external iliac artery is used instead, but there are other contributory factors. In theory, risk for colon necrosis is higher if EVAR occludes a previously patent inferior mesenteric artery, previous colon surgery has interrupted the collateral pathways from the superior mesenteric artery, or the superior mesenteric and celiac arteries are stenotic or occluded. In practice, colon ischemia is more likely to result from embolism to the pelvic circulation than from proximal internal iliac artery occlusion.[166-168] The risk for buttock claudication is probably greater if the deep femoral arteries are severely diseased.

Internal Iliac Occlusion

The presence of a rich cross-pelvic collateral network was the basis for two early principles of common iliac aneurysm management at the time of EVAR. First, the internal iliac artery should be occluded with plugs or embolization coils to prevent retrograde (type II) endoleak. Second, bilateral internal iliac occlusion should be avoided at all cost, whereas unilateral occlusion is relatively benign. Both assumptions have been challenged. Opinions vary widely regarding the dangers of bilateral internal iliac embolization,[169,170] and some authors just cover the internal iliac artery with a stent-graft en route to an external iliac implantation site. Nevertheless, the current standard of practice for EVAR in the presence of an iliac aneurysm involves catheter-based proximal internal iliac artery occlusion (anatomy permitting) and some attempt to preserve flow to at least one internal iliac artery. Occlusion of the internal iliac artery is done as far proximally as possible to preserve distal collateral branches.

When internal iliac aneurysms preclude preservation of the internal iliac, some authors have advocated staged coil embolization in the hope that collateral pathways will develop in the time between interventions.[171] This approach also rests on the assumption that the newly developed collaterals will come from some artery outside the field of repair, such as the deep femoral artery, not some artery that will be occluded when EVAR completes aortoiliac exclusion, such as the inferior mesenteric or contralateral internal iliac.

Preserving Internal Iliac Flow

The problem of internal iliac artery occlusion can be avoided if one of the common iliac arteries is small enough to serve as an implantation site for a wide graft limb.[172] The Zenith stent-graft, for example, has graft limbs up to 24 mm in diameter for use in iliac arteries up to 22 mm in diameter (see Fig. 129-6). Even larger iliac arteries can be treated by substituting an aortic cuff or, in the case of the Zenith, an upside-down aortic converter for the usual limb extension. The use of a dilated common iliac artery as a distal implantation site has the theoretical disadvantage of leaving an aneurysm in the making untreated or only partially treated. However, the potential for further iliac dilatation is rarely realized in practice.[171] More likely the patient will die of something else before an iliac aneurysm large enough to warrant treatment develops. In any case, should an aneurysm develop, a stent-graft extension to the external iliac artery remains an option.

The other options for internal iliac preservation are combined external iliac stent-graft implantation with surgical bypass to the internal iliac artery, combined aortouniiliac stent-graft implantation to the contralateral side with insertion of a covered stent between the ipsilateral external and internal iliac arteries, and insertion of a bifurcated iliac stent-graft with prograde outflow to both the external and internal iliac arteries.

Our preferred approach is a bifurcated common iliac reconstruction with a covered stent as an extension into the internal iliac artery (Fig. 129-10). The necessary bifurcated component (see Fig. 129-10A) has long been available outside the United States for use with the Zenith AAA stent-graft.[173] If the common iliac artery is longer than 5 to

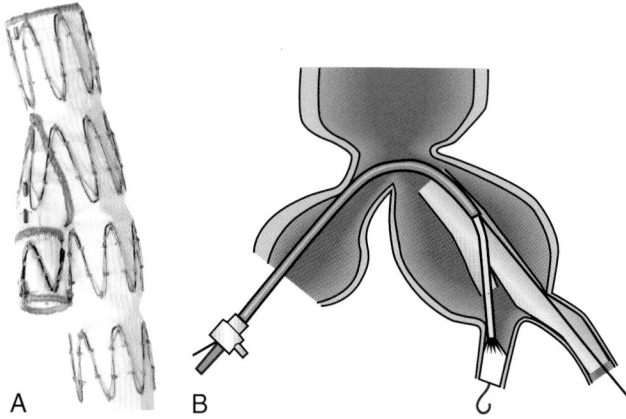

Figure 129-10 A, The bifurcated iliac component has outflow into the external and internal iliac arteries. **B,** The internal iliac branch is usually inserted through a contralateral femoral approach.

6 cm, the covered stent extension to the internal iliac artery is usually inserted over the aortic bifurcation from the contralateral femoral artery (see Fig. 129-10B). Otherwise, the covered stent has to be inserted through a brachial approach, which has become the preferred technique in East Asia, where many patients have short dilated common iliac arteries.

Stent Fatigue

Micromotion of a stent-graft's metallic exoskeleton produces a change in its crystalline structure at points of strain that leads to fracture of the stent struts, barbs, and longitudinal supports, which may or may not affect stent-graft function. Surface irregularities on inadequately polished stents, especially nitinol stents, serve as foci for stress and strain and initiate erosive changes that further degrade stent structure.

Both sources of structural failure were common features in early stent-graft designs and, until recently, the sole source of information regarding the causes of stent fatigue and fracture. Preclinical durability testing in vitro was limited by a lack of information regarding boundary conditions. The standard assumption of 5% cyclic strain bears no relation to the observed behavior of any implanted stent-graft. Serial fluoroscopic studies of the Zenith stent-graft, for example, show a striking reduction in motion of the central portion of the stent-graft as the external pressure falls below the internal pressure throughout the cardiac cycle. At 1 month the pulsatile diameter change was less than 0.5% of systolic diameter.

The Vanguard stent-graft provided examples of every form of structural failure, including stent fracture, stent corrosion, graft erosion, suture line failure, and component separation.[24,25] Others, such as the LifePath and original Ancure, broke in ways that profoundly affected their function.[174] All the currently available stent-grafts are prone to barb separation and stent breakage.[175,176] An analysis of explanted AneuRx

stent-grafts showed multiple stent fractures and fabric holes.[62] However, there is little evidence linking these minor structural failures to adverse outcomes,[62] and the more serious failure modes have been addressed by changes in stent-graft design.

FOLLOW-UP

The primary goal of follow-up is to identify impending failure while it is still amenable to treatment, preferably catheter-based treatment. The failing stent-graft produces no physical signs or symptoms until some catastrophic event occurs, hence the importance of image-based follow-up. The standard recommendations for contrast-enhanced CT at 1, 6, and 12 months and then annually were developed as part of the regulatory approval process. In the absence of any data on long-term outcome, imaging protocols had to be as rigorous as possible. That constraint no longer applies. We now have sufficient information on long-term device performance to make device-specific recommendations regarding follow-up.

Imaging

Follow-up imaging is intended to detect any change in the structure, position, or function of the stent-graft. Possible imaging modalities include MRI, duplex ultrasound, plain abdominal radiography, and CT with or without intravenous contrast enhancement. MRI is expensive and cannot be used to image ferromagnetic stent-grafts such as the Zenith.[124] Moreover, gadolinium contrast is contraindicated in patients with renal failure. Duplex ultrasound is inexpensive and noninvasive but of variable quality, depending on the experience of the technician and patient-related factors such as bowel gas and obesity.[120]

Contrast-enhanced CT scans are nephrotoxic and no better than unenhanced CT scans for the detection of aneurysm dilatation, but when reconstructed in three dimensions, they can be used to assess aneurysm volume, stent-graft position, and luminal narrowing. Three-dimensional images, in the form of volume-rendered displays, maximum image intensity projections, multiplanar reconstructions, and curved planar reconstructions, can be created by using the processing capabilities of the CT scanner, a free-standing workstation (TeraRecon, San Mateo, CA), or an outside service (M2S, Inc., West Lebanon, NH).

The relative merits of duplex ultrasound as a means of detecting endoleak were discussed under "Endoleak Detection." Duplex may also provide noninvasive measurements of aneurysm diameter. Data from the Aneurysm Detection and Management (ADAM) study show a disparity between CT-based measurements and duplex-based measurements of 5 mm or more in about 30% of cases,[101] and the results of duplex ultrasound are certainly dependent on technique. Serial measurements by the same individuals using the same equipment should provide more reliable information in the majority of cases, and patients who are difficult to study by ultrasound can be triaged to another form of aneurysm diameter measurement, such as non–contrast-enhanced CT.

Sac Pressure Measurement

Some authors have recommended sac pressure monitoring[49,50,141,177] as an alternative to image-based follow-up. The pressure measurements obtained with an implantable sensor have been shown to correlate well with the pressure measurements obtained through a catheter in the sac,[50] and low sac pressures predict aneurysm shrinkage however they are measured.[51,52] One potential role for monitoring sac pressure is for cases of known type II endoleak, for which aneurysm dilatation currently stands as the primary indication for re-intervention. This technique might even have a role as the primary means of follow-up, with the following caveats. First, the sensitivity and specificity of early postoperative pressure measurements for the detection of direct endoleak (types I and III) were 94% and 80%, respectively.[49] Some dangerous endoleaks would be missed and some patients would require imaging studies based on false-positive pressure readings. Second, sac pressure varies throughout the sac,[54,142] and the direction of measurement influences the reading.[177] The pressure readings obtained by an implanted sensor in one orientation and one part of the aneurysm may be a poor reflection of overall sac pressure and the risk for dilatation or rupture. Third, pressure monitoring will not identify incipient failure caused by progressive migration or component separation until an endoleak (type I or III) develops and leads to aneurysm pressurization and possible rupture. In the absence of image-based follow-up, the only way to ensure prompt detection and treatment would be very frequent pressure measurement.

Device-Specific Late Failure Modes

Graft limb occlusion is by far the most common late failure mode of the Zenith device.[97,149] In our experience, routine CT-based imaging rarely shows signs of impending occlusion. Patients underwent rigorous contrast-enhanced CT follow-up only to be seen later with signs and symptoms of limb thrombosis. Besides, the majority of cases of limb occlusion occurred within a month of implantation. The other late failure modes of the Zenith device are rare and preventable. Migration, the most common late failure mode of the AneuRx stent-graft, may also be difficult to identify on standard CT scans (see earlier under "Migration") until wall contact is lost and a type I endoleak develops. The same limitation applies to pressure monitoring for the detection of migration. Other widely used devices have migration rates between those of the Zenith and AneuRx devices.[96] Component separation, stent fracture, and fabric erosion used to be common complications of EVAR with first-generation devices,[12,17,26,62,65,102,103] but they have largely been eliminated by improvements in stent-graft design.

Recommendations for Follow-up

Recent data regarding the long-term stability of EVAR have prompted some to reduce the follow-up regimen.[101,178,179] Device-specific modes of late failure require device-specific follow-up. The institutional experience at the University of California, San Francisco (UCSF), reflects the performance of the Zenith stent-graft, which has low rates of migration, component separation, secondary endoleak, and endotension[71,102,180] and a high rate of early limb thrombosis. We agree with the recommendations of Sternbergh and colleagues.[179] In the absence of endoleak on 1-month and 12-month contrast-enhanced CT scans, annual follow-up consists of plain abdominal radiographs in multiple views to monitor stent-graft shape and structure and duplex ultrasound to monitor aneurysm diameter. If duplex is not feasible because of obesity or bowel gas, we monitor aneurysm diameter with non–contrast-enhanced CT.

ENDOVASCULAR ANEURYSM REPAIR IN THE PROXIMAL ABDOMINAL AORTA

Most abdominal aortic stent-grafts are designed for implantation within a segment of nondilated infrarenal aorta, the neck. The lack of a suitable neck is the most common factor precluding standard infrarenal EVAR.[30-34] The minimum neck length depends on the angle, shape, and diameter of the neck. When the neck is clearly inadequate, one has to look to the pararenal, paravisceral, or supraceliac aorta for an attachment site, depending on the proximal extent of disease. Under these circumstances, the stent-graft has to satisfy competing goals: exclude the aneurysmal segment of aorta from the circulation and maintain flow to the aneurysm's renal, superior mesenteric, and celiac branches.

Renal Stents

Renal stents can be inserted after stent-graft implantation to push the margin of the graft down and maintain a channel to one or both renal arteries in the event of partial renal orificial coverage by the covered stent.[181] The technique differs from stent implantation for renal artery stenosis in two regards. First, access to the renal artery may be complicated by the presence of an uncovered suprarenal attachment stent that divides the pararenal aorta into triangles. It is almost always possible to find a route around the stent struts through one of these triangles into the renal artery, but one has to be sure that this route traverses the base of a triangle, which is wide, not the apex of the adjacent triangle, which is narrow. Second, the functioning part of the stent is in the aorta, not the renal artery. The stent can be short, but it has to stick well out of the renal orifice into the aorta.

Another approach is to insert the renal stent through a transbrachial sheath alongside the top of the stent-graft. This type of stent pushes the wall of the stent-graft inward, not

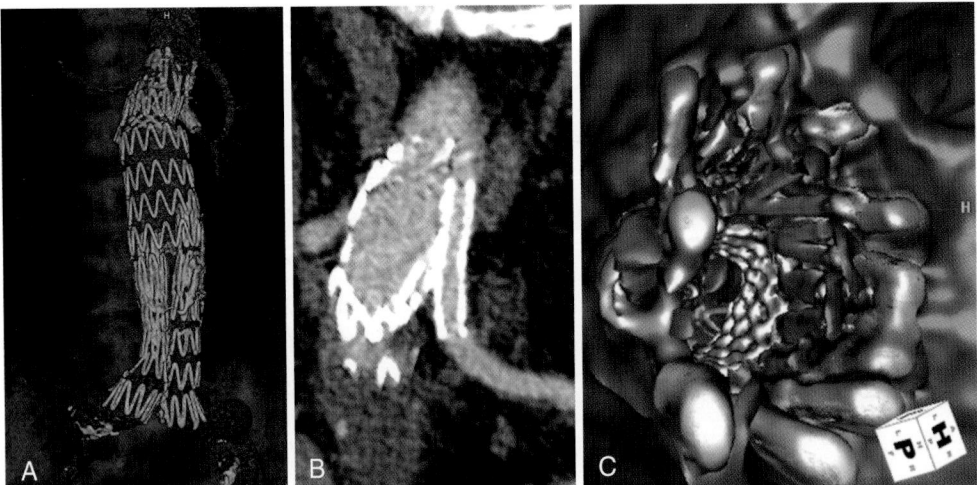

Figure 129-11 Surface-rendered (**A**), thin-slice maximum intensity projection (**B**), and fly-through (**C**) reconstructions of a postoperative contrast-enhanced CT scan after endovascular aneurysm repair with the snorkel technique.

downward, and permits a greater degree of renal coverage. The proximal end of the renal stent extends just beyond the proximal end of the aortic stent-graft (Fig. 129-11) as a "snorkel" or "chimney."[182]

The presence of a renal stent disrupts the seal between the stent-graft and aorta and creates potential routes of leakage into the aneurysm (type I endoleak), hence the importance of close apposition between the stent-graft and the nondilated aorta below the renal arteries. A giant Palmaz stent is sometimes needed to enhance this tenuous rim of contact. This is easier to do at the time of stent-graft insertion than a week later when the CT scan shows an endoleak because one of the prerequisites for Palmaz stent implantation is balloon protection of the renal stent lumen, and renal access may be difficult to re-establish.

There are no data on the long-term results of adjunctive renal stenting, but medium-term endoleak and renal patency rates are encouraging.[181,182] The mere presence of a renal stent does not appear to induce a hyperplastic response. The main problem with this approach is the lack of an alternative plan in the event of persistent endoleak. The only endovascular remedies involve the loss of a renal artery.

Fenestrated Stent-Grafts

The key to successful implantation of a suprarenal fenestrated stent-graft is precise alignment between each fenestration and the corresponding renal artery. This is achieved by staged stent-graft deployment, which affords the opportunity to insert a bridging catheter to guide the last stages of stent-graft expansion.[35,36] The bridging catheter is then replaced with a flared bridging stent to maintain close apposition between the margin of the fenestration and the margin of the renal orifice. No guiding catheters or stents are used with the open-topped fenestrations, or scallops, to the superior mesenteric and celiac artery orifices.

The technique of fenestrated stent-graft implantation may be complicated, yet thousands of these devices have been inserted worldwide with high rates of technical and clinical success.[183,184] The most worrisome complication has been renal artery stenosis or occlusion,[185] yet the results of fenestrated EVAR seem to be improving. The largest published series,[184] consisting of 119 patients, was notable for a 74% rate of aneurysm shrinkage at 2 years with no ruptures, no conversions, and only one instance of migration. Similar findings have been reported from the U.S. pivotal investigational device exemption trial. All 30 fenestrated Zenith stent-grafts were inserted successfully, and with 2 years of follow-up there have been no aneurysm-related deaths, no ruptures, no conversions, no type I endoleaks, no type III endoleaks, and no cases of aneurysm dilatation. The mortality and morbidity rates of both studies compare well with the results of open surgery for juxtarenal aneurysm.[186-188]

Branched Stent-Grafts

Pararenal and thoracoabdominal aortic aneurysms are not amenable to repair with standard fenestrated stent-grafts because the fenestrations would open directly into the aneurysm. The substitution of a covered stent for the usual uncovered bridging stent converts the fenestration into a branch through which blood flows across the aneurysm sac from the trunk of the stent-graft to the lumen of the target artery. This approach has been used to treat pararenal and thoracoabdominal aneurysms.[40,43] The tenuous connection between the margin of the fenestration and the outer surface of the usual balloon-expanded covered stent is hemostatic and stable, provided that the branch is short and the stent-graft's position is stable. However, when the aneurysm is large and the branch is long, hemodynamic and respiratory movements are more likely to distort the covered stent and lead to branch occlusion or a type III endoleak.

At UCSF we prefer self-expanding covered stents to balloon-expandable stents and axially oriented cuffs to fenestrations[41,42] because we believe that cuff-re-enforced intercomponent connections are more robust, more hemostatic, easier to plan, and easier to insert (Fig. 129-12). Axially oriented connections allow intraoperative adjustments to be made in the exact length and orientation of each covered stent. This form of in situ customization is very forgiving. Small errors in stent-graft sizing or implantation are without serious consequences, and in many cases the multibranched stent-graft can be assembled from standard off-the-shelf components. All 48 branched stent-grafts in a series of pararenal and thoracoabdominal aortic aneurysm repairs were inserted as intended. Among the 40 patients with nothing but caudad cuffs, the perioperative mortality rate was 5% and the paraplegia rate was 5%. The sole case of type I endoleak was treated early in the postoperative course with an additional covered stent. There have been no migrations or component separations with follow-up to 3 years. The assisted primary patency rate of the branches was 98%. In view of the fact that 55% of these patients had type II or III thoracoabdominal aortic aneurysms, the mortality and morbidity rates compare well with the results of open surgery[189-192] or hybrid repair.[193,194]

Despite these encouraging results, widespread application of multibranched endovascular aneurysm repair is limited by the high cumulative cost of the components and regulatory barriers to device availability, especially in the United States. There currently exist no viable regulatory pathways for approval of this type of device because it has several components, each from a different manufacturer.

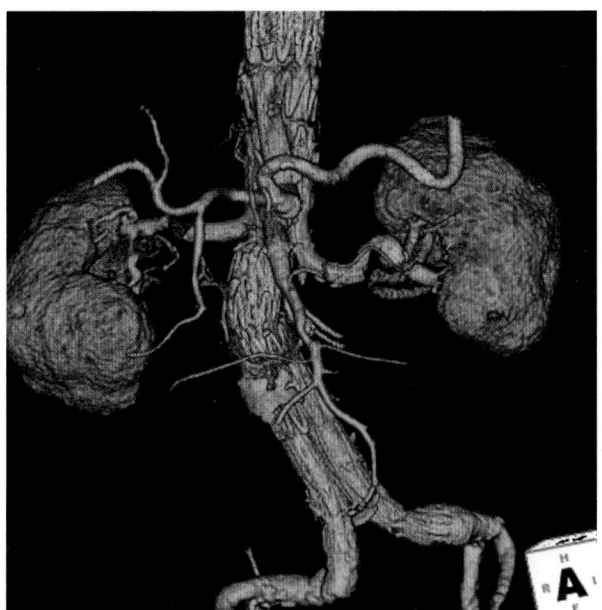

Figure 129-12 Surface-rendered CT after endovascular repair of a thoracoabdominal aortic aneurysm with a multibranched stent-graft.

ENDOVASCULAR REPAIR OF ISOLATED ILIAC ARTERY ANEURYSMS

Epidemiology and Indications

Approximately 20% to 30% of patients who have AAAs also have iliac aneurysms, and approximately 80% who have iliac aneurysms also have AAAs. Isolated iliac aneurysms, most of which affect the common iliac artery, represent only 2% of all intra-abdominal aneurysms.[195]

The relationship between aneurysm diameter and rupture risk is not as clear for iliac aneurysms as it is for aortic aneurysms.[196] In the absence of good data on the natural history of iliac aneurysms, most authors recommend treatment when the diameter exceeds 30 to 40 mm.[197,198] The specific approach to endovascular treatment of an isolated iliac aneurysm depends largely on the state of the proximal and distal ends of the common iliac artery.

Technique

The presence of a nondilated segment of proximal common iliac artery (70% to 80% of cases) permits unilateral repair.[198-200] Although the proximal implantation site may not be frankly aneurysmal, it is often much larger than the distal implantation site, in which case unilateral iliac aneurysm repair requires a tapered stent-graft. Aorto-uniiliac stent-grafts, Zenith uniiliac converters, and reversed graft limbs[199] have all been used in this role. The size disparity between the proximal and distal implantation sites contributes to a high incidence of graft thrombosis. Adjunctive stenting with bare-metal stents is often advisable in cases of external iliac implantation.[149,152] The absence of a nondilated segment of proximal common iliac artery (20% to 30% of cases) necessitates proximal implantation of a bifurcated or uniiliac stent-graft in the aorta, which requires wide-caliber bilateral femoral access.

The presence of a nondilated segment of distal common iliac artery permits preservation of the internal iliac artery. More commonly, the common iliac aneurysm ends at its bifurcation, the only distal implantation site is in the external iliac artery, and prograde flow to the internal iliac is lost.[198-200] The indications for internal iliac embolization or preservation are the same whether endovascular repair of the aneurysmal common iliac artery occurs alone or in association with endovascular repair of an AAA (see earlier under "Pelvic Ischemia").

Internal Iliac Aneurysm. Approximately 40% of isolated iliac aneurysms involve the internal iliac artery, half of which are associated with common iliac aneurysms[200] and the other half are confined to the internal iliac arteries. When the entire internal iliac artery is involved, as it usually is, the aneurysm cannot be excluded from the circulation without occluding internal iliac flow. Effective therapy closes both ends of the internal iliac artery. The distal end is closed with embolization coils. The proximal end is closed with coils, an Amplatzer plug, or a stent-graft between the common and the external iliac arteries.

Results

Several studies have compared the results of endovascular and open surgical repair of isolated iliac aneurysms.[198,199] None were large enough for meaningful comparisons of mortality, but all concluded that endovascular repair was associated with significantly less blood loss (<50 versus 318 mL), shorter operative time (86 versus 143 minutes), shorter hospital stay (2.1 versus 4.8 days), and lower complication rates than open repair,[198,199] at least in the short term.

COST OF ENDOVASCULAR ANEURYSM REPAIR

In the short term, reductions in the cost of perioperative care generally fail to offset the high price of an endovascular stent-graft. The initial in-hospital cost of EVAR is approximately $20,000 in the United States.[201] This is higher than the mean cost of open surgical repair. The same is true in the United Kingdom, as evidenced by the findings of EVAR-1.[64] The exact numbers depends on local costs and practice patterns, both of which are still evolving.

The long-term costs are even more difficult to determine, partly because they depend on device-specific re-intervention rates and follow-up protocols. In the absence of re-intervention, the cost of follow-up to 5 years is approximately $3700,[201] and re-intervention increases the cost almost 10-fold. However, these additional postoperative costs should not be regarded as inevitable consequences of the endovascular approach. Long-term outcomes, re-intervention rates, and follow-up protocols are changing as more stable devices enter widespread use. Recent evidence suggests that the long-term results of EVAR are at least as good as those of open repair,[64,106] that re-intervention is rarely necessary to treat type II endoleak, and that routine CT-based follow-up is a low-yield activity.[101]

IMPACT OF ENDOVASCULAR REPAIR ON THE MORTALITY OF ABDOMINAL AORTIC ANEURYSM REPAIR

The time when EVAR could be described as a failed experiment[202] is long gone. Whatever doubts remain regarding the relative merits of EVAR versus open surgery, vascular surgeons have triaged patients to EVAR in ever-increasing numbers. The selection process is apparent when one compares EVAR and surgical patients.[26,70-73] EVAR patients tend to have less severe arterial disease, whereas surgical patients tend to have less severe cardiopulmonary disease. An overall reduction in the perioperative mortality of aneurysm repair reflects the combined effects of three factors: EVAR has a low mortality rate, the mortality rates of open surgery are better

in healthier patients, and changing skill sets change referral patterns, thereby funneling cases to high-volume centers,[203] where the results of aneurysm repair have always been better.[204,205]

UNRESOLVED ISSUES

The main unresolved issue is how to manage patients who before the advent of EVAR would have been observed. These patients fall into two groups: those with small aneurysms and those with high-risk physiology. In each case there remains enough doubt regarding proper management to warrant a randomized controlled study.

A randomized comparison of EVAR versus observation of high-risk patients with large aneurysms has already been done, but the study (EVAR-2) had serious flaws and the findings are controversial. Another study is needed.

A randomized comparison of open aneurysm repair versus observation of normal-risk patients with small (4.0 to 5.5 cm) aneurysms has also already been done, with open repair in the treatment arm.[99,101] Both studies supported the idea that observation is safe but often ends in treatment. The corresponding EVAR trials are under way, but several complex factors may make them difficult to interpret. In many small aneurysm cases the choice is between early treatment, with a long period of follow-up and possible re-intervention, and late treatment, with a long period of observation. The difference between the two alternatives depends largely on the nature of the follow-up protocol and the rate of re-intervention. An unstable stent-graft requires close follow-up and frequent re-intervention, which may tilt the balance in favor of observation. In addition, early data suggest that various drug regimens (statins, doxycycline, roxithromycin) may reduce the rates of aneurysm dilatation[206-208] and rupture.[66,209] Success in this area will also tilt the balance in favor of observation. These multiple factors suggest that individual patient decision making by informed, experienced surgeons will probably lead to optimal results.

SELECTED KEY REFERENCES

Dias NV, Ivancev K, Malina M, Resch T, Lindblad B, Sonesson B. Intra-aneurysm sac pressure measurements after endovascular aneurysm repair: differences between shrinking, unchanged, and expanding aneurysms with and without endoleaks. *J Vasc Surg.* 2004;39:1229-1235.
These data support the long-assumed connection between endoleak, aneurysm pressurization, and aneurysm diameter change.

Greenhalgh RM, Brown LC, Kwong GP, Powell JT, Thompson SG; EVAR trial participants. Comparison of endovascular aneurysm repair with open repair in patients with abdominal aortic aneurysm (EVAR trial 1), 30-day operative mortality results: randomized controlled trial. *Lancet.* 2004;364:843-848.
This large prospective randomized study compares the results of open surgery with the results of EVAR in good-risk patients. It is one of the few sources of level 1 data on the subject.

EVAR trial participants. Endovascular aneurysm repair and outcome in patients unfit for open repair of abdominal aortic aneurysm (EVAR trial 2): randomised controlled trial. *Lancet.* 2005;365:2187-2192.
Flawed as it is, this study remains the only source of level 1 data on the relative mortality of EVAR and observation in patients considered unfit for surgical repair.

Franks SC, Sutton AJ, Bown MJ, Sayers RD. Systematic review and meta-analysis of 12 years of endovascular abdominal aortic aneurysm repair. *Eur J Vasc Endovasc Surg.* 2007;33:154-171.
This meta-regression analysis showed a steady decline in postoperative mortality, rupture, and endoleak rates between 1992 and 2002.

Schermerhorn ML, O'Malley AJ, Jhaveri A, et al. Endovascular vs. open repair of abdominal aortic aneurysms in the medicare population. *N Engl J Med.* 2008;358:464-474.
This retrospective analysis is one of the few sources of data on the late complications of open surgical aneurysm repair.

van Marrewijk C, Buth J, Harris PL, Norgren L, Nevelsteen A, Wyatt MG. Significance of endoleaks after endovascular repair of abdominal aortic aneurysms: The EUROSTAR experience. *J Vasc Surg.* 2002; 35:461-473.
This review of registry data examines the relationship between endoleak type, failure mode, and outcome. It provides a sound basis for the interpretation of postoperative CT findings.

van Marrewijk CJ, Leurs LJ, Vallabhaneni SR, Harris PL, Buth J, Laheij RJ, for the EUROSTAR collaborators. Risk-adjusted outcome analysis of endovascular abdominal aortic aneurysm repair. *J Endovasc Ther.* 2005;12:417-429.
This analysis of EUROSTAR registry data gives the device-specific risks for various late complications of EVAR.

REFERENCES

The reference list can be found on the companion Expert Consult Web site at *www.expertconsult.com.*

Section **17** Arterial Aneurysms

CHAPTER 130

Abdominal Aortic Aneurysms: Ruptured

Thomas F. Lindsay

Rupture of abdominal aortic aneurysm (RAAA) remains a lethal condition despite almost 60 years since the first reports of successful repair with homografts before the availability of polyester grafts.[1,2] The early report of repair of RAAA from Cooley and DeBakey noted a 50% survival rate, a statistic that has proved stubbornly difficult to improve over 6 decades of effort.[3]

■ MORTALITY OF RUPTURE

A meta-analysis of the first 50 years of RAAA publications noted that the mortality rate for ruptured repair has fallen only 3.5% per decade since the initial successful repairs were reported.[2] A meta-analysis of publications between 1991 and 2006 suggested no significant overall change in mortality with open repair over this period.[1] This conclusion is supported by data from U.S. Veterans Affairs (VA) hospitals and the U.S. National Hospital Discharge database (over the years 1979 to 1997), which have not demonstrated a decline in RAAA mortality.[2] Between 1994 and 2003, mortality after open RAAA repair was unchanged based on U.S. Medicare data.[4] It is estimated that 80% of the mortality from abdominal aortic aneurysms (AAAs) is secondary to rupture. The mortality rate for patients who arrive at the hospital alive ranges between 40% and 70%.[2,5,6] When autopsy data are taken into account, including those patients who die at home before arrival at the hospital or without any hospital care at all, the RAAA mortality rate approaches 90%.[7]

The high postoperative mortality rates after aortic rupture are secondary to a high incidence of myocardial infarction, renal failure, and the development of multiple organ failure (MOF). Aortic rupture and open repair result in a combination of ischemia-reperfusion injuries, hemorrhagic shock, and lower torso ischemia. The synergistic effect of the total-body ischemia caused by hemorrhagic shock and the lower torso ischemia that occurs during repair, followed by reperfusion secondary to resuscitation and aortic unclamping, has been proposed to explain the high incidence of MOF and mortality after repair. This hypothesis is supported by data from both animal experimentation and human clinical studies.[8,9] The application of endovascular techniques to repair ruptured AAAs (rEVAR) reduces the operative and ischemic insult in two ways. First, it avoids a laparotomy, thus reducing the potential for iatrogenic arterial and venous operative injuries and their associated blood loss. Second, it minimizes the duration and severity of the lower torso ischemic insult. Recent data from large administrative databases in the United States have demonstrated increased application of endovascular aneurysm repair (EVAR) to RAAA.[4,5,10,11] Analysis of mortality rates of rEVAR cases between 2000 and 2003 noted a significant reduction in the mortality of RAAA patients treated by EVAR (31.85 versus 50.8%; $P < .001$).[12]

Terminology

AAA rupture is defined as bleeding outside the adventitia of a dilated aortic wall. RAAA is further subclassified into free and retroperitoneal rupture. Free rupture into the peritoneal cavity has a worse prognosis because the rapid, large-volume blood loss overwhelms the ability of retroperitoneal tissue to provide tamponade and thereby reduce the rate and volume of blood loss.[13]

Differentiation between symptomatic and ruptured aneurysms is critical. Symptomatic AAAs are those that have become painful and tender but in which blood has not breached the aortic wall. Symptomatic aneurysms may have symptoms of variable severity ranging from mild tenderness to pain indistinguishable from rupture. The pain is thought to be related to acute expansion of the wall, intramural hemorrhage, wall degeneration, or bleeding into the thrombus and is therefore considered a prelude to actual rupture, which requires urgent repair. Symptomatic aneurysms are not associated with hypotension; however, the prognosis is much better than that of RAAA (but worse than after elective repair).[14] The inclusion of symptomatic aneurysms in data on RAAA will artificially improve the data. Those with symptoms and an AAA require rapid diagnosis and management to prevent rupture and its associated adverse outcomes.[13]

Impact of Endovascular Repair

rEVAR may be the most important innovation in more than 50 years and has the potential to reduce the excessive mortality of RAAA, and published series have begun to show significant mortality benefits with the use of rEVAR.[4,10,11,15,16] This is consistent with the "two-hit" injury hypothesis because the second hit, the lower torso ischemia, is markedly reduced by rEVAR.[9] The importance of several issues remains unresolved, including the rapid availability of preoperative computed tomography (CT) to identify those who are not anatomic candidates for this therapy (estimates range between 33% and 53%). Other logistical considerations include the availability of trained staff and of the devices required to perform rEVAR at all centers at all hours.[17,18] However, in general, more stable patients with RAAA have been selected for rEVAR, whereas less stable patients have been treated by open repair. This potentially biases the comparison, and some have suggested that EVAR and open repair for RAAA have similar mortality in comparable patients.[19]

EPIDEMIOLOGY

The true incidence of RAAA is difficult to determine in different populations because of the measurement methods used. Population-based autopsy data have revealed higher numbers of RAAAs and an overall mortality rate of 90% for RAAA. Those who die outside the hospital would be excluded from national, statewide, and center-based publications, thus resulting in an underestimation of the true incidence of RAAA.

Population statistics from the United States demonstrate that aortic aneurysms account for 15,810 deaths per year (1999 data), with 83.5% of these deaths occurring in patients older than 65 years and 93% in those older than 55.[20] In the United Kingdom there are on average 6800 deaths from RAAA per year, and it accounts for 2.1% of all deaths in men older than 65.[18] RAAA is the 10th leading cause of death in men older than 65 years in the United States. Thus, RAAA remains a significant cause of death and accounts for a similar number of deaths as in prostate, gastric, and esophageal cancer.

Analysis of the U.S. National Inpatient Sample (NIS) database (which is a sample of all ages and payers) has noted a decline in the incidence of RAAAs per year from 9979 in 1993 to 6921 in 2005, a 30% decrease.[5,10,16] The largest decline in RAAA incidence occurred after the 1999 approval of commercial EVAR devices.[16] Medicare data (population >65 years of age) in the United States also suggested a decrease in the number of RAAAs diagnosed from 18.7 to 13.6 per 100,00 population from 1994 to 2003 (Fig. 130-1).[4] A significantly greater decline in RAAA incidence was observed for men

(29%) than for women, in whom the decline was 12% over the decade. A greater proportion of women (21%) than men (16%) had rupture.[11] Women underwent RAAA repair significantly less frequently, 62% versus 79% of men, and the proportion of women with rupture continues to increase. Thus, although a smaller percentage of women have aneurysms, they are more commonly seen with rupture, are on average 2 years older than men when initially evaluated, and have a lower incidence of repair with worse outcomes.

In the Oxford Region of the United Kingdom, the incidence of age- and sex-standardized hospital admission rates for RAAA between 1979 and 1999 increased from 0.3 to 2.2 admissions per 100,000 in women and from 5.2 to 14.9 admissions per 100,000 in men.[21] This represents an increase of 12.1% for women and 8.2% for men. These differences may relate to the number of autopsies performed because many ruptured AAAs are not diagnosed unless an autopsy is performed and death is attributed to other, usually cardiac causes. In general, this leads to an underestimation of the incidence of RAAA.[7] Because fewer autopsies are being performed in recent years, one would predict an apparent decline in RAAA because of failure to diagnose nonoperated cases. Although it is difficult to obtain precise incidence estimates, recent U.S. data do suggest a significant decline in the incidence of RAAA.[12,16]

Impact of Ruptured Abdominal Aortic Aneurysm on Total Abdominal Aortic Aneurysm–Related Mortality

Interestingly, only the most recent NIS data have shown a decline in total AAA-related mortality.[16] This has resulted from an increase in elective AAA repair (with a decline in the mortality rate because of more cases being done by EVAR) and from fewer RAAA repairs and declining overall procedural mortality. The decline in total AAA-related mortality has accelerated since the introduction of EVAR after Food and Drug Administration approval in 1999. Previously, there was little evidence that elective repair resulted in a reduction in the number of RAAAs over the years 1980 to 2000.[22] This change suggests that the ability to detect and treat AAA electively has improved. Recent data from the United Kingdom have demonstrated that a large randomized AAA screening program did reduce aneurysm-related mortality by 53% despite a 6% elective perioperative mortality rate.[23] These data conclusively show that the incidence of RAAA and its attendant death rate can be reduced by screening the population at risk.[23] In the United States, screening for AAA in new male Medicare enrollees began in 2005, and it will take several years to observe its impact on the incidence of RAAA in men. Other large national screening programs have yet to begin.

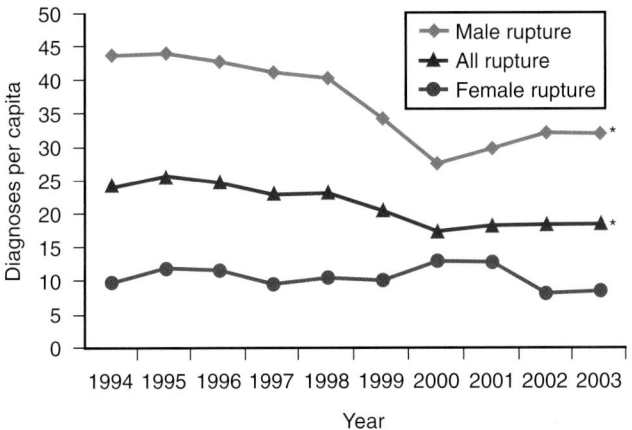

Figure 130-1 Ruptured abdominal aortic aneurysm repairs in men and women from 1994 to 2003 reported as diagnoses per 100,000 Medicare recipients. Rupture repairs are normalized to sex-appropriate populations. *P < .05 versus 1994 totals. *(From Dillavou ED, Muluk SC, Makaroun MS. A decade of change in abdominal aortic aneurysm repair in the United States: have we improved outcomes equally between men and women? J Vasc Surg. 2006;43:230-238.)*

PATHOGENESIS OF AORTIC RUPTURE

Clinical Factors Associated with Rupture

The single best method for predicting RAAA has traditionally been AAA diameter. The 5.5-cm-diameter threshold for

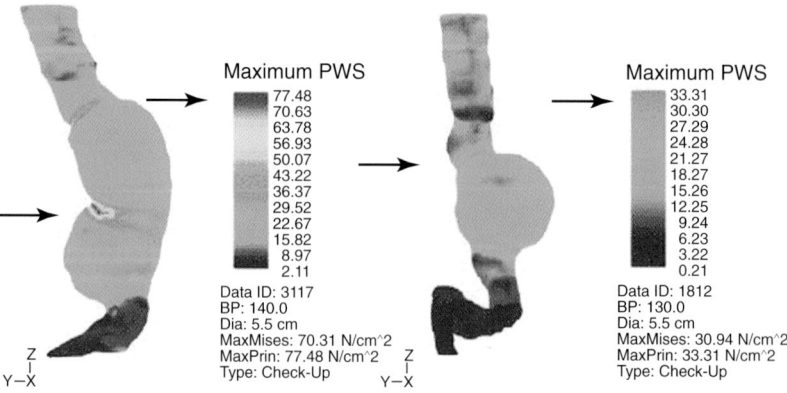

Figure 130-2 Three-dimensional stress distribution for maximum wall stress at peak systolic blood pressure (PWS) for two 5.5-cm aneurysms. Stress is mapped to corresponding colors, with highest stress shown in *red* and lower stress in *blue*. The stress map for the patient on the right has been color-coded to correspond to the stress map for the patient on the left for ease of comparison. *(From Fillinger MF, Marra SP, Raghavan ML, Kennedy FE. Prediction of rupture risk in abdominal aortic aneurysm during observation: wall stress versus diameter. J Vasc Surg. 2003;37:724-732.)*

repair in men is supported by two randomized trials, the Aneurysm Detection and Management (ADAM) trial and the U.K. Small Aneurysm Trial.[25,26] Female sex has also been found to be an independent risk factor for rupture, and a 5-cm threshold for repair in women has been suggested even though large prospective trials have not enrolled enough women to accurately define the optimal threshold for elective repair.[27] The observation that some small AAAs do rupture implies that factors other than size contribute to rupture risk. In addition to AAA diameter, the U.K. Small Aneurysm Trial found that female sex, higher mean blood pressure, hypertension, current smoking, and lower forced expiratory volume in 1 second (FEV_1) were independently associated with an increased risk for RAAA.[28] Female sex was associated with a threefold higher risk for rupture, comparable to the impact of a 1-cm increase in diameter. The association between chronic obstructive pulmonary disease and rupture has been identified in several retrospective studies; however, the association between rupture and lower FEV_1 was apparent only after 1167 nonrandomized patients were included in the analysis in the U.K. Small Aneurysm Trial.[29] Body mass index, age, serum cholesterol, and the ankle-brachial pressure index were not associated with an increased risk for RAAA.

Mechanism of Rupture

Aneurysm rupture represents failure of the aortic wall to bear the load or tension to which it is exposed. When the force of the blood pressure exceeds the ability of the aortic wall to bear that load, the aneurysm wall ruptures and blood extravagates. In vitro testing has demonstrated that the failure strength of human aneurysmal aortic wall is 65 N/cm² versus 121 N/cm² for nonaneurysmal human aortic wall. This indicates that the aneurysmal aortic wall is a weak structure.[30,31] Laplace's law (tension is proportional to radius times pressure) relates wall tension to pressure, thus emphasizing the importance of size. Although this method may be satisfactory for symmetric structures, it does not take into account the complex geometry of individual AAAs. The engineering technique of finite element analysis (FEA) has been applied to AAAs to estimate regional variations in peak wall stress (PWS) throughout the entire aneurysm wall. Using CT scan data, a mesh is applied

to the aortic wall, and FEA is used to calculate PWS for many small segments of the aortic wall to provide a visual representation of PWS (Fig. 130-2). Early three-dimensional representations of PWS noted that the posterior wall of the aorta had higher values corresponding to the site where most AAAs were noted in clinical observations and autopsy studies to have ruptured.[32,33]

Importance of Wall Stress

CT scans of elective, symptomatic, and ruptured AAAs were used to calculate PWS with FEA, and PWS was found to be a better predictor of rupture than Laplace's law.[32] Ruptured and symptomatic AAAs had similar calculated values of PWS (48 ± 6 and 48 ± 4 N/cm²), as opposed to elective cases, in which PWS was lower (37 ± 2 N/cm²).[34] Even when AAA diameters were equal, the PWS of ruptured and symptomatic AAAs was higher than that of asymptomatic ones. Small AAAs with high PWS can have a rupture risk similar to a much larger AAA with lower PWS, which explains the clinical observation that some small AAAs rupture whereas some large AAAs (>6.5 cm) are still able to undergo elective repair (Fig. 130-3).

In asymptomatic individuals, elevated PWS has been shown to identify AAAs that will become symptomatic or rupture.[34] This observation was re-enforced by an analysis of elective, ruptured, and symptomatic AAAs in which there was no difference in AAA diameter among groups; however, there were significant differences in PWS at the systolic blood pressure noted.[35] Analysis of the tensile strength of specimens of the anterior aortic wall harvested from elective and ruptured AAA patients noted significantly reduced aortic wall thickness and lower aortic wall tensile strength in the RAAA group than in elective AAA patients.[36] Other factors that have been investigated for prediction of rupture risk include geometry of the AAA, with ruptured AAAs being less tortuous but having greater cross-sectional diameter asymmetry. Women's AAAs rupture at smaller diameters (5 to 10 mm smaller than men), and current smokers have a higher risk for rupture.[28,37] The role of intraluminal thrombus has also been investigated as a risk factor for rupture secondary to its role in causing wall hypoxia.[38] Currently, several methods of determining patient-

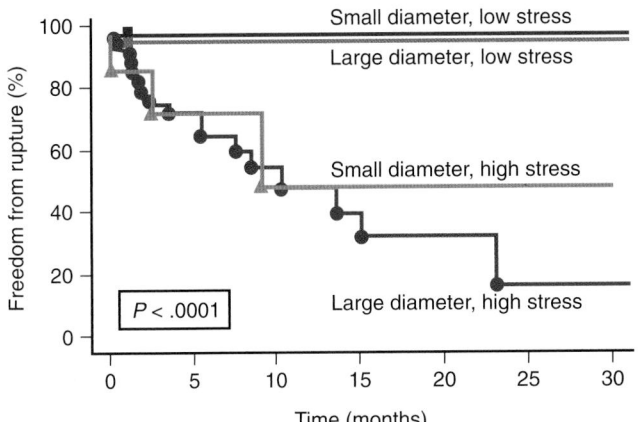

Figure 130-3 Life-table for freedom from rupture or emergency surgery because of acute symptoms. Subgroups were analyzed for combinations of small and large diameter and low and high wall stress, with the same thresholds as used in the other life-tables. Low-stress aneurysms had a low rupture rate whether they were small or large, and high-stress aneurysms had a high rupture rate regardless of size. *(From Fillinger MF, Marra SP, Raghavan ML, Kennedy FE. Prediction of rupture risk in abdominal aortic aneurysm during observation: wall stress versus diameter. J Vasc Surg. 2003;37:724-732.)*

specific rupture risk have been published; however, at present they remain investigational tools, although their validation will be very important for clinical care.[39,40]

Seasonal variability in RAAA rates has been identified, with increased rates during spring and fall. AAAs tend to rupture more frequently when atmospheric pressure is low, especially in those who are hypertensive.[41,42]

Biologic Changes in the Walls of Ruptured Abdominal Aortic Aneurysms

Just as alteration in PWS may be an important predictor of RAAA, the strength of the aortic wall is related to the elastin and fibrillar collagen types I and III content. The content of these components may not be uniform, and tissue failure leading to rupture may occur as a result of local loss of matrix strength secondary to the action of tissue enzymes that regulate proteolysis of matrix components. Comparison of the level of matrix metalloproteinases (MMPs) and tissue inhibitors of MMPs in the anterior aortic wall and at the site of AAA rupture has demonstrated that levels of MMP-8 and MMP-9 are significantly elevated at the site of rupture whereas levels in the anterior wall of the aorta are similar in elective repair and ruptured AAAs.[43] These measurements included both the total and active fractions of these enzymes. The enzymes appeared to be localized in mesenchymal cells at the site of rupture and were independent of the inflammatory infiltrate. Recently, significantly greater elevations in serum MMP-1 and MMP-9 levels were reported in patients with RAAA than in those undergoing elective AAA repair.[44] The mechanisms responsible for the local aortic wall elevations in MMP-8 and MMP-9 remain unclear; however, it is interesting to speculate on a relationship between PWS (a physical measure) and MMP activity in the aortic wall and serum (a biologic variable) and the possible signal transduction mechanisms relating these factors.

CLINICAL FINDINGS

Symptoms and Signs

RAAA is characterized by the classic triad of severe abdominal or back pain, hypotension, and a palpable pulsatile abdominal mass.[45,46] Large abdominal girth or hypotension can frequently obscure palpation of aneurysms. A history of a syncopal episode may indicate hypotension if low blood pressure has not been documented. A clinical history suggesting this combination of symptoms in a patient potentially at risk for AAA mandates that the clinician consider rupture and attempt to rule out this diagnosis. Other common symptoms reported include groin or flank pain, hematuria, and groin hernia (even incarceration) secondary to increased intra-abdominal pressure. Rupture into the vena cava may be manifested as congestive heart failure with distended neck veins, an abdominal bruit, and microscopic or macroscopic hematuria. This is an infrequent but well-recognized clinical scenario of an aortocaval fistula. Other possible communications between the aorta and venous structures include rupture into the iliac or renal vein. Rupture into the renal vein can lead to acute left varicocele and a painful scrotal mass.[47]

Differential Diagnosis and Misdiagnosis

In patients older than 50 years with hypotension or syncope (or both), consideration of RAAA is critical because it has the worst prognosis of conditions included in the differential diagnosis. A rapid, accurate history and examination are critical. The differential diagnosis may include renal colic, diverticulitis, pancreatitis, gastrointestinal hemorrhage, inferior myocardial infarction, and perforated ulcer. Although the signs and symptoms of RAAA can be clear-cut, in the early stages it may be difficult to recognize. Studies have examined the clinical findings in patients in whom RAAA was subsequently diagnosed.[45] In only 23% was a definitive and immediate diagnosis of RAAA made by the first physician who examined the patient.[48] The rate of incorrect diagnosis ranges from 16% to 60%.[49] The most common misdiagnoses were renal colic, perforated viscus, diverticulitis, gastrointestinal hemorrhage, and ischemic bowel. It is important to recall that the initial manifestation of renal colic occurs infrequently in patients older than 50 years. The classic triad of pain, hypotension, and a pulsatile mass was present in only 9% of the misdiagnosed group as compared with 34% of the correctly diagnosed group. The presence of a pulsatile mass was identified in 72% of those correctly diagnosed but in only 26% of the misdiagnosed patients. Thus, the lack of a pulsatile mass frequently confuses the diagnosis. Furthermore, the use of ultrasound in older studies was reported as being consistent with rupture in only 51% of cases.[49]

DIAGNOSTIC EVALUATION

Plain Radiographs

Plain radiography is now less frequently performed than ultrasound or CT in patients with abdominal pain. However, if the aortic wall is sufficiently calcified, an aneurysm not otherwise suspected can be identified on radiographs. A retrospective review of plain films of patients with RAAAs noted evidence of the diagnosis on 90% of the films.[50] Enlargement of a calcified aortic wall beyond normal limits was seen in 65%, and loss of a psoas shadow from retroperitoneal hemorrhage was identified in 75%.

Ultrasound

The introduction of bedside ultrasound in the emergency department and training of emergency physicians in its application for trauma have led to its use for imaging of the abdominal aorta in cases of suspected rupture. FAST (focused assessment with sonography in trauma) ultrasound protocols can rapidly identify fluid collections and direct further trauma care.[51] It has been used in the emergency room to rapidly evaluate aortic diameter in those with a suspicion of RAAA.[52] Ultrasound examination of the abdominal aorta can accurately identify an AAA and frequently takes less than 5 minutes.[53] When ultrasound is used in patients with back pain, abdominal pain, or other suspicion of AAA, it can identify aortic aneurysms with high sensitivity, specificity, and positive and negative predicative values.[54] To date, no large prospective studies have been conducted; however, it appears that with appropriate training of emergency physicians, the use of ultrasound to quickly assess patients for the presence of AAA is probably beneficial because it can rapidly direct further consultation, investigation, and therapy. Although ultrasound can rapidly identify an AAA, it is not accurate for exclusion of rupture.[53,54]

Computed Tomography

Accuracy

The most accurate method of diagnosing RAAA is CT, which also provides important information about associated abnormalities and conditions. CT scanning in patients suspected of having RAAA or other causes of abdominal pain is frequently ordered by the emergency physician when the diagnosis is unclear. A non–contrast-enhanced CT scan can identify retroperitoneal hemorrhage associated with a ruptured AAA and can also provide important anatomic information (Fig. 130-4). In addition, alternative abdominal pathology may be discovered should no AAA be identified. CT scanning with contrast enhancement is required for ideal planning of RAAA repair with commercially available stent-graft devices for the same reasons that it is required for elective repair. The volume of contrast material required can be reduced with proper timing, which can lessen its renal impact, especially if EVAR

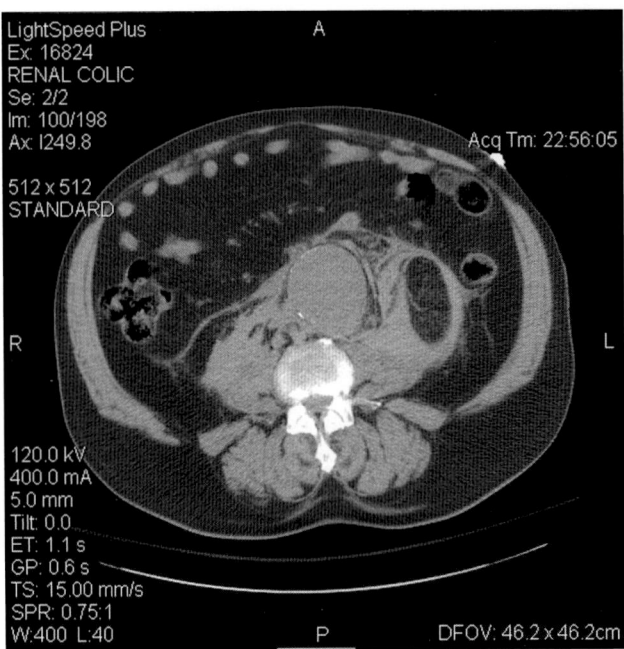

Figure 130-4 CT scan of a ruptured abdominal aortic aneurysm. Note the pattern of stranding of blood into the tissues. No contrast material was used, and the scan was performed for the diagnosis of renal colic.

is performed with additional volumes of contrast agent. Renal dysfunction may be induced by the combination of high dosages of contrast material and renal hypoperfusion.

Evidence of retroperitoneal blood, when used as the "gold standard" to diagnose RAAA on CT, was found to be 77% sensitive and 100% specific in a retrospective series.[55] Its positive predictive value was 100% and its negative predicative value was 89%. The low rate of false-negatives studies (no rupture on CT but RAAA found at surgery) is comforting. Interestingly, the level of agreement of the diagnosis of RAAA based on CT scanning was only moderate in five observers, whereas agreement on suitability for EVAR was only fair in vascular surgeons and radiologists experienced in EVAR from the Amsterdam Acute Aortic trial.[56] Intraobserver agreement on rupture and suitability for EVAR was higher than interobserver agreement. This disconcerting finding remains to be confirmed by others.

Timing of Computed Tomography

Prospective and retrospective studies have examined the delay between the initial manifestation of RAAA and time to death to determine whether sufficient time exists to perform a CT scan and evaluate patients' suitability for EVAR. Patients who were not treated surgically for RAAA because of co-morbidity or advanced age had a median time from onset of symptoms to death of just over 16 hours.[57] Only 13% died within 2 hours of hospital admission, and the median time between admission and death was 11 hours. This suggested that sufficient time exists for most patients to undergo CT scanning and evaluation for EVAR. A prospective analysis from regional U.K. centers identified that 33% of RAAA patients were transferred from other hospitals. The median time from arrival to surgery for operative cases was 159 minutes, and mortality was not affected by the length of delay or CT scanning. Thus, for the majority of patients who are stable on arrival at a center where definitive care will be carried out, a prompt CT scan does not appear to adversely affect mortality.[58]

Although studies show that on average there is sufficient time between arrival at the emergency department and death from RAAA for performance of CT, it is difficult to predict continued hemodynamic stability of individual patients during a CT scan. Thus, CT scans should be performed with a minimum of delay. The patient should be monitored and accompanied at all times because deterioration can occur rapidly. Both the U.K. RAAA randomized trial and the Amsterdam Acute Aneurysm trial identified patients too unstable for CT scanning who required immediate transfer to the operating room.[59,60] In the U.K. RAAA randomized trial, the time to arrival at the operating room was 25 minutes shorter in the EVAR group versus open repair despite the requirement for a contrast-enhanced CT scan. This suggests that the existence of a protocol for management of RAAA may significantly shorten the time to definitive therapy despite the requirement for the scan.[61,62]

■ INITIAL MANAGEMENT

Transfer to an Appropriate Institution

When the diagnosis of RAAA is being considered, emergency vascular surgical consultation is critical. If the patient arrives at a location where definitive management cannot be carried out, urgent transfer to a center with trained individuals who can undertake the repair is required. Further imaging may be obtained before transfer to the operating room where either open repair or EVAR can be performed. The impact of transferring RAAA patients to regional centers where they can be cared for by an experienced vascular team has been studied. Transfer does increase the time between initial hospital admission and arrival in the operating room, but mortality rates were similar in patients who arrived directly and patients who were transferred. Mortality in the first 24 hours was more common in transferred patients; however, the duration of intensive care unit stay and hospitalization was similar in those who survived.[63]

Permissive Hypotension

Preoperative resuscitation of hypotensive patients with RAAA before operative intervention must be judicious.[6,64-66] If resuscitation is aggressive, the elevated blood pressure can lead to further hemorrhage by overcoming the tamponade that stabilized the initial rupture. Further bleeding before the patient arrives in a setting where definitive therapy can be carried out can be lethal. This has led to the recommendation for permissive hypotension, in which resuscitation is minimized to maintain consciousness and prevent ST depression, usually at

a systolic pressure of 70 to 80 mm Hg, and for avoidance of aggressive resuscitation to pressures higher than 100 mm Hg.

Related Trauma-Bleeding Studies

Animal studies have documented increased blood loss and reduced survival in models of arterial injury when resuscitation occurs before control of hemorrhage.[66-68] A 78% mortality rate was noted in a series of RAAA patients treated with aggressive fluid resuscitation, prehospital paramedic care, transport to a trauma center, and prompt open surgical repair.[6] The excessive mortality in this series approached the 90% mortality observed in the Malmö population-based RAAA autopsy series and may reflect the rapid transport of patients who might not otherwise survive to arrive at the hospital alive for therapy in other parts of the country.[7] Significant side effect of overly aggressive fluid resuscitation include increased blood loss and dilutional and hypothermic coagulopathy. A randomized trial in young patients with penetrating trauma and hypotension (systolic blood pressure <90 mm Hg) demonstrated improved survival in those in whom fluid resuscitation therapy was delayed until arrival at the operating room door.[65] Improved survival differences were small (70% in the delayed-resuscitation group versus 62% in those with immediate resuscitation); however, there was also a reduction in complications and shorter hospitals stay. A British consensus statement supports the judicious use of small boluses of fluid titrated to maintain a radial pulse in penetrating trauma victims.[69] Elderly patients who suffer from more co-morbid conditions tolerate hypotension poorly. Thus, application of these results to older patients with RAAA is unclear because there are no randomized data comparing the degree of resuscitation in patients with RAAA.

Clinical Application

Crawford initially suggested minimal fluid resuscitation to maintain systolic blood pressure at 50 to 70 mm Hg in patients with RAAA.[64] Recent algorithms for RAAA care include permissive hypotensive resuscitation.[70] Rather than titrating fluid administration to a specific blood pressure, a balance should be achieved between organ ischemia from inadequate resuscitation and the risk of rebleeding from overaggressive replacement. Thus, moderate resuscitation to retain consciousness and prevent ST-segment depression is currently the preferred approach to preserve the initial tamponade that stabilized the aortic rupture until definitive repair can be carried out.[66] At present there is no evidence that resuscitation is better with blood than with crystalloids. If blood is available without delaying patient transfer, it should accompany the patient and can be given instead of crystalloid solutions to maintain consciousness as just described.

Operative Preparation

At initial evaluation of possible RAAA, blood should be crossmatched so that it will be available at surgery. In the operating room, trained anesthesia, nursing, and technical personnel can prepare the patient for operative intervention. Large-bore access, insertion of an arterial line, and placement of a Foley catheter can be done simultaneously. Hemodynamic deterioration of the patient's condition during preparation can be addressed promptly if one is in the proper location. The patient is prepared and draped awake before anesthesia is induced with agents designed to have a minimal effect on blood pressure. This allows the repair (open or endovascular) to be commenced immediately after induction. Alternatively, local anesthesia and sedation can be used for rEVAR.

OPERATIVE STRATEGIES: ENDOVASCULAR REPAIR

EVAR is rapidly becoming the preferred method of therapy for RAAA, given suitable anatomy and an experienced team that can perform it. Recent U.S. NIS data have demonstrated the increase in EVAR use for RAAA (Fig. 130-5).[10] Data from 2005 show that the proportion of RAAAs treated by EVAR has increased to 17%.[16]

Currently, open surgical repair is reserved for those who are anatomically unsuitable for EVAR, for environments where EVAR is not available, or when EVAR fails to seal the AAA.

Initial Management

To facilitate the use of EVAR for RAAA, protocols for the treatment of RAAA have been implemented locally to expedite the evaluation and transfer of these patients to an operating room where appropriate devices and imaging capability exist[61,62] (Fig. 130-6). Early identification of RAAA patients through protocol implementation should allow time for a CT scan while they are stable and then transfer to the operating room.

Thin-slice CT scanning with contrast enhancement can be accomplished with lower volumes of contrast agent to assess neck diameter, angulation, and iliac size.[71]

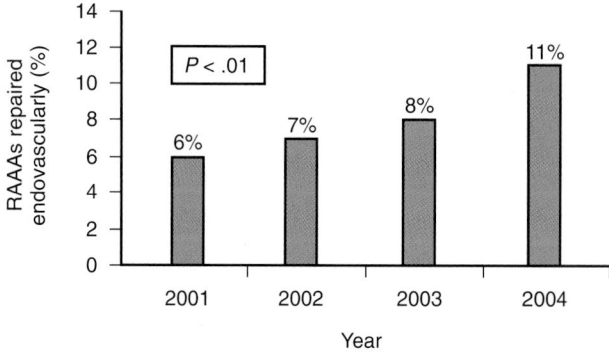

Figure 130-5 Percentage of ruptured abdominal aortic aneurysms (RAAAs) that underwent endovascular repair. *(From Lesperance K, Andersen C, Singh N, et al. Expanding use of emergency endovascular repair for ruptured abdominal aortic aneurysms: disparities in outcomes from a nationwide perspective. J Vasc Surg. 2008;47:1165-1170.)*

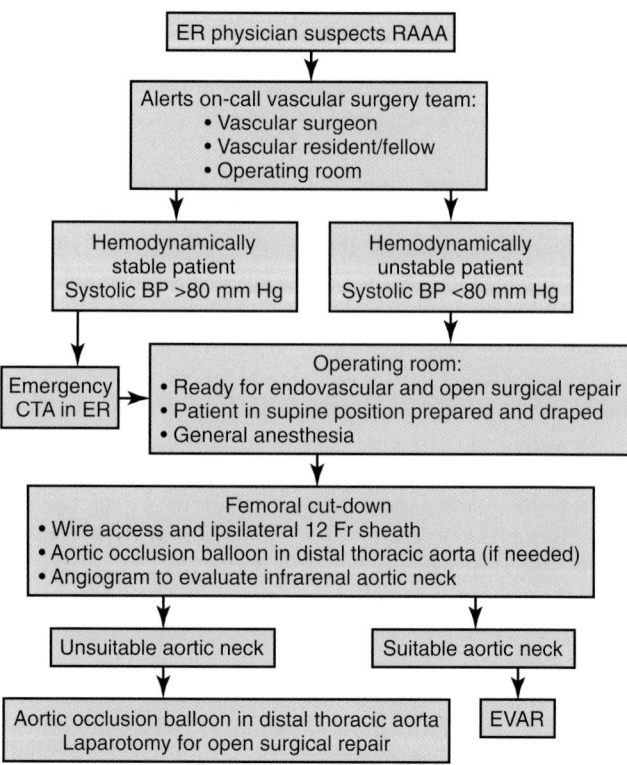

Figure 130-6 Flow chart for initial management to facilitate the use of endovascular aneurysm repair (EVAR) for ruptured abdominal aortic aneurysm (AAA). BP, blood pressure; CTA, computed tomographic angiography; ER, emergency room.

Assessment of Anatomic Suitability

The proportion of RAAAs suitable for EVAR is variable but has been calculated at between 47% and 67% based on two recent meta-analyses.[17,18] Appropriate endovascular candidates can then be selected after prompt review of the CT scan. Unfortunately, RAAAs have a larger infrarenal neck diameter and shorter neck length than do electively repaired AAAs.[72,73] These differences in AAA morphology not only affect the ability to perform EVAR but also have a significant impact on the size of device chosen to repair these aneurysms. A multicenter study noted that the largest diameter main body components were used most frequently in rEVAR.[74]

Operative Technique

In the operating room local anesthesia can be used to allow percutaneous access to the aorta. In stable patients, standard EVAR is then performed (see Chapter 129: Abdominal Aortic Aneurysms: Endovascular Treatment), although an aortouni-iliac device followed by a femorofemoral crossover graft may achieve more rapid control of hemorrhage and is therefore preferred for unstable patients. A compliant balloon may be advanced through a sheath into the lower thoracic aorta for even more rapid control of hemorrhage. Inflation of the balloon above the end of a stabilized sheath prevents aortic pressure from pushing the balloon down into the aneurysm sac, thus allowing proximal control. An alternative approach is to place a balloon via a brachial artery cut-down technique; however, the large sheath required makes this technique less attractive. Both techniques require fluoroscopy and can be complicated by tortuous anatomy. The femoral approach is preferred by most groups. Patients who are unstable can then undergo intraoperative angiography below the level of the occlusion balloon if a CT scan was not performed to allow measurement of aortic and iliac diameter. Once control is achieved, a second femoral cut-down can be performed to allow placement of the main body and the extensions required. Use of aortouniiliac stent-grafts with a contralateral iliac occluder and a femorofemoral crossover is the fastest way to achieve effective aneurysm exclusion (Fig. 130-7). This simplifies the procedure and reduces the number of components required to perform this procedure quickly and safely. Interestingly, even in centers that have championed protocols for rEVAR, patients continue to undergo open repair between 53% and 64% of the time.[61,62]

Local anesthesia has been used so that sympathetic tone, which may sustain blood pressure, is not negated. Although this advantage may be significant, it must be balanced by the difficulty encountered by the patient in remaining sufficiently still to allow the procedure to continue.[61,62] It may be possible to begin the procedure under local anesthesia and convert to general anesthesia to allow accurate positioning and release of the graft. Reports of completely percutaneous RAAA repair have now been published.[75]

Exclusion criteria for rEVAR include neck length less than 1 cm, neck diameter greater than 32 mm, angulation greater than 60 degrees, common iliac diameter greater than 20 mm or less than 6 mm, and inability to preserve at least one internal iliac artery. Preservation of internal iliac flow is critical to reduce the high incidence of colon ischemia seen in both open and endovascular RAAA repair (42% versus 23%, respectively, detected by sigmoidoscopy).[76,77] Other exclusion criteria may include extensive circumferential calcification or the presence of significant thrombus at the landing zones. In the emergency situation there has been a tendency to suggest relaxing the usual EVAR exclusion criteria; however, if this is done and EVAR fails to seal the aorta without a leak, any potential benefit achieved by this approach may be negated.

Endoleaks

Endoleaks pose a unique problem in the ruptured AAA setting because they may result in ongoing hemorrhage. Type Ia leaks can be treated with a large Palmaz stent or extension cuffs, or both, if additional aorta below the renal arteries is available. Type Ib leaks are treated with additional balloon expansion, stenting, or further extension of the graft into the iliac artery. Type II leaks have been observed after resolution of the hematoma, but they have not been reported to result in continued leakage of blood outside the aneurysm. It is surprising that endoleaks have not been reported to be a larger problem after RAAA repair. Ongoing hemorrhage has been reported and therapy can be required. Persistent type I leaks have been reported, one with a 4-month follow-up; however, this is not a recommended approach.[71]

Results of Endovascular Repair of Ruptured Abdominal Aortic Aneurysms

Outcomes of rEVAR appear encouraging, with the most recent U.S. national database reporting that 17% of RAAAs in 2005 were treated by EVAR.[16] Table 130-1 contains the most recent large series that compare open and endovascular repair for RAAA. Use of an endovascular approach appears to reduce 30-day mortality by 10% to 20%. These data are subject to bias secondary to choosing the best anatomic candidates and those who have stable blood pressure for rEVAR. This leaves the less stable, technically more challenging RAAAs for open repair, with its anticipated higher mortality. To date, no large multicenter study reporting on a group of consecutively treated patients is available, which would suggest that this therapy can be offered on a population-wide basis. As noted earlier, rapid access to thin-slice CT scanning, proper equipment, a modest stock of devises, and expertise are required around the clock to make this therapy feasible.

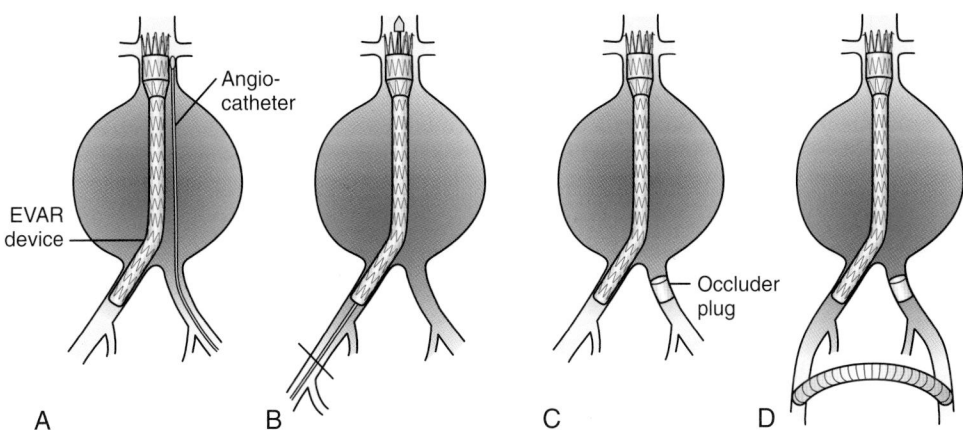

Figure 130-7 Endovascular repair of a ruptured abdominal aortic aneurysm. **A,** Graft inserted and placed below the renal arteries. **B,** Graft deployed. **C,** Occluding plug placed. **D,** Femorofemoral crossover completed.

Table 130-1 Results of Ruptured Abdominal Aortic Aneurysms from Recent Administrative Data, Systematic Reviews, and Meta-analyses

| Series | Year | Source and Date | Open Repair | | rEVAR | | Difference |
			Number of Subjects	30-Day Mortality (%)	Number of Subjects (%)	30-Day Mortality (%)	
Dillavou et al.[12]	2006	CMS, 2003	5,042	52	598 (11.9)	33	P < .001
Greco et al.[15]	2006	4 states, 2000-2003	5,508	47	290 (5.3)	39	P = .005
McPhee et al.[11]	2007	NIS, 2001-2004	18,839	38	2,093 (11.1)	29	
Harkin et al.[18]	2007	Systematic review	5,983	34	891 (14.9)	18	
Hoornweg et al.[1]	2008	Meta-analysis, 1991-2006	60,822	48.5			
Mastracci et al.[17]	2008	Systematic and meta-analysis	3,213		436 (13.6)	21	
Lesperance et al.[10]	2008	NIS, 2003-2004	8,982	42	949 (10.5)	18	P < .001
Giles et al.[16]	2009	NIS, 2001-2005	20,836	40.8	2,499 (10.7)	32.3	P < .001
Totals			**129,225**	**44.6**	**7,756**	**27.7**	

CMS, Centers for Medicare and Medicaid; rEVAR, endovascular techniques to repair ruptured abdominal aortic aneurysms; NIS, National Inpatient Sample.

As EVAR expertise becomes more widespread, this technology has the potential to reduce the mortality rate of RAAA, a development that has been difficult to achieve over the last 60 years.

Deaths and Complications after Endovascular Repair of Ruptured Abdominal Aortic Aneurysms

Deaths after rEVAR are secondary to colon ischemia, MOF, and continued hemorrhage. Postoperative complications include renal failure, arterial ischemia, wound infection, and abdominal compartment syndrome related to the hematoma. Drainage of retroperitoneal hematoma after EVAR has been required because of the development of abdominal compartment syndrome.[78] Renal dysfunction or failure can be due to the combination of the insult induced by hemorrhage and the contrast agent required for the CT scan and/or embolization from the implantation procedure. The incidence of renal dysfunction has been reported to be 28% in one series, with only two patients requiring hemofiltration and none requiring permanent dialysis.[79]

OPERATIVE STRATEGIES: OPEN REPAIR

The first critical element in RAAA repair is safe, rapid, and effective proximal aortic control (Fig. 130-8). Most surgeons prefer a transperitoneal, midline incision because it affords wide exposure to the abdominal aorta and allows rapid supraceliac control if necessary.[64,80] Rather than automatically proceeding to supraceliac control, we prefer to inspect the retroperitoneum after the bowel and duodenum are reflected, unless hypotension requires immediate clamping. If extensive hematoma is not seen in the pararenal area, careful dissection facilitates identification of the left renal vein, an important landmark for achieving infrarenal control. Care must be taken to avoid venous injury because it can increase mortality. Should aortic control be lost after entering the hematoma during dissection and bleeding ensues, supraceliac control is obtained.

Options for Proximal Control

Transperitoneal

A transperitoneal approach has generally been advocated for RAAA repair to reduce the incidence of missed associated abdominal pathology.[80] The supraceliac aorta can be exposed at the diaphragm by retracting the left lobe of the liver to the right (see Fig. 130-8). The gastrohepatic omentum is opened to allow entry into the lesser sac. The nasogastric tube is used to identify the esophagus and proximal part of the stomach, which are retracted to the left. The aorta is identified between the crura of the diaphragm. The crura may need to be split with electrocautery to allow rapid and accurate clamp placement. After clamping of the supraceliac aorta, the clamp may be repositioned to the infrarenal neck if possible, or the proximal anastomosis can be completed from within the aneurysm sac, a clamp placed on the graft, and the supraceliac clamp removed to reperfuse the viscera and kidneys. Supraceliac clamping should be as brief as possible. Unclamping the visceral and renal vessels may result in significant hypotension and therefore requires careful coordination with the anesthesia team to ensure that the proper fluids are administered and that pressor agents and bicarbonate are prepared for use if required. Supraceliac control is beneficial in cases of severe hypotension or uncontrolled bleeding from intraperitoneal rupture. It also helps avoid the renal, gonadal, and inferior mesenteric vein injuries often associated with blind dissection to identify the infrarenal aortic neck if there is substantial hematoma in this area. However, supraceliac clamping has the disadvantage of ischemic injury to the liver, bowel, and kidneys, which in addition to the injury induced by hemorrhagic shock may contribute to the development of MOF (see later under "Multisystem Organ Failure").[8,81] For aneurysms with clear evidence of suprarenal extension identified on CT, a ninth interspace thoracoabdominal incision allows rapid access to the aorta just above the diaphragm. A medial visceral rotation is then carried out to expose the visceral aorta, and standard elective techniques are used to repair and reperfuse the renal and visceral vessels.

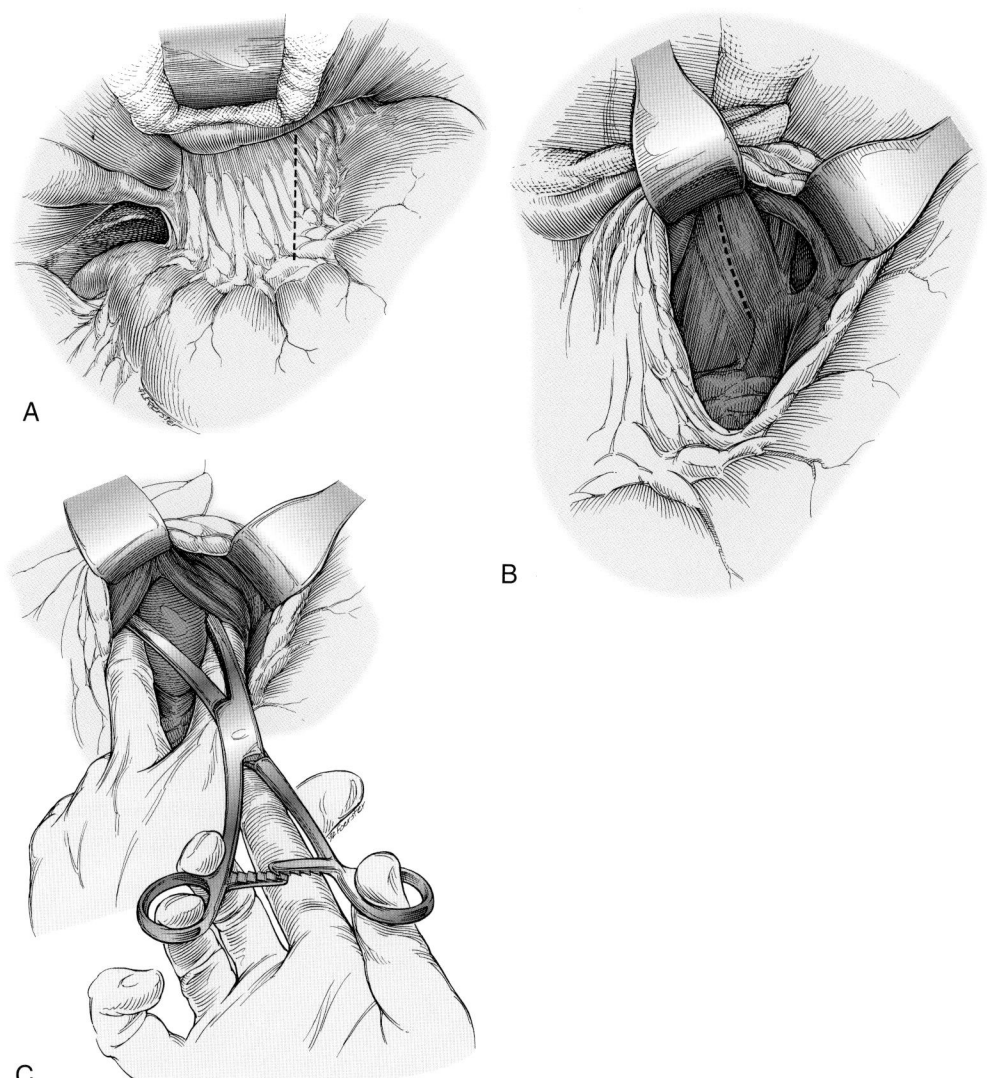

A

B

C

Figure 130-8 Exposure of the supraceliac aorta. **A** and **B,** Initially, the lesser sac needs to be opened to allow opening of the diaphragmatic crura. **C,** Blunt dissection of the aorta then allows a clamp to be placed over the two fingers that are exposing the aorta. *(From Rutherford RB.* Atlas of Vascular Surgery: Basic Techniques and Exposures. *Philadelphia, PA: WB Saunders; 1993:188-189.)*

Retroperitoneal

Others have advocated a retroperitoneal approach based on a large experience with elective, symptomatic, and ruptured AAA repair.[82] The 10th interspace retroperitoneal approach has been recommended by some for RAAA repair. In a retrospective analysis the retroperitoneal approach was associated with less intraoperative hypotension and lower mortality than the transperitoneal approach, although some patients with unusual features were excluded.[83] This series demonstrated that the retroperitoneal approach for RAAA repair is safe when performed by those familiar with its use during elective repair. For those unfamiliar with the retroperitoneal approach, a ninth interspace thoracoabdominal incision as noted earlier can allow rapid aortic control. This approach can be particularly useful in patients with challenging body habitus or for other hostile abdominal situations in which this approach would be recommended for elective repair. If a suprarenal AAA is unknowingly approached via a midline incision—and

this is not recommended—medial visceral rotation is required to expose the suprarenal aorta. In this technique the left colon is mobilized to incise the lateral peritoneal attachments. The colon, pancreas, spleen, and kidney may be elevated to allow access to the diaphragmatic crura that cover the aorta at this level. However, leaving the left kidney in situ is prefered if the initial incision was an anterior laparotomy. Division of the crura allows access to the entire intra-abdominal aorta and visceral and renal vessels.

Additional Options

Other options for proximal aortic control include use of an aortic compressor over the supraceliac aorta to compress it against the lumbar spine if rapid control is required before exposure can be obtained. In addition, direct placement of an aortic balloon through the aneurysm sac has been described, but this method can disrupt the aortic thrombus and lead to embolization, and it is more frequently associated with balloon malposition or movement as the aneurysm sac is opened. Also, a brachial or femoral puncture or cut-down to insert an occlusion balloon supported by a sheath (prevents balloon migration) into the visceral aorta under fluoroscopic guidance is also possible, as discussed earlier.[84] The compressor and balloon techniques are blind and may not provide complete control. Therefore, a direct approach to the infrarenal or supraceliac aorta is recommended in most cases.

Distal control can be achieved with clamps on the iliac arteries or occasionally the distal aorta. When substantial hematoma is present, however, distal dissection can be difficult and associated with iliac vein injury. Routine iliac occlusion balloon placement after opening the aneurysm sac avoids this dissection and reduces the chance of injury.

Operative Technique

In open cases, once proximal control is achieved, it is useful to allow the anesthesia team several minutes for further resuscitation before opening the aneurysm. During this period blood replacement can be initiated to prepare for the blood loss that will occur from the lumbar arteries or unclamped iliac arteries on opening the aneurysm.

Once the aneurysm is opened, retrograde bleeding from the inferior mesenteric and lumbar arteries can be controlled by suture ligation. Bleeding from the proximal aorta will need to be controlled with suction if a supraceliac clamp is used. If bleeding occurs from a proximal infrarenal clamp that is not completely applied posteriorly, it can usually be remedied by posterior pressure on the clamp against the spine while the proximal anastomosis is completed. Systemic heparinization can be avoided to reduce bleeding complications, although heparinized saline can be administered directly into the iliac arteries in an attempt to reduce distal thrombosis. Aggressive retrograde flushing of the iliac artery before distal anastomotic completion is important to remove any soft clot, especially if heparin is not used.

Aortic repair should be accomplished rapidly with a tube graft if possible. Tube grafts have been reported to have better outcomes than bifurcated grafts in older series. Their use will lead to the shortest operation and the least overall systemic physiologic insult. Moderate (up to 3 to 4 cm in diameter) iliac aneurysms can be repaired at a later date unless they are the site of rupture. If aortobiiliac repair is required, the easiest limb should be repaired first to reduce lower torso ischemic time. Rarely, aortobifemoral grafting may be required in patients with extensive iliac occlusive disease. With either of these approaches it is important to ensure that at least one internal iliac artery is reperfused to reduce the risk of pelvic and colon ischemia.

Aortocaval Fistula

Rarely, venous bleeding, which can be secondary to an aortocaval fistula, will continue to fill the opened aneurysm. Direct digital pressure or the use of proximal and distal sponge sticks is recommended for control of the vena cava above and below the fistula. Suture of the fistula from within the aneurysm is then performed. It is important to not generate an air embolism or push thrombus or other aortic debris into the vena cava during this repair. Attempts to dissect the vena cava proximally and distally will greatly increase the chance of a venous injury (see Chapter 71: Acquired Arteriovenous Fistulae).

Autotransfusion

The use of red-cell salvage with a cell saver device has proved beneficial in reducing mortality in RAAA patients undergoing open repair. When red-cell salvage was not used, the odds ratio of postoperative death at 1 month was 25 times higher.[78,85] One study suggested that use of a cell saver increases respiratory complications. However, use of the device was based on surgeon preference and may have been biased toward more complicated cases.[86] Red-cell salvage has become a part of protocols designed to standardize and reduce mortality from ruptured AAAs.[70] Red-cell salvage is now considered an important element in improving survival.[87] It has also been shown to reduce the need for transfusion in the elective situation.[88] A decision analysis of elective AAA repair suggested that routine use is not cost-effective but that its use can be justified when increased blood loss is anticipated.[89] When a red-cell salvage device is used, one must remember to replace the coagulation factors that are removed during processing.

Hypothermia

Hypothermia is associated with an increased incidence of surgical bleeding, wound infection, and morbid cardiac events.[90] Prevention of hypothermia (by 1.3°C) can reduce cardiac events in elective noncardiac surgery. Hypothermia was noted to be a significant factor associated with mortality in RAAA patients transferred to a regional center.[91] Though not prospectively studied in RAAA, prevention of hypothermia with the use of warmed anesthetic gases, warming of all intravenous fluids, and the use of forced air warming devices should be beneficial in this patient population.

Anatomic Abnormalities

Variant anatomy can greatly complicate open repair of a ruptured AAA; however, preoperative CT scanning can identify these abnormalities and allow time for planning. Arterial and venous injuries increase the mortality rate in RAAA repairs. Identification of an inflammatory aneurysm may require suprarenal or supraceliac control. Minimal dissection of the duodenum from the aorta and repair from within the aneurysm will then be critical to achieve success. This issue is described further for the elective situation in Chapter 128 (Abdominal Aortic Aneurysms: Open Surgical Treatment).

Venous Abnormalities

The most common venous abnormalities encountered include a retroaortic renal vein (1% to 3%), circumaortic renal vein

(0.5% to 1.5%), left-sided vena cava (0.15% to 0.5%), and duplicate inferior vena cava (0.4% to 3%).[92] Closure of the aortic clamp can tear a retroaortic renal vein and result in significant venous bleeding. The retroaortic veins tend to cross behind the aorta at a lower level than the anterior renal vein, so care must be taken to ensure that the clamp does not gather the vein and tear it when it is being closed. The best approach to repair of a torn posterior vein is direct venous repair or ligation. Ligation may require division of the aorta after moving the clamp to a more proximal location and retraction of the aorta superiorly to accomplish ligation. In patients with a left-sided vena cava or duplicate inferior vena cava, these structures frequently cross in front of the aorta at the level of the renal vein. This can prevent access to the proximal aorta and complicate repair. Should elevation and mobilization fail to allow sufficient access to repair the aneurysm, the venous structure may need to be divided to permit adequate repair. Reanastomosis can be accomplished at the conclusion of the procedure if required.

Renal Abnormalities

A horseshoe kidney discovered during RAAA repair will present a severe technical challenge. The position of the kidney (high or low) and the number of renal arteries are the key factors that require assessment before proceeding.[93] A kidney at the neck of the aneurysm may prevent adequate exposure for aortic cross-clamping, and a supraceliac clamp site may be required. Once control is achieved, the renal blood supply can be assessed. Should only a fibrous cord be joining the kidneys anteriorly, it can be divided. Unfortunately, the isthmus often contains substantial renal tissue, possibly the renal collecting system and blood vessels. If such is the case, identification of the renal blood supply is critical. Should the blood supply be from the iliac arteries, rapid repair of the aneurysm should be completed. Should the blood supply be from the anterior aortic wall, a patch of aortic wall and separate Carrel patches may be required to reperfuse the kidney. If the diagnosis is made preoperatively, a retroperitoneal approach may be selected. Adjunctive measures for renal protection may include systemic mannitol (3 to 5 mL/kg) or N-acetylcysteine administration (600 mg an as intravenous bolus or as high as 100 mg/kg based on animal studies) and renal cooling.[94,95]

Abdominal Closure after Ruptured Abdominal Aortic Aneurysms

Primary abdominal closure has been the most common approach. However, in 25% to 30% of patients the abdomen cannot be closed without significant tension secondary to swollen bowel, excessive tissue edema, or massive retroperitoneal hematoma.[96]

Abdominal Compartment Syndrome

Abdominal compartment syndrome is caused by increased intraperitoneal pressure and results in hypoventilation, decreased venous return, hypoxemia, increased intracranial pressure, and renal failure. Impairment of organ and capillary bed perfusion leads to mucosal ischemia, which may predispose these patients to the development of multiple organ dysfunction syndrome.[97] A bladder pressure in excess of 30 cm H_2O or 25 mm Hg is diagnostic. Bladder pressure is reflective of intra-abdominal pressure when the bladder volume is between 50 and 100 mL.[98] To measure this pressure the bladder is drained and then filled with 50 to 100 mL of sterile saline. The drainage tubing is clamped beyond the aspiration port and a needle is inserted into the aspiration port and connected to a pressure transducer. The transducer is zeroed at the pubic symphysis. Intra-abdominal pressure has been shown to be higher at the conclusion of RAAA repair than after elective open or endovascular repair.[99] These early measurements were unable to predict organ failure accurately; however, those with higher initial intra-abdominal pressure did have more abnormal physiologic abnormalities than the lower pressure group. Ruptured AAAs repaired by EVAR are subject to the development of abdominal compartment syndrome, which is associated with high mortality.[100]

Delayed Closure

Although delayed closure after RAAA repair has been reported since 1991, it has recently been suggested as a means of reducing the development of subsequent organ failure in both trauma and ruptured AAA patients.[101] Early mesh closure appears to reduce the incidence of MOF and may reduce mortality in comparison to patients who eventually went back to the operating room for decompressive laparotomy and delayed mesh closure. Patients who have severe preoperative anemia, prolonged shock, preoperative cardiac arrest, massive resuscitation, profound hypothermia, and severe acidosis may benefit from early closure with mesh sewn to the fascia. Different types of mesh are available, but nonabsorbable mesh covered with a polyurethane drape to prevent fluid loss is most commonly used.[102] When early mesh closure was compared with late mesh closure, the incidence of colon ischemia was 6% versus 40%.[96] Furthermore, no aortic graft infections have been observed to date. The abdomen was closed after 2 to 5 days, and there was an increase in the wound complication rate. Another approach is vacuum-assisted wound closure with return to the operating room for definitive closure at a later time. Although the data to date are retrospective, early mesh closure to prevent the development of abdominal compartment syndrome leading to MOF appears to be a useful adjunct in the treatment of RAAA in selected patients.

■ COMPLICATIONS OF REPAIR OF RUPTURED ABDOMINAL AORTIC ANEURYSMS

Local Complications

Postoperative bleeding has been shown to develop at a frequency between 12% and 14.4%.[103] The incidence is related to the prevalence of coagulopathy, which can develop secondary to the lack of coagulation factor replacement and hypothermia. Limb ischemia can be related to large- or small-vessel distal occlusion; these in turn are caused by in situ thrombosis (often, patients are not heparinized) and/or embolization of aortic debris. Because many surgeons do not systemically administer heparin, particular attention must be paid to retrograde iliac flushing before completion of the distal anastomosis.

Colonic Ischemia

Colonic ischemia is a lethal consequence of any AAA repair; however, the highest incidence occurs with RAAA repair. The most recent prospective data using sigmoidoscopy note an incidence of 38% with open repair and 23% after rEVAR.[76,77] It can range in severity from patchy mucosal necrosis (grade I), to mucosal and muscularis involvement (grade II), to transmural necrosis, gangrene, and perforation (grade III).[76] If colonic ischemia is suspected during the postoperative period, sigmoidoscopy/colonoscopy to visualize the area is diagnostic. In a prospective analysis of RAAA patients who survived 24 hours postoperatively, a 26% incidence of grades I and II changes was detected with colonoscopy, with 10% having grade III changes. Of those with grade I or II, 11% progressed to grade III within 48 hours. Those with grade III changes were found at surgery to have extensive sigmoid and frequently rectal necrosis and even with surgical management had a mortality rate of 55%. Factors responsible for colonic ischemia include the degree and duration of hypotension, patency of the inferior mesenteric artery, collateral supply from the superior mesenteric and internal iliac branches, and the site of the hematoma. Care must be taken at the conclusion of open aortic repair to examine the colon and evaluate the blood supply by Doppler should its viability be in doubt. Reimplantation of the inferior mesenteric artery may be of benefit even if both internal iliac arteries have been preserved by the repair. A recent analysis has demonstrated that RAAA repair with an aortobifemoral graft was associated with a 22% incidence of colon ischemia versus 4% for tube grafts and 2.7% for aortouniiliac or biiliac grafts.[104] Colonic ischemia is also prevalent after rEVAR. Sigmoidoscopy performed on those surviving beyond 24 hours demonstrated a 23% incidence of colon ischemia after rEVAR versus 38% with open repair.[77] Thus, EVAR does not eliminate the significant incidence of colon ischemia, which remains a deadly complication. This high incidence has led some to recommend routine colonoscopy after RAAA repair to avoid delayed detection.[76]

Spinal Ischemia

Paraplegia and paraparesis are rare complications that have been reported after both open and endovascular repair of ruptured aneurysms. The incidence with open repair was 2.3% versus 11.5% after rEVAR, and both groups experienced a 50% mortality rate.[103,105] After both open repair and rEVAR, interruption of the pelvic blood supply, prolonged aortic cross-clamping (or prolonged functional occlusion during EVAR),

preoperative and intraoperative hypotension, aortic embolization, and internal iliac interruption have all been suggested to be associated with spinal cord injury.[106] Drainage of cerebrospinal fluid has not reversed the paraplegia once symptoms were noted, although it has been effective in some cases after elective EVAR (see Chapter 133: Thoracic and Thoracoabdominal Aneurysms: Endovascular Treatment).

Systemic Complications

RAAA repair is associated with the development of multisystem organ injury remote from the site of the aortic repair. Rupture results in blood loss and hypotension. Repair requires aortic clamping, which results in a second ischemic insult to the lower torso. The most common systemic complications are myocardial infarction, respiratory failure, renal failure, congestive heart failure, arrhythmias, hyperbilirubinemia, sepsis, and multiple organ dysfunction. These data demonstrate that rEVAR is associated with significantly less bleeding, acute renal failure, and respiratory complication than are seen with open repair. The data were derived between 2000 and 2003 from an analysis of four large states with more than 5000 patients studied.[15]

Cardiac Complications

Myocardial infarction, arrhythmias, cardiac arrest, and congestive heart failure all represent life-threatening situations that increase mortality after RAAA.[103] Interestingly, rEVAR has not been demonstrated to reduce the number of cardiac complications.[15] Myocardial infarction develops secondary to the increased demand placed on the heart to compensate for blood loss, resuscitation, and aortic clamping and declamping in the setting of frequent preexisting coronary disease. Cardiac arrest is associated with a mortality rate of 81% to 100% and occurs in up to 20% of cases. Myocardial infarction develops in 14% to 24% and is associated with a mortality rate of 19% to 66%.[15,103] Arrhythmias requiring therapy developed in 23% with an associated mortality rate of 46%. Congestive heart failure developed in 20% and was associated with 41% mortality. If all patients with cardiac events are pooled, 42% of patients sustained a cardiac event, which was associated with a 44% early mortality rate. Rapid detection plus prompt treatment of postoperative myocardial infarction, arrhythmias, or congestive heart failure is required, as discussed in Chapter 38 (Systemic Complications: Cardiac).

Respiratory Failure

Respiratory failure develops in 26% to 47% of cases and is associated with a mortality rate between 34% and 68%.[103,107] It is characterized by high oxygen requirements, increased lung permeability, and a decrease in lung compliance. Administration of large volumes of fluid and blood products, as well as preexisting pulmonary dysfunction and long cross-clamp times, predisposes to the development of this syndrome. Analysis of respiratory complication in 290 rEVAR cases versus 5508 open repairs of RAAA demonstrated a significantly lower incidence after rEVAR than after open repair, 21.7% versus 32.4%.[15] Thus, the lower torso ischemia induced by aortic cross-clamping and the longer duration in open repair than in rEVAR appear to be key factors in the release of mediators that result in the development of respiratory failure. Treatment is discussed in Chapter 39 (Systemic Complications: Respiratory).

Renal Dysfunction

A common theme in large databases and prospective and retrospective studies of RAAA has been demonstration of an important relationship between the development of renal dysfunction and mortality after RAAA repair.[15,103,108] The incidence of renal dysfunction after aneurysm repair is low in elective cases but rises progressively in symptomatic patients and ruptured patients, in whom rates vary between 26% and 42%. Renal failure requiring dialysis has been noted to develop in 11% to 40% of patients. Those who require dialysis have mortality rates between 76% and 89%.[103,107] Renal dysfunction has been found to be increased in those with suprarenal cross-clamping or a longer duration of aortic cross-clamping, preexisting renal dysfunction, shock, and increased age.[109] Although the etiology of the renal dysfunction is multifactorial, individuals in whom it develops have often sustained a greater insult to other organs as well. Suprarenal clamping is used more commonly than AAA elective repair in patients with RAAA and is associated with an increased incidence of renal dysfunction and dialysis.[110] Thus, the development of renal dysfunction after RAAA repair with an infrarenal clamp, especially in those with previously normal renal function, is a reflection of the severity of the systemic insult that the patient has suffered. The incidence of renal dysfunction is significantly reduced after rEVAR (14.8% versus 24.8% after open repair) despite the contrast material required to complete the procedure.[15] Treatment is discussed in Chapter 40 (Systemic Complications: Renal).

Liver Failure

Hepatic failure is a late event after RAAA. Early studies suggested that it occurred after the development of pulmonary, cardiac, and gastrointestinal dysfunction.[111] Jaundice did not become evident until the sixth postoperative day and was associated with a mortality rate of 83%.[112] No hepatic necrosis was noted, and the dysfunction was ascribed to hypoxic hepatic injury. Maziak and colleagues found that hepatic function began to diverge between survivors and nonsurvivors on the 7th postoperative day and became significantly different on the 10th postoperative day.[113]

The liver can sustain a hypoxic injury after hemorrhagic shock but must cope with reabsorption of the hematoma and the increased metabolism that this demands. At present, predictive factors for hepatic failure have not been identified, and the etiology of the dysfunction is poorly understood.

Irreversible Shock

In the late stages of hemorrhagic shock, an irreversible state can develop in which aortic clamping, aggressive fluid resuscitation, and inotropic support can fail to reverse the hypotension.[6] This is also observed in animal models of hemorrhage. These deaths usually occur in the operating room and account for 10% to 15% of RAAA deaths.

Multisystem Organ Failure

Multiple organ dysfunction remote from the site of the aortic repair develops frequently after RAAA and is associated with elevated mortality rates. RAAA results in blood loss and hypotension. Repair requires aortic clamping, which results in a second ischemic insult to the lower torso. This was first reported in a 1973 review of renal failure after RAAA in which progressive organ failure was described.[111] Since that report, MOF has been reported with a postoperative incidence of up to 64%, and in several series it is the most common cause of death after 48 hours, where it accounted for up to 93% of deaths.[113-115] The development of MOF or a systemic inflammatory syndrome has been extensively described in trauma patients and those with pancreatitis and a perforated viscus. It is critical to note that relatively few RAAA patients have positive blood cultures as an initiating event of their MOF, which differentiates them from other intensive care patients with MOF.[113,114] In contrast, young patients who suffer penetrating arterial trauma with hypotension have survival rates between 62% and 70%. These patients had intraoperative blood loss of 2.5 to 3.1 L, yet the incidence of systemic complications in these arterial trauma patients such as acute respiratory distress syndrome (1% to 4%), sepsis syndrome (5%), and renal failure (1% to 4%) was dramatically lower than after RAAA.[65]

The etiologic factors responsible for the development of multiple organ dysfunction syndrome center on the magnitude, number, and timing of the inducing inflammatory insults. Evidence from clinical RAAA data suggests that suprarenal clamping and longer duration of aortic clamping are associated with higher rates of postoperative complications and death.[109] The incidence of MOF was noted to be 3.8% after elective repair, 38% after urgent repair, and 64% after ruptured aneurysm repair.[81] The mortality rate in patients with RAAA and MOF was 69%, versus 0% in those who did not have MOF. Thus, RAAA is a potent stimulus to induce multiple organ dysfunction, which is a lethal condition.

Two-Hit Hypothesis of Multisystem Organ Failure

A hypothesis that may account for the excessive complications and the persistently high and unchanging mortality in the patient population undergoing open RAAA repair is the "two-hit" hypothesis.[8,9] Rupture plus repair of an aneurysm is

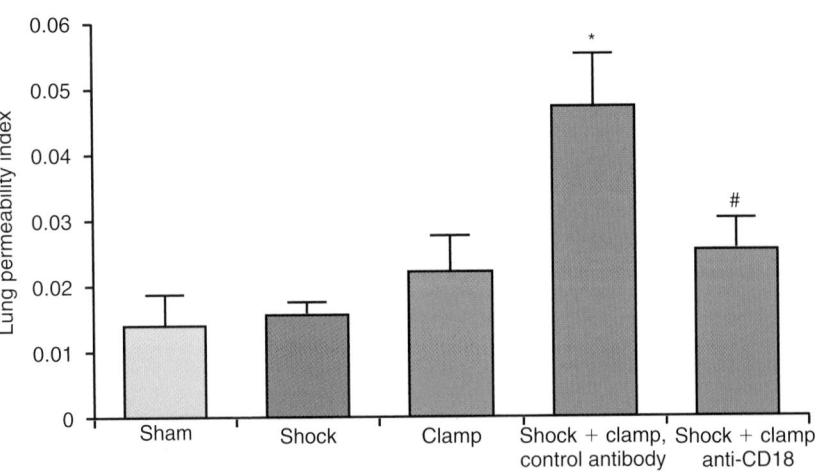

Figure 130-9 Lung permeability index as a measure of systemic lung injury in sham, shock, clamp, and shock-plus-clamp animals treated with control and CD18 monoclonal antibody (anti-CD18). The synergy of the two injuries results in systemic organ injury, which is reduced by neutralization of the CD18 neutrophil adhesion receptor. *P < .5 versus sham, shock, and clamp. #P < .5 versus shock plus clamp (control antibody). *(Modified from Boyd AJ, Rubin BB, Walker PM, et al. A CD18 monoclonal antibody reduces multiple organ injury in a model of ruptured abdominal aortic aneurysm. Am J Physiol. 1999;277:H172-H182.)*

a combination of two ischemic events followed by reperfusion. Hemorrhagic shock is a total-body ischemic event that primes the inflammatory response.[116] This affects the entire body, although the insult to various tissues may be different.[117] Aneurysm repair requires a second ischemic event, aortic clamping, that causes relative lower torso ischemia.[118] Reperfusion occurs as a result of resuscitation and removal of the aortic clamp once the repair is completed. This theory is supported by data from an animal model of ruptured AAA and data collected from clinical cases.[9,119]

In an animal model of RAAA the individual insults of hemorrhagic shock alone or aortic clamping alone were insufficient to result in the development of systemic organ injury.[8] When the events were combined, a synergistic effect resulted in the rapid onset of systemic organ injury that resembled the clinical situation but over a much shorter time course (Fig. 130-9). Animal studies of hemorrhagic shock have demonstrated that cardiac contractile dysfunction develops after resuscitation and may further reduce tissue perfusion, thereby contributing to the high incidence of cardiac events after RAAA.[120]

Studies comparing neutrophil activation in elective and ruptured AAA repair demonstrate that RAAA patients have neutrophils that are primed to respond to ex vivo stimulation on arrival at the emergency department and that further elevation in neutrophil oxidative burst develops in the postoperative period, thus suggesting that the operative repair further activated these cells.[121] When markers of neutrophil lipid peroxidation injury were assessed in elective AAA repair, no oxidative injury was noted.[9] In the RAAA group there was evidence of significant oxidative injury on arrival at the emergency room, and further significant elevations were noted by the third postoperative day. A significant relationship between the level of neutrophil oxidative burst and the level of these products of tissue oxidative injury was identified and suggested a mechanistic link. Inhibition of the complement cascade has been beneficial in animals, but human studies are pending.[122] Thus, data from both a laboratory model and human subjects that RAAA is a "two-hit" model of injury may begin to explain why the mortality after open RAAA repair has failed to drop dramatically despite all the advances in intraoperative and postoperative management. rEVAR, which minimizes lower torso ischemia and is associated with significantly lower mortality, is consistent with this "two-hit" theory. Further advances in therapy for this group of patients may come from the administration of inhibitors that restrict activation of the inflammatory response (see Fig. 130-9).

Other studies have investigated levels of the cytokines interleukin-6 (IL-6), IL-10, and HLA-DR, along with sequential organ failure assessment scores in RAAA patients.[123] High levels of IL-6 and IL-10 were noted in the postoperative period in nonsurvivors, as were high sequential organ failure assessment scores over the first 3 days. Depressed levels of HLA-DR on monocytes in the first few postoperative days were found in nonsurvivors.

■ OUTCOME OF RUPTURED ABDOMINAL AORTIC ANEURYSM REPAIR

Early Survival

The 30-day survival rate of those undergoing open RAAA repair is traditionally quoted at 50% based on a large accumulation of data from statewide audits, community centers, national databases, and tertiary centers.[11,103,108,124] A meta-analysis of the first 50 years of RAAA repair noted an overall operative mortality rate of 48%, with 15% occurring intraoperatively, and the postoperative mortality rate after successful surgery was 40%. Mortality declined 3.5% over each 10-year period of the study. A more recent meta-analysis of studies between 1991 and 2006 that included more than 60,000 patients found an overall mortality rate of 48.5%.[1] Thus, overall progress in reducing RAAA mortality has been stubbornly slow. This suggests that factors other than those easily controlled by the health care team are responsible for the excessive mortality observed in patients with this condition.

Results of Endovascular versus Open Repair of Abdominal Aortic Aneurysms

There is increasing evidence that rEVAR is able to decrease the mortality of RAAA repair with fewer complications (bleeding, renal, and respiratory), shorter hospital stays, and more patients being able to return home rather than going to institutional care after the procedure.[10,12] Conversion from rEVAR to open repair has been reported and seems to be associated with increased mortality, although this is mostly based on anecdotal data and no large series. The following studies summarize diverse publications, and the collective results demonstrate that an increasing number of RAAAs are being treated by EVAR and that it probably has a beneficial impact on early mortality.

Randomized Trial. One prospective randomized trial of open versus endovascular repair of RAAA has been reported.[60] During the study period 103 patients with RAAA were evaluated. Of these, only 32 stable enough to have a CT scan, were fit for open repair, and thus were recruited into the study. The open repair group had a mortality rate of 53% versus 53% in the EVAR group on an intention-to-treat basis. Of those who survived to undergo repair, open repair was associated with a 43% mortality rate versus 46% in the EVAR group. The EVAR group had less blood loss and less blood transfused; however, there were no significant benefits in length of stay or complications suffered. The authors used an aortouniiliac repair and noted that the patients were frequently unable to tolerate the ischemic pain during femoro-femoral crossover grafting when performed under local anesthesia. Thus, this study has not provided any definitive support for EVAR in the ruptured setting.

Meta-analysis. Several meta-analyses and a Cochrane review have been published on rEVAR to determine whether this therapy reduces mortality for RAAA.[10,17,18,125] Single-center studies and other publications with relatively small numbers of patients frequently claim improved mortality with rEVAR, but the generalizability of this conclusion has been in doubt. A pooled estimate of rEVAR mortality was 21% in a meta-analysis with a population of 436 patients.[17] The mortality was noted to be 18% in studies reporting an algorithm for RAAA care versus 32% in those without. An analysis of rEVAR from four large states noted an overall in-hospital mortality of 39% for rEVAR versus 48% for open repair.[15] After controlling for demographic and co-morbid differences by logistic regression, rEVAR was associated with a significantly decreased odds ratio for mortality of 0.78.[15]

Administrative Database Results. Large administrative databases such as the U.S. NIS and the U.S. Centers for Medicare and Medicaid have the advantage of examining larger patient populations over time.[10,12] These large databases confirm two important trends in RAAA therapy. First, the percentage of patients undergoing rEVAR is increasing each year, from 6% in 2001 to 17% in 2005 (see Fig. 130-5).[16] Second, the total RAAA mortality rate is declining secondary to rEVAR, and mortality after open RAAA repair was reduced from 1979 to 1997.[22]

In 2001, mortality after rEVAR was higher than that after open repair (43% versus 40%); however, with each subse-

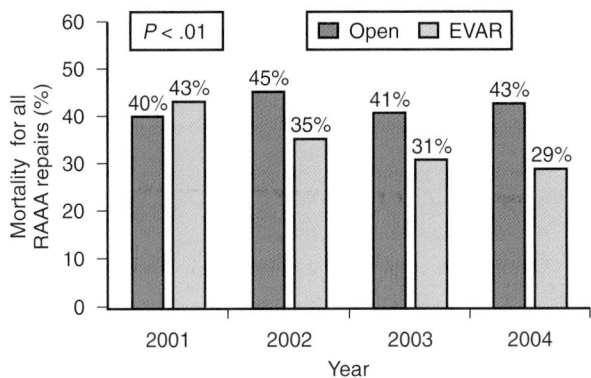

Figure 130-10 Mortality rate of open repair versus endovascular repair (EVAR) of ruptured abdominal aortic aneurysms (RAAAs). *(From Lesperance K, Andersen C, Singh N, et al. Expanding use of emergency endovascular repair for ruptured abdominal aortic aneurysms: disparities in outcomes from a nationwide perspective.* J Vasc Surg. *2008;47:1165-1170.)*

quent year, rEVAR mortality has decreased (in 2004, 29% versus 43% for open repair) (Fig. 130-10).[10] The age, sex, and preexisting co-morbid conditions were similar between the open repair and rEVAR groups, but open repair patients had higher estimated mortality scores and underwent more secondary surgical procedures (tracheostomy and exploratory laparotomy) than did the rEVAR group. Mortality after open repair did not decrease during the study and remained between 40% and 45%. Differences in RAAA outcome were also demonstrated between teaching and nonteaching centers in a univariate analysis. Mortality after both rEVAR and open repair was higher at the nonteaching centers.[10]

Analysis of the U.S. NIS database for 2001 to 2004 included 20,932 ruptured patients with an overall mortality rate of 37.3%.[11] In this sample 10% of patients underwent rEVAR and had a significantly lower mortality rate, 28% versus 38.2% for open repair. This suggests a reduction in mortality from the 48% that was observed between 1979 and 1997 from the National Hospital Discharge survey.[22] Data from the Centers for Medicare and Medicaid Services also noted a significantly lower mortality rate for rEVAR of 32% in 2003 versus 51% for open repair.[12] Overall, the introduction of EVAR has increased elective repair, reduced the mortality associated with RAAA, and probably contributed to the reduced incidence of RAAA in the population[16] (Fig. 130-11).

Thus, there is increasing evidence that rEVAR is able to decrease the early mortality of RAAA repair with fewer complications (bleeding, renal, and respiratory), shorter hospital stays, and more patients being able to return home rather than going to institutional care after the procedure.[10,12]

Predictors of Early Mortality after Ruptured Abdominal Aortic Aneurysm Repair

Prediction of survival after surgical RAAA repair and return to a functional life with a minimum of complications presents a formidable task. Many scoring systems have been devised

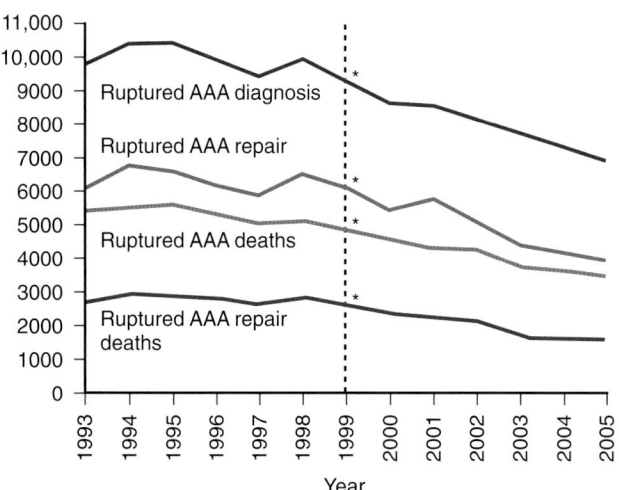

Figure 130-11 Ruptured abdominal aortic aneurysms (AAAs) from 1993 to 2005 after AAA repair (total diagnoses, repairs, total deaths, repair deaths). An *asterisk* indicates that the decline in diagnoses, repairs, and deaths after the introduction of endovascular aneurysm repair (EVAR) was greater than the decline before EVAR (P < .0001). *(From Lesperance K, Andersen C, Singh N, et al. Expanding use of emergency endovascular repair for ruptured abdominal aortic aneurysms: disparities in outcomes from a nationwide perspective.* J Vasc Surg. *2008;47:1165-1170.)*

> **Box 130-1 Risk Factors Associated with an Increased Risk of Mortality in Patients with Abdominal Aortic Aneurysm Rupture**
>
> - Increasing age
> - Women
> - Nonwhite race
> - Insurance status (higher for those who self-pay or are on Medicaid in the United States)
> - Co-morbid conditions
> - Congestive heart failure
> - Renal failure
> - Valvular heart disease

(Hardman Index, Glasgow Aneurysm Score, V and RAAA-POSSUM, Edinburgh Ruptured Aneurysm Score), yet none predict postoperative outcome with sufficient accuracy to deny repair to an individual patient in the emergency department.[126,127] However, there are important variables that have been evaluated to help the surgeon determine the likelihood of survival to better counsel elderly, high-risk patients who may elect not to undergo emergency RAAA repair.

Variables Predicting Outcome

Variables that have been identified to be associated with a reduction in survival include loss of consciousness, preoperatively increased creatinine, preexisting congestive heart failure, low hemoglobin, chronic obstructive pulmonary disease, female gender, nonwhite race, smaller size of the hospital, duration of hypotension, preoperative cardiac arrest, Acute Physiology and Chronic Health Evaluation II (APACHE II) score, base deficit, core temperature, and payer status (Box 130-1).[6,13,95,103,104,107,128-136] Analysis has identified six variables that are most commonly associated with death after RAAA: hypotension, advanced age, cardiac arrest, raised serum creatinine, low hemoglobin/hematocrit, and ischemic heart disease.[126] Female gender has been noted in large North American data to be associated with an increased risk for death after RAAA.[11] In fact, women experience AAA rupture when they are on average 2 to 3 years older than men, rupture at smaller sizes, have a decreased incidence of repair (56% versus 73% for men), and have higher mortality rates (52% versus 44%) than men.[4,11]

Canadian Aneurysm Study. Prospective data from the Canadian aneurysm study of RAAA patients identified individual variables that were statistically significant predictors of 1-month survival.[103] The predictive variables from a univariate analysis that were associated with increased mortality were preinduction systolic blood pressure (≥70 mm Hg, 36% early survival rate; 70 to 119 mm Hg, 38% survival rate; ≥120 mm Hg, 75% survival rate), preoperative serum creatinine (≤1.3 mg/dL [115 μmol/L], 77% survival rate; >1.3 mg/dL [115 μmol/L], 47% survival rate), intraoperative urine output (0 mL, 4% survival rate; 1 to 199 mL, 55% survival rate; ≥200 mL, 69% survival rate), site of the cross-clamp (infrarenal, 56% survival rate; suprarenal, 29% survival rate), and duration of cross-clamping (<60 minutes, 67% survival rate; ≥60 minutes, 43% survival rate). Multiple logistic regression identified that preinduction blood pressure and serum creatinine (variables known in the emergency department) can predict survival. However, even with blood pressure lower than 70 mm Hg and a creatinine level higher than 1.3 mg/dL (115 μmol/L), the survival rate was still 25%. The addition of intraoperative variables to the logistic regression model further enhanced the ability to predict survival. The site of the aortic clamp, the volume of blood administered, and intraoperative urine output also helped predict early survival. Infrarenal clamping with less than 1800 mL of blood administered plus a urine output greater than 200 mL was associated with an 89% survival rate. In a patient who required a suprarenal clamp, needed more than 3500 mL of blood, and had no intraoperative urine output, the survival rate was predicted to be 3%. When the preoperative and intraoperative variables were added to a single model, serum creatinine, clamp site, and intraoperative urine output were predictive of survival. When all preoperative, intraoperative, and postoperative variables were included, early survival was predicted by site of the aortic cross-clamp and occurrence of myocardial infarction, respiratory failure, kidney damage, and coagulopathy.[103]

Postoperative Estimates of Survival

At the conclusion of RAAA repair, the surgeon can review the key variables to give the family an estimate of the expected outcome. Table 130-2 combines the preoperative and intraoperative variables that were significant in a prospective analysis of early survival using a logistic regression model. Postoperative complications further enhance the ability to predict survival as noted by the variables in Table 130-3. Dialysis has a dramatic impact on survival, even when no other complications are present. The development of two complications also has a dramatic impact on mortality, especially if one is a rise in creatinine or dialysis requirement.

Predicting Early Postoperative Death

The multiple organ dysfunction score (MODS) follows the function of six key organ systems (respiratory, renal, hepatic, hematologic, neurologic, and cardiac) over time to determine the relationship between progressive organ dysfunction and mortality.[113] Those who survived had minimal postoperative change in their MODS; however, those who died after 48 hours had significantly larger increases in their MODS. The renal and hepatic components of the MODS were responsible for the progressive increase in total MODS and were significantly higher in those who died after 48 hours than in survivors. Renal dysfunction became significantly different between survivors and nonsurvivors on the third postoperative day, whereas it took until day 10 for the hepatic dysfunction scores to become significantly different. Patients in whom renal dysfunction developed followed by hepatic dysfunction were at the highest mortality risk.

Late Survival
Open Repair

Several studies have examined long-term survival after successful open RAAA repair. Data from the U.S. VA medical centers, the Mayo Clinic long-term study, and the Canadian aneurysm study all demonstrated that survival is lower than in those who undergo elective open AAA repair or in the

Table 130-2 Logistic Regression Model Showing the Interaction of Significant Preoperative and Intraoperative Variables That Predict Early Survival after Repair of Ruptured Abdominal Aortic Aneurysms

Creatinine		Clamp Site	Intraoperative Urine Output (mL)	Probability of Survival (%)
mg/dL	μmol/L			
≤1.3	≤115	Infrarenal	≥200	90
≤1.3	≤115	Infrarenal	1-199	76
>1.3	>115	Infrarenal	≥200	71
≤1.3	≤115	Suprarenal	≥200	65
≤1.3	≤115	Infrarenal	0	52
>1.3	>115	Infrarenal	1-199	46
≤1.3	≤115	Suprarenal	1-199	39
>1.3	>115	Suprarenal	≥200	33
>1.3	>115	Infrarenal	0	23
≤1.3	≤115	Suprarenal	0	18
>1.3	>115	Suprarenal	1-199	15
>1.3	>115	Suprarenal	0	6

Modified from Johnston KW. Ruptured abdominal aortic aneurysm: six-year follow-up results of a multicenter prospective study. Canadian Society for Vascular Surgery Aneurysm Study Group. *J Vasc Surg.* 1994;19:888-900.

Table 130-3 Logistic Regression Model Showing the Interaction of Significant Postoperative Complications That Predicted Early Survival after Ruptured Abdominal Aortic Aneurysm Repair

Postoperative Complications				
Myocardial Infarction	*Respiratory Failure*	*Coagulopathy*	*Renal Dysfunction*	**Probability of Survival (%)**
No	No	No	No	96
No	No	Yes	No	91
No	Yes	No	No	74
Yes	No	No	No	66
No	No	No	↑ Creatinine	66
No	Yes	Yes	No	58
Yes	No	Yes	No	49
No	No	Yes	↑ Creatinine	48
Yes	Yes	No	No	21
No	Yes	No	↑ Creatinine	20
Yes	No	No	↑ Creatinine	15
No	No	No	Dialysis	15
Yes	Yes	Yes	No	11
No	Yes	Yes	↑ Creatinine	11
Yes	No	Yes	↑ Creatinine	8
No	No	Yes	Dialysis	8
Yes	Yes	No	↑ Creatinine	2
No	Yes	No	Dialysis	2
Yes	No	No	Dialysis	2
Yes	Yes	Yes	↑ Creatinine	1
No	Yes	Yes	Dialysis	1
Yes	No	Yes	Dialysis	1
No	Yes	No	Dialysis	0
Yes	Yes	Yes	Dialysis	0

Modified from Johnston KW. Ruptured abdominal aortic aneurysm: six-year follow-up results of a multicenter prospective study. Canadian Society for Vascular Surgery Aneurysm Study Group. *J Vasc Surg.* 1994;19:888.

Section **17** Arterial Aneurysms

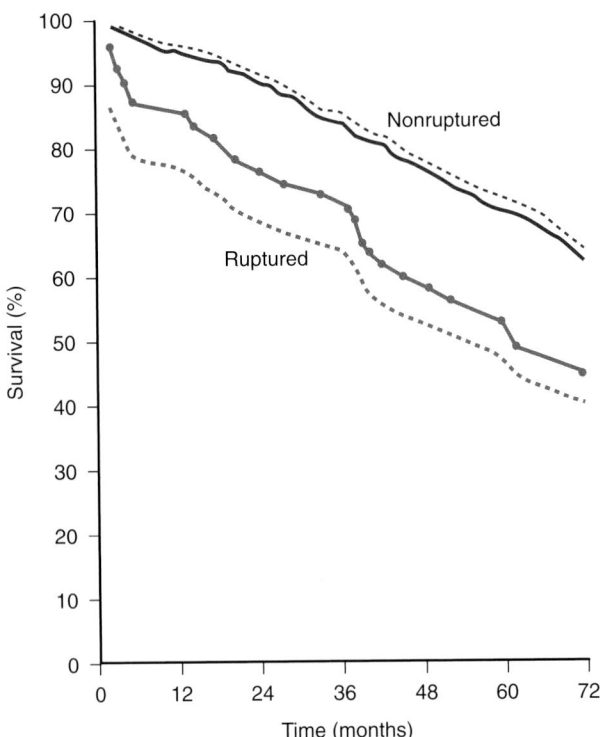

Figure 130-12 Long-term survival after elective (nonruptured) or ruptured abdominal aortic aneurysm repair from the Canadian aneurysm study for patients who survived longer than 30 days. In the ruptured abdominal aortic aneurysm group, survival declines rapidly in the first several months but subsequently begins to parallel the elective abdominal aortic aneurysm group. *Dotted lines* indicate the error associated with the measurement of survival. *(Data from Johnston KW. Ruptured abdominal aortic aneurysm: six-year follow-up results of a multicenter prospective study. Canadian Society for Vascular Surgery Aneurysm Study Group. J Vasc Surg. 1994;19:888-900.)*

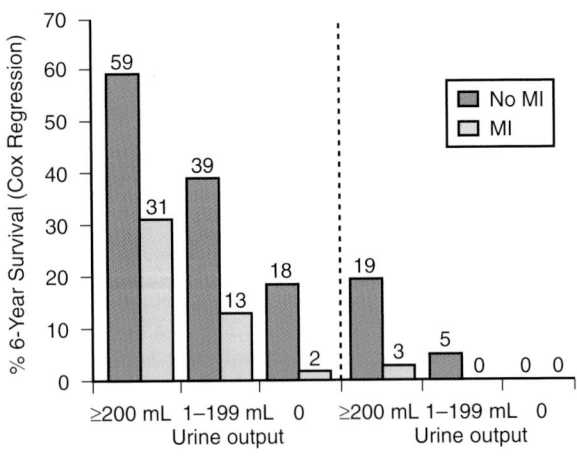

Figure 130-13 Late postoperative survival. When all variables were considered together, intraoperative urine output, respiratory failure, and myocardial infarction (MI) were predictors of late survival in a Cox proportional hazards model. *(Data from Johnston KW. Ruptured abdominal aortic aneurysm: six-year follow-up results of a multicenter prospective study. Canadian Society for Vascular Surgery Aneurysm Study Group. J Vasc Surg. 1994;19:888-900.)*

age- and sex-matched general population that does not have aneurysms.[103,137,138] More recent Finnish data suggest that long-term RAAA survival is equal to that of the age- and sex-matched Finish population, but it is the first study to make this assertion.[139] The survival of patients undergoing elective open AAA repair overlaps that of the age- and sex-matched general population. In the Canadian aneurysm study data, the 5-year survival rate for those alive at 30 days who underwent open RAAA repair was 53% versus 71% in patients who had undergone elective repair[103] (Fig. 130-12). Data from U.S. VA medical centers noted a 5-year survival rate of 54% for RAAA repair and 69% for the elective group.[138] In the Mayo Clinic long-term study the survival rate at 5 years was 64% and 74% for ruptured and elective AAA repair, respectively.[137] Thus, the long-term survival of RAAA patients is significantly less than their elective counterparts.

The Canadian aneurysm study, the Mayo series, and the VA study examined variables associated with late mortality.[103,137,138] The Canadian aneurysm study identified preoperative, intraoperative, and postoperative variables that were associated with late survival. When all the variables were considered together in a Cox model, intraoperative urine output (the lower the urine volume, the lower the survival), the development of respiratory failure, and an identified myocardial infarction were all negative predictors of late survival (Fig. 130-13). The Mayo series found coronary artery disease to be the primary cause of late death.[137] Stepwise logistic regression in the VA study identified increasing age, illness severity, and patient complexity as being independently associated with late mortality after hospital discharge.[138] Complications related to the aortic graft are higher in the RAAA group (6% in the VA study, 17% in the Mayo study) than in the elective group (2% in the VA study, 8% in the Mayo study).[137,138]

In summary, early postoperative survival of RAAA patients is dramatically less than that of those undergoing elective repair; in addition, these patients' survival over the long term is also lower than that of the elective AAA repair and general age-matched population. Late deaths were secondary to coronary artery disease, pulmonary disease, cancer, cerebrovascular disease, and renal failure.

Endovascular Aneurysm Repair

The studies that report late outcomes of rEVAR frequently contain less than 50 patients, and the length of follow-up is variable.[140-144] In one study with a 37% perioperative mortality rate, the median follow-up was 32 months and the 3-year survival rate was 36%.[139] It was concluded that EVAR did not improve long-term survival for RAAA. Others have reached similar conclusions.[144] Currently, there are insufficiently large data sets with long-term follow-up data on rEVAR to determine whether this therapy will reduce the increased long-term death rate observed in the open repair group.

Late Re-interventions

Re-interventions occur in both open and endovascular repair cases. In recent series reporting concurrent open repair and rEVAR, rates of surgical re-intervention ranged from 10% to 28% for open cases versus 19% to 23% for rEVAR cases.[141,143,145] In the rEVAR cases therapy was required for endoleaks, limb occlusions, and rerupture.[138] Thus, careful long-term clinical and imaging follow-up for those undergoing rEVAR is required to identify graft migration, increasing endoleaks, and progression of limb stenosis leading to limb occlusion.

■ QUALITY OF LIFE AFTER RUPTURED ABDOMINAL AORTIC ANEURYSM REPAIR

Quality of life after RAAA repair has been assessed with several different instruments, including the Short Form (36) Health Survey (SF-36), the EuroQoL EQ-D5, and the WHO-QOL-BREF assessment tools.[146-148] With the SF-36, outcomes were similar for elective and ruptured AAA patients, with only the social function component showing lower scores for the elective patients. The overall SF-36 scores compared favorably with the age- and sex-matched general population. When measured in quality-adjusted life years, the mean number was 8.5 for hospital survivors. In hospital survivors it was noted that physical functioning was significantly lower in those who survived RAAA repair than in age- and sex-adjusted population controls. There was no difference in the quality of life of RAAA patients who had major postoperative complications and those who did not. Thus, patients who survive RAAA repair have an acceptable quality of life, which suggests that a continued aggressive approach to repair is indicated.

SELECTED KEY REFERENCES

Bown MJ, Sutton AJ, Bell PR, Sayers RD. A meta-analysis of 50 years of ruptured abdominal aortic aneurysm repair. *Br J Surg.* 2002;89:714-730.
Demonstrates that despite years of effort, RAAA mortality has not been greatly reduced by medical intervention.

Dillavou ED, Muluk SC, Makaroun MS. Improving aneurysm-related outcomes: nationwide benefits of endovascular repair. *J Vasc Surg.* 2006;43:446-451.
Data from the U.S. Medicare database on both elective and ruptured AAAs that suggest a trend toward improvement in outcome of RAAA treated with EVAR.

Giles KA, Pomposelli F, Hamsdan A, Wyers M, Jhevari A, Schermerhorn ML. Decrease in total aneurysm related deaths in the era of endovas-cular aneurysm repair. *J Vasc Surg.* 2009;49:543-550; discussion 550-551.
Most up-to-date analysis of a large data set from the United States suggesting that the introduction of EVAR has reduced RAAA– and total AAA–related mortality.

Hinchliffe RJ, Bruijstens L, MacSweeney ST, Braithwaite BD. A ran-domised trial of endovascular and open surgery for ruptured abdomi-nal aortic aneurysm—results of a pilot study and lessons learned for future studies. *Eur J Vasc Endovasc Surg.* 2006;32:506-513.
Report of the first attempted randomized trial of open RAAA versus EVAR.

Hoornweg LL, Storm-Versloot MN, Ubbink DT, Koelemay MJ, Lege-mate DA, Balm R. Meta analysis on mortality of ruptured abdominal aortic aneurysms. *Eur J Vasc Endovasc Surg.* 2008;35:558-570.
Reviews the last 15 years of RAAA publications and shows little improvement.

Johnston KW. Ruptured abdominal aortic aneurysm: six-year follow-up results of a multicenter prospective study. Canadian Society for Vascular Surgery Aneurysm Study Group. *J Vasc Surg.* 1994;19:888-900.
This classic paper with prospective data collection analyzes risk factors associated with both early and late death with long-term follow-up.

Lesperance K, Andersen C, Singh N, Starnes B, Martin MJ. Expanding use of emergency endovascular repair for ruptured abdominal aortic aneurysm: disparities in outcomes from a nationwide perspective. *J Vasc Surg.* 2008;47:1165-1170; discussion 1170-1171.
Provides data on more than 28,000 RAAA cases from an admin-istrative database and demonstrates a benefit for rEVAR.

Lindsay TF, Luo XP, Lehotay DC, Rubin BB, Anderson M, Walker PM, Romaschin AD. Ruptured abdominal aortic aneurysm, a "two-hit" ischemia/reperfusion injury: evidence from an analysis of oxidative products. *J Vasc Surg.* 1999;30:219-228.
This paper provides the initial evidence for validity of the two-hit hypothesis of organ injury in human RAAA.

McPhee JT, Hill JS, Eslami MH. The impact of gender on presentation, therapy, and mortality of abdominal aortic aneurysm in the United States, 2001-2004. *J Vasc Surg.* 2007;45:891-899.
Administrative database that includes more than 20,000 ruptured AAAs treated by open and endovascular means. Includes patient characteristics and trends over time.

Wilson WR, Anderton M, Schwalbe EC, Jones JL, Furness PN, Bell PR, Thompson MM. Matrix metalloproteinase-8 and -9 are increased at the site of abdominal aortic aneurysm rupture. *Circulation.* 2006;113:438-445.
Provides evidence that a local change in the level of MMPs is associ-ated with aortic wall rupture.

REFERENCES

The reference list can be found on the companion Expert Consult Web site at *www.expertconsult.com.*

CHAPTER 131

Thoracic and Thoracoabdominal Aortic Aneurysms: Evaluation and Decision Making

Gilbert R. Upchurch, Jr., and Himanshu J. Patel

Aortic diseases, including aortic aneurysms, are the 12th leading cause of death in the United States.[1] Although abdominal aortic aneurysms (AAAs) and ascending aortic aneurysms are more common, descending thoracic aortic aneurysms (TAAs) and thoracoabdominal aortic aneurysms (TAAAs) are not rare, with an estimated incidence of 5.9 cases per 100,000 person-years.[2] TAA repair is associated with a high degree of morbidity and mortality. Even though anatomically TAAs, including those of the ascending aorta, aortic arch, and descending aorta, course from the ascending aorta to the diaphragm, the focus of this chapter is on descending TAAs and TAAAs. TAAAs, which can occur from the left subclavian artery to the aortic bifurcation, are defined by anatomic criteria. This chapter provides insight on degenerative TAAAs, excluding the entity of aortic dissection and connective tissue disorders, except when appropriate.

BACKGROUND

History of Open Repair

Because the techniques of open and endovascular TAAA repair are discussed in more detail in Chapter 132 (Thoracic and Thoracoabdominal Aneurysms: Open Surgical Treatment) and Chapter 133 (Thoracic and Thoracoabdominal Aneurysms: Endovascular Treatment), the history of repair will be described only in brief to aid in understanding the evolution of therapy. The goal of treatment of TAAAs is to prevent the attendant excessive mortality associated with aortic rupture. The modern era of thoracic aortic surgery was introduced by Lam and Aram, who used an aortic homograft to replace the thoracic aorta.[3] This was followed 2 years later by surgical repair of a TAAA with insertion of a synthetic vascular graft.[4] Etheredge and colleagues in 1955 were the first to report successful repair of an AAA with visceral vessel involvement.[5] Creech and coworkers are credited with repair of four TAAAs by using a Dacron graft with multiple side arm branches to the visceral and renal vessels.[6] Crawford is credited with developing, over the next 30 years, many of the surgical techniques used today.[7] Over the last 50 years the diagnosis and open surgical treatment of TAAAs have become refined as a result of advances in technology, including the use of distal aortic perfusion and cerebrospinal fluid drainage during repair, improved critical care, and better blood banking, which led to improved surgical outcomes. However, despite these adjuncts, the mortality rate after elective open TAAA repair in the United States is still 22% (Fig. 131-1A).[8] Although elective repair of a TAAA is a difficult undertaking, repair of ruptured TAAAs is associated with a 54% mortality rate and has not improved over time (Fig. 131-1B).[9] Of all operations performed, there is perhaps no other procedure in which specialization and volume have had a more favorable impact on outcomes. In reports by Cowan and others, it was documented that high-volume surgeons and high-volume hospitals have significantly lower mortality rates than do low-volume surgeons and low-volume hospitals for elective and emergency open TAAA repair.[8,9] Given the high perioperative mortality associated with open TAAA repair, regionalization of care to high-volume providers with consistently lower postoperative mortality deserves consideration.

Initial Endovascular Repairs

An alternative technique for the treatment of isolated TAAAs in the form of stent-grafting emerged in the 1990s.[10,11] Volodos and colleagues are credited with placement of the first thoracic aortic endograft.[12] The use of stent-graft technology has exploded in the last decade, and stent-grafts have been used to treat a number of thoracic aortic pathologies, including elective and ruptured (Fig. 131-2) aneurysms, dissections, and transections.[13-15] Thoracic endovascular aortic repair (TEVAR), the specifics of which are covered in Chapter 133 (Thoracic and Thoracoabdominal Aneurysms: Endovascular Treatment), is clearly associated with less physiologic strain on the patient, fewer blood transfusions, fewer hospital and intensive care unit days, and lower in-hospital mortality than seen with open TAAA repair.[16-20] Though approved by the Food and Drug Administration (FDA) only for isolated degenerative descending TAAs, TEVAR has been used as an alternative to open repair to treat ruptured TAAAs, aortic dissections, mycotic aneurysms, and aortic transections.[21-23] Similar to endovascular AAA repair, which was originally developed to treat elderly patients with significant cardiac, pulmonary, and renal co-morbid conditions, an endovascular approach is now considered primary therapy for many patients with TAAAs.[24-26] This may translate into a relative explosion of TAA repair secondary to the introduction of new technology.

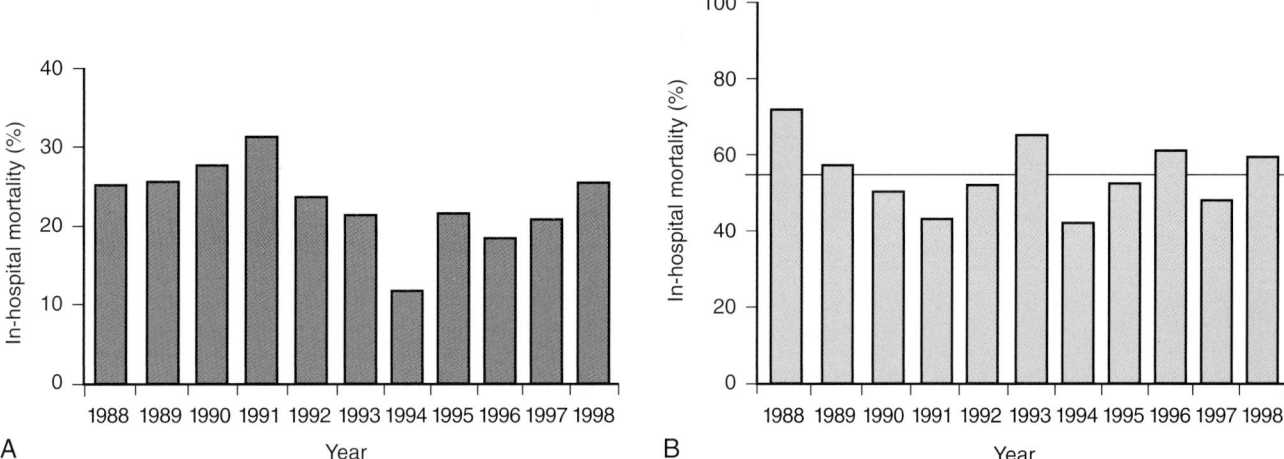

Figure 131-1 A, In-hospital mortality after elective open thoracoabdominal aortic aneurysm (TAAA) repair. Data after repair of intact TAAAs in 1542 patients from 1988 to 1998 were obtained from the Nationwide Inpatient Sample, a stratified discharge database of a representative 20% of U.S. hospitals. Overall mortality was 22.3% and improved over time. **B,** After emergency open TAAA repair, a 54% mortality rate was documented with no change in mortality over time. *(Used with permission from Cowan JA Jr, Dimick JB, Henke PK, et al. Surgical treatment of intact thoracoabdominal aortic aneurysms in the United States: hospital and surgeon volume–related outcomes. J Vasc Surg. 2003;37:1169-1174; and Cowan JA Jr, Dimick JB, Wainess RM, et al. Ruptured thoracoabdominal aortic aneurysm treatment in the United States: 1988 to 1998. J Vasc Surg. 2003;38:319-322.)*

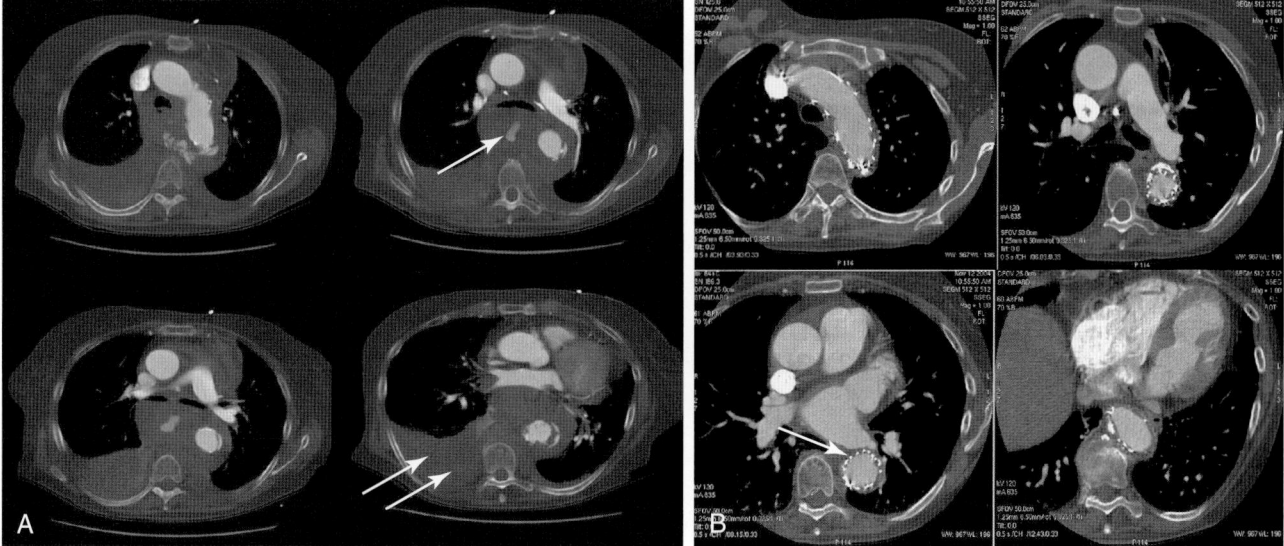

Figure 131-2 A, Multiple CT scan levels documenting a ruptured thoracoabdominal aortic aneurysm (TAAA). The *single arrow* denotes dissection associated with the rupture. The *double arrow* points to a left pleural effusion. **B,** A repeat CT scan 8 months after placement of a thoracic endograft shows resolution of the effusion and exclusion of the TAAA. The *arrow* denotes a stent-graft.

Not commercially available in the United States to date, advanced endovascular technology, including fenestrated and multibranched endografts, is widely used in Europe, Australia, and select investigational sites in the United States.[27,28] Though not compared in a prospective randomized trial with open TAAA repair, mortality is reported to be between 5% and 9% in patients considered high risk for open repair. Hybrid procedures in which extra-anatomic bypasses are performed to the brachiocephalic, visceral, or renal vessels, followed serially by stent-grafting, have also recently been heralded as an alternative to open TAAA repair (Fig. 131-3).[29,30]

Section **17** Arterial Aneurysms

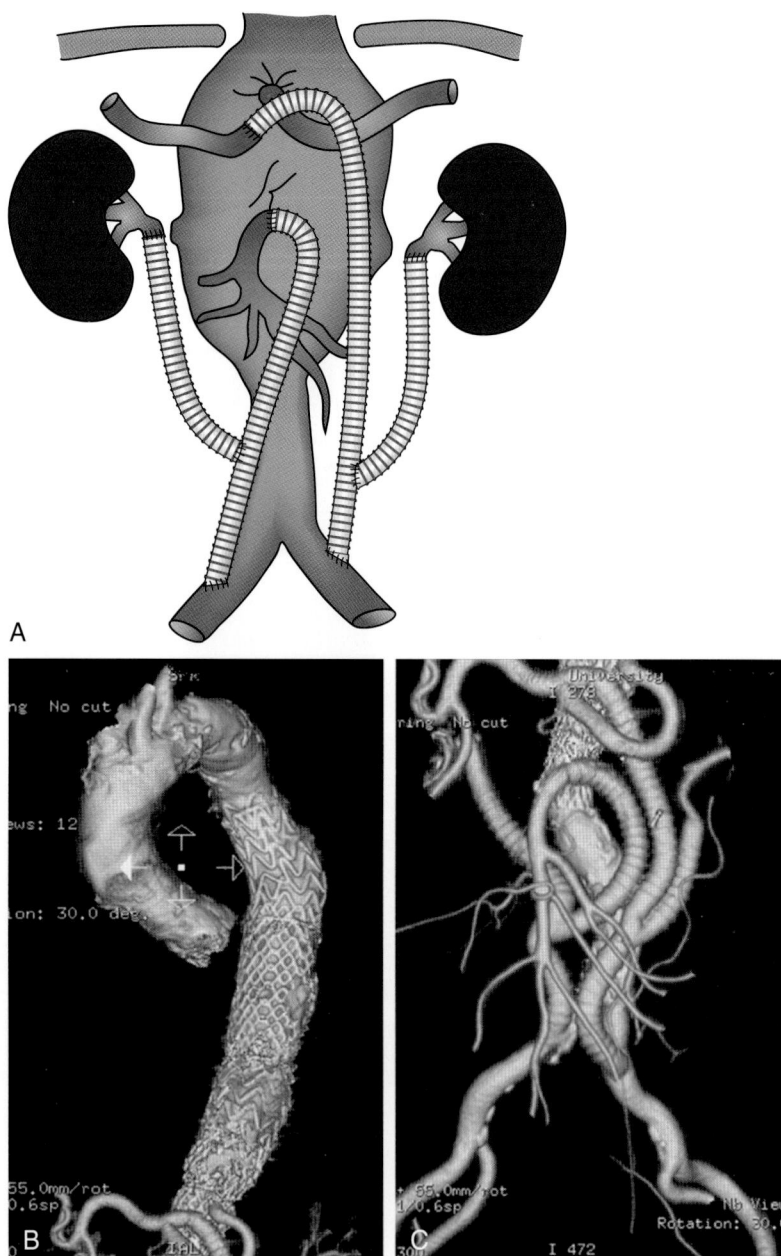

Figure 131-3 A, Schematic drawing of a hybrid procedure, or extra-anatomic bypasses to visceral and renal vessels followed by stent-grafting. Proximal (**B**) and distal (**C**) CTA images are shown after the hybrid procedure.

■ EPIDEMIOLOGY

Definition

TAAAs are localized dilatations in the thoracic and abdominal aorta secondary to weakening and subsequent expansion of the aortic wall. A TAAA by definition is a dilatation at least 1.5 times its normal value.[31] When all aneurysms of the thoracic aorta are considered, those of the ascending aorta are the most common (40%). Aneurysms of the descending thoracic aortic account for 35% of TAAs, whereas aortic arch aneurysms (15%) and TAAAs (10%) account for a smaller percentage (Table 131-1).[2,32] Defining these anatomic aortic sizes appears to be critical to help identify pathologic aortic growth because TAAA diameter is the strongest predictor of

rupture, with a reported mean aortic diameter of ruptured TAAAs of 6.1 cm in one study.[33]

Normal and Pathologic Aortic Size

The aorta normally enlarges as it progresses from the aortic root to the terminal aorta (see Table 131-1).[32] In addition, gender, age, and body surface area influence aortic diameter. Even after adjusting for age and body surface area, mean aortic size is significantly smaller, usually 2 to 3 mm, in women than in men.[34-37] Body surface area is reported to be a better predictor of aortic diameter than height or weight.[37] Normal and pathologic growth rates are also important. A mean increase in TAAA cross-sectional diameter of

Table 131-1 Normal Aortic Diameter and Length by Segment, As Well As Percentage of Thoracoabdominal Aortic Aneurysm Total by Segment

	Mean Aortic Diameter (cm)	Mean Aortic Length (cm)	TAAAs (%)
Ascending aorta	3	5	40
Aortic arch	2.5-3.5	4	15
Descending thoracic aorta	2.3-2	NR	35
Thoracoabdominal aorta	1.7-2.6*	NR	10

*Average 2 mm larger in males than females.
NR, not reported.
Data from Bickerstaff LK, Pairolero PC, Hollier LH, et al. Thoracic aortic aneurysms: a population-based study. *Surgery*. 1982;92:1103-1108; and Vasan RS, Larson MG, Benjamin EJ, Levy D. Echocardiographic reference values for aortic root size: the Framingham Heart Study. *J Am Soc Echocardiogr*. 1995;8:793-800.

0.4 cm/yr has been reported.[33] Importantly, the growth rates of TAAAs are not predictable or linear. However, there is consensus that TAAAs, similar to AAAs, have growth rates that accelerate as they enlarge.[38] For example, TAAAs larger than 5 cm expand at a growth rate of 0.79 cm/yr, whereas TAAAs less than 5 cm experience growth rates of 0.17 cm/yr.[33] Dapunt and associates documented that patients with ruptured TAAAs experienced growth rates of 0.7 cm/yr.[33]

The terms *saccular* and *fusiform* should also be defined for TAAAs because the morphology of an aneurysm will often dictate treatment options, as well as specific causes (i.e., mycotic aneurysms are often saccular and at high risk for rupture).[39] Most TAAAs are fusiform aneurysms, which are a chronic uniform dilatation involving the whole circumference of the aorta. In contrast, saccular aneurysms often represent

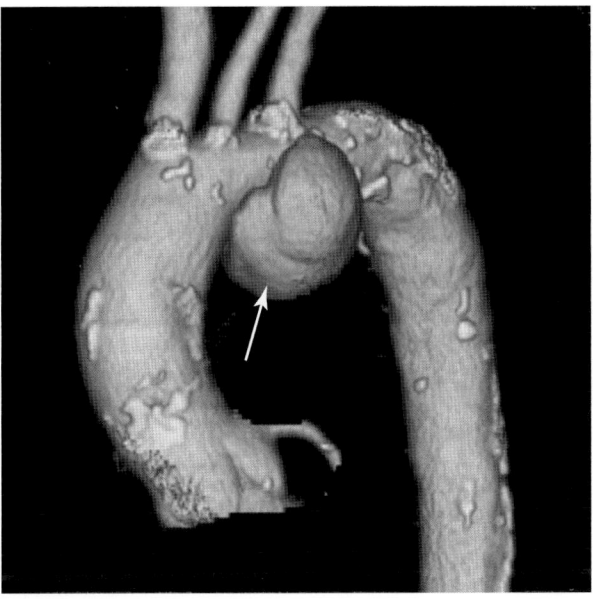

Figure 131-4 Saccular, mycotic thoracoabdominal aortic aneurysm. The patient had bacteremia and was found to have a distal aortic arch/proximal descending thoracic aortic saccular aneurysm (*arrow*).

an eccentric dilatation of the aorta (Fig. 131-4). The size at which eccentric saccular aneurysms are repaired has not been well studied; however, most would concur that a lower threshold is an acceptable indication for repair.

Population Affected

TAAAs are primarily a disease of the elderly. The average age of patients with TAAAs is 65 years, with a male-female ratio of 1.7:1[2]; in contrast, in patients with AAAs whose mean age is 75 years, the male-female ratio is 6:1.[40] TAAAs clearly have a genetic component in that more than 20% of patients will have a first-degree relative affected by aneurysm disease.[41-43]

Risk Factors for Disease and Rupture

Many risk factors common in patients with AAAs, including hypertension, smoking, and atherosclerosis in other arteries, are also common in patients with TAAAs.[2,44-46] Though most often described as degenerative, in up to 20% of patients TAAAs are the sequelae of chronic aortic dissection,[47] wherein aneurysmal dilatation of the outer wall of the false lumen necessitates late aortic repair in up to 40% of patients irrespective of initial medical or surgical treatment of the dissection. Systemic hypertension—in particular, elevated diastolic blood pressure greater than 100 mm Hg—has been associated with aortic growth and rupture.[33,48]

Because most patients with TAAAs are asymptomatic, treatment is aimed at preventing rupture. Natural history studies of TAAAs are rarer than those of isolated infrarenal AAAs, probably related to their much less frequent occurrence. In addition, studies on TAAAs often include patients with both acute and chronic aortic dissection, which serves to complicate natural history data. Initial studies from the 1970s by Pressler and McNamara documented that approximately 40% of patients who did not undergo surgical repair died of TAAA rupture whereas 32% died of other cardiovascular diseases. Mean survival was less than 3 years. During the extended period of observation, more than 90% of patients sustained aortic rupture, with 68% of ruptures occurring more than 1 month after the diagnosis.[49,50] The 5-year survival rate for patients with 6.0-cm TAAAs is 54%, with a risk for rupture of 3.7%/yr and a risk for death of 12%/yr. Median survival in patients with untreated TAAAs is poor at only 3.3 years.[51] In a natural history study of patients who were not candidates for surgery by Crawford and DeNatale, the survival rate was just 24% at 2 years, with over half the deaths related to aneurysm rupture. Chronic obstructive pulmonary disease (COPD) was noted in 80% of the subgroup with rupture.[52] Similar studies in patients with small infrarenal AAAs have confirmed COPD as a significant risk factor for rupture.[53] Cambria and others followed a series of 57 patients with TAAAs who were not considered operative candidates. In addition to COPD, the authors found an association (*P* = .06) between rupture and chronic renal failure.[54] In a study by Griepp and colleagues, 165 patients with TAAAs were monitored after being assigned nonoperative status.

Table 131-2 Risk Factors for Thoracoabdominal Aortic Aneurysm Rupture

Risk Factor	Relative Rate	P Value
Age	2.6*	.02
Pain	2.3	.04
Chronic obstructive pulmonary disease	3.6†	.004
Descending aortic diameter	1.9	.003
Abdominal aortic diameter	1.50‡	.05

*The relative rate increases by a factor of 2.6 for each decade of age.
†The relative rate increases by a factor of 1.9 for each centimeter of descending aortic diameter.
‡The relative rate increases by a factor of 1.5 for each centimeter of abdominal aortic diameter.
From Juvonen T, Ergin MA, Galla JD, et al. Risk factors for rupture of chronic type B dissections. *J Thorac Cardiovasc Surg.* 1999;117:776-777.

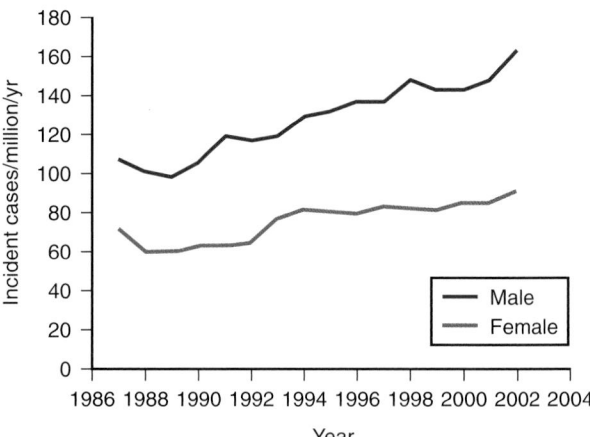

Figure 131-5 Increasing incidence of thoracoabdominal aortic aneurysms and dissection in the Swedish population (men and women), 1987 to 2002 (cases per million). *(Used with permission from Olsson C, Thelin S, Stahle E, et al. Thoracic aortic aneurysm and dissection: increasing prevalence and improved outcomes reported in a nationwide population-based study of more than 14,000 cases from 1987 to 2002. Circulation. 2006;114: 2611-2618.)*

Twenty percent of patients eventually suffered rupture. Important risk factors for rupture included older age, COPD, uncharacteristic continued pain, and aortic diameter. Patients with aortic dissection ruptured at smaller aortic diameters than did those with nondissected degenerative aneurysms.[55]

Aneurysm diameter is the most important risk factor for rupture. Dapunt and coworkers documented that TAAAs greater than 8 cm have an 80% risk for rupture within 1 year of diagnosis.[33] However, the size at which TAAAs rupture is unpredictable. Similar to AAAs, it appears that aneurysm growth rates play a role. The average expansion rate of a TAAA is approximately 0.10 to 0.42 cm/yr.[51,56-58] Coady and associates suggested that expansion by more than 1 cm/yr signals impending rupture.[56] Juvonen and colleagues examined 114 patients with TAAAs in detail.[59] Multivariate analysis suggested that increasing age, pain (even atypical), COPD, descending thoracic aortic diameter, and abdominal aortic diameter were predictive of rupture (Table 131-2).

Incidence/Prevalence

The incidence and prevalence of TAAAs have been increasing over the last several decades.[2] Clouse and coauthors documented that the incidence of TAAAs in the United States is 10.4 cases per 100,000.[60] Olsson and colleagues recently examined the prevalence of TAAA in a large contemporary population. All subjects with thoracic aortic dissections or aneurysms from 1987 to 2002 were identified in the Swedish National Healthcare Registry. Of 14,229 individuals with thoracic aortic disease, the diagnosis was made in 11,039 (78%) before death. The incidence of thoracic aortic disease rose by 52% in men and 28% in women to reach 16.3 and 9.1 per 100,000 per year, respectively. The authors concluded that the prevalence and incidence of thoracic aortic disease were higher than previously reported and increasing (Fig. 131-5).[61] The increasing prevalence of TAAAs has been attributed to a number of factors, including improved imaging techniques, an aging population, and increased patient and physician awareness.[62]

PATHOGENESIS

The development of a TAAA is a multifactorial event that involves a complex interaction of genetic factors, cellular imbalance, and altered hemodynamic factors.[63] The increased incidence of TAAAs in patients with Marfan's syndrome and other connective tissue disorders inherited in a mendelian manner, as well as the familial inheritance of nonsyndromic TAAAs and dissections typically inherited in an autosomal dominant fashion with marked variability in the age of onset and decreased penetrance, suggests a varying genetic role along different segments of the aorta.[64] More recent studies have suggested that genetic variation in extracellular matrix (ECM) actin and myosin may contribute to the development of TAAAs.[65,66] Wang, Elefteriades, and coauthors examined genetic signatures in the peripheral blood of patients with TAAAs (n = 58) and control patients (n = 36). This study documented a number of gene families that were different between the two groups, including those involved in the cell cycle, DNA metabolism, glycolysis, interferon-γ signaling, and transcription factors. The authors concluded that analysis of peripheral blood to determine expression signatures may help identify patients with TAAAs with high accuracy.[67]

TAAA formation therefore is a complicated, dynamic process involving both extracellular and cellular processes, similar to other aneurysms (see Chapter 8: Arterial Aneurysms). Once initiated through a combination of the aforementioned factors, inflammation and pathologic remodeling of the ECM occur. A large body of evidence suggests that ECM degradation by matrix metalloproteinases (MMPs) exceeds matrix production and repair during average function. Although the biomechanical properties and composition of the aorta, including the role of elastin and collagen in the arterial matrix, are discussed in Chapter 8 (Arterial Aneurysms), it is important to emphasize that there are significant differences in the composition of the aortic wall as one progresses from the ascending aorta to the iliac bifurcation. Andreotti and colleagues documented that the ascending aorta has a greater concentration of elastin and is therefore more compliant than the descending aorta. This alteration in elastin concentration leads to a progressive decrease in the elastin-collagen ratio as the aorta progresses from the ascending aorta to the abdominal aorta.[68] The media also becomes thinner as one progresses from proximal to distal along the aorta.[69]

A number of recent studies have documented the overexpression and increased activity of various ECM proteinases, specifically the MMPs, in human TAAAs.[70] These proteolytic enzymes, which have been more extensively studied in AAAs, are clearly critical as well during the formation of TAAAs. Sinha and coworkers documented asymmetric production of MMP-9 in the expanding human TAAA wall, which correlated with increased numbers of macrophages.[71] In contrast, MMP-2 was documented to be increased in the wall of the TAAA that was preserved, in particular, at the point where smooth muscle cells were more abundant and the wall was preserved (Fig. 131-6). Ikonomidis and associates studied the role of MMPs in a murine model of TAAAs.[70] These authors documented that MMP-9 gene deletion attenuated TAA formation despite increases in MMP-2 activity. They concluded that interactions between MMP-9 and MMP-2 are necessary to facilitate TAAA progression.

Aortic Wall Histology

The histology of TAAAs is most closely associated with medial degeneration, formerly known as cystic medial necrosis (Fig. 131-7). Medial degeneration is characterized by fragmentation and loss of elastic fibers, loss of smooth muscle cells, and collections of interstitial collagenous tissue, basophilic ground substance, and proteoglycans.[72,73] Although medial degeneration is considered part of the normal aging process, it is accelerated by certain clinical conditions such as hypertension and atherosclerosis.[74] Given the relative widespread process along the thoracic aorta, medial degeneration is most closely associated with the development of fusiform aneurysms. Genetic abnormalities such as Marfan's syndrome also accelerate aortic medial degeneration.[75] Though TAAAs were originally described as noninflammatory, recent studies have shown that infiltration of leukocytes contributes to the formation and development of TAAAs. The significant difference in the epidemiology and histology of TAAAs and AAAs suggests distinct causes.

■ ETIOLOGY

Eighty percent of TAAAs are secondary to medial degeneration, with approximately 15% to 20% being caused by aortic dissection (Box 131-1) (see Chapter 135: Aortic Dissection). Patients with TAAAs secondary to aortic dissection are typically younger, but the aneurysms involve more extensive aortic segments than do degenerative aneurysms.[76] The aorta

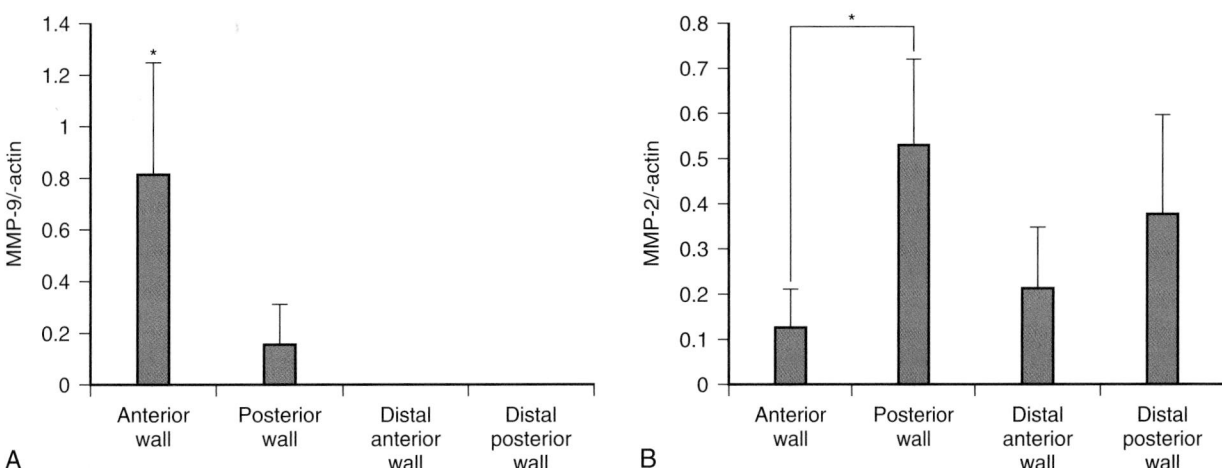

Figure 131-6 A, At the level of the thoracoabdominal aortic aneurysm (TAAA), matrix metalloproteinase-9 (MMP-9) expression is 4.3-fold higher in the anterior wall than in the posterior wall. MMP-9 is minimally detectable in the distal aspects of the aneurysm. (*P <.05.) **B,** At the level of the TAAA, MMP-2 expression is 3.2-fold higher in the posterior wall than in the anterior wall. MMP-2 is present in the distal aspects of the aneurysm, although the level of expression is not significantly different from MMP-2 expression at the level of the aneurysm. (*P < .05.) Data are reported as means ± standard error. *(Used with permission from Sinha I, Bethi S, Cronin P, et al. A biologic basis for asymmetric growth in descending thoracic aortic aneurysms: a role for matrix metalloproteinase 9 and 2. J Vasc Surg. 2006;43:342-348.)*

Section **17** Arterial Aneurysms

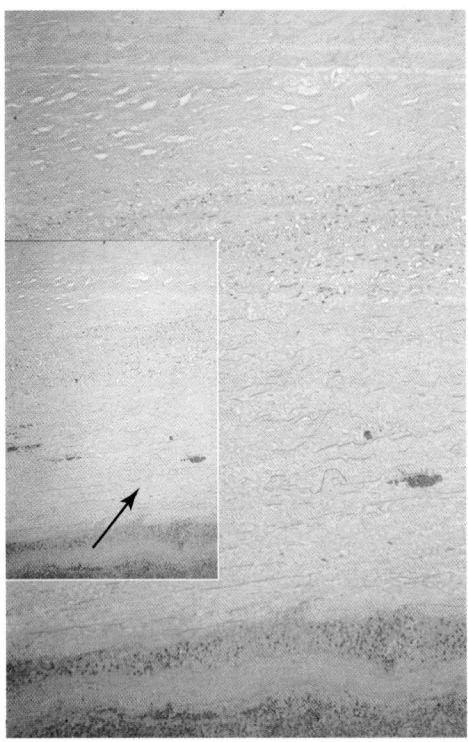

Figure 131-7 Documentation of medial degeneration and fragmented elastin (see *insert, arrow*) by histology (H&E, ×100) of an aortic section in a patient with a thoracoabdominal aortic aneurysm. *(Courtesy of Dr. David Williams.)*

Box 131-1 Etiology of Thoracoabdominal Aortic Aneurysms and the Relative Percentage Contributing to Disease

- Degenerative (associated with atherosclerosis) (80%)
- Dissections (15% to 20%)
- Connective tissue disorders (Marfan's syndrome, Ehlers-Danlos syndrome, etc.)
- Infection (2%)
- Mycotic aneurysms (*Salmonella*, *Haemophilus influenzae*, *Staphylococcus* sp.)
- Syphilis
- Tuberculosis
- Aortitis (2%)
- Takayasu's disease
- Nonspecific variety of giant cell aortitis
- Rheumatoid aortitis
- Ankylosing spondylitis
- Reiter's syndrome
- Relapsing polychondritis
- Postoperative pseudoaneurysms (<1%)
- Associated with unrepaired and repaired aortic coarctations
- Traumatic (<1%)

Data from Panneton JM, Hollier LH. Nondissecting thoracoabdominal aortic aneurysms: Part I. *Ann Vasc Surg.* 1995;9:503-514; and Cambria RP, Davison JK, Zannetti S, et al. Thoracoabdominal aneurysm repair: perspectives over a decade with the clamp-and-sew technique. *Ann Surg.* 1997;226:294-303; discussion 303-305.

---

in patients with Marfan's syndrome is particularly prone to aortic dissection and subsequent TAAA formation.[77] Both systemic autoimmune disorders, such as Takayasu's arteritis, and chronic nonspecific aortitis can destroy the aortic media with progressive aneurysm formation. Aneurysms associated with arteritis are more commonly seen in women than degenerative aneurysms. Aneurysms of the upper thoracic aorta can also be secondary to congenital aortic coarctations, either in unrepaired coarctations or after repair.[78-80]

TAAAs may also form secondary to infection. Although saccular aneurysms have been described as mycotic, these aneurysms are most often bacterial and occur because of hematogenous spread of emboli laden with bacteria. Infected TAAAs usually arise as a result of seeding of atherosclerotic plaque in the aorta, the development of a focal inflammatory process in the aortic wall, and ultimately the formation of a false aneurysm. Infected TAAAs present many challenging dilemmas. The goal of therapy is to debulk the infection and restore arterial continuity. For years this has involved in situ repair with its attendant lifetime risk of reinfection. Recent reports of treatment of infected TAAAs with endovascular prostheses are beginning to accumulate.[81,82]

ANATOMIC CLASSIFICATION

Evaluation of a patient with a TAAA, as well as the technical performance of either open or endovascular repair, is closely aligned with the Crawford classification (Fig. 131-8).[83-85] The classification of TAAAs also has important therapeutic implications for the operation to be performed, as well as the risk for specific complications. Type I TAAAs account for approximately 25% of all TAAAs; they involve the entire descending thoracic aorta and extend only to the upper abdominal aorta. Type II TAAAs (approximately 30% of TAAAs) involve the entire descending thoracic aorta and most or all of the abdominal aorta (Fig. 131-9A). Type III TAAAs (less than 25%) involve variable lengths of the descending thoracic aorta and extend into the abdominal aorta (Fig. 131-9B). Type IV TAAAs (<25%) are limited to most or all of the abdominal aorta, including the visceral and renal arteries.

CLINICAL FINDINGS
History and Physical Examination

Most patients with TAAAs have no symptoms attributable to their disease at the time of diagnosis.[46,50,86] The diagnosis is therefore often made when evaluating the patient for unrelated conditions. Although most patients with TAAAs are often asymptomatic, most aneurysms will become symptomatic before they rupture.[86] Panneton and Hollier documented that 57% of patients with degenerative TAAAs will have symptoms before rupture.

The most common initial symptom in patients with TAAAs is vague pain, which can occur in the chest, back, flank, or abdomen. The differential diagnosis in a patient with a symp-

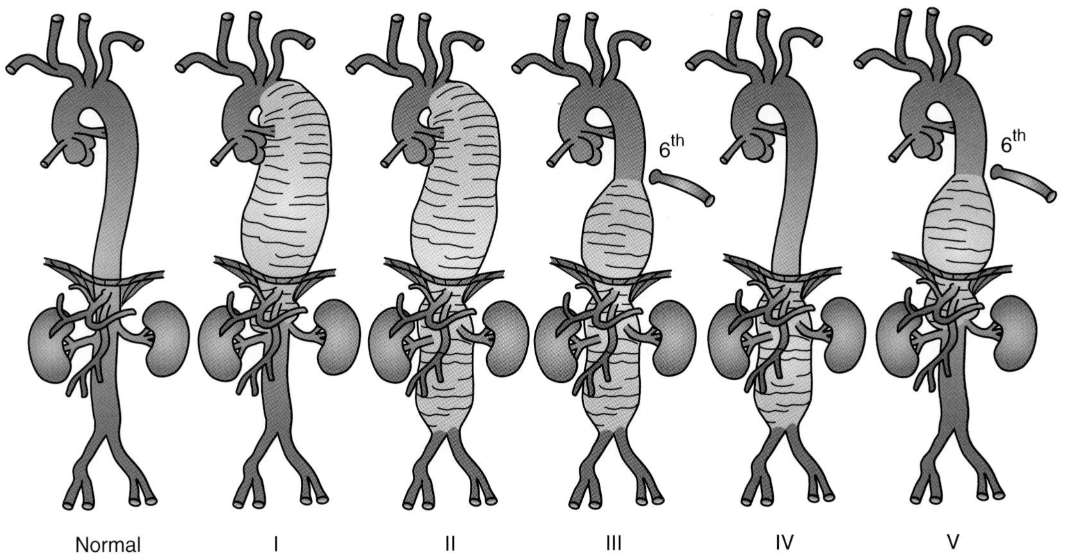

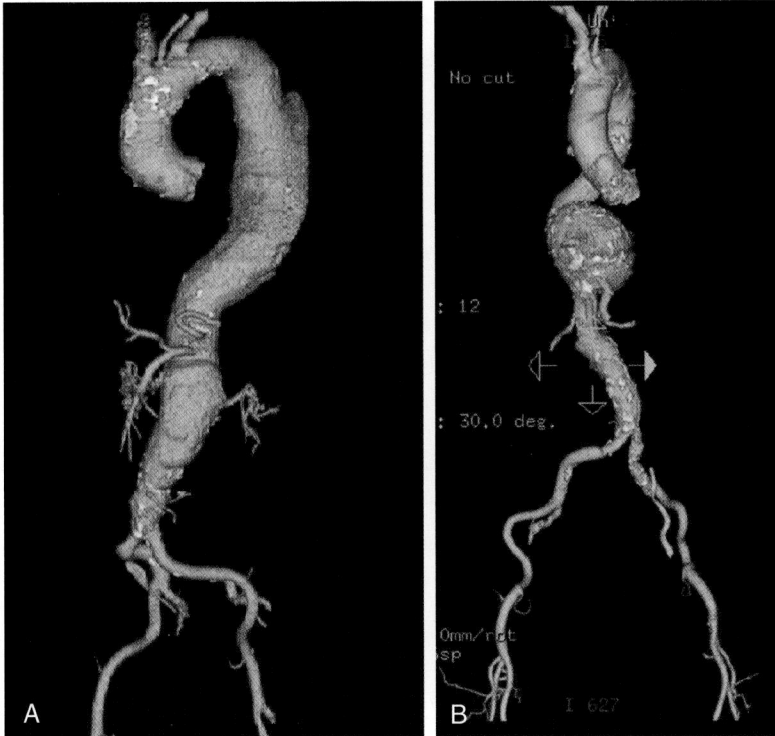

Figure 131-8 Crawford classification of thoracoabdominal aortic aneurysms. Type I, distal to the left subclavian artery to above the renal arteries. Type II, distal to the left subclavian artery to below the renal arteries. Type III, from the sixth intercostal space to the renal arteries. Type IV, from the 13th intercostal space to the iliac bifurcation (entire abdominal aorta). Type V, below the sixth intercostal space to just above the renal arteries.

Figure 131-9 Three-dimensional CTA of a type II thoracoabdominal aortic aneurysm (TAAA) (**A**) with associated dissection and a type III saccular TAAA (**B**).

tomatic TAAA therefore includes angina, aortic dissection, and degenerative disease of the spine. The chronic pain associated with TAAAs may easily be dismissed in patients with TAAAs before the diagnosis of a TAAA has been made. Typical of most aneurysms when enlarging, pain may increase in severity dramatically. Juovenen and coworkers suggested that the back pain associated with a TAAA can indeed be chronic and have a different pattern and implication than noted with AAAs, in which the back pain is more often acute

and suggests pending rupture.[59] Symptoms may also occur in patients with TAAAs from compression of the thoracic aorta by structures in the thoracic cavity. Hoarseness can develop in patients with TAAAs as a result of stretching or compression of the left recurrent laryngeal nerve. Tracheal deviation, persistent cough, or other respiratory symptoms may also be present.[49,87] Dysphagia is an uncommon, nonspecific complaint reported by patients with TAAAs that is due to compression of the aneurysm by the esophagus.[88] Sudden and catastrophic hemoptysis or hematemesis may occur as a result of erosion of the TAAA into the bronchial and pulmonary space or the esophagus, respectively. Patients with TAAAs may rarely have neurologic deficits, including paraplegia. This is much more common in those with aortic dissection. Embolization to the visceral, renal, and lower extremity arteries has been reported.[89] Patients with an abdominal component of their aneurysm may have gastrointestinal hemorrhage, aortoenteric fistulae, or a functional small bowel obstruction secondary to compression of the duodenum. Most patients with symptoms have TAAAs that have attained a diameter greater than 5 cm.

Patients with TAAAs generally have no obvious physical findings in the chest area unless tracheal deviation is present.[90] Patients with an abdominal component of their TAAA may have a pulsatile abdominal mass similar to pure AAAs.

Synchronous Aneurysm Risk

Studies examining the natural history of patients with TAAAs indicate that between 20% and 30% will also have an AAA.[49,91] In a series of 1500 patients Crawford and Cohen documented that 13% harbored aneurysms in other segments.[92] This appears to be true when examining patients who undergo TAAA repair as well, where as many as a third of patients will have undergone previous aortic repair.[93] Most commonly patients with TAAAs have undergone previous infrarenal AAA repair. Patients with TAAAs are also at risk for discontinuous aneurysms or aneurysms proximal to their TAAA. Synchronous proximal ascending and arch aneurysms are noted in 6% to 13% of patients with TAAAs.[86] Even after repair, at least 10% of patients with TAAAs will require subsequent aneurysm repair in noncontiguous aortic segments.[94] Patients with Marfan's syndrome who have suffered a type A dissection appear to be at high risk for this type of manifestation. As discussed in Chapter 133 (Thoracic and Thoracoabdominal Aneurysms: Endovascular Treatment) and Chapter 134 (Aortic Arch Aneurysms and Dissection), there is clearly an increasing trend in treating complex arch aneurysms and TAAAs with sequential open and endovascular therapies.[95-97]

■ DIAGNOSTIC EVALUATION

Patients with TAAAs frequently have significant coexisting medical conditions, including hypertension, coronary artery disease, COPD, congestive heart failure, cerebrovascular occlusive disease, and peripheral vascular occlusive disease. Cross-sectional imaging, mainly by computed tomography (CT), is the primary method to visualize the thoracic and abdominal aorta for determining aneurysm diameter and extent. Because most TAAAs are small when discovered, serial imaging is required; however, level A and B evidence regarding the timing of surveillance is lacking. Serial imaging is typically performed at 6- to 12-month intervals but varies depending on the initial diameter and extent of the aneurysm.

Imaging

Accurate and precise determination of the anatomy of a patient with a TAAA is mandatory in determining both the need for and the details of operative repair, as well as the prescribed follow-up in patients with TAAAs who have not reached a diameter threshold for repair. A chest radiograph (Fig. 131-10) or plain films of the abdomen in patients with TAAA may suggest an enlarged thoracic aorta secondary to a calcified aortic wall. Indirect findings suggestive of TAAA on chest radiography include a widened mediastinum, enlargement of the aortic knob, and tracheal deviation.

Arteriography

Although in the past aortography was routinely performed as part of the preoperative evaluation of patients with TAAAs to define the extent and location of the aneurysm, angiography is presently considered obsolete except for special situations, such as attempting to map the spinal cord circulation. Williams and coworkers used angiography to identify the spinal artery of Adamkiewicz, or the great radicular artery, to help prevent paraplegia by knowing in advance of TAAA repair which intercostal artery is providing this important branch to enable prompt and focused revascularization.[98] Indications for angiography also include evaluation of branch anatomy in a patient with a TAAA and occlusive disease in the cerebrovascular, visceral, renal, or iliac beds when one wants to limit the use of iodinated contrast material in those with chronic renal

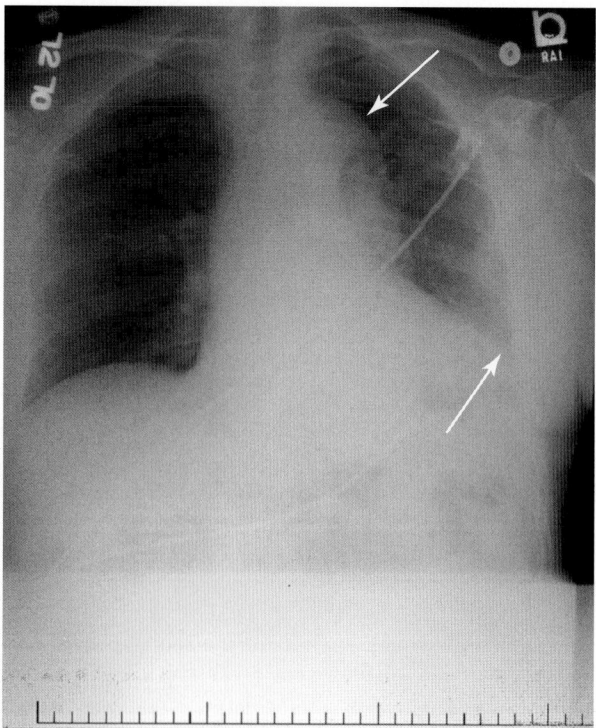

Figure 131-10 Chest radiograph in the posteroanterior projection documenting a rim of calcification outlining the dilated thoracic aorta (*top arrow*), as well as a left-sided pleural effusion (*bottom arrow*) in a patient with a ruptured thoracoabdominal aortic aneurysm.

failure. Selective angiography using dilute contrast or CO_2 might also be used to treat patients with occlusive disease before TAAA repair, even though few specific studies documenting this approach have been performed.

Computed Tomography

Spiral CT scanning with three-dimensional reconstructions is now the "gold standard" for evaluating the aorta in patients with TAAAs. Spiral CT using 360-degree rotation of the x-ray beam source can document the extent of the aortic aneurysm and provide accurate serial measurement of aneurysm diameter. Computer programs can generate sagittal, coronal, and oblique images, as well as three-dimensional renderings that can be used to determine whether a patient is a candidate for a stent-graft (Fig. 131-11).[99] A general assessment of other organs in the chest, abdomen, and pelvis is also obtained with CT, which allows the detection of other pathology, including cancer, that might affect patient management and surgical planning.[100,101] In patients with renal insufficiency, CT without iodinated contrast agents can be useful to determine TAAA size or extent but will not provide accurate data regarding the atherosclerotic burden of branch vessels or the presence of a dissection. It is our general impression, supported by studies,[102] that given the standard use of low-osmolar, smaller boluses of contrast material in performing computed tomographic angiography (CTA), contrast-related acute renal failure after CTA is in fact rare and when it does occur is mild.

CTA also importantly allows other essential information to be obtained, include assessment of occlusive disease in branch vessels. In addition, CTA documents the patency of important intercostals that might be reimplanted into the aortic graft if extensive open TAAA repair is being considered. CTA further documents the presence of thrombus, inflammatory changes, dissection, and retroperitoneal blood suggestive of a ruptured aneurysm. The relative advantages of CT scanning over magnetic resonance imaging (MRI) include its being less expensive, quicker to perform and thus less claustrophobia-inducing, useful in patients with previous implanted ferromagnetic devices, and widely available.

A word of caution is needed regarding CTA and the timing of TAAA repair. Because of the nephrotoxicity of iodinated contrast agents, in the elective surgery and endovascular therapy setting CTA is best delayed for at least 24 hours after CT, especially in patients with chronic renal insufficiency. The administration of *N*-acetylcysteine and intravenous hydration are current strategies used to limit contrast-induced nephropathy.[103,104] If contrast-induced nephropathy does occur, elective repairs should be delayed until renal function returns to baseline.

Magnetic Resonance Imaging and Magnetic Resonance Angiography

MRI/magnetic resonance angiography (MRA) can be considered when evaluating patients with TAAAs, especially those with renal insufficiency, because it avoids the use of iodinated contrast material (Fig. 131-12). MRA has also been used to map the spinal cord circulation before TAAA repair.[105] Although MRI is believed to provide better contrast resolution, its spatial resolution is poorer than that of CT scanning. Initially, there was enthusiastic support for using MRI/MRA to identify the patency of visceral and renal vessels in patients with TAAAs.[106] However, recent concerns over the use of gadolinium in patients with renal insufficiency has made the use of MRA less attractive in those with aortic aneurysms.[107] MRI/MRA is also technically limited in that thrombus and calcium are not prominently displayed. In addition, the increased time required to acquire the images, the associated claustrophobia, the increased cost, and interference from metallic implants make MRA of limited use in the treatment of TAAAs.

Laboratory Testing

At present, there are no available biomarkers to suggest the presence of a TAAA. Initial research in patients with acute aortic dissections has focused on a number of proteins, including lipoprotein (a),[108] S-100B,[109] and calponin.[110] Touat and others have suggested that platelet activation and thrombin generation occur in patients with large dilated ascending aortic aneurysms, particularly in areas of mucoid

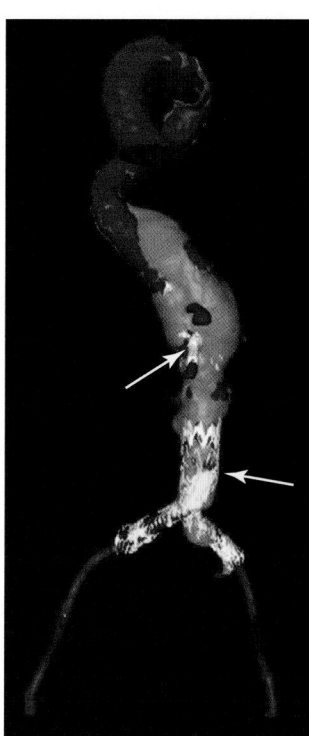

Figure 131-11 Three-dimensional CT scan in patient with Marfan's syndrome and a complicated dissection and thoracoabdominal aortic aneurysm. The patient had earlier undergone placement of a superior mesenteric artery stent (*top arrow*) for mesenteric malperfusion associated with aortic dissection. The patient subsequently underwent endovascular abdominal aortic aneurysm (AAA) repair (*bottom arrow*, infrarenal) for an aortoenteric fistulae after open AAA repair.

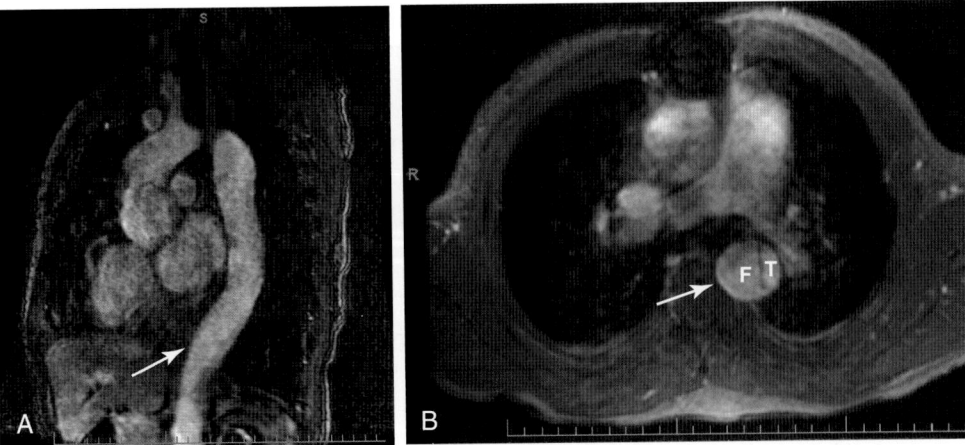

Figure 131-12 MRA of thoracoabdominal aortic aneurysm (TAAA). **A,** Sagittal MRA view with gadolinium enhancement in a patient with a type B aortic dissection and subsequent TAAA formation. The *arrow* denotes an area of maximal aneurysmal dilatation. **B,** Axial cut at same level (*arrow*) documenting the true (T) and false (F) lumen of dissection.

degeneration.[111] Standard laboratory testing, including a complete blood count with platelets, coagulation studies, and determination of blood urea nitrogen and creatinine levels, is standard before TAAA repair. Reports have suggested that the rare patient with a TAAA may have low-grade disseminated intravascular coagulation based on consumptive coagulopathy from the aneurysm.[112]

MEDICAL THERAPY

It is important to acknowledge that there is no level A or B evidence comparing modern medical therapy (aspirin, beta blocker, statin, angiotensin-converting enzyme inhibitor, smoking cessation medications) with open or endovascular TAAA repair. In general, nonoperative management consists of strict blood pressure control with beta blockade, cessation of smoking, and periodic imaging to monitor the size of the TAAA. There are guidelines to help us in the management and preoperative preparation of patients with AAAs, but not specifically for patients with TAAAs. In addition, reports focused on medical therapies to limit or slow the growth of TAAAs are few.

Antihypertensive Medication

Beta Blockers

Wheat and Palmer are credited with documenting that decreasing the force of myocardial contraction (dP/dt) slows aortic growth and may prevent TAAA rupture secondary to aortic dissection, but not degenerative TAAAs.[113] This observation is the basis for prescribing β-adrenergic blocking agents as first-line antihypertensive therapy for patients with TAAAs. Shores and colleagues used propranolol over a 10-year period and showed a significant reduction in growth of the aortic root, aortic events, and mortality in patients with Marfan's syndrome.[114] Results in animal models of AAA have not translated into beneficial effects of slowing AAA growth in humans.[115,116] It is therefore not clear that beta blockers retard aortic growth in patients with degenerative TAAAs.

Regardless, the safety and efficacy of beta blockers in preventing death secondary to myocardial infarction are well documented, and therefore they should be prescribed, especially in the preoperative setting.

Angiotensin-Converting Enzyme Inhibitors or Receptor Blockers

There is increasing evidence that oxidative stress plays an important role in the development of degenerative TAAs. Ejiri and associates documented a role for the renin-angiotensin system in the pathogenesis of TAAAs. Human thoracic aneurysmal (n = 40) and nonaneurysmal (control, n = 39) aortic sections were examined and the results documented markedly increased in situ production of reactive oxygen species throughout the TAAA wall. Multiple regression analysis revealed that medical treatment with angiotensin II type 1 receptor blockers suppressed expression of reactive oxygen species in TAAA.[117] This research suggests that angiotensin-converting enzyme inhibitors or receptor blockers may be of benefit to hypertensive patients with TAAAs.

Statins

A well-studied class of drugs with important cholesterol-lowering properties is the 3-hydroxy-3-methylglutaryl coenzyme A (HMG-CoA) reductase inhibitors. HMG-CoA reductase inhibitors, also known as statins, in addition to lowering cholesterol also have pleiotropic effects that inhibit inflammation.[118,119] Specific to TAAAs, recent studies in human TAAAs have shown a role for p22phox-based reduced nicotinamide adenine dinucleotide/reduced nicotinamide adenine dinucleotide phosphate (NADH/NADPH) oxidase in the pathogenesis of TAAAs. This study suggested that statins might have inhibitory effects on the formation of TAAAs via the suppression of NADH/NADPH oxidase.[117] Although data examining TAAA growth in humans are lacking, Schouten and associates documented that statins inhibit the growth of AAAs.[120] A recent study suggested that statins are effective in lowering mortality after endovascular AAA repair but not after TAAA repair.[121] These authors concluded that this variable response to statins indirectly supports the concept of a distinct pathogenesis of AAAs and TAAAs. Nonetheless, most patients with TAAAs have indications for statin therapy, and this might reduce growth rates.

Smoking Cessation

Patients who smoke or who have COPD are at increased risk for the development of TAAAs. TAAAs also grow faster and rupture more often in smokers.[33,59] Cannon and Read suggested that this was secondary to increased elastolytic activity.[122] Based on the AAA literature, few would argue that patients who smoke are at risk for the development of TAAAs.[123,124] These studies suggest that active pursuit of cessation of cigarette smoking is an important adjunct in those under observation with a TAAA.

■ SELECTION OF TREATMENT

The decision when to operate on a patient with a TAAA involves assessment of the likelihood of aortic rupture versus the operative risk of the individual patient.[125] It is unclear at present what the impact of endovascular therapy will be, with its attendant lower short-term mortality and morbidity, on decision making regarding what aortic diameter should serve as a threshold for TAAA repair. Two major factors, the patient's physiologic reserve and vascular anatomy, play a significant role in determining whether a patient is best suited for open repair or an endovascular approach.[126]

Size Criteria

Size criteria for TAAA repair are not as clearly defined as for infrarenal AAAs because there are no level A or B scientific data regarding the timing of operative intervention.[127,128] This issue is further complicated by the observation that degenerative TAAAs are often not uniform in size and involve aortic segments of varying diameters and morphology. In addition, it is important to recognize the impact of body size on aortic size. Adjustment for body surface area or height needs to be incorporated into decision making about the threshold for repair and risk for rupture.[129] For the average older man (5'6" to 5'10"), the normal proximal descending aorta is 2.8 cm, the mid-descending aorta is 2.7 cm, and the distal descending aorta is 2.6 cm. The authors suggested that the accepted size indications for TAAA repair, independent of etiology, might be a diameter of 5.2 to 5.6 cm or twice the diameter of the normal contiguous aorta, depending on the aortic segment being repaired. Algorithms suggest that 0.6 cm can be added to or subtracted from these figures for individuals taller than 6 feet or shorter than 5 feet.[83,130] Others have suggested that repair of TAAAs should be considered in patients with aortas twice the size of a normal continuous segment or approximately 6 cm in diameter.[90]

Based on natural history studies that have documented an extremely high risk for rupture and death if left untreated, all patients with TAAAs should be considered for repair.[4,49,55,131] The natural history of ruptured TAAAs was first study extensively by Crawford and colleagues.[132] In a series of more than 100 ruptured TAAAs, the authors noted that 80% of ruptures occurred in patients with aneurysms that were less than 10 cm in diameter. The presence of an aortic dissection portended rupture at smaller diameters, with a reported 13% of ruptures occurring in aneurysms smaller than 6 cm. Rupture occurred in the thoracic and abdominal cavity with approximately equal frequency. They concluded by suggesting that because elective surgery was associated with a 92% survival rate, TAAA repair should be considered before rupture when aneurysms are 5 cm or larger in good-risk patients, in patients with symptomatic aneurysms, and in most patients with larger aneurysms. In a large Scandinavian autopsy series, Juvonen and colleagues suggested that 6 cm should be the threshold for open TAAA repair.[59] More recently, Elefteriades suggested that the size criteria for surgical TAAA intervention should be greater than 6.5 cm.[133] The author suggested that this threshold should be lowered for patients with connective tissue disorders, in whom repair should be offered when the aneurysm attains a diameter of 6.0 cm.[133] A positive family history for aortic rupture or dissection might also serve to lower the threshold for repair. Coady and coauthors suggested that in asymptomatic TAAA patients who are monitored longitudinally, there are "hinge points" that demarcate highly dangerous aortic thresholds.[56] For the descending thoracic aorta, the hinge point is 7 cm, where a 43% risk for rupture is encountered. This suggests a "conservative" criterion of 6.5 cm for surgical intervention in TAAAs. Because multiple studies have suggested increased mortality and morbidity for types I and II TAAAs, perhaps a higher threshold for repair (6 cm) should be used in these patients. In contrast, patients with less extensive aneurysms such as type IV TAAAs might be better served to undergo repair at a diameter of 5.5 cm. Although patients with symptoms should undergo TAAA repair even if their aneurysm has not attained a certain diameter threshold, the threshold for repair should be tailored to the individual surgeon and institutional results.

■ PREOPERATIVE EVALUATION

The physiologic stress on a patient undergoing open TAAA repair is unparalleled, and it is to be emphasized that the preoperative evaluation detailed herein will probably differ substantially as a function of the mode of operative repair. The initial evaluation of a patient with a TAAA begins with a thorough history and physical examination focusing on the patient's cardiac, pulmonary, and renal function. Imaging studies are reviewed to determine the operative plan. Standard preoperative laboratory testing, electrocardiography, and chest radiography should be performed.

Cardiac

Because the typical patient undergoing TAAA repair is elderly, impaired myocardial function and the presence of atherosclerotic disease of the coronary arteries are common in patients undergoing aneurysm repair.[134,135] In landmark studies in patients before undergoing AAA repair, Hertzer and colleagues documented that 42% had significant coronary artery disease in the setting of ischemic cardiac symptoms. Importantly, 19% of the patients who were symptom free also had significant coronary artery disease. Given the high prevalence of coronary disease combined with the stress of this operation, cardiac disease is the leading cause of mortality after open TAAA repair.[84,86] Cardiac disease has been reported to be responsible for 49% of early deaths, as well as a third of late deaths after TAAA repair. Therefore, before TAAA repair, all patients should undergo extensive evaluation of their coronary arteries and heart valves. The introduction of endovascular TAAA repair may have an impact on the extensive and invasive nature of this evaluation, but to date data are lacking.

The preoperative electrocardiogram in a hypertensive patient with a degenerative TAAA may suggest left ventricular hypertrophy. There may also be evidence of ischemic heart disease. Although noninvasive stress testing can often predict areas of reversible ischemia and may be useful in an asymptomatic patient, the use of coronary angiography in patients with suspected atherosclerotic coronary disease (e.g., angina, low ejection fraction, previous coronary artery bypass grafting [CABG]) may be indicated (see Chapter 38: Systemic Complications: Cardiac).

In the elective setting, coronary artery revascularization, either by coronary angioplasty/stenting or by CABG, may be indicated. Details about the specifics of coronary revascularization are important. For example, if the patient is to undergo coronary stenting, clopidogrel is used for a minimum of 6 weeks, which will delay TAAA repair. Avoidance of drug-eluting coronary stents, with their attendant lifelong indication for clopidogrel, is also not indicated. In addition, if the patient is to undergo CABG, use of the left internal mammary artery is discouraged, primarily because it serves as an important collateral to the spinal cord, as well as the chest wall.

Echocardiography, most often transesophageal echocardiography (TEE), is helpful in demonstrating left ventricular function and concomitant valvular abnormalities. TEE is also useful in evaluating the ascending and descending thoracic aorta. There are many advantages to TEE over other modalities, including the ability to perform it in the emergency room or operating room. It can also be safely used in patients with renal insufficiency to assess ascending and descending thoracic aortic size, as well as the presence of dissection. However, TEE may not be widely available in the emergency setting and is operator dependent.

Pulmonary

Pulmonary complications after open TAAA repair are common, with the incidence of COPD estimated to be between 30% and 40%. COPD is also associated with increased perioperative mortality after TAAA repair.[84,136] Pulmonary function tests and arterial blood gas analysis are performed routinely. Preoperative maneuvers to improve pulmonary function before TAAA repair include immediate cessation of smoking, use of appropriate bronchodilators, and rarely the administration of preoperative steroids when an acute exacerbation of reactive airway disease occurs (see Chapter 39: Systemic Complications: Respiratory). Patients can also be placed on an exercise program to improve lung capacity and lose weight if obesity accompanies their lung disease. In a study of patients with COPD undergoing elective open AAA repair, fewer prescribed inhalers, lower hematocrit, renal insufficiency, and coronary artery disease were associated with unfavorable outcomes.[137] Preservation of the left recurrent laryngeal and phrenic nerves is an important adjunct to decrease the incidence of pulmonary complications in these patients.

Renal

Much has been written about the impact of renal failure on the outcome of patients undergoing TAAA repair. A large series of patients undergoing open TAAA repair suggested that the rate of renal failure postoperatively ranges from 5% to 40%, with an attendant mortality rate as high as 70%.[138-141] Acute renal failure also predicts increased nonrenal complications postoperatively, including respiratory failure. Second only to aortic rupture, chronic renal insufficiency is the strongest predictor of perioperative acute renal failure and mortality after TAAA repair (Fig. 131-13).[142,143] Therefore, evaluation of renal function before TAAA repair, whether open or endovascular, is imperative.[142] A full 15% of patients with TAAAs will have some degree of chronic renal insufficiency, as defined by a creatinine level of 1.8 mg/dL (159 μmol/L) or greater.[44] Preoperative renal insufficiency is such a strong predictor of poor outcome after type II to type V TAAA repair that it has been suggested to be a relative contraindication to proceed with repair. Renal function is routinely assessed with standard

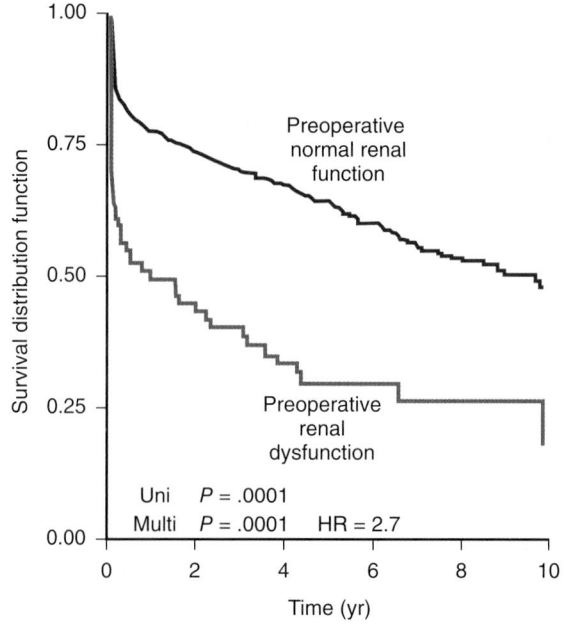

Figure 131-13 Ten-year actuarial survival for patients with and without preoperative renal failure. HR, hazard ratio.

laboratory tests, including blood urea nitrogen and creatinine. Huynh and coworkers documented that calculation of the glomerular filtration rate is a superior predictor of outcome than calculation of creatinine after TAAA repair.[144] Cross-sectional imaging will aid the surgeon in evaluating kidney size and the often associated renovascular atherosclerotic disease. If physiologic testing is required, duplex ultrasonography will provide information regarding the severity of ostial atherosclerotic disease, based on velocities, as well as parenchymal function, based on resistive indices. When performing TAAA repair in renal failure patients, it is imperative that severe renal artery occlusive disease be treated intraoperatively by endarterectomy, stenting, or bypass grafting with the expectation that renal function will not worsen.[145,146] Stenting before TAAA repair to theoretically improve renal function has been reported.[147]

Preoperative intravenous hydration, as well as avoidance of nephrotoxic agents such as iodinated contrast material, is indicated. Although national trends have moved away from admitting patients preoperatively to the hospital, this group of patients, especially if their visceral arteries are to be bypassed, should probably still be admitted to the hospital and undergo both bowel preparation and intravenous hydration. The rationale has to do with attempting to decrease the risk for bacterial translocation, especially in the setting of visceral ischemia during placement of a synthetic graft at the time of TAAA repair.[148]

Functional Status

All surgeons know that the preoperative functional status of patients undergoing TAAA is critical, even though few objective studies in patients with TAAA have examined this subject in detail. Hua and coworkers, using the National Surgical Quality Improvement Program database in patients undergoing AAA repair, suggested that "poor functional status" predicted mortality.[149] Although TAAA repair has been shown to improve survival, a recent report by Zierer and coauthors examined the late functional status and quality of life of asymptomatic patients undergoing elective repair.[150] Over a 5-year period, 110 asymptomatic patients underwent elective thoracic aortic replacement for ascending, descending, or thoracoabdominal aneurysms. Functional status, physical and psychological quality of life (Medical Outcome Study 36-Item Short Form Health Survey, in which 50 represents the normalized age-matched U.S. population), and survival (Kaplan-Meier) were assessed. The results documented that return to normal activity levels was independent of age and procedure. At a mean of 35 months, psychological quality of life was similar between the various surgical groups, but physical quality of life was lower after thoracoabdominal than after ascending or descending aneurysm repair ($P < .02$). Importantly, age did not affect physical quality of life, and interestingly, older patients had improved psychological quality of life. The overall survival rate was 70% at 4 years, but once again it was lower for thoracoabdominal than for ascending or descending aneurysms ($P < .002$). The authors suggested

that advanced age does not impair return to normal functional status and that patients with asymptomatic thoracic aneurysms thus should not be denied elective replacement based on age alone because functional recovery is not significantly impaired.[150]

Addressing quality of life issues between open aortic repair and TEVAR, Dick and associates performed a post hoc analysis of a prospectively collected consecutive series of 136 patients with surgical diseases of the descending aorta between January 2001 and December 2005. Endpoints included perioperative and late mortality rates, as well as long-term quality of life as assessed by the Short Form Health Survey and Hospital Anxiety and Depression Score questionnaires. The study documented no differences in perioperative mortality rates (9% for open repair versus 8% for TEVAR, $P = .254$). Cumulative long-term mortality rates were similar in both cohorts. Overall quality of life scores were 93 (63 to 110) for open repair and 83 (60 to 112) for TEVAR and were not significantly different. Anxiety and depression scores were not increased after open surgery. The authors suggested that both TEVAR and open aortic repair provide excellent long-term results in the treatment of thoracic aortic disease and thus provide little aid in helping us council patients on which type of repair they should seek.[151]

Although most of these studies have focused on perioperative functional status, Rigberg and colleagues documented that late (1-year) survival was poor after TAAA repair and decreased with patient age.[152] Another study by Crawford and coworkers also investigated late (5-year) functional status after TAA repair. These authors concluded that permanent loss of functional capacity occurs only rarely in survivors of TAA repair but noted the difficulty in obtaining appropriate controls for studies such as this.[153]

OPEN VERSUS ENDOVASCULAR REPAIR FOR THORACOABDOMINAL AORTIC ANEURYSMS

Until recently, surgical therapy for elective TAAAs involved major surgery with a significant risk for perioperative mortality and morbidity. Centers of excellence in this procedure report elective mortality and paraplegia rates of 4.8% and 4.6%, respectively.[131] Mortality rates after surgical treatment of ruptured TAAA is extremely high, even though rates of 26% have been reported.[154] In contrast, national mortality rates before the introduction of endovascular technology were 22%.[8] Surviving patients experience many postoperative complications and have lengthy hospital stays. Given the continued high mortality and morbidity in contemporary surgical practice, it is not surprising that new techniques for repair were developed. Data suggest that TEVAR of isolated descending TAAs is a safe alternative to open surgery and is associated with lower mortality and morbidity.[16,155] However, it is important to recognize that long-term results are not yet available.

The decision regarding which therapy is appropriate for a particular patient is an evolving aspect of care of these complicated patients. There are few guidelines on indications for TEVAR versus open TAAA repair as determined in a prospective randomized comparison. However, three industry-sponsored comparative trials are now available. Examination of a few specific population-based rather than single-center studies comparing open and endovascular therapy for TAAs is warranted.

Endovascular Graft Trials

Although all of the device-specific trials are prospective, these trials are not randomized. They also suffer from primary use of historical control patients undergoing open TAA repair. In addition, they were not designed to help us determine which patients are best served by stent-grafting versus open repair and do not include patients with visceral or renal artery involvement. Clearly, this is an evolving field, with branched and fenestrated endografts perhaps being available in the near future. In addition, the hybrid procedure to treat TAAAs is believed by some to be preferable to open repair for Crawford types I to III TAAAs.[156]

Gore TAG Trial

Bavaria's group documented follow-up on the initial multicenter trial involving 140 patients with stent-grafts (Gore TAG Thoracic Endograft, Flagstaff, AZ) versus an open surgical cohort of 94 patients, which included historical and concurrent open controls.[16] Perioperative mortality was significantly lower in the endograft (TEVAR) group than in open surgical controls (2.1% for TEVAR versus 11.7% for open repair, $P < .001$). Perioperative complication rates and intensive care unit and hospital length of stay were also significantly reduced in the TEVAR group. The incidence of endoleaks at 2 years was 9% in the TEVAR group, with three interventions performed in the endograft cohort. At 2 years, Kaplan-Meier analysis revealed no difference in overall mortality.[24]

Cook TX2 Trial

This study compared 160 patients undergoing TEVAR with the Zenith TX2 Endovascular Graft (William Cook Europe, ApS, Bjaeverskov, Denmark) with 70 patients undergoing open TAA repair.[25] The 30-day survival rate was better for the TEVAR group than for the open group (98.1% versus 94.3%, $P < .01$). The TEVAR group also had fewer cardiovascular, pulmonary, and vascular adverse events, although neurologic events were not significantly different. No ruptures or conversions occurred in the first year in the TEVAR group, and re-intervention rates were similar in both groups. At 12 months, aneurysm growth was identified in 7.1% (8/112) of patients (3.9% endoleak rate). The authors concluded that TEVAR with the TX2 endograft is a safe, effective alternative to open surgical repair for the treatment of anatomically suitable descending TAAs at 1 year of follow-up.

Medtronic VALOR Trial

This report summarized the 30-day and 12-month results of endovascular treatment with the Medtronic Vascular Talent Thoracic Stent-Graft System (Medtronic Vascular, Santa Rosa, CA) for patients with TAAs who were also candidates for open repair.[26] Similar to the TAG trial, the study was a prospective, nonrandomized, multicenter trial. TEVAR results were compared with those of a retrospective open surgical cohort from three centers of excellence. In this trial, 195 patients underwent TEVAR and 189 underwent open TAA repair. The 30-day TEVAR group had a perioperative mortality rate of 2.1%. Major adverse advents occurred in 41% of the stent-graft group, including paraplegia in 1.5%, paraparesis in 7.2%, and stroke in 3.6%. At 12 months the TEVAR group had an all-cause mortality rate of 16.1% and an aneurysm-related mortality rate of 3.1%. The Talent Thoracic Stent-Graft System showed statistically superior performance with respect to acute procedural outcomes ($P < .001$), 30-day major adverse events (41% versus 84%, $P < .001$), perioperative mortality (2% versus 8%, $P < .01$), and 12-month aneurysm-related mortality (3.1% versus 12%, $P < .002$) when compared with open TAA repair. The authors concluded by suggesting that the Talent Thoracic Stent-Graft System is a safe and effective endovascular therapeutic alternative to open surgery in patients with TAAs.

Long-term Results

Long-term follow-up data from the preclinical Gore TAG trial were recently published. Makaroun and coauthors reported 5-year follow-up with the Gore TAG device in treating degenerative TAAAs and documented no difference in all-cause mortality between endovascular and open TAAA repair at 5 years (67% versus 68%).[157] Major adverse events at 5 years were significantly reduced in the TEVAR group (57.9% versus 78.7%, $P = .001$). Endoleaks in the TAG group decreased from 8.1% at 1 month to 4.3% at 5 years. Five TAG patients have undergone major aneurysm-related re-interventions at 5 years (3.6%), including one arch aneurysm repair for a type 1 endoleak and migration, one open conversion, and five endovascular procedures for endoleaks in three patients. For the TEVAR patients, sac size at 60 months decreased in 50% and increased in 19% with respect to the 1-month baseline. At 5 years there have been no ruptures, one migration, no collapses, and 20 instances of stent fracture in 19 patients, all before revision of the TAG graft. Although the authors acknowledged that the rates of secondary intervention were much higher in the stent-graft group, they concluded that stent-graft repair of TAAA was superior to open repair at 5 years. It is important to note that even though this study is prospective, it was not randomized. In addition, it was not designed to help us determine which patients are best served by stenting versus open repair.

A meta-analysis reviewing open TAAA repair and stent-grafting by Walsh and colleagues included 17 eligible studies totaling 1109 patients and demonstrated that stenting was associated with a significant reduction in mortality (pooled odds ratio, 0.36; $P < .0001$) and major neurologic injury (pooled odds ratio, 0.39; $P < .0001$), with no difference in the major re-intervention rate after elective TAAA repair. Importantly, there was no effect on mortality in patients with thoracic aortic trauma or rupture. The authors concluded by suggesting that endovascular TAAA repair reduces perioperative mortality and neurologic complications in patients undergoing elective TAAA repair, although they did suggest that there may be less benefit in other thoracic aortic conditions.[158]

Decision Making

Current Status

A recent report from the Society of Thoracic Surgeons Endovascular Surgery Task Force is useful in trying to determine which patients should undergo open TAAA repair versus endovascular stent-grafting.[159] The panel acknowledged that diseases of the thoracic aorta are increasingly being treated by stent-grafts. However, no prospective randomized trials comparing the two types of repair for the same type of pathology have been performed. At present in the United States there are three FDA-approved endografts for the treatment of degenerative TAAAs. First-generation stent-grafts suffered a number of graft-related complications (stent fractures, graft collapse, etc.), as well as complications from the introduction of new technology (increased stroke risk, ascending aortic dissections, etc.). It should be recognized that thoracic stent-grafting is relatively new with little long-term follow-up. The long-term consequences of repeated radiation exposure as a result of serial CT scanning is also unknown. In general, although TAAA is a serious disease, it is also relatively indolent. The authors concluded by emphatically stating that identification of small TAAAs does not justify the use of endovascular stent-grafting because the rates of rupture, dissection, and death with TAAAs less than 5 cm are relatively low.

Contemporary results of open surgical repair of TAAAs are primarily generated at institutions with great expertise in this area. There is little doubt that TAAA repair, despite the disease itself being relatively rare, is one of the few operations where surgeon and hospital volume influence mortality.[8,9] Based on 1898 cases, a mortality rate of 4.8% can be attained after open TAAA repair in centers of excellence,[159] as opposed to a national mortality rate of greater than 20% from administrative data.[8] In addition, the risk for paralysis and stroke is 3.4% and 2.7%, respectively, after open TAAA repair in centers of excellence. Five- and 10-year survival rates are 60% and 38%, respectively.[159]

With the technology presently available, few would argue for treating all thoracic aortic pathology by stent-grafting alone or some combination of stent-grafting and extra-anatomic bypasses to the exclusion of open TAAA repair. Indications for endovascular intervention are not clearly defined at present and instead are based on reports of open TAAA repair from institutions with great expertise. Long-term results after endografting are not yet generally available, with the first 5-year follow-up report of the only FDA-approved endograft

just recently published.[157] Mortality rates after endovascular TAAA repair vary widely between 2% and 26%, depending largely on the nature of the indication for the operation (elective versus urgent versus emergency), patient co-morbid conditions, and the experience of the endovascular specialist.[159] Midterm results suggested that moderate-term survival rates (3 to 8 years) also varied greatly between 25% and 90%. Although there should clearly be enthusiasm for the use of endovascular therapies to treat many thoracic aortic pathologies, it should be recognized that late complications, such as endoleaks, stent fractures, and stent migration, are more common after endovascular TAAA repair than after open repair. The issue of increased cost (initial cost of the stent-grafts, multiple CT scans in follow-up, secondary procedures, etc.) associated with endografting will also need to be figured into the equation when considering which therapy is correct for a particular patient. Importantly, it is also not clear at present whether a more aggressive endovascular approach will affect long-term survival or freedom from aortic complications when compared with open surgical therapy.

Subpopulations Benefiting from Thoracic Endovascular Aortic Repair

There are clear subpopulations of patients best served by TEVAR. It is reasonable to conclude that patients older than 75 years, if anatomically suitable, should be directed toward stent-grafting.[8] The subset of patients with significant COPD is also likely to benefit from stent-grafting when possible to avoid the attendant risks incurred from a thoracotomy. Patients with increasing pain or with ruptured TAAAs should also be considered for TEVAR, which can often be performed more expeditiously than open repair if the anatomy is appropriate for an endovascular approach. Clearly, future studies will help us better discern which subpopulations are best served by stent-grafting for TAAA.

Current Indications for Thoracic Endovascular Aortic Repair

At present, outside of off-label use of thoracic and abdominal stent-grafts or investigational device exemptions, indications for TEVAR are only for degenerative TAAAs with adequate proximal and distal aortic landing zones. Fenestrated and multibranched endografts, which are widely available in Europe and Australia, may in the future ultimately make the hybrid procedure that is performed in the United States today mostly obsolete. As with the evolution of many new technologies, the indication for stent-grafting is based on a lower short-term mortality rate in comparison to open TAAA repair or medical therapy, not necessarily on long-term outcomes. New less invasive therapies such as TEVAR often need to document only clinical equipoise to gain market share. Regardless, the physician caring for a patient with a TAAA should consider a constellation of issues, including age, co-morbid diseases, symptoms, life expectancy, quality of life, aortic diameter, aneurysm morphology and extent, suitability of a landing zone for a stent-graft, cost of therapies, and

THORACIC ENDOVASCULAR AORTIC REPAIR VERSUS OBSERVATION

The issue whether to offer patients with TAAAs endovascular repair when they are not candidates for open repair because of excessive co-morbid conditions has not been addressed in a prospective randomized fashion. In patients with infrarenal AAAs, the EVAR-2 trial suggested that such patients did not benefit in terms of survival when randomized to endovascular repair versus observation, although this was related to the rather high (9%) operative mortality associated with stent-graft repair in this study.[160] Patel and colleagues examined this issue in 46 asymptomatic patients with descending thoracic aortic disease who were considered high risk for open surgery for reasons of age 80 years or older (47.8%) or co-morbid conditions (84.8%). Twenty-one patients underwent TEVAR, whereas another 25 either were excluded from TEVAR on the basis of unfavorable anatomy or refused intervention. All-cause mortality in the entire cohort was 50%. Yet the median actual time to mortality was different between the two groups (control, 9.2 months; TEVAR, 24.9 months; *P* = .01). Life-table analysis demonstrated improved survival with TEVAR at 24 months (*P* = .05) (Fig. 131-14).[161]

In a study by Rosselli and associates, patients with thoracoabdominal aneurysms considered "high risk" for conventional surgery were enrolled in a prospective trial to evaluate a novel endovascular grafting system. Devices were custom-designed for each patient with the use of high-resolution CT. Although there was no control group, the authors treated 73 patients by endovascular repair for type I, II, or III (n = 28) or for type IV (n = 45) TAAAs. Technical success was achieved in 93% of patients (68/73), and the 30-day mortality rate was 5.4% (4/73). Major perioperative complications occurred in 11 (15%) patients, including paraplegia (2.7%, 2/73), new onset of dialysis (1.4%, 1/73), prolonged ventilator support (6.8%, 5/73), myocardial infarction (5.4%, 4/73), and minor hemorrhagic stroke (1.4%; 1/72). The authors concluded that endovascular repair of aortic aneurysms involving the visceral segment in nonsurgical high-risk candidates is feasible with acceptable morbidity and mortality rates. They also suggested that assessment of durability will require longer follow-up.[27]

SELECTED KEY REFERENCES

Barbour JR, Spinale FG, Ikonomidis JS. Proteinase systems and thoracic aortic aneurysm progression. *J Surg Res.* 2007;139:292-307.
Excellent review on the current state of our understanding of the pathogenesis of TAAAs that primarily focuses on the enzymes involved in remodeling of the aorta during aneurysm formation.

Cowan JA Jr, Dimick JB, Henke PK, Huber TS, Stanley JC, Upchurch Jr GR. Surgical treatment of intact thoracoabdominal aortic aneurysms in the United States: hospital and surgeon volume-related outcomes. *J Vasc Surg.* 2003;37:1169-1174.
Large administrative database examination of elective open thoracoabdominal aortic aneurysm repair in the United States documenting a staggering mortality rate of 22% after repair.

Dake MD, Miller DC, Semba CP, Mitchell RS, Walker PJ, Liddell RP. Transluminal placement of endovascular stent-grafts for the treatment of descending thoracic aortic aneurysms. *N Engl J Med.* 1994; 331:1729-1734.
One of first and largest experiences to date using endovascular stent-grafting to treat thoracic aortic aneurysms.

Makaroun MS, Dillavou ED, Kee ST, Sicard G, Chaikof E, Bavaria J, Williams D, Cambria RP, Mitchell RS. Endovascular treatment of thoracic aortic aneurysms: results of the phase II multicenter trial of the GORE TAG thoracic endoprosthesis. *J Vasc Surg.* 2005;41: 1-9.
Report on the Gore TAG endovascular graft that led to its FDA approval in the United States.

McNamara JJ, Pressler VM. Natural history of arteriosclerotic thoracic aortic aneurysms. *Ann Thorac Surg.* 1978;26:468-473.
One of earliest descriptions of the natural history of thoracic aortic aneurysms.

Roselli EE, Greenberg RK, Pfaff K, Francis C, Svensson LG, Lytle BW. Endovascular treatment of thoracoabdominal aortic aneurysms. *J Thorac Cardiovasc Surg.* 2007;133:1474-1482.
Largest experience in the United States with fenestrated and multibranched endografts for TAAAs.

Svensson LG, Crawford ES, Hess KR, Coselli JS, Safi HJ. Experience with 1509 patients undergoing thoracoabdominal aortic operations. *J Vasc Surg.* 1993;17:357-370.
Despite being 15 years old, this report from Dr. Crawford's massive experience with open TAAA repair describes many of the adjuncts and approaches used in modern TAAA repair.

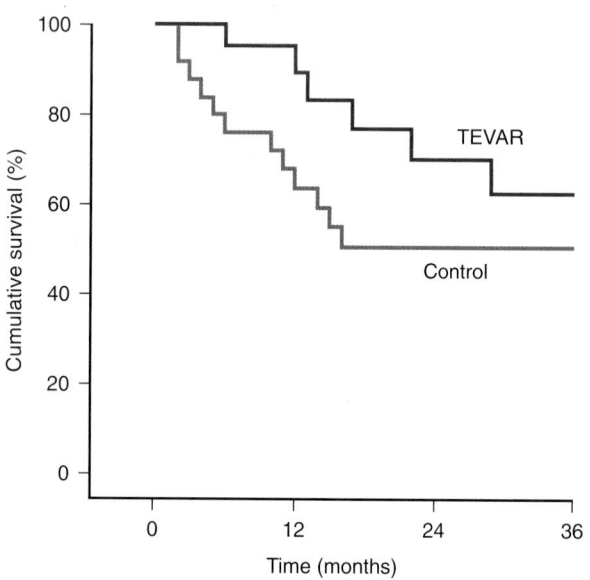

Figure 131-14 Life-table analysis demonstrating that elective thoracic endovascular aorta repair (TEVAR) results in an early-term to intermediate-term survival advantage for high-risk asymptomatic patients with thoracic aortic disease. Note that the 1- and 2-year life-table survival rate for TEVAR is 95% and 70%, respectively; in contrast, the 1- and 2-year life-table survival rates for the control arm are 68% (*P* = .03) and 51% (*P* = .05), respectively. (*Used with permission from Patel HJ, Shillingford MS, Williams DM, et al. Survival benefit of endovascular descending thoracic aortic repair for the high-risk patient.* Ann Thorac Surg. *2007;83:1628-1633; discussion 1633-1624.*)

REFERENCES

The reference list can be found on the companion Expert Consult Web site at *www.expertconsult.com.*

CHAPTER 132

Thoracic and Thoracoabdominal Aneurysms: Open Surgical Treatment

Michael J. Jacobs and Geert Willem Schurink

Based in part on a chapter in the previous edition by Hazim J. Safi, MD; Tam T. Huynh, MD; Anthony L. Estrera, MD; and Charles C. Miller III, PhD.

The first successful end-to-end anastomosis of the thoracic aorta after resection of an aortic coarctation was performed in Sweden.[1] Open repair of a luetic descending thoracic aortic aneurysm (DTAA) with a homograft was first reported by Lam and Aram in 1951.[2] In the first thoracoabdominal aortic aneurysm (TAAA) repair by Etheredge and colleagues in 1954, a temporary shunt was used from the distal thoracic aorta to the distal abdominal aorta.[3] A homograft was inserted and the visceral vessels were implanted in the homograft. Shumacker modified this technique by using the homograft as the permanent bypass, implanting the visceral vessels in the homograft, and subsequently excising the aneurysm.[4] DeBakey and associates developed the polyester tube graft for placement in the descending thoracic aorta, sutured the Dacron graft to the aorta proximal and distal to the aneurysm, and bypassed all visceral arteries one after another.[5] In 1974, Crawford improved the technique for TAAA repair by introducing the principle of the inclusion technique, wherein aortic branches are reconstructed from within the aneurysm via excised patches in the main aortic graft.[6] Furthermore, he started the technique of reattachment of the intercostal arteries into the graft to prevent paraplegia.

Aortic cross-clamp time was the most important predictor of end-organ damage and postoperative paraplegia during DTAA and TAAA repairs. Several adjuncts have since been developed to allow a longer cross-clamp time and improve outcome, including profound hypothermia, neuroprotective medication, epidural cooling, and drainage of cerebrospinal fluid (CSF). Various techniques of distal aortic perfusion further improved the mortality and morbidity after DTAA and TAAA repair. Complications after TAAA repair significantly depend on the extent of the aneurysm. The classification of thoracoabdominal aneurysms by Crawford enables us to adjust the operative strategy according to the various risks for complications (Fig. 132-1).[7] Reconstructive techniques for DTAA and TAAA remain in evolution with the advent of endovascular stent-graft repair in the thoracic aorta, as reviewed in Chapter 133 (Thoracic and Thoracoabdominal Aneurysms: Endovascular Treatment); this evolution is likely to proceed over the next decade or longer. Thus, open surgical repair remains either the best or only option for many patients. In addition, there is little consensus on the application of operative adjuncts, including variations on extracorporeal circulation, spinal cord protection, and renal/visceral perfusates.

INDICATIONS AND CONTRAINDICATIONS

The objective of surgical treatment of DTAA and TAAA is to prevent death from rupture. Natural history data and

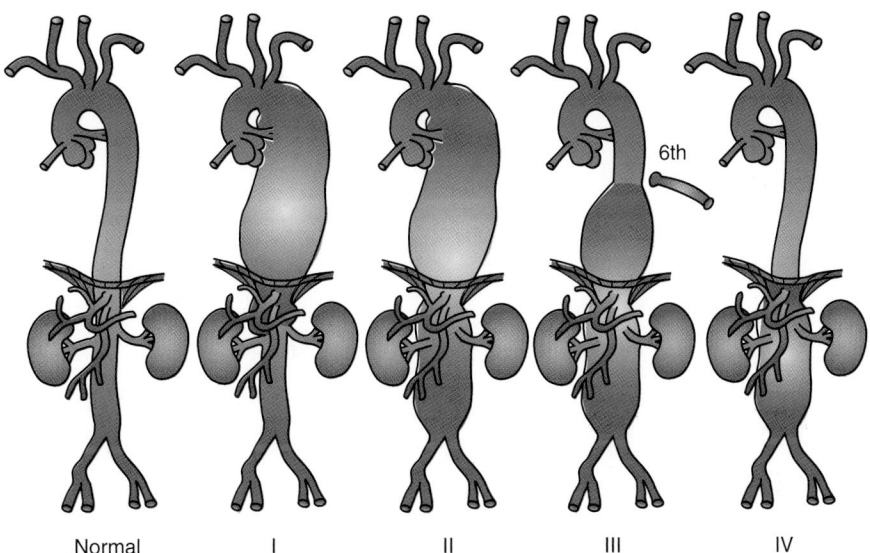

Figure 132-1 Normal thoracoabdominal aorta and aneurysm classification. Type I, distal to the left subclavian artery to above the renal arteries. Type II, distal to the left subclavian artery to below the renal arteries. Type III, from the sixth intercostal space (or variable lengths of the descending aorta) to below the renal arteries. Type IV, from the 12th intercostal space to the iliac bifurcation (total abdominal aortic aneurysm).

Normal   I   II   III   IV

clinical decision making for these lesions are reviewed in Chapter 131 (Thoracic and Thoracoabdominal Aneurysms: Evaluation and Decision Making). Symptoms such as recent chest or back pain in the presence of a thoracic aneurysm have always been considered an indication for surgery because of imminent rupture. However, vague and uncharacteristic pain is also significantly associated with subsequent rupture (odds ratio, 2.3).[8] Furthermore, unlike the more common abdominal aortic aneurysm (AAA), these lesions can produce a chronic pain syndrome, characteristically to the left of the spine and particularly in the circumstance of a very large aneurysm in the region of the hiatus. Uncommon symptoms, such as dyspnea secondary to tracheal or left mainstem bronchial compression between the aneurysm and vertebral spine[9] or dysphagia secondary to esophageal compression at the level of the diaphragm,[10] are indications for treatment. Unlike the case of endovascular treatment, the direct reduction in diameter of the aneurysm after open repair will lead to relief of symptoms. In addition, erosion of the esophagus because of aneurysmal pressure can occur.[11] Perhaps as a result of the major operative insult involved and the reluctance of patients and their physicians to undergo elective surgery, in a significant number of patients surgery is undertaken in something other than elective circumstances, which in turn is associated with increased perioperative risk.

Degenerative Aneurysm

Indications for Repair

Most patients with a DTAA or TAAA are asymptomatic. In this patient group the decision to perform open repair is generally based on the size, extent, and expansion rate of the aneurysm.

For patients with degenerative aneurysms, elective treatment is usually advised if the patient is a suitable candidate and the diameter exceeds 6 cm.[12-14] In contrast to the extensive data on the natural history of AAAs, information on thoracic and thoracoabdominal aneurysms is more scarce and is summarized in Chapter 131 (Thoracic and Thoracoabdominal Aneurysms: Evaluation and Decision Making). The groups of Griepp and Elefteriades performed extensive research on the natural history of thoracic aneurysms.[8,15-20] These natural history studies indicate that beside diameter[18,21-24] and pain,[23] age,[23] the presence of chronic obstructive pulmonary disease (COPD)[8,25] or renal insufficiency,[24,26,27] the extent of the aneurysm,[18,21,24] and the expansion rate of the aneurysm[21,28] are independent risk factors for rupture. Hirose and coworkers found that the average growth rate of DTAAs (0.42 cm/yr) is greater than that of AAAs (0.28 cm/yr).[29] Efforts have been made to put several of these risk factors into a formula to calculate the annual risk for rupture of each individual patient.[8] In daily practice, we use 6 cm as a threshold diameter for the treatment of degenerative DTAA and TAAA. The presence of risk factors for rupture can influence the individual indication for surgery, and certain variables such as the presence of

COPD will also increase the perioperative risk associated with open surgery.

Contraindications

Contraindications to open repair of DTAA or TAAA are mainly determined by operative risk factors such as age, impaired cardiac and pulmonary function, poor functional status, and renal insufficiency. Anatomic considerations such as previous thoracotomy and an abdominal stoma can present prohibitive operative risk; in contemporary practice such features will also influence the choice between open and endovascular surgery (also see Chapter 131: Thoracic and Thoracoabdominal Aneurysms: Evaluation and Decision Making). Anatomic complexity in the form of previous aortic grafting procedures is commonly encountered in patients with thoracic and thoracoabdominal aneurysms. Up to 36% of patients have previously undergone aortic surgery, with abdominal aortic grafts used in 59%, thoracic grafts in 17%, and thoracoabdominal grafts in 21%.[30,31]

Connective Tissue–Related Aneurysm

Aneurysms secondary to inherited connective tissue diseases (CTDs) are discussed extensively in Chapter 140 (Aneurysms Caused by Connective Tissue Abnormalities). Marfan's syndrome and type IV Ehlers-Danlos syndrome are the most significant disorders causing aneurysmal dilatation of the thoracic aorta. In patients with Ehlers-Danlos syndrome, dissection or aneurysms can develop in almost every major artery, including the thoracic and thoracoabdominal aorta. Marfan's syndrome typically causes aortic root dilatation, aortic valve insufficiency, and dissection. The majority of patients with Marfan's syndrome have their first operation on the ascending thoracic aorta (83%).[32] Repetitive surgery is common. DTAAs or TAAAs were the primary site of repair in 14% of cases and the second site of repair in 64%. Risk factors for repeated surgery were the presence of acute or chronic dissection at the time of the initial operation, hypertension after the first operation, and a history of smoking.[32] Patients with Marfan's syndrome are significantly younger than those with degenerative aneurysms.[13,17,33,34] The physical condition of the younger patients with Marfan's syndrome is much better that in the group without this syndrome.[33] Because of the higher incidence of dissection and rupture of descending aortic aneurysms in patients with Marfan's syndrome, the recommended threshold for repair is an aneurysm diameter of 5.0 to 5.5 cm.[13,16]

Postdissection Aneurysm

Chronic type B dissection is the second most common cause of DTAA and TAAA formation. In patients undergoing surgery for TAAA, up to 24% suffer from chronic dissection,[31] whereas up to 39% of patients with DTAA have chronic dissection.[35] Of all patients with aortic dissection, 20% to 40% will require subsequent aortic replacement for aneurysmal degeneration irrespective of the initial medical or surgical treatment (see also Chapter 135: Aortic Dissection).[36] The presence of blood flow in the false lumen is the most significant risk factor for an increase in diameter, with a mean growth rate of 3.3 mm/yr versus 1.4-mm/yr shrinkage in diameter in patients with a thrombosed false lumen. The growth rate of thoracic aortic dissections was significantly faster than that of AAAs (4.1 and 1.2 mm/yr, respectively)[37]; these results are comparable to those of degenerative aneurysms reported by Hirose and Svensson.[38] There are conflicting reports regarding the role of dissection in the likelihood of aneurysm growth and rupture. The growth rate of postdissection aneurysms can be comparable to that of degenerative thoracic aneurysms[25] or faster.[16] Several authors report a higher rupture rate for postdissection aneurysms than for degenerative aneurysms.[8,21,23,39] Female gender and the presence of COPD are factors contributing to a significantly higher growth rate.[37] However, the diameter indication for asymptomatic postdissection DTAA or TAAA is the same as for degenerative aneurysms, except as noted earlier for patients with syndromic conditions such as Marfan's syndrome.

Miscellaneous Etiologies

Infection

Rare causes of thoracic or thoracoabdominal aneurysms are bacterial infections (mycotic aneurysms), which average just 1% to 2% in most major series. With regard to the aortic segment involved, repair by either in situ replacement or extra-anatomic reconstruction can be challenging. In situ replacement with appropriate antibiotic coverage has been reported to result in a survival rate of 86%.[40] Even when surgery has been successful, the prognosis is often very poor because of the weakened health status of the patient in whom this type of aneurysm has developed (see also Chapter 139: Infected Aneurysms).[41]

Vasculitis

Inflammatory diseases of the aortic wall, such as Behçet's disease[42-44] and Takayasu's arteritis,[44,45] can also lead to aneurysm formation (see also Chapter 76: Vasculitis and Other Arteriopathies and Chapter 78: Takayasu's Disease).

Penetrating Ulcers

Penetrating aortic ulcers (PAUs) are frequently observed in the descending thoracic aorta. They are often multiple and frequently accompanied by extensive atherosclerotic changes in the aortic wall. There is debate about whether PAUs should be treated by an aggressive surgical approach[46,47] as opposed to a conservative medical approach.[48] In these studies by Stanson and colleagues, Tittle and colleagues, and Cho and colleagues, late survival was comparable between those operated on and those treated medically, with only rupture at

initial evaluation and maximum aortic diameter, not the dimension of the PAU, being predictive of failure of medical treatment.[46-48] A number of clinical and anatomic variables will influence clinical decision making, as reviewed in Chapter 135 (Aortic Dissection). Such variables include overall aortic size (probably the most important factor) and the clinical circumstances (i.e., whether associated with an acute aortic syndrome). Because of its segmental nature, PAU is preferably treated with an endovascular stent-graft. In case of localization near the visceral and renal arteries, open repair is the treatment of choice.

False Aneurysm

False aneurysms in the thoracic aorta can be the result of previous aortic surgery or trauma. Anastomotic aneurysms can often be treated by endovascular means, provided that major aortic side branches are not involved (see also Chapter 43: Local Complications: Anastomotic Aneurysms). Without previous surgery, false aneurysms can be the result of a PAU or traumatic aortic injury. Kiefer and colleagues showed that low-risk patients with a chronic post-traumatic aneurysm of the aortic isthmus can be successfully treated with excellent long-term results by resection and direct aortoaortic anastomosis without prosthetic interposition.[49]

Endovascular Failure–Related Aneurysm

Failure of endovascular procedures in the thoracic and thoracoabdominal aorta is a new challenging entity in open aortic surgery. Most complications after endovascular stent-graft treatment can be repaired by additional endovascular procedures. However, in the case of type I endoleaks without an adequate additional landing zone for extra cuffs or in the case of retrograde type A dissections, conventional open repair can be the most appropriate treatment.[50] Progression of dilatation after endovascular treatment of postdissection aneurysms can be an indication for open aneurysm repair in a good-risk patient, especially if the visceral and renal arteries are involved in the aneurysm or potential landing zone. In these cases, type IV TAAA repair can be performed by using the distal end of the stent-graft as the site for the proximal anastomosis.

■ RELEVANT ANATOMY

Location and Extent of Aneurysm

Knowledge of the location and extent of thoracic and thoracoabdominal aneurysms is important for predicting patients' outcomes. For this reason, classification systems for DTAA and TAAA have been devised to enable the surgeon to tailor the extent of the incision and the use of various operative techniques and adjunctive measures to the individual patient. Furthermore, it allows more appropriate comparison of surgical outcomes of the different types of thoracoabdominal aneurysms treated with different surgical techniques and adjunctive measures.

Section **17** Arterial Aneurysms

Thoracoabdominal Aneurysm Classification

Crawford and Coselli proposed a classification of thoracoabdominal aneurysms that consists of four types.[51] A type I TAAA starts just distal to the left subclavian artery and includes the total descending thoracic aorta and the proximal abdominal aorta up to the level of the renal arteries. A type II TAAA includes the complete thoracoabdominal aorta from the level of the left subclavian artery to the aortic bifurcation. In many patients with postdissection aneurysms or Marfan's syndrome, the iliac arteries are also affected. A type III TAAA includes variable lengths of the more distal thoracic aorta and ends at the aortic bifurcation or lower. A type IV TAAA includes the total abdominal aorta starting at the level of the diaphragm (T12) to the aortic bifurcation or lower (see Fig. 132-1).

Descending Thoracic Aneurysm Classification

DTAA was classified to distinguish the risk of spinal cord ischemia's developing during open DTAA repair.[35] This classification consists of three types (Fig. 132-2). In type A the DTAA starts at the level of the left subclavian artery and ends at the level of T6. Type B starts at T6 and ends at the level of the diaphragm. Type C covers the total descending thoracic aorta.

Involvement of the Aortic Arch

It is not uncommon for DTAAs and TAAAs to involve, in particular, the distal aortic arch. In degenerative aneurysms the more proximal arch is not usually dilated. However, when the origin of the aneurysm is at the level of the left subclavian artery, cross-clamping proximal to the subclavian artery is often necessary. Girardi and coauthors reported cross-clamping between the left carotid and left subclavian arteries in 42% of their types I and II TAAAs.[52] Aneurysms that develop after previous repair of type A aortic dissection often include both the aortic arch and the thoracic or thoracoabdominal aorta (Fig. 132-3). In these cases, cross-

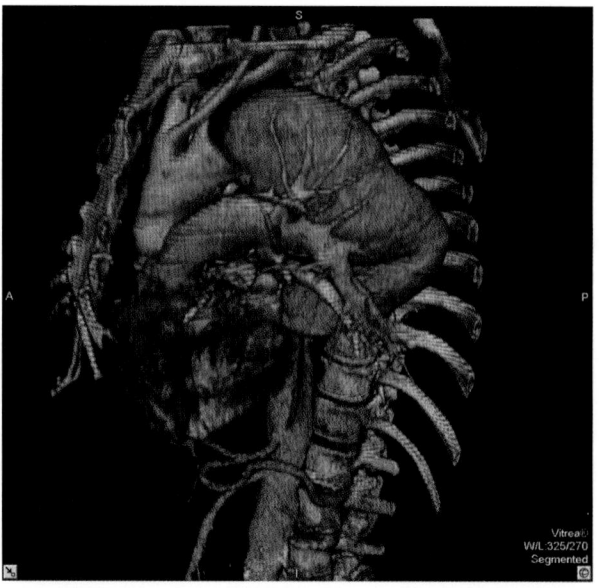

Figure 132-3 Reconstructed computed tomography scan showing a descending thoracic aortic aneurysm with involvement of a distal arch aneurysm, which would not allow proximal cross-clamping distal to the left subclavian artery.

clamping between the innominate artery and left carotid artery is sometimes required.[53] Cross-clamping in this position possibly compromises cerebral perfusion. If the extent of arch involvement is extreme, proximal clamp control may be hazardous or impossible, especially when graft replacement of the ascending arch or hemiarch has previously been performed. In such cases complete cardiopulmonary bypass with associated profound hypothermic circulatory arrest may be required. Although this technique is routine in a variety of ascending/arch operations (see Chapter 134: Aortic Arch Aneurysms and Dissection), it is associated with significant bleeding and pulmonary complication such that most authorities recommend this approach only when no other technical option to repair the aneurysm exists.[54,55] Issues related to cerebral neuromonitoring, brain protection, selective antegrade cerebral perfusion, and other nuances of profound

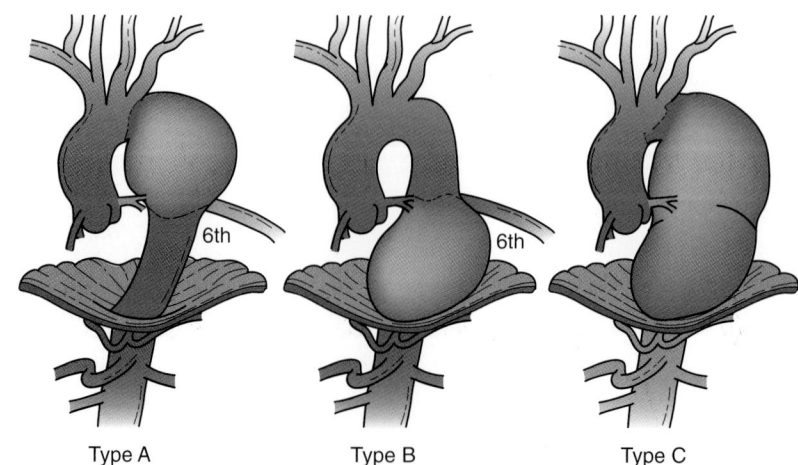

Figure 132-2 Classification of descending thoracic aortic aneurysms: type A, from the left subclavian artery to T6; type B, from T6 to the level of the diaphragm; type C, from the left subclavian artery to the level of the diaphragm. *(From Estrera AL, Miller CC 3rd, Chen EP, et al. Descending thoracic aortic aneurysm repair: 12-year experience using distal aortic perfusion and cerebrospinal fluid drainage. Ann Thorac Surg. 2005;80:1290-1296; discussion 1296.)*

Type A   Type B   Type C

hypothermia are discussed in Chapter 134 (Aortic Arch Aneurysms and Dissection).

Involvement of the Iliac Arteries

Types II, III, and IV thoracoabdominal aneurysms can either terminate at the aortic bifurcation or extend into the iliac arteries. Especially in cases of postdissection aneurysms, iliac involvement is common. However, minor to moderate degrees of iliac aneurysmal or occlusive disease (or both) are best ignored during TAAA resection because extending the operation into the pelvis considerably increases both operative time and complexity and can threaten the integrity of the hypogastric circulation. When distal aortic perfusion is maintained by cannulation of the femoral artery, the extent of the aneurysm into the iliac arteries often prohibits perfusion of both legs and results in prolonged contralateral leg ischemia. To prevent this complication, reconstruction can start with a bifurcated graft on both iliac arteries when temporary sequential infrarenal cross-clamping is possible. Instead of cannulating the femoral artery, the prosthetic graft can be used as arterial inflow for distal aortic perfusion.

■ OPERATIVE PLANNING

Anatomic Assessment

Computed Tomography

Computed tomography (CT) is the most widely used tool for assessment of the descending and thoracoabdominal aorta because it provides information to classify the aneurysm according to location, extent, and diameter (Fig. 132-4). It is a sensitive tool for follow-up of small aneurysms, for determination of the timing of elective surgery, and for postoperative follow-up studies.[20,29,56] In these studies CT is ideally used with intravenous contrast enhancement to image the aortic lumen and its side branches, as well as intraluminal thrombus, intramural hematomas, PAUs, dissection, and atherosclerotic wall changes.[57,58] The degree of mural thrombus (or the lack thereof) in the T8 to L1 region can provide the surgeon with a reasonable representation of whether there will be patent intercostal arteries to deal with intraoperatively. The introduction of spiral CT techniques and 64-slice CT has provided a major improvement in CT imaging quality in the form of better multiplanar reconstructions and maximum intensity projections. Such reconstructions improve assessment of aneurysm morphology, an essential prerequisite for operative planning (e.g., selection of sequential clamp sites when distal aortic perfusion is used). Contraindications to this technique include allergies to ionic contrast media and renal insufficiency. It is generally agreed that renal insufficiency and diabetes are risk factors for contrast-induced nephropathy, particularly when coexisting.[59] Patients whose renal insufficiency would not prohibit surgery can typically be studied with contrast-enhanced CT scanning safely (see also Chapter 21: Computed Tomography).

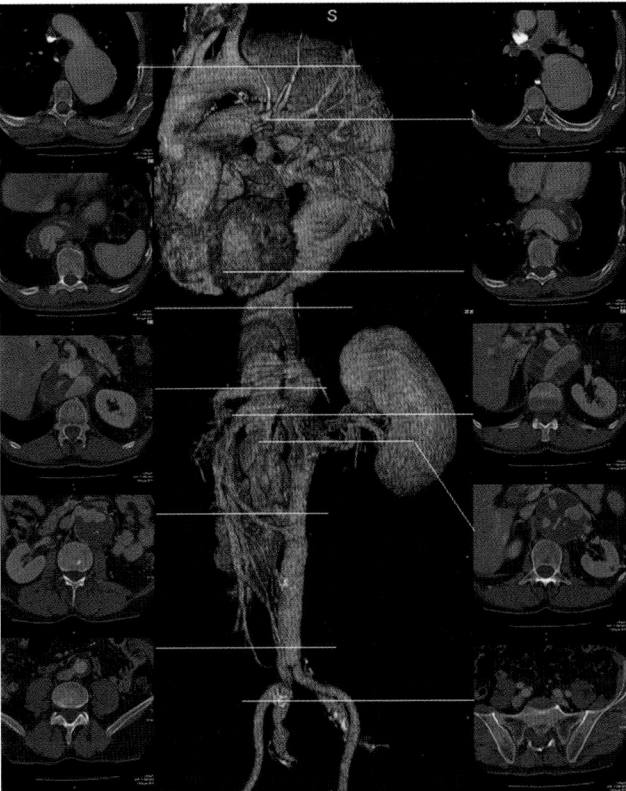

Figure 132-4 Preoperative CT scan showing a type II postdissection thoracoabdominal aortic aneurysm. The dissection starts just distal to the left subclavian artery. In the proximal descending thoracic aorta, both the true and false lumina are without thrombus. The anteriorly positioned true lumen provides blood to the celiac trunk, superior mesenteric artery, and right renal artery. The left renal artery arises from the false lumen, which is partly thrombosed and has multiple flow channels at the abdominal level.

Magnetic Resonance Imaging

Magnetic resonance imaging (MRI) can be used to image most aspects of the DTAA and TAAA, except for aortic wall calcifications.[60] MRI of the aortic wall itself is superior to CT if, for example, the goal is to detect acute inflammatory changes or hemorrhage. This technique can be used without contrast agents, but administration of contrast agents such as gadolinium will provide superb information about the aortic lumen and side branch involvement. The use of MRI will result in a major decrease in radiation exposure from repeated CT, which is especially important in young patients with dissection (e.g., in Marfan's syndrome[61]). The presence of pacemakers and artificial heart valves is a contraindication to the use of MRI. In addition, claustrophobia can be a problem with this imaging technique. Previously, contrast-enhanced MRI was often advised over CT angiography (CTA) in patients with renal insufficiency. However, reports of nephrogenic systemic fibrosis after MRI contrast agents have greatly curtailed their use.[62]

Arteriography

The use of aortography for assessment of aneurysm morphology is outdated in the present CT/MRI era. The absence of information about intraluminal thrombus and aortic wall pathology is the major disadvantage with this invasive procedure. Furthermore, allergies to contrast media and the potential for both renal insufficiency and atheroembolism advise against this technique, except in rare circumstances.

Spinal Cord Circulation

Preserving spinal cord circulation during DTAA and TAAA repair is of eminent importance. Normally, the anterior spinal artery is supplied by several anterior radiculomedullary arteries, which are abundant in the cervical and upper thoracic region, where branches of the vertebral artery contribute medullary components. However, the anterior spinal artery itself becomes narrower in caliber and even discontinuous in some individuals as it courses to the lower thoracolumbar cord. Accordingly, this region is a so-called watershed area, more prone to ischemic injury during thoracic aortic operations, and its circulation is often dependent on the largest extrinsic radiculomedullary artery, known as the artery of Adamkiewicz. In turn, this artery originates from arborizing branches of the posterior components of (often) multiple intercostals vessels, those on the left being more important.[63,64] The artery of Adamkiewicz itself arises in the T8-L2 region in some 72% of patients.[65] In patients with DTAA or TAAA, the segmental artery supplying the artery of Adamkiewicz can be occluded by intraluminal thrombus or atherosclerotic wall changes. Preoperative information about the location and patency of the feeding segmental artery can be important for operative planning and postoperative neurologic outcome. Digital subtraction angiography can be used to localize the artery of Adamkiewicz, but it can also cause iatrogenic paraplegia.[66] Even though advocated by a few groups, preoperative invasive angiography has been supplanted by axial imaging techniques. Both CTA and magnetic resonance angiography (MRA) have been used successfully to provide information about the artery of Adamkiewicz, as well as about the collateral circulation in the case of segmental artery occlusion (Fig. 132-5).[65,67-69] The importance of the lower lumbar and pelvic arteries has been recognized. Both were major contributors to the spinal cord circulation in 16% and 8% of cases, respectively.[70] In addition, the collateral circulation in most patients originated caudal to the distal clamp site (e.g., from the pelvic arteries), which can be perfused by means of extracorporeal circulation during cross-clamping.[71]

Co-morbidity Assessment

Open surgery for DTAA and TAAA, especially type II, poses a major risk for the patient. Because the most frequent complications include myocardial infarction, pulmonary insufficiency, renal failure, and stroke, evaluation of these organ systems is essential for preoperative risk assessment and reduction of risk.[7,13,31,35,72,73] In addition, age and aneurysm extent are important predictors of mortality after open repair.

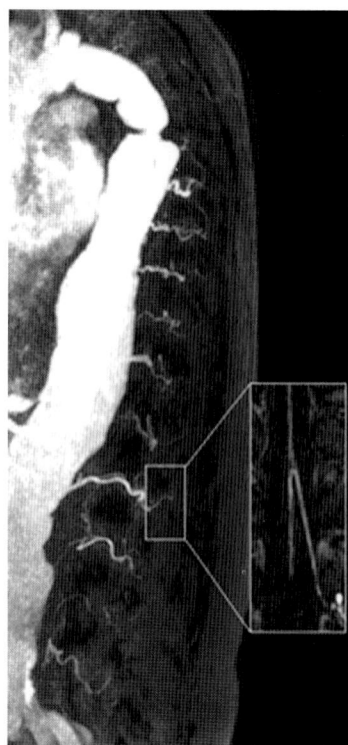

Figure 132-5 Preoperative MRA showing patent intercostal arteries and the main artery connecting with the anterior spinal artery. This information is applied during reattachment of the segmental arteries.

Cardiac

Patients with degenerative aneurysms are known to be older than postdissection patients and have more cardiovascular risk factors. Many patients (34% to 40%) suffer from coronary artery disease.[74,75] In a study by Suzuki and associates addressing cardiac assessment in 854 TAAA patients, impaired left ventricular function appeared to be the strongest predictor of perioperative mortality.[75] Cardiac function can be evaluated by electrocardiography, echocardiography, and stress testing, as discussed in Chapter 30 (Preoperative Management) and Chapter 38 (Systemic Complications: Cardiac). Despite the rather negative posture toward aggressive cardiac evaluation before vascular surgery in general, in TAAA repair the threshold for coronary arteriography and antecedent mechanical intervention for coronary artery disease is lower.[74]

Pulmonary

A history of smoking and the presence of chronic pulmonary disease are important predictors of postoperative pulmonary complications, which are the single most frequent source of perioperative morbidity. Preoperative pulmonary function is impaired in 23% to 36% of patients, which can lead to oxygenation problems during surgery in the case of single-lung ventilation and can elevate the risk for prolonged postoperative ventilation and pneumonia in the postoperative period.[35,76] Spirometric testing and arterial blood gas analysis have to be performed to evaluate pulmonary function. Absolute cessation of cigarette smoking for at least 4 weeks before surgery is mandatory. A period of pulmonary rehabilitation with appropriate medications may be indicated in those with marginal pulmonary reserve, although it is important to emphasize that this should not include the addition of systemic steroids because we have observed steroids to be associated with aneurysm rupture.

Renal

Preoperative renal impairment has been demonstrated in multiple series to be the single most powerful predictor of postoperative renal failure,[77,78] which in turn is a strong correlate of postoperative mortality.[79,80] However, some degree of renovascular/visceral occlusive disease is commonplace in TAAA patients, and in some of these patients the potential for recovery of renal function with concomitant renovascular repair is real. Although renal dysfunction cannot be modified before surgery, identification of the relevant renovascular anatomy can influence the use of adjunctive measures for renal protection during surgery.[81,82]

Cerebrovascular

If cross-clamping in the aortic arch is anticipated, imaging of the carotid arteries (e.g., by duplex ultrasonography or MRA) is advised to minimize the risk for stroke.

■ ADJUNCTIVE MEASURES FOR END-ORGAN PROTECTION

In the initial era of DTAA and TAAA repair, the clamp-and-sew technique was used without adjunctive measures, with subsequent end-organ (viscera, kidneys, and spinal cord) ischemia being the main problem. A clearer understanding of the determinants of operative risk and the major postoperative complications has led to the introduction of several extracorporeal circulation methods and adjunctive measures for end-organ protection. Various combinations of these techniques are used for different extents of DTAA and TAAA. However, use of the various adjuncts, including extracorporeal circulation, is inconsistent even in centers of excellence in TAAA repair. Most have discarded the simple clamp-and-sew technique originally advocated by Crawford for its simplicity and value in hemostasis and have adopted distal aortic perfusion provided by left atriofemoral bypass with a sequential clamping technique, at least for types I and II TAAAs and for the majority of DTAAs. Given amenable anatomy, this intuitively logical approach has been demonstrated to diminish organ-specific postoperative complications.[81,82] Its use for types III and IV TAAAs remains variable; in type III lesions, the amount of descending aorta to be resected will probably influence its use. In type IV lesions, wherein up to 50% of patients can undergo reconstruction with a single beveled anastomosis that incorporates the proximal aorta and visceral vessels, the use of extracorporeal circulation is unnecessary.

Extracorporeal Circulation

Atriofemoral Perfusion

The goal of providing distal aortic perfusion during thoracic aortic cross-clamping is to maintain blood flow through the mesenteric and renal arteries and to the spinal cord. In addition, left ventricular "unloading" is facilitated, particularly when a very proximal aortic cross-clamp is required. After opening the abdominal aorta, this technique provides the opportunity for selective antegrade visceral and renal artery perfusion through multiple sidearm cannulas, although use of these cannulas varies widely among surgeons experienced in TAAA repair. Most frequently used for DTAA and TAAA repair is distal aortic perfusion by partial left heart bypass. In this method, venous cannulation is performed through the left atrial appendage or, more commonly and conveniently, through the left inferior pulmonary vein. Via a centrifugal pump, blood is returned through a left femoral artery cannula. Besides distal aortic perfusion and the possibility of selective side branch perfusion, this method provides decompression of cardiac and cerebral perfusion during thoracic cross-clamping. The bypass flow rate is adjustable for preservation of adequate proximal aortic pressure. Distal mean aortic pressure should be approximately 60 mm Hg, but it can be adjusted according to urine production and spinal cord function monitoring tests (when used).[81] This bypass circuit is simple in concept and execution, can be used with extrapericardial access to the left atrium, and (because it is used with anticoagulant-impregnated tubing) requires only a modest dose of heparin; an in-line heat exchanger can provide moderate systemic hypothermia and rewarming during later stages of the reconstruction. Bleeding complications with this technique are greatly reduced when compared with full cardiopulmonary bypass, for which an oxygenator is required in the circuit and much larger heparin doses. For type IV TAAA, this technique can be changed to venous cannulation of the right atrium via the left femoral vein. However, incorporation of an oxygenator is mandatory, and many surgeons favor a variation of the clamp-and-sew technique for such lesions.

Hypothermic Arrest

Profound hypothermic circulatory arrest with total cardiopulmonary bypass can be established after arterial and venous femoral cannulation and full heparinization. As noted earlier, the majority of surgeons agree that this technique should be used only when no other technical option to repair the TAAA exists. After fibrillation and placement of a left ventricular vent, full cardiopulmonary bypass can be achieved. In DTAA and TAAA repair, this technique is advised in case proximal control is not feasible because of rupture, aneurysm size, or location of the dissection. Furthermore, an open anastomosis without cross-clamping can be indicated in patients with poor aortic tissue quality (e.g., acute type B dissection) or undergoing simultaneous repair of the aortic arch.[55,83,84] According to Kouchoukos and coworkers, the use of other adjunctive measures, such as CSF drainage, monitoring of CSF pressure, epidural cooling, and selective renal and visceral artery perfusion, is not necessary.[84]

Other Perfusion Techniques

Distal aortic perfusion and selective perfusion of the mesenteric arteries can be achieved without pump devices. The Gott shunt[85] and external axillofemoral artery bypass[86] have been used as a passive bypass circuit for repair of DTAA and TAAA. Cambria and associates have substantial experience with an in-line mesenteric shunt technique.[87,88] In this technique, a Dacron sidearm of the aortic graft is connected to a catheter in the celiac trunk or superior mesenteric artery after finishing the proximal aortic anastomosis, which generally restores pulsatile flow to the mesenteric circulation within 25 minutes, even in the absence of distal aortic perfusion. This technique is used in combination with renal artery perfusion with 4°C renal preservation solution and epidural cooling with 4°C saline.

Spinal Cord Protection

Paraplegia secondary to spinal cord ischemia is the most devastating complication after DTAA and TAAA repair. Patients most at risk are those with a type II TAAA and prolonged aortic cross-clamp times.[72,89,90] In patients with DTAA and TAAA, variations of the "normal" anatomy covered earlier, at least at the aortic level, occur commonly, with occlusion of the intercostal arteries by mural thrombus resulting in collateral filling of the anterior spinal artery.[65] It is interesting to note that spontaneous paraplegia, which can develop as a result of acute obliteration of multiple intercostal arteries, as might occur with acute aortic dissection (see Chapter 135: Aortic Dissection), virtually never occurs with chronic intercostal obliteration by a degenerative aneurysm. During open repair a variety of adjunctive measures can be performed to reduce spinal cord ischemia; they can be broadly classified as measures that seek to preserve cord blood supply (e.g., CSF drainage, intercostal artery reconstruction) and neuroprotective adjuncts such as variations of hypothermia and endorphin receptor blockage.[91] Monitoring of spinal cord function with evoked potentials, reattachment of intercostal arteries, distal aortic perfusion, CSF drainage, and systemic or local hypothermia are the principal adjuncts used in contemporary practice to reduce the development of spinal cord ischemia.

Evoked Potential Monitoring

Adequate spinal cord circulation can be assessed by means of monitoring somatosensory evoked potentials (SSEPs) and motor evoked potentials (MEPs) (Fig. 132-6). After stimulating the dorsal tibial nerve in SSEP monitoring, the signal is conducted through the dorsal columns of the spinal cord and is recorded from the scalp. MEPs specifically reflect motor function and motor tract blood supply. MEPs can be stimulated by electrical or magnetic transcranial stimuli and are typically recorded at the level of the anterior tibial muscle and

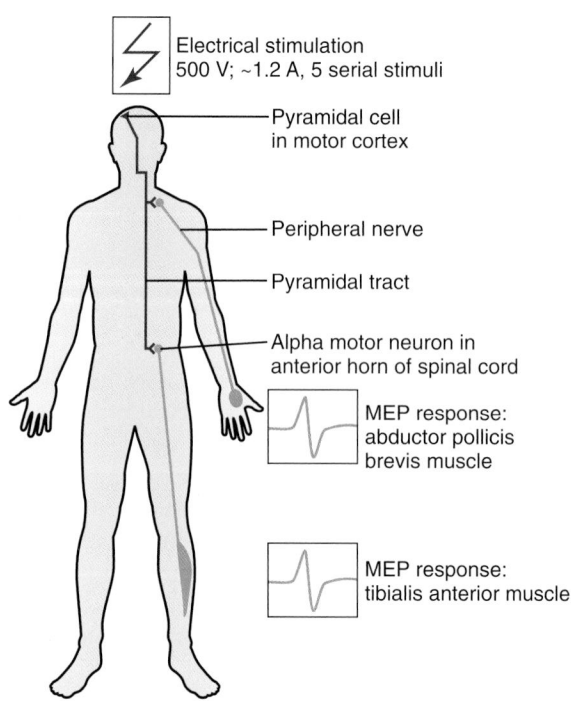

Figure 132-6 Schematic drawing of monitoring motor evoked potentials (MEPs). Transcranial stimuli are conducted via the corticospinal tract and activate the anterior horn motor neuron, thereby resulting in a muscle contraction, which is recorded as a compound muscle action potential.

compared with recordings at the thenar muscles, which are independent of the spinal cord blood supply.[70,92,93] To guide spinal cord protective actions, the monitoring should afford a short interval between the onset and detection of spinal cord ischemia. SSEPs are known for their long delay between the onset and detection of ischemia with respect to MEPs[94,95] and the occurrence of false-negative results.[96] Accordingly, they have largely been discarded in favor of MEPs. MEPs are influenced by neuromuscular blockade, so careful coordination with or modification of anesthetic strategies is necessary to achieve successful monitoring.[97]

Changes in spinal cord function as measured by SSEPs or MEPs influence the operative strategy. Frequently, elevating distal aortic pressure will normalize evoked potentials. Furthermore, decreasing body temperature and accelerated reattachment of the segmental arteries, even outside the standard T8-L1 level, can reverse spinal cord ischemia.[98] Monitoring of spinal cord function can also be used as a guide to sacrifice as many segmental arteries as possible, even prior to cross-clamp application and opening of the aneurysm.[99] With this technique, backbleeding of segmental arteries after opening the aorta and steal from the spinal cord circulation are avoided. Without monitoring of spinal cord function it is advised that all patent intercostal arteries between T8 and L1 be reattached.[88,100,101]

Hypothermia

Reduction of body temperature significantly decreases the incidence of spinal cord ischemic complications. The neuroprotective effect of hypothermia is presumed to be secondary to decreased tissue metabolism. Oxygen demand by neural tissue is known to decrease 6% to 7% per degree centigrade body temperature.[102] Hypothermia for spinal cord protection can be either systemic or regional. Regional epidural cooling was advocated in the past[103] but has largely been abandoned in favor of systemic hypothermia. Profound systemic hypothermia[104] is an option but, as noted above, is used rarely because of its risk for coagulopathy, pulmonary dysfunction, and massive fluid shifts. Passive moderate hypothermia[100,101] by lowering room temperature and active moderate hypothermia with the use of a heat exchanger in the distal aortic perfusion circuit[105] provide additional hypothermia options.

Cerebrospinal Fluid Drainage

CSF drainage during DTAA and TAAA repair has been used for several decades.[106,107] The rationale is that aortic cross-clamping both decreases arterial spinal cord pressure and increases CFS pressure.[108] CFS drainage, both during and after surgery, decreases CSF pressure and increases the relative spinal cord perfusion pressure. In a prospective randomized trial of 145 patients with types I and II TAAA in which the effect of CSF drainage on postoperative paraplegia was studied, CSF drainage was significantly better than control (3% and 13%, respectively).[109] Before this study the evidence base for use of CSF drainage was meager, yet ease of use, a low incidence of complications,[110] and a substantial body of clinical series purporting to show benefit have made CSF drainage nearly universal in operative strategies for thoracoabdominal aortic repair. Delayed paraplegia after DTAA and TAAA repair may be related to reperfusion syndrome with swelling of the spinal cord. Continuation of CSF drainage up to 72 hours postoperatively is thought to be beneficial in preventing delayed paraplegia.[88,100,109] In case of delayed-onset paraplegia, increasing spinal cord perfusion by elevation of systemic blood pressure and CSF drainage can reverse the paraplegia.[111] These observations have led to the empirical conclusion that the spinal cord collateral circulation can be very much in a state of flux in the hours and days after TAAA repair. Delayed deficits can occur even weeks after surgery, often in association with a hypotensive precipitant, such as might occur during a hemodialysis run. Accordingly, strict protocols to avoid and promptly treat perioperative hypotension are important to avoid delayed deficits.

Renal and Visceral Organ Protection

In DTAA repair with a distal cross-clamp above the celiac artery, continuous visceral and renal perfusion is possible when using a distal aortic perfusion method. If this method is combined with moderate systemic hypothermia, the kidneys and intestines should have minimal ischemic insults. Quite a different scenario is presented when opening the visceral aortic segment in TAAA repair; herein, local hypothermic perfusion of the renal arteries in particular is favored by many authors. Although the ingredients of such perfusate have been

debated for decades, most agree that the hypothermic component is the most important,[88,112,113] and this is now supported by randomized trial data.[114] However, negative results of cold perfusion on renal recovery have also been published.[115] An alternative is to provide active blood perfusion of the renal and mesenteric arteries because moderately hypothermic blood has protective effects on hepatorenal function.[81,116] To optimize renal perfusion, flow and pressure in the perfusion catheter can be measured.[81] Renal perfusion is established with 12 or 14 Fr catheters connected to the left-sided heart bypass. Volume flow is assessed with ultrasound, and pressure channels in the catheters enable pressure-controlled perfusion of the kidneys. Mean arterial pressure in the renal artery should be approximately 70 mm Hg and volume flow around 275 mL/min.

■ SURGICAL TECHNIQUE
Descending Thoracic Aortic Aneurysm

A fundamental principle in thoracic and thoracoabdominal aortic surgery is adequate exposure. Because the extent of the aneurysmal disease can vary tremendously, the approach to each case must be individualized according to the involved segment. The techniques described serve as a general guideline in these patients.

Positioning and Incision

After introduction of an intrathecal catheter for CSF drainage, the patient is positioned on a vacuum mattress in a right lateral decubitus position with the shoulders at a right angle (80 to 90 degrees) to the edge of the table and the left hip at 60 degrees to allow access to both sides of the groin. The top end of the vacuum mattress is distal to the right shoulder to avoid venous damming of the arm and head. The left arm hangs over to the right side and leans on an arm support, generally on traction to rotate the left scapula away from the spine and mainly for adequate exposure of lesions involving the proximal descending aorta. In general, a posterolateral thoracotomy via the sixth intercostal space provides excellent access to the entire descending thoracic aorta, although adequate access to the proximal descending aorta requires an approach via the fifth intercostal space, sometimes with resection of the sixth rib. If additional proximal exposure is required, the fifth rib can be shingled posteriorly. Double-lumen endotracheal intubation allows deflation and collapse of the left lung, which is carefully retracted to avoid lung damage and bleeding. If exposure of the aorta is not sufficient, several options exist to improve and extend the proximal and distal access: transecting but leaving the rib dorsally, opening the costal margin, or resecting the entire fifth or sixth rib; such considerations are highly dependent on the patient's body habitus. A self-retaining retractor on the edges of the incision or separate retractors at the proximal and distal ribs are used to maintain full thoracic exposure. Alternatively, strong lace bonds around the left scapula and the dorsal ribs can provide similar surgical access.

Exposure for Clamping

Depending on the extent of the aneurysm, the level of the proximal clamp position is prepared. Usually, the clamp can be positioned just distal to the left subclavian artery. If necessary, the clamp can be placed between the left carotid and left subclavian arteries.

Adequate preparation of the proximal clamp position is crucial and includes the following steps. The vagus and recurrent laryngeal nerves have to be identified and injury avoided. Transection of the ligamentum arteriosum ameliorates access to the inner curve of the distal arch and allows digital encircling of the aorta. If more proximal clamping is required, access can be facilitated by opening the pericardium dorsal to the phrenic nerve and approaching the aortic arch over the pulmonary artery, which offers access to the inner curve of the arch opposite the left carotid artery. Subsequently, the clamp position can be prepared. Afterward, the aorta is dissected from the esophagus and should be completely freed to avoid later prosthetic-esophageal fistula formation. Proximal and medial aortic side branches such as the left bronchial arteries can be clipped and divided.

Preparation of the distal clamp position, either at the level of the diaphragm or higher, requires only a small opening of the parietal pleura covering the aorta to allow sharp or digital encircling of the aorta. Opening of the parietal pleura should be performed as close as possible to the aortic wall and with direct vision of the accessory hemiazygos vein, which runs parallel and lateral to the aorta. The ideal plane for the cross-clamp is between the accessory hemiazygos vein and the aortic wall to avoid significant venous bleeding when transecting the aorta. Damage to the intercostal arteries should also be avoided, and therefore dissection can best be performed at the level of a costovertebral junction, where no intercostal arteries are located. With extensive aneurysms, sequential clamp positions can be prepared to minimize spinal cord ischemia. If feasible, a second proximal cross-clamp position is prepared only a few centimeters lower than the first proximal clamp to allow maximal thoracic aortic perfusion via the left bypass during performance of the proximal anastomosis.

Extracorporeal Perfusion

The next step focuses on extracorporeal circulation. If chosen for femoral artery and femoral vein cannulation, no further intrathoracic steps are necessary. In the case of left heart bypass, the left femoral artery and either the left atrium or the left pulmonary vein are cannulated, the latter being technically easier. The pericardium dorsal to the phrenic nerve is opened, the lower or common pulmonary vein is dissected free, and two purse-string sutures are attached to fixate the cannula; alternatively, an entirely extrapericardial access to the inferior pulmonary vein is favored by many surgeons. Only limited heparinization (0.5 mg/kg) with an active clotting time of approximately 200 seconds is required. Insertion of the cannula into the pulmonary vein should be performed

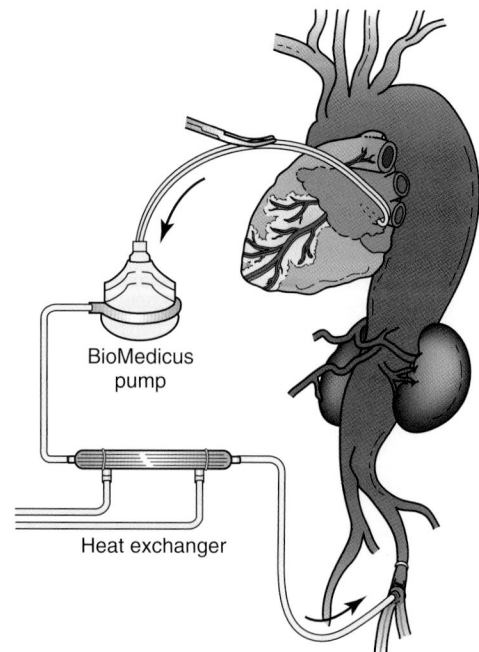

Figure 132-7 Distal aortic perfusion from the left pulmonary vein to the left femoral artery. Side branches can be connected to the system to provide antegrade perfusion of the visceral arteries.

with the patient in the Trendelenburg position while the anesthesiologist maintains positive pressure and apnea to avoid air embolism. The left femoral artery is the most convenient access for arterial inflow, and distal perfusion pressure is monitored with a right femoral artery cannula (Fig. 132-7). Obviously, a careful review of preoperative CTA images is required to ensure that either occlusive disease or chronic dissection will not cause inadequate retrograde flow. With the cannulas connected, the left heart bypass can start, and the patient's pre-bypass cardiac output is used as a rough guide to adequate flow rates.

Anastomoses and Repair

Depending on the anatomy and extension of the aneurysm, the direction of aortic repair can be either from distal to proximal or vice versa. When starting proximally, the clamps are positioned (Fig. 132-8A) and distal aortic perfusion started at a mean arterial pressure of approximately 60 mm Hg. In our experience, distal arterial pressure is adjusted in accordance with the amplitude of the MEPs. The aorta is completely transected to ensure adequate separation from the esophagus (Fig. 132-8B), and the proximal anastomosis is performed with running 3-0 or 4-0 monofilament polypropylene suture (Fig. 132-8C), with or without Teflon support, depending on the quality of the aortic wall. After completion of this anastomosis, the aortic clamp is released and put on the graft. Next, the aorta is cross-clamped more distally and the aortic segment opened. Small arteries above T6 are oversewn and intercostal arteries between T8 and T12 may be reattached to the tube graft (Fig. 132-9).

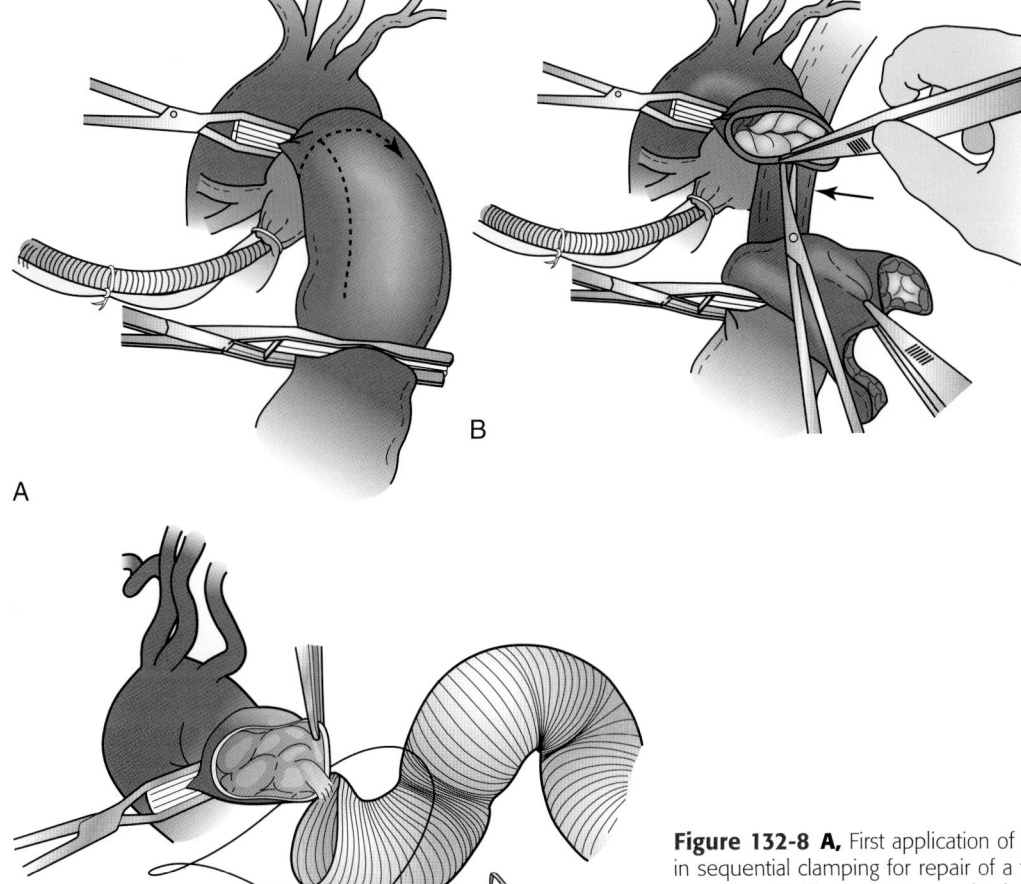

Figure 132-8 A, First application of the proximal and distal clamps in sequential clamping for repair of a thoracoabdominal aortic aneurysm. **B,** The aorta is completely transected and separated from the esophagus (*arrow*). **C,** Proximal anastomosis for repair of a thoracoabdominal aortic aneurysm.

Spinal Cord Protection

With regard to spinal cord protection, several strategies are described. Griepp and coworkers follow the practice of clipping the intercostal arteries before opening the aorta unless the MEPs demonstrate a decrease in spinal cord function.[99,117] The intercostal arteries that are left and considered to be important are subsequently reattached; however, in their experience this is rarely necessary. Others routinely reinsert all intercostal vessels between T8 and T12 if technically feasible.[109,118] We rely entirely on MEPs and have a liberal attitude toward reattachment of intercostal arteries at the T8-T12 level.[98] However, if the MEPs disappear completely and adjunctive measures such as increasing mean arterial pressure and distal arterial pressure do not restore the MEPs, our strategy is to reimplant the arteries between the clamps, irrespective of the anatomic level. We do this because losing MEPs with adequate proximal and distal flow and pressure can indicate only that important arteries are located between the clamps and, in our approach, is an indication of the need for a very aggressive posture toward intercostal revascularization. This implies that the absence of visible vessels prompts us to perform aortic endarterectomy, and in our experience it

is surprising for backbleeding arteries to always become apparent. Because the tissue of this endarterectomized aorta is too thin and fragile to reattach in an end-to-side fashion, we revascularize these intercostal arteries with a sidearm polyester graft. If the MEPs are completely abolished, we insert a selective perfusion catheter in the graft and start selective perfusion (Fig. 132-10A) before anastomosing the graft in the aortic tube prosthesis to limit spinal cord ischemic time (Fig. 132-10B). The fact that MEPs return after reperfusion indicates that these apparently occluded arteries are still interconnected in a collateral network. Figure 132-5 demonstrates a preoperative MRA with visualization of the intercostal arteries and main vessel that connects to the anterior spinal artery; this segmental artery will be reimplanted during surgery.

Intercostal Artery Reimplantation

The aortic tissue around the intercostal arteries to be reimplanted should be excluded as much as possible to avoid aneurysm formation of the reattached button. This means that the sutures should be placed as close as possible to the orifices of the segmental arteries. Three-French Pruitt balloon occlu-

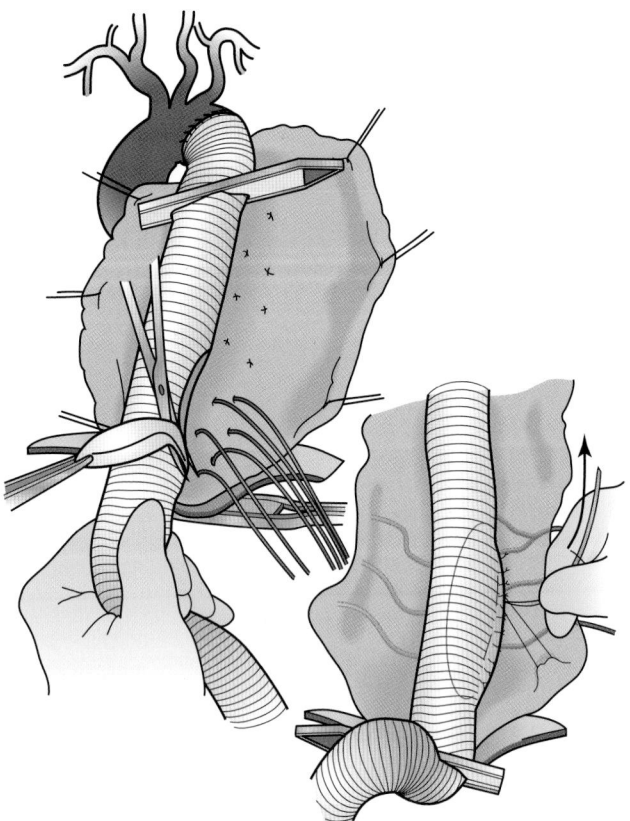

Figure 132-9 An elliptical hole is cut in the graft, and the lower intercostal arteries are reattached as a patch to the graft.

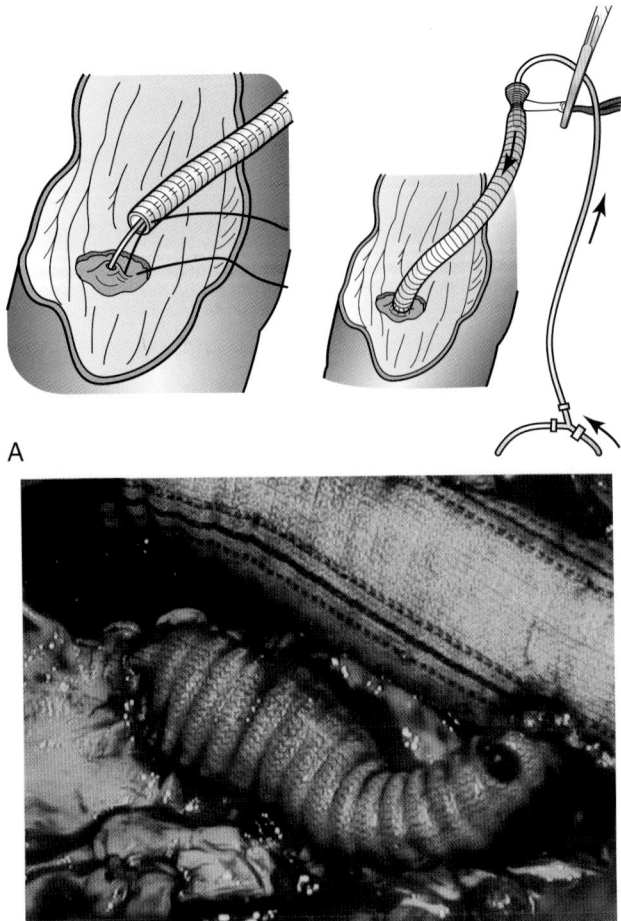

Figure 132-10 A, Schematic drawing of an endarterectomized aortic layer demonstrating a backbleeding intercostal artery that is revascularized by means of a polyester graft. A selective perfusion catheter is inserted in the graft to reperfuse the spinal cord. **B,** Example of a short separate graft from an aortic tube prosthesis to a pair of two intercostal arteries.

sion catheters in the intercostal arteries not only stop backbleeding but can also indicate the anatomic direction and course of the vessels, which vary considerably. During reattachment of the button, identification of the course and direction of the vessels can help in avoiding suturing through such an intercostal vessel. It should be emphasized that in degenerative aneurysms, the majority of intercostal arteries are occluded and spinal cord function largely depends on an extensive collateral network.[70] In many patients the number of patent intercostal arteries is very limited, and frequently, aortic wall quality is too poor for reattachment in the tube graft. In such cases it might also be necessary to use a separate polyester graft to revascularize these segmental vessels. Because the aortic tissue to work with is often thin and fragile, we prefer to use 5-0 RB-1 or RB-2 needles to create a strong rim by involving enough remaining aortic tissue for a firm anastomosis with the polyester graft. Utmost care has to be taken to prevent adventitial tears in the anastomosis because they might lead to subadventitial bleeding, which can subsequently cause the surrounding tissue to swell and threaten spinal cord perfusion.

Completion

The distal anastomosis is performed according to the same principles as the proximal anastomosis, and after the clamps are released, the repair is completed. If necessary, the patient is warmed to 37° C by means of the heat exchanger in the extracorporeal circuit. After extensive hemostasis, the cannulas are removed and the patient receives protamine. If possible, the aortic wall is wrapped around the graft and the left lung is reinflated. Chest tubes are inserted, the ribs attached, and the different layers closed.

Thoracoabdominal Aortic Aneurysm

Positioning and Incision

Preparation of a patient with a TAAA is similar to that described earlier, except that positioning on the vacuum mattress is different: the shoulders and chest are not turned to the right as much (70 to 80 degrees) to allow a smooth transition to the abdominal wall, which is at approximately 60 degrees, and the left hip is positioned at 30 degrees. In types I, II, and III TAAA, the lateral thoracotomy (generally the sixth intercostal space) is extended over the costal margin in an oblique line, and both the caudal extent and the mediolateral position of the incision are dictated by the extent of the aneurysm and body habitus. In type I the abdominal incision can stop at the umbilicus, and in type IV the thoracotomy is performed through the eighth intercostal space and can be limited to the anterior part only, just enough to allow appropriate cross-clamping in the chest.

Aortic Exposure

The costal margin is divided and access to the aorta is achieved by either a retroperitoneal or transperitoneal approach, depending on the surgeon's preference. In any case, the abdominal aorta is approached laterally from the descending colon and dorsal to the spleen and left kidney, which is rotated anteriorly out of its bed; the exception to this approach is a repeat operation wherein left kidney mobilization was done at the initial operation. In these cases the risk of injury to the kidney is such that it is left in situ and the surgeon will need to work around the left renal vein. The diaphragm can be divided completely, but we prefer to cut the anterior, muscular part only to avoid injury to branches of the phrenic nerve (Fig. 132-11). This limited opening of the diaphragm offers better postoperative pulmonary function than does complete division; however, complete division may be necessary to achieve adequate exposure, especially if intercostal reconstruction is required. Such intraoperative judgments about phrenic nerve preservation will be predicated on the status of the patient's pulmonary reserve. At the aortic level the overlying musculature of the crus can be divided in longitudinal fashion; the right index finger can be used to dissect on the anterior side of the distal thoracic aorta toward the abdominal aorta, under and through the muscles of the diaphragm and crus, after division of the median arcuate ligament, which typically courses just cephalic to the left renal artery origin. In very large aneurysms, this musculature has to be freed from the aneurysmal wall over the bilateral edges of the aorta to achieve enough space. A loop is then placed around the diaphragm and can be pulled in all directions to expose the supraceliac and distal descending thoracic aortic segments. Adequate exposure in this region is essential because important intercostal and visceral arteries will have to be managed afterward.

Going further distally, all para-aortic tissue is transected along the line of the intended aortotomy. After the left kidney is rotated anteriorly, a key step is identification of the aortic origin of the left renal artery because it serves as the starting point for division of the retroperitoneal tissue over the infrarenal aorta and the landmark to begin the more cephalad division of the median arcuate ligament and the muscular fibers of the diaphragmatic crura. Frequently, a large posterior branch of the anteriorly located left renal vein will indicate the position of the left renal artery. Veins lateral to the aorta, such as the renal lumbar vein, have to be tied and transected. The left ureter should also be identified to avoid injury while cross-clamping. If the aneurysm involves the iliac arteries, the common, external, and internal iliac arteries are dissected and prepared for cross-clamping.

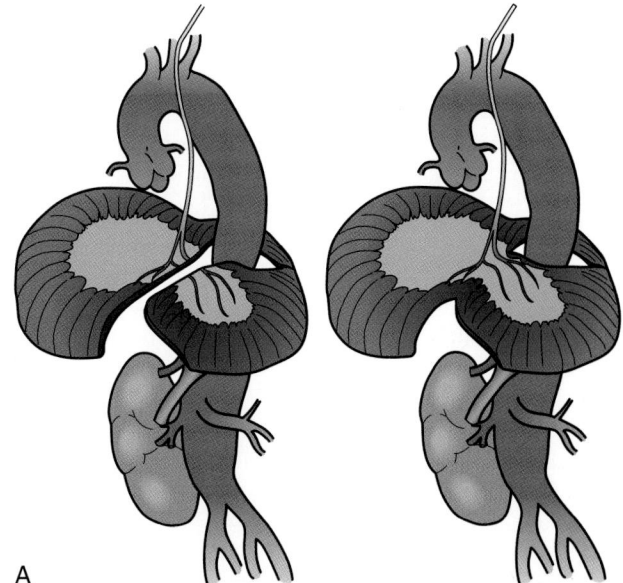

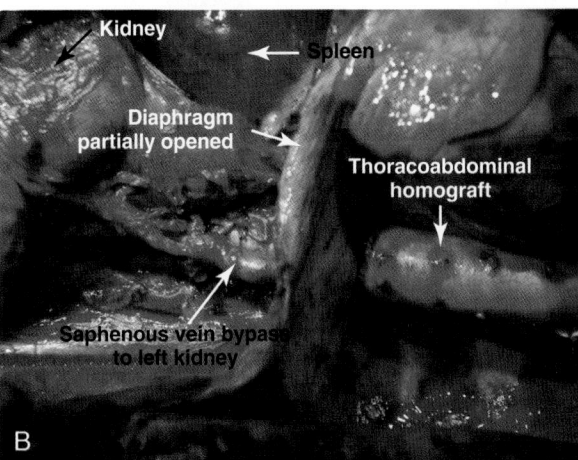

Figure 132-11 A, Previously, the diaphragm was divided (*left*); currently, only the muscular portion of the diaphragm is cut (*right*). **B,** Perioperative image of thoracolaparotomy with a limited incision of the diaphragm in a patient with an infected thoracoabdominal graft undergoing resection of the prosthesis and implantation of a homograft.

Extracorporeal Circulation

In types I, II, and III TAAA, extracorporeal circulation is established by means of femoral artery and femoral vein or left femoral artery and pulmonary vein (or left atrial) cannulation. Our tubing system consists of four integrated catheters connected to 12 Fr or 14 Fr balloon-inflatable catheters for selective perfusion of the celiac axis, superior mesenteric artery, and both renal arteries.[13] Alternatively, the kidneys can be protected by means of continuous perfusion with cold lactated Ringer's solution.[113]

Anastomoses and Repair

In general, the aortic reconstruction is performed from the proximal part to the distal level of the aneurysm. However, repair can also be carried out from the distal side on. This technique is discussed later (under "Postdissection

Thoracoabdominal Aneurysm"). When performing the standard sequence, the thoracic part of the procedure is equivalent to the technique described for descending thoracic aneurysms. Until the level of the celiac axis, the sequential steps are followed under continuous distal aortic perfusion while keeping CSF pressure lower than 10 mm Hg. Temperature is allowed to decrease spontaneously to 32° C to 33° C as a means of general organ and spinal cord protection. If urine output decreases, distal aortic perfusion pressure is increased. Decreased urine output can often occur in patients suffering from arterial hypertension because they are generally used to higher perfusion pressure than the mean pressure of the pump.

After the thoracic portion of the procedure is completed, the visceral and renal arteries come in focus. In most cases of degenerative disease (and indeed many dissection patients), reconstruction of these vessels is by means of the inclusion technique described by Crawford. In type I TAAA, the distal clamp is positioned between the superior mesenteric artery and both renal arteries, if feasible, or distal to the renal arteries. The distal anastomosis is performed at the level of the renal arteries with an oblique technique incorporating the visceral and renal arteries, usually without the need for separate button reimplantation of these vessels. In our experience with types II, III, and IV TAAA, without exception, the left renal artery is treated with a selective 8-mm polyester or polytetrafluoroethylene graft. Therefore, before cross-clamping the abdominal aorta, we first revascularize the left renal artery. After clamping and dividing the artery at the aorta, an 8-mm polyester graft is anastomosed in an oblique, end-to-end fashion and a perfusion catheter is inserted in the graft to provide selective perfusion. Because the kidneys are pressure-dependent organs, we continuously assess pressure at the tip of the catheter in the renal graft and keep it at a minimal mean level of 60 to 70 mm Hg. Ultrasound probes around the selective catheters allow measurement of flow in each artery. Alternatively, the left renal artery can simply be amputated first and a renal cold preservation solution instilled therein, with its reconstruction deferred until the celiac, superior mesenteric, and right renal arteries have been reconstructed.

After completion of the left renal artery reconstruction, the infrarenal aorta is cross-clamped and the aorta opened. Catheters are inserted into the celiac axis, superior mesenteric artery, and right renal artery, and selective perfusion is started at a mean flow of 150 to 300 mL/min in the renal and 200 to 500 mL/min in the visceral arteries, depending on the diameter of the arteries (Fig. 132-12). In general, the destructive atherosclerotic disease saves the origins of the celiac axis and superior mesenteric and right renal arteries, thereby allowing reattachment of these three vessels as an inclusion button in the tube graft (Fig. 132-13).

Visceral and Renal Arteries

Although the original Crawford concept was to minimize dissection and avoid circumferential external control of the celiac and superior mesenteric arteries, we prefer external

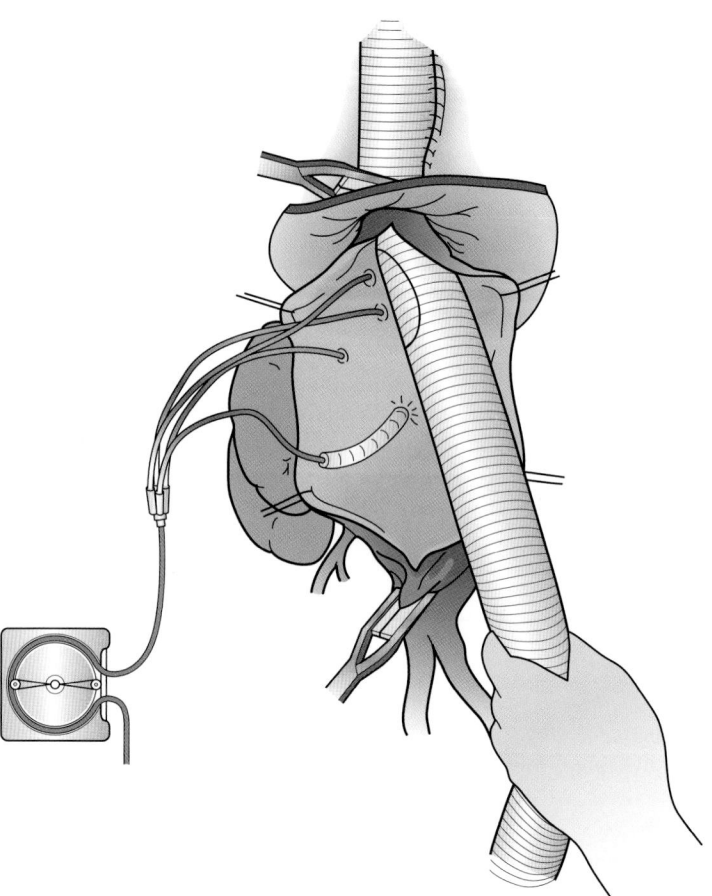

Figure 132-12 Perfusion of the celiac, superior mesenteric, and renal arteries. Note that the left renal artery is perfused via its separate sidearm graft and is subsequently attached to the aortic graft.

control of these vessels because (1) it is usually straightforward except in the case of very large aneurysms, (2) it facilitates placement of perfusion catheters should the surgeon choose to do so, (3) it enables precise orificial endarterectomy if needed, and (4) it allows direct Doppler interrogation of these vessels after repair. In the case of substantial separation of the celiac and superior mesenteric origins, a convenient technique is to amputate the celiac origin as a Carrell patch, defer its reconstruction, and use a single inclusion button for the superior mesenteric and right renal arteries. This results in less superior mesenteric and right renal ischemia and minimizes the potential for subsequent visceral patch aneurysm. To avoid patch aneurysm formation and have adequate material for sewing, it is recommended that the anastomosis be placed as close as possible to the orifices of these arteries and attempts be made to insert the needle into the lumen or at the edge of the lumen and aortic wall. Just before finishing the anastomosis, the catheters are removed to ensure that ischemic time is limited to a few minutes. In case of severely calcified or proximally stenosed visceral or renal arteries, orificial endarterectomy will be required or separate individual bypass can be constructed. Alternatively and in particular reference to the right renal artery, wherein there is never circumferential external access and its course may be such that it is occluded by the inclusion button suture bites, orificial balloon-

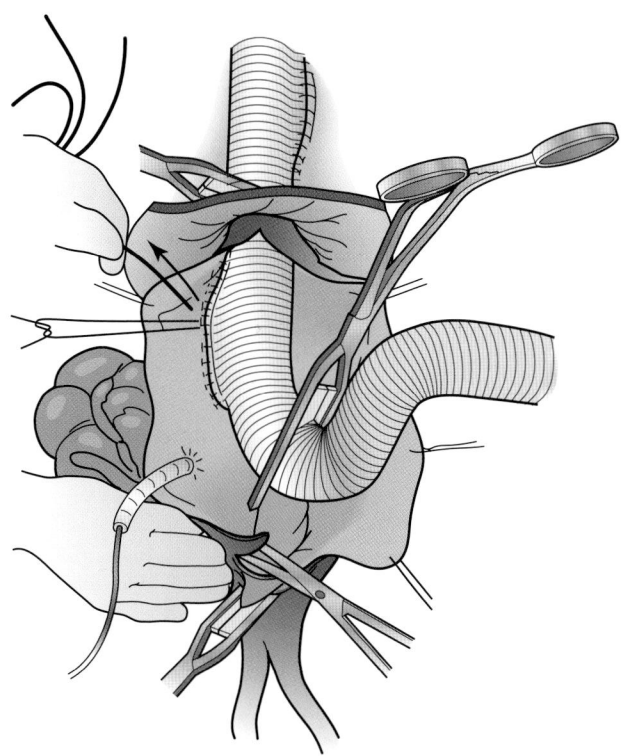

Figure 132-13 Reattachment of the inclusion button reconstruction of the celiac, superior mesenteric, and right renal arteries.

expandable stenting can be a convenient technical expedient (Fig. 132-14). In patients with CTD, especially in young patients with Marfan's syndrome, it is recommended that as little aortic tissue as possible be reimplanted to limit patch aneurysms during follow-up. Depending on both the quality of the aortic wall and the degree of separation of the renal/visceral vessel origins, it may be advisable to revascularize both visceral and renal arteries by means of four individual grafts. When reattaching as a button, the aforementioned technique of suturing a circular Teflon strip at the level of the orifices can be used for re-enforcement of the anastomosis. The same holds for reimplantation of the intercostal and lumbar arteries, where patch aneurysms occur frequently.

Spinal Cord Protection

With regard to spinal cord perfusion, patients with degenerative TAAAs largely depend on collateral blood flow to the anterior spinal artery via lumbar arteries and both hypogastric arteries.[70] Therefore, lumbar arteries at the L1-L5 level might be extremely important to reimplant, which in our experience is based on MEP information. This becomes even more crucial in case no intercostal arteries were found or

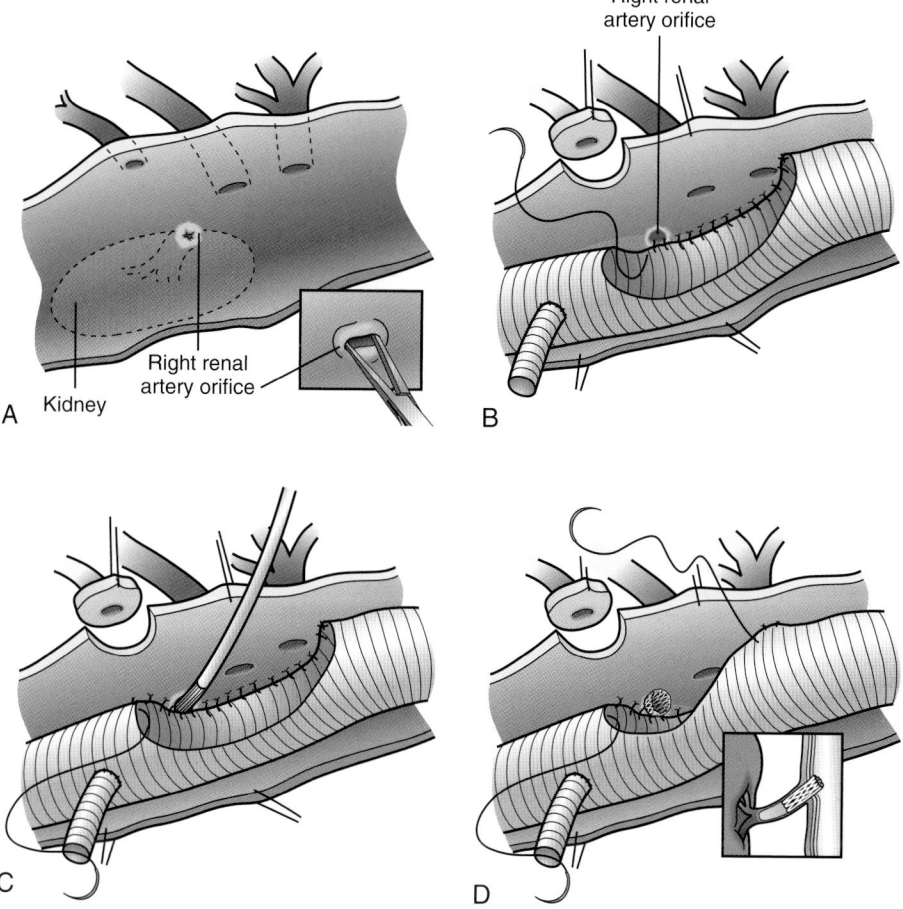

Figure 132-14 A–D, As an alternative to endarterectomizing the renal or mesenteric ostia, a stent can be placed in the vessel ostium to ensure patency. *(From Patel R, Chung TK, Conrad M, et al. Balloon expandable stents facilitate right renal artery reconstruction during complex open aortic aneurysm repair. J Vasc Surg. 2009. In press.)*

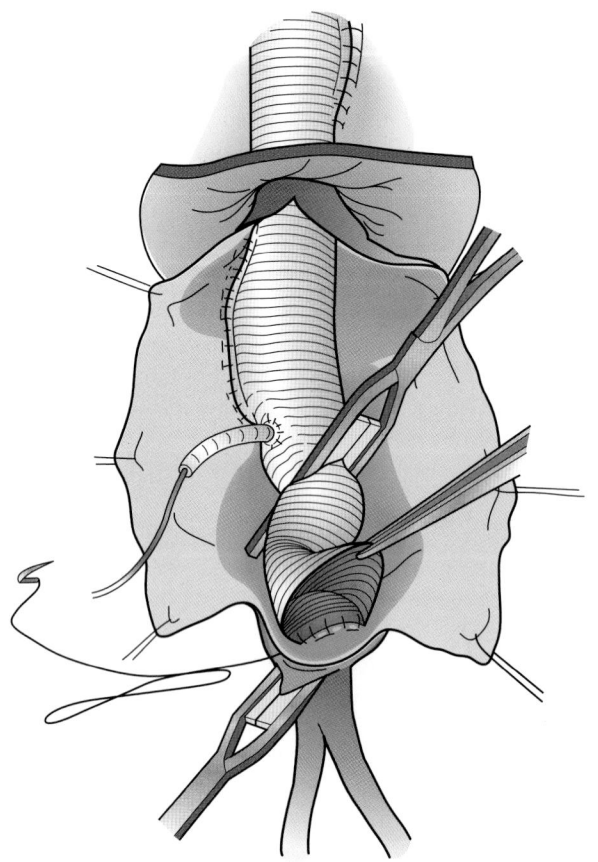

Figure 132-15 Completion of the distal anastomosis for repair of a thoracoabdominal aortic aneurysm.

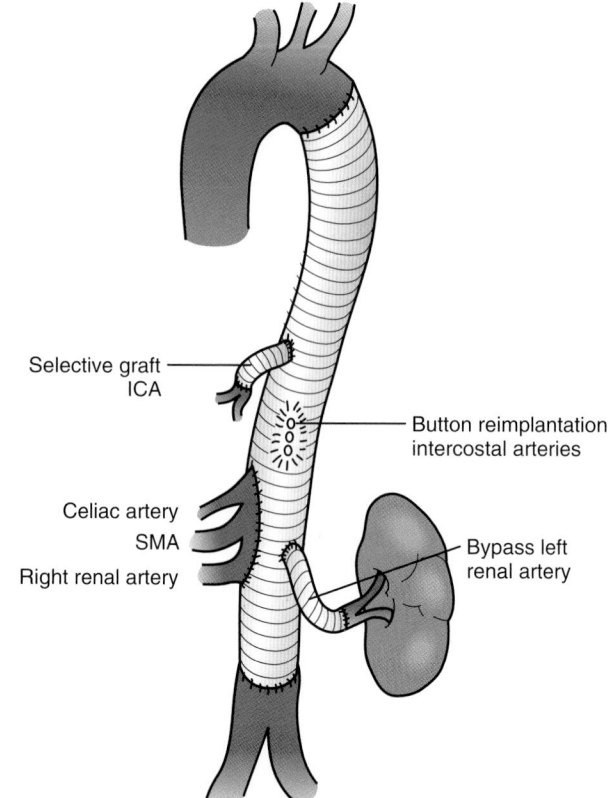

Figure 132-16 Typical final situation after reconstruction of a type II thoracoabdominal aortic aneurysm. In this case the segmental arteries are revascularized by using both a selective graft and button reimplantation. The celiac axis, superior mesenteric artery (SMA), and right renal artery are reimplanted as an inclusion button in the graft and a bypass is used for revascularization of the left renal artery. ICA, intercostal artery.

reimplanted during the thoracic phase of the procedure and spinal cord blood flow becomes dependent on this collateral network.

Completion

Finally, the distal anastomosis is performed, with the level being dependent on the extent of the aneurysm (Fig. 132-15). If the iliac arteries are affected, a bifurcated graft has to be attached to the tube graft and both arteries revascularized, including both hypogastric arteries. A typical situation after reconstruction of a type II TAAA is shown in Figure 132-16.

After the last aortic or iliac anastomosis, the left renal graft (and others if applicable) is implanted in the tube graft while using a side-biting clamp on the main prosthesis. Although this is the strategy when the left renal graft is perfused from the bypass circuit, an alternative is to attach the left renal graft to the main graft before any clamps are placed; in such circumstances the left renal anastomosis is performed before the distal aortic anastomosis. This graft will have enough length to be left in a nice curve to avoid kinking after repositioning the left kidney, although its orientation should be assessed after the left kidney has been returned to its anatomic position. Selective grafts to segmental arteries can be kept short because kinking does not occur. While performing these last

anastomoses, the patient is rewarmed to 37° C and extensive hemostasis is undertaken. Next, the cannulas are removed and protamine administered. Finally, the aneurysmal layer is closed over the graft and the muscular layers of the crus, including the aortic wall, are firmly closed in such a way that herniation cannot occur. After abdominal repositioning, the diaphragm is closed with running suture and attached to the costal margin. Chest tubes are inserted and the thorax and abdomen closed in the usual manner.

Postdissection Thoracoabdominal Aneurysm

Postdissection thoracoabdominal aneurysms can develop after a DeBakey type I (extensive Stanford type A) or a DeBakey type III (Stanford type B) aortic dissection in which longitudinal extension of the dissection involved the descending thoracic and abdominal aorta, most often including the iliac arteries as well. Such late aneurysmal degeneration of the outer wall of the false lumen occurs in 30% to 45% of patients, as noted earlier.[119] Acute type A dissections are always repaired via sternotomy, and in general the proximal part of the ascending aorta is replaced with a tube graft. If the tear extends into the arch, more extensive repair is required;

however, total arch replacement is uncommon in the acute phase. If the nonresected part of the aortic arch dilates over time and the thoracoabdominal diameter progresses as well, the DTAA or TAAA is associated with an arch or distal arch aneurysm.

Technique

One of the main differences between degenerative and post-dissection aneurysms is patency of the intercostal and lumbar arteries: in the latter group almost all segmental arteries are patent, whereas in atherosclerotic aneurysms, the majority of the segmental vessels are occluded.[65,120] In postdissection aneurysms, the important segmental vessels most often originate from the true lumen, which is obviously an advantage for revascularization because the quality of tissue is better than in the false lumen.

The surgical strategy is similar to the technique described earlier; however, some different approaches can be considered. First, sequential clamping, if feasible, enables stepwise aortic reconstruction and limits the sometimes substantial blood loss caused by profound backbleeding from the intercostal arteries because of the distal perfusion; blocking with balloon catheters or oversewing these arteries requires a significant amount of time, and therefore sequential steps are preferred. Second, the direction of aortic reconstruction can be reversed from distal to proximal to avoid insufficient perfusion of the visceral, renal, and segmental arteries as a result of changed flow patterns induced by retrograde perfusion; type B dissections cause a wide range of morphologic changes with different false and true lumina and entries and reentries with subsequent visceral and renal circulation via separate pathways. Cross-clamping the proximal descending aorta and starting retrograde aortic perfusion can change these alternative perfusion channels to the visceral organs and potentially cause malperfusion and subsequent ischemia. Therefore, one can consider starting the reconstruction at the distal portion with either a bifurcated graft to the iliac arteries or a tube graft to the aortic bifurcation, clearly dependent on whether the anatomy would permit such a strategy.

While performing these anastomoses, the aortic cross-clamp is placed distal to the renal arteries and all organs are perfused in an antegrade direction. The arterial cannula is then inserted and fixed in the polyester graft and the venous cannula in the right atrium via the femoral vein to allow extracorporeal circulation and perfusion of the legs. Next, the left renal artery can be reconstructed with a separate graft and perfused via the prosthesis. The visceral and right renal arteries are then reconstructed, either as an island reimplantation or with separate grafts if the dissection injured these arteries as well. Treatment and handling of the dissected layers require utmost care because severe complications can develop if the true lumen is not correctly identified and controlled. The true lumen is often much smaller and can even be compressed in such a way that it might be disregarded. If the aorta is not entirely encircled and cross-clamped, significant bleeding through the incompletely clamped true lumen occurs as soon

as the aorta is opened. An important technical principle of dealing with the dissected aorta is to circumferentially divide the aorta at all suture lines to ensure adequate adventitial purchase of the suture bites; an exception is the posteroinferior aspect of the visceral inclusion button. Careful review of preoperative CTA images will alert the surgeon to these relationships.

Another potential danger of overlooking the small true lumen is leaving the intercostal arteries without reattachment. Therefore, it is essential that the septum between the true and false lumina be opened over the entire length of the aortotomy. The septum is subsequently resected while leaving a small 1- to 2-mm rim of septum between both lumina. Revascularizing segmental arteries originating from the false lumen might be hazardous because the aortic tissue is thin and of inferior quality. The intercostal and lumbar arteries coming from the true lumen are reimplanted while limiting the amount of aortic tissue as much as possible by suturing on the edge of the vessels. In general, most surgeons reimplant segmental arteries between T8 and L1, depending on the patency and quality of the aortic wall. Our strategy of revascularization depends on MEP monitoring.

At the site of the planned proximal anastomosis in post–type B dissections, the origin of the initial intimal tear is often at the level of the left subclavian artery. Moreover, the aortic wall at the tear can be thickened and contain false lumen thrombosis, which can compromise an adequate proximal anastomosis. Therefore, it is frequently necessary to cross-clamp between the left carotid and left subclavian arteries and resect the diseased aortic tissue until adequate and relatively normal aortic material is reached. Finally, an end-to-end anastomosis to a circumferentially divided aorta is performed, either at the edge of the left subclavian artery or distal to the carotid artery with reimplantation or bypass of the left subclavian artery.

Aortic Arch Involvement

Combined aneurysmal disease of the distal aortic arch and descending thoracic and thoracoabdominal aorta is rather common, especially in patients with Marfan's syndrome and those who suffered from type A dissection with longitudinal involvement of the entire aorta. In addition, patients with post–type B dissection requiring aortic repair often have distal aortic arch involvement, which necessitates clamping between the left carotid and subclavian arteries or even more proximally. As noted earlier, in the majority of degenerative lesions, cross-clamp application on either side of the left subclavian is usually feasible. Surgical treatment of genuine incontinuity aneurysms of the ascending arch and descending aorta is a unique surgical challenge[121] that involves adequate protection of the heart, maintenance of brain integrity, and minimization of spinal cord injury and organ failure induced by prolonged circulatory arrest times.[122] In our experience with DTAA and TAAA we identified aortic arch involvement in approximately 15% of patients, which requires total or partial arch repair as well, in addition to the DTAA or TAAA procedure.

Technique

The traditional repair, which requires a two-stage operation with the elephant trunk technique, is described in Chapter 134 (Aortic Arch Aneurysms and Dissection). If feasible, we perform simultaneous repair and use the fifth intercostal space. The technique of extracorporeal circulation depends on the extent of the procedure. If cross-clamping in the arch is possible, left heart bypass is instituted by means of left heart bypass. In patients undergoing aortic arch repair, total extracorporeal circulation is implemented by means of femoral vein and artery cannulation (full heparinization, 3 mg/kg) and a vent via the left pulmonary vein. In these cases, patients are cooled moderately (25°C to 28°C) after the aorta is cross-clamped distal to the left subclavian artery to allow distal aortic perfusion. Next, the aortic arch is opened and a Foley catheter inserted and inflated in the ascending aorta or previously implanted ascending prosthesis to administer cardioplegia. This technique is not possible in the case of aneurysmal disease of the ascending aorta. Selective antegrade brain perfusion is then implemented by connecting catheters placed in the innominate and left carotid artery to the extracorporeal circuit. The standard total antegrade cerebral flow is 10 mg/kg/min with a mean pressure of 60 mm Hg. Continuous transcranial Doppler assessment of both medial cerebral arteries and electroencephalography are used to monitor the adequacy of brain perfusion and guide flow and pressure adjustments, if necessary. Meanwhile, distal aortic perfusion provides spinal cord protection, which is assessed by means of MEPs. This "triple-surveillance," including transcranial Doppler, electroencephalography, and MEPs, is our standard neuromonitoring protocol in patients undergoing combined aortic arch and DTAA or TAAA repair. In patients with Marfan's syndrome and diseased supra-aortic side branches, the innominate and left carotid arteries are reconstructed with selective polyester grafts while continuously being perfused. In other cases these vessels are reattached in the main graft. After arch repair the selective catheters are removed and the heart is filled, de-aired, and reperfused via cannulation of a prefabricated side branch of the arch prosthesis (Y-connection in the arterial tubing system). Subsequently, the DTAA or TAAA is replaced.

Postoperative Management

During the first 24 to 48 postoperative hours, hemodynamic stabilization is essential with respect to cardiac, renal, visceral, and spinal cord function. The documented blood pressure values during the operation required for adequate hemodynamics, urine output, and spinal cord function are integrated into the postoperative orders for the intensive care unit (ICU). This individualized strategy allows hypertensive patients to receive hemodynamic management different from that of normotensive patients. In the latter group, mean arterial pressure in the ICU is kept between 80 and 90 mm Hg, whereas hypertensive patients might require higher pressure to maintain urine output and visceral perfusion. In the ICU we strive for the mean arterial pressures that were necessary during the operation to maintain adequate evoked potentials. Optimizing oxygen delivery, cardiac output, and volume status is crucial and requires continuous monitoring and adjustment, if necessary. Large blood pressure fluctuations should be avoided because medical interventions most often provoke even worse instability and can precipitate ischemic complications such as paraplegia and renal failure during hypotensive phases and bleeding during hypertensive phases. Blood coagulation is intensively controlled and aggressively corrected and anemia treated by transfusion. CSF drainage continues for 72 hours, even in patients without neurologic deficits. Ventilatory support and pulmonary recruitment, including bronchoscopy, are provided for optimal treatment of atelectasis and prevention of pneumonia to allow fast weaning and extubation. In patients with prolonged ventilator support, early tracheostomy is recommended.

■ SURGICAL RESULTS

Descending Thoracic Aortic Aneurysm

When reporting on the surgical outcome of open DTAA repair, several major influencing factors have to be considered. First, it should be emphasized that published results mainly come from centers of excellence in which experience, infrastructure, and dedication lead to better outcomes than those reported by nationwide analyses. Second, surgical outcome greatly depends on preoperative, perioperative, and postoperative conditions, which can vary tremendously.

Morbidity and Mortality

Circumstances other than elective procedures are associated with doubled mortality, even in patients who are hemodynamically stable during preoperative preparation.[72] This is even more the case in patients with acute dissection who are undergoing surgical repair of the descending aorta.[123] The extent of surgical DTAA repair varies widely, from resection of a limited, short aortic segment to extensive replacement from the distal arch to the celiac axis. Reports of surgical outcomes in the literature have never correlated results and the extent of DTAA repair. However, involvement of the distal aortic arch or extensive proximal descending aortic disease precluding placement of a proximal aortic clamp significantly deteriorates surgical outcomes,[54] so when cross-clamping is not feasible, hypothermic circulatory arrest can be performed, but with increased morbidity and mortality rates. Underlying disease also influences surgical outcome: atherosclerotic degenerative aneurysms occur mainly in patients older than 60 years, whereas CTDs affect younger patients, which clearly explains the better survival and long-term results in the latter group.

The largest retrospective series of DTAA repair have been published by Coselli and coauthors[124] and Estera and colleagues.[35] By using propensity scoring and risk stratification analysis, Coselli and associates determined that the use of left heart bypass did not reduce the incidence of paraplegia when compared with the "clamp-and-sew" technique.[124] The overall paraplegia rate was 2.6% and 30-day mortality was 2.8%. Estrera and coworkers demonstrated that CSF drainage and left heart bypass produce beneficial effects by significantly lowering the incidence of neurologic deficits in comparison to patients operated on without adjunctive measures (1.3% versus 6.5%, $P < .02$) and undergoing nonemergency procedures.[35] In their experience, 30-day mortality was 8%. Patel and colleagues used hypothermic circulatory arrest and encountered 30-day mortality of 6% and permanent paralysis in 4.5%.[125] From the results of experienced centers it can be concluded that open surgical repair of DTAA is durable with a low incidence of morbidity, mortality, and secondary aortic interventions. Indeed, a recent consensus document from centers of excellence noted a mean 7.5% mortality with paraplegia occurring in less than 3% of patients.[126] However, recently published material from the National Inpatient Sample administrative database, perhaps more likely reflecting real-world experience, indicated an operative mortality of 10% for all intact DTAA repairs, but this figure increased to 17.6% in patients treated after the age of 75. Mortality with resection of ruptured DTAA was 45%.[127]

Comparison with Endovascular Repair

Recent multicenter studies comparing endovascular and open repair of DTAA report different results for open repair, and these might actually reflect the real-world results of surgical repair. Bavaria and coauthors reported on the results of the first completed multicenter trial directed at gaining approval from the U.S. Food and Drug Administration for endovascular versus open surgical repair of DTAA.[128] In the open surgical control cohort group, perioperative mortality was 11.7%, and spinal cord ischemia occurred in 14%, respiratory failure in 20%, and renal insufficiency in 13%. Unfortunately, details regarding surgical techniques were not described, and it is unknown whether protective measures such as CSF drainage and left heart bypass were applied. Nevertheless, this series probably represents the common practice of open DTAA repair, even more so in view of the fact that this trial was carried out in 16 major U.S. academic centers. Because there are now three published comparative trials of elective endovascular versus open repair for intact aneurysms of the descending thoracic aorta in patients who were candidates for either procedure physiologically, a realistic picture of the contemporary results of surgical DTAA repair is available. In these trials a total of 353 patients treated by open surgery were enrolled; 30-day operative mortality was 8.5%, evidence of any spinal cord ischemic complication was noted in 13%, and major paraplegia occurred in 5.1%. All these endpoints occurred at significantly higher rates in patients treated with open surgery than in those treated by endovascular repair.[128-130] (See also Chapter 133: Thoracic and Thoracoabdominal Aneurysms: Endovascular Treatment)

Thoracoabdominal Aortic Aneurysm

Because of the larger extent of aortic pathology requiring both thoracotomy and laparotomy, TAAA repair has significantly higher morbidity and mortality than isolated DTAA repair. Development of the aforementioned protective measures has contributed to improved surgical outcome; however, postoperative complications remain high. Only a few centers in the world are committed to this complex surgery, which entails substantial resources for infrastructure, equipment, and clinical research. The majority of published experience of open TAAA procedures comes from these specialized centers and does not represent common surgical practice for these complex aneurysms.

Morbidity and Mortality

When analyzing nationwide databases, it becomes apparent that the clinical outcome of open TAAA repair is rather disappointing. In an age-stratified study, Rigberg and associates determined 30-day and 1-year mortality for TAAA repair in 797 electively operated patients in the state of California and showed that 30-day mortality statistics do not really reflect the incidence of death after this procedure: overall mortality was 19% at 30 days and 31% at 1 year.[131] They found a steep increase in mortality with increasing age such that elective, 1-year mortality was 40% in octogenarians. These sobering mortality findings of a statewide database were also encountered by the single-center experience of Rectenwald and coworkers, who found a survival rate at 1 year of 67% and concluded that good functional outcome after TAAA repair is significantly less common than reported in the literature[132]; however their data were skewed by a rather high, nearly 20% operative mortality. Individual high-volume centers demonstrate better outcomes (Table 132-1) that vary between 6% and 10% mortality,[13,88,133-135] but it remains difficult to assess mortality in relation to aneurysm extent, preoperative morbidity, and postoperative complications. Cowan and colleagues addressed the impact of provider volume on surgical outcome of open TAAA repair and correlated annual hospital and surgeon volume with clinical results.[135] They analyzed the results of 1542 patients from 1988 to 1998 and obtained information from the Nationwide Inpatient Sample, which represents 20% of U.S. hospitals. Overall operative mortality for nonruptured aneurysms was 22% and improved over time.

Table 132-1 Thirty-Day Mortality after Thoracoabdominal Aortic Aneurysm Repair

Series	Year	Collective	Mortality (%)
Cowan et al.[135]	2003	Nationwide	22
Rigberg et al.[131]	2006	Statewide	19
Rectenwald et al.[132]	2002	Single center	20
Coselli et al.[133]	2002	Single center	5.7
Kouchoukos et al.[134]	2003	Single center	7.1
Conrad et al.[88]	2007	Single center	8.2

Mortality rates were significantly higher in low-volume hospitals (27% versus 15%) and when performed by low-volume surgeons (26% versus 11%). The authors therefore recommend centralization of these procedures. These clinical results could be poor because the sample was taken more than a decade ago and progress has since been achieved; however, the message of volume-related outcome will still remain. It should be emphasized that patient's outcome not only is determined by surgical skills but also greatly depends on an integrated team effort consisting of high-level anesthesia, extracorporeal support, neuroprotection and neuromonitoring, ICU management, and cardiopulmonary assistance.

Long-term Results

Late aortic-related events after TAAA repair can be defined as aortic disease causing death or necessitating further intervention or graft-related complications after hospital discharge, including infection, pseudoaneurysm, and branch occlusion. Clouse and coworkers analyzed 333 patients over a 15-year interval and reported event-free survival rates of 96% and 71% at 1 and 5 years, respectively.[136] Late aortic events occurred in 10% of patients, with the majority of them being repetitive aortic surgery for native aortic disease in remote or noncontiguous aortic segments. Graft-related complications were uncommon and degeneration of anastomoses was rarely encountered, thus illustrating the anatomic durability of TAAA repair.

Impact of Connective Tissue Disorders

The largest experience of TAAA repair in patients with Marfan's syndrome consists of 137 with confirmed and 163 with suspected Marfan's syndrome.[137] The 30-day mortality rate was 4.3%, and freedom from repair failure was significantly better in patients with confirmed (90% at 10 years) than in those with suspected (82% at 10 years, $P = .001$) Marfan's syndrome. Of these 300 patients, 31 had DTAA and 178 suffered from TAAA. Surgical mortality was less than 6%, and major complications included renal failure in 6% and neurologic deficit in 4%. The authors concluded that operative treatment of aortic pathology in patients with Marfan's syndrome provides excellent results and long-term survival. Dardik and colleagues demonstrated that patients with CTDs have similar perioperative and long-term survival rates after TAAA repair as do patients without CTDs.[138] Patients with CTD suffered from more extensive aneurysms (type I and II) and had an increased risk for paraparesis. In CTD patients, long-term CT surveillance showed no relative increase in aortic size and persistent freedom from recurrent aortic events. The postoperative cumulative 5-year survival rate of TAAA patients with and without CTDs was similar (53%). In our experience, mortality did not occur and major complications such as paraplegia, renal failure, stroke, and myocardial infarction were not encountered.[33] At 38 months' follow-up, all patients were alive and returned to work. Kalkat and associates demonstrated similar outcomes,[34] thus justifying the

conclusion that surgical repair of DTAA and TAAA provides excellent results in patients with Marfan's syndrome.

COMPLICATIONS

Cardiac

In general, morbidity is induced by the extensive tissue trauma and the effects of aortic clamping. Subsequently, complex pathophysiologic mechanisms are initiated that can lead to severe organ dysfunction and multiorgan failure. The direct relationship between aortic cross-clamp times and postoperative complications is well known. First, proximal clamping leads to increased cardiac pressure and stress with subsequent increased myocardial oxygen demand and consumption, which in patients with coronary artery disease can cause (lethal) myocardial infarction. The use of left heart bypass reduces afterload and contributes to fewer cardiac events. Preoperative coronary artery disease is common in that it occurs in 36% to 48% of patients.[31,88] Postoperative cardiac complications, reported in 12% to 25% of patients, include myocardial infarction, arrhythmia, congestive heart failure, and unstable angina.

Myocardial contractility may be depressed by surgical injury, hypothermic damage, anesthetic agents, deterioration of cardiopulmonary bypass function, or infarction. Surgical injury also includes manipulation of the left atrium, which can cause atrial fibrillation with subsequent hemodynamic instability and decreased organ perfusion during and after the procedure. Not only left heart failure but also right heart failure can occur during DTAA and TAAA repair as a result of previous cardiac surgery, coronary artery disease, or right ventricular hypertrophy. Right ventricular dysfunction should be treated by reduction of pulmonary vasoconstriction and maintenance of myocardial contractility.

Pulmonary

Respiratory failure is the most common complication and is probably inevitable after this operation. Svensson and associates prospectively evaluated 1414 patients and identified independent predictors for respiratory failure, defined as ventilatory support exceeding 48 hours: chronic pulmonary disease, history of smoking, and cardiac and renal complications.[139] Pulmonary complications requiring respiratory support with tracheostomy were observed in 112 patients (8%), and 40% of these patients died. The overall incidence of pulmonary complications in the most recent studies ranges between 32% and 49%.[31,88] In our experience, the incidence of any respiratory failure was reduced from 61% to 30%, coincident with avoidance of left hemidiaphragm paralysis. It is obvious that the left lung should be handled with utmost care, especially when it is collapsed. Direct trauma causing air leaks, subcutaneous emphysema, atelectasis, or bleeding will provoke respiratory failure, particularly in the circumstance of "redo" thoracotomy.

Pulmonary function can also be impaired by cytokine-induced multiple-organ dysfunction as part of a systemic inflammatory response to ischemia-reperfusion or the application of circulatory assist techniques.[140] Additional increased endotoxin release from the gastrointestinal (GI) tract can likewise contribute to organ dysfunction and respiratory failure.

The incidence of pulmonary complications after DTAA repair is lower, mainly because of the fact that the diaphragm is not transected and the procedure is less extensive than TAAA repair. Finally, for type IV TAAA, limited diaphragmatic incision and preservation of its phrenic innervation are nearly always feasible.

Renal

Postoperative renal failure predisposes to adverse outcomes. In patients undergoing TAAA repair, renal failure increases the risk for early death nearly 10-fold.[141] The main risk factors for the development of renal failure include aneurysm extent, ischemic time, and preoperative renal impairment. Kidney protection during TAAA operations has been the subject of clinical research for several decades. Besides distal aortic perfusion, two protective measures have proved to be of clinical value: cold crystalloid perfusion and normothermic blood perfusion. Köksoy and coworkers prospectively compared cold crystalloid perfusion and selective blood perfusion and found significantly higher acute renal dysfunction in the blood perfusion group.[113] Multivariate analysis confirmed that the use of cold crystalloid perfusion was independently protective against renal failure. In our experience, blood perfusion of the kidneys by means of selective catheters from side branches of the extracorporeal system provides excellent protection. However, because the kidneys are pressure-dependent organs, we continuously assess intrarenal pressure and keep the mean pressure at a minimal level of 60 mm Hg. Using this technique, renal failure requiring hemodialysis occurred in less than 2%.[98]

When assessing renal outcome it is important to describe the definition of postoperative renal dysfunction. Some define acute renal failure as an increase in serum creatinine (SCr) of 1 mg/dL/day (88 μmol/L/day) for 2 consecutive days or the need for hemodialysis. The glomerular filtration rate is an alternative method of evaluating kidney function. Kashyap and colleagues proposed the following differentiation of renal dysfunction[141]:

- SCr elevation less than 50% above baseline
- SCr elevation 50% to 100% above baseline
- Doubling of the SCr level, but a peak less than 3.0 mg/dL (265 μmol/L)
- Acute renal failure, that is, doubling of the SCr level and the level greater than 3.0 mg/dL
- Acute renal failure necessitating dialysis

Using these criteria, they reported renal failure in 11.5% of patients who underwent TAAA repair. More recently, the same center published their 20-year experience and reported any type of renal failure in 20.9% and renal failure requiring dialysis in 4.6% when using cold kidney preservation solution.[88] Coselli and colleagues assessed clinical outcomes after 2286 TAAA repairs and encountered overall renal failure requiring dialysis in 5.6% and 8.3% in those with type II TAAA.[31]

Gastrointestinal

GI complications after DTAA and TAAA procedures are reported rarely. Achouh and associates addressed 30-day GI complications in these patients and distinguished postoperative biliary disease, hepatic dysfunction, pancreatitis, GI bleeding, peptic ulcer disease, bowel ischemia, and ileus.[142] GI complications occurred in 7% of patients overall, and 30-day mortality was 39.5% in patients in whom GI complications developed, which was significantly higher than the 13.5% mortality in patients without GI complications. Postoperative biliary disease, hepatic dysfunction, and bowel ischemia were significantly associated with higher mortality. Bowel ischemia is the most frequent GI complication and is mainly due to embolization secondary to aortic manipulation, aortic cross-clamping, and associated atherosclerotic disease of the visceral arteries. The etiology of postoperative pancreatitis includes pancreatic trauma secondary to surgical dissection, perioperative resection of the spleen, hypoperfusion, and atheroembolization. Obviously, patients with DTAA are not exposed to abdominal surgery and therefore suffer less from GI complications than do patients undergoing TAAA.

Spinal Cord Injury

Immediate Paraplegia

Despite all described adjunctive measures, spinal cord injury persists. In open DTAA surgery, the combination of CSF drainage, distal aortic perfusion, and reimplantation of intercostal arteries has reduced spinal cord ischemia and subsequent paraplegia significantly. In centers of excellence, the incidence of immediate paraplegia ranges between 0% and 3% if surgery is performed with adjunctive procedures or clamp times are less than 30 minutes.[35,124,134] In TAAA patients these figures are entirely different. Current neurologic outcomes of TAAA repair focus on studies using adjunctive measures because the majority of surgeons have abandoned isolated simple clamp-and-sew techniques to overcome the damaging effects of prolonged ischemia, especially when exceeding 30 minutes' clamp time. Neurologic outcomes after extensive TAAA procedures vary tremendously and are mainly determined by preoperative risk factors, extent of the disease, and experience of the surgeon and center. Neurologic outcome is derived from highly dedicated and specialized centers and does not represent the results in general practice.

Using hypothermic cardiopulmonary bypass and circulatory arrest, Kouchoukos and associates treated 211 patients suffering from DTAA and TAAA without other adjunctive agents.[134] Of the 121 survivors with TAAA, paraplegia occurred in 2.6% with type I, in 4.1% with type II, and in 5.9% with type III aneurysms. Conrad and coworkers used epidural cooling in the majority of cases and a clamp-and-sew technique with adjuncts in 92%.[88] Patent intercostal arteries in the T9-L1 region were reimplanted and CSF drainage was routinely performed with maintenance of pressure at 10 mm Hg. In 455 patients they encountered major paraplegia in 9.5% and paraparesis in 3.7%. The overall incidence of neurologic deficits according to aneurysm extent was 15.7% with type I, 20.3% with type II, 14% with type III, and 2.9% with type IV aneurysms. In the extensive series of Coselli and colleagues, the overall incidence of paraplegia-paraparesis was 3.8%, with an 6.3% incidence in those with type II aneurysms.[31]

Etz and associates follow the protocol of systematic sacrifice of intercostal vessels based on evoked potential monitoring, and arteries are reimplanted only if the evoked potentials disappear.[143] Their surgical protocol included CSF drainage with maintenance of pressure below 10 mm Hg for 72 hours. In a series of 858 TAAA repairs they reported an overall paraplegia rate of 2.7%, and the authors hypothesized that spinal cord perfusion is maintained via collateral circulation. Clinical and angiographic studies have confirmed the importance of this collateral flow, mainly coming from the hypogastric circulation.[70]

In our experience with types I and II aneurysms under MEP monitoring, immediate paraplegia occurred in 2.7% of patients. However, when addressing only type II aneurysms, the paraplegia rate was 4.2%. It is noteworthy that we have not encountered any false-positive or false-negative MEP recordings in a series of more than 400 TAAA repairs.

Delayed Paraplegia

The exact incidence of delayed paraplegia is unknown; however, centers with a large TAAA experience indicate that approximately 25% of all spinal cord injuries are delayed.[144] Preoperative risk factors for delayed paraplegia are emergency procedures, type II aneurysms, number of sacrificed segmental arteries, and renal failure. The main postoperative risk factors include hemodynamic instability secondary to atrial fibrillation, bleeding, multiorgan failure, and sepsis.

Azizzadeh and colleagues could not identify a single risk factor, but the combination of lower mean arterial pressure and drain complications produced the highest odds ratio for neurologic deficit.[145] In our experience with patients in whom delayed paraplegia developed, perioperative problems with spinal cord perfusion were identified by MEP recording. In some patients complete loss of MEPs was encountered during surgery, and reattaching the intercostal arteries, increasing mean arterial pressure, and keeping CSF pressure below 10 mm Hg restored MEP amplitudes to approximately 10% of the initial level. Postoperative hypotensive phases caused irreversible damage and obviously infarcted the spinal cord. This finding indicates that spinal cord perfusion can be critically endangered but still sufficient to allow adequate anterior horn function, as shown by moving legs in an awake patient. However, arterial hypotension in these circumstances can provoke definite and permanent spinal cord infarction. It is therefore extremely important that postoperative management include adequate CSF drainage and optimal hemodynamic equilibrium with elevated mean arterial pressure.

It should be noted that spinal fluid drainage carries significant risks itself, such as subdural hematoma or intraspinal hemorrhage.[146,147]

Graft-Related

Graft-related complications occur rarely; however, aorto-esophageal and aortobronchial fistulae are well-known and feared events.

Aortobronchial or aortoesophageal fistulae seldom occur but can develop after thoracic aortic surgery. In literature many case reports or limited series are described, and therefore the incidence of these complications cannot be assessed.

In patients with an aortobronchial fistula the most common symptom is hemoptysis, which can be limited but also massive and fatal. Because of anatomic reasons the majority of fistulae are communications between the left bronchial tree and the descending aortic graft or anastomosis.[148] The interval between initial aortic surgery and manifestation of the fistula can vary considerably and range from years to decades.[149] This life-threatening situation requires rapid diagnosis and treatment.

The incidence of aortoesophageal fistulae is also unknown, but direct contact between the esophagus and aortic graft can always be shown. The close anatomic relationship between the descending thoracic aorta and esophagus explains the potential risk for fistulae, especially if anastomotic sutures injure or even include the esophagus. Massive GI bleeding can occur, and rapid diagnosis should be followed by prompt intervention. At present, as with postsurgical aortobronchial fistulae, the first option is endovascular coverage of the fistula; however, with esophageal fistulae, infection and recurrent bleeding appear to be a serious problem. Endovascular treatment can be performed as a lifesaving procedure and be considered as a bridge to final treatment, which if necessary, consists of esophageal resection and replacement of the aorta with a homograft or extra-anatomic aortic bypass from the ascending to the descending aorta.

◼ LATE SURVIVAL

Only few recent studies have addressed long-term outcomes after surgical repair of DTAA and TAAA. Generally, only high-volume centers report on late survival in a reliable statistical manner. Table 132-2 summarizes the survival rates of the most recent publications. In patients undergoing open DTAA repair, the survival rate is approximately 64% at 5 years and 35% at 10 years.[35,125,150]

In TAAA procedures, Coselli and colleagues have the largest experience and report an actuarial 5-year survival rate of 66% for repair of type II aneurysm, which was significantly lower than that after the other types (75.4%).[76] Other high-volume centers report 5-year survival rates of 53% after TAAA repair[138] and 54%, 29%, and 21% survival rates at 5, 10, and 15 years, respectively.[88] Miller and coworkers[151]

Table 132-2 Long-term Survival after Open DTAA and TAAA Repair

Series	Year	Disease	Mean Follow-up (yr)	Survival (%)
Patel et al.[125]	2006	DTAA	4	64
Estrera et al.[35]	2005	DTAA	5	64
			10	35
Coselli et al.[76]	2002	TAAA type II	5	66
Dardik et al.[138]	2002	TAAA	5	53
Conrad et al.[88]	2007	TAAA	5	54
			10	29
			15	21

DTAA, descending thoracic aortic aneurysm; TAAA, thoracoabdominal aortic aneurysm.

analyzed 1004 patients who underwent DTAA and TAAA procedures and compared their survival with the outcome of a population based-study published by Bickerstaff and colleagues.[39] This population-based epidemiologic study of the incidence and survival of patients with thoracic aneurysms was conducted over a 30-year period. The 5-year survival rate in the population-based cohort was 13%, as opposed to 61% in the treated group of Miller and associates, a difference of 48%, thus indicating that two patients need to be treated to prevent one death at 5 years.

Surveillance

After DTAA and TAAA repair, lifelong surveillance with imaging is necessary to assess subsequent aneurysm formation in the remaining native aortic tissue and the reattached side branches. Especially in patients with CTD, this native aortic tissue is prone to dilatation. Furthermore, anastomotic aneurysms can develop at suture lines and require open or endovascular repair if necessary. At present, thoracoabdominal aortic assessment can be performed entirely with MRI or CT, and the recommended frequency would be once per year in uncomplicated cases and more intensively in patients with morphologic changes.

SELECTED KEY REFERENCES

Conrad MF, Crawford RS, Davison JK, Cambria RP. Thoracoabdominal aneurysm repair: a 20-year perspective. *Ann Thorac Surg.* 2007;83: S856-S861; discussion S890-S892.
Extensive experience on the outcome of TAAA repair in a modern series.

Coselli JS, Lemaire SA, Köksoy C, Schmittling ZC, Curling PE. Cerebrospinal fluid drainage reduces paraplegia after thoracoabdominal aortic aneurysm repair: results of a randomized clinical trial. *J Vasc Surg.* 2002;35:631-639.
Randomized trial showing the important role of cerebrospinal fluid drainage.

Davies RR, Gallo A, Coady MA, Tellides G, Botta DM, Burke B, Coe MP, Kopf GS, Elefteriades JA. Novel measurement of relative aortic size predicts rupture of thoracic aortic aneurysms. *Ann Thorac Surg.* 2006;81:169-177.
Describes the lethal aspect of descending thoracic aneurysms and the importance of size measurements.

Griepp RB, Griepp EB. Spinal cord perfusion and protection during descending thoracic and thoracoabdominal aortic surgery: the collateral network concept. *Ann Thorac Surg.* 2007;83:S865-S869; discussion S890-S892.
Describes the role and importance of collateral blood flow to the spinal cord.

Jacobs MJ, Mess W, Mochtar B, Nijenhuis RJ, Statius van Eps RG, Schurink GW. The value of motor evoked potentials in reducing paraplegia during thoracoabdominal aneurysm repair. *J Vasc Surg.* 2006;43:239-246.
Technique of monitoring spinal cord integrity during TAAA repair.

Kouchoukos NT, Masetti P, Rokkas CK, Murphy SF. Hypothermic cardiopulmonary bypass and circulatory arrest for operations on the descending thoracic and thoracoabdominal aorta. *Ann Thorac Surg.* 2002;74:S1885-S1887; discussion S1892-S1898.
Profound hypothermia and circulatory arrest as a technique in TAAA repair.

Nijenhuis RJ, Jacobs MJ, Jaspers K, Reinders M, van Engelshoven JM, Leiner T, Backes WH. Comparison of magnetic resonance with computed tomography angiography for preoperative localization of the Adamkiewicz artery in thoracoabdominal aortic aneurysm patients. *J Vasc Surg.* 2007;45:677-685.
Novel techniques to visualize the spinal cord vasculature.

Rigberg DA, McGory ML, Zingmond DS, Maggard MA, Agustin M, Lawrence PF, Ko CY. Thirty-day mortality statistics underestimate the risk of repair of thoracoabdominal aortic aneurysms: a statewide experience. *J Vasc Surg.* 2006;43:217-222; discussion 223.
Describes surgical outcomes of TAAA repair in the "real world," outside centers of excellence.

Svensson LG, Crawford ES, Hess KR, Coselli JS, Safi HJ. Experience with 1509 patients undergoing thoracoabdominal aortic operations. *J Vasc Surg.* 1993;17:357-368; discussion 368-370.
Classic paper with surgical outcomes of TAAA repair in largest patient population ever published (until that time).

Wong DR, Coselli JS, Amerman K, Bozinovski J, Carter SA, Vaughn WK, LeMaire SA. Delayed spinal cord deficits after thoracoabdominal aortic aneurysm repair. *Ann Thorac Surg.* 2007;83:1345-1355; discussion 1355.
Addresses the issue of delayed paraplegia after TAAA repair.

REFERENCES

The reference list can be found on the companion Expert Consult Web site at *www.expertconsult.com*.

Section 17 Arterial Aneurysms

Thoracic and Thoracoabdominal Aneurysms: Endovascular Treatment

Jae Sung Cho and Michel S. Makaroun

Shortly after Parodi and colleagues' first report of endovascular abdominal aortic aneurysm repair (EVAR),[1] Dake and coworkers introduced the same concept of stent-graft exclusion for the thoracic aorta in December 1994.[2] The stent-grafts were custom-designed for each patient and were constructed of self-expanding stainless steel stents covered with woven Dacron grafts. Ten years later, thoracic endovascular aortic repair (TEVAR) for descending thoracic aortic aneurysms (DTAAs) became a mainstream technology with the release of commercial endografts starting with the TAG device (W. L. Gore and Associates, Flagstaff, AZ) in early 2005. Experimental work continues to be aimed at extending the same technique to thoracoabdominal aortic aneurysms (TAAAs). Many concepts had been explored until Chuter and associates used branched grafts in 2001 for the first total endovascular repair of TAAA with preservation of all four visceral arteries.[3-7]

In contrast to EVAR, which has been compared with open surgical alternatives in randomized controlled trials, most clinical information about TEVAR originates from industry-sponsored nonrandomized comparisons to open repair of DTAA, as well as single-center experiences or registry data that combine different pathologies and indications. Nonetheless, TEVAR has emerged as an attractive option for the treatment of DTAA and has shown very good early and midterm results.

■ APPROVED DEVICES FOR THORACIC ENDOVASCULAR AORTIC REPAIR

The pace of development of commercial stent-grafts for the thoracic aorta has lagged behind those for infrarenal abdominal aortic aneurysms (AAAs) because of a lower incidence of DTAA, the need for a larger device profile and delivery sheaths, the hostile hemodynamic forces in the thoracic aorta, and the proximity of the great vessels. Despite these hurdles, steady, albeit slow progress has been made, with several new thoracic devices being released or still undergoing testing. Three commercial devices have completed their regulatory trials and are currently approved for use in the United States, although many more are in use throughout the world. One other device (Relay, Bolton Medical, Inc., Sunrise, FL) is currently undergoing a phase II trial in the United States.

Detailed descriptions of these devices are provided in Chapter 90 (Aortic Stents and Stent-Grafts).

Gore TAG Device

The TAG endoprosthesis is made of an expanded polytetrafluoroethylene (ePTFE) tube re-enforced with an ePTFE/fluorinated ethylene propylene film and an external nickel-titanium (nitinol) self-expanding stent affixed to the graft with ePTFE/fluorinated ethylene propylene bonding tape (Fig. 133-1). This device deploys from the middle of the graft toward each end, a design characteristic intended to prevent a windsock effect at the proximal fixation zone. A circumferential PTFE sealing cuff is located at the base of each flared, scalloped end. The device is constrained by ePTFE tape that is released during deployment from the middle of the device toward both ends. Devices are currently available in 26- to 40-mm diameters and 10-, 15-, or 20-cm lengths, depending on the diameter. The device profile requires 20 Fr to 24 Fr introducer sheaths. A 45-mm-diameter device is under clinical testing. A minimum of a 2-cm neck is required for sealing on both ends, and 7% to 18% oversizing of the device in relation to the native aorta at that level is recommended. The currently available TAG device is a modification of the original device that was introduced when longitudinal wire frac-

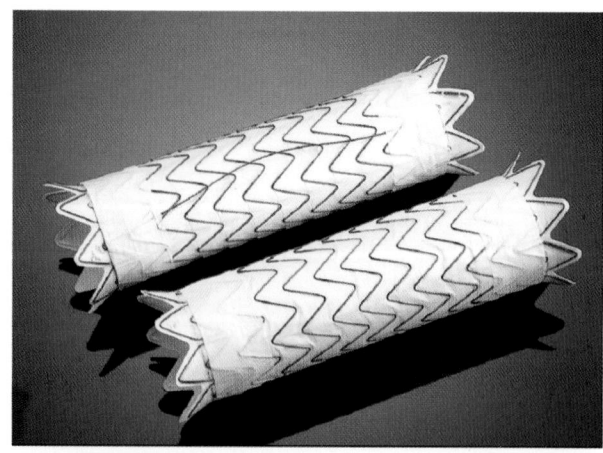

Figure 133-1 Gore TAG thoracic endoprosthesis with a longitudinal spine (*top*) and the modified device with the spine removed (*bottom*).

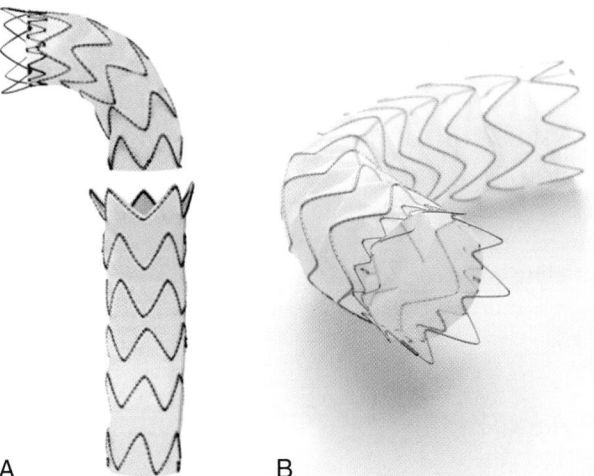

Figure 133-2 Medtronic Valiant stent-graft with increased (eight) stent peaks (**A**) versus the original Talent device with five stent peaks (**B**).

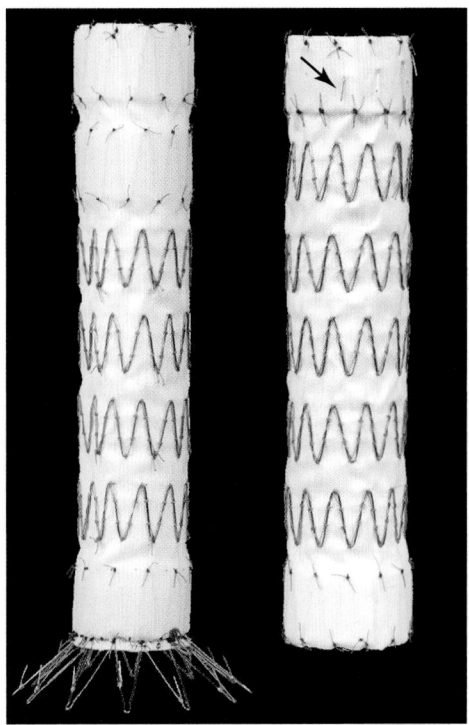

Figure 133-3 Cook TX2 device. Note the caudally oriented barbs intended to provide active fixation (*right, arrow*) at the proximal attachment site. On the *left*, the intended distal component of the intended two- piece construct has a distal bare-metal stent to prevent migration.

tures were discovered. It is constructed from three ePTFE layers to increase strength and reduce porosity.

Medtronic Talent Device

The "Talent" device (Medtronic, Santa Rosa, CA) is composed of a thin woven polyester fabric sewn to a self-expanding nitinol wire frame. The device comes in four different configurations: proximal main, proximal extension, distal main, and distal extension. The proximal stent-grafts and the distal extension are equipped with a bare spring (FreeFlo) to improve fixation and allow deployment across the origins of the great vessels proximally and the celiac axis distally. It has the widest assortment of device diameters, ranging from 22 to 46 mm. The range of lengths is just 112 to 116 mm. Ten percent to 20% oversizing in relation to the aortic neck is recommended, and a 2-cm sealing zone is required in the neck. Tapered grafts are also available to accommodate the differences in diameter along the length of the aorta. The grafts are loaded in a 20 Fr to 24 Fr delivery system. The Valiant device is a modified Talent without a longitudinal bar but with increased stent peaks and closed-web options. It is available in longer lengths of 22 cm and is currently undergoing clinical testing in the United States (Fig. 133-2).[8]

Cook Zenith TX2 Device

The Zenith TX2 is a two-piece modular graft made of woven Dacron fabric sewn to self-expanding stainless steel Z-stents. The stents are on the inside of the graft in the sealing zone but are on the outside in the rest of the endoprosthesis (Fig. 133-3). The device is available in diameters from 28 to 42 mm and in lengths from 120 to 216 mm. Active fixation is provided by barbs on both ends that are oriented caudad in the proximal sealing stent and directed craniad on a bare distal stent; these barbs are specifically intended to prevent graft migration and separation of components during conforma-

tional changes in the aneurysm after TEVAR. The device is contained in an introduction system 20 or 22 Fr in diameter that allows staged deployment. A minimum of a 3-cm landing zone is recommended.

THORACIC ENDOVASCULAR AORTIC REPAIR FOR DESCENDING THORACIC ANEURYSMS

Indications and Contraindications

The indication to treat a thoracic aneurysm depends on the size of the aneurysm, its rate of growth and location, and symptoms and general medical condition of the patient (see Chapter 131: Thoracic and Thoracoabdominal Aneurysms: Evaluation and Decision Making). Similar criteria should be applied for both open and endovascular repair and commonly include a size of 6 cm or larger, a saccular configuration, and symptomatic aneurysms, including rupture. The size recommendations are somewhat variable because no randomized trials exist to guide the decision-making process. The main considerations in the preferential choice of TEVAR over open repair are anatomic. An appropriate landing zone should be available both proximally and distally to allow sealing and exclusion of the aneurysm from the circulation, as well as appropriately sized arterial access to deliver the stent-graft to its desired location. Anatomy, however, is not the only overriding parameter in treatment planning; age and risk assessment also play a significant role in selecting the appropriate treatment modality.

In the presence of suitable anatomy, TEVAR seems to be the logical choice in most patients because of its lower morbidity and mortality. However, even in these patients, the decision should be tempered by the paucity of extended follow-up data for TEVAR and the requirement for lifelong clinical and imaging follow-up. Most current fatigue testing is carried out to 10 years based on International Standardization Organization recommendations. Consideration should be given to thoracotomy in young patients with long life expectancy and apparent low risk for open repair. For high-risk individuals, the decision is simple given that clinical results clearly favor an endovascular approach. As more long-term data become available, more liberal use of TEVAR in lower risk individuals may become easier to justify, particularly in light of the demonstrated significant perioperative reduction in risk with TEVAR (see later).[9] In the absence of level A or B evidence comparing the results of open repair of DTAA and TEVAR, lack of long-term durability data, and potential carcinogenic effects of the repeated radiation exposure necessary for graft surveillance, some investigators advocate TEVAR only when the predicted operative risk is clearly lower than the risk associated with conventional open repair.[10]

The majority of patients, however, do not have perfect anatomy for TEVAR, and the risk-benefit assessment becomes more complex. Many aneurysms impinge on a major arterial branch that must be occluded for adequate sealing. In these situations, the safety of such branch sacrifice must be balanced against further observation of the aneurysm or open repair. The alternative would be surgical bypass or "debranching" to maintain perfusion while extending the sealing zone, as reviewed later. The incremental risks of branch occlusion or the particular surgical bypass involved should be carefully evaluated when considering the TEVAR option and would be appropriate only in case of poor-risk individuals with large aneurysms. This category includes those with cardiac or pulmonary co-morbid conditions that would preclude safe open repair or those with acute manifestations or "high-risk" anatomic conditions such as previous thoracotomy.

Many relative contraindications to stent-graft treatment of DTAA exist. TEVAR should be contraindicated when the anatomy of the aneurysm prevents safe and effective performance of stent-graft exclusion of the DTAA because short- and long-term complication rates are increased in such cases. Aortic size outside the treatment range of available devices should be avoided. Severe tortuosity of the aneurysm or the access vessels can also increase morbidity. Severe aortoiliac occlusive disease, rapid taper of the aorta, and circumferential thrombus at the attachment sites all preclude the safe performance of TEVAR, so TEVAR should be avoided in the presence of these conditions. Severe angulation of the arch of greater than 60 degrees adjacent to the proximal portion of the aneurysm increases the difficulty of tracking and sealing at that level. Endovascular repairs should also be avoided in patients with life-threatening allergic reaction to intravenous contrast material or nickel, patients with significant chronic renal insufficiency (because of precipitation of end-stage renal failure), and those who cannot be monitored reliably.

Relevant Anatomy

Careful assessment of anatomy and meticulous preoperative planning are key to successful TEVAR. Although anatomic requirements can be device specific, adequate arterial access and sealing zones are essential for all. Several anatomic features, when present, may facilitate TEVAR or render it very difficult.

Iliac Anatomy

Most procedures use the common femoral artery as access to the aorta. Both lumen size and degree of tortuosity can have a profound impact on the procedure. The right iliac artery normally provides less of an angle at the aortic junction and thus is favored for device access, whereas the contralateral side is usually reserved for angiography catheters to control deployment. This, however, is not universally true, and individual assessment is required.

An ideal access channel would have a lumen of at least 8 mm to allow larger device sizes to be introduced when needed. The smallest diameter is typically in the proximal external iliac artery, an area that is also more prone to calcified plaque that can restrict delivery of the device. This is particularly the case in women, whose iliofemoral arteries tend to be smaller.[11] When the narrowest part at that level falls below the minimum size required for the planned device, access is generally shifted proximally to the common iliac artery by using an iliac conduit. Rarely, the entire iliac system is hostile to delivery of the device on both sides, and consideration can then be given to access through the distal aorta if the risks associated with thoracotomy are too significant.

The Aortic Channel

The abdominal aorta rarely presents an anatomic hindrance to delivery of the device, but tortuosity of the thoracic aorta can be challenging in the presence of aneurysmal disease because it is frequently associated with elongation and exaggeration of the normal curvatures of the aorta in the chest. As illustrated in Figure 133-4, this is particularly relevant in the case of a large descending thoracic aorta when cephalocaudad elongation causes exaggeration of the posteroanterior course of the aorta as it enters the aortic hiatus. This tortuosity, when combined with increased angulation at the transition from the arch to the proximal descending aorta, may result in difficulty tracking because of bending of the delivery catheter at flexion points as it negotiates severely angulated regions.

Aortic Sealing Zones

Adequate fixation of a stent-graft to both proximal and distal landing zones is essential for successful performance of TEVAR. To standardize comparisons, Ishimaru's group

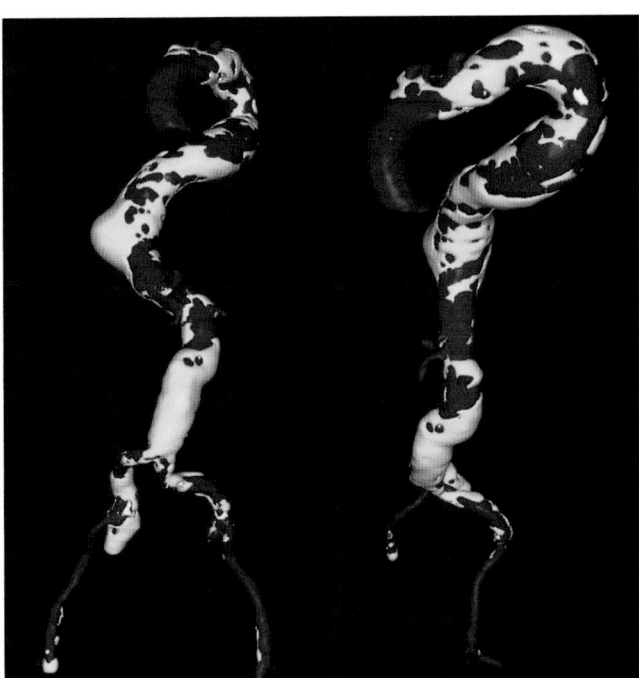

Figure 133-4 Three-dimensional reconstruction of the entire aortoiliac tree demonstrating tortuosity at the level of the aortic arch, descending thoracic aorta, abdominal aorta, and iliac arteries.

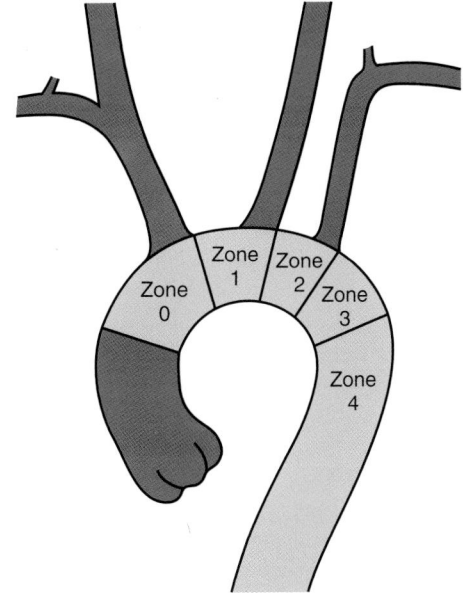

Figure 133-5 Five landing zones of the thoracic aorta.

classified the thoracic aorta into five landing zones (Fig. 133-5).[12] Each zone is bordered by a tangential line aligned with the distal sides of each great vessel. Zone 0 involves the origin of the innominate artery; zone 1, the origin of the left common carotid artery (CCA); zone 2, the origin of the left subclavian artery (SA); zone 3, the proximal descending thoracic aorta down to the T4 vertebral body; and zone 4, the remainder of the descending thoracic aorta. Atherosclerotic aneurysms are typically not limited to one focal area, and the degenerative process usually involves the apparently normal adjacent aorta. This is important in selection of landing zone

length. Although 2 to 3 cm is considered adequate for various devices, a longer seal zone may be preferable, especially at angulated areas to decrease the occurrence of late endoleaks and to protect from late aneurysmal degeneration. This urge to cover more aorta, however, should be tempered by the increased risk for spinal cord ischemia (SCI) with excessive coverage. The landing zone should ideally be parallel in configuration and distal to the left SA (zones 3 and 4) and proximal to the celiac artery (Fig. 133-6). This results in the best outcomes. A sealing zone in a curved portion of the aorta, generally near the left SA (zones 2 and 3), presents added complexity. The longitudinal stiffness of the devices often prevents complete apposition to the inner curve. The minimum sealing length at that zone should apply to the shorter inner curve length rather than the longer outer curve. The proximity of the sealing zones to major branches should be carefully evaluated to avoid occlusion of a necessary artery, or alternatively, a bypass should be planned to maintain patency of the branch. The decision whether to revascularize the left SA is discussed under "Management of the Left Subclavian Artery."

Operative Planning and Options

Imaging

Preoperative planning begins with imaging studies to delineate the anatomic morphology of the aneurysm, its relationship to adjacent arch and mesenteric vessels, and the availability of access vessels. The primary modality for such planning is computed tomographic angiography (CTA), which has mostly supplanted the additional use of catheter angiography in preoperative planning and is capable of providing all preoperative anatomic information. Although fine reconstructions (<2.5 mm) from older-generation scanners are acceptable, the 64-slice computed tomography (CT) scanner is the latest technology and provides fine definition and very fast scan times. It also offers three-dimensional volume rendering, as well as maximum intensity projections and sagittal and coronal reconstructions, which aid in the analysis of angles and relationships to adjacent vessels. Third-party software companies such as M2S (Medical Metrx Software, West Lebanon, NH), Vitrea (Vital Images, Minnetonka, MN), and Aquarius (TeraRecon, Inc, San Mateo, CA) offer additional tools such as reconstructions orthogonal to the line of flow and virtual grafts to aid in measurements and procedure planning. When patients cannot undergo CTA because of severe allergies or renal failure, gated magnetic resonance angiography (MRA) can be substituted for additional information and is usually added to a CT scan without contrast enhancement.

The preoperative CTA should include the chest, abdomen, and pelvis with and without contrast enhancement to fully evaluate the access vessels, as well as the extent of calcification and angulation throughout. Tortuosity is best delineated by a three-dimensional reconstruction. Qualitative evaluation of arch disease for atheromatous burden, as well as the vertebral arteries, is critical to minimize the risk for cerebral ischemic complications when proximal extension

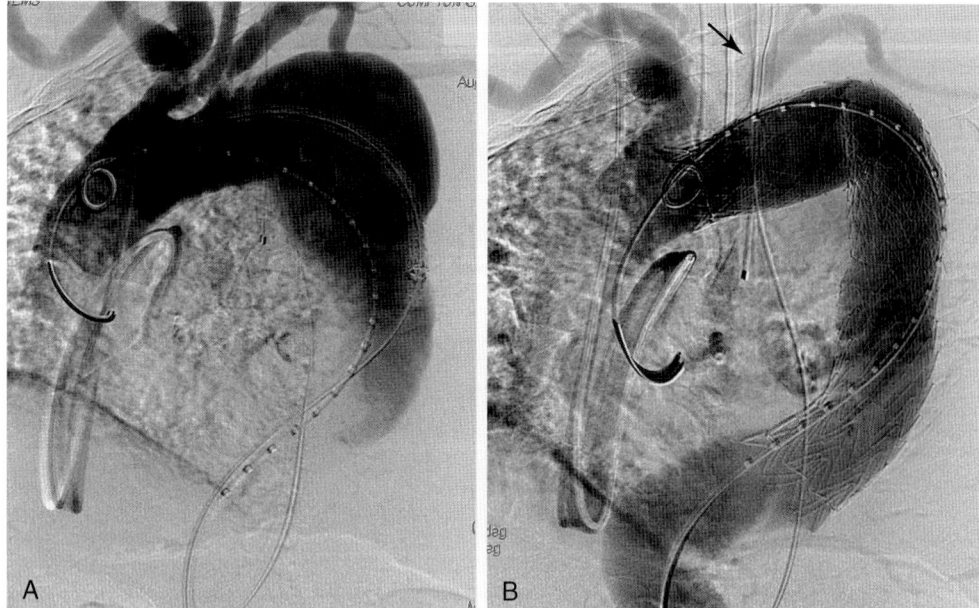

Figure 133-6 A, Operative thoracic aortography demonstrating a large thoracic aortic aneurysm. Note the parallel proximal and distal landing zones. **B,** Completion aortography showing the thoracic endograft deployed proximal to the left subclavian artery with completion exclusion of the aneurysm. Note the retrograde filling of the left subclavian artery without endoleak (*arrow*).

into zone 2 is planned. This can be achieved by extracranial imaging with CTA or MRA and less often by catheter angiography. Determination of pelvic flow can be critical in assessing perfusion to the spinal cord, especially in patients in whom a prior aortic reconstruction exists or when anticipating coverage of a long segment of aorta or the left SA without revascularization.

Sizing

Accurate measurements of the diameter of the access vessels and the sealing zones are important to determine the feasibility of the procedure and appropriate graft sizes, which are typically oversized by 10% to 20%, depending on manufacturers' recommendations. These recommendations should be followed closely because they form the range in which fatigue testing of the stent-grafts was performed in the preclinical assessment phase. Too small a stent-graft can result in an endoleak or migration, whereas excessive oversizing may cause infolding, poor sealing because of gutter formation and excessive radial force with accelerated degeneration of the neck, and possibly earlier material failure. Diameters are best measured on reconstructions orthogonal to the line of flow, especially in areas of tortuosity and angulation, to avoid erroneous measurements. If reconstructions are not available, the short axis is a reasonable estimate of the true diameter, particularly in zone 4.[13] Neck diameters between the proximal and distal sealing zones can be different, which may lead to inappropriate oversizing on the smaller end. Strategies for overcoming this problem include the use of tapered grafts or shorter devices deploying a larger device inside the smaller one to prevent a type III endoleak.

Appropriate length measurements are also necessary to estimate the required device lengths. This is difficult in the thoracic aorta because the aorta moves posterolaterally in its proximal portion and anteromedially near the diaphragm. The presence of a DTAA exacerbates this native tortuosity and adds complexity in that the aorta and aneurysm have both inside and outside measurements that can be different from each other. The best estimate of length is a centerline flow measurement from a three-dimensional reconstruction, although this will commonly underestimate the length of endografts needed because the graft will tend to gravitate toward the greater curvature, especially when a large cavity exists in the aneurysm sac.

Selection of Access

Planning for access clearly depends on device size and access arteries. With TEVAR requiring large device sizes and with DTAA being more prevalent than infrarenal AAA in women,[14] an iliac conduit is often needed, typically in 15% of patients, and is better done prophylactically than after an iliac artery injury.[15]

Identification of Landing Zones

The lack of adequate landing zones both proximally and distally is encountered frequently. Extension into zone 2 to achieve adequate sealing proximally was required at least 20% of the time in some regulatory trials.[15] The decision to cover the left SA or bypass it has undergone a substantial shift over the years. Although all early cases underwent a left carotid–subclavian bypass or transposition, later reports of safe coverage resulted in indiscriminate coverage of the left SA.[16-20] Recently, however, renewed interest in preserving flow in the left SA developed after reports of brainstem stroke and increased risk for SCI or severe arm ischemia.[21,22]

Management of the Left Subclavian Artery

The left SA is an important vessel for perfusion of both the spinal cord and the brain via the left vertebral artery (VA).[23] It also provides blood flow to the spinal cord via the internal mammary and its anterior intercostal branches.[24] When feasible, it should be preserved during TEVAR when deploying a stent-graft at or near the left SA. Placing a transbrachial left SA access wire in these situations can be helpful. It can serve as a guide for safe and precise deployment of the device at the level of the left SA and as a rescue procedure to restore flow should inadvertent coverage of the vessel occur. It can also be used for retrograde salvage of the left SA[25] or embolization at completion of the procedure to prevent a type II endoleak after intentional coverage of the vessel.

Although coverage of the left SA is generally well tolerated because of a rich collateral network,[16-20,26] routine exclusion should be discouraged because both experimental and clinical evidence suggests that not all patients can tolerate the occlusion safely.[26-28] Frequently, however, deployment of a stent-graft into zone 2 is necessary to achieve a proximal seal in the absence of an acceptable landing zone distal to the left SA. Prophylactic left SA revascularization was performed routinely during the early regulatory trials to avoid potential neurologic or upper extremity ischemic complications (Fig. 133-7).[29] The procedure, however, adds an operative intervention with its attendant risks. In addition to death and stroke, recurrent laryngeal and phrenic nerve injuries, as well as thoracic duct injuries, have been reported.[21,30]

When reconstruction is undesirable, careful preoperative imaging should be performed to assess the patency of the right VA into the basilar artery, as well as the circle of Willis, to identify patients who cannot tolerate left SA occlusion. Others can safely undergo coverage as an initial intervention with later revascularization if necessary. Mandatory left SA revascularization is indicated in the presence of a dominant left VA, a patent left internal mammary bypass to a coronary artery, an aberrant right SA, a hypoplastic right VA, or an anomalous origin of the left VA from the arch.[21,26,31] Revascularization should also be considered when an elevated risk for paraplegia exists with extensive coverage of the thoracic aorta combined with previous infrarenal aortic replacement.

Coverage without revascularization has been linked to an increased risk for SCI in a recent review of EuroSTAR (European Collaborators on Stent/Graft Techniques for Aortic Aneurysm Repair) registry data.[22] The incidence of left SA occlusion without revascularization was significantly higher in those with SCI (40%) than in those without (19%). On multivariate analysis, left SA coverage without revascularization was an independent predictor of SCI with an odds ratio of 3.49. A Northwestern series also indicates the importance of selective left SA revascularization when its coverage is necessary.[21] In a series of 30 patients with left SA coverage, 22 with and 8 without periprocedural left SA revascularization, a 63% incidence of acute complications (stroke and subclavian steal syndrome) was noted in patients without left SA reconstruction, whereas only one delayed paraparesis and two vocal cord palsies occurred in those with left SA transposition/bypass grafting. Delayed revascularization can usually be performed in cases of arm ischemia without untoward effects.[21,31] Revascularization of the left SA may be performed by either left CCA–to–left SA bypass grafting or left SA–to–left CCA

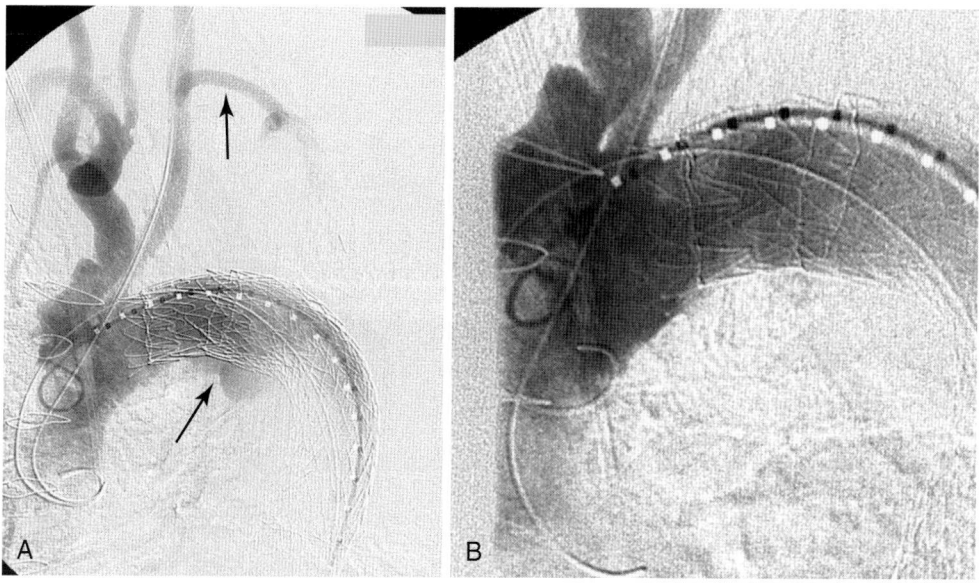

Figure 133-7 A, Left subclavian transposition to the left common carotid artery (*top arrow*) to lengthen the proximal landing zone. Note type I endoleak with filling of the aneurysm sac (*bottom arrow*). **B,** The endoleak resolved after secondary ballooning.

transposition. Although transposition eliminates any source of type II endoleak, it is more difficult and less desirable in these situations because the left SA can be aneurysmal or distorted by the proximity of the descending thoracic aorta; furthermore, preservation of the posteriorly located VA can be difficult, and for this reason most surgeons favor carotid-to-subclavian bypass grafting (see Chapter 117: Upper Extremity Arterial Disease: Revascularization) with ligation of the left SA proximal to the left VA. This also obviates any potential for retrograde type 2 endoleak.

Management of the Celiac Axis

If the distal landing zone is inadequate, the operator faces similar options as with the left SA. When adequate collateral circulation between the celiac axis and superior mesenteric artery (SMA), especially through the gastroduodenal artery, is ascertained by preoperative angiography, the celiac axis may be covered safely to extend the distal landing zone during TEVAR.[32] Criado and coworkers observed no mesenteric ischemic complications with three cases of celiac axis coverage.[11] Vaddineni and associates recently reported seven such cases without any mesenteric or spinal ischemic complications.[33] If the collateral network is not adequate, a bypass to the celiac circulation must be provided before occlusion. At the 2008 annual meeting of the Society for Vascular Surgery, Darling and colleagues presented their series of 21 patients with celiac axis coverage during TEVAR.[34] They observed one fatal hepatic ischemic complication in a patient who had no demonstrable SMA-celiac collaterals, but no late complications were noted. They concluded that celiac coverage can be performed safely in the presence of SMA-celiac collaterals.

Adjunctive Measures for Neuroprotection

As reviewed later, TEVAR is not without risk for SCI complications, and there is consensus that patients with long-segment descending thoracic aortic coverage and antecedent or concomitant abdominal aortic grafting are at particular risk. In such circumstances adjuncts are often used, albeit without a firm evidence base. Such techniques have been evaluated mostly during open repair of TAAA. For a more detailed discussion the reader is referred to Chapter 132 (Thoracic and Thoracoabdominal Aneurysms: Open Surgical Treatment).

One of the most commonly used adjuncts with TEVAR is drainage of cerebrospinal fluid (CSF). Although some use it routinely, most centers use it selectively in patients with an elevated potential for paraplegia, such as extensive coverage of the thoracic aorta and association with abdominal aortoiliac pathology. The drain is typically inserted preoperatively and maintained for around 48 hours while keeping pressure less than 10 cm H_2O. The advantage of selective drain use with TEVAR relates to an obligatory intensive care unit admission, but it is also desirable for arterial line monitoring and maintenance of relative hypertension. The incidence of hemor-

rhagic complications from catheter placement is also not negligible, and such complications are reported in 0% to 3% of patients.[35] Regardless of whether it is used preoperatively, CSF drainage has been shown to be effective in reversal of delayed-onset paraplegia after TEVAR and should be used whenever SCI is suspected.[36]

Besides the anatomic features noted earlier, hemodynamic stability seems to play a pivotal role in spinal cord protection because the underlying pathology appears to be poor collateral flow and decreased perfusion of the spinal cord. A low mean intraoperative arterial blood pressure of 70 mm Hg or less has been linked to SCI in one review.[36] Except for the short time required for endograft deployment, when relatively low blood pressure may be beneficial, an elevated pressure is preferred intraoperatively. Similar to the open DTAA repair paradigm, postoperative hypotension has been noted to precipitate SCI events in patients after TEVAR.

Of pharmacologic adjuncts, naloxone has been studied the most. Intravenous naloxone has been shown to be effective in decreasing circulating levels of excitotoxic amino acids and antagonizing opiate-mediated spinal cord vasoconstriction after open TAAA repair. Its beneficial effects have been observed in open procedures,[37,38] and it may be used in selected cases of TEVAR.

The importance of the artery of Adamkiewicz, which is usually located between T8 and L2, has been debated extensively but has not clearly been linked to SCI. The EuroSTAR review found an association between T10 coverage and SCI: 40% of patients with SCI exhibited T10 occlusion, and only 18% of this 40% did not suffer periprocedural paraplegia or paraparesis.[22] The association, however, was no longer present on multivariate regression analysis. Accordingly, no recommendation can yet be made to avoid covering the T10 region with a stent-graft; the variable origin of this vessel along the length of the thoracic aorta and its multiple contributing collateral vessels form the essence of this position.

Operative Technique
Access

Once the side for entry is chosen based on preoperative imaging, the ipsilateral common femoral artery is exposed via standard surgical technique or is accessed percutaneously after a Perclose suture technique.[39] The contralateral artery is accessed percutaneously for placement of a marker pigtail catheter. Once access is established, a stiff wire (Lunderquist or Meier) is placed in the ascending aorta. It is helpful to mark the back end of the wire on the table to detect any unintentional movement of the wire with potential loss of wire access.

When a conduit is needed, it is constructed through a small retroperitoneal incision in the ipsilateral lower quadrant. A 10-mm Dacron graft is anastomosed to the distal common iliac artery in end-to-side fashion (Fig. 133-8). A large-diameter conduit is needed to accommodate the use of larger sheaths, as well as an additional catheter and wire if access to the contralateral artery is to be avoided. It can be used through that incision or, in large individuals, can be brought out

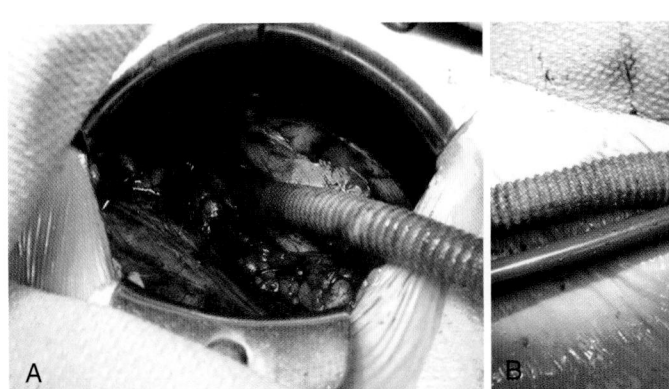

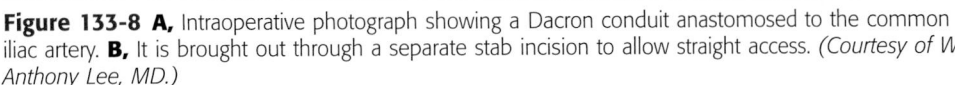

Figure 133-8 A, Intraoperative photograph showing a Dacron conduit anastomosed to the common iliac artery. **B,** It is brought out through a separate stab incision to allow straight access. *(Courtesy of W. Anthony Lee, MD.)*

through a separate stab incision in the lower part of the abdomen or the groin to allow straight access to the iliac artery. It is best to introduce the sheath or catheter through a stab incision in the graft rather than through the open end of the conduit. This provides stability of the sheath during later manipulations. At the end of the procedure, the conduit may be transected at the base or converted to an iliofemoral bypass graft if the femoral pulse is weak or if the external iliac artery had been damaged by earlier attempts at using it for access. The latter would also allow easier access during future interventions, if necessary. This procedure can be done expeditiously, without excessive prolongation of operative time.

Placement of a guide wire or catheter into the celiac axis or SMA, when the celiac axis is to be covered, can serve as a reference guide. In the event that imprecise deployment results in encroachment on the celiac axis or SMA, it can provide ready access to the vessel for possible stent placement. Similarly, the left SA can also be accessed via the left brachial artery to provide access should restoration of flow to the left SA be required, as mentioned earlier.

Imaging and Control of Deployment

Aortography is then performed through a marker pigtail catheter with an appropriate left anterior oblique projection of the image intensifier when the proximal zone is close to the arch. For visualization of the distal landing zone, especially near the celiac axis, a full lateral projection allows the best view. The angiogram serves to locate important branches and landmarks, as well as help confirm the estimated lengths of graft required. As with other methods, this too underestimates the exact length needed. The same information can be obtained by intravascular ultrasound (IVUS) if the patient cannot tolerate significant doses of contrast material. Transesophageal echocardiography (TEE) can also be helpful,

Delivery

Once the landing zones are visualized, the chosen stent-graft is introduced via the delivery catheter/sheath under fluoro-

scopic guidance. The device is usually advanced past the target region and brought back to the target line to eliminate any stored forward energy. Application of steady forward pressure on the wire tends to keep it pushed against the outer curvature of the aorta for more accurate estimation of deployment targets.

Tortuosity of the iliac system can generally be handled with stiff wires, and the newer hydrophilic delivery systems make it less of an issue. Telescoping of the iliac on the stiff delivery system, however, may limit the ability to torque the device and increase the chance for iliac injury. On occasion, excessive tortuosity of the external iliac may best be handled through a more proximal access in the common iliac artery. Acute angles in the descending thoracic aorta may render device tracking very difficult. Various strategies, such as buddy wires, long sheaths, or distal graft deployment first, may be used to negotiate these areas. If this fails, a brachiofemoral wire allows better tracking and delivery of the device to its target. This can be achieved by snaring a long soft glidewire in a relatively healthy proximal aortic zone, introduced via access from the right brachial artery for zone 2 deployment or from one side for more distal landing zones. Once the wire is snared, a long catheter is placed over the wire across the aortosubclavian junction to avoid possible dissection or tearing at this location. The glidewire is then brought through the femoral vessel and exchanged for a Lunderquist wire. When the right brachial artery is used, greater precautionary measures should be taken because the wire is positioned across the great vessels and can result in cerebral embolic complications.

Deployment

When more than one device is being used, the smaller one should be deployed first to allow sealing at the overlap zone. If both are of the same size, strategies depend on the tortuosity of the aorta, and a longer overlap zone should be planned to decrease the chance for a type III endoleak. When more than two devices are needed, the proximal and distal landing zones may be treated first, with the third larger device bridging the gap between the two. For large proximal aneurysms, distal deployment first may be preferable because it stabilizes the proximal graft and allows more accurate placement.

Deployment of the stent-graft follows the instructions for use of each particular device. Strategies for accurate placement are device specific, but all benefit from a temporary reduction in mean arterial pressure to decrease the windsock effect that may result in placement of the endograft more distally than desired. The Talent device is the most susceptible to this effect because it is exposed one stent at a time from proximal to distal. Both adenosine-induced cardiac arrest and rapid pacing of the heart have been used to reduce the high flow rate in the thoracic aorta and improve the accuracy of deployment, but they are rarely necessary in most procedures. Avoiding excessively slow deployment and maintaining forward force on the wire may be helpful. The entire deployment procedure should be performed under fluoroscopic guidance.

The Cook TX2 deploys in a staged fashion with the proximal sealing stent still partially constrained until the device is positioned at the target zone. The TAG device is deployed by releasing the constraining sleeve by turning and pulling the deployment knob, which is a continuation of a deployment line connected to the sleeve. The device is deployed rapidly from the middle toward both ends of the graft. Balloon inflation is used to mold the sealing zones to the aorta and improve apposition at the overlap zones. Because the Talent and TX2 are completely contained in their delivery sheaths, these sheaths must be exchanged between every device placement. The TAG device is introduced through a separate sheath, thus obviating the need for entire sheath exchanges between introductions of multiple stent-grafts, provided that an appropriate sheath size was chosen for the largest device to be used.

Completion angiography is used to confirm accurate placement, as well as the absence of endoleaks (Fig. 133-9). Types I and III endoleaks should be corrected by additional ballooning or extensions as appropriate for each situation. Care

should be exercised when removing the sheath because iliac injury and tearing can still occur at this stage. Using the sheath dilator before withdrawal may help, but maintaining wire access is paramount inasmuch as serious iliac injuries can lead to sudden severe bleeding and hypotension. A pelvic angiogram may be useful after the sheath has been pulled to the distal external iliac artery to evaluate the integrity of the iliac system. Balloon control of the bleeding vessel and even repair of the injury with a stent-graft can be lifesaving procedures.[40]

Results

Despite a large body of literature on the subject in the last 5 years, no randomized trials have compared TEVAR with open surgery for the treatment of DTAA. The availability of late results is limited, and what exists does yet not completely reflect the rapid evolution of devices, refinement in delivery systems, and maturation of both institutional and general learning curves. Most single-center and registry reports include a mixture of anatomic locations, stent-graft types, and varying degrees of urgency, which makes the evaluation of results somewhat difficult. Similar shortcomings are common in the open surgical literature on the topic and prevent accurate comparisons of mortality and morbidity between the two modalities. This is exaggerated by the typically low-risk patients in surgical series, with most patients undergoing TEVAR in such studies usually being in a higher risk category. The proportion of patients falling in the "unfit for open surgery" category ranges from 28% to 77%,[22,41-43] and the proportion in American Society of Anesthesiologists class IV or higher ranges from 16% to 52%.[11,44-46]

The U.S. Food and Drug Administration (FDA) pivotal trials of the three approved devices (TAG, TX2, and Talent) thus provide the best insight on the safety and efficacy of TEVAR because they include a rigid follow-up of a uniform well-defined population. Table 133-1 summarizes results up to 1 year from the three regulatory trials, as well as one large registry from Europe.[15,29,46-50] Patients in the FDA trials were

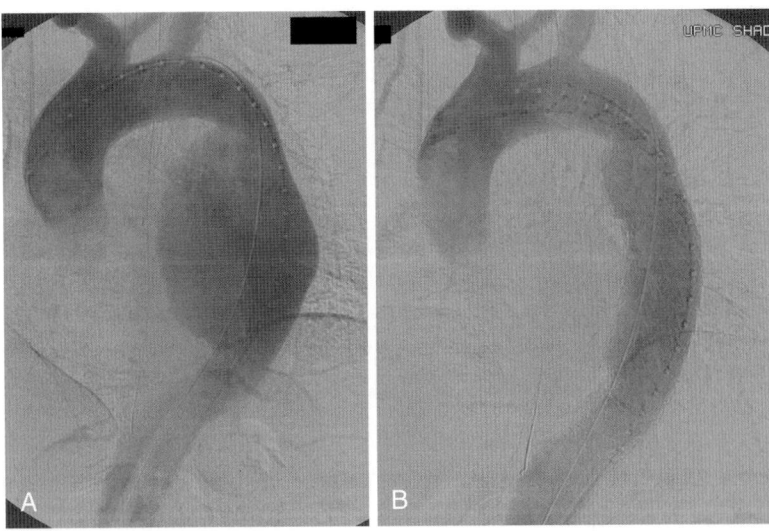

Figure 133-9 A, Intraoperative angiogram showing a large fusiform descending thoracic aortic aneurysm. **B,** Two TAG stent-grafts are deployed to exclude the aneurysm. The aneurysm is well excluded without an endoleak.

Table 133-1 Summary of Results from Three Regulatory Trials and One Large Registry from Europe

	FDA Regulatory Trials				
	Trials			**Combined Open Repair Controls from the Trials**	**EuroSTAR + U.K. Registry***
	Gore TAG Study	*STARZ*	*Valor Medical*		
Stent-graft	TAG	TX2	Talent	—	Multiple
Number of patients	140	160	195	353	249
Males	58%	72%	59%	54%	74%
Mean age (yr)	71	72	70	68	71
Aneurysm (mean size, mm)	DTAA (64)	DTAA (61)	DTAA (55)	63[†]	DTAA + arch (66)
Risk	Good risk	Good risk	Good risk	Good risk	Combined
Type	Elective	Elective	Elective	Elective	75% Elective
Period	1999-2001	2004-2006	2003-2005	—	1997-2003
Procedural Events					
Technical success rate	98%	98.8%	99.5%	N/A	87%
>1 device	56%	59%	>90% (Est)	N/A	66%
Conduit used	15%	9.4%	21%	N/A	16.4%
Deployment zone 2	20%	13.2%	10%-25% (Est)	N/A	17%
LSA revascularization	20%	3.2%	5.2%	N/A	9%
EBL (mL)	250	216	371	2510	—
Hospital stay (days)	3.0	5.0	6.4	14.8	—
Early Results (30 Days)					
Mortality[‡]	1.5%	1.9%	2.1%	7.1 %	5.3%, elective only
SCI (paraplegia/paraparesis)	2.8% (2/2)	5.6% (2/7)	8.7% (3/14)	13.0%	4%
Stroke	3.5%	2.5%	3.6%	6.7%	2.8%
MAE[§]	28%	41.9%	30%	77.3%	—
Vascular complications[§]	14%	22%	9.2%	16.3%	2.4%
Endoleak at 30 days[∣]	3.6%	4.8%	25.9%	N/A	9.2%
Results at 1 Year					
Sac size increase >5 mm[∣]	9%	7.1%	8.5%	N/A	14.6%
Endoleak[∣]	3.9%	3.9%	12.2%	N/A	4.2%
Migration >10 mm	0.7%	2.8%	3.9%	N/A	—
Aneurysm-related survival (KM)	97%	94.2%	96.9%	89%	93% (Est)
All-cause survival (KM)	83%	91.6%%	83.9%	82%	80%
Ruptures	0	0	0.5%	—	0.4%
Reinterventions[¶]	2.1%	4.4%	10.7%	3.7%[†]	5.2%
Conversion	0.7%	0	0.5%	N/A	—
Device integrity issues	12.8%**	0	2%	N/A	—
Thrombosis	0	0	0	0	—

*Combination EuroSTAR and U.K. registry. Patients before 2000 were entered retrospectively. Only the subset of atherosclerotic aneurysms is included here.
[†]Based on the data from TAG and STARZ control patients.
[‡]Thirty-day mortality is reported in the table. Operative mortality, which includes in-hospital deaths beyond 30 days, is higher, especially in the open surgical group.
[§]The definition of adverse events and major complications is variable between studies.
[∣]Source: Core laboratory for STARZ and Valor Medical, investigators for Gore TAG.
[¶]Only repeat interventions on the thoracic aorta are included.
**Longitudinal wire fractures in the original TAG with no significant clinical events. A wire is no longer present in the marketed modified TAG.
DTAA, descending thoracic aortic aneurysm; EBL, estimated blood loss; Est, estimated value from text; KM, Kaplan Meier estimate; LSA, left subclavian artery; MAE, major adverse event; N/A, not available; SCI, spinal cord ischemia; STARZ, Study of Thoracic Aortic Aneurysm Repair with the Zenith TX2 Thoracic TAA Endovascular Graft.

good-risk surgical candidates operated on electively. The European registry is more typical of general practice, with emergency procedures, variable risk, and more diffuse anatomy including more proximal arch disease in 13% of patients. Combined results from open surgery control arms of the three trials are listed. Reporting standards were defined by the Ad Hoc Committee of the Society for Vascular Surgery (SVS)/ American Association for Vascular Surgery (AAVS) in 2002.[51] Unfortunately, not all reports follow the guidelines accurately because of different study design, endpoint definition, and method of data collection. In general, technical success is defined as delivery of the device to the intended location with satisfactory exclusion of the aneurysm and no type I or II endoleaks. Clinical success adds the outcomes of aneurysm-related deaths, rupture, endoleaks, and re-intervention.

Technical Results

The demographics and early results are remarkably similar in all three FDA trials. Male gender dominates in all TEVAR series and accounts for 60% to 70% of patients. The "gender gap" is less prominent than in patients with AAAs because more patients with DTAA are women (40% to 45%) and more are judged to be TEVAR candidates (30% to 40%). The average age at intervention was 71 years. The average aneurysm size was larger than 6 cm in all but one trial. Definitions, procedures, and inclusion criteria were not identical among the studies, thus making blanket comparison of outcomes inappropriate. With minor differences, demographic parameters, as well as risk factors, were in general well matched between the endovascular arms and the control groups.

Successful completion rates of the TEVAR procedure were very high in all three studies (98%) as a result of the expected success when disciplined patient selection and adherence to recommended anatomic requirements are followed, as are typically enforced in most FDA trials. All failures were access-related when reported. Though still respectable, the registry shows a lower degree of technical success because of more liberal use of endografts in clinical practice outside the limits of clinical testing and a more rigid definition of success. The incidence of conduit use was high, ranging from 10% to 20%, averaging nearly one in seven patients. Most of the conduits were to the common iliac artery but a few were to the aorta. Failure to use a conduit or accessing the aorta was the cause of all technical failures in the regulatory trials.

The number of devices used per patient depends on the length of the pathologic area, the length of the devices available, and the tapering requirements of different aortic diameters. Even with long devices that are not tapered, 56% of patients still required more than one device to properly cover the aneurysm and the additional required sealing zones (TAG). Although the Valor trial did not report that statistic, the shortest aneurysm length treated was 8 cm, and because of the additional minimum landing zones of 4 cm and the longest length of devices available, essentially all cases required more than one device, with an average of 2.7 per case. The modified Valiant device will be available in longer lengths, so single devices can be used in many cases.

Use of zone 2 for proximal sealing is common, performed in 15% to 20% of cases because of the high incidence of proximal TAAAs without an acceptable landing zone distal to the left SA. The Valor trial reported deployment of the proximal uncovered stent in zone 1 or 2 in 33% of patients, but the actual number with left SA coverage was not specified. The variable degree of left SA revascularization before coverage reflects the changing practice patterns during different time periods. The TAG study, which finished enrollment in 2001, reported 100% revascularization rates (as was mandated by the protocol); rates dropped to 25% in the STARZ (Study of Thoracic Aortic Aneurysm Repair with the Zenith TX2 Thoracic TAA Endovascular Graft) trial, which was conducted during the period 2004 to 2006.

Perioperative Outcomes

The early experience with first-generation devices and high-risk inoperable individuals was associated with a relatively high early mortality of 9% to 12% with TEVAR but documented its feasibility.[43,52] The more recent trials in Table 133-1 report an enviable 30-day mortality of around 2%, significantly less than the 7% mortality in the open repair

group, as a result of the less invasive nature of the procedure, improved commercial devices, and enrollment of good-risk patients. It is important to note that "operative mortality," which includes all delayed in-hospital deaths beyond 30 days, does affect the open group more than the TEVAR patients and shows a significantly larger benefit with TEVAR (2% versus 12% for the TAG study, 1.9% versus 5.7% for the STARZ trial, and 2.1% versus 7.9% for the Valor trial).[15,48,49,53] In both summarizing and applying statistical analysis to the data displayed in Table 133-1 it can be stated that TEVAR compares favorably with open repair with respect to operative morbidity. In conglomerate, the three comparative clinical trials detailed in Table 133-1 included 495 patients treated by TEVAR for anatomically suitable DTAA and 353 patients managed by open surgery; notably, these procedures mostly were performed in academic medical centers of excellence. Operative mortality for TEVAR was 2% and that for open repair was 8.5% ($P < .001$). With more liberal application of the technology, however, the European registry reported a higher 30-day mortality of 5.3% in elective cases that also included arch aneurysms. In a meta-analysis of 17 studies, Walsh and colleagues found a significant reduction in mortality and major neurologic complication rates with TEVAR.[54]

Late Results

Although many reports give some insight on expectations for the midterm, only the TAG study has reported its 5-year results.[9,43,52,55-59] One-year outcomes, summarized in Table 133-1, underscore an advantage for TEVAR in aneurysm-related survival, which averaged 95% across trials, significantly better than the 89% figure for the combined open repair group. The TAG trial has reported this advantage to persist for at least 5 years because the difference mostly reflects the effect of the perioperative period with few, if any, later aneurysm-related mortalities in both the open and TEVAR groups.[9,48] All-cause late survival, however, showed minimal differences between open and endovascular modalities beyond 1 year, which mirrored the findings of randomized EVAR trials in the abdominal aorta.[9,55,59] At 5 years, overall survival rates in the TEVAR and open groups were 68% and 67%, respectively, thus indicating similar late effectiveness for both procedures.[9]

Late outcomes are not as encouraging in high-risk populations. A Stanford series of 103 patients, 60 of whom were deemed inoperable, reported a low 5-year survival estimate of 31%, as opposed to 78% for those who were open surgical candidates. This brings into question the appropriateness of any treatment in asymptomatic high-risk patients.[43]

Complications

Complications of TEVAR, like all endovascular procedures, can be conveniently divided into a general category common to all significant operative interventions and a procedure-specific category. General complications are not well detailed in most reports, and the FDA trials focused on combined trial-specific safety endpoints, which makes individual complication rates difficult to isolate. At any rate, the incidence of major or serious adverse events strongly favors the TEVAR group over open repair in the three trials that compared similar measures between both modalities (see Table 133-1). As expected in a population with advanced age and atherosclerotic disease, cardiopulmonary complications dominated the early morbidity, although frequency and severity were less than with open repair.[48,50] As an illustration, the STARZ trial reported a cardiovascular complication rate of 15.6% for TEVAR and 44.3% for the open group with an identical incidence of pulmonary complications (15.6% versus 44.3%).[48] At long term, the benefit of TEVAR with respect to the occurrence of major or serious adverse events persisted throughout the 5-year follow-up.[9] The incidence of major or serious adverse events and other secondary measures such as blood loss and hospital stay was strongly in favor of TEVAR over open repair, as illustrated by much lower blood loss and shorter hospital stay.

Vascular Complications

Vascular complications, related for the most part to the use of large sheaths in atherosclerotic arteries, were relatively high in the early TAG trial (14%). They were reduced significantly to 6% in a follow-up confirmatory trial of the modified TAG system in 51 patients in 2004, which reflects the collective learning curve for TEVAR.[15] The spreading awareness of vascular issues has resulted in a reduction in vascular complications to the 5% to 10% range in most recent reports.[15,49,60] The unusually high incidence in the STARZ trial (see Table 133-1) is not as much an indication of a higher complication rate as it is a difference in the definition of vascular events, which was far more inclusive than in the other reports, but the incidence was still considerably lower than that in patients undergoing open surgery (40%). Serious iliac artery injuries, a subset of vascular complications, ranging from a tear to complete avulsion and eversion on the sheath during withdrawal (Fig. 133-10) are less common but potentially life threatening. The prophylactic use of iliac conduits should be encouraged to avoid these injuries.

Neurologic Complications

Neurologic complications can be devastating after DTAA repair by either TEVAR or open thoracotomy. Although stroke receives less attention than SCI, it is just as common and occurs at similar rates during open and endovascular repairs, from 3% to 5%.[15,21,22,48,49] Deployment of the proximal end of the endograft in zone 2 proximal to the left SA shows a strong association with perioperative stroke, probably secondary to manipulation of the arch with catheters, wires, balloons, and stent-grafts at the origin of the cerebral vessels.[11,15,19] In the TAG study, stroke was noted in 14% of patients with zone 2 deployment versus 1% when the stent-graft was completely distal to the left SA.[29] Only the Zenith TX2 study reported dissonant results, with all four strokes in

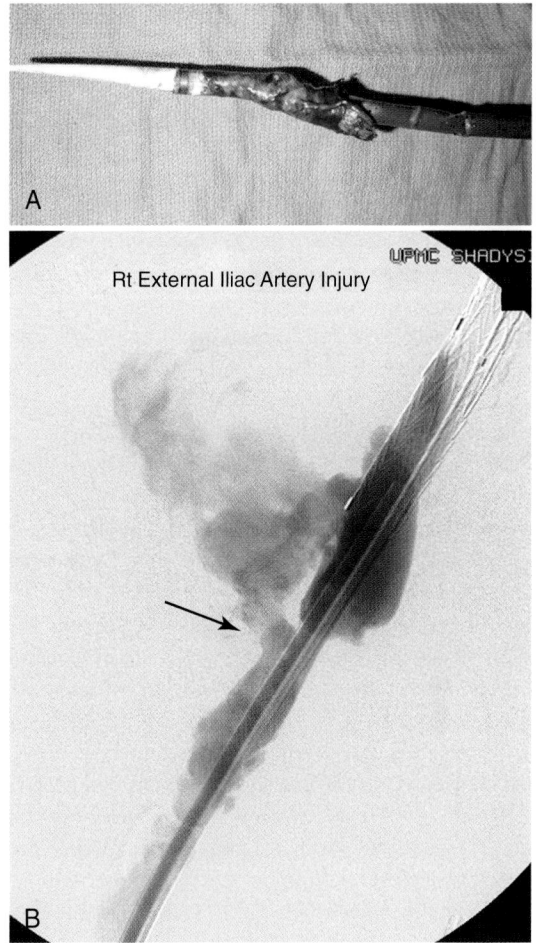

Figure 133-10 A, Torn segment of an external iliac artery on the delivery system. **B,** Angiography illustrating the injury (*arrow*). The stent-graft in the iliac artery is from previously performed endovascular abdominal aortic aneurysm repair.

the study occurring with the graft distal to the left SA.[48] This finding is difficult to explain but may relate to proximal deployment of the TX2, which normally starts more proximally and is then adjusted to its final position. The importance of operator technique, with minimal manipulation, meticulous cleansing of guide wires and catheters, and limited use of balloon molding only inside the grafts, cannot be overemphasized in minimizing the risk for stroke during TEVAR. Other factors that have been identified in the EuroSTAR data as being independent predictors of stroke included female sex and prolonged procedure time (>160 minutes).[22]

As was initially observed with the TAG study, which showed a marked reduction in paraplegia/paraparesis in comparison to open procedures (3% versus 14%), the advantage of spinal cord protection with TEVAR was again evident when the data from all three FDA trials were compared with open controls (6.2% versus 13%, $P < .007$) (see Table 133-1). The high reported incidence of SCI in the control group has been criticized as not being representative of modern series from centers of excellence, which have reported 2.5% to 3% paraplegia rates after open DTAA repair.[61,62] The difference may be due to the retrospective analysis in these reports, exclusion of high-risk patients with anastomoses in the distal arch requiring hypothermic arrest, variable use of neuroprotective adjuncts, and most notably the lack of reporting of paraparesis as part of these series. Both were included in the control group of the FDA trials. Stone and coauthors reported an SCI incidence of 8.6% in a recent open repair cohort when paraparesis was included.[41] If only devastating permanent paraplegia is considered, TEVAR at 1.6% is favored over open surgery at 5.1% ($P < .0037$). The reduced incidence of SCI with TEVAR may be related to avoidance of thoracic aortic clamping and reduced hemodynamic disturbances at the spinal cord level because of lack of blood loss from intercostal backbleeding. It should also be noted that SCI is not confined to the perioperative period. Delayed recurrent SCI and paraplegia have been reported after TEVAR.[63,64]

Several factors have been linked to an increased risk for SCI after TEVAR: concomitant or previous open infrarenal aortic replacement,[11,22,29,44,56,59,65-67] extensive thoracic aortic coverage,[19,22,46,50,52,57,60,66] renal insufficiency,[22,68] intraoperative hypotension (systolic blood pressure <80 mm Hg),[14,36] and coverage of the hypogastric artery and left SA.[21,22,64,69] Some of these risk factors are beyond the clinician's control, but many, such as coverage of the left SA and hypogastric arteries, can be averted by modifying the operative plan. As mentioned earlier, EuroSTAR data showed that coverage of the left SA without revascularization was independently associated with SCI.[22] Recent reports also suggest that left SA revascularization may be required more frequently than was previously recognized for either left upper extremity ischemic symptoms[31] or spinal cord protection.[21,22] Lumbar and pelvic collaterals also account for 25% of the spinal cord blood supply,[70] and compromised hypogastric artery flow contributes to the development of SCI.[69] For this reason, preservation of internal iliac flow and staged repair of synchronous DTAA and AAA to allow collateralization have been advocated.[36,66]

Endoleaks

Early endoleak rates at the 30-day follow-up were inexplicably high in the Valor trial at nearly 26%, whereas they were far less in the TAG (3.6%) and STARZ (4.8%) studies, as well as the EuroSTAR registry (see Table 133-1). This is mostly a definition issue because all endoleaks observed at any time

before 30 days were included in the Valor report, whereas only endoleaks at the 30-day follow-up were included in the other two studies. At 1 year, endoleaks were present in nearly 4% of TAG and TX2 patients and in 12% of Talent patients. During long-term follow-up of the TAG study, approximately 4% of patients continued to have an endoleak at each yearly follow-up up to 5 years.[9,48,49] The incidence of endoleaks is decreasing with second-generation devices, which have design improvements and better conformability.[60]

The distribution of endoleak type is also variable, with the TAG study reporting a majority of types I and III endoleaks and the other two studies a majority of type II endoleaks. This is again most likely a reporting issue because the TAG study relied on investigator reports whereas the other two trials relied on a core laboratory. Endoleaks were in general less common than in comparable EVAR series, with more types I and III endoleaks and fewer type II, and they accounted for most but not all re-interventions.[71,72]

Sac Enlargement

Aneurysm sac shrinkage is a good surrogate marker for successful repair of all aneurysms, including DTAA (Fig. 133-11). Sac enlargement is a concerning finding because it possibly indicates poor exclusion and pressurization of the sac. It may also introduce the potential for progressive outward traction in a larger cavity and possibly result in stent-graft kinking or dislodgement.

Sac enlargement rate of greater than 5 mm is encountered more frequently with TEVAR than with abdominal EVAR and has been reported in 7% to 14% of patients at 1 year, with little variation associated with different devices (see Table 133-1). Only the TAG pivotal trial has thus far reported late results in a longitudinal cohort, and sac enlargement was noted in nearly 20% at 5 years. Shrinkage was observed in 50% and a stable sac was noted in the remaining patients.[9] These rates may or may not apply to other grafts because the ePTFE material in the TAG study graft was somewhat porous with a sac behavior resembling that of the original abdominal Gore Excluder.[73] Both the TAG and Excluder endografts were modified to a less porous ePTFE material, which resulted in a much higher rate of sac shrinkage in the infrarenal

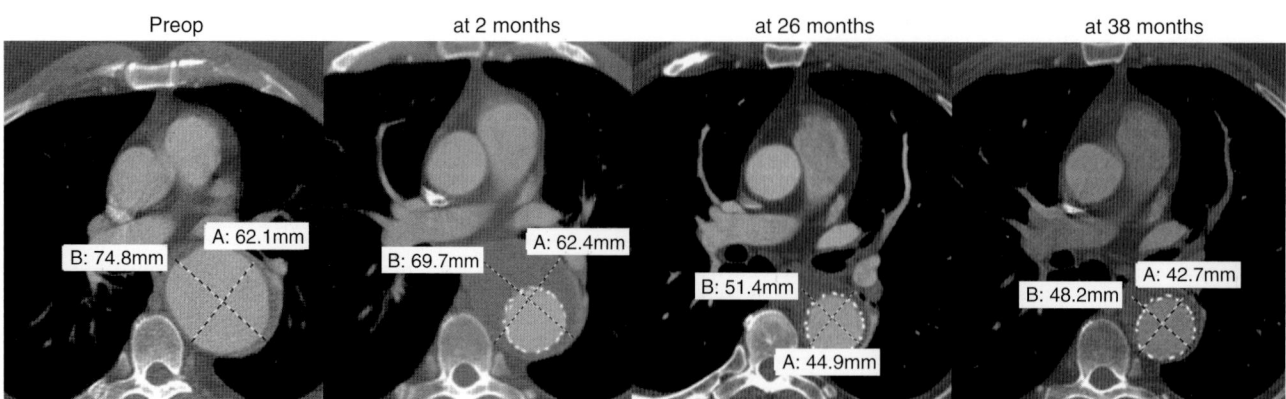

Figure 133-11 Serial follow-up CT scans after thoracic endovascular aortic repair showing progressive sac shrinkage.

position.[74] Similarly, data from the confirmatory trial of the modified TAG device with the low-permeability ePTFE has thus far shown a lower incidence of sac enlargement at 2 years of 2.9% versus 12.9% with the original device (*P* = .11). Long-term follow-up is obviously necessary.

Migration, Device Integrity, and Rupture

Late migration of the device has been reported to occur in 0% to 30% of patients.[46,75] With TEVAR, migration occurring at both ends, with distal migration of the proximal segment and proximal migration of the distal end, was seen frequently with early devices in association with neck dilatation and stent-graft kinking.[46,66,75,76] The current commercial devices tested in the U.S. pivotal trials seem to have a low migration potential ranging from 0.7% to 3.9% (see Table 133-1). At 5 years the TAG trial showed no late migration of greater than 10 mm by investigator reporting.[9] Illustrating the variability in data sources, a core laboratory evaluation of a limited number of patients from the same study reported 97% freedom from migration at 12 months, 87% at 24 months, and 83% at 3 years.[77] None of the migrations were clinically significant except for an early one associated with an arch aneurysm. Migration was noted on both ends of the devices, with the TX2 trial reporting one cranial and two caudal migrations through 1 year. None of them were associated with endoleak or sac expansion or required an intervention.

The early experience with TEVAR in high-risk individuals was associated with significant complication rates, with one study reporting 13% stent fracture and 6% late rupture rates.[78] Current devices suffer few device integrity issues, and complication rates are expected to be less than 2% for the devices marketed in the United States. The original TAG device showed fractures in the longitudinal wire in 14% of patients during 5 years of follow-up, with only one patient suspected of having a type III endoleak undergoing endovascular repair. The wire has been removed from the modified device. No stent fracture, barb separation, stent-to-graft separation, or component separation was observed in the TX2 device in 1 year of follow-up. One patient had a distal bare stent strut entanglement that was detected at discharge. Three Talent devices were noted to have a fracture during follow-up, one in the connecting bar. One device was found to have a fabric abrasion after explantation for rupture. This is the only known case of rupture among the 495 patients enrolled in the pivotal trials. The connecting bar has been removed from the modified investigational Valiant device. No graft thrombosis has been seen in all of these large devices.

Re-interventions

Re-intervention is defined as all procedures performed on patients referable to or as a consequence of the initial procedure. Early re-interventions were reported in only 2.1% in the pivotal TAG cohort during the first year but in 10.7% in the Talent study. Most re-interventions are for the treatment of endoleaks and several are endovascular. TX2 re-interven-

tion rates through 1 year were similar between the two groups (4.4% for TEVAR versus 5.7% for open treatment). At long term, data available from the TAG study showed a total re-intervention rate of 3.6% in treated patients (2.1% for open repair). Two patients underwent surgical conversion, one for an aortoesophageal fistula and the second for an arch aneurysm and migration of the proximal device in a very large neck that did not meet inclusion and exclusion criteria. Both occurred during the first year of follow-up. Three patients had five endovascular revisions for endoleaks. Secondary procedures of any kind during the 5-year follow-up were reported in 15% of the TAG patients and 32% of the open surgical controls. Although most secondary interventions after TAG were endoleak related, those after open repairs were due to wound complications, tracheostomy, and gastrointestinal tract–related problems. This high rate of secondary re-intervention performed in the open surgical group is contrary to a common a priori assumption that most have.[9,41] These rates are different from infrarenal EVAR reports of much lower rates in open procedures and are due in part to the high morbidity associated with thoracotomy and open DTAA repair, for which many early secondary procedures were required.

Postoperative Management

No special management is required after TEVAR unless the patient has a spinal drain that should be monitored closely. CSF pressure should be kept at 10 cm H_2O or lower. If the patient is neurologically intact, the drain can be clamped on the second postoperative day and removed the following day. Maintenance of a modestly elevated mean arterial pressure (>80 mm Hg) as assessed by arterial line is an important adjunct, with an even higher pressure limit if any evidence of neurologic deficit is detected. Prophylactic antibiotics are standard, and no postoperative anticoagulation is needed unless otherwise indicated.

Follow-up

Recommended follow-up schedules typically include a CT scan of the chest with and without contrast enhancement, preferably with delayed imaging to detect slow endoleaks at 1, 6, and 12 months during the first year. Yearly follow-up is then recommended for life. Four-view chest radiographs using a technique modified to identify metallic structures are also recommended at each visit. MRA can be used with most nitinol-based grafts to check for endoleaks in the event of renal failure developing or severe contrast allergy. The frequency of these tests is undergoing critical appraisal with current stable devices to reduce radiation exposure, cost, and patient inconvenience.

■ THORACIC ENDOVASCULAR AORTIC REPAIR FOR THORACOABDOMINAL ANEURYSMS

Endovascular treatment of TAAAs remains a developing technique with limited data to support either of the two available approaches: visceral debranching or investigational branched endografts. Both are currently being evaluated in high-risk individuals. Although commercially available stent-grafts can be used for hybrid procedures, genuine branched grafts are currently limited in the United States to those with physician-sponsored investigational device exemption studies.

Visceral Debranching (Hybrid Procedures)

In patients with an inadequate distal landing zone above the visceral vessels or actual extension of aneurysmal disease into the visceral aortic segment, TEVAR can still be performed by extending the landing zone through relocation of the visceral aortic branches with a bypass procedure. This is usually accomplished by using distal inflow sites such as the common iliac arteries or the infrarenal aorta, depending on anatomic suitability. Exclusion of the TAAA with stent-grafts can then follow via an endovascular approach either simultaneously or in a staged procedure. This hybrid surgical/endovascular procedure has the theoretical advantages of substituting laparotomy for thoracoabdominal exposure, avoiding division of the diaphragm and aortic clamping, and reducing visceral ischemic time. Complication rates are presumed to be lower than those of open thoracoabdominal repair.

Indications and Contraindications

Because experience is still limited with this procedure, clear indications and contraindications are not well characterized. The hybrid approach is entertained for patients with TAAAs who meet the standard criteria for repair, whose physiologic reserves prohibit an open thoracoabdominal procedure, and whose complex anatomy precludes standard TEVAR. Hybrid repair of TAAA remains a significant operation with high potential for postoperative complications, so all patients need to be thoroughly evaluated with preoperative cardiac stress testing and pulmonary function tests. The most appropriate indication would be a patient with significant pulmonary compromise but adequate cardiac and renal function reserve. Forced expiratory volume in 1 second of less than 1.2 L/min forced expiratory flow at 25% to 75% of less than 40% of predicted, and significant retention of carbon dioxide on resting blood gas analysis are indicators of postoperative pulmonary complications that would prevent an open thoracoabdominal incision and favor a hybrid approach.[79] Indeed, advanced COPD commonly presents a management dilemma because of the threat of major pulmonary morbidity with open surgery, yet the presence of such COPD is a well-established risk factor for TAAA expansion and rupture (see Chapter 131: Thoracic and Thoracoabdominal Aneurysms: Evaluation and Decision Making).[80] Patients with a high risk for paraplegia (previous thoracic or abdominal aortic repair), requirement for home oxygen, prior thoracotomy, or preoperative renal insufficiency may also be considered for this approach. Some operators find it preferable in all patients because it provides a better safety profile for extensive TAAA;

their morbidity and mortality rates with standard open repair were unacceptably high.[81]

Poor cardiac function (history of congestive heart failure, reversible myocardial ischemia), lack of a normal, healthy distal aorta or an iliac artery that could serve as an inflow source, and insufficient landing zones both proximally and distally are significant contraindications to a hybrid procedure. There also appears to be little benefit over open repair in patients with type IV TAAA, unless it is a recurrent visceral patch aneurysmal dilatation or the patient has severe COPD. In standard surgery for type IV TAAA, the overall operative insult is similar to that for a visceral debranching operation.

Relevant Anatomy

The presence of landing zones proximally and distally and other anatomic requirements remain similar to TEVAR. In addition, a suitable inflow source for the bypass and adequate target vessels for the procedure are necessary. Multiple renal arteries, severe occlusive disease of the aortoiliac segment, and severe calcifications and tortuosity make this approach more challenging. Access for delivery of the endograft may, however, be easier than with standard TEVAR because direct access through the iliac arteries or aorta is feasible as part of the same procedure. In circumstances in which the surgeon chooses to defer TEVAR to a second stage, a conduit can still be tunneled to the groin region and temporarily buried in subcutaneous tissue; it can be retrieved later, cleared by thrombectomy, and used to introduce the stent-graft.

Operative Planning and Options

Planning for TEVAR is as previously discussed. Additional planning for a hybrid procedure centers around the particular arteries to bypass and the choice of inflow site, which is usually based on the individual patient's anatomy, previous abdominal aortic surgery, and the extent of the aneurysm. The SMA and both renal arteries should be bypassed in all cases if coverage of their origin is anticipated. The need for bypass to the celiac axis depends on the extent of SMA collaterals in the form of a large gastroduodenal artery or a replaced right hepatic artery. Previous infrarenal aortic repair or type IV TAAA repair presents a technical benefit in that the existing graft provides not only a secure landing zone but also a safe clamp and anastomotic site for inflow to the debranching bypass grafts. In cases of an aneurysmal infrarenal aorta, the distal aorta should have at least 2 cm for proper distal sealing of the endograft. If the aneurysmal disease extends to the aortic bifurcation and no landing zone is left in the aorta, a more distal iliac site is chosen for the inflow source of the bypasses and a bifurcated abdominal endoprosthesis may be used with landing of the thoracic endograft in the main aortic section (Fig. 133-12). If the anatomy allows, an isolated infrarenal AAA repair with either a tube or bifurcated surgical graft may be performed first, from which retrograde bypass to the visceral and renal arteries is constructed, followed by stent-grafting (Fig. 133-13). When inflow is

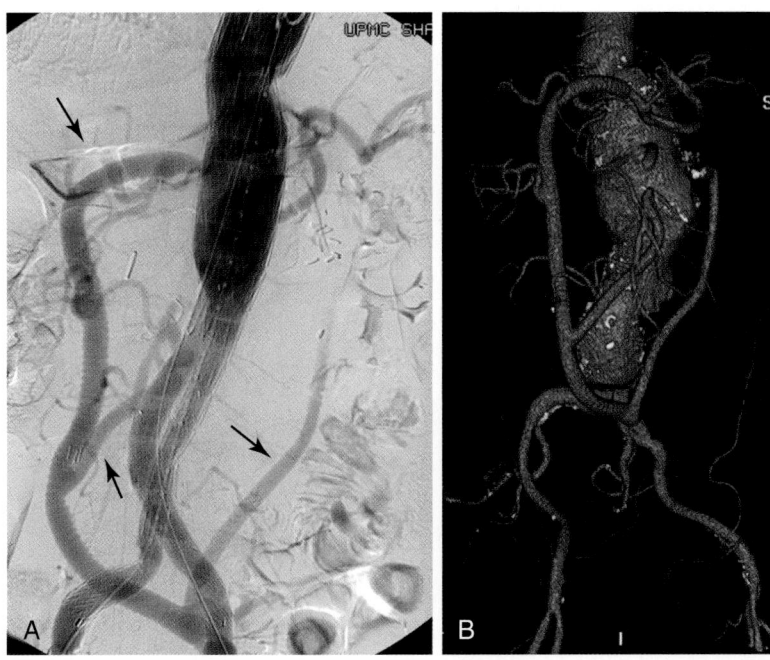

Figure 133-12 A, A thoracic endograft is deployed into a bifurcated abdominal endograft. Retrograde bypass grafts originating from the distal common iliac artery to the celiac axis (*top arrow*), the right renal artery (*bottom left arrow*) and the left renal artery (*bottom right arrow*) are illustrated. **B,** Three-dimensional reconstruction of a postoperative CT scan.

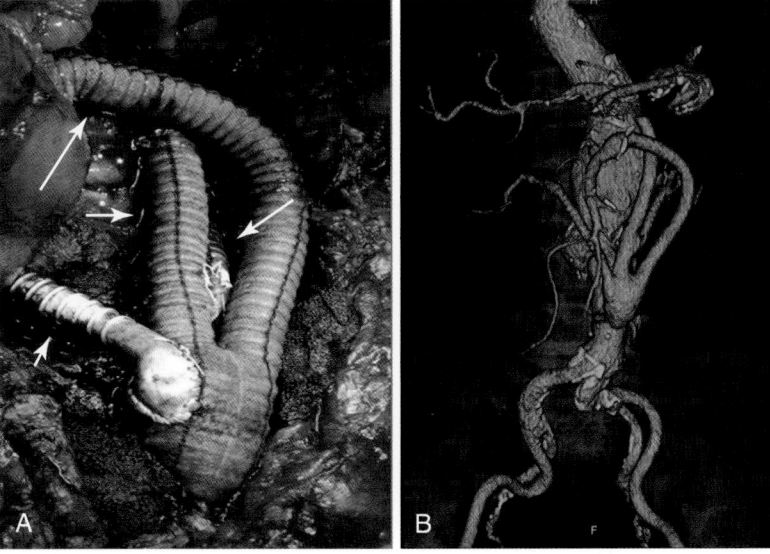

Figure 133-13 A, Intraoperative photograph illustrating visceral debranching with retrograde bypass grafting to all four visceral vessels. The *top arrow* indicates a bypass graft to the superior mesenteric artery, the *middle left arrow* to the celiac axis, the *middle right arrow* to the left renal artery, and the *bottom arrow* to the right renal artery **B,** Postoperative CT reconstruction. Note that the renal parenchyma is not well visualized because these images are surface-rendered three-dimensional reconstructions.

derived from an iliac artery, the contralateral iliac-femoral artery is preferred for an access site to avoid compromising blood flow through the bypass. Alternatively, a side limb may be sewn onto the bypass graft itself and used as conduit; it is divided and ligated on completion of stent-graft deployment.

All antihypertensive medications except for beta blockers should be withheld to help reduce postoperative SCI.[82] CSF drainage can also be used to help prevent SCI, especially in the setting of extensive aortic coverage or previous aortic replacement.

Operative Technique

Under general and epidural anesthesia for postoperative pain control, the infrarenal aorta–aortic graft, the origins of the renal arteries, the SMA, and the celiac axis are exposed through a conventional midline laparotomy. We have found standard inframesocolic aortic exposure to provide adequate access to the visceral vessel origins after division of the dense neurosplanchnic tissue at the origin of the SMA and division of the median arcuate ligament on the anterior surface of the aorta. The iliac arteries are also exposed when they are intended to be the inflow source.

A variety of reconstruction configurations may be used. Bifurcated, trifurcated, two bifurcated grafts, or many variations thereof have been described. Standard synthetic grafts are used with 6- to 8-mm limbs to the recipient vessel in either end-to-end or side-to-end fashion. The celiac bypass is usually routed via either a retrocolic or retropancreatic tunnel and anastomosed end to end to the celiac axis or end to side to the common hepatic artery. To avoid kinking, the lengths of all grafts are determined under arterial pressure and the visceral grafts routed in a "lazy C" fashion. The proximal end of the recipient vessels must be ligated to prevent type II endoleaks. Use of clips is not recommended.[81] The grafts are then covered with an omental flap to minimize the risk for late graft-enteric erosion. After revascularization of the visceral and renal arteries, endovascular exclusion of the TAAA is carried out. This may be done in a single setting or in a staged fashion. The endograft is deployed via standard endovascular techniques and principles in a sequential manner beginning with the smallest diameter.

Results

The literature is limited on this subject and does not allow any serious comparison to open repair because only a handful of series consist of more than 10 patients.[81,83-86] The results are varied, mostly because of small numbers, different selection criteria, different levels of acuity, and different lengths of coverage. Reported technical success rates, defined by exclusion of the aneurysm without a type I or III endoleak, range from 77% to 100%. In addition to standard TEVAR issues, causes of failure include myocardial instability and flow through the bypass grafts that may be insufficient to provide blood flow to the visceral organs.[81] Procedural time is not short, ranging from 239 to 368 minutes, and blood loss can average 2000 mL per procedure.[83] Mean hospital length of stay was 26 and 27 days in the two largest series with a median 9-day intensive care unit length of stay.[81,84] In a study that used a staged approach, the mean length of stay after TEVAR alone was 12 days.[76] The mean/median organ ischemic time ranged from 15 to 20 minutes.[81,84]

Data on intermediate-term outcomes are limited but suggest acceptable results. Chiesa and coauthors reported no aneurysm-related or procedure-related complications with a median follow-up of 15 months.[83] With similar follow-up, Zhou and colleagues noted no late aneurysm-related mortality, whereas Resch and coworkers reported two late aneurysm-related deaths in 13 patients.[85,86] Böckler and associates reported an overall survival rate of 70% at 3 years.[84]

Complications

Despite its perceived theoretical advantage, hybrid visceral debranching is associated with high mortality and complication rates. Mortality has been reported to vary from 13% to 23%,[81,83-85] although one report noted no deaths in a series of 15 patients.[86] As expected, elective procedures are associated with lower mortality rates than emergency cases are. The incidence of complications ranges widely from 19% to 59%.[84,86] A main concern is patency of the visceral grafts and its consequences should graft thrombosis occur (Fig. 133-14). Indeed, graft thrombosis is not uncommon (11% and 6.4%) and results in mesenteric ischemia and renal insufficiency.[84,86] Transient renal insufficiency requiring hemodialysis as a result of either atheroembolization or contrast-induced nephrotoxicity is reported in up to 32% of patients.[84] In one study,

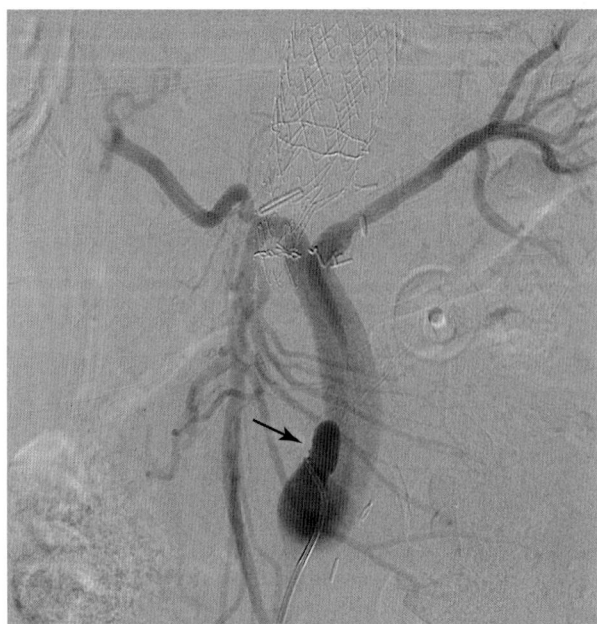

Figure 133-14 Follow-up arteriography demonstrating occlusion of the right renal bypass graft (*arrow*).

no graft-related complications were noted at a median follow-up of 15 months.[83]

The incidence of SCI varies widely from 0% to 31%, with Resch and coauthors reporting the highest rate with two cases of paraplegia and two cases of paraparesis in 13 patients after staged procedures.[85] The acuity and extent of coverage, however, are significant variables. In one series with a 16% SCI rate, 30% of the patients were treated on an emergency basis, and all but 3 of the 26 patients had the entire thoracoabdominal aorta covered.[84] Two studies reported no paraplegia or stroke at all.[85,86]

The reported overall incidence of endoleaks ranges from 0% to 62%. Unless the endoleak originates from a nonligated branch vessel, most type II endoleaks appear to resolve without intervention.[81-86] Type I endoleaks, as usual, require treatment by extension endografts or additional procedures. The presence of multiple visceral grafts in the retroperitoneal cavity juxtaposed to bowel also portends a late risk for graft-enteric erosion.[87]

Postoperative Management

Standard principles of surgical management after open vascular reconstructive procedures should apply. Acute graft thrombosis may cause either acute renal failure or mesenteric ischemia. Prompt diagnostic testing followed by exploration and revision of the graft is indicated should there be any suspicion of graft occlusion. Lower extremity motor function should be carefully checked at frequent intervals. Any change should prompt insertion of a CSF drain unless one is already present or the patient is coagulopathic. Permissive hypertension should be used.

Follow-up

The established surveillance principles after TEVAR described in the previous section also apply for these patients. In addition, duplex evaluation may be used for any suspicious graft occlusion.

Branched Endograft for Thoracoabdominal Aortic Aneurysm Repair

Complete endovascular repair of TAAA with avoidance of aortic cross-clamping and spinal cord ischemic time and with minimal renal and visceral ischemic time is an attractive concept for high-risk patients who cannot tolerate any open cavitary incision. This can be achieved with the use of branched/fenestrated endografts, which remain investigational at this stage but may provide the least invasive option for treating TAAAs (Fig. 133-15).

Indications and Contraindications

Currently, branched grafts remain the domain of very few centers in the United States, with these procedures being performed on high-risk individuals with large TAAAs under physician-sponsored institutional investigational device exemption protocols. Although many design features such as the configuration of side branches and bridging stent-grafts are not well settled, these grafts are more widely available in

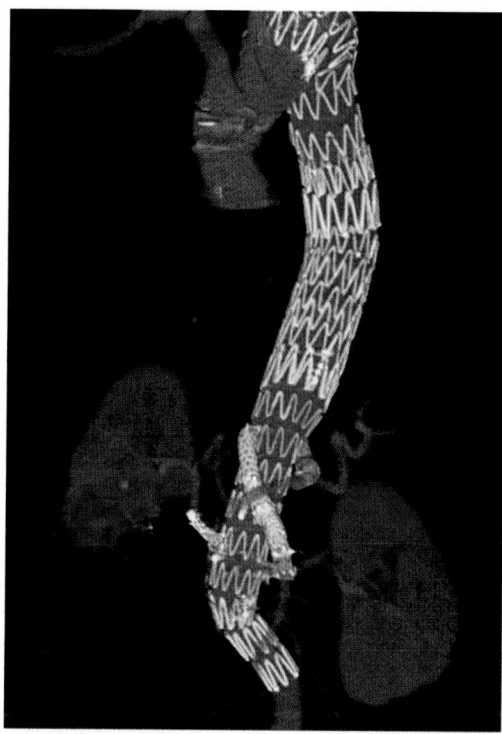

Figure 133-15 Follow-up CT reconstruction demonstrating exclusion of the thoracoabdominal aorta with branch grafts to the celiac axis and superior mesenteric and bilateral renal arteries. *(Courtesy of Roy K. Greenberg, MD.)*

Europe, Australia, and South America.[82,88-91] Even though the application of these branched grafts is currently restricted to individuals who cannot tolerate the open procedure, the indications are expected to broaden as the technology matures and long-term results become more widely available. Patients with an expected mortality rate of greater than 20% with open surgical treatment and whose life expectancy is longer than 2 years may soon be regarded as suitable candidates.[82] Groups with the highest risk for SCI (TAAA types I and II) or who have previously undergone infrarenal or thoracic aortic surgery may also benefit from this technology.

Unsuitable anatomic conditions, characterized by lack of proximal or distal landing zones and significant angulation or stenosis of the visceral arteries precluding access and stent-grafting of the branches, are contraindications to total endovascular treatment of TAAA. Symptomatic or ruptured aneurysms are not currently suitable for this technique because of the lengthy planning process, construction of the devices, and performance of the procedure. Other contraindications to exposure to radiation and intravenous contrast material would also apply.

Relevant Anatomy

Apart from the standard landing zone requirements, the deployment of branched endografts depends on an adequate luminal space in the distal thoracic aorta and visceral aorta to allow expansion of the branch-bearing segment, as well as adequate space for manipulation and deployment of the bridging grafts. Multiple suitable access sites, including brachial and femoral access, are typically required. Excessive tortuosity of either the aneurysm or the access vessels limits the ease of catheterization of the visceral arteries and may render the procedure difficult, if not impossible to conclude.

Operative Planning and Options

The planning of all TEVAR procedures is key to success, but more so for branched endografts. Meticulous planning is necessary to align the fenestrations and branches with their respective targets. The aneurysmal space allows flexible bridging grafts to reach the branches from semi-standard re-enforced or directional branches (Fig. 133-16).[88] Proper overlap in the artery as well as in the branched segment is very important to avoid disconnections with remodeling of the aneurysm. Short straight segments or longer spiral branches have been used successfully in this area and have replaced the original designs with simple fenestrations (see Fig. 133-16).

Operative Technique

The endograft consists of a segment with multiple short side branches or fenestrations (or both) of variable design, one for each visceral artery to be reconstructed. It is introduced from a femoral or iliac approach followed by catheterization of the

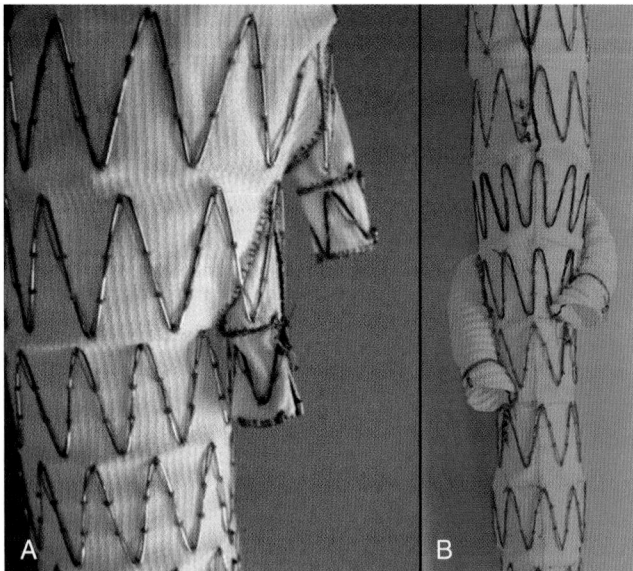

Figure 133-16 Stent-grafts with multiple side branches (**A**) and long spiral branches (**B**). *(A, courtesy of Timothy Chuter, MD; B, courtesy of Roy K. Greenberg, MD.)*

visceral arteries through the endograft branches, typically from a brachial approach. The gap is then bridged by available flexible self-expanding or balloon-expandable stent-grafts. Balloon-expandable grafts are flared on the inside to improve sealing. Proximal or distal extensions are added before or after the branch-bearing segment, depending on the anatomy of the aneurysm.[82,90,91] The procedure can be involved and can last from 6 to 12 hours.

Results

Since Chuter and colleagues' first report of a successful, completely endovascular repair of TAAA with preservation of all four visceral vessels via a branched stent-graft in 2001,[6] only a few series and case reports have been published.[82,89,90,92,93] Although the patient suffered delayed paraplegia, it provided proof of feasibility of the concept. Anderson and coauthors reported a series of four patients with TAAA treated by implantation of fenestrated and branched stent-grafts into 13 target visceral vessels.[89] There was one perioperative death and one renal artery occlusion. At 1-year follow-up, complete aneurysm exclusion with patency of all visceral arteries was noted in the three surviving patients. A report by Muhs and associates in 2006 included eight patients with TAAA.[90] No perioperative deaths or SCI was observed in this subgroup of patients. The two largest reports, from Chuter and coworkers[82] and Greenberg and Lytle,[88] included 22 and 73 patients, respectively, and documented promising results in a group unfit for open repair. Technical success rates were 93% to 100%, and branch revascularization was successful in 95% to 100% of patients. Mean blood loss was 714 mL in one study with the mean contrast use being slightly greater than 200 mL. Mean hospital stay was 9 to 11 days. Operative mortality was

5.5% to 9.1%, and SCI was noted in 3% to 13%. The survival rate at 1 year was nearly 90%.

Complications

Branch occlusion was noted rarely in both large studies at midterm follow-up. No stent-graft migration, component separation, or fractures were reported. The renal dysfunction described after fenestrated grafts[94,95] has been rare with branched TAAA repair.[82,90] Potential causes of renal dysfunction include intravenous contrast–induced nephrotoxicity, embolization during stent-graft insertion or deployment, and kinking or thrombosis of the covered stent-graft. Endoleaks were present early in 9% to 11% and required few late reinterventions for correction. No ruptures or aneurysm sac expansion have been observed in limited follow-up.

Postoperative Management

Postoperative management and follow-up are identical to that for other TEVAR procedures, with special attention paid to possible visceral branch ischemia as a result of kinking and type III endoleaks from branch disconnections. Because of long thoracoabdominal segment coverage, the previously reviewed precautions with respect to delayed SCI should be routine practice.

■ THORACIC ENDOVASCULAR AORTIC REPAIR FOR AORTIC-ARTERIAL EMBOLIZATION

Atheroembolism resulting from plaque fragments or platelet debris in ulcerated plaque can result in significant morbidity and mortality.[96] Mobile thrombi in the aorta occur less frequently but are no less dangerous.[97-100] Emboli may originate at any level from the arch to the aortoiliac segment and can result in strokes, limb loss, or visceral infarcts, most notably renal failure.[101] Events can occur spontaneously or complicate endovascular interventions, cardiac procedures with arch clamping, or thoracic and abdominal aortic operations. The diagnosis is usually made by contrast-enhanced CT angiography or TEE. Exclusion of the offending plaque or thrombus is necessary to avoid serious complications.[96,101-103] The thoracic aorta is the source of embolism in 10% to 15% of patients and is associated with nearly a 60% recurrence rate and significant mortality if untreated because visceral ischemia and renal failure are common.[96]

Operative Technique

Standard techniques are used for placement of the endograft. However, because the offending plaque is hard to identify in a usually diffusely diseased aorta, IVUS is especially helpful in identifying the exact location of the most mobile and threatening components. The use of IVUS also helps in reducing the contrast load in these patients with compromised kidney function. Care must be taken to minimize

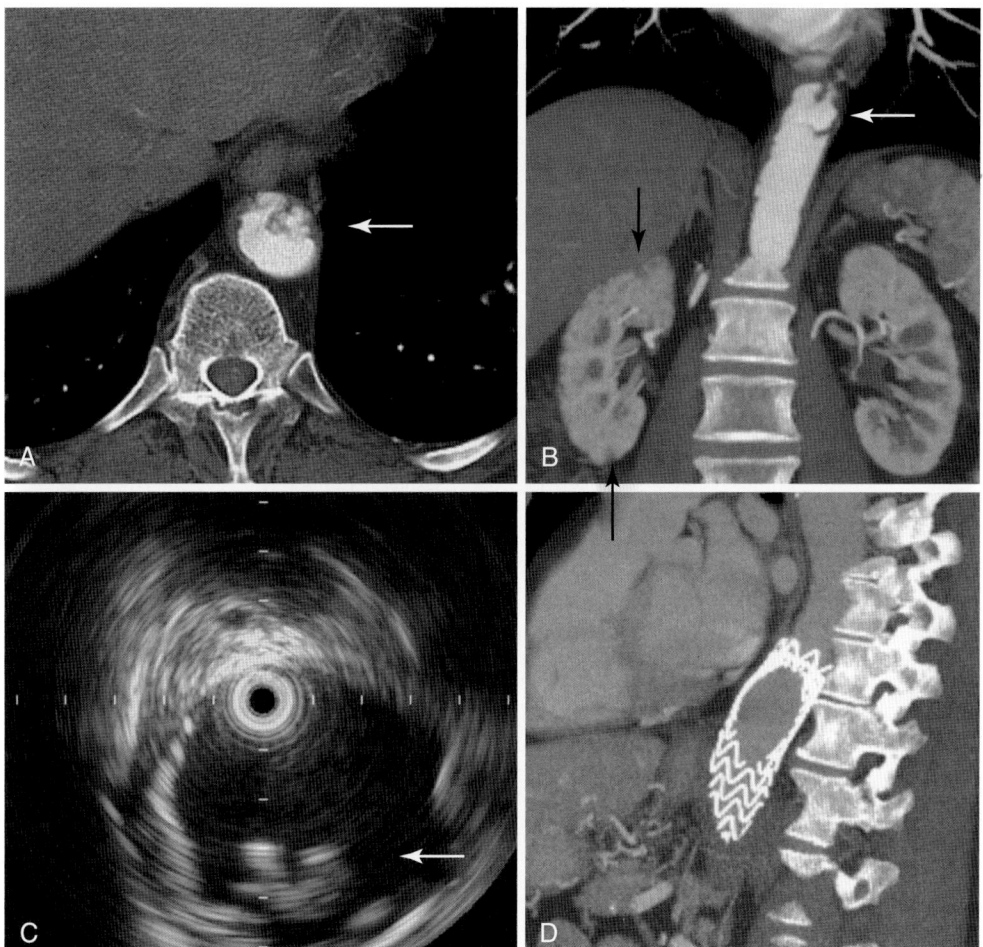

Figure 133-17 A, Cross-sectional view of an atheroma in the thoracic aorta (*arrow*). **B,** Coronal view of the kidneys with multiple areas of infarcts (*arrows*). **C,** Atheroma visualized on intravascular ultrasound intraoperatively (*arrow*). **D,** TAG exclusion of the lesion.

manipulations to avoid precipitating an embolic shower. We did not encounter any in our four cases, and very few reports suggest that it is a major complicating factor. TEE can also be helpful to localize the lesion in conjunction with or when IVUS is not available.

It is not clear what should be an appropriate follow-up for these patients because the absence of an aneurysm makes migration or endoleak formation a nonissue. Contrast-enhanced CT scans are probably not needed yearly, but the appropriate follow-up schedule is uncertain. Additional episodes of embolization should be evaluated in the same manner.

Results

There have been sporadic reports of endovascular treatment of embolizing lesions from the iliac to the thoracic aorta to prevent further embolization and reduce the significant mortality and morbidity associated with expectant management or open procedures.[104-108] The number of cases is limited, although they do demonstrate the feasibility and relative effectiveness of the technique. No summary of results is yet feasible, but recurrent embolization has not been described,

which may be a testament to proper selection of cases. We have successfully treated one mobile thoracic aortic thrombus and three atherosclerotic thoracic aortas with generalized embolization to the viscera and lower extremities. The description is unpublished as of yet (Fig. 133-17). The reader will note that the illustrated cases represent examples of focal pathology in which a reasonable assessment that this was the offending lesion could be made. Stent-graft exclusion in such cases is logical and has been curative. It must be acknowledged, however, that many patients referred for consideration of such therapy will demonstrate diffuse long-segment atheromatous degeneration of the thoracic and thoracoabdominal aorta, clearly not amenable to such focal therapy; a fear of inducing life-threatening atheromatous embolization often results in noninterventional treatment in such cases.

SELECTED KEY REFERENCES

Black SA, Wolfe JH, Clark M, Hamady M, Cheshire NJ, Jenkins MP. Complex thoracoabdominal aortic aneurysms: endovascular exclusion with visceral revascularization. *J Vasc Surg.* 2006;43:1081-1089.
This is one of the two largest articles reporting early results on hybrid repairs of thoracoabdominal aortic aneurysm and chronic aortic dissections with aneurysmal degeneration.

Böckler D, Kotelis D, Geisbüsch P, Hyhlik-Dürr A, Klemm K, von Tengg-Kobligk H, Kauczor HU, Allenberg JR. Hybrid procedures for thoracoabdominal aortic aneurysms and chronic aortic dissections—A single center experience in 28 patients. *J Vasc Surg*. 2008;47: 724-732.
This is the second of the two largest articles reporting early results on hybrid repairs of thoracoabdominal aortic aneurysm and chronic aortic dissections with aneurysmal degeneration.

Chuter TA, Rapp JH, Hiramoto JS, Schneider DB, Howell B, Reilly LM. Endovascular treatment of thoracoabdominal aortic aneurysms. *J Vasc Surg*. 2008;47:6-16.
This article provides a short-term report of the first author's pioneering work on total endovascular repair of thoracoabdominal aortic aneurysm in patients unfit for open repair.

Fairman, RM, Farber M, Kwolek, CJ, Matsumoto A, Garrett EH, Sicard G, Mehta M, White R, Lumsden A, Lee WA, Tuchek JM, Criado R. Pivotal results of the Medtronic Vascular Talent Thoracic Stent Graft System for patients with thoracic aortic disease: the VALOR trial. *J Vasc Surg*. 2008;48:546-554.
This article reports early and 1-year outcome data on the VALOR trial (an FDA-run trial comparing TEVAR with open repair of DTAAs).

Leurs LJ, Bell R, Degrieck Y, Thomas S, Hobo R, Lundbom J. Endovascular treatment of thoracic aortic diseases: combined experience from the EUROSTAR and United Kingdom Thoracic Endograft registries. *J Vasc Surg*. 2004;40:670-679.
This article summarizes the European experience and provides perioperative and 1-year data from both the EUROSTAR and U.K. registries.

Makaroun MS, Dillavou ED, Wheatley GH, Cambria RA. Five-year results of endovascular treatment with the Gore TAG device compared to open repair of thoracic aortic aneurysms. *J Vasc Surg*. 2008;47:912-918.
This is the only article that provides long-term performance and durability data from the TAG study (an FDA-run trial comparing TEVAR with the Gore TAG device and open repair of DTAAs).

Matsumura JS, Cambria RP, Dake MD, Moore RD, Svensson LG, Snyder S. International controlled clinical trial of thoracic endovascular aneurysm repair with the Zenith TX2 endovascular graft: 1-year results. *J Vasc Surg*. 2008;47:247-257.
This article provides early and 1-year outcome data from the STARZ trial (an FDA-run trial comparing TEVAR and open repair of DTAAs).

Walsh SR, Tang TY, Sadat U, Naik J, Gaunt ME, Boyle JR, Hayes PD, Varty K. Endovascular stenting versus open surgery for thoracic aortic disease: systematic review and meta-analysis of perioperative results. *J Vasc Surg*. 2008;47:1094-1098.
This meta-analysis compares the results of open surgical repair of thoracic aortic pathology and endovascular repair.

REFERENCES

The reference list can be found on the companion Expert Consult Web site at *www.expertconsult.com*.

CHAPTER 134

Aortic Arch Aneurysms and Dissection

Roy K. Greenberg and Lars G. Svensson

The aortic arch is defined as the curved portion of the aorta from the proximal origin of the innominate artery to the distal origin of the left subclavian artery. This area gives rise to the upper extremity and cerebral vessels. When diseased, this region is associated with typical aortic challenges such as rupture or dissection or may lead to end-organ problems such as stroke, upper extremity embolization, or compromised distal aortic perfusion. It is rare for aortic disease to be isolated to the aortic arch (approximately 4% of all aortic aneurysms); more commonly, the arch is involved in pathology that includes the ascending aorta, the descending thoracic aorta, or both. However, treatment of lesions that involve the arch requires specific expertise because of the complex aortic morphology, pathology, and risk for stroke. Common conditions that affect the arch include aneurysms, dissections, and atherosclerotic disease. Such conditions frequently challenge even experienced surgeons regardless of the intended choice of treatment, which includes endovascular options and open surgery. Irrespective of the type and extent of disease, a well-thought-out strategic approach is required before embarking on any sort of arch procedure. Considerations must include assessment of the proximal and distal extent of the disease, risk for embolic stroke, risk for stroke resulting from inadequate cerebral perfusion, and the methods by which flow will be restored to the arch branches and distal aorta. The durability of the repair must be assessed in the context of the overall health of the patient along with the patient's projected life expectancy. Additionally, one should be mindful of the effect of the intended treatment on the ascending and descending thoracic aorta. Finally, it also behooves patients and their physicians to be educated with respect to all treatment options irrespective of individual clinician preference. In this manner, educated decisions can be made with regard to the best treatment options for a given patient.

ANATOMY AND CONGENITAL ANOMALIES

Embryologically, the aortic arch is formed from a complex series of events centering around the aortic sac, dorsal aortas, and five aortic arches that connect the two structures (see Chapter 2: Embryology). The adult aortic arch is derived from the aortic sac (proximal arch, innominate artery, and ascending aorta), left fourth aortic arch (midarch), and left dorsal aortas (distal arch and descending thoracic aorta). The supra-aortic trunk vessels are formed from the aortic sac

(brachiocephalic or innominate artery), paired third arches (common carotid arteries), right fourth arch (proximal right subclavian), and seventh intersegmental artery (left subclavian artery and distal right subclavian artery). Therefore, when applying the most commonly accepted surgical definition of the aortic arch, which includes the 270- to 330-degree curve that connects the cranially directed ascending aorta with the caudally oriented descending aorta, we must recognize that such tissue represents an embryologic mix of tissue derived from various segments. Three vessels originate from the mid-portion of the curve, including the brachiocephalic (innominate) trunk, left common carotid artery, and left subclavian artery.

Congenital Anomalies

Given the complexities of the morphologic changes that occur during embryologic development of the aortic arch, it comes as no surprise that architectural anomalies are commonly encountered in this region. Most frequently the arch has three branches, referred to as a type A arch. Type B arches, also called bovine arches, have only two arteries arising from the aorta, with the left common carotid artery originating from the proximal portion of the innominate artery (Fig. 134-1A) rather than from the aorta proper (10% to 15% of the population).[1] In a type C arch, the left vertebral artery originates from the aorta rather than the left subclavian artery (4% of the population).[1] Numerous other variations exist, but only those that may relate to the development of specific pathology are discussed here.

Aberrant Subclavian Artery

An aberrant right subclavian artery usually arises immediately proximal to the aortic isthmus and distal and posterior to the left subclavian artery. When the proximal portion of the aberrant right subclavian artery or aorta surrounding the anomalous takeoff dilates, it is termed a *diverticulum of Kommerell* (Fig. 134-1B). Many variations of this abnormality may occur. A common theme among the symptoms is compression of the esophagus, worsening dysphagia ("lusoria natural"), and compression of the left bronchus resulting in asthma-like symptoms (see Chapter 137: Upper Extremity Aneurysms). Other variations, such as common origins of the carotid arteries, are sometimes associated with other genetic abnormalities and, when appropriate, should prompt further evaluation.

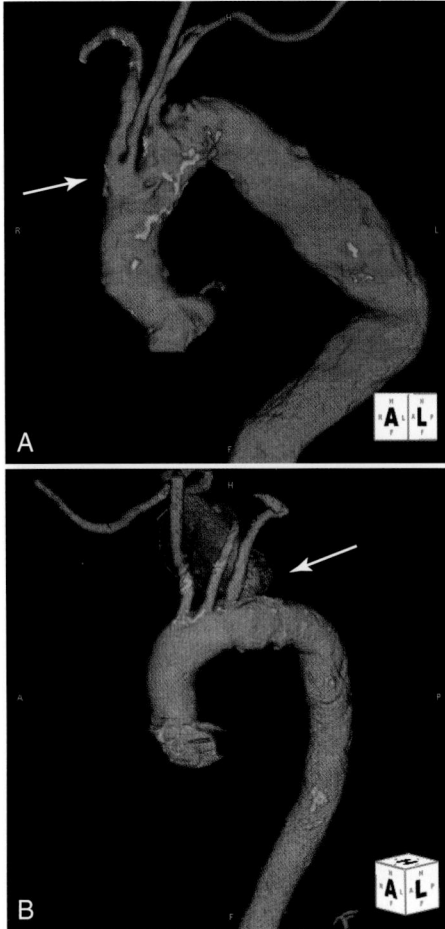

Figure 134-1 Congenital arch anomalies. **A,** A bovine arch (*arrow*) is the most commonly found congenital variant of the supra-aortic trunk vessels. Although there is no pathology associated with this finding, it must be evaluated in the context of the planned operation because it may create challenges in endovascular access to the left common carotid artery. The left vertebral artery may also arise directly from the aortic arch between the left carotid and subclavian arteries. This must also be taken into consideration, specifically when intending to cover the origin of the vessel, because the status of the contralateral vertebral artery and circle of Willis should be understood. Aberrant right subclavian arteries frequently become aneurysmal and typically arise immediately distal and posterior to a normal left subclavian origin. This abnormality is termed a *diverticulum of Kommerell* (*arrow*) (**B**). Other variations, such as common origins of the carotid arteries, are also described.

Right-Sided Arch

Two variations of true right-sided arches were initially described by Felson and Palaew.[2] In type I anomalies, the ascending aorta and aortic arch are right sided, and the aortic arch crosses behind rather than in front of the trachea and esophagus into the left side of the chest. The left subclavian in this situation typically arises from the ascending aorta, as does the left carotid and innominate artery. Should the descending aortic segment enlarge, compressive symptoms of the esophagus and trachea may develop. These symptoms result from a vascular ring that surrounds the trachea and esophagus and consists of the anomalous aortic arch and branches, the pulmonary artery, and the descending aorta

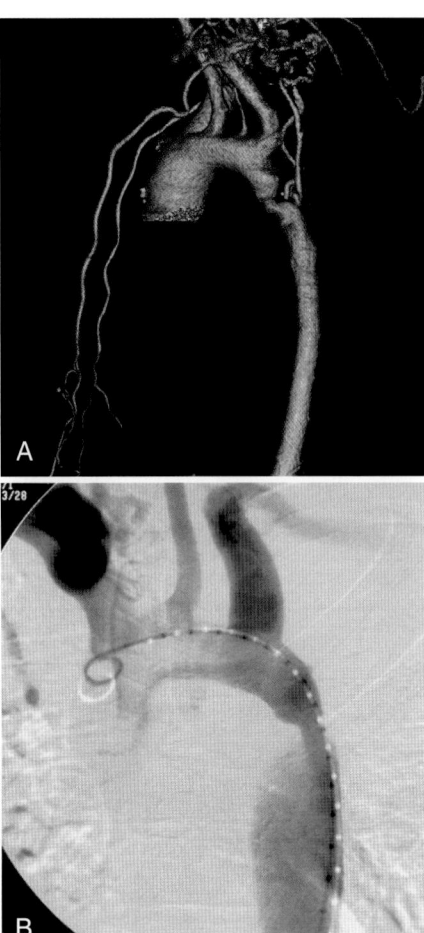

Figure 134-2 Aortic coarctation. These images demonstrate the appearance of a postductal aortic coarctation. **A,** Three-dimensional reconstruction of a computed tomography scan that nicely depicts the rich collateral network typically accompanying all manifestations of adults with coarctation. **B,** Angiogram demonstrating the post-stenotic dilatation, in addition to the dilated left subclavian artery, that is frequently associated with aortic coarctation.

along with the ductus arteriosus. A type II anomaly involves a right-sided arch in conjunction with an aberrant left subclavian origin that traverses from the right side of the chest behind the trachea into the left side of the chest to supply a left subclavian artery.

Coarctation

Aortic coarctation, or narrowing of the aorta, is also a manifestation of congenital arch disease and is anatomically described in relation to the ductus arteriosus (ligamentum arteriosum). The narrowing can be preductal, postductal, or ductal. Most commonly, in adults an aortic coarctation is immediately distal to the atrophied ductus (postductal), but such cases are often associated with a hypoplastic, more proximal aortic arch (Fig. 134-2). Rarely, the arch or descending aorta is completely interrupted in adults, and flow to the distal aorta must be maintained through collaterals. This defect can occur between the left subclavian artery and descending tho-

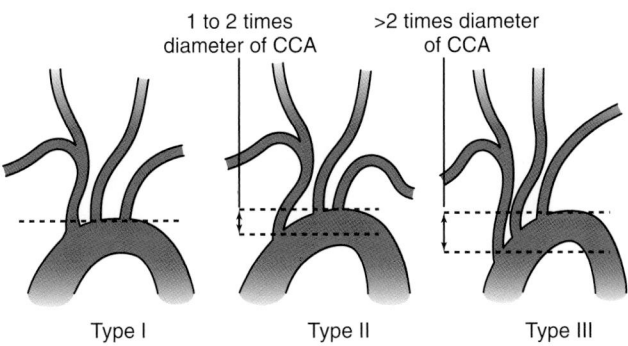

Figure 134-3 Types of aortic arch configuration with respect to origins of arch vessels. CCA, common carotid artery.

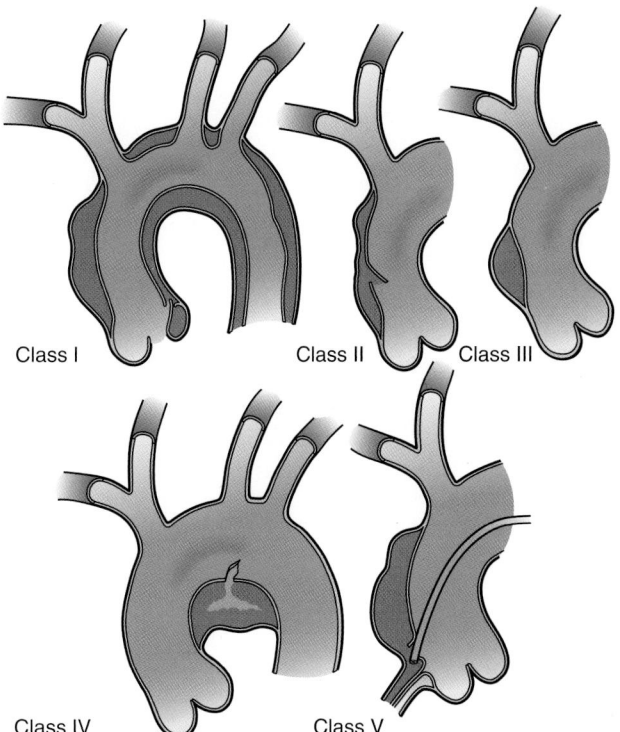

Figure 134-4 Classification of arch dissection tears.

racic aorta (type A), the left subclavian and carotid arteries (type B), or the left carotid and brachiocephalic arteries (type C).[3] Although surgical correction of all the aforementioned congenital defects has been well documented and several other anomalies have been described and associated with many genetic conditions, the details are beyond the scope of this chapter.

Anatomic Classification

Irrespective of the specific architecture of the arteries supplying the upper part of the body, the location of the supra-aortic trunk vessel island may vary as well. Typically, in a young healthy individual the vessels are centered on the arch; however, with age, aneurysm formation, or aortic elongation, the arch vessel island is pushed proximally. A classification system was developed describing the location of the island of supra-aortic trunk vessels as type I, II or III, in an effort to help predict the difficulty that may be encountered when attempting to achieve endovascular access to these vessels. Such a description also has implications with respect to surgical accessibility of the vessels via either median sternotomy or left lateral thoracotomy (Fig. 134-3).

◼ ETIOLOGY OF ANEURYSMS AND DISSECTIONS

Degenerative Aneurysms

The etiology of degenerative aneurysms involving the aortic arch is not entirely clear in many patients. Frequent associated factors include smoking, chronic pulmonary disease, Takayasu's disease, giant cell arteritis, polymyalgia rheumatica, temporal arteritis, and other connective tissue disorders and syndromes. A growing list of genetic mutations and spontaneous mutations has been linked to familial patterns of aneurysmal disease. Included among these genetic mutations are Marfan's syndrome, bicuspid aortic valves, Ehlers-Danlos syndrome, Loeys-Dietz syndrome, familial thoracic aneurysmal disease, Erdheim's deformity, polycystic kidney disease, trisomy, Turner's syndrome, and Noonan's syndrome.[4,5] Nonspecific aneurysms of the arch can be manifested as isolated saccular outpouchings, can exist as the terminal segment

of an ascending aortic aneurysm or the proximal portion of a descending thoracic aneurysm, or simply bridge ascending and descending aneurysmal disease.

Arch Dissection

Aortic dissection is typically classified according to the Stanford or DeBakey classification systems (see Chapter 135: Aortic Dissection). We prefer to classify patients as having a tear either proximal or distal to the innominate artery, in keeping with the indications for urgent surgical repair. However, tears in the aortic arch have been grouped into five separate classes (Fig. 134-4).[6] Each class may have implications for surgical management of the defect.

Class I Tears. Class I tears originate in the aortic arch. This type accounts for about 10% of patients with aortic dissections and results in the classic two-lumen aortic dissection with a septum or flap between the two lumina (Fig. 134-5).

Class II Tears. Class II tears are those with intramural hematomas of the aortic arch in which the tear cannot be imaged on preoperative imaging studies. The tear is virtually always found during surgery but is not visible with preoperative imaging methods because of the clot obscuring the tear.

Class III Tears. Localized tears of the intima in the aortic arch without extensive undermining of the intima or propagation of the dissection into two lumina are considered class III tears. Although this type of dissection is rare, it is most commonly seen in the ascending aorta in patients with Marfan's syndrome and is only occasionally seen in the aortic arch.

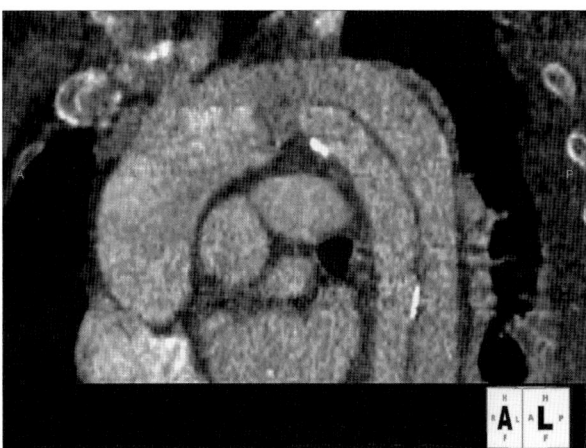

Figure 134-5 This image demonstrates the presence of a dissection originating within the aortic arch (class I). Such dissections pose some clinical dilemmas should they become complicated because they are not readily treated with stent-grafts, and open surgery is complex and requires arch replacement in the setting of an acute injury to the aortic wall.

Class IV Tears. Class IV tears are associated with penetrating ulcers and are not infrequently associated with an area of calcification or an atheromatous ulcer. The dissection plane penetrates into the medial layer and causes an intramural hematoma.

Class V Tears. Class V tears are associated with iatrogenic maneuvers; for example, we have seen them after cardiac catheterization, in association with aortic stent-grafting, or from stents placed in the origin of the innominate, carotid, or subclavian arteries.

Repair of an arch dissection is carried out in accordance with the pathology. However, prevention of retrograde dissection into the ascending aorta, malperfusion, and rupture constitutes the primary objective of both endovascular and open therapy. These objectives must be viewed in the context of the magnitude of the required operation and the fragility of the aortic tissue at the time of the acute manifestation.

Infections

Areas of calcium deposition within the aortic arch may often be found to be the origin of aortic infections (see also Chapter 139: Infected Aneurysms). Most frequently, mycotic aneurysms affecting the aortic arch are located on the lesser curvature. Commonly, the organisms include *Staphylococcus*, *Streptococcus*, *Pseudomonas*, and *Salmonella* species. Less frequently, tuberculosis and syphilitic infections of the arch or ascending aorta (or both) have been reported; these may not involve frank pus or false aneurysm formation but cause systemic symptoms in patients who have some degree of immune dysfunction. Patients who have previously undergone aortic repair may also be prone to infection. This problem is always complex and fraught with danger. As with any type of arterial infection, these patients require wide excision and débridement of all foreign material along with aortic replacement

involving either homografts or extra-anatomic reconstruction. Such operations are extensive and frequently require the placement of multiple homografts in series. After such an endeavor, the large infected cavities must be filled with either omentum or a muscle flap. Similarly, if graft material must be used, consideration should be given to using an omental flap to wrap around the graft material and gel-impregnated grafts soaked in an aminoglycoside, in rifampicin, or in amphotericin B in an attempt to add further protection against reinfection.

■ PATIENT EVALUATION

As recently as 30 years ago, the typical patient with an arch aneurysm was initially seen because of either dissection or rupture and severe chest and back pain. In the modern era, most such patients coming to the attention of surgeons have asymptomatic aneurysms of the aortic arch that were detected by chest radiography, echocardiography, magnetic resonance imaging, or computed tomography (CT) scans obtained for unrelated purposes. In such cases, a detailed preoperative evaluation is required, which should include imaging, cardiac evaluation, pulmonary evaluation, and neurologic evaluation.

Imaging

Aortic imaging with a high-resolution CT scan should be obtained in all patients without contraindications to a moderate dose of contrast material. The CT scan should be reconstructed at intervals no greater than 2 mm to offer the best resolution for visualizing the arch pathology. Furthermore, all CT scan machines today can acquire data in a gated fashion, and retrospective gating can be used to provide clear images of the highly mobile proximal aorta. These techniques will help differentiate pathology isolated to the aortic arch from that involving the ascending aorta or critical arch branches.

Cardiac Evaluation

Echocardiography is useful to confirm the status of the ascending aorta but not useful for assessment of the aortic arch because of shadowing from the trachea and lungs. Cardiac dysfunction and valvular abnormalities are commonly identified by echocardiography in patients with arch or ascending aortic pathology. The systolic and diastolic function of the left ventricle can be well assessed with these studies, in addition to gathering information regarding pulmonary hypertension and right-sided heart failure. Cardiac catheterization is routinely performed before open arch surgery and is selectively performed in the setting of endovascular procedures, particularly in patients with evidence of cardiac dysfunction (i.e., symptoms, reversible ischemia on stress analysis, or concerns related to echocardiography). The information gained provides details about the status of the coronary anatomy and valvular or left ventricular dysfunction, as well as selective aortic images.

Pulmonary Evaluation

Assessment of pulmonary status largely revolves around the evaluation of pulmonary function tests so that the patient's pulmonary condition can be improved preoperatively. Chronic obstructive pulmonary disease is common in patients with aortic pathology, and pulmonary function tests are primarily used as a measure to predict the risk for respiratory problems after the procedure. Although most open arch repairs are performed through a median sternotomy, which is less debilitating to pulmonary function than is a left thoracotomy, considerable risk exists. Forced expiratory volume exhaled during the first second is used to assess obstructive airway disease, whereas forced expiratory flow at 25% to 75% of forced vital capacity is used to assess small-airway disease and effort-independent expiration, two factors that have been linked to ventilator-weaning difficulties.[7] These tests are particularly important when one is considering staged treatment of complex aneurysmal disease involving the arch and descending thoracic aorta.

Neurologic Evaluation

A complete neurologic examination is necessary as a baseline for each patient before any arch intervention. Duplex ultrasonography is performed to assess the status of the origin of all arch branches, any stenoses within the carotid bulb, and distal internal carotid flow, in addition to flow direction, dominance, and the presence of occlusive disease of the vertebral arteries. Cross-sectional imaging studies of the brain (usually magnetic resonance angiography/imaging) are routinely obtained before open surgical arch repair and selectively in endovascular cases. These studies provide information about the morphology of the circle of Willis, as well as previous neurologic events. A remarkably high proportion of patients show evidence of previous strokes or brain scarring or atrophy. Such lesions have been associated with a greater risk for stroke or delayed neurologic recovery after surgery. Prospective analyses have noted that up to 38% of patients will have neurocognitive deficits on preoperative neurocognitive testing that correlate with lesions detected by magnetic resonance imaging.[8]

■ NATURAL HISTORY AND INDICATIONS FOR INTERVENTION

Aneurysms

The natural history of isolated arch disease is poorly documented. Aneurysm size and shape anywhere in the aorta will relate to the risk for rupture and dissection, and the available data must be viewed in the context of potential growth rates and balanced against the risk for complications or death

resulting from an intervention. Although no data exist to define the growth rate of arch aneurysms, it has been reported that aneurysms of the ascending aorta grow at a rate of about 0.07 cm/yr and those of the descending aorta at a rate of 0.19 cm/yr.[9] It seems logical that aneurysms of the arch enlarge at a rate somewhere between the two. The presence of aortic dissection tends to cause accelerated growth, which increases the range to 0.14 to 0.28 cm/yr.[10] It also has been noted that larger aneurysms grow faster than smaller aneurysms.[10] The average size of rupture or dissection for ascending aneurysms is 6 cm and that for descending aneurysms is 7.2 cm, so the indication for intervention for these two aortic segments is 5.0 to 5.5 cm and 5.5 to 6.5 cm, respectively, depending on patient age and co-morbid conditions.[11] Several factors can influence the clinician to alter the size at which an intervention is indicated. Marfan's syndrome, bicuspid aortic valves, and a strong family history of aneurysmal disease or rupture may prompt earlier interventions, whereas serious co-morbid diseases may result in a more conservative approach. Little data exist to support early intervention for small penetrating ulcers of the aortic arch. Most are detected incidentally when CT scans are obtained for unrelated pathologies, and others are manifested as rupture, most typically into the mediastinum. Although treatment is always indicated if possible for ruptured arch aneurysms, anti-impulse therapy and medical management of such lesions have been successful in nonsurgical candidates.

Dissection

The most common manifestations of aortic arch dissection are the residual flaps after surgical repair of a proximal dissection with an ascending graft. After repair of ascending dissections, the unrepaired and thus vulnerable aorta should be serially monitored. Aortic dilatation in such a setting should be considered for intervention. In contrast, dissections originating within the arch or distal to the left subclavian artery followed by retrograde propagation into the arch pose a poorly defined risk for further complications, including involvement of the ascending aorta or root, coronary artery dissection, and cardiac tamponade. Many clinicians have argued that urgent repair of such lesions is required, whereas others may elect to treat these lesions medically, analogous to uncomplicated distal dissections. The prognosis of de novo dissections originating in the arch is probably different from that of the more grave outcomes resulting from retrograde arch and ascending dissection after endovascular repair.[12]

In summary, treatment is recommended for patients with arch aneurysms that exceed 5.5 to 6 cm, depending on the lesion's morphology and etiology and the extent of co-morbid conditions. Chronically dissected arches and patients with Marfan's syndrome may require earlier intervention.[13] Dissections originating within the aortic arch may be treated surgically in good-risk candidates or handled akin to uncomplicated distal dissections. Symptomatic penetrating ulcers and large ulcers (>2 cm) are best repaired in patients without extensive co-morbid conditions.

OPEN SURGICAL REPAIR

The decision to intervene on an arch aneurysm must be accompanied by a well-thought-out surgical plan. Attention to concomitant disease, such as coronary artery disease, is crucial for planning such procedures. The status of the ascending and descending thoracic aorta is also critical. Ascending repair can be performed along with arch repair through a median sternotomy, but access to the descending aorta is limited, and thus staged procedures or a clamshell incision may be required. Isolated arch disease, particularly focal defects, can simply be resected and replaced with a patch, whereas more extensive disease requires more formal aortic repair. Regardless of the type of operation that will be conducted, the heart, brain, recurrent laryngeal nerve, and kidneys must be protected.

Cerebral Protection

Deep Hypothermic Circulatory Arrest

The use of deep hypothermic circulatory arrest was originally described by Griepp and colleagues in 1975,[14] and today, most patients undergoing open aortic arch surgery benefit from this method of brain protection.[8,15-17] The neuroprotection conveyed is hypothesized to occur as a result of a reduction in cerebral metabolism, as well as slowing of several ischemic injury cascades. In addition to the overall higher morbidity and mortality inherent in surgeries that require deep hypothermic circulatory arrest, hypothermia has relatively specific detrimental effects on the coagulation cascade[18-20] that result in increased bleeding, as well as a higher risk for wound infections.[21] There is still controversy regarding the required degree of hypothermia, the method of cannulation, and the use of brain perfusion adjuncts (antegrade or retrograde) intended to limit cerebral ischemia time.[22] Animal research, retrospective studies, and prospective randomized trials have assessed various aspects of cooling, the use of heart-lung machines, and acid buffering,[8,23-25] which has resulted in several protocols allowing deep hypothermic circulatory arrest.[26]

The essential features of most protocols include methods to cool patients below 20° C, electroencephalographic monitoring of brain activity, the use of pentothal before circulatory arrest, the administration of neuroprotective pharmacologic agents, the use of membrane oxygenators, filtration on pump tubing, and the speed with which warming occurs.[27] The most common site of cannulation for deep hypothermia and circulatory arrest has historically been the common femoral artery, although today many surgeons prefer using the axillary, subclavian,[28,29] or even the innominate artery.[30] A marked reduction in the incidence of stroke was noted when using a conduit anastomosed to the axillary or subclavian artery as opposed to

direct aortic cannulation, cannulation of the femoral artery, or direct introduction of the cannula into the subclavian or axillary artery. Such a technique also facilitates the use of antegrade brain perfusion by simply occluding the proximal innominate artery (with a balloon) while allowing infusion into the side graft. This has been shown to generate very few microemboli[31] and can be supplemented with an additional catheter placed in the left common carotid artery to achieve bilateral antegrade brain perfusion, a technique that is particularly useful if it is known that the circle of Willis is not complete (required in approximately 14% of patients). The technique is also used for distal arch aneurysms that involve the descending thoracic aorta when it is not possible to safely clamp the proximal aorta. Success has been reported in such circumstances, but with a higher incidence of complications, including renal issues, bleeding, stroke, and cardiac problems.[32]

Antegrade and Retrograde Cerebral Perfusion

The use of antegrade versus retrograde brain perfusion has been controversial.[16,17,26,33-35] Antegrade perfusion maintains physiologic flow and pressure through arterial access, whereas retrograde perfusion relies on venous access and flow reversal for perfusion. The benefits of antegrade perfusion (Fig. 134-6) are obvious, and the attributes of retrograde cerebral perfusion include a certain amount of perfusion in addition to the ability to evacuate any air and debris that may have accumulated in the cerebral vascular system during a circulatory arrest procedure. To accomplish retrograde cerebral perfusion, the superior vena cava must be encircled and cannulated and serves as the means to deliver flow in a retrograde manner into the cerebrovascular system. Animal studies have demonstrated that the initial pressure required to overcome the valve system in the jugular veins is relatively high and that the degree of perfusion is perhaps suboptimal. In our analysis of more than 900 patients undergoing retrograde brain perfusion, we have been unable to demonstrate a reduction in stroke incidence when compared with patients undergoing deep hypothermia and circulatory arrest alone.[36] However, randomized trials have failed to definitively identify an optimal method for adjunctive cerebral perfusion.[37] Extended and complex methods of providing brain perfusion in the setting of hypothermic circulatory arrest may serve to lengthen the arrest period, thus offsetting any potential benefit of the perfusion.[8] However, based on our current level of understanding, we do not recommend any form of brain perfusion for most patients undergoing hemiarch replacement. If there is a concern regarding embolic issues arising from arch debris or endarterectomy, retrograde perfusion may be used, particularly during the terminal portion of the reconstruction. Patients requiring total arch replacement are subjected to hypothermic circulatory arrest supplemented with either antegrade or retrograde perfusion to safely conduct the operative repair. These strategies are summarized in Table 134-1.

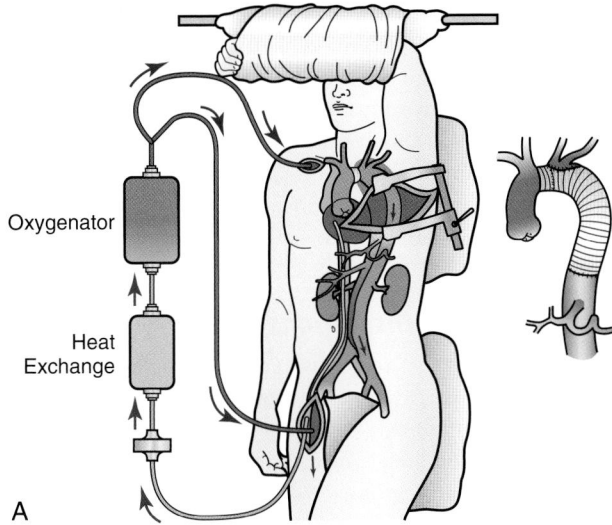

Table 134-1 Perfusion Techniques in Total Arch Replacement

Procedure	Hypothermia	Antegrade Perfusion	Retrograde Perfusion
Hemiarch	<20°C	No	No
+ Aortic dissection	<20°C	No	No
+ Endarterectomy	<20°C	No	Only if embolic concern
+ Innominate branch	Moderate	Yes	No
+ Severe aortic incompetence	Moderate	Yes	No
Total arch	<20°C	Yes*	Yes*
+ Branches (2-3)	<20° or moderate	Yes	No
+ Elephant trunk	<20°C	Yes*	Yes*
Saccular aneurysm			
Option 1	<20°C	No	Yes
Option 2	Moderate	Yes	No

*Indicates that either antegrade or retrograde brain perfusion is used for the procedure.

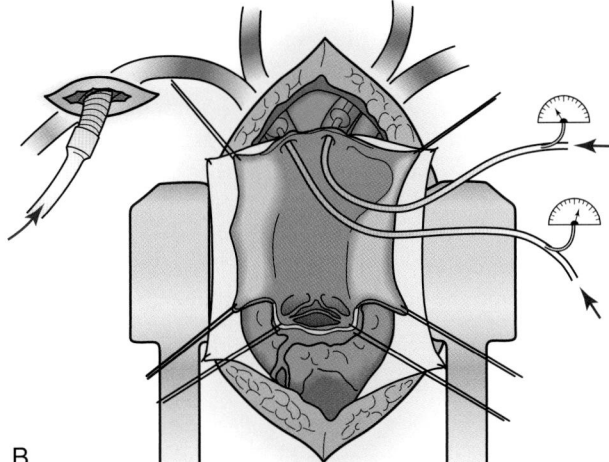

Figure 134-6 Perfusion techniques. **A,** Antegrade perfusion is delivered to the axillary artery via a conduit. Blood acquired from a venous cannula is oxygenated and then recirculated into the arterial system via a femoral arterial line and, if desired, an axillary line. The axillary line is typically inserted through a conduit, and when antegrade perfusion is used, the origins of the supra-aortic trunk vessels must be occluded. This can be done with clamps or with balloon catheters as depicted in **B.**

Open Repair Techniques

Total Arch Replacement

Total arch replacement without an elephant trunk graft (ETG) procedure is fairly uncommon and accounts for only about 10% of our arch operations, given the likelihood that the disease will extend into the descending thoracic aorta despite the presence of a neck at the isthmus and distal arch. Isolated total arch replacement involves an end-to-end anastomosis to the proximal descending thoracic aorta while ensuring that such an anastomosis occurs 2 to 3 cm distal to the origin of any of the supra-aortic trunk vessels (Fig. 134-7). This construct will facilitate any future repairs that are required to address pathology of the descending thoracic

aorta. After construction of the distal anastomosis (which is performed under hypothermic circulatory arrest), the arch vessels are reimplanted as an island or via individual grafts. The patient is then rewarmed while the proximal anastomosis is completed to a segment of nondiseased ascending aorta, which is most commonly the sinotubular junction, or to a root graft.

Hemiarch Repairs

This subgroup of patients typically has aortic root and ascending aneurysms that extend into the aortic arch. Surgical decisions for such patients revolve around the need to replace the aortic valve or the aortic root with coronary reimplantation and the distal extent of arch involvement. In general, patients younger than 80 years can tolerate hypothermic circulatory arrest relatively well, in contrast to older patients, in whom the risk for stroke becomes higher.[16] Thus, patients younger than 80 years will typically undergo a single procedure that is intended to address the ascending aortic and arch pathology concomitantly, with or without valve and aortic root repair. When the arch component is limited to the proximal arch in the region of the innominate artery, a simple hemiarch replacement can be done by transecting the aorta at the distal end of the diseased segment in a beveled manner to incorporate the innominate or left common carotid artery, or the vessels can be reimplanted as an island or via individual prosthetic grafts. During such a repair, a variable amount of arch tissue can be replaced by tailoring the prosthesis to incorporate a segment of the proximal descending thoracic aorta. As mentioned previously, such procedures can be done without the use of antegrade or retrograde cerebral perfusion, assuming that there is limited concern for the generation of atheroembolic material. Distal

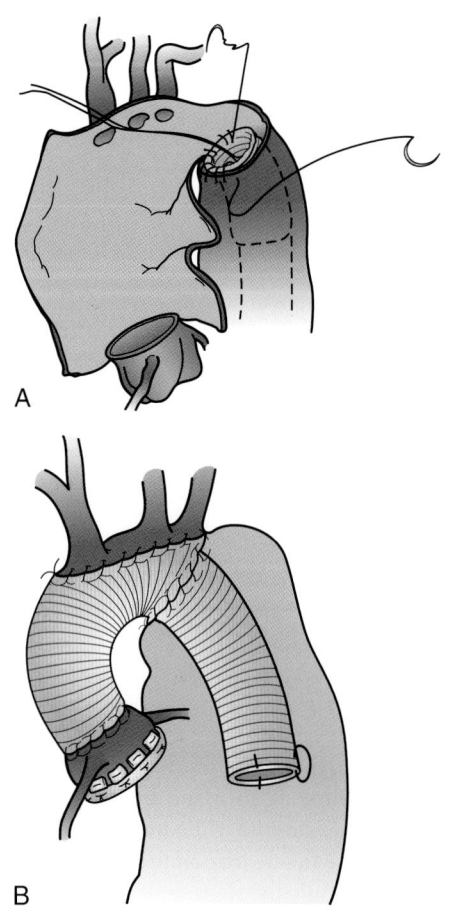

Figure 134-7 Total arch elephant trunk procedure. The repair is typically performed in a distal-to-proximal fashion. The desired graft material is involuted on itself to create a double-layered graft. The aortic arch is opened and the graft is placed in the descending thoracic aorta. An anastomosis is then constructed either distal to the left subclavian artery or between the left carotid and subclavian arteries (**A**). This anastomosis typically has to be re-enforced with pledgeted sutures as well. The inner layer is then withdrawn and the supra-aortic trunk vessels are attached as an island to the graft, with the proximal anastomosis sewn to healthy aorta or, as in this case, to the sinotubular junction (**B**).

arch aneurysms may also be approached via a left thoracotomy. Although this is a reasonable option for select patients (such as individuals with multiple previous median sternotomies), the risk for stroke and neurocognitive deficit is somewhat higher than with an anterior staged ETG strategy, particularly if deep hypothermic circulatory arrest is required for a proximal anastomosis[32] and in the era of endovascular completion of ETG.[38]

Segmental Arch Repair

For localized aneurysms of the aortic arch or proximal descending aorta, the repair can be simplified by using techniques involving aortic débridement and prosthetic patching. Isolated saccular aneurysms can be repaired in this manner after induction of circulatory arrest by opening the aneurysm, removing the surrounding calcium from the aneurysm neck,

and closing the defect with a polyester patch. In patients with mycotic aneurysms, it is preferable to use either homograft or pericardial tissue and thoroughly débride the area. If this is not available, a gel-infiltrated graft can be used, and if the organism is known, an antimicrobial agent such as gentamicin (against gram-negative organisms and *Staphylococcus*), rifampin (against gram-positive organisms), or amphotericin B (against fungal infections) can used to soak the graft.

Repair of Aortic Dissections

In most patients with acute dissections involving the ascending aorta or the aortic arch, the aorta can be transected at the innominate artery during circulatory arrest to allow construction of the distal anastomosis, followed by the proximal anastomosis in the region of the sinotubular junction during rewarming. In approximately 10% of patients with proximal dissection the tear originates in the aortic arch, and some controversy exists regarding the most appropriate management and repair strategy. In the absence of a rupture or dilatation the tear may simply be closed with two layers of running 4-0 polypropylene suture and pledgets. Although this is not an optimal procedure for these patients, in some circumstances it offers the fastest means to repair the proximal extent of the dissection and have the patient survive the operation. Alternatively, if the arch is aneurysmal, total arch repair or ETG repair may be carried out, depending on the extent of the disease and the acuity of the symptoms.

Elephant Trunk Grafts

The ETG procedure was originally described by Hans Borst and associates.[39] The first stage of this procedure involves an arch repair with placement of a polyester graft, a portion of which is left dangling in the aneurysmal proximal thoracic aorta (see Fig. 134-7). The technique has evolved into anastomosis of a double layer of graft by inverting the graft into itself, pushing the invaginated graft into the descending aorta, and then sewing the distal anastomosis to the most suitable segment of aorta distal to the left subclavian artery or between the left subclavian and carotid arteries. This anastomosis is frequently supplemented with a second layer of pledgeted sutures. The inner graft is withdrawn through the completed anastomosis, and the great vessels are attached followed by the reconstruction of the proximal anastomosis. The ETG can be used in concert with a total arch repair or in isolation during other cardiac procedures to facilitate later treatment of distal arch or proximal descending aortic aneurysms.

Management of such extensive aortic aneurysms is associated with considerable risk. Safi and coauthors reported 218 ascending arch repairs by ETG with a mortality of 9% for the first stage and 10% for the second stage, in addition to other morbid events.[40] We reported a 2% mortality rate for the first stage with a 5% stroke rate and an interstage mortality of 12%. Of the patients who underwent the second stage (57%), 4% died.[41] The second stage of the

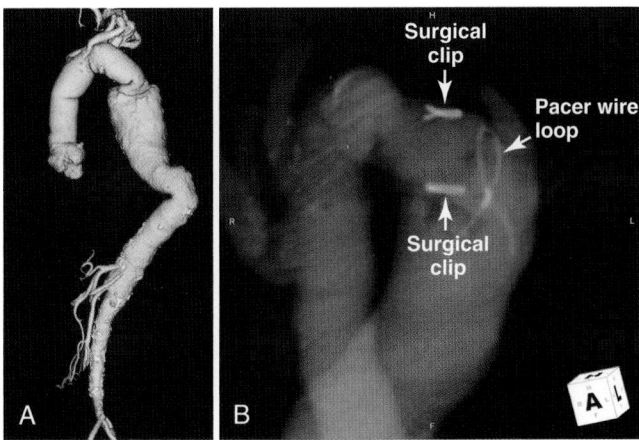

Figure 134-8 Elephant trunk graft (ETG) completion. **A,** After placement of an ETG it is often helpful to repeat a CT scan to delineate the status of the ETG in terms of expanded diameter and tortuosity. Specific views of the repair can be created to visualize the terminal end of the graft. We prefer to place hemoclips in two locations at the end of the graft and often attach a wire loop more proximally on the outer graft aspect. **B,** The loop can be cannulated and retracted after snaring it to apply countertraction should it prove to be challenging to advance the endovascular graft into the ETG.

procedure has historically been performed through a left thoracotomy and aortotomy with rapid retrieval and clamping of the ETG.[39] The distal end of the ETG serves as the site for the proximal anastomosis of the second-stage repair. The completion, or second-stage, procedure is arguably more difficult for patients to tolerate than the initial procedure. The advent of endovascular techniques to treat the descending thoracic aorta has allowed the second-stage procedure to be completed in a less invasive manner, presuming that the distal descending aorta is an appropriate seal zone for endograft repair. If consideration is given to endo-

vascular completion of the ETG, the first-stage procedure should be modified accordingly. The length of the ETG must be carefully tailored to the extent of the distal aneurysm, tortuosity of the aorta, and the presence of a distal dissection. Metallic clips placed onto the terminal end of the ETG and dangling within the proximal descending thoracic aneurysm will allow fluoroscopic visualization of the length of graft material (Fig. 134-8). Additionally, a pacing wire sewn 1 cm from the distal end of the ETG can provide a means of applying traction to the ETG while advancing an endovascular device.[38,41]

HYBRID STRATEGIES

Several methods have been proposed to limit the invasiveness of open surgery involving the aortic arch and ameliorate the morbidity associated with hypothermic circulatory arrest. All involve the use of endovascular stent-grafts and most commonly extra-anatomic bypass, yet they differ in the manner in which the stent-grafts are introduced, procedure timing, the location of fixation and sealing, and the necessity for multiple stages. Table 134-2 summarizes the results of hybrid arch repair strategies in the context of the type of repair used and the risk for stroke or death.

Hybrid Elephant Trunk Completion
Endovascular Completion

The traditional ETG operation involves two stages, the first via a median sternotomy. The completion procedure is most frequently done in a staged fashion through a left thoracotomy or thoracoabdominal incision. There is a significant number of patients who die as a result of rupture before

Table 134-2 Hybrid Aortic Arch Repair Results

Type of Repair	Series	Number of Patients	Perioperative Mortality (%)	Neurologic Deficit (%)
Extra-anatomic bypass	Melissano et al.[42]	37	6.3	3.1 stroke 3.1 paraplegia
	Szeto et al.[43]	8	13	25 cerebral 0 paraplegia
	Schumacher et al.[44]	25 (16 hemiarch, 9 total arch)	20 elective, 36 emergency cases	0 paraplegia 5 stroke
	Bergeron et al.[45]	25 (15 total arch)	8	4
	Akasaka et al.[46]	12	0	16 (1 stroke, 1 paraplegia)
	Czerny et al.[47]	27 (10 total arch)	7.4	0
Frozen elephant trunk graft	Baraki et al.[48]	39 (18 arch aneurysms, 21 dissections)	13	13
	Gorlitzer et al.[49]	7 (5 dissections, 2 aneurysms)	0	14
	Mizuno et al.[50]	9	22	33 (2 paraplegia, 1 stroke)
	Chavan et al.[51]	22	4.5	13.6
	Usui et al.[52]	24	0	17
	Kato et al.[53]	19	5.3	15.8 (2 paraplegia, 1 stroke)
Retrograde elephant trunk graft completion	Greenberg et al.[38]	22	4.5	13.6 (paraplegia all with thoracoabdominal + arch repairs)
Arch branch	Inoue et al.[54]	15	0	6.7
	Ferreira et al., Schneider et al[55,56]	2	0	0

the second-stage ETG completion, in addition to a subset of patients who simply do not return for their second-stage operation.[41,57] For these reasons, several attempts have been made to modify the conventional operation so that it becomes a single-stage procedure or a less invasive multistage procedure. The purpose of the ETG is to facilitate a safe and durable proximal anastomosis that is accessible from the left side of the chest. This readily lends itself to endovascular completion. In fact, the surgical graft dangling within the descending thoracic aorta provides an optimal location to seal and fixate an endovascular device. The first hybrid ETG completion was reported in 2001.[58] The Cleveland Clinic series remains the largest to date and described several fundamental modifications that have proved useful in cases intended for hybrid therapy.[38,41]

Technique. It is important to ensure that the distal end of the ETG is visible with fluoroscopy. Placement of metallic hemoclips along the distal end provides markers that can readily be identified during the completion procedure (see Fig. 134-8). The length of the ETG is critical. Excessively long ETGs become overly tortuous, complicate introduction of the endovascular graft, and potentially create problems during follow-up because of graft lengthening (Fig. 134-9). Furthermore, it appears that the risk for paralysis from long ETGs is increased as well. The proximal anastomosis of the ETG to the aortic arch cannot be constrictive or provide an inflow source between sutures into the distal aneurysm sac. If the anastomosis is flow restrictive, thrombus can develop and the ETG can occlude. Next, through-and-through access into the ETG should be established via a right brachial approach. This will prevent the need for excessive manipulation within the aneurysm sac and alongside the dangling ETG, a region that is frequently lined with thrombus. Next, adequate overlap into the ETG with only mild oversizing should be ensured. Optimally, the endovascular graft will not transcend the arch curvature but reside entirely within the relatively straight segment of the ETG in the proximal descending thoracic aorta. Finally, the endovascular graft should be fixated within the ETG. Considerable morphologic changes in polyester grafts occur during follow-up. The crimps straighten and the graft lengthens, which results in unexpected tortuosity. The joint between the ETG and stent-graft is modular and therefore subject to dislocation.

Frozen Elephant Trunk

The use of intraoperative stented ETGs, also termed *frozen ETG*, has been proposed as a means of treating arch aneurysms that extend into the proximal to mid-descending thoracic aorta. To accomplish this, the distal component of the repair must be delivered through an open aortic arch in the beginning of the procedure. The technique most commonly used to do so differs from other conventional endovascular options. Blunt-tipped delivery systems that can be inserted directly into the proximal descending thoracic aorta without

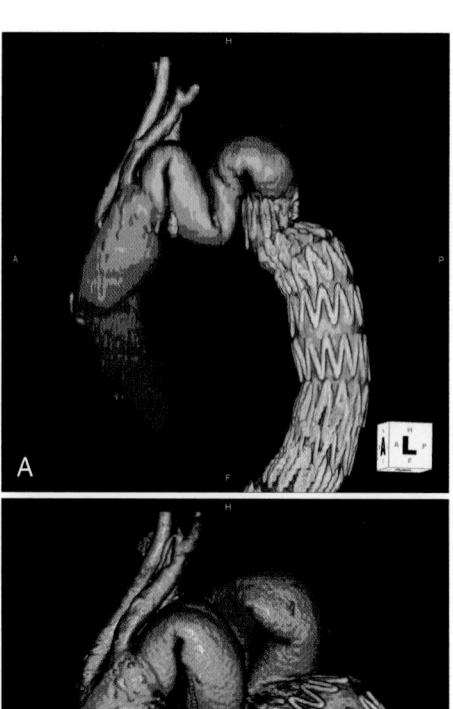

Figure 134-9 Elephant trunk graft (ETG) follow-up. Long ETGs have been noted to be disadvantageous. Two primary issues have been cited. The first is a higher risk for paraplegia, and the second relates to the tortuosity that develops as the ETG lengthens over time. **A** and **B,** ETG repair before discharge (**A**) and after 3 years of follow-up (**B**). The centerline length of the ETG has increased by approximately 7 cm, which has imposed added tortuosity and morphologic changes in the proximal aspect of the stent-graft.

the use of a wire have been used. The advantage of this method is the speed with which it can be accomplished and the fact that it obviates the need for fluoroscopy. This technique has been used to treat both aneurysms and dissections with success.[48-53,59,60] This technique cannot be performed safely in the setting of more distal disease and in patients with complex dissections resulting in fenestrations and lumina in the proximal descending aorta. Modifications of this technique have been used, including fluoroscopically guided placement with over-the-wire devices and the use of femoral access, simply to provide a true lumen wire on which a device can be delivered from the arch. Challenges with these procedures include the potential for prolonging circulatory arrest time and the risk for paraplegia. The latter was noted to be a serious issue when longer distal components of the ETG were used.[58] The high incidence of paraplegia in these cases has been attributed to a "multiple-hit" hypothesis whereby the blood supply to the cord is detrimentally nonpulsatile flow while on pump (often with low pressures); intercostals covered by the stent-graft are lost; and a period of hypothermic circulatory arrest is needed. For these reasons, the frozen ETG technique is commonly restricted to proximal lesions only.

Reverse Elephant Trunk

In certain circumstances it may be advantageous to complete the endovascular portion before performance of an open arch procedure. This may be considered if the fixation and sealing region is questionable, and in the absence of a secure device that excludes the aneurysm, the proximal end of the stent-graft can serve as the distal anastomosis for an open arch repair or can simply be sutured to the surrounding aorta in a manner similar to a conventional ETG (Fig. 134-10). To accomplish this, the stent-graft must be deployed into the arch, frequently proximal to the left subclavian artery, or it may be difficult to use as a distal site for the anastomosis.

■ ARCH-DEBRANCHING OPERATIONS

To treat an aneurysm involving the aortic arch with a stent-graft it is necessary to "debranch" the great vessels that would need to be covered for effective proximal sealing of the endograft. There are several options for revascularization, depending on which great vessels need to be covered.

Bypass Grafting via Median Sternotomy

This method is used when the origins of all three great vessels need to be moved to the proximal ascending aorta. It requires at least a partial sternotomy but avoids the use of circulatory arrest. To accomplish this technique, a side-biting clamp is carefully applied to an acceptable region of the ascending aorta, and a bifurcated, trifurcated, or large tubular graft is anastomosed in an end-to-side fashion (Fig. 134-11). Placement of this anastomosis within the ascending aorta is critical because the region immediately distal to it will be the required seal zone for the endovascular graft. Each of the supra-aortic trunk vessels is then ligated proximally and the distal end is attached in an end-to-end or end-to-side fashion in a sequential manner to eliminate significant cerebral ischemia. After construction of the bypass graft, the endovascular graft can be inserted via either an antegrade side graft or a retrograde femoral approach. If an antegrade approach is desired, a side arm is attached to the extra-anatomic bypass graft near the ascending aortic anastomosis to allow device delivery.[61] If a retrograde femoral approach is desired, it can be performed in a staged or single-setting fashion. Clearly, with any extra-anatomic bypass approach, fluoroscopy must be used to ensure proper positioning of the endografts.

Cervical Bypass Grafts

This method is used when only the left subclavian and left common carotid arteries need to be debranched. The use of

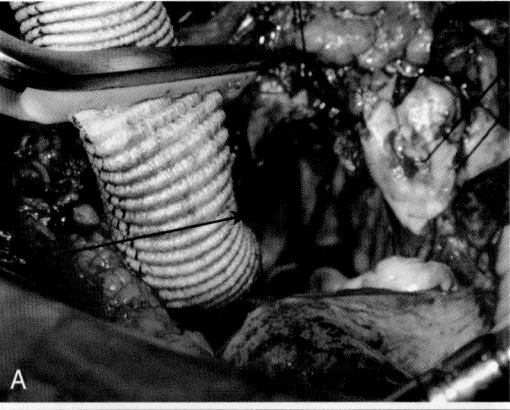
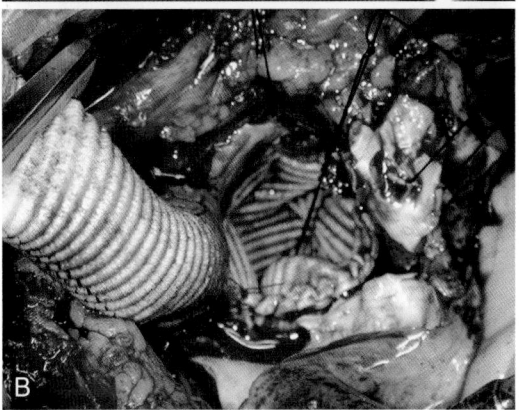
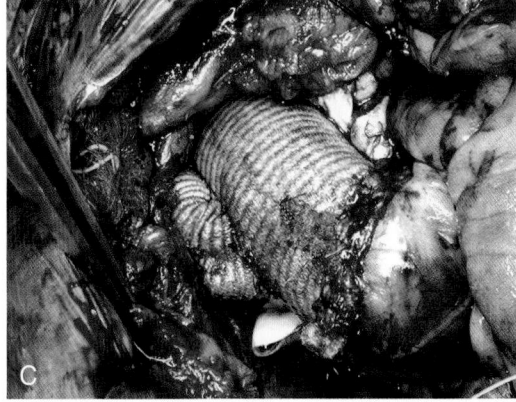

Figure 134-10 Reverse elephant trunk graft (ETG). In some circumstances it may be beneficial to implant the stent-grafts before an arch procedure. **A,** Picture taken through an open arch. The *arrow* points to the stent-grafts within the descending thoracic aorta. The graft material has been sewn to the island of the supra-aortic trunk vessels for purposes of antegrade perfusion. The ETG is then pushed into the stent-grafts and sewn to the proximal edge (**B**). The inner layer of graft is then withdrawn and the arch vessels anastomosed. The proximal anastomosis is constructed to healthy ascending aorta (**C**).

cervical bypass grafts has historically been relegated to the treatment of occlusive disease and combined with stent-grafts as originally described by Buth and colleagues.[62]

Left Carotid-Subclavian Bypass

The most commonly performed bypass is from the left common carotid artery to the left subclavian artery when

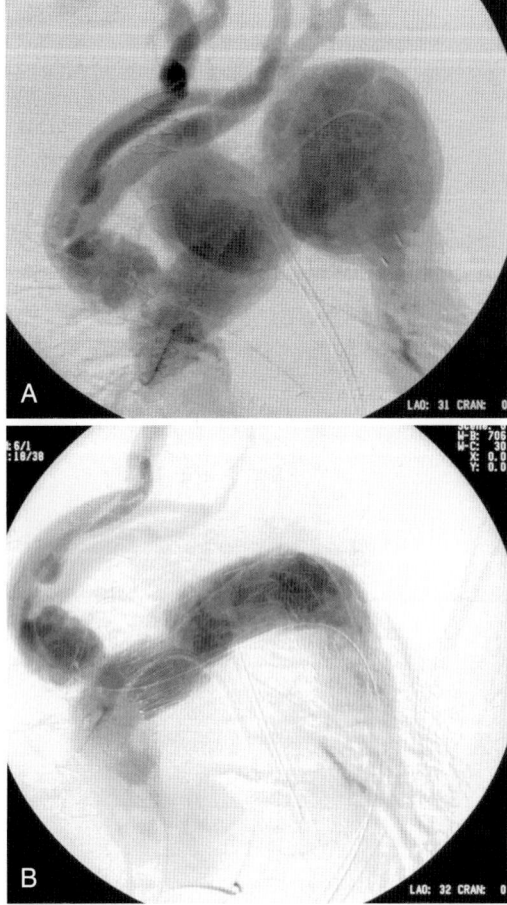

Figure 134-11 Ascending aortic bypass. Transthoracic bypass requires an anastomosis sewn to the ascending aorta. This can be done through a conventional or partial median sternotomy. Techniques using a bifurcated graft (**A**) and tubular constructs have been described. Imaging after bypass is essential, although this may be accomplished during the same procedure. The endovascular device can then be inserted in a traditional retrograde femoral manner or through an additional side arm sutured to the ascending aortic bypass graft. The endograft is placed so that it abuts the proximal anastomosis of the bypass to ensure maximal aortic coverage (**B**).

only the left subclavian orifice needs to be covered with an aortic stent-graft. Although the left subclavian artery was initially considered to be somewhat superfluous (in the absence of internal mammary–based coronary circulation or dominant vertebral flow) and was covered with an aortic endograft proximally without much risk, recent literature has demonstrated the importance of the vessel.[63-65] When the left subclavian artery is occluded proximally in the absence of a bypass graft, vertebral artery blood flow is usually reversed and provides inflow for the arm and upper part of the chest. By providing antegrade flow to the left subclavian from the carotid, antegrade left vertebral and internal mammary flow is maintained. Consideration must also be given to preserving vertebral arteries arising directly from the arch. In this situation, reimplantation of the vertebral onto the common carotid can readily be performed simultaneously with a carotid-

subclavian bypass. Preservation of antegrade vertebral flow may be beneficial to the spinal cord circulation and help diminish the risk for paraplegia in the setting of long descending thoracic grafts that extend into the arch. The risks associated with such a bypass are minimal, particularly when proximal dissection and ligation of the subclavian are not performed but completed with endovascular coils or plugs. As an alternative to bypass, subclavian-to-carotid artery transposition can also be performed (see Chapter 100: Brachiocephalic Artery Disease: Surgical Treatment).

Carotid-Carotid Bypass

Carotid-carotid bypasses were rarely needed before endovascular grafting of the aortic arch. The technique involves bilateral midneck incisions with a prosthetic graft sewn end to side to both vessels, followed by proximal ligation of the left common carotid artery. The bypass graft is usually extended to the left subclavian artery as well in this circumstance. The graft can be tunneled in front of or behind the esophagus, although many prefer the anterior approach to avoid complaints regarding pulsatile flow along the posterior of the esophagus during eating. The patency of these bypass grafts is generally good,[66,67] and surgical complications are rare. The procedure is fairly well tolerated, even by patients with considerable co-morbid conditions; however, the amount of distance gained for coverage on the aorta is relatively small. The distance between each of the supra-aortic trunk vessels is typically 1 to 2 cm, and the arch, in that region, is generally tortuous. Thus, careful assessment of the anatomy must be made to determine whether a bypass graft based on anything other than the ascending aorta will provide an adequate region for sealing and fixation. Endovascular grafts can be deployed immediately after extra-anatomic bypass procedures or in a staged manner.

Double-Barrel Endovascular Debranching

Recently, some authors have described a method of preserving arch vessel patency while covering the target vessel ostium with an aortic stent-graft and simultaneously placing a parallel graft from the target arch branch. Such a technique has been used in the infrarenal aorta in the setting of short proximal necks to protect the renal arteries.[68] To accomplish this technique in the arch, retrograde wire and sheath access must be obtained from the desired supra-aortic trunk vessels into the ascending aorta before stent-graft deployment. Then, after placement of the aortic stent-graft, a second stent or stent-graft is placed in such a manner that it extends from the proximal sealing region of the aortic stent-grafts well into the supra-aortic trunk vessel. The length of this stent runs in parallel with the aortic graft to the level of the proximal seal. The supra-aortic trunk stent thus acts as a "snorkel" and creates a "double barrel" that allows blood to flow into the arch vessel alongside the aortic stent-grafts. A small number of cases using such a technique have been reported, but most consider this a bailout procedure.[69-71] The primary problems with such a strategy relate to incomplete mating of the two parallel stent-grafts. Thus, although this approach may be applicable for certain focal arch aneurysms, its use for fusiform aneurysms of the arch is probably limited because the aortic seal zone is compromised and the deformation of both the aortic stent-grafts and parallel stent is concerning from a biomechanical standpoint (Fig. 134-12). Further concern is raised by the potential for intimal injury and subsequent retrograde dissection in the setting of unequal wall apposition and disparate motion between the two devices.

BRANCHED AND FENESTRATED ENDOVASCULAR GRAFTS

Branched Stent-Grafts

The first successful deployment of a branched graft for the supra-aortic trunk vessels was reported by Inoue and colleagues in 1996[72] and then the data supplemented in 1999.[54] The device used consisted of a unibody graft with multiple (up to three) limbs that are snared and pulled into each of the aortic trunk vessels. Surprisingly, this was accomplished with local anesthesia in 14 of the first 15 patients treated. Some issues, including stroke risk and graft material durability, were encountered during development of the devices and have slowed refinement of the device and technique considerably. Chuter and coauthors reported successful treatment of an arch aneurysm with the first modular branched device in 2003 (Fig. 134-13).[73] The device used is functionally a bifurcated endograft that is deployed from a conduit sewn to the innominate or proximal right carotid artery. The proximal portion of the implant resides within the mid-ascending aorta, and the ipsilateral limb is deployed into the innominate artery. After deployment of the proximal component, cannulation of the "contralateral limb" is achieved from a retrograde femoral access site, and the distal thoracic device is inserted into the overlap segment and deployed. Two reports of this technique have been published.[55,73]

Fenestrated Stent-Grafts

The use of fenestrations for arch vessels has been described, but no large published series exist. Although this is a direct extension of abdominal fenestrations,[74] they pose a different set of challenges. Alignment of the fenestrations in the abdominal segment is aided by the relatively straight morphology of the visceral aorta, in contrast to the aortic arch. Consequently, alternative techniques have been used to orient the fenestrations. Methods have included the use of precurved delivery systems, preloaded catheters and wires, and torque-controlled flexible devices (Fig. 134-14). Placement of mating stents or stent-grafts is typically done via one or more of the brachial vessels, which in the setting of a left carotid branch will require a carotid-subclavian bypass graft or direct left carotid artery access. The concept of fenestrating a stent-graft from a retrograde approach has been termed *in situ fenestration*. Although this technique has been described

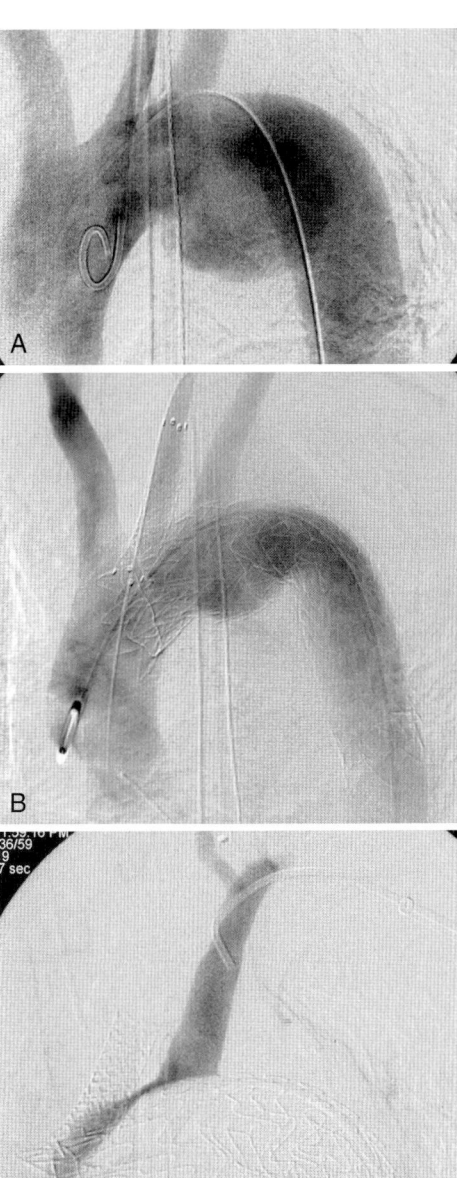

Figure 134-12 Chimney grafts for arch aneurysms. This series of images from 2003 demonstrates the use of chimney grafts to treat a ruptured arch aneurysm in a pulmonary cripple. The initial angiogram (**A**) shows the arch aneurysm abutting the left common carotid origin. The aortic stent-grafts were intentionally placed so that they covered the left subclavian and the left common carotid arteries, and a stent was placed inside the left common carotid artery, alongside the aortic stent, and terminated at the proximal sealing region (**B**). Although this sealed the rupture that was on the inferior aspect of the aneurysm, the incomplete nature of the seal is readily apparent when an injection is performed from the left subclavian artery (**C**). The contrast material tracks proximally from the left subclavian, between the left carotid stent and aortic stent-grafts, through a channel that is created from the deformity caused by the carotid stent.

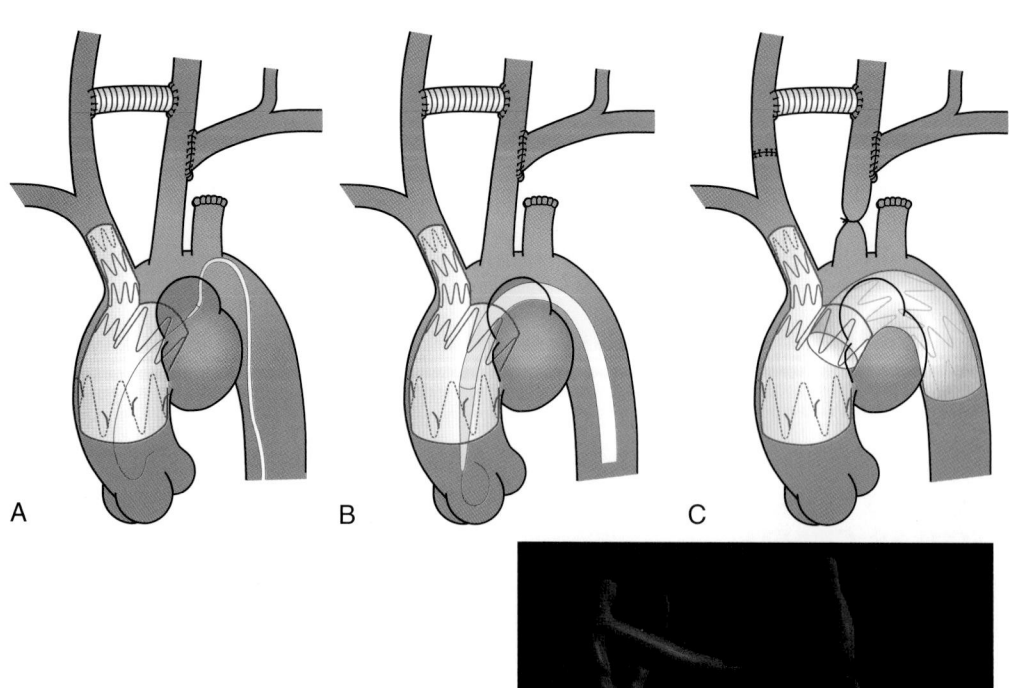

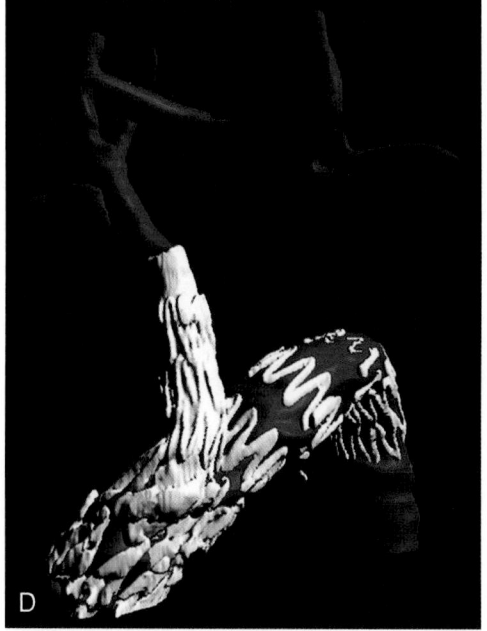

Figure 134-13 Arch branch techniques. This method of treating arch aneurysms involves the use of a bifurcated endograft. The device is deployed via a conduit sewn to the right carotid or innominate artery. The "contralateral" limb is intended to reside within the proximal arch and is cannulated from the groin (**A**). A thoracic extension component is inserted (**B**) and then deployed to complete the repair (**C**). Carotid-carotid-subclavian bypasses maintain the circulation to the remainder of the supra-aortic trunk vessels. A completion CT scan is depicted in **D**.

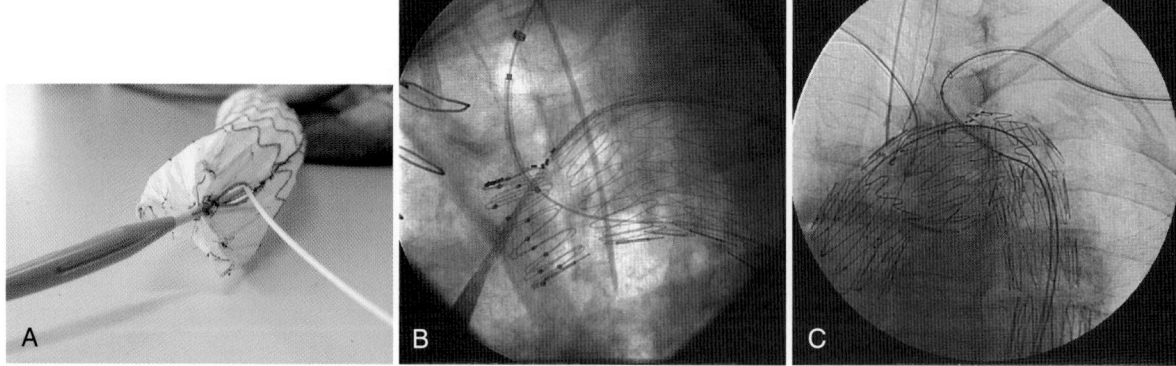

Figure 134-14 Fenestrated and branched arch grafts. The ability to incorporate the supra-aortic trunk vessels into an endovascular repair without a hybrid procedure is challenging given the complex three-dimensional relationship between the branches and the aorta. The inability to rotate a device adequately within the arch without subjecting the patient to a high risk for neurologic insults precludes much device movement. Preloaded wires and catheters have been used to mitigate the risk of improper fenestration/branch alignment along with minimal device movement within the arch. These figures depict an example of a catheter loaded through the fenestration of a thoracic device. After introduction of the device, a wire inserted through the catheter is snared from the desired branch artery. This technique provides through-and-through access into a fenestration or scallop. The device can then be properly positioned with the branch or fenestration immediately below the target vessel, and the delivery sheath can then be withdrawn. Small final modifications in device positioning remain possible given that the endograft remains fixed to the delivery system by the trigger wires (**A**). One (**B**) or two (**C**) branches may be incorporated in this manner.

in animal studies[75] and a few human cases, it is not commonly performed.[76]

Few published series describing fenestrated arch devices exist, and the available data largely relate to case reports.[77] The Najuta endograft system originated from the Tokyo Medical University.[78] Several geometric shapes of the graft exist and are tailored to fit the individual patient arch anatomy. The device is constructed with longitudinally connected Z-stents covered with expanded polytetrafluoroethylene that is sutured only at the proximal and distal ends of the device. The device has been used in hundreds of patients, yet there are no published reports in the English literature.

SELECTED KEY REFERENCES

Appoo JJ, Augoustides JG, Pochettino A, Savino JS, McGarvey ML, Cowie DC, Gambone AJ, Harris H, Cheung AT, Bavaria JE. Perioperative outcome in adults undergoing elective deep hypothermic circulatory arrest with retrograde cerebral perfusion in proximal aortic arch repair: evaluation of protocol-based care. *J Cardiothorac Vasc Anesth*. 2006;20:3-7.
Perhaps the state-of-the-art study indicating an operative mortality of 7.6% and a stroke rate of 3.8% in a series of 79 consecutive patients managed with hypothermic arrest and retrograde cerebral perfusion. The study emphasized the importance of a uniform protocol for the application of brain protective techniques.

Byrne J, Darling RC, III, Roddy SP, Mehta M, Paty PS, Kreienberg PB, Chang BB, Ozsvath KJ, Sternbach Y, Shah DM. Long term outcome for extra-anatomic arch reconstruction. An analysis of 143 procedures. *Eur J Vasc Endovasc Surg*. 2007;34:444-450.
Comprehensive results (i.e., perioperative and long-term follow-up data) on the spectrum of arch vessel reconstructions; operative mortality was less than 1%, and the primary patency rate at 1 year was 98%.

Coady MA, Rizzo JA, Hammond GL, Mandapati D, Darr U, Kpft GS, Elefteriades JA. What is the appropriate size criterion for resection of thoracic aortic aneurysms? *J Thorac Cardiovasc Surg*. 1997;113: 476-491.
This report documented the annual growth rate of degenerative and dissection-related thoracic aneurysms. Intervention for descending lesions was recommended at 6.5 cm.

Greenberg RK, Haddad F, Svensson L, O'Neill S, Walker E, Lyden SP, Clair D, Lytle B. Hybrid approaches to thoracic aortic aneurysms: the role of endovascular elephant trunk completion. *Circulation*. 2005; 112:2619-2626.
Largest and among the first reports of endovascular completion stage 2 elephant trunk repair, even including adjunctive surgical repairs of abdominal aortic branches. A notable reduction in mortality when compared with standard surgical completion stage 2 was demonstrated.

Melissano G, Civilini E, Bertoglio L, Calliari F, Setacci F, Calori G, Chiesa R. Results of endografting of the aortic arch in different landing zones. *Eur J Vasc Endovasc Surg*. 2007;33:561-566.
Large series of thoracic endovascular aneurysm repair implants at various levels of the aortic arch; it details the nature of the debranching procedures needed at the various levels of proximal sealing.

Safi HJ, Miller CC, III, Estrera AL, Huynh TT, Porat EE, Allen BS, Sheinbaum R. Staged repair of extensive aortic aneurysms: long-term experience with the elephant trunk technique. *Ann Surg*. 2004; 240:677-684.
Largest series of elephant trunk operations in the literature with excellent 5-year survival in patients who complete both stages. The article is nicely illustrated with the technical components of the operation. Perhaps most impressive (and relative to Greenberg et al., above), fully 50% of patients did not return for the stage 2 completion operation.

Svensson LG, Husain A, Penney DL, Swanson RA, Margolis DS, Kimmel WA, Nadolny E, Shahian DM. A prospective randomized study of neurocognitive function and S-100 protein after antegrade or retrograde brain perfusion with hypothermic arrest for aortic surgery. *J Thorac Cardiovasc Surg*. 2000;119:163-167.
Fifteen patients were randomly assigned to three different strategies for brain protection during ascending arch surgery. A battery of neurocognitive function studies and a marker of brain injury revealed no difference in the three approaches.

Svensson LG, Kim KH, Blackstone EG, Alster JM, McCarthy PM, Greenberg RK, Sabik JF, D'Agostino RS, Lytle BW, Cosgrove DM. Elephant trunk procedure: newer indications and uses. *Ann Thorac Surg*. 2004;78:109-116.
Large clinical series emphasizing the range of pathology potentially treated with this approach and the impressive long-term survival advantage in those able to complete the second-stage operation versus those who do not.

REFERENCES

The reference list can be found on the companion Expert Consult Web site at *www.expertconsult.com*.

CHAPTER 135

Aortic Dissection

Mark F. Conrad and Richard P. Cambria

Acute aortic dissection is the most common catastrophic event affecting the aorta, with an incidence exceeding that of ruptured abdominal aortic aneurysm. The first report of aortic dissection and the concept of a true and a false lumen are attributed to Shekelton in the early 1800s.[1] The term *anurysme dissequant*, or dissecting aneurysm, introduced by Laennec in 1819,[2] remains a source of confusion because acute dissections can occur in both dilated diseased aortas and aortas of normal diameter in seemingly healthy individuals. Accordingly, the terms *dissection* and *aneurysm* should not be used interchangeably; although dissection can occur in a pre-existing degenerative aneurysm and aneurysms can complicate chronic dissections, the presence of one is not dependent on the other. An additional source of diagnostic confusion is the presence of other pathologies of the thoracic aorta such as intramural hematoma and penetrating aortic ulcer, which have clinical and radiographic similarity with acute dissection.

Aortic dissection is a lethal disease. Early studies indicated that without treatment, the majority of patients died within 3 months of diagnosis and few survived the chronic phase more than 5 years because of aneurysmal degeneration and rupture of the outer wall of the false lumen.[3,4] Despite improvements in both medical and surgical therapeutic options, the overall mortality associated with acute dissection remains significant. In a population-based epidemiologic study by Clouse and coworkers, 38% of aortic dissections were diagnosed at autopsy.[5] This substantial mortality rate in undiagnosed patients underscores the importance of early diagnosis and initiation of appropriate therapy. Indeed, Khan and Nair predicted that the mortality rate for acute dissection left untreated will exceed 22.7% within 6 hours, 50% within 24 hours, and 68% within the first week.[6] Death from acute dissection of the ascending aorta is usually secondary to the central cardio-aortic complications of aortic rupture into the pericardium, acute aortic regurgitation, and coronary ostial compromise,[7,8] whereas descending aortic dissections are more commonly associated with death from end-organ compromise secondary to obstruction of visceral or extremity vessels.[9,10]

The International Registry of Acute Aortic Dissection (IRAD) is a multinational registry that began enrolling patients in January 1996. It initially included 12 centers in 6 countries and has grown to 24 referral centers in 11 countries. All patients with acute aortic dissection confirmed by diagnostic imaging studies, by direct visualization in the operating room, or at autopsy are included in the registry. Data are entered from a prospectively collected questionnaire consist-

ing of 290 variables that have been externally validated at each site.[11] This project has provided contemporary insight into the short- and now long-term outcomes of acute dissection and proposed therapeutic options and consequently is referenced often herein.[12,13]

In this chapter we review the classification, pathologic anatomy, pathogenesis, clinical findings, and diagnostic and treatment modalities for acute aortic dissection, with emphasis on the role of the vascular/endovascular surgeon. Although a thorough understanding of all components of acute dissection seems requisite for those who propose to treat aortic dissection, the technical principles of graft replacement of the ascending aorta, being the province of cardiac surgeons, is not detailed. Because open graft replacement for the treatment of descending aortic dissection is rarely indicated, it is anticipated that the vascular/endovascular surgeon will become the primary interventionalist in the care of patients with acute dissection of the descending aorta and the complications of peripheral vascular compromise. Finally, treatment of the principal late complication of acute aortic dissection—the development of thoracoabdominal aneurysms—is considered in Chapter 131 (Thoracic and Thoracoabdominal Aneurysms: Evaluation and Decision Making).

■ CLASSIFICATION

Aortic dissections are classified according to the anatomic location of the entry tear and the time between the onset of symptoms and patient evaluation.

Temporal

A dissection is considered acute when the diagnosis is made within 2 weeks of the initial onset of symptoms and thereafter becomes chronic. Although such designation appears arbitrary, it is based on autopsy studies showing that 74% of patients who die of aortic dissections do so in the first 14 days.[14] Accordingly, such temporal classification combined with the anatomic location of the entry tear can have immediate therapeutic implications.

Anatomic

The anatomic classification of aortic dissection is based on the location of the intimal tear and the extent of the dissection along the aorta. Two classification schemes are used to describe aortic dissections. The original, proposed by DeBakey

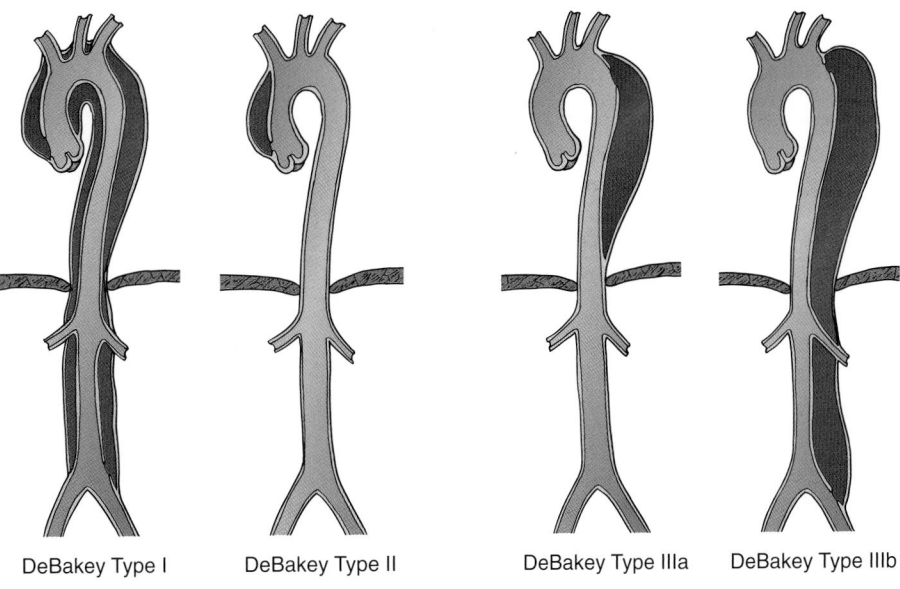

DeBakey Type I   DeBakey Type II   DeBakey Type IIIa   DeBakey Type IIIb

Stanford Type A   Stanford Type B

Figure 135-1 Acute aortic dissection can be classified by the original DeBakey system (*darker color*) based on location of the proximal tear and distal extent of the dissection flap or on the Stanford system (*lighter color*), which uses location of the proximal tear alone.

and colleagues in 1965, delineates both the origin of the entry tear and the extent of the descending aortic dissection.[15] The scheme (Fig. 135-1) uses the following classification:

- Type I: The dissection originates in the ascending aorta and extends through the aortic arch and into the descending aorta or abdominal aorta (or both) for a varying distance.
- Type II: The dissection originates in and is confined to the ascending aorta.
- Type IIIa: The dissection originates in the descending aorta and is limited to the same.
- Type IIIb: The dissection involves the descending and variable extents of the abdominal aorta.

The Stanford classification, described by Daily and associates in 1970, simplified the anatomic classification according to the origin of the entry tear alone.[16]

- A Stanford type A dissection originates in the ascending aorta and therefore encompasses DeBakey types I and II dissections.
- A Stanford type B dissection originates in the descending aorta distal to the origin of the left subclavian artery (DeBakey types IIIa and IIIb; see Fig. 135-1).

Because the origin of the entry tear is the key predictor of early outcomes, most patients are now stratified into Stanford type A or B at diagnosis to direct initial therapy. Prompt graft replacement of the ascending aorta is the appropriate treatment for the majority (for exceptions, see "Open Surgical Treatment of Ascending Aortic Dissection") of patients with Stanford type A dissections because they are associated with a high risk for lethal cardioaortic complications (principally, aortic rupture or myocardial ischemia from extension into the coronary arteries) in the hours and days after symptom onset. Alternatively, patients with Stanford type B dissections are managed initially with medical therapy unless one or more

complications develop (reviewed under "Pathogenesis of Malperfusion Syndromes").

EPIDEMIOLOGY

Recent population-based studies have estimated the incidence of acute aortic dissection to range from 2.9 to 3.5 per 100,000 person-years.[5,17] Factors that predispose to the development of aortic dissection include older age, hypertension, and structural abnormalities of the aortic wall.[6,11] Men are more frequently affected, with a male-female ratio of 4:1 reported in a recent IRAD series.[18] In our cumulative experience, type A dissections account for 60% of cases, which is consistent with the IRAD data, wherein 62.5% of 1417 patients had type A dissections.[12] The incidence of type A dissection peaks between 50 and 60 years, whereas type B dissections occur more frequently between 60 and 70 years of age.[11] Hypertension is the rule and was present in 70% of patients in the IRAD database (Table 135-1).[18]

Table 135-1 Demographic and Clinical Features of combined MGH and IRAD Experience with Acute Aortic Dissection

Variable	MGH*	IRAD[36]	Total
Patients	512	1078	1590
Age (mean)	62 years	62.4 years	—
Male	347 (67.8%)	732 (67.9%)	1079 (67.9%)
Type A	278 (54.3%)	674 (62.5%)	952 (59.9%)
Hypertension	361 (70.5%)	755 (70%)	1116 (70.2%)
VC/pulse deficit	159 (31%)	259 (24%)	418 (26.3%)

*Unpublished data.
IRAD, International Registry of Acute Aortic Dissection; MGH, Massachusetts General Hospital; VC, vascular complication.

Risk Factors for Dissection

Cardiovascular Conditions

Cardiovascular conditions such as acute myocardial infarction and sudden death have been shown to demonstrate certain chronobiologic patterns of occurrence,[19,20] and the same is true of acute aortic dissection.[21] The onset of dissection occurs most frequently in the morning hours between 6 AM and 12 noon and more often in the winter (28%) than the summer (20%), independent of the endogenous climate.[21,22] Aortic wall structural abnormalities and the presence of a bicuspid aortic valve with or without its accompanying aortic root dilatation are well-established risk factors for ascending aortic dissection. Indeed, the presence of a bicuspid aortic valve has been documented in 7% to 14% of all aortic dissections.[11,23] Other aortic diseases, such as coarctation of the aorta, annuloaortic ectasia, chromosomal abnormalities (Turner's syndrome and Noonan's syndrome), aortic arch hypoplasia, and hereditary conditions (Marfan's syndrome and Ehlers-Danlos syndrome), are also risk factors for the development of acute aortic dissection.[24] Marfan's syndrome accounts for 50% of cases of acute aortic dissection in patients younger than 40 years (see Chapter 134: Aortic Arch Aneurysms and Dissection).[18]

Pregnancy

It has previously been reported that in women younger than 40 years, 50% of aortic dissections occur during pregnancy[25]; however, a recent review of the IRAD data showed an incidence of 13%.[18] Preeclampsia with resultant hypertension is the most common cause of peripartum aortic dissection, but pregnant women with Marfan's syndrome are also at high risk; the presence of a dilated aortic root (>4 cm) is the best predictor of dissection in a pregnant patient with Marfan's syndrome.[26] The most common site of aortic dissection in young (<40 years) patients is the ascending aorta involving the sinuses of Valsalva or the sinotubular junction, whereas type A dissections in older patients are more likely to originate in the ascending aorta.[18]

Cocaine Abuse

Cocaine ingestion, a rare cause of acute aortic dissection in otherwise healthy individuals, has an incidence as high as 37% in an urban setting but was present in less than 1% of the IRAD population.[18,27,28] Recently, Daniel and coauthors reviewed the characteristics of 16 patients who had used cocaine within 24 hours of the onset of acute aortic dissection. They found that the prototypical patient was a young (average age, 47 years), male (75%) smoker (100%) with a history of hypertension (70%) and no particular trend toward dissection type.[28] One possible mechanism is related to catecholamine release, which causes the triad of profound hypertension, vasoconstriction, and increased cardiac output. This creates a dramatic, acute increase in ventricular contraction (shearing) force (dP/dt) on the aortic wall. The intimal tear occurs most often at the ligamentum arteriosum, where the aorta is rela-tively fixed and unable to tolerate the accelerating aortic pressure wave generated by the profound tachycardia and malignant hypertension.[28,29]

PATHOLOGIC ANATOMY OF ACUTE AORTIC DISSECTION

Intimal Tear

The process of aortic dissection is dynamic, and it can occur anywhere along the course of the aorta and result in a wide spectrum of clinical manifestations. The pathognomonic lesion is an intimal tear followed by blood surging either antegrade (typically) or retrograde (depending on the hemodynamic gradient between the true and false lumina) and cleaving the intimal and medial layers of the aortic wall longitudinally for a variable distance.[6,30] The typical tear is transverse, not circumferential, and the intimomedial layer can be cleaved both longitudinally and circumferentially.[6] The adventitially bound blood-filled space created between the dissected layers of the aortic wall becomes the false lumen. Fenestrations (connections between the true and false lumina) occur within the intimal flap downstream, usually at branch vessel ostia, and are cleaved by the dissection process; they serve as sites of reentry of blood flow into the true lumen and thus maintain false lumen patency. The presence of an "intimal flap," which represents the intimomedial septum between the true and the false lumen, is the most characteristic pathology in acute aortic dissection. The intimal flap/tear originates in the ascending aorta in 65%, in the descending aorta in 25%, and in the arch and abdominal aorta in 10% of patients.[11] In the descending aorta, the intimal tear typically originates within a few centimeters of the left subclavian artery because this segment of the aorta is subject to the greatest pressure fluctuations.[14,31,32] In the usual pattern of a Stanford type B dissection, the cleavage plane will progress with the distal false lumen on the left posterolateral aspect of the aorta (80% of patients); the celiac, superior mesenteric, and right renal arteries typically emanate from the true lumen, and the left renal artery arises from the false lumen.[14] However, variations in this pattern are frequently encountered.

Cystic Medial Necrosis

One pathologic process that is associated with increased risk for aortic dissection is medial degeneration of the aortic wall (cystic medial necrosis), which diminishes the structural integrity of the aortic layers.[32,33] The central lesion appears to be deterioration of medial collagen and elastin fibers through elastolysis; this is considered to be a factor in most cases of aortic dissection.[34] In particular, classic cystic medial necrosis appears to be an essential feature of several hereditary conditions such as Ehlers-Danlos syndrome and Marfan's disease,[24] yet specific connective tissue diseases account for only 10% to 15% of all acute aortic dissections.[11] Even in "normal individuals," in whom dissections occur without any antecedent diagnosis of syndromic diseases, the degree of medial degeneration still tends to be greater than expected as part of normal aging. The exact cause of this medial degeneration remains unclear, but advanced age and hypertension appear to be the most important factors.[21,34,35]

Atherosclerosis

Atherosclerosis has not been considered to be an important etiologic feature of acute aortic dissection and was present in only 31% of patients in the IRAD registry.[36] However, Jex and coworkers noted either gross or microscopic atheroma in 83% of patients in their series.[37] Atherosclerotic plaque may, in fact, be protective, serving to terminate the dissection process, because the transmural inflammatory nature of atherosclerosis may fuse the aortic layers.[38] The presence of an atherosclerotic aneurysm with concurrent aortic dissection occurred in only 14% to 15% of patients in recent series.[36,39] The unusual coexistence of an aortic dissection that originates in or involves a preexisting atherosclerotic aneurysm appears to change the natural history, and rupture is the probable scenario. For instance, in a review of 325 patients with aortic dissection, rupture in the abdomen occurred only in the setting of antecedent degenerative, atherosclerotic aneurysm.[38] These findings support the posture of treating such type B dissections as "complicated," and initial surgical priority should be given to the aorta where both entities are present (usually the infrarenal abdominal aorta).

◼ PATHOGENESIS OF MALPERFUSION SYNDROMES

Consistent over several series, aortic branch compromise is present in up to 31% of patients with acute aortic dissection,[10,36,40,41] with progression to malperfusion syndrome correlating with early mortality.[9,10,36] Malperfusion syndrome occurs when there is end-organ ischemia secondary to aortic branch compromise from the dissecting process. It can involve one or more vascular beds simultaneously, with early symptoms often being subtle and of varying severity over the hours and days after initial symptom onset. The terms *aortic branch compromise* and *malperfusion syndrome* should not be used interchangeably because the obstruction is often subtotal and produces variable degrees of end-organ ischemia, and certain affected vessels (e.g., the subclavian and celiac arteries) may not produce critical ischemia, even with total occlusion, as a result of the presence of collateral circulation. Virtually any aortic branch can be affected, and as intuitively suspected, the morbid clinical events will vary as a function of the vascular territory involved. Mesenteric involvement is associated with intestinal infarction, whereas subclavian and lower extremity occlusive events are often well tolerated (Fig. 135-2).

Mechanism

Identifying the mechanisms of branch compromise is a critical step in formulating effective treatment plans. The anatomic and physiologic variables underpinning any compromised

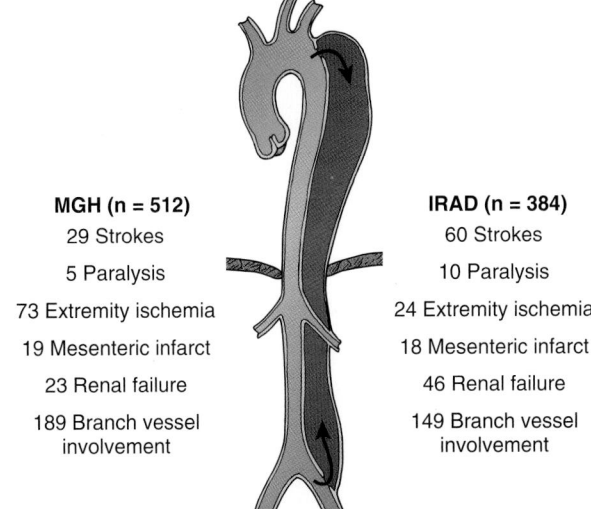

MGH (n = 512)	IRAD (n = 384)
29 Strokes	60 Strokes
5 Paralysis	10 Paralysis
73 Extremity ischemia	24 Extremity ischemia
19 Mesenteric infarct	18 Mesenteric infarct
23 Renal failure	46 Renal failure
189 Branch vessel involvement	149 Branch vessel involvement

Figure 135-2 Comparison of the Massachusetts General Hospital (MGH) and the International Registry of Acute Aortic Dissection (IRAD) experience with peripheral vascular complications after acute aortic dissection. Differences between the number of branch vessels involved and clinical events represent asymptomatic lesions.

vascular bed include (1) the percentage of aortic circumference dissected, (2) the presence of a distal reentrant focus in false lumen or true lumen outflow, and (3) the topography of branch ostia to the true versus the false lumen.[7] In the minutes after an aortic dissection is initiated, the true lumen (representing the remnant of the original aortic lumen) collapses to a variable degree and the false lumen expands.[42] The adventitially bound outer wall of the false lumen must expand to a larger diameter to accommodate the same wall tension at a given blood pressure, as governed by the law of Laplace. In contrast, the true lumen, which contains the majority of the elastic components of the aortic wall, undergoes radial elastic collapse.[42] Therefore, the degree to which the true lumen recoils and the false lumen expands (i.e., their respective cross-sectional areas) depends on the percentage of the total aortic circumference involved with the dissection. In the presence of a deep proximal tear and the absence of distal fenestrations, mean false lumen pressure increases and results in compression of the true lumen[43] (Fig. 135-3). A compressed true lumen will lead to impaired perfusion of distal structures and should increase the index of suspicion for visceral and renal ischemia. Finally, the topographic relationship of the true and false lumina and the potential for extension of the dissection into the aortic branch itself are the anatomic factors that determine the mechanism of the malperfusion syndrome (see Fig. 135-3).

Two mechanisms for aortic branch vessel compromise have been identified, each of which has specific treatment implications in the management of malperfusion syndromes as originally described by Williams and colleagues.[42]

Dynamic Obstruction

In *dynamic obstruction*, the compressed true lumen is unable to provide adequate volume flow, or the dissection flap may

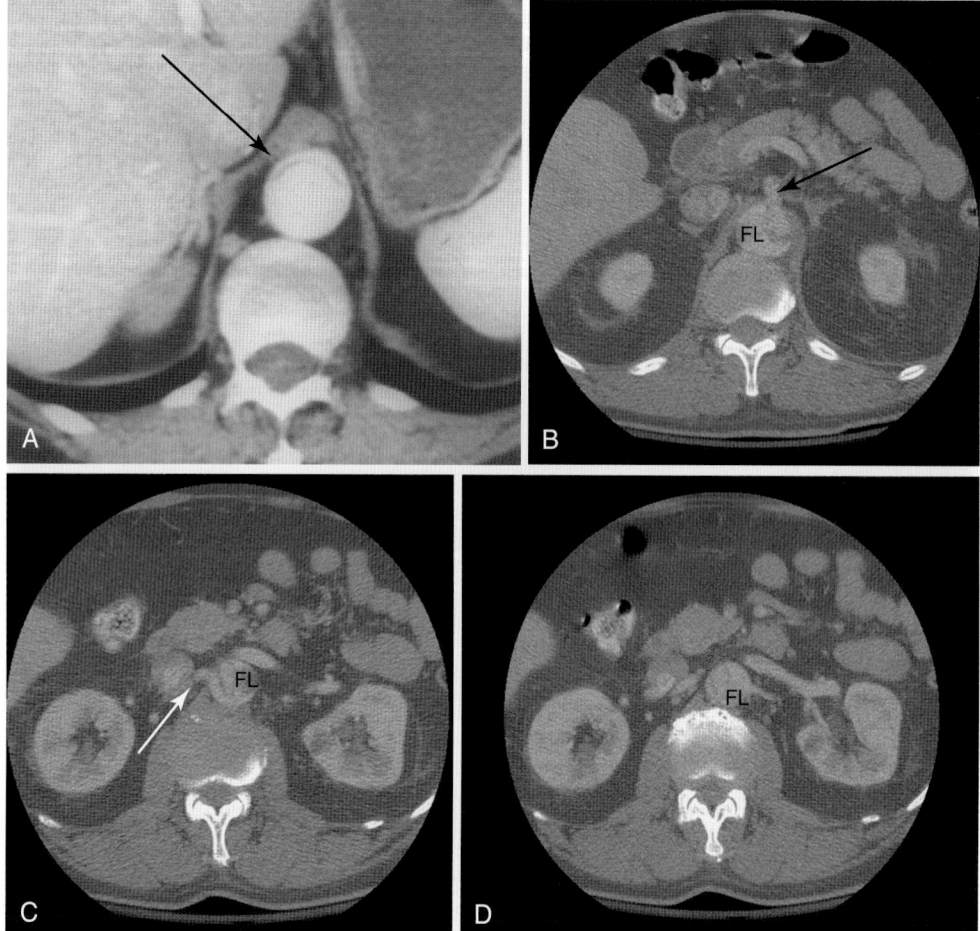

Figure 135-3 Computed tomographic angiographic findings of acute aortic dissection. **A,** Axial image of aortic dissection with a compressed true lumen (*arrow*). **B,** Axial image of aortic dissection with the superior mesenteric artery arising from the true lumen (*arrow*). **C,** Axial image of aortic dissection with the right renal artery (*arrow*) arising from the compressed true lumen. **D,** Axial image of aortic dissection with the left renal artery originating from the false lumen (FL).

prolapse into the vessel ostium, which remains anatomically intact (Fig. 135-4A and B). This is the more common mechanism of branch compromise and is responsible, at least in part, for some 80% of malperfusion syndromes.[44] The severity of the true lumen collapse and the degree of aortic-level ostial vessel occlusion are determined by the circumference of the dissected aorta, cardiac output, blood pressure, heart rate, and peripheral resistance of the outflow vessel.[45] Pulse deficits based on dynamic obstruction may wax and wane over time because of variability in the aforementioned factors.[7,46] Chung and associates modeled the anatomy and physiologic conditions of a Stanford type B aortic dissection in vitro to study the hydrodynamic effects that worsen true lumen collapse. In conditions of equal outflow from each lumen in pulsatile flow, increasing the size of the aortic entry tear from 10 to 30 mm (i.e., increasing the amount of aortic circumference involved) significantly aggravated the degree of true lumen collapse. On the basis of these observations, they concluded that movement of the dissection flap to produce dynamic obstruction of any branch vessel is related to the size of the entry tear, the limita-

tion in false lumen outflow, and the increased true lumen outflow produced by falling peripheral resistance.[45]

Static Obstruction

In acute dissection, the false lumen is highly thrombogenic as a result of the exposed adventitial and medial layers. Thrombus formation may occur in the blind end of the dissection column; more often, however, "reentrant" foci maintain false lumen flow.[47] If the blind end or the propagating end of the dissection column enters and constricts the ostium of a branch vessel, organ injury can occur as a result of thrombosis or hypoperfusion of the involved vessel. This mechanism for malperfusion syndrome involves the dissecting process extending into the branch vessel proper and narrowing it to a variable degree and has been termed *static obstruction* (Fig. 135-4C to E).[44] This obstruction is unlikely to resolve with restoration of aortic true lumen flow alone, and some manipulation of the vessel itself (e.g., stent, bypass graft) will typically be required. Alternatively, the more common scenario occurs

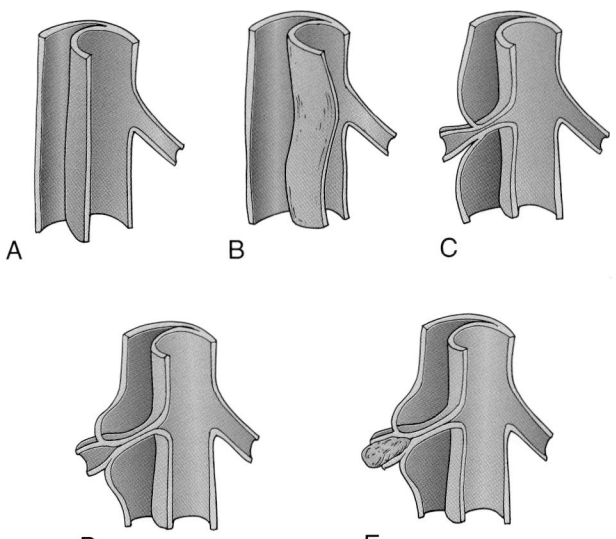

Figure 135-4 Mechanisms of aortic branch obstruction in acute dissection. **A** and **B,** In dynamic obstruction, the septum may prolapse into the vessel ostium during the cardiac cycle, and flow in the compressed true lumen is inadequate to perfuse the branch vessel ostia, which remain anatomically intact. **C–E,** Nearly complete circumferential dissection with static obstruction—the cleavage plane of the dissection extends into the ostium and compromises inflow. Thrombosis beyond the compromised ostia may further worsen perfusion.

when the dissection process shears the aortic intimomedial layer around the vessel ostium and the vessel anatomy itself remains intact, with flow provided by the false lumen. Accordingly, most false lumen branches rarely show evidence of ongoing malperfusion[47] (see Fig. 135-4B).

■ CLINICAL FINDINGS

Pain

The most common symptom of acute aortic dissection is pain (located in the back, abdomen, or chest), reported in more than 93% of patients, with 85% specifying an abrupt onset.[11,48] The pain is typically (in 78% of patients) described as anterior in location in type A dissections, whereas for type B dissections the pain is more often experienced in the back (in 64% of patients).[11,23] Although the classic description of the pain associated with aortic dissection is ripping or tearing (50%), patients more frequently complain of sharp, stabbing pain (68%) and less often experience migratory symptoms (19%).[11] Pain has been localized to the abdomen in up to 21% of patients with type A and 43% with type B dissection.[11] In such patients a high index of suspicion for mesenteric vascular compromise is warranted. Typically, the pain is severe and causes the patient to seek medical attention within minutes to hours of onset; it has been described as "the worst ever" by nearly 90% of patients.[11] Control of the pain with antihypertensive therapy is a mainstay in the early management of acute aortic dissection, and recurrence of the pain implies failure of medical therapy and warrants repeat imaging to direct therapy.

However, in the absence of clinical or radiographic signs of pathoanatomic changes, medical therapy remains appropriate management of patients with early recurrent pain after type B dissection.[49]

Syncope

Syncope may complicate the manifestation of acute aortic dissection in 5% to 10% of patients, and its presence often indicates the development of cardiac tamponade or involvement of the brachiocephalic vessels.[50] Overall, patients in IRAD with syncope were more likely to have type A than type B dissection (19% versus 3%, $P < .001$) and more likely to have cardiac tamponade (28% versus 8%, $P < .001$).[51] Similarly, they were more likely to have a stroke (18% versus 4%, $P < .001$) and more likely to die in the hospital (34% versus 23%, $P = .01$). Although patients with syncope had a higher rate of severe complications (tamponade, stroke, death), in almost half, these complications were not the cause of their loss of consciousness. The mechanisms underlying this fact may be related to other pathophysiologic perturbations, such as vasovagal events or direct stretching of baroreceptors in the aortic wall.[52,53]

Neurologic Symptoms

Spinal cord ischemia from the interruption of intercostal vessels is clearly more common with type B aortic dissections and occurs in 2% to 10% of all patients.[54] Direct compression of any peripheral nerve can occur rarely and result in paresthesias (lumbar plexopathy), hoarseness of voice (compression of the recurrent laryngeal nerve), or Horner's syndrome (compression of the sympathetic ganglion).[55-57]

Hypertension

On initial physical examination, hypertension is present in 70% of patients with type B dissection but in only 25% to 35% of those with type A dissection. The presence of hypotension complicating type B dissection is rare (<5% of patients), but it may accompany 25% of dissections that involve the ascending aorta, potentially as a result of aortic valve disruption or cardiac tamponade.[11] The malperfusion of brachiocephalic vessels by the dissection may falsely depress brachial cuff pressure.[58] Hypertension refractory to medical management is common in type B dissections and occurs in 64% patients.[59] However, because this refractory hypertension is not usually associated with renal artery compromise or aortic dilatation, continued medical management is warranted.

Peripheral Vascular Complications

Peripheral vascular complications are common and occur in 30% to 50% patients in whom the aortic arch, the thoracoabdominal aorta, or both are involved.[10,40,41] Cambria and colleagues were the first to quantify the contribution of said complications to overall mortality. They noted that in patients with peripheral vascular complications not involving the ascending aorta, the brachiocephalic trunk was involved in 14% of patients, the common carotid arteries in 21%, the left subclavian in 14%, and ileofemoral arteries in 35%.[10] This distribution was again borne out by the IRAD data 15 years later.[60] Patients with pulse deficits more often exhibit neurologic deficits, coma, and hypotension, and a deficit of the carotid pulse strongly correlates with fatal stroke.[9] In this population, mortality is clearly linked to the number of pulse deficits at initial evaluation. Indeed, within the first 24 hours, 9.4% of patients with no deficits died, 15.8% with one or two deficits died, and 35.3% with three or more deficits died.[60] Not surprisingly, it is uncommon for isolated lower extremity pulse deficits to cause mortality as a result of lower extremity ischemia or its sequelae.[10] Despite this seemingly favorable prognosis, leg ischemia caused by acute dissection remains a marker for extensive dissection and may be accompanied by other compromised vascular territories, and the clinical course of lower extremity ischemia can be variable in that up to a third of this group may demonstrate spontaneous return of pulses.[10]

■ DIAGNOSTIC EVALUATION

In the United States, acute chest pain is the chief complaint in 8.2% of all emergency department visits. This translates to almost 4.6 million patients annually.[61] The majority of these patients do not have an aortic dissection, and it would be inefficient, unrealistic, and costly to perform axial imaging on all patients with acute chest pain. Indeed, the indiscriminate application of thoracic imaging to patients with a low pretest probability of having an aortic dissection has been predicted to yield an 85% false-positive rate.[62] However, aortic dissection often affects younger patients (in their 50s) and thus is often not readily apparent. Indeed, physicians correctly suspect the entity in only 15% to 43% of cases, and aortic dissection is often identified as an incidental finding during evaluation for another pathologic process.[17,63] Historically, retrograde aortography was considered the reference standard for the evaluation of acute aortic dissection. However, improvement in other techniques such as contrast-enhanced computed tomographic angiography (CTA), transesophageal echocardiography (TEE), and magnetic resonance imaging (MRI) has shifted the role of aortography from diagnostic to adjunctive during endovascular management. An evaluation of the IRAD data showed that worldwide from 1996 to 1999, CTA was the initial test performed in 63% of patients, and 75% underwent CTA as part of the evaluation.[64] TEE was also routinely used (72%), although it was the first test obtained in only 32% of patients. More than two thirds of patients required two or more imaging tests, with MRI (19%) and aortography (19%) being used at the same frequency.[64] Although the choice of diagnostic modality may be predicated on local availability/practice patterns, certain essentials exist. First, the diagnosis of acute aortic dissection must be confirmed or refuted. Second, the extent of the dissection, the

potential involvement of branch vessels, and the presence of immediate life-threatening complications such as tamponade should be provided.

Imaging

Plain Radiography

Plain chest radiography is often the first imaging study obtained during the evaluation for acute chest pain, but the findings of aortic dissection on chest radiography are nonspecific and never diagnostic. Such findings include widening of the cardiac or aortic silhouette, displacement of aortic calcifications, and effusions.[11,23] Widening of the mediastinum is the most common finding, whereas displaced aortic calcifications are usually seen with type A dissections.[11] Pleural effusions occur most frequently in patients with type B dissection and are usually secondary to an inflammatory reaction of the mediastinal pleura.[65] Because these findings are not diagnostic, additional imaging is required.

Aortography

Aortography has a sensitivity of 86% to 88% and a specificity of 75% to 94% for the diagnosis of thoracic aortic dissection, but false-negative angiograms can occur when the false lumen has thrombosed.[66-69] The aortographic findings considered supportive of a diagnosis of aortic dissection include distortion of the normal contrast column, flow reversal or stasis into a false channel, failure of major branches to fill, and aortic valvular regurgitation.[68] Most contemporary diagnostic paradigms have de-emphasized the role of aortography because it is time-consuming and invasive, incurs a risk for contrast-induced nephropathy, and is expensive. Therefore, in contemporary practice, aortography is considered unnecessary before surgical repair of proximal dissection.[64,70] In the management of distal dissection it is used as part of treatment (see "Endovascular Treatment of Aortic Dissection") rather than as a diagnostic modality.

Computed Tomographic Angiography

As shown by the IRAD data, computed tomography (CT) was part of the diagnostic evaluation in 75% of patients.[48] CT scanning is readily available, is noninvasive, and has a reported sensitivity of 83% to 95% and a specificity of 87% to 100% for the diagnosis of acute aortic dissection.[71-73] The chief limitation of imaging is the ascending aorta, where the sensitivity may drop to less than 80%, but this is readily overcome by the addition of TEE.[58] A dedicated protocol to image the entire aorta is usually sufficient to provide the necessary diagnostic information. A helical CT dissection protocol will yield excellent aortic imaging of the true and false lumina and approximate entry tear sites and will aid in planning interventions (Fig. 135-5). In most cases, the true lumen may be localized by its continuity with an undissected segment of the aorta.[74] However, in circumferential dissection of the aortic root or when imaging of the aortic arch is omitted, this rule

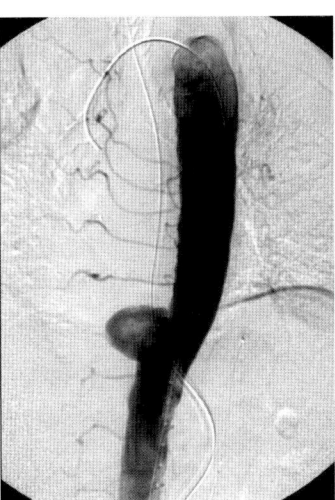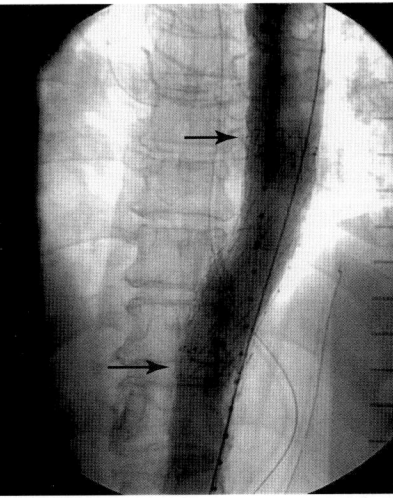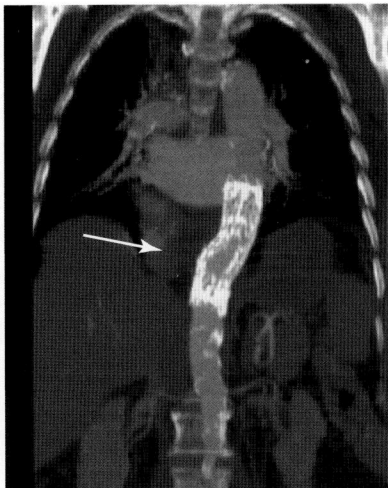

Figure 135-5 Stent-graft (*arrows*) treatment of a mid-descending thoracic aorta penetrating aortic ulcer.

may be difficult to apply. The presence of intraluminal thrombus is a fairly good marker of the false lumen, but in patients with a concomitant degenerative aneurysm, thrombus may be present in the true lumen.[74] The finding of greatest significance is that in the descending thoracic aorta, the false lumen is larger than the true lumen in more than 90% of cases ($P < .05$).[74]

The orientation and mobility of the dissection flap can be assessed with CTA, and if the dissection flap is concave toward the false lumen, a true lumen pressure deficit can be predicted with 91% sensitivity and 72% specificity.[47] The dissection flap is more often noted to be in a curved orientation (63% of cases) in the acute phase, whereas the flap was flat in 75% of cases of chronic dissection.[74] As displayed in Figure 135-3A, a slitlike compressed true lumen is perhaps the key radiographic finding that should substantially raise the index of suspicion for renal/visceral/lower extremity malperfusion syndrome.

Three-dimensional CT scan reconstructions can aid treatment planning, but axial imaging affords the best opportunity to detect topographic relationships of the true and false lumina and potential aortic branch compromise. Although it is appropriate to operate on acute type A dissections based on CT findings alone, IRAD data show that most patients undergo preoperative CT (71%) and TEE (77%) (either preoperatively or intraoperatively) in circumstances in which the clinical or laboratory signs (or both) dictate the need for urgent revascularization.[75] In comparison to other modalities, CT scanning is the least operator dependent, provides useful anatomic correlates for surgical and endovascular therapy, and most reliably collects information for follow-up analysis and measurement.

Echocardiography

The sensitivity and specificity of transthoracic echocardiography (TTE) range from 35% to 80% and 40% to 95%, respectively.[76,77] The chief technical limitations of TTE, whether performed in suprasternal or subcostal views, are narrow intercostal spaces, obesity, and emphysema. In addition, false positives have been reported in TTE imaging of the ascending aorta as a result of artifacts.[78]

TEE overcomes the limitations of surface echocardiography by the anatomic proximity of the esophagus to the aorta. The sensitivity of TEE has been reported to be as high as 98%, and its specificity ranges from 63% to 96%.[79-81] Advantages of TEE include wide availability, ease of use, and bedside capability. In addition, TEE possesses the ability to reveal entry tear sites, false lumen flow/thrombus, involvement of the arch or coronary arteries, degrees of aortic valvular regurgitation, and pericardial effusions. The addition of color-flow Doppler patterns may decrease false positives by recognizing differential flow velocities in the true and false lumina.[82] The chief limitations of TEE are its anatomic blind spot in the distal ascending aorta and arch secondary to the air-filled trachea and left mainstem bronchus and its inability to document extension of dissection beyond the diaphragm.[83] Despite these shortcomings, TEE can be particularly useful in delineating dissection and relevant surgical pathology in the ascending aorta, and therefore it is chiefly applied in this territory.[84] Moreover, in an unstable patient with a suspected acute dissection in the ascending aorta, TEE may be performed in the operating room to expedite diagnosis and definitive therapy.

Magnetic Resonance Imaging

MRI has an overall sensitivity and specificity for the diagnosis of aortic dissection in the range of 95% to 100%.[64,85,86] MRI can detect the site of the entry tear, the extent of the dissection, potential branch vessel involvement, and differential true versus false lumen flow. The overall sensitivity and specificity for the diagnosis of branch vessel involvement are 90% and 96%, respectively.[87] The chief limitations of MRI include the lack of immediate availability, long examination times, and lack of monitoring for critically ill patients. In addition, patients who have pacemakers, aneurysm clippings, or ocular implants are not candidates for MRI.

TREATMENT

Optimal treatment of acute dissection is predicated on timely diagnosis and thorough understanding of the anatomic extent of the pathology. Prompt institution of intravenous antihypertensive medications to lower systemic blood pressure and pulse (dP/dt) is a key element of initial therapy for all patients, with the goal of stabilizing the extent of the dissection, reducing intimal flap mobility, relieving dynamic aortic branch obstruction, and decreasing the risk for rupture. Mortality in the acute phase of a proximal dissection may exceed 1% per hour as a result of the central cardioaortic complications of tamponade, acute aortic valvular insufficiency, and coronary obstruction. Thus, prompt ascending aortic graft replacement with or without aortic valve repair/replacement is the treatment of choice for the majority of patients with acute type A aortic dissection. For patients with type B dissections, the catastrophic complication of rupture is uncommon, except in those with advanced false lumen dilatation or the equivalent of aneurysm formation at the aortic entry site.[7] Furthermore, in patients with uncomplicated type B dissections, surgical therapy (i.e., graft replacement of the aortic entry tear site) has not demonstrated superiority over medical or interventional therapy for stable patients.[48]

Aortic branch compromise by the propagating false lumen and subsequent malperfusion syndrome may complicate the initial manifestation in patients with extensive type B dissections. A complication-specific approach involving open surgical and endovascular options to treat such malperfusion syndromes remains the standard of care and is reviewed subsequently. The application of stent-graft repair at the entry tear may alter this paradigm in the near future.

Medical Treatment

Medical treatment of aortic dissection was first advocated in the 1960s by Wheat and Palmer (ironically, surgeons) as an alternative for patients too ill to undergo surgical therapy.[88] Currently, medical management in an intensive care unit is the initial therapy for virtually all patients with the tentative diagnosis of aortic dissection. Immediate management of acute aortic dissection is directed toward reducing the hemodynamic forces that have initiated and propagated the intimal tear and cleavage of the aortic wall. The goal of medical therapy is to reduce systolic blood pressure and dP/dt and thereby reduce the forces predisposing the dissected aorta to rupture or compromise of branch vessels.[58] Intravenous antihypertensive therapy should be started in all patients in whom acute aortic dissection is suspected, with the exception of those with hypotension.[58] For patients with hypotension in the setting of acute dissection, expeditious evaluation for tamponade is warranted, but percutaneous pericardiocentesis as a temporizing measure is not advised because it often accelerates bleeding or shock.[89]

In contemporary practice, the combination of a beta blocker and a vasodilator is standard medical therapy. The beta blocker should be initiated before the direct vasodilator (i.e., sodium nitroprusside); otherwise, the reflex sympathetic stimulation from direct vasodilation will stimulate catecholamine release and resultant increases in dP/dt, opposite the desired effect. The cornerstone of medical therapy is reduction of *both* dP/dt and arterial blood pressure. For acute reduction of dP/dt, an intravenous beta blocker is infused in incremental doses until evidence of effective beta blockade is achieved, usually indicated by a heart rate of 60 to 80 beats/min. Beta blockers that achieve both α- and β-adrenergic blockade (such as labetalol) may provide both dP/dt reduction and blood pressure lowering. Short-acting beta blockers (such as esmolol) may be particularly useful as a test of beta blockade tolerance in patients at risk for bronchospasm or flaring of chronic obstructive pulmonary disease. In these patients, a cardioselective beta blocker such as atenolol or metoprolol may be desirable. For acute reduction of arterial pressure, the direct vasodilator sodium nitroprusside is very effective and should be used after beta blockade is achieved.

Patients should be placed in the intensive care unit during the acute period with continuous blood pressure monitoring via an intra-arterial catheter, telemetry monitoring of cardiac rhythms, and hemodynamic surveillance involving a Foley catheter and pulmonary artery catheter if necessary. Once the patient's blood pressure has been controlled to a systolic pressure of 105 to 120 mm Hg (or a mean arterial pressure of 60 to 70 mm Hg) and the pain has resolved, he or she can be transitioned to oral antihypertensives. Patients managed medically should be monitored with serial surveillance imaging studies that should consist of contrast-enhanced CTA. The first study should be obtained before discharge from the initial hospitalization and then at 6-month intervals. Once a dissection has been stable for two scans, follow-up imaging can be performed on a yearly basis.[90]

Open Surgical Treatment of Ascending Aortic Dissection

A complete review of the surgical literature and state-of-the-art management of acute type A dissection is beyond the scope of this chapter. Medical therapy has been associated with 60% in-hospital mortality in patients with type A dissection, and urgent surgical repair is the treatment of choice unless major neurologic deficits or peripheral vascular complications of the dissection pose greater overall risk (i.e., visceral ischemia) than the threat of proximal rupture (Fig. 135-6). Patel and coworkers have shown improvement in early mortality with percutaneous restoration of end-organ perfusion followed by delayed operative repair in patients with acute type A dissection and peripheral malperfusion syndrome. Although 33% of these patients died before operative repair, there was no difference in mortality between those with malperfusion and those without who underwent operative repair.[91] Conversely, Fann and colleagues showed that after repair of the ascending thoracic aorta, 92% of patients with type A dissection and peripheral vascular compromise had resolution of their peripheral symptoms and did not require additional vascular

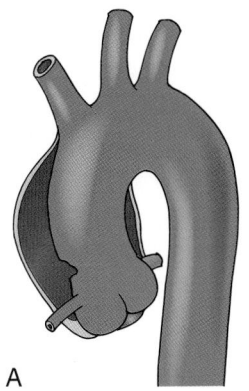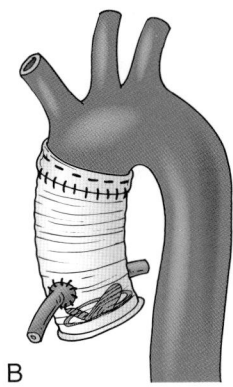

Figure 135-6 A and **B,** Repair of type A dissection with replacement of the ascending aorta. The anatomic goals of replacement include (1) resection of the aortic tear, (2) resuspension/repair or replacement of the aortic valve as necessary, (3) routine use of circulatory arrest to perform at least the distal anastomosis, and (4) reconstruction of the aortic layers so that flow is redirected into the true lumen and false lumen flow is eliminated (this is successful only 50% of time).

Table 135-2 Results of Graft Replacement for Acute Type A Aortic Dissection

Series	Year	Number of Patients	Adjuncts (%)	Results (%)	
				Preoperative Shock	Mortality
Bakhtiary et al.[97]	2008	120	ACP (100)	34	5
Knipp et al.[98] (NIS)	2007	3013	NA	NA	26
Rampoldi et al.[75] (IRAD)	2007	682	HCA (92) RCP (51)	31	24
Apaydin et al.[99]	2002	108	HCA (99)	12	25
Mehta et al.[100]	2002	437	HCA (87) RCP (56)	28	26
Bavaria et al.[95]	2001	104	HCA(100) RCP (100) EEG (66)	10	9

ACP, antegrade cerebral perfusion; EEG, neurocerebral monitoring; HCA, hypothermic circulatory arrest; IRAD, International Registry of Acute Aortic Dissection; NA, not available; NIS, National Inpatient Sample; RCP, retrograde cerebral perfusion.

procedures.[92] A second cohort of patients who may benefit from delayed operative repair are those initially seen more than 2 days after the onset of symptoms. Davies and associates showed that patients in whom such delay occurs have already survived the initial high-risk period, and 43% were treated nonoperatively with a trend toward improved long-term survival in comparison to those who underwent immediate operative intervention.[93]

The IRAD study group found an overall operative mortality of 25% in patients with proximal aortic dissection and noted a significant difference between stable patients and those who were unstable at initial evaluation (17% versus 31%, $P < .001$).[11,94] One of the main determinants of poor outcome is neurologic status at diagnosis. In a series of 104 consecutive patients who underwent repair of type A aortic dissection, mortality was universal in patients who were neurologically unresponsive and intubated. In addition, a 45% death rate was reported when patients who had a stroke underwent otherwise successful repair of type A dissection.

Since the first report of successful repair of type A dissection in 1963 by Morris, substantial improvements in cardiac surgical techniques, including intraoperative TEE, cerebral protection by profound hypothermic circulatory arrest, advanced prostheses for managing the dissected aorta or aortic valve (or both), and avoidance of extensive arch resections, have led to improvements in outcomes.[95] However, despite the advances in surgical techniques and perioperative care, operative mortality remains significant, with rates of 9% to 26% in representative large series (Table 135-2).[9,75,94-100] The anatomic goal of open repair is resection of the aortic intimal tear with graft replacement and reconstruction of the aortic wall layers in the distal anastomosis so that false lumen flow is eliminated. Persistent false lumen flow continues in many patients after ascending aortic graft replacement despite the liberal use of circulatory arrest and technical adjuncts such as glue aortoplasty.[101]

Selection of patients who require aortic valve replacement in concert with repair of ascending aortic dissection is now directed by intraoperative TEE, and valve replacement can be avoided in up to 80% of patients.[102,103] Indications for aortic valve replacement include Marfan's syndrome, sinus of Valsalva aneurysm, a bicuspid valve or other leaflet pathology, and extension of the tear and dissection into the annulus.[95] A second technical issue involves the extent of arch replacement, with 20% to 30% of patients with type A dissection having intimal tears that extend into the arch or descending aorta.[104] A recent report from the Stanford group indicated that although arch involvement increases the risk for future distal aortic degeneration, an aggressive posture toward arch replacement has not improved long-term outcomes.[96,103] The type A dissection arm of the IRAD registry was recently used to develop a risk model for prediction of surgical mortality.[75] They reported an in-hospital mortality of 23.9% and identified age older than 70 years, previous cardiac surgery, hypotension/shock at initial evaluation, cardiac tamponade, any pulse deficit, and myocardial ischemia as independent predictors of poor outcome.[75]

Open Surgical Treatment of Descending Aortic Dissection

Threatened or actual rupture at the aortic intimal tear in the proximal descending aorta in our view remains the only indication for acute open graft replacement in patients with distal dissection. Unless an extensive aneurysm is present, resection should be confined to the proximal descending aorta because mortality and spinal cord ischemia dramatically increase the risk in patients with extensive aortic replacement in the setting of acute dissection.[105] Although an anatomic goal of central aortic replacement is reconstruction of the aortic wall layers in the distal anastomosis and obliteration of false lumen flow, 25% to 50% of patients with type B aortic dissection who are treated surgically can be expected to have persistent false lumen flow.[106,107] In addition to a significant incidence of persistent false lumen flow, other reasons for abandonment of central aortic repair in patients with acute type B dissection include substantial surgical morbidity, the equivalent results of medical therapy, and its variable success in relieving distal malperfusion. The mortality rate for open repair of acute type B aortic dissection has ranged from 6% to 69% in several large series.[108-112] In a recent IRAD review of 476 patients with type B dissection, 82 (17.2%) were treated surgically with descending aortic replacement (70%), partial arch replacement (21%), or total arch replacement (8%).[111] Their in-hospital mortality was 29.3%, with the highest death rate in patients who required surgery within 24 hours of admission. In addition, central aortic grafting alone may be unsuccessful in alleviating distal malperfusion syndromes, depending on the mechanism of obstruction and the anatomic complexity of the dissection, thus making additional revascularization of the visceral and lower extremity vessels potentially necessary. Given the variable results with open repair, it seems logical that thoracic endovascular aortic repair will be preferred over open repair even in circumstances in which the indication includes actual or threatened aortic rupture.

Though presently rarely indicated, central aortic graft replacement for type B aortic dissection presents significant technical challenges. To ensure anastomotic integrity, strips of Teflon felt can be placed inside the true lumen and outside the aortic wall and sewn together with the aortic wall "sandwiched" in between.[113] In contradistinction, the introduction of glue aortoplasty is an important contribution to modern-day aortic dissection surgery. With the aorta transected and a sponge inserted in the true lumen to protect its diameter, the glue is applied for a length of 2 cm between the dissected layers at a thickness of 2 mm. After 2 minutes, the aortic layers are fused and strengthened to accept a collagen-impregnated woven Dacron graft with a running polypropylene suture. The complexity of repair of the friable proximal aorta will lead to prolonged cross-clamp time such that distal aortic perfusion with partial left heart bypass should be used to maintain visceral and spinal cord blood flow. Indeed, in a series of 22 patients undergoing graft replacement of the descending aorta for acute type B dissection, spinal cord ischemic complications were reported in 7 (32%), and acute dissection was a significant predictor of postoperative neurologic deficit (odds ratio, 10.59; 95% confidence interval, 2.45 to 45.82; P = .002).[105]

Endovascular Treatment of Aortic Dissection

Goal of Treatment

Stent-graft repair of the aortic entry tear may ultimately provide the means to accomplish the intuitively logical short- and long-term goals of central aortic repair of the entry tear

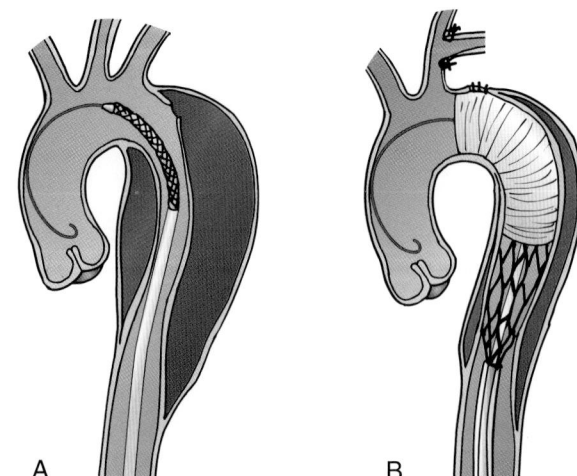

Figure 135-7 A and **B,** Stent-graft deployment to cover the proximal entry tear in the hope of inducing false lumen thrombosis and true lumen re-expansion. The latter should also alleviate the "downstream" branch compromise caused by dynamic obstruction mechanisms. False lumen thrombosis in the thoracic aorta should, in theory, minimize subsequent aneurysmal expansion of the outer wall of the false lumen.

while obviating the substantial morbidity associated with conventional surgical repair. In 1999, the endovascular treatment of acute type B dissections with stent-graft technology was described in two sentinel reports.[114,115] Such an approach may lessen the incidence and severity of malperfusion syndromes and reduce late aortic-related complications by minimizing the incidence of aneurysmal degeneration of the outer wall of the false lumen. Medical therapy remains the current standard of care for uncomplicated type B aortic dissections, with operative therapy (open or endovascular) being reserved for patients who experience complications such as malperfusion syndromes. The concept of inducing false lumen thrombosis by sealing the aortic tear with an aortic endograft has the potential to reduce both early and late complications of type B dissection.[116] When indicated, the goals of thoracic endovascular aortic repair (TEVAR) for acute type B dissection include coverage of the proximal entry tear, expansion of the true lumen with restoration of flow to the visceral vessels, and obliteration of false lumen flow with subsequent complete thrombosis (Fig. 135-7). When these components of therapy are successfully achieved, aortic remodeling should occur with subsequent prevention of future aneurysmal degeneration of the outer wall of the false lumen.

False Lumen Thrombosis

From a practical perspective, stent-graft repair of acute dissection in the United States has been available only since April 2005, coincident with initial Food and Drug Administration (FDA) approval of a commercially available thoracic stent-graft. To date, the application of available endovascular devices for acute dissection constitutes off-label use because such devices are currently FDA approved in the United States only for the treatment of degenerative thoracic aneurysms.

Dake and colleagues were able to achieve complete or partial thrombosis of the false lumen in 100% of patients, with relief of corresponding symptoms in 76% of patients and morbidity/mortality rates that compared favorably with those after open surgery.[114] In the natural history of medically managed type B dissections, continued patency of the false lumen is an independent risk factor for progression of chronic dissections to aneurysmal dilatation.[117] During the first 4 to 7 years after acute aortic dissection managed medically, aneurysmal degeneration of the false lumen in the thoracic aorta may develop in 14% to 40% of patients treated with medical therapy alone.[11,118,119]

Persistent false lumen patency is an independent risk factor for aneurysmal degeneration of chronic dissections.[38,114,120-123] Indeed, Sueyoshi and coworkers showed that a patent false lumen will enlarge 3.3 mm/yr even in stable, uncomplicated cases.[124] In a review of the IRAD data, Tsai and associates showed that partial thrombosis of the false lumen is an independent predictor of postdischarge mortality (patent, 13.7%; partial thrombosis, 31.6%; complete thrombosis, 22.6%).[123] The proposed mechanism is that formation of thrombus may occlude the distal outflow tears and lead to a significant increase in mean arterial and diastolic pressure as compared with that in a patent lumen with adequate outflow.[123] Although most late deaths are related to co-morbid conditions, subsequent complications such as late rupture and aneurysm development have been estimated to occur in 20% to 50% of patients.[32,119,125] Thus, the concept of inducing false lumen thrombosis by sealing the aortic tear with an aortic endograft has the potential to reduce both early and late complications of type B dissection (Fig. 135-8).

Technical Details

Particular technical points of stent-graft repair of aortic dissection deserve emphasis. First, placement of uncovered stents over the entry tear within the proximal true aortic lumen is ill advised. The ability of an uncovered stent to direct flow away from the false lumen relies on sheer radial force, and tolerance of the acutely dissected intimal flap to accommodate aggressive oversizing in an effort to compress the false lumen is unknown. In addition, the eccentricity of true and false lumen geometry may also place demands on radial force distribution and result in overdistention of the true lumen in tortuous portions of the aorta. By these two mechanisms, deployment of such uncovered stents may cause aortic rupture or create new entry tears. These observations on the poor performance of uncovered stents in an acutely dissected aorta have been confirmed in multiple animal studies.[126-128] Finally, the indiscriminate use of uncovered stents in the true or false lumen may compromise later interventions by limiting sheath access or device deployment.[129]

Overall, in a patient being considered for stent-graft treatment, the location of the entry tear and proper recognition of the proximal zone of fixation are fundamental to procedural success. Once selected, stent-graft repair of acute aortic dissection should be performed in an operating room with adequate fluoroscopic imaging. True lumen access should be obtained from either a brachial or femoral approach; typically, because the tear in type B dissection is distal to the left subclavian artery, rapid true lumen access is easily obtained through a right transbrachial approach. Proper true lumen position should then be confirmed with intravascular ultrasound, which is also useful for confirming the relationship of branch vessels to the dissection flap (Fig. 135-9). It is essential that the operator be comfortable with intravascular ultrasound when performing endovascular repair of the aortic entry tear because it can prevent inadvertent deployment in the false lumen. If device tracking is difficult because of tortuosity or associated occlusive aortic disease, "through-and-through" access from the brachial to the femoral artery can be achieved with intravascular snares to facilitate device delivery. The operator should have definitive knowledge of the three-dimensional aortic topography displayed on the preintervention CT scan before embarking on endovascular therapy. Induction of hypotension or bradycardia by pharma-

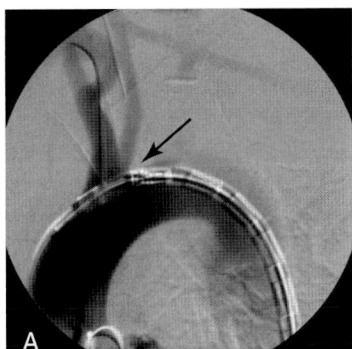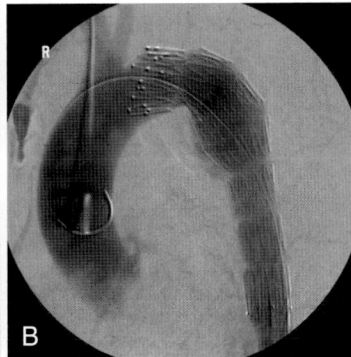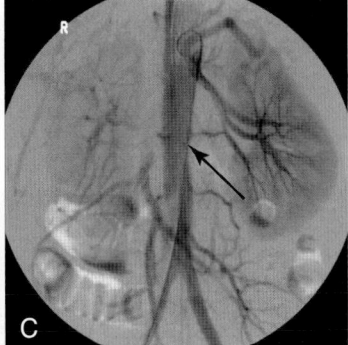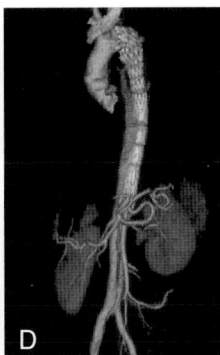

Figure 135-8 Endovascular repair of acute type B aortic dissection. **A,** Thoracic aortography showing a stent-graft in the descending thoracic aorta. The proximal portion of the graft (*arrow*) is placed at the level of the left common carotid artery so that it covers the left subclavian artery to obtain a proximal seal in normal aorta. **B,** Thoracic aortography showing the stent-graft deployed with obliteration of the proximal false lumen. **C,** Abdominal aortography after proximal stent-grafting showing true lumen expansion (*arrow*) with persistent false lumen flow. **D,** Three-dimensional aortic reconstruction after endovascular repair showing obliteration of the false lumen in the thoracic aorta, persistent flow in the abdominal aorta, expansion of the true lumen, and perfusion to all visceral vessels.

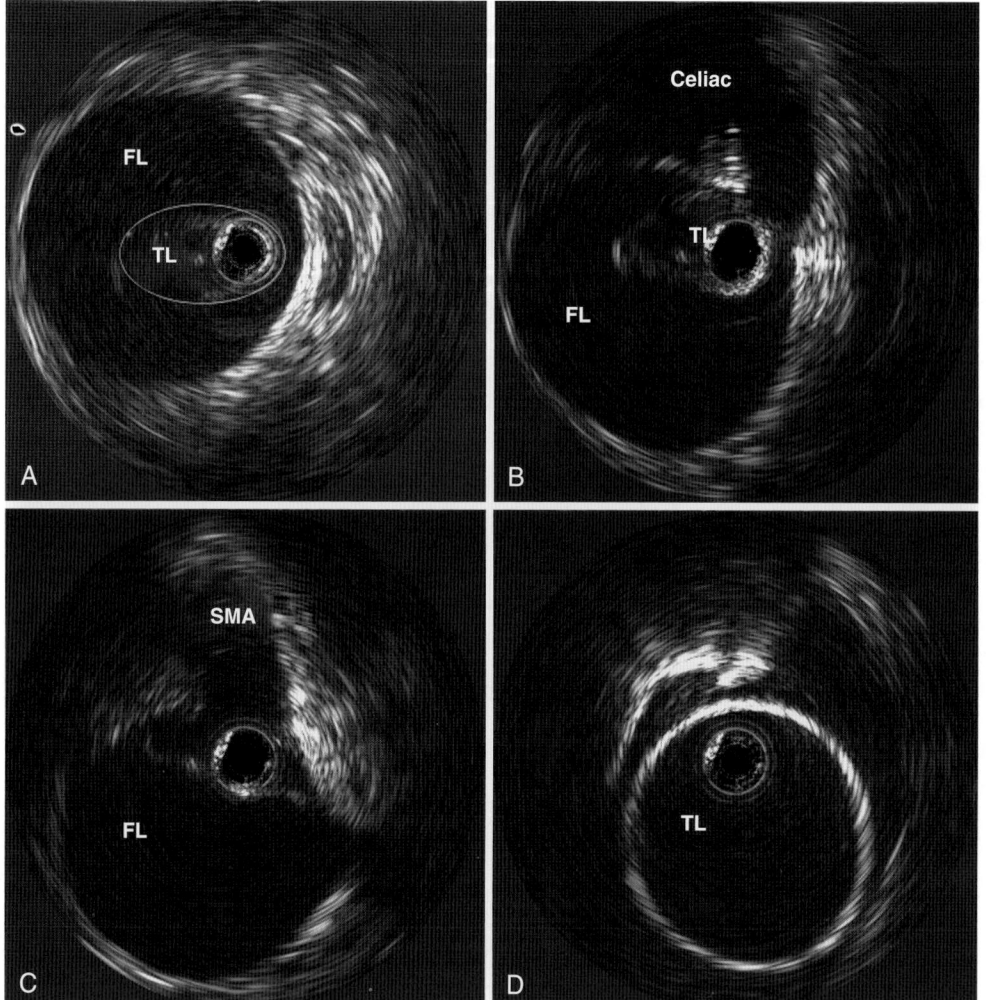

Figure 135-9 Intravascular ultrasound (IVUS) of acute aortic dissection. **A,** IVUS of acute type B dissection with a "floating" true lumen (TL, enhanced by the *circle*). FL, false lumen. **B,** IVUS of acute type B dissection at the level of the celiac artery that originates from the compressed true lumen. **C,** IVUS of acute type B dissection at the level of the superior mesenteric artery (SMA) that originates from the compressed true lumen. **D,** IVUS of the expanded true lumen after endovascular repair of acute type B dissection.

cologic means may increase the accuracy of entry tear sealing during deployment. Furthermore, if a compliant, large-diameter (33 to 40 mm) aortic occlusion balloon is needed to ensure adequate apposition of the device to the aortic wall, it should be used cautiously within the stent-graft (not the native aorta) to avoid aortic disruption.

Early Outcomes

Multiple small studies have detailed their short-term experience with endovascular repair of type B aortic dissections (Table 135-3).[114,130-134] The EuroSTAR (European Collaborators on Stent/Graft Techniques for Aortic Aneurysm Repair)/U.K. Registry report is the largest compendium of patients treated with thoracic aortic stent-grafts to date. In the combined registry, 131 patients with aortic dissection (5% proximal, 81% distal, 14% not classified) were treated with stent-grafts; 57% had symptoms of rupture, aortic expansion,

Table 135-3 Results of Endovascular Treatment of Acute Type B Aortic Dissection

Series	Number of Patients	Indications (%)	Therapy (%)	Mortality (%)
Greenberg et al.[171]	31	MS (77) AR (23)	Stent (94) Fen (6)	29
Slonim et al.[134]	40	NA	Stent (60) Fen (5) Both (35)	25
Lopera et al.[172]	10	NA	Stent (100)	0
Duebener et al.[133]	10	MS (50) AR (30)	Stent (100)	20
Dake et al.[111]	15	NA	Stent (100)	20
Schoder et al.[134]	28	MS (50) AR (11)	Stent (100)	11

AR, aortic rupture; Fen, fenestration; MS, Marfan's syndrome; NA, not available;

or side branch occlusion. Although no meaningful long-term data are available, primary technical success was achieved in 89% and 30-day mortality was 8.4%.[135] Paraplegia occurred in 0.8% of those treated, and survival at 1 year after treatment was reported in 90% of 67 patients who had such follow-up.

A recent meta-analysis of all published series of stent-graft repair for aortic dissection before 2005 identified 609 patients with a procedural success rate of 98.2%. Thirty-day mortality was 5.3% (it was threefold higher in patients with acute dissection), and the neurologic complication rate was 2.9%.[136] A study from China looked at 63 patients with acute dissection who underwent stent-graft placement within 2 weeks of symptoms. They reported a clinical success rate of 95.2% with a 30-day mortality of 3.2%, no paraplegia, and a 1-year false lumen thrombosis rate of 98.4%.[137]

These preliminary data suggest that stent-graft repair may ultimately become the treatment of choice for the majority of patients with distal dissections; the available data consisting largely of registry and single-center retrospective reviews permit only the conclusion that stent-graft repair of the aortic entry tear can provide effective treatment of complicated type B dissections with the inherent advantages of a minimally invasive approach. However, the available data are insufficient to make treatment plans, in particular with regard to patients with uncomplicated distal dissections (those typically treated with medical therapy). Indeed, medical therapy in such patients has usually produced favorable results, perhaps not a surprising finding because these patients do not have immediately threatening anatomic complications of their dissection.

To potentially clarify (although it has not) the role of stent-graft treatment of type B aortic dissection, the Investigation of Stent-Grafts in Aortic Dissection (INSTEAD) trial was designed as a prospective, randomized, multicenter trial performed in Europe that compared stent-grafting with medical therapy for the treatment of chronic, uncomplicated type B aortic dissection. However, because all-cause 1-year mortality was the study's principal endpoint in patients with chronic type B dissection, the 1-year results have not provided conclusive data. Most patients were randomized to medical versus stent-graft therapy 2 weeks after the onset of symptoms. Thus, patients with early complications (those who would most likely benefit from endovascular therapy) were essentially subtracted from the study cohort. Not surprisingly, the investigators found no difference in 30-day mortality between the two groups. However, 1-year mortality was higher in the TEVAR patients (3% for medical versus 8.6% for TEVAR patients) as a result of a periprocedural mortality rate of 3%. The encouraging data reported in this trial involved aortic remodeling, which may be considered a surrogate for prevention of late aneurysm formation. To wit, the stent-graft group experienced false lumen thrombosis in more than 90% of patients at 1 year (significantly higher than in the medically treated group).

The use of stent-graft repair for the treatment of acute dissections holds promise to reduce both early complications and progression over time to aneurysmal degeneration. The instantaneous and dramatic occurrence of false lumen thrombosis by coverage of the aortic entry tear appears to be a key determinant in the process; the significance of small distal fenestrations remains unknown. Furthermore, early treatment in the window of acute type B dissection appears to be associated with improved technical outcomes, consistent with the hypothesis that true lumen/septum malleability may diminish in the chronic phase of the disease. Clearly, comparative clinical trials are needed to clarify the role of stent-graft repair of acute distal dissections.

Other Endovascular Approaches

Mossop and coworkers from Australia described their experience with staged thoracoabdominal and branch vessel endoluminal repair in 25 patients. Initial treatment involved endograft closure of the proximal entry tear and bare-metal, self-expanding Z-stenting of the true lumen, thereby supporting the true lumen and stabilizing the dissection flap. At the 1-week follow-up, secondary reentry tears were sealed by a variety of endovascular approaches, including placement of branch vessel covered stents, placement of short-segment covered aortic endografts, and coil embolization of the false lumen (Fig. 135-10). In their series spanning more than 4 years, they reported no Z-stent migration or stent-related intimal trauma resulting in rupture. Induction of false lumen thrombosis was achieved in 85%. The survival rate at a mean follow-up of 2.5 years was 100%.[138]

Treatment of Malperfusion Syndrome

Malperfusion syndromes may complicate the initial manifestation of acute aortic dissection in 25% to 40% of patients.[10,139,140] When type A dissections that extend into the thoracoabdominal aorta are repaired by open replacement of the ascending aorta, ischemic complications persist in up to 25% of patients.[139] As expected, surgical management of aortic branch compromise in this instance leads to excessive morbidity and mortality, often related to failure to recognize subtle signs and symptoms during the early postoperative period. In this setting, an endovascular approach such as fenestration of the aortic septum and branch orifice stenting is promising because the mortality after open repair of aortic dissection in patients with renal ischemia is 50% to 80% and as high as 87% in those with mesenteric ischemia[10,60]; in contrast, several series of surgical fenestration of the dissection flap in the setting of malperfusion syndromes have reported mortality rates of 20%.[131,141] Current indications for aortic fenestration or branch vessel stenting are dependent on the anatomic extent of the dissection as determined by CT scanning.[140]

Endovascular Treatment

In the initial endovascular management of a patient with an acute aortic dissection complicated by malperfusion, true and

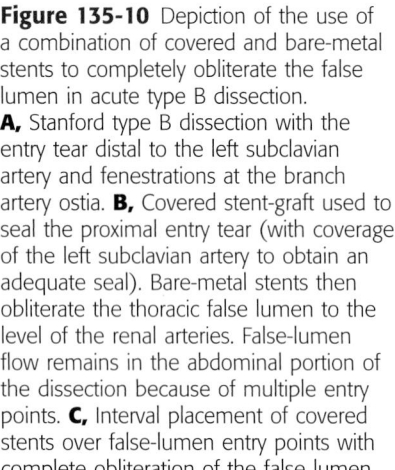
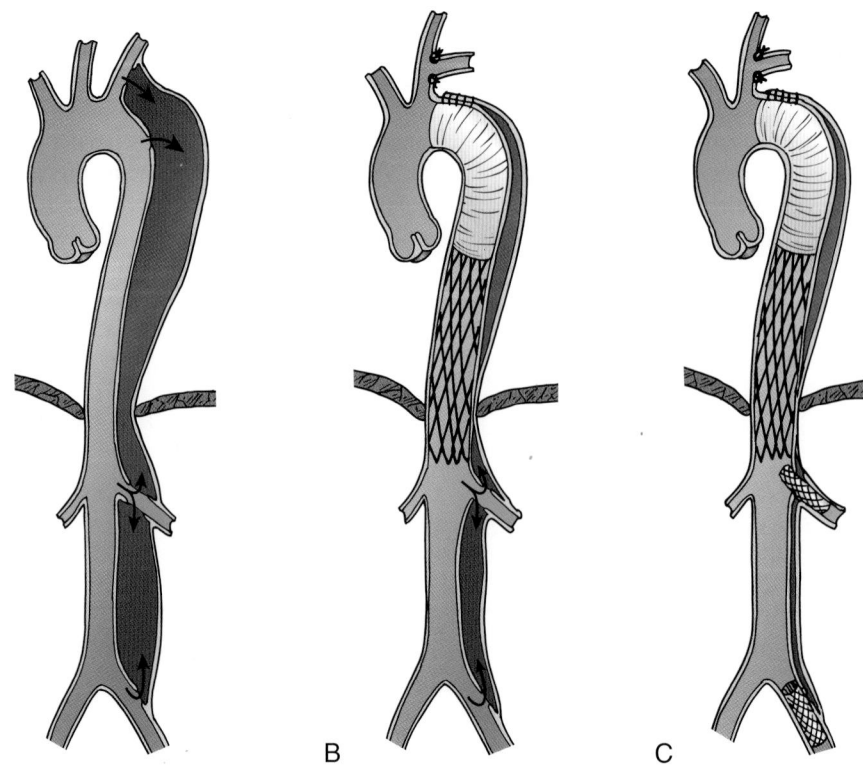

Figure 135-10 Depiction of the use of a combination of covered and bare-metal stents to completely obliterate the false lumen in acute type B dissection. **A,** Stanford type B dissection with the entry tear distal to the left subclavian artery and fenestrations at the branch artery ostia. **B,** Covered stent-graft used to seal the proximal entry tear (with coverage of the left subclavian artery to obtain an adequate seal). Bare-metal stents then obliterate the thoracic false lumen to the level of the renal arteries. False-lumen flow remains in the abdominal portion of the dissection because of multiple entry points. **C,** Interval placement of covered stents over false-lumen entry points with complete obliteration of the false lumen.

A   B   C

false lumen access must be obtained. Intravascular ultrasound should be performed from the ascending aorta to the iliac vessels to define the relationship of the dissection flap to the visceral and renal arteries.[39,142,143] Angiography can often be limited to hand injections of selected branch arteries to prove that the catheter/wire is beyond the dissection and in "normal" artery. This practice limits the contrast load during the procedure and thus avoids further insult to the kidneys.[39] In addition, power injection into the true lumen of the dissected aorta may give the false impression of adequate perfusion to branch vessels compromised by dynamic obstruction. Similarly, demonstrating equal catheter-derived pressures in the true and false lumina does not ensure adequate perfusion in particular branches, for the reasons reviewed earlier. Such pressure measurements have meaning only if obtained in the vessel of inquiry as opposed to the aortic lumen. Indeed, Barnes and colleagues define objective evidence of malperfusion as the presence of a pressure gradient between the aortic root and branch (not aorta) end-hole catheter.[39] All aortic branches should be visualized before intervention because changes in flap mobility secondary to relief of obstruction in any single vessel may alter perfusion in other aortic side branches. If compromise of any aortic branch vessel is uncovered by the dissection, wire access into the distal true lumen of the vessel should be secured. In general, placement of self-expanding stents in a potentially compromised aortic branch should precede aortic fenestration because fenestration may unpredictably alter aortic flow and make it extremely difficult to regain endovascular access to compromised vessels.[140]

Percutaneous Fenestration. Fenestration of the intimal flap may be performed by several techniques under the combined guidance of ultrasound and fluoroscopy. Most commonly, fenestration is performed from the smaller (usually the true lumen) to the larger lumen. Using a Rösch-Uchida needle, Brockenbrough needle, Colopinto needle, or the back end of a 0.014-inch wire, a fenestration is created close to the compromised aortic branch. After the needle and a stiff wire are advanced from the true to the false lumen, a 5 Fr catheter is advanced into the alternate lumen. Confirmation of position across the membrane is performed by injection of contrast material. Subsequently, an angioplasty balloon at least 12 to 15 mm in diameter and 20 to 40 mm in length is used to create a fenestration tear (Fig. 135-11). An alternative technique of fenestration has been termed the "scissors technique."[144] Stiff guide wires are placed in each lumen from a single femoral access, and a single long sheath is advanced over the two wires, thus dividing the membrane over this distance. Those familiar with use of the "scissors technique" have reported both clean longitudinal tears (the ideal result) and circumferential separation of the flap from the aortic wall with aortoaortic intussusception (not ideal).[145] Finally, the use of a snare to deliver a wire from one femoral access through the flap and down the contralateral femoral access has been described. By pulling this "U" down the distal aorta, a fenestration defect may be created with the same potential risk for intimal dehiscence described earlier. In light of these dramatic and unpredictable alterations in intimal flap anatomy and flow dynamics incurred by overly aggressive fenestration in the visceral aorta, investigators with the largest series of patients

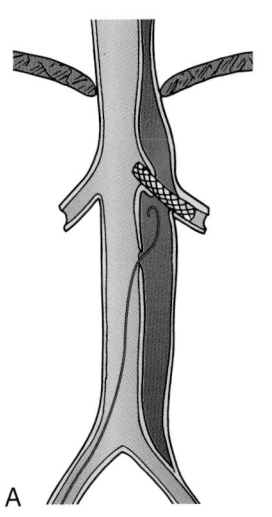 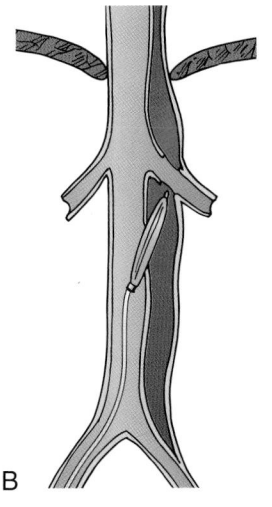 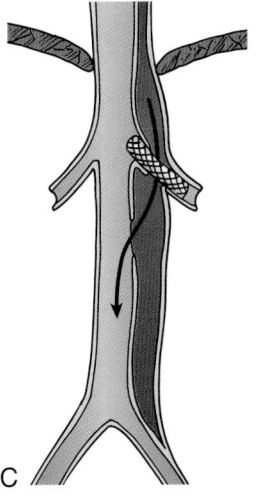

Figure 135-11 Depiction of endovascular fenestration. **A,** The left renal artery (coming off the false lumen) is made to originate from the true lumen. This requires stenting with either a covered or bare-metal stent. **B,** A balloon is then used to enlarge natural fenestrations in the dissection flap to allow flow through the open fenestration (**C**).

currently recommend that percutaneous fenestration be limited to the distal aorta.[131] The ideal hemodynamic result for fenestration of the dissected intima is realized when peak systolic pressure is equalized between the two lumina in the aorta and the false lumen is decompressed.[45,140,146]

In a series of 40 patients with malperfusion syndromes, 14 underwent combined stenting and balloon fenestration, 24 underwent stenting alone, and 2 underwent fenestration alone.[131] The location of the balloon fenestration was in the thoracic aorta in eight patients, in the upper abdominal aorta in three patients, and just above the aortic bifurcation in seven patients. Flow was restored to the ischemic territories in 37 of 40 patients (93%), but the 30-day survival rate was 75%. In follow-up past the 30-day perioperative period, five additional patients died, with one of these deaths being related to false lumen rupture and two of unknown etiology. This 30-day death rate of 25% compares favorably with the historical surgical series wherein operative mortality was reported to be up to 50%.[147] However, contemporary surgical series have demonstrated substantially improved operative mortality, even for patients with mesenteric compromise,[9] and thus it is worth emphasizing that mortality in such patients is more often referable to delayed diagnosis than to the morbidity associated with the intervention itself.

The effect of fenestration on the long-term outcome of false lumen expansion in patients with distal dissections is unknown because the false lumen remains pressurized and therefore at risk for continued progression to aneurysm. Beregi and coauthors reported a series of 46 patients treated by either stent-graft therapy (n = 12) or balloon fenestration (n = 34) for peripheral ischemic complications of acute aortic dissection and found that a decrease in aortic diameter occurred in patients treated with stent-grafts whereas the diameter in those with balloon fenestration increased.[148] Indeed, it is likely that as further experience with TEVAR of the proximal entry tear is gained, fenestration and stenting of branch vessels will be used as an adjunct to stent-grafting rather than as definitive therapy.

Open Surgical Treatment

Because dynamic obstruction at the aortic level is the most common mechanism of malperfusion syndromes, surgical fenestration has been the most frequently applied procedure (Fig. 135-12).[7] This operation at the abdominal aortic level was first described by Robert Shaw from the Massachusetts General Hospital in a 1955 case report.[149] Later that year, Cooley and DeBakey reported initial graft replacement of the proximal thoracic aorta for acute dissection, and the fenestration procedure was rapidly eclipsed.[150] However, inasmuch as several series before the endovascular era have documented unpredictable relief of malperfusion syndromes and substantial morbidity and mortality of open graft replacement (obliteration of the false lumen may lead to ischemia of organs, usually the left kidney, whose vessels originate in the false lumen), surgical fenestration has regained favor.[15,151-153] Indeed, for this reason and because the threat of proximal aortic rupture is rare, many surgeons have favored a complication-specific approach in which the intervention is directed toward restoring flow to acutely affected organs.[9,154]

Technique. The fundamental technique of surgical fenestration is wide resection of the dissected septum to relieve aortic obstruction by equalizing flow between the true and false lumina. A primary consideration is whether aortic clamping and the fenestration are confined to the infrarenal aorta. It may be desirable to extend the septectomy into the visceral segment to permit direct inspection/repair of the ostia of the mesenteric and renal vessels.[155] Experience has demonstrated that the duration of supraceliac clamping can be limited to the 20-minute range, with repositioning of the clamp to an infrarenal location after closure of the visceral segment aortotomy. Interposition of a short-segment polyester graft in the infrarenal aorta facilitates reconstruction of the aortic layers at the distal anastomosis with the double-layer Teflon felt technique. Our posture relative to extending the fenestration/septectomy into the visceral aortic segment is dictated by the anatomic complexity displayed on the CT scan. Small aortic diameter, total absence of visceral artery flow, extension

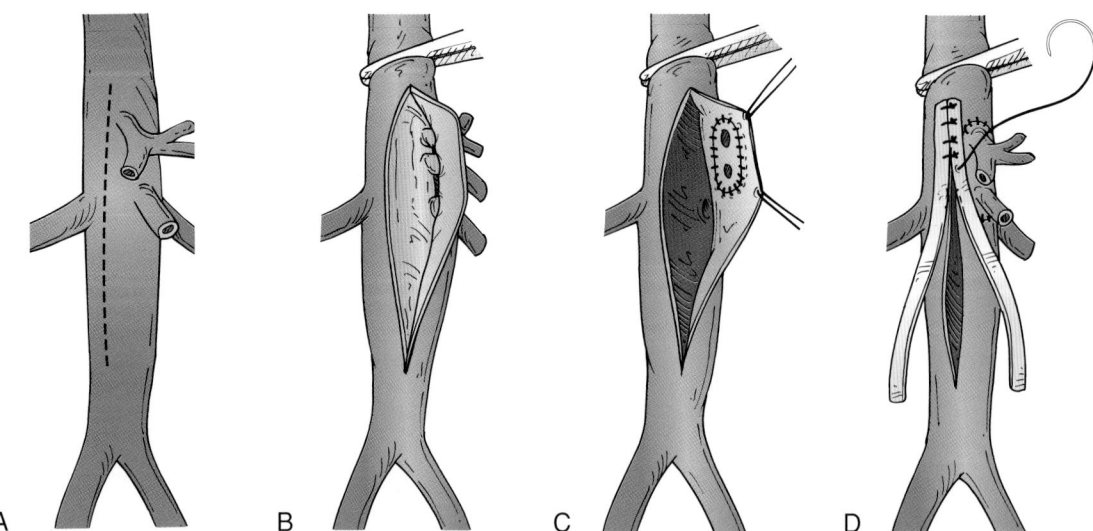

Figure 135-12 Technique of surgical abdominal aortic fenestration. **A,** Dissection involving the visceral segment of the aorta. **B,** If static obstruction of the renal or visceral vessels is suspected from axial imaging studies, the fenestration can be carried onto the visceral aortic segment. The left kidney has been swept anteriorly, and note that the left renal artery is perfused from the false lumen. The septum is incised to expose the origins of the celiac/superior mesenteric/right renal artery perfused via the true lumen. **C,** Direct suture repair of the vessel ostium may be required, herein shown at the left renal origin, whose orifice abuts the circumferential terminus of the dissection. **D,** After septectomy in the visceral segment, the outer aortic wall is closed over Teflon felt and the clamp is moved to the infrarenal aorta, which is most conveniently reconstructed with a tube graft.

of the dissected septum directly to or beyond a vital branch orifice, and radiographic evidence of a septum intussuscepted into a renal/mesenteric vessel are all considerations that prompt extension of the aortotomy into the visceral segment. Such an approach also permits direct repair of a static obstruction (i.e., in which the branch vessel itself is dissected). This can be accomplished by circumferential suturing of the vessel intima to the aortic wall at the ostia. Because continuous exposure of the visceral segment is desirable in the surgical treatment of malperfusion syndrome, we prefer left flank approaches for this procedure. Depending on body habitus, a 9th or 10th interspace thoracoabdominal approach is used to allow complete infradiaphragmatic aortic exposure, transperitoneal inspection of the viscera, and palpation of the superior mesenteric artery pulse caudal to the mesocolon. At a median follow-up of 19 months, no significant aortic dilatation occurred with such aortic tailoring as a surgical technique.[155] Advocates of surgical fenestration for malperfusion syndromes have asserted that the "surgical" morbidity and mortality rates quoted to support endovascular therapies are outdated and strongly influenced by delays in diagnosis and treatment.[156]

Results. Eleftriades and coauthors reported in 1992 their experience using a "complication-specific" approach to acute aortic dissection. The overall survival rate for the total population was 65% at 1 year, 57% at 3 years, 50% at 5 years, and 28% at 10 years. Of the 14 patients in the total experience treated by fenestration, their actuarial survival rate was 77%, 77%, and 53% at 1, 3, and 5 years, respectively. None of the surgically fenestrated patients were found to have expansion of their aortic diameters on follow-up. Surgical fenestration

was performed in the infrarenal aorta and resulted in relief of ischemia in 13 of 14 patients (93%). The authors concluded that the relative simplicity of surgical fenestration allows subsequent survival almost uniformly unless the patient's preoperative overall status had been severely compromised.[141]

A recent report from the Mayo Clinic affords perspective on both the infrequent need for and the durability of surgical fenestration.[157] From their database of 857 patients with a diagnosis of aortic dissection, only 321 underwent surgical intervention of any kind. Clinical or radiographic evidence of malperfusion was observed in 81 patients (25%). Fourteen patients underwent surgical fenestration during the study period, thus representing 1.6% of the total study population. Four patients had organ or limb malperfusion after proximal aortic replacement for aortic dissection, a finding similar to other reports. The mean interval between onset of malperfusion and fenestration was 19 hours (range, 3 to 48 hours). Surgical fenestration relieved malperfusion syndrome in all 10 patients with organ or limb ischemia. Operative mortality was 43% (3/7) in the acute dissection group; seven patients were treated in the chronic phase of the disease with no mortality. Follow-up at a mean of 5.1 years for the 11 survivors revealed no evidence of aneurysm formation at the site of fenestration. The authors note that in comparing surgical fenestration with series of endovascular fenestration, the likelihood of subsequent aortic complications related to expansion or rupture of the false lumen may be greater in patients treated by endovascular means. Therefore, although endovascular fenestration may offer more rapid restoration of perfusion, its durability would seem to be less than that of surgical fenestration techniques.[157]

Our cumulative experience affords a perspective over a 35-year period involving some 200 patients with acute aortic dissection treated during the 1990s and in part clarifies the role of open surgical fenestration and peripheral endovascular intervention in patients with malperfusion syndromes.[9] Nearly a third of the patients had evidence of branch occlusion; 17 (32%) of these 53 patients underwent peripheral vascular intervention to restore circulation. The overall mortality rate in the interval 1990 to 1999 was significantly lower than in an earlier report from 1965 to 1986 (18% versus 37%, P < .006).[9] In discerning the factors associated with improved results over time, three variables were important. First, aortic rupture occurred in just 6% of patients versus 18% in the previous interval. Presumably, dissection was being diagnosed and patients referred more promptly. Second, the impact of branch occlusion on mortality was no longer significant, thus implying that recognition and treatment of malperfusion syndromes had improved the overall results. Third, mortality in patients with mesenteric ischemia had improved to 37%, whereas an 87% mortality rate was observed in our earlier report. Recently, the IRAD data implicated mesenteric ischemia as being responsible for 15% of all deaths related to acute dissection.[11] For patients with mesenteric or renal malperfusion syndromes, surgical fenestration was used in nine patients. Restoration of flow was successful in all patients, and all patients thus treated survived, whereas two deaths occurred in those with mesenteric ischemia managed by percutaneous fenestration. Open aortic fenestration is an excellent method of restoring circulation to vascular territories affected by malperfusion syndromes, especially when the mesenteric and renal beds are involved, and it affords the opportunity to assess bowel viability and plan second-look procedures. Treatment priority should be assigned to the most life-threatening condition in patients with acute aortic dissection. The presence of mesenteric ischemia assumes such priority in virtually all patients and constitutes an exception to prompt central aortic repair in those with type A dissection.

■ NATURAL HISTORY AND FOLLOW-UP

The primary late complication of aortic dissection is aneurysmal dilatation of the outer wall of the false lumen; of patients surviving acute dissection, 25% to 40% will progress to aneurysmal dilatation of the dissected aorta despite medical management (Fig. 135-13).[158,159] In most clinical series of thoracoabdominal aneurysms, approximately 20% of cases are the sequelae of chronic dissection, for which conventional open repair is typically the only treatment option in contemporary practice.[160] Indeed, a variety of technical and anatomic considerations indicate that stent-graft repair of aneurysms of chronic dissection etiology remains a major challenge.[161] Factors that appear to have a significant impact on chronic aneurysm development after dissection include poorly controlled hypertension, a maximal aortic diameter of at least 4 cm in the acute phase, and continued patency of the false lumen.[121] Furthermore, some 10% to 20% of those with dissection will subsequently experience late rupture of the aneu-

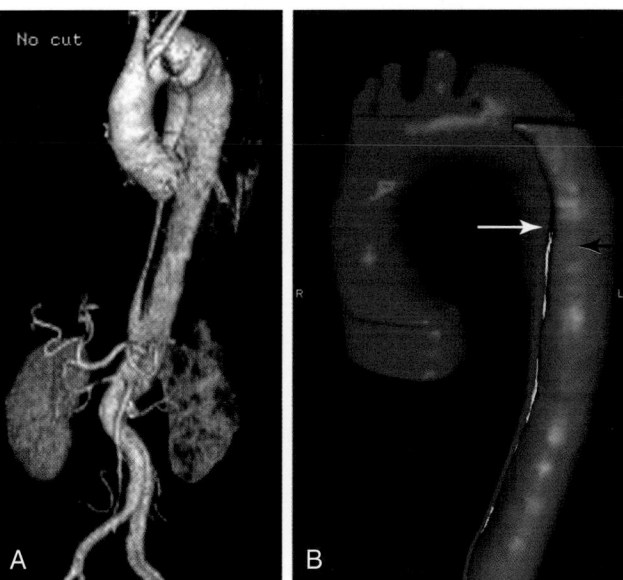

Figure 135-13 CT angiogram depiction of aneurysmal degeneration of chronic aortic dissection. **A,** Three-dimensional reconstruction of chronic dissection with false lumen enlargement and aneurysm formation in the thoracic aorta. **B,** M2S reconstruction of chronic aortic dissection showing the enlarged false lumen (*black arrow*) and narrow true lumen (*white arrow*).

rysm,[121] and conventional surgical repair of such lesions is considerably more complex than repair of degenerative aneurysms (see Chapter 131: Thoracic and Thoracoabdominal Aneurysms: Evaluation and Decision Making).

Long-term Survival

A recent review of the IRAD data focused on long-term survival of patients with acute aortic dissection. In an examination of 242 consecutive patients discharged alive after type B dissections, Tsai and coworkers found that the 3-year survival rate was 77.6% for patients treated medically, 82.8% for those treated surgically, and 76.2% for those treated by stent-graft repair.[13] Independent predictors of long-term mortality included female gender, previous aortic aneurysm, atherosclerosis, renal failure, and in-hospital hypotension/shock.[13] Examination of the 273 type A dissection patients discharged alive found that the survival rate in patients treated with surgery was 90.5% at 3 years versus 68.7% for those treated medically.[12] Independent predictors of mortality in this cohort included atherosclerosis and previous cardiac surgery.[12] These studies show that although post-hospital survival is excellent after type A dissection, nearly a quarter of those with type B dissection died within 3 years, thus suggesting that current treatment strategies are inadequate.

Late Therapy

Aneurysms that are the sequelae of chronic dissection tend to be more extensive than degenerative aneurysms and occur in younger patients. Treatment with effective beta blockade is an essential feature of long-term therapy and follow-up. The rationale for such therapy is based on the recognition that patients with aortic dissection have a systemic illness that places their entire aorta at risk for further dissection, aneurysm, or rupture. Guidelines recommend progressive upward titration of beta blockade to achieve a blood pressure lower than 125/80 mm Hg in usual patients and lower than 120 in those with Marfan's syndrome. In addition, aggressive beta blockade has been shown to retard growth of the aortic root in patients with Marfan's syndrome and may have a similar effect on the thoracoabdominal aorta.[162] Serial imaging is the cornerstone of long-term follow-up, and axial imaging modalities should encompass the entire aorta. Though in developmental stages at present, branched stent-graft technologies will probably have an important role in the future management of patients with aneurysms of chronic dissection etiology.[163]

INTRAMURAL HEMATOMA AND PENETRATING AORTIC ULCER

Two aortic entities related to aortic dissection deserve mention. An intramural hematoma (IMH) represents a collection of blood that is confined to the aortic media, whereas a penetrating aortic ulcer (PAU) is a defect in the elastic lamina of the aortic wall that leads to localized medial disruption and potential rupture. These are two closely related (possibly the same) aortic conditions that commonly cause diagnostic confusion with classic aortic dissection (Fig. 135-14). Such confusion is related to the fact that these entities share the feature of intimal violation with the flowing blood gaining entry or propagating (or both) between the aortic wall layers (usually within the media), and IMH and PAU may be present concurrently. PAU is often noted as a radiographic curiosity on CT scans obtained for evaluation of the thoracic aorta, whereas IMH is a dissection process wherein the defining features include absence of an "intimal flap" and (as implied by the name) a thrombosed false lumen.

Etiology and Diagnosis

In both conditions, symptomatic patients have an abrupt onset of severe pain in the chest, neck, back, abdomen, or various combinations thereof that is typical of acute aortic syndrome. Paradoxically (and unlike classic aortic dissection), both are manifestations of degenerative aortic pathology that typically occurs in older patients with significant hypertension and often with diffuse degenerative atherosclerotic disease of the thoracic aorta. IMH of the thoracic aorta has been characterized as a distinct clinical entity whose distinguishing radiographic features are the absence of direct communication between the thrombus in the false lumen and the true lumen and the absence of a definable intimal flap (as seen with classic aortic dissection) or penetrating ulcer.[164,165] IMH extent is variable in terms of both the length and circumference of the aorta involved and the direction of propagation. The etiology of IMH was initially thought to involve spontaneous rupture of the vasa vasorum within the medial layers of the aortic wall that will occasionally evolve into a PAU (a rare event). More consistent with our own observations, a PAU phenomenon is usually the origin of IMH, and whether the ulcer-like projection is radiographically demonstrated is merely serendipity.[166] Indeed, in the Mayo Clinic series, approximately 80% of patients with PAU had an associated IMH.[167] PAU is used to describe lesions when a cap-like projection of contrast material is seen (on CT scan) beyond

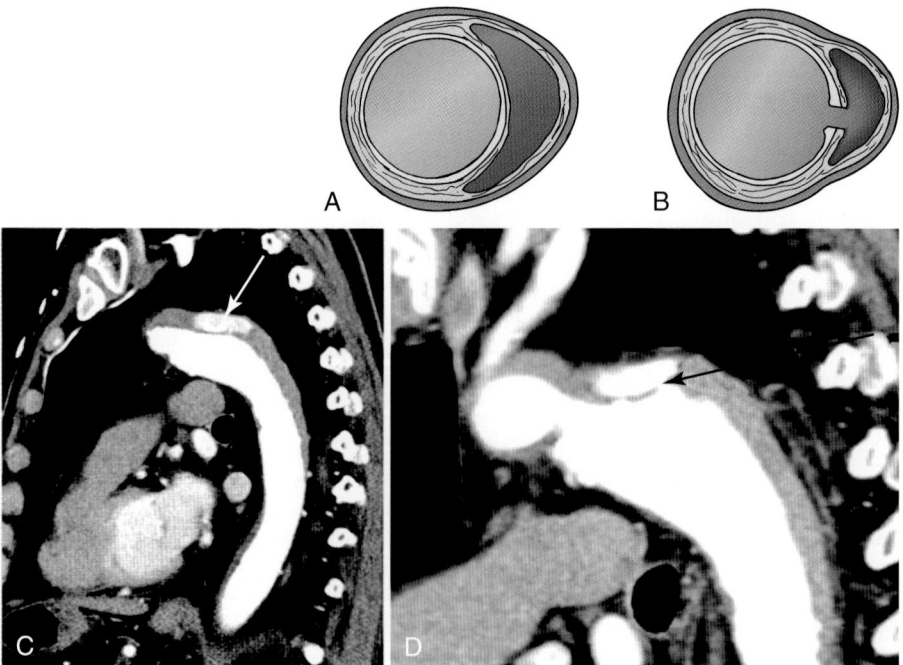

Figure 135-14 Penetrating aortic ulcer and intramural hematoma. **A,** Depiction of an intramural hematoma. **B,** Depiction of a penetrating aortic ulcer. **C,** CT angiogram of a penetrating aortic ulcer (*arrow*) in the descending thoracic aorta. **D,** CT angiogram of a penetrating aortic ulcer showing the entry point in the true lumen.

the usual luminal aortic boundary (see Fig. 135-14). In this instance, the atherosclerotic lesion penetrates the internal elastic lamina and facilitates hematoma formation within the media. Further propagation of this flap is thought to be prevented by the presence of atherosclerotic disease in the aorta (a rare finding in classic aortic dissection).[168]

Treatment

Although the natural history of asymptomatic type B IMH and PAU has been complete resolution in 50% to 80% of patients,[168] progression to classic dissection or aneurysmal degeneration of the aorta can occur.[166,169] The IRAD database examined 1010 patients with symptoms of acute aortic syndrome and identified a 5.7% incidence of IMH. The descending aorta was affected in 60% of cases, whereas classic aortic dissection more commonly affected the ascending aorta (65% of cases). The overall mortality of IMH was similar to that of classic aortic dissection, 20.7% versus 23.9%, both for proximal (39.1% versus 29.9%) and distal (8.3% versus 13.1%) locations. Among the 51 patients whose initial diagnostic study revealed IMH, 8 (16%) progressed to aortic dissection on a second imaging study. A normal aortic diameter in the acute phase was the best predictor of IMH regression without complications. The IRAD investigators recommended prompt surgical therapy for IMH involvement of the ascending aorta. Intense medical therapy (goal of systolic blood pressure <120/80, heart rate <60) with serial imaging was recommended for involvement of the arch and descending aorta.[170]

A recent report of 35 patients with IMH detailed a significant correlation between disease progression and initial aortic diameter or hematoma thickness (or both). Patients with an initial aortic diameter greater than 40 mm had a 30-fold increased risk for progression to either aneurysm formation or rupture. In addition, hematoma thickness greater than 1 cm was associated with a ninefold increased risk for progression. This suggests that the degree of separation of the aortic wall layers may contribute to chronic aneurysmal degeneration.[171]

Although such focal pathology may be ideally suited for stent-graft repair (see Fig. 135-5), patients with incidental asymptomatic IMH or PAU of the descending aorta are currently managed with medical therapy. Tittle and colleagues detailed their experience in 45 patients with symptomatic PAU and IMH. In this cohort, 33% had rupture on admission and 53% required surgery. Patients with lesions involving the ascending aorta were more likely to undergo surgical repair (83%), whereas only 50% of patients with involvement of the descending thoracic aorta were operated on.[172] Indications for intervention included aortic diameter greater than 6 cm, rupture, impending rupture, or major progression in size despite medical therapy.[166] Patients with involvement of the ascending aorta are usually treated surgically because of the high risk for cardioaortic complications. Surveillance imaging of patients with IMH or PAU treated medically should be frequent, especially in those with evidence of aneurysmal dilatation.

SELECTED KEY REFERENCES

Clouse WD, Hallett JW Jr, Schaff HV, Spittell PC, Rowland CM, Ilstrup DM, Melton LJ 3rd. Acute aortic dissection: population-based incidence compared with degenerative aortic aneurysm rupture. *Mayo Clin Proc.* 2004;79:176-180.
An excellent review of the natural history of untreated aortic dissection in a contemporary patient population.

Lauterbach SR, Cambria RP, Brewster DC, Gertler JP, Lamuraglia GM, Isselbacher EM, Hilgenberg AD, Moncure AC. Contemporary management of aortic branch compromise resulting from acute aortic dissection. *J Vasc Surg.* 2001;33:1185-1192.
This article characterizes the manifestations of malperfusion syndrome and details a complication-specific approach to surgical intervention.

Mossop PJ, McLachlan CS, Amukotuwa SA, Nixon IK. Staged endovascular treatment for complicated type B aortic dissection. *Nat Clin Pract Cardiovasc Med.* 2005;2:316-321; quiz 322.
Details a new frontier in endovascular management of acute aortic dissection. This technique/graft design is currently part of a prospective, multicenter trial.

Sueyoshi E, Imada T, Sakamoto I, Matsuoka Y, Hayashi K. Analysis of predictive factors for progression of type B aortic intramural hematoma with computed tomography. *J Vasc Surg.* 2002;35:1179-1183.
Excellent review of the dissection-related entity of intramural hematoma.

Tsai TT, Evangelista A, Nienaber CA, Myrmel T, Meinhardt G, Cooper JV, Smith DE, Suzuki T, Fattori R, Llovet A, Froehlich J, Hutchison S, Distante A, Sundt T, Beckman J, Januzzi JL Jr, Isselbacher EM, Eagle KA. International Registry of Acute Aortic Dissection. Partial thrombosis of the false lumen in patients with acute type B aortic dissection. *N Engl J Med.* 2007;357:349-359.
This article details new hemodynamic theories regarding the contribution of false lumen flow to eventual aneurysmal degeneration after aortic dissection.

REFERENCES

The reference list can be found on the companion Expert Consult Web site at *www.expertconsult.com.*

Section **17** Arterial Aneurysms

CHAPTER 136

Lower Extremity Aneurysms

Frank B. Pomposelli and Allen Hamdan

Aneurysms occurring in the arteries of the lower limb are the most common after aneurysms of the infrarenal aorta. They can be classified as true arterial aneurysms caused by degeneration of the entire arterial wall or false aneurysms caused by focal disruption as a result of trauma, infection, or anastomotic disruption. In clinical practice, the majority of popliteal aneurysms encountered are true aneurysms, whereas those of the femoral artery are false aneurysms. Regardless of etiology, all lower extremity aneurysms can be considered either asymptomatic or symptomatic. Asymptomatic aneurysms may be detected on physical examination as a painless pulsating mass in the groin or behind the knee or can be undetectable without the aid of an imaging study. Symptomatic aneurysms can be manifested as local pain, neuralgia, or swelling from compression of adjacent nerves or veins (including the development of deep venous thrombosis) or as ischemia secondary to either distal embolization or aneurysm thrombosis. Frank rupture is also seen, albeit infrequently, in contrast to aneurysms of the aorta.

A strong association exists between the presence of true aneurysms of the femoral or popliteal arteries and those of the contralateral extremity, as well as the aortoiliac segment. Consequently, the discovery of a lower extremity aneurysm mandates careful observation, evaluation, or both for associated aneurysms in the opposite limb and abdominal aorta.

The objectives of treatment of lower extremity aneurysms are straightforward: exclude the aneurysm from the circulation while maintaining distal arterial perfusion and relieve any existing symptoms. It is preferable to treat aneurysms while asymptomatic because such treatment results in less morbidity and higher rates of limb salvage and graft patency than when treating acute manifestations such as popliteal aneurysm thrombosis with critical limb ischemia. Unfortunately, the natural history of both femoral and popliteal aneurysms is unclear, thus making decisions about their treatment, especially when small and asymptomatic, controversial. Moreover, determining their natural history is difficult in that their true incidence in the general population is not known. The definition of what constitutes a lower extremity aneurysm is problematic because the diameter of normal arteries can vary with the age, size, and gender of the patient. These issues become more complex in the subset of the patients with arteriomegaly (see Chapter 8: Arterial Aneurysms), when the normal diameter of the arteries may be impossible to determine. Because true aneurysms of the lower extremity are relatively uncommon, most studies involve the experience of individual centers

and usually include fewer than 100 patients. In our own tertiary referral practice, where more than 4000 lower extremity reconstructions have been performed in a recent 10-year period, we treated only 51 aneurysms in 39 patients.[1]

Definitive treatment of lower extremity arterial aneurysms is usually accomplished by ligation/exclusion with bypass or an interposition graft. In recent years, endovascular treatment with self-expanding stent-grafts has evolved as a viable alternative in some circumstances. As with other catheter-based interventions in the lower extremity, the resultant reduction in perioperative complications and the shorter recovery times with endovascular therapy must be weighed against the higher likelihood of graft failure and need for reintervention. This chapter focuses on the evaluation and management of true aneurysms of the lower extremity and iatrogenic femoral false aneurysms. Although popliteal aneurysms are of most clinical significance, the lower extremity aneurysms will be discussed in anatomic sequence.

FEMORAL ARTERY ANEURYSMS

Common Femoral Artery Aneurysms

True aneurysms of the common femoral artery (CFA) are relatively rare and usually associated with aortic or popliteal artery aneurysms. A CFA aneurysm is defined as a focal dilatation of the artery to 1.5 times the normal diameter of the adjacent segment of artery.[2] As with popliteal aneurysms, the diameter of the normal femoral artery varies with the size, girth, and gender of the patient. The normal diameter is reported to range from 0.78 to 1.12 cm in men and 0.78 to 0.85 cm in women.[3] In clinical practice, the minimum threshold for treatment of an asymptomatic femoral aneurysm is 2.5 cm. (False aneurysms caused by infection are discussed in Chapter 139: Infected Aneurysms, those secondary to anastomotic disruption in Chapter 43: Local Complications: Anastomotic Aneurysms, and those caused by trauma in Chapter 155: Vascular Trauma: Extremity).

The classification scheme for femoral aneurysms devised by Cutler and Darling is simple and relevant in planning treatment.[4] Type 1 aneurysms involve only the CFA and end proximal to the femoral bifurcation, whereas type 2 aneurysms extend into the origin of the deep femoral artery. Type 1 aneurysms account for 44% to 85% of all femoral artery aneurysms.[4,5]

Epidemiology

CFA aneurysms are predominantly found in older men who smoke and have hypertension. The vast majority are degenerative, but they have also been reported in a variety of other conditions, including Behçet's syndrome,[6-8] acromegaly,[9] and arteriomegaly.[10] They are the second most common peripheral aneurysm after popliteal aneurysms. The mean age at diagnosis is 65, with a male-female ratio of 28:1 to 30:1. Bilateral aneurysms are present in 50% of patients.[4,5,11-15] Femoral aneurysms are frequently found in the presence of other aneurysms. Aortic aneurysms have a reported prevalence of 50% to 90% in patients with femoral aneurysms,[4,5,15,16] and 27% to 44% will have an associated popliteal artery aneurysm.[4,5] In early retrospective series relying on physical examination or arteriography, femoral aneurysms were considered to be a relatively uncommon occurrence in patients with aortic aneurysm. In a more recent prospective study using routine duplex surveillance in all patients with aortic aneurysms, Diwan and colleagues found that 14% of men with aortic aneurysms had femoral or popliteal aneurysms whereas none were found in women.[17] The frequent occurrence of aortic and popliteal aneurysms in patients with femoral aneurysms suggests that there may be a systemic or genetic defect affecting arterial wall integrity that places the patient at lifelong risk for aneurysm formation in multiple locations (see Chapter 8: Arterial Aneurysms). Consequently, any patient in whom a peripheral aneurysm has been discovered and all men with aortic aneurysms should undergo routine screening by duplex ultrasonography for aortic and popliteal aneurysms and lifelong follow-up for further aneurysm formation.

Clinical Findings

Approximately 30% to 40% of patients are asymptomatic at initial evaluation,[4,5] usually with a painless pulsating femoral mass discovered on physical examination. Approximately 30% to 40% have local pain or tenderness and may have symptoms of femoral neuralgia or limb edema from compression of the adjacent femoral vein or nerve.

In reported series, 10% to 65% have complications of ischemia, including claudication[18] or critical limb ischemia from acute thrombosis, especially when the deep femoral artery and the superficial femoral artery (SFA) are involved.[4,5,11] Acute thrombosis occurs in approximately 15% of reported cases. Distal embolization causing blue toe syndrome does occur, albeit infrequently. Rupture is exceedingly uncommon and generally occurs only in aneurysms larger than 5 cm in diameter.[13,19]

Diagnosis

Femoral aneurysms may be detected by physical examination, although 20% to 30% are missed by this method alone.[5,17] Duplex ultrasonography reliably detects the presence of femoral artery aneurysms and provides additional important information regarding their diameter, the presence of luminal thrombus, and involvement of the femoral bifurcation,[20,21] and it can simultaneously be used to rule out occult aneurysms in the aortic or popliteal arteries. Magnetic resonance angiography[22] (MRA) and computed tomographic angiography[23,24] (CTA) are accurate imaging modalities that can provide additional precise and detailed anatomic information when planning treatment, especially information on patency of the external iliac artery and SFA. Both have largely supplanted contrast-enhanced arteriography for this purpose.

Natural History

Precise information regarding the behavior of femoral aneurysms is unknown because of their relatively infrequent occurrence. Most reports evaluating the natural history are biased by the fact that they largely represent patients who have been treated, many of whom were symptomatic at initial evaluation.

In one of the largest reported series of 172 femoral aneurysms in 100 patients, 40 were asymptomatic, and 105 small (<2.5 cm) aneurysms were managed nonoperatively.[5] Of this nonoperative group, limb-threatening ischemic symptoms developed in only three patients over a period of 28 months. Surprisingly, the mean diameter of symptomatic and asymptomatic aneurysms was identical at 2.8 cm. In other series, thrombosis or other major complications have been reported to occur in 43% to 47% of cases.[4,25] Although no clear threshold diameter for treatment has been established, complications are infrequent with small aneurysms and occur in no more than 1% to 2% of patients per year. Consequently, small femoral aneurysms less than 2.5 cm in diameter are generally considered to have a benign natural history and can be managed expectantly, provided that they do not continue to enlarge or cause symptoms.[5,11]

Indications for Treatment

All symptomatic femoral aneurysm should be repaired. Even though no correlation has been made between aneurysm diameter and likelihood of complications, most surgeons recommend repairing asymptomatic aneurysms larger than 2.5 cm,[18,26] although this recommendation is not evidence based and others have advocated a more conservative approach.[27] For patients being observed without treatment, a baseline ultrasound and pulse examination should be undertaken. Intervention should be considered for subsequent expansion or the onset of symptoms. The loss of previously present distal pulses in a patient with a femoral aneurysm is indicative of occult distal embolization and is generally considered an indication for elective repair.

Surgical Treatment

CFA aneurysms may be managed by a variety of surgical techniques, depending on their extent, associated occlusive disease, and the presence of other aneurysms.

Surgical reconstructions are performed through a vertical groin incision over the CFA. If the aneurysm is large and proximal control cannot be obtained safely in the groin, the external iliac artery can be controlled through a separate retroperitoneal incision or by dividing the inguinal ligament. Alternatively and less invasively, balloon occlusion of the external iliac artery can be performed by contralateral femoral artery percutaneous access.

Type 1 aneurysms are treated with a short interposition graft of Dacron or polytetrafluoroethylene (PTFE). Small aneurysms can be fully excised, whereas larger aneurysms can be treated from within the aneurysm sac by using the graft inclusion technique, analogous to that done for aortic aneurysms (Fig. 136-1). This technique avoids potential injury to adjacent structures, which can be densely adherent to the surface of the aneurysm sac. Type 2 aneurysms are more complex and require placement of an interposition graft from the proximal CFA to either the deep femoral artery or the SFA with either a separate jump graft to the other branch or implantation of the other branch into the primary graft (Fig. 136-2). Several authors have emphasized the importance of preserving the patency of the deep femoral artery to reduce the likelihood of subsequent ischemic complications.[4,11,26] Determining which technique to use is based on local geometry and the quality of the femoral arterial branches. Whenever the SFA is occluded, an end-to-end common femoral–to–deep femoral interposition graft can be created with simultaneous division and ligation of the origin of the SFA.

Prosthetic grafts are preferred in this location because their size most closely matches that of the femoral vessels and their performance has generally been excellent in this loca-

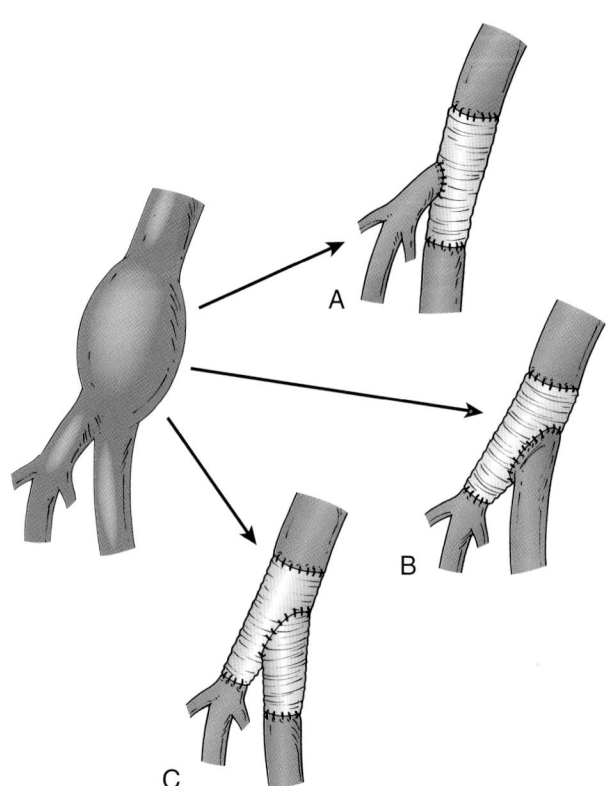

Figure 136-2 Surgical reconstruction of a type 2 femoral artery aneurysm can be accomplished by different configurations, depending on local anatomy. The initial interposition graft can be placed between the common femoral and either the superficial femoral (**A**) or the profunda femoris artery (**B**) with reimplantation of the other branch into the side of the graft. **C,** If the origin of the artery to be implanted is diseased or not long enough to reach the interposition graft, a short graft can be used to facilitate reimplantation. It is important to preserve flow to the profunda femoris artery in all type 2 aneurysm repairs. *(From O'Hara P. Treatment of femoral and popliteal artery aneurysms. In Zelenock GB, Huber TS, Messina LM, et al, eds.* Mastery of Vascular and Endovascular Surgery. *Philadelphia, PA: Lippincott Williams & Wilkins; 2006.)*

tion. Autologous vein conduit is used only in instances in which infection is present.

Results. The results of surgical treatment have generally been excellent. Five-year patency rates average 85% for isolated femoral aneurysms. Mortality has generally ranged from 0% to 5% in most series.[26]

Iatrogenic Femoral Artery False Aneurysms

Iatrogenic femoral pseudoaneurysms are the most common complication resulting from arterial puncture of the CFA for diagnostic and interventional procedures. It is estimated that they occur in 0.6% to 6% of femoral catheterization procedures.[28-30] Risk factors include large sheath size, anticoagulation or coagulopathy, puncture site not in the CFA, arterial wall calcification, and inadequate manual compression for hemostasis after sheath removal. Obesity, female gender, and

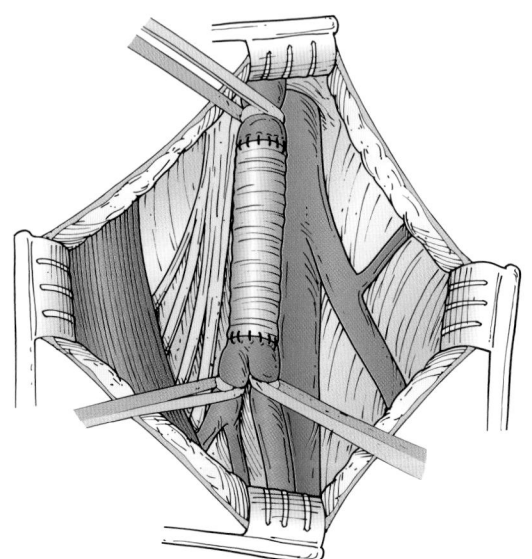

Figure 136-1 Surgical repair of a type 1 femoral artery aneurysm is accomplished with a simple interposition graft through a vertical groin incision. Small aneurysms can be excised, whereas larger aneurysms can be repaired with the graft inclusion technique used for aortic aneurysm repair. *(From Ouriel K, Rutherford RB, eds.* Atlas of Vascular Surgery. *Philadelphia, PA: WB Saunders; 1998.)*

chronic renal failure requiring hemodialysis are other risk factors.[30-33]

Clinical Findings and Natural History

The most common clinical manifestation is a painful pulsating mass in the groin, usually with an associated hematoma. Femoral bruits are heard frequently, and if an arteriovenous fistula is present, the bruits have a characteristic continuous to-and-fro quality. Patients may also complain of femoral neuropathic pain, paresis of hip flexion, or edema from compression of adjacent structures. Progressive enlargement can result in overlying skin ischemia and necrosis. In our experience, distal embolization or limb ischemia is rare. Rupture can lead to cardiovascular collapse and death from hemorrhagic shock and is a surgical emergency.[32] Significant bleeding can occur without overt clinical findings if the initial puncture is in the external iliac artery or through the inguinal ligament and results in occult bleeding into the retroperitoneal space.

Aneurysm size and the presence of anticoagulation determine which pseudoaneurysms require treatment. Most aneurysms less than 3 cm in diameter will thrombose spontaneously and may be safely observed with periodic duplex examination. Continued anticoagulation greatly decreases the likelihood of spontaneous closure.[34,35] In our own prospective series, 18 pseudoaneurysms were identified out of 1838 femoral catheterizations over an 8-month period (0.98% incidence). Aneurysms that were smaller than 1.8 cm in diameter and causing no symptoms were observed. Surgical repair was carried out if the aneurysms enlarged by 100% or did not close within 2 months. Of the 16 that were managed expectantly, half thrombosed spontaneously and the other half required repair. Although the difference did not reach statistical significance, the likelihood of spontaneous closure was lower for aneurysms smaller than 1.8 cm in diameter, and no aneurysm closed spontaneously in the presence of continued anticoagulation regardless of size.[36]

Diagnosis

Duplex ultrasonography is the preferred imaging method. The sensitivity and specificity of duplex ultrasonography for femoral false aneurysms are 94% and 97%, respectively.[37] Duplex ultrasonography also provides important information on diameter, morphology, and anatomy of the neck and location of the femoral artery defect. On B-mode imaging, the aneurysms will appear as an echolucent mass adjacent to the artery with compression of adjacent tissues.[33] A characteristic "jet" of blood flow through the neck and into the aneurysm sac is often seen on color-flow Doppler imaging and confirms the diagnosis (Fig. 136-3).

Surgical Treatment

Before 1991, femoral pseudoaneurysms were treated surgically. More recently, the development of effective minimally

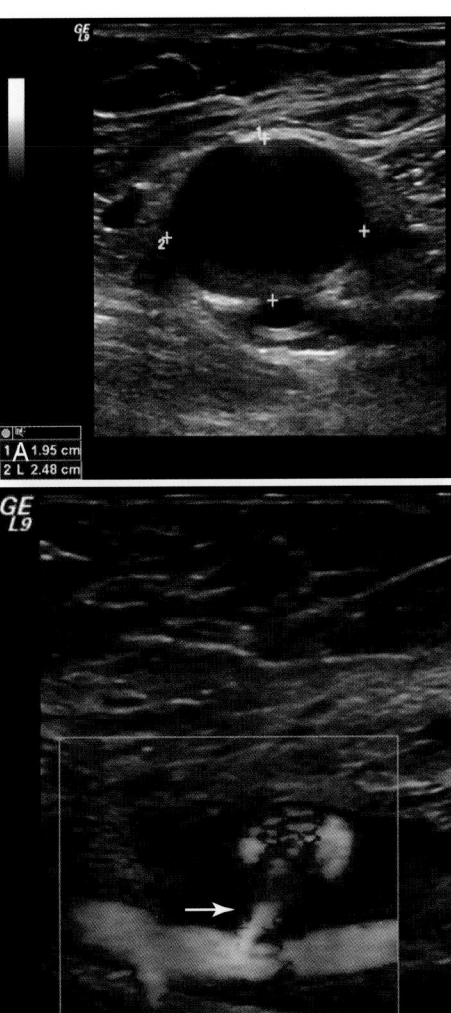

Figure 136-3 A, Duplex ultrasonography of a femoral false aneurysm demonstrating a large echolucent mass anterior to the femoral artery. The *cursor* marks outline the dimensions of the aneurysm cavity. **B,** Color-flow imaging demonstrating a "jet" of blood entering the aneurysm sac through a relatively long neck (*arrow*), an important anatomic requirement for safe thrombin injection. **C,** Real-time color-flow imaging revealing characteristic flow as blood enters and leaves the aneurysm sac through the neck with each cardiac cycle (see the Expert Consult Web site for the video in part **C**).

invasive therapies has resulted in performance of surgical repair most frequently for contraindications to or failure of less invasive therapies. Open repair is still the primary therapy for patients with rupture, for aneurysms with overlying skin ischemia or necrosis, when associated with an arteriovenous fistula, or when the puncture is proximal to the inguinal ligament. In patients with iatrogenic false aneurysms who require urgent or emergency cardiac surgery, surgical aneurysm repair is usually performed in conjunction with the cardiac surgery.

The principles of surgery are straightforward: obtain control proximal and distal to the site of puncture, open and evacuate the aneurysm sac, identify the puncture site, and

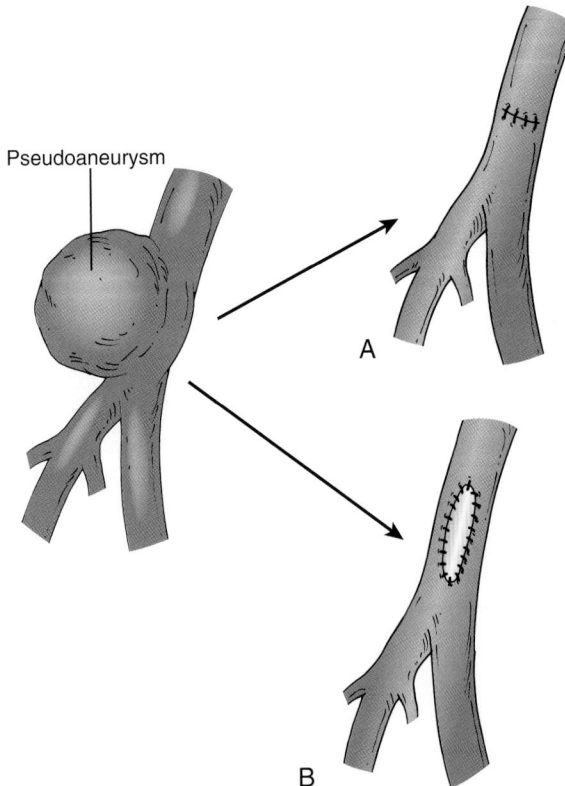

Pseudoaneurysm

A

B

Figure 136-4 Surgical repair of an iatrogenic femoral artery false aneurysm. After obtaining proximal and distal control, the sac is opened and the arterial defect exposed. Repair can be accomplished in most cases by direct suture repair (**A**), although patch repair may occasionally be needed (**B**). (*From O'Hara P. Treatment of femoral and popliteal artery aneurysms. In Zelenock GB, Huber TS, Messina LM, et al, eds.* Mastery of Vascular and Endovascular Surgery. *Philadelphia, PA: Lippincott Williams & Wilkins; 2006.*)

repair with interrupted sutures in a horizontal fashion. In rare circumstances, femoral endarterectomy or patch angioplasty (or both), preferably with a segment of saphenous vein, may be required (Fig. 136-4). Procedures can be performed under local, regional, or general anesthesia. In our opinion, local anesthesia offers few advantages over general anesthesia in most cases. With very large aneurysms, obtaining proximal control below the inguinal ligament may be difficult or impossible. In this circumstance, a distal retroperitoneal approach can be used to gain access to the external iliac artery, or the inguinal ligament can be divided. If appropriate facilities are available, percutaneous balloon occlusion via the contralateral femoral artery is an alternative, less invasive method to obtain iliac control. In the event of rupture or rapid expansion, especially in patients with hypotension and shock, the aneurysm sac is opened immediately with no attempt at proximal control. The hematoma is evacuated and hemostasis achieved by direct digital manual compression of the bleeding puncture site. Proximal and distal control can then be obtained in standard fashion.

Open repair has the advantage of allowing decompression of the hematoma cavity at the time of repair. We prefer the use of a large closed-suction drain in the hematoma cavity,

which is left in place until drainage decreases to less than 30 mL/day. Complications are not infrequent and include infection, seroma formation, delayed discharge, and increased cost.[38] Deaths are uncommon except in patients with rupture and shock.[32]

Ultrasound-Guided Compression

Compression of false aneurysms to induce thrombosis was proposed as a less invasive alternative to surgery in 1991.[39] Duplex ultrasound is used to locate the aneurysm, and suitable pressure is applied with the transducer to stop flow within the aneurysm cavity while maintaining flow in the adjacent femoral artery. Excessive pressure can result in femoral artery thrombosis.[40] Compression is maintained for 10 to 20 minutes, after which time flow is reassessed. If flow persists, the procedure is repeated one or more times until flow within the aneurysm cavity is noted to have stopped. Patients are maintained on bed rest for 6 hours and duplex re-evaluation is performed 24 and 48 hours after the procedure to rule out recurrence.

Success rates for ultrasound-guided compression (UGC) range from 66% to 86%, with compression times required averaging 30 to 44 minutes.[39-41] Recurrence has been reported in 4% of cases.[40] The presence of anticoagulation greatly reduces the likelihood of success to less than 40%.[40-42] UGC is contraindicated in patients with ischemic skin changes or infection and when the puncture site originates above the inguinal ligament. Moreover, UGC is not usually possible in patients with severe pain and very large hematomas. Imaging and compression are technically more difficult in obese patients, thus decreasing the likelihood of success. Aneurysm rupture, femoral vein thrombosis, limb ischemia from femoral arterial thrombosis, and hypotension from vasovagal events are all potential complications that have occurred in 2% to 4% of cases.[40,41,43]

From a practical standpoint, UGC has the disadvantage of being time-consuming and placing demands on the vascular laboratory, time, equipment, and personnel. Operator and patient fatigue and management of the often significant pain that patients experience during compression are common problems.[44] Use of mechanical compression devices can obviate some of these issues but requires a cooperative and immobile patient and repeated re-evaluation during compression.[45] Such devices offer little advantage and have not generally been widely accepted.

Ultrasound-Guided Thrombin Injection

Angiographically directed thrombin injection via percutaneous means into the aneurysm cavity to induce immediate thrombosis was first described by Cope and Zeit more than 20 years ago.[46] Kang and associates modified the technique by performing direct percutaneous aneurysm puncture under duplex ultrasound guidance.[47] Thrombin directly converts fibrinogen to fibrin, thereby leading to immediate clot formation and "short-circuiting" the upstream mechanism of the coagulation cascade where heparin and warfarin interact. Consequently, thrombin injection is effective even in patients receiving anticoagulation. Bovine and human thrombin is commercially available in powder form that is reconstituted in normal saline immediately before use.

Ultrasound-guided thrombin injection (UGTI) is quick, simple, and relatively painless. Duplex ultrasonography is used to identify the aneurysm cavity. After infiltration with local anesthetic, the cavity is punctured with either a 22-gauge catheter or a 25-gauge hypodermic needle. Spinal needles can be used for deeper aneurysms. Identification of the needle or catheter within the aneurysm sac is a critical step (Fig. 136-5) and can be facilitated with the use of a commercially available echodense needle.[48-50] The needle is filled with thrombin, which when inserted causes a small clot to form at the needle tip that is readily visualized on ultrasonography.[47] Once proper positioning of the needle is confirmed, thrombin (1000 IU/mL) is injected slowly through a 3-mL syringe for

a period of about 10 to 15 seconds until flow within the cavity ceases. In our experience and that of others, approximately 1000 units of thrombin are required to induce thrombosis. It is important to inject slowly and stop immediately once thrombosis has occurred to minimize the chance of thrombin's entering the circulation. A second injection is sometimes required.[47] Patients are placed on bed rest for 1 hour. Duplex ultrasonography is repeated 24 hours later to confirm permanent thrombosis of the aneurysm.

UGTI has a success rate of 93% to 100% in reported series.[47,48,51-54] Its simplicity and efficacy in anticoagulated patients make it the procedure of choice for treating femoral false aneurysms. In a recent Cochrane database meta-analysis comparing the two techniques, Tisi and Callam found that UGTI was more effective than UGC (relative risk, 7.50; $P = .002$).[55]

Complications with UGTI are infrequent and include distal embolization of thrombin,[49] groin abscess,[56] and femoral artery[57] and vein[58] thrombosis. Allergic reactions, including anaphylaxis in patients previously exposed to bovine thrombin, have been reported.[59] Distal embolization occurs in 2% of cases and can be minimized by slow injection. In cases of thromboembolism, anticoagulation with intravenous heparin should be started immediately. In patients with severe ischemia not responding to heparin, angiography and thromboembolectomy or lytic therapy may be required.[49,51] UGTI should not be used in aneurysms with short, wide necks because embolization is more likely to occur. It is contraindicated in patients with infection or overlying skin necrosis or with allergy to bovine thrombin, in the presence of an arteriovenous fistula, in ischemic extremities, and in pregnant patients.

Profunda Femoral Artery Aneurysms

Isolated aneurysms of the profunda femoral artery are rare and account for 0.5% of all peripheral aneurysms and just 1% to 2.6% of femoral artery aneurysms (Fig. 136-6).[4,60] Precise information regarding their natural history and behavior is not known, and the information available is largely based on very small series or isolated case reports. A high complication rate (58%) is common at initial evaluation.[61] It is postulated that this phenomenon occurs because of their location beneath the muscles of the thigh. Consequently, asymptomatic aneurysms often escape detection and are usually found only after a complication has occurred. Synchronous aneurysms at other locations are common and occur in up to 81% of reported cases.[4,60,62] In a recent series from the Mayo Clinic, 11 of the 15 (73%) patients had aneurysms at other locations.[63]

Rupture appears to occur more frequently with profunda femoral aneurysms, with rates ranging from 30% to 45% of reported cases.[62,64-67] Whether rupture is truly more common than in other peripheral aneurysms is impossible to determine and may be a result of publication bias of this unusual complication. In the Mayo Clinic series, rupture occurred in only 13% of cases.[63]

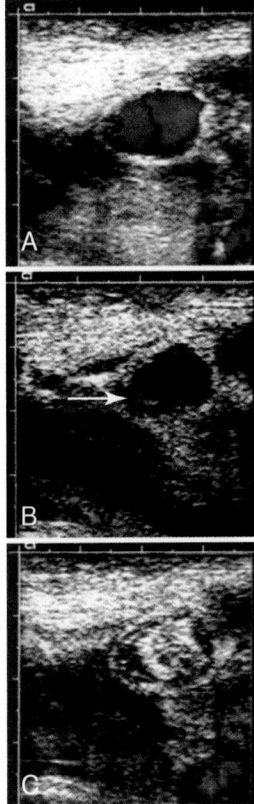

Figure 136-5 Duplex ultrasound of a femoral pseudoaneurysm. **A,** Color-flow image demonstrating typical swirling flow in the pseudoaneurysm cavity. **B,** This image, taken 18 seconds later with color flow turned off, shows the tip of a 22-gauge needle in the left lower portion of the pseudoaneurysm (*arrow*). After placement of the needle, color flow is turned back on and thrombin is injected. **C,** Color-flow image 21 seconds later demonstrating that the pseudoaneurysm cavity is completely filled with echogenic thrombus. (*From Kang SS, Labropoulos N, Mansour MA, Baker WH. Percutaneous ultrasound guided thrombin injection: a new method for treating postcatheterization femoral pseudoaneurysms. J Vasc Surg. 1998;27:1032-1038.*)

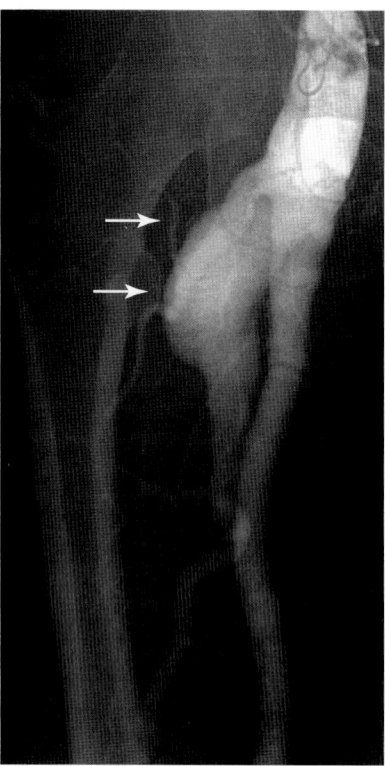

Figure 136-6 Arteriogram of a large symptomatic aneurysm of the profunda femoris artery (*arrows*). The aneurysm originates at the origin of the profunda femoris artery. Note the ectasia of the common femoral and proximal superficial femoral arteries.

Surgical Treatment

Surgical repair is carried out through a vertical groin incision. In most cases, aneurysmectomy within an interposition graft of either saphenous vein or prosthetic material is preferred. In constructing interposition grafts, large branches of the profunda femoral artery should be preserved whenever possible. Dissection is usually started at the CFA bifurcation and extends inferiorly and slightly laterally over the course of the deep femoral artery. The SFA is retracted medially, and as the dissection extends more distally, the sartorius and rectus femoris muscles are reflected laterally. Larger crossing branches of the deep femoral vein are encountered and must be carefully divided and suture ligated. Branches of the femoral nerve are also encountered and must be preserved and protected from injury by self-retaining retractors or cautery. Gentle dissection is necessary to avoid troublesome venous injury. Proximal control is usually obtained at the level of the CFA, although in instances of rupture with massive hematoma in the groin, control of the distal external iliac artery may be necessary. Distal arterial control can be accomplished with silicon rubber vessel loops or by balloon catheter occlusion.

Although graft replacement is generally preferred, for aneurysms confined to the distal branches of the deep femoral artery, simple ligation may be a reasonable treatment.[61] Proximal profunda femoral ligation may be also reasonable in patients with rupture, especially when the SFA is patent; however, such ligation may place the patient at risk for future limb ischemia and amputation.[63] In highly selected cases

of aneurysms involving distal branches of the profunda femoral artery, embolization may be a reasonable nonsurgical alternative.[68,69]

Superficial Femoral Artery Aneurysms

Isolated aneurysms of the SFA are rare. Most are found in the presence of diffuse arterial enlargement from arteriomegaly or as a proximal extension of a popliteal artery aneurysm (Fig. 136-7). In their recent report of 13 SFA aneurysms, Jarrett and coworkers could find only 34 cases in the literature, including their own.[70] In their series, 46% of patients had evidence of distal ischemia, 31% of the aneurysms were manifested as an asymptomatic thigh mass, and 23% were discovered during vascular evaluation for other problems. In their review of the literature they estimated the incidence of rupture to be 34%, although they had no ruptures in their own experience. Thrombosis or embolism was present in 26% and other aneurysms were present in 39% of patients, the majority of whom were male. In an earlier review of 17 cases, Rigdon and Monajjem found that 65% had complications, including rupture in 35%, thrombosis in 18%, and distal embolism in 18%.[71] Limb salvage rates were excellent (94%). Similar to popliteal aneurysms, SFA aneurysms demonstrate a high male preponderance ranging from 75% to 85%.[70,71] Surgical treatment has been recommended for most SFA aneurysms because of the propensity for symptoms to develop.

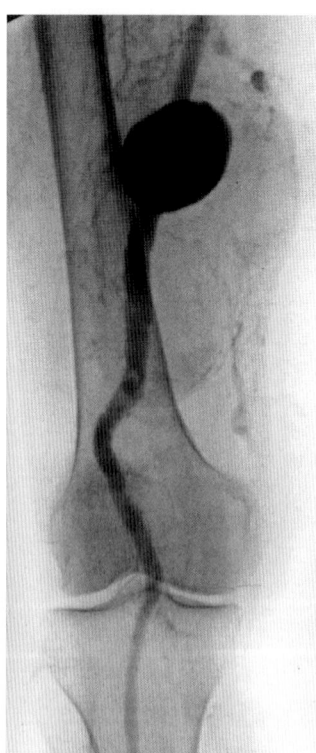

Figure 136-7 Arteriogram of a massive, isolated aneurysm of the distal superficial femoral artery. Calcification in the wall of the aneurysm can be seen faintly. The true size of the aneurysm is greatly underestimated by the angiogram, which is outlining only the flow channel within the sac; the flow channel is lined by extensive intraluminal thrombus.

Surgical Treatment

Preoperative arteriography is performed to evaluate the inflow and outflow vessels. Either saphenous vein or prosthetic graft can be used. Prosthetic grafts work well in the groin or thigh and can usually be matched to the diameter of the artery. Vein grafts are preferred for any reconstruction crossing the knee joint, which may be necessary with distal occlusive disease or if the aneurysm is being treated in conjunction with a popliteal artery aneurysm. Exposure is obtained in either the groin or midthigh or at both sites, depending on the extent of the aneurysm. The surgical approach is nearly identical to that for popliteal aneurysm repair. Focal aneurysms are treated by opening the sac, evacuating thrombus, and creating an end-to-end interposition graft. For more extensive aneurysms, proximal and distal ligation can be performed, followed by a bypass graft. Although long-term follow-up is not available, Rigdon and Monajjem[71] reported a limb salvage rate of 94% with no deaths, whereas Jarrett and coauthors[70] reported successful bypass in 11 cases with no mortality. Two patients underwent primary amputation for unsalvageable ischemia at initial evaluation.

■ POPLITEAL ARTERY ANEURYSMS

Definition

The definition of what constitutes a popliteal artery aneurysm varies in the contemporary literature. The normal diameter of a popliteal artery varies with the size and gender of the patient and ranges from approximately 0.5 to 1.1 cm.[2,20] Recent anatomic studies have shown that the popliteal artery itself differs in diameter from proximal to distal, with the proximal portion more closely approximating the diameter of the SFA and the distal popliteal artery tending to be smaller.[72] Most aneurysms appear to occur in the proximal part or midportion of the popliteal artery. An aneurysm may be considered to be present if the total enlargement is 1.5 times the diameter of a normal adjacent segment of artery.[2] Others consider a diameter of 1.5 cm or greater in the "average" patient an aneurysm, although in clinical practice most surgeons use 2 cm as the threshold diameter.

Epidemiology

Popliteal artery aneurysm is almost exclusively a disease of men. In most series, 95% to 100% of patients treated are male. Aneurysms are frequently bilateral and often accompanied by aortic aneurysms. In a large review of the English literature that included 1673 patients, 97% of the patients were male.[73] Contralateral aneurysms were found in 50% and aortic aneurysms in 36%. In a recent single-center series consisting of 289 patients spanning 20 years at the Mayo Clinic, Huang and colleagues reported that 97% of their patients were male, 54% of aneurysms were bilateral, and aortic aneurysms were present or had been treated in 51%.[74]

Although popliteal aneurysms are the most common aneurysms of the lower extremity and account for 70% of all lower extremity aneurysms, they are relatively uncommon. Lawrence and coworkers estimated that the incidence of femoral and popliteal aneurysms in hospitalized patients was 7.4 per 100,000 men and 1 per 100,000 women.[75] The prevalence of popliteal aneurysms in patients being evaluated for aortic aneurysms averages about 8% (range, 3% to 12%).[3,76,77] Conversely, in patients being evaluated for popliteal aneurysms, the prevalence of aortic aneurysms averages 40%,[73] and it may be as high as 70% in patients with bilateral popliteal aneurysms.[74] Moreover, in patients treated for isolated popliteal aneurysms, the likelihood of another aneurysm developing at a remote site over a 10-year period is estimated to be as high as 50%, thus mandating careful scrutiny of all patients at initial encounter and continued surveillance for life after treatment.[78]

Clinical Findings

Popliteal aneurysms may be manifested as an asymptomatic pulsating mass behind the knee or cause symptoms of either chronic or acute ischemia. A minority of patients will have symptoms attributable to compression, including pain or pressure behind the knee, distal limb swelling, and occasionally deep venous thrombosis of the popliteal vein.[73] Compressive injury to the common peroneal nerve resulting in footdrop has also been reported.[79] In most series there is a correlation between the size of the aneurysm and the presence of symptoms (Fig. 136-8). Aneurysms less than 2 cm are rarely symptomatic, presumably because they seldom contain thrombus, although this has not been proved. Huang and associates noted that asymptomatic aneurysms averaged 2.6 cm as opposed to 3.0 cm in patients with chronic or acute ischemic symptoms ($P < .05$).[74] In a series of 200 popliteal aneurysms, Varga and coworkers found that the median diameter of symptomatic aneurysms was 3 cm versus 2 cm in those without symptoms ($P = .0004$).[80]

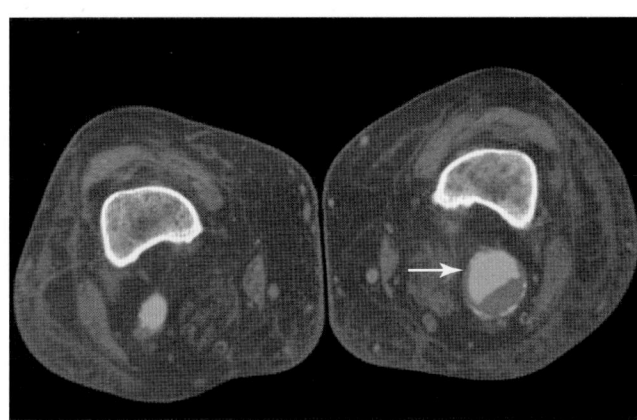

Figure 136-8 Axial images on a CT angiogram of an elderly man with bilateral popliteal artery aneurysms. The patient was being evaluated for critical ischemia of his left foot. Note the intraluminal thrombus, especially in the larger left aneurysm (*arrow*).

In most series, less than 40% of treated patients had no symptoms.[73,80,81] However, approximately 40% of asymptomatic patients will have absent distal foot pulses, which appears to adversely affect the natural history. Dawson and colleagues found that the likelihood of symptoms developing in untreated asymptomatic patients with absent foot pulses was 86% at 3 years as compared with 34% in asymptomatic patients with intact pulses.[82] Symptoms of ischemia can be chronic or acute and are due to thrombosis of the aneurysm itself or emboli to the distal circulation. Manifestations of chronic limb ischemia, including mild to moderate claudication and ischemic rest pain, are present in 40% of symptomatic patients.[73,74] Blue toe syndrome from distal emboli to the digital vessels is also seen occasionally.[83]

Acute Ischemia

Acute limb ischemia is the most feared complication of popliteal aneurysms. Its occurrence can complicate treatment, and it is associated with significant risk for limb loss. In recent years, the liberal use of thrombolytic therapy coupled with distal arterial reconstructive surgery has decreased the likelihood of major limb amputation with acute ischemia; however, it remains a significant problem. In recent series, acutely ischemic patients have accounted for 21% to 35% of treated patients. Thrombolytic therapy has been used in 30% to 45% of acutely ischemic limbs to improve outflow.[1,74,84-86] Patients with acute ischemia but viable limbs and no sensory or motor symptoms can often be stabilized with intravenous heparin and treated semi-electively. Others will have an acutely threatened limb requiring emergency surgical treatment. Patients may occasionally have unsalvageable limbs for which major amputation is the only treatment option. Considerable surgical judgment is necessary in determining whether a patient needs to be treated immediately or can be temporized in the hope of improving the situation with thrombolytic therapy.

Rupture is an unusual complication that occurs in 0% to 7% in published series[73] with an average of about 2%. Patients with rupture will most commonly be seen initially with severe swelling and pain in the popliteal space and distal limb edema. Approximately 14% will have an associated popliteal vein thrombosis. Hemorrhagic shock is rare, probably because of containment of the hematoma by the small confines of the popliteal space.

Diagnosis

Detecting popliteal aneurysms is critical before symptoms or complications occur, especially acute limb ischemia. The results of surgical treatment are best in asymptomatic patients and progressively worse in those with either chronic ischemic symptoms or critical limb ischemia.[74] As discussed previously, patients most likely to harbor occult popliteal aneurysms are those with known aortic and femoral aneurysms or a contralateral popliteal aneurysm. During physical examination, a popliteal aneurysm should be suspected whenever a prominent pulsation is felt in the popliteal space, especially with the knee in a moderate degree of flexion. Thrombosed aneurysms may be manifested as a firm nonpulsating mass. Physical examination has been proved to be unreliable, with both false-positive and false-negative results.[76] Duplex ultrasonography has been shown to be superior to physical examination in detecting popliteal aneurysms.[77] Beyond detection, duplex ultrasonography provides critical information relevant to treatment, including the diameter, presence of intraluminal thrombus, velocity of blood flow, and patency of outflow arteries.

Imaging

Once the decision has been made to treat, additional anatomic information is usually required. Traditionally, contrast-enhanced arteriography (Fig. 136-9) has been used to identify points of inflow and suitable outflow target arteries for bypass grafts. It is also critical in the use of thrombolytic therapy. MRA may also be used, and increasingly, spiral CTA has taken on a more prominent role. MRA and CTA have the additional advantage of providing three-dimensional information in the coronal and sagittal planes (Fig. 136-10) about the aneurysm itself, as well as the popliteal space, both of which may be important, particularly when considering endovascular therapy (see "Endovascular Popliteal Aneurysm Repair").

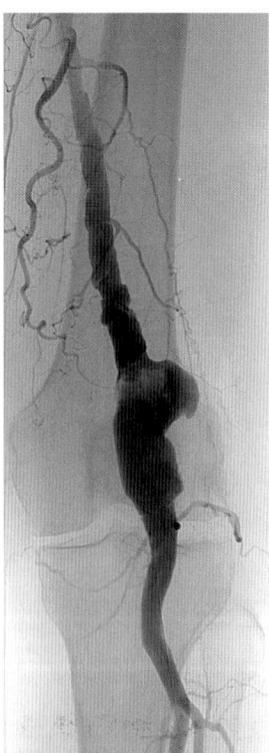

Figure 136-9 Contrast-enhanced arteriogram of a left popliteal aneurysm involving the above-knee popliteal artery. The true diameter of the aneurysm may be underestimated by contrast-enhanced arteriography because of the presence of nonvisualized intraluminal thrombus obscuring the true diameter of the arterial wall, similar to aortography for aortic aneurysms.

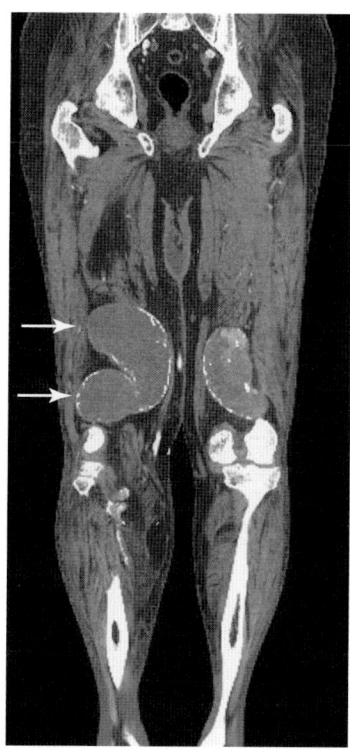

Figure 136-10 Coronal reconstruction of both lower extremities of an arterial-phase CT scan of an elderly man with massive bilateral popliteal artery aneurysms. Note the extreme tortuosity and kinking of the aneurysm in the right lower extremity (*arrows*). The aneurysm in the left leg, though smaller, is still quite large. Both were causing symptoms of limb ischemia. CT angiography has proved to be a useful adjunct or alternative to conventional angiography in the evaluation of patients for surgical treatment. (*Courtesy of Benjamin Starnes, MD.*)

Natural History

Like aortic aneurysms, popliteal aneurysms are an insidious process that may cause no symptoms for an extended period. Frequently, the first evidence of their presence is an ischemic complication. Without widespread screening, it is not possible to determine the prevalence or natural history of popliteal aneurysms in the general population. Although it is likely that many small popliteal aneurysms may never enlarge, cause symptoms, or be recognized, the natural history of many others is one of progressive enlargement with the ultimate development of symptoms or ischemic complications, or both. The most feared complication is irreversible leg ischemia requiring amputation secondary to either sudden aneurysm thrombosis or extensive distal embolic occlusion. Several studies,[80,87] including a large review article[73] encompassing patients treated over a 40-year period, have underscored the danger of critical limb ischemia and amputation in untreated popliteal artery aneurysms. On average, the risk for development of thromboembolic complications was 35% at 3 years, with an amputation rate of 25%. In patients with nonpalpable foot pulses at initial evaluation, the likelihood of complications was far higher (86%). On this basis it has been recommended that all aneurysms 2 cm or greater in diameter be repaired when feasible. Vigilance and a high index of suspi-

cion are necessary for making the diagnosis, especially in high-risk patient populations, who should undergo screening duplex ultrasound examination whenever an aneurysm is suspected. In patients with simultaneous aortic and popliteal artery aneurysms, treatment of the abdominal aortic aneurysm before repair of the popliteal aneurysm may put the patient at increased risk for popliteal aneurysm thrombosis. Dawson and coauthors reported three episodes of popliteal aneurysm thrombosis within 24 hours of abdominal aortic aneurysm repair.[82]

Indications for Treatment

The decision to intervene with a popliteal aneurysm requires weighing the risks and results of treatment against the risks of continued follow-up. The argument for early intervention for small aneurysms is based on several factors.[88-91] With small asymptomatic aneurysms, long-term graft patency and limb salvage rates are usually greater than 95%, and perioperative mortality with treatment is low, usually around 1% to 2%. Mortality rates can be three to four times higher in patients treated with critical limb ischemia. Even small aneurysms can thrombose and cause severe symptoms. Ascher and associates found a higher incidence of thrombosis, clinical symptoms, and distal occlusive disease in smaller aneurysms, although only two were less than 2 cm in diameter.[92]

Others have suggested that asymptomatic aneurysms even 3 cm in diameter can be safely observed.[27,93-95] The arguments for this approach are based on the observation that asymptomatic aneurysms without intramural thrombus or distortion from excessive tortuosity and with intact distal pulses rarely cause symptoms. Moreover, although results with surgery have generally been excellent, complications and deaths have occurred, especially in patients with severe co-morbid conditions or those who are very elderly. With the advent of modern techniques of thrombolysis and distal arterial bypass, excellent rates of graft patency and limb salvage can be obtained, even in patients in whom critical limb ischemia develops, thus suggesting that the consequences of a wrong decision to monitor a patient are not as dire as previously considered. In our own study of 51 popliteal aneurysms treated over a period of 10 years, when the results of elective versus emergency treatment were compared, 14 of the 51 limbs were treated on an emergency basis for the acute onset of critical ischemia and one was treated for rupture. Only one patient ultimately required an early amputation, and the second patient had an amputation 5 years after initial treatment for recurrent ischemic complications. There were no other amputations in the emergency group. The limb salvage rate was 93% in the group treated on an emergency basis versus 100% in nonemergency cases over the 5-year period. The difference was not statistically different.

Without the results of a multicenter prospective randomized trial, the decision regarding treatment remains one of surgical judgment and must be individualized to the specific patient and clinical situation. Moreover, many of the previous arguments were based on results in the era before endovascular therapy. Our approach is to offer elective repair for all asymptomatic aneurysms 2.5 cm or larger unless we believe that the risks associated with treatment are excessive because of the health status of the patient. For frail patients in poor health or with limited life expectancy, we observe even larger aneurysms, provided that the estimated risk for complications is low (minimal intraluminal thrombus, palpable distal pulses, and no evidence of continued expansion). When treatment is required in this subset of patients, endovascular repair has become our preferred method of treatment (see "Endovascular Popliteal Aneurysm Repair").

Elective Surgical Treatment: Open Repair

The primary objective of treatment of popliteal artery aneurysms is to exclude them from the circulation. In 1785, John Hunter ligated the popliteal artery of a coachman with a large popliteal aneurysm in the canal that now bears his name. He correctly postulated that collateral circulation would maintain the viability of the limb.[96] In the modern era, arterial bypass with ligation or interposition grafting has replaced simple ligation and remains the "gold standard" for treatment.

As with any lower extremity arterial reconstruction, proper treatment requires careful planning and starts with a comprehensive arteriogram of the entire extremity from the groin to the toes. Alternatively, this information can be obtained with MRA or spiral CTA, as previously described. In our practice, duplex ultrasonography is used for screening and diagnosis and has a limited role in terms of anatomic imaging for bypass, although it is very useful for vein mapping in preparation for bypass. The information obtained from contrast-enhanced angiography or MRA is used to determine the location of the proximal and distal anastomotic sites. MRA and CTA can also provide information about the size, shape, and extent of the aneurysm, which is helpful in determining whether to use a medial or posterior approach. Small or fusiform aneurysms are best approached medially by conventional bypass with aneurysm ligation. For large, saccular aneurysms, particularly those with symptoms attributable to compression of adjacent structures, direct exposure from the posterior approach with interposition grafting from within the sac is preferable, unless the aneurysm extends too far proximally. The posterior approach is also advantageous to decompress an aneurysm that has continued to enlarge after bypass and ligation because of backfilling from geniculate branches.

Medial Approach

The patient is positioned supine and the saphenous vein is exposed as the first step in the procedure, starting in the groin, midthigh, or ankle, depending on the procedure. Once the vein has been mobilized and harvested, the same incision can be used to expose the popliteal artery above and below the knee joint in a fashion identical to that used for femoropopliteal bypass. Similarly, the same incision can be used to expose the posterior tibial and peroneal arteries. For the ante-

rior tibial and pedal arteries or if a lateral approach is planned for the distal peroneal artery, separate incisions will be required. Arterial exposure of the above-knee or below-knee popliteal artery can be difficult with large aneurysms or in the presence of arteriomegaly. Compression of the popliteal veins can lead to venous engorgement and venous hypertension. Extensive kinking, tortuosity, and lateral displacement, especially of the distal popliteal artery, can occasionally make exposure challenging. In cases of arteriomegaly, even the inflow and outflow arteries may be unusually large and make separation from the adjacent structures more difficult. Vessels are isolated with conventional silicone rubber vessel loops. In most cases a tunnel is then created from the above-knee to the below-knee popliteal space between the heads of the gastrocnemius muscle. This may be difficult in patients with large popliteal aneurysms filling most of the popliteal space. Decompression of the aneurysm sac and endoaneurysmorrhaphy may be required before tunneling can be performed safely. The patient is administered intravenous heparin at a dose of 80 to 100 U/kg or at a dose to prolong the activated clotting time to 250 to 300 seconds.

Arterial bypass is performed in standard fashion with either an end-to-side or an end-to-end anastomosis. There is frequently a size discrepancy between vein graft and the popliteal arteries, especially above the knee, thus making the end-to-side technique preferable. Either reversed or nonreversed vein grafts can be used, depending on surgeon preference and experience. In bypasses extending from the CFA to a distal tibial vessel, in situ bypass is an alternative. For occluded aneurysms, the procedure is conducted like any other lower extremity arterial bypass. If the aneurysm is patent, ligation must be performed in conjunction with the bypass procedure. The inflow and outflow arteries to the aneurysm sac should be ligated as close to the aneurysm as possible. In focal aneurysms confined to the proximal and mid-popliteal artery, the aneurysm is ligated just distal to the proximal anastomosis and just proximal to the distal arterial anastomosis. If an in situ bypass to a more distal target is performed, separate exposure of the two points of ligation will be required. The aneurysm should always be ligated both proximally and distally as close to the sac as possible to promote aneurysm thrombosis and decrease the likelihood of continued expansion from collateral filling. Jones and colleagues demonstrated that proximal ligature alone or ligature of the inflow and outflow arteries remotely from the aneurysm sac increases the likelihood of continued aneurysm expansion.[97] Completion arteriography, angioscopy, or duplex ultrasonography is performed before closure.

The medial approach is our preferred technique for most popliteal aneurysm repairs and the only logical option for bypass grafts that need to extend to the distal tibial or pedal vessels. The medial approach has the advantages of being familiar to all vascular surgeons and providing easy access to the entire great saphenous vein. Virtually all of the procedure is performed at some distance from the aneurysm, thus reducing the likelihood of operative injury to structures adherent to the surface of the popliteal aneurysm. The principal disadvantage of the medial approach is that it is generally used in conjunction with aneurysm ligation but without decompression. Numerous studies have shown that even with proximal and distal ligation, as many as 30% of aneurysms will not ultimately thrombose and may continue to enlarge if collateral blood flow into the aneurysm sac persists in a situation analogous to that of a type 2 endoleak with endovascular aneurysm repair.[97-99] Continued expansion can result in pain, compression symptoms, and even rupture.[100] To avoid this problem, most authors are proponents of opening all but the smallest popliteal aneurysms in order to suture ligate backbleeding side branches. This can usually be done from the above-knee or below-knee popliteal space. A thigh tourniquet can decrease bleeding from collaterals once the aneurysm sac is opened.[74] In some cases it may be necessary to divide the tendon of the medial head of the gastrocnemius muscle to facilitate access to the popliteal aneurysm. The tendon can then be reattached after decompression with a heavy-gauge monofilament suture. In our experience, this rarely leads to disability.

Posterior Approach

For large aneurysms confined to the popliteal space that are causing symptoms from compression or in which the aneurysm has caused distortion and displacement of the normal anatomy as a result of tortuosity, elongation, and kinking, the posterior approach is preferred. This is also an appropriate approach for a smaller aneurysm, but it is not applicable for aneurysms that extend proximally beyond the popliteal space.

The patient is placed prone. An S-shaped incision is made with the superior end starting on the medial side of the thigh to expose the proximal popliteal artery and great saphenous vein. The incision extends laterally across the flexion crease of the knee and ends on the lateral aspects of the proximal part of the calf directly over the proximal small saphenous vein (Fig. 136-11). If the small saphenous vein is of adequate size for bypass, the incision can be continued for harvest of the vein. Alternatively, the great saphenous vein can be harvested relatively easily from the thigh with the patient prone. Preoperative vein mapping should always be performed before popliteal aneurysm repair to avoid extending incisions only to find the vein to be inadequate in caliber or quality.

The proximal popliteal artery is identified by palpation distal to the adductor canal and exposed by separating the semimembranosus and semitendinosus muscles medially from the long head of the biceps femoris laterally. Circumferential control is obtained with silicone rubber vessel loops. Dissection is continued distally on the anterior surface of the aneurysm sac to avoid injury to the tibial and peroneal nerves, which may be encountered coursing lateral and slightly posterior to the aneurysm. The distal popliteal artery is identified and circumferentially controlled. If exposure of the tibioperoneal trunk or proximal tibial vessels is required, access from this approach is possible, although we prefer to use the medial approach if tibial bypass is required.

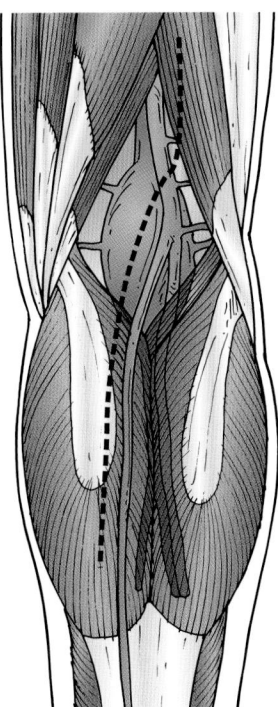

Figure 136-11 Placement of a "lazy S" incision for the posterior approach to a popliteal artery aneurysm. *(From Ouriel K, Rutherford RB, eds.* Atlas of Vascular Surgery. *Philadelphia, PA: WB Saunders; 1998.)*

After the administration of intravenous heparin, proximal and distal control is obtained and the aneurysm sac is opened. Thrombus is removed and backbleeding geniculate collaterals are oversewn from within, analogous to the approach used for aortic aneurysms. Circulation can be restored by either bypass or an interposition graft. If an interposition vein graft is planned, the graft can be beveled to facilitate end-to-end anastomosis to the transected popliteal artery (Fig. 136-12). Alternatively, a standard end-to-side bypass can be performed and is preferable when there is a significant size discrepancy between the popliteal artery and the bypass graft, which commonly occurs when using vein conduit. For interposition prosthetic grafts, an end-to-end anastomosis can be created from within the aneurysm sac by applying the graft inclusion technique used for abdominal aortic aneurysm repair. This approach has the advantage of requiring less dissection of the popliteal artery. Some surgeons prefer the routine use of prosthetic conduits for the posterior approach because the diameter of the graft can be more closely matched to the diameter of the popliteal artery and the complications associated with vein harvest are avoided. Excellent short-term results with prosthetic popliteal bypass have been reported in some series, especially when good outflow exists.[101]

Emergency Surgical Treatment: Open Repair

Patients with acute limb ischemia require urgent intervention to avoid amputation. In a patient with a viable limb and no

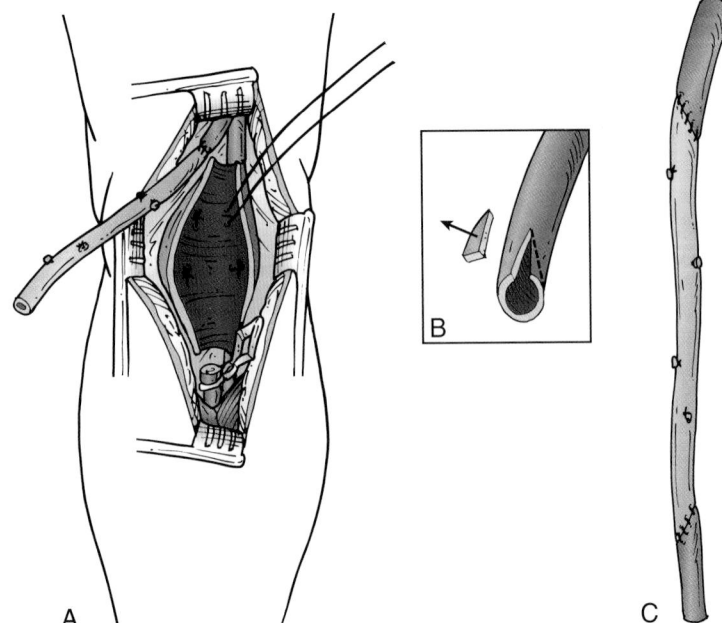

Figure 136-12 Technique for placing an interposition vein graft from the posterior approach for a popliteal artery aneurysm. **A,** After the aneurysm is opened and thrombus removed, backbleeding geniculate branches are oversewn from within the sac, analogous to aortic aneurysm repair. **B,** The vein graft and artery can be beveled to facilitate end-to-end anastomosis. **C,** The completed repair. *(From Ouriel K, Rutherford RB, eds. Atlas of Vascular Surgery. Philadelphia, PA: WB Saunders; 1998.)*

symptoms of sensory or motor dysfunction, intravenous heparin can be administrated to stabilize the patient. Arteriography and surgery are performed during the same admission. If the aneurysm is fully occluded and a patent distal outflow vessel is identified on arteriography, a vein bypass to the patent outflow vessel is performed as described previously. If no outflow vessel is identified and the patient's limb is not immediately threatened, intra-arterial thrombolysis is started with the objective of restoring flow to potential outflow target vessels (see "Thrombolysis").

In cases in which the patient's limb is immediately in jeopardy because of sensory and motor dysfunction and there is no time for thrombolysis, surgery should be performed immediately. If no outflow vessel was identified on the arteriogram, thromboembolectomy of the distal popliteal or tibial vessels (or both) should be attempted. Embolectomy or thrombectomy of the popliteal artery is relatively straightforward and best approached from the below-knee popliteal artery. For embolectomy of individual tibial arteries, blind passage of embolectomy catheters from the popliteal artery usually fails and is ill advised. The region of the trifurcation of the popliteal artery should be exposed to gain access to all three arteries. A No. 2 Fogarty balloon embolectomy catheter can then be passed into each of the three tibial vessels. This must be done with utmost care to avoid potential intimal injury, perforation, or rupture. Alternatively, tibial vessels can be exposed at the ankle and retrograde passage of Fogarty catheters attempted.[102] Bypass grafts can then be extended to this level via the same arteriotomy, or a vein patch angioplasty of the distal arteriotomy can be performed with bypass to the more proximal portion of the artery. Intra-arterial thrombolysis in conjunction with bypass and embolectomy has been described

in some cases to further clear residual thrombus from the outflow vessels.[103,104] After bypass, patients may exhibit signs of reperfusion injury, including rhabdomyolysis, and may require fasciotomy.

Thrombolysis

Approximately 30% of patients with popliteal aneurysms have acute ischemic symptoms at initial evaluation. When studied with angiography, 25% to 45% of acutely ischemic patients will have thrombosis of the aneurysm with either no visible runoff vessel or severely compromised runoff thought to be unsuitable for bypass because of embolization. In these cases, pre-bypass catheter-directed intra-arterial thrombolysis has been shown to be effective in improving the likelihood of limb salvage in this challenging group of patients. Considerable judgment is required to determine whether a patient is suitable for thrombolysis, and the need to delay surgery for 12 to 24 hours for thrombolysis must be taken into account. Moreover, the potential risk for serious or life-threatening bleeding complications must be considered, and these may vary from patient to patient. Ultimately, the decision to perform thrombolysis must be individualized according to patient factors and clinical circumstances.

Technique. The decision to perform thrombolysis is usually made at the time of the diagnostic arteriogram. Intraoperative thrombolysis can also be used as adjunct to emergency surgery. The details of thrombolysis are described in Chapter 85 (Technique: Endovascular Therapeutic) and will be described here only briefly.

Percutaneous access using a single-puncture technique is obtained in the contralateral femoral artery. We prefer an ultrasound-guided micropuncture technique for gaining access. A 6 Fr sheath is delivered over the bifurcation and placed into the mid to distal SFA. An attempt is made to cross the clotted popliteal or distal outflow vessel (or both) with a guide wire. We prefer 0.018- or 0.014-inch wires. If access is achieved, a standard thrombolysis infusion catheter is placed over the wire. In some cases a coaxial multi-side-hole infusion catheter and wire can be used to lyse the distal popliteal artery and tibial runoff simultaneously. Either tissue plasminogen activator or urokinase can be delivered, first as a bolus into the clot and then by an infusion. In some cases, mechanical thrombectomy devices may be useful as an adjunct to thrombolysis. Patients are re-imaged in 6 to 24 hours, depending on improvement or worsening of clinical ischemia. If a suitable outflow target artery is visualized, lysis is stopped and the patient is immediately prepared for surgery (Fig. 136-13). Total clearance of all thrombus is not needed for successful bypass to the popliteal artery; however, if the popliteal artery is poorly visualized but a more distal tibial or pedal vessel is seen, bypass is performed to that level without delaying surgery longer in an attempt to further clear the popliteal

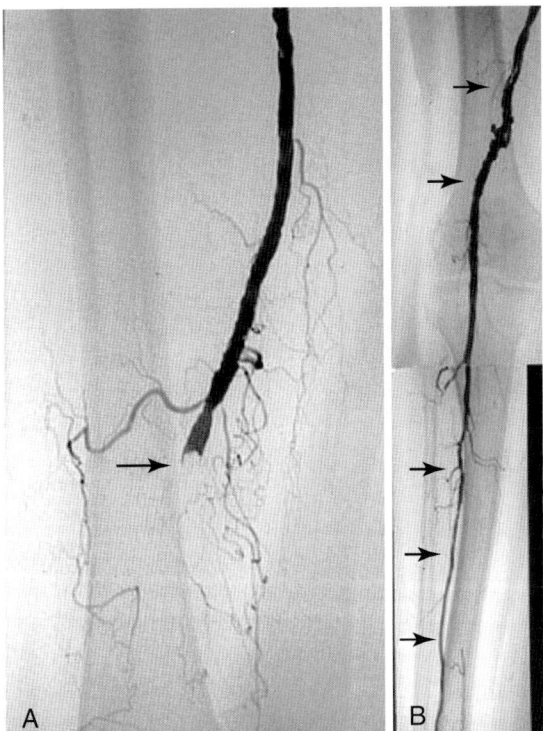

Figure 136-13 Acute thrombosis of a popliteal artery aneurysm. **A,** No outflow artery is visualized on the initial arteriogram. Note the reverse meniscus caused by thrombus in the popliteal artery (*arrow*). The aneurysm is not seen because of thrombosis. **B,** After 12 hours of thrombolysis with tissue plasminogen activator, the aneurysm (*double arrows*), as well as the entire popliteal artery with patent runoff into the peroneal artery (*triple arrows*), is now seen.

artery. Endovascular repair may be appropriate after lysis, provided that the anatomy is favorable (see "Endovascular Popliteal Aneurysm Repair").

If no clinical improvement in seen in 24 hours and no suitable runoff vessel is identified, patients are continued on intravenous heparin in the hope of recruiting enough collaterals to maintain limb viability. Most patients, though, will ultimately require amputation. Continuing thrombolysis beyond 24 hours is unlikely to result in an improved outcome in most patients and greatly increases the risk for bleeding complications.

Results. Several series, including our own,[1] have demonstrated the value of preoperative thrombolysis started at the time of diagnostic arteriography for improving outflow before bypass in 29% to 45% of patients with acute ischemia.[74,84,85,105] Marty and associates found that thrombolysis restored one- or two-vessel runoff in 77% of cases and predicted short- and long-term limb salvage, whereas failure of thrombolysis resulted in the need for amputation.[106] In our own series, 13 patients had acute ischemia. In the emergency group the cumulative primary and secondary patency rates were 85% and 100% at 1 and 5 years.[1] In the four patients who underwent thrombolysis, none required amputation. Tibial or pedal arteries were the outflow artery in 57% of the bypasses performed in the emergency group. In another series from the Mayo Clinic,[74] of the 74 patients with an acute manifestation, 34 underwent thrombolysis, 24 preoperatively and 14 during surgery. Thirty-day results were 94% primary patency and 91% limb salvage for those with lysis, and 87% primary patency and 92% limb salvage for those without lysis. Preoperative thrombolysis appeared to reduce the amputation rate from 96% to 69% in the group of patients presenting with severe critical limb ischemia.

The largest report on thrombolysis for popliteal aneurysms comes from the Swedish Vascular Registry,[86,103] which included treatment of 743 limbs for popliteal artery aneurysms over a 15-year period. Acute ischemia was present in 235 limbs, 100 of which (43%) were treated by preoperative thrombolysis, whereas 135 other patients went directly to surgery. In the immediate surgery group 32 patients underwent intraoperative thrombolysis. Based on review of preoperative and postoperative arteriograms, thrombolysis significantly improved runoff in 87% and remained unchanged in 13%, all of whom ultimately required amputation.

Our own experience agrees with that of the series previously discussed in that when properly applied, intra-arterial thrombolysis can uncover outflow target arteries suitable for bypass, thereby improving the chance of limb salvage. However, the decision to use thrombolysis in cases of critical ischemia is never straightforward and must be individualized to the specific clinical situation. If surgeons do not possess the requisite endovascular skills and expertise to perform it themselves, they must have the immediate support of a committed interventionalist. The importance of adhering to the principles of treatment of acute limb ischemia must be remembered;

most important is that any patient in whom the use of thrombolysis is being considered must be able to withstand another 12 to 18 hours of ischemia. It should never be used in marginally viable or nonviable limbs or in patients with specific contraindications to its use.

Results of Open Surgical Treatment

Overall, results of the treatment of popliteal artery aneurysms are affected by the absence or presence of symptoms, whether the repair is done electively or on an emergency basis, and whether the conduit used is saphenous vein or a prosthesis. Equally good results have been reported with either the medial or posterior approach.[86,107] In most series, saphenous vein grafts have generally been superior regardless of the approach used and may be most indicated in disadvantaged situations. Huang and colleagues divided patients into three groups on the basis of the severity of symptoms: group 1, asymptomatic; group 2, chronic ischemia; and group 3, acute ischemia.[74] All early deaths and amputations occurred in group 3, and early graft thrombosis was seen more than twice as frequently in group 3 as in groups 1 and 2 combined. Patency of the saphenous vein was superior to prosthetic conduit overall (94% versus 63%). No patient in group 1 or 2 suffered limb loss when a reconstruction was performed with saphenous vein. The impact of saphenous vein on outcome was most dramatic in group 3, where the patency rate at 1 year was 96% versus 67% for prosthetic grafts. Pulli and associates evaluated a 20-year experience of 159 popliteal aneurysms.[85] The risk for amputation at 30 days was 6.5% and 1.4% in symptomatic and asymptomatic patients, respectively. The limb salvage rate at 5 years was 93.4% and 80.4% for symptomatic versus asymptomatic patients, respectively, although in patients with claudication alone the results were nearly identical to those without symptoms (limb salvage rate of 90.5%). Patients with critical ischemia at initial evaluation had a dismal 5-year limb salvage rate of just 59%. In the large series on popliteal aneurysm repair from the Swedish Vascular Registry, in which 717 limbs were included, Ravn and coauthors reported an overall limb salvage rate of 89% in follow-up to 15 years. In a Cox regression model, age (odds ratio [OR], 1.06), emergency procedure (OR, 2.67), and prosthetic graft for bypass (OR, 2.02) were all independent correlates of the need for amputation.[86]

A few authors have been proponents of the primary use of a prosthetic graft for popliteal aneurysm repair, especially in the circumstance of short grafts and excellent outflow. Pulli and colleagues found no difference in patency at 6 years in 118 PTFE and 34 vein grafts (72% versus 80% rates, respectively). Beseth and Moore reported a 96% secondary patency rate at 22 months' follow-up in 30 prosthetic grafts, 25 of which had two- or three-vessel runoff at the time of treatment.[101] Blanco and coworkers demonstrated that short-segment PTFE grafts from the above-knee to the below-knee popliteal artery had comparable patency to vein grafts; however, longer PTFE grafts originating from the CFA had significantly worse patency rates than vein did (86% versus

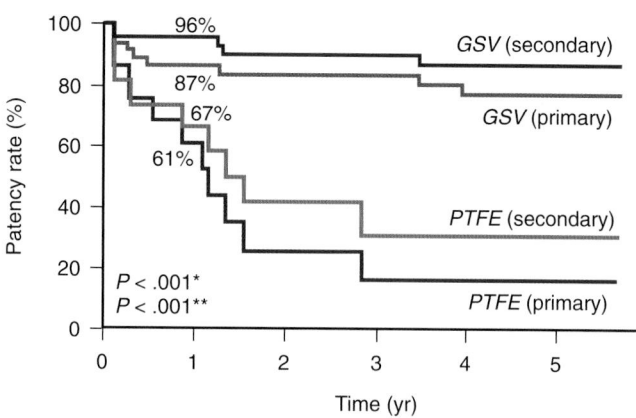

Figure 136-14 Life-table analysis of the patency rates of the great saphenous vein (GSV) and polytetrafluoroethylene (PTFE) grafts for repair of popliteal artery aneurysms with critical limb ischemia. Vein grafts remained patent more than twice as frequently as PTFE at 5 years and were nearly identical to the results reported for elective aneurysm repair. (*Primary patency; **secondary patency.) *(From Huang Y, Gloviczki P, Noel AA, et al. Early complications and long-term outcome after open surgical treatment of popliteal artery aneurysms: is exclusion with saphenous vein bypass still the gold standard? J Vasc Surg. 2007;45:706-713; discussion 713-715.)*

57%, *P* = .02).[108] Nonetheless, most authors are proponents of the routine use of saphenous vein. In Dawson and colleagues' systematic review of 2445 popliteal aneurysms in the literature, the patency rate at 5 years ranged from 77% to 100% for saphenous grafts versus 29% to 74% for prostheses.[73] The secondary patency rate at 5 years was 94% for saphenous vein and 63% for PTFE in the Mayo Clinic series.[74] Life-table analysis demonstrated that vein was especially advantageous in the most compromised patients with critical ischemia and suboptimal outflow (Fig. 136-14).

Endovascular Popliteal Aneurysm Repair

Marin and coauthors reported the first endovascular popliteal aneurysm repair (EPAR) with a "homemade" device created from a 6-mm PTFE bypass graft attached to two balloon-expandable stents.[109] A number of small series using other types of "homemade" stent-grafts were subsequently published,[24,110] and with the introduction and improvement in commercially available self-expanding stent-grafts and delivery systems, EPAR has become less cumbersome and more standardized, thus allowing more widespread application.

Indications

The indications for treatment are identical to those discussed previously for open surgical repair. The rationale for choosing endovascular treatment over conventional surgery is predicated on the concept that the resultant reduction in complications associated with open surgery, including more lengthy recovery, can be achieved while maintaining similar rates of limb salvage without an excessive need for re-intervention. Currently, the long-term results of EPAR are unknown and the short-term results generally demonstrate patency rates inferior to those of open surgery and a higher rate of re-intervention. Consequently, the use of EPAR for small, asymptomatic aneurysms should be undertaken with some circumspection. Most surgeons have generally reserved EPAR for patients in whom the risks related to anesthesia and surgery are prohibitive and who have appropriate anatomy for endograft implantation.

Focal aneurysms are most suited for EPAR. As with endovascular aortic aneurysm repair, there should be a segment of relatively normal artery both proximal and distal to the aneurysm to allow attachment and creation of a watertight seal.[111] The caliber of the attachment site should be 10% to 20% smaller than the diameter of the stent-graft and free of excessive calcification, thrombus, tortuosity, or angulation[112,113] The aneurysm itself should not contain excessive amounts of thrombus or debris.

Contraindications

As with endovascular aortic aneurysm repair, EPAR is constrained primarily by anatomy. Patients with thrombosed aneurysms or occluded SFAs cannot have a stent-graft placed and require conventional surgical bypass. Access arteries must be of adequate caliber to accept an introducer sheath, which can range in size from 9 to 11 Fr with current devices. If percutaneous access is planned, sites of puncture should be free of excessive wall calcification or intraluminal thrombus.

EPAR is probably ill advised in patients with distal embolization because placement and deployment may dislodge debris and worsen the situation. Crossing the knee joint with a device does not appear to be a contraindication[114] (see "Planning: Anatomic Requirements"); however, very diffuse aneurysms extending proximal to the adductor hiatus or involving the entire below-knee popliteal artery or SFA should be treated surgically.

Early experience has demonstrated that many EPAR patients require re-intervention for graft thrombosis, thus making careful follow-up and access to repeat treatment mandatory. A relative contraindication is the inability of the patient to comply with the required follow-up or living in a location where prompt return to the treating facility is not possible. Many surgeons believe that until more complete follow-up data are available, EPAR should not be performed in young healthy patients without contraindications to conventional surgical treatment.

Planning: Anatomic Requirements

EPAR requires careful preoperative planning. Crucial information includes the location, diameter, length, and shape of the aneurysm, as well as the diameter and quality of both the access vessels and attachment sites. Additionally, the patency and quality of the runoff vessels must be evaluated. Arterial-phase spiral CTA is currently the imaging modality of choice for EPAR. CT data can be reformatted into three-dimensional images oriented on the centerline of flow by

using commercially available software packages to aid in planning and measuring. Anatomic requirements have not yet been standardized, and the decision regarding which patients are most suited for EPAR varies with the experience and judgment of the surgeon or interventionalist.

One of the principal objections to EPAR is the need for stent-grafts in most cases to cross the knee joint, which are subject to kinking and stent fracture from knee flexion. However, some authors have suggested that it may actually be better to fully cross the knee joint with a stent-graft.[114] Dynamic anatomic studies using magnetic resonance imaging to study movement of the popliteal artery with flexion have revealed that points of fixation of the artery at the origin of the anterior tibial artery distally and at the origin of descending geniculate artery proximally do not allow kinking of the artery at the level of the knee joint. Because of the points of fixation, bending of the knee joint causes flexion of the popliteal artery *proximal* to the articular surface, whereas the middle and distal segments of the artery move posteriorly with little or no flexion (Fig. 136-15).

Technique

With the commercial development of low-profile devices, many procedures can be performed percutaneously under local anesthesia with moderate intravenous sedation. Percutaneous access usually requires a closure device after sheath removal. Deployment of a closure device at the time of sheath placement, the Preclose technique popularized with endovascular aortic aneurysm repair, is an alternative.[115]

Depending on patient anatomy and surgeon preference, access can be accomplished from the contralateral or ipsilateral CFA. For tall patients, long sheaths up to 11 Fr must be available if contralateral access is planned. The steps of the procedure are not unlike deployment of a self-expanding stent in the SFA and are outlined in Box 136-1. Most aneurysms can be treated with a single graft, but if more than one stent-graft is needed, overlap of at least 3 cm is suggested.

After surgery most patients can be discharged home the next day. Aspirin and clopidogrel are continued indefinitely.[111] Warfarin is not used routinely with the exception of treatment of stent-graft thrombosis. Most surgeons evaluate the repair with CTA in the early follow-up period. Stent-graft function can then be monitored with duplex ultrasonography. We prefer follow-up intervals of 3 months in the first year and every 6 months thereafter.

Results

An analysis of currently published series of EPAR demonstrates that it is technically feasible and easy to perform in most subjects with appropriate anatomy. Complications and mortality rates have been low. Because of the rarity of popliteal aneurysms, most series contain relatively small numbers of patients with limited follow-up. Table 136-1 shows the results of some of the larger experiences with EPAR.[24,110-112,114] The weighted average for primary and secondary patency

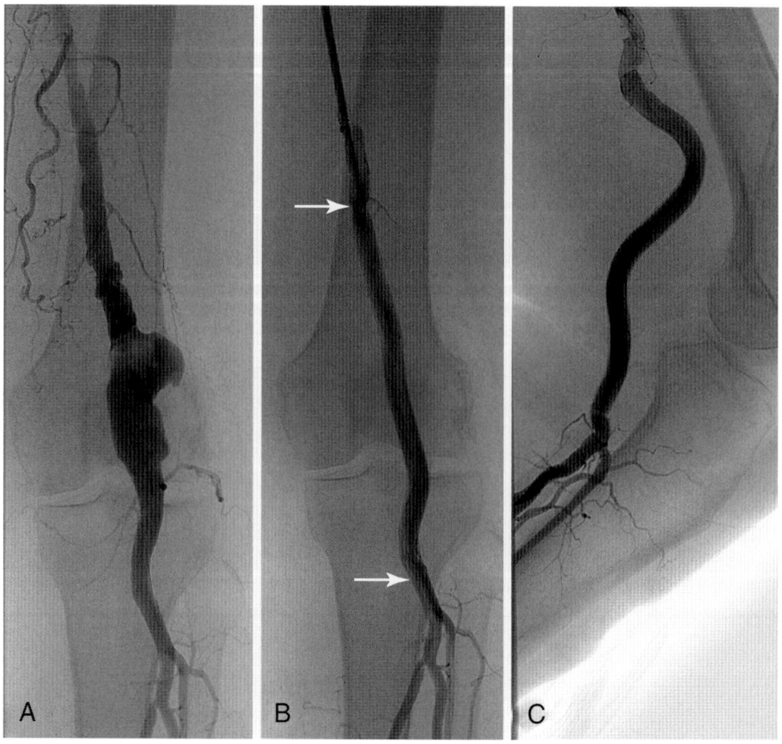

Figure 136-15 Endovascular repair of a popliteal artery aneurysm. **A,** Initial arteriogram demonstrating that the aneurysm involves most of the above-knee popliteal artery. The below-knee popliteal artery is normal and will be the distal attachment site for the stent-graft, which necessitates crossing the knee joint with the device. **B,** Completion arteriogram through the introducer sheath demonstrating the stent-graft in place across the knee joint (*arrows*). **C,** A lateral projection with the knee flexed 90 degrees demonstrates that the point of maximal flexion is actually proximal to the joint and does not result in kinking of the graft. Minimal bending and some posterior deflection of the graft are evident at the level of the articular surface of the joint (see text).

Box 136-1 Steps in Deployment of an Endograft for a Popliteal Aneurysm

1. Pretreat with clopidogrel.
2. Perform contralateral femoral puncture with delivery of an appropriately sized sheath over the bifurcation into the superior femoral artery.
3. Heparinize to an activated clotting time of greater than 250 seconds.
4. Cross the aneurysm into the distal popliteal artery or tibial vessels with a 0.035- or 0.018-inch wire, depending on the instructions for use of the device. Create a road map angiogram.
5. Deploy the graft from the distal to the proximal landing zone and overlap with additional grafts as needed. Postdilate the entirety of the graft to "iron out" any kinks or stenoses.
6. Perform a completion angiogram to evaluate for endoleak and preservation of runoff without embolization. In addition, an angiogram with the knee in extreme flexion should be performed to identify potential areas of kinking. A fluorographic save image to serve as a baseline for structural integrity of the graft is helpful.
7. Prescribe clopidogrel postoperatively indefinitely.

Table 136-1 Results of Endovascular Treatment of Popliteal Artery Aneurysms

Series	Number of Patients	Graft Types	Results (%)	
			Primary Patency	*Secondary Patency*
Curi et al.[112]	15	Viabahn	83 (2-yr)	100 (2-yr)
Teilliu et al.[111]	57	Hemobahn, Viabahn	77 (2-yr)	87 (2-yr)
Lagana et al.[24]	17	Hemobahn, Wallgraft	63 (1-yr)	73 (1-yr)
Gerasimidis et al.[110]	9	Various	47 (1-yr)	75 (1-yr)
Antonello et al.[114]	15	Hemobahn	87 (1-yr)	100 (1-yr)

poor runoff, patency rates 30 days after the procedure were 100% in the operative group and 93% in the endovascular group, with one thrombosis occurring the day after the procedure.[114] The primary patency rate in the stent-graft group at 1 and 4 years was 87% and 80%, respectively, versus 100% and 80% for surgery. Both groups had a 100% secondary patency rate at 4 years. Although this study suggests that patients with excellent anatomy can achieve results with EPAR that are comparable to those of surgery, a final conclusion cannot be reached without larger trials and longer follow-up.

◼ TIBIAL ARTERY ANEURYSMS

Tibial artery aneurysms are occasionally encountered in practice. Most are pseudoaneurysms occurring as a result of

rates is 65% and 76%, respectively, at 1.5 years, which is inferior to the rates for open surgery. In a recent meta-analysis, EPAR resulted in a decrease in overall length of stay and recovery when compared with surgery but had a significantly increased rate of early thrombosis resulting in the need for repeat interventions.[116] Anatomy may influence the outcome and durability of EPAR. In the only small, randomized trial, which consisted of 26 patients undergoing surgery or EPAR and excluded patients with unfavorable anatomy and penetrating trauma,[117] long-bone fractures, or iatrogenic injury during fracture fixation[118] or in association with bone tumors.[61] A major cause is direct injury as a result of thromboembolectomy with balloon catheters[119,120] or other catheter-based interventions.

Symptoms are rare, although some patients may have local pain or swelling of the calf.[121] Duplex ultrasonography can be used to identify tibial pseudoaneurysms and the diagnosis confirmed by contrast-enhanced arteriography.

Surgical treatment usually consists of simple ligation if the other tibial vessels are normal. Reconstruction with saphenous vein may be necessary and should always be performed if no other tibial artery is patent. Coil embolization with thrombin injection has been reported.[120] For very small aneurysms, spontaneous thrombosis may occur, and expectant observation with subsequent follow-up may be all that is required.

SELECTED KEY REFERENCES

Antonello M, Frigatti P, Battocchio P, Lepidi S, Cognolato D, Dall'Antonia A, Stramanà R, Deriu GP, Grego F. Open repair versus endovascular treatment for asymptomatic popliteal artery aneurysm: results of a prospective randomized study. *J Vasc Surg.* 2005;42: 185-193.
The only major randomized trial comparing open surgery and endovascular repair for popliteal aneurysms.

Corriere MA, Guzman RJ. True and false aneurysms of the femoral artery. *Semin Vasc Surg.* 2005;18:216-223.
An excellent review article of the current management of both atherosclerotic and femoral artery false aneurysms.

Dawson I, Sie RB, van Bockel JH. Atherosclerotic popliteal aneurysm. *Br J Surg.* 1997;84:293-299.
Large review of the behavior and treatment of popliteal aneurysms encompassing more than 2400 patients over a 15-year period.

Diwan A, Sarkar R, Stanley JC, Zelenock GB, Wakefield TW. Incidence of femoral and popliteal artery aneurysms in patients with abdominal aortic aneurysms. *J Vasc Surg.* 2000;31:863-869.
This prospective analysis identifies the high incidence of lower extremity aneurysms in patients with aortic aneurysms.

Graham LM, Zelenock GB, Whitehouse WM Jr, Erlandson EE, Dent TL, Lindenauer SM, Stanley JC. Clinical significance of arteriosclerotic femoral artery aneurysms. *Arch Surg.* 1980;115:502-507.
Classic and often quoted reference on degenerative femoral aneurysms.

Harbuzariu C, Duncan AA, Bower TC, Kalra M, Gloviczki P. Profunda femoris artery aneurysms: association with aneurysmal disease and limb ischemia. *J Vasc Surg.* 2008;47:31-34; discussion 34-35.
Largest single-center series of an unusual and infrequently seen aneurysm.

Huang Y, Gloviczki P, Noel AA, Sullivan TM, Kalra M, Gullerud RE, Hoskin TL, Bower TC. Early complications and long-term outcome after open surgical treatment of popliteal artery aneurysms: is exclusion with saphenous vein bypass still the gold standard? *J Vasc Surg.* 2007;45:706-713; discussion 713-715.
Updated single-center series with important details on the results of emergency and elective treatment, the behavior of vein and prosthetic grafts, and thrombolytic therapy.

Kang SS, Labropoulos N, Mansour MA, Baker WH. Percutaneous ultrasound guided thrombin injection: a new method for treating postcatheterization femoral pseudoaneurysms. *J Vasc Surg.* 1998;27: 1032-1038.
Original report on the technique of ultrasound-guided thrombin injection.

Perry MO. John Hunter—triumph and tragedy. *J Vasc Surg.* 1993; 17:7-14.
In his 1992 presidential address to the Society for Vascular Surgery, Dr. Perry provides an excellent historical account of the life of John Hunter.

Ravn H, Bjorck M. Popliteal artery aneurysm with acute ischemia in 229 patients. Outcome after thrombolytic and surgical therapy. *Eur J Vasc Endovasc Surg.* 2007;33:690-695.
This largest series on the treatment of popliteal aneurysms looks at results of treatment of emergency cases.

REFERENCES

The reference list can be found on the companion Expert Consult Web site at *www.expertconsult.com.*

CHAPTER 137

Upper Extremity Aneurysms

Carlos H. Timaran

Based in part on a chapter in the previous edition by G. Patrick Clagett, MD.

Upper extremity aneurysms are uncommon in comparison to other peripheral arterial aneurysms.[1] Unlike aortoiliac and most visceral aneurysms, whose growth can result in rupture, most upper extremity aneurysms, when symptomatic, cause limb ischemia from thrombosis or embolization with potential digit or even major amputations. Proximal aneurysms of the great vessels, however, can result in either death from rupture and exsanguination or a myriad of complications, including upper extremity ischemia from thromboembolism, neuromuscular and sensory dysfunction from compression of the brachial plexus, dysphagia from esophageal compression in cases of aberrant right subclavian artery aneurysms, and neurologic deficits secondary to thromboembolism in the vertebral and carotid circulations. In contrast, more distally located upper extremity aneurysms are manifested almost exclusively by thromboembolic complications of the hand and digits.

The first attempted surgical correction of an arch vessel aneurysm, the most frequent type of upper extremity aneurysm, was performed in 1818 by Mott in New York, who ligated the innominate artery.[2] The first successful treatment of a subclavian artery aneurysm was achieved in 1864 by Smyth in New Orleans, who ligated the right common carotid artery and the innominate artery.[3] The aneurysm recurred and ruptured 10 years later. Halsted was the first to successfully combine ligation with resection of a subclavian artery aneurysm in 1892 at the Johns Hopkins Hospital.[4] In 1913, Matas reported 225 cases of treatment of aneurysms by endoaneurysmorrhaphy, and 7 of them were subclavian aneurysms.[5]

◼ ARCH VESSEL ANEURYSMS

Epidemiology and Etiology

Innominate, common carotid, and subclavian artery aneurysms usually arise from degenerative disease; less commonly, these aneurysms can result from trauma, fibromuscular dysplasia, syphilis, cystic medial necrosis, invasion of the vessel wall by contiguous tuberculous lymphadenitis, and idiopathic congenital causes. Only 1% of all peripheral arterial aneurysms involve the subclavian and innominate arteries. Thirty percent to 50% of patients with nonspecific degenerative arch vessel aneurysms have aortoiliac or other peripheral aneurysms.[6,7] Patients with these aneurysms should therefore be thoroughly evaluated for concurrent aneurysms.

Arch vessel aneurysms usually occur in patients of either sex older than 60 years, but they seem to be more common in men. Aneurysms of the distal subclavian artery, frequently with extension into the first portion of the axillary artery, are generally associated with thoracic outlet obstruction, cervical rib, and other bony abnormalities that result in arterial compression and subsequent degenerative changes causing poststenotic dilatation. This specific type of aneurysm is discussed in Chapter 124 (Thoracic Outlet Syndrome: Arterial).

Subclavian Artery Aneurysms

True subclavian aneurysms, typically seen in elderly patients, are usually degenerative. Pairolero and coauthors reported the treatment of 31 patients with subclavian artery aneurysms over a 20-year period.[6] True degenerative aneurysms were repaired in 12 patients, traumatic pseudoaneurysms in 10, and aneurysms secondary to thoracic outlet obstruction in 6. McCollum and associates also reported their 25-year experience with subclavian aneurysm repair in 15 patients, over half of which were true degenerative aneurysms.[7] Pseudoaneurysms frequently occur as a result of blunt and penetrating trauma. Iatrogenic injury from inadvertent cannulation of the subclavian artery with pseudoaneurysm formation is uncommon but increasing in frequency because of the common requirements for invasive monitoring and hemodialysis via the subclavian vein. The recent preferential use of ultrasound-guided central venous access may result in reduced arterial injuries or pseudoaneurysms.[8] In most cases, simple removal of the misplaced catheter and careful compression are all that is necessary. Many patients with this problem are unstable and coagulopathic, however. This situation, along with the inability to compress the artery effectively when the injury is beneath the clavicle, may result in significant hemorrhage and false aneurysm formation. Recent reports have described the successful use of endovascular techniques with endografts or percutaneous closure devices to repair arterial injuries occurring during central venous access.[9-11]

Innominate Artery Aneurysms

True aneurysms of the innominate artery are rare. Kieffer and colleagues reported six degenerative aneurysms in 27 patients with innominate artery aneurysms that also included mycotic, dissecting, connective tissue, and extension of arch aneurysms, as well as traumatic and iatrogenic pseudoaneurysms.[12]

Similarly, Bower and associates reported their 40-year experience that included only 4 patients with true aneurysms of the innominate artery among 73 patients treated surgically for brachiocephalic aneurysms.[13] Although most patients have thromboembolic complications involving either the upper extremity or the cerebral circulation, rupture occurred in one patient reported by Kieffer and colleagues.[12] Because of the devastating consequences of untreated innominate artery aneurysms, Bower and coworkers have recommended operative treatment of all symptomatic and asymptomatic affected patients fit for surgical repair to avoid the natural history that inevitably leads to rupture or thromboembolism.[13]

Common Carotid Artery Aneurysms

True aneurysms of the common carotid arteries are very rare. In fact, pseudoaneurysms of the carotid arteries are considerably more frequent and usually result from complications of carotid reconstructions, blunt or penetrating trauma, or carotid dissections or infections.[14,15] The vast majority of true aneurysms of the carotid arteries are degenerative[16]; other less frequent causes include fibromuscular dysplasia, Marfan's syndrome, Behçet's disease, and Takayasu's arteritis.[15,17] Bilateral common carotid artery aneurysms are extremely unusual and generally associated with Takayasu's arteritis.[18] Carotid bifurcation and internal carotid artery aneurysms are discussed in Chapter 98 (Carotid Artery: Aneurysms).

Clinical Findings

Symptoms

The initial symptoms of arch vessel aneurysms include (1) chest, neck, and shoulder pain from acute expansion or rupture; (2) upper extremity acute and chronic ischemic symptoms from thromboembolism; (3) upper extremity pain and neurologic dysfunction from brachial plexus compression; (4) hoarseness from compression of the right recurrent laryngeal nerve; (5) respiratory insufficiency from tracheal compression; (6) transient ischemic attacks and stroke from retrograde thromboembolism in the vertebral and right carotid circulations; (7) dysphagia from esophageal compression in cases of aberrant right subclavian artery; and (8) hemoptysis from erosion into the apex of the lung. Tracheobronchial or esophageal fistulization as a result of contiguous arch vessel aneurysms can also occur.

Signs

In patients without symptoms, the diagnosis may be made by imaging studies for unrelated conditions. In cases of subclavian artery aneurysms, patients may note the presence of a supraclavicular pulsatile mass. Most asymptomatic pulsatile masses in this area, however, represent tortuous and elongated common carotid and subclavian arteries and not necessarily aneurysmal degeneration (Fig. 137-1). These masses can usually be distinguished from true aneurysms by duplex

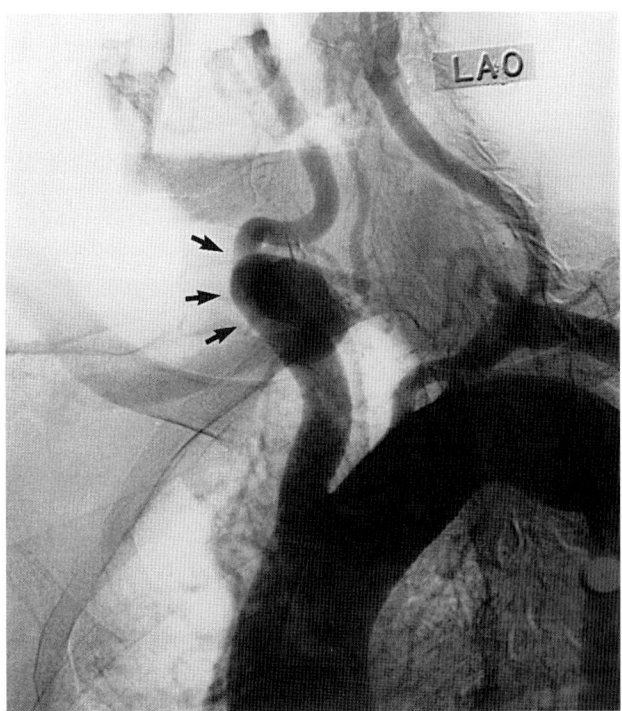

Figure 137-1 The confluence of elongated and tortuous innominate, subclavian, and common carotid arteries gives rise to a pulsatile mass in the right supraclavicular fossa and base of the neck (*arrows*). This common condition is harmless but is frequently confused on physical examination with a subclavian or common carotid aneurysm. Ultrasonography can usually differentiate between them; however, arteriography is sometimes required. LAO, left anterior oblique view.

ultrasonography or other noninvasive imaging studies. In addition to a supraclavicular mass, physical signs may include (1) a supraclavicular bruit, (2) absent or diminished pulses in the upper extremity, (3) normal pulses with signs of microembolization (blue finger syndrome), (4) sensory and motor signs of brachial plexus compression, (5) vocal cord paralysis, and (6) Horner's syndrome resulting from compression of the stellate ganglion and other contributions to the cervical sympathetic chain at the base of the neck.[19]

Imaging

Plain films of the chest may reveal a superior mediastinal mass that may suggest the presence of a neoplasm. Ultrasonography, magnetic resonance (MR) imaging, or computed tomography (CT) establishes the diagnosis. Conventional arch and upper extremity angiography and MR or CT angiography are important to delineate the extent of the aneurysm, to assess sites of vascular occlusion in cases complicated by thromboembolism, to note the competency of the contralateral vertebral circulation if the ipsilateral vertebral artery originates from an aneurysmal vessel, and to assess anatomic suitability for endovascular repair. These points are essential in planning appropriate management (i.e., surgical reconstruction or endovascular repair).

Open Surgical Repair

Contemporary surgical repair of arch vessel aneurysms involves resection or endoaneurysmorrhaphy and re-establishment of arterial continuity with an end-to-end anastomosis (for very small aneurysms) or, more commonly, an interposition arterial prosthetic graft. Although proximal and distal ligation of arch vessel aneurysms has occasionally been successful in the past, ligation without direct or extra-anatomic reconstruction should not generally be performed because ischemic symptoms develop in 25% of cases so treated.[6]

Innominate Artery Aneurysms

An anatomic classification of the extent of the aneurysm has been proposed by Kieffer and colleagues to guide surgical repair of aneurysms of the innominate artery (Fig. 137-2).[12] Group A is confined to the innominate artery distal its origin. Group B is the most common and involves the innominate artery and its origin. Group C involves both the innominate artery and the ascending aorta.

The innominate and proximal subclavian arteries are usually exposed through a median sternotomy extended into the right side of the neck. Proximal control of the innominate artery is obtained at the aortic arch. The right subclavian and right common carotid arteries are exposed and dissected for distal control. The aneurysm is resected, and reconstruction with a prosthetic graft is generally performed. For types A and B aneurysms, the proximal graft anastomosis is usually performed in the native ascending aorta proximal to the innominate origin. The graft is then anastomosed to the unin-

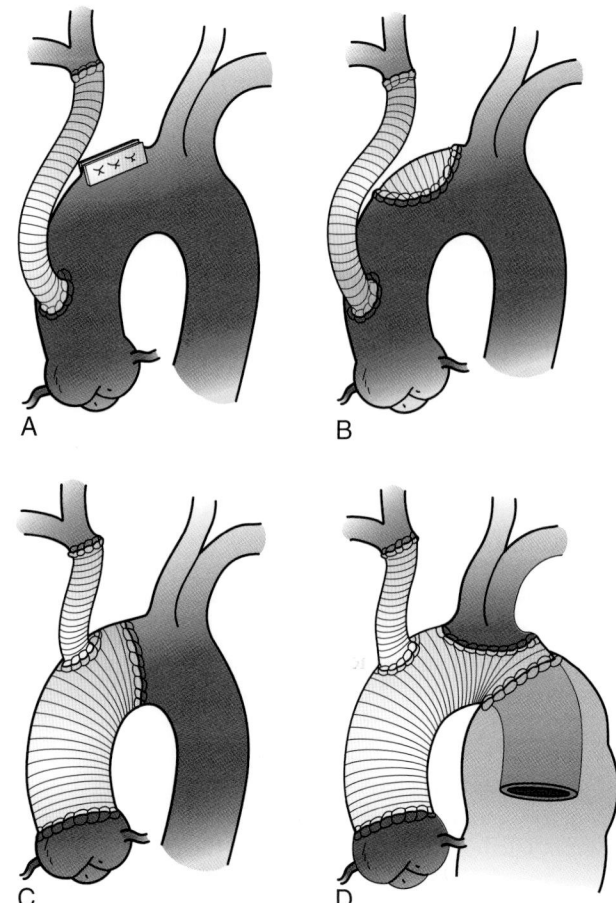

Figure 137-3 Techniques used for the treatment of aneurysms of the innominate artery. **A,** Lateral suture of the aorta. **B,** Patch angioplasty of the aorta. **C,** Replacement of the ascending aorta. **D,** Replacement of the ascending aorta and transverse aortic arch in association with a distal elephant trunk prosthesis. *(From Kieffer E, Chiche L, Koskas F, Bahnini A. Aneurysms of the innominate artery: surgical treatment of 27 patients. J Vasc Surg. 2001;2:222.)*

volved distal innominate artery (Fig. 137-3). The origin of the innominate artery is oversewn with a running suture, or patch angioplasty of the aorta may occasionally be required. For lesions extending into the origins of the right subclavian or common carotid artery, a bifurcated graft can be used or a branch graft to the subclavian artery can be sewn onto the graft going into the common carotid artery. The bifurcated configuration may sometimes be prone to compression or kinking when the sternum is closed, so caution should be exercised when performing the proximal anastomosis in the lateral aspect of the ascending aorta. In cases of a bovine arch, additional graft reconstruction of the left common carotid artery may be necessary. Type C innominate artery aneurysms usually require aortic arch and innominate artery prosthetic graft replacement with cardiopulmonary bypass and hypothermic circulatory arrest.

Subclavian Artery Aneurysms

Subclavian artery aneurysms can be divided into proximal, which are typically degenerative, or distal, which are gener-

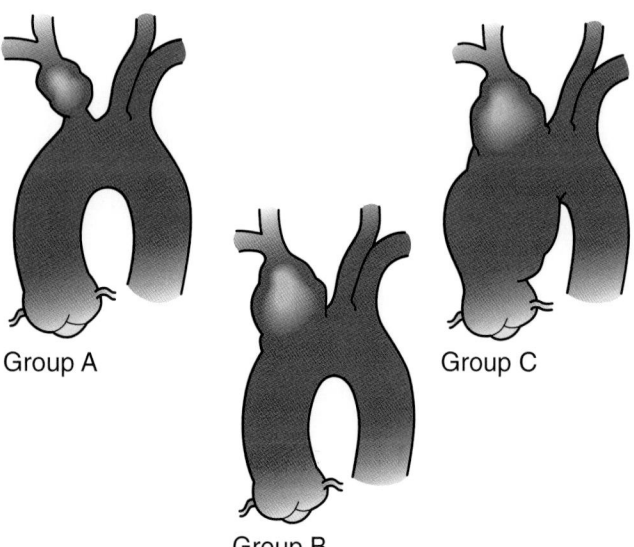

Figure 137-2 Classification of aneurysms of the innominate artery according to the extent of involvement. Group A, no involvement of the origin of the innominate artery. Group B, involvement of the origin of the innominate artery but not the aorta. Group C, involvement of the innominate artery and aorta. *(From Kieffer E, Chiche L, Koskas F, Bahnini A. Aneurysms of the innominate artery: surgical treatment of 27 patients. J Vasc Surg. 2001;2:222.)*

ally related to thoracic outlet syndrome. For proximal right subclavian aneurysms, median sternotomy with extension into the supraclavicular fossa is usually necessary to gain adequate exposure for proximal control. Supraclavicular and infraclavicular incisions may be used to mobilize the proximal and distal subclavian artery. Resection of the clavicle also offers excellent exposure of the subclavian artery. Partial medial clavicular resection is rarely necessary, although it may helpful for proximal subclavian artery exposure when median sternotomy is not feasible. The supraclavicular incision is extended medially, and the fascia and periosteum are incised. The origins of the sternocleidomastoid and pectoralis major muscles are reflected subperiosteally, the first superiorly and the second inferiorly. The medial third of the clavicle is disarticulated and subperiosteally resected with care taken to avoid injury to the subclavian vein. In cases of proximal left subclavian aneurysm, a left thoracotomy combined with supraclavicular exposure may be necessary.

Extra-anatomic reconstruction combined with proximal and distal ligation of the aneurysm has also been described in unusual circumstances.[20] For aneurysms involving the mid and distal subclavian artery, a supraclavicular incision often provides adequate exposure and may be complemented by an infraclavicular incision for distal control. Alternatively, proximal and distal control may be achieved endovascularly with balloon occlusion catheters placed angiographically. Division or resection of the midportion of the clavicle may be necessary to gain additional exposure, and if so, the clavicle may be reconstructed at the completion of the operation. If the aneurysm involves the origin of the vertebral artery, reconstruction by reimplantation or other means is appropriate, particularly if this is the dominant vertebral artery or for cases in which the contralateral vertebral artery is hypoplastic or diseased.

Results

Aneurysm resection with graft replacement is durable and yields excellent long-term results. In one of the largest reported series, normal upper extremity circulation was maintained, and there were no procedure-related complications during a mean follow-up of 9.2 years.[6] Although open repair frequently results in durable and excellent long-term outcomes, considerable associated morbidity and mortality have been reported. In fact, in-hospital mortality could be as high as 11% according to a recent report of open repair of innominate artery aneurysms, in which 18% of patients required prolonged ventilation.[12] Because many patients with true aneurysms are unfit for open repair as a result of their advanced age and multiple co-morbid conditions, careful patient selection is mandatory to improve outcomes. Relative contraindications to open repair also include severely compromised pulmonary function, previous sternotomy or left thoracotomy, and hemodynamic instability secondary to multiple trauma.

Endovascular Repair

Endovascular repair is an attractive option for patients unfit for open repair because it is associated with lower morbidity and mortality. In fact, there are many reports of endovascular repair of arch vessel aneurysms, particularly those involving the innominate and subclavian arteries.[21-26] This approach is particularly suitable for unstable patients and those with multiple medical morbidities that make them unfit for open repair. It may also be helpful in actively bleeding, coagulopathic patients with iatrogenic, catheter-induced, or other penetrating injury of the arch vessels.[27-32] In addition, aneurysm secondary to connective tissue disorders may be more suitable for endovascular repair to avoid direct resection and anastomoses to diseased vessels.[33]

Anatomic Considerations

The proximal portion and midportion of the subclavian artery are most amenable to endovascular treatment. However, several anatomic limitations exist. It is unusual for true subclavian or innominate aneurysms to have adequate proximal and distal landing zones. Moreover, coverage of branch vessels such as the right carotid artery, vertebral arteries, and left internal mammary artery (when it has been used for coronary bypass) may not be feasible. Endografts crossing the first rib may be subject to extrinsic compression. The distal subclavian artery is located between the clavicle and the first rib, and endografts in this location are subject to compression, deformation, and fracture.[30,31,34,35] Another potential complication of endograft placement in the right subclavian artery is stroke from embolic debris dislodged into the right common carotid artery.[32] The origin of the vertebral artery is vulnerable on both sides and may be covered during stent-graft deployment. This is usually well tolerated when the contralateral vertebral artery is patent and of adequate size. Posterior circulation stroke may occur, however, when the contralateral vertebral artery is highly stenotic, hypoplastic, or occluded. In this circumstance, the ipsilateral vertebral artery should be revascularized by end-to-side anastomosis to the common carotid artery or other means. Whenever the origin of the vertebral artery is involved by the aneurysm, coil embolization of the ipsilateral vertebral artery is desirable to prevent future branch vessel endoleaks.

Technique

Endovascular repair of subclavian or innominate artery aneurysms is usually performed through a transbrachial or transfemoral approach. A transaxillary approach has occasionally been necessary.[33] Both balloon-mounted and self-expanding endografts have been used for endovascular repair of arch vessel aneurysms. The most frequently used endografts include the Wallgraft (Boston Scientific, Natick, MA), Viabahn (W.L. Gore & Assoc., Flagstaff, AZ), and Fluency (C.R. Bard, Inc., Murray Hill, NJ). Most contemporary endografts generally require 8 or 9 Fr delivery sheaths, depending on endograft diameter. Larger endografts, however, such as those required for endovascular repair of innominate artery aneurysms, still require large introducer sheaths, usually 11 or 12 Fr. The more flexible Viabahn endograft may be more suitable in cases of considerable arterial tortuosity. Lower profile devices, such as the balloon-mounted iCast endograft (Atrium Medical, Hudson, NH), which is available up to 10-mm diameter, can be delivered through a 7 Fr sheath. Of note, the largest iCast endograft can potentially be dilated up to 12 mm in diameter. Because of the discrepancy in proximal and distal landing zone diameters, a combination of endografts of different size may be necessary. Furthermore, given the rigidity of balloon-mounted endografts, they may be used for accurate proximal deployment at the level of the ostium of the vessel and combined with more flexible distal self-expanding endografts.

Hybrid Operations

Another innovative approach that is minimally invasive and avoids placement of an endograft combines coil embolization of the subclavian artery aneurysm and carotid-subclavian bypass.[36] Complete exclusion of the subclavian aneurysm is facilitated by ligation of the subclavian artery proximal to the distal anastomosis of the carotid-subclavian bypass. These procedures can be staged or combined in an operating room equipped with high-resolution imaging equipment. As with endograft placement, care must be taken to preserve flow in the vertebral artery if the contralateral vertebral artery is inadequate.

With the introduction of endografts specific for endovascular treatment of thoracic aortic aneurysms, hybrid procedures have become feasible for more proximal aneurysms of the great vessels and those extending into the aortic arch. In these procedures, exclusion of the orifice of aneurysmal arch vessels is combined with thoracic endovascular aortic aneurysm repair and extra-anatomic arch vessel revascularization

(i.e., carotid-carotid, subclavian transposition, and carotid-subclavian bypass).[37]

Results

The long-term durability of endografts in the subclavian artery is unknown. Short-term patency rates range from 83% to 100% over a mean follow-up of 7 to 29 months.[25,29-31,38] Endograft compression, deformation, and fracture and stenosis from intimal hyperplasia have been reported and may limit the applicability of endovascular repair in this location.[27-29] For these reasons, open surgical repair remains the preferred approach for good-risk patients with innominate and subclavian aneurysms.

ABERRANT SUBCLAVIAN ARTERY AND KOMMERELL'S DIVERTICULUM ANEURYSMS

Anatomy

Aberrant Subclavian Artery

An aberrant right subclavian artery arising from the proximal portion of the descending thoracic aorta is the most common congenital anomaly of the aortic arch and occurs in 0.5% to 1% of the population.[39] It was first described in 1735 at autopsy by Hunauld. In 1794, Bayford described "dysphagia lusoria," or difficulty swallowing caused by impingement of the aberrant vessel on the esophagus. The anomalous right subclavian artery originates distal to the left subclavian origin, typically posterior and inferior on the arch, and crosses the midline between the esophagus and the spine (Fig. 137-4). Alternatively, in individuals with a right-sided aortic arch, an aberrant left subclavian artery may originate distal to the origin of the right subclavian, and this may also become aneurysmal. During embryologic development, the left fourth arch becomes part of the aortic arch, whereas the right fourth arch becomes the root of the right subclavian artery. An aberrant

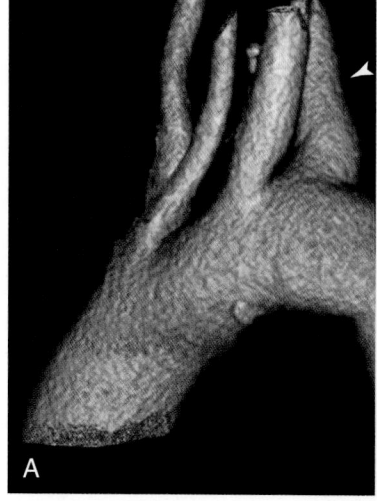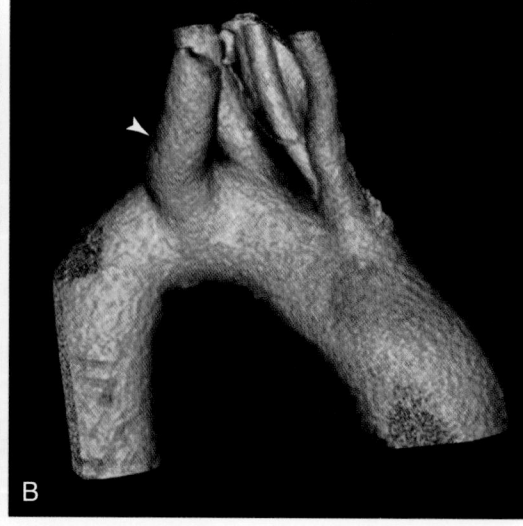

Figure 137-4 Anterior (**A**) and posterior (**B**) three-dimensional CT angiographic views of the aortic arch reveal that the anomalous right subclavian artery (*arrowhead*) originates both distal and posteroinferior on the arch relative to the left subclavian origin.

right subclavian artery occurs when the right fourth aortic arch and right dorsal aorta involute cranial to the seventh intersegmental artery.

Aberrant Subclavian Artery Aneurysm

Aneurysms of an aberrant subclavian artery are encountered most frequently in adults older than 50 years of either sex. Most patients with this anomaly are asymptomatic, and the aberrant subclavian artery is of no clinical consequence. Rarely, the vessel compresses the esophagus against the posterior trachea and gives rise to difficulty swallowing, a condition termed *dysphagia lusoria*.[40]

Kommerell's Diverticulum

Degenerative aneurysmal changes in the proximal portion of the aberrant subclavian artery or its aortic origin may occur in up to 60% of patients.[41] This condition has been termed *Kommerell's diverticulum* after Kommerell, who in 1936 described a diverticulum of the aorta at the origin of the anomalous subclavian artery.[39] McCallen and Schaff first called attention to the clinical significance of aneurysmal change in an anomalous right subclavian artery in a 1956 report.[42] The largest experience to date with this condition was reported by Kieffer and associates, who surgically treated 33 adults with aberrant subclavian arteries, 17 of whom had a Kommerell diverticulum or aneurysmal change of the thoracic aorta at the origin of the aberrant subclavian artery.[43]

Clinical Findings

Aberrant Right Subclavian Artery

A nonaneurysmal aberrant right subclavian artery may result in dysphagia and symptomatic arterial occlusive disease. According to Kieffer and colleagues, 11 of 33 patients without aneurysmal degeneration exhibited dysphagia, whereas upper right limb ischemia developed in 5 because of either arterial occlusive disease or embolism originating from the nonaneurysmal aberrant right subclavian artery.[43]

Aberrant Subclavian Artery Aneurysm

Though it is sometimes discovered incidentally, patients with aneurysm of an aberrant right subclavian artery usually have dysphagia from esophageal compression, dyspnea and coughing from tracheal compression, chest pain from expansion or rupture, or symptoms of right upper extremity ischemia secondary to thromboembolism. Patients may also be seen on an emergency basis with aneurysm rupture or dissection. According to Austin and Wolfe, 19% of patients were found to have rupture at initial evaluation, all of whom died.[39] More recently, Cina and coauthors reported that 53% of patients were initially seen with either rupture or dissection.[44] Aneurysm rupture in these cases seems to be unrelated to the size of the aneurysm. Many reported cases occurred in asymptomatic

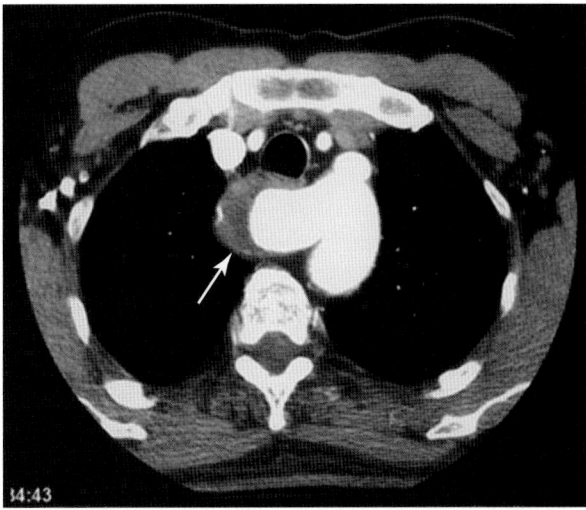

Figure 137-5 Contrast-enhanced axial CT scan at the level of the aortic arch. An aneurysm of the aberrant right subclavian artery (*arrow*) is demonstrated passing posterior to the trachea and esophagus. *(From Munneke GJ, Loosemore TM, Belli AM, et al. Aneurysm of an aberrant right subclavian artery successfully excluded by a thoracic aortic stent graft with supra-aortic bypass of three arch vessels. Cardiovasc Intervent Radiol. 2005;5:653.)*

patients whose aneurysm was found on chest radiography and interpreted as a superior mediastinal mass. Chest CT can detect this condition noninvasively, but CT or digital subtraction angiography is necessary to plan surgical treatment or endovascular repair (Fig. 137-5). Approximately a fifth of reported patients with this anomaly have an associated abdominal aortic aneurysm.[39]

Surgical Treatment

Aberrant Right Subclavian Artery

Open repair is usually performed through a supraclavicular incision. The aberrant right subclavian artery is divided via a right supraclavicular incision after dissecting it to the left of the esophagus. The distal end of the subclavian artery is then anastomosed to the right common carotid. Ligation to the left of the esophagus relieves local pressure symptoms. This approach is satisfactory when the more proximal aberrant subclavian artery is not aneurysmal.[40,45]

Aberrant Subclavian Artery Aneurysm

Because of the propensity of these aneurysms to cause symptoms and because of the possibility of lethal rupture, resection or exclusion of the aneurysmal artery with vascular reconstruction of the subclavian artery is recommended. Multiple procedures and reconstructions for open repair of these aneurysms have been described. The best approach depends on the anatomic characteristics of the lesion, patient fitness, and acuity of the symptoms. In the elective setting, open repair consists of staged extra-anatomic bypass to reconstruct the aberrant subclavian artery, followed by thoracotomy to oversew the origin of Kommerell's diverticulum. Simple side-biting clamp exclusion may be possible, although interposition graft resection of the aorta itself may be necessary in up to 30% of patients with aortic involvement.[43] Considerations for the procedure are similar to those for open repair of an atherosclerotic proximal left subclavian aneurysm. The repair may be accomplished via a right or left posterolateral thoracotomy (depending on the position of the aortic arch) or a median sternotomy.[39,43,46,47] The subclavian artery is reconstructed by interposition arterial grafting in which the proximal anastomosis may be performed to the ascending aorta. Alternatively, a left posterolateral thoracotomy for proximal resection of the aneurysm coupled with a right supraclavicular incision for reconstruction of the subclavian artery by end-to-side anastomosis to the right common carotid artery has been described.[48] A staged approach consisting of right carotid–subclavian bypass or transposition (end-subclavian to side-carotid) (see Chapter 98: Carotid Artery Disease: Aneurysms) preceding left thoracotomy and resection of the aneurysm with oversewing of the origin from the aortic arch is attractive because the risk for cerebral and right upper extremity embolization is minimized. Extra-anatomic reconstruction of the right subclavian artery has also been described. Because it is necessary to resect the aneurysmal vessel near its origin from the aorta, the modified extrathoracic approach alone, as described for the treatment of dysphagia lusoria with non-aneurysmal aberrant subclavian vessels, would not be effective.

Endovascular-Hybrid Treatment

Open repair may be associated with high rates of neurologic complications and mortality, particularly in patients unfit for open major vascular reconstruction. Because the thoracotomy and aortic clamping are the most morbid portions of open repair, which has a reported mortality rate of up to 30%,[43] the combination of aortic endografting and extra-anatomic bypass is particularly appealing for management of this condition. In addition, open repair may be contraindicated after previous thoracotomy.

Hybrid Approach

Endovascular occlusion of a symptomatic aberrant right subclavian artery, with or without aneurysm, by means of thoracic aortic endografts combined with distal ligation is an alternative to open repair. Alternatively, because exposure to the proximal aberrant right subclavian artery is limited through a cervical approach and to avoid leaving a stump that may evolve into an aneurysm, a hybrid approach to the proximal end of the artery may be necessary. For this purpose, an occlusion device may be placed in antegrade or retrograde fashion at the origin of the aberrant right subclavian artery (Fig. 137-6).[49] The antegrade approach may be preferable to have better control of the deployment and to avoid emboliza-

tion of the occluder into the aortic arch, which may occur when a retrograde approach is used.

A thoracic endograft can effectively exclude antegrade flow into an aberrant right subclavian artery aneurysm (Fig. 137-7).[50-52] With current devices, however, endovascular repair alone is insufficient for the treatment of most lesions. Thoracic aortic endografting usually needs to be combined with revascularization of one or both subclavian arteries (Fig. 137-8).[51,53] In the majority of cases, the orifices of the aberrant right and left subclavian arteries are situated at the same level or in close proximity. To effectively occlude the origin of the aberrant vessel with a thoracic endograft, its placement usually requires exclusion of both subclavian arteries.[51] Although single subclavian artery coverage may be feasible during thoracic aortic endografting, bilateral occlusion is not recommended because of the possible development of not only subclavian steal syndrome or upper limb ischemia but also spinal ischemia or stroke.[54] To reduce these complications, bilateral subclavian transposition or carotid-subclavian bypass procedures may need to be performed before endovascular treatment.[55] In some cases the left common carotid artery can also arise from the aortic arch very near the origins of the left subclavian and aberrant right subclavian artery. Transposition and revascularization of two or three arch vessels to provide an adequate neck for thoracic endografting may be necessary.[50]

The combination of endovascular and subclavian revascularization procedures significantly reduces the morbidity and mortality associated with repair of these aneurysms and, if effective and durable, could become standard treatment. Long-term outcomes of such therapy, however, are not established, and more importantly, it remains unclear whether covering the aortic origin of the aneurysm with an aortic endograft can effectively relieve compressive symptoms of the diverticulum and prevent rupture.

Endovascular Approach

Other endovascular techniques for the treatment of an aberrant right subclavian artery aneurysm have been described. Davidian and associates reported a case in which aneurysm exclusion was performed by intraluminal placement of an endograft confined to the aberrant vessel.[23] A similar approach has been used to seal the entry site of an aortic dissection originating from an aberrant right subclavian artery.[56] In this case, dissection involved the aortic arch and the distal aorta. A Wallgraft endograft was deployed in the aberrant right subclavian artery to seal the main intimal tear. Alternatively, Hoppe and coworkers chose to occlude an aberrant subclavian artery aneurysm with two Amplatzer septal occluders (AGA Medical, Golden Valley, MN) at the proximal and distal ends of the aneurysm, thereby preserving antegrade flow in the left common carotid, subclavian, and vertebral arteries while excluding the aneurysm.[57] The eventual need for revascularization of the right upper extremity could be assessed after the procedure.

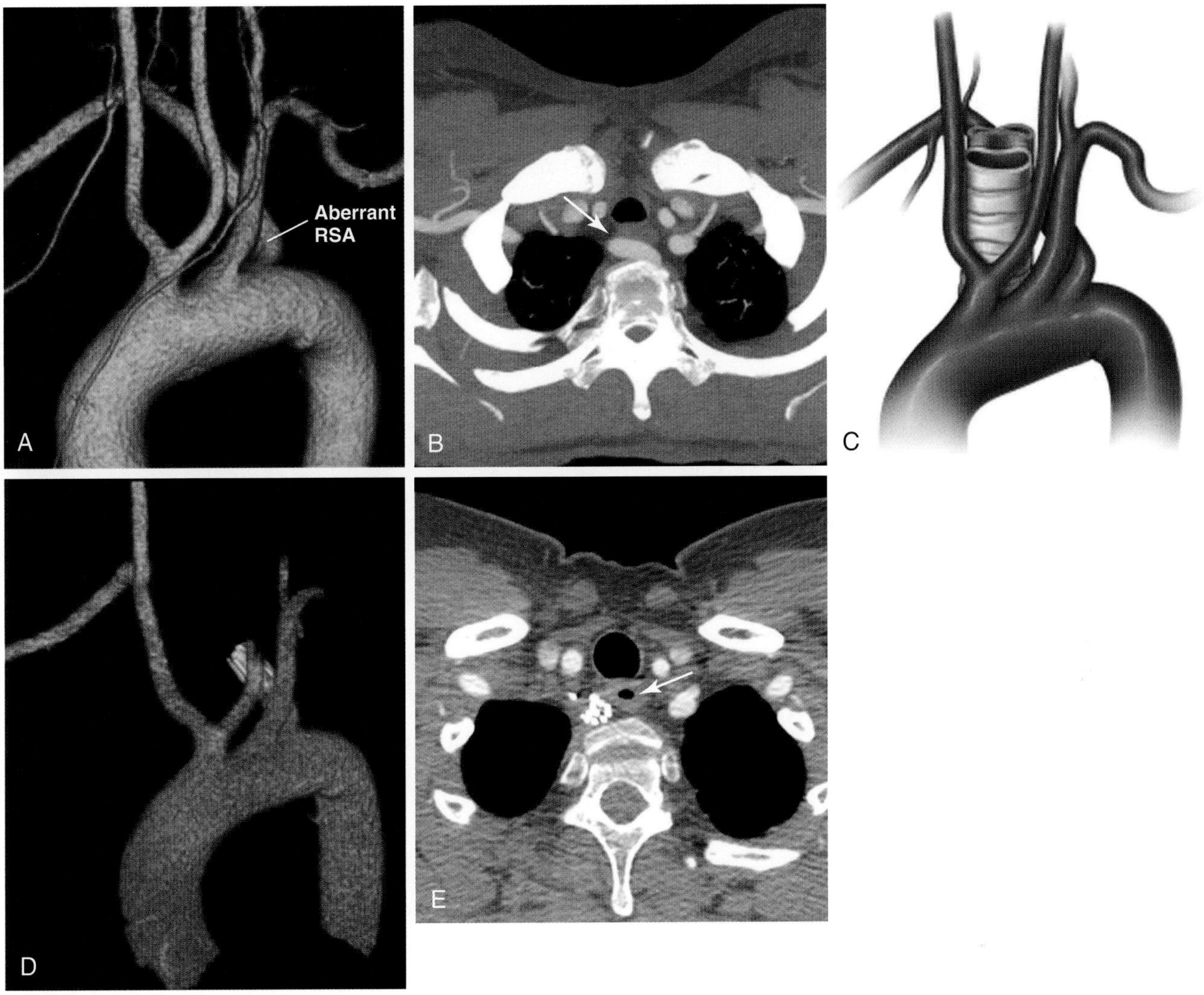

Figure 137-6 A, Three-dimensional CT angiography shows the aberrant right subclavian artery (RSA) arising from the distal arch and running posterior. **B,** An axial CT scan shows an aberrant right subclavian artery (*arrow*) compressing the esophagus through a posterior course. **C,** Illustration of the aberrant origin and course of the right subclavian artery. **D,** Postoperative CT angiography shows the right carotid-subclavian bypass and occlusive device within the aberrant subclavian artery, **E,** A postoperative axial CT scan at same level as in the preoperative CT shows decompression of the esophagus. *(From Shennib H, Diethrich EB. Novel approaches for the treatment of the aberrant right subclavian artery and its aneurysms. J Vasc Surg. 2008;47:1066.)*

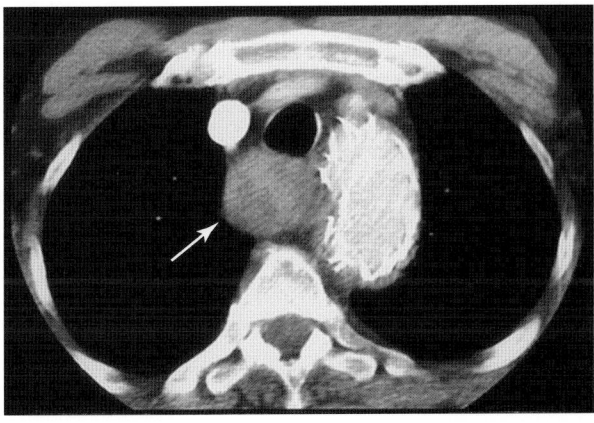

Figure 137-7 A contrast-enhanced CT scan performed 6 weeks after endovascular repair demonstrates a thrombosed right subclavian artery aneurysm (*arrow*). *(From Munneke GJ, Loosemore TM, Belli AM, et al. Aneurysm of an aberrant right subclavian artery successfully excluded by a thoracic aortic stent graft with supra-aortic bypass of three arch vessels. Cardiovasc Intervent Radiol. 2005;5:653.)*

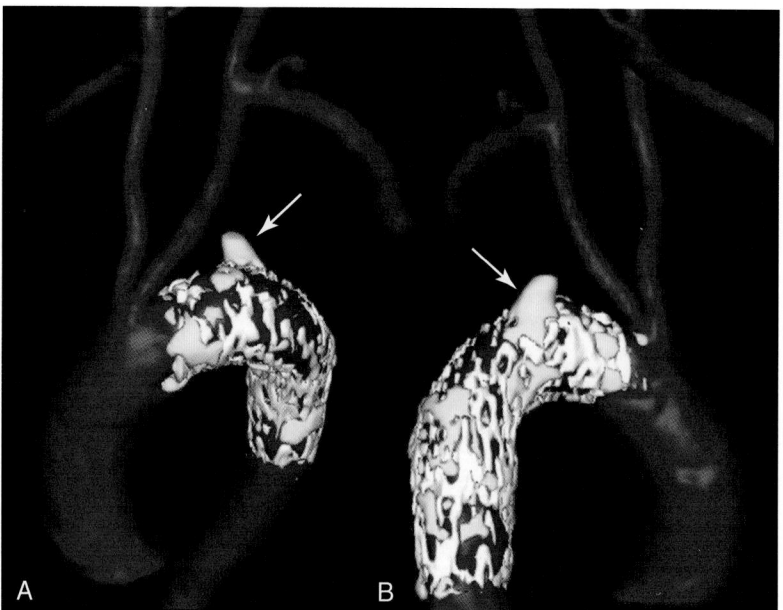

Figure 137-8 Anterior (**A**) and posterior (**B**) three-dimensional CT angiographic views after thoracic aortic endografting combined with bilateral subclavian-to-carotid transposition reveals thrombosis of the proximal aberrant right subclavian artery (*arrows*).

AXILLARY ARTERY ANEURYSMS

Etiology and Pathology

Axillary artery aneurysms are rare and usually caused by blunt or penetrating trauma.[58] Congenital axillary aneurysms have infrequently been reported.[59,60] Most post-traumatic axillary aneurysms typically occur in young men involved in athletic activities that are associated with repetitious, forceful extension of the upper extremity.[61,62] The mechanism of injury is probably related to repeated abduction and external rotation of the upper extremity with downward displacement of the humeral head. The circumflex humeral arteries that generally arise from the third portion of the axillary artery encircle the surgical neck of the humerus and create a tethering effect on the axillary artery, which is in a fixed position relative to the humerus. The repeated compression of the axillary artery can lead to intimal damage, thrombosis, and aneurysm formation of the circumflex humeral arteries or the axillary artery. Post-traumatic axillary artery aneurysms have primarily been reported in baseball pitchers, but such aneurysms should be suspected in any athlete with signs and symptoms suggestive of digital ischemia.

False Aneurysms

False aneurysms of the axillary artery usually occur with penetrating trauma (Fig. 137-9) but may also occur with blunt trauma in the form of humeral fractures and anterior dislocation of the shoulder.[63,64] In the latter instance, the mechanism may be avulsion of the tethered thoracoacromial, subscapular,

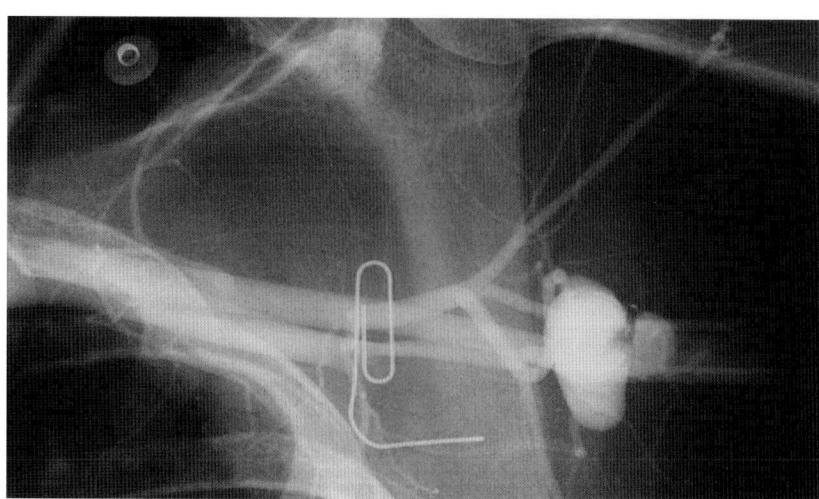

Figure 137-9 False aneurysm of the axillary artery as a result of a stab injury.

or circumflex humeral vessels at the time of dislocation. These aneurysms are often manifested late as chronic false aneurysms because the diagnosis is delayed. Given the excellent collateral circulation in this area, distal perfusion may be adequate despite extensive axillary artery injury. These aneurysms can lead to serious and permanent neurologic disability, however, because of hemorrhage into the axillary sheath and compression of the brachial plexus.

Arteriography should be considered in all cases of significant penetrating trauma to the shoulder or arm, blunt trauma with abnormal pulse examination, and blunt trauma with normal pulse examination but brachial plexus palsy because the likelihood of concomitant vascular injury is high in these cases. Duplex ultrasonography may also allow accurate diagnosis. Arteriography, CT angiography, or MR angiography should be performed in patients with blunt trauma to the shoulder or axilla with a normal neurovascular examination initially but with signs of brachial plexus neuropathy on follow-up. The presence of an expanding chronic false aneurysm should be suspected in such cases.[63]

Crutch-induced blunt trauma producing aneurysmal dilatation of the axillary artery usually occurs in older patients. These lesions were first described by Rob and Standeven[65] in 1956, with subsequent cases reported by Brooks and Fowler[66] and Abbott and Darling.[67] Pathologic examination of these aneurysms reveals markedly thickened walls and wrinkled, roughened intima. Instead of the typical changes of degenerative aneurysms, severe fragmentation of medial elastic fibers and marked periadventitial fibrosis suggestive of chronic trauma are present.[67] Thrombus, usually loosely adherent to the damaged intima, may become dislodged by further trauma from crutches and is the source of acute, chronic, or repetitive emboli. In many cases the aneurysm thromboses completely when symptoms begin. The most common initial complaints relate to upper extremity ischemia, and these aneurysms should be suspected when a patient who has been using crutches for a prolonged period has an absent brachial pulse.

Treatment

Open Surgery

Surgical treatment of axillary artery aneurysms is straightforward and involves resection of the aneurysm and interposition vein grafting. The brachial plexus and surrounding vascular structures should be protected during dissection of the aneurysm. Prosthetic reconstruction of the axillary artery may be performed when adequate vein conduits are not available. Autogenous vein grafts are preferred for upper extremity reconstructions because of improved patency rates with these conduits.[68] Occasionally, an adjacent segment of the axillary or brachial vein has been used to reconstruct the artery (Fig. 137-10A). This vein is extremely thin walled, however, and may itself become aneurysmal with time (Fig. 137-10B and C). For this reason a segment of saphenous vein is the conduit of choice. Perioperative morbidity is usually minimal. Long-term results are excellent, with a 100% graft patency rate in

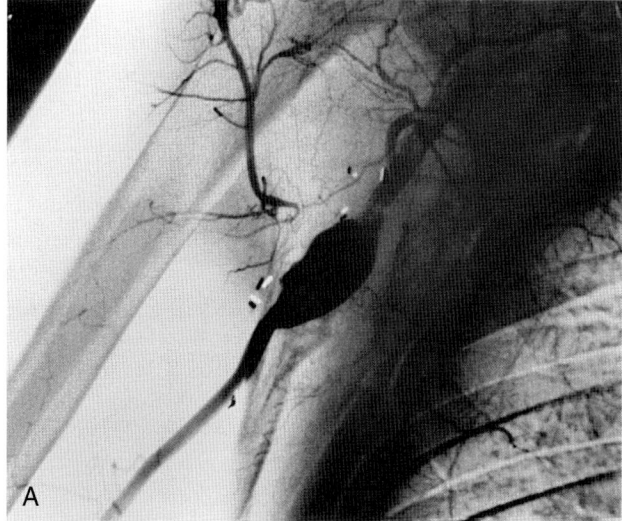

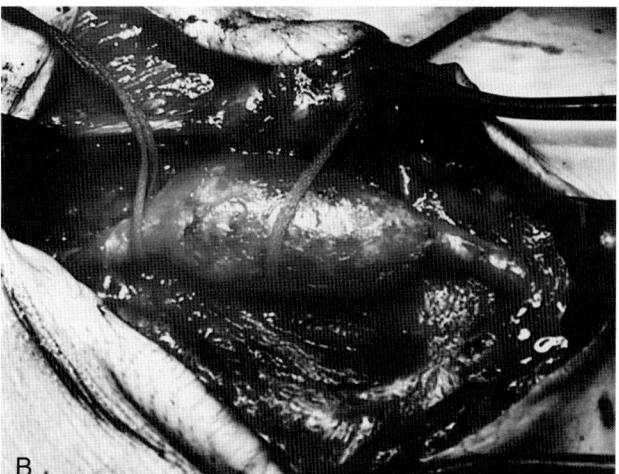

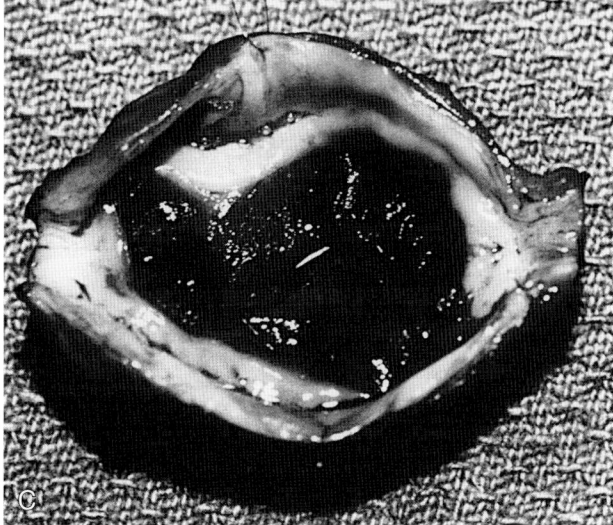

Figure 137-10 A, Aneurysmal dilatation of an interposition brachial vein graft used to reconstruct the axillary artery at the time of penetrating trauma 4 years previously. **B,** Operative dissection of the aneurysmal interposition brachial vein graft. **C,** Mural thrombus lining the aneurysmal interposition brachial vein graft.

one report at a mean follow-up period of 3.2 ± 0.41 years.[69] The initial symptoms usually resolve, except for paralysis related to concomitant nerve injury.

Endovascular Treatment

Endovascular repair of axillary artery aneurysms and pseudoaneurysms has been reported.[70] In most cases, endograft placement is sufficient to achieve complete exclusion of the aneurysm cavity. Occasionally, embolization of the avulsed branch vessel with microcoils to isolate the sac and prevent retrograde endoleak may be required.[71] Case series of endovascular treatment are small, however, with limited follow-up. Primary endograft patency rates of 100% up to 1 year have been reported. Endovascular repair of axillary aneurysms should be considered an alternative to surgical treatment in patients with major co-morbid conditions and high surgical risk.

■ BRACHIAL ARTERY ANEURYSMS

Etiology

Most aneurysms of the brachial artery are false aneurysms caused by repetitive trauma or iatrogenic complications. Occupational and recreational activities have also been implicated. In many instances, however, no specific cause can be identified and these aneurysms are classified as idiopathic.[72] Matas was the first to recognize a traumatic aneurysm of the brachial artery in a young laborer, which was repaired with his classic endoaneurysmorrhaphy technique.[73] Repetitive blunt trauma can lead to aneurysm formation by compression of the arterial wall and contusion of the arterial media. Penetrating trauma can also cause partial arterial wall laceration and pseudoaneurysm formation. Intravenous drug abuse is currently a frequent cause of infected pseudoaneurysms in the antecubital fossa.[74] Similarly, frequent arterial catheterization contributes to an increased incidence of false aneurysm formation. Other uncommon causes of true aneurysms of the brachial artery include congenital connective tissue abnormalities, such as those found in association with type IV Ehlers-Danlos syndrome,[75,76] Kawasaki's syndrome,[77] Buerger's disease,[78] Kaposi's sarcoma,[79] and cystic adventitial disease.[80] Another uncommon cause of brachial artery aneurysm is dissection.

Clinical Evaluation

Most patients with brachial artery aneurysms have symptoms of median nerve compression or local pain, given the close proximity of the two structures. Other symptoms include hand and digital ischemia as a result of thrombosis of the aneurysm or distal embolization (or both). The diagnosis of brachial artery aneurysm can be made on physical examination. The presence of an obvious pulsatile mass is also frequently recognized by patients. Duplex ultrasonography can establish the diagnosis. Upper extremity arteriography,

however, is usually necessary to delineate the extent of the aneurysm, assess sites of vascular occlusion in cases complicated by thromboembolism, and determine whether there are anatomic variants that might affect reconstruction. Simple iatrogenic brachial artery false aneurysms can generally be repaired without the need for angiography.

Treatment

Although brachial artery aneurysms have been safely monitored nonoperatively, it is impossible to predict which aneurysms are more likely to become symptomatic and lead to complications. Because of the high incidence of symptoms and complications and the minimal morbidity associated with operative treatment, aneurysm repair should be offered to all patients.

Open Surgical Treatment

Open surgical repair is the preferred method of treatment and can be performed under local, regional, or general anesthesia. It usually consists of resection with either patch or interposition vein grafting, resection and primary anastomosis, or in the case of iatrogenic false aneurysms, simple suture repair.

Endovascular Treatment

Although a few reports have described the use of endografts for repair of traumatic brachial artery injuries, only two case reports have described their use for the treatment of brachial artery aneurysms. In one case, a mycotic brachial pseudoaneurysm developed secondary to a wound infection with methicillin-resistant *Staphylococcus aureus* after emergency brachial artery bypass grafting with a segment of the great saphenous vein. This pseudoaneurysm was successfully treated with an endograft and antibiotics. In a second case, a brachial artery aneurysm was treated with an endograft in a patient who had sustained a gunshot wound to the left arm.[81] This patient had a complex open humeral fracture and brachial plexus injury initially treated by wound débridement, skin grafting, external fixation, and physical therapy. Two months after the initial injury, acute left arm pain and a pulsatile mass developed in the upper part of the patient's arm. Arteriography demonstrated nearly total transection of the proximal left brachial artery. The origin of the pseudoaneurysm was successfully excluded with an endograft.[82]

Iatrogenic Injury

Clinical Findings

Brachial artery pseudoaneurysms secondary to access injuries during peripheral angiography, cardiac catheterization, or endovascular interventions are common indications for upper extremity arterial repair.[83] Brachial artery thrombosis, however, is more frequent and occurs in 1% to 7% of cases.[84-87] Although percutaneous brachial access for peripheral and cardiac angiography or interventions has largely replaced brachial artery cutdown, the frequency of brachial artery pseudoaneurysm formation continues to be low (0.3% in one large series[84]) and not different from pseudoaneurysm rates with the femoral artery approach.[83] Distal (near antecubital) access to the brachial artery is recommended because the artery is less mobile and easier to puncture at this point than more proximally and because improved compression against the distal end of the humerus is possible here.[85] The presence of a pseudoaneurysm may be suggested by a mass at the puncture site, evidence of distal occlusion or embolization, or neurologic complications related to compression. The diagnosis can usually be made with duplex ultrasonography.

Treatment

Nonoperative treatment of brachial artery pseudoaneurysms can be considered when they are small, asymptomatic, and likely to thrombose spontaneously. In most instances, however, symptomatic iatrogenic brachial artery pseudoaneurysms should be repaired surgically under local or regional anesthesia because it is difficult to predict which ones will continue to expand and require more difficult repair later. Direct suture repair with evacuation of the hematoma is generally sufficient. Though reported, injection of thrombin into pseudoaneurysms of the brachial artery may be considered less favorable because the superficial location of the vessel is usually associated with pseudoaneurysms with relatively short necks.[88,89] If deemed appropriate, small-gauge needles can be used and lesser amounts of thrombin than typically used in the femoral artery may be injected in the brachial artery pseudoaneurysm under duplex ultrasound guidance.

SELECTED KEY REFERENCES

Chambers CM, Curci JA. Treatment of nonaortic aneurysms in the endograft era: aneurysms of the innominate and subclavian arteries. *Semin Vasc Surg.* 2005;4:184.

Review article about endovascular repair techniques for innominate and subclavian artery aneurysms.

Gray RJ, Stone WM, Fowl RJ, Cherry KJ, Bower TC. Management of true aneurysms distal to the axillary artery. *J Vasc Surg.* 1998;4:606.
Case series describing the clinical findings and management of brachial and distal upper extremity artery aneurysms.

Kieffer E, Bahnini A, Koskas F. Aberrant subclavian artery: surgical treatment in thirty-three adult patients. *J Vasc Surg.* 1994;1:100.
Observational study on open repair of aberrant right subclavian artery aneurysms.

Kieffer E, Chiche L, Koskas F, Bahnini A. Aneurysms of the innominate artery: surgical treatment of 27 patients. *J Vasc Surg.* 2001;2:222.
Largest series about the clinical manifestations and open repair of innominate artery aneurysms.

Munneke GJ, Loosemore TM, Belli AM, Thompson MM, Morgan RA. Aneurysm of an aberrant right subclavian artery successfully excluded by a thoracic aortic stent graft with supra-aortic bypass of three arch vessels. *Cardiovasc Intervent Radiol.* 2005;5:653.
Case report describing the alternatives for endovascular repair of aberrant right subclavian artery aneurysms.

Pairolero PC, Walls JT, Payne WS, Hollier LH, Fairbairn JF. Subclavian-axillary artery aneurysms. *Surgery.* 1981;4:757.
Observational study on open repair of subclavian artery aneurysms.

Sullivan TM, Bacharach JM, Perl J, Gray B. Endovascular management of unusual aneurysms of the axillary and subclavian arteries. *J Endovasc Surg.* 1996;4:389.
Observational study about endovascular repair of axillary and subclavian artery aneurysms.

REFERENCES

The reference list can be found on the companion Expert Consult Web site at *www.expertconsult.com.*

Section **17** Arterial Aneurysms

CHAPTER 138

Splanchnic Artery Aneurysms

Caron B. Rockman and Thomas S. Maldonado

Aneurysms of the splanchnic arteries are a relatively rare but clinically important vascular condition. These interesting lesions have been recognized for more than 200 years.[1,2] The first successful operation for a splanchnic aneurysm, surgical repair of a mycotic aneurysm of the superior mesenteric artery (SMA), was reported by DeBakey and Cooley in 1953.[3] Nonetheless, the natural history of splanchnic aneurysms and their potential for rupture or other complications are relatively poorly defined because of their overall scarcity. The great majority of reports in the literature are accounts of only one or two cases. Impressive institutional case series have been documented but rarely consist of more than a compilation of several dozen cases. The recent increase in the number of articles in the literature involving splanchnic aneurysms is mainly related to a rise in the use of novel and varied catheter-based techniques for their treatment. Even though much valuable information may be gained from reading these individual reports, they may be inherently predisposed toward a representation of unusual manifestations and successful outcomes. However, it is clear even from these numerous case reports that a significant proportion of splanchnic artery aneurysms come to medical attention because of rupture; therefore, an aggressive approach to their diagnosis and management certainly seems warranted.

PREVALENCE AND ETIOLOGY

Splanchnic artery aneurysms encompass intra-abdominal aneurysms that are not part of the aortoiliac system and include aneurysms of the celiac artery, the superior and inferior mesenteric arteries, and their branches (see Chapter 145: Renovascular Disease: Aneurysms and Arteriovenous Fistulae). Of all intra-abdominal aneurysms, only approximately 5% affect the splanchnic arteries.[4] The prevalence of splanchnic artery aneurysms in the general population has been estimated at 0.1% to 2%.[5] As of 2002, it was estimated that there were slightly more than 3000 cases reported in the literature.[6] The frequency of the anatomic distribution of aneurysms of the splanchnic vessels is estimated to be the following: aneurysms of the splenic artery, 60% (Fig. 138-1); hepatic artery, 20%; SMA, 6%; celiac artery, 4%; gastric and gastroepiploic arteries, 4%; jejunal, ileal, and colic arteries, 3%; pancreaticoduodenal and pancreatic arteries, 2%; gastroduodenal artery (GDA), 1.5%; and inferior mesenteric artery, less than 1%.[7] As many as a third of splanchnic artery aneurysms may be associated with other coexisting nonsplanchnic aneurysms.

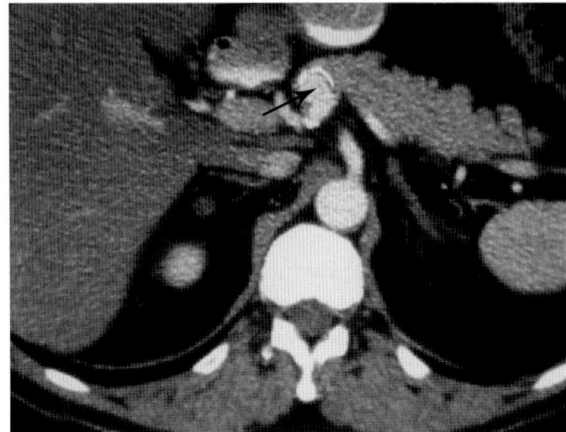

Figure 138-1 Splenic artery aneurysm. A calcified proximal splenic artery aneurysm is noted adjacent to the pancreas on computed tomography (*arrow*).

In recent years, several authors have reported an increased proportion of hepatic artery aneurysms (HAAs) that has surpassed the prevalence of splenic artery aneurysms (SPAAs) in some cases. This increase is thought to be secondary to an increasing number of hepatic and intrahepatic pseudoaneurysms related to either trauma or the escalating number of interventional procedures related to biliary disease.[8,9]

The underlying causes and pathophysiologies associated with these lesions are diverse, and there is a wide spectrum of anatomic locations within the splanchnic vessels. Approximately a third of splanchnic artery aneurysms may be associated with other aneurysmal disease, including disease in the distribution of the thoracic aorta, abdominal aorta, renal arteries, iliac arteries, lower extremity arteries, and intracranial arteries, in decreasing order of frequency.[10] Splanchnic artery aneurysms include both true aneurysms and false aneurysms, or pseudoaneurysms. Many true splanchnic artery aneurysms are degenerative or atherosclerotic, with histologic specimens demonstrating reduced smooth muscle, disruption of elastic fibers, and deficiency of the arterial media.[8] Other common causes associated with true splanchnic artery aneurysms include fibromuscular dysplasia, collagen vascular diseases, inflammatory conditions, and other rare inherited illnesses such as Ehlers-Danlos syndrome.[11] In contrast to the causes of true aneurysms of the splanchnic vessels, splanchnic artery pseudoaneurysms are most commonly related to trauma, iatrogenic injury, local inflammatory processes, or infection.

RUPTURE RISK

The clinical significance of splanchnic artery aneurysms is mainly related to their potential for rupture and the extreme challenge of emergency diagnosis and treatment of these uncommon aneurysms once rupture has occurred. Nearly a fourth of splanchnic artery aneurysms reported in the literature have initially been evaluated for rupture, and the reported mortality rate of these diagnosed ruptures is at least 10% and likely to be much higher.[7,10] The mortality reported after ruptured celiac artery aneurysms (CAAs) and ruptured SPAAs in pregnant women approaches 100%. However, because of the increased use of sophisticated forms of intra-abdominal imaging, including magnetic resonance imaging and angiography (MRI, MRA) and computed tomography scans and angiography (CT, CTA), occult splanchnic artery aneurysms are being diagnosed with increased frequency (Fig. 138-2). These detailed imaging studies are allowing improved awareness of asymptomatic lesions by vascular surgeons and enhanced potential for preoperative or preprocedural planning and elective treatment of these aneurysms. Improvements in endovascular therapies have also led to an enhanced ability to treat these often anatomically complex lesions with a large variety of individualized and precise catheter-based therapies.

Although precise rates of rupture are difficult to characterize, reported figures of the risk for rupture are 20% to 44% for HAAs, 13% for CAAs, and 90% for gastric artery aneurysms (GAAs) and gastroepiploic artery aneurysms (GEAAs).[12-14] SPAAs are thought to have a particular tendency for rupture, especially during the third trimester of pregnancy.[15] It is difficult to precisely characterize which factors in an individual aneurysm will predispose to rupture. Splanchnic artery pseudoaneurysms certainly have a higher rupture potential than true aneurysms do. Although larger size would certainly seem to imply a higher chance for rupture, very small splanchnic aneurysms can rupture as well, particularly in the jejunal, ileal, or colic artery distribution. There is no firm evidence that calcification in a splanchnic artery aneurysm protects against rupture. Splanchnic artery aneurysms can rupture into the peritoneal cavity, retroperitoneal space, gastrointestinal tract, or biliary tract. Free rupture into the peritoneal cavity resulting in hemoperitoneum is often termed "abdominal apoplexy." Rupture of splanchnic artery aneurysms may also be manifested as life-threatening gastrointestinal hemorrhage.

GENERAL TREATMENT PRINCIPLES

Traditionally, splanchnic artery aneurysms were managed by either close serial observation or open surgical repair, depending on their size, the underlying clinical scenario, and the anatomic location. Surgical options include aneurysm exclusion or ligation, excision, revascularization, or any combination of these therapies, depending on the location of the lesion and the collateral vascular anatomy. The development of endovascular techniques now provides clinicians with an alternative method of treatment that is generally associated with low morbidity and recurrence rates. General principles are discussed in this section, whereas details on specific aneurysm types are discussed later.

Elective Repair

Though not directed by randomized prospective trials, general principles of management of splanchnic artery aneurysms do exist. Because of their potential for rupture, nearly all splanchnic artery pseudoaneurysms and many true aneurysms warrant intervention. Indications for intervention in true aneurysms are generally related to the size of the aneurysm or associated symptomatology. Anecdotally, many asymptomatic small splanchnic aneurysms can be managed conservatively by serial observation with good outcomes. When required, treatment can usually be accomplished by either open surgical or endovascular approaches. The goal of treatment is to prevent aneurysm expansion and potential rupture by excluding it from the arterial circulation while maintaining necessary distal or collateral bed perfusion. Depending on the location of the aneurysm, this can be accomplished in a variety of ways. In areas of the splanchnic circulation with an abundance of collateral flow, such as the splenic artery, proximal and distal ligation of the aneurysm segment is a viable surgical option. This can also be accomplished by endovascular isolation of the aneurysmal segment, either by placement of a stent-graft or by coil embolization of the proximal and distal arterial segments. Successful endovascular embolization of even frankly ruptured splanchnic aneurysms has been reported.[16]

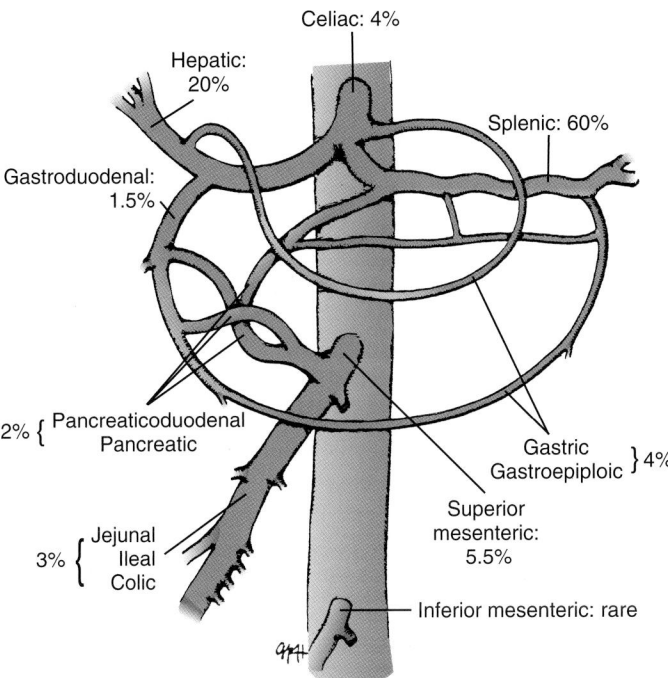

Figure 138-2 Relative incidence of aneurysms affecting the arteries of the splanchnic circulation as reported in the literature.

Emergency Repair

For ruptured splanchnic artery aneurysms discovered at laparotomy, ligation of the aneurysm without vascular reconstruction is the preferred treatment when feasible. Patients with ruptured SPAAs are usually treated with concomitant splenectomy. Ligation without revascularization can generally be performed for common HAAs proximal to a normal GDA and is preferred for emergency treatment of GAAs, GEAAs, and pancreaticoduodenal artery aneurysms (PDAAs).[1,10] Emergency surgical treatment of mesenteric branch arterial aneurysms may occasionally require concomitant intestinal resection for bowel ischemia or infarction. Percutaneous treatment is a viable option for ruptured splanchnic aneurysms discovered preoperatively by CT, MRI, or arteriography. In most reported series of splanchnic aneurysms, no consistent risk factors predisposing to rupture were identified. Although large size would certainly imply an increased potential for rupture, even very small splanchnic artery aneurysms have occasionally been manifested as life-threatening hemorrhage secondary to rupture.[10] Therefore, size criteria as an indication for intervention are not always specifically defined.

Special Considerations for Associated Conditions

Knowledge of the association of unusual aneurysms in the setting of rare conditions is important. In addition to many collagen vascular diseases and inflammatory conditions, splanchnic aneurysms can occur in conjunction with von Recklinghausen's disease.[17] Multiple splanchnic aneurysms are usually associated with connective tissue disease, systemic arteritis, or endocarditis with resultant diffuse septic embolization.[9,18] They have also been associated with excessive oral amphetamine use.

Periarteritis Nodosa

Two associated medical conditions deserve particular mention. Periarteritis nodosa is a progressive inflammatory disease of small and medium-sized arteries.[19] It is considered to be a type of systemic necrotizing vasculitis. Patients with this illness commonly have small multiple aneurysm of the mesenteric, hepatic, and renal arteries, and spontaneous rupture can occur. If rupture does occur, ligation of the bleeding vessel is usually adequate treatment of small aneurysms of the distal splanchnic arterial tree. When intact asymptomatic aneurysms are diagnosed in patients with periarteritis nodosa, initial treatment with immunosuppressive or cytotoxic agents is appropriate. Actual regression of these aneurysms after pharmacologic management is well documented.[20]

Ehlers-Danlos Syndrome

Patients with the inherited connective tissue disorder Ehlers-Danlos syndrome are susceptible to both aneurysm formation and spontaneous rupture of nonaneurysmal vessels because of their fragility.[4] Splanchnic aneurysms reported in patients with Ehlers-Danlos syndrome appear to be equally distributed among the hepatic, splenic, renal, and celiac arteries. Surgical repair in these patients is exceedingly difficult, and ligation is preferable to vascular reconstruction when possible. Endovascular techniques may have a significant advantage in these patients, although arteriography itself has been noted to be associated with high morbidity (see also Chapter 140: Aneurysms Caused by Connective Tissue Abnormalities).[21]

■ SURGICAL AND ENDOVASCULAR TECHNIQUES

Preoperative imaging is critical in determining whether the aneurysm and arterial anatomy favor open surgery or endovascular intervention. Although angiography remains the imaging "gold standard" and allows concomitant endovascular interventions, less invasive imaging such as MRA and CTA play an equal and arguably superior role in evaluating patients with splanchnic artery aneurysms. MRA and CTA postprocessing using volume-rendering techniques allows excellent three-dimensional reconstruction of the aneurysm in relation to its afferent and efferent branches, whereas axial images enable one to visualize mural thrombus that may not be apparent on conventional angiography. This knowledge is critical for determining proper landing zones in the proximal and distal nonaneurysmal segments of the artery for stent-grafts, as well as for determining whether the neck morphology is adequate for coil embolization.

Open Surgery

Treatment of splanchnic artery aneurysms has evolved significantly over the past few decades. Conventional open surgical repair can include simple ligation, aneurysmorrhaphy with preservation of end-organ perfusion, or aneurysmectomy and revascularization via bypass. The open surgical approach is durable and thus may not require as vigilant follow-up as the endovascular approach. Moreover, open surgical repair may allow treatment of associated conditions such as pancreatic pseudocysts, as well as direct visualization to assess end-organ ischemia, such as intestinal viability when applicable. Simple ligation of the proximal and distal branches is often best when performed in cases of hemodynamic instability and rupture. However, this can be done safely only in the presence of adequate collateral flow to the distal vascular bed. For example, the splenic artery can usually be ligated without consequence because of the rich collateral supply to the spleen provided by the short gastric arteries and pancreaticoduodenal arcade.[7] The celiac trunk, SMA, and common hepatic artery may also be ligated, provided that collateral flow exists via the pancreaticoduodenal artery and GDA. Simple ligation is not possible, however, when collateral flow is absent or inadequate. Aneurysms of the proper hepatic artery, celiac artery, and SMA most often require ligation or resection (or both) with concomitant revascularization.

The open surgical approach can be accomplished under general anesthesia via a midline, transverse, or bilateral subcostal incision. Alternatively, laparoscopic repair may offer a minimally invasive approach, perhaps best suited for treating SPAAs.[22,23] An Endo-GIA stapler (Autosuture, Norwalk, CT) can be used to transect the splenic artery proximal and distal to the aneurysm (or across the base of a saccular aneurysm if possible). Even though the laparoscopic technique has been touted as resulting in less postoperative pain and shorter hospital stay, it should be reserved for hemodynamically stable patients who do not have evidence of rupture. In addition, laparoscopic repair is relatively contraindicated in a pregnant patient with an asymptomatic SPAA because of the potential risk for hypercapnia and acidosis in the patient and fetus.[23]

Endovascular Treatment

The evolution of endovascular therapies has provided a minimally invasive approach to treating splanchnic artery aneurysms and has some clear benefits such as shorter hospital stay and quicker recovery. Endovascular interventions may also be preferable to open surgery in certain clinical scenarios. In particular, a hostile abdomen, such as in the setting of pancreatitis-related splenic artery pseudoaneurysms or abdominal sepsis, and intraparenchymal aneurysms are better served with an endovascular approach. Furthermore, patients with severe co-morbid conditions that are prohibitive for open surgery may also be ideal candidates for endovascular interventions. The endovascular approach has its own unique set of complications and concerns, however, including access-related injuries, contrast-induced toxicity and anaphylaxis, arterial dissection and thrombosis, and embolization of nontarget structures. The goal of all endovascular treatment is to isolate the aneurysm from the arterial circulation, which can be done in a number of ways, such as coil embolization, placement of a covered stent-graft, and injection of thrombin, "glue," or particles. When considering an endovascular approach, one must take into consideration the vessel involved, the underlying etiology, and the status of the end organ. Furthermore, aneurysm morphology and location can often dictate the optimal type of endovascular approach.

Embolization

Coil embolization techniques are often used to "trap'" the aneurysm between coils placed proximally and distally within the normal part of the parent artery. This technique is well suited for aneurysms in larger arteries but requires adequate collateral circulation to the end organ. SPAAs can often be excluded from the circulation in this way by coil embolization of first the distal and then the proximal segment of the parent artery. For smaller arteries, coils or particles placed in distal branches can be used successfully.[24,25] Indeed, endovascular embolization of intraparenchymal SPAAs or HAAs offers a significant advantage over open surgical approaches, where definitive surgical treatment may require sacrificing the spleen or part of the liver. Small-caliber microcatheters are used to achieve superselective catheterization in small third- and fourth-order intraparenchymal vessels. Coaxial microcatheters are positioned in the afferent artery, and embolizing material (thrombin or cyanoacrylate "glue") is injected into the sac. This allows minimal parenchymal ischemia and maximal organ preservation of the liver, spleen, or kidney.[26]

Aneurysm morphology often dictates the preferred type of endovascular treatment. Saccular aneurysms can be embolized with coils, thrombin, or both, particularly if they have a narrow neck.[27,28] Aneurysms with wider necks may require stent-assisted embolization. This technique uses a stent to cage the aneurysm and permits coils to be delivered into the sac through the interstices of the stent. Glue or thrombin can also be used to facilitate thrombosis of the sac.

Covered Stent-Grafts

Covered stent-grafts are ideal for treating splanchnic aneurysms when flow to the end organ via the parent artery must be preserved. They are best suited for larger arteries and may be limited by bulky, stiff delivery systems, which often preclude placement of the covered stent in more distal tortuous branches. Covered stent-grafts also risk compromising secondary or tertiary vessels and should not generally be used to treat aneurysms that involve a branch point. Finally, self-expanding stent-grafts rely on a similar proximal and distal target vessel caliber to ensure a proper seal. Oversizing of these devices can result in endoleak or in-stent thrombosis. In patients with size discrepancies in seal zone diameters, balloon-expandable stent-grafts offer a subtle advantage over self-expanding stents. Balloon-expandable stent-grafts can be dilated proximally (or distally if needed) to achieve a funneled or tapered configuration that may accommodate small differences in vessel caliber. Nevertheless, aneurysms with large discrepancies in proximal and distal diameter are probably not well suited for treatment with balloon-expandable stent-grafts and should be considered for coil embolization or open repair.

Despite these limitations, covered stent-grafts are an important adjunct to the endovascular armamentarium for treating splanchnic artery aneurysms, and their use is likely to increase with the development of lower profile, more flexible devices.[29-33] A significant advantage of stent-grafts over embolization techniques is that follow-up imaging is not confounded by artifact from radiopaque coils or glue; most liquid adhesive embolic materials require dilution with a contrast agent to be used under fluoroscopic guidance. This can result in significant artifact on subsequent surveillance imaging studies. Furthermore, sac size may be more meaningful when monitored on postprocedural imaging if a stent-graft is used to exclude the aneurysm. Coils and glue act as a space-occupying cast and therefore prevent shrinkage of the aneurysm sac, thus making follow-up imaging relevant only in the event of sac growth. Indeed, Rossi and colleagues described four cases of splanchnic artery aneurysms successfully treated with stent-grafts and demonstrated complete exclusion and sac shrinkage in all the patients available for follow-up at 16 to 24 months.[31]

SPECIFIC SPLANCHNIC ANEURYSMS

Splenic Artery Aneurysms

Prevalence and Epidemiology

SPAAs are the most common of the splanchnic artery aneurysms and account for as many as 60% of all reported splanchnic aneurysms. They are recognized for their significant potential to rupture. Despite their relatively high prevalence in comparison to other splanchnic aneurysms, there are few large series in the literature. The prevalence of the lesions in the general population is low. A large general autopsy study estimated their overall incidence to be 0.01%,[34] whereas more specific examination of the splenic arteries in an autopsy study of patients older than 60 years revealed an incidence of 10%.[35] The prevalence of incidentally noted aneurysmal changes in the splenic artery on arteriographic studies was reported to be 0.78%, and such changes have been found incidentally in 0.1% to 10% of autopsies.[7] In contrast to routine atherosclerotic or degenerative aneurysmal disease, SPAAs are found much more commonly in women than men at an approximate ratio of 4:1.[7,15] They are also noted to occur in younger patients at a mean age of 52 years.[15,36]

SPAAs are usually saccular and less than 2 cm in diameter, with the majority being located in the mid or distal splenic artery or at bifurcation points.[15,18] Giant SPAAs with diameters larger than 10 cm have been reported, and in contrast to smaller SPAAs, these lesions appear to be more common in men.[37]

Pathogenesis and Risk Factors

The most common clinical risk factors reported in association with SPAAs are female gender, a history of multiple pregnancies, and portal hypertension.[15,38] In one reported series, it was noted that 80% of patients with SPAAs were women who had an average of 4.5 pregnancies.[39] Other authors have reported that nearly 50% of women with SPAAs had had more than six pregnancies.[18,40] Portal hypertension may be present in as many as a quarter of patients with SPAAs,[41] and approximately 10% of patients awaiting liver transplantation may have splenic artery lesions.[42] SPAAs have also been noted to occur concomitantly with less common conditions, including polyarteritis nodosa, systemic lupus erythematosus,[15,43] and anomalous origin of the splenic artery.[15,44,45] Blunt splenic trauma and pancreatitis have frequently been reported in association with splenic artery pseudoaneurysms, and trauma-related pseudoaneurysms of the splenic artery are often being managed with endovascular techniques. The increased frequency of these reports may be a result of the overall recent trend toward nonoperative management of blunt splenic injuries.[46]

Local hemodynamic aspects, hypertension, hormonal factors, and medial degeneration have all been mentioned as causative factors in the development of SPAAs.[39] During pregnancy, hemodynamic and physiologic changes consisting of increased blood volume, increased cardiac output, and portal congestion are thought to be related to an increase in splenic artery flow, which contributes to aneurysm formation.[16] Hormonal changes during pregnancy may be associated with impaired elastin formation and degeneration of the internal elastic lamina. In addition to the effects of estrogen and progesterone, a late-pregnancy hormone called relaxin may alter the elasticity of the arterial wall.[47] Relaxin is also responsible for the elasticity of the symphysis pubis to facilitate delivery. However, the splenic artery appears to be more susceptible to these changes than other vessels.[24]

Histologic changes noted on microscopic examination of SPAAs have included typical atherosclerotic changes, calcifications, intimal hyperplasia, arterial dysplasia, fibromuscular dysplasia, and cystic medial degeneration.[15,34,48]

Clinical Findings and Diagnosis

Before the 1980s it was reported that approximately 10% or more of SPAAs were ruptured at the time of diagnosis.[15,40,49] Currently, most SPAAs are found incidentally during abdominal imaging performed for other unrelated symptoms. A classic calcified ring may be noted in the left upper quadrant on a plain x-ray film of the abdomen (Fig. 138-3). Although a small proportion of patients may have an abdominal bruit, the majority of physical examinations are normal in patients with asymptomatic lesions. Rare large aneurysms may produce vague abdominal pain or symptoms related to compression of adjacent structures, but most patients with significant pain are experiencing rupture or acute aneurysm expansion. When rupture occurs, patients usually complain of acute left-sided abdominal pain. Shock, abdominal distention, and death can result from free intraperitoneal rupture of an SPAA.[34]

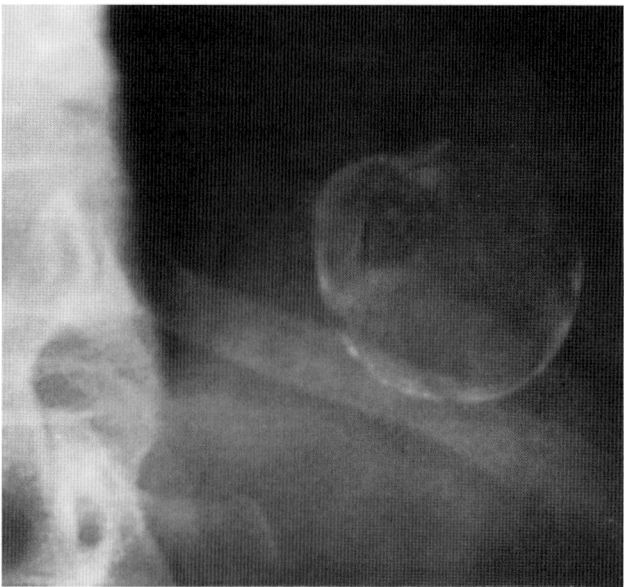

Figure 138-3 Splenic artery aneurysm. The curvilinear, signet ring–like calcifications in the left upper quadrant are characteristic of the radiologic appearance of splenic artery aneurysms on plain radiographs.

However, an initially contained rupture into the lesser sac may occur and provide a window of opportunity for treatment if the proper diagnosis is made. This "double-rupture" phenomenon may be seen in 20% to 30% of cases and allows an important chance for diagnosis and treatment before free intraperitoneal rupture, which usually occurs within 48 hours.[8,48,49] In addition to lesser sac or peritoneal cavity rupture, SPAAs may occasionally rupture into adjacent structures, including the gastrointestinal tract, pancreatic ducts, or splenic vein.[1,50-52] Splenic artery pseudoaneurysms secondary to pancreatitis may rupture into a pancreatic pseudocyst[46] or into the pancreatic duct, a condition called hemosuccus pancreaticus.[53]

The overall mortality of ruptured SPAAs is as high as 25%.[18,49] Pregnancy may be associated with 20% to 50% of all ruptures.[36,39] The association of SPAA and pregnancy is well documented. Rupture of an SPAA during pregnancy, which usually occurs during the third trimester, has devastating maternal and fetal mortality rates of 80% and 90%, respectively.[54,55] The frequent occurrence of rupture in the third trimester and the clinical findings of abdominal pain and shock often lead to the understandable misdiagnosis of the situation as an obstetric emergency. Portal hypertension may be associated with an additional 20% of SPAA ruptures.[36,39]

Indications and Technique for Treatment

SPAAs that have ruptured or are symptomatic require urgent treatment. Additionally, aneurysms in pregnant women or those of childbearing age also absolutely warrant treatment. Less stringent indications for treatment include aneurysms that are noted to be enlarging or those greater than 2 cm in diameter, but these size criteria are not absolute. Several authors have recommended consideration of treatment in patients with portal hypertension or in candidates for liver transplantation.[8] Clearly, the age and medical condition of the patient also play a role in determining whether intervention is an option. A large review of SPAAs from the Mayo Clinic involving 207 patients included a report of more than 150 who were treated nonsurgically and observed for a mean period of 75 months.[56] The conservatively managed SPAAs ranged from 0.8 to 5 cm in diameter. Aneurysm enlargement was noted in 10% of cases; however, there were no cases of aneurysm rupture or complications related to conservative management.[56] Despite the generally favorable outcome of conservatively managed SPAAs in this particular series, it is clear that patients treated initially by surveillance were carefully selected and rigorously monitored. In addition to the particular clinical scenarios delineated earlier that clearly warrant treatment of SPAAs, most vascular surgeons would consider appropriate elective intervention for asymptomatic patients with lesions whose diameter is greater than 2 cm when the procedural risk is thought to be appropriately low. If one estimates the incidence of rupture to be 2% with a mortality of at least 25% when rupture has occurred, operative mortality rates should be less than 0.5% to justify elective surgical therapy, in one author's opinion.[18]

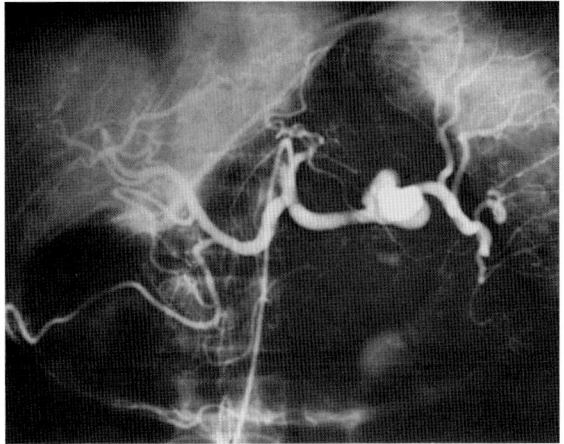

Figure 138-4 Splenic artery aneurysm. Splanchnic angiography reveals a mid–splenic artery aneurysm.

Traditional surgical management of SPAAs includes proximal and distal ligation or aneurysmectomy (or both) for lesions in the proximal or middle portion of the splenic artery (Fig. 138-4). Revascularization of the distal splenic artery is not generally warranted because collateral flow to the spleen is maintained by the short gastric arteries (Fig. 138-5). For more distal lesions adjacent to the splenic hilum, splenectomy has been the most commonly performed operation. This is required when the aneurysm involves intrasplenic branches

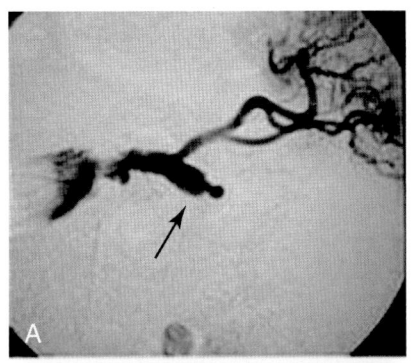

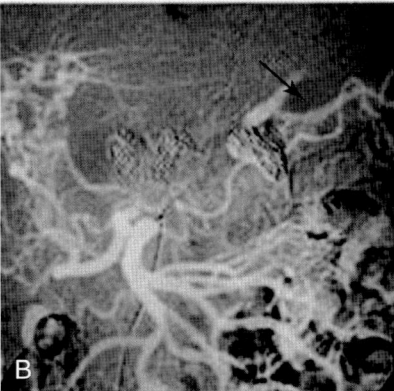

Figure 138-5 Successful coil embolization of another splenic artery aneurysm, this time located in the proximal splenic artery. **A,** The *arrow* denotes a saccular aneurysm of the proximal splenic artery. **B,** Postprocedure selective injection of the superior mesenteric artery reveals filling of the distal splenic artery (*arrow*) via collaterals.

Section **17** Arterial Aneurysms

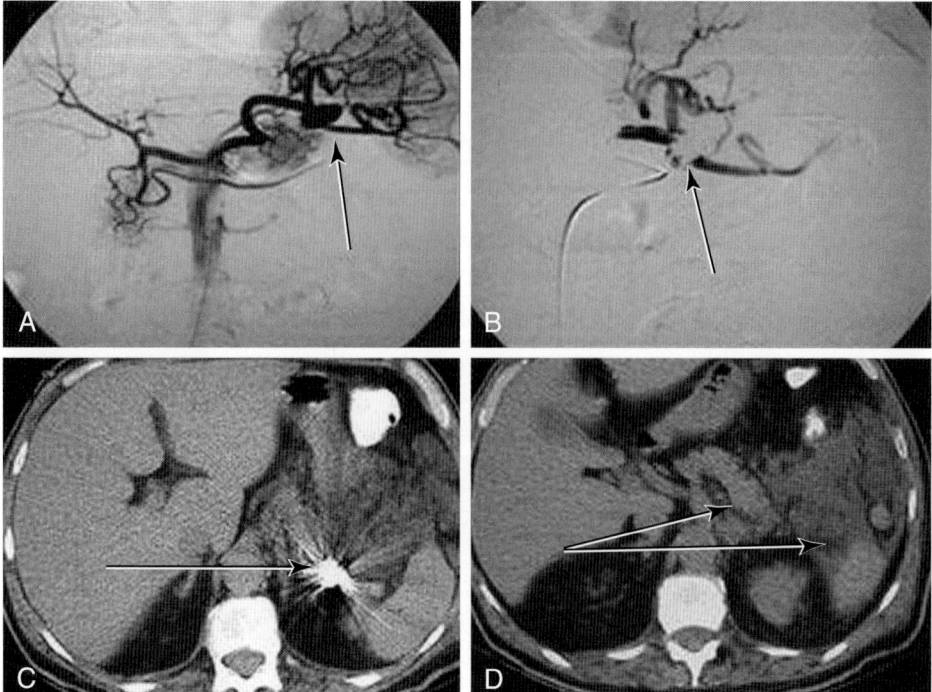

Figure 138-6 Coil embolization of a distal splenic artery aneurysm. **A,** Saccular aneurysm of the splenic artery (*arrow*). **B,** Successful coil embolization with no flow in the aneurysm (*arrow*). **C,** Artifact on CT secondary to coils (*arrow*). **D,** Postembolization CT scan revealing a splenic infarct and pancreatitis (*arrows*).

within the splenic parenchyma. Distal pancreatectomy may occasionally be warranted for the treatment of these distal lesions as well.[7,8,56] Laparoscopic repair of SPAAs by clipping or exclusion has been reported; intraoperative ultrasonography is believed to be an important adjunct to this procedure.[23] Laparoscopic occlusion combined with coil embolization has been proposed as a treatment method for aberrant SPAAs located in the retropancreatic position, for which traditional surgical exposure would be exceedingly difficult.[57]

Endovascular exclusion of SPAAs has been used more recently with general success. Treatment options include coil embolization of the splenic artery both proximal and distal to the aneurysm itself, thereby effectively "trapping" the lesion. Other options for a saccular-type aneurysm include embolization of the aneurysm sac with coils or cyanoacrylate glue (or both) or occlusion of the lesion with percutaneous or open thrombin injection.[58] In addition, stent-grafting has been performed, particularly for saccular lesions of the mid splenic artery. There has been some concern regarding splenic infarction and pancreatitis when embolization of very distal splenic artery lesions has been performed.[5,59] In a review of 48 endovascular procedures for splanchnic artery pseudoaneurysms, 20 interventions on the splenic artery were performed.[60] Six end-organ infarcts were identified in this series; all were within the splenic bed. Two additional patients displayed splenic atrophy on CT scanning after previous embolization of the splenic artery, without obvious clinical evidence of initial splenic infarction. In another report, one episode of splenic infarction associated with severe pancreatitis was noted after embolization of a distal splenic artery lesion

(Fig. 138-6).[5] However, other authors have reported splenic infarction after embolization of even more proximal SPAAs as well.[61]

Hepatic Artery Aneurysms

Prevalence and Epidemiology

After the splenic artery, the hepatic artery is the second most common location for aneurysmal degeneration in the splanchnic circulation, and HAAs represent 20% of all splanchnic artery aneurysms.[9,62] Although the true prevalence of HAAs is unknown, they appear to be rare, with approximately 500 cases reported in the literature. In large autopsy series, the prevalence of HAAs is 0.1%.[63,64] Nevertheless, the number of asymptomatic HAAs appears to have increased significantly in recent years because of more prevalent use of cross-sectional imaging modalities such as CT and MRI (Figs. 138-7 and 138-8), iatrogenic injuries resulting from endoscopic and percutaneous interventions for the treatment of hepatobiliary disease, and the adoption of nonoperative management of blunt liver trauma. Indeed, in the decade from 1985 to 1995, HAAs were the most frequently reported aneurysms in some centers.[9,65] Approximately half of these reported HAAs were pseudoaneurysms found in the intrahepatic parenchyma (Fig. 138-9). Unlike SPAAs, which are more commonly found in women, HAAs have a male preponderance of 2:1[9] and are typically seen in individuals at a mean of 60 years of age if traumatic aneurysms are excluded, which are more likely to occur in younger patients.[62]

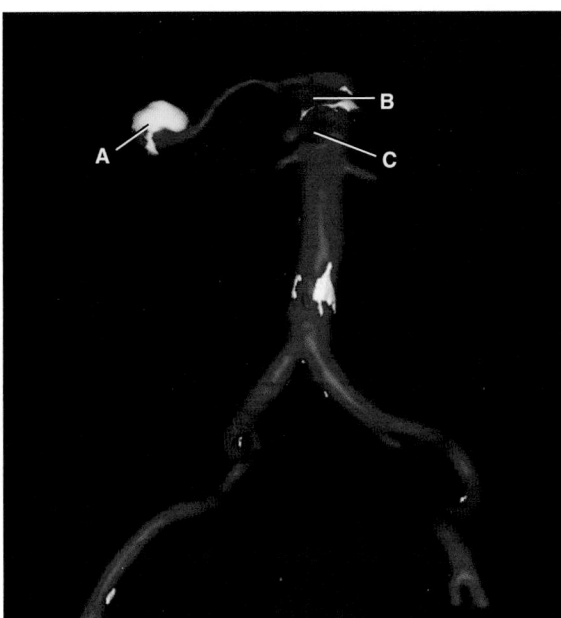

Figure 138-7 CT angiogram demonstrating a hepatic artery aneurysm. A, hepatic artery aneurysm; B, celiac trunk; C, proximal superior mesenteric artery.

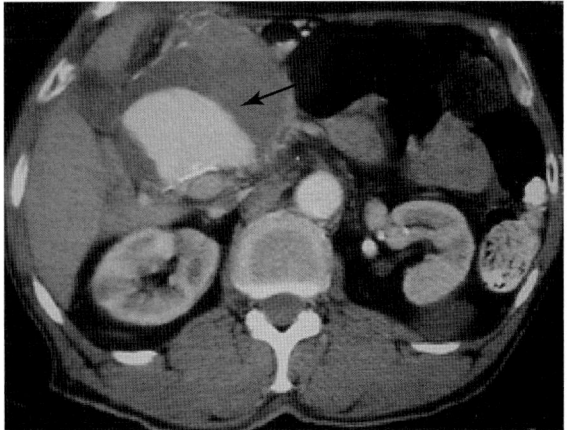

Figure 138-8 CT scan demonstrating a hepatic artery aneurysm (*arrow*).

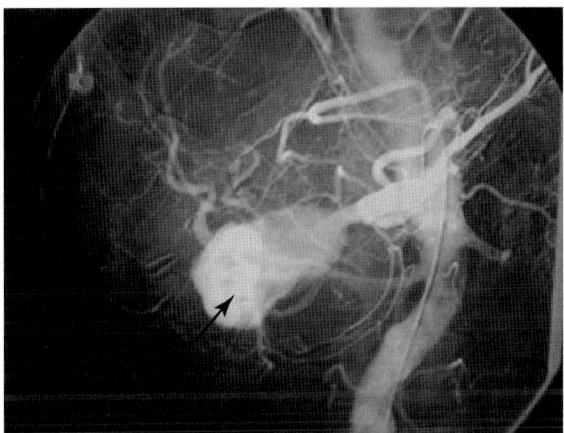

Figure 138-9 Hepatic artery aneurysm. Splanchnic arteriography demonstrates a large intraparenchymal pseudoaneurysm of the hepatic artery (*arrow*).

Pathogenesis and Risk Factors

The causes of HAA are numerous, with degenerative ("atherosclerotic") causes accounting for approximately 30% of cases.[64] In addition, medial degeneration, fibrodysplasia, trauma, infection, biliary diseases and percutaneous or endoscopic procedures, polyarteritis nodosa, and congenital disorders have all been described.[66] Approximately 80% of HAAs are extrahepatic, with 63% being found in the common hepatic artery, 28% in the right hepatic artery, 5% in the left hepatic artery, and 4% in both the right and left hepatic arteries.[66,67] Concomitant aneurysms are seen in the splanchnic and nonsplanchnic circulation in 31% and 42% of patients, respectively.[62] In a report of 36 HAAs, concomitant abdominal aortic aneurysms were noted in 20% of cases.[67]

Clinical Findings and Diagnosis

Although many HAAs are asymptomatic and found only incidentally, they have the highest rate of rupture (44%) among all splanchnic artery aneurysms and frequently become symptomatic (60%).[68] Symptoms can include epigastric or right upper quadrant pain and subsequent gastrointestinal hemorrhage and jaundice. The classic triad of Quincke consisting of abdominal pain, hematobilia, and obstructive jaundice is uncommon and seen in less than a third of cases.[62,69]

Risk factors associated with rupture are not well defined; however, reported mortality rates range from 21% to 40%.[8,67,70] Abbas and colleagues reported the Mayo Clinic experience of 22 patients with HAAs (mean aneurysm diameter, 2.3 cm; range, 1.5 to 5 cm) monitored nonoperatively for a mean of 68 months.[67] There were no ruptures in this group, but an increase in aneurysm size was noted in 27% of patients; the maximum growth rate was 0.8 cm over a 34-month period. As is the case with SPAAs, despite the fact that nonoperative management may be appropriate in some cases, these patients must be carefully selected and meticulously monitored. Most practitioners would consider elective intervention for lesions larger than 2 cm in diameter, provided that the patient's medical condition is appropriate and the potential risks of intervention are anticipated to be low. The risks associated with either endovascular or open surgical intervention for HAAs may be dependent on the location and etiology of the lesion.

The distinction between true and false aneurysms may prove to be an important prognostic factor when assessing risk for rupture of HAAs. Among the largest series of endovascular treatment of splanchnic artery aneurysms, a recent study from the Cleveland Clinic Foundation found that false aneurysms were more likely to be symptomatic than true aneurysms and more often required urgent intervention as a result.[60] The significant majority of HAAs in this series were false aneurysms (11 of 12), whereas only a minority of treated SPAAs were false aneurysms (5 of 20). The authors concluded that all splanchnic false aneurysms should be treated irrespective of size because of their unpredictable natural history and higher risk for rupture than true aneurysms.

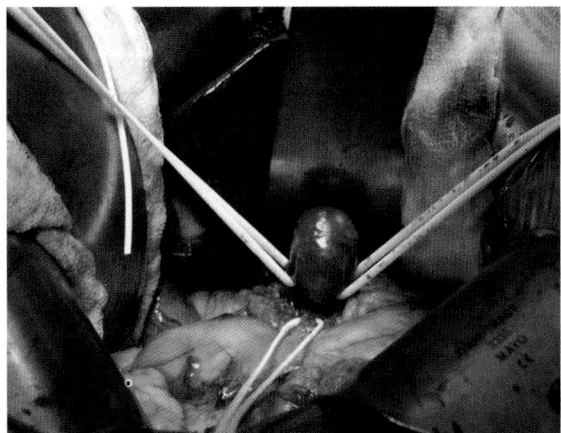

Figure 138-10 Hepatic artery aneurysm. An intraoperative photograph demonstrates an aneurysm of the common hepatic artery proximal to the gastroduodenal artery. The aneurysm was treated by simple proximal and distal ligation and aneurysmectomy.

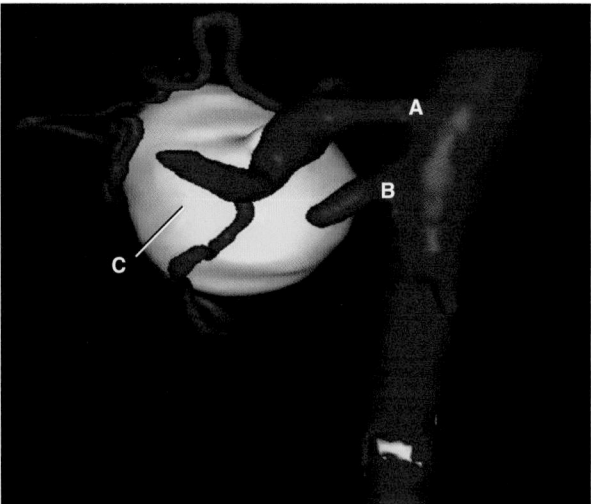

Figure 138-11 Celiac artery aneurysm. A CT angiogram demonstrates a large aneurysm of the celiac artery. A, celiac trunk; B, superior mesenteric artery; C, celiac artery aneurysm.

Indications and Technique for Treatment

Intervention for HAAs should be considered in all patients who are symptomatic and in asymptomatic patients with true aneurysms larger than 2 cm in diameter or with rapid growth on serial imaging studies. As mentioned previously, intrahepatic false aneurysms, commonly seen after iatrogenic injury or trauma, should be repaired irrespective of size (see Fig. 138-9). Finally, HAAs in patients with periarteritis nodosa or known fibromuscular dysplasia are considered to be at increased risk for rupture and should be repaired.[60,66]

Treatment options depend to a large extent on the anatomic location and morphology of the HAA, underlying etiology, and status of the end organ. Common HAAs can be treated by open ligation or exclusion by coil embolization because the GDA generally provides sufficient collateral flow to the liver (Fig. 138-10). In cases in which the GDA is diminutive or inadequate, open arterial reconstruction or covered stent-grafts may be necessary to preserve hepatic arterial flow. Hepatic artery ligation should never be performed in patients with cirrhosis or other evidence of liver disease because even a slight degree of ischemic compromise can be catastrophic. Aneurysms distal to the GDA arising in the proper hepatic artery generally require arterial reconstruction. Intrahepatic aneurysms or pseudoaneurysms are ideal candidates for coil or particle embolization techniques because these aneurysms are often difficult to access surgically. Moreover, treatment with embolization avoids the need for hepatic parenchymal resection.

Celiac Artery Aneurysms

Prevalence and Epidemiology

CAAs probably account for approximately 5% of all splanchnic artery aneurysms (Figs. 138-11 and 138-12). Their prevalence has been reported to be 1 in 8000 autopsies.[71] Only

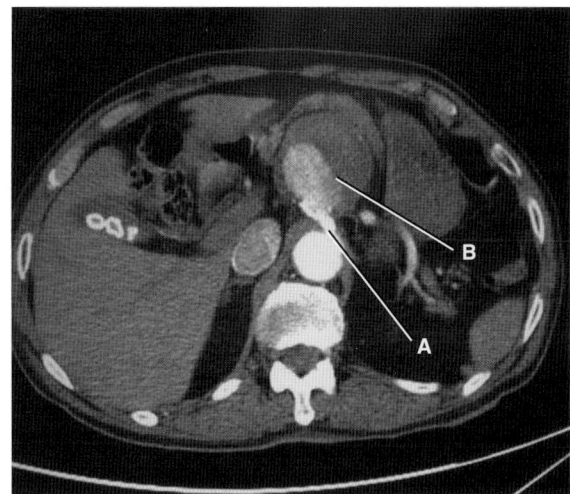

Figure 138-12 Celiac artery aneurysm. A conventional CT scan demonstrates a large aneurysm of the celiac artery. A, celiac origin; B, celiac artery aneurysm.

slightly more than 130 cases had been reported in the medical literature as of the mid-1990s.[9,72] They are associated with other splanchnic artery aneurysms in 40% of cases and with aortic aneurysms in 20% of cases.[73,74]

In contrast to SPAAs, CAAs are more commonly found in men (66%) than women.[7] In a review of 306 splanchnic artery aneurysms, true CAAs were identified in only 18 cases (5.9%).[75] Pathologic findings noted in CAA specimens include atherosclerotic changes and medial degeneration. Most CAAs are thought to be atherosclerotic.[75] However, as in the case of other splanchnic artery aneurysms, the mean age of patients with CAAs has been reported to be 56 years, considerably younger than the typical atherosclerotic patient population.[7,75,76]

Pathogenesis and Risk Factors

Historically, many CAAs were caused by syphilis, although this is currently an uncommon cause of celiac lesions.[72] Contemporary CAAs are likely to be related to medial degeneration or atherosclerotic disease. Less common causes include trauma, collagen vascular disease, arterial dissection, anomalous splanchnic circulation, and mycotic aneurysms. As with SMA aneurysms (SMAAs), CAAs have been reported to occur in the setting of spontaneous isolated dissection of the celiac artery.[77] An association between the development of CAAs and anomalous mesenteric vasculature has frequently been reported.[78] The most commonly reported associated configurations include anomalous origins of the right or left hepatic arteries or a common celiacomesenteric trunk.[78,79] Interestingly, other splanchnic artery aneurysms, in particular PDAAs, have been associated with both congenital absence and occlusion of the celiac axis.[80]

Clinical Findings and Diagnosis

CAAs have a strong tendency to rupture with a resultant high mortality rate; it was reported that 33 of 34 patients with CAAs diagnosed in 1943 died of rupture.[81] The overall contemporary reported risk for rupture appears to range from 10% to 20%, with an associated mortality of 50%.[18,72,75] The natural history of these lesions remains poorly defined; hypertension, aneurysm etiology, and the presence or absence of calcification do not appear to influence the potential for rupture. In one series, the size of ruptured lesions ranged from 2 to 6 cm and was no different from diagnosed intact lesions.[72] The majority of patients reported with CAAs have been symptomatic at initial encounter, although occult aneurysms are more likely to be diagnosed radiologically in the current era. Symptoms related to CAAs can include epigastric abdominal pain or hemorrhagic shock related to rupture. Patients may also exhibit gastrointestinal hemorrhage or jaundice related to biliary obstruction. Many patients with CAAs are found to have other concomitant splanchnic aneurysms.[7] Like SPAAs, CAAs may rupture initially into the lesser sac and cause localized epigastric pain and mild hypovolemia. The patient will decompensate when free rupture into the peritoneal cavity through the foramen of Winslow occurs. This "double-rupture" sequence may have occurred in nearly 25% of reported cases.[1]

Indications and Technique for Treatment

The mortality rate associated with ruptured CAAs may be 50% or higher.[9,18] Therefore, it is reasonable to consider treatment appropriate for all patients in whom a large or symptomatic CAA is diagnosed, unless medical co-morbid diseases absolutely preclude effective treatment. There are no absolute size criteria with which to direct the indication for treatment; however, treatment of lesions larger than 1.5 cm seems appropriate. Nonetheless, in a reported series of 18 CAAs in which eight asymptomatic patients were managed nonoperatively, only one subsequent rupture was noted to occur.[75] The other observed CAAs had no evidence of enlargement or rupture during a mean 91-month follow-up period.[75] Therefore, the decision to treat must be individualized on the basis of size, anatomy, etiology, and the potential morbidity associated with the proposed procedure. The availability of applicable endovascular techniques, as with other splanchnic aneurysms, has expanded the armamentarium of treatment options for these cases. Splanchnic arteriography is required to precisely define the anatomy of the aneurysm and the distal arterial tree and the nature of the collateral circulation. Occult coexisting splanchnic artery occlusive disease is an important factor in the decision to undertake particular treatment options and decide whether revascularization is warranted. Other anatomic features, including the presence of a suitable proximal aneurysm neck, may weigh into the consideration of endovascular options for treatment.

Historically, surgical treatment of these aneurysms was the only feasible option for management. Open surgical options included aneurysmectomy, aneurysmorrhaphy, and ligation.[7,72,82] The necessity for celiac or celiac branch revascularization depends on a number of factors, including the location of the aneurysm itself and the nature of the collateral mesenteric circulation. Simple ligation of the celiac artery is a viable option in a meaningful proportion of cases and has been undertaken in as many as 35% of reported surgically treated cases in the literature.[9,72] Ligation of the celiac artery is reportedly well tolerated in most cases, but it may be problematic in patients with underlying hepatic disease. When the artery is ligated, collateral flow is provided by the SMA, pancreaticoduodenal artery, and GDA.[1] The standard surgical approach involving revascularization is celiac aneurysmectomy with aortoceliac bypass grafting, most commonly using prosthetic material.[83] In one reported series of nine patients undergoing elective open surgical repair, revascularization was performed in 89%.[75] Aneurysmorrhaphy for isolated saccular lesions of the celiac artery has also been reported.[18] Successful endovascular techniques have included coil or glue embolization, percutaneous or open thrombin injection, and endovascular stent-grafting.[1,80,84-88] One report of five cases of endovascular occlusion of CAAs revealed no ischemic sequelae and uniformly good technical results.[89] Late development of coil migration into the stomach and development of a fatal aortogastric fistula have been reported after coil embolization of a CAA.[90]

Superior Mesenteric Artery Aneurysms
Prevalence and Epidemiology

SMAAs represent only 5.5% of all splanchnic artery aneurysms and appear to have an equal gender distribution.[9,91] Most commonly found within the first 5 cm of the artery, these aneurysms are particularly dangerous because complications such as aneurysm rupture, acute thrombosis, or distal embolization may jeopardize the entire small bowel.

Pathogenesis and Risk Factors

Unlike SPAAs or HAAs, SMAAs are thought to be associated with an infectious etiology in the majority of cases. Mycotic aneurysms account for 60% of cases and are thought to occur most commonly as a result of subacute bacterial endocarditis with infection by nonhemolytic *Streptococcus*. The predilection for mycotic aneurysms to be manifested in the SMA is incompletely understood but may be related to the orientation and size of the origin of the SMA as it arises from the aorta; this geometric configuration may predispose to lodging of septic cardiac emboli in this anatomic location (see also Chapter 139: Infected Aneurysms). Other causes include local connective tissue disease or atherosclerosis, as well as false aneurysms secondary to pancreatitis, dissection, or trauma.[83,91,92]

Clinical Findings and Diagnosis

Though uncommon, these aneurysms are associated with high mortality and should be treated expeditiously when diagnosed, irrespective of size. The majority of SMAAs, 70% to 90%, are symptomatic at initial evaluation.[91] Patients usually have general abdominal pain that can often be mistaken for much more common conditions, and thus a high index of suspicion is required for diagnosis. Shanley and coauthors reported a large series of 52 patients with SMAAs over a period of 3 decades and found the most frequent symptoms to be abdominal pain, nausea, vomiting, and gastrointestinal hemorrhage. A tender pulsatile mass can often be appreciated, and fever is present in up to 20% of patients.[9] Rupture is thought to occur in as many as 50% of patients[83,91,93] and is associated with a mortality rate (30% to 90%) that is significantly worse than that in patients undergoing elective repair (<15%).[91] High mortality is usually a result of intestinal ischemia or free rupture and exsanguination into the peritoneal cavity.

Indications and Technique for Treatment

Treatment of SMAAs should be considered regardless of size or symptomatology because of the high mortality risk associated with potential rupture. However, as with other splanchnic aneurysms, there are no definitive factors associated with rupture other than increasing size. SMA false aneurysms, especially when mycotic, often have some element of contained rupture at the time of diagnosis, and in these cases treatment is certainly warranted. Nonetheless, observation and conservative management may also be reasonable for small, noninfected SMA true aneurysms without associated symptoms or complications. As with other splanchnic aneurysms, treatment must be individualized and based on the etiology, size, and anatomic location of the lesion; co-morbid conditions of the patient; and the potential morbidity of the proposed procedure.

When surgical therapy is considered, some SMAAs can be ligated and excised safely because of the extensive collateral flow to the intestines via the celiac artery and the inferior

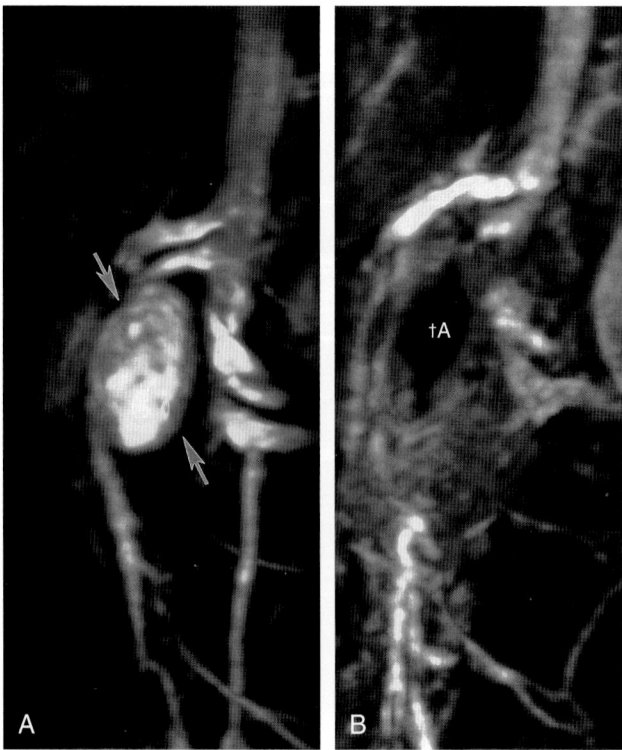

Figure 138-13 Superior mesenteric artery aneurysm. **A,** MRA documenting a large saccular aneurysm in a patient with Ehlers-Danlos syndrome. **B,** Postoperative MRA documenting a thrombosed aneurysm after proximal and distal ligation.

mesenteric artery (Fig. 138-13). Saccular aneurysms of the SMA, in particular, can be treated by aneurysmorrhaphy. Alternatively, arterial reconstruction using great saphenous vein or prosthetic conduits is possible. Severe atherosclerosis of the proximal SMA and splanchnic aorta, as is often present in cases of SMAA, can make revascularization procedures especially challenging. The current era of endovascular therapy has provided an important alternative treatment option for such challenging cases. Embolization techniques using coils, particles, or "glue" have been used successfully. Likewise, aneurysm exclusion with covered stent-grafts has the advantage of preserving the enteric circulation, which may be especially important in cases in which the normally robust collaterals have been compromised as a result of splanchnic occlusive disease or previous bowel resection.[33] In cases of mycotic aneurysms involving the SMA, some have recommended intravenous antibiotics before endovascular interventions.[94] As is true with CAAs, endovascular techniques for the treatment of SMAAs are largely dictated by the anatomic location of the disease. Because these aneurysms typically occur in the very proximal portions of the parent artery, a landing zone for coil embolization or stent-graft seal is often not feasible and open repair may be necessary.[95]

Spontaneous Superior Mesenteric Artery Dissection

Isolated spontaneous dissection of the SMA is a rare entity, but it is the most common location for dissection occurring

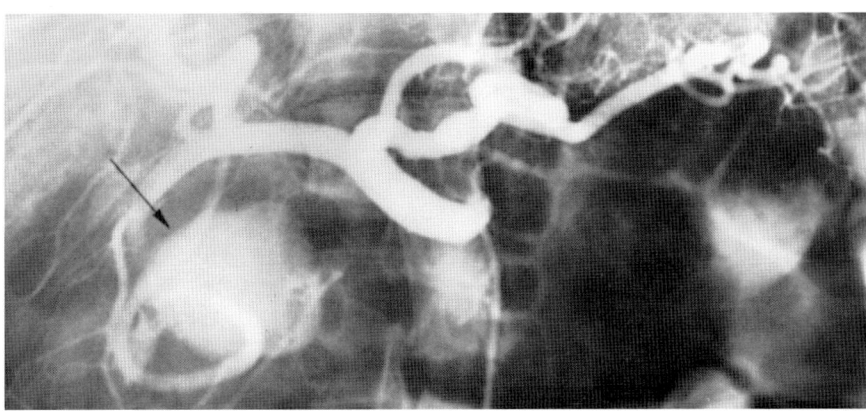

Figure 138-14 Gastroduodenal artery aneurysm (*arrow*) shown on a selective celiac arteriogram. *(From Eckhauser FE, Stanley JC, Zelenock GB, et al. Gastroduodenal and pancreaticoduodenal artery aneurysms: a complication of pancreatitis causing spontaneous gastrointestinal hemorrhage.* Surgery. *1980;88:335.)*

in a splanchnic vessel independent of the aorta. Among the complications of SMA dissection is aneurysmal degeneration. It had been suggested in the early literature that isolated spontaneous dissection of the SMA was associated with cystic medial degeneration,[96] atherosclerosis,[97] and fibromuscular dysplasia.[98,99] However, in the vast majority of cases an underlying cause of the dissection cannot be identified. Solis and associates reported that the dissection often begins 1.5 to 3 cm from the SMA ostium, with sparing of the origin of the SMA.[96] It is postulated that this is the location where the SMA exits from the inferior border of the pancreas and thus is more susceptible to shearing stress; the situation may be analogous to that seen at the ligamentum arteriosum during rapid deceleration injuries causing aortic transection. Most patients have acute-onset abdominal pain that is usually localized to the epigastrium; however, with the increased sensitivity of CT scans it is apparent that a small subset of patients will be asymptomatic at diagnosis. Physical examination findings are nonspecific, and abdominal bruits were found in just 14% of cases. Numerous open surgical approaches have been advocated for arterial reconstruction, as well endovascular stent placement for the treatment of SMA dissection.[100-102] Intervention for spontaneous SMA dissection is not universally endorsed, however. Anticoagulation alone is considered by some to be the preferred treatment, with numerous case reports and series describing resolution of pain with stabilization of the dissection flap. Close monitoring with serial imaging studies should be performed in such cases.

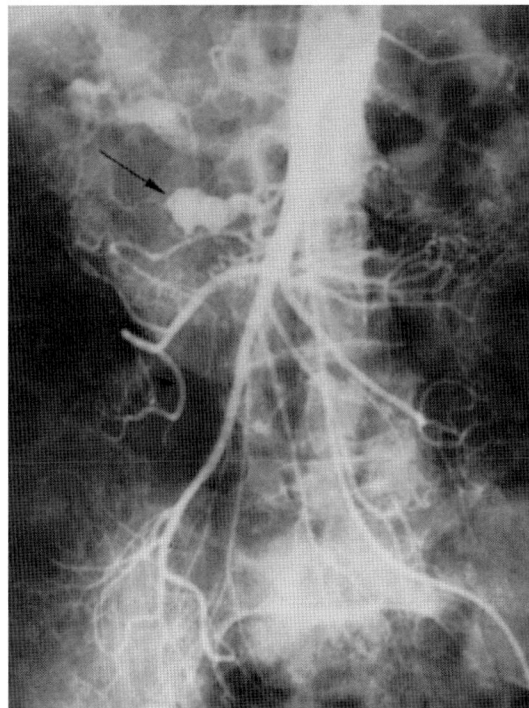

Figure 138-15 Inferior pancreaticoduodenal artery aneurysm. Selective injection of the superior mesenteric artery shows a pseudoaneurysm (*arrow*) that evolved as a complication of pancreatitis. *(From Stanley JC, Frey CF, Miller TA, et al. Major arterial hemorrhage: a complication of pancreatic pseudocysts and chronic pancreatitis.* Arch Surg. *1976;111:435.)*

Pancreaticoduodenal and Gastroduodenal Artery Aneurysms

Prevalence and Etiology

Gastroduodenal artery aneurysms (GDAAs), PDAAs, and aneurysms of their branches are among the most uncommon of all splanchnic artery aneurysms and are almost always associated with pancreatic or biliary tract disease (Figs. 138-14 and 138-15). GDAAs account for 1.5% of all splanchnic artery aneurysms, and PDAAs represent another 2%.[103-105] A distinction between true and false aneurysms in the pancreaticoduodenal distribution is noteworthy because they are

probably secondary to different causes and may carry different prognoses. False aneurysms account for roughly a third of all aneurysms of the pancreaticoduodenal artery and are often associated with pancreatic necrosis or pseudocyst expansion and erosion, septic emboli, and abdominal trauma. Such trauma may include iatrogenic injuries after pancreatic or biliary surgery or intervention.[106,107] Patients with PDAAs tend to initially be seen in their 50s, with men affected more often than women by a ratio of approximately 4:1. It has been postulated that the increased prevalence in men may reflect an increased incidence of alcoholic pancreatitis leading to false aneurysmal degeneration.[108-110] True degenerative

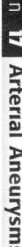

PDAAs are less common and thought to develop as a result of increased flow through the pancreatic arcades in association with celiac trunk occlusive disease or, occasionally, median arcuate ligament syndrome. In detailed arteriographic examination of five cases of PDAA associated with celiac artery stenosis, conspicuously developed collateral arteries were noted on SMA injection. The authors hypothesized that hemodynamic changes in the splanchnic arterial networks were the possible cause of the associated aneurysms.[111] This has prompted some surgeons to treat the celiac stenosis or occlusion and the aneurysm at same time, thus correcting for this underlying etiology.[104,107,112] These noninflammatory true aneurysms do not appear to have the same gender predilection as pseudoaneurysms of the pancreaticoduodenal arcade.[113]

Clinical Findings and Diagnosis

The clinical findings in patients with GDAA and PDAA can be vague and nonspecific. The majority of patients are symptomatic with abdominal pain that is epigastric or radiating to the back.[114,115] The pain is often sudden in onset and can correspond to rupture into the gastrointestinal tract or peritoneum. Gastrointestinal hemorrhage is likely to occur into either the duodenum or pancreatic duct.[104,116,117] Nearly 60% of all GDAAs and 30% of all PDAAs are related to pancreatitis, thus making symptoms from the aneurysm often indistinguishable from those of the underlying inflammatory state.[108] Although up to 75% of PDAAs can be manifested as rupture, the routine use of CT and MRA may allow earlier detection and intervention.[118] A recent series of PDAAs by Bageacu and coworkers found that 62% of aneurysms were diagnosed when the aneurysm ruptured, with a resulting mortality of 21%.[104] Ruptures can be contained by the retroperitoneal location of the peripancreatic arcades, similar to a retroperitoneal hematoma. Once the peritoneum proper is violated, free rupture usually leads to massive hemorrhage and shock. The reported mortality after rupture of GDAAs is significantly higher than that for PDAAs and approaches 50%.

Arteriography is a critical component of the evaluation of patients suspected of having a symptomatic gastroduodenal, pancreaticoduodenal, or pancreatic arterial aneurysm.[119] It allows important imaging of aneurysm location and its efferent and afferent arteries, as well as the possibility of endovascular intervention. CTA is also of great value in evaluating PDAAs and the nature of coexisting gastroduodenal or pancreatic disease.

Indications and Techniques for Treatment

Unlike some other splanchnic artery aneurysms, there does not appear to be a clear correlation between the size of true PDAAs and rupture, thus supporting a consideration of prompt intervention for all such aneurysms, irrespective of size.[104,120] Likewise, false aneurysms of the GDA should be treated promptly because of their significant risk for rupture.

Although these aneurysms may be approached surgically, their anatomic location can be challenging, especially in cases of rupture. Ligation without revascularization is often necessary in the setting of a ruptured PDAA and hemodynamic instability. Several reports describe more aggressive approaches, including partial pancreatectomy or pancreaticoduodenectomy.[104,121] Even in hemodynamically stable patients without evidence of rupture, it may be difficult to identify the aneurysm within the substance of the pancreas. The presence of pancreatitis may also add to the degree of difficulty when performing open surgical repair of these aneurysms. Simple ligation may be difficult or ineffective because of the numerous branches that usually supply PDAAs. Ligation of all branches is essential for adequate aneurysm exclusion and can often best be achieved from within the aneurysmal sac. The surgical approach for ligation of GDAAs is usually more straightforward.

The advent of endovascular techniques has provided an attractive alternative for these often surgically inaccessible lesions. Angiography allows precise localization of the aneurysm, as well as identification of the numerous small branches that often feed the PDAA. Similar to endovascular interventions for other splanchnic artery aneurysms, successful treatment of GDAAs, PDAAs, and pancreatic aneurysms requires complete exclusion of the sac from the arterial circulation. Coil embolization techniques have been used with excellent procedural success rates; however, sac reperfusion can occur and thus requires vigilant postoperative monitoring with regular imaging studies.[59,60,119,122] Boudghene and coauthors reported definitive success in 25 of 32 patients (78%) treated by coil embolization, with reperfusion and occasionally rupture occurring in cases in which initial embolization was inadequate.[119] Definitive treatment of true PDAAs by endovascular techniques can be limited by the fact that concomitant celiac artery occlusion requiring revascularization may not be possible without an open approach. Combined open and endovascular interventions to permit coil embolization, as well as celiac revascularization, have been reported.[107,114] Percutaneous and ultrasound-guided intraoperative thrombin occlusion of GDAAs and pancreatic arterial aneurysms has also been described and may be useful in the treatment of selected patients, including those with acute pancreatitis.[80,123]

Gastric/Gastroepiploic Aneurysms
Prevalence and Etiology

GAAs and GEAAs are rare, together accounting for approximately 4% of all splanchnic artery aneurysmal disease. The underlying causes of these aneurysms are reported to be degenerative in 30%, traumatic in 25%, and inflammatory in 15%.[124,125] Histologic examination of a successfully treated 8-cm GEAA revealed medial fibrosis and atherosclerosis.[12] Other common related inflammatory processes include pancreatitis, peptic ulcer disease, and vasculitis.[10,18] Less common causes include infectious aneurysms secondary to septic emboli, inflammatory conditions, and medial dysplasia.

GEAAs are less frequent than aneurysms of the main gastric arteries, with a ratio of approximately 1:10.[12,18,125] These lesions are reported to occur in elderly men in the sixth or seventh decade of life.

Clinical Findings and Diagnosis

More than 90% of reported GEAAs have been ruptured on initial evaluation, with the patient exhibiting hemoperitoneum and hemorrhagic shock.[124] The diagnosis, therefore, is commonly made on laparotomy in hemodynamically unstable patients. There may be a 10% to 40% chance of concomitant intra-abdominal aneurysmal disease.[124] Surgical management generally consists of resection and ligation, most commonly without arterial reconstruction. Embolization via an endovascular approach would be technically feasible in an incidentally noted GAA or GEAA that is diagnosed before rupture.

Indications and Techniques for Treatment

Early diagnosis plus treatment of recognized GAAs and GEAAs is warranted because 70% of patients in whom rupture occurs die.[18] If the diagnosis is established before rupture, an endovascular option, generally consisting of embolization of the artery, is feasible.[126] Successful percutaneous thrombin injection in the emergency setting has also been reported.[127] However, the diagnosis is usually established only at laparotomy for hemoperitoneum and shock. When GAAs and GEAAs occur in a location outside the stomach, ligation of the involved vessel with or without aneurysmectomy is appropriate treatment.[128] Intramural GAAs located within the wall of the stomach can be excised simultaneously with the involved portion of the stomach wall.

Jejunal, Ileal, and Colic Artery Aneurysms

Prevalence and Etiology

Aneurysms of these mesenteric branch vessels are extremely rare (Figs. 138-16 and 138-17). In one large review of the literature, only 2% of all reported splanchnic artery aneurysms were located in the distribution of the jejunal, ileal, or colic arteries.[76,129] The pathogenesis of these unusual aneurysms is incompletely characterized. Occasionally, they are found to be multiple in a patient with periarteritis nodosa or other inherited inflammatory or connective tissue disorders. The great majority of lesions are solitary, except for lesions associated with periarteritis nodosa or other connective tissue disorders.[18] In a report from the Mayo Clinic consisting of a 2-decade experience with splanchnic artery aneurysms in more than 300 patients, only eight cases of these mesenteric branch aneurysms were encountered.[6] One of these patients had an associated abdominal aortic aneurysm, and two other patients were noted to have additional concomitant splanchnic vessel aneurysms. There was an equal gender distribution among the patients.[18] Three patients were initially seen with

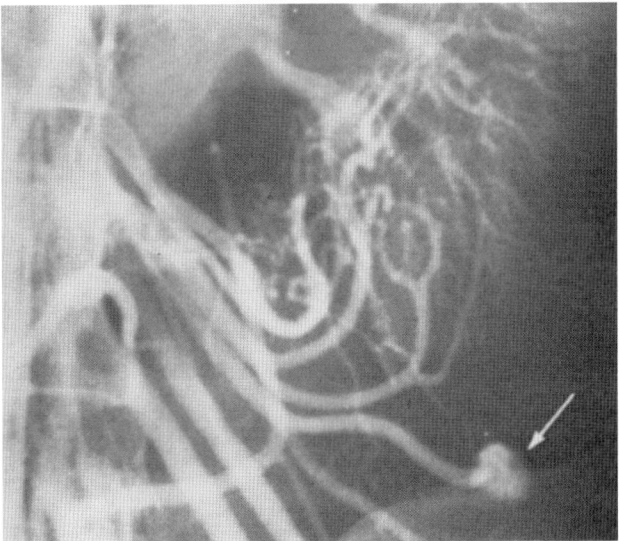

Figure 138-16 Ileal artery aneurysm. A mesenteric arteriogram documents the presence of a saccular aneurysm (*arrow*) of a distal ileal artery.

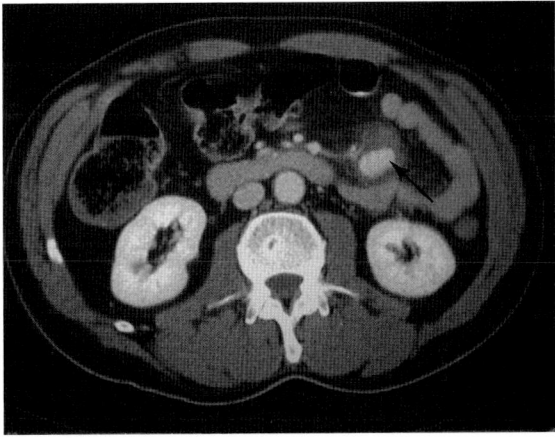

Figure 138-17 CT scan demonstrating a mycotic aneurysm (*arrow*) of a jejunal artery branch secondary to septic emboli.

rupture, and all three of these cases involved colic artery aneurysms, as opposed to jejunal or ileal vessel aneurysms. Two of the three patients with ruptured colic artery aneurysms were women with a history of multiple pregnancies. In contrast to the colic artery lesions, rupture of jejunal lesions is thought to be extremely rare.[129] Inferior mesenteric artery aneurysms are among the most uncommon of these aneurysms.[130] They have occasionally been reported in association with concomitant stenosis of the SMA and celiac axis.[130-132]

A variety of causes have been proposed for these uncommon lesions. As with other splanchnic artery aneurysms, atherosclerosis, medial degeneration, infection, inflammation, and trauma all represent possible causes.[129] If none of these risk factors exist, the presence of a congenital aneurysm may be considered, especially in a younger patient.[129] Among seven mesenteric branch vessel aneurysms in a larger series examining aneurysm etiology, one was thought to be atherosclerotic and three infectious, and three aneurysms were considered to be iatrogenic and related to recent abdominal surgery.[122]

Indications and Techniques for Treatment

Jejunal, ileal, and colic artery aneurysms can rupture freely into the peritoneal cavity or can rupture into adjacent intestinal segments and cause gastrointestinal hemorrhage. Most reported ruptured mesenteric branch artery aneurysms are small, less than 1 cm in diameter.[6,7,133] Intraoperative identification of a ruptured jejunal branch aneurysm can be exceedingly difficult.[129] Preoperative arteriography, when feasible, can be helpful in identifying and locating the aneurysm. Most open surgical treatment has consisted of ligation of the aneurysm with concomitant colectomy or small bowel resection if necessary. Endovascular treatment has consisted of embolization with microcatheter techniques.[6,134] Embolization must completely exclude the aneurysms on both sides of the feeding vessel to prevent backbleeding and consistent pressurization of the aneurysm sac. Colonic ischemia after endovascular coil embolization for an inferior mesenteric artery aneurysm has been reported.[122] Care must be taken to prevent unnecessary occlusion of adjacent mesenteric vessels supplying the small or large intestinal tract; otherwise, intestinal ischemia and infarction are potential complications of this technique.[6] Management of larger and more proximal mesenteric branch vessel aneurysms would probably require revascularization to prevent significant bowel resection.

TREATMENT RESULTS FOR SPLANCHNIC ANEURYSMS

Open Surgery

The results of open surgical therapy are greatly dependent on whether the procedure is performed electively or on an emergency basis and to a further extent on the anatomic complexity of the lesion and the nature of the required surgical repair. As previously stated in the sections on specific aneurysmal locations, emergency treatment of ruptured splanchnic aneurysms carries mortality that is greater than 50% in many reported series. Electively treated splanchnic aneurysms clearly have significantly lower perioperative morbidity and mortality. In a comparatively large case series reported by Pulli and coworkers involving 53 elective open surgical procedures for asymptomatic splanchnic aneurysms, the perioperative mortality rate was 1.8%.[135] The single death was due to acute pancreatitis in a patient with a giant SPAA. Two major operative complications were recorded, one retroperitoneal hematoma and one case of pancreatitis. During a mean follow-up period of 82 months, two aneurysm-related complications occurred, and the 10-year survival rate was 80%. In an additional retrospective series of splanchnic aneurysms, patients with electively treated lesions (n = 27) had no early mortalities, whereas the overall mortality of patients with ruptured aneurysms (n = 15) was 23%.[118] The morbidity rate for elective cases was 12% for open surgical repair and 18% for patients treated by embolization in this series, with the most common complication being limited splenic infarction after embolization. In another report consisting of 24 open surgical repairs and 35 endovascular repairs, there were no differences in mortality or complications between the two groups; there were no mortalities among patients with electively treated lesions.[61]

Endovascular Treatment

Technical success after percutaneous coil embolization of splanchnic artery aneurysms is acceptable and ranges from 81% to 98%.[5,59-61,136-138] Tulsyan and colleagues, reporting on 48 patients treated by coil embolization, showed that endovascular management of splanchnic artery aneurysms can yield excellent results with low overall periprocedural morbidity.[60] In this large series, a procedural indication of rupture appeared to confer significant risk for periprocedural morbidity when treating these patients with endovascular techniques. Four of 22 unstable patients (18%) who underwent urgent or emergency repair died, but there were no deaths in patients treated electively. Nevertheless, open repair of ruptured splanchnic artery aneurysms also carries significant risk and has been reported to be associated with a mortality of 10% to 25%[48] for SPAAs and up to 40% for HAAs.[67] Others have shown that the presence of hemodynamic instability should not preclude endovascular management. Sachdev and associates treated 35 patients by endovascular interventions with an overall mortality of 2.9%. All 10 patients with rupture were managed successfully via an endovascular approach.[61]

Complications of Endovascular Intervention

The risk for end-organ ischemia appears to be an especially salient concern with regard to endovascular repair. Ischemia can result from complications directly related to the intervention, such as arterial dissection, acute thrombosis, or embolization of nontarget tissue, or from inadequate collateral circulation after deliberate vessel occlusion. In the series by Tulsyan and coworkers, postembolization syndrome, manifested as left-sided abdominal discomfort or other evidence of splenic ischemia, occurred in 40% of patients treated for splenic aneurysms, although all were self-limited.[60] Only one occurred as a result of nontarget embolization, where *n*-butylcyanoacrylate "glue" was found to embolize to the hilum of the spleen. Others have reported a similar incidence of end-organ ischemia after endovascular interventions, although the clinical significance remains to be determined. Sachdev and colleagues demonstrated some evidence of splenic infarction in 6 of 15 SPAAs treated endovascularly.[61] One of them was a result of splenic dissection and complete thrombosis requiring splenectomy. The remaining infarctions were detected on follow-up imaging but were of no clinical consequence. Anatomic considerations may also play a role in determining the best treatment option. Saltzberg and coauthors reported major endovascular procedure–related complications in 4 of 11 patients with distal SPAAs (36.4%).[5] One late recurrence, two major splenic infarcts, and one episode of severe pancreatitis occurred. The authors concluded that patients with aneurysmal disease at the splenic hilum may be better managed by open repair and splenectomy.[5]

Late Failure after Endovascular Intervention

Although initial technical success rates with an endovascular approach for treating splanchnic artery aneurysms approach 100%, long-term success is less well defined. Lagana and associates studied 25 patients with 29 splanchnic artery aneurysms treated by sac embolization (n = 9), endovascular exclusion (n = 6), coil/thrombin embolization of the afferent artery (n = 10), stent-graft placement (n = 2), and percutaneous ultrasound-guided thrombin injection (n = 2).[28] Follow-up over a mean period of 19 months revealed that 10% of patients had signs of reperfusion at 1 month. All of them were treated successfully with additional endovascular procedures. Others have shown similar early recanalization rates.[118] Sachdev and coworkers found that 7 of 59 patients (12%) required one or more re-interventions after an initial endovascular procedure, with a mean time to re-intervention of 2.1 months.[61]

Thrombin Injection for Failed Interventions

Ultrasound-guided percutaneous thrombin injection appears to be a viable method for treating failed endovascular interventions or even an alternative to initial endovascular treatment.[139-142] Similar to thrombin injections for femoral artery pseudoaneurysms, this technique uses ultrasound or CT guidance (or both) to help deliver thrombin to the nidus of an aneurysm, thus facilitating thrombosis. This technique is particularly applicable to saccular aneurysms with a narrow neck arising from the parent vessel. Even though larger splanchnic aneurysms in thinner patients have been successfully injected with thrombin under ultrasound guidance transabdominally, CT guidance may be preferable in cases in which bowel gas and body habitus limit sonographic visualization of the lesion. Moreover, CT-guided percutaneous injections can be approached via the flank with the patient in the lateral decubitus position.

Surveillance after Endovascular Intervention

Continued surveillance, even after secondary technical success, is imperative because the natural history of splanchnic artery aneurysms after endovascular treatment remains unclear. This is especially true of saccular aneurysms treated by coil or thrombin embolization; unlike formal exclusion with a covered stent, these aneurysms are not technically "excluded" from the arterial circulation. Indeed, sac thrombosis may not protect the aneurysm sac from pressure transmitted through thrombus, and eventual sac growth or rupture may still occur.[143,144] Reports of reperfusion and even rupture after "successful" embolization of splanchnic aneurysms support the notion that a thrombosed aneurysm may not represent the definitive treatment in all cases.[128,145]

SELECTED KEY REFERENCES

Abbas MA, Stone WM, Fowl RJ, Gloviczki P, Oldenburg WA, Pairolero PC, Hallett JW, Bower TC, Panneton JM, Cherry KJ. Splenic artery aneurysms: two decades experience at Mayo clinic. *Ann Vasc Surg.* 2002;16:442-449.
  A 20-year institutional review of splenic artery aneurysms.

Carr SC, Pearce WH, Vogelzang RL, McCarthy WJ, Nemcek AA Jr, Yao JS. Current management of visceral artery aneurysms. *Surgery.* 1996;120:627-633; discussion 633-634.
  A large institutional review of 40 patients with a focus on newer endovascular forms of treatment and changes in management strategies over time.

Carroccio A, Jacobs TS, Faries P, Carroccio A, Jacobs TS, Faries P, Ellozy SH, Teodorescu VJ, Ting W, Marin ML. Endovascular treatment of visceral artery aneurysms. *Vasc Endovascular Surg.* 2007; 41:373-382.
  A large institutional review of contemporary endovascular management of splanchnic artery aneurysms.

Graham LM, Stanley JC, Whitehouse WM Jr, Zelenock GB, Wakefield TW, Cronenwett JL, Lindenauer SM. Celiac artery aneurysms: historic (1745-1949) versus contemporary (1950-1984) differences in etiology and clinical importance. *J Vasc Surg.* 1985;2:757-764.
  An institutional and literature review focusing on changes in clinical findings, etiology, and management of celiac artery aneurysms between the historical and modern surgical eras.

Messina LM, Shanley CJ. Visceral artery aneurysms. *Surg Clin North Am.* 1997;77:425-442.
  An excellent overall review of splanchnic artery aneurysms.

Pulli R, Dorigo W, Troisi N, Pratesi G, Innocenti AA, Pratesi C. Surgical treatment of visceral artery aneurysms: a 25-year experience. *J Vasc Surg.* 2008;48:334-342.
  A large series reporting early and late outcomes of elective open surgical repair.

Sachdev U, Baril DT, Ellozy SH, Lookstein RA, Silverberg D, Jacobs TS, Carroccio A, Teodorescu VJ, Marin ML. Management of aneurysms involving branches of the celiac and superior mesenteric arteries: a comparison of surgical and endovascular therapy. *J Vasc Surg.* 2006;44:718-724.
  A large institutional review of 61 treated visceral aneurysms along with comparison and analysis of open surgical and endovascular therapies.

Saltzberg SS, Maldonado TS, Lamparello PJ, Cayne NS, Nalbandian MM, Rosen RJ, Jacobowitz GR, Adelman MA, Gagne PJ, Riles TS, Rockman CB. Is endovascular therapy the preferred treatment for all visceral artery aneurysms? *Ann Vasc Surg.* 2005;19:507-515.
  An institutional review of open, endovascular, and conservative management of visceral artery aneurysms.

Shanley CJ, Shah NL, Messina LM. Common splanchnic artery aneurysms: splenic, hepatic, and celiac. *Ann Vasc Surg.* 1996;10: 315-322.
  A large institutional review of the most common splanchnic artery aneurysms: splenic, hepatic, and celiac.

Stanley JC, Wakefield TW, Graham LM, Whitehouse WM Jr, Zelenock GB, Lindenauer SM. Clinical importance and management of splanchnic artery aneurysms. *J Vasc Surg.* 1986;3:836-840.
  A large institutional review of splanchnic artery epidemiology and management.

Tulsyan N, Kashyap VS, Greenberg RK, Sarac TP, Clair DG, Pierce G, Ouriel K. The endovascular management of visceral artery aneurysms and pseudoaneurysms. *J Vasc Surg.* 2007;45:276-283; discussion 283.
  A large institutional review of 48 patients who underwent endovascular management of visceral artery aneurysms and pseudoaneurysms.

REFERENCES

The reference list can be found on the companion Expert Consult Web site at *www.expertconsult.com.*

CHAPTER 139

Infected Aneurysms

Mitchell R. Weaver and Daniel J. Reddy

Infected aneurysms have been reported in practically every arterial segment, and although these aneurysms represent only a very small proportion of all aneurysms, they are among the most difficult to treat. The vascular surgeon is often faced with a patient compromised by sepsis, artery rupture, and challenging anatomic locations of aneurysms, which may obviate simple excision as a viable treatment option.

BACKGROUND

During the 19th century several authors predated Osler's landmark work with case reports associating endocarditis, septic emboli, arterial abscesses, and ruptured infected aneurysms of the superior mesenteric and popliteal arteries (see the Appendix on the Expert Consult Web site). In 1885, Osler presented the first comprehensive discussion of an infected aneurysm and remarked on the "anatomical characters..., clinical features, and ... etiological and pathological relations."[1] In 1923, Stengel and Wolferth described 4 patients and reviewed another 213 infected aneurysms with the finding that in 30 patients there was no evidence of bacterial endocarditis, thus showing that infected aneurysms can occur in connection with a variety of other septic conditions.[2] Sommerville and colleagues, in 1959, reported on the existence of a third type of arterial infection—one occurring in preexisting atherosclerotic aneurysms—and found six infected aneurysms in a series of more than 20,000 Mayo Clinic autopsies.[3]

In more recent years, the incidence of arterial infections and infected aneurysms has increased in response to the increasing prevalence of immunosuppressed hosts,[4-6] invasive hemodynamic monitoring,[7] angiography,[8,9] and drug addiction.[10-14] This change in pathogenesis has been noted by other authors, who emphasize that a fourth type of infected aneurysm has emerged as a significant clinical entity—post-traumatic infected false aneurysm (pseudoaneurysm).[15] The greatest number of such infected aneurysms has been associated with intravenous or intra-arterial drug injection.[11] As a result of developing treatment modalities that use catheter-based percutaneous approaches for a variety of occlusive or aneurysmal vascular lesions, iatrogenic infected false aneurysms seem to be increasing in frequency.[16] In contemporary practice, the option of in-line (in situ) arterial reconstruction after resection of an infected aneurysm has become closer to an everyday reality because of preserved homografts, innovative vein conduits, early detection, and effective antimicrobial therapies.[17,18]

CLASSIFICATION

On the basis of etiology, there are four types of infected aneurysm: mycotic aneurysms from septic arterial emboli, microbial arteritis with aneurysm formation, infected preexisting aneurysms, and post-traumatic infected false aneurysms (Table 139-1). Excluded are aneurysms resulting from contiguous infection, spontaneous aortoenteric fistulae, and infections of synthetic vascular prostheses.

Mycotic Aneurysms

Prevalence and Location

Mycotic aneurysms develop when septic emboli of cardiac origin lodge in the lumen or the vasa vasorum of peripheral

Table 139-1 Clinical Characteristics of Infected Aneurysms

	Mycotic Aneurysm	Microbial Arteritis	Infection of Existing Aneurysm	Post-traumatic Infected False Aneurysm
Etiology	Endocarditis	Bacteremia	Bacteremia	Narcotic addiction, trauma
Age	30-50 yr	>50 yr	>50 yr	<30 yr
Incidence	Rare	Common	Unusual	Common
Location	Aorta	Aorta	Infrarenal	Femoral
	Visceral	Iliac artery	Aorta	Carotid
	Intracranial	Intimal defects		
	Peripheral			
Bacteriology	Gram-positive cocci	*Salmonella*	*Staphylococcus*	*Staphylococcus aureus*
		Others	Others	Polymicrobial
Mortality	25%	75%	90%	5%

From Wilson SE, Van Wagenen P, Passaro E Jr. Arterial infection. *Curr Probl Surg.* 1978;15:5.

arteries. Mycotic aneurysms can occur in both normal and abnormal arteries and have developed in virtually every named artery: intracranially; the great vessels; the thoracoabdominal aorta; and the visceral, extremity, pulmonary, and coronary arteries. In the pre-antibiotic era, approximately 90% of all infected aneurysms were mycotic aneurysms.[2,19,20] The century following Osler's initial description of this entity saw antibiotic therapy, the advancement of microbiologic techniques allowing identification and treatment of specific bacterial infections, and the development of open heart surgery to permit replacement of the infected cardiac valve. These advances have sharply lowered the prevalence of mycotic aneurysms in absolute terms and as a percentage of infected aneurysms.[3,10,15,19,21,22]

Even though mycotic aneurysms may occur in multiple sites in a given patient, certain anatomic locations predominate[1]—the aorta and the intracranial, superior mesenteric, and femoral arteries.[2,22] The predilection of mycotic aneurysms for certain anatomic sites relates to their pathogenesis. In larger arteries such as the aorta, infected emboli may lodge in the relatively large vasa vasorum and cause vessel wall ischemia and infection. As the medial layer is destroyed by this process, an aneurysm forms. In smaller arteries, the infected macroscopic emboli may lodge in the vessel lumen or wall and initiate a similar pathologic process. Sites predisposed to the formation of mycotic aneurysms are bifurcations, arteriovenous fistulae, and coarctations.[19,23] Reports of mycotic aneurysms occurring in the tibioperoneal trunk, the common hepatic artery, the ascending aorta, the carotid artery, and the cerebral artery represent the variety of arterial segments in which mycotic aneurysms are found.[24-29]

Bacteriology

In 1923, Stengel and Wolferth reported that the predominant organisms found were nonhemolytic streptococci, pneumococci, and staphylococci.[2] In 1986, Magilligan and Quinn reported that the dominant infecting organisms in patients with no history of drug abuse (n = 55) but with native valve endocarditis leading to infected aneurysms were *Streptococcus viridans* (22%), *Staphylococcus aureus* (20%), *Streptococcus faecalis* (14%), and *Staphylococcus epidermidis* (11%).[30] Exotic bacteria, such as *Eikenella corrodens* and *Propionibacterium acnes*, and the fungus *Aspergillus* were also noted. In narcotic addicts (n = 36) with endocarditis leading to infected aneurysms, the infecting organisms were *S. aureus* (36%), *Pseudomonas* species (16%), polymicrobial species (15%), *S. faecalis* (13%), and *S. viridans* (11%). Exotic organisms such as *Micrococcus* species, *Corynebacterium* species, and *Candida albicans* were also isolated. The organisms responsible in each of the six intracerebral mycotic aneurysms among these 91 patients were *S. faecalis* (3), *S. viridans* (1), *Pseudomonas* (1), and *C. albicans* (1).[30] In 1984, Brown and colleagues reported that *S. aureus* and various streptococcal species accounted for 38% of infected aneurysms of all types.[31] In six large published series of aortoiliac aneurysms, *Staphylococcus* and *Streptococcus* species accounted for 28% of infected aneurysms (Fig. 139-1).[32-37]

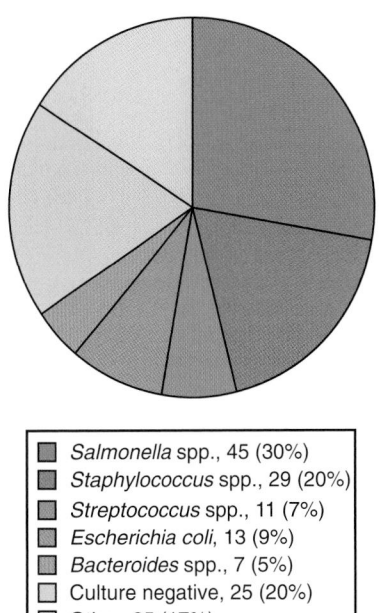

Salmonella spp., 45 (30%)
Staphylococcus spp., 29 (20%)
Streptococcus spp., 11 (7%)
Escherichia coli, 13 (9%)
Bacteroides spp., 7 (5%)
Culture negative, 25 (20%)
Other, 25 (17%)

Figure 139-1 Reported organisms recovered from combined series of 143 aortoiliac aneurysms, 1996 to 2002. Data are from Hsu,[32] Moneta,[33] Muller,[34] Oderich,[35] Sessa,[36] Sriussadaporn,[37] and their colleagues. Other organisms include *Clostridium* spp., *Enterococcus* group, *Acinetobacter* spp., *Enterobacter* spp., *Listeria monocytogenes*, *Pseudomonas* spp., *Campylobacter fetus*, *Corynebacterium* spp., *Aspergillus*, *Coccidioides immitis*, *Candida* spp., *Mycobacterium avium* complex, *Haemophilus influenzae*, and *Mycobacterium tuberculosis*.

Microbial Arteritis with Aneurysm

Prevalence and Location

In the pre-antibiotic era, microbial arteritis with aneurysm occurred in approximately 14% of patients with infected aneurysms.[2] In modern times, as a result of the decline in rheumatic fever and bacterial endocarditis, microbial arteritis with aneurysm is more prevalent than mycotic aneurysm.[31] This increase is due to the aging of the population and the corresponding increase in atherosclerosis, an important factor predisposing arteries to infection.

The prevalence in adults of infected aneurysms produced by microbial arteritis is estimated to be 0.06% to 0.65%.[38,39] Diseased intima, which when normal is highly resistant to infection, allows blood-borne bacteria to inoculate the arterial wall. Once infection is established, suppuration, localized perforation, and false aneurysm formation follow (Fig. 139-2). Supporting atherosclerosis as the principal predisposing factor in the pathogenesis of microbial arteritis is the fact that the aorta, the most frequent site of atherosclerosis, is also the most frequent location of these lesions (by a 3:1 margin over peripheral sites).[40-44] In our series, microbial arteritis accounted for 77% of infected aortoiliac aneurysms.[39]

Patients undergoing hemodialysis are thought to be particularly vulnerable to *Staphylococcus* bacteremia and resulting microbial arteritis.[45] Microbial arteritis of the subclavian artery after irradiation for breast cancer,[46] aortic infection after gastrointestinal endoscopy in an immunosuppressed

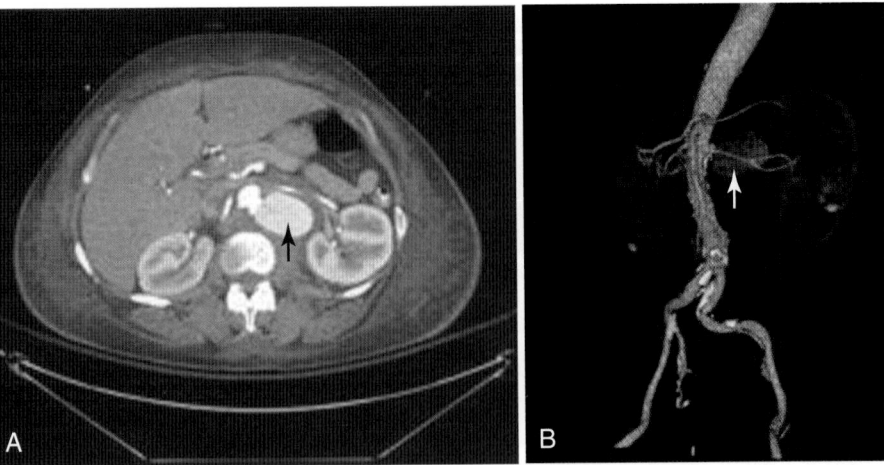

Figure 139-2 Axial and reconstructed computed tomographic angiography (CTA) images of a patient with *Salmonella* microbial aortitis and an aneurysm. **A,** CTA showing contained rupture of the infected aneurysm (*arrow*). **B,** Three-dimensional reformatting showing a saccular eccentric infected aneurysm of the juxtarenal aorta (*arrow*).

patient, and appendicitis and lumbar osteomyelitis have been reported.[47-49] Overall, co-morbid conditions associated with at least a degree of immunosuppression are common and reported in up to 70% of patients with infected aneurysms.[32,33,35]

Bacteriology

The predominant microorganisms associated with microbial arteritis leading to aneurysms are *Escherichia coli* and *Salmonella* and *Staphylococcus* species.[15] *Bacteroides fragilis* aneurysms of the suprarenal aorta have also been reported, thus highlighting the necessity of culturing for anaerobes in these cases.[39,50] The overall 25% culture-negative rate may indicate a deficiency in obtaining anaerobic cultures.

The importance of *Salmonella* species in microbial arteritis, particularly microbial aortitis, has been mentioned in many reports and were cited in our own review at the Henry Ford Hospital.[39] The diseased aorta has a unique vulnerability to *Salmonella* (see Fig. 139-2). The most virulent *Salmonella* species are *S. choleraesuis* and *S. typhimurium*, which account for 62% of reported cases of *Salmonella* arteritis.[15] Although *Salmonella* species are the predominant organisms reported worldwide,[51-54] other organisms (e.g., *Listeria monocytogenes*,[55,56] *Klebsiella pneumoniae*,[57] *Clostridium septicum*[58-60]) and fungal species (e.g., *Aspergillus niger*[61]) have also been reported.

Infected Preexisting Aneurysms
Prevalence and Location

The prevalence of infection in preexisting atherosclerotic aneurysms was estimated by Sommerville and associates to be 3.4%.[3] Bennett and Cherry[40] and Jarrett and coauthors[21] reported parallel findings and noted the relative rarity of this lesion and its propensity for rupture.

The related entity of aortic aneurysms colonized by bacteria had been identified in two nearly simultaneous reports by Ernst and colleagues[62] and Williams and Fisher.[63] Patients undergoing abdominal aortic aneurysmectomy were studied

prospectively, and bacterial cultures were performed on samples of the aneurysm wall and its contents and on bowel bag fluid. Overall, 15% of cultures yielded positive results. There was a higher prevalence of positive cultures in patients with ruptured aneurysms (38%) than in those with asymptomatic (9%) and symptomatic (13%) aneurysms.[62] Although the clinical significance of these findings is unknown, it seems that colonized aneurysms do not pose the same threat to patients as infected aneurysms. Steed and colleagues concluded that significant contamination of intraluminal thrombus in aneurysms is rare.[64] Other authors have confirmed this report and advise that routine culture of aneurysm contents or wall is not necessary when the clinical picture does not suggest aneurysm infection.[65] Just as the abdominal aorta is the most common site for true aneurysms, the abdominal aorta is the predominant site reported for secondary infection of aneurysms (Fig. 139-3). Lesions have been discovered in other locations, and in earlier times, bacterial overgrowth in luetic aneurysms of the thoracic aorta was encountered.[15]

Bacteriology

Some authors have noted that the index of suspicion for infected abdominal aortic aneurysms (AAAs) is generally low, and consequently these lesions may have been underreported.[63] The study of infected preexisting AAAs by Jarrett and associates documented a predominance of gram-positive organisms (59%) over gram-negative organisms (35%).[21] The most prevalent organism was *Staphylococcus* (41%). Though less common, gram-negative infections were more virulent than gram-positive infections from the standpoint of aneurysm rupture (84% versus 10%) and patient mortality (84% versus 50%).

In another study, colonized aneurysms yielded 81% gram-positive and 19% gram-negative organisms.[62] The most prevalent organism was *S. epidermidis*, which accounted for 53% of positive cultures. Coliform sepsis in a preexisting AAA has been associated with an appendiceal abscess.[66]

As emerging technologies based on percutaneous or minimally invasive endovascular repairs gain popularity, infection

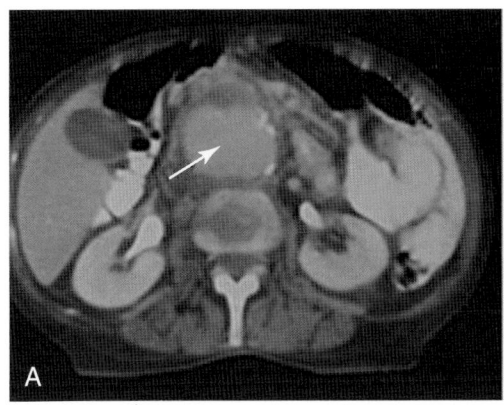
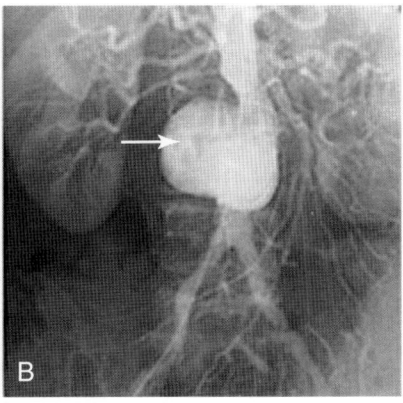

Figure 139-3 Diagnostic radiology studies of a patient with *Salmonella* infection of a preexisting small atherosclerotic aneurysm. **A,** Contrast-enhanced computed tomography scan showing a saccular aneurysm with calcification (*arrow*). **B,** Transfemoral aortogram showing a saccular atherosclerotic infrarenal aneurysm (*arrow*).

in a previously existing aneurysm and microbial arteritis may be associated with postimplantation infection, particularly when synthetic prostheses are used.[67] Unintentionally, grafts may be placed in a septic field that would otherwise have been subject to débridement in the course of a conventional open procedure. In clinical practice, however, this does not appear to be a significant issue inasmuch as midterm reports on several endografts either do not report graft infection as a complication or at most find it in 1% of cases in follow-up.[68]

Post-traumatic Infected False Aneurysms

Prevalence and Location

Post-traumatic infected false aneurysms have become a prevalent type of infected aneurysm in recent decades in clinical practice. The primary factor in this shifting emphasis in pathogenesis is drug addiction. The femoral triangle, used by narcotic addicts for repeated attempted vein injections, is the most common site in which these lesions occur (see Fig. 139-8A). Other locations, such as the external iliac and carotid arteries and the subclavian arteries, have also been reported (Fig. 139-4).[11,19,69]

Another factor contributing to the increasing incidence of these lesions is the proliferation of various invasive testing and monitoring procedures. In susceptible individuals, percutaneous arterial puncture may result in an iatrogenic post-traumatic infected false aneurysm.[7,8] Along with the increase in percutaneous endovascular procedures has come the increased use of percutaneous femoral artery closure devices, which may be associated with an increased incidence of infected pseudoaneurysms.[70]

Malanoski and coworkers reported that 55 of 102 patients (54%) with blood cultures positive for *S. aureus* at the New England Deaconess Hospital over a 2-year period had bacteremia attributable to an intravascular catheter.[53] Five of these patients had *Staphylococcus* sepsis after undergoing percutaneous coronary intervention (PCI). Two of the five patients also manifested a post-traumatic infected false aneurysm of the accessed femoral artery.

Samore and colleagues, reporting on catheter-related bacteremia in 3473 PCI patients from the Beth Israel Deaconess Medical Center, noted a low frequency (0.24%) of PCI-related bacteremia.[16] They reported significant morbidity, however, including post-traumatic infected false aneurysms of the punctured femoral artery. Independent risk factors for the development of septic complications after PCI were duration of the procedure, number of

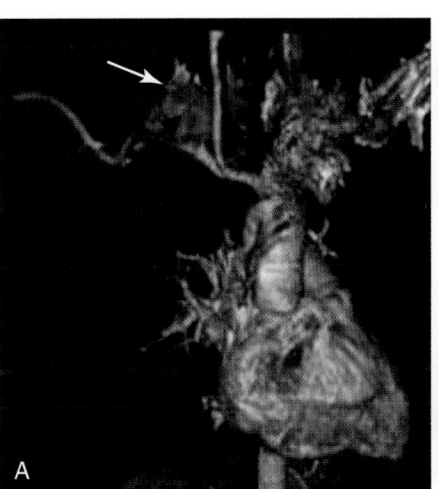
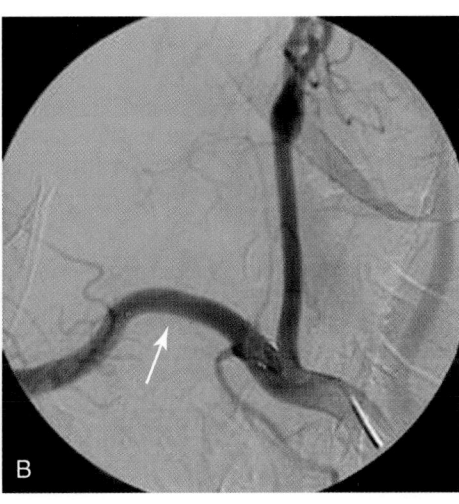

Figure 139-4 A, Computed tomographic angiography image with three-dimensional reconstruction in a patient with a polymicrobial post-traumatic false aneurysm of the right subclavian artery caused by repeated percutaneous cervical injection of illegal narcotics (*arrow*). **B,** Treatment with a covered stent-graft for control of hemorrhage (*arrow*). Adjuvant therapy included open débridement and irrigation along with intravenous antimicrobial therapy.

catheterizations at the same site, difficult vascular access, arterial sheath in place longer than 1 day, and associated congestive heart failure

Bacteriology

Since 1965, when the most prevalent form of infected aneurysm was a post-traumatic infected false aneurysm, the predominant infecting organism has been *S. aureus* (30%).[31,71] In our report of infected femoral artery false aneurysms in drug addicts, 35 of 54 patients (65%) had pure cultures of *S. aureus* from the aneurysm. Seventeen of these 35 staphylococcal cultures (48%) were found to be methicillin resistant. An additional eight patients had mixed polymicrobial cultures, including *S. aureus*, *E. coli*, *S. faecalis*, *Pseudomonas aeruginosa*, and various *Enterobacter* organisms.[14] Johnson and coauthors, reporting on drug-related infected false aneurysms in a variety of anatomic locations, isolated *S. aureus* from a high percentage of blood (71%) and wound (76%) cultures.[11]

■ CLINICAL FINDINGS

The clinical manifestation of infected aneurysms depends on the etiologic mechanism and the anatomic site involved. The clinical characteristics of various aneurysm types are summarized in Table 139-1. Although infected aneurysms occur in all age groups, including neonates[72,73] and children,[74] when there is no antecedent history of arterial injury, the typical patient is older and has atherosclerosis.[3,75] Infected aneurysms of the femoral or carotid arteries or other superficial peripheral locations are readily appreciated, however, and 90% are palpable.[42] Post-traumatic infected false aneurysms are often easily identified by physical examination. These often femoral false aneurysms are characterized by a tender pulsatile mass (indicative of contained rupture), some other manifestation of sepsis, or bleeding in almost every patient.[12-14] In patients with infected aneurysms secondary to microbial arteritis or infection of preexistent aneurysms, the principal signs and symptoms of an aneurysm and sepsis may be subtle (Table 139-2). Patients with infected aortic aneurysms usually have fever of unknown origin. Because of the insidious signs and symptoms

Table 139-2 Infected Aortoiliac Aneurysms: Clinical Findings

Clinical Marker	Number of Patients (%)
Abdominal pain	12 (92)
Fever	10 (77)
Leukocytosis*	9 (69)
Positive blood cultures	9 (69)
Palpable abdominal mass	6 (46)
Rupture	4 (31)

*Leukocyte count greater than 10×10^9/L.
From Reddy DJ, Shepard AD, Evans JR, et al. Management of infected aortoiliac aneurysms. *Arch Surg*. 1991;126:873. Copyright 1991, American Medical Association.

of infected aneurysms, a high index of suspicion is needed in the following situations: a positive blood or tissue culture, erosion of lumbar vertebrae, female gender, the presence of uncalcified aneurysms, and initial manifestation of an aneurysm after bacterial sepsis, particularly in immunocompromised patients.[21,41,72,76]

Of infected AAAs, 40% might not be palpable and may go unrecognized until rupture.[42,77-79] Pain is a common symptom, with either back or abdominal pain reported in several series in 40% to more than 90% of patients.[32,35,39] In addition, several series report fever and chills in 77% to more than 90% of patients with infected aneurysms.[32,35,39] Some series report co-morbid conditions associated with immunosuppression in up to 70% of patients.[35] Fungal arterial infections are rare but characteristically occur in patients with chronic immune suppression[4] or diabetes mellitus[80] or after treatment of a disseminated fungal disease.[81] The clinical manifestation of these rare infections may be limited to fever or malaise or may be more apparent, such as gangrene in an extremity after distal embolization.

Although infected aneurysms can occur in virtually any artery and may be accompanied by a variety of clinical signs and symptoms, they are similar in that they all eventually lead to sepsis or hemorrhage. Consequently, whenever the surgeon suspects this diagnosis, it must be assumed that the patient's life or limb is in jeopardy, and confirmation of the diagnosis and urgent surgical therapy are required.

■ DIAGNOSIS
Laboratory Studies

In most patients, leukocytosis is a sensitive but nonspecific indicator of an infected aneurysm.[14,21,38,39,82] The sensitivity of this finding may be limited, however, by intercurrent antimicrobial therapy that has suppressed but not cured the infection.[81] A lack of specificity is also underscored by reports of sealed ruptures of bland, uninfected, atherosclerotic aneurysms that may simulate sepsis and exhibit leukocytosis.[83] Likewise, an elevated erythrocyte sedimentation rate is often present but nonspecific. These limitations underscore the need for more specific and sensitive tests to confirm the presence of an infected aneurysm.

Positive blood cultures in a patient with an aneurysm are considered specific for an infected aneurysm until proved otherwise, although positive cultures do lack sensitivity. Anderson and colleagues found positive cultures in only 50% of such patients.[10] It follows that negative blood cultures alone are not sufficiently sensitive to rule out the diagnosis of an infected aneurysm.

When the diagnosis of an infected aneurysm is first entertained during surgery, as prompted by unexpected findings of purulence or other abnormal tissue appearance suggesting more than bland atherosclerotic changes, samples of the aneurysm wall and contents should be obtained for culture with a search for aerobic and anaerobic bacteria and fungi. Additional information may be gained by Gram stains. These studies should not be considered sufficient, however, to ensure that the aneurysm is not infected because neither negative blood cultures nor intraoperative Gram stains are sufficiently sensitive to exclude the diagnosis of infected aneurysm.[31] Culture results of the aneurysm wall and contents are not available during the operation and can be used only to direct postoperative antimicrobial therapy; even final culture results may be misleading in patients treated with antibiotics. Some authors have advocated wider use of aneurysm content and wall cultures in routine operations for aortic aneurysm.[21,62] It is important to underscore that the mere demonstration of positive cultures of the aneurysm wall and contents does not confirm the presence of an infected aneurysm without the constellation of clinical findings tempered by clinical judgment and experience. In our experience with infected aortoiliac aneurysms, 69% of patients had positive preoperative blood cultures and 92% had positive aneurysm wall cultures. Operative Gram stains were positive in 50% of patients with ruptured infected aneurysms but in only 11% of patients with unruptured but infected aneurysms.[39]

Imaging

Ultrasonography of the abdominal aorta is safe and noninvasive and will provide general information about aneurysm size and location, but it is less reliable for detecting the presence or extent of arterial infection. Ultrasonography has proven utility in the diagnosis of femoral artery false aneurysms, but the ability of duplex scanning to detect infection is uncertain, and we do not use it for this purpose.[14]

As spiral computed tomography (CT) scan technology with multiplanar reconstruction has become readily available, CT angiography (CTA) has become the diagnostic test of choice. Findings can include saccular or eccentrically configured aneurysms in an otherwise normal aorta, soft tissue inflammation or a mass around the aorta, and rupture or penetration. Other findings may include saccular aneurysm in an otherwise normal-appearing vessel, multilobulated aneurysm, and eccentric aneurysm with a relatively narrow neck that is specifically found in infected aneurysms from microbial arteritis inasmuch as these are false aneurysms.

Although CTA is valuable in determining the etiology and assessing the presence or absence of aneurysm rupture (see Figs. 139-2 and 139-3), it may still often fail to give a definitive answer to the question of the presence or absence of infection.[84-87] Short-interval serial CT scans may be valuable in suspected cases when the initial CT findings are nondiagnostic. Short-interval studies revealing rapidly enlarging or changing aneurysms are highly suggestive of infection. The previously noted findings suggestive of an infected aneurysm should prompt a complete "downstream" study because so-called satellite or multifocal lesions can occur.

Magnetic resonance imaging (MRI) may prove helpful for screening certain anatomic sites or when radiography or contrast media are contraindicated. The use of MRI is being reported with increasing frequency.[88,89] Specific MRI sequences can reveal active inflammation, a particular advantage over CT scanning. Although some investigators have found indium 111–labeled white blood cell scanning useful in diagnosing prosthetic graft infection, this modality has not always been accurate in confirming the diagnosis of an infected aneurysm.[90,91] It may be of use when other imaging studies are equivocal. Australian investigators have reported on the utility of bone and leukocyte scintigraphy to show the extent of adjacent soft tissue and lumbar osteomyelitis in a case of ruptured infected AAA.[92]

Though not used as frequently since the development of CTA technology, digital subtraction angiography has been used in the treatment of infected aneurysms for diagnosis and planning of repair. The arteriographic criteria for infection in an aneurysm are as follows: saccular aneurysm in an otherwise normal-appearing vessel, multilobulated aneurysm, and eccentric aneurysm with a relatively narrow neck. An infected aneurysm may not exhibit any arteriographic characteristics indicative of infection, however.[93]

SURGICAL TREATMENT

Preoperative Care

When an infected aneurysm is suspected, broad-spectrum antibiotic therapy should be initiated and continued until the organism is isolated, and then the antimicrobial therapy should be tailored to organism-specific antimicrobial sensitivities. Drug therapy is begun before surgery and continued postoperatively and, in certain circumstances, for life.[41,94] Multidrug-resistant strains pose a serious risk and have been associated with clinical cases originating from livestock vectors.

Treatment of narcotic addicts should include active and passive tetanus prophylaxis. Although organism-specific antibiotic therapy is an essential element of successful surgical management of an infected aneurysm, patient survival depends on prompt diagnosis and surgery.[21,39] Ruptures of infected aneurysms have been reported in patients undergoing antibiotic therapy while awaiting surgery and in those who have completed antibiotic therapy and are thought, erroneously, to have bland aneurysms sterilized by antibiotics.[3,95,96] Undue delay in operative intervention must be avoided. Reported spontaneous cures of infected aneurysms are exceptions.[9] In cases of a ruptured or symptomatic aneurysm, surgery should be undertaken urgently.

Operative Principles

Six general principles have traditionally been applied in the operative management of infected aneurysms:

1. Control of hemorrhage
2. Confirmation of the diagnosis, including tissue smears for Gram stains and culture of specimens for aerobic and anaerobic bacteria and fungi
3. Operative control of sepsis, including aneurysm resection and ligation of healthy artery, followed by wide débridement of all surrounding infected tissue along with antibiotic irrigation and placement of drains when needed

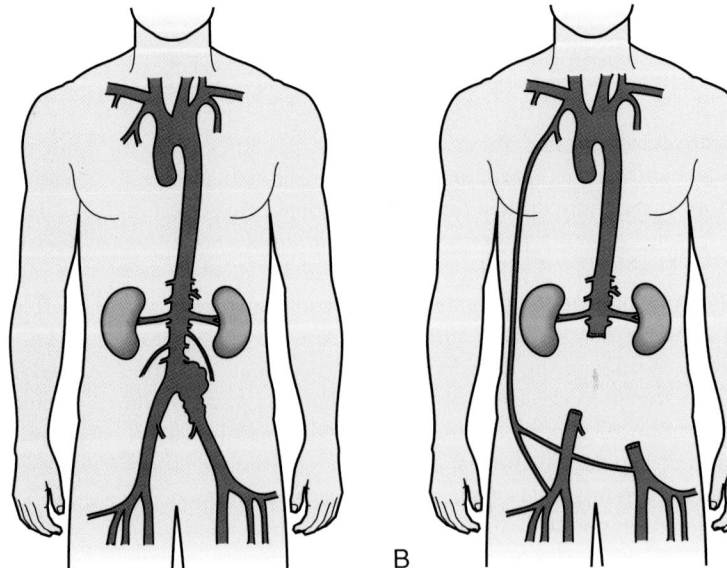

Figure 139-5 Treatment of an infected infrarenal aortoiliac aneurysm by ligation of heathy infrarenal aorta, wide débridement of all surrounding infected tissue, and arterial reconstruction through uninfected planes with axillobifemoral bypass. Note preservation of right internal iliac artery. **A,** Preoperative. **B,** Postoperative.

4. Thorough postoperative wound care, including frequent dressing changes and débridement as needed

5. Continuation of antibiotics for a prolonged period after surgery

6. Arterial reconstruction of vital arteries through uninfected tissue planes with selected use of interposition grafting through the bed of the resected aneurysm, soft tissue coverage such as omental wrap if possible, and the use of autologous tissue for reconstruction

The first five principles are established, uncontroversial surgical tenets. Controversy exists, however, about the selection of patients for in situ arterial reconstruction and the timing and methods of reconstruction, particularly when the infected aneurysm involves the aorta, the femoral artery, or the carotid artery.[11,12,14,17,18,31,41,82,97-103] Classically, resection plus extra-anatomic revascularization has been the treatment; however, in certain cases ligation and excision without reconstruction may be a viable option, whereas in other locations, such as the more proximal aorta, in situ reconstruction with prosthetic graft may be the only option. Cryopreserved homografts are being reported as reasonable alternatives for grafting. In contemporary practice, the option of in situ reconstructions versus excision with extra-anatomic bypass will be contingent on a variety of factors, including the nature and virulence of the infection and, perhaps most important, the anatomic location, as described under "Allografts."

Aorta

Extra-anatomic Reconstruction

The classic approach to management of an infected AAA when limited to the infrarenal segment is similar to the treatment of an infected aortic prosthesis. The entire aneurysm is resected, the infected tissues are thoroughly débrided, drainage is established, and arterial reconstruction by axillobifemoral bypass is carried out through uninfected planes (Fig. 139-5).[21,82,98,104] This approach avoids the risks related to placement of a graft in the infected retroperitoneum, which is reported to be associated with an overall 23% reoperation rate that increases to 63% when the infecting organism is gram negative.[98] Axillobifemoral bypass is a less durable reconstruction, however, than successful interposition aortic grafting.[39,103,105] In one of the larger multicenter studies of patients treated with this method, Bacourt and Koskas reported an early mortality rate of 24% and an overall mortality rate of 42%.[106] Complications specific to this method include aortic stump rupture, which has been reported to have an incidence as high as 50% when cultures at the site are positive, and infection of the axillobifemoral bypass, which is reported at a rate of 6% to 20% in different series.[21,82,98,104,107,108]

In Situ Reconstruction

Because of limitations of the "resection and extra-anatomic bypass" approach, some surgeons advocate in situ interposition aortic grafts after resection of an infected aortic aneurysm.[31,41,99,100,103,109] This is specifically applicable when the infected aneurysm involves the suprarenal or thoracoabdominal component of the aorta, where direct repair may be the only option.[110] Options that have been used for conduit for this reconstruction include femoral-popliteal vein, cryopreserved homograft, and prosthetic grafts with or without antibiotic impregnation.[17,18,109,112-118] When performing in situ reconstruction, just as for extra-anatomic reconstruction, thorough debridement of infected tissue is required until healthy artery is present to which an anastomosis can be performed. Once completed, the graft should be covered with a viable omental flap (Fig. 139-6). Prolonged antibiotic therapy is recommended by most authors; however, the duration necessary has not been defined, but suggested lengths of treatment range from 4 to 6 weeks to lifelong therapy.

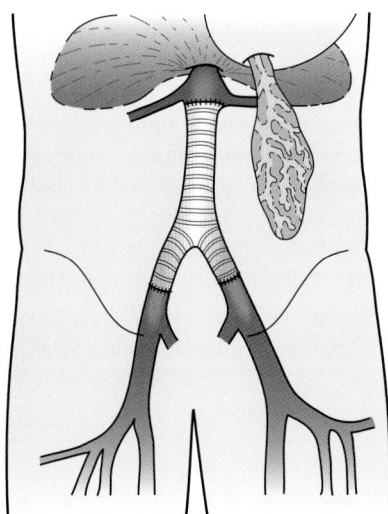

Figure 139-6 Illustration demonstrating in situ repair of an infected aneurysm of the abdominal aorta with a prosthetic graft after resection of the aneurysm and thorough débridement of the bed of the aneurysm. A pedicle of viable gastrocolic omentum is used to cover the graft. The omental pedicle is diverted through the transverse mesocolon to lessen the risk of its causing future bowel obstruction.

Femoral-Popliteal Vein. Clagett and colleagues reported a prospective study suggesting the feasibility and durability of autogenous aortoiliac or aortofemoral vein grafts to treat prosthetic infections.[119] This method may have application in the treatment of infected aneurysms and is gaining wider clinical acceptance and application.[120] The durability of this procedure has been reported by Beck and coauthors in a series of 240 neo-aortoiliac system reconstructions using femoral popliteal vein; they cited primary patency rates of 87% and 82% at 2 and 5 years, respectively, along with primary assisted patency rates of 96% and 94% at 2 and 5 years, respectively.[121] However, drawbacks include longer operative times required for harvesting and preparation of the deep veins, as well as lower extremity morbidity from the dissection and removal of the deep venous system. Nonetheless, the development of chronic venous insufficiency and venous ulceration in survivors over time has been reported to be low (15%) after deep vein harvest.[122] Clagett's group reported the intermediate and late follow-up CT image findings after neo-aortoiliac reconstruction and confirmed its utility in the management of patients with aortofemoral prosthetic graft infections.[123] Beck, writing for the same group of investigators, recently concluded that risk factors for restenosis included small graft size, history of coronary artery disease, and smoking, although primary patency rates at 2 and 5 years were 87% and 82%, respectively, and assisted primary patency rates were 96% and 94%, as stated previously.[124]

Allografts. Allografts have been used as conduit in the presence of infection. Experimental data in a canine model suggest that in situ arterial allografts are less vulnerable to infection than commonly available synthetic prostheses.[125] If this sug-

gestion is true, this decreased infectability may make arterial allografts an appropriate choice when circumstances require re-establishment of aortic continuity in a contaminated field. Even though fresh allografts have been associated with a significant number of complications, clinical reports from many centers in the United States and Europe have detailed the use of cryopreserved arterial homografts for in situ replacement of infected aneurysms of various aortic segments.[17,18,109,112-118] Vogt and associates reported a series of 72 patients with either mycotic aneurysms or graft infections of the thoracic or abdominal aorta; comparison of the group treated with prosthetic graft (extra-anatomic or in situ) and the group treated with in situ cryopreserved allografts showed superior disease-related survival free of reoperation in the allograft group.[18] Noel and colleagues, in a review of the U.S. cryopreserved aortic allograft registry, reported a 30-day mortality rate of 13% and an overall mortality rate of 25% during a mean follow-up period of 5.3 months (range, 1 to 22 months).[17] Mortality in 4% of the cases was specifically attributed to the graft. Graft-related morbidity included perianastomotic hemorrhage in 9%, graft limb occlusion in 9%, pseudoaneurysm in 2%, and amputation in 5%. The authors concluded that the preliminary data failed to justify the preferential use of cryopreserved allografts for use in arterial reconstructions for the treatment of infected aneurysms and graft infections over other established techniques.[17] The lack of readily available cryopreserved grafts of the appropriate diameter and length has also limited its wider application.

Prosthetic Grafts. Several series have also reported satisfactory outcomes with in situ repairs using prosthetic graft, which may be the only option for some paravisceral or thoracoabdominal aneurysms. In these cases, adjunctive use of antibiotic-releasing beads implanted in the perigraft tissue, omental coverage, and rifampin-bonded polyester (Dacron) grafts have been used.[101,126,127] Oderich and coworkers described creating an antibiotic-soaked, gelatin-impregnated Dacron graft by soaking it at room temperature in a 60-mg/mL solution of rifampin in sterile saline for 30 to 60 minutes.[35] Muller and colleagues have added coverage of graft with gentamicin-soaked gauze.[34] Oderich and coauthors reported on 43 patients, 27 of whom had aneurysms involving the juxtarenal aorta or more proximal aorta, and 35 of the 43 patients underwent in situ reconstruction with prosthetic graft. Operative mortality was 21% with no significant difference between in situ and extra-anatomic reconstructions. In addition, at 5 years the incidence of graft-related infection was 6%. Variables that they found to be associated with increased aneurysm-related death included extensive periaortic infection, female gender, *S. aureus* infection, rupture, and suprarenal location.[35] Muller and coworkers reported on 33 mycotic aneurysms, 17 of which were suprarenal or involved the more proximal aorta. Each of the 17 of the more proximal aneurysms and 8 of the remaining 16 more distal aneurysms were treated by in situ reconstruction. An overall in-hospital mortality rate of 36% with in situ reconstruction has compared favorably with extra-anatomic reconstruction. Aneurysm rupture rather than its proximal location was associated with a significant increase in mortalitly.[34]

Endovascular Treatment

Endovascular treatment methods, devices, and experiences have increased over the last decade, and successful endoluminal management of these challenging aneurysms has been reported as well. When successful, this therapy has the advantage of being less invasive and less physiologically stressful in an already compromised patient. The concern, however, is that such intervention omits the principles of drainage of sepsis and wide débridement, which have been established as cornerstones in the effort to eradicate these arterial infections. Nonetheless, endoluminal repairs have been accomplished with standard endovascular techniques and stent-grafts intended for both aortic and thoracic aneurysm repair; in addition, non–commercially available fenestrated grafts have been reported for repair of paravisceral aneurysms. Perhaps as expected, reinfection and late failures have been emphasized by several authors (Fig. 139-7).[128-132] Several of the reported interventions have included adjunctive procedures such as soaking the graft in antibiotics before deployment and percutaneously placed drainage catheters, as well as open surgical débridement.

Outcome data and long-term results are very limited. Kan and coworkers in 2007 reviewed the relevant literature on endoluminal management of infected aortic aneurysms.[128] They reported an 89.6% ± 4.4% 30-day survival rate and an 82% ± 5.8% 2-year survival rate in 48 cases via life-table analysis. Multivariate logistic regression analysis revealed rupture and fever to be associated with persistent infection. Those with persistent infection did poorly. Typically, endovascular stent-grafting was combined with long-term antibiotic therapy. Even when long-term antibiotic therapy has been provided, adverse outcomes such as persistent or recurrent infections have appeared.[128] Reoperation for these infected aneurysms, after having been inadequately treated by

endovascular means, is more likely to be unsuccessful or even complicated by patient mortality.[128,132-134] Our group believes that the role of endovascular therapy for the treatment of infected aneurysms is emerging but remains undefined. The clinical findings, microbiologic studies to determine the virulence and susceptibility of the organisms and tolerable and practical antimicrobial therapy, the degree of sepsis, and local contamination will probably also contribute to this therapy's success or failure. The questions to be addressed by investigators are (1) When is endovascular repair only palliative therapy? (2) When does it serve as a bridge to staged definitive surgical therapy? and (3) When is endovascular repair the preferred, definitive therapy?

Selection of Treatment

In selected patients, in situ repair through the bed of the resected aneurysm may be justified when there is no gross sepsis, but in situ repair should be avoided when the retroperitoneum is grossly purulent.[36,135] Even complex reconstruction of the suprarenal aorta may be accomplished with extra-anatomic techniques.[105,136] Some reports have emphasized that recognition of organism virulence and the severity and extent of the aortic infection is more important than strict adherence to any single operative approach or method of arterial reconstruction.[37,137,138] Proper patient selection and surgical judgment are among the prime determinants of management success. In infected aneurysms of the aortic arch, thoracic aorta, thoracoabdominal aorta, and suprarenal abdominal aorta, interposition grafting may be the only feasible approach.[41,97,139-141] An endovascular approach may be an attractive treatment option because of its minimally invasive character, and it may therefore be the better choice for patients with infected aneurysms who are critically ill with hostile or impractical operative exposure or as an expedient to halt hemorrhage. Because this approach challenges the tenets of surgical débridement for control of sepsis and remote arterial bypass, it is the probable explanation for the persistent infections encountered during follow-up. Nonetheless,

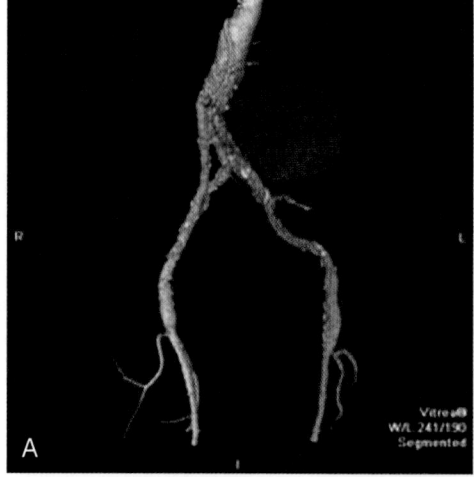
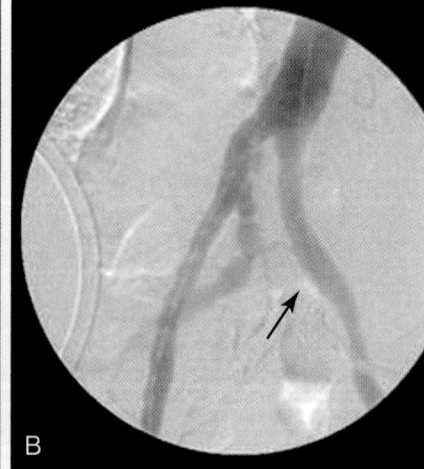

Figure 139-7 A, CTA findings in an 80-year-old debilitated woman demonstrating a large infected false aneurysm of the left common iliac artery. **B,** Digital subtraction angiogram revealing exclusion of the pseudoaneurysm after emergency stent-graft (*arrow*) deployment for control of hemorrhage.

reports of successful endovascular treatment beyond 2 years' follow-up are appearing in the literature with increasing regularity.[142]

Femoral Artery

Management options for the treatment of infected femoral artery aneurysms are (1) arterial excision alone and (2) arterial excision followed by arterial reconstruction. The various operative techniques for arterial reconstruction include an interposition vein autograft with a sartorius muscle flap, obturator bypass, lateral femoral bypass, and axillary–to–distal femoral bypass (Fig. 139-8). If the cause of the infected aneurysm is other than drug injection, obturator bypass or interposition grafting usually seems to be the preferred treatment.[143,144] Drug addicts are unsuitable candidates for arterial reconstruction with synthetic arterial prostheses because continued drug use carries a high risk for graft infection (Table

139-3).[10,12,14] In this select group of patients, when reconstruction of the femoral artery is considered desirable, it is necessary to control groin sepsis and to use autogenous grafts. Great saphenous vein from the midthigh is usually available, even in patients with a long history of drug abuse.[14]

Although selection criteria and methods of femoral arterial reconstruction in drug addicts are controversial, there is general agreement that most patients do not require reconstruction to avoid amputation.[5,12,14,101] The collateral circulation is usually sufficient to maintain limb viability even after the femoral artery bifurcation has been ligated (Fig. 139-9). Amputation is almost never necessary when femoral artery ligation-excision is limited to a single femoral artery segment—the common, superficial, or deep femoral artery (see Table 139-3). Patients at risk for amputation are those in whom the femoral artery bifurcation must be excised. In these circumstances, reconstruction by autogenous vein interposition may be considered when local wound conditions are

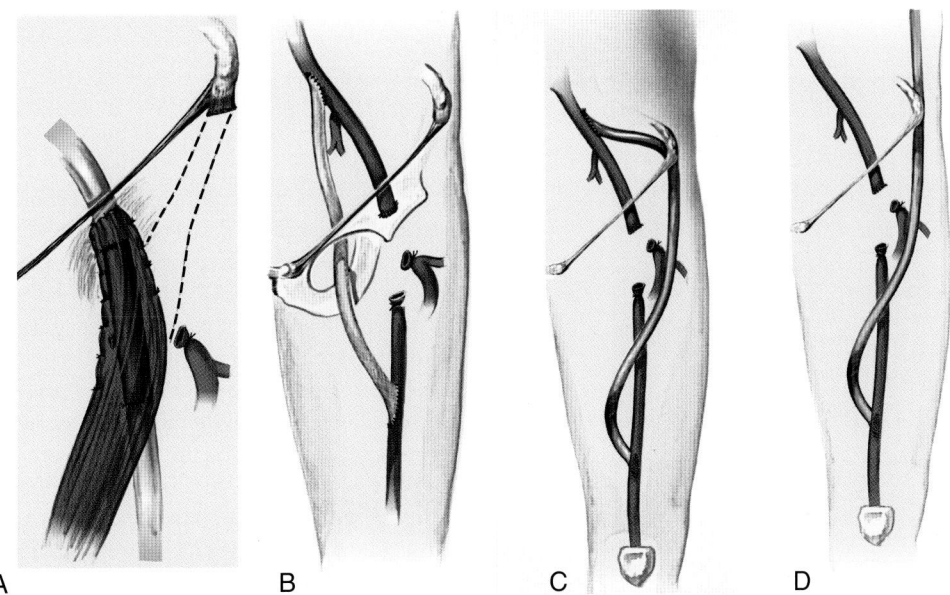

A   B   C   D

Figure 139-8 Methods of femoral artery reconstruction. **A,** Interposition vein autograft covered by rotated sartorius muscle. **B,** Obturator bypass. **C,** Lateral femoral bypass. **D,** Axillary–to–distal femoral bypass. (**A, B,** and **D,** From Reddy DJ, Smith RF, Elliott JP Jr, et al. Infected femoral artery false aneurysms in drug addicts: evolution of selective vascular reconstruction. J Vasc Surg. 1986;3:718.)

Table 139-3 Treatment Method and Results of Infected Femoral Artery False Aneurysms Secondary to Drug Addiction

Type of Aneurysm and Treatment	Number of Aneurysms	Number of Viable Limbs	Cases of Graft Sepsis (%)	Number of Amputations (%)
Common femoral artery: ligation-excision	14	14	—	0
Deep femoral artery: ligation-excision	11	11	—	0
Superficial femoral artery: ligation-excision	4	4	—	0
Common femoral bifurcation				
Ligation-excision	21	14	—	7 (33)
Reconstruction with autogenous vein	6	6	1	0
Reconstruction with synthetic prosthesis	3	3	3 (100)	0
Reconstruction by primary anastomosis	1	1	0	0
Total	**60**	**53**	**4**	**7 (12)**

From Reddy DJ, Smith RF, Elliott JP Jr, et al. Infected femoral artery false aneurysms in drug addicts: evolution of selective vascular reconstruction. *J Vasc Surg.* 1986;3:718.

favorable, although experience with this technique is limited.[14] When ligation of the femoral bifurcation is required but reconstruction is not feasible, we empirically instill a concentrated heparin-sodium solution antegradely into the ligated femoral artery in an effort to preserve all possible arterial collaterals. Unless there is a specific indication, however, anticoagulation therapy is not continued in the postoperative period.

The optimal management of these lesions is a matter of debate.[13,14,101,102,145-149] It is generally agreed that surgical therapy is required and prolonged use of antibiotics is inappropriate.

Lower extremity amputation rates after treatment of infected femoral artery false aneurysms have ranged from 11% to 25%.[10-12,14,101] The above-knee amputation rate after ligation-excision of the femoral artery bifurcation in drug

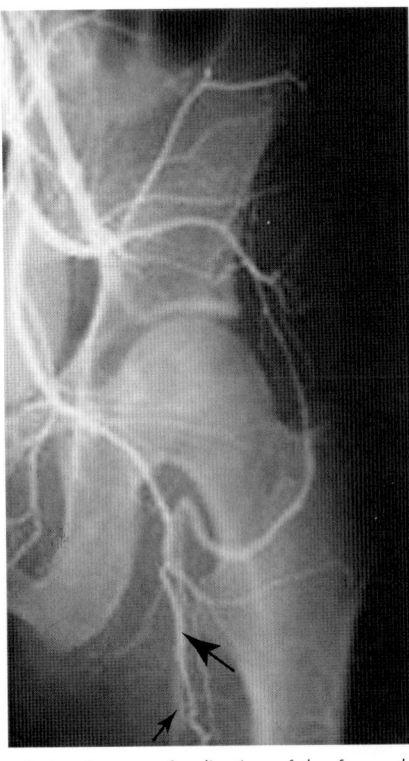

Figure 139-9 Arteriogram after ligation of the femoral artery bifurcation showing prompt reconstitution of the deep femoral artery by numerous collaterals (*large arrow*) with faint visualization of the slightly more distal superficial femoral artery (*small arrow*).

addicts approximates 33%. When groin sepsis is not controlled, revascularization in an attempt to prevent amputation may pose an unnecessary and potentially lethal risk for graft sepsis and should be undertaken with caution. Amputation may be unavoidable in patients with infected femoral false aneurysms.

Carotid Artery

Although ligation without arterial reconstruction is often safe in the treatment of infected aneurysms of the innominate, common carotid, or upper extremity vessels, there is a major risk for stroke or death after ligation of the cervical internal carotid artery, which of course mandates anticoagulation to prevent stroke from thrombus propagating up the internal carotid, as well as maintenance of appropriate postligation systemic blood pressure. Although ligation-excision without reconstruction is controversial, many authors favor it and prefer to avoid the potential disastrous consequences of graft sepsis and hemorrhage after reconstruction.[150,151] Other authors favor primary reconstruction of the carotid artery with autogenous vein[69,152] or progressive clamp occlusion of the internal carotid artery while observing the awake patient for clinical signs of cerebral ischemia.[153]

Data providing a rational basis for selection of patients for carotid artery ligation versus reconstruction have been reported by Ehrenfeld and colleagues.[154] They found ligation of the internal carotid artery to be safe if carotid stump systolic pressure exceeded 70 mm Hg. This was a selected group of patients who had received anticoagulation therapy and in whom systemic blood pressure had been maintained at defined levels, but this group may not be representative. The rarity of these lesions highlights the need for individualized patient management.[29,155,156] In the special circumstance of cerebral mycotic aneurysms, stereoscopic synthesized brain-surface imaging with magnetic resonance angiography for anatomic localization has emerged as a useful modality.[26,92]

Visceral Arteries

Although visceral arterial aneurysms are uncommon, a high percentage are infected, in particular those of the superior mesenteric artery.[157] Treatment must be individualized and directed by angiography (Fig. 139-10). When feasible,

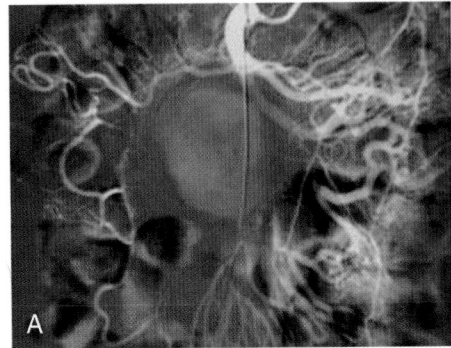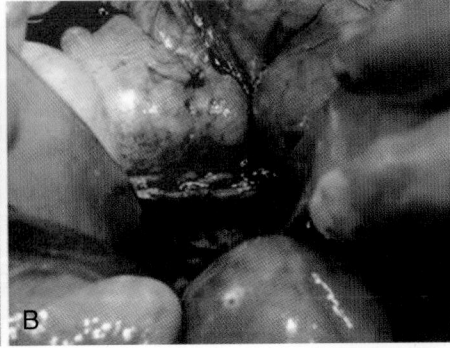

Figure 139-10 A, Arteriogram demonstrating a large infected aneurysm of the superior mesenteric artery. **B,** Operative photograph of a ligated and débrided superior mesenteric artery aneurysm. The causative organism was *Klebsiella pneumoniae.*

aneurysm ligation-excision is desirable, but arterial reconstruction with saphenous or femoral vein autografts or other innovations may be required to preserve organ or bowel viability (see also Chapter 138: Splanchnic Artery Aneurysms).[29,158,159]

SELECTED KEY REFERENCES

Anderson CB, Butcher HR Jr, Ballinger WF. Mycotic aneurysms. *Arch Surg.* 1974;109:712.
The first modern clinical series that established the important clinical findings and management scheme.

Brown SL, Busuttil RW, Baker JD, Machleder HI, Moore WS, Barker WF. Bacteriologic and surgical determinants of survival in patients with mycotic aneurysms. *J Vasc Surg.* 1984;1:541.
Comprehensive catalog of the important microbiologic correlates with these disease entities.

Clagett GP, Valentine RJ, Hagino RT. Autogenous aortoiliac/femoral reconstruction from superficial femoral-popliteal veins: feasibility and durability. *J Vasc Surg.* 1997;25:255.
This is a large clinical experience with a novel and successful autogenous reconstruction approach to complex arterial infections.

Kan C, Lee H, Yang Y. Outcome after endovascular stent graft treatment for mycotic aortic aneurysm: a systematic review. *J Vasc Surg* 2007;46:906.
Recent review of infected aneurysms treated with endovascular stent-grafts.

Oderich GS, Panneton JM, Bower TC, Cherry KJ Jr, Rowland CM, Noel AA, Hallett JW Jr, Gloviczki P. Infected aortic aneurysms: aggressive presentation, complicated early outcome but durable results. *J Vasc Surg.* 2001;34:900.
Large recent clinical series on the management of infected aortic aneurysms.

Osler W. The Gulstonian lectures on malignant endocarditis. *BMJ.* 1885;1:467.
This is the classic study that provides the foundational clinical understanding and nomenclature with which every vascular surgeon should be conversant.

Oz MC, Brener BJ, Buda JA, Todd G, Brenner RW, Goldenkranz RJ, McNicholas KW, Lemole GM, Lozner JS. A ten-year experience with bacterial aortitis. *J Vasc Surg.* 1989;10:439.
This paper established the extent and configuration of microbial arteritis in the aortoiliac segment.

Reddy DJ, Shepard AD, Evans JR, Wright DJ, Smith RF, Ernst CB. Management of infected aortoiliac aneurysms. *Arch Surg.* 1991; 126:873.
This is a comprehensive large medical center review of the open management of this challenging pathologic entity.

Reddy DJ, Smith RF, Elliott JP Jr, Haddad GK, Wanek EA. Infected femoral artery false aneurysms in drug addicts: evolution of selective vascular reconstruction. *J Vasc Surg.* 1986;3:718.
Unique clinical experience that permitted a rational approach to life and limb salvage based on the anatomic location of the post-traumatic infected false aneurysm.

Vogt PR, Brunner-LaRocca HP, Lachat M, Ruef C, Turina MI. Technical details with the use of cryopreserved arterial allograft for aortic infection: influence on early and mid term mortality. *J Vasc Surg.* 2002;35:80.
This paper reports a large series on the use of cryopreserved arterial allografts for the treatment of infected aortic aneurysms.

REFERENCES

The reference list can be found on the companion Expert Consult Web site at *www.expertconsult.com.*

Section **17** Arterial Aneurysms

CHAPTER 140

Aneurysms Caused by Connective Tissue Abnormalities

James H. Black, III

The primary structural proteins of connective tissue are composed of collagen and elastin, which vary in type and amount within each of the body's tissues; those constitutive of blood vessels are displayed in Table 140-1. A connective tissue disease is a genetic disease in which the primary target is either collagen or elastin protein assembly, disruption of which leads to an inherent predisposition to degeneration, loss of structural integrity, and consequent aneurysm formation or spontaneous vascular dissection and rupture. Although inflammation may affect these proteins and induce structural damage in some patients, such conditions often imply some element of autoimmune disorder and are termed *collagen vascular diseases* or *mixed connective tissue diseases*. Such conditions and arteritides related to the vascular tree are considered in Chapters 76 (Vasculitis and Other Arteriopathies), 77 (Thromboangiitis Obliterans), and 78 (Takayasu's Disease) and may have genetic profiles that predispose to their development. Although clustering of aneurysms in multiply affected family members within these arteritides may indicate some element of an inheritance pattern, there are often greatly varying levels of expression and penetrance and no defined genetic test available to assist treatment. For the sporadic occurrence of degenerative aneurysms within kindreds, the underlying mechanisms are considered in Chapter 126 (Arterial Aneurysms: General Considerations). Herein we seek to define the common connective tissue diseases affecting the arterial tree, which have a studied natural history, a defined basis for genetic inheritance, and sufficiently understood pathophysiologic mechanisms to guide treatment paradigms. These "heritable disorders of connective tissue"[1] have severe vascular manifestations and most commonly include Marfan's syndrome, the vascular type of Ehlers-Danlos syndrome (EDS IV), Loeys-Dietz syndrome (LDS), and familial thoracic aortic aneurysm and dissection (TAAD).

Table 140-1 Structural Elements of Blood Vessels

Structural Proteins	Approximate Amount (% Dry Wt)	Function
Type I collagen	20-40	Fibrillar network
Type III collagen	20-40	Thin fibrils
Elastin, fibrillin	20-40	Elasticity
Type IV collagen, laminin	<5	Basal lamina
Types V and VI collagen	<2	Function unclear
Proteoglycans (>30 types)	<3	Resiliency

■ MARFAN'S SYNDROME

Antonin-Bernard Marfan was a Professor of Pediatrics in Paris who in 1896 encountered a 5-year-old girl with congenital deformation of all four limbs.[2] By the age of 11 years, thoracolumbar kyphoscoliosis, pectus carinatum, and signs of tuberculosis had developed.[3] She died at age 16 from infection, and no autopsy was performed to document any vascular involvement. The first description of aortic pathology in Marfan's syndrome was published in 1943, a year after the death of Professor Marfan.[4] Although Marfan correctly identified the many mendelian features of the condition that would eventually bear his name, the pleiotropic disorder has benefited from decades of further description of clinical manifestations, molecular pathogenesis, and emerging therapeutic options.

Epidemiology and Natural History

The incidence of Marfan's syndrome is about 2 to 3 per 10,000 individuals, but this estimate relies on proper recognition of all affected and genetically predisposed individuals.[5] A population-based study in Scotland found an incidence of 1 in 9802 live births,[6] although this number would underestimate the true incidence inasmuch as the features of Marfan's syndrome, particularly the skeletal ones, become more apparent with growth. Furthermore, even though the disorder is passed as a dominant mendelian trait, about 25% of cases are due to sporadic de novo mutations.[7] The disease has no gender predisposition. Its incidence is increased in athletes, particularly in basketball and volleyball players, because the characteristic tall stature with long-bone overgrowth (dolichostenomelia) confers a competitive advantage. In a screening study of 415 high-school basketball and volleyball athletes performed with standard echocardiography, 4 (1%) of these subjects exhibited aortic root enlargement greater than 4.6 cm, and Marfan's syndrome was diagnosed in 2.[8]

The life span of individuals with Marfan's syndrome was significantly shortened before the widespread and successful refinement of aortic root surgery. Before adoption of thresholds for aortic root replacement, the cause of death was cardiovascular (aortic rupture, aortic dissection, or valvular disease) in 90% of cases.[9] A report in the 1970s on the life expectancy of patients with Marfan's syndrome described longevity as only two thirds that of unaffected individuals, with life-table mortality curves deviating in infancy.[9] However, a more recent assessment of longevity in patients with Marfan's syndrome describes a nearly normal life expectancy as a result of improvement and refinement in diagnosis and treatment, particularly of the cardiovascular manifestations of the disorder.[10]

Pathogenesis

As early as 1955 it was suggested that the basic structural defect in Marfan's syndrome was localized to the elastic fiber,[11] with skin and aorta from affected patients showing decreased elastin content and fragmentation of elastic fibers.[12,13] Yet the elastin gene and molecule were a poor target to explain the clinical manifestations of Marfan's syndrome in tissues that are devoid of elastin, such as bone and the ciliary zonules in the eye. Further histochemical analysis demonstrated that the amorphous fragmented elastin tissues were surrounded by a rodlike material with a distinct staining pattern and distinguishable susceptibility to enzymatic digestion.[14,15] These so-called microfibrils are 10 to 14 nm in diameter and are constituents of all connective tissue.[15] Sakai and colleagues first identified fibrillin-1 (FBN1) as the principal component of the extracellular matrix microfibril, present in all tissues with the phenotypic manifestations of Marfan's syndrome.[16] Additional linkage analysis mapped the Marfan's syndrome locus to 15q21.1.[17] To date, all of the mutation analyses have identified the *FBN1* gene as the sole locus for classic Marfan's syndrome, and most families have unique or private mutations. More than 550 mutations have been reported within the *FBN1* gene.[18] Neither the location of the mutation or the type of amino acid altered is sufficient to predict phenotype in any individual patient. An exception is mutations within exons 24 to 32, which are associated with a severe form of Marfan's syndrome diagnosed in early childhood.[19] The mutation is passed in an autosomal dominant manner with complete penetrance, so 50% of the offspring of an affected individual can inherit a genetic predisposition to the disorder.[5]

Role of Fibrillin

The *FBN1* gene contains 65 exons spanning 235 kilobases of genomic DNA.[20,21] The gene encodes a 350-kD glycoprotein that is highly conserved among different species, thus suggesting its critical homeostatic importance.[21] Initial findings suggested that the defect in Marfan's syndrome was caused by activity of the mutant protein on the deposition, stability, or function of the neighboring normal protein—the "dominant negative effect." This would, of course, bode poorly for the development of productive treatment strategies because it implied that patients had an immutable structural predisposition to tissue failure later in life.[5] However, the association between a mutant fibrillar protein exerting a dominant effect and severity of disease was refuted by the discovery of patients with severe disease and nearly absent levels of mutant protein because of a premature termination codon created by their specific mutation.[22] To reconcile, murine models of Marfan's

syndrome have provided the opportunity to study the earliest pathogenetic abnormalities in elastogenesis and aortic aneurysm formation.[23,24] These models demonstrated that normal FBN1 molecules are not needed to assemble an elastic fiber; rather, microfibrils are required to maintain normal elastic fibers during postnatal life. If proper connections among elastic fibers and vascular smooth muscles cells are not suitably maintained, cells adopt matrix-degrading enzymes such as matrix metalloproteinase types 2 and 9. Thereafter, aortic wall homeostasis is perturbed, and inflammation and elastic fiber calcification and structural weakening may ensue. This pathology has been observed in large muscular arteries from patients with Marfan's syndrome,[25] which led to appreciation of the classic lesion of cystic medial necrosis in large arteries of individuals with Marfan's syndrome. Verhoeff–van Gieson staining of elastic fibers in the aorta demonstrates classic lamellar disorganization in Marfan's syndrome secondary to errant elastic fiber maintenance (Fig. 140-1).

Interaction with Transforming Growth Factor-β

Recent discovery of the role of microfibrils in regulating cytokines has further advanced our understanding of the pathogenesis of Marfan's syndrome and raised the possibility of a new treatment paradigm. FBN1 shares a high degree of homology with the latent transforming growth factor-β (TGF-β) binding proteins. The TGF-β cytokines are secreted as large latent complexes consisting of TGF-β, a latency-associated peptide, and one of three latent TGF-β binding proteins (Fig. 140-2).[26] In normal trafficking, the large latent complex is sequestered and bound to microfibrils, and TGF-β cytokine signaling is prevented. Once the mature cytokine is released from the binding proteins, interactions with cell surface receptors and downstream signaling can occur via the well-defined SMAD (nuclear proteins involved in signal transduction for TGF-β ligands) transcription factor pathways, which modulate the effects of TGF-β. The homology between fibrillins and latent TGF-β binding proteins prompted the hypothesis that microfibrils may play a role in the trafficking of TGF-β and its activation. Credence has been lent to this hypothesis with the demonstration of elevated TGF-β activity and free TGF-β levels in FBN1-deficient mice during developmental septation of the lung[27] and the development of myxomatous cardiac valvular changes.[28] As depicted in Figure 140-2, without proper microfibrils the TGF-β complex cannot form, thereby leaving TGF-β in the milieu to incite excess signaling. This pathogenetic mechanism of dysregulated TGF-β activity seems more plausible in explaining the clinical features of Marfan's syndrome that are poorly reconciled with structural failure, such as long-bone overgrowth, craniofacial abnormalities, and muscle hypoplasia.[28]

Clinical Manifestations and Diagnostic Evaluation

Marfan's syndrome is a multisystem disorder with manifestations principally within the cardiovascular, ocular, and skeletal

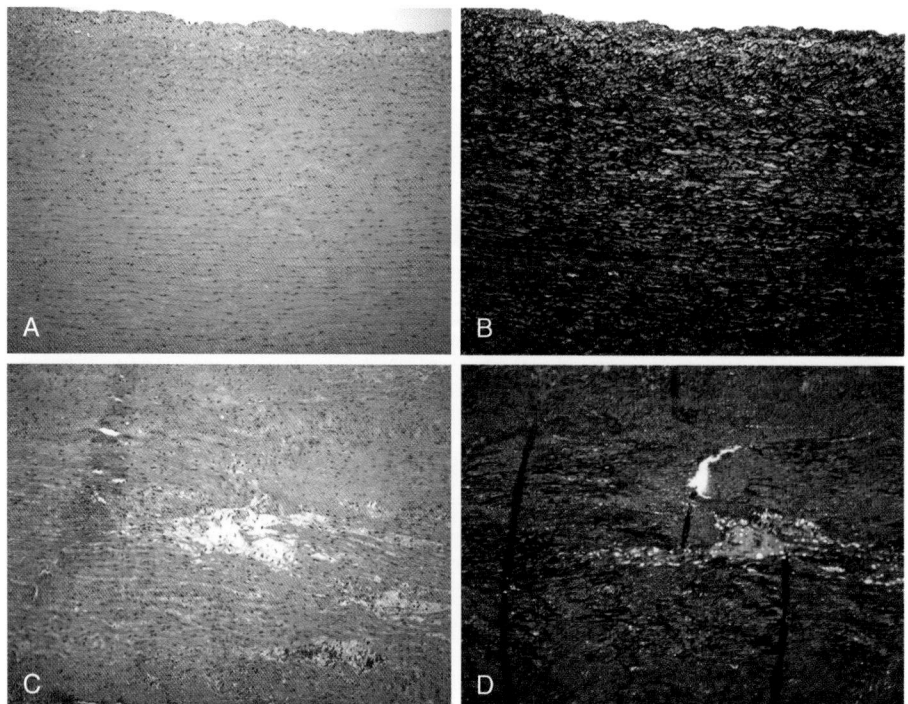

Figure 140-1 A and **B,** Photomicrographs illustrating the regular and parallel nature of the elastic lamellae found within the media of the normal ascending aorta. The lamellae are composed of elastic fibers running in parallel with intervening smooth muscle, ground substance, and collagen. The Verhoeff–van Gieson (VVG) stain highlights these major elastic fibers (*black*) (A, hematoxylin-eosin [H&E], ×100; B, VVG, ×100). **C** and **D,** Photomicrographs showing profound fragmentation of the elastic fibers, with spaces left within the media of the ascending aorta. Though often referred to as cystic medial degeneration, the spaces created by this fragmentation lack a lining and hence are not truly "cysts." These spaces often contain increased amounts of glycoproteins. The VVG stain further highlights the severe elastic fiber (*black*) fragmentation. The *vertical black lines* are fixation artifacts from folding of the elastic sheet (C, H&E; D, VVG). *(Plates courtesy of Joseph Maleszewski, MD, Johns Hopkins Hospital Department of Pathology.)*

systems. The disorder occurs worldwide, with no gender or race predilection. However, the cardinal manifestation of aortic root aneurysm and its risk for life-threatening aortic dissection or rupture led to a shortened life expectancy. Consequently, the leading cause of mortality was cardiovascular in more than 90% of cases (aortic dissection, valve disease, or congestive heart failure), which decreased life expectancy to approximately two thirds that of unaffected individuals.[5] Improvements in recognition of Marfan's syndrome and surgical advances have returned life expectancy to the nearly normal range by addressing the most threatening manifestations of Marfan's syndrome—aortic catastrophe in the form of dissection or rupture of the ascending aorta.

Diagnostic Criteria

Ghent Criteria.
Clinical diagnostic criteria for Marfan's syndrome were outlined at the International Nosology of Heritable Connective Tissue Disorders in 1986 during the Connective Tissue Meeting in Berlin.[29] Thereafter, the recognition that many individuals diagnosed under these original criteria did not have the *FBN1* mutation (genetic testing

became possible after 1986) led to a focused revision in 1996.[30] Termed the *Ghent criteria,* greater emphasis was placed on diagnostic use of clinical findings and the family history, with differentiation into major and minor criteria (Box 140-1). A "major criterion" is one that carries high diagnostic specificity because it is so infrequent in the general population.[31] In practice, if a patient sustains an ascending aortic dissection (a major criterion in the cardiovascular system) and is the index case in the family, positive genetic testing and identification of any minor involvement of another body system would fulfill the diagnosis of Marfan's syndrome. For diagnosis of Marfan's syndrome in patients in whom genetic testing is not available or the family history is not contributory, major criteria must be fulfilled in two organ systems and a third system must have at least minor involvement. Once Marfan's syndrome is diagnosed in an individual, all first-degree relatives should be evaluated for the presence of the condition. In children, this may require repeated evaluations to avoid missing the disorder in evolution.

Genetic Testing.
The role of clinical genetic testing in establishing a diagnosis remains limited because more than

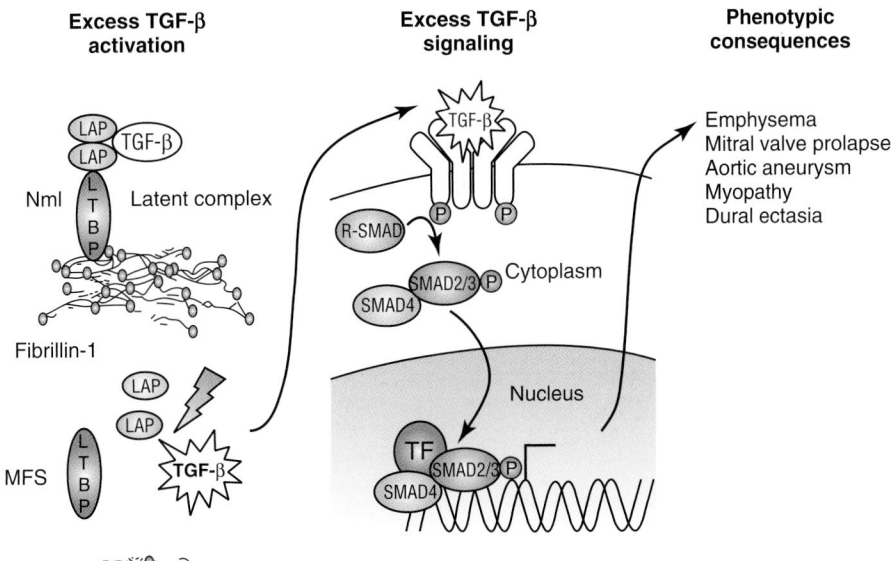

Figure 140-2 Excess activation of transforming growth factor-β (TGF-β) causes many of the features of Marfan's syndrome. Normal TGF-β metabolism requires binding of the cytokine to several proteins, including microfibrils, to prevent excess signaling. In Marfan's syndrome, lack of normal microfibrillar assembly allows TGF-β to remain unsequestered in the extracellular space. As a consequence, excess TGF-β signaling can occur on the cell surface of TGF-β receptors. Once the TGF-β binds to its receptor, downstream receptor-associated SMAD proteins translocate to the nucleus to modulate transcriptional activity, alter protein expression, and yield phenotypic change. LAP, latency-associated peptide; LTBP, latent TGF-β binding protein; Nml, normal; MFS, Marfan's syndrome; TF, tissue factor.

500 mutations have been found and 90% of the mutations are unique within a pedigree.[18] Even within families in which the same mutation is shared, phenotypic variation is prominent. Thus, exacting a genotype-phenotype correlation is difficult.[32] Furthermore, approximately 25% of patients with the disorder have a de novo mutation, thereby limiting the feasibility of a more focused analysis. In addition, it is estimated that 10% of the mutations in the *FBN1* gene that cause Marfan's syndrome are missed by conventional screening methods.[33] At present, the diagnosis of Marfan's syndrome rests primarily on physical clinical assessment based on the Ghent criteria.

Differential Diagnosis

Other conditions also associated with *FBN1* mutations may be considered in the differential diagnosis of Marfan's syndrome. The MASS phenotype is based on the association of *m*itral valve prolapse, myopia, mild *a*ortic root dilatation, *s*triae, and mild *s*keletal changes.[34] The skeletal features of MASS often include the mild manifestations of tall stature, mild dolichostenomelia (long-bone growth), and scoliosis. Occasionally, a major Ghent criterion from the skeletal system may be met but no other major criteria are noted. For patients with MASS, mutations in the *FBN1* gene have generally created premature termination codons and the mutant transcript can be easily and rapidly degraded.[35]

Shprintzen-Goldberg syndrome is characterized by craniosynostosis, facial hypoplasia, anterior chest deformity, arachnodactyly (long, spider-like fingers), and aortic root dila-

tation. Developmental delay is also common. Point mutations in *FBN1* have been found in some affected individuals, but phenotypic heterogeneity, specifically regarding development, retardation, and aortic root involvement, probably indicates substantial genotypic variation.[36] The aortic root enlargement in Shprintzen-Goldberg syndrome is similar to that in Marfan's syndrome.

Homocystinuria is caused by a deficiency of cystathionine β-synthase. Patients with homocystinuria often have tall stature, long-bone overgrowth, and ectopia lentis, but no aortic enlargement. The inheritance is autosomal recessive, and affected individuals often have mental retardation, a history of thromboembolism, and coronary artery disease. Plasma homocysteine levels are typically markedly elevated, which easily distinguishes this disease from Marfan's syndrome.[5]

Congenital contractural arachnodactyly shares many skeletal features with Marfan's syndrome, but no ocular and cardiovascular manifestations are present. The mutation in the few patients reported in the literature is located in the *FBN2* gene,[37] and physical therapy is key to maintaining joint range of motion.

The overlap of LDS and Marfan's syndrome is considered later in this chapter.

Surveillance

Marfan's syndrome is a pleiotropic disorder, and surveillance of the many systems at risk for abnormality is

Box 140-1 Ghent Criteria for the Diagnosis of Marfan's Syndrome

INDEX CASE

- If the family/genetic history is not contributory, major criteria in two or more different organ systems and involvement of a third organ system are required.
- If a genetic mutation known to cause Marfan's syndrome in others is identified, one major criterion in an organ system and involvement of a second organ system are required.

RELATIVE OF AN INDEX CASE WHO HAS MET THE CRITERIA FOR DIAGNOSIS

- With the presence of a major criterion in the family history, one major criterion in an organ system and involvement of a second organ system are required.

GENETIC/FAMILY HISTORY

Major criteria (any one of the following):

- Having a parent, child, or sibling who meets these diagnostic criteria independently
- Presence of a mutation in *FBN1*, which is known to cause Marfan's syndrome
- Presence of a haplotype around *FBN1*, inherited by descent, that is known to be associated with unequivocally diagnosed Marfan's syndrome in the family

Minor criteria:

- None

ORGAN SYSTEMS

Cardiovascular

Major criteria (either):

- Dilatation of the ascending aorta, with or without aortic regurgitation, and involving at least the sinuses of Valsalva
- Dissection of the ascending aorta

Minor criteria (only one need be present):

- Mitral valve prolapse with or without mitral valve regurgitation
- Dilatation of the main pulmonary artery in the absence of valvular or peripheral pulmonic stenosis and age younger than 40 years
- Calcification of the mitral annulus and age younger than 40 years
- Dilatation or dissection of the descending thoracic or abdominal aorta and age younger than 50 years

For involvement of the cardiovascular system, only one of the minor criteria must be present.

Skeletal

Major criteria (at least four of the following constitute a major criterion in the skeletal system):

- Pectus carinatum
- Pectus excavatum requiring surgery
- Reduced upper segment–to–lower segment ratio or arm span–to–height ratio >1.05
- Wrist and thumb signs (wrist: ability to overlap the fifth finger and thumb around the wrist; thumb: extends across the ulnar border of the hand when folded inward)

- Scoliosis of >20 degrees or spondylolisthesis
- Reduced extension at the elbows (<170 degrees)
- Medial displacement of the medial malleolus causing pes planus (flatfeet)
- Protrusio acetabuli (medial socket wall protrudes/bows into the ring of the pelvis)

Minor criteria:

- Pectus excavatum of moderate severity
- Joint hypermobility
- High arched palate with dental crowding
- Facial appearance (dolichocephaly: long and narrow face, malar hypoplasia, enophthalmos, retrognathia, down-slanting palpebral features)

For involvement of the skeletal system, at least two features contributing to major criteria or one feature from the list contributing to the major criterion and two minor criteria must be present.

Ocular System

Major criterion:

- Ectopia lentis (lens dislocation)

Minor criteria:

- Abnormally flat cornea
- Increased globe length
- Hypoplastic iris or ciliary muscle causing decreased miosis (leading to nearsightedness)

For involvement of the ocular system, at least two minor criteria must be present.

Pulmonary System

Major criteria:

- None

Minor criteria:

- Spontaneous pneumothorax
- Apical blebs

For involvement of the pulmonary system, only one minor criterion must be present.

Skin and Integument

Major criteria:

- None

Minor criteria:

- Striae atrophicae (stretch marks) without marked weight gain, pregnancy, or repetitive stress)
- Recurrent hernia

For involvement of the skin and integument, only one minor criterion must be present.

Dura

Major criterion:

- Lumbosacral dural ectasia

Minor criteria:

- None

---

prudent. The cardinal manifestations are ocular, skeletal, and cardiovascular. Regular examinations by an ophthalmologist for slit-lamp testing, a cardiologist for imaging of the aortic root, and an orthopedist for the development of scoliosis should be performed on an annual basis. In this section, focus is placed on aortic and vascular pathology. For recommendations with regard to the other body systems, the reader may find useful information at the National Marfan Foundation website (www.marfan.org). The clinical manifestations within the cardiovascular system that require preventive attention involve the atrioventricular valves, annuloaortic valve mechanism, and the aortic root and ascending aorta.

Valvular Disease

Thickening of the atrioventricular valves is very common and often associated with mitral or tricuspid valve prolapse.[5] In about 25% of patients, the mitral valve prolapse may progress to severe mitral regurgitation.[38] Mitral regurgitation is the most common indication for cardiac surgery in infants and children with the disorder.[38] In children with early onset of Marfan's syndrome, congestive heart failure, pulmonary hypertension, and death may result from this mitral insufficiency, which is the leading cause of morbidity and mortality in young children with the disorder.[38] Interestingly, progression of mitral valve prolapse to severe regurgitation occurs in twice as many women as men.[38] Calcification of the mitral annulus in individuals younger than 40 years constitutes a minor criterion in the cardiovascular system.

Aortic valve dysfunction probably represents a late event in the continuum of annuloaortic ectasia secondary to root degeneration. The aortic valve, like the mitral valve, may also be susceptible to calcification at an early age.[38] Dilated cardiomyopathy beyond explanation by the associated valvular incompetence is likewise seen in patients with Marfan's syndrome. The mutant FBN1 protein in the cardiac ventricles has been implicated, but overall, rates of cardiomyopathy are low. In a study of 234 patients with Marfan's syndrome but without significant aortic or atrioventricular valvular disease, 17 (7.3%) had left ventricular enlargement, but none had an ejection fraction less than 25%.[39]

Aortic Disease

Aortic aneurysm and dissection are the most life-threatening manifestations of Marfan's syndrome. The threat is dependent on age, with rupture and dissection rates increasing as the aortic root dilates.[40,41] Because root dilatation at the sinuses of Valsalva can begin in utero, lifelong transthoracic echocardiography is needed. For patients in whom the aortic root and ascending aorta are poorly visualized as a result of anterior chest deformity, computed tomographic angiography or magnetic resonance angiography (to avoid radiation exposure) is a viable substitute. In contrast to degenerative aneurysm, the dilatation may be confined to just the aortic root and not the ascending aorta. Normal aortic dimensions can vary widely with both age and size, and thus proper interpretation in patients affected by Marfan's syndrome requires age-dependent nomograms.[40] Absolute thresholds for replacement of the aortic root in children have not been established given the observation that dissection is very rare in the young.[5] However, if the aortic root is noted to grow more than 1 cm over consecutive annual assessment or if significant aortic regurgitation is present, early surgery may be necessary.[31] In children and teenagers, this nomogram reflects the number of standard deviations of the patient's aortic root from the mean aortic root diameter in the population and is termed a

Z-score. If the child's Z-score deviates rapidly from the population (>2 to 3 SD) under surveillance, aortic root repair may be justified to prevent rupture. In adults, surgical repair of the aortic root and ascending aorta to prevent aortic rupture and dissection is recommended when its greatest diameter exceeds 50 mm.[31,41] Earlier intervention may be warranted with a family history of aortic dissection at lesser diameter.

Prevention

Lifestyle modifications are routinely recommended once the diagnosis of Marfan's syndrome is established. On the basis of data from the United States, genetic cardiovascular diseases account for 40% of deaths in young athletes.[42,43] A recent consensus document stated that "burst" exertion such as sprinting, weightlifting, basketball, and soccer should generally be avoided. Favored are recreational sports in which energy expenditure is stable and consistent over long periods, such as informal jogging, biking, and lap swimming.[44] Symptoms potentially referable to a cardiovascular cause, such as shortness of breath, presyncope, and chest discomfort, should prompt immediate withdrawal from activity and evaluation. Recent litigation suggests that physician reliance on consensus statements to determine medically reasonable levels of activity in patients with cardiovascular abnormalities is appropriate.[45]

Medical Treatment

Medical treatment with β-adrenergic receptor blockade to delay aortic root growth or prevent aortic dissection in patients with Marfan's syndrome is currently considered a standard of care.[5,31] General recommendations are a resting heart rate lower than 70 beats/min and a heart rate less than 100 beats/min with submaximal exercise. The rationale for this treatment paradigm is focused on decreasing proximal aortic shear stress and dP/dt. The only randomized trial assessing the effect of beta blockade studied 70 patients, 32 of whom received propranolol.[46] Treated patients were titrated via an open-label approach to keep the heart rate at 100 beats/min during exercise or a 30% rise in the systolic time interval. Serial echocardiograms were performed and correlated with age, height, and weight over a mean follow-up of 7 years. Fewer patients in the propranolol-treated group reached the primary endpoint of aortic regurgitation, aortic dissection, surgery, heart failure, or death (five in treatment group and nine in control group). Aortic growth after normalization was lower in the propranolol-treated group (0.023 cm/yr) than in the control group (0.084 cm/yr, $P < .001$).[46] For patients with increased body weight or an end-diastolic aortic diameter greater than 40 mm, the response to beta blockade was worse, thus suggesting that beta blockers must be given at an adequate dose and early in the course of the disorder to optimize benefit.[31,46] Approximately 10% to 20% patients will be intolerant of beta blockade because of asthma, fatigue, or depression. For these patients, a calcium channel blocker may be justified.[47]

Recent publication of the ability of losartan, a Food and Drug Administration–approved antihypertensive medication and selective angiotensin II receptor antagonist, to inhibit aortic aneurysm in murine models of Marfan's syndrome[48] has opened a potential new medical treatment paradigm. The exact mechanisms by which losartan inhibits TGF-β in the aortic wall are not completely understood, but a variety of feedback mechanisms are likely.[49] A multicenter trial comparing beta blockade and losartan therapy for control of aortic root growth in children and young adults with Marfan's syndrome has been initiated through the National Institutes of Health. Currently, there are no specific recommendations for losartan dosing or long-term therapy in individuals with Marfan's syndrome.

Surgical Treatment

The traditional threshold for prophylactic surgical repair of the aortic root is 5 cm in patients with Marfan's syndrome. The association between aortic diameter and risk for aortic catastrophe is clearly established, and aortic aneurysm size greater than 6 cm predicts a fourfold increase in risk for aortic rupture or dissection in patients with Marfan's syndrome.[50] For patients with acute manifestations—rupture in the aortic root or type A dissection—the goal of the surgery is preservation of life, and the most expedient repair may be placement of a graft with a mechanical valve (composite root replacement, Bentall procedure), as opposed to the more erudite repairs offered in elective scenarios to preserve the aortic valve by resuspension or remodeling techniques. Historically, aortic root catastrophe was the suspected culprit in 90% of Marfan-associated deaths,[10] but once a dissection has occurred, degeneration to aneurysm may affect other segments of the aorta or its branches in survivors. Operations on the arterial tree outside the ascending aorta have been reported (Fig. 140-3) and can have acceptable outcomes.[51] Indeed, as the life expectancy of individuals affected by Marfan's syndrome has increased with prophylactic root replacement, it is plausible that the remaining aorta, or other large arteries, may progress to require repair in the absence of antecedent dissection. For aortic arch and descending thoracic or thoracoabdominal aneurysms, standard criteria for repair generally follow that of atherosclerotic aneurysms—a threshold of 5.5 to 6.0 cm.[31]

Aortic Root

Composite surgical replacement of the aortic root and valve was pioneered by Bentall and De Bono in 1968.[52] Previously, the outlook for repair of dissection or aneurysms in the aortic root in patients with Marfan's syndrome was dismal, with high bleeding rates and excessive mortality. The Bentall technique has proved to be safe and durable. In 1999, Gott and coauthors reported the outcome of 675 patients with Marfan's syndrome who underwent root and valve replacement between 1968 and 1996 at 10 centers with special expertise.[41] Eighty-nine percent of patients received a composite valve graft (CVG), with 30% of the operations performed for acute type

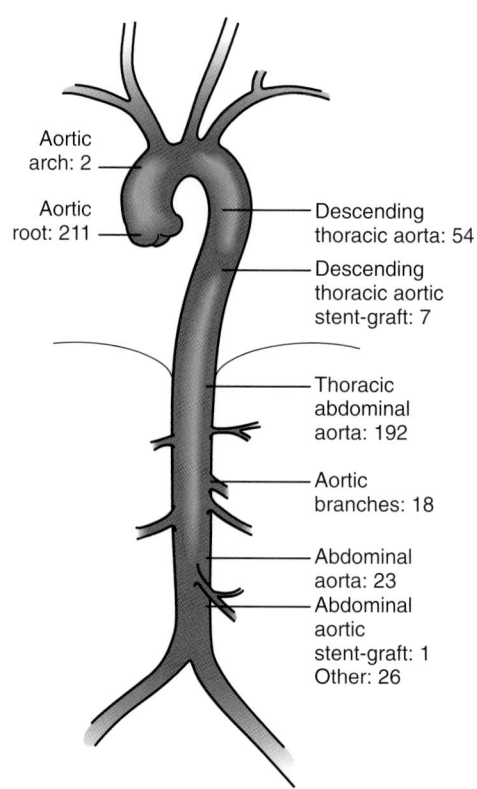

Figure 140-3 Distribution of vascular repairs in 300 patients with Marfan's syndrome. *(From Neglén P, Hollis KC, Olivier J, Raju S. Stenting of the venous outflow in chronic venous disease: long-term stent-related outcome, clinical, and hemodynamic result. J Vasc Surg. 2007;46:979-990.)*

A dissection. Emergency surgery was performed on 103 patients (within 24 hours), urgent surgery on 117 (1 to 7 days), and elective repair on 455. Thirty-day mortality was lowest for elective CVG surgery (1.5%) and highest for emergency repairs (11.7%). Long-term survival was significantly improved when compared with the natural history of aortic disease, with a 10-year survival rate of 91%. At a follow-up of 6.7 years, 36% of the deaths were attributable to the "downstream" aorta. Although reoperative root replacement was rare after CVG surgery, 10% of patients required distal aortic surgery, typically for the consequences of chronic dissection.

Because of the risk for thromboembolism and the lifetime requirement for anticoagulation with warfarin, recent effort had been directed at maintaining the native aortic valve. This valve-sparing root replacement approach has the additional benefit of avoiding warfarin embryopathy in women with Marfan's syndrome who may later desire pregnancy. To date, there has been no randomized trial comparing CVG surgery and valve-sparing root replacement techniques, but the available data are encouraging and have shown low rates of valve dysfunction (20% to 25% with significant aortic regurgitation) and few reoperations (Fig. 140-4).[53,54]

Descending Thoracic and Thoracoabdominal Aorta

The first successful replacement of the thoracoabdominal aorta in a patient with Marfan's syndrome was performed by

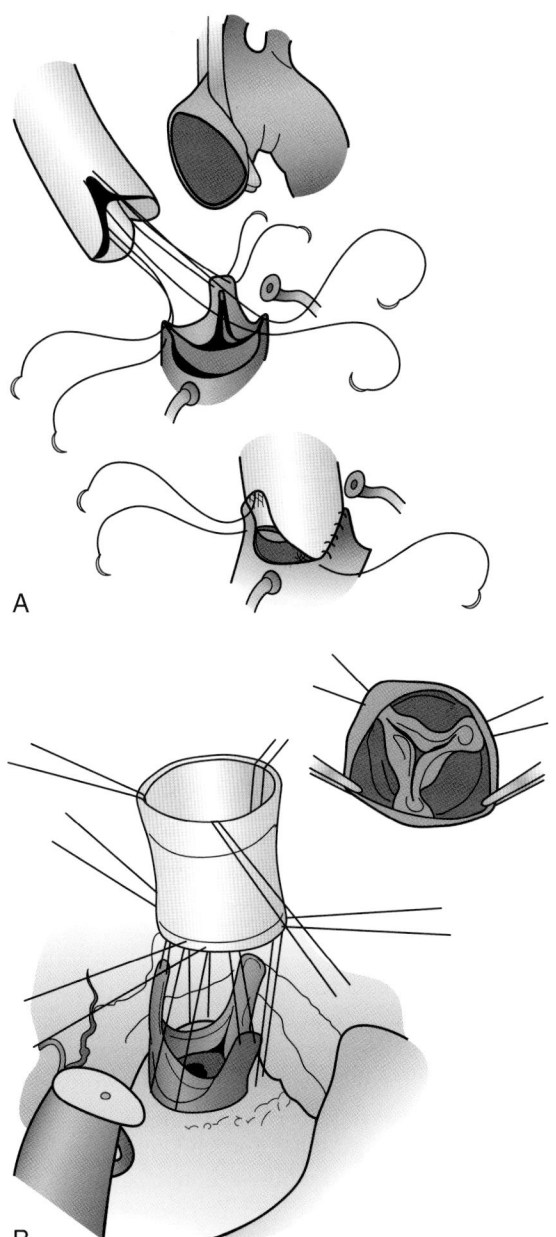

A

B

Figure 140-4 Valve-sparing techniques have reduced the need for composite valve graft replacement of the aortic root, thus avoiding the need for long-term anticoagulation **A,** Remodeling technique for valve-sparing aortic root replacement. The Dacron tongues allow some billowing of the sinuses of Valsalva, but incorporation of the aortic wall at the intercommissural triangles may be associated with a higher incidence of later aortic regurgitation. **B,** Reimplantation of the valve leaflets into a sinus of Valsalva graft to circumferentially re-enforce the entire root and valvular scaffold appears to be associated with a reduced incidence of late aortic valve regurgitation.

Crawford in the 1980s.[55] Elective surgical repair of descending thoracic aortic aneurysm and thoracoabdominal aortic aneurysms (TAAAs) in Marfan's syndrome has benefited from the general refinements and introduction of adjuncts to reduce spinal cord injury and other major complications in a manner similar to standard atherosclerotic aneurysms (see Chapter 132: Thoracic and Thoracoabdominal Aneurysms: Open

Surgical Treatment). Prophylactic aortic replacement is indicated when the aortic diameter reaches 5.5 to 6.0 cm or if symptoms related to the aneurysm occur. Because of the frequent involvement of the descending and thoracoabdominal aorta with aneurysms of chronic dissection etiology, the extent of repairs in Marfan's syndrome tend to be greater, with 42% to 78% of all TAAAs being DeBakey type II.[51,56] As expected, the mean age of patients with Marfan's syndrome undergoing such repair is 34 to 48 years, younger than patients with non–connective tissue diseases.[51,56,57] In comparison to patients undergoing repair of degenerative TAAAs, the rate of acute development of dissection or rupture in patients with Marfan's syndrome and TAAAs was not higher (6% to 8% for each).[51,57] Paraparesis and paraplegia rates after TAAA repair in Marfan's syndrome compare favorably with non–connective tissue disease results when matched for the extent of repair required.[51,56,57] Because of the very young mean age of patients with Marfan's syndrome undergoing TAAA repair versus the older mean age of patients with degenerative TAAA, overall long-term survival was better in those with Marfan's syndrome.[51]

Given the preponderance of type II TAAA repairs in the available series, freedom from further aortic repair is high because little aorta remains to degenerate. However, secondary aortic procedures after TAAA repair in patients with Marfan's syndrome are often performed for pseudoaneurysm or for aneurysm degeneration of the inclusion or Carrel patch (Fig. 140-5). Indeed, in the series of Lemaire and coworkers, 95% of reoperations (19 of 20) after previous TAAA repair (n = 178) in Marfan's patients were performed for visceral patch aneurysm.[51] In our series of 107 patients who underwent TAAA repair, including creation of visceral patches, 17 were known to have a connective tissue disease.[58] With a mean time to diagnosis of 6.5 years, 3 of these 17 patients (17.6%) returned with aneurysmal degeneration of the visceral patch. By comparison, visceral patch aneurysms were noted after only 5.6% of atherosclerotic TAAA repairs.[58] All of these Marfan's patients had inclusion patches that encompassed the celiac axis, superior mesenteric artery, and both renal arteries, thus suggesting that the visceral patch should have been greatly reduced in all patients with connective tissue diseases to prevent late degeneration. I, along with many surgeons, will avoid patch inclusion entirely and use a prefabricated four-branch graft to perform individual bypasses to the renal and visceral aortic branches. Intercostal inclusion patches that degenerate to aneurysms may be treated with stent-graft therapy, although paraplegia concerns are paramount. Given the morbidity associated with repair of the patch aneurysm (two intraoperative deaths in five patients taken to the operating room), Dardik and colleagues recommend maintaining an indication for repair of 6.0 cm or greater.[58]

Abdominal aortic aneurysms (AAAs) can occur in patients with Marfan's syndrome as a result of antecedent aortic dissection or degenerative disease with aging. Thresholds for repair are generally more aggressive than those of the wider nonsyndromic AAA population, with aneurysms greater than 5.0 cm requiring repair. Rapid progression to AAA after pre-

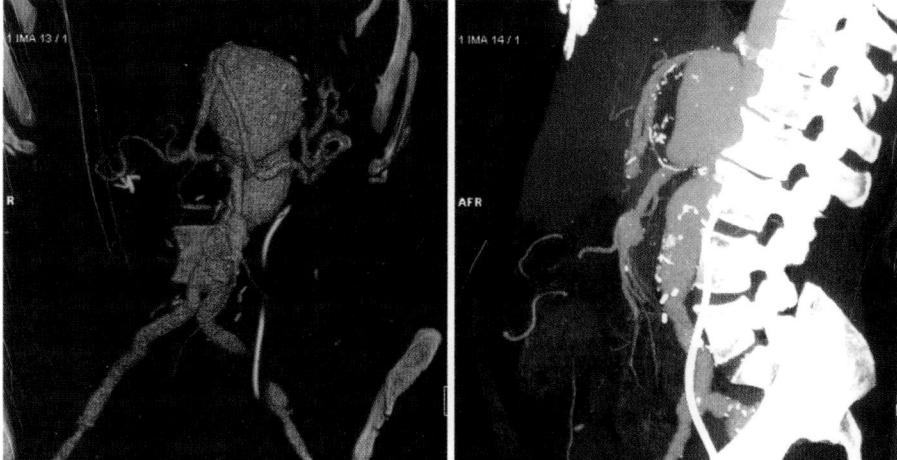

Figure 140-5 Ten-centimeter visceral patch aneurysm 7.5 years after a type II thoracoabdominal aortic aneurysm repair in a 48-year-old woman with Marfan's syndrome. A hybrid open/endovascular stent-graft approach was used to repair the region.

vious aortic dissection should also be monitored after any proximal dissection event. Freedom from recurrent AAA after open surgical repair was reported in 23 Marfan's patients, thus suggesting that satisfactory results can be achieved without higher rates of major complications.[51]

Endovascular Treatment

In general, aortic stent-grafts should not be used in the native thoracic or abdominal aorta in patients with Marfan's syndrome or in those with other connective tissue diseases. The currently approved devices have never been studied in the fragile milieu of the Marfan aorta (connective tissue disease was an exclusion criterion), and the question of persistent radial force on the aorta remains unanswered. A recent publication recommended endovascular repair *only* in instances of late localized pseudoaneurysm and stenting across native tissue aneurysm from "graft to graft."[31] A recent consensus statement recommended strongly against endovascular repair unless operative risk was deemed truly prohibitive by a center experienced in the management of complex aortic disease.[59] This opinion is shared by the majority of surgeons experi-

enced in central aortic surgery. A recent report of thoracic endovascular repair in eight patients with connective tissue diseases (six with Marfan's syndrome, two with EDS) demonstrated initial success with few major complications, but the authors narrowly propose that the technique may be justified in emergencies as a "bridging" method.[60] No long-term follow-up is provided.

VASCULAR-TYPE EHLERS-DANLOS SYNDROME

EDS is a heterogeneous group of heritable disorders of connective tissue characterized by joint hypermobility, skin hyperextensibility, and tissue fragility affecting the skin, ligaments, joints, blood vessels, and internal organs. There are many subtypes of the disorder (see Table 140-2 or www.ednf. org), with classic EDS (types I and II) being the most common; it is inherited as an autosomal trait and gained some repute from the "Elastic Man" and "India Rubber Man" of the late 19th century sideshows and Barnum circuses.[61] The importance of identifying the correct type cannot be overstated

Table 140-2 Subtypes of Ehlers-Danlos Syndrome

Nomenclature (New Terms)	Type	Skin (0-4+) (Elastic/Fragile)	Joint Laxity (0-3+)	Features	Inheritance
Classic	I, II	+++/+++	+++	Vascular complications rarely	AD
Hypermobile	III	+/+	+++	Arthritis	AR
Vascular	IV	−/++++	+	Rupture of arteries, uterus, intestine; thin skin	AD
Kyphoscoliotic	VIA, VIB	+++/++	+++	Hypotonia, osteoporosis, kyphoscoliosis; rupture of arteries, globe of eye	AR
Arthrochalasic	VIIA, VIIB	++/+	+++	Hip subluxation, osteoporosis	AD
Dermatosparactic	VIIC	−/++++	+	Skin doughy and lax	AR
Other	V	++/++		Skin lax	X-linked
	VIII	+/++	++	Periodontal disease	AD
	IX	+/−	+	Lax skin, osteoporosis, bladder diverticula, retardation	X-linked
	X	+/+	++	Petechiae	?

AD, autosomal dominant; AR, autosomal recessive.

because the natural history and modes of inheritance differ among the subtypes. Historically, the older literature did not clearly differentiate among the types, and the severe complications of the vascular type of EDS were cited as being representative of the whole syndrome, thereby creating unnecessary anxiety. The current nomenclature (i.e., naming the vascular phenotype as vascular EDS) attempts to reenforce this important separation from other subtypes. In this review the focus will be on the vascular type (EDS IV), its pathogenesis (defective type III procollagen encoded by the *COL3A1* gene leading to extreme vascular fragility), and its management.

Epidemiology and Natural History

The prevalence of EDS IV is currently estimated to be 1 in 50,000, and it is inherited in an autosomal dominant manner.[62] Approximately 50% of cases represent new mutation that occur sporadically and without an antecedent family history. As a rule, each patient or family carries a unique mutation in the *COL3A1* gene, which codes for type III procollagen.[63] There have been documented cases of parental mosaicism in which a healthy parent passed a mutation resulting in an affected offspring; the white cells and fibroblasts of the offspring had different proportions of mutant alleles, thus suggesting that allocation of the mutant progenitor cell occurred differentially in embryogenesis.[64]

The overall life expectancy of patients with EDS IV is dramatically shortened, largely as a result of vascular rupture, with a median life span of 48 years (range, 6 to 73 years).[65] Vascular rupture is largely unpredictable and can occur in the presence of nearly normal vessel diameters. In a study of 220 patients with EDS IV confirmed by abnormal type III procollagen molecules and 199 relatives with a clinical diagnosis of EDS IV, major complications in childhood were rare, but 25% of the subjects suffered medical or surgical complications by the age of 20. By 40 years of age, major complications in the vascular or gastrointestinal systems (men and women) or reproductive system (women, e.g., uterine rupture in pregnancy) had developed in 89%.[65] Death occurred in 131 subjects, with rupture of thoracic or abdominal vessels in 78 (60%), central nervous system hemorrhage in 9 (7%), and an unspecified bleeding source in 16 (12%). Organ rupture (heart, uterus, spleen, liver) caused death in 13 (10%) of the patients, and intestinal rupture led to death in 10 (8%) (Fig. 140-6).[65]

Pathogenesis

EDS IV is due to mutations in the *COL3A1* gene, which encodes a protein for type III collagen assembly. Because most arteries and arterioles have significant amounts of type III collagen, defects in *COL3A1* lead to inherent weakness of these vessels. The gene encodes a procollagen molecule, proa1(III), and basic collagen synthesis requires three polypeptide procollagen chains, referred to as α chains, to be folded tightly into a triple helix.[61,65,66] The abnormal collagen III molecule cannot fold stably into a triple helix, is slowly

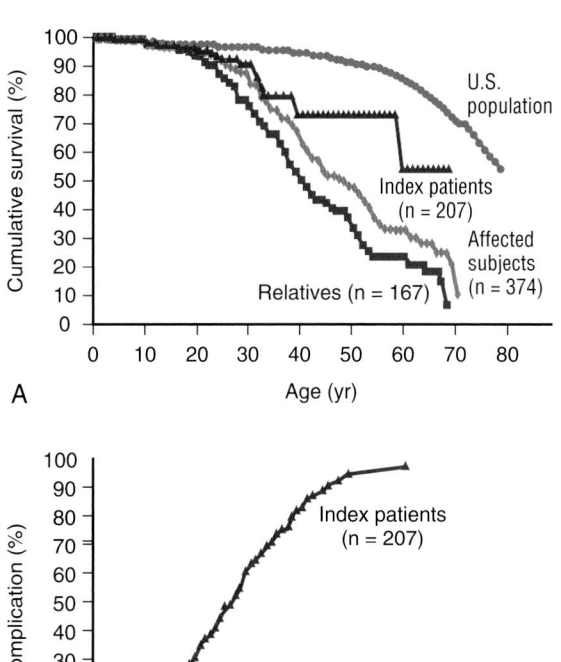

Figure 140-6 A, The survival curve of patients with type IV Ehlers-Danlos syndrome (EDS IV) is appreciably lower than that of population controls. Index patients and their relatives accounted for the total number of affected subjects studied. The index patients were identified younger than their affected relatives, as would be expected when family histories are used to identify affected members of previous generations. **B,** The time of first complication (vascular, gastrointestinal, or uterine) in index patients with EDS IV rises progressively with time. *(From Pepin M, Schwarze U, Superti-Furga A, Byers PH. Clinical and genetic features of Ehlers-Danlos type IV, the vascular type. N Engl J Med. 2000;342:673-680.)*

degraded in the rough endoplasmic reticulum of the fibroblast, and is never secreted extracellularly.[67] The central concept of heterozygous mutations leading to structural defects of collagen α chains and instability or nonsecretion of the mutant protein has proved correct in several collagen disorders and has been termed "protein suicide."[67]

Morphologically, proa1(III) mutations result in greatly reduced amounts of collagen III, with 10% to 25% of normal levels noted in the lung, skin, and vessels.[68,69] Although collagen III is a minor component of adult skin, its deficiency has a dramatic effect, probably because of its presence as the dominant collagen in fetuses less than 20 weeks old. It seems likely that collagen III is the primary scaffold in the developing fetus for subsequent matrix deposition by dermal fibroblasts.[70] The skin in individuals with EDS IV may measure only a quarter of the normal thickness, so it appears translucent and reveals the extensive network of subcutaneous veins, a major criterion of affected individuals.[71] Medium and large arterial vessels are also appreciated to have a thin wall with a markedly reduced collagen content.[72] The average collagen fibril cross-sectional area is decreased in the media of all arteries, and the adventitia is thinned, thus greatly diminishing tensile strength.[72]

Clinical Evaluation

Common Manifestations

EDS IV has the worst prognosis among the types of EDS, and for this reason, proper diagnosis is essential because the physical findings may mimic other EDS subtypes or other connective tissue diseases (Box 140-2).[73] The presence of any two or more of the major criteria (easy bruising, translucent skin, facial features, and history of arterial, uterine, or intestinal rupture) is highly indicative of the diagnosis, and collagen testing is strongly recommended. Such testing is both labor-intensive and time-intensive but should strongly be considered before any treatment course is chosen for the suspected affected individual. The diagnosis of EDS IV is most commonly confirmed by demonstration of structurally abnormal collagen III.[74] Direct molecular genetic analysis of the *COL3A1* gene is also possible from a blood or serum sample, but this approach is not widely used because of the labor-intensive mutation analysis.

Differential Diagnosis

The differential diagnosis of EDS IV includes disorders of bruisability and wound healing such as von Willebrand's disease, platelet disorders, and scurvy. Bruisability is often elicited in children and may mimic nonaccidental injury ("battered child").[75] Indeed, excessive bruising with hematoma formation is a common first manifestation. In EDS IV, rupture or dissection of arteries occurs most often in medium-sized vessels, as opposed to the predominant occurrence of rupture and dissection in the aorta of patients with Marfan's

syndrome. The vessel tortuosity and elongation may be similar to findings in the arterial tortuosity syndrome or LDS, but vascular surgery is often much better tolerated in the latter. Multiple aneurysms through the visceral vessels may also be noted in polycystic kidney disease and hereditary forms of cerebral cavernous malformations.[76] Varicose veins and venous aneurysms are commonly seen in EDS IV but have little clinical significance.

Selection of Treatment

Although no specific medical therapies exist for EDS IV, knowledge of the diagnosis can influence management strategies, assist in reproductive counseling, and direct the treatment of major complications. All patients with a confirmed diagnosis of EDS IV should carry a medical attention bracelet, papers noting information on the condition, and their blood group. General recommendations for anesthesia also exist, including crossmatching of adequate blood, avoidance of intramuscular injection, adequate peripheral access, avoidance of arterial lines and central venous catheters, and gentle intubation maneuvers.[77] If central access is required, ultrasound-guided access (i.e., "sono-site") is mandatory.

True Aneurysms

True aneurysms in EDS IV are rare and occurred in only 14% of patients in one series.[82] Overall, vascular catastrophe in EDS IV is not predictable, and vessel rupture can occur at any vessel diameter. Given the difficulty of handling the fragile tissues and vessels, management of spontaneous bleeding should be conservative as long as possible, especially in the interstitial (muscular, retroperitoneal) spaces.[78,79] Bleeding within the peritoneal cavity usually requires immediate transfusion; if surgery is required, vessel ligation with umbilical tape appears to be the safest course versus direct repair.[78] Direct reconstructions must be tensionless, often pledgetted to reduce suture trauma, and re-enforced circumferentially (Fig. 140-7). Angiography should be avoided because of

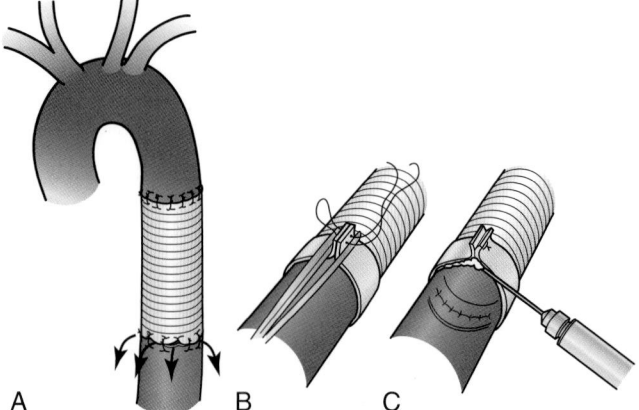

Figure 140-7 Lack of adventitial and medial thickness in type IV Ehlers-Danlos syndrome promotes suture line bleeding (**A**), and buttressing with felt (**B**) and application of BioGlue (**C**) may reduce suture line tension and promote hemostasis.

Box 140-2 Diagnostic Criteria for Ehlers-Danlos Syndrome, Vascular Type

MAJOR DIAGNOSTIC CRITERIA
- Thin, translucent skin
- Arterial/intestinal/uterine fragility or rupture
- Extensive bruising
- Characteristic facial appearance (thin delicate nose, thin lips, hollow cheeks)

MINOR DIAGNOSTIC CRITERIA
- Acrogeria (taut, thin skin)
- Hypermobility of small joints
- Tendon and muscle rupture
- Talipes equinovarus (clubfoot)
- Early-onset varicose veins
- Arteriovenous, carotid-cavernous sinus fistula
- Pneumothorax/pneumohemothorax
- Gingival recession
- Positive family history, sudden death in one or more close relatives

Data from Beighton P, De Paepe A, Danks D, et al. Ehlers-Danlos syndromes: revised nosology, Villefranche, 1997. *Am J Med Genet.* 1997;77: 31-37.

severe morbidity and risk for vessel dissection or perforation (or both) during selective catheterization or from the puncture site itself. In one study, the major complication rate from arteriography was 67% with 12% mortality,[79] although the benefit of more contemporary lower profile catheter and endovascular devices may have a favorable impact on this historically high percentage. If endovascular and arteriographic approaches are needed, direct repair of the femoral artery should be strongly considered. With the advent of high-quality three-dimensional imaging, diagnostic arteriography can be minimized and saved for subsequent endovascular therapies when indicated.

Vascular Complications

The vascular complications are typified by arterial dissection, often associated with minor aneurysmal degeneration. When confronted with bleeding from vascular rupture, the recommendation of avoiding any operation until faced with imminent risk of death remained axiomatic for many decades. This axiom further complicated patients with known aneurysms, whose vessels were allowed to dilate progressively under regular surveillance, which caused much angst between surgeon and patient. For the individual patient, elective aneurysm repair must be considered, especially if previous operative therapies did not report excessive fragility. EDS IV patients at highest risk for inoperable tissue fragility can be suspected if seen at a very early age (<20 years) or multiple asymptomatic dissections or aneurysms are noted, apart from the index vascular lesion.

Nonvascular Complications

Gastrointestinal perforations account for 25% of all EDS IV complications.[65] The sigmoid colon is the location of most perforations, and prompt diagnosis and immediate colostomy are favored.[65] For small bowel intestinal rupture, ostomy is also preferred, and most patients undergo restoration of bowel continuity in a staged fashion without complication.[65] Recurrent bowel perforation is always a risk and occurred between 2 weeks and 26 years after the first event in 17% of patients.[65]

Uterine and pregnancy-related complications are discussed under "Pregnancy in Patients with Type IV Ehlers-Danlos Syndrome."

Medical Treatment

No effective medical therapy exists for EDS IV. Prophylactic measures to control blood pressure (ideal systolic blood pressure <120 mm Hg) and reduce atherosclerotic risk factors are recommended, but no studies have demonstrated an impact on the natural history of the disease or time to first major complication. Lifestyle modifications for EDS IV follow the general recommendations for other genetic disease. as reviewed in the section on Marfan's syndrome earlier in this chapter.[44] Daily doses of ascorbic acid (vitamin C) have been offered on the theoretical basis of improving procollagen sta-

bility by conversion of proline residues in the Y position within Gly-X-Y sequences to hydroxyproline via prolyl hydroxylase. This enzyme requires ascorbic acid as a cofactor, and the resulting hydroxylation event allows the mature collagen molecule to fold into a triple helix stably at body temperature.

Surgical Treatment

Surgical management of EDS IV is a formidable challenge. The traditional risk assessment paradigm cites invasive procedures so fraught with complications that intervention should be performed only when faced with imminent risk of death.[80,81] The findings in patients with EDS IV can include arterial manifestations throughout the entire vascular tree (Fig. 140-8).

The outcomes of 31 patients over a 30-year period were studied retrospectively at the Mayo Clinic.[82] Among 24 patients, there were 132 vascular complications that prompted evaluation. Although 85 of the 132 complications were present before or during the first evaluation, 47 additional complications arose during a 6.3-year median follow-up. Fifteen of 31 patients underwent a vascular intervention, with two operative deaths (one death in a patient after ascending aortic repair, and one death, after a series of eight operations, by anastomotic rupture of a carotid-subclavian graft). Emergency or urgent operations were undertaken in 70% of

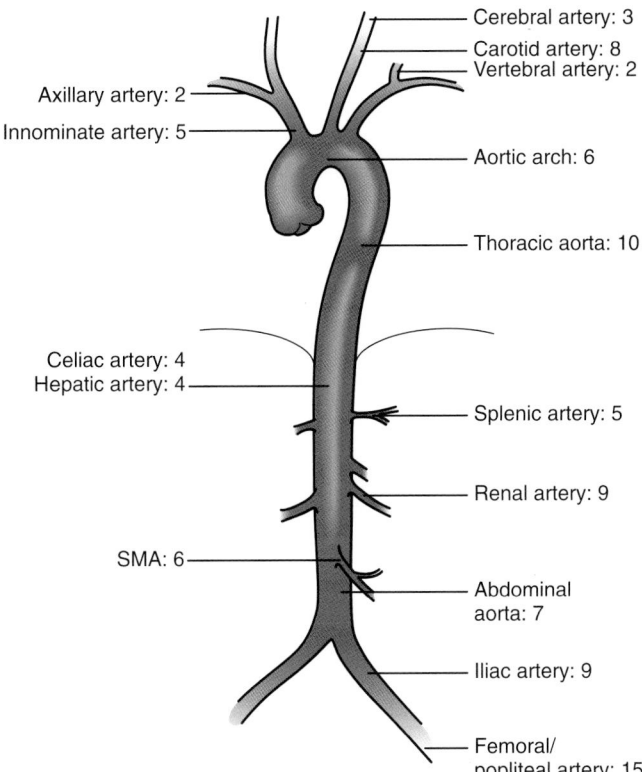

Figure 140-8 Arterial distribution of vascular complications in 24 patients with a clinical diagnosis of type IV Ehlers-Danlos syndrome. SMA, superior mesenteric artery. *(From Oderich GS, Panneton JM, Bower TC. The spectrum, management and clinical outcome of Ehlers-Danlos syndrome type IV. A 30 year experience. J Vasc Surg. 2005;42:98-106.)*

patients. The overall procedure-related morbidity rate was 46%, including a 37% incidence of postoperative bleeding and a 20% re-exploration rate. Late graft-related complications occurred in 40% of arterial reconstructions and included anastomotic aneurysm, anastomotic disruption, and graft thrombosis. The Mayo Clinic authors recommend a high threshold for elective repair, and urgent operative therapies are reserved for acute symptomatic aneurysms after a trial of conservative medical treatment.

Ultimately, patient risk-benefit assessment compels any decision to proceed with a major surgical intervention. It is worthwhile noting that genetic analysis of specific mutations and collagen III biochemical assay do not predict the clinical course.[61,82] However, like most connective tissue diseases, the clinical history can be informative. Complications can be expected in patients with severe phenotypic features (e.g., severely affected skin, facial morphology), those with onset at an early age, and those with previous complicated courses. Furthermore, because the median survival is 48 to 54 years,[65,82] older patients may become intolerant of procedural manipulations, as opposed to previous uncomplicated medical or surgical events at younger ages, and assume a higher risk profile as vessel fragility worsens over a lifetime of EDS IV.

Endovascular Treatment

Endovascular approaches for coil embolization of aortic branch vessels and other medium-sized arteries have been successful in patients with hemorrhage.[82] Such approaches should be strongly considered for spontaneous splenic and hepatic arterial tears, 90% of which occur without previous trauma.[82] Arterial access can precipitate femoral rupture and pseudoaneurysm formation, especially when large devices are necessary. Consideration should be given to open repair of any access puncture (see Fig. 140-7), particularly when a larger French size is introduced, given the rate of complications reported.[79] Accordingly, stent-graft therapy for aortic aneurysms has not been reported in a significant sample, and long-term durability and threat to the fixation zones in the setting of chronic outward radial force may increase the frequency of secondary interventions. Consequently, it is generally agreed that stent-graft therapy for EDS IV (and other connective tissue diseases) should be avoided.[59] Carotid-cavernous fistula is a classic complication of EDS IV that is amenable to coil embolization in selected patients. It may be manifested as subtle, progressive proptosis or headache, and high-quality imaging is key to determine whether the fistula can be addressed without risk of internal carotid sacrifice and resultant major stroke.

Pregnancy in Patients with Type IV Ehlers-Danlos Syndrome

Pregnancy in women in EDS IV should be closely monitored. Whether elective cesarean section is warranted before labor or spontaneous vaginal delivery should be allowed is not known.[83] In the largest study of 220 patients with EDS IV, 81

women had 183 deliveries. Twelve women (15%) died during the peripartum period or within 2 weeks after delivery.[65] The cause of death in these women was uterine rupture in five, vessel rupture during labor in two, and death in the postpartum period from vessel rupture in five. Women with EDS who become pregnant should be considered high risk and managed at high-risk centers. Genetic counseling is also mandatory because the disorder is inherited as autosomal dominant trait and 50% of offspring of an affected individual would be expected to manifest the disorder in their lifetime.

■ LOEYS-DIETZ SYNDROME

LDS is a newly described aortic syndrome typified by aortic aneurysm and vascular tortuosity, the characteristic craniofacial abnormality of a bifid uvula or cleft palate, and finally, hypertelorism.[84] The disease is caused by heterozygous mutations in the genes encoding TGF-β receptors 1 and 2 (TGFBR1 and TGFBR2). Since the original report, two subtypes of LDS have been delineated. LDS type I has both severe craniofacial features and aortic aneurysms. LDS type II is characterized by less severe craniofacial abnormality, usually only a bifid uvula or high palate, and aortic aneurysms. Although the primary aneurysm involves the aortic root, the aggressive nature of the root aneurysm to dissect or rupture (or both) at small diameter and in childhood separates this condition from Marfan's syndrome and EDS IV. Identification of affected patients and testing of all first-degree relatives are of paramount importance to motivate individuals for prophylactic surgery.

Epidemiology

In a study of 52 probands and 38 relatives, the median survival of the cohort was 37.0 years. Of these 90 patients, 27 deaths occurred before or during the study interval at a mean age of 26.0 years (range, 0.5 to 47.0). The leading cause of death was thoracic aortic dissection in 67%, followed by abdominal aortic dissection in 22% and cerebral hemorrhage in 7%. The mean age at the first vascular dissection was 26.7 years, and the mean age at the first vascular surgery, usually for ascending aortic pathology, was 19.8 years.[84]

Comparison of survival in the two subtypes of LDS was also reported.[84] In LDS type I, the mean age at death was lower (22.6 years) than in LDS type II (31.8 years, $P = .06$). The mean age at the first surgery was 10 years younger in LDS type I than in type II (16.9 years versus 26.9 years, $P = .03$). Craniofacial abnormalities, when scored according to a craniofacial severity index, correlated inversely with the time of first surgery (more severe craniofacial abnormality indicated more aggressive aortic pathology).[84]

Pathogenesis

Ultrastructural analysis of the aortic wall demonstrates disorganized collagen deposition in LDS patients, in excess of that appreciated in Marfan's syndrome. Elastin fibers are disarrayed and fragmented with reduced total elastin content noted.[85] Two major genetic perturbations leading to LDS have been described in the TGF-β signaling pathway.[84,85] Approximately two thirds of LDS patients have mutations in the gene encoding TGFBR2, and the remainder have mutations in the gene encoding TGFBR1.[84] With rare exception, the mutations were heterozygous missense mutations affecting amino acids in the functionally critical intracellular domain of the receptor.[85] Indeed, truncation of the intracellular domain of the TGF-β receptor would be expected to preclude signal transduction, yet a paradoxical increase in TGF-β activity is observed,[84] and tissues from affected individuals show nuclear enrichment of SMAD2, which suggests increased TGF-β signaling.[85] The mechanism by which mutations in the TGF-β receptor cause the multisystem manifestations of LDS is poorly understood and remains to be fully elucidated, but it probably involves the receptor signaling cascade for TGF-β and dysregulated feedback mechanisms. There are no firm genotype-phenotype correlations to predict more aggressive aortic pathology.

Clinical Evaluation

LDS is a multisystem disorder with a classic triad of craniofacial abnormality (90%), hypertelorism (wide-set eyes, 90%), and arterial tortuosity/aneurysm (98%). In 40 LDS patients who underwent anthropometric evaluation, besides the classic triad there were also additional findings throughout the craniofacial, skeletal, and cutaneous systems.[84] Developmental delay was infrequent (15%) and occasionally associated with craniosynostosis, hydrocephalus, or Arnold-Chiari malformation, thus suggesting that learning disability is a rare primary manifestation.[84]

Common Manifestations

The craniofacial manifestations encountered are most commonly hypertelorism and cleft palate or bifid uvula (Fig. 140-9). Craniosynostosis was present in 48%, malar hypoplasia (flat midface) in 60%, and blue sclerae in 40%. In contradistinction to Marfan's syndrome, lens dislocation (ectopia lentis) was not recorded in any patient with LDS.[84]

Skeletal manifestations included arachnodactyly in 70% and pectus deformity (excavatum or carinatum) in 68%. Club-foot malformations were noted in 45%, and joint laxity occurred in 68% of subjects.[84] Importantly, this joint laxity was also noted in the cervical spine, and cervical spine–atlas instability could make standard intubation maneuvers a threat for spinal cord compression. Accordingly, flexion and extension views of the cervical spine are recommended, with greater than 30% slip indicating a need for cervical fusion for safety. Dolichostenomelia (long-bone overgrowth), seen often in Marfan's syndrome, was infrequently noted in LDS (18%).[84]

Cardiovascular involvement is a hallmark of LDS, but aneurysms are not limited to the aortic root and can occur throughout the vascular tree. Arterial tortuosity, particular of the supra-aortic vessels, should prompt consideration of the

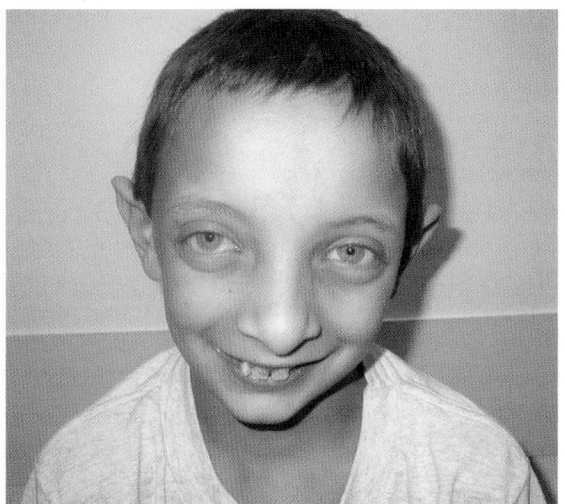

Figure 140-9 Hypertelorism is noted in 90% of patients with Loeys-Dietz syndrome. In addition, this patient demonstrates malar hypoplasia (underdeveloped and flattened midface/zygomatic arches) and retrognathia (the mandible recedes under the maxilla). *(From Williams JA, Loeys BL, Nwakanma LU, et al. Early surgical experience with Loeys-Dietz: a new syndrome of aggressive thoracic aortic aneurysm disease. Ann Thorac Surg. 2007;83: S757-S763.)*

disease.[86] Vessel elongation within tortuous segments can be difficult to diagnose without three-dimensional imaging (Fig. 140-10) and centerline measurement.

Patients, especially children, affected by LDS have high rates of severe allergy, with food allergy and inflammatory bowel disease noted in many. There is no distinct mechanistic insight into this preponderance, which is not seen in any other connective tissue disease. Increased levels of TGF-β are proposed to interfere with normal CD4+ T-helper cell differentiation, thereby yielding T-helper cells that produce

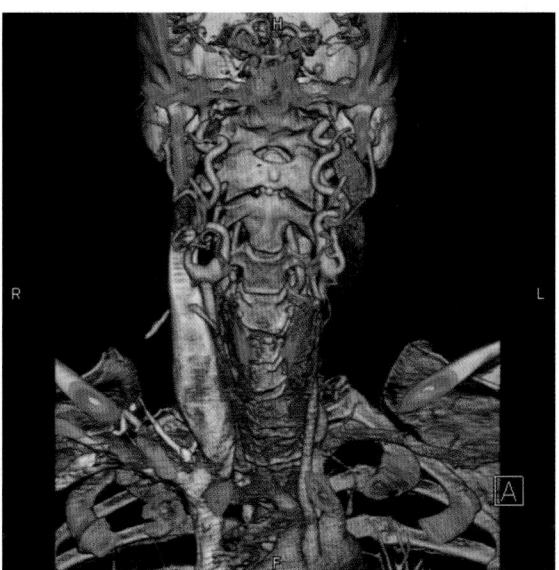

Figure 140-10 Bilateral carotid and vertebral tortuosity is a common peripheral vascular finding in patients with Loeys-Dietz syndrome.

interleukin-17. These cells have been implicated in the development of autoimmune inflammatory conditions (personal communication, Harry Dietz, MD).

Differential Diagnosis

The differential diagnosis of LDS includes arterial tortuosity syndrome wherein medial degeneration of elastic fibers can lead to elongation, stenosis, tortuosity, and eventual aneurysm formation. Interestingly, arterial tortuosity syndrome is an autosomal recessive disorder caused by mutation of the glucose transporter GLUT10 and is the only connective tissue disease recognized to stem from defective glucose metabolism. GLUT10 deficiency is associated with upregulation of TGF-β in the arterial wall, also observed in LDS.[87] The cardiovascular prognosis seems much more favorable in arterial tortuosity syndrome than in LDS.[87] Because of the early age of appearance of dramatic pathology, vascular-type EDS is often considered along with LDS. It could not be more critical to differentiate the two, either by clinical examination to determine the LDS triad or by biochemical testing to confirm EDS IV, because surgical management and tissue fragility are dramatically more challenging in patients with EDS IV than in those with LDS.

Selection of Treatment

Risk assessment for prophylactic repair in patients with LDS must account for the aggressive nature of the aneurysms in this disorder. For adults, aneurysms of the thoracoabdominal and infrarenal aorta are repaired when they are 4.0 cm or greater. Certainly, each patient should be evaluated individually, and for those with marked craniofacial abnormality, an aggressive posture toward repair should be maintained because arterial rupture at lesser diameter may be expected. A new diagnosis of LDS should prompt a head-to-toe computed tomography or magnetic resonance imaging study to determine the presence of arterial pathology outside the aortic root (Fig. 140-11).[87] Because involvement of the supra-aortic trunks and vertebral vessels is not uncommon, surgical exposure may be difficult, and embolization approaches should be considered. Given the widespread involvement of the arterial pathology in this disorder, multiple operations or interventions on a single patient are not uncommon.[84,88,89]

In a review of the peripheral vascular findings in 68 patients with LDS at Johns Hopkins, asymptomatic carotid tortuosity, without aneurysm, was the most common peripheral finding in 44 patients (65%). Subclavian or vertebral artery tortuosity, without aneurysm, was appreciated in 14 patients (21%), and aneurysm in 6 patients (9%). Proximal descending thoracic aortic aneurysm with an average growth rate of 1.8 mm/yr was noted in 24 patients (35%). Abdominal aortic tortuosity was noted in 9 patients (13%), with combined aneurysm in 5 patients (7%). Infrarenal aortic centerline measurements were increased 1.4- to 2.0-fold (range, 130 to 160 mm). Iliac and femoropopliteal aneurysms were infrequent and encountered in 6 patients and 2 patients (9% and 3%, respectively).[90]

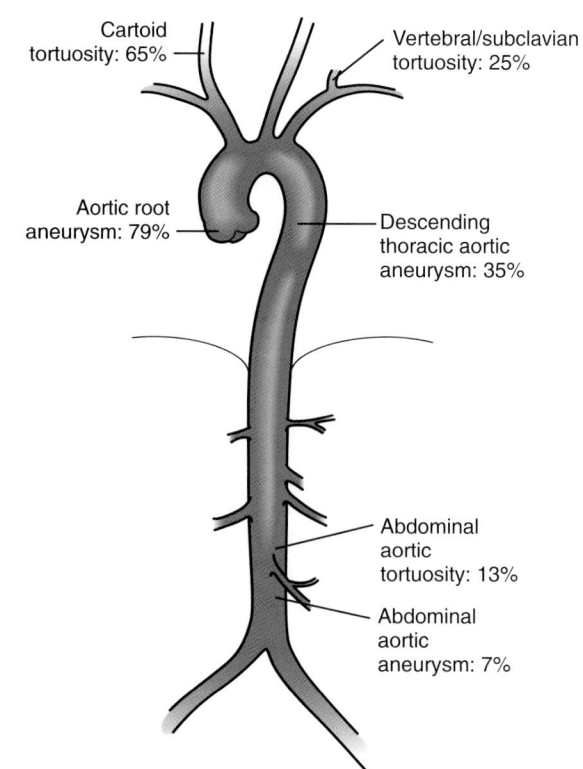

Figure 140-11 Vascular involvement of the supra-aortic branches and entire aorta is common in patients with Loeys-Dietz syndrome. *(From Coucke PJ, Willaert A, Wessels MW, et al. Mutations in the facilitative glucose transporter GLUT10 alter angiogenesis and cause arterial tortuosity syndrome. Nat Genet. 2006;38:452-457.)*

Medical Treatment

Current recommendations for medical management and surveillance in LDS are predicated on the beta-blockade regimen recommended for patients with Marfan's syndrome, with the threshold for repair being more aggressive in LDS. Nonetheless, the pathophysiologic mechanism of increased TGF-β activity in the vessel wall compels some to initiate losartan therapy for the disease based on the mechanisms demonstrated in the pathophysiology of Marfan's syndrome. However, randomized trials are lacking, and preliminary data for losartan therapy are not conclusive to date. Lifestyle modifications should also restrict "burst" activity per Marfan's syndrome restrictions.[44]

Surgical Treatment

Early results after surgical treatment of aneurysm in LDS are now emerging because of the recent characterization of clinical and genetic features specific to the disease. Tissue handling and aortic anastomoses are favorable, and a small series of aortic root replacement in adults and children demonstrated no operative mortality, but 3 of 21 patients died in follow-up of thoracic aortic (n = 2) and abdominal aortic (n = 1) rupture.[86] In my institution, there have been five patients who returned for descending thoracic aortic replacement after previous ascending aortic aneurysm repair or valve-sparing aortic root aneurysm repair. Three of these patients returned

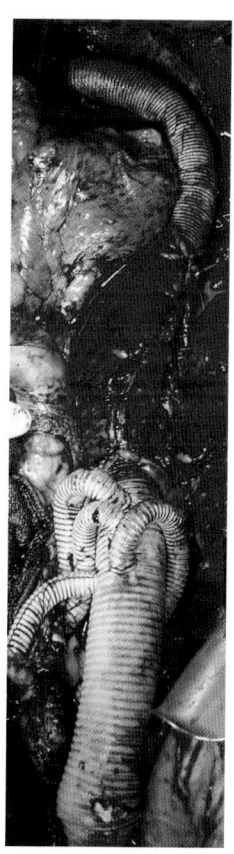

Figure 140-12 Complete replacement of a thoracoabdominal aorta with branched Dacron grafts individually to the renovisceral vessels to avoid an inclusion patch technique.

thereafter with patch aneurysms after previous thoracoabdominal repairs and were confirmed as having LDS on subsequent TGFBR testing. As in Marfan's syndrome, this limited experience suggests that inclusion patch size should be limited or preferably avoided by direct anastomosis to the renal and visceral origins with prefabricated, branched Dacron grafts (Fig. 140-12) to the renal and visceral vessels. Based on experience in the aortic root with premature rupture at small diameters, a general recommendation for repair of any aortic segment in adults would be 4 cm or growth of aneurysm more than 0.5 cm in 1 year.[86,88] Recommendations for repair of peripheral aneurysms in LDS have not been determined, but both the rate of growth and absolute size factor into the decision, thus making regular surveillance with high-quality imaging critical. Vessel tortuosity may also be progressive, yet arterial dissection or degeneration in the vascular hairpins has not been appreciated.

FAMILIAL THORACIC AORTIC ANEURYSM AND DISSECTION

Although it has been recognized that TAAD occurs in individuals with known genetic syndromes, a genetic basis for patients with TAAD who do not have a defined connective tissue disease has recently been investigated. These patients typically exhibit minimal or no outward anthropometric evi-

dence of Marfan's syndrome, EDS IV, or LDS yet often relate an impressive history of aortic catastrophe in antecedents. Familial studies suggest that 11% to 19% of all nonsyndromic TAAD patients have a first-degree relative with TAAD.[90,91] Pedigree analysis suggests that familial TAAD is inherited as a predominantly autosomal dominant disorder with decreased penetrance and variable expression that yields considerable clinical heterogeneity.[92] Genetic mapping of loci in familial TAAD has provided new insight into the pathogenesis of aneurysms throughout the aorta.

Pathogenesis

Five loci have been mapped for familial TAAD to date, including three identified genes. Despite locus heterogeneity, the final common pathologic change in the aortic wall is medial degeneration.[92,93] Smooth muscle cell disarray and proteoglycan accumulation are also typically present.[93] The first locus mapped for familial TAAD was the *TAAD1* locus at 5q13-14.[94] The initial genetic screen identified the location of the defective gene by using two families with similar phenotype for mapping. Subsequent to this mapping, 15 other families with familial TAAD patterning were found to carry the same gene defect, which was segregated as an autosomal dominant disease. In families with this gene, women seemed to be less affected, thus suggesting reduced penetrance of expresssion.[95] Involvement of the ascending aorta is the primary finding.[95]

A second locus for familial TAAD was mapped to 11q23-24 and designated *FAA1*. Linkage to this region was established by using a single large family.[96] In contrast to *TAAD1*, *FAA1* was associated with more diffuse vascular disease involving both thoracic and abdominal aortic aneurysms, as well as other arteries. *FAA1* appears to be rare as a cause of familial TAAD inasmuch as no additional families have been linked to the *FAA1* locus.[95]

A third locus for familial TAAD, termed *TAAD2*, was mapped to 3p24-25, and it was determined that *TGFBR2* is the mutant gene at this locus.[97,98] The *TGFBR2* gene was screened in 80 unrelated families with familial TAAD, and mutations were discovered in the *TGFBR2* gene in just 4 (5%), thus suggesting that *TGFBR2* mutations are an uncommon cause of familial TAAD. All four affected families carried mutations that affected arginine at amino acid 460 in the intracellular kinase domain, a finding suggesting a "hot spot" for familial TAAD and mutations. Ascending aortic pathology developed in these families, in addition to aneurysms and dissections in the descending aorta and other vessels.[98]

A fourth locus was mapped to 16p12.2-13.13 in a family with TAAD associated with patent ductus arteriosus.[99] The defective gene was identified as smooth muscle cell myosin heavy-chain 11 (*MYH11*). MYH11 is a major contractile protein specific to smooth muscle cells. Affected individuals heterozygous for *MYH11* mutations have marked aortic stiffness with a substantial decrease in aortic compliance.[99] Pathologic examination of the aortic wall in *MYH11* heterozygous individuals demonstrates a marked decrease in smooth muscle content and resultant weakness of the aortic wall. Growth factor analysis failed to demonstrate TGF-β mRNA changes in MYH11 smooth muscle cells versus age-matched controls, but insulin-like growth factor 1 (IGF-I) expression was noted in the aortic media and vasa vasorum.[93] IGF-I expression is known to increase in cyclic stretch as an adaptive response to maintain vessel tone. Pathways downstream from IGF-I include extracellular signal–regulated kinase (ERK), which can result in smooth muscle cell proliferation.[93] Enhanced expression of angiotensin-converting enzyme and markers of angiotensin II, which would potentiate smooth muscle cell proliferation, were also noted in MYH11 samples.[93] It is estimated that *MYH11* mutations account for approximately 2% of cases of familial TAAD.[100]

α-Actin mutations have recently been discovered to cause 14% of cases of familial TAAD.[100] The actin proteins are highly conserved and are critical cytoskeletal elements. Aortic tissue demonstrates cystic medial degeneration with focal areas of marked vascular smooth muscle proliferation. Interestingly, familial TAAD patients with *ACTA2* mutations are also noted to have significant livedo reticularis, a physical finding not encountered in the other connective tissue diseases. The overall penetrance to express aneurysm or dissection in individuals with familial TAAD and *ACTA2* mutations was low (0.48) and did not change with age. This fact distinguishes *ACTA2* mutations from other genes in familial TAAD, where penetrance is clearly age related.[100]

Clinical Manifestations

Patients with familial TAAD are seen at a younger age than those with sporadic thoracic aortic aneurysms (mean age, 58.2 versus 65.7 years), thus suggesting a more aggressive clinical entity.[90] In familial TAAD, thoracic aneurysms are the most common (66%), followed by AAAs (25%) and cerebral aneurysms (8% to 10%).[90] Although the ascending aorta is more commonly affected by aneurysm (82%) than by dissection (18%), an equal distribution of aortic dissections and aneurysms is appreciated in the descending thoracic aorta (50% each) in affected individuals. In comparison to Marfan's syndrome and sporadic thoracic aortic aneurysm, the proportion of descending thoracic aortic dissections was highest in familial TAAD.[90]

Selection of Treatment

Selection of treatment for patients with familial TAAD is complicated by the variable penetrance and expressivity of the disorder and the lack of an established genotype-phenotype correlation. In some families, the clinical history may suggest aortic catastrophe at very minimal aortic diameter dilatation, and treatment thresholds should be considered in the context of the pedigree history. For patients with a minimal contributory family history, treatment recommendations should follow typical sporadic thresholds of 6.0 cm for thoracic aortic aneurysms and 5.5 cm for AAAs. Thoracic aortic growth rates in familial TAAD are comparatively higher than those of sporadic aneurysms, on average 0.21 versus 0.16 cm/yr, respectively.[90] Endovascular stent-grafting approaches have not been reported in familial TAAD, but like other connective tissue diseases, concerns about the inherent weakness and fragility of the aortic wall are paramount. Consensus on stent-graft therapy for patients with familial TAAD is not available, but one should follow the previous documents advising against such approaches for connective tissue diseases.[59]

SELECTED KEY REFERENCES

Guo DC, Pannu H, Tran-Fadulu V, Papke CL, Yu RK, Avidan N, Bourgeois S, Estrera AL, Safi HJ, Sparks E, Amor D, Ades L, McConnell V, Willoughby CE, Abuelo D, Willing M, Lewis RA, Kim DH, Scherer S, Tung PP, Ahn C, Buja LM, Raman CS, Shete SS, Milewicz DM. Mutations in smooth muscle α-actin (ACTA-2) lead to thoracic aortic aneurysms and dissections. *Nat Genet.* 2007;39:1488-1493.
  First description of the novel discovery of the importance of the smooth muscle cell machinery in maintenance of aortic wall homeostasis.

Habashi JP, Judge DP, Holm TM, Cohn RD, Loeys BL, Cooper TK, Myers L, Klein EC, Liu G, Calvi C, Podowski M, Neptune ER, Halushka MK, Bedja D, Gabrielson K, Rifkin DB, Carta L, Ramirez F, Huso DL, Dietz HC. Losartan, an AT-1 antagonist, prevents aortic aneurysm in a mouse model of Marfan syndrome. *Science.* 2006;312:117-121.
  Landmark publication implicating TGF-β in Marfan's syndrome and the experimental evidence for losartan therapy.

Judge DP, Dietz HC. Marfan's Syndrome. *Lancet.* 2005;366:1965-1976.
  An excellent review of the comprehensive management strategies used in Marfan's syndrome.

Loeys BL, Schwarze U, Holm T. Aneurysm syndromes caused by mutations in the TGF-β receptor. *N Engl J Med.* 2006;355:788-798.
  Natural history of Loeys-Dietz syndrome and initial experience in surgical intervention.

Milewicz DM, Dietz HC, Miller C. Treatment of aortic disease in patients with Marfan syndrome. *Circulation.* 2005;111:e150-e157.
  Review of indications for arterial repairs in Marfan's syndrome.

Pepin M, Schwarze U, Superti-Furga A, Byers PH. Clinical and genetic features of Ehlers-Danlos type IV, the vascular type. *N Engl J Med.* 2000;342:673-680.
  Widely quoted paper on the natural history of EDS IV.

Zhu L, Vranckx R, Khau Van Kien P, Lalande A, Boisset N, Mathieu F, Wegman M, Glancy L, Gasc JM, Brunotte F, Bruneval P, Wolf JE, Michel JB, Jeunemaitre X. Mutations in myosin heavy chain 11 cause a syndrome associating thoracic aortic aneurysm/aortic dissection and patent ductus arteriosus. *Nat Genet.* 2006;38:343-349.

REFERENCES

The reference list can be found on the companion Expert Consult Web site at *www.expertconsult.com.*

Renal and Mesenteric Disease | *Section* **18**

James Seeger

CHAPTER 141

Renovascular Disease: General Considerations

Bryan W. Tillman and Randolph L. Geary

Based in part on chapters in the previous edition by Kimberley J. Hansen, MD, FACS; Joshua W. Bernheim, MD; K. Craig Kent, MD; David B. Wilson, MD; and Richard H. Dean, MD.

Renal artery disease encompasses a range of disorders affecting blood flow to the kidneys and is much more prevalent than is generally recognized, affecting 6.8% of elderly Americans.[1] Atherosclerosis is the most common cause of renal artery stenosis (RAS) and the primary focus of this chapter (Fig. 141-1). Other lesions affecting renal blood flow include fibromuscular dysplasia (FMD; see Chapter 144: Renovascular Disease: Fibrodysplasia), dissection and trauma (see Chapters 135: Aortic Dissection; 146: Renovascular Disease: Acute Occlusive Events; and 154: Vascular Trauma: Abdominal), and congenital hypoplastic syndromes of the aorta and renal arteries.[2,3] The importance of RAS is related primarily to its two major clinical manifestations—hypertension and impaired renal function—and to their contributions to adverse cardiovascular events, dialysis dependence, and mortality.[4,5]

HISTORICAL BACKGROUND

In 1899, Tigerstedt and Bergman isolated a substance from rabbit kidneys with pressor effects and called it *renin*,[6] but not for decades was its role in renovascular disease established. Katzenstein in 1905 linked experimental renal artery constriction to hypertension,[7] and Goldblatt in 1934 published elegant

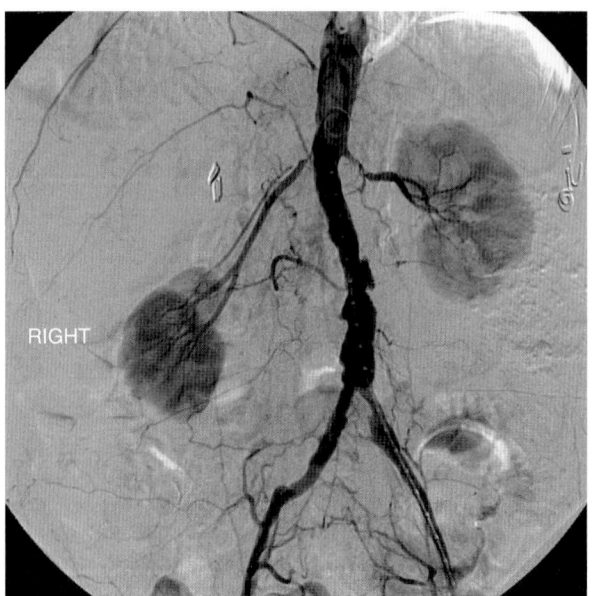

Figure 141-1 Digital subtraction angiography illustrating bilateral atherosclerotic renal artery stenosis.

experiments linking renal artery constriction to kidney atrophy and hypertension that could be cured by nephrectomy.[8] Goldblatt also showed that the physiology of hypertension differed, depending on whether one or both renal arteries were occluded, which he described as "renin-dependent" and "volume-dependent" hypertension, respectively.

The first successful treatment of renovascular hypertension was reported in 1938 by Leadbetter and Burkland, who removed an ischemic ectopic kidney from a hypertensive child.[9] Nephrectomy subsequently became a common treatment for hypertension in patients with an associated small kidney, but the results were unpredictable, with only one in four patients actually cured of hypertension.[10] The first cure of hypertension by direct renal artery reconstruction was reported by Freeman and colleagues in 1954, who performed an endarterectomy for bilateral ostial lesions.[11] Enthusiasm for renal revascularization increased dramatically after the introduction of aortography, and numerous reports of improved blood pressure control followed.[12-15] By 1960, however, a critical reappraisal showed that blood pressure was improved in less than half of patients undergoing surgery,[13,16] and this inability to predict who would benefit led to pessimism about the utility of repair.

Ultimately, the results of renal revascularization would improve only after the biochemical regulation of blood pressure was understood. Once the renin-angiotensin-aldosterone axis was characterized and its role in renovascular hypertension defined,[17-20] assays became available to accurately measure plasma renin activity. These and other functional tests ushered in the modern era of renal artery surgery in which physicians can more reliably identify patients likely to benefit from repair.

Although hypertension has historically been the primary trigger for screening and intervention in renovascular disease, and it remains so today, impaired renal excretory function from renal artery disease has a far greater impact on patient survival.[21] Experiments early in the 20th century showed that the kidney was intolerant of warm ischemia and that renal artery constriction caused renal atrophy in dogs.[8] In 1962, in a study of eight patients with bilateral RAS, Morris and coworkers showed that azotemia could be reversed by renal artery reconstruction.[15] Similar reports followed from Dean and others who coined the term *ischemic nephropathy* to describe renal insufficiency from impaired renal artery flow.[22-26] Even more provocative were early reports of patients being removed from dialysis following renal artery reconstruction.[27-29] Selecting azotemic patients who would benefit from surgery proved to be difficult, but recent studies have identified clinical characteristics predictive of improved or stabilized renal function after repair.[30,31]

Finally, since the introduction of percutaneous angioplasty of the renal arteries by Gruntzig and associates in 1978[32] and balloon-expandable stents in 1989,[33] endovascular treatment of anatomic renal artery disease has increased exponentially. In the United States, more than 21,660 renal revascularization procedures were performed under Medicare in 2000, the bulk of which were endovascular.[34] Enthusiasm for endovascular reconstruction of the renal arteries has outpaced clinical research to establish its niche in the contemporary management of renovascular hypertension or ischemic nephropathy (see Chapter 143: Renovascular Disease: Endovascular Treatment).

■ EPIDEMIOLOGY

Prevalence of Anatomic Renal Artery Disease

Independent-Living Elderly

The prevalence of RAS, independent of associated hypertension or renal failure, can be estimated from contemporary population-based studies. In a community-based study of 870 independently living adults aged 65 years or older, the prevalence of critical RAS on duplex ultrasound screening was 7%.[35] Of those, 12% had bilateral stenoses and 12% had complete occlusion. Risk factors associated with stenosis included increasing age, systolic hypertension, and reduced high-density lipoprotein cholesterol. Importantly, only slightly more than half of affected individuals were clinically hypertensive, and in contrast to previous studies in high-risk populations,[36] the prevalence was not significantly impacted by ethnicity or gender.[35]

Autopsy Series

Additional estimates of the prevalence of RAS in the general population have come from autopsy series. These studies represent the only data currently available from unselected low-risk individuals of a variety of ages. In 1964, Schwartz and White reported a series of 154 consecutive autopsies in which

the aorta and renal arteries were examined specifically for RAS.[37] They found that the prevalence of significant stenosis was 6% in patients younger than 55 years and 40% in patients older than 75. Bilateral stenoses were common, found in approximately half of affected individuals, and the proximal renal artery was the most common lesion location. That same year Holley and coworkers reported on 295 autopsies, but they excluded individuals with known intrinsic kidney disease.[38] They found that overall, 22% had significant RAS, most commonly involving the proximal renal arteries.

Prevalence of Renal Artery Stenosis in High-Risk Populations

Atherosclerotic Coronary Artery and Peripheral Arterial Disease

The prevalence of RAS has been estimated to be 15% to 45% in angiographic series characterizing atherosclerosis in other arterial beds, but these rates are heavily biased by the systemic nature of atherosclerosis (Table 141-1).[35,39-43]

The incidence of RAS in patients with coronary artery disease (CAD) ranges from 15% to 22%.[44] Jean and colleagues performed aortography in 196 patients undergoing heart catheterization and found that 18% of those with CAD had coexisting RAS.[39] Harding and associates demonstrated an association between RAS and increasing angiographic severity of CAD.[45] Some series have found a lower prevalence of RAS in African Americans[36] and in women, but these observations contrast with population-based studies in which race and gender have little effect on the prevalence of RAS.[1]

The prevalence of RAS is high among patients with severe peripheral and carotid atherosclerosis (see Table 141-1). In patients being treated for carotid stenosis, the prevalence of RAS is reportedly 20% to 27%.[46,47] Miralles and colleagues screened 168 consecutive patients undergoing elective treatment of aortoiliac occlusive disease for concomitant RAS and found that 40% had a critical lesion of one or both renal arteries.[40] The percentage increased to greater than 50% for the subset that also had carotid disease.[40]

Renal Insufficiency

Renal parenchymal injury in patients at risk for RAS can be complex, and the contribution of hypoperfusion from the

Section 18 Renal and Mesenteric Disease

Table 141-1 Prevalence of Renal Artery Stenosis (RAS) in High-Risk Populations

Series	Year	Number of Patients	Risk Factor	Patients with RAS (%)	Comments
Hansen et al.[35]	2002	834	Age	6.8	Free-living elderly
Jean et al.[39]	1994	196	Coronary artery disease (CAD)	22	Suspected CAD, undergoing angiography
Miralles et al.[40]	1998	168	Peripheral arterial disease	40	Aortoiliac occlusive disease
Appel et al.[41]	1995	45	Dialysis	22	New-onset dialysis
Davis et al.[42]	2009	434	Hypertension (adult)	32	
Lawson et al.[43]	1997	74	Hypertension (children)	78	

lesion itself is difficult to fully characterize.[48] Moreover, risk factors for renal failure (e.g., hypertension, diabetes, hyperlipidemia) overlap significantly with those for atherosclerosis, the primary cause of RAS. Thus, it is not surprising that the prevalence of RAS is high in patients with chronic renal insufficiency (14%).[49]

RAS has been reported in 9% to 22% of patients with end-stage renal disease (ESRD) requiring dialysis,[41,50,51] but the prevalence varies significantly by age, ethnicity, and gender. It is highest in older Caucasian men and surprisingly infrequent among African Americans with ESRD.[40,41,49-51] In our experience, virtually all patients with ischemic nephropathy also present with severe hypertension.[28] Those who are normotensive or only mildly hypertensive on presentation likely have another cause for their azotemia.

Hypertension

Although not all patients with RAS exhibit hypertension,[1,35] this is the most common clinical manifestation leading to diagnostic screening. When hypertension is present, it tends to be more severe and refractory to medical therapy compared with essential hypertension.[1] This point is illustrated by a study of 500 patients undergoing intervention for renovascular disease in whom the average systolic blood pressure was 200 mm Hg and the average number of antihypertensive medications was 2.6 (additional demographics are provided in Table 141-2).[52]

Using duplex ultrasonography to screen 629 adults presenting with newly diagnosed hypertension, we found that 25% had incident RAS. This doubled in patients older than 60 years with severe hypertension (diastolic blood pressure >110 mm Hg) and rose to 71% for the subset that also had renal insufficiency (serum creatinine >2.0 mg/dL [177 μmol/L]). Similarly, Holley and coworkers reported an extremely high prevalence of RAS (62%) in older patients with severe hypertension.[38] Atherosclerotic RAS is not found in children, but hypertension in this age group can result from other anatomic lesions that reduce renal perfusion. In a review of hypertensive children younger than 5 years, Lawson and associates reported that 78% had a correctable renin-mediated etiology.[43]

Table 141-2 Demographics of Patient Population Undergoing Renal Revascularization

Parameter	Value
Age	65 ± 9 yr
Gender	49% male, 51% female
Systolic blood pressure	200 ± 35 mm Hg
Diastolic blood pressure	104 ± 21 mm Hg
Number of antihypertensive medications	2.6 ± 1.1
Creatinine (mean)	2.6 mg/dL (230 μmol/L)
Co-morbid extrarenal atherosclerosis	90%
Coexisting coronary artery disease	70%
Diabetes	16%

Natural History of Renal Artery Stenosis
Anatomic Progression

Critical to decision making in the treatment of RAS is an understanding of the natural history of lesions managed expectantly. Many patients whose lesions are identified incidentally or by screening are asymptomatic or have hypertension that is effectively controlled with medications. Some clinicians have argued that even in these patients, the risk of lesion progression and its consequences is great enough to warrant prophylactic repair. Even in patients with more severe symptoms of hypertension and renal insufficiency, an understanding of the risk of lesion progression is critical to a proper risk assessment in individuals being considered for invasive treatment.

Earlier studies using serial angiography in high-risk populations reported that the risk for anatomic progression of renovascular disease ranged from 11% to 35%.[53-56] In these studies approximately 10% of arteries progressed to complete occlusion, but only when a severe stenosis preexisted.[53,55] Duplex surveillance has also been employed in high-risk populations. Zierler and coworkers performed serial examinations of 80 patients with renovascular hypertension whose arteries were initially classified as normal, less than 60% stenotic, or greater than 60% stenotic.[57] After 3 years' follow-up, 8% of arteries initially classified as normal and 43% initially classified as less than 60% stenotic had progressed to greater than 60% RAS. Progression to complete occlusion was observed in 7% of arteries, but again, only when a significant preexisting lesion (>60%) was present on prior examination. Factors associated with lesion progression included older age, higher systolic pressure, smoking, female gender, and poorly controlled hypertension.

Functional Progression

Individuals with RAS may or may not have severe hypertension or reduced renal function, but progression of renal artery disease has been associated with these functional measures of renal hypoperfusion. Moreover, their clinical consequences (cardiovascular morbidity and progression to dialysis) provide the rationale for treatment. For instance, among 41 patients with renovascular hypertension who were randomized to medical therapy, Dean and associates found that 46% showed a significant rise in serum creatinine and 37% lost more than 10% of renal length.[53] Schreiber and colleagues also reported that a significant number patients with greater than 60% RAS lost renal function, estimated by a rise in creatinine, even when the degree of stenosis remained stable.[54]

In another series of 122 patients with renovascular hypertension followed prospectively, Caps and coworkers reported that 21% of kidneys with greater than 60% stenosis at baseline had shrunk by more than 1 cm after 2 years, with an associated rise in creatinine.[58] Risk of atrophy correlated with the degree of stenosis and systolic hypertension. Others have confirmed that medical management of RAS results in a relatively high rate of progression of stenosis, accompanied by kidney shrinkage, loss of excretory function,[56] and even progression to dialysis in 7% to 12% of patients within 3 to 4 years.[59,60]

The only prospective longitudinal population-based study of the natural history of atherosclerotic RAS was recently published by Pearce and colleagues.[61] They found that among the 119 patients (235 kidneys) studied, none of the 13 with significant RAS identified at initial screening had progressed to occlusion. However, nine kidneys without disease at baseline developed critical RAS on follow-up, including one occlusion. The overall incidence of progression to significant (>60%) RAS after 8 years of follow-up was only 4%, a markedly reduced rate than that observed in studies of highly selected high-risk patients.

Taken together, these studies demonstrate that progression of anatomic RAS is unlikely in low-risk patients in whom RAS is found incidentally. In high-risk groups with severe lesions, accelerated hypertension and loss of renal function are more common. Additionally, the risk of progression is highest in the elderly with advanced, preexisting renal artery disease.

Morbidity

The major risks of RAS are the extent to which hypertension and loss of excretory renal function translate to excess morbidity and mortality from cardiovascular events or dialysis dependence. A significant increase in end-organ damage has been reported in patients with renovascular hypertension compared with those with essential hypertension, as revealed by left ventricular hypertrophy, elevated creatinine, and proteinuria.[62] These differences were found despite matching patients for hypertension severity. Mailloux and coworkers projected that renal artery disease accounts for 10% to 18% of incident dialysis dependence among the elderly. This is especially troublesome, given the profound reduction in quality of life, high mortality (median survival, 25 months), and expense associated with the onset of dialysis in the elderly.[50]

Appel[41] and Valentine[63] have shown an association between RAS and a previous history of cardiovascular events, including stroke. Valentine also showed that RAS was a risk factor for increased perioperative cardiovascular events.[63] In 1235 patients with arteriographic documentation of CAD, Conlon and associates showed that those with greater than 50% RAS had a markedly reduced 4-year survival (88% versus 67%), primarily from excess cardiovascular events.[64]

These and other groups have speculated on the potential mechanisms linking renovascular disease to cardiovascular events, including accelerated progression of existing atherosclerosis, altered lipid metabolism associated with renal insufficiency, and adverse systemic cardiovascular influences of excess renin and angiotensin II.[41] Until recently, however, no prospective or population-based studies had looked specifically at this question. Edwards and coworkers from our center recently documented the risk of adverse coronary events among 870 independently living individuals older than 65 years in a cohort of the Cardiovascular Risk in Communities Study.[65] All were screened for greater than 60% RAS by duplex ultrasound. During a mean follow-up of only 14 months, the risk of cardiovascular events doubled for the 6.8% of participants with RAS, even after controlling for coexisting risk factors, including hypertension and prevalent cardiovascular disease.

PATHOGENESIS

Etiology of Renal Artery Lesions

As noted earlier, the most common pathology underlying renal artery disease is atherosclerosis. This is particular true for RAS of clinical significance. To illustrate this point, 91% to 98% of patients undergoing percutaneous treatment for RAS have atherosclerotic lesions.[66,67] Endovascular series, however, are likely to show a significant bias toward atherosclerosis because procedures are often performed in patients being studied or treated for atherosclerosis in other arterial beds. We recently reviewed our experience in 840 patients undergoing open renal artery reconstruction from 1987 to 2008, excluding patients who underwent combined renal repair during the repair of aortic aneurysms or occlusive disease. Consistent with the literature, we found that 81% of lesions were atherosclerotic in origin, 14% were caused by FMD, and 1% were dissections. Children accounted for 3% of this cohort, and most presented with hypoplastic renal arteries, midaortic syndrome, or dissection.

Atherosclerotic renal artery disease commonly involves the renal ostia, but stenoses may occur at any level within the renal arteries, including small intraparenchymal vessels.[37,38] Cross-sections of renal artery plaques show histology typical of atherosclerotic lesions in other vascular beds, with variable accumulation of monocytes and lymphocytes, smooth muscle cells, lipid, mineralization, and so forth (see Chapter 4: Atherosclerosis). Peculiar to ostial renal artery lesions, however, and relevant to their treatment, is the finding that the first few millimeters of stenotic lumen is often formed by contiguous aortic plaque oriented perpendicular to the renal artery. This plaque is typically very thick and heavily calcified, creating a rigid sheet that resists balloon dilatation. For this reason, most authorities recommend primary stenting if an endovascular repair is planned for ostial RAS.[68] Further, when performing a transaortic thromboendarterectomy for ostial lesions, a sleeve of aortic plaque is generally removed in continuity with the renal lesions (Fig. 141-2).

Pathophysiology of Renovascular Hypertension

Renovascular hypertension is initiated by progressive kidney hypoperfusion, which activates the neuroendocrine-renin-angiotensin-aldosterone system. This leads to vasoconstriction and volume expansion. If this state persists, adaptive remodeling of the heart and vasculature contributes to the sustained and accentuated hypertension of chronic renovascular disease.

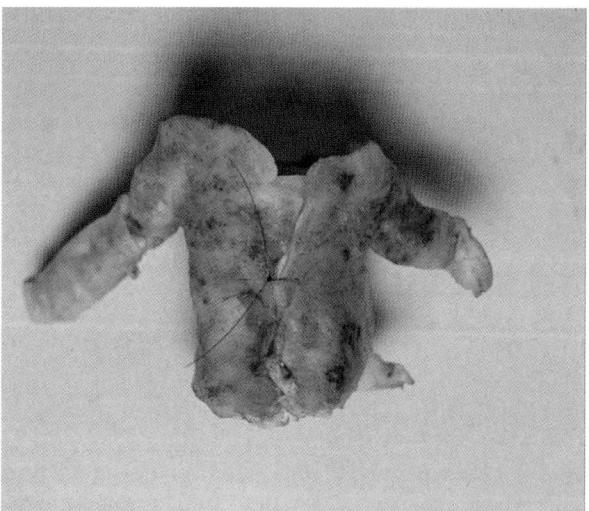

Figure 141-2 Operative specimen from transaortic sleeve endarterectomy illustrating proximal renal artery plaque contiguous with aortic disease.

In response to reduced pressure, juxtaglomerular cells release renin, which catalyzes the cleavage of angiotensinogen, an α_2-globulin synthesized in the liver. The resulting decapeptide angiotensin I then undergoes a second cleavage event catalyzed by angiotensin-converting enzyme (ACE) to form the octapeptide angiotensin II, a primary effector of renin-induced hypertension.[69] This cascade occurs locally within the kidney, within the systemic circulation, and within many extrarenal tissues. ACE is present at high levels in the lung but is also active in the glomerulus, endothelium, heart, and brain.[70,71] Therefore, angiotensin II is also formed in a number of extrarenal tissues through local renin-angiotensin systems. Additional proteases have been identified that cleave angiotensin, including tonin, cathepsin, chymase, and kallikrein.[69,72]

Angiotensin II is the primary effector of renovascular hypertension through arteriolar vasoconstriction and sodium and water reabsorption. These effects are mediated by activation of the angiotensin type 1 receptor (ATR1), a G protein–coupled receptor that directly activates vasoconstrictor and mitogenic signaling in blood vessels through the protein kinase C pathway. Cross-talk between ATR1 and other receptor classes can amplify signaling by important smooth muscle cell constrictors and mitogens, including platelet-derived growth factor (PDGF),[73] and ATR1 activation upregulates expression of the potent vasoconstrictors norepinephrine and endothelin-1.[74,75]

Angiotensin II acts on the adrenal cortex to stimulate aldosterone release, leading to volume expansion in response to renal tubular sodium absorption.[76] It can also stimulate tubular sodium absorption directly via ATR1 activation. If a functional contralateral kidney is present, sodium retention is blunted by natriuresis from the normal kidney.[77,78] In contrast, a patient with only one functional kidney or with contralateral RAS cannot mount the compensatory natriuresis, resulting in so-called volume-dependent or Goldblatt hypertension.

The importance of angiotensin II can be easily demonstrated through pharmacologic inhibition of ACE or the ATR1 using specific antihypertensive medications. ACE inhibitors (ACEIs) and angiotensin receptor blockers (ARBs) are very effective in treating renovascular hypertension from unilateral disease; they also provide an indirect, if unintentional, diagnostic intervention when prescribed to patients with bilateral RAS: the loss of arteriolar tone leads to an acute decompensation in glomerular filtration that is reversible when the medication is stopped.[79]

The mechanism of elevated arterial pressure in renovascular hypertension changes over time. Though initially mediated by the effects of angiotensin II, as outlined earlier, subsequent remodeling in both the heart and resistance vessels contributes to continued pressure elevations and associated cardiovascular embarrassment.[80-82] The nature of vascular remodeling seen in RAS-dependent hypertension is distinct from that observed in essential hypertension. In essential hypertension, resistance vessels exhibit eutrophic remodeling, with no significant change in wall mass; in contrast, in patients with chronic hyperreninemia as in RAS, remodeling is hypertrophic, with expansion of the medial layer,[83] and is responsive to ACEIs.[84] Negative effects of chronic activation of the renin-angiotensin system are also being elucidated in other organs, where blocking angiotensin II production has been found to improve cardiac remodeling and inhibit vascular hypertrophy, endothelial dysfunction, thrombosis, and platelet aggregation.[85,86]

Pathophysiology of Ischemic Nephropathy

The term *ischemic nephropathy* has been used for decades to describe renal insufficiency from RAS, but its molecular basis remains incompletely defined.[87] Hypoperfusion results in impaired glomerular filtration,[88] but the role of frank ischemia is less well established than the name suggests.[31,89] Certainly, rapid progression to renal artery occlusion causes ischemia and atrophy of the affected kidney, but a chronic decrease in flow leads to impaired excretory function through a number of pathways.

Clinically, the relationship between renovascular disease and loss of excretory function is strongly associated with elevated blood pressure.[21] Mechanistically, as for renovascular hypertension, angiotensin II appears to play a central role. By increasing efferent arteriolar tone,[90] angiotensin II increases glomerular capillary pressure to maintain filtration in the presence of reduced renal perfusion. However, secondary effects of chronic angiotensin II excess within the kidney include ATR1-induced expression of several profibrotic cytokines and growth factors.

Angiotensin II increases the expression of transforming growth factor-β (TGF-β), a master regulator of extracellular matrix production, and PDGF, a potent mitogen for smooth muscle cells, renal fibroblasts, and the mesangial cells essential for normal glomerular function. Angiotensin II also induces nuclear factor-κB, a potent inducer of proinflammatory gene expression. Increases in aldosterone have also been shown to activate TGF-β and thereby contribute to glomerulosclerosis and tubulointerstitial injury.[91-97] Evidence is also emerging that renal artery lesions themselves contribute to the loss of excretory function. Atherosclerotic plaques spontaneously release atheroembolic debris, causing significant damage to the kidney.[98]

CLINICAL PRESENTATION
History and Physical Examination

As noted earlier, roughly half of individuals with anatomic renal artery disease have no associated symptoms. Those with functional lesions typically present with severe hypertension, with or without reduced excretory renal function. Other symptoms, physical findings, and laboratory abnormalities are typically nonspecific, so practitioners need to be aware of which individuals are at greatest risk. Advanced age, severe hypertension refractory to multiple antihypertensive agents, and history of coexisting coronary artery or peripheral arterial disease should also raise suspicion. Although renal artery disease often leads to impaired renal function, in our experience, virtually all patients with ischemic nephropathy have severe coexisting hypertension. Therefore, azotemia without hypertension, even in a patient with documented RAS, should prompt an evaluation for other intrinsic renal pathology. Renal artery disease should be in the differential diagnosis of any child with unexplained hypertension.[99]

A scenario frequently diagnostic of bilateral RAS is a patient who presents in acute renal failure upon starting treatment with an ACEI or ARB.[79] Increased efferent arteriolar tone induced by angiotensin II is a critical compensatory mechanism to maintain filtration pressure in bilateral renal artery disease. Pharmacologic blockade of efferent arteriolar constriction by ACEIs or ARBs leads to an acute decompensation in filtration. When the effect of the medication is recognized early, simply stopping the culprit medication results in a return of renal function to baseline. Subsequent imaging confirms the presence of bilateral renal lesions.

Individuals with acute exacerbations of unrecognized or poorly controlled renovascular hypertension may present in "hypertensive crisis." This is more common when long-standing hypertension has led to compensatory end-organ remodeling, such as myocardial hypertrophy with abnormal diastolic relaxation. Patients often present in congestive heart failure from "flash" pulmonary edema or with neurologic symptoms ranging from headache and visual disturbances to overt stroke. The severe increase in hydrostatic pressure drives fluid into the extravascular space, causing edema of the extremities and internal organs, including the brain. Acute hypertension can also damage the kidney, resulting in proteinuria and elevated creatinine. As blood pressure is normalized, proteinuria and azotemia resolve and return to baseline. In this setting, it is important to allow a patient with acute renal damage to recover before performing imaging with iodinated contrast agents, using resolution of proteinuria and creatinine as a guide to recovery.

On examination, patients may have severe elevation of systolic and diastolic blood pressure, abdominal bruits, and nonspecific stigmata of heart and vascular disease.[30,100] Diminished lower extremity pulses may be present in children with coarctation or midaortic syndromes. Pulse deficits may also be found in young adults with Takayasu's arteritis[101] or in patients presenting with aortic dissection and malperfusion.

Laboratory Findings

Though nonspecific, blood chemistries may show elevated urea nitrogen and creatinine. The electrocardiogram may show a strain pattern with increased voltage, consistent with ventricular wall thickening in response to chronic hypertension. Echocardiography can confirm ventricular hypertrophy with impaired diastolic relaxation. Specialized biochemical assays such as plasma renin levels are rarely useful in the contemporary diagnosis of renovascular disease unless they are combined with selected invasive renal vein renin sampling (see "Renal Vein Renin Assays"). Measuring plasma aldosterone in patients with hypokalemia may identify those with primary hyperaldosteronism, and assays of urine metanephrines or serum catecholamines can identify metabolically active adrenal tumors leading to hypertension, such as Conn's disease and pheochromocytoma.[102]

DIAGNOSTIC EVALUATION
Noninvasive Imaging
Duplex Ultrasonography

The ideal imaging modality for renal artery disease would be a rapid, noninvasive study with excellent resolution, accuracy, and reproducibility. It would carry minimal risk to the patient and be inexpensive. Of all the tools presently available, color duplex ultrasonography best fits this profile and has become the primary method of screening for renal artery disease in a number of centers. Duplex avoids ionizing radiation and the potential for allergic or nephrotoxic reactions to iodinated contrast agents. Ultrasound does not require intravenous access and is safe in patients with medical implants. The primary limitation of renal duplex is that it is technically demanding relative to other studies performed in the average vascular laboratory. Study times can range from 10 to 60 minutes, depending on the patient's body habitus and the technician's experience. Factors that may interfere with insonation of the renal artery include excessive bowel gas, obesity, and altered flow from advanced kidney disease. In our experience, these factors contribute to incomplete examinations in about 4% of studies.[103]

At our institution, the examination begins after the patient has fasted overnight to reduce bowel gas. With the patient supine, an anterior examination of the aorta and main renal arteries is performed using color-flow imaging to exclude aneurysm, stenosis, or occlusion of the perirenal aorta. Velocity waveforms are then recorded from the proximal, mid, and distal renal arteries at a 60-degree angle of insonation. The patient is then placed in the left and right lateral positions, and velocity waveforms are recorded again from the proximal, mid, and distal renal arteries at an angle of insonation approaching 0 degrees. Velocity waveforms are also recorded from the renal parenchyma of superior, mid, and inferior poles to calculate a resistive index (peak systolic velocity–end-diastolic velocity/peak systolic velocity) and acceleration time (interval from onset of systole to peak systole in milliseconds). The examination is completed by recording kidney length.

When validated against conventional arteriography, the accuracy of duplex ultrasonography in detecting significant RAS can exceed 90% in experienced hands.[103-106] Although a number of criteria have been shown to predict critical stenosis, the most consistent is increased peak systolic velocity in the main renal artery (>1.8 to 2.0 m/sec),[103,105,107] with associated post-stenotic turbulence.[108] In 74 consecutive patients undergoing renal arteriography, duplex ultrasonography correctly identified stenosis of greater than 60% with a sensitivity of 93%, a specificity of 98%, and an overall accuracy of 96% in kidneys with single renal arteries.[103] Sensitivity decreased to 86% in kidneys with multiple renal arteries (present in 15% of kidneys), but specificity remained high at 98%.[103] Some centers rely on the ratio of renal artery to aortic peak systolic velocity, with a ratio greater than >3.5 defining stenosis of greater than 60%.[109] Similar data have been reported from a number of centers,[46,105,107,110-112] but others have been unable to reproduce these excellent results.[113,114]

Attempts to simplify the duplex diagnosis of critical RAS include indirect studies of the distal renal vasculature. A flank approach is used to record Doppler arterial waveforms from the hilum or parenchyma. Blunted waveforms with delayed systolic upstroke are indicative of a proximal stenosis. Acceleration time is used to estimate this delay by calculating the period between the onset and peak of systole. Acceleration time greater than 100 msec indicates a critical stenosis within the proximal renal artery.[108] A number of investigators have documented a reasonable correlation between elevated acceleration time and stenosis on conventional angiography.[106,115] Our own published experience suggests that although acceleration time has a high positive predictive value (97%), it does not provide adequate sensitivity to be used as the sole screening examination.[108]

The resistive index has also been used to indirectly identify critical RAS. A normal value is less than 0.7. Values greater than 0.8 may indicate critical RAS, but abnormal results are nonspecific and are often caused by intrinsic medical renal disease in which scarring and fibrosis lead to elevated resistance to flow within the parenchyma (e.g., nephrosclerosis, glomerular sclerosis). Radermacher and colleagues showed that in 131 patients undergoing renal revascularization, a resistive index greater than 0.8 was predictive of a poor hypertension response and progression of renal insufficiency, consistent with irreversible intrinsic medical renal disease not improved by the restoration of blood flow.[116] Conversely, 94% of patients with an index less than 0.8 had improved blood pressure and lack of progression to dialysis after reconstruction. Despite these data, the role of the resistive index in managing patients with RAS remains controversial.

Computed Tomographic Angiography

Advances in the speed, resolution, and postprocessing of computed tomography (CT) have contributed to the widespread application of computed tomographic angiography (CTA) for vascular imaging (see Chapter 21: Computed Tomography). Modern multichannel scanners can acquire volumetric data of the arterial system at high spatial resolution, which permits precise three-dimensional visualization and quantification of vascular abnormalities that are not possible with digital subtraction angiography (DSA).[117] CTA is noninvasive and widely available, and image acquisition and formatting are less technically demanding than for duplex ultrasonography or contrast-enhanced magnetic resonance angiography (MRA) of the renal arteries.

Disadvantages of CTA include exposure to ionizing radiation and iodinated contrast agents. Radiation exposure is typically greater than is generally appreciated (see Chapter 20: Radiation Safety and Chapter 21: Computed Tomography), with the patient receiving a 5.2-mSv dose for a typical renal artery examination using a four-slice scanner.[118] To put this in context, a typical chest x-ray delivers 0.02 to 0.06 mSv, or 87- to 260-fold less than CTA. The volume of iodinated contrast agent for typical renal CTA, 120 to 140 mL, can also be problematic, given the increased frequency of renal insufficiency in patients with RAS.[119]

CTA data sets are now generally evaluated on modern workstations capable of reformatting axial sections into two- or three-dimensional images that can be viewed from any angle. Post-processing techniques include multiplanar reformatting, maximum intensity projection, volume rendering, and shaded surface display algorithms (see Chapter 21: Computed Tomography), which are helpful in localizing and characterizing renal artery pathology and invaluable in planning interventions. Reformations orthogonal to a stenosis may significantly increase diagnostic accuracy,[120] but as with MRA, a review of source images is critical before drawing conclusions about the extent of pathology.

A number of studies have compared CTA with DSA in the diagnosis of atherosclerotic RAS. Sensitivity, specificity, and accuracy in defining stenosis of the main renal artery approach 100% in contemporary series (Table 141-3).[103,105,110,111,117,121-127] In sharp contrast, however, a large prospective multicenter study from the Netherlands compared CTA and contrast-enhanced MRA with DSA in 356 patients suspected of having RAS. Overall, sensitivity ranged from 61% to 69% for CTA and 57% to 67% for MRA; specificity ranged from 89% to 97% for CTA and from 77% to 90% for MRA.[128] Explanations for these disparate results include suboptimal image capture protocols, a low prevalence of disease in the study population, a relatively high proportion of RAS patients with FMD, and a suboptimal standard of reference. Others may argue that these

Table 141-3 Accuracy of Duplex Ultrasonography, Computed Tomographic Angiography (CTA), and Magnetic Resonance Angiography (MRA) for the Evaluation of Renal Artery Stenosis

Series	Year	Modality	Number of Kidneys	Sensitivity (%)	Specificity (%)
Hansen et al.[103]	1990	Duplex	122	93	98
Olin et al.[111]	1995	Duplex	102	98	98
Mollo et al.[110]	1997	Duplex	53	75	100
Hua et al.[105]	2000	Duplex	58	91	75
Kaatee et al.[121]	1997	CTA	71	95	97
Equine et al.[122]	1999	CTA	50	94	95
Wittenberg et al.[123]	1999	CTA	82	96	99
Fraioli et al.[117]	2006	CTA	50	100	98.6
Korst et al.[124]	2000	MRA	75	100	85
Bongers et al.[125]	2000	MRA	43	100	100
De Cobelli et al.[126]	2000	MRA	45	100	93
Voiculescu et al.[127]	2001	MRA	36	96	86

data are closer to "real-world" expectations than those reported from highly specialized imaging centers. Among the noninvasive imaging methods discussed in this section, CTA is less accurate at identifying stenoses of accessory and polar vessels. In addition, although CTA is generally considered better than contrast-enhanced MRA in distinguishing RAS from FMD, few large studies have assessed the accuracy of CTA versus DSA in detecting FMD.[129]

Another distinct advantage of CTA is the detailed information about surrounding tissues and organs obtained from the same imaging sequences. Important examples include kidney length and cortical thickness and quality of the adjacent aorta and visceral arteries. The latter may help in planning surgical reconstruction of RAS by identifying locations suitable for cross-clamping and inflow sources for bypass procedures. This information is generally not derived from renal duplex ultrasonography or MRA. The presence of adrenal tumors may suggest other secondary sources of hypertension such as pheochromocytoma or aldosterone-secreting tumor (Conn's disease). CTA can also characterize the lumen of stented renal arteries without significant image distortion, unlike MRA. Improved visualization of lumen dimensions in calcified vessels has been demonstrated with newer post-processing protocols such as curved planar reconstructions (see Chapter 21: Computed Tomography).

Magnetic Resonance Angiography

MRA has been studied extensively for imaging of the vasculature in general and the renal arteries in particular.[130,131] Its advantages are that it is noninvasive and does not require ionizing radiation or iodinated contrast agents; as with CTA, data sets can be reformatted into two- or three-dimensional images of the vasculature capable of being viewed from virtually any projection. Magnetic resonance imaging (MRI) also has a number of limitations (discussed in detail in Chapter 22:

Magnetic Resonance Imaging), including long scan times, which predispose to movement artifact, and the tight confines of closed scanners, which may cause claustrophobia. The magnetic field is disturbed by metal, so images of structures adjacent to implants (e.g., vascular stents, surgical clips, prostheses) are distorted, and MRI is contraindicated in patients with implants or foreign bodies that could move in response to the magnetic force, with dire consequences (e.g., intracranial clips, cardiac pacemakers, implantable cardioverter-defibrillators, intraocular metal fragments).[132]

Although noncontrast MRA protocols can provide excellent imaging of the aorta and its branches (e.g., time-of-flight and phase contrast sequences), most contemporary protocols for imaging the renal arteries employ contrast-enhanced MRA performed with a field strength of 1.5 T. The renal arteries are imaged in the coronal plane during a 15- to 20-second breath-hold after the infusion of gadolinium. Three-dimensional volumetric reformations of the source images provide an excellent view of the renal artery lumen, and their accuracy in identifying significant RAS approaches that of CTA, using DSA as the "gold standard" (see Table 141-3). MRA is slightly more prone to overestimate the degree of stenosis,[133] but the negative predictive value is excellent; therefore, a normal study can help exclude atherosclerotic stenosis of the main renal artery. However, contrast-enhanced MRA has not performed well in the setting of multiple renal arteries or in patients with FMD.[119]

A recent problem associated with contrast-enhanced MRA is the uncommon but potentially fatal complication of nephrogenic systemic fibrosis. This is a scleroderma-like syndrome associated with the use of gadolinium in patients with severe renal insufficiency.[134] Fibrosis is most common in the extremities but may involve the lung, diaphragm, esophagus, heart, and vasculature.[135] The pathogenesis is ill defined, but most patients have ESRD,[136] and a dose effect is likely. Broome and coworkers reported that 12 of 207 dialysis patients receiving

0.2 mmol/kg gadolinium developed nephrogenic systemic fibrosis, while none of 94 patients receiving 0.1 mmol/kg were affected.[137] The Food and Drug Administration has issued a black-box warning to avoid the administration of gadolinium to patients with ESRD or a glomerular filtration rate less than 15 mL/min per 1.73 m^2 unless absolutely necessary.[138] Those who are exposed should be dialyzed immediately afterward to reduce the risk of nephrogenic systemic fibrosis,[139] but this does not provide complete protection.[137]

Invasive Imaging

Digital Subtraction Angiography

As noted earlier, DSA is the gold standard against which all other imaging for renal artery disease is compared. Its major strengths are high resolution and accuracy in defining renal artery disease and its role in enabling endovascular renal reconstructions. Major drawbacks are that it is invasive, with a risk of access site complications that are occasionally limb or life threatening. DSA also exposes patients to ionizing radiation and nephrotoxic contrast agents; it is labor intensive, requiring a team of trained specialists; and it is expensive (see Chapter 18: Arteriography).

Images acquired by DSA are in planar format and thus lack the additional image information obtained with three-dimensional CTA and MRA (Fig. 141-3). New equipment has been developed to create CT reconstructions from DSA data in the interventional suite,[140,141] but this technology is not widely available nor particularly useful in defining renal artery pathology. Resolution with DSA imaging is extremely high and generally exceeds that required for diagnostic and therapeutic applications. However, image quality can be negatively impacted by a number of factors, including obesity, bowel gas, retained gastrointestinal contrast material from preceding examinations, and movement (see Chapter 18: Arteriography). A number of technical considerations that can help optimize patient safety and image quality are discussed in detail in Chapters 18 (Arteriography) and 143 (Renovascular Disease: Endovascular Treatment).

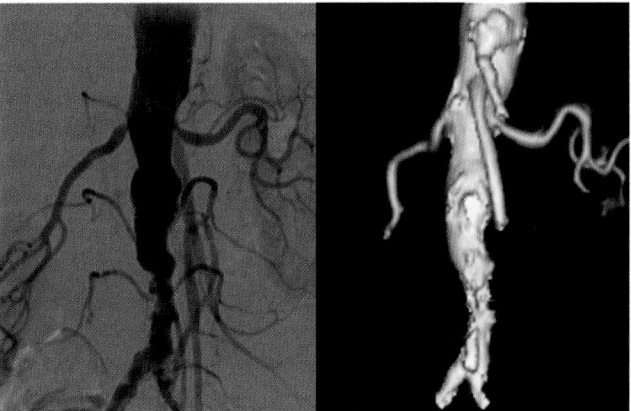

Figure 141-3 Comparison of digital subtraction angiography (*left*) and volume-rendered CTA (*right*) in a patient with bilateral proximal renal artery stenosis.

A minority of patients referred for screening for secondary causes of severe hypertension will be found to have RAS. Thus, screening for RAS using DSA would needlessly expose more than half of patients to unnecessary risks.[142,143] Given the wide availability of noninvasive screening studies for RAS, we generally reserve DSA for patients undergoing endovascular or open renal artery reconstructions. In the latter group, it is important to define the patient's entire perirenal vascular anatomy, including accessory arteries, branch vessel disease, blood supply to the contralateral kidney, and status of the adjacent aorta and visceral vessels as potential inflow sources.

We generally perform diagnostic and interventional renal arteriography from a femoral approach; however, we may use a brachial approach in patients with severe aortoiliac disease or when the arteries arise at difficult angles from the aorta. When DSA is performed to plan an open reconstruction, we begin with anteroposterior and lateral aortography, including the origin of the visceral vessels. We then adjust the angle of imaging to accommodate renal anatomy as needed. Many patients have had prior abdominal CT or MRI demonstrating the orientation of the renal ostia on the aorta. Most commonly, an anteroposterior or slight left anterior oblique projection is optimal because the right renal ostium frequently arises slightly anteriorly on the aorta and the left ostium arises posteriorly (i.e., 10 o'clock and 4 o'clock, respectively, if viewed axially by CT). This information can help in selecting a projection angle to display the most proximal segment of the renal arteries without the overlap of contrast within the aorta. This is relevant because most atherosclerotic renal artery disease is ostial. Planning from prior axial imaging may also help reduce the radiation and contrast exposure needed to complete an examination.

Many patients who require intervention have renal insufficiency and are at high risk for contrast-induced nephropathy. Preprocedural hydration and reducing the exposure to iodinated contrast agents can greatly reduce this risk. Strategies used in our practice to minimize contrast exposure include the use of carbon dioxide (CO_2) aortography (Fig. 141-4). Gadolinium has also been used,[144,145] but we have found that the resolution is superior with CO_2. Subsequent focused imaging is then done with small volumes of dilute (one-third strength) iso-osmolar nonionic contrast agents to complete the study or intervention. If an azotemic patient is being treated for bilateral disease, treatment should be staged to minimize contrast exposure. Recent data also suggest that atheroemboli dislodged during endovascular treatment of atherosclerotic stenoses contribute to impaired renal function or lack of improvement after treatment.[146] To investigate this hypothesis, prospective studies have been initiated to determine whether distal embolic protection devices can improve the results of endovascular renal interventions (see Chapters 18: Arteriography and 143: Renovascular Disease: Endovascular Treatment).

Functional Studies

Although each imaging modality discussed earlier can detect RAS, all are inconsistent at identifying a "functional" lesion

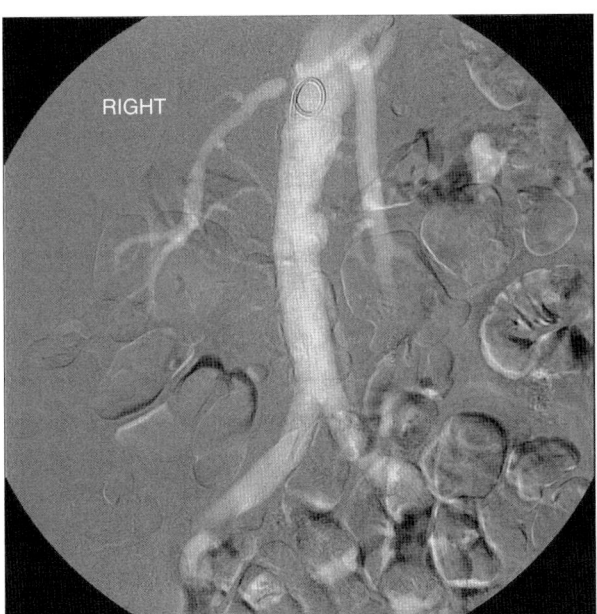

Figure 141-4 Strategies to limit nephrotoxic contrast exposure during renal angiography include the use of alternative contrast agents such as carbon dioxide (shown) and gadolinium.

causally linked to hypertension or impaired renal function that can be cured or stabilized by revascularization. A variety of additional tests have been used to define functional lesions. These include a significant pressure gradient across a lesion documented by direct pull-back measurements or the indirect analysis of distal arterial duplex waveforms showing increased acceleration times.[106] Kidney length has been used as a surrogate for functional renal mass, with loss of length ipsilateral to a stenosis attributed to ischemic nephropathy. Split renal function studies using radionuclide renography can also measure kidney excretory function ipsilateral to a stenosis. Although each of these methods can help support the clinical assessment in a patient with RAS, none has proved consistent in identifying those who will benefit from revascularization.

New assays are being developed to identify functional lesions causing renovascular hypertension with or without ischemic nephropathy. These include plasma brain natriuretic peptide levels, more commonly used as a marker of heart muscle stretch in congestive heart failure. Brain natriuretic peptide is also produced in the kidney and upregulated in response to renal hypoperfusion from critical RAS. In patients with normal heart function, plasma brain natriuretic peptide levels correlate with functional outcomes following the treatment of RAS.[147] Functional MRI has also been introduced as a method of defining altered excretory function in patients with RAS.[148] Whether these results will be validated in larger prospective studies of patients managed medically and with reconstruction remains to be seen. Two functional assays that have been studied extensively and remain in use in some centers today are captopril renography and selective renal vein renins.

Radionuclide Renography

Split renal function can be measured by quantifying the uptake and excretion of specific radiolabeled molecules such as technetium 99m–labeled mercaptoacetyltriglycine. Abnormal uptake and excretion may localize to a kidney beyond the site of RAS, suggesting a causal relationship to loss of function. However, normal renography is common in patients with hypertension who benefit from revascularization. Moreover, in azotemic patients with unilateral RAS, abnormal renography is as common in the contralateral kidney as in the one with the stenosis.[149]

ACEI renography, more commonly known as captopril renography, combines renography with pharmacologic manipulation of the renin-angiotensin system. Inhibiting angiotensin II production or receptor activation in a patient with RAS suspected of having renovascular hypertension can unmask intrinsic renal compensation specific to a functionally active lesion. With critical unilateral renal artery disease, the affected kidney compensates for reduced glomerular perfusion by constricting efferent arterioles to maintain filtration pressure. This vasoconstriction is caused by angiotensin II, which is excessive in kidneys in which hypoperfusion has led to excess renin production (see earlier under "Pathophysiology of Renovascular Hypertension"). Thus, when renography is repeated after the pharmacologic blockade of ACE, a decline in excretory function is seen due to loss of compensatory efferent arteriolar constriction as angiotensin II levels fall. If the contralateral kidney is normal, renography may show enhanced excretory function after ACE inhibition, as efferent arteriolar dilatation leads to increased glomerular filtration in the setting of normal perfusion.[150]

The goal of ACEI renography is to detect renovascular hypertension, not RAS per se. Prior studies have shown that this assay is inferior to standard imaging (e.g., duplex, CTA, MRA) for screening hypertensive patients for RAS.[151,152] Conversely, in patients with documented RAS, ACEI renography is good at distinguishing between renovascular and essential hypertension and thus at identifying patients likely to benefit from revascularization.[153] A normal study effectively excludes renovascular hypertension, but the assay is less accurate in patients with severe azotemia or those with small, poorly functioning kidneys. In these settings, an abnormal baseline renogram is less likely to change significantly with ACE inhibition, causing false-negative or indeterminate results.[154] However, Erbsloh-Moller and associates studied 20 azotemic patients with serum creatinine levels greater than 1.8 mg/dL (159 μmol/L) and reported that the sensitivity and specificity of a positive study exceeded 90% in predicting blood pressure response to revascularization.[155]

Renal Vein Renin Assays

Selective renal vein renin assays have been used to document the functional significance of known RAS, but the invasive nature of the procedure makes it inappropriate as a screening tool. Major limitations include the extent of patient preparation and standardization required to derive meaningful results. Short-term changes in renin production can be introduced by a number of variables. It is our practice to stop medications likely to alter renin release (i.e., all except diuretics and calcium channel blockers) 5 days before the assay, if possible, and to initiate a low-sodium diet. Oral furosemide (40 mg) is given the evening before the assay, and the following morning, patients are placed flat and supine on strict bed rest 4 hours before and during the assay. Separate catheters are inserted percutaneously into the left and right renal veins and the inferior vena cava (IVC). A reference "systemic" sample is drawn from the IVC, followed by simultaneous aspiration of the right and left renal vein catheters, repeated two or three times at 5-minute intervals. A final systemic IVC sample is collected, and the procedure is concluded.

Reporting standards vary, but a ratio (or index) of renal vein renin to systemic renin is most useful for defining patients likely to benefit from reconstruction.[156] A ratio of 1.5 or greater is considered positive, linking ipsilateral RAS to excess renin production.[157] The ratio for the opposite uninvolved kidney may be low because of compensatory renin suppression.[158] Lateralizing renins are generally informative, predicting a blood pressure benefit from revascularization, but they may not predict cure.[159] In contrast, failure to lateralize has a low negative predictive value for benefit from revascularization.

In our experience, the renin ratio's ability to predict response to reconstruction in patients with ischemic nephropathy is unclear.[160] A renin ratio is also of limited value in patients with severe bilateral renal artery disease or disease limited to a solitary kidney.[159] Accessory renal artery lesions present a challenge as well, because superselective catheterization of accompanying vein branches is generally impractical. In these circumstances, the decision for intervention is based on the severity of stenosis, hypertension, and renal insufficiency.

TREATMENT SELECTION

A diagnosis of RAS carries a high risk for cardiovascular morbidity in low-risk populations[161] and for progression to occlusion (Table 141-4),[53-58,162-166] dialysis dependence, and death in selected high-risk populations.[53-56,58-61] Despite these compelling statistics, few level I data exist to help guide the management of affected patients. In fact, no prospective randomized trial comparing renal artery reconstruction (open or endovascular) to medical management has shown improved survival, increased freedom from dialysis, or reduction in adverse cardiovascular events with intervention. Certainly, no data are available to justify "prophylactic" repair in patients with asymptomatic RAS. For these reasons, patients with renal artery disease should be approached conservatively, and interventions should be offered only to those with severe disease who fail medical management. When an intervention is deemed appropriate, the approach should be tailored to local expertise and guided by local results until further guidelines are forthcoming from clinical trials.

At Wake Forest University School of Medicine, it is our practice to reserve intervention for patients with severe, poorly controlled hypertension; those with hypertension associated with ischemic nephropathy; and those with severe hypertension contributing to cardiopulmonary or neurologic embarrassment. Given the relatively inferior durability of endovascular reconstructions (see Chapter 143: Renovascular Disease: Endovascular Treatment), we advocate open surgery for good-risk patients with bilateral disease, patients undergoing concomitant aortic reconstruction for aneurysms or occlusive disease, patients with disease in multiple ipsilateral renal arteries or branch vessels, and children with congenital lesions.

Table 141-4 Natural History of Renal Artery Stenosis: Selected Series

Series	Year	Number of Patients	Imaging Modality	Anatomic Progression (%)	Occlusion (%)
Wollenweber et al.[162]	1968	1109	Angiography	59	—
Meaney et al.[163]	1968	39	Angiography	36	4
Dean et al.[53]	1981	41	Angiography	17	12
Schreiber et al.[54]	1984	85	Angiography	44	11
Tollefson and Ernst[55]	1991	48	Angiography	53	9
Zierler et al.[57]	1994	80	Duplex ultrasonography	8	3
Zierler et al.[164]	1996	76	Duplex ultrasonography	20	7
Crowley et al.[56]	1998	1178	Angiography	11	0.3
Caps et al.[58]	1998	170	Duplex ultrasonography	31	3
Webster et al.[165]	1998	30	Angiography	13	0
Van Jaarsveld and Krijnen[166]	2000	50	Angiography	20	5

From Corriere MA, Edwards MS, Hansen KJ. Abdominal aortic aneurysm and renal artery stenosis. *Vasc Dis Management*. 2008;5:16.

Medical Management of Renovascular Disease

Risk Factor Modification

All patients with atherosclerotic RAS should be treated aggressively to control hypertension and risk factors associated with the progression of atherosclerosis or renal insufficiency. As for other forms of peripheral vascular disease (e.g., carotid artery and peripheral arterial disease), even patients with silent lesions are at increased risk for adverse cardiovascular events.[161] Patients should be monitored regularly for changes in blood pressure and renal function, and kidney length should be measured yearly using noninvasive imaging. In centers experienced at renal duplex imaging, progression of stenosis can be assessed annually in both the index vessel and nonstenotic renal arteries, given the high incidence of new lesions developing over time.[167]

Approaches to lowering atherosclerosis risk factors are covered in detail in Chapters 25 through 29 (Atherosclerotic Risk Factors: General Considerations; Atherosclerotic Risk Factors: Smoking; Atherosclerotic Risk Factors: Diabetes; Atherosclerotic Risk Factors: Hyperlipidemia; and Atherosclerotic Risk Factors: Hypertension), but in general, patients with renovascular disease should be encouraged to stop smoking, consume a heart-healthy diet, and exercise regularly. Diabetes control is essential because this disease not only contributes to atherosclerosis progression but also directly damages the renal parenchyma, causing loss of excretory function. Control of hypertension and hyperlipidemia is also essential.

Blood Pressure Control

Given that the renin-angiotensin system mediates hypertension and end-organ dysfunction in renal artery disease, ACEIs and ARBs are first-line therapy to control blood pressure in patients with RAS.[79] Many patients require more than one class of medication to achieve a normal blood pressure, and occasionally, ACEIs and ARBs are not tolerated or precipitate acute renal failure in the setting of severe bilateral RAS. A number of other classes of antihypertensives can be added or substituted, based on specific patient factors and cost considerations. Choices include diuretics, beta blockers, calcium channel blockers, and others (see Chapter 29: Atherosclerotic Risk Factors: Hypertension). Diuretics, particularly loop and thiazide diuretics, can be particularly useful in patients with bilateral RAS, in whom fluid retention from aldosterone excess is most pronounced. Spironolactone should be used cautiously in the setting of impaired renal function or in combination with ACEIs to avoid hyperkalemia.[168]

Target systolic and diastolic pressures are generally the same as for patients with essential hypertension. Blood pressure should not be maintained at an elevated level because of theoretical concerns that an abrupt normalization of pressure could precipitate renal failure. In the rare patient with marginally compensated renal function, control of hypertension

may be associated with a rise in serum creatinine. If the renal dysfunction is attributed to ischemic nephropathy rather than intrinsic renal disease, this may indicate a medical failure, and if it is progressive, consideration should be given to revascularization.

Hyperlipidemia

Lipid lowering, specifically with the use of statins, is beneficial in patients with atherosclerotic renovascular disease. Cheung and colleagues found that the risk for progression of RAS decreased by 72% in 79 patients treated with a statin.[169] Statins have also been associated with regression of atherosclerotic RAS.[169,170] The role of statins in reducing the risk of coronary, carotid, and lower extremity atherosclerotic disease has been clearly established (see Chapter 25: Atherosclerotic Risk Factors: General Considerations and Chapter 28: Atherosclerotic Risk Factors: Hyperlipidemia).[171-173]

Surgical Management

Open Repair

Fewer open surgeries are being performed for symptomatic RAS, but not only because of the availability of less invasive alternatives. Refinements in patient selection have emerged from the analysis of outcomes after open repair[52,174] and from a better understanding of the natural history of RAS treated medically.[61] Prospective case series by our group and others have helped shift the focus of surgery in renovascular disease away from blood pressure control and toward the preservation of excretory renal function.[52,160] As outlined at the beginning of this section, we currently perform open renal repair primarily in hypertensive patients with ischemic nephropathy. We also consider repair in good-risk patients with bilateral RAS or branch vessel disease who have failed medical treatment of their hypertension.

Open repair of atherosclerotic RAS is very durable. We have reported clinical patency rates as high as 97% at a mean follow-up of 3 years[52] and 96% in patients followed for 2 years postoperatively by serial duplex imaging.[175] Blood pressure responses have varied in the literature, but in our experience, 85% of patients are improved or cured following complete repair.[52,176] Operative renal artery repair carries a risk of significant morbidity, ranging from 7% to 24% in experienced hands, and mortality varies from 2.6% to 8%.[52,160,176-181] In our experience, operative mortality approaches 1% for unilateral reconstruction and 3% for bilateral repair,[52] but this increases significantly when renal repair is combined with aortic reconstruction.[182]

In an analysis of 500 patients undergoing open repair of atherosclerotic RAS, the severity of preexisting hypertension correlated with improved late dialysis-free survival. Curiously, survival correlated poorly with the effect of surgery on hypertension.[52] In contrast, increased survival was associated with improved or stabilized excretory renal function in the early postoperative period.[52,167] Patients who appeared to benefit most included those with a recent rapid decline in glomerular filtration rate who also had severe bilateral RAS or occlusion and severe hypertension.[52,160,176,181,183] To illustrate this point, among 45 ESRD patients who met these criteria, 70% were permanently removed from dialysis after open renal repair.[52]

Nephrectomy is largely of historical significance among patients with renovascular disease, given the effectiveness and diversity of available antihypertensive medications. In our practice, we take an aggressive approach toward the revascularization of kidneys with greater than 15% excretory function on radionuclide renography, even when the ipsilateral renal artery is completely occluded; this has also been described by others.[184] Nephrectomy is reserved for the small subset of patients with poorly functioning kidneys and unreconstructable arteries who have failed medical management of hypertension. Other select populations in which the risks of open repair are justified are discussed in detail in Chapter 142: Renovascular Disease: Open Surgical Treatment.

Endovascular Repair

The development of angioplasty balloons and vascular stents has led to an exponential increase in the number of RAS patients treated by endovascular means. An increasingly common scenario is the incidental finding of RAS on aortography performed during the evaluation for unrelated vascular pathology, and in some centers, "drive-by" renal artery interventions have become common, irrespective of preprocedural evidence of functional renal artery disease. As noted earlier, however, randomized trials comparing endovascular therapy and medical management of RAS fail to show a clear benefit in mortality, dialysis dependence, or adverse cardiovascular events with intervention.[185-187] Blood pressure control is roughly equivalent to that reported for surgery, but in our view, a major limitation is the failure of angioplasty or stenting to consistently improve or stabilize excretory renal function.[188] Although the reasons for this are likely multifactorial, some investigators suggest that atheroemboli released during the procedure cause permanent kidney damage,[146] adding to the more obvious effects of nephrotoxic contrast agents and high rates of restenosis.

Angioplasty alone is effective at treating nonostial stenoses of the main renal artery caused by atherosclerosis or medial fibroplasia, whereas stenting has proved superior in the management of ostial lesions. Van de Ven and coworkers randomized patients with ostial RAS to either angioplasty or primary stenting and reported superior technical success and primary patency with stenting.[189] Stenting was also associated with a lower rate of restenosis at 6 months (14% versus 48%); complications and responses of hypertension and renal function were similar. Because the majority of RAS patients have ostial lesions, rates of stenting have increased dramatically.

Restenosis remains the primary mode of failure following technically successful endovascular reconstruction for RAS.

A meta-analysis from Leertouwer and associates found the average rate of restenosis after angioplasty and primary stenting in RAS to be 26% and 17%, respectively.[190] At present, a few risk factors have been identified that predict which patients are likely to develop restenosis after renal artery reconstruction. These include small renal artery caliber, incomplete revascularization (i.e., residual stenosis after endovascular treatment), and a history of prior restenosis at the site being treated. The pathogenesis is the same as in other sites, with intimal hyperplasia being the primary culprit in stented vessels (see Chapter 5: Intimal Hyperplasia).

Given the limitations of endovascular reconstruction and the lack of a clear benefit over medical management, we generally reserve renal artery angioplasty and stenting for high-risk patients with severe hypertension who have failed medical management or shown progressive loss of renal function attributable to ischemic nephropathy. For a complete discussion of the endovascular management of renovascular disease, see Chapter 143: Renovascular Disease: Endovascular Treatment.

SELECTED KEY REFERENCES

Balk EM, Raman G. *Comparative Effectiveness of Management Strategies for Renal Artery Stenosis: 2007 Update.* Comparative Effectiveness Review No. 5 Update. (Prepared by Tufts-New England Medical Center under Contract No. 290-02-0022.) Rockville, MD: Agency for Healthcare Research and Quality; November 2007.
Articulates the limitations of the methods of treating RAS, challenging the evidence for stenting.

Cherr GS, Hansen KJ, Craven TE, Edwards MS, Ligush J Jr, Levy PJ, Freedman BI, Dean RH. Surgical management of atherosclerotic renovascular disease. *J Vasc Surg.* 2002;35:236-245.
Approach to and results of open surgery for renal artery disease from a high-volume center.

Crowley JJ, Santos RM, Peter RH, Puma JA, Schwab SJ, Phillips HR, Stack RS, Conlon PJ. Progression of renal artery stenosis in patients undergoing cardiac catheterization. *Am Heart J.* 1998;136: 913-918.
Defines the anatomic progression of angiographically defined RAS.

Edwards MS, Craven TE, Burke GL, Dean RH, Hansen KJ. Renovascular disease and the risk of adverse coronary events in the elderly: a prospective, population-based study. *Arch Intern Med.* 2005;165: 207-213.
Defines the strong link between renal artery and coronary disease.

Hansen KJ, Edwards MS, Craven TE, Cherr GS, Jackson SA, Appel RG, Burke GL, Dean RH. Prevalence of renovascular disease in the elderly: a population-based study. *J Vasc Surg.* 2002;36:443-451.
Defines the scope of renal artery disease in a free-living population.

Leertouwer TC, Gussenhoven EJ, Bosch JL, van Jaarsveld BC, van Dijk LC, Deinum J, Man In 't Veld AJ. Stent placement for renal arterial stenosis: where do we stand? A meta-analysis. *Radiology.* 2000;216: 78-85.
Summarizes the effects of stenting on blood pressure, renal function, and rates of restenosis.

Mailloux LU, Napolitano B, Bellucci AG, Vernace M, Wilkes BM, Mossey RT. Renal vascular disease causing end-stage renal disease, incidence, clinical correlates, and outcomes: a 20-year clinical experience. *Am J Kidney Dis.* 1994;24:622-629.
Estimates the contribution of renal artery disease to progression to dialysis.

Marone LK, Clouse WD, Dorer DJ, Brewster DC, Lamuraglia GM, Watkins MT, Kwolek CJ, Cambria RP. Preservation of renal function with surgical revascularization in patients with atherosclerotic renovascular disease. *J Vasc Surg.* 2004;39:322-329.
Approach to and results of open surgery for renal artery disease from a high-volume center.

Nordmann AJ, Logan AG. Balloon angioplasty versus medical therapy for hypertensive patients with renal artery obstruction. *Cochrane Database Syst Rev.* 2003;CD002944.
Cochrane review of renal angioplasty.

REFERENCES

The reference list can be found on the companion Expert Consult Web site at *www.expertconsult.com.*

CHAPTER 142

Renovascular Disease: Open Surgical Treatment

Christopher J. Godshall and Kimberley J. Hansen

■ HISTORICAL BACKGROUND

Renovascular Hypertension

In 1937, Goldblatt demonstrated that constriction of the renal artery produced atrophy of the kidney and hypertension in a canine model.[1] As a clinical pathologist, Goldblatt noticed that extensive vascular disease was often present at autopsy in patients with hypertension and was frequently severe in the renal arteries. His innovative work defined a causal relationship between renovascular disease and hypertension. Goldblatt's elegant experiments introduced a new era by showing that renal artery stenosis could produce a form of hypertension correctable by nephrectomy.

In 1938, Leadbetter and Burkland described the first successful treatment of renovascular hypertension.[2] These authors removed an ischemic ectopic kidney in a 5-year-old child, resulting in cure of severe hypertension. This procedure and associated photomicrographs represented the first clinical documentation of a renovascular origin of hypertension. Thereafter, nephrectomy was introduced as a treatment for patients with hypertension and a small kidney demonstrated by intravenous pyelogram. Smith in 1956 reviewed 575 such cases and found that nephrectomy cured only one quarter of patients with hypertension.[3] This finding led him to suggest that nephrectomy be limited to strictly urologic indications.

Freeman in 1954 performed a transaortic bilateral renal artery thromboendarterectomy in a hypertensive patient, which resulted in the first cure of hypertension by renal revascularization.[4] The subsequent widespread use of aortography was accompanied by enthusiastic support for renal revascularization and the description of its blood pressure benefits.[5-8] However, by 1960 it became apparent that renal revascularization in all hypertensive patients with renal artery stenosis resulted in blood pressure benefits in less than half. These clinical results fostered general pessimism regarding the value of operative renal artery reconstruction for the treatment of hypertension.

The introduction of functional tests of physiologic significance ushered in the contemporary operative management of renovascular hypertension. Studies by Howard and Connor,[9] Stamey and associates,[10] Page and Helmes,[11] and others[12-14] identified the role of the renin-angiotensin-aldosterone system in blood pressure control and described the pathophysiology of renovascular hypertension. With accurate assays for plasma renin activity, physicians could accurately predict which renal artery lesion produced hypertension.

Renovascular Renal Insufficiency (Ischemic Nephropathy)

Until the early 1960s, the management of renovascular disease focused solely on hypertension. In 1962, Morris and associates reported on eight azotemic patients with global renal ischemia who had improved blood pressure and renal function after renal revascularization.[15] Dean and coworkers,[16,17] Libertino and Zinman,[18] and Novick and associates[19] found a similar beneficial functional response when bilateral renal artery lesions were corrected in azotemic patients.

Although it is well accepted that renovascular hypertension is caused by increased activity of the renin-angiotensin-aldosterone system in the acute state and sustained through adaptive cardiovascular changes in the chronic state, the pathophysiology of ischemic nephropathy is incompletely understood. The earliest clinical reports suggested a glomerular filtration failure based on decreased perfusion pressure within the kidney.[20] However, the cellular and subcellular basis for ischemic nephropathy is poorly defined. Similar to renovascular hypertension, the renin-angiotensin system likely contributes to ischemic nephropathy through its paracrine effects, with intrarenal angiotensin peptides affecting arteriolar tone.[21] Angiotensin peptides have also been shown to promote tubular interstitial injury in the presence of renal artery stenosis.[22] This observation is supported by an increase in interstitial platelet-derived growth factor-β, which is associated with increased extracellular matrix and interstitial fibrosis.[23-26] In addition to the potentially reversible contributors to excretory renal insufficiency, an atherosclerotic renovascular lesion may serve as a source of atheroemboli.[27] Distinguishing potentially reversible ischemic nephropathy from irreversible renal parenchymal disease has enormous clinical relevance because the recovery of renal function after open surgical repair of renal lesions associated with ischemic nephropathy is the single strongest predictor of dialysis-free survival.[28,29]

■ INDICATIONS FOR SURGICAL REPAIR

The rationale for the treatment of renovascular disease by any method is to improve event-free survival. In the past, hypertension response was the primary outcome measure for the vast majority of interventions for renovascular disease. However, experience in 500 consecutive patients treated for atherosclerotic renovascular disease demonstrated a lack of association between improved hypertension response and cardiovascular morbidity or mortality.[29] Moreover, when all patients with atherosclerotic disease were considered, increased severity of preoperative hypertension was associated with improved dialysis-free survival. This observation suggests a possible shift in the paradigm for the evaluation and management of atherosclerotic renal artery disease. In this altered paradigm, severe hypertension could be viewed as a key preoperative characteristic favoring clinical benefit, and renal function after operation could be considered the key response. Examination of patients with atherosclerotic renal artery disease, as well as those with ischemic nephropathy, has demonstrated that an early incremental increase in excretory renal function is the primary determinant of dialysis-free survival.[28,29]

Unfortunately, once renovascular disease is identified in combination with severe hypertension or excretory renal insufficiency, discriminating predictors of blood pressure and renal function response are lacking. Use of a renal vein systemic renin index has been proposed to predict hypertension cure.[30] Although results from selective renal vein renin assays are useful to guide management in selected cases of unilateral renal artery disease, whether considered as an index or a ratio value, lateralizing renin assays can predict blood pressure benefit but not blood pressure cure.[31] Moreover, renal function response in patients with ischemic nephropathy is uncertain after renal artery intervention.[28] Studies have also described a significant correlation between parameters derived from segmental renal artery Doppler spectral analysis (i.e., resistive index) and response to intervention, as well as progression to dialysis dependence.[32,33] However, despite extensive experience with renal duplex sonography, we have not been able to reproduce these results for open operative management of renal artery disease.[34] Rather, in our clinical experience with more than 700 patients with atherosclerotic renal artery disease undergoing open operative repair, factors favoring postoperative recovery of renal function include severe preoperative hypertension, bilateral or global atherosclerotic renovascular disease due to high-grade (>90%) stenosis or renal artery occlusion, and rapidly deteriorating renal function before surgery.[28,31,35-37] When each of these favorable features was present in patients considered permanently dialysis dependent, 70% of those who underwent open operative repair were permanently removed from dialysis.[28,38] Given the relationship of renal function to both quality and quantity of life, predictors of functional response after renal artery intervention should be a primary focus for future investigation.

Until recently, there were no prospective, population-based reports that defined the natural history of renovascular disease. Available information was extrapolated from angiographic case series and ultrasound examinations from retrospective reviews or from prospective studies of select hypertensive patients.[19,35,39-47] The quality of these studies and their interpretation have varied widely. Most commonly, authors have considered anatomic progression of atherosclerotic renovascular disease a certainty, with an inevitable decline in kidney size and kidney function. This view has been cited to support intervention for renal artery disease whenever it is discovered, even in the absence of hypertension or renal insufficiency.

Based on a recent prospective, population-based study of progression of atherosclerotic renovascular disease in the elderly,[48] we do not favor prophylactic intervention for asymptomatic renovascular disease. In a longitudinal cohort study that included 119 Cardiovascular Health Study participants with 235 kidneys, no kidney progressed to occlusion over a mean follow-up of 8.5 years. In the participants with mild to moderate hypertension, progression to hemodynamically significant renal artery stenosis was observed in only 4%, an annualized rate of 0.5% per year.[48]

Although we do not recommend prophylactic renal revascularization in the absence of hypertension or renal insufficiency, empirical renal artery repair is appropriate in select circumstances. The term *empirical repair* implies that hypertension, excretory renal dysfunction, or both are present, although a causal relationship between the renal artery lesion and these clinical sequelae has not been established. Open repair of a unilateral renal artery lesion may be appropriate as an independent procedure or combined with aortic repair in the presence of negative functional studies or when such studies have not been performed, if hypertension remains severe and uncontrollable despite maximal drug therapy, and if the patient is relatively young and lacks significant risk factors for operation. In these circumstances, correction of a renal artery lesion may be justified; however, because the probability of blood pressure benefit is lower in such patients, morbidity from the open procedure must also be predictably low.[49] Empirical unilateral repair in individuals with ischemic nephropathy has been associated with functional improvement in only a small proportion of patients, and it cannot be recommended as a clinically proven therapeutic intervention.[28,38]

When a patient has bilateral renal artery stenoses and hypertension, the decision to perform empirical open renal artery repair alone or in combination with correction of aortic disease is based on the severity of hypertension and the severity of the renal artery lesions. When disease consists of severe stenosis of one renal artery and only mild to moderate contralateral disease, the patient is treated as if he or she has a unilateral lesion. If both renal artery lesions are moderately severe (60% to 80% diameter-reducing stenosis), revascularization is undertaken only if associated hypertension (and renal insufficiency) is severe. In contrast, if both renal artery lesions are severe (>80% stenosis) and the patient has severe hypertension, bilateral simultaneous renal revascularization is performed, especially when excretory renal insufficiency is present. However, because the degree of azotemia usually parallels the severity of hypertension, a patient who presents with severe excretory renal insufficiency but only mild hypertension usually has concomitant renal parenchymal disease. Characteristically, renovascular disease contributing to severe azotemia or dialysis dependence is associated with severe hypertension and severe bilateral stenoses or renal artery occlusions.[29]

Section 18 Renal and Mesenteric Disease

OPEN OPERATIVE STRATEGY

As noted earlier, the presence of hypertension is considered a prerequisite for renal artery intervention, and functional studies are generally used to guide the management of unilateral lesions. Empirical renal artery repair is performed without functional studies when hypertension is severe, renal artery disease is bilateral, or the patient has ischemic nephropathy.[29,31,50] Prophylactic renal artery repair in the absence of hypertension, whether as an isolated procedure or combined with aortic reconstruction, is not recommended. During surgical reconstruction, all hemodynamically significant renal artery disease is corrected in a single operation, with the exception of disease requiring bilateral ex vivo reconstructions, which are staged. Having observed beneficial blood pressure and renal function responses regardless of kidney size or histologic pattern on renal biopsy, we reserve nephrectomy for unreconstructable renal artery disease in a nonfunctioning kidney (i.e., <10% function by renography).[28,35,42] Direct aortorenal reconstructions are preferred over indirect methods because concomitant disease of the celiac axis is present in 40% to 50% of patients, and bilateral repair is required in half.[28,31] Failed renal artery repair is also associated with a significantly increased risk of dialysis dependence.[50] To minimize these failures, intraoperative duplex is used to evaluate the technical results of surgical repair.[51]

MANAGEMENT OPTIONS

There are no prospective randomized trials comparing best medical management, open operative repair, and percutaneous intervention with or without endoluminal stenting. Consequently, the question of optimal management of renovascular disease contributing to hypertension or renal insufficiency is unanswerable. In the absence of level I data, advocates of each form of management cite selected clinical data to support their particular view.

Without doubt, percutaneous intervention for renovascular disease has increased dramatically over the past decade. Answers regarding the contribution of percutaneous management to event-free survival and freedom from dialysis dependence must await the completion of several large, prospective, randomized trials that are currently under way.[52] Our experience with percutaneous management as a substitute for open operative repair has demonstrated only modest hypertension and renal function response.[53] Consequently, we continue to advocate open operative repair for select patients. These include children with hypoplastic lesions[54,55] and adults with dysplastic lesions other than medial fibroplasia or with medial fibroplasia involving branch and segmental renal arteries when complicated by renal artery aneurysm.[56] We advocate open operative repair for atherosclerotic renovascular disease in good-risk patients younger than 65 years who demonstrate

global renal ischemia manifested by critical stenosis and renal artery occlusion, especially when severe hypertension is associated with excretory renal insufficiency and rapidly deteriorating excretory function.[28,29,38] Selection criteria for the repair of renal artery aneurysms are discussed in Chapter 145 (Renovascular Disease: Aneurysms and Arteriovenous Fistulae), but we continue to favor open operative repair as opposed to coiling, stenting, or stent-grafting these lesions.[56]

A variety of open operative techniques have been used to correct renal artery disease, but three basic operations are most frequently used: aortorenal bypass, renal artery thromboendarterectomy, and renal artery reimplantation. No single approach achieves optimal repair of all types of renovascular lesions in all patients. Aortorenal bypass using saphenous vein is probably the most versatile technique; however, transaortic thromboendarterectomy is especially useful for orificial atherosclerosis involving multiple renal arteries. Occasionally the renal artery demonstrates sufficient redundancy to allow for reimplantation, which is probably the simplest technique and is particularly appropriate for hypoplastic renal artery lesions in children.[54,55]

PREFERRED SURGICAL TECHNIQUES
Preoperative Preparation

Antihypertensive medications are reduced during the preoperative period to the minimum necessary for blood pressure control. Frequently, patients who normally require large doses of multiple medications for hypertension management have reduced requirements while hospitalized on bed rest. If continued therapy is required, vasodilators (e.g., amlodipine) and selective β-adrenergic blocking agents (e.g., atenolol, metoprolol) are useful. There are few adverse effects on hemodynamics when these agents are combined with general anesthesia. If an adult's diastolic blood pressure exceeds 120 mm Hg, surgery should be postponed until the pressure is brought under control. In this case, a combination of intravenous nicardipine and esmolol is administered in an intensive care setting with continuous intra-arterial blood pressure monitoring. Similarly, if the patient has significant heart disease, the pulmonary artery wedge pressure and cardiac index are monitored to maintain optimal cardiac performance before and after operation.

Certain measures are used in almost all open renal artery operations. Mannitol is administered intravenously in 12.5-g doses early in the operation during aortic and renal artery dissection. Repeated doses are administered before and after periods of renal ischemia, up to a total dose of 1 g/kg body weight. Just before renal artery cross-clamping, heparin 100 units/kg body weight is given intravenously, and systemic anticoagulation is verified by activated clotting time. Unless required for hemostasis, protamine is not routinely administered for the reversal of heparin at the completion of the operation.

Mobilization and Dissection

Midline Exposure

A midline abdominal incision is made when bilateral renal artery repair or combined aortorenal repair is planned. The patient is positioned supine, with the umbilicus at the level of the table break, and the operating table is flexed 10 to 15 degrees. To obtain full exposure of the upper abdominal aorta and renal branches, it is important that the last 1 or 2 cm of the proximal incision is made coursing to one side of the xiphoid (Fig. 142-1). Some type of fixed mechanical retraction is also advantageous, particularly when combined aortorenal procedures are required. Otherwise, extended flank and subcostal incisions are reserved for the correction of unilateral branch renal artery lesions or splanchnorenal bypass.

When the midline xiphoid-to-pubis incision is used, the posterior peritoneum overlying the aorta is incised longitu-

dinally, and the duodenum is mobilized at the ligament of Treitz. During this maneuver it is important to identify and spare visceral collaterals that course at this level. Finally, the duodenum is reflected to the patient's right to expose the left renal vein. By extending the posterior peritoneal incision to the left along the inferior border of the pancreas, an avascular plane posterior to the pancreas can be entered (see Fig. 142-1) to expose the entire left renal hilum. This exposure is especially important when there are distal renal artery lesions to be managed (Fig. 142-2A). The left renal artery lies posterior to the left renal vein. In some cases, the vein can be retracted cephalad to expose the artery; in other cases, caudad retraction of the vein provides better access. Usually, the gonadal and adrenal veins, which enter the left renal vein, must be ligated and divided to facilitate exposure of the distal artery. Frequently a lumbar vein enters the posterior wall of the left renal vein, and it can be easily injured unless special care is taken (Fig. 142-2B). The proximal portion of the right renal artery can be exposed through the base of the mesentery by retracting the left renal vein cephalad and the vena cava to the patient's right (Fig. 142-2C). However, the distal portion of the right renal artery is best exposed by mobilizing the duodenum and right colon medially; the right

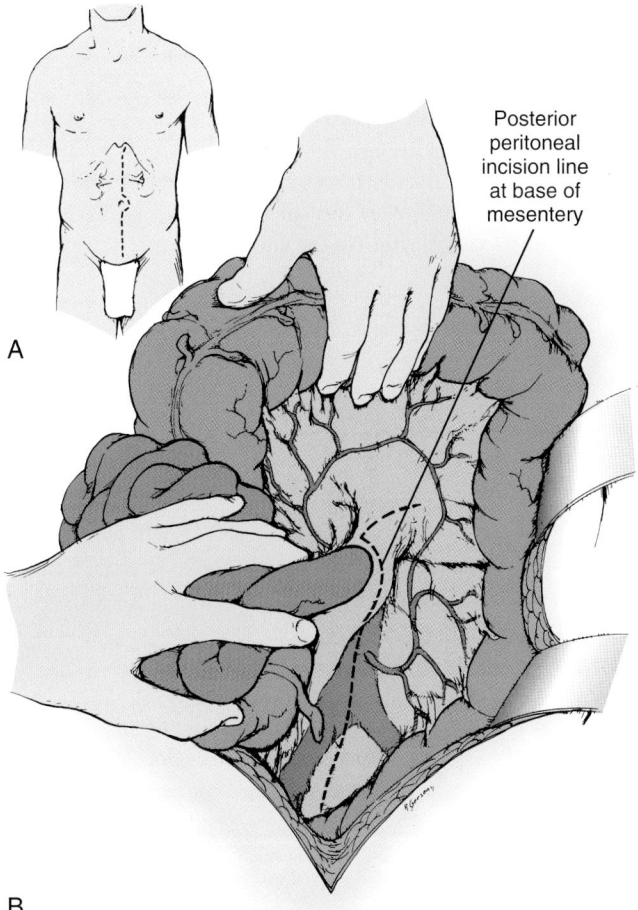

Figure 142-1 A and **B,** Exposure of the aorta and left renal hilum through the base of the mesentery. Extension of the posterior peritoneal incision to the left, along the inferior border of the pancreas, provides entry to an avascular plane posterior to the pancreas. This allows excellent exposure of the entire left renal vein and hilum as well as the proximal right renal artery. *(From Benjamin ME, Dean RH. Techniques in renal artery reconstruction: Part I. Ann Vasc Surg. 1996;10:306-314.)*

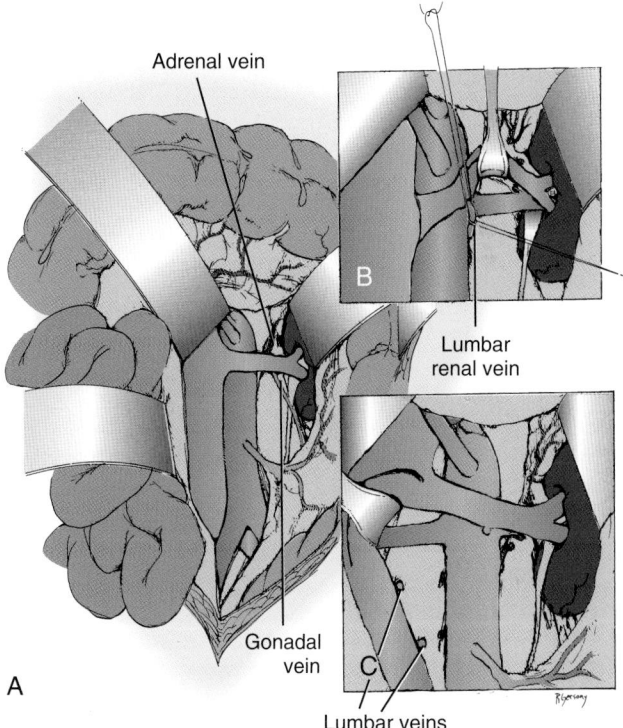

Figure 142-2 A, Exposure of the proximal right renal artery through the base of the mesentery. **B,** Mobilization of the left renal vein by ligating and dividing the adrenal, gonadal, and lumbar renal veins allows exposure of the entire left renal artery to the hilum. **C,** On occasion, lumbar veins are ligated and divided to allow retraction of the vena cava to the right. Often, adequate exposure of the proximal renal artery disease can be obtained without this maneuver. *(From Benjamin ME, Dean RH. Techniques in renal artery reconstruction: Part I. Ann Vasc Surg. 1996;10:306-314.)*

renal vein is mobilized and usually retracted cephalad to expose the artery.

Flank Exposure

When a branch renal artery repair is required, especially when an ex vivo technique is used or when the supraceliac aorta is the inflow source for aortorenal bypass, an extended flank incision is useful. With the ipsilateral flank elevated, the incision extends from the opposite semilunar line into the flank, bisecting the abdominal wall between the costal margin and iliac crest. A left or right visceral mobilization allows access to the renal vasculature and the aortic crus. The crus can be divided, and an extrapleural dissection of the descending thoracic aorta can provide access to the T9-T10 thoracic aorta for proximal control and anastomosis.[57,58]

Whether right or left branch renal artery exposure is required, the key is creation of the correct dissection plane between the mesentery anteriorly and Gerota's fascia posteriorly. The renal vein is identified first and mobilized from the caval origin to the renal hilum. On the right, small venous branches at the junction with the cava require ligation. The adrenal, gonadal, and lumbar branches on the left can be sacrificed to facilitate exposure.

Branch renal artery exposure on the right is achieved by colonic and duodenal mobilization. First, the hepatic flexure is mobilized at the peritoneal reflection (Fig. 142-3). With the

right colon retracted medially and inferiorly, a Kocher maneuver mobilizes the duodenum and pancreatic head to expose the inferior vena cava and right renal vein (Fig. 142-4). Typically, the right renal artery is located just inferior to the accompanying vein, which can be retracted superiorly to provide the best exposure. Although accessory vessels may arise from the aorta or iliac vessels at any level, all arterial branches coursing anterior to the vena cava should be considered accessory right renal branches and carefully preserved (Fig. 142-5).

When bilateral renal artery lesions are to be corrected, and when correction of a right renal artery lesion or bilateral lesions is combined with aortic reconstruction, these exposure techniques can be modified. Extended aortic exposure can be provided by mobilizing the base of the small bowel mesentery to allow complete evisceration of the entire small bowel, right colon, and transverse colon. For this extended exposure, the posterior peritoneal incision begins with division of the ligament of Treitz and proceeds along the base of the mesentery to the cecum and then along the lateral gutter to the foramen of Winslow (Fig. 142-6A). The inferior border of the pancreas is fully mobilized to enter a retropancreatic plane, thereby exposing the aorta to a point above the superior mesenteric artery. Through this modified exposure, simultaneous bilateral renal endarterectomies, aortorenal grafting, or renal artery attachment to the aortic graft can be performed with complete visualization of the entire aorta and its branches.

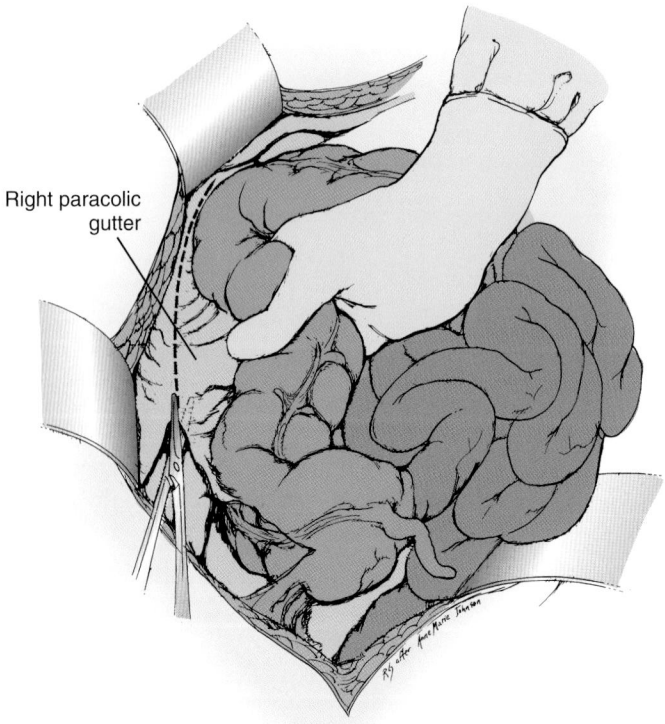

Figure 142-3 Exposure of the distal right renal artery begins with mobilization of the ascending colon and hepatic flexure. *(From Benjamin ME, Dean RH. Techniques in renal artery reconstruction: Part I. Ann Vasc Surg. 1996;10:306-314.)*

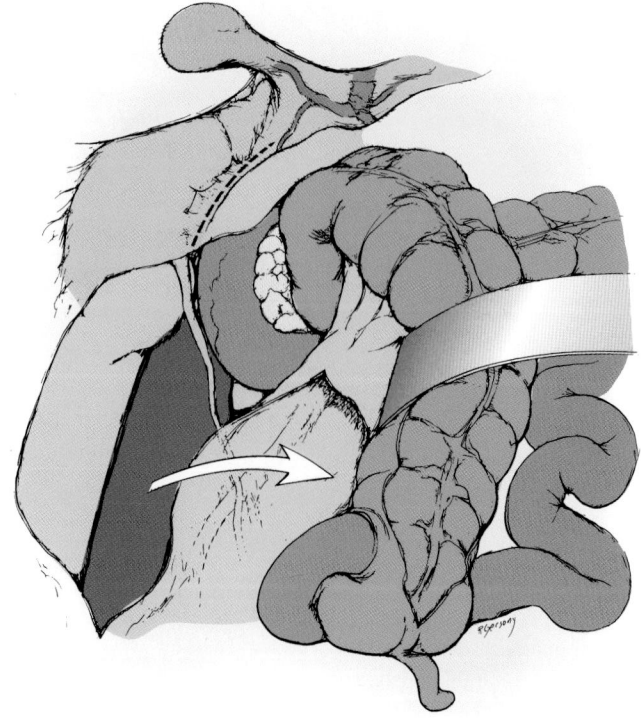

Figure 142-4 With the right colon mobilized medially, a Kocher maneuver exposes the right renal hilum. *(From Benjamin ME, Dean RH. Techniques in renal artery reconstruction: Part I. Ann Vasc Surg. 1996;10:306-314.)*

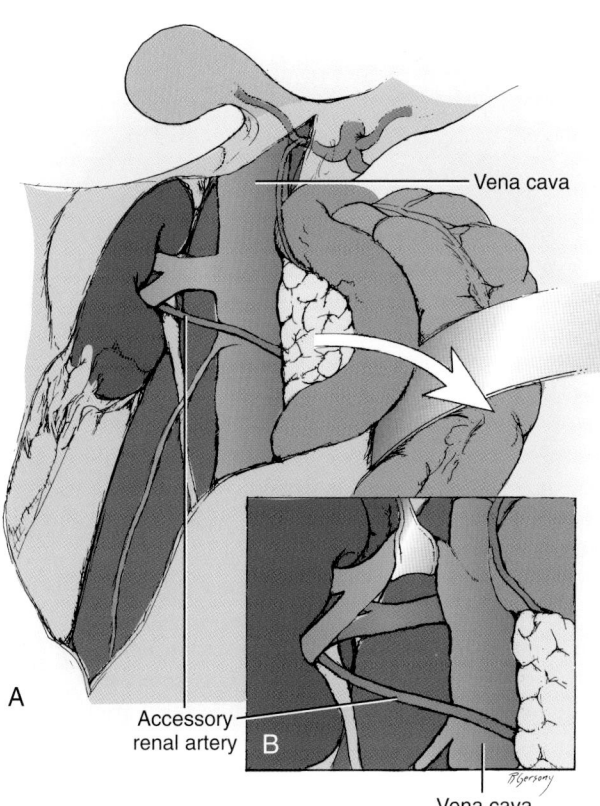

Figure 142-5 A, Arteries encountered anterior to the vena cava should be considered accessory renal arteries and preserved. **B,** The right renal vein is typically mobilized superiorly for exposure of the distal right renal artery. *(From Benjamin ME, Dean RH. Techniques in renal artery reconstruction: Part I.* Ann Vasc Surg. *1996;10:306-314.)*

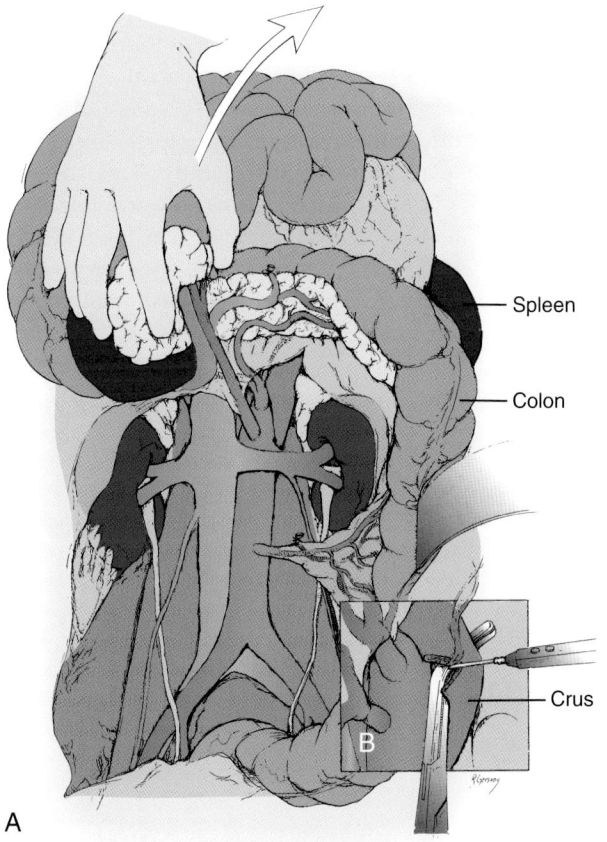

Figure 142-6 A, For bilateral renal artery reconstruction combined with aortic repair, extended exposure can be obtained by mobilizing the cecum and ascending colon. The entire small bowel and right colon are then mobilized to the right upper quadrant and retracted superiorly. **B,** Partial division of the diaphragmatic crus exposes the origin of the mesenteric vessels. *(From Benjamin ME, Dean RH. Techniques in renal artery reconstruction: Part I.* Ann Vasc Surg. *1996;10:306-314.)*

Another useful technique for suprarenal aortic exposure is to partially divide both diaphragmatic crura as they pass behind the renal arteries to their paravertebral attachment. This partial division of the crus allows the aorta above the superior mesenteric artery to be easily visualized and mobilized for suprarenal cross-clamping (Fig. 142-6B).

Aortorenal Bypass

Three types of materials are available for aortorenal bypass: autologous saphenous vein, autologous hypogastric artery, and synthetic graft. The decision regarding which graft to use depends on a number of factors. In most instances, we prefer the saphenous vein for older adults. However, if the vein is small (<4 mm in diameter) or sclerotic, the hypogastric artery or a synthetic graft may be preferable. In addition, vein enlargement can be anticipated in virtually all young adults. Although structural immaturity has been cited as the cause of enlargement and aneurysmal degeneration when the saphenous vein is used for renal artery reconstruction in children,[55] it should be remembered that the normal renal blood flow in the young resembles an arteriovenous fistula with continuous forward flow. This fact alone may account for vein enlargement in a young patient with normal renovascular resistance.

In lieu of vein, a 6-mm, thin-walled polytetrafluoroethylene (PTFE) graft is satisfactory when the distal renal artery is of sufficient caliber (>4 mm). Hypogastric artery autograft is preferred for aortorenal bypass in children when reimplantation is not possible.[54,55,59,60]

Occasionally, end-to-side distal anastomoses are used to include polar renal arteries. In this instance, end-to-side anastomosis between the polar renal artery and the graft is performed after the proximal aortic anastomosis. After the end-to-side anastomosis is completed, the most distal main renal artery reconstruction is made in an end-to-end fashion (Fig. 142-7).

In creating the distal anastomosis, the length of the arteriotomy should be at least three times the diameter of the smaller conduit to guard against late suture-line stenosis. An anastomosis is created with 7-0 monofilament polypropylene continuous sutures using loupe magnification. Just before completing the renal artery anastomosis, the occluding clamps are temporarily removed to flush air and small debris. When renal artery bypass can be accomplished without cold perfusion preservation, the aortic anastomosis is performed first, removing an ellipse of the anterolateral aortic wall. This is especially important when the aorta is relatively inflexible owing to atherosclerotic involvement. A 5.2-mm aortic punch applied two or three times creates a satisfactory ellipse in most instances. In combined aortorenal reconstructions, the proximal anastomosis is performed first using polyester aortic graft, with a thin-walled 6-mm PTFE graft attached in an end-to-side fashion for renal artery bypass. The distal aortic reconstruction is completed, and the distal renal anastomosis is created as the last step.

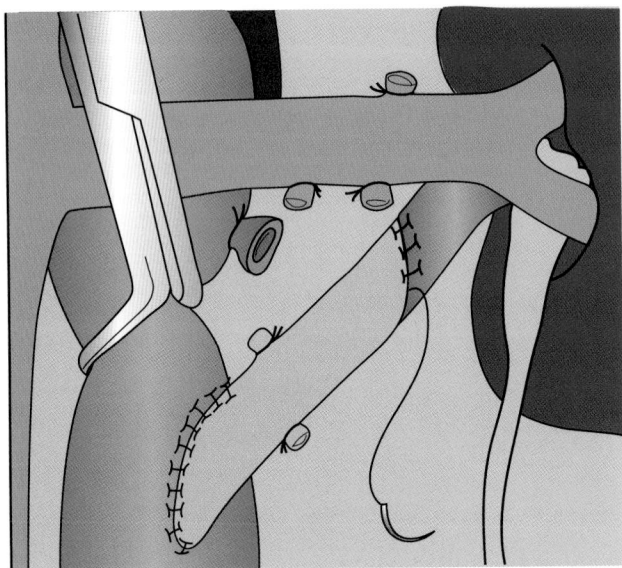

Figure 142-7 Technique for end-to-end aortorenal bypass grafting. The length of arteriotomy is at least three times the diameter of the artery to prevent recurrent anastomotic stenosis. For the anastomosis, 6-0 or 7-0 monofilament polypropylene sutures are placed in continuous fashion with loupe magnification. If the apex sutures are placed too deeply or with excess advancement, stenosis can be created, posing a risk of late graft thrombosis. *(From Benjamin ME, Dean RH. Techniques in renal artery reconstruction: Part I. Ann Vasc Surg. 1996;10:306-314.)*

Renal Artery Thromboendarterectomy

In cases of ostial atherosclerosis of both renal artery origins, simultaneous bilateral endarterectomy may be the most suitable procedure. Endarterectomy can be either transaortic or transrenal. In the transrenal procedure, the aortotomy is made transversely and carried across the aorta and into the renal artery to a point beyond the visible atheromatous disease (Fig. 142-8A and B). With this method, the distal endarterectomy can be assessed and tacked down with mattress sutures under direct vision if necessary. Following completion of the endarterectomy, the arteriotomy is closed. In most patients, this closure is performed with a synthetic PTFE or polyester patch to ensure that the proximal renal artery is widely patent (Fig. 142-8C).

For the majority of renal endarterectomies, the transaortic technique is used.[29] The transaortic method is particularly applicable in patients with multiple renal arteries that demonstrate ostial disease. In this case, all visible and palpable renal artery atheroma should end within 1 cm of its aortic origin. Transaortic endarterectomy is performed through a longitudinal aortotomy, with sleeve endarterectomy of the aorta and eversion endarterectomy of the renal arteries (Fig. 142-9). The aortotomy is closed with 5-0 polypropylene as a continuous suture. When combined aortic replacement is planned, the transaortic endarterectomy is performed through the transected aorta. Whether a longitudinal aortotomy is used or an endarterectomy is performed through the divided aorta, it is important to mobilize the renal arteries extensively to allow eversion of the artery into the aorta. This allows the distal endpoint to be completed under direct vision. When the aortic atheroma is divided flush with the adventitia using scissors, tacking sutures are usually not required.

As is the case for thromboendarterectomy at any site, the procedure is contraindicated by the presence of preaneurysmal degeneration of the aorta and the presence of transmural calcification. The latter condition can be subtle and may be missed unless the aorta is carefully and gently palpated. Aortic

Figure 142-8 A, Exposure of the juxtarenal aorta and renal arteries in preparation for transrenal endarterectomy. **B,** When the renal atheroma extends more than 1 cm from the aortic origin, a transverse aortotomy is used, with care taken to carry the incision out onto the renal artery to a point beyond the stenosis. **C,** After completion of the endarterectomy, the arteriotomy is usually closed with a prosthetic patch angioplasty beyond the endarterectomy endpoint. *(From Benjamin ME, Dean RH. Techniques in renal artery reconstruction: Part I. Ann Vasc Surg. 1996;10:306-314.)*

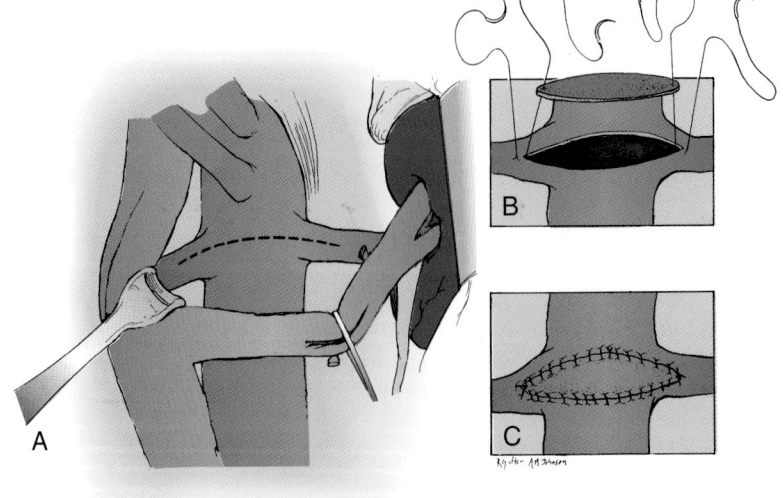

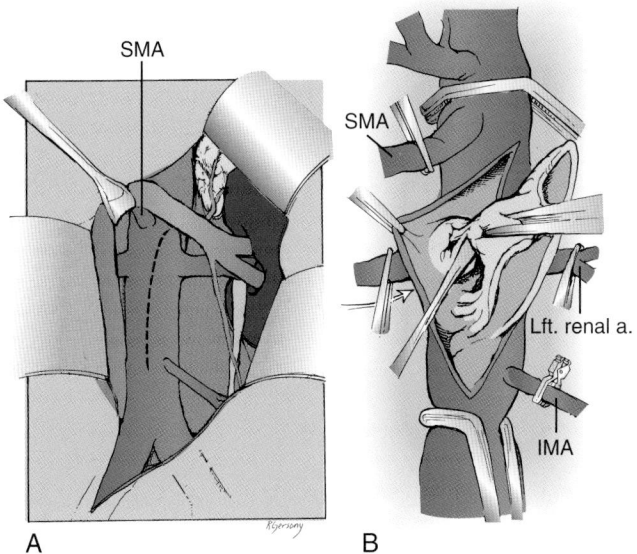

Figure 142-9 Exposure for a longitudinal transaortic endarterectomy is obtained by the standard transperitoneal approach. The duodenum is mobilized at the ligament of Treitz in standard fashion, or for more complete exposure, the ascending colon and small bowel are mobilized. **A,** *Dotted line* shows the location of the aortotomy. **B,** The plaque is transected sharply, and with eversion of the renal arteries, the atherosclerotic plaque is removed from each renal ostium. The aortotomy is typically closed with a running 4-0 or 5-0 polypropylene suture. IMA, inferior mesenteric artery; SMA, superior mesenteric artery. *(From Benjamin ME, Dean RH. Techniques in renal artery reconstruction: Part I.* Ann Vasc Surg. *1996;10:306-314.)*

atheroma complicated by transmural calcification resembles fine-grade sandpaper on palpation. Endarterectomy in this setting is characterized by numerous sites of punctate bleeding after blood flow is restored.

Renal Artery Reimplantation

After the renal artery has been dissected from the surrounding retroperitoneal tissue, the vessel may be somewhat redundant. When the renal artery stenosis is orificial and there is sufficient vessel length, the renal artery can be transected and reimplanted into the aorta at a slightly lower level. The renal artery must be spatulated, and a portion of the aortic wall must be removed as in renal artery bypass (Fig. 142-10). This technique has particular application in children with orificial lesions, where the need for graft material is avoided[54,55]; however, it is suitable for selected atherosclerotic lesions as well.[61] Unlike prosthetic bypass performed during combined aortic replacement in adults, the renal artery–to–graft anastomosis is usually performed immediately after the proximal aortic anastomosis, followed by distal aortic reconstruction.

■ OTHER SURGICAL TECHNIQUES

Splanchnorenal Bypass

Splanchnorenal bypass and other indirect revascularization procedures have received increased attention as alternative methods of renal revascularization.[62] We do not believe that these procedures demonstrate the same durability as direct aortorenal reconstructions, but they are useful in a highly select group of high-risk patients.[29,63]

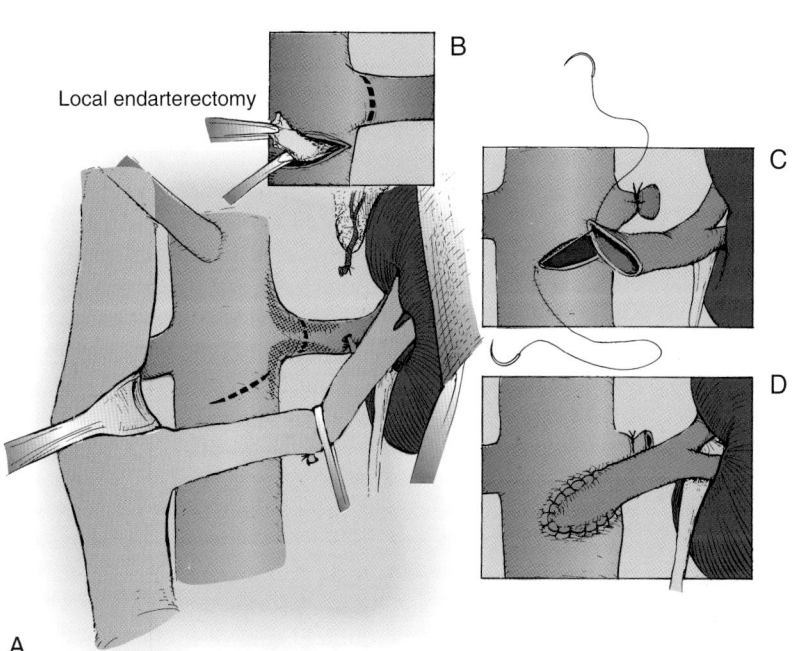

Figure 142-10 When the renal artery is redundant, the vessel can be reimplanted at a lower level (**A**). Local endarterectomy (**B**) allows placement of the monofilament suture in the aortic wall (**C**). The native renal artery is then ligated, proximally spatulated, and reimplanted (**D**). *(From Benjamin ME, Dean RH. Techniques in renal artery reconstruction: Part II.* Ann Vasc Surg. *1996;10: 409-414.)*

Hepatorenal Bypass

A right subcostal incision is used to perform hepatorenal bypass.[62] The lesser omentum is incised to expose the hepatic artery both proximal and distal to the gastroduodenal artery (Fig. 142-11). Next, the descending duodenum is mobilized by a Kocher maneuver, the inferior vena cava is identified, the right renal vein is identified, and the right renal artery is exposed either immediately cephalic or caudal to the renal vein.

A great saphenous vein graft is usually used to construct the bypass. The hepatic artery anastomosis of the vein graft can be placed at the site of the amputated stump of the gastroduodenal artery; however, this vessel may serve as an important collateral for intestinal perfusion. Therefore, the proximal anastomosis is usually made to the common hepatic artery, routing the graft through the foramen of Winslow. The renal artery is then transected and brought anterior to the vena cava for anastomosis end to end to the graft (Fig. 142-12).

Splenorenal Bypass

Splenorenal bypass can be performed through a midline or a left subcostal incision.[62,63] The posterior pancreas is mobilized by reflecting the inferior border cephalad. A retropancreatic plane is developed, and the splenic artery is mobilized from

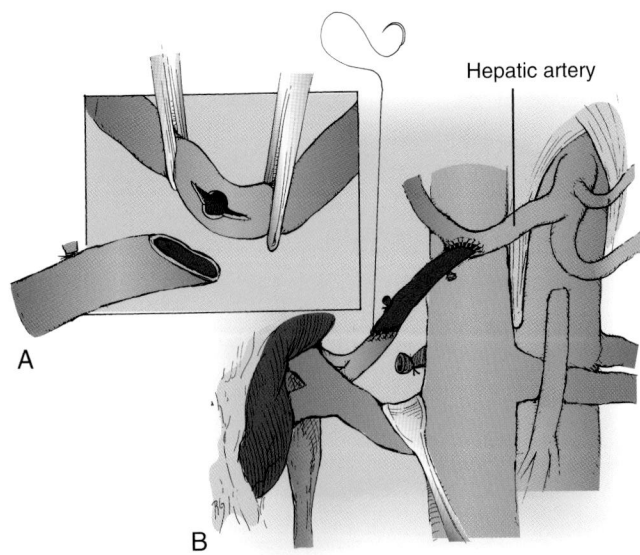

Figure 142-12 The reconstruction is completed using a saphenous vein interposition graft between the side of the hepatic artery (**A**) and the distal end of the transected right renal artery anterior to the vena cava (**B**). *(From Benjamin ME, Dean RH. Techniques in renal artery reconstruction: Part II. Ann Vasc Surg. 1996;10:409-414.)*

the left gastroepiploic artery to the level of its branches. The left renal artery is exposed cephalic to the left renal vein after division of the adrenal vein. After the splenic artery has been mobilized, it may be divided proximally, spatulated, and anastomosed end to end to the transected renal artery (Fig. 142-13). Alternatively, a segment of saphenous vein may be used as a bypass.

Branch Renal Artery Reconstruction

Owing to the widespread use of percutaneous techniques for main renal artery pathologies, a significant proportion of open renal artery reconstructions requires branch exposure and branch reconstruction. These procedures may require a complex repair, culminating in prolonged renal ischemia. Available data suggest that when more than 40 minutes of warm renal ischemia is required for renal revascularization, measures to protect renal function should be instituted.[64-67]

Several pharmacologic therapies have been promoted to provide protection during renal ischemia; however, to date, no therapy has surpassed hypothermia for protection when renal ischemia exceeds 1 hour.[66,68-71] Surface cooling and hypothermic perfusion have been proposed, but their advantages are not well defined. Renal tolerance to ischemia is related in part to the duration of ischemia, the adequacy of collateral circulation, and the method of vascular control. Unprotected warm renal ischemia is best tolerated when only the renal artery is controlled.[66] Control of both renal artery and vein is associated with greater dysfunction than isolated arterial control, as is intermittent control with repeated renal perfusion.

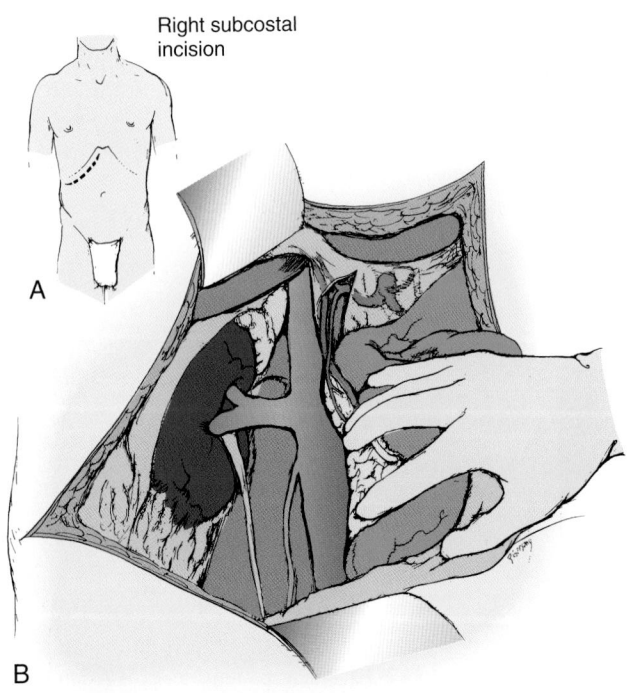

Figure 142-11 A and **B,** In preparation for extra-anatomic reconstruction of the right renal artery, the common hepatic artery and proximal gastroduodenal artery are exposed in the hepatoduodenal ligament. Exposure is typically through an extended right flank skin incision (**A**). *(From Benjamin ME, Dean RH. Techniques in renal artery reconstruction: Part II. Ann Vasc Surg. 1996;10:409-414.)*

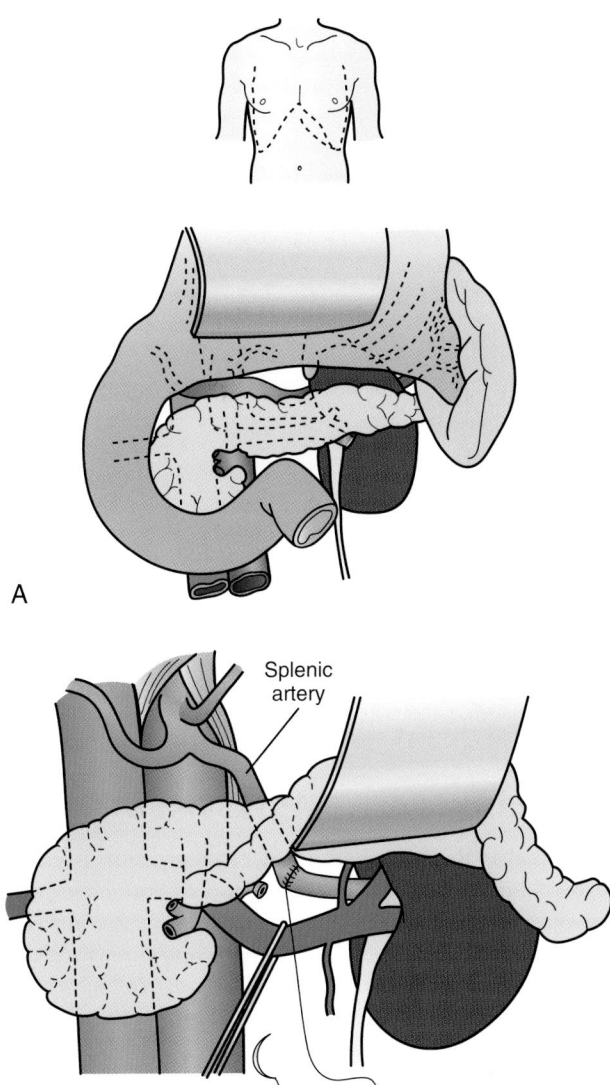

A

B

Splenic artery

Figure 142-13 Exposure of the left renal hilum in preparation for splenorenal bypass (**A**). The pancreas has been mobilized along its inferior margin and retracted superiorly (**B**). The transected splenic artery may be anastomosed end to end to the transected left renal artery. A splenectomy is not routinely performed. *(From Benjamin ME, Dean RH. Techniques in renal artery reconstruction: Part II.* Ann Vasc Surg. *1996;10:409-414.)*

Numerous methods for renal cooling and hypothermia during branch renal artery repair have been described, but our preference is intermittent hypothermic perfusion with topical ice slush. Otherwise, several steps are common to every branch renal artery reconstruction. To promote renal cortical perfusion, small doses of intravenous mannitol are administered throughout renal artery exposure and reperfusion.[71-73] Before the division of the renal artery, intravenous heparin (100 units/kg) is administered and monitored as described earlier.

Hypothermia appears to be more important than the composition of the perfusate; however, we prefer a perfusate with an intracellular composition of electrolytes. This composition theoretically limits ion exchange and intracellular volume

shifts that contribute to organelle dysfunction associated with the decreased activity of membrane-bound sodium-potassium adenosine triphosphatase.[66,74,75] Regardless of whether there is division and reattachment of the renal vein, branch renal artery repairs using cold perfusion preservation are made in an orthotopic fashion, with the kidney returned to the renal fossa rather than autotransplanted into the pelvis.

Several exposures for hypothermic branch renal artery reconstructions are available. When isolated branch renal artery repair is performed with orthotopic replacement, an extended flank incision is made from the lower rib margin and carried to the posterior axillary line as described earlier. This method is our preferred approach for ex vivo reconstruction. The ureter is mobilized to the pelvic brim with a large amount of periureteric soft tissue. An elastic sling is placed around the ureter to control ureteric collaterals and prevent subsequent renal rewarming.

Gerota's fascia is opened with a cruciate incision; the kidney is completely mobilized, and the renal vessels are divided (Fig. 142-14). The kidney is placed in a plastic sling and perfused with a chilled renal preservation solution. Continuous perfusion during the period of total renal ischemia is possible with perfusion pump systems and may be superior for prolonged renal preservation.[76] However, simple intermittent flushing with a chilled preservation solution provides equal protection during the shorter periods (2 to 3 hours) required for ex vivo dissection and branch renal artery reconstructions. For this technique, we refrigerate the preservative overnight, add additional components (Table 142-1) immediately before use to make up 1 L of solution, and hang the chilled (5°C to 10°C) solution at a height of at least 2 m. We flush 300 to 500 mL of solution through the kidney immediately after its removal from the renal fossa, until the venous effluent is clear and all segments of the kidney have blanched. As each anastomosis is completed, the kidney is perfused with an additional 100 to 200 mL of chilled solution. In addition to maintaining satisfactory hypothermia, periodic perfusion demonstrates suture-line leaks that can be repaired before reimplantation. With this technique, renal core temperatures are maintained at 10°C or below throughout the period of reconstruction.

Even though it is an accepted method after ex vivo reconstruction, autotransplantation to the iliac fossa is unnecessary for most ex vivo reconstructions. This technique was adopted from renal transplantation. Reduction in the magnitude of the operative exposure, ability to manually palpate the transplanted kidney, and ease of removal when treatment of rejection fails are all practical reasons for placing the transplanted kidney in the recipient's iliac fossa. However, none of these advantages applies to patients requiring autogenous ex vivo reconstruction. Because many ex vivo procedures are performed in relatively young patients, the durability of the operation must be measured in terms of decades. For this reason, attachment of the kidney to the iliac arterial system within or below sites susceptible to subsequent atherosclerosis subjects the repaired vessels to disease that may threaten their long-term patency. Moreover, subsequent management of

Section 18 **Renal and Mesenteric Disease**

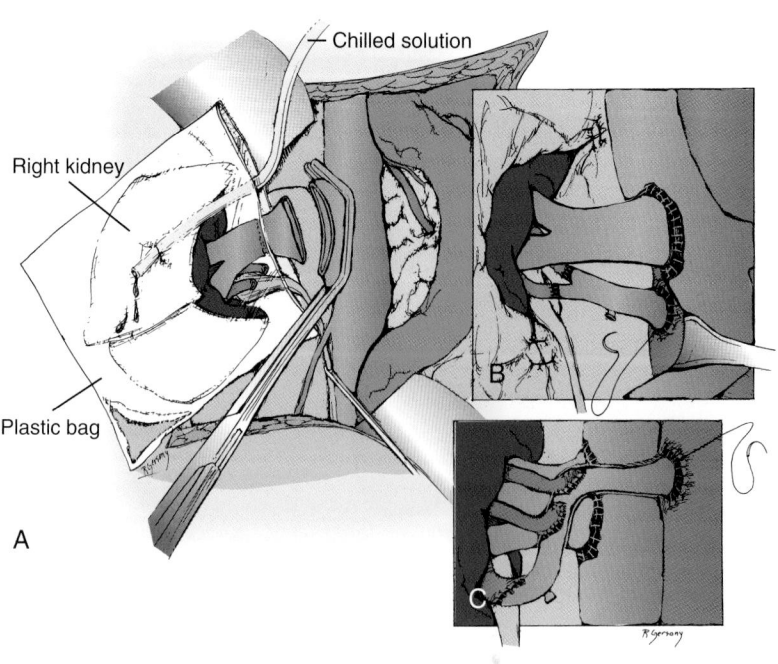

Figure 142-14 An ellipse of the vena cava containing the renal vein origin is excised by placement of a large partially occluding clamp (**A**). After ex vivo branch repair, the renal vein can be reattached without risk of anastomotic stricture (**B**). The kidney is returned to its native bed after ex vivo repair. Gerota's fascia is reapproximated to provide stability to the repaired kidney. Arterial reconstruction can be accomplished via end-to-end anastomoses after syndactylizing the distal branch or combined with end-to-side anastomoses (**C**). *(From Benjamin ME, Dean RH. Techniques in renal artery reconstruction: Part II. Ann Vasc Surg. 1996;10:409-414.)*

Table 142-1 Solution for Cold Perfusion Preservation of the Kidney

Composition	
Component	**Amount (g/L)**
K₂HPO₄	7.4
KH₂PO₄	2.04
KCl	1.12
NaHCO₃	0.84

Ionic Concentration	
Electrolyte	**Concentration (mEq/L)**
Potassium	115
Sodium	10
Phosphate (HPO₄⁻)	85
Phosphate (H₂PO₄⁻)	15
Chloride	15
Bicarbonate	10

Additives at Time of Use to 930 mL of Solution
70 mL 50% dextrose; 2000 units sodium heparin

Electrolyte solution for kidney preservation supplied by Travenol Labs, Inc., Deerfield, IL

peripheral vascular disease may be complicated by the presence of the autotransplanted kidney. Finally, if the kidney is replaced in the renal fossa and the renal artery graft is properly attached to the aorta at a proximal infrarenal site, the result should equal that of the standard aortorenal bypass and carry a high probability of technical success and long-term durability.

INTRAOPERATIVE ASSESSMENT

Provided that the best method of reconstruction is chosen for renal artery repair, the short course and high blood flow rates characteristic of direct renal reconstruction favor their patency. Consequently, flawless technical repair plays a dominant role in determining postoperative success.[77-79] The negative impact of technical errors unrecognized at operation is implied by the fact that we have observed no late thromboses of renovascular reconstructions free of disease after 1 year.[80]

Angiography

Intraoperative assessment of most arterial reconstructions is made by angiography.[81,82] This method has serious limitations, however, when applied to upper aortic and branch aortic reconstruction. Angiography provides static images and evaluates the anatomy in only one projection.[83,84] In addition, arteriolar vasospasm in response to contrast injection may falsely suggest distal vascular occlusion. Finally, coexisting renal insufficiency is present in 75% of patients with atherosclerotic renovascular disease,[29] increasing the risk of postoperative contrast nephropathy.

Duplex Sonography

The risks and inherent limitations of completion angiography are not applicable to intraoperative duplex sonography.[51] Because the ultrasound probe can be placed immediately adjacent to the vascular repair, high carrying frequencies can be used to provide excellent B-scan detail sensitive to 1-mm defects. Once imaged, defects can be viewed in a multitude of

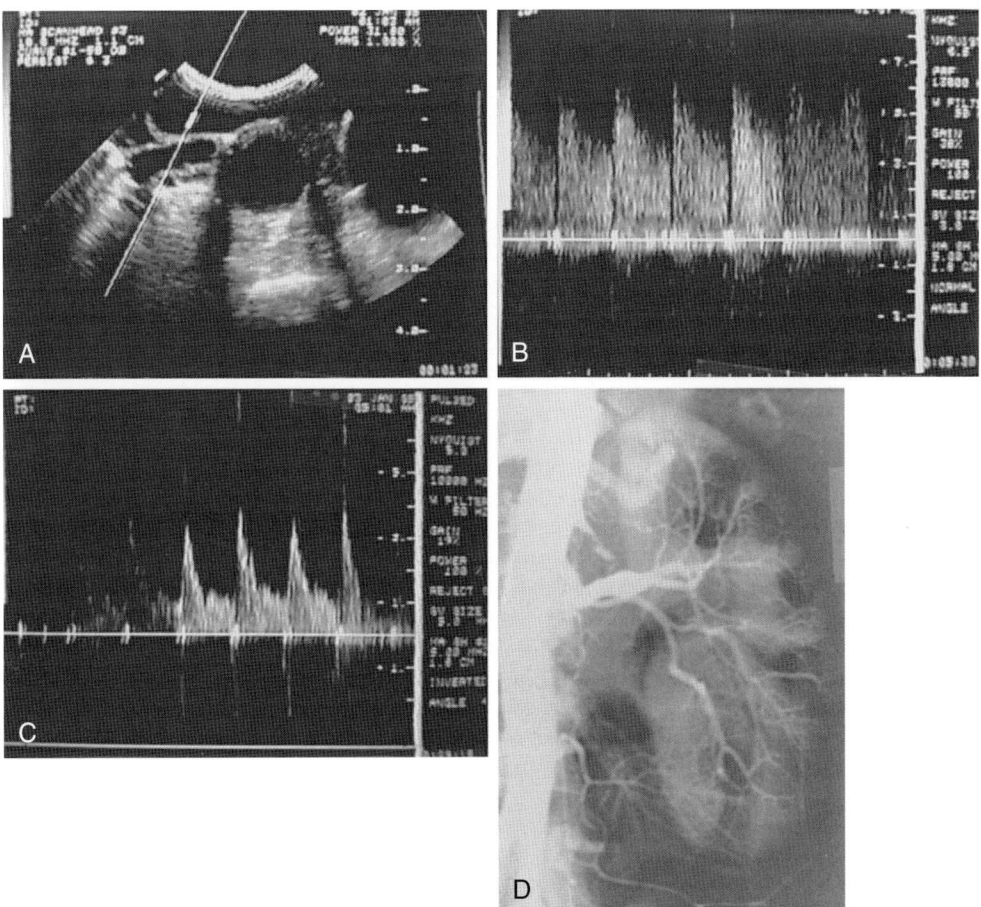

Figure 142-15 A, Sagittal image of a major B-scan defect. **B,** The intimal flap at the proximal anastomosis demonstrates a focal increase in renal artery peak systolic velocity (3.1 m/sec). **C,** After revision, peak systolic velocity is decreased (1.1 m/sec). **D,** Follow-up angiogram demonstrates a widely patent anastomosis. This patient was cured of hypertension. *(From Hansen KJ, O'Neil EA, Reavis SW, et al. Intraoperative duplex sonography during renal artery reconstruction. J Vasc Surg. 1991;14: 364-374.)*

projections during conditions of uninterrupted, pulsatile blood flow. In addition to providing excellent anatomic detail, important hemodynamic information is obtained from the spectral analysis of the Doppler-shifted signal proximal and distal to the imaged defect (Fig. 142-15).[51] Freedom from static projections, the absence of potentially nephrotoxic contrast material, and the hemodynamic data provided by Doppler spectral analysis make duplex sonography a useful intraoperative method to assess both renovascular and mesenteric repairs.

To realize these advantages of intraoperative duplex, close cooperation between the vascular surgeon and the vascular technologist is required for accurate intraoperative assessment. Although the surgeon is responsible for manipulating the probe head to acquire optimal B-scan images of the vascular repair at likely sites of technical error, proper power and time gain adjustments are best made by an experienced technologist. Close cooperation is likewise required to obtain complete pulse-Doppler sampling associated with abnormalities on B-scan images. While the surgeon images areas of interest at an optimal insonating angle, the technologist sets

the Doppler sample depth and volume and estimates blood flow velocities from the Doppler spectrum analyzer. Finally, the participation of vascular technologists during intraoperative assessment enhances their ability to obtain satisfactory surveillance duplex studies during follow-up. Intraoperative duplex assessment with the routine participation of a vascular technologist has yielded a scan time of 5 to 10 minutes and a 98% study completion rate.[43,51]

Currently, we use a 10/5.0 MHz compact linear array probe with Doppler color flow designed specifically for intraoperative assessment. The probe is placed within a sterile sheath with a latex tip containing sterile gel. After the operative field is flooded with warm saline, B-scan images are first obtained in a longitudinal projection. Care is taken to image the entire upper abdominal aorta and renal artery origins along the entire length of the repair. All defects seen in the longitudinal projection are imaged in the transverse projection to confirm their anatomic presence and estimate the associated luminal narrowing. Doppler samples are then obtained just proximal and distal to imaged lesions in the longitudinal projection, determining their potential contribution to flow disturbance. Our criteria for major B-scan defects associated with greater than 60% diameter-reducing stenosis or occlusion have been validated in a canine model of graded renal artery stenosis.[51] They also proved valid in a retrospective study when preoperative radiographic studies were compared with intraoperative duplex before surgical repair.[43]

With the application of these criteria in more than 800 open renal artery repairs, intraoperative duplex has been 86% sensitive and 100% specific for technical defects associated with postoperative stenosis and occlusion of direct aortorenal reconstruction. These anatomic results have been supported by the clinical response to open operation. Eighty-six percent of hypertensive patients have demonstrated a favorable hypertension response, and 63% of patients with renal insufficiency have demonstrated improved renal function after surgery.[28,29,38]

The designation of B-scan defects according to Doppler velocity criteria provides accurate information to guide decisions regarding intraoperative revision. However, there are special circumstances that deserve comment. Unlike surface duplex sonography, where the Doppler sample volume is large relative to the renal artery diameter, a small Doppler sample volume can be accurately positioned within the mid-center stream flow. Despite a small, centered Doppler sample, renal artery repairs demonstrate at least moderate spectral broadening. Transaortic endarterectomy gives the audible Doppler signal an oscillating characteristic, which is normal and not associated with anatomic defects. In addition, an infrequent intraoperative study demonstrates peak systolic velocities that exceed the criteria for critical stenosis when no anatomic defect exists. In these cases, the peak systolic velocities are uniformly elevated throughout the repair, there is no focal velocity change, and there is no distal turbulent waveform. This scenario is most commonly encountered immediately after renal artery reconstruction for nonatherosclerotic renovascular disease. Moreover, renovascular repair to a solitary kidney frequently demonstrates increased velocities throughout. Finally, an increase in peak systolic velocity is observed in transition from the main renal artery to the segmental renal vessels after branch renal artery repair; however, no distal turbulent waveform is observed.

In addition to these systolic spectral abnormalities, changes may be observed in the diastolic Doppler spectra in the absence of technical error. Abnormal diastolic spectra may be observed after revascularization of chronic renal ischemia. Reflecting increased vascular resistance in response to reperfusion, these spectra demonstrate abbreviated systolic flow, short systolic acceleration times, and decreased diastolic flow. This picture can mimic distal embolic catastrophe; however, it is distinguished from embolization by spectral changes observed after the intra-arterial administration of papaverine. In the case of functional vasospasm, the Doppler spectral signature characteristic for the renal artery usually appears within 5 minutes.

Finally, some B-scan abnormalities observed in conjunction with renal endarterectomy deserve comment. Infrequently, an irregular B-scan abnormality evolves during the performance of a completion scan. This B-scan finding may be associated with either increased or decreased (blunted) peak velocities but reflects the formation of intra-arterial thrombus. Unlike acute venous thrombus, which is usually echo lucent, acute arterial platelet aggregates are characterized by irregular echogenic material. Regardless of the associated velocity estimates, the endarterectomy site should be reopened and revised immediately. Last, a B-scan defect that is minor by velocity criteria may be revised based on its location and appearance. A mobile flap longer than 2 mm at the distal endpoint of an endarterectomy site is usually revised owing to its mere presence and the potential for dissection or thrombosis.

RESULTS OF OPEN OPERATIVE MANAGEMENT

Anatomic Results

Our center's cumulative open operative experience from January 1987 through June 2007 includes more than 1500 renal artery repairs in more than 900 patients. This consecutive operative experience is described in Table 142-2.[50] Over this 10.5-year period, 720 renovascular reconstructions and 57 primary nephrectomies were performed in 534 patients, applying the management philosophy and operative techniques described. Postoperative stenosis or thrombosis occurred in 3.3% of renal artery repairs, resulting in recurrent hypertension and declining renal function in 3.7% of patients at a mean follow-up of 36 months.[29] However, because complete anatomic failure of repair (i.e., thrombosis) may result in blood pressure benefit equivalent to nephrectomy, anatomic failure is potentially more common than the rate of recurrent hypertension or reoperation.[51] To examine the rate of anatomic failure, the results of 277 postoperative duplex studies in 128 consecutive patients were reviewed.[50] Over a mean follow-up of 22 months, 6 of 177 operative renal artery repairs (3.4%) stenosed, whereas 7 of 59 contralateral, unoperated arteries (11.9%) developed hemodynamically signifi-

Table 142-2 Summary of Operative Management (N = 543 Patients)

Operations		Number of Operations
Total renovascular reconstructions		720
Aortorenal bypass		445
Vein	288	
PTFE	127	
Dacron	19	
Hypogastric artery	11	
Ex vivo	33*	
Reimplantation		52
Thromboendarterectomy		223
Total nephrectomies		57
Total kidneys operated		777

*Total includes vein reconstructions.
PTFE, polytetrafluoroethylene.
From Hansen KJ, Deitch JS, Oskin TC, et al. Renal artery repair: consequence of operative failures. *Ann Surg.* 1998;227:678-690.

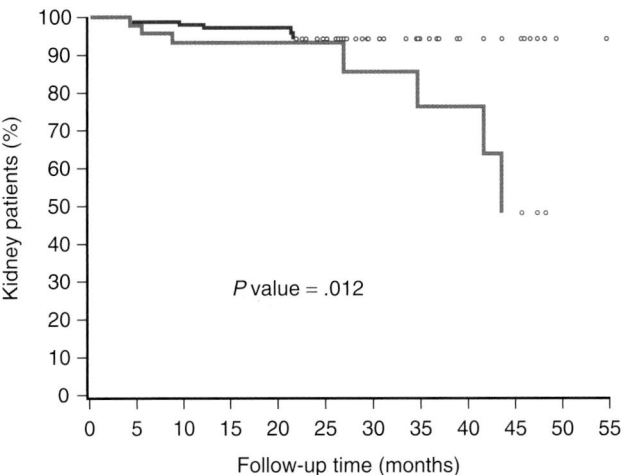

Figure 142-16 Estimated patency of direct aortorenal repair (*red line*) compared with the development of significant disease in unrepaired native renal arteries (*blue line*). (*From Hansen KJ, Deitch JS, Oskin TC, et al. Renal artery repair: consequence of operative failures.* Ann Surg. *1998;227:678-690.*)

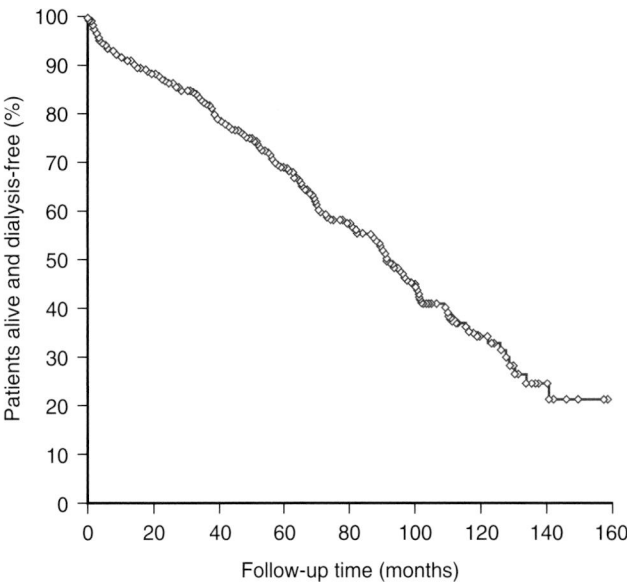

Figure 142-17 Product-limit estimates of time to death or dialysis for all patients with atherosclerotic renovascular disease (N = 477). (*From Cherr GS, Hansen KJ, Craven TE, et al. Surgical management of atherosclerotic renovascular disease.* J Vasc Surg. *2002;35:236-245.*)

cant disease. Overall, the incidence of follow-up stenosis was significantly greater for unoperated renal arteries than for operative repairs (*P* = .12) (Fig. 142-16). Compared with other reports describing the failure of renovascular repair,[79,85] these results support the techniques of operative management described here.

Operative Morbidity and Mortality

Perioperative morbidity accounting for prolonged hospital stay has been observed in 15% to 20% of patients.[28,29] Less than one half of 1% of patients with ischemic nephropathy have undergone operation that resulted in permanent dialysis dependence within 1 month of repair.[28] In these patients, serum creatinine and estimated glomerular filtration rate averaged 3.4 mg/dL (301 μmol/L) and 20.2 mL/min per 1.73m^2, respectively. Perioperative mortality, defined as in-hospital death or death within 30 days of surgery, varies with the patient and the complexity of reconstruction. Patient characteristics demonstrating a significant and independent association with perioperative mortality include advanced age and depressed left ventricular systolic function (i.e., ejection fraction <25%).[29] Overall, over the past 10 years, mortality following isolated renal artery repair has averaged 0.8%, compared with 1.6% for bilateral renal artery repair and 3.3% for bilateral repair combined with aortic repair for atherosclerosis. This compares with a 6.9% mortality rate when visceral, renal, and aortic repair are combined in one procedure.[49]

Hypertension Response

Based on criteria that consider both blood pressure measurements and medication requirements at least 1 month after operation, 85% of surgical survivors were cured or improved, and 15% were considered to have blood pressure failure after open reconstruction for atherosclerotic renal artery disease.[29]

When patients with atherosclerosis were stratified according to hypertension response and dialysis-free survival, only resolution of hypertension was significantly associated with improved estimated survival (Fig. 142-17).[29]

Renal Function Response

When all patients treated for atherosclerotic renovascular disease are considered, renal function improved significantly. When only patients with atherosclerotic renovascular disease and ischemic nephropathy—defined by a preoperative serum creatinine greater than 1.8 mg/dL (159 μmol/L)—are considered, 58% of patients demonstrated improved renal function 3 weeks after repair.[28,29] When 45 patients considered permanently dependent on dialysis were examined, 70% were permanently removed from dialysis dependence after open operation.[28,38] Although other authors consider that recovery of renal function is limited by elevated serum creatinine, when patients are selected based on severe hypertension and rapidly deteriorating renal function, the proportion of patients improved increases with increasing severity of preoperative renal dysfunction. This association between increased preoperative serum creatinine and improved postoperative renal function is independent and highly significant (*P* < .0001).[28,29]

Blood Function and Renal Function Benefit: Clinical Outcome

Progression to death or dialysis among patients with atherosclerotic renovascular disease has demonstrated significant associations with both preoperative parameters and postoperative blood pressure and renal function response. Preoperative factors that have demonstrated a significant association with death or dialysis include diabetes mellitus, severe aortic occlusive disease, and poor renal function.[29] Postoperatively, significant associations were noted for "blood pressure cured" compared with "blood pressure improved" or "blood pressure failed" (Fig. 142-18). Moreover, improved postoperative renal function demonstrated significant associations with increased dialysis-free survival compared with unchanged renal function. The relationship between each category of renal function response and dialysis-free survival demonstrated significant interaction with preoperative renal function. For patients whose renal function was unchanged, an increased risk for death or dialysis was observed in patients with poor preoperative renal function.[28] For patients whose renal func-

tion worsened, an increased risk for death or dialysis was significant among those with preoperative renal function at median values of estimated glomerular filtration rate or greater. These significant interactions are shown for predicted dialysis-free survival according to preoperative renal function response in Figure 142-19.

Consequence of Failed Open Renal Artery Repair

A review of our experience with 720 renal artery reconstructions and a mean follow-up of 27 months demonstrated anatomic failure of the reconstruction in 24 renal arteries among 20 patients.[50] Secondary management included 10 "redo" reconstructions and 10 nephrectomies for unreconstructable renovascular disease.

Secondary management was influenced by the type of primary repair, the presence of postoperative stenosis or thrombosis, and whether clinical failure occurred early or late after the primary operation. All three early failures required nephrectomy. Of the remaining 21 repairs that failed between 2 and 36 months, 9 were associated with thrombosis and 12 were secondary to stenosis. Thrombosis was significantly more common in the first postoperative year compared with recurrent stenosis (89% versus 10%); two early thromboses were ex vivo reconstructions. Two ex vivo reconstructions failed after recurrent branch stenosis, and each was treated with redo ex vivo repair and patch angioplasty. In each failure treated by nephrectomy, the kidney provided less than 5% of renal function by preoperative isotopic renography.[50]

Regardless of the type of management (redo reconstruction versus nephrectomy), and regardless of the renal function or blood pressure benefit after re-intervention, the product-limit estimates of dialysis-free survival for patients experienc-

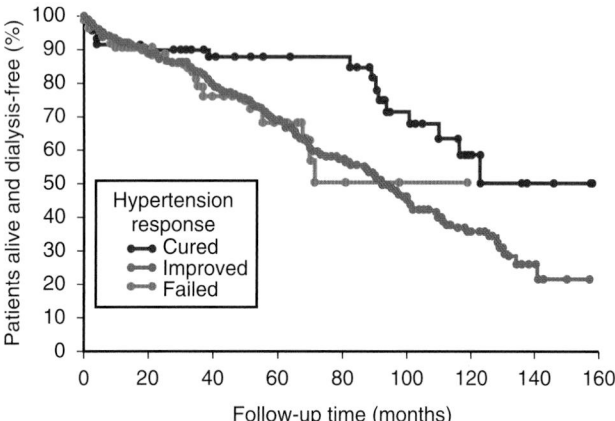

Figure 142-18 Product-limit estimates of time to death or dialysis according to hypertension response to operation. *(From Cherr GS, Hansen KJ, Craven TE, et al. Surgical management of atherosclerotic renovascular disease. J Vasc Surg. 2002;35: 236-245.)*

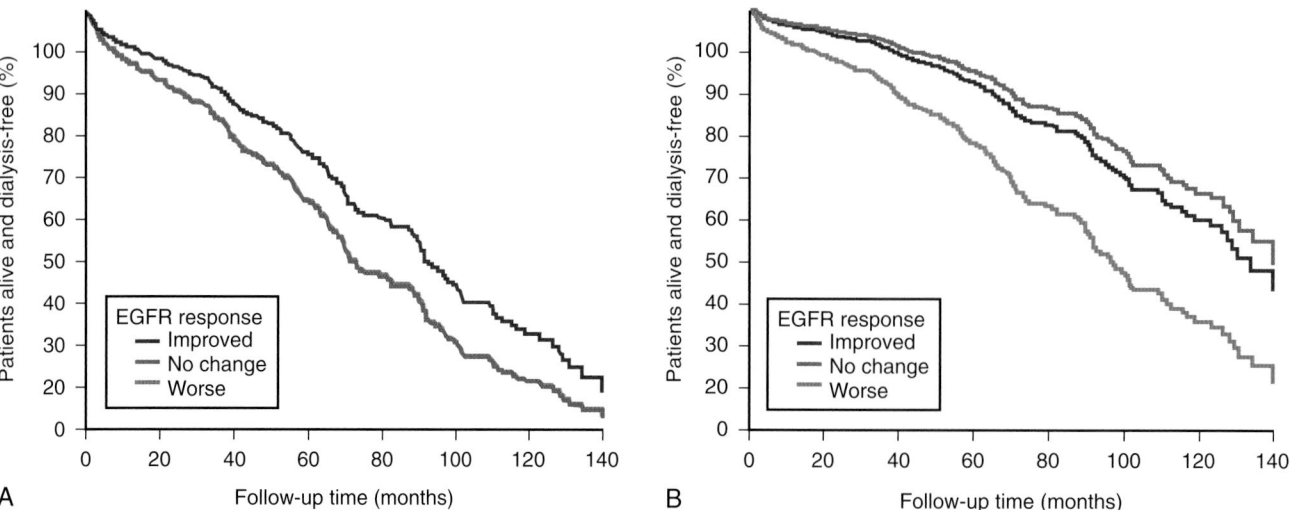

Figure 142-19 Predicted dialysis-free survival according to postoperative renal function response for patients with a preoperative estimated glomerular filtration rate (EGFR) of 25 mL/min/m^2 (25th percentile, **A**) or 39 mL/min/m^2 (median value, **B**). The interaction between preoperative EGFR and renal function response for dialysis-free survival was significant and independent. *(From Cherr GS, Hansen KJ, Craven TE, et al. Surgical management of atherosclerotic renovascular disease. J Vasc Surg. 2002;35:236-245.)*

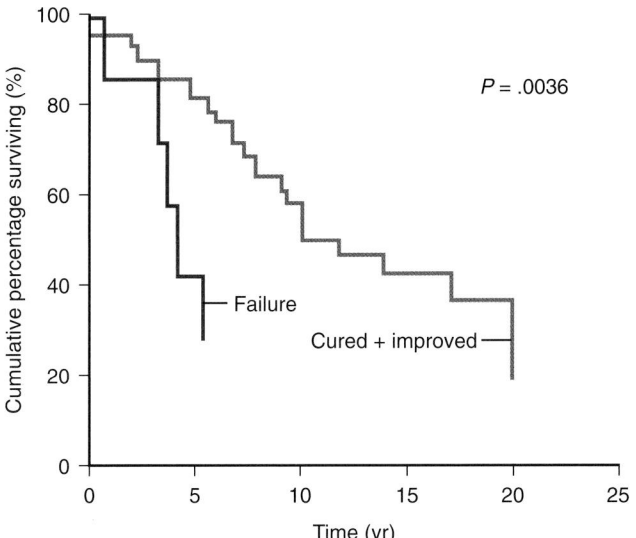

Figure 142-20 Product-limit estimates of dialysis-free survival for 20 patients requiring a second renal artery operation (*red line*) and 514 patients having primary renal artery repair only (*blue line*), with an adjusted *P* value. Operative failure was associated with a significant and independent decrease in dialysis-free survival. *(From Hansen KJ, Deitch JS, Oskin TC, et al. Renal artery repair: consequences of operative failures.* Ann Surg. *1998;227:678-690.)*

ing failure of open operative renal artery repair were decreased compared with patients who obtained primary patency (Fig. 142-20). Patients requiring secondary intervention also demonstrated a significant and independent risk of eventual dialysis dependence (relative risk, 12.6; confidence interval, 4.5-34.9; *P* < .001) and decreased dialysis-free survival (relative risk, 2.4; confidence interval, 1.1-5.4; *P* = .035).[50] Whether failed balloon angioplasty with endoluminal stenting demonstrates similar significant associations with eventual dialysis dependence or death is not known.

This experience with failed open renal artery repair re-enforces two management strategies. First, irretrievable loss of excretory renal function observed after failed renal artery repair supports the view that renal revascularization should be performed for clear indications, not as a prophylactic procedure in the absence of either hypertension or renal insuf-ficiency.[29,31,49] Second, the direct aortorenal reconstruction used in the majority of these patients is durable.[50] The short length and high blood flow characterizing aortorenal repair favor prolonged patency.

SELECTED KEY REFERENCES

Cherr GS, Hansen KJ, Craven TE, Edwards MS, Ligush J Jr, Levy PJ, Freedman BI, Dean RH. Surgical management of atherosclerotic renovascular disease. *J Vasc Surg.* 2002;35:236-245.
Management of atherosclerotic renovascular disease has focused solely on hypertension. Along with the article by Hansen and colleagues (later in this list), this work establishes an incremental increase in excretory renal function as the dominant determinant of dialysis-free survival on follow-up. Among patients with severe hypertension and renal insufficiency, changing renal function at 3 weeks predicts dialysis-free survival—a relationship that is stable at 10 years follow-up.

Dzau VJ, Re R. Tissue angiotensin system in cardiovascular medicine. A paradigm shift? *Circulation.* 1994;89:493-498.
The renin-angiotensin system has been demonstrated in virtually every tissue studied. This report summarizes the classic experiments of Goldblatt and provides an overview of the importance of tissue renin and angiotensin in both health and disease.

Hansen KJ, Cherr GS, Craven TE, Motew SJ, Travis JA, Wong JM, Levy PJ, Freedman BI, Ligush J Jr, Dean RH. Management of ischemic nephropathy: dialysis-free survival after surgical repair. *J Vasc Surg.* 2000;32:472-481.
See the annotation for Cherr and colleagues.

Rimmer JM, Gennari FJ. Atherosclerotic renovascular disease and progressive renal failure. *Ann Intern Med.* 1993;118:712-719.
This overview summarizes data related to the progression of atherosclerotic renovascular lesions and their contribution to excretory renal insufficiency.

Stanley JC, Criado E, Upchurch GR Jr, Brophy PD, Cho KJ, Rectenwald JE, Michigan Pediatric Renovascular Group, Kershaw DB, Williams DM, Berguer R, Henke PK, Wakefield TW. Pediatric renovascular hypertension: 132 primary and 30 secondary operation in 97 children. *J Vasc Surg.* 2006;44:1219-1229.
This contemporary classic defines the management of renovascular disease in children. It is a must-read for surgeons considering open operative repair in this age group.

REFERENCES

The reference list can be found on the companion Expert Consult Web site at *www.expertconsult.com.*

Renovascular Disease: Endovascular Treatment

Matthew A. Corriere and Matthew S. Edwards

The treatment of renovascular disease (RVD) is currently in a state of evolution. Surgical treatment represents the "gold standard" for durable renal revascularization. Unfortunately, the morbidity and mortality associated with surgical revascularization are significant, even when performed in centers with extensive experience. As a result, endovascular techniques for renal revascularization, including percutaneous transluminal angioplasty (PTA) with or without endoluminal stent placement, have emerged as another option for the revascularization of occlusive lesions of the renal artery. These endovascular techniques offer the potential benefits of decreased morbidity, mortality, patient recovery time, and hospital resource use compared with conventional open surgical revascularization. However, they also offer the potential drawbacks of decreased effectiveness and durability. Predictably, controversy persists regarding the appropriate application of surgical and endovascular therapy in the treatment of RVD, with proponents of each modality citing selected literature to support their position. This chapter provides an overview of the technical aspects involved in the performance of endovascular renal revascularization, as well as current data concerning the technical results, clinical outcomes, and associated complications.

DECISION MAKING

In general, decisions about open or percutaneous renal artery revascularization should be based on identical principles with regard to clinical manifestations and symptoms.

Indications

Although no level I evidence currently exists to definitively guide treatment decisions, there is broad consensus that decisions to treat should be based on the presence of hemodynamically significant stenosis in the setting of severe, difficult-to-control hypertension with or without associated renal dysfunction.

Hypertensive manifestations of RVD include a spectrum of clinical presentations ranging from chronic, severe hypertension refractory to pharmacologic management to hypertensive emergencies involving acute blood pressure elevations associated with target organ damage, including flash pulmonary edema, hypertensive encephalopathy, myocardial infarction, and acute renal failure.[1] Given the recent evidence

demonstrating a lack of survival benefit with blood pressure improvement alone,[2,3] our group now limits renal revascularization to those patients with truly uncontrollable hypertension and those whose hypertension is complicated by documented end-organ effects.

Renal dysfunction in patients with hemodynamically significant atherosclerotic RVD is commonly referred to as *ischemic nephropathy*,[4] although the establishment of a definitive causal relationship between anatomic RVD and renal dysfunction can be challenging in individual patients, despite extensive diagnostic testing. The diagnostic evaluation and pathophysiology of atherosclerotic RVD are discussed in detail in Chapter 141 (Renovascular Disease: General Considerations). Conditions that support a causal relationship between anatomically defined renal artery stenosis and disease manifestations are based primarily on reported predictors of response to intervention and include a precipitous decline in renal function over a short period,[2,5] severity of hypertension,[6-8] and presence of anatomic disease affecting perfusion to the entire functioning renal mass.[3,7,9] In truth, a causal relationship can be proved only by a physiologic response following revascularization. Given the data presented in Chapter 141 (Renovascular Disease: General Considerations), our group strongly believes that RVD associated with renal dysfunction is the most appropriate contemporary indication for renal artery revascularization.

Contraindications

Contraindications to the treatment of RVD by endovascular means can be broadly classified as anatomic contraindications, cases in which open revascularization is optimal, and cases undertaken for prophylactic revascularization.

Anatomic contraindications involve situations in which the diseased renal arteries cannot be easily treated with existing endovascular devices or, more commonly, those arteries cannot be treated with any reasonable expectation of a durable result. For instance, when RVD extends into the terminal portion of a main renal artery or involves a very short main renal artery, treatment with currently available devices may be problematic. RVD in the branch arteries beyond the main bifurcation, lesions in multiple small renal arteries (Fig. 143-1), diffuse aortic atherosclerotic disease (e.g., coral reef atheroma), and lesions in children (which are most often hypoplastic) are all poor candidates for endovascular treatment owing to durability concerns. In these situations, open

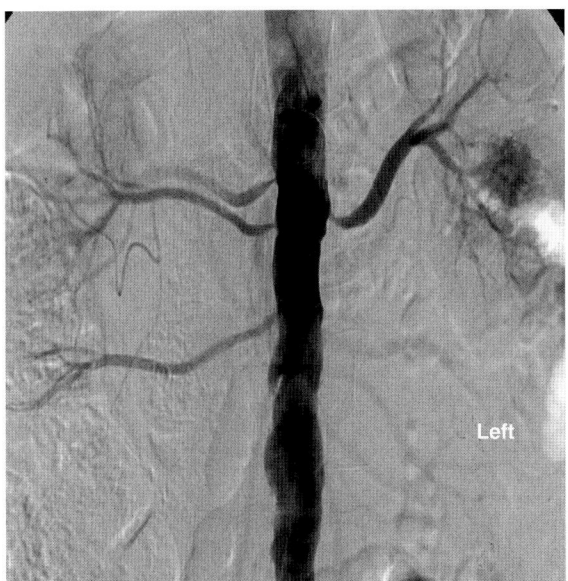

Figure 143-1 Abdominal aortogram demonstrates hemodynamically significant stenoses involving multiple right renal arteries.

surgical revascularization is likely the better treatment, unless the patient is a prohibitive surgical risk.

Surgical revascularization is also preferred in patients with indications for renal revascularization who require open aortic surgery. The addition of renal revascularization in these patients does not require a significant modification of exposure, and both pathologies can be treated in a single procedural setting. Existing data regarding open renal revascularization demonstrate that results are superior to endovascular treatment in terms of durability and renal function. We therefore consider it the treatment of choice in patients who require open aortic exposure for other reasons. We also consider open revascularization the initial treatment of choice for appropriate-risk patients, particularly young or fit patients with ischemic nephropathy.

With regard to prophylactic revascularization, the high rate of technical success and low incidence of periprocedural complications associated with endovascular renal artery revascularization have led to an increasingly aggressive application of this technique in recent years.[10,11] There is currently no evidence, however, supporting prophylactic renal revascularization (i.e., endovascular treatment of renal artery stenosis in patients with normal renal function whose blood pressure is either normal or well controlled with medical therapy). The natural history of atherosclerotic renal artery stenosis is associated with anatomic progression in only 8% to 31% of patients and progression to occlusion in 0% to 7%.[12-18] Further, when anatomic disease progression does occur, it is not consistently associated with longitudinal increases in blood pressure or serum creatinine.[16] Considering the benign clinical course of asymptomatic renal artery stenosis in the majority of patients, together with the risk of a deterioration in renal function associated with intervention (discussed under "Results"), we support a nonoperative management

strategy for asymptomatic patients with normal renal function and normal or easily controlled blood pressure and condemn prophylactic renal artery intervention, given the existing evidence.

■ PLANNING AND OPTIONS
Relevant Anatomy

The renal arteries originate laterally from the abdominal aorta and commonly assume an oblique orientation in their proximal course relative to the aortic axis (Fig. 143-2). Because aortography performed in a straight anteroposterior position can produce contrast overlap between the aorta and the proximal renal arteries, resulting in inadequate visualization of ostial disease, oblique imaging is frequently optimal for renal arteriography or intervention. Because multiple renal arteries, present in 18% of patients, may not be accurately characterized with duplex ultrasound,[19] accessory arteries may be an unanticipated finding in patients imaged with duplex ultrasound alone before intervention, and they must be assessed for occlusive disease during procedural planning. Distal renal artery diameter in patients undergoing endovascular intervention is usually 5 to 6 mm.[20,21] Post-stenotic renal artery dilatation is common[21] and may result in a size mismatch between the luminal diameter and the stent or protection device; small-diameter arteries (<3.5 mm) increase the technical difficulty of ostial engagement and endovascular treatment. Endovascular treatment of atherosclerotic disease is most often performed for lesions of the ostial or proximal main renal artery.[22-28] Branch vessel atherosclerosis is encountered less frequently and is seldom an ideal candidate for endovascular management.

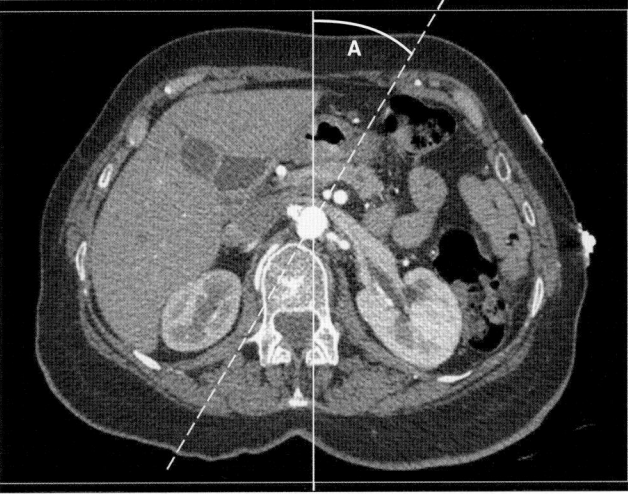

Figure 143-2 Oblique orientation of proximal renal arteries. Computed tomographic angiography demonstrates the axis perpendicular to the proximal renal arteries (*dashed line*) relative to the axis perpendicular to straight anteroposterior imaging (*solid line*). The resulting angle (A) indicates the oblique correction needed to avoid artifact resulting from contrast overlap between the aorta and the proximal renal artery, which could result in underestimation of the degree of renal artery stenosis.

Contrast-Related Considerations

Angiographic visualization of the arterial anatomy is a fundamental element of both diagnosis and endovascular treatment of atherosclerotic RVD. Accordingly, procedural planning should incorporate an assessment of the likelihood of contrast-induced nephropathy and the implementation of protective measures for high-risk patients. In addition to associated renal dysfunction and hypertension, common conditions among patients with RVD that may predispose to contrast-induced renal function impairment include diabetes mellitus, congestive heart failure, anemia, and shock[29-37]; chronic volume depletion may represent an additional risk factor in patients on diuretic medications. Procedure-related risk factors for contrast-induced nephropathy include the volume, osmolality, and viscosity of the contrast agent administered.[33,38-42]

Strategies to prevent contrast-induced nephropathy may include a variety of measures directed at maximizing renal perfusion, reducing oxidative stress, and inhibiting vasoconstriction. Hydration is a generally accepted prophylactic measure, but evidence supporting the routine use of *N*-acetylcysteine, sodium bicarbonate, or ascorbic acid is inconsistent.[33,43] Currently, we prepare all patients for aortorenal arteriography with preoperative hydration using isotonic saline (reduced in the setting of significant congestive heart failure), the administration of *N*-acetylcysteine, and the routine use of iso-osmolar, non-ionic contrast (iodixanol) at the lowest volume possible. For patients with renal dysfunction, we also administer sodium bicarbonate and ascorbic acid before the intervention. In the setting of severe renal dysfunction (estimated glomerular filtration rate [eGFR] <30 mL/min/1.73m^2), we employ carbon dioxide as an adjunctive contrast agent during initial aortography and selective cannulation to reduce the volume of iodinated contrast material.[44,45]

Medical Management

In the setting of acute, symptomatic presentations of RVD, such as hypertensive emergency or acute renal failure, clinical stabilization is usually possible through aggressive medical management, allowing intervention to be performed in a lower risk, elective setting. Acute renal failure in the setting of RVD is frequently precipitated by the initiation of angiotensin-converting enzyme inhibitors or angiotensin receptor antagonists in patients with bilateral disease or hypovolemia.[46-48] Deferring renal intervention until functional recovery is complete in these patients avoids additional renal insult from the administration of nephrotoxic contrast agents. For elective revascularization, nonsteroidal anti-inflammatory drugs, diuretics, metformin, and warfarin are withheld during the periprocedural period. Preoperative aspirin and statin therapy are initiated in all patients without contraindications. With the exception of angiotensin-converting enzyme inhibitors and angiotensin receptor antagonists, routine antihypertensive medications can be taken by the patient on the morning of the procedure with a sip of water.

Primary Angioplasty versus Angioplasty and Stenting

Although primary angioplasty is currently considered appropriate endovascular management for renal artery fibromuscular dysplasia (see Chapter 144: Renovascular Disease: Fibrodysplasia), primary endoluminal stenting for the treatment of ostial atherosclerotic RVD is associated with superior technical success and a lower incidence of recurrent stenosis than is angioplasty alone.[22,28,49] Contemporary endovascular management of ostial atherosclerotic RVD therefore consists of renal artery percutaneous transluminal angioplasty with primary endoluminal stenting (RA-PTAS); primary angioplasty is more commonly reserved for the management of recurrent disease. Nonostial atherosclerotic lesions may also respond well to angioplasty alone, but secondary stent placement should be considered if primary angioplasty is unsuccessful owing to elastic recoil, residual stenosis, persistent pressure gradient, or arterial dissection.

Bilateral Atherosclerotic Renovascular Disease

In patients with bilateral, hemodynamically significant atherosclerotic RVD, we proceed initially with unilateral treatment and assess how renal function or hypertension responds to intervention. If the clinical response is inadequate (renal function is unchanged or worse; blood pressure has not improved) and there is no evidence of recurrent stenosis, contralateral RA-PTAS is performed. In patients who achieve improved blood pressure control or renal function, medical management is continued with duplex ultrasound surveillance. We believe that this staged approach, compared with simultaneous bilateral RA-PTAS, reduces the contrast volume administered during a single procedure and decreases the likelihood of acute renal failure due to bilateral technical complications (e.g., flow-limiting dissection, atheroembolization).

■ DESCRIPTION OF TECHNIQUE

Access

Common femoral artery access is safe, versatile, and our preferred site for RA-PTAS. When selective renal artery cannulation is planned, selection of a femoral access location contralateral to the targeted renal artery facilitates ostial cannulation owing to the catheter's tendency to preferentially track along the contralateral aortic wall (Fig. 143-3). The brachial artery is an alternative access site that may be preferable in patients with aortoiliac occlusive disease, in renal arteries with significant inferior angulation relative to the main axis of the aorta, or when selective cannulation via a femoral approach has been unsuccessful. Compared with the femoral artery, disadvantages of brachial access include a higher incidence of access-related complications and catheter or sheath diameter limitations.[50,51]

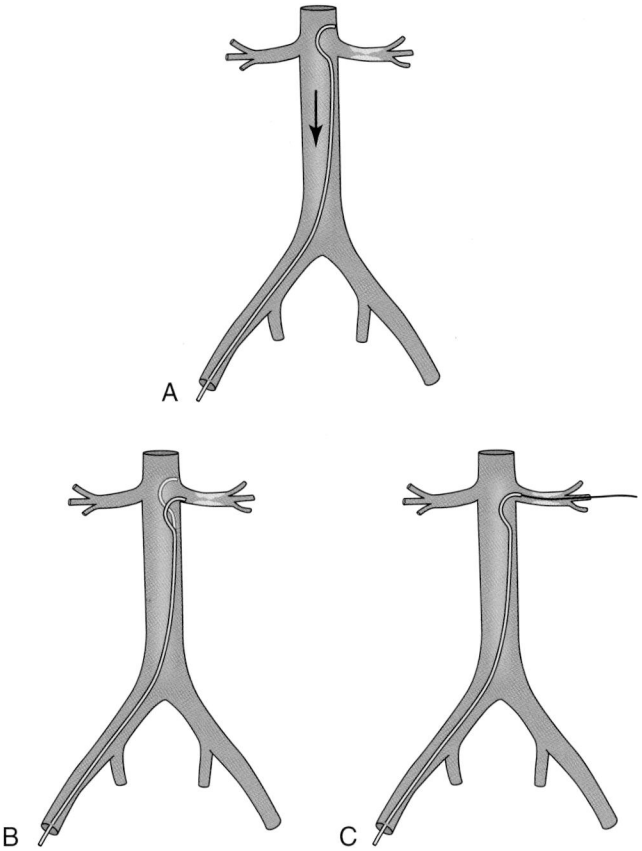

Figure 143-3 A–C, Contralateral femoral access often facilitates selective renal cannulation. *(From Schneider PA. More about how to get where you are going: selective catherization. In: Campbell B, ed. Endovascular Skills: Guidewires, Catheters, Arteriography, Balloon Angioplasty, Stents. St. Louis: Quality Medical Publishing; 1998:71.)*

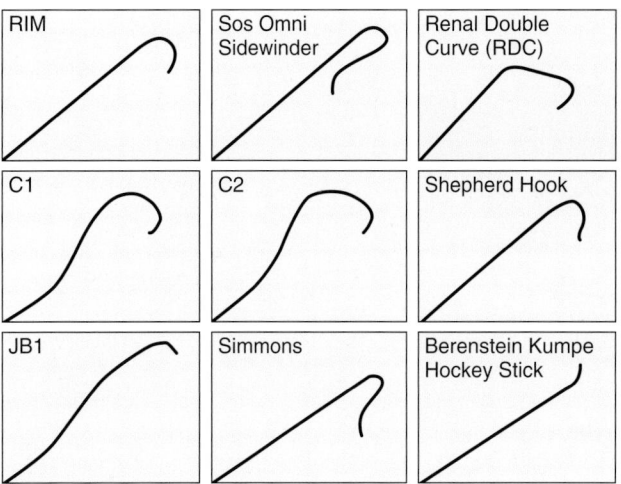

Figure 143-4 Various selective catheters commonly used to cannulate a renal artery.

Angioplasty and Stenting

A discussion of diagnostic angiography is included in Chapter 18 (Arteriography). Following initial diagnostic aortography, the patient is systemically heparinized, and the target renal artery is accessed using a selective catheter (Fig. 143-4). The selective catheter and sheath are exchanged over a 0.035-inch guide wire for a guide sheath or guide catheter. Either of these access platforms provides mechanical support during guide wire exchange and facilitates the delivery of therapeutic devices to the targeted lesion or lesions. Multiple device configurations are commercially available, and a luminal diameter of 6 Fr accommodates the majority of angioplasty and stenting systems. The tip of the guide sheath or catheter is positioned at or within the orifice of the targeted renal artery; then a guide wire is passed across the stenotic lesion. We believe that smaller wire systems minimize renal artery trauma and have technical advantages when crossing critical lesions. We prefer a 0.14-inch guide wire with a floppy, radiopaque tip for lesion passage. Once guide wire access across the stenotic lesion has been obtained, care must be taken to avoid advancement of the nontapered guide sheath or catheter, which could result in injury to the luminal surface of the renal artery.

Atheroembolization occurs during RA-PTAS and may affect renal function responses to intervention. We have demonstrated relationships between the quantity of embolic material liberated and stent diameter, stent oversizing, lesion predilatation, black race, and preoperative use of antiplatelet medications.[52] Although these findings provide hypothetical support for the concept of distal embolic protection during RA-PTAS, patient benefit from this procedural modification has not been prospectively demonstrated. A recent randomized trial by Cooper and coworkers reported that distal embolic protection combined with glycoprotein IIb/IIIa inhibition offered protection against a postoperative decline in eGFR; however, no protective effect was demonstrated for either of these treatment modifications when used alone.[53] At present, no commercially available distal embolic protection device is approved by the U.S. Food and Drug Administration for use in the renal circulation. If renal artery distal embolic protection is desired, a wire system incorporating a distal renal artery occlusion balloon or filter is used for crossing the lesion and subsequently deployed distally. If an occlusion balloon device is used, complete renal artery occlusion is confirmed by the hand injection of contrast material (Fig. 143-5). Angioplasty and stenting are then performed, followed by aspiration of the static column of blood distal to the treated lesion, irrigation with heparinized saline, and repeat aspiration. The distal occlusion balloon is then deflated, and completion angiography is performed. Filter devices permit ongoing distal renal artery flow in their deployed configurations and use a porous membrane to trap embolic material. Following angioplasty and stenting, the filter is collapsed back into its nondeployed state to trap any captured embolic material before device withdrawal. Most filter protection devices have membrane porosities of 100 μm or greater[54] and are therefore inadequate for capturing the majority of particulate debris liberated during RA-PTAS.[52,55] We therefore prefer balloon occlusion devices for distal protection.[56]

Both coaxial systems (which require assisted exchange and advancement of the entire catheter over the wire) and

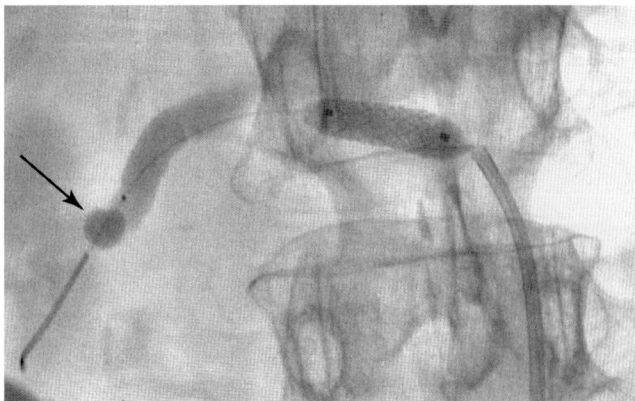

Figure 143-5 Renal angioplasty and stenting with distal renal artery balloon occlusion for embolic protection. A static column of contrast material is visible proximal to the occlusion balloon (*arrow*) during stent deployment.

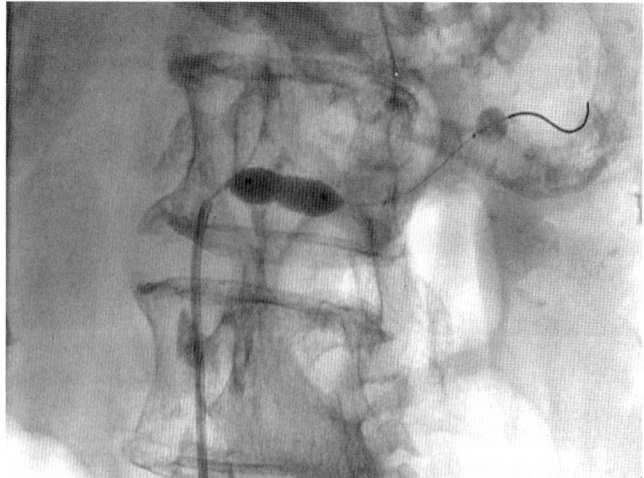

Figure 143-6 "Waisting" of an endoluminal stent being treated with postdeployment dilatation. The distal renal artery occlusion balloon is also visible.

monorail systems (which allow more rapid catheter exchange and wire control by a single operator) are available for RA-PTAS. For critical lesions, initial predilatation angioplasty may be necessary to permit subsequent endoluminal stenting. The angioplasty balloon diameter should be based on quantitative angiographic measurements; we select angioplasty balloons sized to match the adjacent normal artery for primary RA-PTAS and select smaller balloons if predilatation is required (we commonly use a 3- by 20-mm low-profile balloon for predilatation). For predilatation, the angioplasty balloon should be inflated to nominal pressure for 30 to 45 seconds before deflation; noting the location of the balloon's "waist" before full inflation is helpful for subsequent endoluminal stent positioning. Patients commonly experience pain or discomfort during angioplasty, but this usually resolves with balloon deflation; symptoms persisting after deflation suggest renal artery injury. Guide wire access is maintained during balloon deflation and removal, and completion angiography is performed if endovascular stenting is not planned (i.e., in the setting of treatment of recurrent disease or non-ostial atherosclerotic lesions).

RA-PTAS is most commonly performed using balloon-expandable stents, which have greater radial strength and can be deployed with relative precision; self-expanding stents offer greater flexibility but are used less frequently. For the treatment of ostial or proximal disease, stents are placed so that the proximal 1 to 2 mm extends into the aorta; more distal stent placement frequently fails to support the true renal artery orifice, is associated with an increased risk of both technical failure and recurrent stenosis,[25,26,57,58] and increases the technical difficulty of subsequent surgical revascularization (if necessary).[59] The shortest stent that adequately covers the lesion should be used, and positioning can be guided by the frequent hand injection of small volumes of contrast material into the catheter or sheath. A balloon-expandable stent is deployed by fully inflating the angioplasty balloon; currently available stents are premounted on low-profile delivery systems that often permit primary RA-PTAS without predilatation. If a residual "waist" is visible on fluoroscopy or com-

pletion angiography following stent deployment, the narrowed area can be dilated with an angioplasty balloon (Fig. 143-6).

Following RA-PTAS, technical results can be assessed with completion angiography, intravascular ultrasound, or pressure gradient measurements. When RA-PTAS has been performed with distal renal artery balloon occlusion protection, we find it useful to measure pressure gradients through the aspiration catheter, which has already been positioned distal to the treated lesion before balloon deflation. Using the aspiration catheter to check pressure gradients during its withdrawal avoids the need to pass an additional catheter past the newly stented lesion, which could lead to stent deformation or migration and loss of guide wire access. Once a satisfactory result has been obtained, the guide wire and sheath are removed, and hemostasis is obtained. An adequate result includes a residual stenosis less than 30% on angiography, peak renal artery systolic velocity less than 1.8 m/sec, or a pressure gradient less than 10 mm Hg between the distal renal artery and the aortic lumen.

POSTPROCEDURE MANAGEMENT

Following intervention, patients are monitored overnight for access site problems and hemodynamic instability. We routinely check the serum creatinine the day after the procedure before hospital discharge. Clopidogrel is initiated post intervention and continued for a minimum of 30 days; aspirin and statin therapy are continued indefinitely. Clinical follow-up with surveillance renal duplex ultrasound is performed at 1 month after intervention, then at 6-month intervals for 2 years, and annually thereafter. We consider a renal artery peak systolic velocity of greater than 180 cm/sec suggestive of disease recurrence. All anatomically identified recurrent lesions are evaluated in combination with their clinical manifestations. For patients with anatomic recurrence in the setting of maintained blood pressure or renal function response to intervention, we increase the frequency of clinical

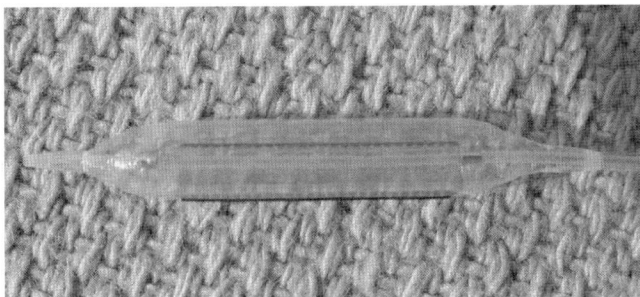

Figure 143-7 Cutting balloon.

follow-up and imaging surveillance but do not intervene unless clinical manifestations occur. When repeat intervention for recurrent disease is required, an endovascular approach is most often chosen. In-stent stenosis due to intimal hyperplasia should be suspected with early disease recurrence; this pathology is difficult to manage with routine balloon angioplasty alone, and technical results may be improved with initial dilatation using a cutting balloon (Fig. 143-7).[60]

■ COMPLICATIONS

Reported major complications include hemorrhage, access site pseudoaneurysm, bowel or extremity ischemia, myocardial infarction, renal artery thrombosis, and acute renal failure.[61,62] Hemodynamic instability following endovascular renal intervention must be presumed to be hemorrhagic until proved otherwise. Computed tomography is a useful tool for identifying and localizing bleeding. Hemorrhage is most commonly related to bleeding at the site of arterial access, but potentially fatal bleeding can also occur at the site of renal artery rupture secondary to angioplasty balloon or guide wire perforation.[63] Retroperitoneal or perinephric hematoma accumulation undetectable on physical examination may be identified using noncontrast computed tomography (Fig. 143-8). If no apparent bleeding is identified, other causes (e.g., myocardial infarction, heart failure, contrast reaction) should be investigated.

Femoral artery duplex ultrasound is a useful screening tool when access site pseudoaneurysm is suspected. Bleeding due to renal artery perforation can be managed with endovascular techniques (e.g., covered stent deployment) or conservative measures in the majority of patients; surgical exploration is less commonly required. Successful endovascular treatment of procedure-related renal artery thrombosis using thrombolysis has also been described.[62] We favor prompt surgical exploration for patients with access site bleeding and hemodynamic instability that persists despite appropriate volume resuscitation and reversal of anticoagulation.

■ RESULTS

Definitions of Success

Following endovascular treatment of atherosclerotic RVD, the criteria for technical success include a reduction in steno-

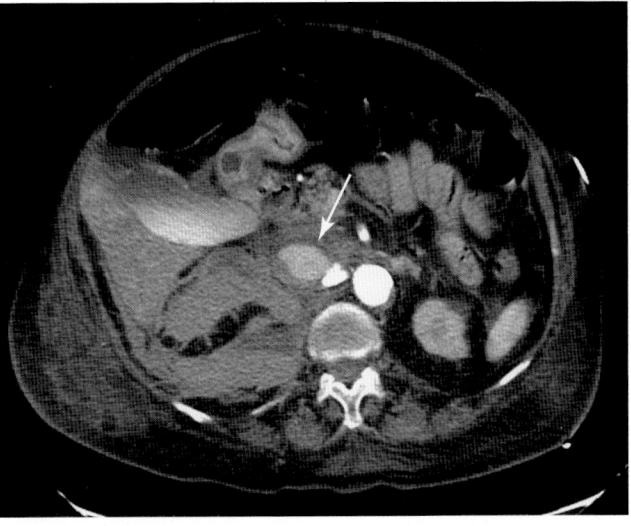

Figure 143-8 Right renal artery rupture resulting from angioplasty and stenting. A retroperitoneal pseudoaneurysm (*arrow*) is visible adjacent to the deployed right renal artery stent on a contrast-enhanced computed tomography scan. The patient required surgical exploration to achieve hemostasis.

sis as assessed by completion angiography and, when endoluminal stenting has been performed, complete coverage of the stenotic lesion by the deployed stent. Postintervention residual stenosis less than 30% has been suggested as a threshold for technical success versus failure.[64] When contrast angiography demonstrates anatomically successful treatment of the stenotic lesion, these findings should be confirmed with transduced pressure measurements immediately proximal and distal to the treated lesion. We consider a persistent pressure gradient greater than 10 mm Hg suggestive of inadequate treatment and perform repeat angioplasty in this setting in the absence of residual stenosis on the completion angiogram.

Whereas technical success implies delivery of the intended treatment with satisfactory anatomic and hemodynamic results, determination of whether the patient has derived any benefit requires a consideration of the indications for intervention and the clinical responses observed. Assessment of the response of hypertension to endovascular renal intervention includes an evaluation of systolic, diastolic, and mean blood pressure and the number of antihypertensive medications as continuous outcome measures. Alternatively, hypertension response can be assessed in a categorical fashion using a combination of blood pressure and medication criteria.[64,65] These methods generally describe the hypertension response as "cure," "improvement," or "failure" and are of value in assessing the clinical relevance of observed responses, particularly when continuous changes in individual measures are statistically significant but quantitatively minor. Serum creatinine, cystatin c, eGFR, and renal length all represent continuous outcome measures indicative of renal function response to intervention; renal response based on these measures is generally categorized as "improved," "unchanged," or "worse," based on postintervention change within a predefined range.

Section 18 Renal and Mesenteric Disease

We generally use a greater than 20% increase or decrease in eGFR to define improvement or worsening of renal function, respectively, with all other patients categorized as unchanged. Alternative analytic approaches have evaluated the impact of renal revascularization on the rate of decline in renal function, defining worsened or unchanged rates of eGFR decline as failure and attributing procedure-related benefit to patients experiencing improvement, stabilization, or slowed rates of decline in eGFR.[64]

Although hypertension and renal function responses to revascularization are relevant clinical endpoints reflecting clinical manifestations of RVD, these measures do not assess the impact of intervention on patient morbidity or survival. Survival free from dialysis or cardiovascular morbidity therefore represents an outcome that provides a more direct means of assessing the true benefit of intervention. Effects of endovascular treatment of RVD on these survival outcomes have not been prospectively characterized, but several randomized trials with survival endpoints are active or have been recently completed, and these results are eagerly anticipated.[66-68]

Early Outcomes

Table 143-1 summarizes outcomes associated with primary RA-PTAS from select contemporary series of adult patients.[5-8,20-23,25-27,49,51,52,56,57,69-87] Technical success rates range from 88% to 100% and exceed 95% in the majority of reports.* Periprocedural 30-day mortality is 0% to 5% in most recent series (see Table 143-1). Procedure-related complications associated with RA-PTAS are most commonly related to arterial access, contrast agent administration, or atheroembolization and occur in 0% to 43% of patients.

Late Outcomes

Late outcomes associated with endovascular renal artery intervention can be considered in terms of hypertension, renal function, anatomic durability (either renal artery patency or rate of disease recurrence), and survival free of dialysis or cardiovascular morbidity. Interpretation of the influence of RA-PTAS on these outcomes is challenging owing to the limitations of available clinical evidence. To date, the results of five prospective, randomized clinical trials evaluating endovascular renal artery intervention have been published. Three of these trials randomized patients to renal artery angioplasty (without stenting) or to medical management,[18,91,92] one compared renal artery angioplasty (without stenting) to surgical revascularization,[93] and one compared RA-PTAS with angioplasty alone.[49] Endpoints for comparisons between RA-PTAS and medical or surgical therapy included blood pressure changes,[18,91-93] renal artery patency,[93] change in serum creatinine,[18,93] or change in eGFR.[93]

With the exception of improved primary patency with surgical revascularization versus renal angioplasty,[93] none of

these studies observed significant differences in primary outcomes between groups randomized to renal artery angioplasty or to medical or surgical therapy. However, the demonstration of technical success and patency advantages associated with RA-PTAS versus angioplasty alone by van de Ven and colleagues[49] was followed by the widespread incorporation of endoluminal stenting into standard endovascular management of ostial RVD.

Lack of routine stenting as part of endovascular therapy, in combination with high crossover rates between treatment groups[91-93] and the exclusion of patients with severe renal dysfunction,[18,93] has limited the ability to generalize the findings of published randomized comparisons of angioplasty and medical or surgical therapy to current practice.[94] This gap in evidence led to the initiation of several prospective randomized comparisons of RA-PTAS and contemporary medical management that either remain active or recently completed follow-up.[66-68,95] Results from these trials will provide insight into the value of RA-PTAS, but at present, the available evidence is limited to retrospective cohort studies that are heterogeneous in their patient selection and outcome measures.

Hypertension Response

Hypertension response to RA-PTAS is most often either improvement or failure; cure is uncommon (see Table 143-1). In several studies, the number of patients categorized as hypertension response failures (i.e., no significant reduction in blood pressure or use of antihypertensive medications) outnumbered the combined patients experiencing cure or improvement.[20,22,27,52,56,70,73,77,85] Reported predictors of hypertension response include severity or duration of preoperative hypertension,[6-8] patient age,[28] percentage of angiographic stenosis,[6] bilateral disease,[7,9] female gender,[8] and preoperative brain natriuretic peptide.[90] Although durable hypertension responses have been reported by several authors,[25,69,73,86] others have observed a loss of initial hypertension response at 6-month follow-up, associated with a return to the preoperative number of blood pressure medications.[77,96] Following RA-PTAS performed at our center, we have observed reductions in blood pressure and antihypertensive medications that are statistically significant,[20,52,56] but blood pressure effects have been quantitatively modest and inconsistent in durability. We therefore have limited enthusiasm for RA-PTAS for the management of hypertension in the setting of normal renal function; in this scenario, we intervene primarily in patients with severe hypertension associated with target organ damage. A similar approach incorporating the presence of target organ damage into clinical decision making for patients with RVD has been described by Hanzel and coworkers.[97]

Renal Function Response

Although several series have reported improvement as the most frequent categorical renal function response to RA-PTAS,[8,75,81] others have observed postoperative deterioration with equal or greater frequency.[21,49,69,76,78,79,82,86] In the

---

*See references 5, 7, 8, 21-23, 25, 26, 28, 49, 51, 56-58, 69, 71-73, 76-78, 80, 81, 84-86, 88-90.

Table 143-1 Outcomes of Primary Renal Artery Percutaneous Transluminal Angioplasty and Stenting

Series	Year	Number of Patients	Bilateral Treatment (%)	Preoperative Renal Dysfunction	Renal Function Response (%) Improved	Unchanged	Worsened	Hypertension Response (%) Cured	Improved	Failed	Perioperative Mortality (%)	Perioperative Complications (%)
MacLeod et al.[70]	1995	29	29	57	25	75		0	40	60	3	18
van de Ven et al.[71]	1995	24	17	NR	33	58	8	0	73	27	0	13
Dorros et al.[69]	1995	76	21	38	28	28	45	6	46	48	5	11
Henry et al.[57]	1996	59	8	17	20	80		18	57	24	NR	3
Iannone[27] et al.	1996	63	22	91	36	46	18	4	35	61	3	32
Harden et al.[72]	1997	32	0	100	35	35	29		NR		13	19
Blum et al.[25]	1997	68	9	29	0	100	0	16	62	22	0	0
Boisclair et al.[26]	1997	33	6	51	41	35	24	6	61	33	0	21
Rundback et al.[76]	1998	45	24	100	18	53	30		NR		4	4
Fiala et al.[74]	1998	21	19	43	0	100			53	47	NR	19
Dorros et al.[73]	1998	163	39	39	33 (unilateral) 38 (bilateral)	33 (unilateral) 42 (bilateral)	34 (unilateral) 21 (bilateral)	1	42	57	2	14
Tuttle et al.[77]	1998	129	15	57	16	75	9	2	46	52	3	23
Gross et al.[75]	1998	30	23	40	55	27	18	0	69	31	3	0
Henry et al.[23]	1999	210	NR	23	29	67	2	19	61	20	<1	4
Rocha-Singh et al.[7]	1999	150	NR	NR	23	70	7		55	45	1	3
Rodriguez-Lopez et al.[78]	1999	108	16	30	0	96	4	13	55	32	4	7
van de Ven et al.[49]	1999	42	24	71	17	55	28	15	43	42	0	43
Baumgartner et al.[22]	2000	64	NR	NR	33	42	25		43	57	2	9
Burket et al.[51]	2000	127	NR	29	43	57			NR		2	4
Giroux et al.[6]	2000	30	NR	70		76	24	24	53	47	NR	NR
Lederman et al.[21]	2001	300	41	37	9	78	14		70	30	<1	2
Yutan et al.[100]	2001	76	22	65		88	12		68	32	3.8	5
Bush et al.[88]	2001	73	16	68	23	51	26		NR		1.4	9
Henry et al.[80]*	2001	28	14	43	18	82	0	14	54	32	0	4
Rocha-Singh et al.[81]	2002	51	55	100	77	18	5		91	9	0	14
Kennedy et al.[84]	2003	261	NR	36		61	39		NR		NR	NR
Gill and Fowler[82]	2003	100	26	75	31	38	31	4	79	17	2	18
Zeller et al.[8]	2003	215	23	52	52	48			76	24	0	5
Henry et al.[89]*	2003	56	14	32	18	82	0	18	59	23	NR	NR
Holden and Hill[83]*	2003	37	24	100		100	0	0	57	33	NR	NR
Zeller et al.[85]	2004	456	NR	52	34	39	27		46	54	<1	NR
Nolan et al.[86]	2005	82	NR	59	23	53	24	NR	81	NR	0	7
Edwards et al.[56]*	2006	26	15	92	53	47	0	0	35	65	0	3
Holden et al.[87]*	2006	63	92	100		97	3	0	55	45	NR	NR
Kashyap et al.[5]	2007	125	36	100	42	23	25		NR		1.6	6
Edwards et al.[52]*	2007	27	4	74	36	64	0	0	48	52	0	0
Corriere et al.[20]*	2008	99	11	75	28	65	7	1	21	78	0	6

*Denotes studies using embolic protection.
NR, not reported.

majority of patients, postintervention renal function is unchanged (see Table 143-1). Reported rates of postintervention improvement versus deterioration in renal function vary widely, and these heterogeneous results may be partly attributable to different patient selection criteria, particularly with regard to the percentage of patients with baseline renal dysfunction (those with normal baseline renal function have no prospect for improvement through intervention). Weighted averages across series of unprotected RA-PTAS demonstrate renal function improvement in approximately 25% of patients, with a roughly equal proportion experiencing postintervention decline (see Table 143-1).

Rather than assessing renal function response as a mean or categorical change in outcome measures, several studies have analyzed renal responses to RA-PTAS using breakpoint analysis based on the slope of either eGFR or the reciprocal of serum creatinine, with effects categorized as improvement, stabilization, or failure.[64] Although these studies have demonstrated that RA-PTAS can reduce the rate of renal function decline,[5,72,81,96] the interpretation of clinical benefit based on breakpoint analysis is controversial. Although patients with increased postoperative eGFR (or decline in serum creatinine) clearly experience a beneficial renal function response, the clinical benefit resulting from the stabilization of renal function or the reduction in the rate of decline is not clear. Although no evidence demonstrating a relationship between renal function stabilization and survival following endovascular renal artery intervention is available, Hansen and associates observed improved dialysis-free survival following open surgical revascularization in patients with early postoperative renal function improvement, but no similar survival effect was noted in patients with unchanged renal function.[3] Similar associations with renal function improvement have been demonstrated following RA-PTAS.[5,84] We therefore believe that when interpreting either categorized changes in eGFR or breakpoint analysis data, patient benefit can be assumed only for those with improvement; presuming a benefit in patients with unchanged or stable renal function may be conceptually flawed.

Reported predictors of renal function response to RA-PTAS include bilateral disease,[9,85] elevated baseline serum creatinine,[8,85] rapid preoperative decline in renal function,[5] and impaired left ventricular function.[8] Series using distal embolic protection during RA-PTAS have reported improved postintervention renal function in 18% to 53% of patients, while renal function deterioration was observed in 0% to 7%.[20,52,56,80,83,87,89] We believe that the decreased frequency of postintervention renal function decline in these series compares favorably with results from cohorts managed without embolic protection.

Disease Recurrence

Restenosis following RA-PTAS has been defined based on angiography,[21,71,77] duplex ultrasound,[86] or both.[78,82,98] Reported rates of restenosis following RA-PTAS range from 5% to 66% and vary with the duration of follow-up and the criteria

for repeat imaging.* As described previously, angioplasty without stenting for ostial RVD is associated with increased rates of restenosis compared with RA-PTAS. Other factors associated with restenosis include preoperative blood pressure,[100] preoperative renal dysfunction,[100] diabetes,[100] small renal artery or stent diameter,[101-103] and smoking.[104] Anatomically identified recurrent stenosis must be considered in combination with clinical manifestations when formulating a management strategy. Acute worsening of hypertension or decline in renal function should prompt the suspicion of disease recurrence. Lederman and colleagues identified recurrent disease twice as frequently when anatomic imaging was performed in the setting of clinical suspicion as opposed to routine postintervention screening (42% versus 21%).[21] The relatively frequency of recurrent disease should be considered when contemplating primary intervention, particularly in asymptomatic patients, and it raises additional concerns regarding the long-term benefits achieved in patients with unchanged renal function following RA-PTAS.

Survival

Survival results following RA-PTAS are limited to retrospective cohort studies that lack medically managed controls. Dorros and associates observed a 74% 3-year survival rate following RA-PTAS; although renal failure was not a frequent cause of death, they observed decreased survival among patients with both baseline renal dysfunction and bilateral disease.[73] Similar overall survival was reported by Kashyap and colleagues, who observed a 63% rate of dialysis-free survival; lack of postintervention improvement in renal function was associated with subsequent dialysis in this series.[5] Similar relationships among baseline renal dysfunction, renal function response, and survival have been described by Kennedy and coworkers.[84] A survival benefit associated with statin use following RA-PTAS has also been described.[105] Preoperative congestive heart failure, coronary artery disease, and chronic obstructive pulmonary disease are additional factors that adversely affect postintervention survival.[21,105]

SELECTED KEY REFERENCES

Balk E, Raman G, Chung M, Ip S, Tatsioni A, Alonso A, Chew P, Gilbert SJ, Lau J. Effectiveness of management strategies for renal artery stenosis: a systematic review. *Ann Intern Med.* 2006;145:901-912.
  Review of contemporary data regarding medical, surgical, and endovascular management of renal artery stenosis.

Cooper CJ, Haller ST, Colyer W, Steffes M, Burket MW, Thomas WJ, Safian R, Reddy B, Brewster P, Ankenbrandt MA, Virmani R, Dippel E, Rocha-Singh K, Murphy TP, Kennedy DJ, Shapiro JI, D'Agostino RD, Pencina MJ, Khuder S. Embolic protection and platelet inhibition during renal artery stenting. *Circulation.* 2008;117:2752-2760.
  Randomized evaluation of distal embolic protection or glycoprotein IIb/IIIa inhibition during renal angioplasty and stenting.

Edwards MS, Corriere MA, Craven TE, Pan XM, Rapp JH, Pearce JD, Mertaugh NB, Hansen KJ. Atheroembolism during percutaneous renal artery revascularization. *J Vasc Surg.* 2007;46:55-61.

---

*See references 21-23, 25, 49, 57, 69, 71, 72, 75, 77-79, 82, 98-100.

Analysis of atheroembolization during RA-PTAS and associations with procedural outcomes.

Garovic VD, Textor SC. Renovascular hypertension and ischemic nephropathy. *Circulation.* 2005;112:1362-1374.
Summarizes the epidemiology, pathophysiology, diagnostic approach, and management of renal artery stenosis.

Leertouwer TC, Gussenhoven EJ, Bosch JL, van Jaarsveld BC, van Dijk LC, Deinum J, Man In't Veld AJ. Stent placement for renal arterial stenosis: where do we stand? A meta-analysis. *Radiology.* 2000;216: 78-85.
Meta-analysis of renal artery stent placement versus angioplasty for renal artery stenosis.

Pearce JD, Craven BL, Craven TE, Piercy KT, Stafford JM, Edwards MS, Hansen KJ. Progression of atherosclerotic renovascular disease: a prospective population-based study. *J Vasc Surg.* 2006;44: 955-962.
Duplex ultrasound–based evaluation of the natural history of atherosclerotic RVD.

REFERENCES

The reference list can be found on the companion Expert Consult Web site at *www.expertconsult.com.*

CHAPTER 144

Renovascular Disease: Fibrodysplasia

Bengt Lindblad and Anders Gottsäter

Based in part on chapters in the previous edition by Darren B. Schneider, MD; James C. Stanley, MD; Louis M. Messina, MD; and Thomas W. Wakefield, MD.

Fibromuscular dysplasia (FMD) (also known as arterial fibrodysplasia) is a nonatherosclerotic, noninflammatory angiopathy of unknown cause. It affects medium-sized arteries—most commonly the renal arteries—and can cause renovascular hypertension. FMD of the renal arteries was first described in 1938 by Leadbetter and Burkland in a 5-year-old boy.[1] Involvement of other arteries was subsequently recognized, and carotid FMD was reported by Palubinskas and Ripley in 1964.[2]

EPIDEMIOLOGY

Symptomatic fibrodysplastic renal artery stenosis reportedly occurs in 0.4% of the population,[3] but the prevalence of asymptomatic FMD in potential renal donors is around 4%.[4,5] The true prevalence is difficult to ascertain because there are no easily applicable screening tests. FMD is most often diagnosed in patients aged 15 to 50 years,[6] but it has been reported from infancy[7,8] to age 89.[9-11] The medial type of FMD is most common and is more than four times more prevalent in females than in males.[3,4] In contrast, the less common intimal type is more prevalent in men.[3,12] In the studies summarized in Tables 144-1 and 144-2, 81.7% of patients in both endovascular and open surgery series were female, for a male-female ratio of 1:4.5. Lesions are bilateral in about 39% of cases and unilateral in about 61%, most often affecting the right renal artery.[13] In our summary of 1880 adult FMD patients (see Tables 144-1 and 144-2), 23.6% had bilateral lesions, with no difference noted between endovascular and open surgery series. In the case of bilateral lesions, it was not always possible to ascertain whether both lesions required treatment. Stanley and coworkers reported bilateral lesions in 65% of patients; however, in only 15% of cases did this significantly influence the management of patients.[14] In series that reported treated sides in unilateral disease (see Tables 144-1 and 144-2), the right renal artery was affected in 72%

Table 144-1 Results of Percutaneous Transluminal Renal Angioplasty for Fibromuscular Dysplasia in Adults

Series	Year	Number of Patients	Gender		Side(s) Affected		Results (%)				Follow-up (mo)
			Male	Female	Unilateral	Bilateral	Technical Success	Cure	Improvement	Failure	
Sos et al.[109]	1983	31	4	27	28	4	87	59	34	7	16
Martin et al.[156]	1985	21	0	21	13	8	100	25	60	15	16
Lüscher et al.[23]	1986	31	7	24	NA	NA	90	50	39	11	15
Hägg et al.[35]	1987	19	3	16	17	2	100	33	22	44	23
Baert et al.[157]	1990	22	4	18	14	10	86	82	0	19	25
Tegtmeyer et al.[158]	1991	66	7	59	32	34	100	41	57	2	39
Simonetti et al.[115]	1993	442	NA	NA	NA	NA	91	64	25	11	93
Rodriguez-Pérez et al.[159]	1994	27	6	17	23	4	100	43	48	10	96
Cluzel et al.[103]	1994	20	5	15	NA	NA	90	65	30	5	19
Bonelli et al.[106]	1995	105	14	91	76	29	89	22	41	37	43
Jensen et al.[107]	1995	30	10	20	29	1	97	39	47	14	12
Davidson et al.[101]	1996	24	1	22	16	8	96	52	22	26	>6
Jagose et al.[160]	1998	6	0	6	2	4	80	50	50	0	108
Klow et al.[161]	1998	49	9	40	34	15	98	25	43	29	61
Lovaria et al.[162]	1999	69	19	50	52	12	82	45	23	32	112
Birrer et al.[108]	2002	27	5	22	23	4	96	37	37	26	12
Fremuth et al.[163]	2002	97	8	89	NA	NA	NA	6	68	32	18
Surowiec et al.[114]	2003	14	0	14	14	3	95	36	43	21	24
De Fraissinette et al.[9]	2003	70	20	50	54	16	94	14	74	12	39
Kumar et al.[164]	2003	20	8	12	18	2	96	85	5	10	68
Hughes et al.[165]	2004	35	12	23	24	11	94	35	58	8	15
Alhadad et al.[29]	2005	59	5	47	54	13	95	24	39	37	84
Tanaka et al.[112]	2007	15	5	10	NA	NA	100	33	47	20	60
Kim et al.[21]	2008	16	8	8	13	3	79	6	74	20	24
Totals		**1315**	**160**	**701**	**536**	**183**					

NA, not available.

Table 144-2 Results of Open Surgery for Fibromuscular Dysplasia

Series	Year	Number of Patients	Gender Male	Gender Female	Unilateral (Right / Left)	Bilateral	Cure	Improvement	Failure	Follow-up (mo)
Buda et al.[130]	1976	42	NA	NA	29 (NA / NA)	13	76	14	10	72
Stoney et al.[136]	1978	24	2	22	21 (NA / NA)	3	38	52	10	36
Bergentz et al.[131]	1979	40	NA	NA	34 (24 / 10)	6	66	24	10	36
Lawrie et al.[166]	1980	113	NA	NA	78 (NA / NA)	35	43	24	33	49
Jakubowski et al.[134]	1981	75	11	64	70 (49 / 21)	5	50	22	3	36
Stoney et al.[150]	1981	78	14	64	78 (58 / 20)	0	66	32	1	67
Stanley et al.[14]	1982	144	11	133	50 (NA / NA)	94	55	39	6	60
Novick et al.[120]	1987	120	29	91	114 (NA / NA)	6	63	30	7	36
Van Bockel et al.[133]	1987	53	13	40	41 (NA / NA)	12	53	34	13	77
Hägg et al.[35]	1987	22	1	22	20 (NA / NA)	2	55	36	9	36
Hansen et al.[167]	1992	43	12	31	37 (NA / NA)	6	43	49	8	24
Murray et al.[127]	1994	68	7	61	68 (NA / NA)	0	74	23	2	90
Andersen et al.[25]	1995	40	5	35	34 (NA / NA)	6	33	57	10	40
Wong et al.[117]	1999	19	1	18	17 (8 / 9)	2	31	58	11	56
Reiher et al.[132]	2000	101	21	80	62 (NA / NA)	39	36	31	33	66
Chiche et al.[119]	2003	30	11	19	5 (NA / NA)	25	96	0	4	62
Marekovic et al.[129]	2004	72	16	56	70 (NA / NA)	2	80	10	10	132
Carmo et al.[122]	2005	26	4	22	20 (13 / 7)	6	27	60	13	29
Lacombe and Ricco[121]	2006	25	10	15	22 (NA / NA)	3	84	12	4	69
Crutchley et al.[71]	2007	37	7	30	29 (NA / NA)	8	15	65	20	34
Totals		**1172**	**175**	**803**	**899 (153 / 67)**	**273**				

NA, not available.

of 461 cases. However, the frequency of unilateral disease affecting the right renal artery differed between open surgical series (68%) and endovascular series (82%).

FMD is more likely to be present in patients with treatment-resistant or malignant hypertension[15,16] than in the general hypertensive population and accounts for up to 10% of all cases of renovascular hypertension[17,18]; the remainder of renovascular hypertension cases are caused mainly by atherosclerosis. Compared with patients with atherosclerotic renal artery stenosis, FMD patients are younger and have both fewer risk factors for atherosclerosis and a lower occurrence of atherosclerosis in other vessels.

FMD is diagnosed most often in Caucasians and is reported less frequently in Hispanic and Asian populations. Only a few reports have been published from Africa and South America.[7,19-21] The true prevalence of renovascular hypertension is unknown, but it may account for 1% to 2% of all cases of hypertension in adults.[3] The prevalence of renovascular hypertension among black hypertensive patients is probably even lower.[22] Because diagnostic criteria vary and prevalence data are often derived from autopsy studies, the prevalence of renovascular hypertension might be overestimated because of the difficulty of estimating the clinical significance of a morphologic stenosis.

Other vessels such as the carotid and coronary arteries can also be affected (Table 144-3),[23] and FMD should be excluded in young people presenting with acute carotid artery dissection or occlusion (see Chapter 97: Carotid Artery Disease: Fibromuscular Dysplasia). Multiple-organ involvement with FMD and cerebral or cardiac ischemia may be associated with

Table 144-3 Arterial Involvement in Fibromuscular Dysplasia

Artery	Frequency of Involvement (%)
Renal arteries	75-89
Bilateral renal arteries	23-65
Unilateral—right renal artery	68-82
Unilateral—left renal artery	18-32
Carotid or vertebral arteries	3-26
Multiple vascular involvement (aorta, iliac, popliteal, splanchnic, hepatic, coronary, subclavian, superficial femoral, tibial, peroneal arteries)	8-28

Based on Lüscher TF, Keller HM, Imhof HG, et al. Fibromuscular hyperplasia: extension of the disease and therapeutic outcome. Results of the University Hospital Zurich Cooperative Study on Fibromuscular Hyperplasia. *Nephron.* 1986;44(Suppl 1):109-114, and data from studies in Tables 144-1 and 144-2.

an increased risk of complications and death.[24] Multiple arterial involvement has been reported in 8 of 34 and 9 of 102 renovascular FMD patients.[25,26]

In childhood, renovascular hypertension is a more important cause of hypertension. It is found in 8% to 10% of all hypertensive children and in up to 25% of those with secondary hypertension. FMD is the most common cause of pediatric renovascular hypertension in North America and Western Europe, whereas Takayasu's arteritis dominates in Asia and Africa.[8] The causes of pediatric renovascular stenosis differ in different populations.[7,19,27] In Turkey (71 million inhabitants) 45 pediatric patients with renovascular hypertension were recorded during a 15-year period.[8] Of these 45 patients, 14 had FMD and 12 had Takayasu's disease. In the largest series reported from the University of Michigan Pediatric Renovascular Group, led by Stanley, nearly all of the 97 children had FMD or arterial dysplasia consisting of complex medial and perimedial dysplastic disease, with secondary intimal hyperplasia in some cases; only a few children had primary intimal dysplasia.[7] Coarctation or hypoplasia of the aorta affected 32 patients, and 19 had celiac or superior mesenteric artery ostial stenosis. Because the number of pediatric FMD patients is small, evaluation and treatment should be centralized.

PATHOGENESIS

Etiology

The fact that FMD is more common among women suggests that hormonal factors may be important.[4,28] Of the 57 women in one study, 9 (16%) had a previous diagnosis of hypertension during pregnancy, compared with 4% to 5% of pregnancies in the general population.[29] The number of pregnancies and the frequency of oral contraceptive use did not differ between patients with FMD and the general population, however.[28,30]

Vessel wall ischemia may also be important for the development of FMD.[31] The vasa vasorum of muscular arteries, which supply oxygen and nutrients to the arterial wall, originate from branch points of the parent arteries. Occlusion of the vasa vasorum induces the formation of dysplastic lesions in animal studies.[32] The vessels most commonly affected by FMD, such as the renal, internal carotid, and external iliac arteries, have long segments that lack branches and thus have few vasa vasorum. Mechanically, both the internal carotid and renal arteries are subjected to repeated stretching during motion and respiration; this may injure the sparse vasa vasorum, causing arterial wall ischemia and the subsequent development of FMD. This hypothesis is supported by the observation that FMD is more common in the right renal artery,[26] which is longer than the left. This makes the right kidney more subject to renal ptosis,[33] which is also common among patients with renal FMD.[34] Vasospasm in the vessel wall might also induce ischemia in the vasa vasorum, and cases of FMD combined with Raynaud's disease have been reported.[35]

FMD is associated with cigarette smoking.[30] The prevalence of smoking is higher in patients with FMD than in matched controls,[28,30,36] and FMD patients who smoke have more severe arterial disease than nonsmokers.[37] The mechanisms by which smoking contributes to FMD have not been elucidated.

The occurrence of renal FMD in siblings and identical twins suggests the possible inheritance of the disease.[38] Rushton suggested that FMD is transmitted in an autosomal dominant manner, with incomplete penetrance and variable clinical symptoms.[39] A French study of renal FMD showed that 11% of patients had at least one sibling with renal FMD[12]; the presence of FMD can be easily overlooked in relatives because it may be associated with only mild hypertension or even normotension. Subclinical dysplasia of the common carotid artery also occurs in renal FMD patients,[40] in accordance with a possible autosomal dominant transmission.[41]

Associations with polymorphisms in the angiotensin-converting enzyme (ACE) allele ACE-I have been reported,[42] and an autoimmune origin of FMD has been suggested by genetic associations with HLA-Drw6.[30]

FMD might coexist with other diseases of the vessel wall and endocrine system. Ehlers-Danlos syndrome type IV has been associated with medial fibroplasias[43] and should be suspected in patients with multiple aneurysms and FMD. FMD has also been reported in association with pheochromocytoma,[44] Marfan's syndrome,[45] Alport's syndrome,[46] and Takayasu's arteritis.[47]

Differential Diagnosis

Important differential diagnoses are type 1 neurofibromatosis,[48,49] vascular Ehlers-Danlos and Williams syndromes, and vasculitis. The diagnosis of these conditions relies on associated phenotypic traits: characteristic skin lesions in type 1 neurofibromatosis[50]; acrogeric dysmorphism, skin elasticity, and distal joint laxity in vascular Ehlers-Danlos syndrome[51]; and facial dysmorphism, supra-aortic stenosis, and particular behavior in Williams syndrome.[52] Genetic tests can also be used to rule out these conditions as alternative diagnoses.

Table 144-4 Classification of Dysplasias

Classification	Gender/Age	Cases (%)	Pathologic Features	Angiographic Appearance
Intimal fibroplasia	Often young; no gender difference	5	Irregularly arranged subendothelial mesenchymal cells with a loose matrix of fibrous connective tissue Collagen deposition frequent; internal elastic lamina may be disrupted	Long, irregular tubular stenosis or ringlike stenosis in children; smooth focal stenosis in adults
Medial dysplasias Medial fibroplasia	Adolescents and females 20-50 yr; female-to-male ratio 5-9:1	80	Areas of thinned media alternating with thickened fibromuscular ridges containing collagen Internal elastic lamina can be fragmented and adventitia intact Advanced medial dysplasia, especially in children, also shows secondary intimal hyperplasia (see Fig. 144-2)	"String of beads" appearance, with the "bead" larger than the proximal vessel Normally involves distal two thirds of main renal artery but can also extend into branches (25%) (see Fig. 144-1)
Perimedial fibroplasia	Young girls and women up to 50 yr	10-15	Patchy collagen deposition between media and adventitia External elastic lamina intact (see Fig. 144-3)	Can also result in "string of beads" appearance, but diameter of "beads" does not exceed diameter of proximal artery (see Fig. 144-4)
Medial hyperplasia	Women 40-50 yr	1	True smooth muscle cell hyperplasia without fibrosis	Mimics appearance of intimal fibroplasia, with smooth concentric stenosis
Adventitial fibroplasia	No gender difference	<1	Dense collagen replaces normally loose connective tissue of adventitia and may extend into surrounding tissue	Long stenosis

Because FMD is, by definition, a noninflammatory process, it is not associated with anemia, thrombocytopenia, or the increased acute phase reactants that often occur in patients with vasculitis. Large-vessel vasculitis sometimes occurs in the absence of changes in acute phase reactants, however.[53] Therefore, it might be difficult to distinguish FMD from inflammatory vessel disease in the absence of tissue samples or laboratory markers confirming inflammation.

Pathology

In vitro studies have demonstrated increased production of collagen, hyaluronate, and chondroitin sulfate in arteries exposed to cyclic stretching.[54] Mural ischemia due to functional defects in the vasa vasorum, possibly in association with developmental renal malposition, has also been postulated as a cause of FMD.[55]

FMD has not been found in other species except for domestic turkeys, where it was reported in 24 of 31 examined turkeys, with no sex differences.[56]

Classification

Three main types of dysplasias have been identified and are classified according to the dominant arterial wall layer involved: intimal, medial, and adventitial (Table 144-4, Figs. 144-1 to 144-4).[26,57-59] It is important to distinguish among the different types of FMD because they warrant special considerations for optimal treatment when the renal artery is affected. Especially in children, dysplastic or hypoplastic developmental lesions involving the aorta and other visceral arteries, secondary dysplasia after inflammatory events, vas-

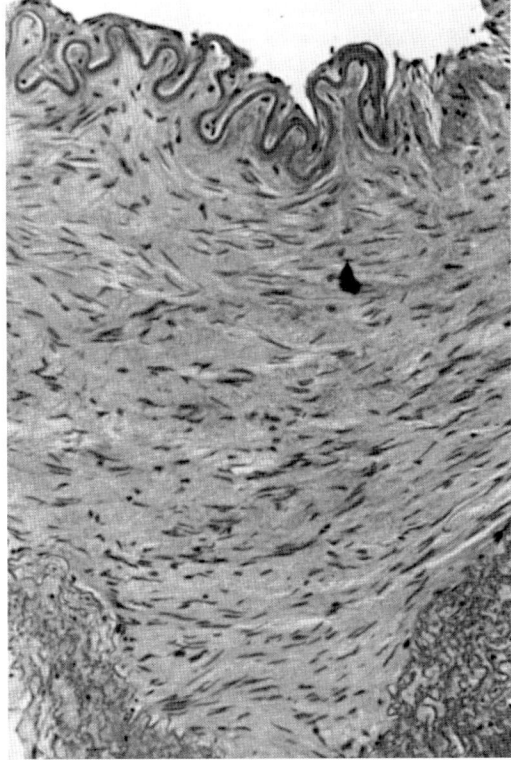

Figure 144-1 Medial fibrodysplasia with dense fibrous connective tissue in the outer media, disordered inner medial smooth muscle, and normal intimal tissues.

culitis, dissection, and post-traumatic lesions need to be differentiated from FMD. Complications of arterial dysplasia, such as aneurysm formation, dissection, and arteriovenous fistula, should be classified as secondary events and differentiated from primary dysplastic lesions.

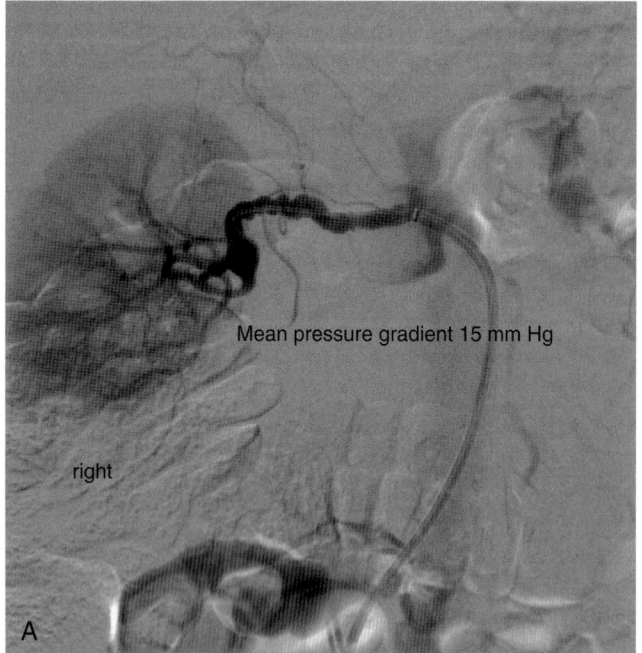

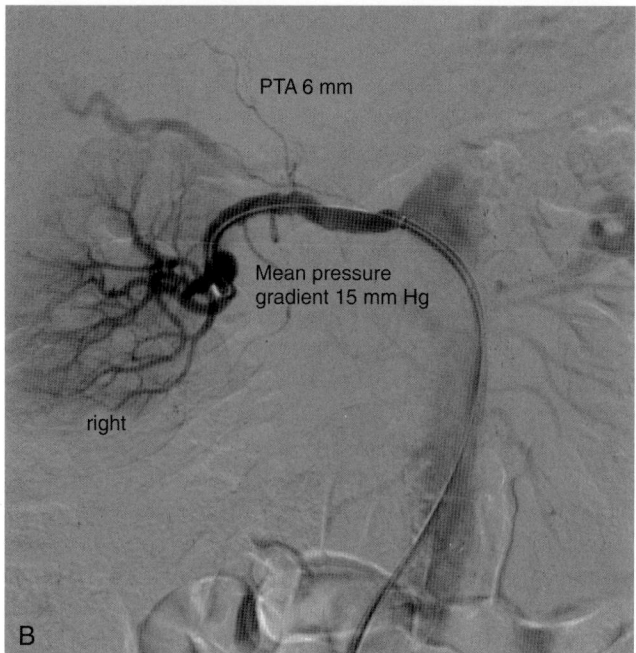

Figure 144-2 Typical selective angiographic appearance of medial fibrodysplasia with the "string of beads" in the distal main artery before (**A**) and after (**B**) dilatation. PTA, percutaneous transluminal angioplasty.

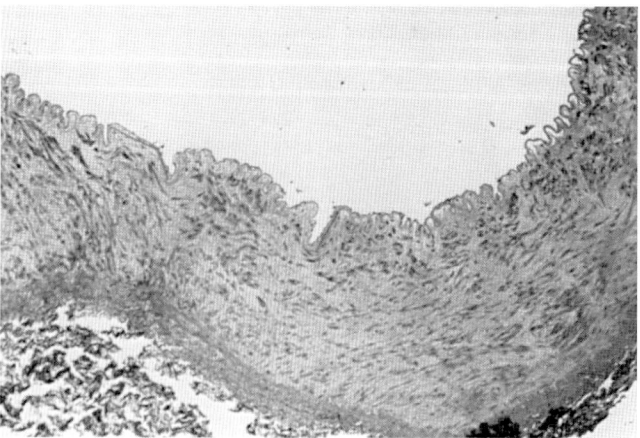

Figure 144-3 Histologic appearance of perimedial dysplasia, in which a homogeneous collar of elastic tissue adjacent to the outer media dominates the examination.

Pathophysiology

When it affects the renal arteries, the changes associated with FMD might lead to luminal narrowing, causing renal artery stenosis and a subsequent pressure gradient in the artery, resulting in renovascular hypertension. Renovascular hypertension is defined as hypertension that is the direct consequence of renal artery stenosis caused by either FMD or, more commonly, atherosclerosis.

Reduction of arterial perfusion pressure in the stenosed kidney leads to activation of the renin-angiotensin-aldoste-rone (RAA) system, resulting in volume expansion and hypertension. Several mechanisms, including increased endothelin-1 (ET-1) production, local RAA activation, arterial wall remodeling, and oxidative stress, help sustain the hypertension,[60] which is no longer dependent only on the RAA system but also on local vasoconstrictive proliferative effects in the arterial wall, gradually leading to resistance to therapy.[61] Inflammatory mediators such as high-sensitivity C-reactive protein, tumor necrosis factor-α, interleukin-6, and neopterin and vasoconstrictive mediators such as ET-1 are increased in patients with renovascular hypertension.[62] A separate analysis of patients with FMD, however, showed that neopterin and ET-1 were lower in patients with renovascular hypertension caused by FMD than in those with renal artery stenosis of atherosclerotic origin.[62] This suggests that inflammatory activation might be less important for the pathophysiology of renovascular hypertension caused by FMD than for that caused by atherosclerosis.

Luminal narrowing leads to renal parenchymal damage and ischemic nephropathy in patients with FMD.[63] This seems to be less important in FMD patients than in those with atherosclerotic renal artery stenosis, however; the latter show more pronounced reductions of total kidney and cortical perfusion compared with FMD patients.[64] In addition, renal perfusion correlates inversely with the degree of stenosis in FMD but not in atherosclerotic renal artery stenosis,[64] further emphasizing that FMD hypertension is more truly renin dependent than is hypertension caused by atherosclerosis.[65]

The contralateral kidney may be damaged by exposure to hypertension in FMD.[63] Deterioration of renal function in a patient with FMD affecting one renal artery suggests the development of bilateral stenosis, parenchymal disease, or both.

◼ NATURAL HISTORY

Data with regard to stenosis progression and risk of deteriorating renal function in patients with FMD do exist,[4,66-69] but

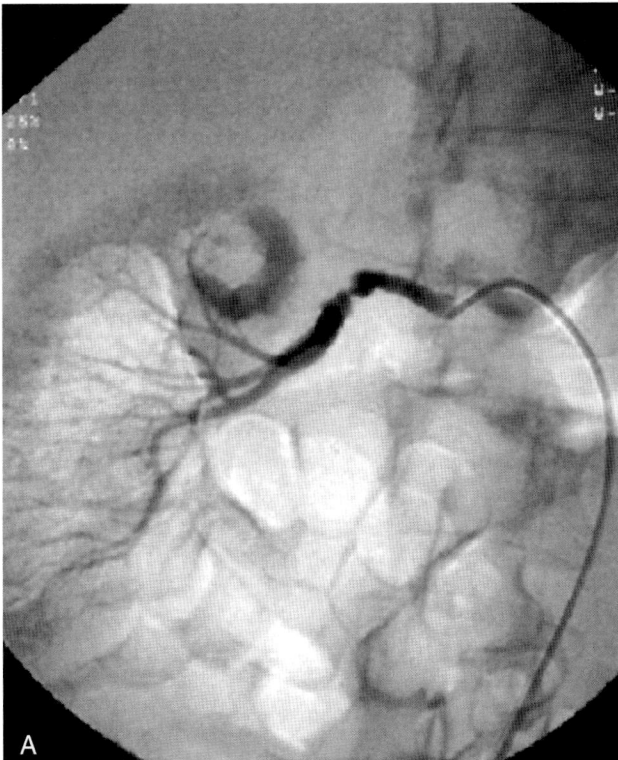

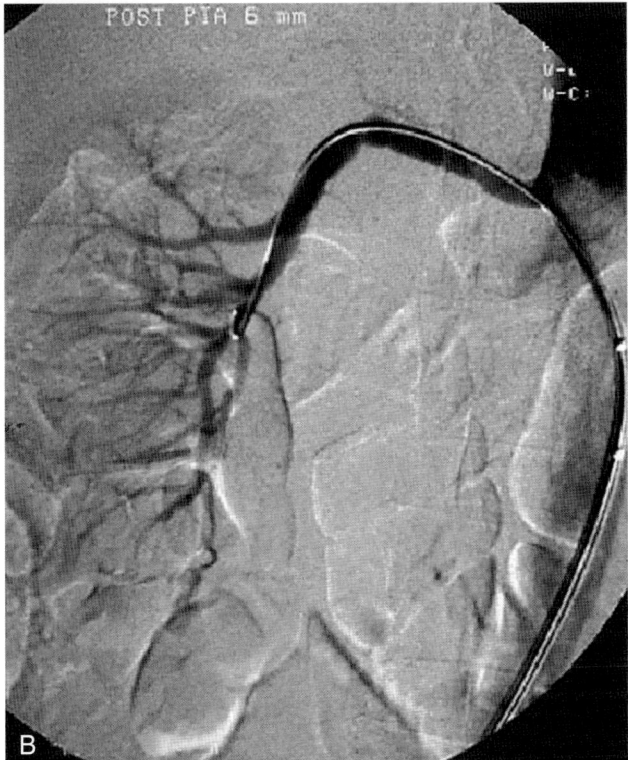

Figure 144-4 Short focal stenosis of the distal main artery, perhaps of the perimedial dysplastic type, before (**A**) and after (**B**) balloon dilatation.

they are scarcer than in patients with atherosclerotic renal artery stenosis. Progression is less severe in FMD than in atherosclerotic stenosis.[3] Between 26% and 28% of subjects with asymptomatic FMD develop hypertension within 4 years,[4,5] and serial angiograms confirm FMD progression in

up to 40% of cases.[67,68] In one angiographic follow-up study of 42 patients, some degree of progression occurred in all patients.[69] Because angiography is not routinely performed in FMD patients with favorable clinical outcomes, these progression rates may be overestimated. FMD might also result in a decreasing renal size[69] and deterioration of renal function, although less often than in patients with atherosclerotic renal artery stenosis.[18,65,70,71] Complete vessel occlusion,[72] renal infarction,[69,73] and severe renal insufficiency,[29,74] as well as regression of stenosis,[75] have been infrequently reported in FMD patients.

CLINICAL PRESENTATION

History and Physical Examination

Arterial hypertension of acute onset or high blood pressure that is increasingly difficult to treat suggests the presence of secondary hypertension—that is, a specific cause of blood pressure elevation, which can be identified in about 5% of adult hypertensive patients.[15] Renovascular hypertension caused by one or more stenoses of the extrarenal arteries is the second most common cause of secondary hypertension (after renal parenchymal disease) and occurs in approximately 2% of adult patients with blood pressure elevation assessed in specialized centers.[76] A physical sign suggesting renal artery stenosis is abdominal bruit with lateralization. In patients with either high-grade stenosis of a single kidney or bilateral disease, often with one renal artery occluded and the other stenosed, acute pulmonary edema may occur, with or without renal failure.[77,78] Typically, these patients present with severe and rapid-onset "flash" pulmonary edema, which can also occur in FMD and may be confused with coronary syndromes.[79] Among patients with renal artery stenosis, the absence of general atherosclerosis suggests that the stenosis is caused by FMD, whereas signs of atherosclerotic disease in other vessels indicate a greater possibility of an atherosclerotic cause.

Screening for Secondary Hypertension

The patient history can reveal acute-onset hypertension, concomitant flushing, or other paroxysmal symptoms. Physical examination may reveal abdominal bruits, and routine laboratory investigations may show signs of renal disease, hypokalemia, or hyperthyroidism. Secondary hypertension is also suggested by a severe blood pressure elevation, a sudden onset or worsening of hypertension, and blood pressure that responds poorly to appropriate doses of at least three drugs, including a diuretic.[15,80] In these cases, specific diagnostic procedures for the evaluation of potential secondary hypertension should be considered, as outlined in Box 144-1.

DIAGNOSTIC EVALUATION

In patients with suspected renovascular hypertension caused by FMD, the following tools can be used for diagnosis.

Renal Ultrasound

Ultrasonography allows a determination of the longitudinal diameter of the kidney, which can be used as a screening test for renal artery stenosis. A difference of more than 1.5 cm between the two kidneys is usually considered diagnostic and is found in 60% to 70% of patients with renovascular hypertension.[81]

Color Doppler ultrasonography can often directly detect stenosis of the renal artery, particularly when localized close to the origin of the vessel.[82] In addition, it can be used to determine the resistance index, which can be predictive of outcome from angioplasty and stenting in atherosclerotic renal artery stenosis.[83] An increased resistance index suggests structural abnormalities in the small blood vessels of the kidney. Patients likely to benefit from renal revascularization can be identified by a resistance index of less than 80, calculated with the following equation:[83]

$$[1 - \text{End-diastolic velocity (cm/sec)/Maximal systolic velocity (cm/sec)}] \times 100$$

This index has not been evaluated in FMD patients, however.

Limitations of renal artery duplex ultrasonography include its dependence on operator skill, the fact that it may be unsuccessful in 20% of patients because of problems visualizing branches or accessory renal arteries, and the difficulty or impossibility of imaging obese patients or those with intervening bowel gas.[84] Because of these limitations and the fact that distal renal artery lesions are not optimally diagnosed by ultrasound, this technique should be restricted to the screening of patients with possible FMD.

Intravascular ultrasound has also been studied and is useful for distinguishing renal FMD from vasculitis and hypoplasia.[85] This method is in limited clinical use, however.

Captopril Renography

Captopril renography is a functional test to detect the angiotensin II dependence of renal function. In a positive test, the oral preadministration of 25 to 50 mg of the ACE inhibitor captopril delays the uptake of tracer, reduces peak uptake, prolongs parenchymal transit, slows excretion, and affects separate function in unilateral disease.[86] The sensitivity and specificity of captopril renography decrease in the presence of renal failure, bilateral disease, branch artery lesions, and a solitary functioning kidney. Although data exist from studies of patients with renal artery stenosis due to FMD, captopril renography is no longer recommended as a first-line method for the diagnosis of FMD owing to its low sensitivity and specificity.[87,88]

Magnetic Resonance Angiography

Magnetic resonance angiography (MRA) is a noninvasive imaging technique. A negative result with contrast-enhanced MRA probably excludes significant renal artery stenosis, but false-positive results due to turbulence are common, and MRA may overestimate the degree of renal artery stenosis.[62,89] MRA can identify vessels as small as 2 to 2.5 mm and therefore has limited resolution for distal and intrarenal arteries.[13] In terms of specificity and sensitivity, gadolinium-enhanced MRA is better than ultrasound and scintigraphy and equal to computed tomographic angiography (CTA) for the detection of renal artery stenosis.[87,88] However, because the resolution of MRA is inadequate for the visualization of branch vessel involvement, its usefulness for the diagnosis of FMD has been questioned.[6] Gadolinium toxicity also precludes the use of MRA in patients with severe renal impairment.

Computed Tomographic Angiography

Spiral CTA has comparable sensitivity to MRA, but it has the disadvantages of requiring a radiation dose and the infusion of a potentially nephrotoxic contrast substance. CTA depicts both the lumen and the vessel wall but has limited resolution for distal and intrarenal arteries.[13] The specificity and sensitivity of CTA for detecting renal artery stenosis are better than for ultrasound and scintigraphy and equal to gadolinium-enhanced MRA,[88] and technical optimization reportedly increases the diagnostic accuracy to 100%.[90] In some centers, MRA or CTA is used as a second-line test after a positive screening test with duplex ultrasonography or captopril renography when the index of clinical suspicion is high. In 25% of FMD patients with intrarenal stenosis, none of these methods is reliable.

Renal Angiography

When one of the aforementioned screening examinations results in a strong suspicion of renal artery stenosis, or when an FMD patient is evaluated and there is a clinical indication to proceed to revascularization, intra-arterial digital subtraction angiography should be performed for confirmation. This invasive procedure is still the "gold standard" for the detection of renal artery stenosis, including that caused by FMD (Fig. 144-5).[6] FMD lesions are typically truncal or distal,

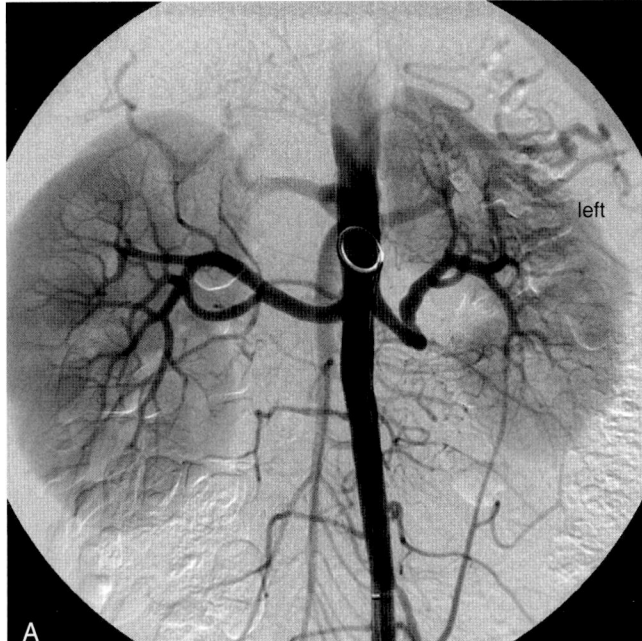

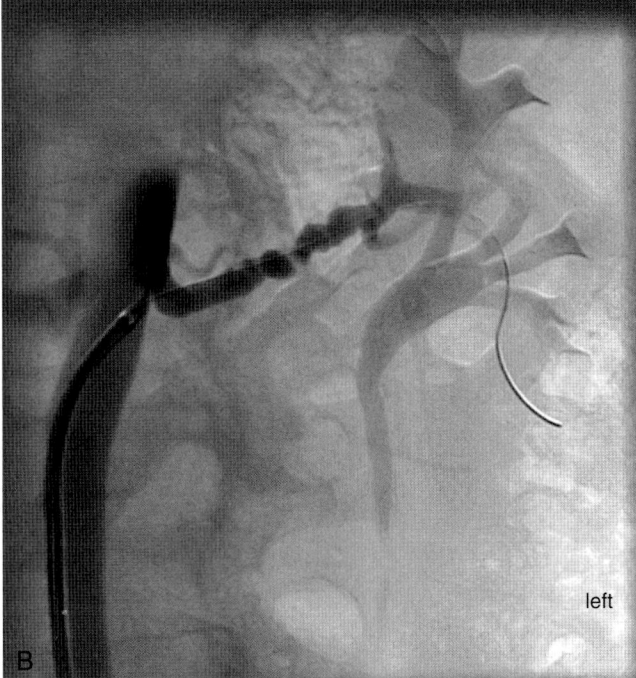

Figure 144-5 A, Aortogram in a hypertensive young man reveals only minor findings in the left renal artery. **B,** Selective angiogram from another angle shows the fibromuscular dysplastic lesion, over which a 60 mm Hg pressure gradient was noted. The patient's hypertension was cured by percutaneous transluminal renal angioplasty.

whereas atherosclerotic lesions are more often proximal or ostial.[3] In medial fibroplasia, the combination of fibromuscular ridges alternating with areas of aneurysm leads to the classic "string of beads" appearance (see Fig. 144-2).[13] Angiography is especially useful in the evaluation of branch vessel disease. Sometimes it is difficult to distinguish FMD from vasculitis, however.

Invasive Testing: Pressure Gradients and Renin Levels

Intra-arterial measurement of the pressure gradient over the stenosis, such as that performed before percutaneous transluminal angioplasty in the iliac arteries,[91] is recommended for renal artery stenosis[92] and as a complement to angiography to select patients for invasive treatment. Different methods have been used for such assessments,[93,94] and there is no consensus regarding what level of mean or systolic pressure gradient indicates a hemodynamically significant renal artery stenosis. A distal-aortic pressure ratio less than 0.90 has been correlated with increased renin levels in the renal vein,[95] suggesting a physiologically relevant stenosis. Pressure measurements have been used to determine the significance of renal artery stenosis caused by FMD,[29,96] and a mean pressure gradient over the stenosis of greater than 10 mm Hg predicts a favorable response to dilatation. Further, pressure measurements have been used to detect FMD lesions responding to therapy in patients without significant signs of renal artery stenosis on angiography.[96] A persistent pressure gradient after an endovascular procedure indicates a higher risk of restenosis.

The determination of the renal vein–renin ratio requires multiple catheterizations, and its invasiveness and complexity are not compensated by an acceptable level of sensitivity or specificity. It is therefore no longer recommended as a diagnostic procedure.[15]

■ TREATMENT SELECTION

The treatment options in renal artery FMD are medical, endovascular, and surgical. Treatment of patients with all forms of renovascular hypertension is controversial owing to the limited number of randomized, long-term-outcome trials comparing different therapeutic approaches, as well as the difficulty of predicting the blood pressure response to renal revascularization procedures in individual patients.[76] In FMD, invasive endovascular or surgical treatment should be considered in patients whose hypertension cannot be controlled with antihypertensive drugs, in those who are intolerant of or noncompliant with medications, and in patients with impaired renal function or ischemic nephropathy.[6] To identify progressive disease in patients on medical therapy only, blood pressure and renal function should be followed regularly. Some authors also recommend that renal size be monitored by regular ultrasound examinations and that revascularization be recommended if it decreases by 1 cm or more.[3]

■ MEDICAL TREATMENT

Prevention

In atherosclerotic renovascular disease, treatment with lifestyle modification, low-dose aspirin, and statins is warranted because of the high risk of progression of atherosclerotic lesions. In patients with FMD, who might have varying degrees of concomitant atherosclerosis or none at all, the indications for such treatment must be evaluated in each individual patient. The most important medical treatment in these patients is antihypertensive drugs.

Medication

Many controlled trials have convincingly shown that lowering blood pressure reduces cardiovascular morbidity and mortality.[97] All patients with renovascular hypertension caused by FMD are therefore candidates for antihypertensive treatment in accordance with current European[15] and American[80] guidelines. In all hypertensive patients, blood pressure should be reduced to less than 140/90 mm Hg, and to lower values if tolerated.

Current guidelines specify five different groups of first-line antihypertensive treatment: ACE inhibitors, angiotensin II receptor blockers (ARBs), beta blockers, calcium channel blockers, and diuretics.[15,80] All of these drugs can be used in the treatment of renovascular hypertension caused by FMD.

Thiazide diuretics and calcium antagonists can be used in appropriate doses, with the possible addition of a blocker of the renin-angiotensin system (ACE inhibitor or ARB). ACE inhibitors and ARBs should not be taken during pregnancy, however. This treatment lowers blood pressure in the majority of patients with renovascular hypertension. In bilateral disease or stenosis of a single kidney, blockade of the renin-angiotensin system requires caution because these drugs' dilatory effects on the efferent arterioles can compromise renal function, leading to a reduction in perfusion pressure beyond the stenosis. This can reduce the capillary pressure within the glomerulus to below the critical perfusion pressure.[98] Slight increases in serum creatinine are common, but they normally revert when treatment is withdrawn. Acute renal failure occurring 1 to 14 days after the initiation of treatment has been described.[99]

ENDOVASCULAR TREATMENT IN ADULTS

At most institutions, open surgical procedures to optimize renal artery blood flow were the dominant invasive treatment for renovascular hypertension in FMD patients until the beginning of the 1990s. Since then, percutaneous transluminal renal angioplasty (PTRA) has become the treatment of choice for renovascular hypertension due to FMD.[100] Unlike patients with atherosclerotic renovascular hypertension, progressive loss of renal function is uncommon in FMD patients.[101] Thus, the main reason for treating FMD is unsatisfactorily controlled hypertension, and treatment often leads to cure or improvement.

Technical Considerations

The technique for PTRA in FMD is basically the same as that used to treat atherosclerotic renal artery lesions. To reduce the number of "minor" complications after PTRA, many recommend a micropuncture technique of the common femoral artery, normally the right one. The puncture site position is controlled angiographically before catheters and guiding catheters are advanced. This ensures optimal compression of the puncture site after the procedure.

Heparinization is the same as for other endovascular procedures. However, FMD patients are often younger and have more pronounced vasoreactivity than those with atherosclerotic renal artery stenosis.

Many FMD patients are already receiving antihypertensive treatment with calcium channel blockers; if not, premedication with short-acting dihydropyridines as nifedipine can be used to reduce the risk of vasospasm. Even so, vasospasm in the kidney vasculature is so frequent in FMD patients that one normally infuses 0.15 mg nitroglycerin into the renal artery just after catheterization in hemodynamically stable patients. If required, this can be repeated during the procedure.

For puncture of the common femoral artery, most centers are using guide wire systems based on 0.014- or 0.018-inch guide wires to reduce vasospasm. All the components in such systems are thin and have a low profile. In FMD patients the right renal artery often takes off from the aorta proximally. Even in the right renal artery, which is often longer than normal in FMD patients, the diversity of available guiding catheters usually allows catheterization from a femoral puncture. A brachial approach is seldom needed to get a better angle for renal catheterization. Both a diagnostic aortogram and selective renal angiograms at different angles are obtained (see Fig. 144-5). In addition, many centers routinely measure pressure gradients. Because there is no optimal tip-pressure catheter, pressure measurements are usually made through a 4 Fr catheter. Balloons for 0.014- or 0.018-inch guide wire systems are thin and normally pass easily into the renal artery.

In FMD patients the stenotic lesion is most often located in the middle part of the main renal artery. The diameter of the selected balloon is normally the same as the diameter of the unaffected proximal part of the renal artery. If the distal part of the renal artery or its branches are affected, the use of multiple guide wires may be necessary. A kissing balloon technique can be used in branches.[102] However, multiple guide wires or kissing balloons are normally not required, and ballooning the main artery first, followed by the branches, often achieves good results.[103] If a cardiac catheterization laboratory equipped with a large inventory of microcatheters, guide wires, and balloons is available, such equipment can be useful for complex FMD stenoses. This may obviate the need to stock a large inventory, but knowledge of how to use these tools in the peripheral vessels is required.

Stenting

In FMD the stenotic lesion is normally located in the distal part of the main renal artery and is therefore highly amenable to PTRA. Balloon angioplasty enlarges the arterial lumen in FMD by breaking the septa causing the narrowings and by stretching the arterial wall, resulting in separation of the intima from the media, fracture of the media, and stretch of the adventitia beyond its elastic recoil.[104] Subsequent changes include smooth muscle cell necrosis, fibrosis, and some degree of neointimal formation.[105] In the vast majority of cases, PTRA provides good results; pressure gradients are completely abolished, and there is no indication for stent placement. Also, given the relative youth of these patients, stenting should be avoided. Surgical intervention may be more appropriate in cases of complex stenosis and should not be made more difficult with stent placement.

Indications to stent FMD lesions include severe procedural complications, suboptimal results with persistent pressure gradients after repeated angioplasty attempts, or small aneurysms in the renal artery.

Procedure-Related Complications

Puncture site hematoma is the most common complication and is reported in 3% to 26% of cases.[9,106-108] The trend toward using micropuncture to optimize puncture site location and the fact that smaller introducers can be used further reduce this risk. Normally, there is no reason to optimize the hemostatic seal with endovascular sutures or plugs, but such adjunctive procedures can be considered. Careful placement of punctures and optimization of initial compression are imperative.

Dissection occurs infrequently (1.4% to 6.7%) if the balloons are not too much oversized.[9,29,106,109] The majority of these dissections are small, and few require treatment. Repeated and prolonged ballooning is recommended, and dissections that are not hemodynamically significant can be left alone without jeopardizing the kidney. However, an extensive dissection that is increasing or limiting flow may, as a last resort, be treated with stent deployment and fixation.[21]

Rupture of the renal artery is uncommon in medial or perimedial dysplasia. Rupture is reported to occur in 2% to 6% of cases,[21,29,106] and it is more common in FMD patients with complex stenoses. Some of these small ruptures stop leaking after prolonged ballooning; others require stents, covered stents, or emergent open surgery after the balloon provides initial hemostasis.

The use of cutting balloons is definitely not a first choice in FMD patients, because ruptures have been reported.[110,111] If cutting balloons are required, it is wise to start with an undersized balloon. Good results have been reported with the use of cutting balloons in complex lesions.[112,113] Before a cutting balloon is used in a "redo" procedure, CTA or MRA may yield information about whether the lesion is dysplastic or hypoplastic. A hypoplastic lesion is a narrowing of the entire vessel with thin walls, which implies a higher risk of rupture. Intravascular ultrasound may add information on wall thickness, and in the future, improved imaging may optimize the selection of patients in whom cutting balloons are a good alternative. Both endovascular rescue equipment and resources for emergent operative repair must be available if complex stenoses are being treated.

Branch occlusion can be caused by the incautious use of guide wires or by dissection during ballooning close to a branch takeoff. This has also been reported as a cause of renal embolism or thrombosis in noncatheterized branches. Branch occlusion is seen in 1% to 5% of FMD patients after PTRA procedures.[9,29,106] Still, most of these patients seem to have a favorable outcome.

Thrombosis of the renal artery after endovascular reconstruction in adults is very rare. Bonelli and colleagues reported a minor occurrence of thrombotic material in the renal artery after PTRA in 5 of 105 FMD patients.[106] Main artery occlusions have not been reported, but embolism might occur to both the kidney and the lower extremity.[106,107]

Early Outcome

The published series on the endovascular treatment of FMD encompass more than 1300 patients (see Table 144-1). When analyzing these reports, it is hard to determine which types of FMD have been treated, however. This probably has an effect on outcome. In addition, recommendations on how to present outcome criteria have changed over time, making the interpretation of results even more difficult. The reports also differ in terms of age and gender distribution.

In the combined material, the male-female ratio was 1:4.35, and 179 of 717 cases (25%) involved bilateral FMD. Some studies also reported on the side involved in unilateral disease.[9,29,114] The right renal artery was affected in 83% of cases, and the left renal artery in 17% (left to right ratio, 1:4.6). Only two nonrandomized studies have reported more than 100 patients.[106,115]

The favorable results of endovascular treatment of main artery FMD lesions are obvious in most reports (see Table 144-1). However, it is often difficult to analyze whether branch artery changes were present or whether one or multiple renal arteries were treated. With the smaller balloons and better catheter techniques available today, PTRA can be performed with good results even when branch arteries are affected.[29,106] However, patients with branch artery involvement show less pronounced blood pressure responses and less optimal long-term effects after PTRA.[29]

Comparisons of published series are difficult because of the large variation in selection criteria and length of follow-up. Further, "cure," "improvement," and "benefit" are not always defined according to current guidelines.[116] In the guidelines published by Rundback and associates, "cure" is defined as diastolic blood pressure (DBP) less than 90 mm Hg and systolic blood pressure (SBP) less than 140 mm Hg while not taking antihypertensive medication; "improvement" is defined as DBP less than 90 mm Hg or SBP less than 140 mm Hg on the same or a reduced number of medications, or a reduction in DBP of at least 15 mm Hg with the same or a reduced number of medications; and "benefit" is defined as cure or improvement.[116] Another limitation when comparing series is that it may be unclear whether diuretics and nitrates were considered to be blood pressure–lowering drugs. When evaluating treatment, attention to 24-hour blood pressure measurements is essential, because effects on nocturnal blood pressure are important.

Late Outcome

Follow-up information varies from less than 1 year up to 7 years in the different series (see Table 144-1), and the interpretation of results depends on how they are reported. Some patients with bilateral stenosis were initially treated unilaterally, with the contralateral lesion treated later, in which case the latter should be reported as a redo procedure. Bonelli and colleagues reported that 6% of their 105 patients required redo procedures.[106] Alhadad and coworkers found that 34% of their patients required a second PTRA procedure; however, the majority of these were either planned contralateral PTRAs or redo operations within 6 months of an initial suboptimal PTRA.[29] Only two patients required late redo PTRA after 4 or more years of follow-up. The restenosis rate is between 7% and 23% in series with control angiography during follow-up[107,108]; however, in the majority of cases, restenosis lacked clinical significance. Today most centers perform control angiography only if the initial PTRA procedure was suboptimal or if branches were treated.[9,29] In summary, in patients with a main artery "string of beads" appearance and a good initial effect after PTRA, the long-term durability is good; for more complex and branch lesions, redo procedures are needed more frequently.

◼ SURGICAL TREATMENT

Patient Selection

Surgical revascularization is currently reserved for patients with severe PTRA complications such as thrombosis, perforation, or dissection that cannot be handled with endovascular techniques. Another option in most of these cases is the use of a stent or a stent-graft; the choice of treatment depends on the extension of the lesion and the current renal flow situation. It is therefore important that PTRA procedures be performed only in institutions where such complications can be handled; the treatment of especially complex FMD lesions should be centralized in such institutions. Open surgery should also be considered after repeated failure of PTRA, recoil, and no effect on stenosis or after repeated restenosis following endovascular treatment. In a series of 19 FMD patients with failed PTRA, Wong and associates reported one emergent surgical revascularization due to thrombosis.[117] Among the remaining patients, two underwent nephrectomy and one was revascularized with aortorenal bypass. Among groups experienced with operative treatment after PTRA failure, the results are favorable.[7,71,117-119] FMD patients with large aneurysms should also be considered for open surgery, and in cases of pediatric renal artery stenosis (see "Pediatric Renal Artery Stenosis and Arterial Dysplasia"), a careful choice between open and endovascular treatment should be made.

Techniques

Aortorenal Bypass

Ostial lesions are normally seen in atherosclerotic disease, and the technique for the operative repair of these lesions is covered elsewhere (see Chapter 142: Renovascular Disease: Open Surgical Treatment). In FMD patients, lesions are most commonly located in the distal portion of the main artery, often combined with branch artery stenosis. These can normally be repaired openly with in situ techniques. Many institutions use transverse, subcostal incisions and expose the kidney retroperitoneally or transperitoneally, depending on how much exposure of the aorta is required (Fig. 144-6). In most FMD patients the aorta or iliac arteries can be used for proximal anastomosis without atherosclerosis limiting its placement.

The renal vessels are exposed, and the intended reconstruction is confirmed to be the best option. Thereafter, graft material for the reconstruction, normally either saphenous vein or arterial homograft, needs to be harvested. In the treatment of FMD, autologous vein grafts are usually preferred for reconstructions in adults,[14] and autologous hypogastric artery grafts are favored for bypass in children.[7,120] The hypogastric artery may also be used in adults, especially if several branches must be reconstructed.[71,119,121] Dacron or expanded polytetrafluoroethylene grafts can be used in renal artery lesions but are not the first choice. After resection of a short part of a renal artery, direct anastomosis is often not possible in adult FMD patients.

A generous anastomotic circumference of the saphenous vein can be achieved by using a branch for widening the anastomotic area (Fig. 144-7). For left renal artery reconstruction, mobilization of the renal vein cephalad normally

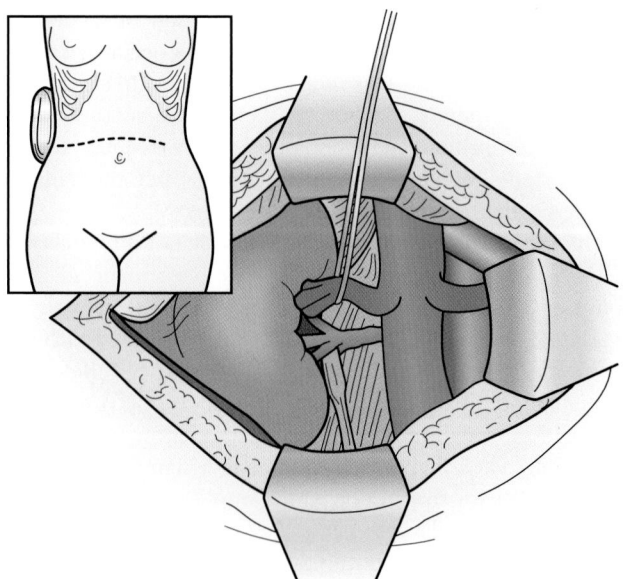

Figure 144-6 Operative approach through a transverse supraumbilical abdominal incision, with an extraperitoneal dissection and reflection of the colon and foregut structures providing exposure of the renal and great vessels.

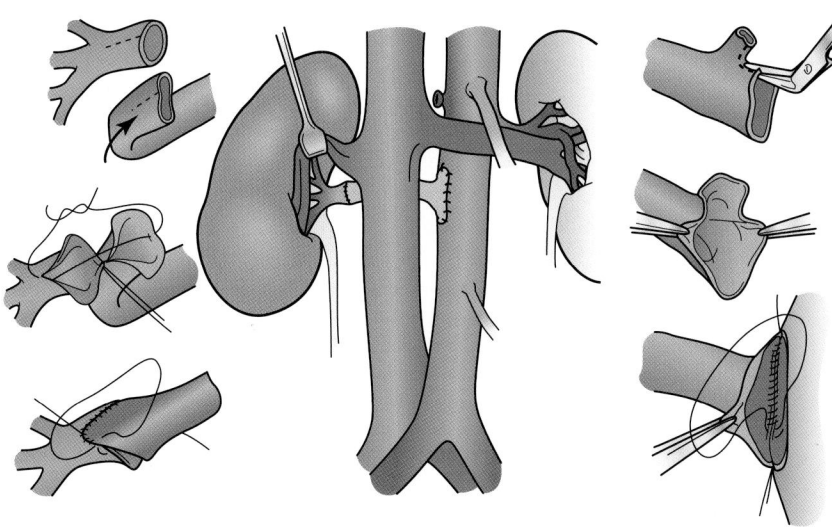

Figure 144-7 Techniques of an end-to-end spatulated renal artery anastomosis and retrocaval placement of the vein graft, with use of a branch of the vein graft to create a wide posteriorly oriented aortic anastomosis.

gives the best exposure of the renal artery. If retrocaval bypass is planned for right renal artery repair, the aortic anastomosis should be constructed on the posterior part of the aorta to avoid the risk of kinking of the graft (see Fig. 144-7). The choice of retrocaval or antecaval positioning of the right renal bypass should be made on a case-by-case basis. Some authors prefer not to pressurize the proximal anastomosis until reconstruction is complete.[70] In patients undergoing in situ reconstructions, some surgeons use cool perfusion during renal ischemia.[71] However, it is hard to maintain such cooling intra-abdominally, and such an effort does not convincingly optimize the outcome for the kidney. If cooling is used, clamping of the renal vein and a small venous incision prevent the cool perfusate from having systemic effects. Thereafter the renal anastomosis is made. Before renal circulation is clamped proximally, adequate diuresis must be established. Many centers use mannitol 12.5 to 20 g intravenously before renal ischemia to optimize diuresis. Mannitol also acts as a specific hydroxyl free radical scavenger. Vascular clamps are placed gently on the distal renal artery. An end-to-end anastomosis is preferred, and it is spatulated to reduce the risk of stricture (see Fig. 144-7). Intraoperative assessment is imperative. Many surgeons assess the reconstruction by measuring the volume of blood flow with ultrasound techniques. If the volume of flow is good, no further intraoperative assessment is required. Intraoperative duplex ultrasonography is reported to be valuable.[71,122] Many centers do not routinely perform an early postreconstruction angiography.

In hypertensive FMD patients in whom an aneurysm constitutes part of the indication for surgery, suturing of the aneurysm (aneurysmorrhaphy) is normally not adequate. A saphenous vein graft interposition is usually required.[123,124]

Autotransplantation

Autotransplantation and renal repair in FMD patients should be considered in the following situations: reoperation for failed renal artery repair, failed endovascular reconstruction after several attempts, multisegmental arterial dysplasia, and a single kidney and stenosis in several renal arteries.

Current indications for autotransplantation and ex vivo repair have changed somewhat owing to refinements in endovascular techniques. PTRA has shown acceptable results in branch artery stenoses. Autotransplantation of the kidney was originally devised as a method for managing patients with high ureteric injury,[125] and it was first used in renovascular hypertension in 1964.[126] Today, fewer patients with FMD are treated surgically, implying that an increasing proportion of patients requiring surgical management have more complex disease, with a multisegmental distribution in not only first-order but also second-order branches. Ex vivo repair and autotransplantation, placing the kidney in the iliac fossa, are often required in the same manner as in renal homotransplantation.[71,119,127-129]

Many institutions preferentially use transverse left or right subcostal retroperitoneal exposure for mobilization of the kidneys. Good access is also obtained with a median or paramedian incision. The renal vasculature is exposed, and the ureter with its surrounding small vessels is freed to at least the level of the iliac vessels. The ureter can be divided and reimplanted in the bladder. This allows optimal separate benchwork after the renal vessels are divided and the kidney is cooled with perfusate. The right kidney has a shorter vein, and a small patch of surrounding vena cava facilitates later vein anastomosis, without causing any significant stenosis of the vena cava. The right renal artery is exposed on the backside of the vena cava as long as required. The artery is ligated first; thereafter the vein is controlled.

The kidney is perfused with saline, Ringer's solution, or Wisconsin solution, normally at a temperature of 4°C, until the venous effluent is clear. This normally requires 300 to 500 mL of perfusate. All renal arteries should be perfused. The kidney is kept in Ringer's solution at 4°C and some ice slush; thereafter, further meticulous dissection can be undertaken.

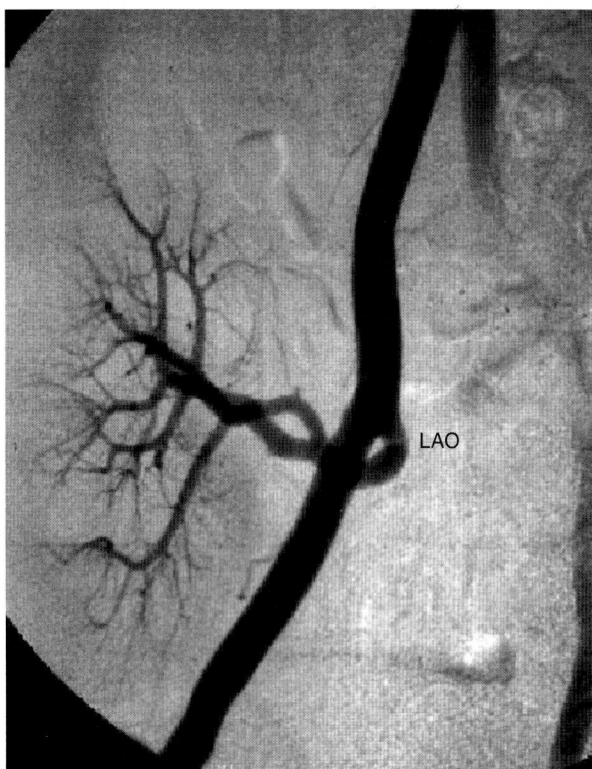

Figure 144-8 Control angiogram after autotransplantation with an arterial allograft (internal iliac artery) and three-branch reconstruction. Slight, insignificant hemodynamic stenosis is seen at the proximal reanastomosis of the internal iliac artery.

Dissection into the renal hilum should be avoided if possible, because the numerous small veins may constitute a challenge. Depending on what type of repair that is planned, further autologous material for vessel repair has to be harvested: parts of the proximal "healthy" renal artery, saphenous vein with or without branches, or internal iliac artery with several branches. The risk of unidentified renal arteries is reduced today with better imaging, but during cool perfusion of the kidney especially, the renal poles should be controlled so that blanching of the entire kidney is achieved.

After reconstruction of the renal vessels, reimplantation of the kidney in the left or right iliac fossa is performed. If the ureter has not been divided, it is important to avoid rotating the kidney when positioning it in the iliac fossa. Normally the vein anastomosis is performed first, and the reconstructed renal artery is then anastomosed either end to side to the external or common iliac artery or end to end to the internal iliac artery (Fig. 144-8).

Results of Open Surgery

The published series on open surgery (see Table 144-2) encompass more than 1100 reconstructed patients and include reports on aortorenal bypass,[25,70,121,122,130-132] branch artery reconstructions,[71,127] and autotransplantation.[119,121,129,133] In spite of these different methods, the early outcome is excellent.

The proportion of cured patients has been somewhat lower during the last 10 years, however, owing to older patients, longer duration of hypertension before surgery, and more complex lesions because PTRA is now used for main artery lesions. The different failure rates among series can be explained by the varying complexity of the cases reported but may also reflect an overly optimistic expectation that reconstruction should be successful in patients with small kidneys with branch artery or multisegmental lesions. The number of nephrectomies required is low.[132-134]

Complications of Open Surgery

Only a few fatal outcomes have been reported after FMD surgery in adults.[71,132,133] The overall morbidity from surgery is between 19% and 28%, mainly caused by minor complications such as urinary tract infection and postoperative pneumonia.[25,132]

Early postoperative occlusion after FMD is seen in 3.8% to 13% of cases, and it occurs more often with venous grafts than with arterial autografts.[25,70,120,132,134] It is more frequent after the repair of renal arteries with small dimension or branches with low flow. Optimal intraoperative assessment of the reconstruction is of the utmost importance to ensure that no technical defects will induce graft thrombosis.[70,71,122]

If pain over the kidney increases, diuresis is reduced (which is often hard to evaluate because mannitol has been given and ischemia time differs), or episodic hypertension occurs during the postoperative course, graft occlusion should be ruled out. This can be achieved with ultrasound performed by an experienced ultrasonographer, conventional angiography, or, perhaps as a first choice today, contrast CTA or MRA. Symptoms may be minor, however, which is reflected by the fact that Reiher and coworkers found 9 unsuspected thromboses in 90 reconstructed patients on routine postoperative angiography.[132] Re-establishment of the renal circulation should be attempted, depending on both the time elapsed between the supposed occlusion and its diagnosis and the collateral circulation, which often helps in delaying total, nonreversible ischemia. Rescue surgery can be considered several days after an occlusion if the renal parenchyma is enhanced by contrast examinations.

Late restenosis has become less common because most anastomoses are now made in an ovoid shape. Restenosis has been reported in 0% to 16% of patients[25,120,121,132] and in less than 8% of vein graft bypasses.[70,135] It is even rarer in arterial allografts[127,136]; branch artery reconstructions also show low rates of restenosis.[71,127]

The need for redo procedures in FMD patients differs, depending on the technique used and the complexity of the initial lesion. After mainly aortorenal bypasses, Novick and associates reported on one redo reconstruction among 120 patients.[120] Reiher and coworkers reported redo procedures in 15 of 101 patients during a 3-year follow-up.[132] Andersen and colleagues reported mainly on branch reconstructions in 40 patients and performed six redos—three on the contralateral kidney and three revisions of the bypass.[25] Chiche and

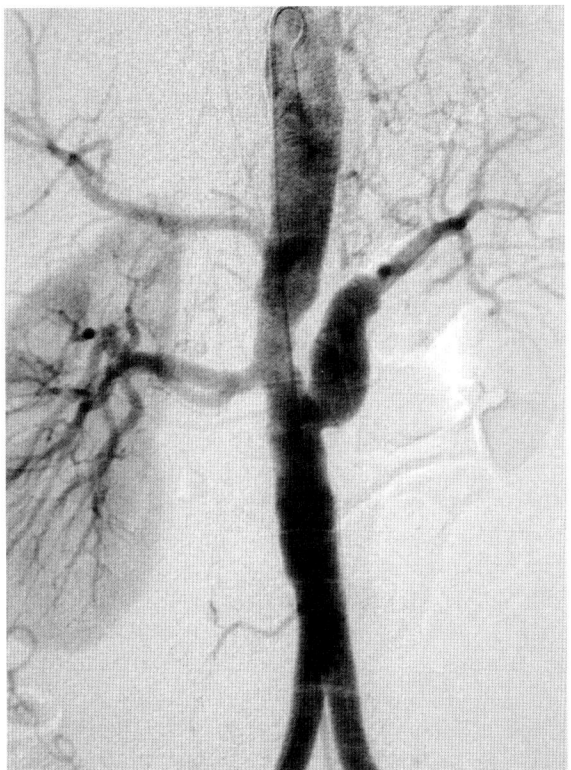

Figure 144-9 Ectatic vein bypass after an aortorenal bypass 6 years earlier. No further dilatation has occurred during the 10-year follow-up.

associates had a redo frequency of 3 out of 30 autotransplanted FMD patients.[119] Secondary treatment using endovascular technology has shown good results because a restenosis treated by a redo is more fibrotic.[29,71,122,132]

Late vein graft dilatations were documented in 20% to 44% of patients in early series of aortorenal bypasses in adults.[135,137] Normally, a nonprogressive increase in vein diameter is seen (Fig. 144-9). Vein graft dilatation has not been reported in series from the last decade,[71,122,132] perhaps reflecting the fact that FMD patients are now older and have a longer duration of hypertension before diagnosis and treatment than in early series.

Renal failure is very uncommon after surgery in FMD patients.[25,70,71,117,122,133]

PEDIATRIC RENAL ARTERY STENOSIS AND ARTERIAL DYSPLASIA

Renovascular disease is the most common cause of hypertension in children after thoracic aortic coarctation and renal parenchymal disease (Fig. 144-10).[7] Approximately 8% to 10% of all pediatric cases of secondary hypertension are due to renovascular disease, and pediatric renal artery stenosis may occur in many different conditions, including FMD, developmental renal artery stenosis, vascular neurofibromatosis type 1, Moyamoya, vasculitis such as Takayasu's disease, Alagille syndrome, and Williams syndrome.[7,19,138,139]

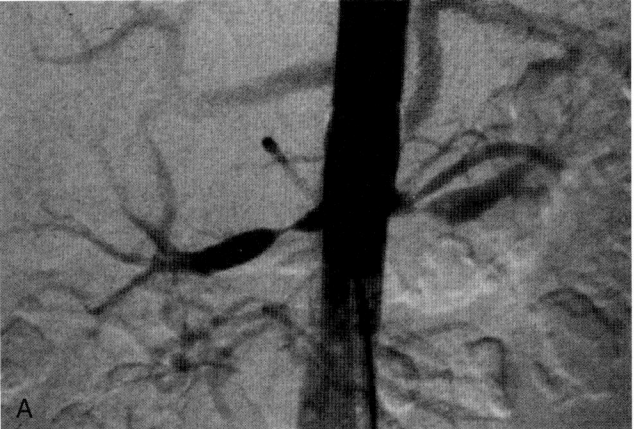

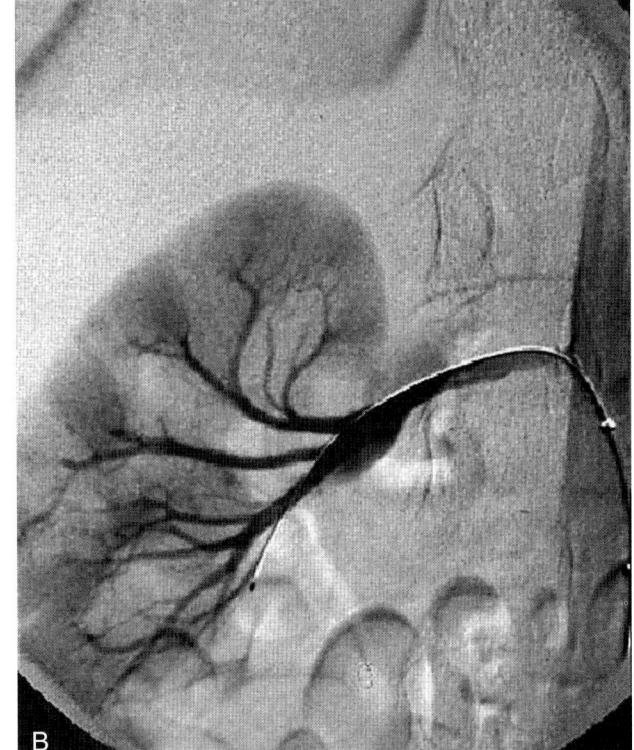

Figure 144-10 A, Bilateral renal artery stenosis in a 6-year-old boy with tapered narrowings close to the takeoff from the aorta. Hypoplasia was ruled out. **B,** He was treated first on the right side, after which the left stenosis was treated. He required a redo of the right lesion 4 years after the initial treatment.

Developmental Renal Artery Stenosis

Up to 40% of children with renovascular hypertension have developmental renal artery lesions with midaortic syndrome and coexisting lesions in both the mesenteric and carotid arteries.[7,139-142] Midaortic dysplastic syndrome is a narrowing of the most distal thoracic and first abdominal part of the aorta. Midaortic changes can also be seen in pediatric patients

Section **18** Renal and Mesenteric Disease

with vascular neurofibromatosis type 1[49] or Takayasu's disease.[19,21,143] In African Americans, Africans, and Asians, arterial dysplasia and developmental midaortic syndrome are uncommon. In Caucasians, congenital causes are considered important in the development of arterial dysplasia and mid-aortic syndrome. Histology of most of these lesions reveals abnormalities in more than one of the three layers of the vessel, with sparse medial tissue and intimal fibroplasia being most common.[7,118]

During the fourth week of embryologic development, the paired dorsal aortas fuse, and all but one of the lateral branches to each kidney regress, normally leaving a solitary renal artery. Events occurring at this time that alter the transition of mesenchyma to medial smooth muscle tissue or its later condensation and growth may cause aortic or visceral artery abnormalities (see Chapter 2: Embryology). Operative treatment of fibrodysplastic renovascular hypertension associated with aortic hypoplasia or midaortic dysplastic syndrome consists of complex thoracoaortic bypasses with concomitant renal artery reconstruction.[7,118,141,144]

Endovascular Treatment in Children

Published series on endovascular treatment in children and adolescents total 230 individuals, the majority having dysplastic lesions, but a few having diseases other than FMD are included (Table 144-5). The gender distribution in children is equal, in contrast to the female preponderance in adults.

Technical success rates are high in published series, with cure or improvement reported in about 90% of cases. Because children have a greater tendency than adults for vasospasm during endovascular procedures, many centers give small doses of nitroglycerin at every exchange of catheters or wires to minimize this problem. In contrast to adult renal artery procedures, thrombosis or embolization into the renal parenchyma occurs in children,[27] making heparinization mandatory.

The majority of patients in the published series have medial or perimedial dysplasia (see Table 144-4); however, the "string of beads" type of lesion is not frequent in children. As reported by Shroff and colleagues, long-segment stenosis occurs in 60%, ostial stenosis in 22%, ostial and long-segment stenosis in 12%, aneurysmal dilatation in 6%, and webs in 6%.[27] McTaggert and coworkers reported on 17 children, 8 of whom had ostial lesions; the main renal artery was affected in 8, and 3 lesions were seen in branches.[145]

After ballooning of a stenosis, the frequency of recoil is high. If this persists after more prolonged dilatation, oversized or cutting balloons should not be used until it has been determined whether the artery is dysplastic or hypoplastic. The use of oversized or cutting balloons may lead to an increased risk of rupture, especially in a hypoplastic artery. Patients with a suspected hypoplastic renal artery or a complex stenosis should be considered for open surgical repair. In very young children, cure should not always be the aim. PTRA can be repeated when the artery is larger, facilitating later rescue with open surgical repair if catastrophic complications occur.

Long-term data on PTRA in children, based on follow-up from 13 months to 12 years, demonstrate variations in outcome (see Table 144-5). Benefit is reported with a high frequency, and restenosis is reported in 27% to 33%.[27,138] Shroff and colleagues reported an especially high rate of restenosis in 10 stented children.[27] They also reported that repair of 7 of 33 main artery lesions failed, and 12 of 14 branch lesions required redo PTRA. These findings are supported by other groups.[146] Follow-up examinations are recommended, especially if the initial treatment was for a complex or branch stenosis. A high rate of failure is also reported after treatment of multisegmental stenosis.[138] These results are encouraging

Table 144-5 Results of Percutaneous Transluminal Renal Angioplasty for Fibromuscular Dysplasia in Children

| Series | Year | Number of Patients | Gender | | Results (%) | | | | Follow-up (mo) |
			Male	Female	Technical Success	Cure	Improvement	Failure	
Fallo et al.[168]	1985	5	1	4	100	80	20	0	15
Mali et al.[146]	1987	12	4	8	100	42	25	33	12
Simunic et al.[169]	1990	4	3	1	100	25	75	0	60
Casalini et al.[170]	1995	36	NA	NA	94	94	0	6	24
Sharma et al.[171]	1996	24	13	11	92	92	0	8	33
Tyagi et al.[19]	1997	35	11	24	91	34	57	7	41
Courtel et al.[138]	1998	16	12	4	94	56	13	19	30
O'Neill[141]	1998	10	5	5	100	30	10	60	96
McTaggart et al.[145]	2000	2	1	1	100	0	50	50	18
Fossali et al.[172]	2000	3	1	2	100	33	66	0	60
Estepa et al.[143]	2000	5	2	3	100	100	0	0	78
Hughes et al.[165]	2004	9	7	2	100	33	44	22	13
Alfonzo et al.[173]	2006	11	7	4	100	37	45	18	138
Shroff et al.[27]	2006	33	22	11	79	21	57	21	144
Bayazit et al.[8]	2007	16	6	10	100	31	50	19	(84)*
Towbin et al.[174]	2007	4	0	4	100	50	50	0	21
Huang et al.[152]	2008	5	3	2	100	100	0	0	57
Totals		**230**	**98**	**96**					

*Estimated.
NA, not available.

but must be weighed against the results of open surgical repair in children. Because series are small, centralization of treatment is recommended. Treatment of very young children to achieve a moderate improvement may allow open surgery to be delayed until they are older, when the procedure can be performed with more perfection and produce better long-term results.

Open Surgery for Pediatric Renovascular Hypertension

A high proportion of pediatric FMD patients has ostial lesions. In the University of Michigan Pediatric Renovascular Group's report, 12 of 97 children undergoing open operation had multisegmental disease, 6 had aneurysms, 70 had ostial lesions, 15 had main artery changes, and 18 had branch involvement.[7] Unilateral stenosis was seen in 65 children and bilateral stenosis in 47 children. Few girls younger than 10 years were treated; at that age, boys were three times more likely than girls to be affected. For children between the ages of 10 and 17, no gender difference was noted.

Midaortic syndrome is frequent in many reported series on renal artery surgery in children: 17 of 50,[141] 20 of 78,[139] 4 of 10,[142] and 32 of 97.[7] Patch aortoplasty or thoracoabdominal bypass has been performed with about the same frequency. Many of these children have renal artery ostial lesions facilitating direct reimplantation into the aorta.[7,118]

Table 144-6 reports on published series covering 404 children and adolescents undergoing open surgery. Early series included a large proportion of patients (40% to 50%) who underwent nephrectomy,[147-149] whereas Stanley and coworkers recently reported on 97 children with irreparable renal disease (n = 11) or unplanned nephrectomy (n = 1) due to technical failure of a planned reconstruction.[7] The University of Michigan group has avoided aortorenal bypass with saphenous vein grafts owing to aneurysm formation in 6 of 25 pediatric vein bypasses.[150,151] Lacombe reported on three cases of aneurysmal dilatation requiring redo surgery and another two cases under observation out of 23 pediatric vein bypasses.[118] Huang and colleagues recently reported on one case of aneurysm development among 12 pediatric venous bypasses

requiring redo procedures.[152] Centers of excellence advocate direct aortorenal anastomosis if feasible, and the University of Michigan experience showed that direct anastomosis was possible in 41 of 58 recent reconstructions.[7] In 83 children, Lacombe used direct anastomosis in 17 cases and splenorenal anastomosis in 22.[118] Arterial allograft is recommended, and the internal iliac artery is usually preferred over a saphenous vein bypass.[144]

The procedural mortality after renal surgery in children is low, and few children develop renal impairment requiring dialysis. Long-term (1 to 10 years) follow-up shows excellent results, with surgery beneficial in about 95% of patients and a minimal restenosis rate following reconstruction, in spite of children's growth (see Table 144-6). In recent series, the number of redo procedures is low. In 83 children, Lacombe reported redos of three aneurysmal vein bypasses, two contralateral cases of renal artery stenosis requiring surgery, and two patients with restenosis 3 and 12 years after the initial reconstruction of aortorenal ostial stenosis.[118] Piercy and associates reported on 25 operated children, 2 of whom required early redos; there was one nephrectomy and one saphenous vein bypass revision, both of which had a favorable effect on hypertension.[144] No late failures were seen. Stanley and coworkers reported 19 redo procedures among 97 operated children, 9 being nephrectomies.[7] Three of Huang and associates' 22 patients required redo procedures—one with PTRA and two with open surgery.[152] Centralization of the operative treatment of children is required.

FIBROMUSCULAR DYSPLASIA AND ANEURYSM

A large proportion of FMD patients exhibit the "string of beads" appearance, with small aneurysmal areas interspaced by webs in the renal artery. "Macroaneurysms" with obvious aneurysmal development are not infrequent, however. The University of Düsseldorf group reported on 11 cases of renal artery aneurysm among 101 FMD patients with renovascular hypertension and 48 FMD patients treated for renal artery aneurysm.[123,132] Murray and coworkers observed aneurysms in

Table 144-6 Results of Open Surgery for Fibromuscular Dysplasia in Children

| Series | Year | Number of Patients | Gender | | Results (%) | | | Follow-up (mo) |
			Male	Female	Cure	Improvement	Failure	
Stoney et al.[147]	1975	14	8	6	86	7	7	120
Lawson et al.[148]	1977	25	12	13	68	24	8	48
Novick et al.[149]	1978	27	13	14	60	19	19	120
Martinez et al.[175]	1990	56	33	23	66	23	11	91
O'Neill[141]	1998	50	24	26	70	26	4	96
Lacombe[118]	2003	83	49	34	87	5	8	112
Chalmers et al.[142]	2000	10	5	5	70	20	10	24
Piercy et al.[144]	2005	25	12	13	36	56	8	46
Stanley et al.[7]	2006	97	39	58	70	27	3	50
Huang et al.[152]	2008	17	(9)*	(8)*	57	39	4	68
Totals		**404**	**204**	**200**				

*Estimated.

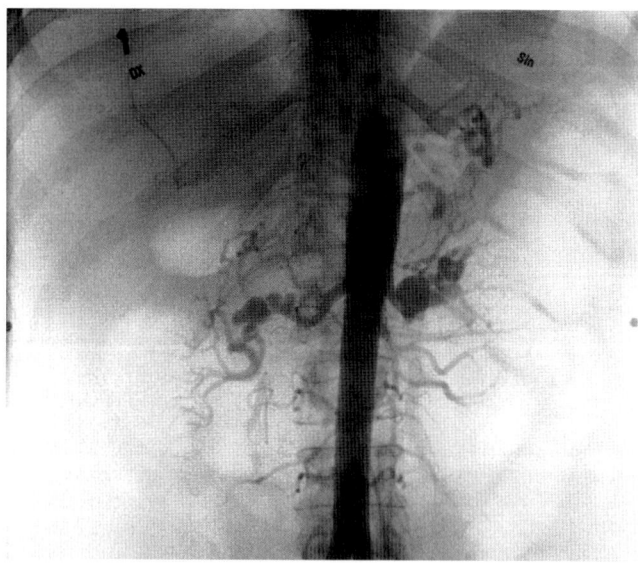

Figure 144-11 Bilateral fibromuscular dysplasia and aneurysm formation in both renal arteries. Hypertension was fairly well controlled on two drugs. No progression of the aneurysms or hypertension has been seen during 15 years of conservative treatment.

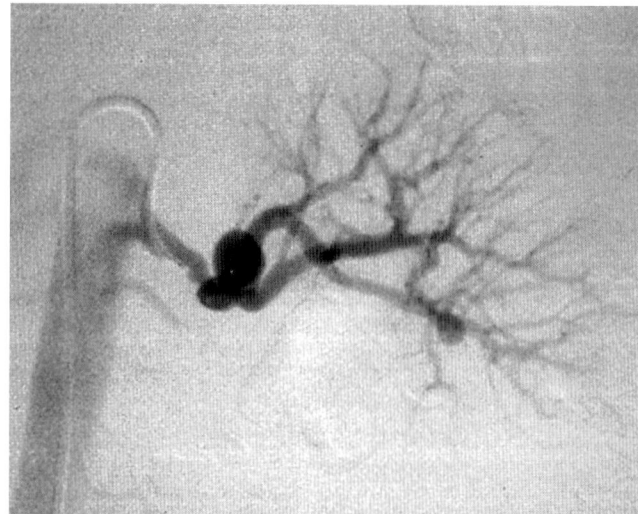

Figure 144-12 Female patient with a fibromuscular dysplastic lesion treated with endovascular dilatation. The medium-sized aneurysm at the branch site has decreased in size during follow-up, and the hypertension has clearly improved.

12 of 68 FMD patients.[127] Vuong and associates found that of 131 histologically examined renal arteries in FMD patients, 35 specimens showed aneurysms measuring 0.5 to 2 cm.[26] Most renal artery aneurysms have a low risk of rupture, however (see Chapter 145: Renovascular Disease: Aneurysms and Arteriovenous Fistulae), and only a few ruptured FMD lesions have been reported.[104,138] How FMD-related aneurysms measuring 1 to 2 cm should be handled is uncertain. Conservative treatment may be successful (Fig. 144-11). If additional risk factors are present, treatment may be justified. Aneurysms larger than 2 cm should probably be excluded.[71,122,132] Among pediatric FMD patients undergoing open surgery, renal artery aneurysms are reported in 5% to 12%.[7,118,144]

Endovascular experience is limited. In some patients with renovascular hypertension, small aneurysms may shrink after successful PTRA of stenotic areas (Fig. 144-12). Favorable outcomes have been reported with both embolization[49,153] and the use of stent-grafts.[154,155]

SELECTED KEY REFERENCES

Bonelli FS, McKusick MA, Textor SC, Kos BS, Stanson AW, Johnson CM, Sheedy PF II, Welch TJ, Schriger A. Renal artery angioplasty: technical results and clinical outcome in 320 patients. *Mayo Clin Proc.* 1995;70:1041-1052.
Large, well-reported series of the endovascular treatment of FMD.

Crutchley TA, Pearce JD, Craven TE, Edwards MS, Dean RH, Hansen KJ. Branch renal artery repair with cold perfusion protection. *J Vasc Surg.* 2007;46:405-412.
Open surgery in complex cases can achieve good results in experienced hands.

Lacombe M, Ricco J-B. Surgical revascularization of renal artery after complicated or failed percutaneous transluminal renal angioplasty. *J Vasc Surg.* 2006;44:537-544.
Open surgery after failed endovascular treatment is possible, with good results.

Slovut DP, Olin JW. Fibromuscular dysplasia. *N Engl J Med.* 2004; 350:1862-1871.
Excellent review of FMD.

Stanley JC, Criado E, Upchurch GR Jr, Brophy PD, Cho KJ, Rectenwald JE; Michigan Pediatric Renovascular Group, Kershaw DB, Williams DM, Berguer R, Henke PK, Wakefield TW. Pediatric renovascular hypertension: 132 primary and 30 secondary operations in 97 children. *J Vasc Surg.* 2006;44:1219-1229.
Largest series of arterial fibrodysplasia in children.

REFERENCES

The reference list can be found on the companion Expert Consult Web site at *www.expertconsult.com.*

Renovascular Disease: Aneurysms and Arteriovenous Fistulae

Keith D. Calligaro and Matthew J. Dougherty

Renal artery aneurysms and renal arteriovenous fistulae (AVFs) are rare entities, but they are encountered frequently enough that vascular surgeons need to be well acquainted with the natural history, diagnosis, and management of these lesions. Endovascular interventions represent the newest advances in the treatment of some of these lesions. Aneurysms and AVFs are discussed separately because they rarely occur concomitantly and their clinical course and treatment differ.

■ RENAL ARTERY ANEURYSMS

Epidemiology

Even in referral centers, few vascular surgeons have extensive experience with the clinical management of renal artery aneurysms.[1,2] Autopsy studies have revealed an incidence of 0.01% to 0.09%, which is probably an underestimation, because renal artery aneurysms may be small, intrarenal, or not specifically sought.[1,3] In two angiography studies, renal artery aneurysms were documented in 0.73% (7 of 965) to 0.97% (83 of 8525) of arteriograms; in a more recent computed tomographic angiographic study, the incidence was 0.7% (6 of 862).[4-6] Conversely, these reports may overestimate the prevalence of these lesions. If renal artery aneurysms were present in almost 1% of patients undergoing abdominal aortography, vascular surgeons would be expected to have a far greater experience diagnosing and treating these lesions than has been reported to date. At Pennsylvania Hospital in Philadelphia, we documented renal artery aneurysms in only 0.12% (1 of 845) of abdominal aortograms. Renal artery aneurysms are bilateral in about 10% of cases.[1,5] If fibrodysplastic cases are omitted, there is an equal incidence in males and females.[1,2,7]

Because of the lack of controlled data, controversy persists regarding the indications for repair of asymptomatic renal artery aneurysms. The optimal method of repair is also controversial. Types of renal artery aneurysms, their clinical manifestations, indications for repair, and techniques of both traditional surgical and newer endovascular interventions are reviewed here.

Pathogenesis

Types of renal artery aneurysms include true (saccular and fusiform), false, dissecting, and intrarenal aneurysms.

True Aneurysms

More than 90% of true renal artery aneurysms are extraparenchymal.[2,8-10] The peak incidence is in patients between the ages of 40 and 60 years. Stanley and colleagues have suggested that true aneurysms are probably due to either atherosclerosis or a congenital defect.[2,10] Although arteriosclerotic changes have been identified in most aneurysms in patients with multiple lesions, this is not a uniform finding, suggesting that arteriosclerosis may not be the most important factor in the genesis of renal artery aneurysms. These aneurysms are more likely due to a congenital medial degenerative process with weakness of the elastic lamina.[7,10] Lesions typically occur at the primary or secondary renal artery bifurcations and are rarely confined only to the main trunk of the renal artery. As discussed later, this finding makes surgical repair challenging.

Approximately 75% of true renal artery aneurysms are saccular. This type of renal artery aneurysm is usually less than 5 cm in diameter,[11] although some as large as 9 cm have been reported.[9,12,13] Saccular aneurysms occur almost invariably at the main renal artery bifurcation.[14] Fusiform aneurysms are usually associated with atherosclerosis or are a result of a post-stenotic dilatation distal to a hemodynamically significant renal artery stenosis, the latter resulting from atherosclerosis or fibromuscular disease.[7,8,14,15] Fusiform aneurysms are generally less than 2 cm in diameter and usually affect the main renal artery trunk.[8]

Arterial fibrodysplasia is often a direct contributor to the development of an aneurysm.[2,10] Medial fibroplasia is typically associated with multiple stenoses and post-stenotic dilatation of the distal two thirds of the renal artery. Renal artery aneurysms in association with fibromuscular dysplasia are generally only a few millimeters in diameter. The typical angiographic appearance of a renal artery involved with medial fibroplasia is a "string of beads." Larger aneurysms can also occur, however, and in one study, renal artery macroaneurysms were found in 9.2% of adults with fibromuscular dysplasia.[10]

A rare cause of renal artery aneurysms is Ehlers-Danlos syndrome. This disorder is associated with extreme arterial fragility and spontaneous rupture and is discussed in Chapter 76 (Vasculitis and Other Arteriopathies).[16]

False Aneurysms (Pseudoaneurysms)

False aneurysms of the renal artery arise from blunt or penetrating trauma and occasionally from iatrogenic causes such as renal artery catheterization. They represent contained ruptures of the renal artery, with only inflammatory and fibrous tissue encasing the leak.

Dissections

Spontaneous dissections confined to the renal artery that do not arise from the adjacent aorta are rare; however, primary dissections causing pseudoaneurysms affect the renal arteries more than any other peripheral artery.[2,14,17-20] Poutasse[14] and Stanley and coworkers[10] reported that 14 of 57 cases of renal artery aneurysms were due to spontaneous dissection. An intimal defect of the renal artery due to atherosclerosis is probably the underlying cause of spontaneous renal artery dissection causing aneurysm, along with dysplastic renovascular disease and trauma.[8] The incidence of dissection in patients with fibrodysplastic renal arteries ranges from 0.5% to 9.0%.[2,17] Dissection often extends into the branches of the renal artery and may pose particularly challenging reconstruction problems.

Traumatic renal artery dissection can occur secondary to blunt abdominal trauma or catheter-induced injury. Blunt trauma accounts for the higher prevalence of dissection in men and is more likely to result in right-sided injuries, possibly because of ptosis-related physical stresses affecting the renal pedicle.[2] Blunt trauma can cause renal artery dissection by either severe stretching of the artery, with fracture of the intima, or compression of the artery against the vertebra. Renal artery dissection caused by guide wires or catheters can occur but is rare, being observed in only 4 of 2200 selective renal artery arteriograms.[17]

Intrarenal Aneurysms

Fewer than 10% of renal artery aneurysms are intraparenchymal.[9,10] Intrarenal aneurysms are usually multiple and may be congenital, associated with collagen vascular disease, or post-traumatic. They may be associated with AVFs, possibly as a result of spontaneous closure of a fistula. Intrarenal aneurysms can occur with polyarteritis nodosa and are usually in the renal cortex.[21,22]

Clinical Manifestations and Diagnosis

Most renal artery aneurysms are asymptomatic and are found on imaging studies such as arteriography, ultrasonography, or computed tomography (CT) performed to investigate other intra-abdominal pathology.[2,13,23] Magnetic resonance angiography (MRA) can also delineate renal artery aneurysms.[92] Clinical manifestations of renal artery aneurysms include rupture, hypertension, pain, and hematuria. In one series, only 11 of 32 patients (34%) who underwent surgery for renal artery aneurysms presented with symptoms.[13]

The most dreaded complication of renal artery aneurysm is rupture. Patients with this complication present with manifestations similar to those of other intra-abdominal arterial ruptures, including syncope, abdominal or flank pain, abdom-

inal distention, and possibly a pulsatile mass. Occasionally, an intact renal artery aneurysm presents with abdominal or flank pain, discomfort, or fullness—symptoms that are presumed to reflect acute aneurysmal expansion.

Renal artery aneurysms may be associated with severe hypertension. Macroaneurysms were found in 2.5% of arteriograms performed for the evaluation of hypertension.[10] Renal artery aneurysms may cause renovascular hypertension by distal embolization with segmental hypoperfusion and renin-mediated vasoconstriction and fluid retention. Compression of an adjacent renal artery branch or luminal stenosis due to extensive thrombus may also lead to renin-mediated hypertension. Frequently, significant renal artery stenosis causes a post-stenotic fusiform aneurysm, and the renal artery stenosis is responsible for the hypertension. Saccular and intrarenal aneurysms are much less likely to be associated with hypertension.

Patients with renal artery aneurysms caused by dissection may present with severe flank pain, hematuria, or acute hypertension, although most dissections are asymptomatic. An intravenous pyelogram may reveal nonfunction or diminished function of the involved kidney, but this is rarely the first test ordered unless urolithiasis is considered a likely cause of the symptoms. Contrast angiography or MRA is essential to detect dissection.

Intrarenal aneurysms may rupture into calices.[3] In addition to pain, microscopic or gross hematuria may occur. Similarly, renal artery aneurysms may rarely cause obstruction of the collecting system. Although main renal artery aneurysms may be large, they are usually not near enough to the caliceal system to cause obstruction. Intrarenal aneurysms tend to be too small to cause significant collecting duct obstruction. However, a 9-cm renal artery aneurysm has been documented to cause hydronephrosis.[12]

Indications for Intervention

Indications to repair a renal artery aneurysm are related to the risk of rupture, hypertension, acute dissection, and other clinical symptoms.

Rupture

Rupture of a renal artery aneurysm is an indication for emergency intervention, as it is for virtually any arterial aneurysm. Probably less than 3% of renal artery aneurysms rupture.[2,10] This complication is associated with a mortality rate of approximately 10% in males and nonpregnant females.[2,10,24,25] In a hemodynamically stable patient, an emergent CT scan may reveal the pathology and allow the surgeon to plan the operative repair. However, if a hypotensive elderly patient presents to the emergency department with abdominal pain and a tender, distended abdomen and does not respond to fluid resuscitation, emergency exploration for a presumptive ruptured abdominal aneurysm may be indicated.

Prevention of rupture is the most common indication for intervention in cases of asymptomatic renal artery aneurysms.

Traditionally, repair has been recommended for renal artery aneurysms greater than 2 cm in diameter.[8,15] The likelihood of rupture of a renal artery aneurysm is controversial because the natural history has not been delineated. Most reports are retrospective reviews of incidentally discovered intact renal artery aneurysms in autopsy series or collections of ruptured aneurysms that lack full details concerning their size and the presence or absence of calcification. Harrow and Sloane reported one of the highest rates of rupture of renal artery aneurysms, noting 14 ruptures in 100 cases.[26] In another series of 126 renal artery aneurysms, 6 ruptured.[27] Many authorities believe that there are no good data to support the belief that the larger the renal artery aneurysm, the more likely it is to rupture.[1,2,8,10,28]

Most other series of asymptomatic renal artery aneurysms in men and nonpregnant women report a much lower incidence of rupture. Only 1 of 62 patients with aneurysms 4 cm in diameter or smaller ruptured after follow-up from 1 to 17 years.[37] None of 19 small aneurysms in another series ruptured.[24] A group of 21 patients was observed for an average of 3 years without rupture.[23] In another series of 18 patients with renal artery aneurysms less than 2.6 cm who were followed for 1 to 16 years, none ruptured.[1] There were no ruptures in a series of 32 patients (who eventually underwent surgery) with renal artery aneurysms that ranged from 0.7 to 9 cm.[13] Of 83 renal artery aneurysms found on arteriography and followed up without surgery,[28] none ruptured or became symptomatic after a mean of 4.3 years.[5] In a pooled analysis, there were no ruptures in more than 200 renal artery aneurysms observed for up to 17 years.[7] One must keep in mind that there was an obvious selection bias in the follow-up of many of these aneurysms (i.e., small size), and many of the larger aneurysms were repaired.

Besides size, other factors may play a role in the consideration of elective surgery for asymptomatic renal artery aneurysms. Calcification of the aneurysm has been thought to protect against rupture. Poutasse suggested that a heavily calcified renal artery aneurysm may be less likely to rupture than a noncalcified or minimally calcified one.[15] In a review of cases through 1959, 14 of 100 noncalcified aneurysms ruptured.[26] In a more recent series, 15 of 18 ruptured renal artery aneurysms were noncalcified.[29] In a series of 62 solitary aneurysms less than 4 cm in diameter, however, one third were not calcified, and only one aneurysm in the entire series ruptured in 1 to 17 years of follow-up.[25] Because of these conflicting data, some authorities believe that the presence or absence of calcification is not relevant when predicting the risk of rupture.[2]

Most authorities agree, however, that pregnancy is associated with a significantly increased risk of rupture of a renal artery aneurysm.[2,10,13,30] Pregnancy may increase the risk of rupture because of the hyperdynamic state, with increased blood volume and cardiac output; hormonal influences on the aneurysm; and increased intra-abdominal pressure due to the gravid uterus.[1,10] Cohen and Shamash reported 18 cases of rupture during pregnancy.[30] In another series of 18 patients having surgery for renal artery aneurysms, the only two rup-

tures were in females at childbirth; both of these aneurysms measured only 1 cm in diameter.[1] In a review of 43 ruptured renal artery aneurysms, 81% occurred in women; 21 of the 35 women in this series were younger than 40 years, and 18 were pregnant. Of the 18 aneurysms of known size, 3 ruptured when they were smaller than 2 cm..[36]

Of note, rupture of renal artery aneurysms in pregnancy has been associated with a maternal mortality rate of 55% and a fetal death rate of 85%.[30,31] Risk of renal artery rupture is small, however, even in pregnant women. In a series of 19,600 autopsies of pregnant women, no ruptured renal artery aneurysms were found.[27] This report did not indicate the number of unruptured renal artery aneurysms found in this population, so the risk of rupture remains uncertain. Regardless, we agree with others that there are enough data to support an aggressive surgical approach for pregnant women with renal artery aneurysms of any size.

Essentially all false renal artery aneurysms of recent onset should be repaired because of the high likelihood of rupture.[8] In the rare case of a chronic, contained rupture of a small false aneurysm that is found months or years later, and the pseudoaneurysm has thrombosed, careful follow-up is probably all that is warranted. Similarly, renal artery aneurysms due to fibrodysplastic disease may be associated with a higher risk of rupture because of the thin-walled nature of these aneurysms, although firm data are lacking.[8] Certainly, renal artery aneurysms in men or in women beyond childbearing age that are less than 2 cm in diameter and associated with fibrodysplastic disease should be studied closely.[8]

In summary, our recommendation concerning the elective repair of asymptomatic renal artery aneurysms in men and in women beyond childbearing age is based on the data just presented and on the well-documented history of other abdominal arterial aneurysms. General guidelines for the repair of asymptomatic abdominal aneurysms include (1) infrarenal aortic aneurysms greater than 5 to 5.5 cm in diameter, (2) common iliac aneurysms greater than 3 cm, and (3) splenic artery aneurysms greater than 3 cm.[22] Surgery is recommended for visceral artery aneurysms of any size.[32] Although various hemodynamic factors may play a role in other intra-abdominal aneurysms, and despite the relative paucity of data suggesting a high risk of rupture, it seems prudent to recommend the repair of renal artery aneurysms greater than 3 cm in diameter in good-risk patients when there is reasonable certainty that nephrectomy will not be required.[26,28] This guideline remains controversial, and others have taken a more conservative approach, reserving repair for aneurysms larger than 4 cm.[33] As previously mentioned, any renal artery aneurysm in women of childbearing age should be repaired.

Hypertension

Although the prevalence of hypertension in patients with renal artery aneurysms is approximately 80% in several series, there is no conclusive evidence that the aneurysms themselves are the direct cause of hypertension unless there is an associated stenosis or compression of an adjacent artery.[1,10,13] In a series of 39 patients with renal artery aneurysms, 26 had diastolic hypertension, but in only 9 (23%) did the hypertension prove to be of renovascular origin.[1] In a more recent series of 16 patients with extraparenchymal renal artery aneurysms, 75% had renovascular hypertension.[35] The indication for surgical intervention for renovascular hypertension due to renal artery stenosis secondary to atherosclerosis continues to be the failure of medical management—namely, diastolic blood pressure greater than 90 to 100 mm Hg despite three antihypertensive medications—and the same criterion should probably be applied when a renal artery aneurysm is present. Both the stenotic artery and the aneurysm must be repaired. Our current evaluation of these patients relies primarily on the clinical scenario, the exclusion of other causes of secondary hypertension, the documentation of significant renal artery stenosis, and, occasionally, the use of captopril renal scans.[36]

Dissection

Emergent intervention is required for dissections that cause renal artery aneurysms and threaten the viability of the kidney. Nephrectomies are frequently required, however, because of the extensive damage to the renal branch vessels and the limited time available to salvage a previously healthy kidney that cannot tolerate prolonged periods of ischemia. If hypertension is the only manifestation of a chronic dissection and the hypertension is well controlled by blood pressure medications, or if the patient is asymptomatic and a renal artery dissection is found incidentally (without an associated aneurysm), surgery is probably not justified.[10]

Other Clinical Manifestations

If a patient with an intact renal artery aneurysm, as documented by CT or magnetic resonance imaging (MRI), is symptomatic—that is, experiences abdominal or flank pain or fullness—repair is indicated regardless of the previously mentioned criteria. Symptoms may be a harbinger of impending rupture, but even if they are not, medical treatment will not relieve these symptoms. Embolization to the renal parenchyma may also account for these symptoms.[9]

Treatment: Medical, Endovascular, Surgical

Repair of a Ruptured Renal Artery Aneurysm

If emergent surgery is required for a ruptured renal artery aneurysm, a midline approach and supraceliac aortic control are generally required. A sizable juxtarenal hematoma does not allow safe aortic exposure and clamping immediately above the renal arteries. If proximal control of the renal artery itself can be obtained, the supraceliac clamp can then be removed. If the bleeding is quickly controlled and the patient is clearly hemodynamically stable, and if the proximal and distal renal arteries lend themselves to a relatively quick and straightforward bypass, consideration can be given to reconstruction. In most cases, however, nephrectomy is required because of the instability of the patient, the prolonged ischemia of the kidney, and the technical and time-consuming nature of surgical repair with a bypass.[2,10,14,37] If the aneurysm extends into the renal parenchyma or if a "bench" repair of the kidney is required, the patient is generally best treated by nephrectomy, as long as the contralateral kidney is known to be intact with normal function. It is possible that a stable patient with a ruptured true or false renal artery aneurysm can be treated with newer endovascular techniques. Routh and associates reported thrombosis of a leaking saccular aneurysm using Gianturco coils, thrombin, and bucrylate.[38]

Elective Repair of Renal Artery Aneurysm

Even in the case of elective surgery, repair of a renal artery aneurysm is usually more challenging than revascularization for renal artery stenosis. Most renal artery aneurysms extend past the bifurcation of the main renal arteries and frequently extend into the renal parenchyma. Associated renal artery stenosis may need to be repaired in conjunction with the aneurysm. For in situ repairs of a renal artery aneurysm, the left kidney can be exposed through a retroperitoneal approach with a transverse left supraumbilical incision. The right kidney can be exposed through a transperitoneal approach with a Kocher maneuver to reflect the right colon and duodenum medially or, occasionally, with a subcostal incision.

Several methods have been used to repair renal artery aneurysms. The most straightforward technique for saccular aneurysms involves aneurysmorrhaphy with primary repair or patching. In three combined series of patients undergoing surgical repair of renal artery aneurysms, about one third (6 of 18, 3 of 10, and 6 of 23) of the aneurysms were able to be repaired in this manner.[1,9,13] If this technique is not possible, we and others prefer autologous tissue bypasses, such as a saphenous vein bypass, if the graft can be anastomosed to the distal part of the main trunk of the renal artery or to the most proximal branches.[8,13] The most common renal arterial reconstruction is an end-to-side anastomosis of a small renal artery branch to the main renal artery or a side-to-side anastomosis of two small renal arteries to create a common inflow channel with a single, larger diameter lumen, which can then be anastomosed to the renal artery or vein. Because the small branches of the main renal artery are often involved with the aneurysm, a branched autologous graft is preferred to reconstruct these lesions. The internal iliac artery is an excellent choice in these reconstructions because of its multiple small side branches.[28,39] Alternatively, the saphenous vein also functions well. The proximal anastomosis of the graft is usually the infrarenal aorta. Useful alternative reconstructions include a splenorenal bypass for a left-sided renal artery aneurysm and hepatorenal bypass for a right-sided aneurysm.

If multiple branch vessels are involved, and especially if the cause of the renal artery aneurysm is dissection, resulting in a friable vessel, extracorporeal or bench surgery may be required.[40,41] This technique is recommended when renal ischemia is projected to exceed 45 minutes or when exposure of small renal branches is required. Ex vivo surgery requires nephrectomy, followed by hypothermic perfusion of the kidney with a heparinized renal preservation solution. The kidney can then be autotransplanted to its original bed, as Dean and associates prefer,[42] or to the iliac fossa. For renal autotransplantation into the iliac fossa, a flank incision with a retroperitoneal approach is used for exposure of the kidney, ureter, and iliac artery. Gonadal and adrenal veins are divided to obtain an adequate length of renal vein. If the reconstruction can be safely performed by placing the kidney on the anterior abdominal wall, the ureter does not need to be divided. The procedure is occasionally best performed at a separate table after dividing the ureter and removing the kidney from the operative field. Perfusion is carried out through the main renal artery to preserve the kidney while selected branches are individually repaired and other branches are perfused. The kidney may be perfused with a heparinized crystalloid solution, such as Collins solution or lactated Ringer's solution with heparin 1000 units/L with 12.5 g of mannitol, while the kidney is wrapped with gauze and placed in a chilled solution at 4°C.[8,38,43] The use of continuous pulsatile perfusion is controversial.[38] Ex vivo repair is also discussed in Chapter 142 (Renovascular Disease: Open Surgical Treatment).

When performed for proper indications by well-trained surgeons, repair of renal artery aneurysms should be associated with low morbidity and mortality.[2,9,43,44] English and colleagues reported a 1.7% perioperative mortality rate for surgical repair in 62 patients with 72 renal artery aneurysms, with 4-year patency of 96% and cured or improved hypertension in three quarters of patients.[45] Pfeiffer and colleagues from Germany reported similar excellent long-term surgical results in a series of 94 patients.[46] In another series of 12 patients operated on for renal artery aneurysms, there was no mortality, and only 1 patient required reoperation for ureteral stenosis.[44] Ex vivo repairs have been shown to be safe and effective by Dean and associates[42] and others.[40] Murray and coworkers reported a series of 11 patients with renal artery aneurysms successfully treated using ex vivo repair.[39] In another series of eight aneurysms, all were successfully repaired with the ex vivo technique, without deaths or complications.[46] In a review of ex vivo repairs, postoperative mortality rates ranged from 0% to 9.6%.[47] Use of bifurcated internal iliac artery autografts was also highly successful in a series of 11 patients, most with fibrodysplastic aneurysms, treated by in situ or bench repair.[39] Finally, in a series of 35 repairs of renal artery aneurysms treated by in situ repair, ex vivo repair, or nephrectomy, there was no mortality and only one postoperative graft occlusion.[13] Recent technologic and surgical developments have also allowed less invasive surgical repair of complex renal artery aneurysms, and both laparoscopic and robot-assisted techniques have been described.[48,49]

An exciting new approach to the treatment renal artery aneurysms includes the use of endovascular techniques.[28,50-52] Degenerative renal artery aneurysms have been treated with transcatheter embolization with detachable platinum coils, which occlude the aneurysms but maintain renal flow.[51-53] One patient in whom a renal artery aneurysm occurred after percutaneous renal biopsy was also successfully treated by embolization.[55] In one of the largest reported series of endovascular repairs, Klein and coworkers treated 12 renal artery aneurysms using selective endovascular embolization with nondetachable microcoils or Guglielmo's detachable coils.[51] Eight aneurysms were located in the bifurcation of the main renal artery, two were in the main renal artery, and two were intrarenal. All 12 aneurysms were successfully occluded, with only two minor complications. These authors concluded that endovascular treatment of renal artery aneurysms with microcoils is as safe as surgical treatment and less invasiave.[51] Alternatively, several authors have recently reported using ethylene vinyl alcohol copolymer to ablate renal artery aneurysms.[56,57] With this technique, the main renal artery is protected with an angioplasty balloon while the polymer is infused into the aneurysmal sac, achieving controlled exclusion.

Over the past 5 years there have also been more numerous reports of endovascular stent-graft exclusion as definitive treatment for renal artery aneurysms. Many aneurysms extend to branch vessels, making this approach risky, but it may be ideal for aneurysms of the main renal artery not involving the branches. Advances in covered stent and stent-graft technology, with smaller diameter devices and lower profile delivery systems, have made definitive treatment of saccular aneurysms feasible. Although most published series have been small, results have been excellent, and this approach will undoubtedly become more common as technology improves.[58-62]

Fibromuscular Dysplasia

Post-stenotic dilatation resulting from fibromuscular disease can be treated by balloon angioplasty of the stenotic lesion; in these cases, the primary indication for treatment is the stenotic lesion. When the lesion extends into the branches of the main renal artery, surgery can yield excellent results. Dean and coworkers reported 24 patients with fibromuscular disease, many of whom had branch aneurysms; all but one did well.[42]

Intrarenal Aneurysms

Intrarenal aneurysms represent particularly challenging lesions. Frequently, a partial nephrectomy is required.[47] Intrarenal aneurysms in association with polyarteritis nodosa have also been successfully treated with renal artery embolization, with preservation of the kidney.[64]

RENAL ARTERIOVENOUS MALFORMATIONS AND FISTULAE

Arteriovenous malformations (AVMs) and AVFs are uncommon lesions that can be associated with hematuria, hypertension, renal dysfunction, high-output congestive heart failure, and even rupture. More than 200 cases have been reported since the first description in 1928.[65] Fistulae may be congenital or acquired. Multiple diagnostic modalities are now available, although conventional selective arteriography remains the standard. Many asymptomatic lesions do not require treatment. In the past, symptomatic lesions were treated surgically, but endovascular treatment has now supplanted surgery in most cases.

Epidemiology and Pathogenesis

Congenital Arteriovenous Malformations

True congenital AVMs of the kidney are rare, with an incidence of only 0.04%.[66] In a large series, only one congenital AVM was noted in 30,000 autopsies.[75] These lesions represent approximately one fourth of all renal AVFs.[67,68] The right kidney is involved more often than the left, and although multiple lesions can occur, a single focus is more common.[40] The angiographic appearance of the lesions is similar to that of AVMs elsewhere, with large coils of dilated vessels. Piquet and colleagues described a single artery feeding all but advanced cases[69]; others described multiple connections of arterial branches and venous tributaries.[65]

An early "blush" is noted and correlates with the degree of arteriovenous shunting, which is variable. These lesions have been described as cirsoid, or varix-like, and are generally focal and located in the renal medulla. AVMs are not neoplastic, but enlargement presumably can occur owing to vessel dilatation and hypertrophy associated with high-flow volume from arteriovenous shunting. Symptomatic AVMs have been reported in pregnancy,[65,70] and it is thought that the hyperdynamic state of the gravida leads to increased AVM flow and symptoms. Histologically, involved vessels have irregular fibrosis or intimal hyperplasia as well as medial hypertrophy. Focal intraparenchymal hemorrhage may be noted in the lamina propria beneath the transitional epithelium of the collecting system.[71]

Acquired Arteriovenous Fistulae

Acquired AVFs may occur spontaneously. Spontaneous AVFs have been documented in association with fibromuscular dysplasia[72] and are thought to develop when a dysplastic or aneurysmal renal artery erodes into a neighboring vein.[73] This may also occur with renal malignancy, and indeed, significant arteriovenous shunting is a hallmark of renal cell carcinoma.[74] With arteriography, it can be difficult to differentiate a renal malignancy from a congenital or acquired AVF, although CT and MRI generally reveal a mass distinct from the renal parenchyma in malignancy. As with AVMs, symptoms depend on the degree of shunting.

Traumatic AVFs are the most common lesions, accounting for more than 70% of all renal AVFs.[65] These lesions may occur after nephrectomy, related to erosion of the arterial stump into the vein with mass ligature[75-77]; after renal artery angioplasty[65]; after blunt[78] or penetrating[76] trauma; after

nephrostomy[78]; and, most commonly, after percutaneous renal biopsy. With the routine use of needle biopsy for the diagnosis of rejection in renal allografts, the incidence of acquired AVFs has grown, although only 1% to 2% of patients who undergo needle biopsy develop symptomatic AVFs.[80,81] However, the true incidence of AVF is 15% to 18% when arteriography is routinely used.[82,83] Similarly, Ozbek and colleagues found AVFs in 8 of 64 patients (12.5%) monitored by color duplex ultrasonography,[84] whereas only 5% developed AVFs in the study of Rollino and associates.[85] In the prospective study of Merkus and colleagues, who used routine color duplex surveillance, 10% of patients undergoing biopsy developed AVFs.[82] In their series, the development of AVFs correlated with bleeding dysfunction (elevated bleeding time or diminished platelet count), supporting the idea that inadequate intraparenchymal hemostasis leads to the development of a channel between artery and vein that subsequently enlarges. Others have reported fewer fistulae and bleeding complications with the use of automated small-gauge needles rather than the standard 14-gauge core biopsy technique.[86,87]

Clinical Presentation

The majority of both congenital and acquired AVFs do not produce clinical symptoms, and many lesions are noted incidentally in studies done for other reasons. Indeed, some patients are discovered to have AVFs when undergoing radiographic evaluation for vague abdominal or flank symptoms. The most common symptom of congenital AVM is hematuria, occurring in 72% of cases.[75] Hematuria occurs when subepithelial varices erode transitional epithelium into the collecting system. A dramatic presentation with massive hematuria can occur,[34,70,88] although minor or microscopic hematuria is more common. Hypertension occurs in congenital AVMs and is also the primary abnormality in most acquired AVFs described as symptomatic. The hypertension is renin mediated, based on diminished glomerular filtration pressure distal to the fistula because of arterial "steal."[68,79,89] Renal dysfunction is usually not noted except in transplant patients, in whom diminished parenchymal flow in the solitary kidney is not masked by a functional contralateral kidney.[90]

Although AVFs are generally painless, intermittent perilumbar discomfort has been reported in some patients.[74,77] This discomfort is generally associated with hematuria and may represent renal colic. Additionally, dyspnea and other symptoms of congestive heart failure may be the primary complaint in some patients; this is more common with acquired lesions, and only with those having a large communication between the artery and vein. This "high-output" type of heart failure is manifest by tachycardia, left ventricular hypertrophy and cardiomegaly, and a palpable thrill in the flank. A continuous abdominal bruit is a hallmark of acquired AVFs and is frequently noted with congenital AVMs as well. Retroperitoneal or intra-abdominal hemorrhage rarely occurs with AVMs and AVFs.[34,91] However, patients with rupture present with severe abdominal and flank pain and shock, a clinical picture indistinguishable from ruptured abdominal aortic aneurysm.

Diagnosis

Excretory urography is performed in many patients presenting with hematuria or flank pain. A filling defect may be noted in the kidney, and dilated vessels can compress the collecting system, although these findings are not specific. Although intravenous pyelography is helpful to exclude more common causes of hematuria, such as nephrolithiasis, it is of limited use in the diagnosis of AVFs.

CT can usually define AVFs and AVMs within the kidney, but it is not always possible to differentiate these lesions from other hypervascular abnormalities such as renal cell carcinoma. Similarly, radionuclide imaging can demonstrate early augmented perfusion, but differentiation from malignancy is not possible.[92] In contrast, ultrafast CT with angiographic reconstruction has significantly improved the noninvasive imaging of AVFs and AVMs.[93] Likewise, contrast-enhanced MRA allows three-dimensional reconstruction that can provide visualization not possible with conventional angiography.[94]

Color duplex imaging is also of growing importance in the diagnosis of AVMs and AVFs. Because it is inexpensive and noninvasive, it is the ideal study for screening purposes. Color duplex imaging has been used liberally to assess for AVFs after percutaneous renal biopsy.[82,95,96] Marked turbulence is noted on color examination, and Doppler spectral analysis reveals an elevation of peak systolic flow velocity and a larger increase in end-diastolic flow velocity compared with the normal renal artery, with a resultant low resistive index.[84,95]

Arteriography has been and remains the definitive diagnostic modality for renal AVMs and AVFs. Rapid opacification of the inferior vena cava is noted. Depending on the size of the fistula, the nephrogram may be diminished distal to the AVF. With congenital AVMs, multiple segmental and interlobar arteries communicate with varix-like veins, whereas a single arterial communication is generally present with acquired AVFs.[75] Although it is a relatively expensive and invasive diagnostic study, arteriography alone offers the opportunity for definitive therapy.

Treatment: Medical, Surgical, Endovascular

The majority of both congenital and acquired AVFs do not cause symptoms and do not require treatment. However, patients may become symptomatic many years after the occurrence or diagnosis of AVFs and should be closely observed for the development of hypertension, hematuria, or high-output cardiac failure. Additionally, most AVFs occurring after percutaneous renal biopsy close spontaneously.[79,82,84,96,97] This is particularly true of AVFs discovered early after biopsy by color duplex ultrasonography. Thus, periodic duplex surveillance along with clinical follow-up for the development of hypertension or renal insufficiency is indicated. If a postbiopsy AVF persists at 1 year, it is not likely to close spontaneously,[80] although intervention should still be delayed until the development of symptoms.[82,89] Although hypertension related to an AVF may be readily controlled with angiotensin-converting enzyme inhibitors.[72] the long-term effect on renal function is not known. In most published reports, patients with hypertension have undergone surgical or endovascular therapy; thus, the natural history of medically treated patients with hypertension secondary to AVFs remains undefined.

For patients with symptomatic AVFs, surgery has been the standard treatment for many years and may still be the best option in certain circumstances.[98,99] Except for very peripheral lesions, a transperitoneal approach is preferred to establish proximal arterial and venous control at the renal pedicle. Owing to the frequent presence of thin-walled, dilated veins and channels, surgery can be challenging. Ex vivo repair for a large, complex renal artery aneurysm causing an AVF in a patient with fibromuscular dysplasia has been reported.[100] With surgery, ligation of the feeding vessel or vessels alone is often not possible, and partial or total nephrectomy is often required. The resultant loss of functional renal mass, as well as the morbidity of the operation itself, makes endovascular treatment an attractive approach.

There are now more than 2 decades of experience with percutaneous arterial embolization therapy for congenital and acquired AVFs.[101] Because renal arteries are "end arteries," they are especially amenable to therapeutic occlusion. In earlier reports, autologous clot was used as the embolic material, but recanalization and recurrence of AVFs are possible, and thrombus has been supplanted by other materials, including gelatins, glues, alcohols, silicon, steel and platinum coils, and detachable balloons.[25,67,91,96,102,103] The development of coaxial catheter systems has allowed highly selective embolization, which can preserve renal function; loss of functional renal parenchyma is reportedly between 0% and 30% with modern techniques. In general, smaller AVFs are treated with glues or macroparticles, whereas coils and balloons are used for larger vessel fistulae (Fig. 145-1).[104] Because Gelfoam and autologous clot resorb, recanalization with recurrence of symptoms can occur in up to 50% of cases.[105,106] For this reason, and because of the perception that microcoils are associated with less indiscriminate embolization than glues and alcohols, recent trends favor the use of microcoils even for smaller AVFs and AVMs.[25,91,96]

Very large AVFs may present a technical challenge owing to the risk of central embolization, and some authors recommend surgery in this setting.[98,99,107,108] Others have reported success in this setting using the Amplatz "spider" device to provide a scaffolding that can then engage other embolic materials.[67,76] Staging the procedure—beginning with large coils, followed weeks later by smaller coils and other materials to close off persistent flow channels—may also be an effective strategy.[109] Because very large arteriovenous communications tend to be at the renal pedicle rather than intraparenchymal, surgical treatment is feasible and probably preferable for good-risk patients.

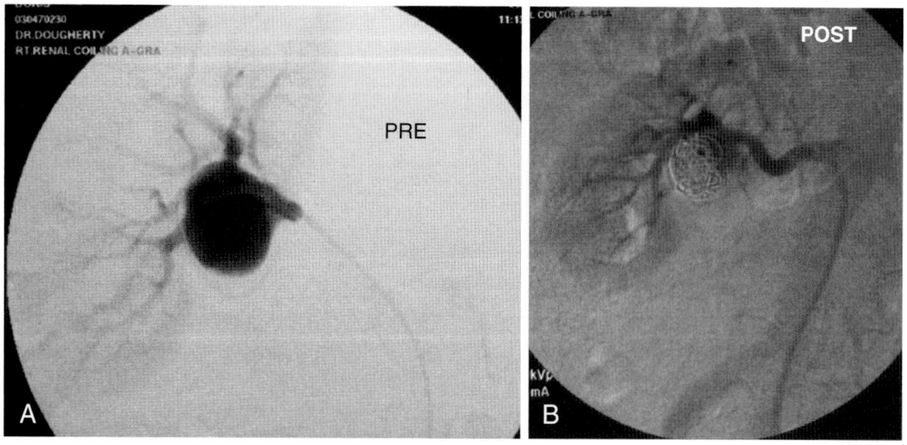

Figure 145-1   A, Arteriogram showing a post-traumatic arteriovenous fistula. This patient suffered a stab wound to the flank and presented with hematuria. **B,** After Gianturco coil embolization of multiple arterial branches, venous communication is no longer present. Hematuria resolved, and the patient recovered uneventfully.

Complications of embolization are unusual but not insignificant. In addition to arterial access site morbidity and contrast agent toxicity, pulmonary or peripheral arterial embolization can occur. This is usually related to the improper selection and delivery of embolic materials. Large AVFs require large devices such as coils or detachable balloons, but even these can embolize centrally. Gelfoam, alcohol, and various glues may be more appropriate for very small communications, but the delivery is less precise, and renal parenchymal infarction seems to be greater with these materials.[79] It is common for patients to have fever, leukocytosis, and even hypertension after embolization, but these are transient and presumed to be secondary to renal infarction.[83] Embolization itself was reported to cause massive collecting system hemorrhage in one case, but this was successfully managed with further embolization.[110] With modern techniques, endovascular treatment is successful in more than 80% of patients[90] and is clearly the treatment of choice for symptomatic congenital or acquired AVFs.

SELECTED KEY REFERENCES

Crotty K, Orihuela E, Warren M. Recent advances in the diagnosis and treatment of renal arteriovenous malformations and fistulas. *J Urol.* 1993;150:1355.
Good overall review of renal AVMs.

Huppert PE, Duda SH, Erley CM, Roth M, Lauchart W, Dietz K, Claussen CD. Embolization of renal vascular lesions: clinical experience with microcoils and tracker catheters. *Cardiovasc Intervent Radiol.* 1993;16:361.
Good review of endovascular intervention for renal artery aneurysms and AVFs.

Lacombe M. Ex situ repair of complex renal artery lesions. *Cardiovasc Surg.* 1994;2:767.
Good review of surgical technique.

Lumsden AB, Salam TA, Walton KG. Renal artery aneurysm: a report of 28 cases. *Cardiovasc Surg.* 1996;4:185.
Large review of one center's experience with renal artery aneurysms.

Stanley JC. Natural history of renal artery stenosis and aneurysms. In: Calligaro KD, Dougherty MJ, Dean RH, eds. *Modern Management of Renovascular Hypertension and Renal Salvage.* Baltimore: Williams & Wilkins; 1996:15.
Large series describing the natural history of renal artery aneurysms.

Takebayashi S, Hosaka M, Kubota Y, Ishizuka E, Iwasaki A, Matsubara S. Transarterial embolization and ablation of renal arteriovenous malformations: efficacy and damages in 30 patients with long-term followup. *J Urol.* 1998;159:696.
Large series of endovascular intervention for AVMs.

REFERENCES

The reference list can be found on the companion Expert Consult Web site at *www.expertconsult.com.*

CHAPTER 146

Renovascular Disease: Acute Occlusive Events

J. Hajo van Bockel and Jaap F. Hamming

An acute renovascular event is defined as a sudden interruption of the arterial or venous blood flow to or from one or both kidneys. Because the renal arteries are considered "end arteries," an interruption of the arterial blood flow, particularly if it occurs acutely, threatens the function and viability of the kidney and can lead to serious consequences such as immediate or late renal replacement therapy. Thus, immediate and adequate management of this emergency is mandatory.

Sudden interruption of renal arterial blood flow may be caused by an embolus, arterial thrombosis (usually in the presence of preexisting stenosis), spontaneous dissection of the renal artery, or trauma. Accidental or intentional occlusion of the main renal artery or accessory renal arteries can also occur during endovascular aneurysm repair; this is covered in Chapter 129 (Abdominal Aortic Aneurysms: Endovascular Treatment). Similarly, other iatrogenic injuries of the renal artery, such as complications that can occur during angioplasty, are covered in Chapter 143 (Renovascular Disease: Endovascular Treatment); acute renal events and visceral ischemia associated with aortic dissection are dealt with in Chapter 135 (Aortic Dissection).

Venous occlusion is also considered an acute renovascular event. Occlusion of the venous circulation may be the result of venous thrombosis and is often associated with coagulation disorders or with dehydration. Venous occlusion is usually less dramatic than arterial occlusion; its course may even be insidious, with symptoms limited to peripheral edema, for example. Because acute renovascular events are rare, the literature provides information on only small series and case reports and occasionally larger series and reviews. This chapter is based mainly on such reports.

HISTORICAL BACKGROUND

The first case of an embolic occlusion of the renal artery was reported in 1856.[1] Von Recklinghausen reported a traumatic occlusion of the renal artery in 1861.[2] Vascular surgical interventions were developed in the 1950s, and the first report of successful surgical intervention for acute and acute-on-chronic renal artery occlusion came in the mid-1950s, when diagnostic methods and vascular surgical techniques to repair renovascular problems became available.[3] The first case of bilateral renal artery thrombosis in which revascularization was established 18 hours after the occlusion, resulting in the return of sufficient renal function to maintain life, was reported in 1972.[4] Thereafter, reconstruction for acute vascular occlusive events became more common.[5,6] The next major step was the improvement in diagnostic imaging heralded by helical computed tomographic angiography (CTA), followed by catheter-based interventions such as angioplasty,[7] with or without stent placement, and the addition of fibrinolytic therapy of thrombotic occlusion.

EPIDEMIOLOGY AND PATHOGENESIS

Acute events involving the renal vessels are unusual, and certain types of renal artery occlusion present specific clinical pictures in particular patient groups and have specific causes. For example, embolism is traditionally associated with heart disease, thrombosis with generalized atherosclerosis, and trauma with young adults. Although each of these diseases and events is rare, they may have serious consequences. Significant loss of kidney function is relatively frequently associated with these acute events compared with chronic diseases (both vascular and parenchymal) of the kidney.

Embolic Occlusion

Patients with heart valve disease or atrial fibrillation may occasionally be affected by emboli occluding the visceral vessels. Renal emboli in the main renal artery are rare. Smaller emboli in distal branches occur more often, resulting in infarction of parts of the kidney; in these cases, it is often impossible to differentiate between embolic and thrombotic events. Renal embolus occurs mainly in patients older than 60 years, some of whom have had previous embolic events. The prevalence of renal infarction, by either emboli or thrombi, in autopsy studies has been estimated at approximately 1.5%.[1] However, in a 3-year period, Korzets and coworkers observed an incidence of acute renal infarction of only 0.007%.[8] The mean age of the patients in that study was 67 years, and 70% had an increased risk for thromboembolic events. Similarly, in an 18-year period, Hazanov and colleagues identified 44 cases of renal infarction in patients with atrial fibrillation and an average age of 69 years; the 30-day mortality was significant at 11%.[9]

The occurrence of multiple small renal emboli due to cholesterol debris is both more common and more important than embolic occlusion of the main renal artery. This complication is associated with both acute and chronic renal impairment. The prevalence of chronic cholesterol crystal embolization (CCE) has been estimated from autopsy reports

2251

at 6.2 cases per million per year. It occurs predominantly in elderly men with a history of atherosclerotic disease and hypertension; the primary CCE site is the kidney, followed by the skin and gastrointestinal tract.[10] CCE is commonly associated with arterial catheterization, particularly cardiac catheterization, and frequent changes of catheters and wires in a severely atherosclerotic suprarenal aorta, which can mobilize atherosclerotic debris that embolizes to the kidneys, gastrointestinal tract, skin, muscles, and toes. Acute embolic renal syndromes have also been recognized after cardiovascular surgery, and fibrinolysis and anticoagulation are triggering factors.[11] Further, distal microembolization to the kidneys in combination with nephrotoxic contrast agents may result in acute renal failure and even permanent dialysis dependency. Therefore, CCE is associated with both poor renal and patient survival. After a mean follow-up of 2 years in one series, more than 30% of patients were on dialysis.[11]

Renal Artery Thrombosis

Thrombotic occlusion is a more common cause of renal artery occlusion than embolic occlusion. Older patients, usually those older than 55 years, are affected by acute thrombosis of a renal artery based on preexisting atherosclerotic stenosis—that is, an acute-on-chronic occlusion (Fig. 146-1). These patients usually have a history of cardiovascular events, including peripheral arterial occlusive disease, cardiac disease, or cerebrovascular disease. Although stenoses are relatively common in older patients with atherosclerotic disease, subsequent complete renal artery occlusion is relatively rare, with a cumulative 5-year incidence of about 5%. Risk factors for thrombosis are high-grade stenosis, systolic hypertension, and diabetes mellitus.[12] In the case of two functioning kidneys, a thrombotic occlusion may occur without symptoms and go unnoticed. However, if both kidneys or a functional single kidney is involved, such an event may result in anuria and the need for renal replacement therapy.

Other miscellaneous causes of renal artery occlusion include coagulation disorders such as antiphospholipid antibody syndrome[13] or factor V Leiden mutation.[14] Such disorders may cause thrombosis in any location within the renal vasculature—the renal artery trunk or branches, intraparenchymal arteries and arterioles, glomerular capillaries, and renal veins. The spectrum of findings associated with antiphospholipid antibody syndrome includes renal artery stenosis or malignant hypertension, renal infarction, renal vein thrombosis, thrombotic microangiopathy, and increased allograft vascular thrombosis.[15] Behçet's disease should also be considered in the differential diagnosis of acute renal infarction in young adults.[16] Finally, renal transplant patients may occasionally suffer from arterial occlusion of the iliac artery—the inflow site for the transplant renal artery—leading to acute renal ischemia. The incidence and prevalence of these rare clinical events are unknown and cannot even be estimated.

Spontaneous Dissection

Spontaneous dissection of the renal artery resulting in renal artery stenosis or occlusion is very rare. The clinical presentation is often dramatic and can be accompanied by severe hypertension and renal failure. Patients are relatively young, and both sexes are affected. In approximately 20% to 25% of patients, spontaneous renal artery dissection is a bilateral event resulting in a threat to the whole renal mass (Fig. 146-2). The underlying disease may be arterial fibrodysplasia, but spontaneous renal artery dissection is also associated with atherosclerosis, in which case a single renal artery is usually affected. Early recognition of the symptoms and signs of acute dissection is important because of the major risk of cardiovascular complications and target organ damage, including significant loss of renal mass.[17]

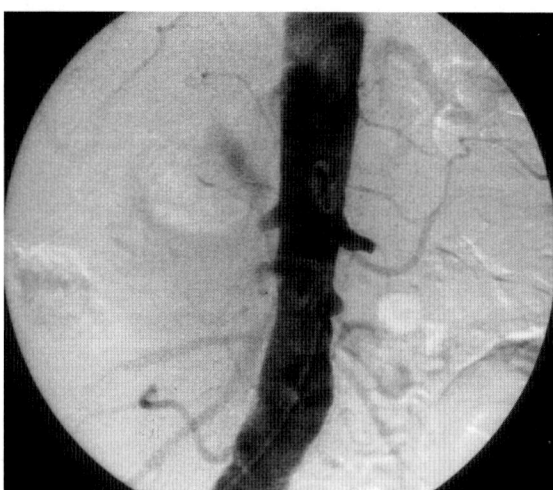

Figure 146-1 Thrombotic occlusion of both renal arteries. The patient had no urine production, and renal function was absent. Nuclear studies showed perfusion, indicating viability of the kidneys by means of collateral circulation.

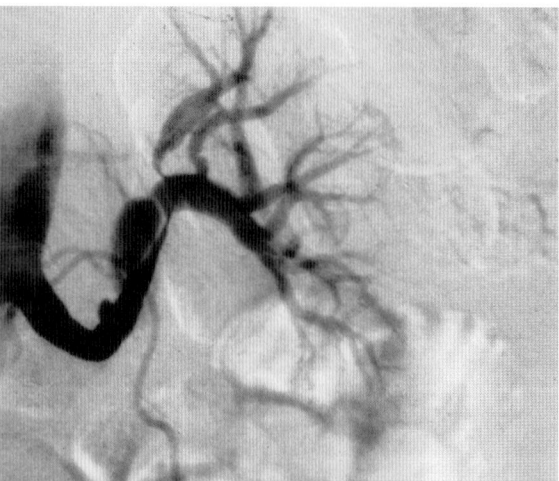

Figure 146-2 Spontaneous renal artery dissection extending into hilar branches of the left kidney. The patient presented with bilateral dissection, severe hypertension, and renal failure. *(From van Rooden CJ, van Baalen JM, van Bockel JH. Spontaneous dissection of renal artery: long-term results of extracorporeal reconstruction and autotransplantation.* J Vasc Surg. *2003;38:116-122.)*

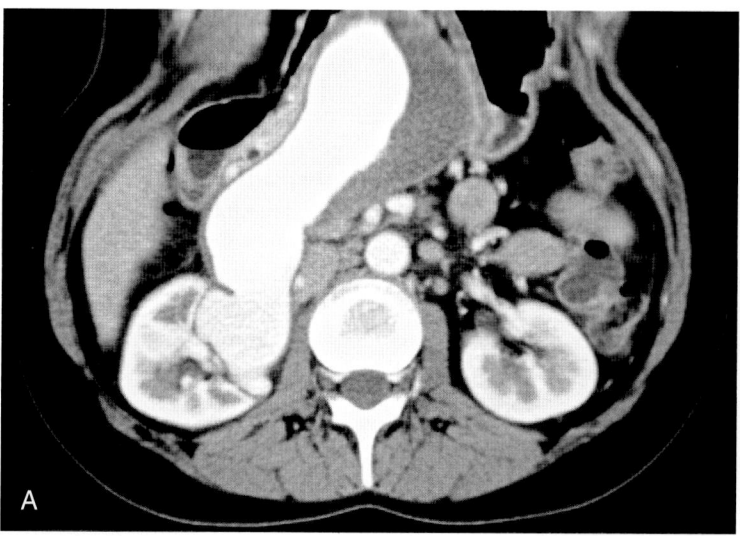
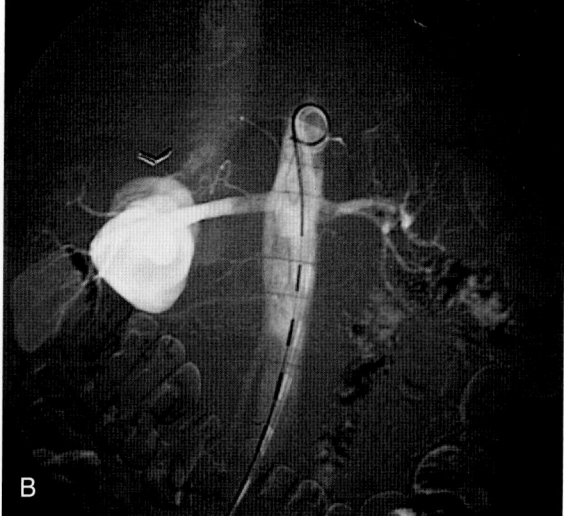

Figure 146-3 Large false aneurysm and arteriovenous fistula involving the right renal artery, renal vein, and vena cava after penetrating trauma by a trocar during laparoscopy. **A,** Computed tomographic angiogram. **B,** Angiogram.

Renovascular Trauma

Renal artery trauma is also rare. It may be caused by direct or indirect trauma and had a prevalence of approximately 4% in a major trauma hospital.[18] A renal injury is present in 7% of all patients with penetrating wounds of the abdomen. Additionally, trocar injuries from laparoscopic trauma can result in renovascular events (Fig. 146-3). Most direct renovascular trauma caused by gunshot and stab wounds is associated with other injuries.[18]

Half of traumatic renal artery injuries are from blunt mechanisms. In crush abdominal injury (seen in motor vehicle accidents), the renal artery may be injured when it is compressed against the vertebral column.[19] In contrast, in indirect renal artery injury, the mechanism is a rapid acceleration and deceleration injury displacing the mobile kidney, resulting in a tear in the elastic intima while the adventitia remains intact. The resulting hemorrhage into the vessel wall leads to thrombosis, resulting in minor or major perfusion defects, most of which are caused by pedicle injuries rather than by injuries of the main renal artery. Blunt trauma may also cause renal artery dissection with formation of a pseudoaneurysm.[20] Blunt injuries, observed as perfusion defects, are usually diagnosed on computed tomography (CT) performed for the evaluation of polytrauma patients. The injuries are often unilateral, rarely bilateral.[21]

Major traumatic renovascular injuries are frequently associated with a poor outcome. In addition to renal dysfunction, post-traumatic renovascular hypertension may result, although the true incidence of this complication is unknown. Some authors have observed that patients with blunt injuries are two times more likely to have a poor outcome than those with penetrating injuries.[22] In contrast, others have reported both high nephrectomy (74%) and high mortality (16%) rates in series with mainly penetrating wounds.[18]

Renal Vein Thrombosis

Occlusion due to thrombus in the major renal veins or tributaries is very rare. It occurs primarily in adults, with an incidence of approximately 0.05%. However, it is probably not as rare as was previously believed; the course may go unnoticed owing to the absence of specific symptoms or because it is a complication of systemic disease. In addition, and in contrast to the arterial circulation, renal veins (particularly those on the left side) have a generous collateral network both inside and outside the kidney. This anatomy may reduce symptoms, and spontaneous recanalization or resolution may also occur.[23] In neonates the prevalence of renal vein thrombosis may be higher, around 0.5%, and it may be initiated by a period of severe or prolonged hypotension. Renal vein thrombosis in both adults and children is associated with renal diseases and nephrotic syndrome.[23] In neonates it is also associated with various other underlying risk factors and carries a poor prognosis.[24] The kidney's reaction to venous occlusion is determined by the acuteness of the disease, extent and timely development of collateral circulation, involvement of one or both kidneys, and origin of the underlying disease.[25]

■ PATHOGENESIS AND PATHOPHYSIOLOGY

In acute renal arterial occlusive events, the duration of warm ischemia time is crucial to the decision whether to intervene. The kidney's tolerance of complete ischemia before the occurrence of permanent damage is not known exactly, but it is reported to vary from 30 minutes[26] to 1 hour at normothermia.[27] Although some have reported tolerance up to approximately 8 hours,[2] it is known that 60 minutes of warm ischemia results in a 70% to 80% immediate loss of function, with complete recovery within weeks; extension of ischemia to 120 minutes results in immediate loss of function and only incomplete recovery (30% to 50%).[26] Warm ischemia up to 90 minutes is associated with complete recovery of function at 14 days.[28] It is also inferred from animal studies that the kidneys will infarct within 3 hours of warm ischemia after complete devascularization.[29]

However, collateral circulation plays an important role in maintaining kidney viability.[30] The renal collateral vessels originate from lumbar, internal iliac, gonadal, renal capsular, and intercostal arteries (Fig. 146-4).[31] The adrenal and lumbar arteries contribute four times more frequently than the periureteric arteries to the collateral circulation.[32] Occasionally, the inferior mesenteric artery contributes as well.[33] These collaterals communicate either prerenally into the hilus or intrarenally via perforating arterioles of the capsule. The capsular and extracapsular tissue also contains small vessels with cross-segmental anastomoses. In any case, 80% of the anastomotic channels are independent of the renal artery.[29] Interestingly, these collateral patterns appear to be similar in dog and human.[34]

The contribution of this collateral circulation to kidney viability in acute and chronic renal artery occlusion is essential. In dogs, acute occlusion from 6 to 48 hours with and without collateral circulation was studied. In the dogs without collateral circulation, the kidneys became infarcted, whereas

all dogs in which the collateral circulation was preserved regained some renal function when revascularized. However, pathologic findings showed extensive tubular necrosis and interstitial fibrosis with glomerular degeneration. Thus, in acute occlusions, collateral circulation appears to be sufficient to maintain renal viability beyond 3 hours of warm ischemia (which causes infarction when collateral circulation is absent), but it is not sufficient to prevent progressive loss of renal function.[29] Furthermore, in a solitary kidney, early incomplete recovery from ischemic injury may result in late deterioration of renal function caused by widespread tubulointerstitial disease.[35]

In contrast, slow renal artery occlusion in dogs over a 7-week period resulted in sufficient collateral circulation development to maintain kidney viability and provide adequate filtration to maintain life.[34] Other experiments have confirmed that the gradual reduction of renal perfusion pressure produces functional and morphologic consequences that are different from those observed with acute ischemic injury. Acute reduction of perfusion pressure resulted in tubular necrosis and glomerular collapse with a 40-fold elevated urinary N-acetyl-glucosaminidase excretion, whereas gradual reduction resulted in reduced renal blood flow by 30% without evidence of disruption in tubular function, reflected by low fractional excretion of sodium levels and normal excretion of N-acetyl-glucosaminidase, although the glomerular filtration rate and filtration fraction were reduced.[36] Experiments have also confirmed that risk factors for damage in acute ischemic injury are age and diabetes mellitus. Aging appeared to increase the susceptibility to severe ischemic acute renal failure in the rat.[37] Furthermore, acute ischemic kidney injury in animals with experimental diabetes mellitus was associated with a more severe deterioration in renal function than in nondiabetic animals.[38]

Renal vein occlusion is caused by the factors known as Virchow's triad, which are related to deep venous thrombosis: damage to the endothelium, stasis of blood flow, and factors and diseases associated with increased coagulability of blood. Heavy proteinuria during nephrotic syndromes may result in a hypercoagulable state with an increased risk of renal vein thrombosis. Although the cause of spontaneous isolated renal vein occlusion by thrombosis is not clearly known, it is probably due to reduced velocity of renal vein blood flow. Regardless, a thrombotic process is likely initiated in the interlobular venules and propagates in the larger veins until it reaches the renal vein. Thrombosis of the renal vein can also be secondary to thrombosis of the inferior vena cava, but extension of caval thrombosis to or above the renal vein is rare. Finally, renal vein occlusion can be caused by malignant diseases, especially renal cell carcinoma; this tumor may extend directly into the lumen of the renal vein, whereas other tumors can cause compression or involvement of the vein. Similarly, inadequate placement of a caval filter can cause a mechanical occlusion of the renal vein. Renal vein occlusion can also develop secondary to primary renal disease. Finally, thrombosis of the renal vein can occur after division of the vein for surgical exposure, but the incidence is not known.[23,25]

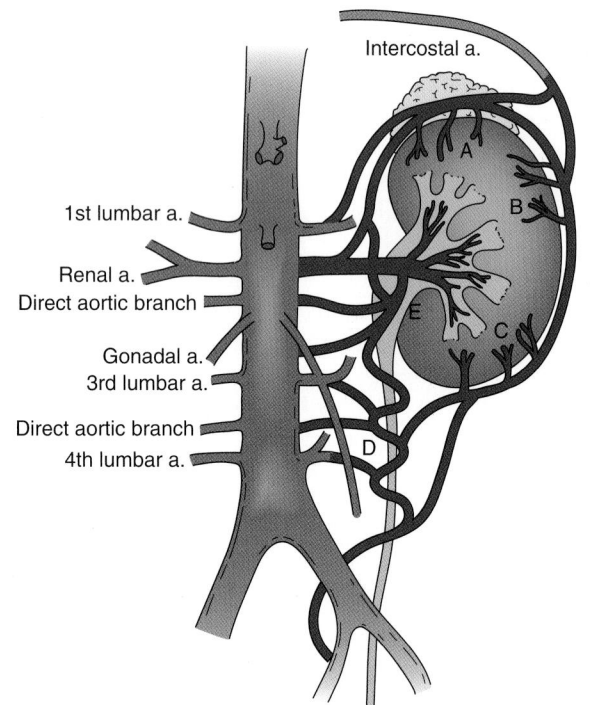

A. Superior capsular complex
B. Lateral capsular complex
C. Inferior capsular complex
D. Periureteric complex
E. Peripelvic complex

Figure 146-4 Collateral circulation of the kidney. (*From Flye MW, Anderson RW, Fish JC, Silver D. Successful surgical treatment of anuria caused by renal artery occlusion. Ann Surg. 1982;195: 346-353.*)

CLINICAL PRESENTATION

Because most individuals have two functioning kidneys, the loss of a kidney is almost immediately and adequately compensated for by the contralateral kidney if it is healthy.[39] Thus, an acute renal occlusive event may go unnoticed if significant symptoms are absent. Often, only nonspecific abdominal symptoms are associated with renal artery occlusion. However, the clinical presentation may vary from pain, usually in the flank, to anuria. The signs and symptoms of acute renal artery occlusion also mimic those of many more common diseases; thus, an occlusive renovascular event may not be suspected, resulting in postponement of adequate treatment. The diagnosis of renal artery occlusion should always be suspected, especially in cases of coexistent cardiopathy or general vascular sclerosis.[40] Unfortunately, no routine laboratory test can diagnose renal artery occlusion, and prompt imaging is required to confirm the diagnosis.[41]

Acute renovascular occlusion can also be associated with (partial) renal infarction. Symptoms associated with such events are more specific and may include pain in the flank, abdomen, or back; hypertension; hematuria; and nausea and vomiting. These symptoms can easily be misdiagnosed as ureteral colic, but vascular occlusion should be considered in the differential diagnosis of acute flank pain.[42,43] In a large series of patients with segmental renal infarction, three quarters had abdominal pain, and hematuria was present in half the patients.[9] In particular, unilateral flank pain in a patient with an increased risk for thromboembolism should raise the suspicion of renal infarction.[8] If a solitary kidney or both kidneys are affected, anuria and acute renal failure may develop. Renovascular injury in trauma patients may also go unnoticed because of associated injuries, and renal perfusion defects are often diagnosed on CT performed for the overall evaluation of abdominal trauma.

The spectrum of symptoms associated with renal vein thrombosis varies from no or minimal symptoms to an acute condition with swelling and hemorrhagic infarction requiring immediate nephrectomy.[25] The clinical presentation depends on the cause and the rapidity and completeness of the occlusion, on the one hand, and whether collateral venous circulation is present, on the other. Like renal artery occlusion, a hemorrhagically infarcted kidney causes flank pain, microscopic hematuria, and rapid deterioration of renal function; however, milder symptoms such as peripheral edema are also common. Symptoms may be absent or may be seen as part of another condition, in which case the diagnosis of renal vein occlusion will not be suspected. Furthermore, when the occlusion is not acute, collateral vessels can develop and provide venous drainage for the kidney so that renal insufficiency does not develop.

DIAGNOSTIC EVALUATION

Laboratory evaluation in patients with acute renovascular events may reveal microscopic or macroscopic hematuria and leukocytosis. Urinalysis may reveal erythrocytes and proteinuria. In the case of cholesterol microemboli, eosinophilia may be present. Indeed, in a review of the literature, 80% of patients had eosinophilia in association with atheroembolic disease.[44] In cases of renal infarction, laboratory testing may show increased levels of lactate dehydrogenase (LDH).[45] More than 90% of patients with embolic occlusion of the renal artery had serum LDH levels greater than 400 U/L (6.7 µkat/L), and mean LDH was 1100 U/L (18.4 µkat/L) in the series of Hazanov and colleagues.[9] Usually, serum creatinine levels are not immediately increased, but they may rise rapidly in the days after the event, depending on the extent of the injury.

Additional diagnostic imaging has included intravenous pyelography (now seldom used), angiography, contrast-enhanced CT, duplex ultrasound, and renal nuclear medicine investigations. In embolic occlusions, renal isotope scans were abnormal in 97% of cases and contrast-enhanced CT in 80%, whereas ultrasound was abnormal in only 11%; angiography provided the best information and was positive in all cases.[9] Despite its accuracy, renal nuclear imaging is now restricted mainly to the evaluation of kidney viability in acute-on-chronic occlusive renal disease; if the kidney is still perfused, often by collateral capsular vessels, an attempt at revascularization may be undertaken.

Duplex ultrasound is a valuable technique in most acute vascular events, but its role in acute renal events is limited. Renal duplex is technically demanding because of the deep location of the renal arteries; it is also limited by obesity and by excessive bowel gas when proper preparation is not possible, such as in an acute situation. As noted, ultrasound was diagnostic in only 11% of embolic events,[9] and false-negative results because of misinterpretation of collateral vessels as the main renal artery have been reported. Additionally, detection of flow in the renal hilum or parenchyma does not exclude renal artery occlusion.[46] The same limits hold true for duplex ultrasound evaluation of renal vein occlusion, in which case the diagnosis relies heavily on direct visualization of the renal vein and direct visualization of a thrombus within the venous lumen.[46]

Currently, CTA provides fast and precise information on the aorta, renal artery, renal parenchymal perfusion defects, renal infarction, and other pathology. Additionally, a normal renal CTA virtually excludes the presence of significant renal artery stenosis.[47] Alternatively, magnetic resonance angiography (MRA) can be performed, although it is well known that MRA tends to overestimate stenosis; however, a normal scan virtually excludes renal artery stenosis. Regardless of the method used, on the basis of the information obtained, additional (more specific) diagnostic information can be sought, and an intervention, either endovascular or open surgery, can be performed. In trauma, CTA has the additional advantage of allowing a complete evaluation for blunt abdominal trauma, and it can accurately identify lesions in both the main renal artery and its branches (Fig. 146-5).[48-50]

Regarding renal vein thrombosis, there are no laboratory investigations that are specific for the diagnosis. However, the coagulation system should be evaluated, particularly antiphos-

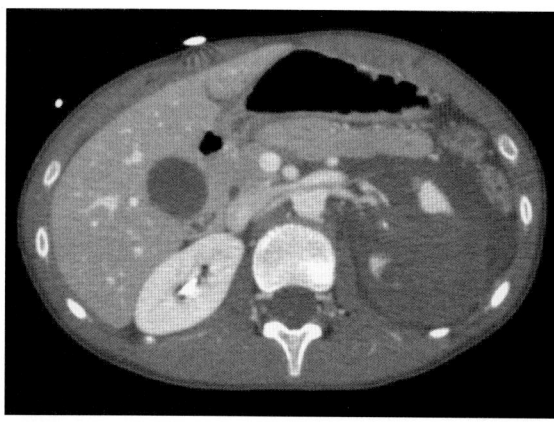

Figure 146-5 CT of left kidney injury. Note the perfusion defect caused by acceleration-deceleration trauma of the renal pedicle, resulting in vascular injury and rupture of the kidney and urinary collecting system.

pholipid antobodies.[15] As in renal artery occlusion, CTA is currently the imaging tool of choice because it is widely available, noninvasive, and accurate; MRA is an alternative. Venography is still considered the final diagnostic test if more details of filling defects are required.

■ TREATMENT

A major dilemma in acute renal artery occlusion is the decision whether to attempt revascularization. Often the period in which the function of embolized or traumatized kidneys can be preserved has passed by the time the diagnosis of renal artery occlusion is made.[51] Yet many case reports and small series have reported reconstructive therapy of an acute embolic or thrombotic occlusion resulting in partial or complete return of renal function, irrespective of the delay in treatment. Therefore, the decision to intervene and the time of intervention should be individualized and based on the warm ischemia time, the patient's condition, the type of lesion or injury, the presence of a normal contralateral kidney, the presence of collateral circulation, and the results of imaging studies. Basically, three treatment modalities are available: medical treatment and intervention by either catheter techniques or open surgery.

Medical Treatment

Medical treatment alone cannot be more than supportive. If an acute renovascular occlusion has been diagnosed, heparinization seems a logical first step, particularly if an embolic event is suspected. Experimentally, several medications, including diuretics, mannitol, dopamine, and prostaglandin E_1, have been studied to reduce the injury caused by ischemia and reperfusion of the affected kidney.[52-56] However, evidence of their clinical effectiveness has never been supported by studies in patients. Additionally, most medical interventions were administered before, not after, the renal circulation was interrupted; therefore, the relevance of this information in the context of acute renovascular occlusive events is doubtful. Regardless, many clinicians use medications such as dopa-

mine, furosemide, and mannitol,[57,58] whose effects have been demonstrated before renal ischemia is induced, during and after re-establishment of the circulation. Regarding renal vein thrombosis, anticoagulation therapy should be started as soon as possible and continued in the same manner as for deep venous thrombosis.[59] In bilateral renal vein thrombosis, extensive thrombus, and transplanted kidneys with renal vein thrombus, treatment with thrombolysis either systemic or locally may be considered.

Interventional Treatment

The selection of patients for intervention depends on the cause, duration, extent, and severity of renal ischemia. If occlusion has been caused by trauma or dissection, it can be assumed that the collateral circulation, if any, is not well developed. Consequently, renal infarction can be expected. In patients with dissection of the renal artery, the occlusion may not be complete; in acute-on-chronic occlusion, collateral circulation may be present. This may be sufficient to keep the kidney viable, although without treatment, function will cease and patients will require renal replacement therapy. If collateral circulation is present, successful revascularization may be possible even after prolonged ischemia times (several days to weeks), and the viability of the kidneys can be deduced from isotope studies with nuclear imaging. Lacombe reported on surgical repair after an interval of up to 68 days after renal artery occlusion.[60] Revascularization was achieved in all cases, and only three nephrectomies were necessary because of renal infarction. However, although the kidney salvage rate was 64%, the postoperative mortality rate was 15%. Thus, endovascular treatment, if feasible, seems preferable to open surgery; when the latter is required, preoperative correction of metabolic derangements and fluid resuscitation are mandatory.

Endovascular Treatment

Successful catheter-directed fibrinolytic therapy for renal artery emboli has been reported. Local fibrinolysis was begun from 1 day to 5 weeks after the event; an average loading dose of 250,000 units of urokinase was infused over 30 minutes, followed by a urokinase infusion of 60,000 units/hour for 8 to 50 hours. In some patients, fibrinolytic therapy was followed by balloon angioplasty to correct residual renal artery stenosis. Although perfusion was restored in almost all kidneys, function was restored in only 3 of the 10 kidneys treated.[61] Other case reports and small series have noted some success using thrombolysis.[62-65] However, from all observations, it is clear that there is a small window of opportunity to restore renal function. The ischemic tolerance of the kidney appears to be approximately 90 minutes, after which the results of intervention are poor[66]; occasionally, success after 72 hours of ischemia has been reported.[67] Generally, the results are encouraging only in selected cases if blood flow can be restored promptly.[68]

In traumatic occlusions, several case series have reported successful catheter-based interventions for thrombotic and embolic occlusion of the renal artery and its branches. If thrombotic occlusion occurs in the presence of collateral circulation, satisfactory results using balloon angioplasty, with direct restoration of urine production, have been observed even after several days of anuria.[69] Several cases of thrombosuction with an aspiration catheter and stenting have also been reported after traumatic occlusion.[70,71] Similarly, small series have demonstrated successful treatment of thrombotic occlusions that occurred after complicated angioplasty with the use of thrombolysis with or without an additional stent.[72] Case studies of percutaneous catheter-directed thrombectomy with or without thrombolysis for acute renal vein thrombosis also indicate satisfactory results, including the re-establishment of urine flow and early improvement in renal function.[73]

In summary, catheter-based intervention for acute renal artery occlusion usually restores perfusion, but mainly when the duration of ischemia is less than 90 minutes. Thereafter, restoration of renal function is probably restricted to those with thrombotic occlusion and previous stenosis, in whom collateral circulation has already developed. In renal vein occlusion, anticoagulation is the primary option, and catheter-directed thrombectomy with or without thrombolysis can be applied in selected cases.

Surgical Treatment

The decision for reconstructive surgery and the choice of technique for an acute renovascular event depends on the underlying pathology (embolic, thrombotic, traumatic, or spontaneous dissection), the duration of ischemia, and the condition of the patient. A wide variety of techniques are available, including thromboembolectomy, endarterectomy, bypass or interposition grafts, extra-anatomic bypass grafting, and extracorporeal repair and autotransplantation. (For further discussion of these techniques, see Chapter 142: Renovascular Disease: Open Surgical Treatment.) In general, older patients, who often have heart disease, should be considered at high risk and should be carefully prepared for open surgical procedures. Additionally, extra-anatomic revascularization techniques without clamping of the aorta may be preferable to aortorenal bypass or endarterectomy that requires clamping of an atherosclerotically diseased aorta.

Renal Emboli. Patients with macroemboli confined to the main renal artery usually have cardiac arrhythmias with or without valvular disease and may have simultaneous emboli in other peripheral arterial sites (mesenteric, lower limb). When multiple emboli are present, an open surgical approach may seem particularly appropriate, but these patients are at high surgical risk. The surgical technique includes exposure of the renal artery by a flank approach or midline incision.[74,75] The renal vein and, subsequently, the renal artery are mobilized, and vessel loops are applied. If the aorta is opened, exposure allowing suprarenal clamping of the aorta is required. After systemic heparinization, embolectomy can be performed transrenally by opening the renal artery with a transverse or longitudinal incision. The clot is carefully and slowly removed

with the help of a Fogarty embolectomy catheter, if necessary, which can be carefully inserted in both the aortic and renal directions. The arteriotomy can be closed primarily with 6-0 sutures or with a venous patch with the help of loupe magnification. Intraoperative duplex ultrasound is used to evaluate the patency of the renal artery after closure.[76]

Results of open embolectomy are not uniformly successful. In one series covering a 20-year period, 13 patients were treated for acute renal artery occlusion as a result of embolism. Embolectomy was successful in the relief of hypertension but was ineffective in the restoration of renal function.[51] Similarly, Lacombe indicated that surgical treatment appeared to be superior to medical treatment with heparin, although the mortality with both treatments was very high (25%).[77] Satisfactory results after surgical embolectomy were also reported from a small series of 10 patients by Bouttier and associates.[78] In the five patients with anuria, four regained satisfactory renal function, and the fifth patient died. In contrast, in the five patients without anuria, renal function returned to normal in four, and one patient required nephrectomy.

Acute Thrombosis. Unlike with an acute embolic occlusion, with a thrombotic occlusion with underlying stenosis, the kidney may remain viable by means of a preexisting collateral circulation from capsular, urethral, lumbar, or adrenal vessels. In this clinical setting, if the kidney is viable and the patient is fit for operation, an attempt to re-establish adequate blood flow should always be considered. The procedure should be carefully timed, because kidney viability allows an adequate cardiovascular inventory and proper preparation to reduce the operative risks. Successful repair after almost a month's delay has been described since the 1980s.[31,79]

Surgical exposure is similar to that for restoration of circulation after an embolic event (see Chapter 142: Renovascular Disease: Open Surgical Treatment).[74,75] Usually, the aorta and the orifices of its branches are diseased from atherosclerosis, which makes clamping and aortorenal bypass surgery difficult; the thickened aortic wall may be problematic for a venous or prosthetic bypass anastomosis. In addition, clamping of the aorta in an azotemic patient is an important risk factor for postoperative cardiovascular morbidity and mortality. The same applies to transrenal or transaortic endarterectomy. Therefore, an extra-anatomic renal bypass construction should be considered. For repair of the right kidney, hepatorenal, mesenteric-renal, or ileorenal bypass is suitable. In all these cases, the patency of the donor vessels should be carefully evaluated. For repair of the left kidney, a splenorenal anastomosis is an excellent solution. Urine flow may start directly after successful revascularization, but postoperative recovery of renal function may take weeks or occasionally longer than expected (Fig. 146-6).[31] Although autotransplantation has been recommended for the repair of complete occlusion, nephrectomy disrupts much of the essential collateral circulation, and a poor outcome has been reported.[80]

Several small series have reported selected patients who underwent repair after acute renal failure caused by acute nontraumatic occlusion of the renal artery.[31] In one series, 20 patients were operated on for acute obstruction of their main

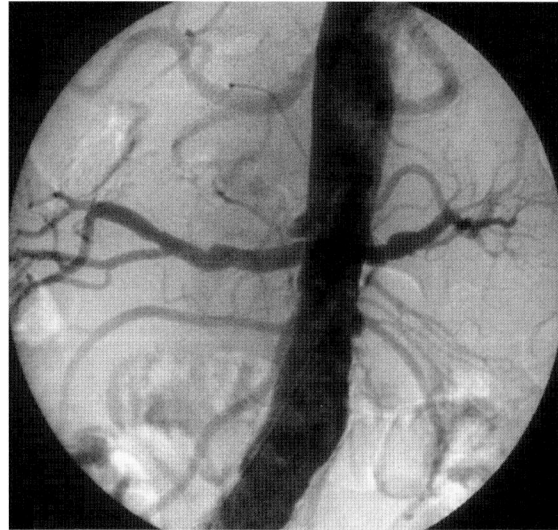

Figure 146-6 Bilateral venous bypass after bilateral thrombotic occlusion (same patient as in Fig. 146-1). Renal biopsy showed partial infarction, but renal function was recovered immediately after repair and gradually improved to normal within several months.

renal arteries (25 kidneys at risk) 18 hours to 68 days after the onset of obstruction.[60] Revascularization was possible in all but three cases; however, the postoperative mortality rate was 15%, and the kidney salvage rate was 64% with satisfactory function. In a second series covering the period 1983 to 1993, eight patients were operated on for occlusive renal artery disease as a cause of acute renal failure requiring preoperative hemodialysis.[81] Oliguria or anuria had lasted from 12 hours to 3 weeks. Revascularization restored urine flow immediately in six patients, with no further need for dialysis in four. These results confirm that retrieval of function is possible, even if repair is delayed for several days to weeks, but mortality is high (15% to 25%) after such procedures.

Trauma. Surgical repair of traumatic occlusions of the renal artery is difficult because most of these injuries are not isolated. Blunt abdominal trauma may result in branch occlusions from pedicle injuries, resulting in perfusion defects rather than occlusion of the main renal artery. Arterial revascularization is seldom indicated in patients with normal contralateral kidneys who have multiple associated injuries. In contrast, an attempt at renal artery revascularization is justified with bilateral injuries, when only one kidney is present, or when a solitary renal artery injury can be simply repaired. High nephrectomy and mortality rates have been reported with repair, however.[18] In a 2000 review by Knudson and coworkers, of 20 patients with bilateral renal artery occlusion, surgical revascularization was attempted in 16 and successful in only 9 (56%).[22] Similarly, of the 139 patients with unilateral renal artery occlusion, surgical revascularization was attempted in 34 and successful in only 9 (26%). Evidence of decreased renal function was noted in 67% of those patients who had successful revascularization, and hypertension developed in only 33% of the patients in whom revascularization was not attempted.[22] Results in children with blunt abdominal trauma were similar: the time to surgical

intervention was longer than 10 hours on average, and only minimal function could be restored.[82]

In summary, surgical revascularization for traumatic unilateral renal artery occlusion rarely results in a successful outcome. Revascularization is indicated in patients with bilateral main renal artery occlusion and in those with injury to a solitary kidney. After either surgical or conservative treatment, patients should be followed closely for the development of hypertension.[83]

Spontaneous Dissection. Spontaneous dissection of the renal artery is very rare. Dissection may be confined to the main renal artery (Fig. 146-7), or it may extend into the branches of the renal artery. When this occurs, alternative reconstructive surgical techniques such as extracorporeal repair and autotransplantation may be required (Fig. 146-8).

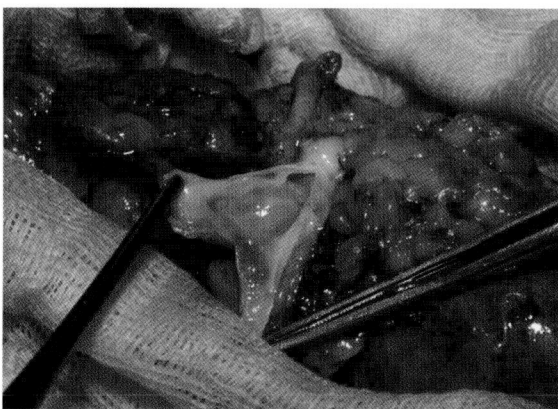

Figure 146-7 Intraoperative photograph of renal artery dissection confined to the main renal artery, repaired with in situ reconstruction.

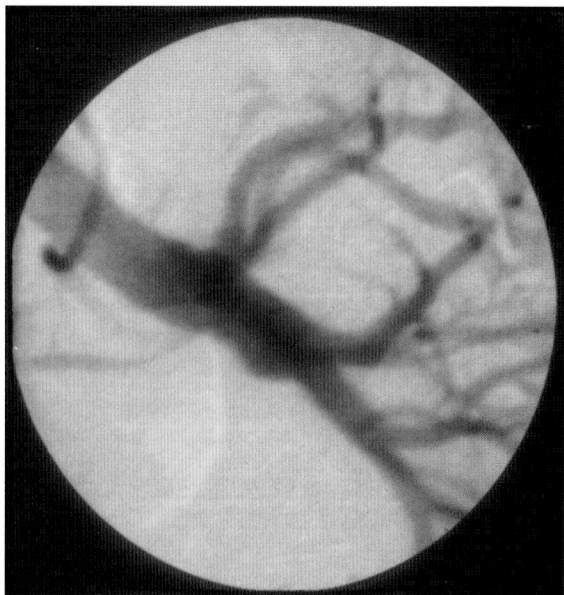

Figure 146-8 Postoperative angiogram after successful extracorporeal repair and autotransplantation for dissection of the left renal artery (same patient as in Fig. 146-2). *(From van Rooden CJ, van Baalen JM, van Bockel JH. Spontaneous dissection of renal artery: long-term results of extracorporeal reconstruction and autotransplantation. J Vasc Surg. 2003;38:116-122.)*

Briefly, this surgical procedure consists of three parts: (1) nephrectomy and renal preservation, (2) extracorporeal reconstruction, and (3) autotransplantation of the kidney as described in Chapter 142 (Renovascular Disease: Open Surgical Treatment).[84] Several small series have reported satisfactory results with in situ and extracorporeal techniques for the repair of spontaneous renal artery dissection.[17,84-87]

Renal Vein Thrombosis. The role of surgery in the treatment of renal vein thrombosis is limited. In the past, surgical thrombectomy was attempted, but rethrombosis was common, probably because the thrombosis originates primarily in smaller renal venules in combination with systemic disease. Nephrectomy may be indicated in rare cases of hemorrhagic infarction of the kidney with rupture and bleeding.

SELECTED KEY REFERENCES

Asghar M, Ahmed K, Shah SS, Siddique MK, Dasgupta P, Khan MS. Renal vein thrombosis. *Eur J Vasc Endovasc Surg.* 2007;34:217-223.
Extensive overview of renal vein thrombosis, including the causes, diagnosis, and treatment options.

Blum U, Billmann P, Krause T, Gabelmann A, Keller E, Moser E, Langer M. Effect of local low-dose thrombolysis on clinical outcome in acute embolic renal artery occlusion. *Radiology.* 1993;189:549-554.
Balanced study of the anatomic and functional outcome of local thrombolysis in acute renal occlusion. In short, the anatomic results were better than the functional outcome.

Hazanov N, Somin M, Attali M, Beilinson N, Thaler M, Mouallem M, Maor Y, Zaks N, Malnick S. Acute renal embolism. Forty-four cases of renal infarction in patients with atrial fibrillation. *Medicine (Baltimore).* 2004;83:292-299.
Largest and most recent experience with the diagnosis and treatment of renal embolism.

Kim HS, Fine DM, Atta MG. Catheter-directed thrombectomy and thrombolysis for acute renal vein thrombosis. *J Vasc Interv Radiol.* 2006;17:815-822.
Small retrospective series evaluating the percutaneous treatment of acute renal vein thrombosis, describing anatomic and functional success.

Knudson MM, Harrison PB, Hoyt DB, Shatz DV, Zietlow SP, Bergstein JM, Mario LA, McAninch JW. Outcome after major renovascular injuries: a Western Trauma Association multicenter report. *J Trauma.* 2000;49:1116-1122.
Retrospective review of patients with severe renal injuries covering a 16-year period and six U.S. university trauma centers. The authors describe diagnostic methods and the functional outcomes of various treatment modalities and propose an algorithm for treatment.

Lohse JR, Shore RM, Belzer FO. Acute renal artery occlusion: the role of collateral circulation. *Arch Surg.* 1982;117:801-804.
Study dealing with acute renal artery occlusion and the compensatory collateral circulation that may preserve kidney viability.

Scolari F, Ravani P, Gaggi R, Santostefano M, Rollino C, Stabellini N, Colla L, Viola BF, Maiorca P, Venturelli C, Bonardelli S, Faggiano P, Barrett BJ. The challenge of diagnosing atheroembolic renal disease: clinical features and prognostic factors. *Circulation.* 2007;116:298-304.
Excellent overview of the risk factors for, causes of, and contributing factors to atheroembolic events, which are an important but usually unrecognized factor in impaired renal function.

van Rooden CJ, van Baalen JM, van Bockel JH. Spontaneous dissection of renal artery: long-term results of extracorporeal reconstruction and autotransplantation. *J Vasc Surg.* 2003;38:116-122.
One of the larger experiences with extracorporeal repair and autotransplantation for spontaneous dissection into the distal renal artery and hilar branches, with satisfactory results.

REFERENCES

The reference list can be found on the companion Expert Consult Web site at *www.expertconsult.com.*

CHAPTER 147

Mesenteric Vascular Disease: General Considerations

Juan Carlos Jimenez and William J. Quinones-Baldrich

Mesenteric ischemia occurs when perfusion of the visceral organs fails to meet normal metabolic requirements. This disorder is categorized as either acute and chronic, based on the duration of symptoms. Acute mesenteric ischemia (AMI) occurs rapidly over hours to days and frequently leads to acute intestinal infarction requiring resection (see Chapter 149: Mesenteric Vascular Disease: Acute Ischemia). The most common causes are embolization to the mesenteric arteries or acute thrombosis related to a preexisting plaque. Chronic mesenteric ischemia (CMI) is a more insidious process and progresses over weeks to several months (see Chapter 148: Mesenteric Vascular Disease: Chronic Ischemia). The most common cause is progressive occlusive disease of the visceral arteries, usually related to atherosclerosis. It is often unrecognized by physicians and is frequently misdiagnosed as a gastrointestinal disorder.

Antonio Beniviene wrote the first description of mesenteric ischemia in the 15th century in Florence, Italy. A scholar of Greek medicine and a busy medical practitioner, he took notes on various gastrointestinal ailments, including gallstones, inflammatory bowel disease, and mesenteric venous thrombosis (MVT). His brother discovered these concise notes after Beniviene's death, and they were subsequently published.[1] Centuries later, the first case of AMI was diagnosed and treated successfully with intestinal resection and reanastomosis by Elliott in 1895. Goodman first described chronic intestinal angina as a clinical disorder in 1918.[2] In 1926, Cokkinis commented on mesenteric ischemia—"the diagnosis [is] impossible, the prognosis hopeless, and the treatment almost useless"—after reporting a series of 12 deaths caused by mesenteric venous occlusion.[3] Dunphy, a surgical resident at the Peter Bent Brigham Hospital in 1936, reported a case of a patient with weight loss and pain out of proportion to abdominal findings who subsequently died and was found to have mesenteric occlusive disease on autopsy. After reviewing the medical records of 12 patients who died of intestinal angina, he found that 7 of the 12 (58%) had a history of chronic abdominal pain, thus introducing the potential for early intervention to prevent disease progression and death.[4] Warren and Eberhard were the first to describe MVT as a distinct cause of intestinal infarction in 1935, differentiating it from occlusion of the mesenteric arteries.

In the modern era, Klass performed the first superior mesenteric artery (SMA) embolectomy in 1950.[5] Intestinal resection was not required. Although the patient died several days later of a heart-related condition, autopsy revealed the bowel to be normal. In 1958, Shaw and Maynard performed the first successful thromboendarterectomy of the SMA at the Massachusetts General Hospital.[6] Morris and colleagues performed the first successful retrograde bypass graft from the infrarenal aorta to the SMA in 1962.[7] Stoney and Wylie at the University of California, San Francisco, first described antegrade aortovisceral bypass and transaortic visceral thromboendarterectomy in 1966. They reported the results of 14 patients treated for symptomatic obstruction of the visceral vessels.[8] One patient died postoperatively, but four patients remained asymptomatic for a mean follow-up of 3½ years. Furrer and coworkers published the initial report of endovascular dilatation of the SMA in 1980 and thus ushered in the current era of percutaneous treatment of visceral arterial occlusive disease.[9]

ANATOMY OF THE VISCERAL ARTERIES

The primitive dorsal aorta gives rise to the abdominal aorta during fetal development. Ventral segmental arteries emerge from the primitive ventral aorta, which disappears around the fourth week of gestation. Multiple segmental branches from the primitive ventral aorta—the 10th, 13th, and 21st—persist and develop into the celiac artery, SMA, and inferior mesenteric artery (IMA), respectively. Disparity in the regression of the primitive ventral aorta and its segmental branches infrequently causes deviations in the visceral arterial anatomy.

The celiac artery arises from the abdominal aorta just caudal to the diaphragm at the level of L1 and is bordered by the median arcuate ligament at the aortic hiatus superiorly and the superior border of the pancreas inferiorly. Traditionally, the three branches from this common trunk include the left gastric, splenic, and common hepatic arteries. However, multiple variations of the true "trifurcation" can exist. Most frequently, the common hepatic artery and its branches arise from the SMA or directly from the abdominal aorta.

Exposure of the celiac trunk is best achieved through a midline transabdominal incision, which also allows visual assessment of bowel viability during surgical revascularization. The celiac trunk and its branches are surrounded by the celiac plexus of nerves, which must be divided for proximal exposure. A midline laparotomy is performed, and the triangular ligament is divided. The gastrohepatic ligament is then divided longitudinally to the level of the posterior parietal peritoneum. The liver is carefully retracted to the right of midline using a self-retaining retractor. Placement of a nasogastric tube facilitates identification of the esophagus. The posterior peritoneum overlying the diaphragmatic crus is divided sharply to expose the celiac trunk. The first vessel encountered is usually the common hepatic artery traversing to the right of midline toward the liver. The hepatic artery can be exposed back to the origin of the celiac trunk, which is covered by lymphatic tissue and the celiac nerve plexus.

The SMA arises a few centimeters caudal to the celiac trunk, and its origin is crossed by the neck of the pancreas and the splenic vein. It arises at a less acute and downward-sloped angle than the celiac trunk and lies superior to both the uncinate process of the pancreas and the third portion of the duodenum. The superior mesenteric vein runs parallel adjacent to the artery, usually along its right border. The first important branch of the SMA is usually the inferior pancreaticoduodenal artery, which supplies collateral circulation with the celiac artery through the gastroduodenal and superior pancreaticoduodenal arteries. The second major branch of the SMA is frequently the middle colic artery, which arises at the inferior border of the pancreas. The right colic, ileocolic, and third-order mesenteric branches arise distally, supplying the small bowel within the mesentery.

During surgical exposure, the SMA can be approached either anteriorly at the base of the transverse colon mesentery or lateral to the fourth portion of the duodenum. Anterior SMA exposure involves lifting the transverse colon superiorly to clearly expose the base of its mesentery. The small intestine is covered in a moist towel or a bowel bag and retracted to the right. A horizontal incision is made through the posterior peritoneum at the base of the mesentery at the level of the proximal jejunum and extended to the right of midline. The middle colic artery can be used as a landmark within the transverse colon mesentery and to localize the main SMA trunk. Palpation often aids in localizing the SMA. Often the superior mesenteric vein is visualized first, and the SMA can be palpated adjacent and to the left of it. This approach provides excellent exposure of the SMA. Exposure of the more proximal SMA to the left and lateral to the fourth portion of the duodenum can also be achieved. The ligament of Treitz is divided, and the lateral wall of the duodenum is mobilized off the anterior surface of the aorta. The SMA can be identified just distal to its origin from the aorta.

The IMA is usually located 3 to 4 cm cephalic to the aortic bifurcation, just to the left of midline, and usually arises at the level of the third lumbar vertebra. The main trunk frequently divides into sigmoidal branches and the left colic artery. The ascending left colic artery forms the inferior marginal artery of Drummond. Sigmoidal branches lead to the left and right superior rectal arteries, which collateralize with branches of the hypogastric arteries in the pelvis.

PHYSIOLOGY OF SPLANCHNIC BLOOD FLOW

Normal intestinal function and nutrient absorption rely on adequate perfusion and oxygenation to the microvascular splanchnic circulation. Various autoregulatory mechanisms ensure adequate gut circulation through both vasoconstriction and relaxation of arterial smooth muscle. The degree of visceral artery dilatation and constriction determines the relatively large fluctuations in splanchnic blood flow during fasting and postprandial states. Visceral blood flow can vary dramatically during resting and postprandial periods, ranging from 10% to 35% of cardiac output.[10] The severely diminished blood flow observed in patients with nonocclusive mesenteric ischemia results from severe vasospasm related to this process. Duplex studies demonstrate moderate to high arterial resistance in the SMA circulation, with low diastolic flow and slight flow reversal during fasting states. In the postprandial period, low-resistance signals are noted throughout both systole and diastole, indicative of dilated splanchnic arteriolar beds; flow reversal does not occur. In contrast, low arterial resistance signals are noted in the celiac artery circulation regardless of feeding, likely due to the influence of the low-resistance hepatic vascular bed. Perko and colleagues also noted that in fasting subjects performing submaximal exercise, splanchnic vascular resistance doubled and exhibited a 50% reduction in hepatosplenic blood flow and a 25% reduction in mesenteric blood flow.[11]

Many extrinsic factors regulate these various flow states. Sympathetic efferent nerves in the prevertebral celiac and mesenteric ganglia, which initiate stimuli for arterial vasoconstriction, perform neural regulation. Hormonal pathways also contribute to extrinsic regulation of splanchnic blood flow. The renin-angiotensin feedback mechanism causes mesenteric vasoconstriction through the direct action of angiotensin II during hypovolemic states. Low volume states and hyperosmolarity also stimulate the neurohypophysis, which causes the release of vasopressin.[12] This hormone causes splanchnic vasoconstriction, reduction in portal venous pressure, and venodilatation.[12] Intrinsic regulation also occurs through metabolic and myogenic pathways.[12] Mucosal ischemia prompts the release of metabolic byproducts, causing vasodilatation in arteriolar smooth muscle and preferentially shunting increased blood flow to the intestinal mucosa. Mucosal perfusion and integrity are maintained in this fashion during periods of relative ischemia.

EPIDEMIOLOGY

Asymptomatic occlusive disease of the visceral arteries is a common finding in elderly patients. Wilson and coworkers demonstrated that 17.5% of 553 consecutive patients older than 65 years examined with duplex ultrasonography had a critical stenosis of at least one visceral vessel.[12] Additionally, autopsy studies have estimated the prevalence of atherosclerosis involving the mesenteric arteries to be between 6% and 10%.[13] Despite these findings, the extensive collateral network within the mesenteric arterial circulation allows most patients to maintain adequate visceral perfusion and remain symptom free. Indeed, in Wilson's study population, asymptomatic disease of the celiac trunk and SMA was not associated with

AMI or CMI, gastrointestinal tract interventions, excessive cardiovascular events, or increased mortality.[12]

In contrast, AMI is a rapidly progressive and morbid condition that is frequently associated with intestinal infarction. Patients with AMI represented 1 in 1000 hospital admissions in a series reported by Stoney and Cunningham in 1993.[14] Similarly, patients with AMI represented 0.1% of annual hospital admissions in the 1997 report by McKinsey and Gewertz.[15] Prompt revascularization and resection of necrotic bowel are often required, and the mortality rate is reportedly 24% to 96%.[16] Elderly patients are most severely affected, and AMI carries a relative risk for mortality of 3.0 in patients older than 60 years.[13]

The exact incidence of CMI is not known; however, it has been estimated to be 1 in 100,000 of the general population per year.[17] Despite the high prevalence of individuals with asymptomatic mesenteric arterial occlusive disease, patients usually demonstrate involvement of two or more mesenteric vessels before symptoms arise. Frequently the celiac trunk, SMA, and IMA have significant atherosclerotic disease before symptomatic presentation. The variability of symptoms in patients with chronic abdominal pain often makes the diagnosis challenging, resulting in treatment delays and increased morbidity.

PATHOPHYSIOLOGY

Acute Mesenteric Ischemia

Embolism

Diminished intestinal perfusion resulting in mesenteric ischemia can develop through various mechanisms. The most common cause of AMI is embolization to the SMA. Arterial emboli are responsible for 40% to 50% of cases of AMI.[18] The proximal source of the embolus is frequently intracardiac mural thrombus. Potential initiating factors include atrial tachyarrhythmias, myocardial infarction, cardiomyopathy, structural heart defects, and cardiac tumors. Endocarditis can result in septic emboli from affected valve leaflets. Mural thrombus in proximal aneurysms in the thoracic or proximal

abdominal aorta can also serve as embolic sources. Because the SMA arises at a less acute angle from the abdominal aorta compared with the other mesenteric vessels, it appears to be the most common final destination for mesenteric emboli. Additionally, such emboli tend to lodge several centimeters from the vessel's origin, usually distal to the middle colic artery (Fig. 147-1A). The angiographic finding of abrupt occlusion of the SMA distal to the middle colic artery with minimal collateralization is virtually diagnostic of AMI due to an embolus.

Arterial Thrombosis

Arterial thrombosis constitutes the next most common cause of AMI and occurs in 20% to 35% of cases.[19,20] Preexisting atherosclerotic plaque affecting all visceral vessels is the most common finding. Hypercoagulability syndromes can also predispose to acute visceral artery thrombosis. The affected segment of artery is usually its origin at the level of the aorta. Patients with acute arterial thrombosis frequently have preexisting symptoms of CMI. Schoots and associates reviewed 45 observational studies encompassing 3692 patients with AMI and found that mortality from acute thrombosis of a mesenteric artery was 77.4%, compared with 54.1% for patients with acute arterial embolism to visceral vascular beds.[21] This increased mortality is likely due to the more proximal location of the occlusion, with more vessels occluded and a larger segment of bowel affected (Fig. 147-1B). Acute extension of an aortic dissection can also serve as a mechanism for abrupt mesenteric vessel occlusion and thrombosis.

In a Swedish study, 213 patients with acute thromboembolic occlusion of the SMA and intestinal infarction were examined post mortem.[22] The degree of intestinal infarction was significantly greater in patients with SMA thrombosis compared with embolus. The cause of occlusion was embolic in 57.3% of patients and thrombotic in 41.3% (indeterminate in 1.4%). Synchronous emboli were found in 68% of patients with primary embolus to the SMA. Cardiac thrombi were found in 48% of patients with an SMA embolus, compared with 11% of patients with thrombotic occlusion.

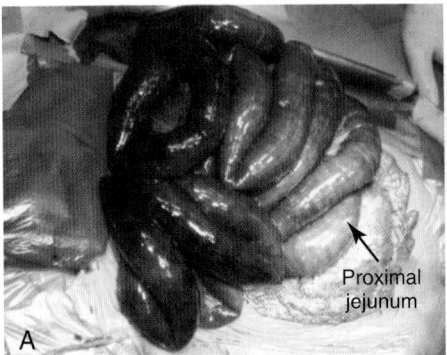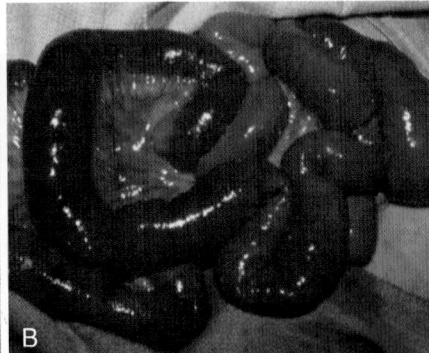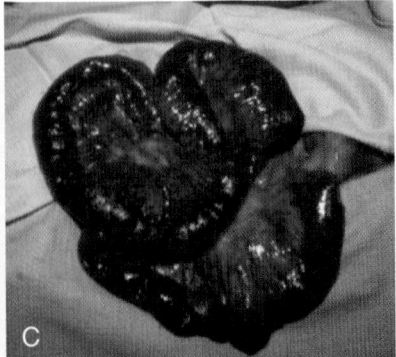

Figure 147-1 A, Operative findings typical of acute mesenteric ischemia secondary to an embolus. Note that the first portion of the jejunum is spared because the embolus lodged distal to the middle colic artery. **B,** Operative findings typical of acute mesenteric ischemia secondary to arterial thrombosis. Note that the entire bowel is affected. **C,** Appearance of the small bowel at second-look surgery after revascularization. Note the hemorrhagic changes in the mesentery.

Nonocclusive Mesenteric Ischemia

Impaired intestinal perfusion in the absence of thromboembolic occlusion is termed nonocclusive mesenteric ischemia (NOMI). Symptomatic patients are frequently found to have extensive atherosclerosis, with involvement of all three visceral arteries. The disease pattern frequently involves the vessel origin, with extension of plaque from the abdominal aorta. However, NOMI can also occur in patients without mesenteric arterial occlusive disease. Thomas and colleagues reviewed patients with angiographic evidence of greater than 50% stenosis of the mesenteric arteries.[23] Fifteen patients were found to have significant three-vessel arterial disease, and 27% of these patients developed symptoms of CMI during 2 to 6 years of follow-up. In contrast, no symptoms were seen in patients without severe three-vessel disease. However, 29 of 72 patients (40%) in whom follow-up was available died during the study. Overall, there was a mean survival of 1.9 years, highlighting the significant morbidity associated with this disorder.

Visceral ischemia can occur due to low-flow states, especially in conjunction with intestinal atherosclerotic disease. NOMI most commonly occurs secondary to cardiac disease, particularly severe congestive heart failure. Atrial fibrillation, commonly a cause of cardiac thrombi and visceral embolization, can also induce NOMI by reducing left ventricular function and causing low cardiac output. Other risk factors for NOMI include hypovolemia, systemic vasoconstrictors, vasoactive drugs (e.g., digoxin, α-adrenergic agents, β-receptor blocking agents, cocaine), aortic insufficiency, cardiopulmonary bypass, abdominal and cardiovascular surgery, and liver failure.[18] Deitch and colleagues also found that bacterial translocation from mucosal injury can occur as early as 2 hours after a 30-minute episode of hypovolemic shock in a rat model of NOMI.[24]

Mesenteric Venous Thrombosis

MVT constitutes 5% to 15% of all cases of mesenteric ischemia.[25,26] Involvement is usually limited to the superior mesenteric vein but can also involve the inferior mesenteric vein and portal vein. MVT is classified as either primary (idiopathic) or secondary. Secondary MVT occurs when an underlying disease process is present; this type accounts for 75% of all patients with this disorder. Inherited or acquired hypercoagulable diseases, including protein-C and -S deficiency, polycythemia vera, antithrombin III deficiency, antiphospholipid antibody syndrome, and factor V Leiden mutation, are frequent causes.[27] Malignancy, trauma, abdominal surgery, hepatic failure, pancreatitis, and oral contraceptive use can all initiate MVT.[24]

The extent of bowel ischemia depends largely on the degree of venous involvement. The transition from normal to ischemic intestine is slower with MVT than with arterial occlusive disease.[18] Edema and hemorrhage of the intestinal wall are frequently seen, followed by focal sloughing of the mucosa.[18] The origin of thrombosis varies, depending on the etiologic process. When an intra-abdominal process is the cause, thrombosis begins in the larger mesenteric veins and progresses to involve the smaller venous arcades and arcuate channels.[24] MVT caused by hypercoagulable conditions usually begins in the smaller mesenteric veins. Symptomatic acute MVT is associated with a 20% to 50% mortality rate.[24] Long-term survival is dependent on the cause of MVT, and recurrence rates are high without long-term anticoagulation. Rhee and associates reviewed the clinical outcomes of 72 patients treated for this disorder and found a 30-day mortality rate of 27% and a recurrence rate of 36%.[28] The long-term survival for patients with chronic MVT was significantly better than for those who presented acutely (83% versus 36%). The survival for patients with this disease did not improve over the 22-year follow-up period. Acute anticoagulation with heparin remains the primary treatment, with surgical exploration reserved for failures of anticoagulation or clinical deterioration (acute abdomen).

■ CLINICAL PRESENTATION

Acute Mesenteric Ischemia

The most common symptom of AMI associated with arterial thromboembolic disease is the sudden onset of abdominal pain. Lack of collateral flow to the visceral organs leads to a more dramatic presentation in AMI, with severe, rapid clinical deterioration. Nausea, vomiting, diarrhea, emptying symptoms, and abdominal distention can also occur. Classically, the pain is out of proportion to the findings on physical examination. Initially, bowel sounds are hyperactive as the failure to relax the bowel smooth muscle leads to emptying symptoms. Bowel sounds are typically diminished in the later stages. Abdominal guarding and rebound tenderness are absent in the early stages of AMI; however, as intestinal ischemia and infarction progress, these signs become more pronounced. They are typically late findings, so their absence should not delay the diagnosis and treatment of AMI. Other late findings include fever, oliguria, dehydration, confusion, tachycardia, and shock.[18] Metabolic abnormalities can include leukocytosis, metabolic acidosis, hyperamylasemia, elevated liver function values, and lactic acidemia.

Patients with NOMI or MVT typically present with a slower clinical course. Frequently, patients with NOMI are critically ill, hospitalized, intubated patients who experience a sudden deterioration in their clinical condition. These patients are often administered intravenous pressors, worsening mesenteric vasoconstriction and thus decreasing splanchnic perfusion. In patients with MVT, fever, abdominal distention, and bloody stools are the most common findings. Dehydration and profound fluid shifts lead to bloody ascites and a hypovolemic state, causing further propagation of venous thrombosis.[18]

Chronic Mesenteric Ischemia

Postprandial abdominal pain and progressive weight loss are the most common symptoms in patients with CMI. Pain is

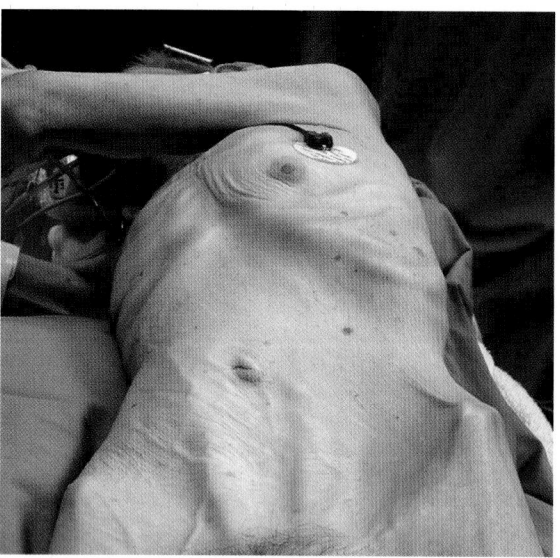

Figure 147-2 Typical patient with chronic mesenteric ischemia with significant weight loss and cachexia. The patient is placed in a right semilateral decubitus position in preparation for retroperitoneal transaortic endarterectomy.

often described as dull and crampy and located in the mid-epigastric region. The course of symptoms can be equated with intestinal claudication. Lack of energy leads to failure of the intestinal smooth muscle to relax, which intensifies the cramping pain. Pain often occurs 15 to 45 minutes after a meal, and the severity varies according to the size and type of meal. Patients typically develop "food fear" and decrease their oral intake in anticipation of severe pain after meals. Changes in bowel habits, nausea, and vomiting are less common findings. CMI is believed to be more prevalent in elderly women. The variable nature of symptoms often makes the diagnosis confusing and can result in delayed treatment. The traditional risk factors for atherosclerosis are usually present. A heavy smoking history is frequently obtained. The majority of patients also have a history of symptomatic manifestations in other vascular beds, most commonly cerebrovascular, coronary, and peripheral arteries.[29]

Physical examination findings are usually nonspecific. Patients are commonly undernourished and cachectic (Fig. 147-2). An abdominal bruit can sometimes be auscultated but is not always present. Bowel sounds are frequently hyperactive. Guarding and rebound tenderness are usually absent. Low prealbumin and albumin levels are often seen, owing to the patient's chronic malnourished state.

DIAGNOSTIC EVALUATION

Noninvasive Evaluation

Duplex ultrasonography is a useful tool for the early, noninvasive diagnosis of visceral ischemic syndromes. Color Doppler scanning can be used to assess the flow velocities and resistance index in the splanchnic arteries and their arterial

beds, as well to evaluate end-organ vascularity. The intestinal wall can also be assessed with a high degree of accuracy using high-resolution transabdominal ultrasound.[30] Transmural hemorrhage, inflammation, and necrotic thickening in the bowel wall can be imaged sonographically. Asymmetric wall thickening with associated ileus can be seen in patients with AMI as well as ascites and free peritoneal air.[28]

Moneta and colleagues performed blinded duplex ultrasound studies in 100 patients who previously underwent arteriography of the celiac trunk and SMA.[31] They hypothesized that lack of flow or a peak systolic velocity (PSV) in the SMA of greater than 275 cm/sec, or no flow or a PSV of greater than 200 cm/sec in the celiac trunk, was a reliable indicator of 70% or greater angiographic stenosis.[32] Using these criteria, duplex sensitivity for detecting lesions in the SMA and celiac artery was 92% and 87%, respectively. Overall accuracy for detection of a 70% lesion in the SMA and celiac artery was 96% and 82%, respectively.

Limitations of transabdominal duplex scanning include the wide variation in examination quality, which is operator dependent. Patient-related factors such as obesity, excessive intraluminal bowel gas, variation in local anatomy, and effects of respiration can affect image quality.[33] Care must be taken to clearly define the origin of each vessel to avoid inaccurate measurements.

Computed tomography (CT) is an accurate, noninvasive imaging modality for diagnosing mesenteric ischemia. Rosow and coworkers were able to predict ischemia with 92% sensitivity in a porcine model using multidetector CT and computed tomographic angiography (CTA).[34] Kirkpatrick and colleagues reported that CTA diagnosed AMI with a sensitivity of 96% and a specificity of 94%.[35] Advantages over conventional angiography include the relative ease and speed of performance, the rapid infusion of contrast agent through peripheral intravenous lines, and the ability to simultaneously image the mesenteric arteries, veins, and visceral organs. Common radiographic findings in the bowel wall related to AMI include increased thickening, dilatation, and attenuation, which can be easily detected using CT. Pneumatosis intestinalis, mesenteric edema, and ascites can also be detected. During the arterial phase of contrast infusion, the mesenteric vessels can be evaluated for thrombosis, embolus, dissection, and aneurysm.

Disadvantages of CT include the risk of contrast nephropathy and hypersensitivity reactions to iodinated contrast agents. Inaccurate timing of contrast infusion during the arterial phase may provide indeterminate images and delay diagnosis. Because calcification at the vessel origins enhances in a similar fashion to intravenous contrast material, it is possible to underestimate the degree of stenosis. Therefore, the non–contrast-enhanced images should be reviewed. Last, CT serves strictly as a diagnostic modality; treatment must be performed via a separate angiographic procedure or laparotomy.

Magnetic resonance angiography (MRA) is useful for diagnosing mesenteric occlusive disease. Because MRA takes significantly longer to perform than CTA, its role in evaluating patients with AMI is limited. Recent studies have shown excellent correlation between conventional angiography of the mesenteric circulation and MRA in patients with CMI, especially of the larger branches.[36] MRA avoids the radiation exposure associated with CTA. However, CTA allows the identification of calcified plaques, giving it a distinct advantage. Patients with hypersensitivity to iodinated contrast agents may also benefit from MRA.

Invasive Evaluation

Conventional angiography remains the "gold standard" in the diagnosis of mesenteric ischemia. Anteroposterior and lateral views of the visceral aorta (Fig. 147-3), as well as selective catheterization of the celiac trunk, SMA, and IMA, provide the most accurate and specific localization of stenotic and

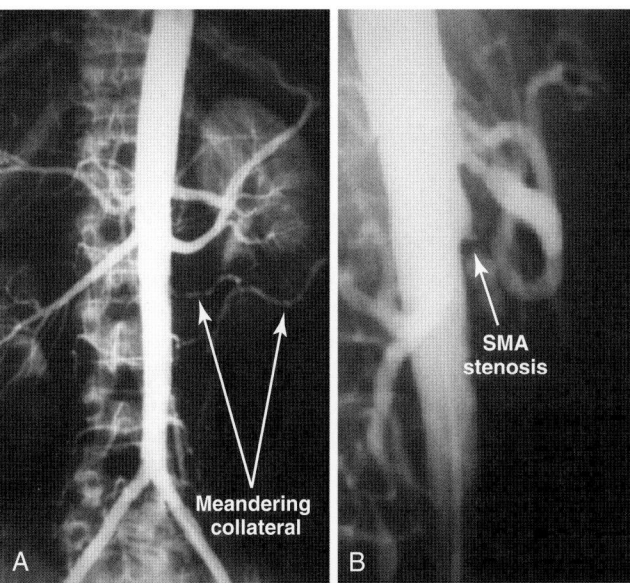
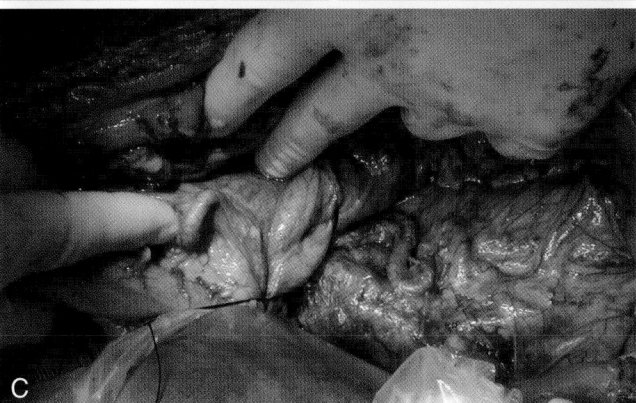

Figure 147-3 A, Anteroposterior angiogram of a patient with chronic mesenteric ischemia. Note the meandering collateral vessels. **B,** Lateral aortogram of a patient with chronic mesenteric ischemia. Lesions are typically located at the origin of the vessel and often protrude into the aortic lumen. SMA, superior mesenteric artery. **C,** Meandering collateral vessels in a patient with chronic mesenteric ischemia at the time of exploration. In patients undergoing surgery for other reasons, this finding should raise the suspicion of significant mesenteric occlusive disease.

occlusive lesions. Therapeutic alternatives such as balloon angioplasty, stenting, and thrombolysis and percutaneous thrombus extraction can all be used to restore luminal visceral blood flow. These options are discussed in more detail in the next section.

TREATMENT OF ACUTE AND CHRONIC MESENTERIC ISCHEMIA

The goal of therapy for patients with mesenteric ischemia is the prompt restoration of blood flow to the visceral organs. Specifics of the treatment of AMI and CMI are also discussed in Chapter 148 (Mesenteric Vascular Disease: Chronic Ischemia) and Chapter 149 (Mesenteric Vascular Disease: Acute Ischemia).

Medical Treatment

Medical treatment alone is not effective in these patients. Preventive risk factor modification helps control the progression of atherosclerosis in the mesenteric circulation as well as other vascular beds. Patients with known risks for inheritable hypercoagulable disorders should undergo screening and should be treated with systemic anticoagulation if indicated.

Before operation, aggressive fluid resuscitation with restoration of adequate urine output is required, owing to the frequent finding of severe dehydration on presentation. Electrolyte abnormalities and metabolic acidosis should also be corrected. Patients with CMI are frequently malnourished, so albumin, prealbumin, and C-reactive protein levels should be checked before revascularization. Preoperative total parenteral nutrition or enteral nutrition should be considered in severely malnourished patients. Finally, because the intestinal mucosa is damaged during periods of prolonged ischemia, bacterial translocation can occur, contributing to systemic sepsis. Broad-spectrum intravenous antibiotics with aggressive fluid resuscitation can lead to decreased mortality in these patients.[37] Treatment against gram-negative and anaerobic organisms is especially important.

Endovascular Treatment

General Principles

Advances in endovascular techniques have greatly expanded the role of percutaneous interventions for patients with mesenteric ischemia in recent years. However, endovascular management remains largely limited to patients with CMI. Balloon angioplasty and stenting are the most common interventions, and recent reports have documented excellent technical results with low patient morbidity.[38-40] Because patients with AMI frequently require intestinal resection, laparotomy with open revascularization is the preferred method of treatment. In those with short-segment stenoses, cardiac and pulmonary co-morbidities, prior abdominal surgery, coagulopathy, or malnutrition, endovascular therapy is often favored. More complex lesions and complete arterial occlusions traditionally favor open revascularization.

Efficacy

Sarac and colleagues at the Cleveland Clinic recently treated 87 mesenteric vessels with percutaneous angioplasty and stenting, including 18 complete occlusions.[41] The vessels were recanalized with 0.035-inch glide wires and stented with either balloon-expandable stents for orificial lesions (80 vessels) or self-expanding nitinol stents for nonorificial lesions associated with curvature (7 vessels). The primary patency and survival at 1 year were equivalent in patients treated for stenosis and occlusion. Overall, primary patency was 65%, primary assisted patency was 97%, and secondary patency was 99%. The cumulative survival at 1 year was 89%.[39]

Silva and associates reviewed the results of 59 consecutive patients who underwent angioplasty and stenting of 79 stenotic (>70%) mesenteric arteries.[38] Procedural success and symptom relief were 96% and 88%, respectively. The restenosis rate at 14 months was 29%, and 17% of patients had recurrent symptoms. All patients with in-stent restenosis underwent successful percutaneous revascularization. At a mean follow-up of 38 months, survival was 79%.

Sharafuddin and colleagues performed stent-assisted angioplasty in 25 consecutive patients with 26 stenosed and occluded mesenteric vessels.[40] Ninety-six percent of the procedures were technically successful. Immediate symptomatic benefit was obtained in all but three patients (88%). Of the three failures, one patient was believed to have extrinsic compression by the median arcuate ligament and refused open surgical repair. One of the remaining two patients underwent surgical bypass, followed by persistent symptoms. The remaining patient's symptoms were attributed to delayed gastric emptying, and placement of a gastric pacemaker provided some relief. Primary and primary assisted stent patencies at 6 months were both 92%.

Although no randomized controlled trials exist, recent retrospective comparisons have suggested high rates of early restenosis in patients treated with balloon angioplasty and stenting.[42-44] Kasirajan and coworkers reviewed 28 patients who underwent balloon angioplasty and stenting of 32 mesenteric vessels over a 3½-year period at the Cleveland Clinic.[42] Five vessels (18%) were treated with balloon angioplasty alone, and 23 vessels (82%) were treated with stent-assisted angioplasty. Outcomes were compared with the results of 85 patients (130 vessels) managed with open surgical revascularization. There was no significant difference in length of hospital stay, overall incidence of perioperative complications, or survival. At 3 years, occlusion and recurrent stenosis were documented in 27% of patients in the endovascular group. Symptomatic recurrence in the endovascular group was 28% at 1 year and 34% at 3 years. The rate of symptomatic recurrence in the open surgery group was 13% at 3 years.

Brown and colleagues reported a restenosis rate of 10% and recurrent symptoms in 9% of patients who underwent mesenteric stenting over a 3-year period at Dartmouth Hitch-

cock Medical Center.[43] At 13 months, 53% of patients required re-intervention. When compared with patients undergoing open revascularization, patients in the stented group were 7 times more likely to develop restenosis, 4 times more likely to develop recurrent symptoms, and 15 times more likely to need re-intervention.

In a similar study by Atkins and coworkers, 42 mesenteric vessels treated with angioplasty (with stenting in 87%) were compared with 88 vessels treated with open revascularization.[44] Mean follow-up was 15 months in the percutaneous transluminal angioplasty (PTA) group and 42 months in the open surgery group. No difference was noted in major morbidity or morality. Radiographic primary patency and primary assisted patency in the PTA group at 1 year were significantly lower (58% and 65%, respectively) compared with the open surgery group (90% and 96%, respectively). PTA with stenting was also associated with the need for earlier re-intervention. Surprisingly, the rates of symptomatic recurrence requiring re-intervention were high in both groups, with no significant difference noted.

Retrograde Mesenteric Stenting

Although angioplasty and stenting have largely been reserved for patients with CMI, techniques for retrograde mesenteric stenting during laparotomy for AMI have recently been described (Fig. 147-4).[45-47] During laparotomy, the SMA is dissected at the base of the transverse mesocolon, and a sheath is inserted in the vessel either percutaneously or via arteriotomy. Wyers and colleagues described placing a longitudinal arteriotomy in the SMA, performing a local thromboendarterectomy if required, and performing patch angioplasty.[46] The sheath is then placed through the distal end of the patch for access to the SMA. Hand-injected lateral aortography is

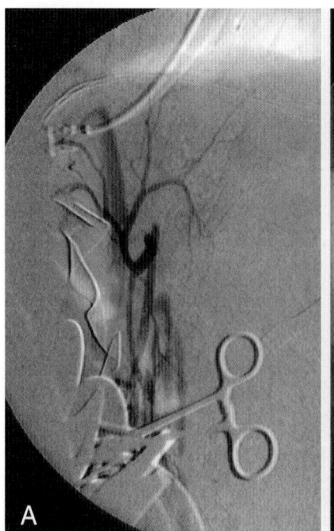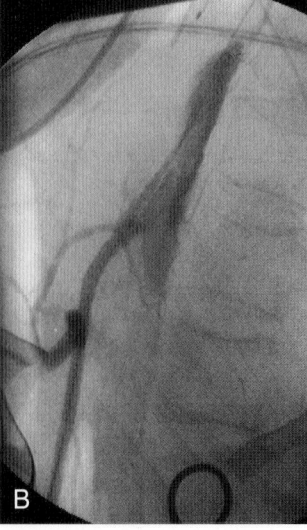

Figure 147-4 A, Retrograde superior mesenteric arteriogram during exploration in a patient with acute mesenteric ischemia secondary to arterial thromboses. Note the proximal occlusion of the superior mesenteric artery. **B,** Intraoperative placement of a proximal superior mesenteric artery stent for acute revascularization of the small bowel.

performed, and a wire is placed retrograde across the lesion into the aorta. A balloon-expandable stent is positioned and deployed to allow protrusion of the stent 1 to 2 mm into the aorta. In the Wyers group's review, they compared patients treated in this manner with patients who underwent antegrade stenting and traditional surgical bypass for AMI. Mortality was 17% for the patients who underwent retrograde stenting, compared with 100% for the antegrade stenting group and 80% for those who underwent surgical bypass. The technical success rate for the retrograde stenting group was 100%.[46] In a study by Moyes and coworkers, four patients were treated similarly with retrograde stenting of the SMA for AMI.[47] Two of the patients were alive at 2 years. One patient experienced stent thrombosis on day 14 and required surgical bypass. The remaining patient died on postoperative day 6 due to multiorgan failure.

Although early results demonstrate good technical success, the long-term efficacy of retrograde mesenteric stenting has not been established. The main advantage of this technique is the ability to inspect the bowel before and after reperfusion, unlike antegrade percutaneous balloon angioplasty. It also has the potential to decrease operative times because the exposure of proximal inflow vessels (aorta, iliac) and the harvest of autogenous conduit for surgical bypass are avoided. Potential disadvantages include inadvertent injury to the vessel or aortic dissection during wire manipulation, and restenosis due to intimal hyperplasia.

Limitations

Endovascular therapy should be the treatment of choice in high-risk patients with CMI. High technical success rates and decreased patient morbidity and mortality rates have been reasonably well established in such individuals. However, in patients who are good surgical candidates, the advantage is not so clear. Restenosis and symptomatic recurrence rates remain relatively high, as documented in the current literature, and re-intervention is often required earlier than with open surgery. Placement of stents in the mesenteric arteries may also complicate future surgical intervention, especially in the celiac trunk, which is relatively short prior to branching. Because the origins of the visceral arteries are angulated downward, especially the SMA, percutaneous access from the femoral arteries may be difficult and result in suboptimal stent placement. Thus, a brachial approach is often preferred. One recent study found a significant improvement in primary patency in patients who underwent treatment through the brachial artery compared with a femoral approach.[39] Finally, with the increasingly aggressive treatment of more complex stenotic lesions and total occlusions, the risk of distal embolization increases, although its extent is unclear. Distal protection, such as that used during carotid stenting, can be considered. Other potential disadvantages of endovascular therapy include access site complications (hematoma, arterial dissection, peripheral embolization), contrast nephropathy, inability to visualize the bowel, and vessel perforation. Stent fracture producing restenosis and recurrent ischemia has been

documented.[48] Reperfusion hemorrhage, traditionally associated with open surgical revascularization, has also been described following balloon angioplasty.[49] Despite these limitations, the role of endovascular techniques will continue to expand for patients with mesenteric ischemia. Early restenosis rates are likely to improve with the development of new balloons, drug-eluting stents, and stent-grafts.

Recommendations

At our institution, we perform mesenteric angiography for all patients with CMI and attempt balloon angioplasty with selective stenting as first-line therapy. The brachial approach is preferred for selective catheterization of the SMA owing to its acute downward angle at its origin. Femoral access is preferred for celiac artery interventions. Patients with isolated stenosis of the celiac artery due to extrinsic compression by the median arcuate ligament undergo laparoscopic lysis of the median arcuate ligament first (Fig. 147-5). Balloon angioplasty and stenting are avoided initially in these patients

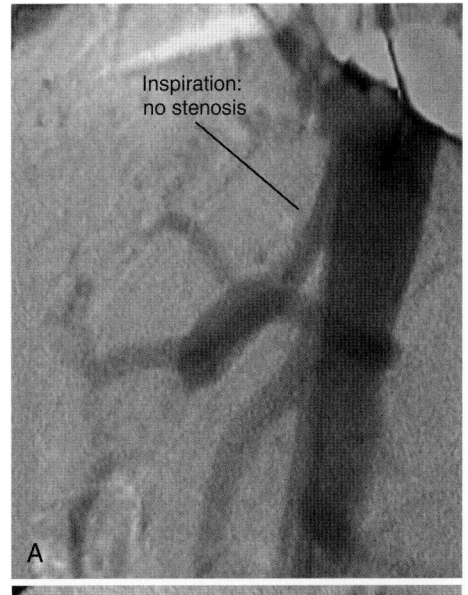

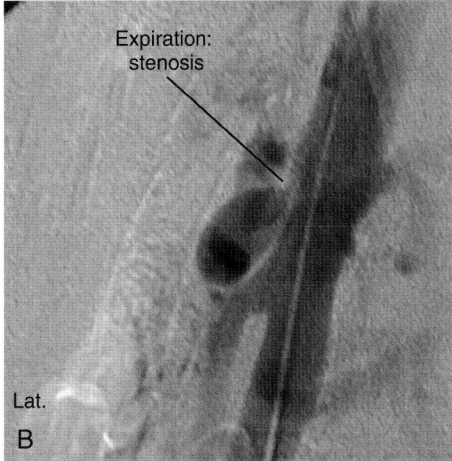

Figure 147-5 A and **B,** Angiographic documentation of extrinsic compression of the celiac artery by the median arcuate ligament. Note that the stenosis is more severe on expiration.

but may be used after median arcuate ligament release in patients with persistent abdominal symptoms. Patients are discharged home and instructed to take daily antiplatelet medications (clopidogrel [Plavix], aspirin) indefinitely following all endovascular procedures if no contraindications exist. We conduct duplex surveillance 1 month after the initial procedure and then at 6-month intervals to assess for continued vessel patency.

Surgical Treatment

General Considerations

Laparotomy with visceral revascularization can be used to treat patients with both AMI and CMI. Patients presenting with signs and symptoms of AMI require urgent abdominal exploration, assessment of bowel viability, and revascularization. Several techniques for the restoration of intestinal perfusion are available to the vascular surgeon, and familiarity with a variety of options is crucial. Before revascularization, large segments of both small and large intestine may appear dusky, ischemic, or necrotic. Because SMA emboli typically lodge distal to its origin, the middle colic artery and ileocolic branches may remain patent. Thus, the pattern of bowel necrosis following embolus may be less extensive and spare the proximal jejunum and transverse colon distribution from ischemia (see Fig. 147-1A). Acute thrombosis usually occurs at the orifice of the SMA, and a more extensive pattern of hypoperfusion and necrosis is present owing to the involvement of proximal SMA branches (see Fig. 147-1B).

Following vascular reconstruction and reperfusion, the bowel should be reassessed. Segments of bowel that otherwise would have been resected may be spared owing to improvement following revascularization. We recommend administering 1 to 2 ampules (500 to 1000 mg) of intravenous fluorescein, followed by evaluation of the bowel with a Wood's lamp. A "patchy" pattern of fluorescein distribution is highly predictive of the need for bowel resection (Fig. 147-6).[50] Doppler evaluation of the mesenteric arteries should also be performed (Fig. 147-7). Intraoperative angiography following vascular reconstruction may be performed to accurately assess the restoration of mesenteric flow. Most patients should undergo "second-look" laparotomy in 24 hours to reassess bowel viability and the need for further resection (see Fig. 147-1C). The decision to perform a second-look laparotomy should be made during the initial procedure and should not be changed based on subsequent clinical improvement.

Acute Mesenteric Ischemia

Detailed descriptions of the techniques of surgical visceral revascularization for AMI are highlighted in Chapter 149 (Mesenteric Vascular Disease: Acute Ischemia).

SMA Embolectomy. Perfusion of the mesenteric arteries is assessed by palpation and Doppler evaluation. In cases in which the obstruction is caused by an embolus, a proximal

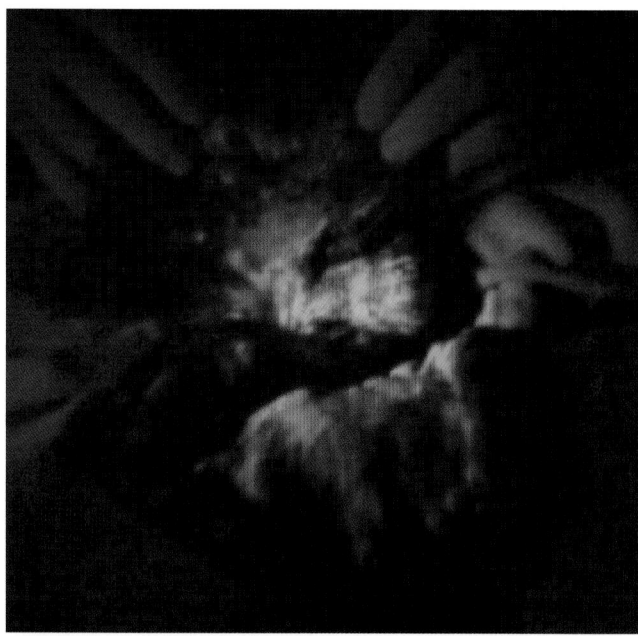

Figure 147-6 Patchy appearance of the distribution of fluorescein in a patient with acute mesenteric ischemia. Note that the fluorescein does not reach the bowel wall and is limited to the mesentery.

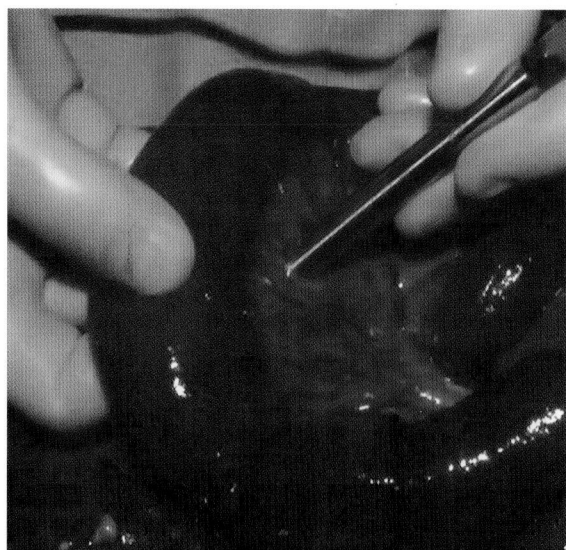

Figure 147-7 Doppler examination of the intestine should be done both at the mesentery and at the antimesenteric border. This is most useful following revascularization.

SMA pulse is often appreciated. Systemic heparinization is established. If the artery feels relatively soft and free of atherosclerotic disease, a transverse arteriotomy is performed distal to the area of obstruction, and the arterial lumen is assessed for thrombus. Balloon-tipped embolectomy catheters are gently passed proximally and distally until no more clot can be removed. Care must be taken not to overinflate the balloons and dissect the arterial intima. Distally, mesenteric vessels are very thin, and overinflation can result in rupture and intramesenteric extravasation. The transverse arteriotomy is then closed primarily with simple interrupted Prolene sutures if no endarterectomy is necessary. In cases in which a flow-limiting plaque is present, the arteriotomy is converted to a longitudinal one, and a local thromboendarterectomy is performed. Patch angioplasty with autogenous vein is the preferred method of revascularization owing to potential contamination from concomitant bowel resection. The arteriotomy site can also be used for distal anastomosis of an antegrade or retrograde bypass if necessary.

Chronic Mesenteric Ischemia

Detailed descriptions of the techniques of surgical visceral revascularization for CMI are highlighted in Chapter 148 (Mesenteric Vascular Disease: Chronic Ischemia).

Transaortic Endarterectomy.
Stoney and Wylie first described the "trapdoor" approach for transaortic endarterectomy (Fig. 147-8) in 1966 at the University of California, San Francisco.[8] It has been performed over the past 4 decades with acceptable morbidity and mortality rates and proven durability. Advantages of this operation include removal of atheroma from the aorta and both visceral arteries simultaneously. Limitations include the need for extended exposure of the upper abdominal aorta via medial visceral rotation and incomplete plaque removal if the atheroma extends to the distal artery or if transmural calcification is present. It is suitable for selected patients with CMI undergoing elective revascularization.

Cunningham and associates compared the results in 48 patients revascularized with transaortic endarterectomy (TEA) with the results in 26 patients who underwent antegrade surgical bypass over a 30-year period.[50,51] Mean follow-up was 71.1 months for the TEA group. Perioperative mortality was 14.6% in the TEA group but was not significantly different from that in the bypass group. Early in this study a thoracoretroperitoneal approach was used for TEA, which likely contributed to the high number of patients with perioperative pulmonary complications (11 of 48, 23%). The percentage of patients who remained symptom free following TEA was 95.8% at 1 year and 86.5% at 5 years. Visceral ischemia times were similar in the TEA and bypass groups (30.5 and 26.0 minutes, respectively). Lau and colleagues performed 14 TEAs for CMI through a retroperitoneal approach over a 10-year period.[52] The technical success rate was 93%. One patient required urgent SMA embolectomy on the second postoperative day. There were no perioperative deaths. Mean follow up was 2.4 years. The overall symptom-free survival rates were 85% and 77% at 1 and 3 years, respectively.

Antegrade Mesenteric Bypass.
Historically, antegrade bypass has demonstrated efficacy and durability.[50,53,54] Jimenez and colleagues reviewed the results of 47 patients with CMI who underwent antegrade synthetic aortoceliac and aorto-mesenteric bypass over a 14-year period.[54] The in-hospital mortality rate was 11%, and the mean length of hospital stay was 32 ± 30 days. At a mean follow-up of 37 months, 100% of surviving patients were symptom free, and 86% had significant weight gain. Primary, primary assisted, and secondary graft patency rates at 5 years were 69%, 94%, and 100%, respectively. Actuarial survival was 74%. Although antegrade bypass was associated with significant perioperative morbidity and mortality, it was also associated with excellent durability and symptom-free survival.[54] Cunningham and Reilly found similar results in their review of 26 antegrade bypasses for CMI.[50,51] They reported a slightly lower perioperative mortality rate (7.7%). The percentage of patients who were symptom free at 1 and 5 years was 96% and 86%, respectively. English and coworkers performed antegrade revascularization for CMI in 80 mesenteric vessels.[55] Their in-hospital mortality rate was 29%. The presence of intestinal gangrene correlated significantly with perioperative death and escalation of symptoms before bypass (acute-on-chronic). Symptom-free survival at 70 months was 57%. This type of bypass is best suited for elective revascularization of CMI.

Retrograde Mesenteric Bypass.
Wylie and associates first described retrograde mesenteric bypass (Fig. 147-9), and the debate continues regarding its efficacy compared with antegrade bypass.[56] Despite this controversy, no convincing evidence favors one approach over the other, and no randomized controlled trials have been conducted. Foley and colleagues from Oregon Health Sciences University examined their results with 50 bypass grafts to the SMA alone for

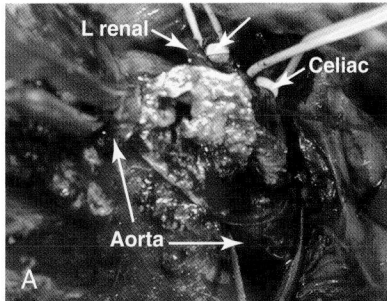
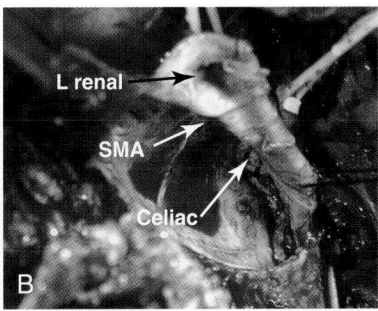
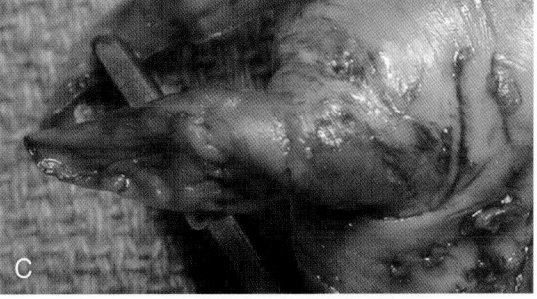

Figure 147-8 A, Transaortic endarterectomy using a trapdoor incision in a patient with severe aortic, mesenteric, and renal occlusive disease. **B,** Appearance of the visceral vessel orifice after transaortic endarterectomy. The aortotomy is usually closed with pledgeted sutures because the arterial wall is very thin following endarterectomy. **C,** Typical specimen after transaortic endarterectomy of an orificial lesion. Note the tapered endpoint. Patients selected for this technique should have lesions limited to the proximal segment of the artery. Failure to obtain an endpoint can be corrected by intraoperative placement of a stent under direct vision. L, left; SMA, superior mesenteric artery.

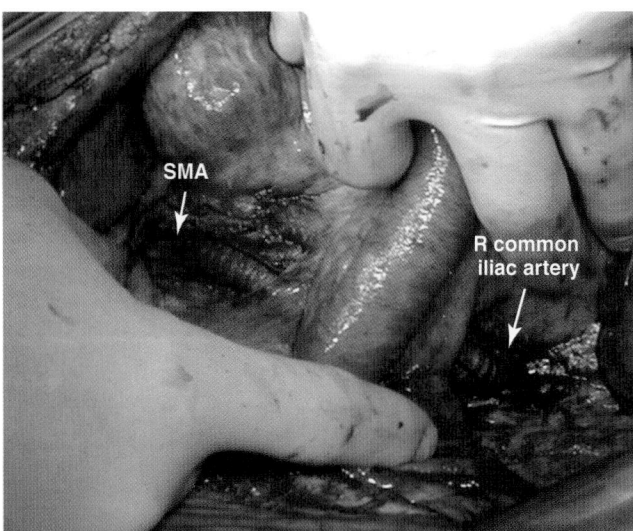

Figure 147-9 Right iliomesenteric bypass for retrograde revascularization of the superior mesenteric artery (SMA). The graft is passed between the leaves of the base of the mesentery to avoid contact with the intestines.

both AMI and CMI.[13] All grafts originated from either the infrarenal aorta or the iliac artery. Perioperative mortality was 3% in patients with CMI and 24% in patients with AMI. All survivors had relief of symptoms in the postoperative period. There were two late deaths related to graft occlusion. Nine-year primary assisted graft patency was 79%, and the 5-year survival was 61%.

In a combined study from Beth Israel Deaconess Medical Center and University of California, Los Angeles, the results of 39 mesenteric bypass procedures were reviewed over a 9-year period.[57] Symptom-free survival following antegrade (n = 21) and retrograde (n = 18) bypass was compared using the Kaplan-Meier life-table method. No significant difference was found between the two techniques. Although the overall incidence of postoperative complications was higher in the antegrade group, the number of major complications in both groups was similar. The 30-day mortality was higher in the antegrade group (14.3%) than in the retrograde group (0%), and none of the patients who died was revascularized for acute ischemia.

Outcomes of Open Repair

Acute Mesenteric Ischemia.
Mortality remains high in patients with AMI despite successful surgical revascularization. One of the contributing factors is ischemia-reperfusion intestinal injury. Although the exact mechanism is not completely understood, ischemia-reperfusion injury has been linked to postoperative myocardial depression,[58,59] sepsis,[60] acute lung injury,[61] and multiorgan failure.[62] Immediately following reperfusion, direct injury to the intestinal wall occurs and triggers a series of events, including the release of various inflammatory mediators, activation and aggregation of neutrophils, and bacterial translocation.[58] The intestine may take several weeks to months to recover, and patients may experience prolonged diarrhea and periods of malabsorption.[62]

The production of toxic oxygen radicals plays an important role in the pathogenesis of mucosal injury and structural integrity following ischemia-reperfusion of the intestine.[60] The mucosal barrier sustains damage, and increased permeability leads to impaired intestinal function and absorption of bacteria and endotoxin.[62] Oxygen-induced free radical production contributes significantly to diminished contractile function. Horton and White found that administering a free radical scavenger (superoxide dismutase and catalase) and a neutrophil stabilizer (pentoxifylline) prevented contractile depression and improved left ventricular function in an animal model of ischemia-reperfusion.[58]

Systemic physiologic effects following AMI are frequently life threatening. Cardiac dysfunction, manifested by arrhythmia and decreased contractility, frequently occurs after intestinal ischemia followed by reperfusion. Neutrophil-related acute lung injury has also been observed after intestinal ischemia and reperfusion.[63] Gerkin and colleagues observed that circulating humoral factors depleted pulmonary endothelial cell adenosine triphosphate in vitro following reperfusion injury.[61] Thus, systemic inflammatory mediators lead to increased microvascular permeability, pulmonary sequestration of neutrophils, and decreased energy stores, which contribute to acute lung injury and clinical pulmonary failure.

Aside from ischemia-reperfusion effects, many factors can contribute to complications following mesenteric revascularization. Kougias and colleagues reviewed the records for 72 patients who underwent surgical visceral revascularization for AMI.[64] The overall 30-day mortality was 31%. Factors associated with increased mortality were renal insufficiency, age older than 70 years, metabolic acidosis, symptom duration, and need for bowel resection during second-look operations. Increased age and prolonged symptom duration were independent predictors of mortality, with relative risks of 3.64 and 4.62, respectively.

In a review of 58 patients with AMI, age older than 60 years was associated with increased mortality.[27] In direct contrast to Kougias' study,[64] bowel resection during first- and second-look operations was associated with increased survival. Interestingly, the percentage of patients undergoing second-look operations was similar in both studies. Overall, the 30-day mortality was 31%, but for NOMI it was 80%.

Chronic Mesenteric Ischemia.
Mateo and colleagues performed a review of 85 patients who underwent revascularization for CMI over a 20-year period.[65] The early postoperative death rate was 8%, and the cumulative 5-year survival rate was 64%. Factors associated with increased mortality were advanced age at operation, existing cardiac disease, hypertension, and additional occlusive disease in other vascular beds. Factors associated with major postoperative morbidity included concomitant aortic replacement, preoperative renal disease, and, interestingly, complete revascularization. Table 147-1 presents the results of revascularization for CMI from selected series.

Table 147-1 Review of Contemporary Series of Elective Revascularization for Chronic Mesenteric Ischemia

Series	Year	Number of Patients	Number of Vessels	Results (%)						Mean Follow-up (mo)
				Immediate Technical Success	Complications	In-Hospital Mortality	Patency at 12 Months	Symptomatic Recurrence		
Kruger[a]	2007	39	41	97	12.2	2.5	95	5.1		39
Atkins et al.[44]	2007	49	88	100	39	2	90	22		42
English et al.[55]	2004	50	80	NA	62	29	97	6		42
Park[29]	2002	98	179	97	20	3	NA	5		23
Jimenez et al.[54]	2002	47	92	100	66	11	69	9		31
Cho[b]	2002	25	25	NA	60	0	57	41		60
Mateo et al.[65]	1999	85	130	94	33	8	76	24		36
Kihara[c]	1999	42	66	97	30	10	65	35		33

NA, not applicable.
[a]Kruger AJ, Walker PJ, Foster WJ, et al. Open surgery for atherosclerotic chronic mesenteric ischemia. *J Vasc Surg.* 2007;46:941-945.
[b]Cho JS, Carr JA, Jacobsen G, et al. Long-term outcome after mesenteric artery reconstruction: a 37-year experience. *J Vasc Surg.* 2002;35:453-460.
[c]Kihara TK, Blebea J, Anderson KM, et al. Risk factors and outcomes following revascularization for chronic mesenteric ischemia. *Ann Vasc Surg.* 1999;13:37-44.

TREATMENT OF NONOCCLUSIVE MESENTERIC ISCHEMIA

NOMI represents an insidious disease process that is distinct from thromboembolic AMI but has a similarly high mortality. Severe congestive heart failure and low-flow states are the most common causes of this disorder, and treatment is directed toward improving circulatory support and increasing cardiac output. Selective mesenteric angiography remains the best invasive diagnostic modality, which can be followed by catheter-based interventions. These include direct infusion of intra-arterial vasodilators such as papaverine and nitroglycerin, as well as angioplasty and stenting if necessary.[20] In a model of cardiac tamponade–induced acute NOMI, Kang and associates demonstrated that low doses of intra-arterial iloprost (prostacyclin), a potent inhibitor of platelet aggregation with fibrinolytic activity, exhibited a significant vasodilatory effect on mesenteric blood flow.[66]

Prostaglandin E_1 (PGE_1) is a potent smooth muscle relaxant that inhibits platelet aggregation, reduces erythrocyte deformation, and inhibits the production of reactive oxygen. A recent study examined the role of multidetector CT in the early diagnosis of NOMI and the subsequent infusion of intravenous high-dose PGE_1.[67] Twenty-two patients with NOMI were investigated over 13 years. Based on the first 13 cases, elderly patients were diagnosed with NOMI if they met three of four criteria after cardiovascular surgery or dialysis: (1) ileus with abdominal pain or nausea, (2) requirement for catecholamine treatment, (3) episode of hypotension, and (4) slow elevation in transaminase level. If a diagnosis of NOMI was established, patients underwent multidetector CT instead of abdominal angiography. If vasospasm of the mesenteric arteries was visualized without evidence of obstruction or stenosis, high-dose intravenous PGE_1 (0.01 to 0.02 µg/kg/min) was initiated for 5 days, with aggressive monitoring for hypotension. In the group of 13 patients who did not receive high-dose PGE_1, nine patients (69%) died. However, nine patients were subsequently diagnosed with CT instead of angiography and underwent intravenous prostaglandin infusion. Seven of nine patients (78%) in this group survived and were discharged from the hospital. Thus, the avoidance of angiography and the avoidance of potential delays in vasodilator infusion with prompt CT diagnosis led to improved outcomes.

TREATMENT OF MESENTERIC VENOUS THROMBOSIS

A detailed discussion of the diagnosis and treatment of MVT is contained in Chapter 150 (Mesenteric Vascular Disease: Venous Thrombosis). The mainstay of treatment for acute and subacute MVT is the prompt initiation of systemic anticoagulation, which improves survival and reduces the risk of recurrence.[24] A bolus injection of heparin followed by a continuous infusion is indicated. We recommend monitoring the partial thromboplastin time and maintaining it between 50 and 70 seconds. Intravenous antibiotics should be administered to decrease bacterial translocation from the intestinal mucosa. Aggressive fluid resuscitation and circulatory support should be performed because of severe bowel edema and shifting of fluid into the peritoneal cavity. Nasogastric decompression and bowel rest are also instituted.

Patients with suspected peritonitis require abdominal exploration and resection of nonviable bowel. We frequently perform a second-look laparotomy 24 hours after the initial operation, which helps avoid resection of viable bowel during the initial operation. Several authors have reported the successful use of direct percutaneous thrombolytic infusion into the mesenteric veins.[68-70] However, Grisham and colleagues reviewed the outcomes of 24 patients with MVT and noted a significantly higher mortality rate in those treated with thrombolytic therapy compared with those receiving systemic anticoagulation alone.[71] There was no significant difference in length of hospital stay between the two groups. In contrast, Semiz-Oysu and colleagues performed multiple percutaneous interventions for prehepatic MVT, including venous recanalization (n = 19), thrombolysis (n = 1), and mechanical thrombectomy (n = 5).[72] They noted an improvement in symptoms in 83% of patients treated, with relatively low mortality (13.6%).

SELECTED KEY REFERENCES

Acosta S, Ogren M, Sternby NH, Bergqvvist D, Bjorck M. Clinical implications for the management of acute thromboembolic occlusion of the superior mesenteric artery: autopsy findings in 213 patients. *Ann Surg.* 2005;241:516-522.
Highlights the increased morbidity associated with SMA embolus in AMI.

Foley MI, Moneta GL, Abou-Zamzam AM Jr, Edwards JM, Taylor LM Jr, Yeager RA, Porter JM. Revascularization of the superior mesenteric artery alone for treatment of intestinal ischemia. *J Vasc Surg.* 2000;32:37-47.
Landmark paper supporting the acceptability of results of retrograde mesenteric bypass for CMI.

Jimenez JG, Huber TS, Ozaki CK, Flynn TC, Berceli SA, Lee WA, Seeger JM. Durability of antegrade synthetic aortomesenteric bypass for chronic mesenteric ischemia. *J Vasc Surg.* 2002;35:1078-1084.
Provides evidence supporting the excellent durability and symptom-free survival associated with antegrade mesenteric bypass.

Sarac TP, Altinel O, Kashyap V, Bena J, Lyden S, Sruvastava S, Eagleton M, Clair D. Endovascular treatment of stenotic and occluded visceral arteries for chronic mesenteric ischemia. *J Vasc Surg.* 2008;47:485-491.
Supports the efficacy of endovascular management of complete occlusions of the visceral arteries.

Stoney RJ, Wylie WJ. Recognition and surgical management of visceral ischaemic syndromes. *Ann Surg.* 1966;164:714-722.
Landmark paper describing novel surgical techniques for the treatment of mesenteric ischemia.

REFERENCES

The reference list can be found on the companion Expert Consult Web site at *www.expertconsult.com.*

Mesenteric Vascular Disease: Chronic Ischemia

Thomas S. Huber and W. Anthony Lee

Chronic mesenteric ischemia is a life-threatening problem that can result in death from inanition or bowel infarction. Fortunately the prevalence is low, and it has been estimated that only about 340 open revascularizations for chronic mesenteric ischemia are performed annually in nonfederal hospitals throughout the United States.[1] The treatment of patients with chronic mesenteric ischemia has evolved over the past several years, paralleling improvements in imaging and an increased emphasis on endovascular or less invasive treatments. Unfortunately there has been little progress with regard to the open surgical approach and our overall understanding of the underlying pathophysiology. Indeed, many of the issues debated during the 1980s and 1990s (e.g., type of open procedure, number of vessels to be revascularized) remain unresolved. Despite these limitations, it is incumbent on vascular surgeons to expedite the diagnosis and treatment of patients with chronic mesenteric ischemia owing to the severity of the underlying problem and the frequency of diagnostic delay before referral.

PATHOPHYSIOLOGY AND ETIOLOGY

The underlying pathophysiology of chronic mesenteric ischemia is failure to achieve postprandial hyperemic intestinal blood flow. In normal individuals, intestinal blood flow increases after eating, with the maximal increase occurring in 30 to 90 minutes.[2,3] This hyperemic response lasts between 4 and 6 hours and varies with the size and composition of the meal.[3,4] The majority of the hyperemic blood flow goes to the small bowel and pancreas, with only a small increase to the stomach and colon.[5] Correspondingly, there is a marked increase in end-diastolic flow velocities in the superior mesenteric artery (SMA), with little change in velocities in the celiac axis, presumably owing to the relatively low resistance in the splenic and hepatic circulations at baseline. In the presence of a hemodynamically significant arterial stenosis, the postprandial hyperemic response is attenuated. This results in a relative imbalance between the tissue supply and demand for oxygen and other metabolites, leading to the onset of postprandial pain or "mesenteric angina." Not surprisingly, the changes in postprandial hyperemic flow and corresponding velocities return to normal after successful mesenteric revascularization.[6]

There is an extensive collateral network between the three visceral vessels (celiac axis, SMA, inferior mesenteric artery [IMA]) and the internal iliac arteries (Fig. 148-1). The celiac

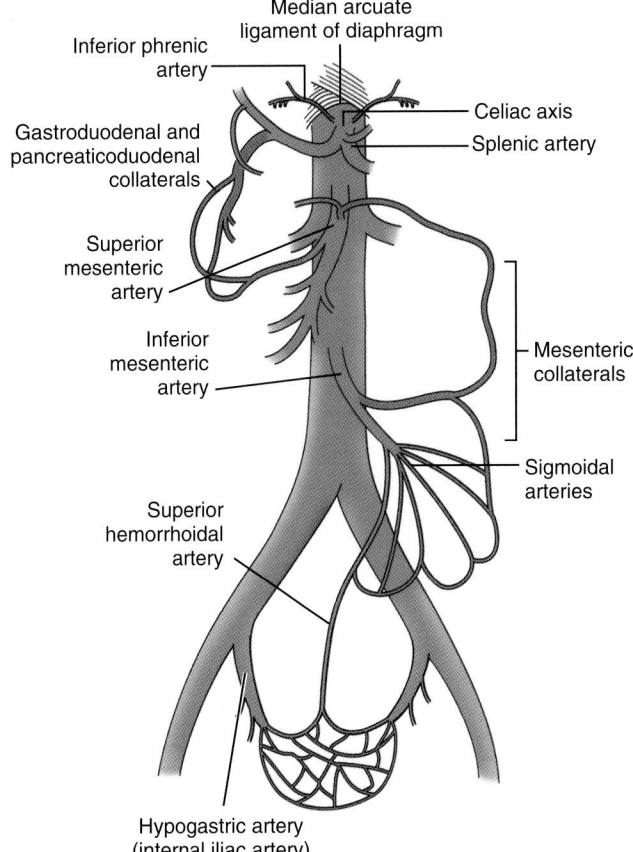

Figure 148-1 Diagram of collateral pathways for the mesenteric vessels. The celiac axis and superior mesenteric arteries communicate through the superior and inferior pancreaticoduodenal arteries, respectively. The superior and inferior mesenteric arteries communicate through the meandering artery and the marginal artery of Drummond, with the former serving as the dominant collateral. The inferior mesenteric artery communicates with the internal iliac artery through the hemorrhoidal vessels. *(From Zelenock GB. Visceral occlusive disease. In: Greenfield LJ, ed. Surgery: Scientific Principles and Practice. Philadelphia: Lippincott, Williams, and Wilkins; 2001:1691.)*

axis and SMA collateralize through the superior (celiac axis) and inferior (SMA) pancreaticoduodenal arteries, with the direction of flow contingent on the location of the significant stenosis. The SMA and IMA collateralize through both the meandering artery and the marginal artery of Drummond. The meandering artery is the most significant collateral vessel and connects the ascending branch of the left colic artery with the middle branch of the middle colic artery. It lies at the base of the mesentery and is at risk of being ligated along with the inferior mesenteric vein during exposure of the infrarenal aorta. The IMA communicates with the internal iliac artery via the hemorrhoidal branches and may represent a more important collateral than was originally appreciated.[7] This collateral pathway may be disrupted during sigmoid colectomy or infrarenal aortic aneurysm repair.

Given the extensive collateral network, patients usually do not become symptomatic unless two of the three visceral vessels have hemodynamically significant lesions. However, this is not an absolute requirement, despite the myth propagated in many surgical textbooks.[8,9] It is possible to become symptomatic in the presence of isolated celiac axis or SMA disease if the collateral pathways are insufficient.[10] This usually occurs owing to a hemodynamically significant lesion in the SMA, as might be predicted from the postprandial hyperemic response. Notably, more than 90% of patients undergoing open surgical revascularization for chronic mesenteric ischemia had a significant stenosis or occlusion of the SMA, and more than 80% had a significant disease in both the celiac axis and the SMA in several large clinical series.[11]

Atherosclerosis is the leading cause of the visceral artery occlusive disease responsible for chronic mesenteric ischemia. A variety of other causes, including fibromuscular disease, aortic dissection, isolated SMA dissection, neurofibromatosis, rheumatoid arthritis, Takayasu's arteritis, giant cell arteritis, polyarteritis nodosa, radiation injury, Buerger's disease, systemic lupus, and drugs (e.g., cocaine, ergots), have been incriminated and merit investigation in the appropriate clinical setting, although collectively, they are significantly less common. Patients with visceral artery occlusive disease often have concomitant renal artery occlusive disease or a pattern consistent with "central aortic" disease. However, visceral artery occlusive disease is relatively common, in contradistinction to mesenteric ischemia. Wilson and colleagues conducted a population study using duplex ultrasound and found that 18% of individuals older than 65 years had a critical stenosis of at least one of the visceral vessels (celiac, 15%; celiac-SMA, 1%; SMA, 1%).[12] Unselected autopsy studies have reported that the incidence of a stenosis greater than 50% in at least one of the three visceral vessels ranges from 6% to 10%.[13] In addition, 27% of patients undergoing arteriography before peripheral arterial reconstruction had comparable stenosis in the SMA or celiac axis.[14]

The natural history of chronic mesenteric ischemia is presumably death from inanition or bowel infarction. Admittedly, the natural history has not been well characterized because patients usually undergo revascularization after diagnosis, so there is no untreated or control group. The natural history of asymptomatic mesenteric artery occlusive disease is even less well characterized. In their population study, Wilson and colleagues reported that none of the patients with visceral artery occlusive disease developed chronic mesenteric ischemia or bowel infarction during follow-up.[12] However, it is important to emphasize that the SMA was

involved in less than 2% of their cases. Thomas and associates attempted to define the natural history of asymptomatic stenoses among 980 patients undergoing mesenteric arteriography during a 7-year period.[15] They reported that 4 of 15 patients with significant (>50%) stenoses in all three visceral arteries developed mesenteric ischemia during a mean follow-up of 2.6 years. Conversely, mesenteric ischemia did not occur in any of the patients who did not have significant disease in all three vessels. They concluded that prophylactic revascularization should be considered in this high-risk group with triple-vessel disease, and it should be routine before aortic reconstruction. Additional justification for prophylactic revascularization is provided by the observation that 15% to 50% of patients with acute mesenteric ischemia secondary to visceral artery occlusive disease do not have any antecedent warning signs.[16,17] Infarction of the bowel after aortic surgery in patients with preexisting visceral artery occlusive disease has also been reported[18] and has been used to justify staged or simultaneous visceral artery revascularization and aortic repair.

DIAGNOSTIC EVALUATION
Clinical Presentation

The clinical presentation of patients with chronic mesenteric ischemia is fairly typical, and the diagnosis is often suggested by their overall appearance. The characteristic patient is a cachectic, middle-aged woman with a long smoking history who presents with abdominal pain and weight loss. Indeed, chronic mesenteric ischemia is one of the few cardiovascular disorders more common in women than in men. A study from the Nationwide Inpatient Sample examining the outcome after revascularization for chronic mesenteric ischemia reported that the mean patient age was 66 ± 11 years and that 76% of patients were women—both within the range of the multi-institution series.[1]

Although abdominal pain is usually the symptom that precipitates presentation to a primary care physician or gastroenterologist, the pain associated with chronic mesenteric ischemia has no specific characteristics. It often involves the midepigastric region and can radiate to the back. It is described as either dull or colicky, but it is distinctly different from the pain associated with peritonitis. The pain usually occurs 15 to 30 minutes after eating and lasts 1 to 3 hours. This is consistent with the underlying pathophysiology and the abnormal postprandial hyperemic response. The cause of the pain itself is unclear and has been attributed to arterial "steal" from the gastric circulation and various ischemic mediators.[19] The pain may progress from intermittent pain associated with certain types or quantities of food to consistent, unremitting pain that likely forebodes bowel infarction. Pain may be absent at the time of presentation because patients develop adaptive strategies to relieve or reduce it.

The net effect of the abdominal pain is that patients avoid certain types of food or eating altogether and lose weight. Indeed, the mean weight loss in many of the large clinical series ranges from 20 to 30 pounds.[7,20-22] This specific behavioral response has been termed "food fear." The weight loss is due to inadequate nutritional intake rather than an absorption problem, as might be hypothesized.[23] Many affected individuals are thin at the onset of their symptoms and cachectic at the time of definitive diagnosis and treatment. Unfortunately, there are no consistent bowel patterns associated with chronic mesenteric ischemia; some patients develop constipation as a result of their food avoidance, while others develop intermittent diarrhea. Notably, acute mesenteric ischemia is a profound cathartic.

Physical examination is not particularly enlightening in terms of diagnosing chronic mesenteric ischemia, with the obvious exception of patients' typical general appearance. They often have evidence of systemic vascular disease and abdominal bruits, although both are fairly nonspecific. The apparent absence of systemic vascular disease on physical examination does not preclude the diagnosis. As noted earlier, the patient's vascular disease may be isolated to the central aortic region.

Diagnostic Imaging

Patients with chronic mesenteric ischemia usually undergo an extensive medical evaluation before the ultimate correct diagnosis. This usually includes an esophagogastroduodenoscopy, colonoscopy, ultrasound, and computed tomography (CT); it is not uncommon for patients to undergo cholecystectomy as well. Usually more than one calendar year passes between the onset of symptoms and the correct diagnosis,[24-27] and the patient undergoes a mean of 2.8 diagnostic tests.[26] The diagnostic evaluation is confounded by the fact that chronic mesenteric ischemia may lead to gastroparesis, gastric ulceration, gastroduodenitis, and gallbladder dysmotility. Further, it is not uncommon for a patient's abdominal pain, weight loss, and generalized "failure to thrive" to be attributed to any one of these pathologic processes during the course of the diagnostic evaluation. Indeed, gastric ulceration is almost pathognomonic for chronic mesenteric ischemia.[7,20,28] The ulcers are likely sequelae of gastric ischemia because they occur in areas of reduced perfusion,[29,30] are refractory to medical management, and resolve after revascularization.

The diagnosis of chronic mesenteric ischemia requires the proper clinical scenario, a confirmatory imaging study, and the exclusion of other potential causes of abdominal pain. The majority of patients referred for evaluation of chronic mesenteric ischemia have already undergone an extensive, prolonged workup, and the diagnosis is usually obvious if not already confirmed. However, the differential diagnosis of abdominal pain is extensive, and chronic mesenteric ischemia is fairly low on this list. Foremost in the differential diagnosis of abdominal pain and weight loss is an intra-abdominal malignancy until proved otherwise. Patients should undergo esophagogastroduodenoscopy, colonoscopy, abdominal ultrasound, and abdominal CT scan early in the evaluation to exclude the more common potential causes of their complaints.

Mesenteric Duplex Ultrasound

Mesenteric duplex ultrasound is an excellent screening tool for occlusive disease in the celiac axis and SMA, with sensitivities, specificities, and predictive values greater than 80% relative to catheter-based contrast arteriography (Fig. 148-2).[31,32] Indeed, a negative mesenteric duplex scan essentially excludes the diagnosis of chronic mesenteric ischemia or visceral artery occlusive disease. The IMA is difficult to visualize and is not routinely included in the examination. Unfortunately, mesenteric duplex ultrasound is technically challenging, operator dependent, and not universally available. It is complicated by the deep location of the vessels, respiratory variation, strict need for a Doppler angle of 60 degrees, and presence of intra-abdominal gas. Moneta and coworkers reported that peak systolic flow velocities greater than 275 cm/sec in the SMA and greater than 200 cm/sec in the celiac axis correspond to

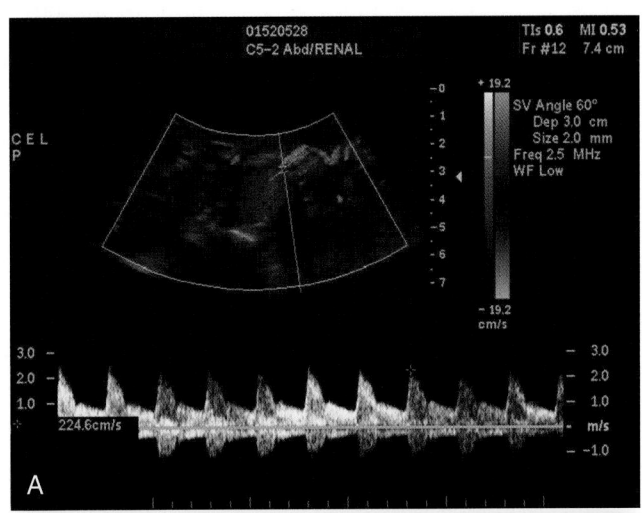

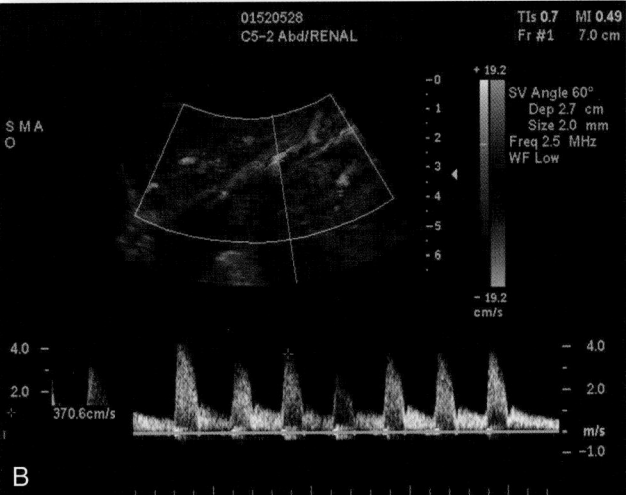

Figure 148-2 A, Color-flow duplex ultrasound of the celiac axis. Note the high-grade stenosis at the origin of the celiac axis. Its peak systolic velocity (PSV) of 224 cm/sec corresponds to a greater than 70% stenosis in our vascular laboratory (celiac axis PSV >200 cm/ sec = >70% stenosis). **B,** Corresponding image of the superior mesenteric artery. A similar high-grade stenosis is seen at the origin, reflected by the PSV of 371 cm/sec (superior mesenteric artery PSV >275 cm/sec = >70% stenosis).

greater than 70% stenoses.[31] Similarly, Zwolak and associates reported that end-diastolic velocities greater than 45 cm/sec in the SMA and greater than 55 cm/sec in the celiac axis correspond to greater than 50% stenoses.[33] Despite these publications, each institution must develop and validate its own criteria for significant stenoses. Several groups have attempted to develop a duplex-based "stress test" for mesenteric artery occlusive disease by imaging the vessels after a mixed-composition meal, but its clinical utility remains unclear.[34,35] Not surprisingly, mesenteric duplex ultrasound has also proved to be an excellent surveillance tool after open and endovascular revascularization.[36-38]

Catheter-Based Contrast Arteriography

Catheter-based contrast arteriography has been the traditional "gold standard" diagnostic study for patients with chronic mesenteric ischemia (Fig. 148-3). It has been used to confirm the mesenteric duplex findings, plan the operative procedure, and facilitate therapeutic interventions. Mesenteric atherosclerotic occlusive disease is essentially "aortic spillover" disease; accordingly, the origins of the celiac axis and SMA are involved, whereas the more distal aspects are spared or preserved. This usually holds true in the presence of complete orificial occlusions, even when the distal vessels are not visualized with the catheter-based arteriogram. Involvement of the distal vasculature suggests a nonatherosclerotic process such as cocaine or ergot ingestion. The presence of well-developed collaterals between the visceral vessels further supports the diagnosis of mesenteric ischemia and attests to the hemodynamic significance of ostial lesions. As

noted earlier, it is relatively common to see renal artery occlusive disease, given the central aortic atherosclerotic process. It is imperative that a lateral arteriogram be obtained, given the orientation of the celiac axis and SMA relative to the aorta. Visceral artery aneurysms are occasionally seen on the arteriogram in the collateral branches—specifically, the pancreaticoduodenal artery. These are presumably flow-related aneurysms similar to those seen in the splenic artery in patients with portal hypertension.[39] It is usually not necessary to selectively catheterize the visceral vessels, given the orificial distribution of the occlusive disease. Rarely, mesenteric angioplasty and stenting may serve as a diagnostic study for patients with mesenteric artery occlusive disease and atypical symptoms.

Multidetector CT Arteriography and Magnetic Resonance Arteriography

Multidetector CT arteriography (Fig. 148-4) and, to a lesser extent, magnetic resonance arteriography have recently supplemented or replaced mesenteric duplex ultrasound and catheter-based contrast arteriography as the imaging study of choice for patients with chronic mesenteric ischemia.[40-47] CT arteriography can accurately identify significant stenoses in the celiac axis and SMA, identify significant visceral collaterals, and exclude other potential intra-abdominal processes in concert with traditional CT images.[40,43,44] In contrast to mesenteric duplex ultrasound, CT arteriography is almost universally available and far less technician dependent. Magnetic resonance arteriography affords many of the same advantages as CT arteriography but is not universally available and has

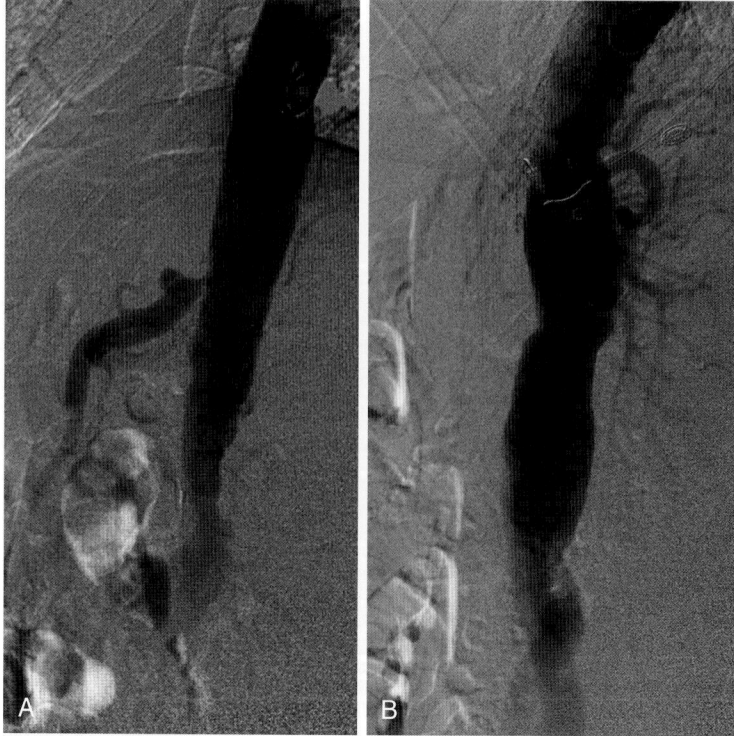

Figure 148-3 A, Catheter-based contrast arteriogram of the aorta in the lateral projection. Note the high-grade stenosis at the origin of the celiac axis. The superior mesenteric artery is not visualized owing to its orificial occlusion. **B,** A second catheter-based contrast arteriogram of the aorta in the lateral projection. Neither the celiac axis nor the superior mesenteric artery is visualized in this patient with a "naked" aorta.

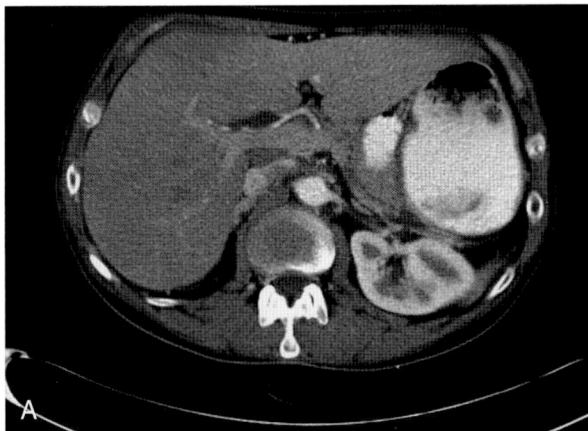

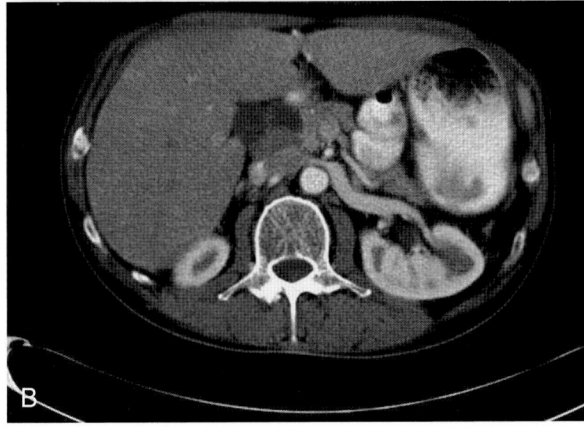

Figure 148-4 A, CT arteriogram of the upper abdomen. The superior mesenteric artery, immediately anterior to the aorta and left renal vein, is occluded, as demonstrated by the absence of contrast material within its lumen. **B,** CT arteriogram a few millimeters caudal to the image in **A.** Note that the superior mesenteric artery is patent at this level, as emphasized by the contrast material within its lumen.

not been used as commonly in this setting.[41,42] CT arteriography also appears to be replacing catheter-based arteriography for the planning of therapeutic interventions; the image quality is more than sufficient to plan an open operative procedure, and a separate catheter-based diagnostic arteriogram is irrelevant for endovascular procedures because the diagnostic and therapeutic components are usually performed simultaneously. Not surprisingly, CT arteriography is also an excellent tool to assess graft and vessel patency in both the early and late postintervention or postoperative periods.[40,43,44] Admittedly, it may not be as cost-effective as mesenteric duplex ultrasound, and it is associated with a small incidence of complications. Further, significant vessel calcification may preclude an accurate assessment of the luminal diameter.

INDICATIONS AND TREATMENT STRATEGIES

Despite the theoretical appeal, there is no role for chronic parenteral alimentation and noninterventional therapies, even in patients at high risk for revascularization owing to co-morbidities. Admittedly, postprandial pain can be relieved by not eating, and parenteral nutrition may allow patients to regain weight. However, the potential for bowel infarction is not alleviated, and lifetime dependence on parenteral nutrition is not practical in terms of convenience, expense, and the risk of catheter-related complications. Indeed, Rheudasil and colleagues reported that a significant percentage of their patients with chronic mesenteric ischemia developed acute mesenteric ischemia in the hospital while on parenteral nutrition awaiting revascularization.[48]

Indications for Revascularization

All patients with chronic mesenteric ischemia should undergo revascularization. The goals of treatment are to reduce pain, prevent bowel infarction, and restore nutritional status. The indication for revascularization in asymptomatic patients with known visceral artery occlusive disease remains unresolved. As noted earlier, Thomas and associates reported that patients with significant occlusive disease in all three visceral vessels represent a high-risk group for bowel infarction,[15] and other anecdotal reports have documented adverse outcomes after aortic reconstruction in a similar subset of patients.[18] Revascularization should be considered in these settings even though the justification in the literature is somewhat weak, and all prophylactic interventions need to be balanced against treatment-associated mortality and morbidity. Patients with untreated visceral artery occlusive disease should be followed closely and counseled regarding the types of symptoms that merit urgent presentation. All episodes of significant abdominal pain in this setting require investigation and should be associated with a low threshold for intervention.

Endovascular versus Open Treatment

The optimal treatment (endovascular versus open) for patients with chronic mesenteric ischemia remains unresolved. Significant changes have occurred over the past several years, with an increased emphasis on the endovascular approach, paralleling changes in our overall discipline. Indeed, endovascular treatment has become first-line therapy in many institutions. However, there have been no randomized controlled trials comparing the two approaches, and these are unlikely to occur in the near future, given the relative infrequency of the problem. The overwhelming majority of outcome studies come from single centers and have been performed in a retrospective fashion. Accordingly, they are subject to a tremendous amount of selection bias. Further, many of the reports are complicated by the inclusion of patients with both acute and chronic mesenteric ischemia, a mixture of operative procedures (e.g., antegrade bypass, retrograde bypass, endarterectomy), a mixture of endovascular procedures (e.g., SMA angioplasty, SMA stent, celiac-SMA stent), and a lack of objective follow-up data. Collectively, these differences make the comparison of treatment strategies difficult.

Similar to its role in other vascular beds, the endovascular approach offers the theoretical advantages of a shorter hospital stay (or outpatient procedure), reduced morbidity, reduced mortality, and improved quality of life. However, the long-term vessel patency rates appear to be inferior to those obtained with open revascularization, and the need for remedial procedures is increased. Biebl and coworkers succinctly summarized the status of the two treatment options, stating, "surgical treatment has superior long-term patency, but it is also more invasive with greater morbidity and mortality compared to endovascular treatment."[49] Importantly, recurrent stenosis after endovascular treatment does not necessarily equate with recurrent symptoms or precipitate acute mesenteric ischemia,[37,50,51] although these adverse outcomes are clearly possible, underscoring the importance of long-term follow-up.[52] The unanswered question is whether the decreased patency rates (and the attendant risk of developing recurrent symptoms or acute mesenteric ischemia) associated with the endovascular approach offset the increased operative morbidity and mortality associated with open repair. Notably, several recent trials comparing the outcomes after endovascular and open treatment for chronic mesenteric ischemia suggested that the endovascular approach should be used selectively and restricted to higher risk patients who cannot tolerate open repair.[52-54] Brown and associates proposed that the endovascular approach can serve as a "bridge" to open revascularization by allowing time to optimize the patient's co-morbidities and nutritional status.[52] In our own practice, we recommend open revascularization for younger, good-risk patients; those whose disease is not amenable to the endovascular approach for anatomic reasons (e.g., flush aortic occlusion of the SMA); and those with recurrent, refractory stenoses after endovascular therapy. The latter two indications account for the majority of patients in our practice. It is our anecdotal impression that patients undergoing revascularization today are both older and sicker than in the pre-endovascular era. Not surprisingly, it is also our anecdotal impression that there has been a concomitant increase in perioperative morbidity and mortality after open repair.

Choices in Open Vascularization

Although the endovascular approach to chronic mesenteric ischemia has become popular over the past few years, there are several ongoing issues with regard to open revascularization that remain unresolved. These include the type of revascularization, the number of vessels to be revascularized, and the optimal conduit. The techniques of reimplantation, endarterectomy, and bypass have all been used successfully, and each possesses theoretical advantages. Mesenteric bypass, either antegrade from the supraceliac aorta or retrograde from the infrarenal aorta or common iliac artery, has emerged as the most common treatment, with the current debate focusing on the specific configuration. The theoretical advantages of antegrade bypass include the facts that the supraceliac aorta is usually uninvolved with atherosclerosis and that the limbs of the graft follow a direct path while maintaining prograde flow. The theoretical advantages of retrograde bypass include the fact that infrarenal aorta–common iliac artery can be exposed more easily and faster and is generally more familiar to most vascular surgeons. Further, there is less hemodynamic instability and potential for distal embolization with infrarenal aortic–iliac clamp application. Admittedly, it is usually possible to partially occlude the supraceliac aorta while performing the proximal anastomosis of the antegrade bypass. One major disadvantage of the retrograde bypass is the obligatory course of the graft and its potential to kink, which is particularly problematic for venous conduits. Indeed, the graft must transition from the aorta, which sits posterior in the abdomen, to the SMA, which sits more anterior and includes a near 180-degree turn.

Inherent to the debate about the type of bypass procedure to perform is the number of vessels to revascularize. Multivessel revascularization offers the theoretical advantage that if one of the graft limbs (or stents) occludes, the patient does not necessarily develop recurrent symptoms or acute intestinal ischemia. Indeed, Hollier and colleagues reported in 1981 that the recurrence rate after open revascularization was inversely related to the number of vessels revascularized and that it exceeded 50% only if a single vessel was repaired.[25] Proponents of isolated retrograde bypass to the SMA emphasize that the procedure revascularizes the primary vessel of concern, that multivessel reconstructions add to the complexity of the procedure, and, most important, that recent series have not shown a significant clinical advantage of multivessel bypass. Indeed, Park and coworkers reported a follow-up study from the same institution as the original report by Hollier's group and stated that they have "maintained a degree of faithfulness" to the multivessel revascularization concept, although they no longer believe that reconstructing the IMA is essential.[55] Similar concerns about the number of vessels to be revascularized have been raised for the endovascular approach, with Silva and associates suggesting that complete revascularization (SMA and celiac axis) plays a role in preventing recurrent symptoms.[51]

Both prosthetic and autogenous conduits have been used with the various mesenteric bypass procedures, although reports comparing their long-term patency rates have been somewhat inconclusive.[26,56-58] Notably, Kihara and colleagues reported that patency rates for vein grafts were significantly lower than those for prosthetic grafts by univariate analysis, but multivariate analysis demonstrated that patient gender was responsible for the observed difference (patency greater in females than in males).[56] Saphenous vein conduits may be at increased risk for developing stenoses, given the relatively high flow rate through the visceral vessels. Modrall and associates reported that the symptomatic recurrence rate after mesenteric bypass was lower in patients who underwent reconstruction using the femoral vein compared with saphenous vein.[58] Indeed, the femoral vein may represent an ideal conduit for mesenteric bypass when a prosthetic conduit is contraindicated, given its mean diameter of 7 mm and relatively thick wall.[59] However, harvesting the femoral vein adds a significant amount of time and complexity to the procedure. In our own practice, we routinely use a Dacron graft unless there is concern about enteric contamination from ischemia or infarction, in which cases we use the femoral vein.

OPERATIVE TECHNIQUE AND PERIOPERATIVE MANAGEMENT

Endovascular Revascularization

Preoperative Evaluation

The preoperative evaluation before endovascular treatment of mesenteric occlusive lesions in patients with chronic mesenteric ischemia is essentially the same as that for any other peripheral endovascular procedure. Patients with a contrast allergy should be treated with an appropriate steroid preparation. Patients with elevated serum creatinine levels (1.5 to 2 mg/dL [133 to 177 μmol/L]) who are considered candidates for standard contrast agents should receive gentle hydration, acetylcysteine, and sodium bicarbonate, although their benefits are somewhat unsubstantiated. If the endovascular approach is unsuccessful and open revascularization is required, the patient should undergo the more extensive preoperative evaluation outlined later. It is very unusual for a failed endovascular procedure to require emergent revascularization, however.

Diagnostic and Interventional Technique

Percutaneous access can be obtained through either the femoral or brachial artery. The primary consideration for the particular approach should be the a priori likelihood of a therapeutic intervention, with the exception of those patients with known anatomic limitations such as iliofemoral or subclavian artery occlusive disease. The femoral approach is more familiar to most operators, is associated with a lower incidence of vascular injury, and is closer to the target artery, thereby allowing the use of shorter guide wires and catheters. However, it should generally be used only when the possibility of a therapeutic intervention is unlikely, owing to the orientation of the mesenteric vessels. Notably, the angle between the mesenteric vessels and the aorta is fairly acute and directed caudad. The vector forces of a catheter directed from the femoral artery are opposite to the angle of the mesenteric vessels; therefore, pushability is compromised. The brachial approach overcomes these limitations, and the change in catheter mechanics is sufficient to overcome the increased physical distance and the need for longer devices. Additional disadvantages of the brachial approach (other than those cited as advantages of the femoral approach) include the limited maximal sheath size possible without a surgical cut-down (i.e., 7 Fr for men, 6 Fr for women), risk of embolic stroke, and difficulty gaining access to the descending thoracic aorta in patients with a tortuous arch. Although aortic access can be obtained from either brachial artery, the left brachial approach is preferred owing to the risk of carotid embolization with prolonged catheterization across the innominate artery. Notably, Sarac and coauthors reported superior outcomes for the endovascular treatment of visceral artery lesions using the brachial approach.[60]

Endovascular treatment is initiated by accessing the left brachial artery near the medial head of the humerus using a micropuncture technique (21-gauge needle, 0.018-inch guide wire) and a short 5 Fr introducer sheath. A combination of a floppy-tipped guide wire (e.g., Bentson) and a pigtail angiographic catheter is used to direct the catheter into the descending thoracic aorta because an undirected guide wire passes into the ascending aorta in the majority of cases. All catheters and guide wires should have a working length of greater than 80 cm and 240 cm, respectively. The initial diagnostic arteriogram is obtained by positioning a pigtail catheter at the level of the 12th thoracic vertebral body, and a flush aortogram is performed in the anteroposterior and lateral projections. Because most lesions in the SMA and celiac axis are orificial (Fig. 148-5) and located in the proximal 2 cm, selective catheterization is usually not necessary unless a distal lesion is suspected or the extent of the lesion cannot be determined. In the presence of severe lesions or frank occlusions, the acquisition interval should be prolonged to allow for delayed filling via the collateral pathways. Provided that either the SMA or the celiac axis is patent, further visualization of the stenotic or occluded vessels can be obtained as needed by selectively catheterizing the patent vessel because of the extensive collateral network. When both the SMA and the celiac axis are severely stenotic or occluded, their distal extent can be further visualized by selectively catheterizing the IMA. The median arcuate ligament may extrinsically compress the proximal celiac axis. This can be differentiated from an intrinsic lesion by obtaining provocative inspiratory and expiratory phase images. A reduction in diameter of greater than 50% in the SMA is usually considered clinically significant, regardless of whether the celiac axis is involved. In contrast, the diagnosis of chronic mesenteric ischemia should be questioned in the presence of an isolated celiac axis stenosis.

Symptomatic stenoses of the visceral vessels can be treated at the time of the diagnostic arteriogram. We prefer to treat both the celiac axis and the SMA if feasible, given the theoretical advantages of multivessel revascularization. Similar to renal artery lesions, the orificial stenoses in the mesenteric vessels are refractory to angioplasty alone, and primary stenting is recommended. Balloon angioplasty with selective stenting is reserved for midsegment lesions. Balloon-expandable stents are preferred over self-expanding ones owing to their superior radial force and controlled deployment. Most currently available balloon-expandable and nitinol self-expanding stents foreshorten only minimally, so stents can be reliably sized and positioned based on the extent and location of the lesion. Similar to the case in other peripheral vascular beds, technologic advances have facilitated the use of smaller systems, as demonstrated by the report of Schaefer and coworkers, who used a monorail system over an 0.018-inch guide wire.[50]

After a decision to proceed with intervention is made, a 90-cm straight 6 Fr guiding sheath is advanced to the orifice of the SMA (or celiac axis, depending on the target vessel) over a stiffer guide wire (e.g., Rosen). The SMA is usually treated before the celiac axis, even in the presence of

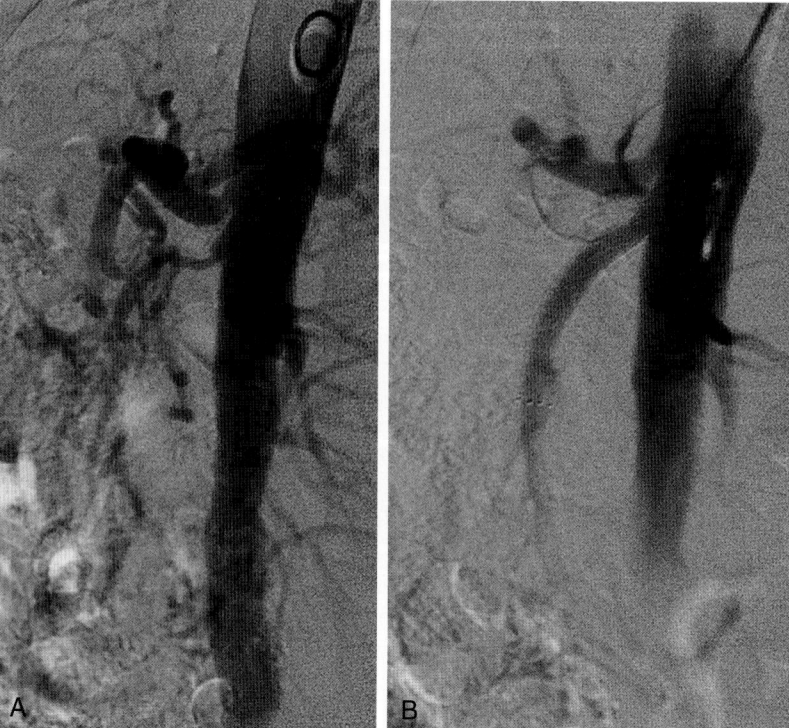

Figure 148-5 A, Lateral arteriogram of the celiac axis and superior mesenteric artery. Note the mild orificial stenosis in the celiac axis and the severe stenosis in the proximal superior mesenteric artery. **B,** Completion study after angioplasty and stenting of the superior mesenteric artery stenosis. Note the widely patent superior mesenteric artery, with no evidence of stenosis.

significant disease in both vessels. The patient is systemically heparinized; typically, a single intravenous bolus (5000 units) suffices, without the need to monitor the activated clotting time or make weight-based dose adjustments. A combination of a 100-cm 5 Fr angled catheter (e.g., multipurpose angiographic [MPA]) and an angled hydrophilic guide wire (e.g., Glidewire) is used to cross the stenosis. The guide wire is removed, and a selective arteriogram is performed using only manual injection to rule out a tandem lesion and, more important, to confirm that the catheter is intravascular and that the vessel has not been injured by the guide wire or catheter manipulations. Intra-arterial nitroglycerin (200 to 400 μg) or papaverine (10 to 15 mg) may be administered to relieve any vasospasm and dilate the distal bed, although this is usually not necessary.

Pressures in the target artery and aorta can be measured by exchanging the 5 Fr MPA catheter for a 4 Fr catheter and simultaneously transducing this coaxial catheter and the 6 Fr guiding sheath if the lesion's hemodynamic significance is questionable; a mean gradient greater than 5 mm Hg or a peak systolic gradient greater than 10 mm Hg is considered significant.

A nonhydrophilic guide wire is re-introduced through the catheter after the selective arteriogram or pressure measurements, and its tip is advanced as far distally as possible. It is imperative that the position of the guide wire tip be closely monitored throughout the procedure because it may inadvertently perforate or dissect the target vessel. This is particularly problematic during celiac axis interventions because the guide wire is positioned in either the hepatic or splenic artery in the

anteroposterior projection while the actual intervention is performed in the lateral projection. A control arteriogram is obtained through the guiding sheath to localize the lesion. It is critical to optimize the projection angle (lateral versus anterior oblique) in order to properly locate the true orifice of the vessel relative to the aorta. Although a dilator and the guiding sheath can be used to "dotter" the stenosis, predilation with a 5- by 20-mm angioplasty balloon is easier and potentially less traumatic. The guiding sheath is gently advanced over the balloon beyond the stenosis. Although the target artery diameter can be estimated using electronic calipers or preoperative CT arteriography, this can underestimate the true diameter owing to depressurization of the artery from the proximal stenosis. In general, a minimum of a 7- or 8-mm-diameter stent should be used. Most balloon-expandable stents are mounted on semicompliant balloons, and an additional diameter expansion up to 0.5 mm can be achieved (depending on the manufacturer) by increasing the inflation pressure over its working range (nominal burst pressure). As a general rule, the segment of the target vessel beyond any post-stenotic dilation should be used as the reference diameter. A 15- to 20-mm-long balloon-expandable stent of appropriate diameter is delivered to the site of the predilated lesion, and the sheath is retracted just proximal to the balloon. A repeat control arteriogram is obtained, and the stent is deployed with its proximal extent protruding roughly 2 mm into the aortic lumen to ensure complete coverage of the proximal extent of the "aortic" lesion. Adjunctive techniques, including proximal molding or funneling of the stent with larger balloons, have been described but are rarely necessary.

Recanalization of occluded mesenteric vessels is similar to that for other arterial beds and may be attempted, although the anticipated technical success rates are somewhat lower. Notably, Sarac and coauthors reported that both patency and survival rates were comparable after endovascular treatment of visceral artery stenoses and occlusions.[60] Although the occlusions are almost always orificial, it is important to determine that the distal artery is patent and to establish the extent of the occlusion using the techniques outlined earlier, because the extent of the occlusion impacts the probability of successful recanalization. A "stump" is beneficial because the orifice of the vessels may be hard to localize in the presence of a flush aortic occlusion. In addition, it is difficult to engage a supporting catheter to facilitate guide wire entry in the presence of a flush occlusion. Provided that the occlusion is amenable to recanalization, a hydrophilic guide wire with a medium-stiff shaft (e.g., Roadrunner) in combination with an angled selective or guiding catheter is used to gently probe the occluded orifice. After guide wire access is obtained, it is critical to pass a catheter (e.g., 4 Fr Glidecatheter) across the occlusion and obtain an arteriogram to confirm that it is actually within the lumen of the vessel. The remaining portions of the procedure are as outlined earlier.

Robken and Shammas described a novel approach in patients with SMA occlusions that involves accessing the vessel retrograde using a wire passed through the celiac axis and the superior pancreaticoduodenal artery.[61] The wire is subsequently passed into the aorta (i.e., retrograde through the SMA) and snared, thereby facilitating subsequent stent placement.

Postoperative Care

The postoperative care after mesenteric angioplasty and stenting is comparable to that for other peripheral endovascular procedures. Patients are traditionally admitted to the hospital for overnight observation and started on clopidogrel for 30 days (75 mg/day), with the first dose (150 mg) given in the recovery room. However, the procedure can be performed on an outpatient basis. Patients are allowed to resume a regular diet within 4 to 6 hours. Most notice a marked improvement in their postprandial symptoms shortly after the procedure. A fasting mesenteric duplex ultrasound scan is obtained on the morning after the procedure to serve as a baseline. Elevated velocities are occasionally noted in the duplex scan despite a technically satisfactory arteriographic result (<30% residual stenosis) and complete resolution of preoperative symptoms. The explanation for these abnormal duplex findings is unclear. In this setting, we follow the patient's clinical course and repeat the arteriogram or intervention only if there is a significant change. A repeat duplex examination is performed at 1 month, and aspirin (325 mg/day) is substituted for clopidogrel at that time. The subsequent follow-up with serial duplex examination is comparable to that outlined later for open revascularization.

Open Revascularization

Preoperative Evaluation

The preoperative evaluation for patients undergoing open mesenteric revascularization is similar to that for other major vascular surgical procedures. All active medical conditions should be optimized, although extensive medical evaluations are likely unnecessary given the relative sense of urgency and life-threatening nature of the underlying problem. Patients with visceral artery occlusive disease, like all patients undergoing peripheral revascularization, usually have concomitant coronary artery disease, as demonstrated by the landmark study by Hertzer and associates.[62] Extensive cardiac evaluation is likewise unnecessary but should be dictated by institutional preference or the American College of Cardiologists' published algorithm for noncardiac surgery.[63] Regardless of the specific preoperative cardiac evaluation, all patients should probably be taking aspirin, a beta blocker, and a cholesterol-lowering agent (preferably a statin–HMG-CoA reductase inhibitor).[64]

Operative planning is facilitated by a CT or catheter-based arteriogram of the aorta and visceral vessels (if not already done). A CT scan of the supraceliac aorta should be obtained if an antegrade bypass from the supraceliac aorta is planned to confirm that the inflow site is adequate (i.e., free of significant atherosclerotic occlusive disease or aneurysmal degeneration). Ankle-brachial indices and a survey of the saphenous and femoral veins are routinely obtained to document the presence of any peripheral arterial occlusive disease and to identify all potential autogenous conduits in the event a prosthetic conduit is contraindicated. Management of oral and enteral feedings in the preoperative period is dictated by the severity and extent of the patient's abdominal pain. Patients with minimal postprandial pain are allowed to continue to eat but are counseled to avoid large meals or the specific types of food that exacerbate their symptoms. Patients with continuous abdominal pain should take nothing by mouth, with the exception of medications. Patients are started on total parenteral nutrition if their preoperative course is expected to be prolonged. However, the operative procedure is not delayed in an attempt to replete the nutritional stores, given the ongoing risk of acute mesenteric ischemia. No specific bowel preparations (e.g., cathartics, enemas) are used in the immediate preoperative period owing to the theoretical risk of precipitating acute mesenteric ischemia.

Antegrade Aortoceliac–Superior Mesenteric Artery Bypass

The procedure can be performed using either a midline or a bilateral subcostal incision; the choice is contingent on surgeon preference and the patient's body habitus. The midline incision is slightly easier and faster to close, and both the inflow source and the outflow vessels are oriented along the midline. However, a bilateral subcostal incision with a midline extension to the xiphoid provides optimal exposure of the upper abdomen. It is particularly helpful in larger men owing to the location of the supraceliac aorta in the postero-superior abdomen. The abdomen should routinely be explored to rule out any other intra-abdominal pathology and to assess the status of the bowel. However, we do not persist too long with this maneuver or take down an extensive number of adhesions if the bowel is viable, unless there is some uncertainty about the diagnosis.

The supraceliac aorta is exposed by incising the left triangular ligament of the liver and reflecting the left lateral segment of the liver to the patient's right. This is facilitated by using a self-retaining retractor such as a Bookwalter and placing the patient in a modest amount of reverse Trendelenburg. The gastrohepatic ligament is then incised, though caution should be exercised during this maneuver because a replaced left hepatic artery (originating from the left gastric artery and coursing through the ligament) is seen approximately 25% of the time.[65] The esophagus and stomach are then retracted to the patient's left. Care should be used throughout the procedure to avoid injuring the esophagus, although it can usually be identified by palpating the nasogastric tube or transesophageal echocardiography probe that passes through its lumen. The posterior peritoneum is then incised, and the aorta is exposed directly. This is facilitated by incising the median arcuate ligament and the crus of the diaphragm. Occasionally the pleura of the lung is entered during this step. This is usually obvious and of little consequence, although a chest radiograph should be obtained in the immediate postoperative period to confirm that the lungs are fully expanded. A sufficient length of supraceliac aorta should be dissected free to facilitate clamp application. It is usually not necessary to dissect the aorta circumferentially over the full extent of the segment in which the clamp will be applied. However, it can be helpful to place an umbilical tape circumferentially around the aorta to serve as a handle should difficulties arise.

The celiac axis can then be exposed by dissecting caudad along the anterior surface of the aorta. This requires incising the remaining fibers of the diaphragm and the dense, fibrous neural tissue known as the celiac ganglion that surrounds the vessel. We prefer to dissect the origin of the celiac axis and its proximal branches circumferentially to facilitate an end-to-end anastomosis. Alternatively, the common hepatic, proper hepatic, and gastroduodenal arteries can be dissected circumferentially and the distal anastomosis performed in an end-to-side fashion. However, it is more difficult to obtain the correct orientation of the limb with this configuration.

A suitable segment of the SMA for the distal anastomosis can be exposed using a variety of techniques. In our preferred approach, the artery is dissected immediately caudal to the inferior border of the pancreas. This is facilitated by entering the lesser sac after incising the gastrocolic ligament. The SMA sits somewhat deep within the retroperitoneal tissue in patients with a moderate amount of retroperitoneal fat and should not be confused with the smaller collateral vessels that run more superficially. Locating the artery is facilitated by identifying the adjacent superior mesenteric vein that courses to the patient's right side. Approximately 2 to 3 cm of the

artery should be dissected to facilitate the anastomosis, but caution should be used during this step because its small branches are friable and easily injured. The SMA can also be approached by elevating the transverse colon and incising the root of its mesentery on the caudal side. The artery lies adjacent to the superior mesenteric vein within the mesenteric fat and can be identified by tracing the middle colic artery retrograde. Last, the SMA can be approached by completely mobilizing the fourth portion of the duodenum after incising the ligament of Treitz and the other peritoneal attachments. After exposing the SMA, a retropancreatic tunnel is created to facilitate passing the limb of the graft. It is usually possible to create this tunnel using gentle, bimanual finger dissection. This maneuver should be performed with caution because the tunnel courses adjacent to the superior mesenteric vein and beneath the splenic vein. A straight aortic clamp can be passed through the tunnel and left in place until the proximal anastomosis is completed.

The anastomosis to the supraceliac aorta can usually be performed by partially occluding the vessel using a side-biting clamp. We use a Lambert-Kaye clamp that has been modified with a clamp-locking device that secures the tips. When it is not possible to partially occlude the aorta owing to the extent of calcification or atherosclerotic involvement, complete occlusion can be obtained with two straight aortic clamps. Before clamp application, the patient is systemically anticoagulated with heparin (100 units/kg) and given 25 g of mannitol, with the latter serving as an antioxidant and diuretic. Our conduit of choice is a bifurcated Dacron graft with a body diameter of 12 mm and limb diameters of 7 mm (12 by 7 mm). However, grafts this size are not universally available and can be substituted with grafts measuring 12 by 6 mm or 14 by 7 mm. An arteriotomy is made along the longitudinal axis of the aorta, and the graft is spatulated in such a fashion that its limbs are oriented on top of each other (Fig. 148-6); in contrast, in the case of an aortobifemoral graft, the limbs are oriented side by side. The body of the graft should be as short as possible, with the heel of the anastomosis essentially being the start of the caudal limb. This is necessary because the distance between the aortic anastomosis and the celiac anastomosis (i.e., the aortoceliac limb) is very short. Occasionally it is necessary to perform a limited endarterectomy on the aorta to facilitate the anastomosis; caution should be exercised to avoid making the aorta so thin that it will not hold sutures. The proximal anastomosis can be somewhat challenging in large patients in whom the aorta is very deep relative to the abdominal wall. These difficulties can be partially reduced by placing stay sutures in the lateral aspects of the aortotomy (3 and 9 o'clock positions) and by placing the sutures using single, sequential bites through the aorta and graft ("two-bite" technique).

The anastomoses to both the celiac axis and the SMA are performed using standard techniques. The cephalic limb of the graft is used for the celiac anastomosis, and the caudal limb is tunneled deep to the pancreas with the assistance of the previously placed aortic clamp. The celiac anastomosis is usually performed in an end-to-end fashion after suture

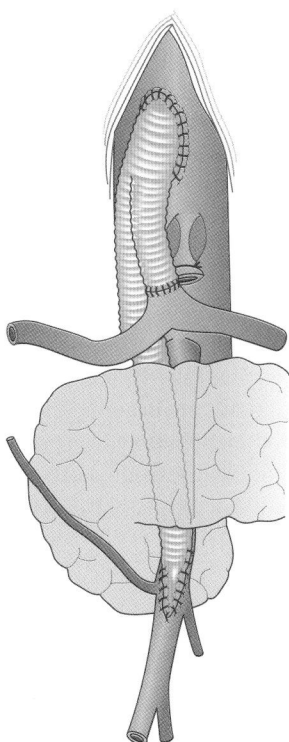

Figure 148-6 Antegrade aortoceliac–superior mesenteric artery bypass. The proximal anastomosis originates from the supraceliac aorta, and the limbs of the graft are oriented on top of each other. The celiac anastomosis is actually performed in an end-to-end fashion, and the superior mesenteric anastomosis is performed end to side. The body of the graft should be left as short as possible because the distance from the aorta to the celiac anastomosis is so short. The inferior limb to the superior mesenteric artery is tunneled deep to the pancreas.

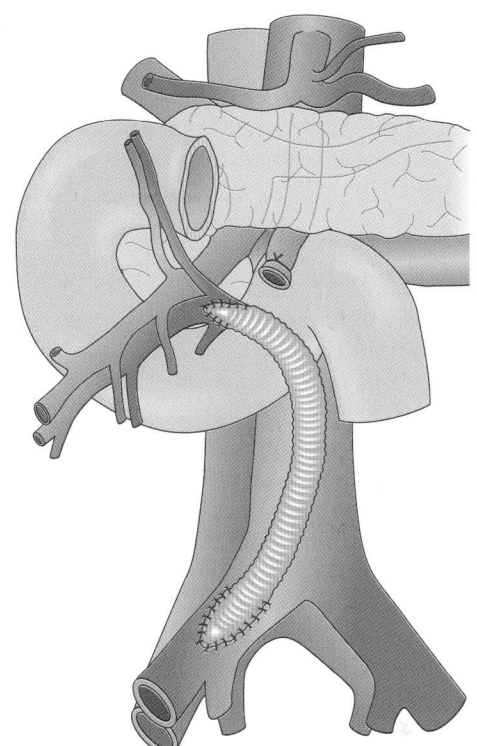

Figure 148-7 Retrograde aorta–superior mesenteric artery bypass. The proximal anastomosis is performed in an end-to-side fashion to the proximal right common iliac artery. The distal anastomosis is performed in an end-to-end fashion to the superior mesenteric artery after mobilization of the ligament of Treitz and the other duodenal peritoneal attachments. The bypass graft takes a gentle curve or C loop as it transitions both posteroanterior and caudocephalad.

ligation of the stump at its origin; the anastomosis to the SMA is usually configured in an end-to-side fashion. We use only continuous wave Doppler to interrogate the completed bypasses, and this approach has been justified by our excellent long-term outcomes.[21] However, Oderich and coworkers advocate intraoperative duplex ultrasound and have reported that unrepaired anastomotic abnormalities are associated with risk of early graft failure, re-intervention, and death.[66] The retroperitoneal tissue over the SMA anastomosis is closed, although we do not routinely attempt to cover the proximal anastomosis. We do not routinely revascularize the IMA.

Retrograde Aorta–Superior Mesenteric Artery Bypass

The principles outlined for the antegrade bypass are also relevant to the retrograde approach (Fig. 148-7). However, several technical points merit further comment. The proximal anastomosis can be positioned on the proximal right common iliac artery, the infrarenal aorta, or the proximal left common iliac artery, in order of our preference. The ultimate choice is contingent on the actual orientation or configuration of the graft and the degree of atherosclerotic occlusive disease in the vessels. The inflow vessels are exposed by incising the overly-

ing retroperitoneal tissue in the standard fashion for an infrarenal abdominal aortic aneurysm repair. The anastomosis is frequently hooded down the right common iliac artery, with its heel placed on the distal aorta immediately proximal to its bifurcation. Foley and colleagues described cutting off one limb of a bifurcated graft and using the body to construct a generous hood for the proximal anastomosis.[11] The proximal anastomosis is usually performed first, but some authors have proposed the opposite order to simplify tunneling the graft.[67]

The SMA is exposed by reflecting the fourth portion of the duodenum after incising the ligament of Treitz and the other peritoneal attachments, as outlined earlier. The distal anastomosis can be performed in either an end-to-end or end-to-side fashion, but the anatomic course of the graft is often more favorable if an end-to-end configuration is used. Either a 6- or 7-mm-diameter Dacron graft is a suitable conduit, although a comparably sized externally supported polytetrafluoroethylene graft is a good alternative and has some theoretical appeal owing to its ability to avoid kinking. The graft should be tunneled in such a fashion that it forms a gentle curve or C loop between the two anastomoses as it traverses caudal to cephalic and posterior to anterior. The loop should be configured such that the SMA anastomosis can be constructed in an antegrade fashion. It is imperative that the graft does not kink and that the anastomoses are tension free. The retroperitoneal tissue over the aorta, the ligament of Treitz, and the peritoneum over the SMA are all reapproximated to exclude the graft from contact with the intestine. Some authors have suggested that the graft be covered with omentum.[68]

Postoperative Care

The immediate postoperative course for patients undergoing open revascularization is frequently complicated by the development of multiple organ dysfunction. Further, the course is distinctly different from that associated with most other abdominal vascular procedures, such as aortic reconstruction for aortoiliac occlusive disease. This propensity to develop multiple organ dysfunction likely accounts for the prolonged intensive care and lengthy hospital stay that are often required and is one of the leading causes of death in the postoperative period.[69] The responsible mechanism is likely the visceral ischemia and reperfusion phenomenon inherent to revascularization. This process induces a complex response involving several interrelated inflammatory mediators that have the potential to cause both local and distant organ injury.[67] In a detailed study, Harward and colleagues characterized the individual organ system dysfunction after revascularization for both acute and chronic mesenteric ischemia.[69] They reported that serum hepatic transaminases increased 90- to 100-fold immediately after surgery and did not normalize for 7 to 10 days, platelet counts fell below 40,000 units within 12 to 24 hours and remained abnormal for the first 3 to 6 days, and the prothrombin and partial thromboplastin times increased and remained elevated for 3 to 6 days. Perhaps most notably, they reported that the overwhelming majority of patients developed a significant pulmonary injury characterized by an elevated mean shunt fraction and a radiographic picture of acute respiratory distress syndrome that manifested 1 to 3 days postoperatively and persisted for 5 to 8 days. A more recent report from Jimenez and associates[21] documented a 64% incidence of multiple organ dysfunction and a 53% incidence of prolonged mechanical ventilation after antegrade revascularization for chronic mesenteric ischemia, supporting the findings of Harward's group.[69]

The optimal patient management strategy after mesenteric revascularization is to support the individual organ systems until the dysfunction resolves. Admittedly, not all patients develop organ dysfunction, but the incidence is quite high and somewhat unpredictable. The optimal ventilator management remains unresolved. We generally extubate patients in the early postoperative period when they satisfy the standard weaning criteria; we are reluctant to maintain them on mechanical ventilation for fear that they may develop a lung injury. However, it is not uncommon for patients to require reintubation and mechanical ventilation. Thrombocytopenia and coagulopathy are usually managed expectantly, with platelet or plasma transfusions reserved for those with severely depressed platelet counts or clinical evidence of bleeding. Notably, the report by Harward and colleagues suggested that the inherent coagulopathy after mesenteric revascularization is not responsive to vitamin K.[69] Patients should be maintained on total parenteral nutrition throughout the postoperative period until their bowel function returns. This is particularly important, given the fact that the majority of patients are severely malnourished. Unfortunately, patients may have a prolonged ileus after revascularization and require parenteral nutrition for some time. The bypass should be interrogated with either a mesenteric duplex or CT arteriogram before discharge to confirm the technical adequacy of the reconstruction. Patients with significant acute changes in their clinical status should also be imaged to confirm that their bypasses are patent. It can be difficult to differentiate the multiple organ dysfunction that is a predictable sequela of ischemia-reperfusion injury from acute mesenteric ischemia secondary to graft thrombosis. Serum lactate levels may be helpful in this setting.

Long-term Follow-up after Endovascular and Open Revascularization

All patients who undergo revascularization for chronic mesenteric ischemia require long-term follow-up because both endovascular and open approaches are subject to the usual host of problems, including anastomotic intimal hyperplasia, in-stent restenosis, stent fracture, and graft thrombosis that can lead to recurrent symptoms and acute mesenteric ischemia. Patients are seen frequently in the early postoperative period until all their active issues resolve; thereafter they are seen at 6-month intervals, with mesenteric duplex ultrasound used to confirm that the graft and vessels are patent and to identify any graft- or anastomosis-related problems. Objective assessment of graft patency is critical and is significantly better than the "return of symptoms" that has been used as a surrogate marker.[57] Needless to say, all recurrent symptoms merit urgent or emergent evaluation with duplex ultrasound or CT arteriography.

All abnormalities on duplex ultrasound should be investigated with a CT or catheter-based arteriogram. The treatment of restenosis after angioplasty and stenting or an anastomotic graft stenosis is essentially the same as that of a de novo lesion.[70,71] The rare lesions that were treated with angioplasty alone during the initial procedure should be stented. Previously stented lesions and anastomotic graft lesions can be treated by angioplasty, with stenting or restenting reserved for refractory lesions.[51] Admittedly, angioplasty of the anastomosis of a prosthetic graft could theoretically disrupt the suture line, although this has not been particularly problematic in other vascular beds.

All endovascular failures can be treated by open repair with either patch angioplasty or bypass. Indeed, endovascular failure constitutes one of the most common indications for mesenteric bypass in our practice. Brown and coworkers stated that remedial open revascularization was not complicated by prior stent placement in their series.[52] It is our anecdotal impression that stents can lead to an inflammatory response in the involved segment of the vessel, which can complicate the subsequent operative dissection. Fortunately, visceral artery occlusive disease is predominantly orificial and is thus separated anatomically from the anastomotic target in the case of the SMA.

Diarrhea is a common complaint after open revascularization and can persist for several months. It is more common in patients with preoperative diarrhea and can be so severe that it necessitates total parenteral nutrition. Jimenez and associates reported that 33% of the patients in their series experienced significant postoperative diarrhea and that it persisted longer than 6 months in 24%.[21] Kihara and colleagues reported that patients had almost 2 stools/day (1.9 ± 0.4) after revascularization for chronic mesenteric ischemia.[56] The cause of the diarrhea is unclear but may be related to intestinal atrophy, bacterial overgrowth, or disruption of the mesenteric neuroplexus.

OUTCOME AFTER ENDOVASCULAR AND OPEN REVASCULARIZATION

Assessment of the perioperative and long-term outcomes after both open and endovascular revascularization for patients with chronic mesenteric ischemia is somewhat limited by the aforementioned concerns about the quality of the underlying studies. However, several conclusions can be drawn from a review of the literature. First, the technical success rates for both approaches are excellent. Success rates exceed 90% in the most recent endovascular series[49-54,60,72-74] and are essentially 100% for open repair,[21,23,49,52-55,75,76] although this endpoint is somewhat irrelevant, given the nature of open procedures.

Second, the perioperative morbidity and mortality rates are significantly lower for the endovascular approach. The reported morbidity and mortality rates for the endovascular approach range from 0% to 19% and 0% to 21%, respectively, with estimated aggregate values of approximately 15% for morbidity and 3% for mortality.[49-54,60,72-74] Silva and associates reported two complications (3%) and a single death (2%) from one of the largest endovascular series (59 patients).[51] The corresponding morbidity and mortality rates after open revascularization range from 4% to 66% and 2% to 15%, respectively, with an estimated aggregate morbidity of approximately 30% and a mortality of approximately 8%.[21,23,49,52-55,75,76] Kruger and colleagues recently reported a 12% morbidity and 2.5% mortality after open revascularization in 39 consecutive patients and concluded that it represented the gold standard of treatment for chronic mesenteric ischemia.[23] The magnitude and types of complications associated with the two approaches are distinctly different, with the endovascular approach associated predominantly with access- or contrast-related events, as would be predicted. The outcomes from these institutional series are comparable to the 45% complication rate and 15% mortality rate for open revascularization for the United States as a whole reported by Derrow and coworkers from a 20% U.S. sample.[1] Mateo and colleagues reported that the complication rates after open

repair, including mortality, were significantly increased by simultaneous aortic reconstruction, complete revascularization, and the presence of preoperative renal insufficiency.[26]

Third, both the endovascular and open approaches are very successful in terms of relieving symptoms, with early clinical success rates exceeding 80% for endovascular treatment[50,51,73,74] and 90% for open revascularization.[21,55] Jimenez and associates reported that patients were able to gain weight after open revascularization and had achieved 103% of their ideal body at 6 months; this compared favorably to a preoperative value of 87%.[21]

Fourth, the total hospital length of stay appears to be dramatically shorter after endovascular treatment. This is highlighted by recent reports comparing endovascular and open approaches in the same institution: Sivamurthy's group[54] reported 1 day (endovascular) versus 23 days (open); Brown,[52] 0 versus 10 days; Atkins,[53] 6 versus 17 days; and Biebl[49] 1 versus 12 days.

Fifth, the objectively documented patency rates are significantly lower after endovascular treatment. Although the duration of follow-up is variable, the estimated aggregate primary patency rate after endovascular repair is approximately 70% at 1 year, with a corresponding primary assisted rate of 85%.[49-54,60,72-74] Sarac and associates[60] reported a 1-year primary and primary assisted rate of 65% and 97%, respectively, while Silva and coworkers[51] reported rates of 71% and 83%, respectively, at 14 months. In contrast, the 5-year primary patency rates for the open approach range from 57% to 92%, and the corresponding primary assisted rates range from 89% to 96%.[21,23,53,75,76] The 5-year primary (69% ± 17%) and primary assisted (96% ± 7%) patency rates from the series reported by Jimenez and associates, encompassing only antegrade bypasses, are shown in Figure 148-8.[21] The estimated aggregate primary and primary assisted patency rates for all open procedures are approximately 80% and 90%, respectively, at 5 years.[21,23,53,75,76]

Sixth, long-term survival after both endovascular and open revascularization appears to be comparable, with an estimated aggregate rate of approximately 70% at 5 years.[21,51] These survival rates are comparable to those in the much larger group of patients with peripheral arterial occlusive disease and claudication.[77] A representative 5-year survival curve (74% ± 12%) from the report by Jimenez and associates is shown in Figure 148-9.[21]

ADDITIONAL CONSIDERATIONS

Mesenteric Infarction

Occasionally patients with a presumed diagnosis of chronic mesenteric ischemia have dead bowel at the time of open revascularization. This usually occurs in patients who have had an exacerbation or acute change in their chronic symptoms. Management principles include revascularization prior to bowel resection, with exception of the obviously dead bowel. Indeed, it is impressive how much marginally

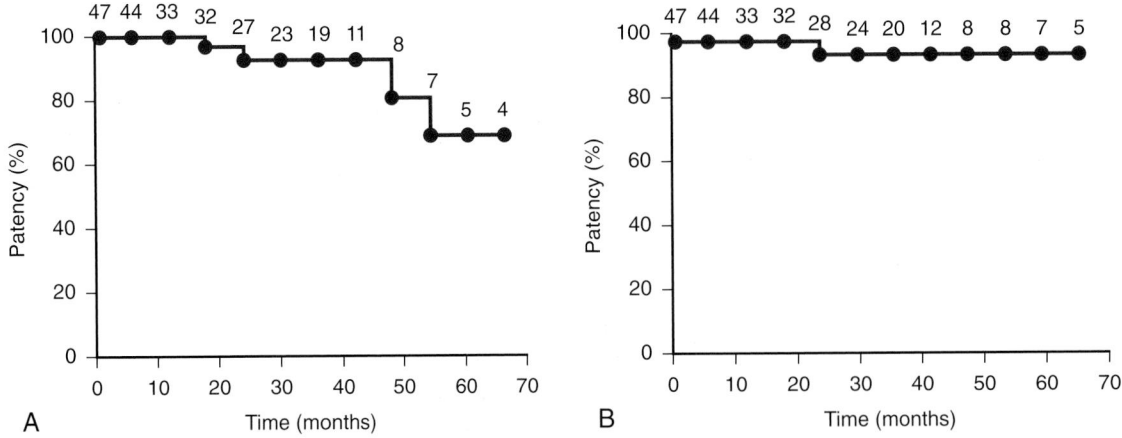

Figure 148-8 A, Primary patency after antegrade aortoceliac–superior mesenteric artery bypass graft using life-table analysis. The number of patients at risk at the beginning of each time interval is shown above the curve. Note that beginning at 42 months, there is a standard error greater than 10%. **B,** Corresponding primary assisted patency rates. *(From Jimenez JG, Huber TS, Ozaki CK, et al. Durability of antegrade synthetic aortomesenteric bypass for chronic mesenteric ischemia. J Vasc Surg. 2002;35:1078-1084.)*

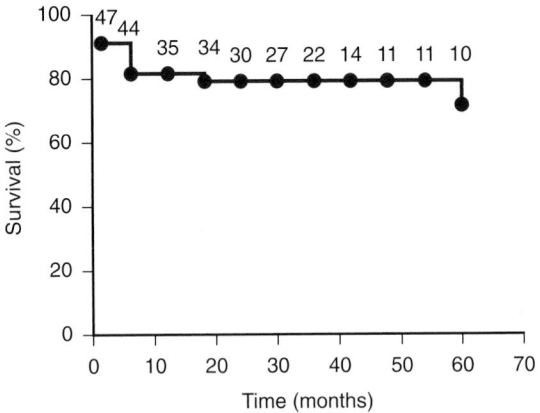

Figure 148-9 Patient survival after antegrade aortoceliac–superior mesenteric artery bypass using life-table analysis. The number of patients at risk at the beginning of each time interval is shown above the curve. Note that beginning at 42 months, there is a standard error greater than 10%. *(From Jimenez JG, Huber TS, Ozaki CK, et al. Durability of antegrade synthetic aortomesenteric bypass for chronic mesenteric ischemia. J Vasc Surg. 2002;35:1078-1084.)*

appearing bowel improves after revascularization. Further, there is little downside to deferring bowel resection until after revascularization, unless there is gross spillage of the enteric contents. Differentiating viable from nonviable bowel may be challenging. Simple adjuncts include visual inspection for peristalsis, use of continuous wave Doppler to detect arterial signals within the mesentery, and intravenous fluorescein in combination with a Wood's lamp. A "second-look" operation 24 to 48 hours after the index procedure can be very helpful to assess the viability of the bowel, and the decision to perform the second procedure should be made at the time of the original operation. A recent retrospective review has questioned the role of the second-look operation and reported that survival was actually greater in patients in whom it was not

performed.[78] However, there was a tremendous selection bias in this review, and the authors conceded that the experience of the surgeon was likely the key factor in the decision to perform the second-look operation.

In the setting of marginal-appearing bowel, resection with the construction of abdominal wall stomas is preferred over primary anastomoses. Admittedly, this commits patients to an additional procedure to restore intestinal continuity. However, the viability of the stoma (and the bowel) can be assessed at the bedside, and the potential for the enteric anastomosis to break down is avoided. Indeed, breakdown of a bowel anastomosis in this setting is potentially catastrophic because the diagnosis can be delayed or confounded by the multiple organ dysfunction that is a common sequela of ischemia-reperfusion injury. Revascularization should be performed using an autogenous conduit in the presence of dead bowel, and both the saphenous and femoral veins have been used. We share some of the concerns expressed by Modrall and colleagues that the patency rates of saphenous vein bypass are inferior.[58] Cadaveric femoral vein may also be an option in this setting, given its use in other infected fields. The bypass itself can be performed in either an antegrade or retrograde configuration, and the same arguments outlined earlier about the relative benefits of each apply. Our preference is to construct an antegrade bypass to the SMA alone using the femoral vein, although we occasionally reimplant the celiac axis on top of the graft.

Aortic Reconstruction and Mesenteric Revascularization

Patients with visceral artery occlusive disease who require aortic reconstruction represent a relatively high-risk population in terms of the potential for an adverse postoperative outcome. In this subset of patients, consideration should be given to revascularization before aortic reconstruction, even in asymptomatic patients. Simultaneous open aortic reconstruction and mesenteric revascularization should be avoided unless absolutely necessary. As noted earlier, Mateo and coworkers reported that the complication rate, including mortality, was increased when aortic reconstructions were performed simultaneously with mesenteric revascularizations.[26] McAfee and colleagues reported that the majority of the deaths in their series occurred after combined procedures.[79] A reasonable alternative approach is staged procedures, with either endovascular or open mesenteric revascularization performed as the initial step; endovascular revascularization may be ideal in this setting owing to its purportedly lower complication rates. In the few instances when simultaneous open revascularization and aortic reconstruction are necessary, the procedure should likely be performed using the retrograde technique owing to its comparative simplicity and minimal additional dissection. Foley and associates reported that combined retrograde mesenteric bypass and aortic reconstruction were not associated with an increased mortality rate.[11]

Median Arcuate Ligament Syndrome

The median arcuate ligament of the diaphragm compresses or narrows the origin of the celiac axis in a significant proportion of individuals, and this compression is augmented or exacerbated by full expiration.[80,81] The contribution of this celiac axis compression to the development of chronic mesenteric ischemia or chronic abdominal pain is uncertain and has been debated for many years.[82] Though feasible, it is unlikely that such compression alone causes ischemic symptoms, given the rich collateral network between the celiac axis and the SMA and the fact that the SMA is the most significant visceral vessel in terms of gut perfusion. The diagnosis of symptomatic celiac axis compression by the median arcuate ligament is truly a diagnosis of exclusion. Reilly and coworkers identified several criteria that may predict relief after surgical therapy for median arcuate ligament syndrome, including female gender, postprandial pain, weight loss greater than 20 pounds, absence of psychiatric or drug abuse history, and the arteriographic findings of celiac axis compression with poststenotic dilatation or collateral flow.[83] These are fairly typical findings in chronic mesenteric ischemia secondary to atherosclerotic occlusive disease. Effective treatment requires decompression of the median arcuate ligament and visceral artery bypass. Endovascular treatment alone is ineffective and likely contraindicated owing to the refractory extrinsic compression of the celiac origin by the ligament. Laparoscopic decompression of the median arcuate ligament may play a role in equivocal patients without obvious atherosclerotic occlusive disease.[84]

Remedial Procedures after Open Surgical Mesenteric Revascularization

Remedial open surgical revascularization for recurrent symptoms of chronic mesenteric ischemia is rare, given the excel-

lent graft patency rates. When necessary, the surgical options include both antegrade and retrograde bypasses, with the choice contingent on the distribution of the occlusive disease and the original procedure. A failed retrograde bypass from the infrarenal aorta to the SMA can usually be remediated with a traditional antegrade bypass from the supraceliac aorta to both the celiac axis and the SMA. This usually requires locating the SMA anastomosis distal to the original one and obviates the concern about the course of the retrograde graft that may have contributed to the initial failure. A failed antegrade bypass can usually be redone or converted to a retrograde bypass. Clearly, this option is much simpler, but the overriding principle in this setting is to optimize the potential long-term success and graft patency rather than minimize the operative procedure. It is distinctly unusual for both limbs of an antegrade bypass to fail. This scenario suggests a problem at the proximal aortic anastomosis. In the more common scenario in which a single graft limb occludes, it is usually due to a stenosis at the distal anastomosis from intimal hyperplasia or a technical problem from tunneling or kinking of the graft. The anastomotic problem can be corrected by graft thrombectomy and revision of the anastomosis with a vein patch or a new interposition graft. Problems related to tunneling of the graft usually require excising the redundant segment or replacing the limb. "Redo" mesenteric bypass—and particularly a "redo" antegrade bypass—may be technically challenging owing to the previous dissection and the interval adhesions. In addition to locating the visceral artery anastomosis more distally, the procedure can be simplified by using the original cuff of the main body to avoid placing additional sutures in the supraceliac aorta. Giswold and coworkers reported an impressive series of 22 patients who underwent 33 repeat (or redo) mesenteric bypasses, with a 6% mortality rate and a 62% primary patency rate at 4 years.[85]

In the very unusual scenario in which traditional antegrade and retrograde bypasses are not feasible, a variety of potential bypass configurations or alternatives are possible. The axillary artery,[86] ascending thoracic aorta,[87] and descending thoracic aorta can all serve as an alternative inflow source; alternative distal targets include the hepatic artery, splenic artery, distal SMA, and named branches of the SMA. Schneider and associates reported a small series of isolated IMA revascularizations for chronic mesenteric ischemia.[88] They stated that the revascularization was sufficient to relieve the symptoms and prevent bowel infarction, although it required a well-developed collateral pathway.

Nonatherosclerotic Causes of Chronic Mesenteric Ischemia

Nonatherosclerotic causes of chronic mesenteric ischemia are rarely encountered, so the clinical experience is limited. Fibromuscular dysplasia may involve the visceral vessels. Symptomatic stenoses are reportedly amenable to balloon angioplasty, with a reasonable outcome.[89] Several of the inflammatory arteritides may involve the visceral vessels and cause chronic mesenteric ischemia. Effective treatment in this setting is contingent on controlling or arresting the underlying inflammatory process and requires a multidisciplinary approach, including a rheumatologist. Revascularization should be delayed until the underlying disease process is arrested or at least controlled. The stenotic lesions may be more distal on the arterial tree than the more common ostial atherosclerotic lesions. Open surgical revascularization may require dissecting the distal SMA in the small bowel mesentery, well beyond the takeoff of the middle colic artery. The distal anastomosis can be facilitated at this level by patching the artery with saphenous vein and then implanting the prosthetic graft on the generous vein patch. Every attempt should be made to preserve the small, friable branches of the SMA.

Aortic and Visceral Artery Dissections

Dissections can occur in the visceral vessels as an extension of an aortic dissection or, less commonly, as an isolated event.[90-93] Aortic dissections with visceral involvement commonly present with visceral malperfusion and acute mesenteric ischemia, although it is conceivable that they could lead to chronic mesenteric ischemia. Endovascular treatment is first-line therapy, but the overall approach is complicated by the presence of the dissection within the aorta, and this approach is discussed in Chapter 135 (Aortic Dissection).

Isolated dissections can occur in any of the visceral vessels, although the SMA appears to be the most common.[93] The majority of patients with spontaneous dissections are male, with an average age of 55 years.[94] The underlying cause remains unknown, although atherosclerosis, medial degeneration, trauma, fibromuscular disease, pregnancy, and a host of arteriopathies have been implicated. Patients may present with abdominal pain that progresses to acute mesenteric ischemia. However, the majority of the patients reported by Takayama and colleagues—one of the largest series in the literature—were actually asymptomatic, and the findings were discovered on imaging studies performed for other reasons.[93] CT arteriography appears to be the diagnostic study of choice. Not surprisingly, the optimal treatment for these isolated dissections remains unresolved. Intervention is indicated for mesenteric ischemia (either acute or chronic), aneurysmal degeneration, and rupture. Both open[93] and endovascular[90] treatments have been reported, although the latter may be optimal, given the fact that the dissection can extend distally in the vessel, unlike the more common scenario with atherosclerotic occlusive disease. Expectant, conservative treatment is likely adequate for asymptomatic or minimally symptomatic patients. Anticoagulation may be indicated in this subset of patients, analogous to its role in the treatment of spontaneous carotid dissections.[91-93] However, the excellent outcomes reported by Takayama and colleagues among asymptomatic patients treated without anticoagulants or antiplatelet agents suggest that these drugs may not be necessary.[93] Patients should be followed with serial CT arteriograms to monitor for aneurysmal degeneration of the affected vessel.[92,93] Similar

to other vascular beds, these dissections can actually "heal" or resolve over time.

SELECTED KEY REFERENCES

Derrow AE, Seeger JM, Dame DA, Carter RL, Ozaki CK, Flynn TC, Huber TS. The outcome in the United States after thoracoabdominal aortic aneurysm repair, renal artery bypass, and mesenteric revascularization. *J Vasc Surg.* 2001;34:54-61.
Defines the outcome across the United States for patients undergoing mesenteric artery bypass using an administrative discharge database.

Foley MI, Moneta GL, Abou-Zamzam AM Jr, Edwards JM, Taylor LM Jr, Yeager RA, Porter JM. Revascularization of the superior mesenteric artery alone for treatment of intestinal ischemia. *J Vasc Surg.* 2000;32:37-47.
Defines the outcome for patients undergoing retrograde mesenteric artery bypass for chronic mesenteric ischemia.

Harward TR, Brooks DL, Flynn TC, Seeger JM. Multiple organ dysfunction after mesenteric artery revascularization. *J Vasc Surg.* 1993; 18:459-467.
Documents the multiple organ dysfunction associated with mesenteric bypass for chronic mesenteric ischemia.

Jimenez JG, Huber TS, Ozaki CK, Flynn TC, Berceli SA, Lee WA, Seeger JM. Durability of antegrade synthetic aortomesenteric bypass for chronic mesenteric ischemia. *J Vasc Surg.* 2002;35:1078-1084.
Defines the outcome for patients undergoing antegrade mesenteric artery bypass for chronic mesenteric ischemia.

Kruger AJ, Walker PJ, Foster WJ, Jenkins JS, Boyne NS, Jenkins J. Open surgery for atherosclerotic chronic mesenteric ischemia. *J Vasc Surg.* 2007;46:941-945.
Describes the contemporary outcome for patients undergoing mesenteric bypass for chronic mesenteric ischemia.

Moneta GL, Lee RW, Yeager RA, Taylor LM Jr, Porter JM. Mesenteric duplex scanning: a blinded prospective study. *J Vasc Surg.* 1993; 17:79-84.
Describes one set of duplex criteria for mesenteric artery stenosis.

Sarac TP, Altinel O, Kashyap V, Bena J, Lyden S, Sruvastava S, Eagleton M, Clair D. Endovascular treatment of stenotic and occluded visceral arteries for chronic mesenteric ischemia. *J Vasc Surg.* 2008;47:485-491.
Describes the outcome for patients undergoing endovascular treatment of chronic mesenteric ischemia.

Silva JA, White CJ, Collins TJ, Jenkins JS, Andry ME, Reilly JP, Ramee SR. Endovascular therapy for chronic mesenteric ischemia. *J Am Coll Cardiol.* 2006;47:944-950.
Describes the outcome for patients undergoing endovascular treatment of chronic mesenteric ischemia.

Thomas JH, Blake K, Pierce GE, Hermreck AS, Seigel E. The clinical course of asymptomatic mesenteric arterial stenosis. *J Vasc Surg.* 1998;27:840-844.
Attempts to define the natural history of asymptomatic visceral artery occlusive disease.

Zwolak RM, Fillinger MF, Walsh DB, LaBombard FE, Musson A, Darling CE, Cronenwett JL. Mesenteric and celiac duplex scanning: a validation study. *J Vasc Surg.* 1998;27:1078-1087.
Describes one set of duplex criteria for mesenteric artery stenosis.

REFERENCES

The reference list can be found on the companion Expert Consult Web site at *www.expertconsult.com.*

CHAPTER 149

Mesenteric Vascular Disease: Acute Ischemia

Mark C. Wyers

Based in part on chapters in the previous edition by Erin M. Moore, MD; Eric D. Endean, MD, FACS; Tina R. Desai, MD; and Hisham S. Bassiouny, MD.

Klass was the first surgeon to focus on the restoration of arterial blood supply in an attempt to salvage acutely ischemic bowel. He reported the first operative superior mesenteric artery (SMA) embolectomy for acute mesenteric ischemia (AMI) in 1951.[1] The next 2 decades produced more such reports and increasing success with SMA thromboembolectomy and thromboendarterectomy[2] for the treatment of acute SMA thrombosis. Unfortunately, successful outcomes after the treatment of acute thrombotic SMA occlusion remained elusive, with mortality rates of 70% to 90%. Early and liberal use of angiography was championed by Boley[3,4] and Clark[5,6] and their respective coauthors in the early 1970s. With an aggressive approach, including the use of vasodilators, they demonstrated a reduction in the AMI mortality rate to approximately 50%. This mortality rate has not been reproduced or improved on, despite all the major advances that have taken place in the subsequent 35 years. In fact, more contemporary reviews still report mortality rates between 60% and 80%.[7,8] Treatment for acute mesenteric arterial occlusions has traditionally been surgical, with intensive medical support, as well as some limited interventional options for nonocclusive mesenteric ischemia (NOMI). There are, however, increasing reports of endovascular or hybrid endovascular-surgical treatments for all forms of AMI that can be applied to the treatment of well-selected patients.

The pathologic causes of abdominal pain and tenderness in the elderly population are protean, and all too frequently, AMI is not included in the initial differential diagnosis. Two reviews in the past decade suggested that only one third of AMI patients were correctly identified before surgical exploration or death.[9,10] Any delay in diagnosis and treatment remains the greatest challenge to reducing morbidity and mortality for all forms of this disease entity.[11] SMA embolism usually results in the most rapid clinical decline because of the lack of established collateral circulation. In this subgroup of patients, survival is approximately 50% when the diagnosis occurs within 24 hours after the onset of symptoms, but it drops sharply to 30% or less when the diagnosis is delayed.[12] Bowel necrosis is probably the best surrogate for delay in diagnosis, and together with advanced patient age it has been linked to higher mortality rates.[11] A high index of suspicion in the setting of a compatible history and physical examination serves as a cornerstone of prompt treatment. Once AMI is suspected, the clinician should quickly move to appropriate testing to confirm the diagnosis, keeping in mind that the best first test may be an operation or arteriography.

CHANGING PARADIGMS IN DIAGNOSIS AND TREATMENT

Before the more detailed discussion of diagnostic tests that follows, it is worth introducing the idea that there has been a paradigm shift in the diagnostic algorithm for AMI. The older model, as championed by Boley and associates,[4,13] advocated early and aggressive use of diagnostic angiography. Today, computed tomographic angiography (CTA) has supplanted diagnostic angiography when occlusive AMI (but not necessarily NOMI) is suspected. With nearly universal 24-hour access to high-resolution CTA, the diagnosis of SMA embolus or thrombotic occlusion can be confirmed, and the bowel can be evaluated concomitantly to support or refute the diagnosis.

Angiography still plays an important role in the diagnosis and treatment of AMI, however. In fact, with an ever-expanding list of endovascular treatments or adjuncts, its therapeutic role is, in many ways, strengthened. Only its timing and application may be somewhat changed. Gone are the days when an arteriogram was performed and the patient returned hours later, after the study had been read. Increasingly, vascular surgeon–interventionalists are able to combine the final steps of diagnosis and treatment on one table in the operating room environment. This allows general and vascular surgeons to work together to provide definitive treatment. In a well-designed treatment pathway, this coupling of angiography and definitive surgical treatment can save precious time in the treatment of these challenging patients.

INCIDENCE AND RISK FACTORS

AMI is uncommon, accounting for less than 1 of every 1000 hospital admissions.[14] Females are affected three times as frequently as males. Patients typically present in their 60s to 70s and often have a number of medical co-morbidities. Clinical risk factors may provide some clue as to the specific pathophysiology. Patients with a history of atrial fibrillation, recent myocardial infarction, congestive heart failure, or peripheral arterial emboli are at risk for an SMA embolus. In contrast, a careful history may reveal postprandial abdominal pain, weight loss, and food intolerance, all of which clearly raise the suspicion of an acute SMA thrombotic occlusion. Finally, a patient with NOMI is likely to be critically ill and to have suffered a significant hemodynamic insult in the preceding hours to days. Cardiac surgery and hemodialysis patients are classically at highest risk for NOMI. The diagnostic algorithm should be tailored based on the suspected cause—arterial embolization, arterial thrombosis, or nonocclusive ischemia.

PATHOPHYSIOLOGIC CLASSIFICATION

Arterial Embolism

Arterial embolism is the most common pathophysiology of AMI, accounting for 40% to 50% of cases.[15] Most embolic events are thromboembolic and arise from a cardiac source. The historical elements that place a patient at risk for a thromboembolic event include atrial tachyarrhythmia, low ejection fraction (congestive heart failure, cardiomyopathy), recent myocardial ischemia or infarction, and ventricular aneurysm. Though less common, more proximal arterial sources of atheroembolic material should also be considered. In these instances, a previous history of cardiac valvular disease, endocarditis, proximal aneurysm, or recent catheter-based angiography may be elicited.[16] Nearly one third of patients with an SMA embolus have had an antecedent embolic event. There is some speculation that the overall incidence of thromboembolism is declining owing to better guidelines for and compliance with anticoagulation in patients with atrial fibrillation.[17]

The SMA is the most common mesenteric vessel to undergo embolism because of its oblique origin from the visceral aortic segment. Thromboemboli tend to be the right size to lodge in the proximal SMA, just beyond the first few jejunal branches as the SMA tapers. A minority (15%) may lodge at the SMA origin, but 50% lodge distal to the middle colic artery,[12] creating a classic pattern of ischemia that spares the first portion of the small intestine and the ascending colon (Fig. 149-1). Atheroembolic emboli, in contrast, tend to be smaller and therefore lodge in the more distal mesenteric circulation. As a result, these emboli are likely to affect bowel perfusion less often and in more localized areas.

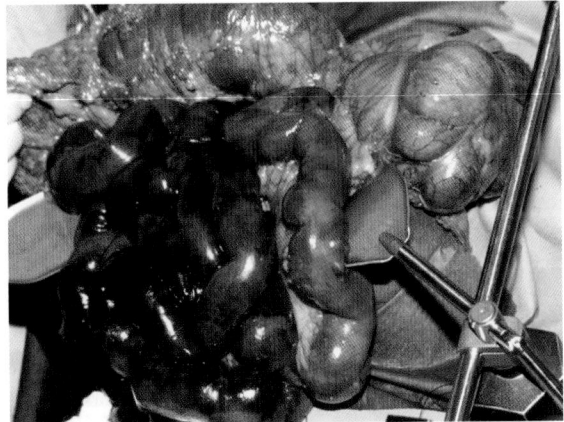

Figure 149-1 Intraoperative photograph of a patient with a superior mesenteric artery embolus. Note the relative sparing of the proximal jejunum and proximal transverse colon. (*Courtesy of R. M. Zwolak.*)

Arterial Thrombosis

Acute arterial thrombosis superimposed on preexisting severe atherosclerotic disease accounts for 25% to 30% of cases.[15,18] Autopsy studies have shown that 6% to 10% of the population has a greater than 50% stenosis in at least one mesenteric artery.[19] Further, the incidence of asymptomatic celiac artery or SMA stenosis greater than 50% in patients undergoing arteriography for other peripheral vascular disease may be as high as 27%.[20] Bowel infarction is more insidious in onset because extensive collaterals are able to maintain viability until there is final closure of a critically stenotic vessel or collateral. Consideration must also be given to how vascular collaterals, interrupted by previous abdominal surgery or bowel resection, may affect the region of bowel involvement. Once established, however, the pattern of infarction is more confluent, unlike that seen with embolic causes. There is no sparing of the proximal jejunum or right colic distribution because the SMA origin is almost uniformly occluded.[21,22]

Acute-on-chronic presentations are not uncommon. Endean and coworkers suggested that up to 20% of AMI patients have a history of postprandial abdominal pain, food avoidance, or weight loss.[23] Even for patients with asymptomatic mesenteric arterial lesions, the natural history of mesenteric occlusive disease is progressive and potentially morbid. In one report, 86% of patients with more advanced three-vessel mesenteric atherosclerosis experienced vague abdominal discomfort, had frank mesenteric ischemia, or died during a 2.6-year mean follow-up interval.[24] Therefore, a history of symptoms of chronic mesenteric ischemia should be elicited.

Nonocclusive Mesenteric Ischemia

NOMI was initially described as a postmortem observation of small intestinal gangrene in patients who had shown no evidence of arterial or venous occlusive disease.[25] Early reports by Cohen,[26] Wilson and Qualheim,[27] and Ende[28] and subsequent ones by Boley and colleagues[3,12,29,30] described this diagnosis in patients with severe cardiac failure. These observations formed the basis for the hypothesis that cardiac failure, peripheral hypoxemia, paradoxical splanchnic vasospasm, and reperfusion injury may all contribute to the development of NOMI.

Mesenteric vasospasm, usually in the distribution of the SMA, is the sine qua non of NOMI. This form of AMI accounts for approximately 20% of presentations and carries the highest mortality rates because of its frequent association with multisystem organ failure.[31,32] Perhaps resulting from excessive sympathetic activity during cardiogenic shock or hypovolemia, the vasospasm represents a homeostatic mechanism that attempts to maintain cardiac and cerebral perfusion at the expense of visceral and peripheral organs. Vasopressin and angiotensin are the likely neurohormonal mediators of this process.[33,34] In the current era, vasoactive medications such as epinephrine, norepinephrine, and vasopressin have also been associated with the development of NOMI.[33-35]

Once mesenteric vasospasm is initiated, it may persist even after correction of the initiating event. Although intestinal autoregulation may initially offset reductions in blood flow, the autoregulatory capacity is exceeded after several hours.[29]

The exact mechanism of persistence of vasospasm is unknown, but it plays an important role in the development and maintenance of occlusive and nonocclusive mesenteric ischemia as well as reperfusion phenomena complicating mesenteric revascularization.[36] The degree of ischemia-reperfusion injury appears to be related to the frequency as well as the duration of ischemic episodes. Clark and Gewertz demonstrated that two 15-minute periods of low flow followed by reperfusion resulted in more severe histologic injury than a single 30-minute period of ischemia.[37] NOMI results in an analogous scenario, whereby hypoperfusion may be partial and occasionally repetitive. Episodic reperfusion is thought to prime the ischemic tissue with leukocytes that are attracted to and produce reactive oxygen species.[38] This concept is supported by studies demonstrating attenuation of ischemia-reperfusion injury by reperfusion with leukopenic blood or blockade of endothelial cell surface receptors for leukocyte adherence.[39,40] Reports of NOMI after elective mesenteric revascularization further support reperfusion injury in the pathogenesis of NOMI.[36]

FINAL COMMON PATHWAY OF BOWEL ISCHEMIA

The degree of reduction in blood flow that the bowel can tolerate without permanent cellular damage is remarkable. Only one fifth of the mesenteric capillaries are open at any given time, and normal oxygen consumption can be maintained with only 20% of maximal blood flow.[41] Proposed mechanisms that result in the preservation of splanchnic tissue perfusion include direct arteriolar smooth muscle relaxation and a metabolic response to adenosine and other metabolites of mucosal ischemia.[42] In addition, the intestinal mucosa is able to extract increasing amounts of oxygen during hypoperfusion[43] to preserve mucosal integrity during periods of metabolic insult. Prolonged ischemia, whatever the pathophysiologic cause, leads to disruption of the intestinal mucosal barrier, primarily through the actions of reactive oxygen metabolites and polymorphonuclear neutrophils.[8] The mucosal surfaces are affected first because the mucosal metabolic demand is much higher than that of the serosa. Clinically, this may present with malabsorption and heme-positive diarrhea before the onset of other symptoms.

DIAGNOSTIC EVALUATION
Clinical Presentation

Many of the signs and symptoms of AMI are easily mistaken for other, more common intra-abdominal pathologies such as pancreatitis, cholecystitis, appendicitis, diverticulitis, and bowel obstruction. The classic description of early symptoms is pain that is greater than expected based on physical examination findings. Depending on the exact cause of AMI and the timing of presentation, this classic presentation may be absent in 20% to 25% of cases.[31] That is, until there is transmural involvement of the bowel, there is relatively little peritoneal irritation, so tenderness to palpation may be minimal. For patients who present with SMA embolism, the onset is more abrupt, without a prodrome, and the progression is rapid. Occasionally, as in Klass' original description, there may be sudden and forceful bowel evacuation shortly after the onset of pain.[1] An intermediate rate of progression can be seen with SMA thrombosis because many of these patients have developed collaterals. Their subacute presentation may start weeks before the final acute insult that prompts them to seek medical attention. Patients may have abdominal pain, distention, diarrhea, acidosis, sepsis, or gastrointestinal bleeding, singly or in combination. NOMI patients may have the most insidious onset and a protracted clinical course. They are least able to offer any history because they are already critically ill, frequently in a hospital critical care setting. The pain associated with NOMI can be variable in location as well as in character.

Laboratory Evaluation

The most common laboratory abnormalities are hemoconcentration, leukocytosis, a high anion gap, and possibly lactic acidosis in more advanced cases. High amylase, aspartate aminotransferase, and lactate dehydrogenase can also be observed. All these serum markers, however, are insensitive and nonspecific for the diagnosis of mesenteric ischemia.[44,45] D-dimer elevation after 2 hours has been correlated with the presence of AMI in a rat model.[46] Similarly, Acosta and colleagues showed elevated D-dimer levels in AMI patients who presented within 24 hours of the onset of symptoms, in contrast to patients with inflammatory conditions or bowel obstruction.[9] No patient with a D-dimer concentration of 0.3 µg/mL (1.6 nmol/L) or less had acute SMA occlusion, suggesting this as a possible exclusionary test.[9] One blood test that holds promise as a future diagnostic test for AMI is an enzyme immunoassay for elevated levels of intestinal fatty acid binding protein. This protein was first discovered in rodents,[47] and the human homologue was found to be elevated in cases of documented bowel infarction.[48] Clinical experience with this test is very limited, and it needs further evaluation.

Diagnostic Imaging
Abdominal Plain Radiographs

Abdominal plain radiographs are normal in up to 25% of patients with AMI.[49] However, ileus may be an early finding consistent with mesenteric ischemia, and advanced cases of intestinal ischemia may show evidence of bowel wall edema ("thumbprinting") or pneumatosis. Plain abdominal radiography is most useful in excluding other causes of abdominal pain such as bowel obstruction or perforation.

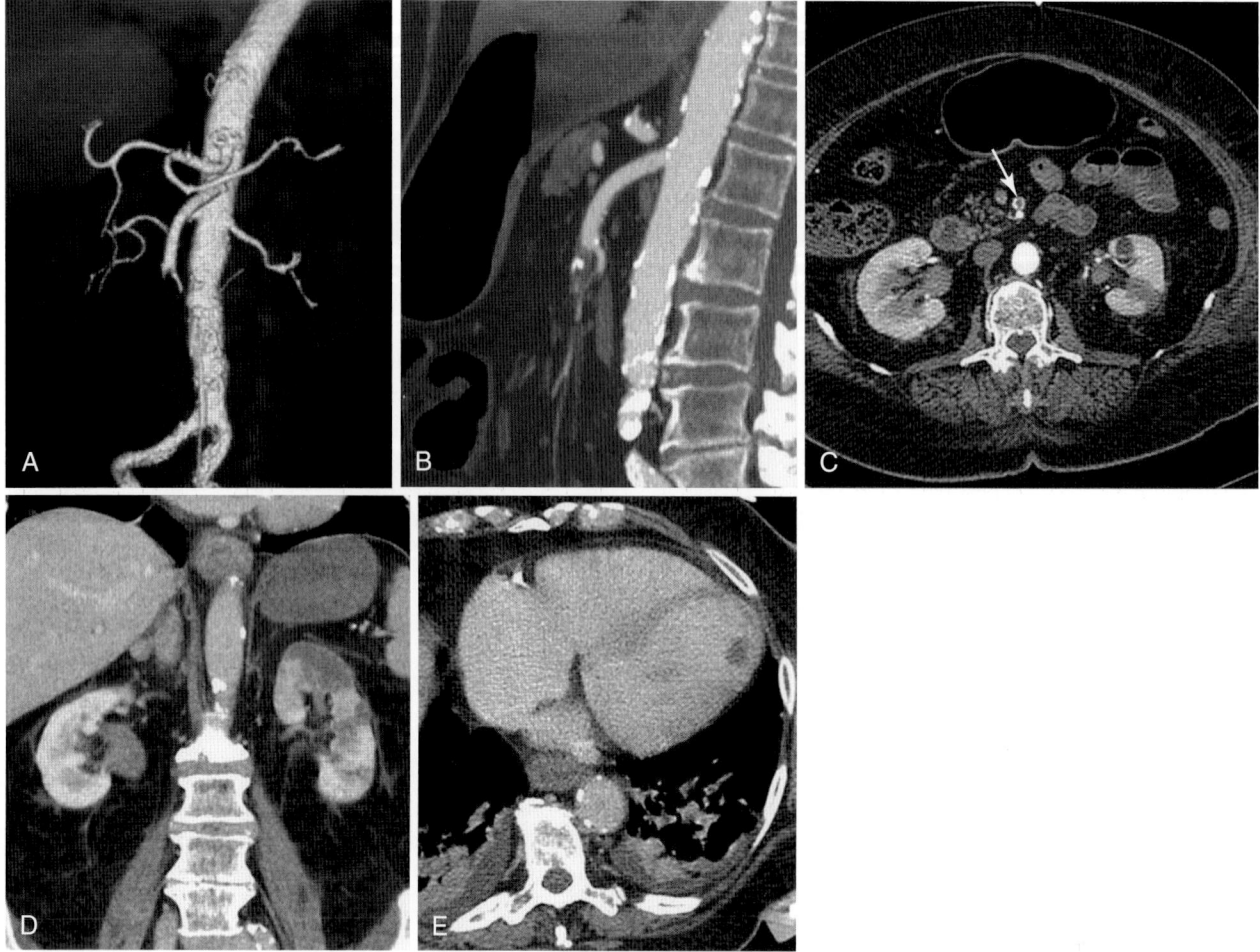

Figure 149-2 A, Three-dimensional volume rendering of arterial-phase MDCTA shows an abrupt mid–superior mesenteric artery (SMA) occlusion consistent with embolus. **B,** Sagittal multiplanar reformat shows the same occlusion. **C,** SMA occlusion seen on an axial CTA slice (*arrow*). **D,** Coronal multiplanar reformat reveals left kidney infarction. **E,** Transverse portal venous-phase MDCTA depicts thrombus in the left ventricle as the likely embolic source. *(From Aschoff AJ, Stuber G, Becker BW, et al. Evaluation of acute mesenteric ischemia: accuracy of biphasic mesenteric multi-detector CT angiography. Abdom Imaging. 2009;34:345-357.)*

Duplex Ultrasonography

Duplex ultrasonography accurately identifies high-grade stenoses of the celiac artery and SMA. It is the noninvasive diagnostic study of choice in patients with symptoms suggesting chronic mesenteric ischemia but has little or no role in the diagnosis of AMI for several important reasons. It is highly technologist dependent, and many hospitals do not have ready access to such specialized vascular laboratory testing, especially during off-hours. The presence of intestinal gas—which is the rule in any nonfasting patient, let alone someone suspected of having AMI—can easily obscure visualization of the mesenteric vessels. Any abdominal tenderness also compromises the study and adds to the patient's suffering.

Computed Tomography

Several authors have described the use of ultrafast multidetector CTA (MDCTA) for the evaluation of both acute and chronic mesenteric ischemia.[50-53] The widespread availability

of this newest generation of CT scanners represents a potential change in the diagnostic algorithm for AMI and offers greater speed than angiography. Using high-resolution MDCTA, a significant amount of information can be obtained about the central arterial and venous circulations. Accurate timing of contrast injection and fine slices through the upper abdomen usually provide excellent visualization of the celiac artery and SMA (Figs. 149-2 and 149-3). CT can also exclude other causes of abdominal pain and assess bowel perfusion to some extent. The timing of intravenous contrast administration is tailored to the specific clinical question. The use of traditional oral "positive" contrast agents detracts from image quality, and most visceral CTA protocols recommend the use of a "negative" oral contrast agent such as water (500 to 750 mL) given immediately before the scan. This prevents image artifact from pooled areas of high opacification within the intestinal tract and also enhances the ability to see bowel wall enhancement (or the lack thereof) in the late arterial phase of the arterial contrast bolus.[51] Main branches of the celiac artery and SMA are seen remarkably well using MDCTA

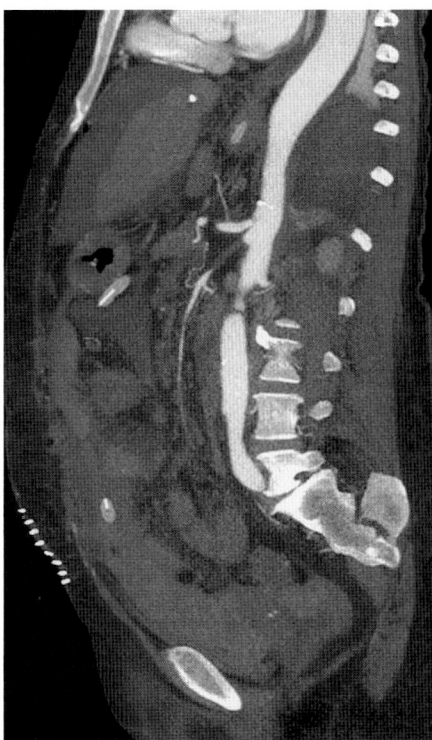

Figure 149-3 CTA sagittal multiplanar reformat shows an acute thrombotic occlusion of the proximal superior mesenteric artery. Bowel resection was performed 3 days before this image was obtained. The concomitant celiac stenosis suggests an acute-on-chronic presentation of acute mesenteric ischemia. *(From Aschoff AJ, Stuber G, Becker BW, et al. Evaluation of acute mesenteric ischemia: accuracy of biphasic mesenteric multi-detector CT angiography.* Abdom Imaging. *2009;34:345-357.)*

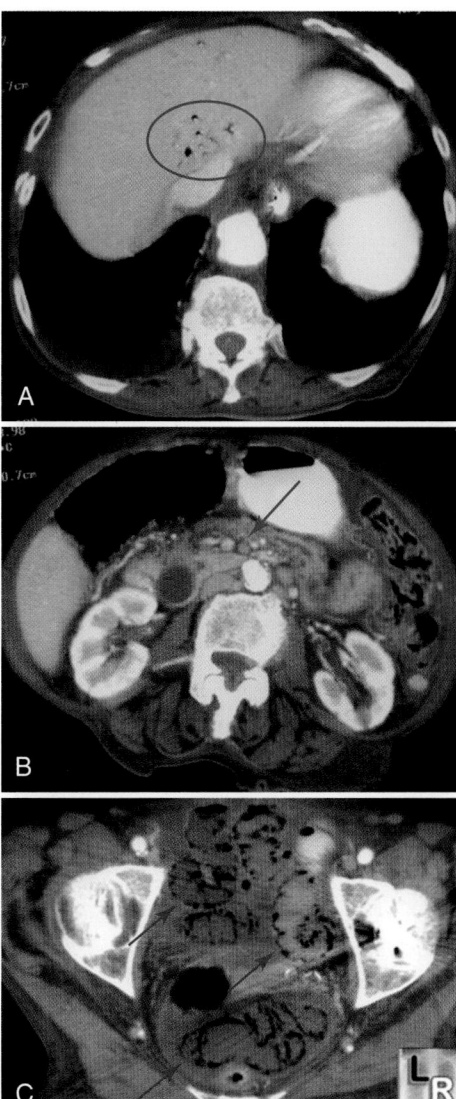

Figure 149-4 A, CTA demonstrating hepatic venous air (*circle*). **B,** The superior mesenteric artery is occluded (*arrow*). **C,** There is extensive colonic pneumatosis and ascites (*arrows*). *(From http://www.learningradiology.com/notes/ginotes/mesentericischemiapage.htm.)*

because of thinner collimation (0.5 to 1.5 mm) and overlapping data acquisition. This reduces the amount of volume averaging and creates higher quality three-dimensional (3D) volume sets for reformatting and interpretation.

Initial interest in so-called biphasic CT was generated in the evaluation of pancreatic and hepatic lesions; it includes an arterial phase and a delayed phase, allowing timed-based visualization of the portal venous system. This method has been applied more recently to detect the early findings of AMI. That is, the same scan is used to detect arterial narrowings or occlusions and to assess associated changes in bowel wall thickness, pneumatosis, and mucosal or bowel wall enhancement patterns that support the diagnosis of AMI (Fig. 149-4). Kirkpatrick and coworkers[54] sought to improve on a previous retrospective report that used single-detector helical CT.[55] Sixty-two patients suspected of having AMI underwent biphasic MDCTA and were evaluated prospectively. As in the previous study, no single CT finding was both sensitive and specific (Table 149-1). Twenty-six patients, however, had AMI confirmed at surgical exploration or based on pathologic examination, and all these patients had been correctly identified by the interpreting radiologist as having AMI. An additional four scans interpreted as demonstrating AMI turned out to be false positives, with the ultimate diagnosis of Crohn's disease (2), neutropenic enterocolitis (1), and infectious

enterocolitis (1). Thus, the initial interpretation had a sensitivity of 100% and a specificity of 89% for the diagnosis of AMI. In the same study, CTA visualization was judged to be satisfactory in all cases up to second-order branches of both the celiac artery and the SMA. Angiography was available in only three patients but correlated well with the CTA findings. In a more recent retrospective chart review using similar MDCTA protocols and even higher resolution CT, Aschoff and associates were able to duplicate Kirkpatrick's findings in terms of overall accuracy.[56] Again, no one CT finding was perfectly sensitive or specific for AMI, but using a combination of CT criteria (pneumatosis, bowel edema, other solid-organ infarction) to generate an overall impression, these authors were able to achieve positive and negative predictive values of 100% and 96%, respectively.

Table 149-1 Analysis of Computed Tomography Findings

Finding	Patients with AMI (n = 26)	Control Group (n = 36)	Sensitivity (%)	Specificity (%)
Pneumatosis intestinalis	11	0	42	100
SMA or combined celiac and IMA occlusion*	5	0	19	100
Arterial embolism	3	0	12	100
SMA or portal venous gas	3	0	12	100
Focal lack of bowel wall enhancement	11	1	42	97
Free intraperitoneal air	5	2	19	94
Superior mesenteric or portal venous thrombosis	4	2	15	94
Solid organ infarction	4	2	15	94
Bowel obstruction	3	2	12	94
Bowel dilatation	17	6	65	83
Mucosal enhancement	12	7	46	81
Bowel wall thickening	22	10	85	72
Mesenteric stranding	23	14	88	61
Ascites	19	24	73	33

*Patients with both celiac and IMA occlusion also had evidence of distal disease in the SMA distribution.
AMI, acute mesenteric ischemia; IMA, inferior mesenteric artery; SMA, superior mesenteric artery.
From Kirkpatrick ID, Kroeker MA, Greenberg HM. Biphasic CT with mesenteric CT angiography in the evaluation of acute mesenteric ischemia: initial experience. *Radiology.* 2003;229:91-98.

Arteriography

Traditional catheter-based arteriography (Fig. 149-5) has been supplanted by MDCTA as the definitive diagnostic study for occlusive forms of AMI. Patients with strongly suspected NOMI may still benefit from a more traditional angiographic approach, as long as there is no immediate need for exploration based on the physical examination. Arteriography's role in the therapy of all forms of AMI, however, has been strengthened. It offers several complementary or stand-alone treatment options, depending on the specific pathology, including injection of intra-arterial vasodilators,[57] thrombolysis,[58] and angioplasty with or without stenting.[59] These are discussed in more detail under "Treatment of Nonocclusive Mesenteric Ischemia" and "Endovascular Treatment." As vascular surgeons become accomplished interventionalists and as intraoperative fluoroscopy improves, the confirmatory diagnostic arteriogram can be accomplished in the operating room, followed by immediate surgical exploration. This unified approach can limit the delay in surgical exploration and revascularization. With respect to the evaluation for chronic mesenteric ischemia, angiography still remains the "gold standard" for preoperative planning, based on its superior image resolution, visualization of collateral flow direction, and identification of disease in the more distal portions of the splanchnic arterial bed.

Magnetic Resonance Angiography

Magnetic resonance angiography (MRA) of the splanchnic vessels is an evolving technology. It is theoretically appealing because it is noninvasive, avoids the risk of allergic reaction and nephrotoxicity associated with iodinated contrast agents, and may not be as operator dependent as duplex ultrasound. Magnetic resonance imaging of the mesenteric vasculature can incorporate both functional and anatomic evaluations, which hold promise for the diagnosis of chronic mesenteric ischemia.[19,60]

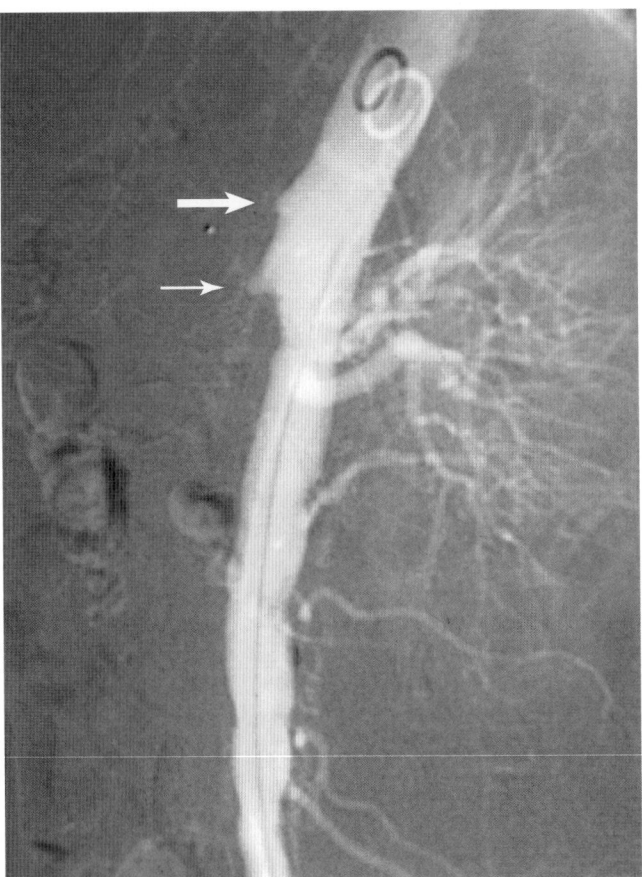

Figure 149-5 Lateral aortogram of a patient with acute mesenteric ischemia due to superior mesenteric artery thrombosis (*small arrow*). Note the chronic occlusion of the celiac artery (*large arrow*).

Anatomic imaging of the visceral vessels relies on contrast-enhanced techniques; noncontrast 3D phase-contrast MRA identifies only 66% of angiographic stenoses and gives some false-positive results.[61] Rapid intravenous bolus administration of a T1-shortening agent such as gadolinium DTPA

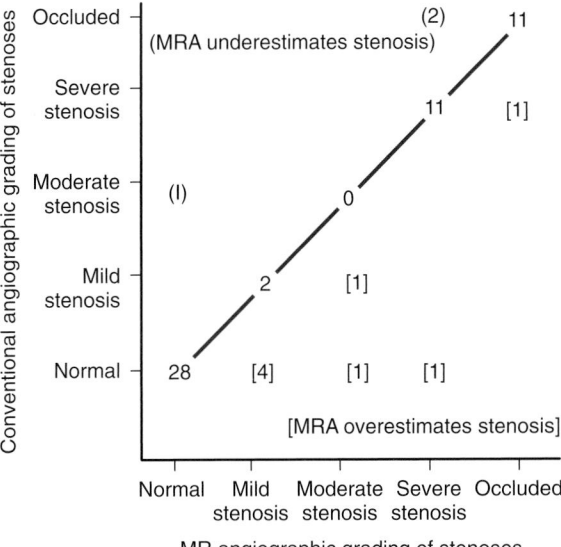

Figure 149-6 Magnetic resonance grading accuracy for the celiac artery, superior mesenteric artery, and inferior mesenteric artery (n = 63) in 26 patients with prospective conventional angiographic correlation. Numbers along the graph line represent the number of arteries in which the results of gadolinium-enhanced magnetic resonance angiography (MRA) and conventional angiography agreed. Numbers in parentheses represent the number of arteries in which MRA underestimated the degree of stenosis. Numbers in brackets represent the number of arteries in which MRA overestimated the degree of stenosis. *(From Carlos RC, Stanley JC, Stafford-Johnson D, Prince MR. Interobserver variability in the evaluation of chronic mesenteric ischemia with gadolinium-enhanced MR angiography. Acad Radiol. 2001;8:879-887.)*

paired with a rapid, 3D, gradient-recalled echo sequence allows consistent imaging of the splanchnic circulation with minimal flow artifact. Commercially available data acquisition protocols are available, and the 3D data set can be post-processed with techniques such as maximum intensity projection, curved planar reformation, and volume rendering, which distill the data into more readily comprehensible images. The most common error in a recent study of the use of 3D contrast-enhanced MRA in the evaluation of mesenteric stenosis was overestimation of the stenosis (Fig. 149-6).[62] The weakness of MRA is its relatively poor spatial resolution, which, even on the best systems, is limited to 1 mm³. Gadolinium-enhanced MRA does not currently provide sufficient resolution to demonstrate distal emboli, nonocclusive low-flow states, small vessel occlusion, or vasculitis.[62] MRA evaluation of the mesenteric arteries is limited to the proximal celiac artery and SMA; the evaluation of SMA branches or the inferior mesenteric artery is limited by the spatial resolution of MRA techniques. In addition, the secondary signs of AMI such as indurated fat or bowel wall thickening, which are routinely delineated by CT, are more difficult to assess with MRA.

Diagnostic Laparoscopy

Laparoscopy in the setting of AMI has limited ability to assess bowel viability. Serosal color can be difficult to judge and can be distorted significantly by a malfunctioning or improperly calibrated camera. Furthermore, segmental ischemia can be missed because of the difficulty in "running" the bowel along its entire length and over all surfaces. To increase the sensitivity of diagnostic laparoscopy, some authors have successfully used fluorescein with a laparoscopic ultraviolet light.[64-66] Nevertheless, diagnostic laparoscopy for this indication has not been widely accepted[67] because it may still miss areas of nonviable bowel.

■ TREATMENT

Initial Resuscitation and Critical Care

Fluid resuscitation of a patient with AMI should begin immediately with isotonic crystalloid solution and continue with blood, if necessary. Electrolyte imbalances (hyperkalemia) should be monitored and corrected. Invasive monitoring (hourly urine output, continuous central pressure and arterial pressure monitoring) is advisable from the beginning to ensure that all parameters are optimized before intravenous contrast administration or operative exploration. Broad-spectrum antibiotics should be given to guard against translocated bacteria and sepsis. If there are no contraindications, intravenous heparin should also be administered to maintain a partial thromboplastin time greater than twice normal.

The presentation of sepsis and organ dysfunction in these patients is common, and for the most part, these disorders are managed as they would be in other situations. Vasopressors, however, may worsen ischemia in marginally viable bowel and exacerbate visceral vasospasm. Before the initiation of any vasopressor, volume resuscitation must be confirmed by the presence of adequate right heart filling pressures. Because of the large and ongoing fluid sequestration in these patients, 24-hour crystalloid requirements in excess of 15 L are not uncommon. When necessary, better vasopressor options include low- to mid-dose dopamine (3 to 8 μg/kg/min) and epinephrine (0.05 to 0.10 μg/kg/min). Pure α-adrenergic agents should be avoided if possible, even after successful revascularization.[8]

Treatment of Nonocclusive Mesenteric Ischemia

NOMI accounts for more than 10% to 20% of cases of acute mesenteric circulatory disorders and leads to extensive irreversible intestinal necrosis. The prognosis is poor, despite the absence of organic obstruction in the principal arteries. The primary treatment for NOMI is medical, with extensive critical care support and prompt arteriography. Operative exploration is reserved for signs of peritonitis that suggest the presence of gangrenous bowel that requires excision.

Interventional therapies can be initiated at the time of the diagnostic arteriogram and are targeted at relieving vasospasm using intra-arterial infusions of vasodilator medications (Fig. 149-7). The angiographic appearance of NOMI

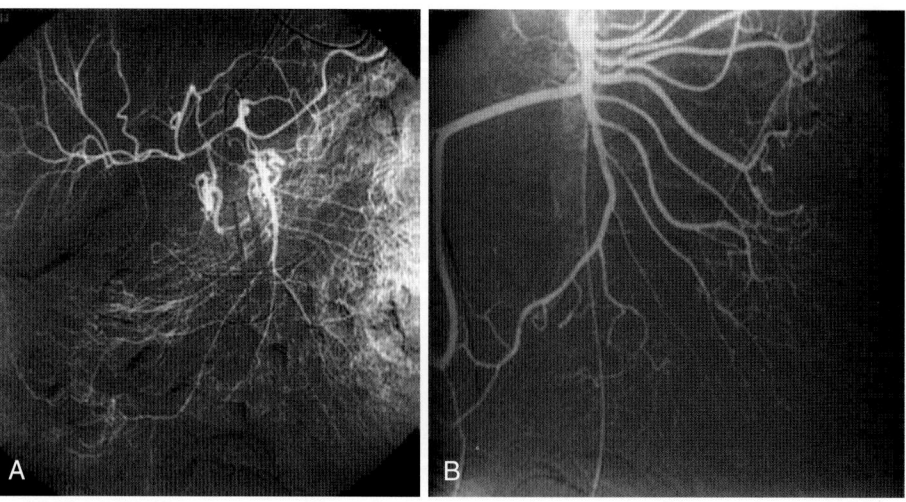

Figure 149-7 Arteriogram with selective superior mesenteric artery (SMA) injections. **A,** Severe SMA vasospasm with narrowing of all SMA branches. Intramural vessels are not seen owing to severe ischemia. **B,** There is significant improvement after several hours of vasodilator administration. *(From Trompeter M. Non-occlusive mesenteric ischemia: etiology, diagnosis, and interventional therapy. Eur Radiol. 2002;12: 1179-1187.)*

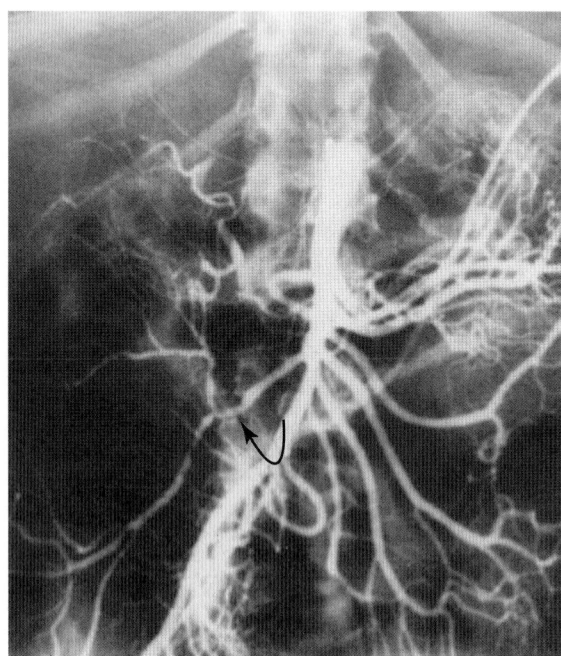

Figure 149-8 Selective superior mesenteric artery arteriogram in a patient with nonocclusive mesenteric ischemia. Note the "string of sausages" appearance of some of the ileocolic branches *(arrow)*. *(From Clark RA, Colley DP, Jacobson ED, et al. Superior mesenteric angiography and blood flow measurement following intra-arterial injection of prostaglandin E1. Radiology. 1980;134:327-333.)*

can be subtle, but Siegelman and associates described four reliable arteriographic criteria for the diagnosis of mesenteric vasospasm: (1) narrowing of the origins of multiple branches of the SMA, (2) alternate dilatation and narrowing of the intestinal branches—the "string of sausages" sign (Fig. 149-8), (3) spasm of the mesenteric arcades, and (4) impaired filling of the intramural vessels.[68] The most common intra-arterial agent used in the majority of reports is the phosphodiesterase inhibitor papaverine. There are multiple case reports of the local infusion of vasodilators—either papaverine[22,69,70] or prostaglandin analogues[71]—leading to improvement.

Boley and coworkers reported favorable mortality rates of 40% to 50% with the aggressive use of intra-arterial vasodilators and suggested that the extent of bowel resection during laparotomy (whatever the cause of ischemia) could be significantly reduced if vasodilatation were performed preoperatively.[4] Once the angiographic diagnosis of NOMI is made and other causes of acute abdomen are excluded, intra-arterial papaverine is initiated at a dose of 30 to 60 mg/hr and often continued for several days as long as the patient's condition remains stable or until there is improvement. Because papaverine is metabolized primarily in the liver, hypotension is uncommon as long as the catheter remains in the SMA, but careful monitoring of the blood pressure, heart rate, and rhythm is appropriate. If a sudden decrease in blood pressure is noted, the papaverine infusion should be substituted with saline, and a plain abdominal radiograph should be obtained to confirm the position of the catheter. Finally, heparin sodium is chemically incompatible with papaverine and should not be infused simultaneously through the same catheter. In the case of resolved abdominal symptoms, a second arteriogram is advisable before the cessation of papaverine, unless the risk of contrast nephropathy precludes it (see Fig. 149-7B).

In a recent report by Mitsuyoshi and colleagues, eight of nine patients with MDCTA evidence of NOMI (Fig. 149-9) who were treated promptly with high-dose intravenous or intra-arterial prostaglandin E$_1$ (PGE$_1$) survived.[71] Intravenous dosing was 0.01 to 0.03 µg/kg/min and was continued for a mean of 4.8 days. In contrast, in the group that was not imaged with MDCTA or treated with PGE$_1$, 9 of 13 patients died. Although these results are admirable, it is not clear whether they are ascribable to PGE$_1$ treatment or to a heightened awareness of the problem, earlier imaging with MDCTA, and prompt diagnosis and supportive treatment.

Surgical Treatment

Surgical exploration is required for all patients who have evidence of any threatened bowel, regardless of the underly-

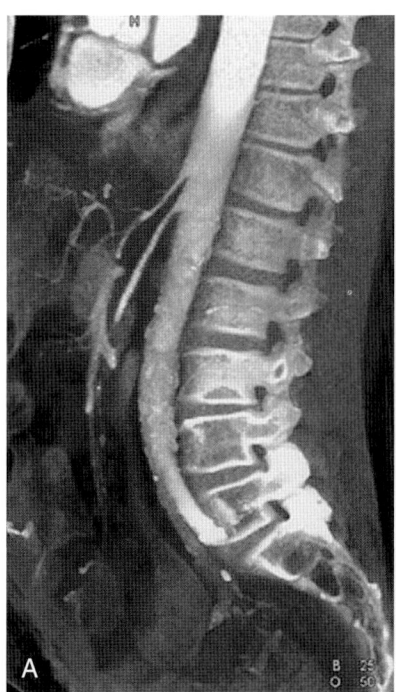 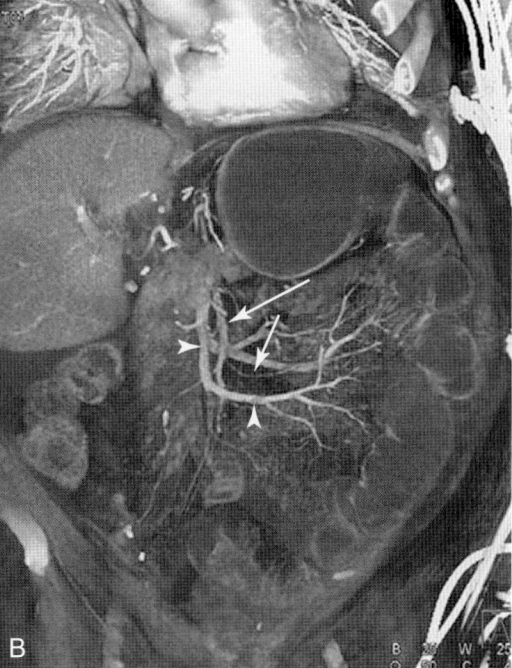

Figure 149-9 CTA appearance of nonocclusive mesenteric ischemia. **A,** Sagittal volume-rendered image shows diffuse narrowing of the main celiac and superior mesenteric arteries. **B,** Coronal oblique volume-rendered image of the same patient shows pruning of the superior mesenteric artery branches (*arrows*). Note the dilated, fluid-filled small intestine and the superior mesenteric vein (*arrowheads*). *(From Horton KM, Fishman EK. Multidetector CT angiography in the diagnosis of mesenteric ischemia. Radiol Clin North Am. 2007;45:275-288.)*

ing cause. The intraoperative appearance of the bowel can be deceiving. Bowel that is nearing irreversible necrosis can be deceptively normal in appearance; conversely, bowel that appears severely ischemic may be viable after revascularization. Thus, in all cases the surgeon should proceed with revascularization before resecting any intestine unless faced with an area of frank necrosis or perforation and peritoneal soilage. In this case, resection of the affected bowel without reanastomosis and with containment of the spillage should be achieved rapidly before revascularization. Only in a very few patients—those who are already in extremis and present with massive bowel necrosis—can revascularization conscionably be withheld. Preparation and draping of all patients undergoing laparotomy for presumed AMI should include both lower extremities at least to the knee to allow the harvest of saphenous or femoral vein for bypass.

The abdomen is best explored via a vertical midline incision (Fig. 149-10). There are two variations in the technique for exposing the SMA below the pancreas. Selection between the two is based on the surgeon's level of confidence regarding the need for simple embolectomy or more complex arterial repair with or without bypass. In the case of a confirmed embolus and a more normal-appearing SMA, the artery can be approached anteriorly at the base of the transverse mesocolon without formal mobilization of the fourth portion of the duodenum or ligament of Treitz. If the SMA is diseased or thrombosis is the cause, a more lateral approach to the SMA above the fourth portion of the duodenum is preferred to facilitate a retrograde bypass, if necessary. These techniques are described in the sections that follow and are depicted in Figures 149-10 and 149-11.

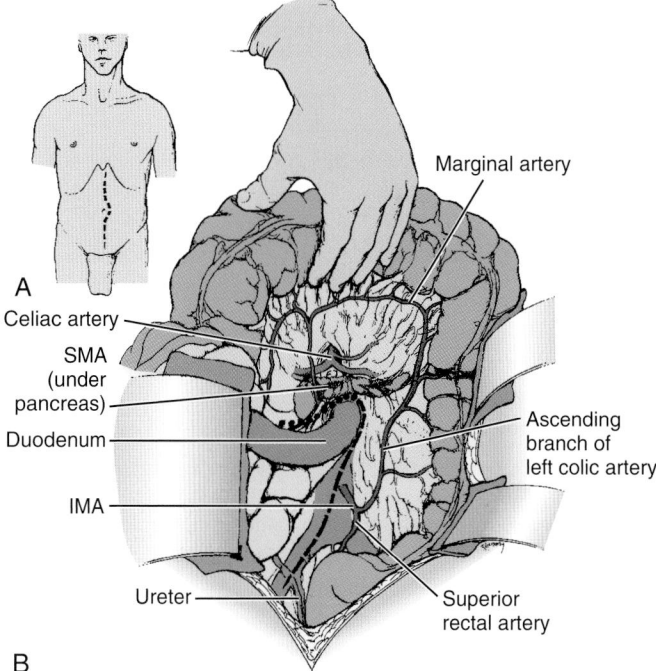

Figure 149-10 A and **B,** Operative exposure of the infrapancreatic superior mesenteric artery (SMA). IMA, inferior mesenteric artery. *(From Kazmers A. Operative management of acute mesenteric ischemia. Ann Vasc Surg. 1998;12:187-197.)*

Superior Mesenteric Artery Embolectomy

Anterior exposure of the SMA for straightforward embolectomy is achieved by elevating the omentum and transverse colon; the small intestine is wrapped in moist laparotomy pads and retracted to the right. A horizontal incision is made in

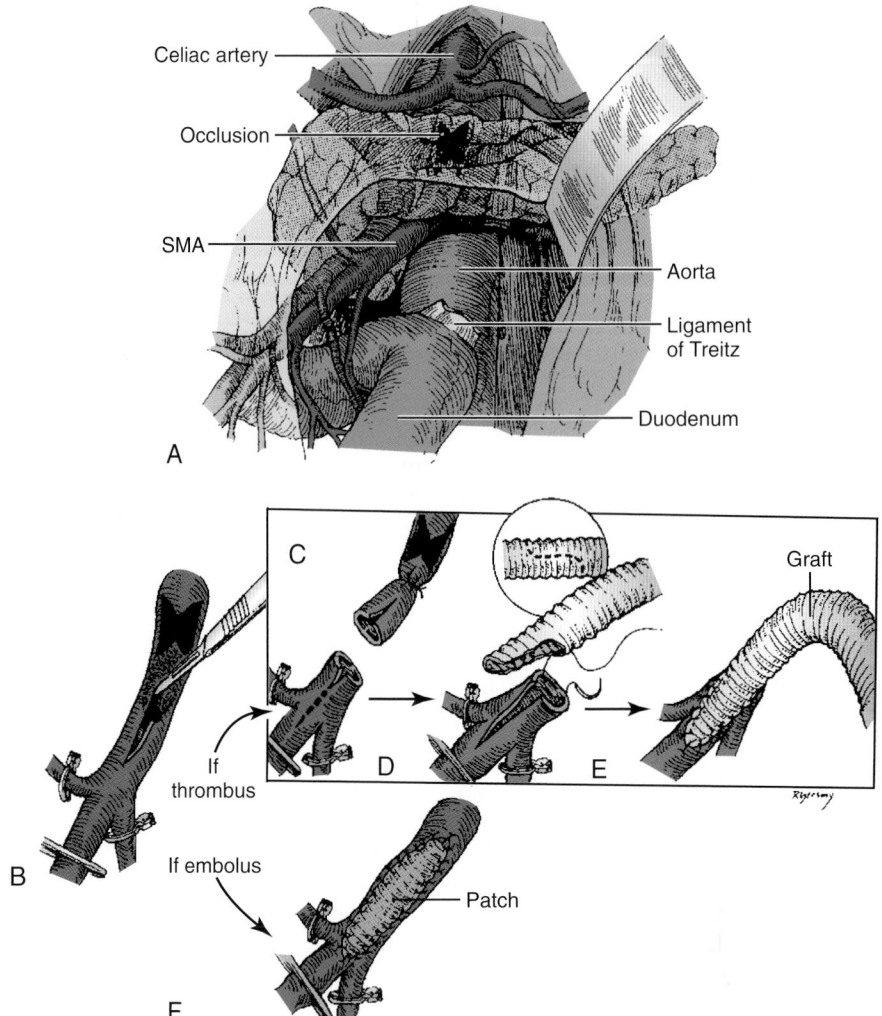

Figure 149-11 A, Operative exposure and preparation of the superior mesenteric artery (SMA) for bypass or patch. **B,** Linear arteriotomy. **C–E,** Creation of a beveled, end-to-end anastomosis. **F,** Patch closure of the SMA. *(From Kazmers A. Operative management of acute mesenteric ischemia. Ann Vasc Surg. 1998;12:187-197.)*

the peritoneum at the base of the transverse mesocolon (see Fig. 149-10B, dotted line). Careful dissection in the mesentery initially uncovers venous tributaries of the superior mesenteric vein, autonomic nerve fibers, and small lymphatics that are divided to gain exposure of the SMA. The SMA lies to the left of the superior mesenteric vein and can be fragile. Exposure of the more proximal segments is possible by judicious mobilization of the inferior pancreatic border (exercise caution when dealing with the pancreas), the nearby splenic vein, and its tributaries from the pancreas.

A segment of the proximal SMA between the middle and right colic branches is isolated. Near-circumferential dissection is frequently required to isolate and control any of the jejunal branches in this segment. After systemic hepariniza-

tion, the artery is opened transversely (Fig. 149-12) in a segment of sufficient diameter to allow direct repair. For diminutive vessels, a short longitudinal arteriotomy with patch closure may be considered. The proximal SMA is vented to allow any clot to be expelled without the use of an embolectomy catheter if possible. When necessary, catheter embolectomy is typically performed with 3 or 4 Fr balloon catheter. With extraction of the embolus, torrential and pulsatile inflow should be expected.

Distally, a smaller embolectomy catheter, typically 2 or 3 Fr, is employed. Great care must be taken to avoid damage or rupture of the fragile mesenteric arteries. Difficulty passing a catheter down multiple small branches adds to the complexity of the distal embolectomy. An alternative or adjunct to

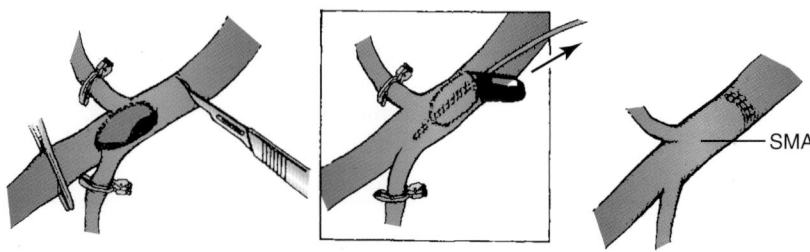

Figure 149-12 Traditional transverse arteriotomy for superior mesenteric artery (SMA) embolectomy. *(From Kazmers A. Operative management of acute mesenteric ischemia. Ann Vasc Surg. 1998;12:187-197.)*

balloon embolectomy of the distal mesenteric vessels is for the surgeon to place a hand on either side of the mesentery and "milk" thrombotic material out of the vessels. After all macroscopic clot is cleared, consideration can also be given to the administration of a small, one-time dose of a thrombolytic agent (recombinant tissue plasminogen activator or urokinase) into the distal vessels. When all thrombus is removed, the arteriotomy is closed primarily with interrupted sutures or with vein patch, and flow is re-established.

Superior Mesenteric Artery Bypass

As mentioned previously, when bypass is considered, the lateral portion of the SMA is exposed rather than the more limited exposure provided by a strictly anterior approach. The peritoneum is opened lateral to the duodenum, down over the aorta, and onto the left or right common iliac artery (see Fig. 149-10B, *dashed line*). Several combinations of graft orientation and conduit are available. The decision is influenced largely by the suitability of potential inflow vessels for a proximal anastomosis and by the presence or absence of peritoneal soilage, respectively. In the emergent setting, a single bypass to the SMA is all that is required. The preference for two-vessel revascularization,[72] which most surgeons espouse in the performance of elective bypass for chronic symptoms, does not apply.

Graft orientation is influenced mainly by the degree of atherosclerosis and occlusive disease present in the inflow vessels and by the overall lie of the graft. Given the choice, most surgeons prefer a retrograde graft orientation, with its origin from the right common iliac artery in a "lazy C" configuration (Fig. 149-13A). This avoids any aortic clamping and usually provides a good lie to prevent kinking. Second-choice inflow sources for retrograde bypasses involve similar

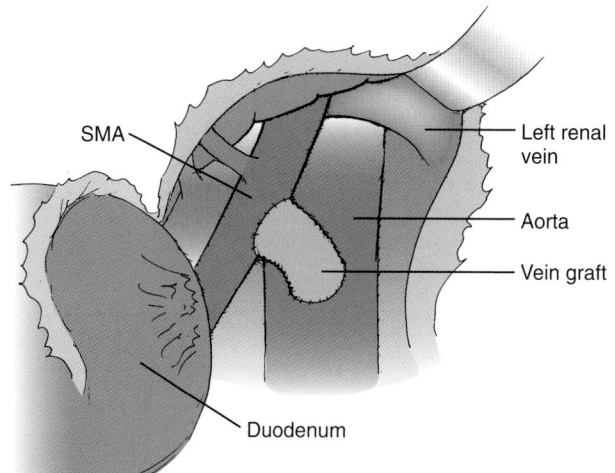

Figure 149-14 Short retrograde aorta–superior mesenteric artery (SMA) bypass. *(From Valentine RJ, Wind GG. Anatomic Exposures in Vascular Surgery. 2nd ed. Philadelphia: Lippincott Williams and Wilkins; 2003:281.)*

lazy C grafts from the left iliac artery or distal infrarenal aorta. With any of these configurations, the graft lie tends to be improved by increasing the graft length slightly and performing an end-to-end graft-to-SMA anastomosis, as pictured in Figure 149-11C to E. Alternatively, a very short retrograde bypass using a larger diameter graft (8 to 10 mm) can be configured from the immediately infrarenal aorta (Fig. 149-14), but the potential for kinking with shorter grafts can be more difficult to anticipate until all the retractors are removed. When distal inflow sources are unclampable, heavily diseased, or aneurysmal, an antegrade bypass can be considered. Advantages of the antegrade bypass include the fact that the supraceliac aorta is often relatively free of disease and that the straighter graft orientation is less prone to kinking. Dissection of the supraceliac aorta is technically more demanding, however; it requires more time and adds a hemodynamically and physiologically stressful aortic cross-clamp if a partial occluding clamp is not possible.

Synthetic bypass grafts of 6- to 8-mm Dacron or externally supported polytetrafluoroethylene are preferred because of the better size match, ease of handling, availability, kink resistance, and general perception that long-term patency is better. The superior patency of prosthetic mesenteric bypasses, however, is not well documented. Therefore, the choice of conduit is heavily influenced by the degree of abdominal contamination and the perceived risk of subsequent graft infection. The actual rate of mesenteric graft infection is not known with certainty, but when present, it is potentially catastrophic and likely to involve virulent organisms. Therefore, if good-quality vein is available, it is preferred in the presence of significant peritoneal soilage. Great saphenous vein and thigh femoral vein are the primary options. Modrall and colleagues reported that symptomatic recurrences were less common in patients bypassed with femoral vein conduit compared with great saphenous vein.[73] In practice, however, the additional time and expertise required to harvest a deep leg vein is too much to consider in such critically ill patients. Great caution

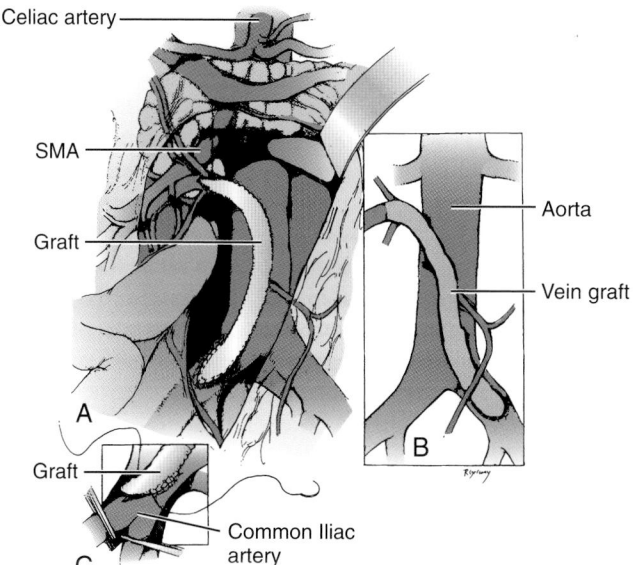

Figure 149-13 Optimal orientation for retrograde superior mesenteric artery (SMA) bypass. **A,** Prosthetic. **B,** Vein. **C,** Proximal iliac graft anastomosis. *(From Kazmers A. Operative management of acute mesenteric ischemia. Ann Vasc Surg. 1998;12:187-197.)*

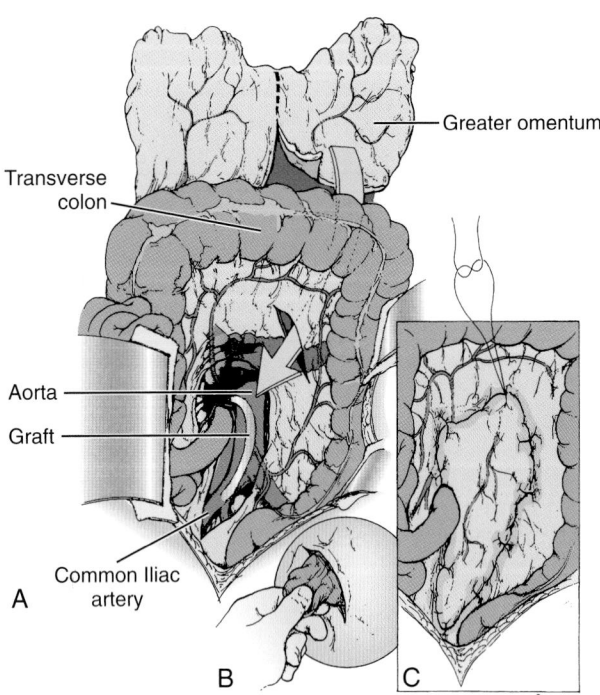

Transverse colon

Greater omentum

Aorta

Graft

Common Iliac artery

A

B

C

Figure 149-15 A-C, Technique for omental flap coverage of a retrograde superior mesenteric artery bypass. *(From Kazmers A. Operative management of acute mesenteric ischemia.* Ann Vasc Surg. *1998;12:187-197.)*

must be used in fashioning a vein graft because their smaller diameter and thin-walled nature make veins more prone to kinking and external compression than synthetic grafts. When prosthetic graft use is unavoidable, Kazmers and colleagues illustrated a useful technique to provide coverage of a retrograde bypass by bringing an omental flap through the transverse mesocolon (Fig. 149-15).[74]

Assessment of Bowel Viability

After revascularization has been accomplished, the viability of the bowel must be reassessed. If possible, 20 to 30 minutes of reperfusion time should be permitted while retractors are being repositioned before making a decision about viability.[74] The initial clinical evaluation of the bowel consists of assessment for visible and palpable pulsations in the mesenteric arcade, normal color and appearance of the bowel serosa, peristalsis, and bleeding from cut surfaces. Each of these is subjective and prone to inaccuracy; with the use of clinical criteria alone, bowel viability can be successfully determined with a sensitivity of only 82% and a specificity of 91%.[75]

Wright and Hobson reported that absence of pulsatile signals on the antimesenteric border of the intestine as detected with a continuous wave 9- to 10-MHz Doppler ultrasound probe implies a nonviable segment.[76] The clinical practicality of this technique combined with surgical judgment has been demonstrated in multiple studies.[75,77,78] As a stand-alone method of determining intestinal viability,

however, Doppler assessment has its limitations because it may miss weak signals in small vasoconstricted vessels in otherwise viable bowel.[79] Other adjunctive methods of bowel viability assessment have been proposed. Highly accurate quantification of perfusion is possible using fluorescein and a perfusion fluorometer[80] or a laser Doppler flowmeter,[81] but special equipment requirements and technical considerations make this less practical for routine clinical use. Whitehill and associates found that Doppler ultrasound evaluation, photoplethysmography, and fluorescein injection may be too sensitive in some cases for an accurate determination of bowel viability, yielding false-positive results by detecting levels of flow below that needed to sustain tissue viability.[82]

Ultimately, accurate determination of intestinal viability is the product of clinical judgment and timely re-evaluation. The need to preserve as much bowel length as possible should deter the surgeon from being overly aggressive in resecting any questionably viable bowel. The option of deferring extensive bowel resection and re-anastomosis underscores the fundamental importance of a mandatory second-look procedure.

Endovascular Treatment

Superior Mesenteric Artery Embolization

Acute arterial occlusion caused by thromboembolization progresses to bowel necrosis faster than either NOMI or mesenteric venous thrombosis. Restoration of flow must be accomplished within a few hours to prevent bowel necrosis and the incipient downward spiral that frequently results in death. Based on this, one would suspect that thrombolysis takes too long to achieve timely revascularization. Nevertheless, there are increasing numbers of successful, single-patient case reports of percutaneous endovascular procedures using mechanical and chemical thrombectomies.[83-91] It is difficult to determine the technical failure rate from such small case reports, which by their nature focus on positive results.

If more broadly applied, one could easily surmise that revascularization failure is more common with endovascular lysis than with direct surgical embolectomy. Wang and coworkers offered a retrospective report of seven patients with SMA emboli who were treated with catheter-based thrombolysis, which was successful in only four.[92] Despite a shorter time to diagnosis and initiation of treatment in the lysis group compared with a similar cohort of nine surgically treated patients, there was no survival difference. Even when technically successful, percutaneous catheter thrombectomy and certainly chemical thrombolysis can be very time-consuming compared with a straightforward open embolectomy.

Schoots and colleagues reviewed 20 case reports and 7 small series published over a 47-year span for a total of 48 patients.[14] Interestingly, only 33% of patients demonstrated total or near-total arteriographic occlusion of the SMA before treatment. Technical resolution of thrombus was achieved in

43 patients, but 18 patients still required operative exploration for bowel resection. Only one surgical embolectomy was performed. Forty-three of the patients survived. This review does not give any credence to the use of percutaneous thrombolysis as an efficacious or even safe mode of therapy for acute SMA embolism. It only serves to magnify the enormous publication bias inherent in the literature on this topic.

Another shortcoming of a less invasive approach to SMA embolism is the lack of a built-in assessment of bowel viability. Surgical treatment incorporates open embolectomy with a thorough assessment of intestinal viability. Patient mortality is closely associated with bowel necrosis, and when resection is necessary, it cannot be delayed. Therefore, a significant weakness of a less invasive approach is that there is often no direct evaluation of intestinal viability. To avoid abdominal exploration, the patient's overall clinical condition, laboratory markers, and occasionally laparoscopy are substituted. These substitutes are unreliable, however, and diagnostic laparoscopy for this indication has not been widely accepted because it may miss areas of nonviable bowel.[67]

Superior Mesenteric Artery Thrombosis

Terminal thrombosis of an atherosclerotic SMA is perhaps the most challenging AMI cohort to treat endovascularly. Successful treatment requires revascularization, meaning that some method must be used to quickly recanalize an elongated occlusion that, unlike with embolic presentations, typically occupies the origin and initial 3 to 6 cm of the SMA. As described previously, operative bypass to the SMA is traditionally required. The operation can be complex, and recovery is challenging in these very ill patients. Thus, a less invasive option for SMA revascularization is theoretically appealing.

Endovascular treatment for mesenteric ischemia has been well described for subacute or chronic presentations, especially in patients at high operative risk or as a bridge to elective surgical bypass after the acute illness has resolved.[93-96] Endovascular treatment has not generally been applied to patients with AMI, however, who need emergent revascularization and potential resection of nonviable bowel. The reason is that a percutaneous procedure does not allow an assessment of bowel viability, requires advanced endovascular skills, and, even in the most experienced hands, can take substantial time, which might delay revascularization. Nevertheless, a few case reports of percutaneous interventional treatment for AMI have been published.[83,84,86,87,89,97] Widespread experience is lacking, and this approach has shortcomings similar to those discussed for the endovascular treatment of SMA embolism. Indeed, our own experience with percutaneous stenting in acutely ischemic patients has been very disappointing in terms of both technical success and patient outcome.[98] It was this experience that led directly to a more efficacious hybrid technique. In our practice, we now reserve percutaneous mesenteric stenting for patients with chronic or subacute presentations who do not require a detailed assessment of bowel viability.

Hybrid Procedure: Retrograde Open Mesenteric Stenting

Wyers and coauthors from Dartmouth recently reported a hybrid open-interventional approach for the treatment of acute atherosclerotic SMA thrombosis that involves an efficient, less invasive mesenteric revascularization without compromising important general surgical principles.[98] In fact, the general surgical principles of thorough abdominal exploration, sepsis control, and a low threshold for second-look operations must be honored to increase the chances of a favorable outcome. Similar to a technique in an earlier case report by Milner and associates,[99] the Dartmouth authors described retrograde open mesenteric stenting (ROMS) of the SMA in six patients. In this ROMS approach, the visceral peritoneum is incised horizontally or longitudinally at the base of the transverse mesocolon, the SMA is controlled, and a local thromboendarterectomy of the SMA is performed if necessary. Placing a patch angioplasty then facilitates retrograde cannulation of the SMA with a long, flexible sheath directed toward the aorta (Fig. 149-16). Because of the superior pushability with sheath access so close to the obstruction, technical success was 100%, even in the five patients who had previous unsuccessful attempts to cross the SMA from a percutaneous antegrade approach. Often, more than one balloon-expandable stent is required to fully treat these SMA lesions, which are typically 3 cm or longer (Fig. 149-17).

This was a small series with no statistically significant results, but the ROMS outcomes were promising. The ROMS

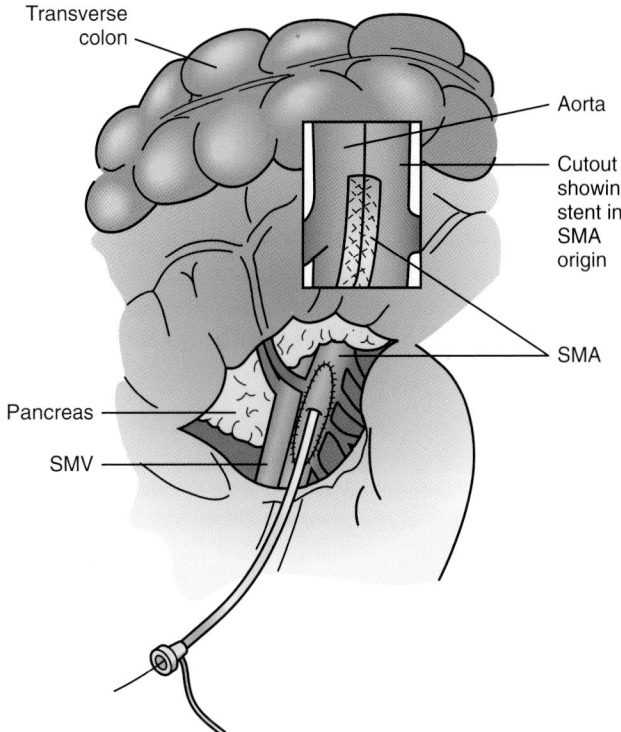

Figure 149-16 Retrograde open mesenteric stenting with a long 6 Fr sheath placed through the patched superior mesenteric artery (SMA). The *inset* illustrates a stent deployed in the proximal SMA. SMV, superior mesenteric vein.

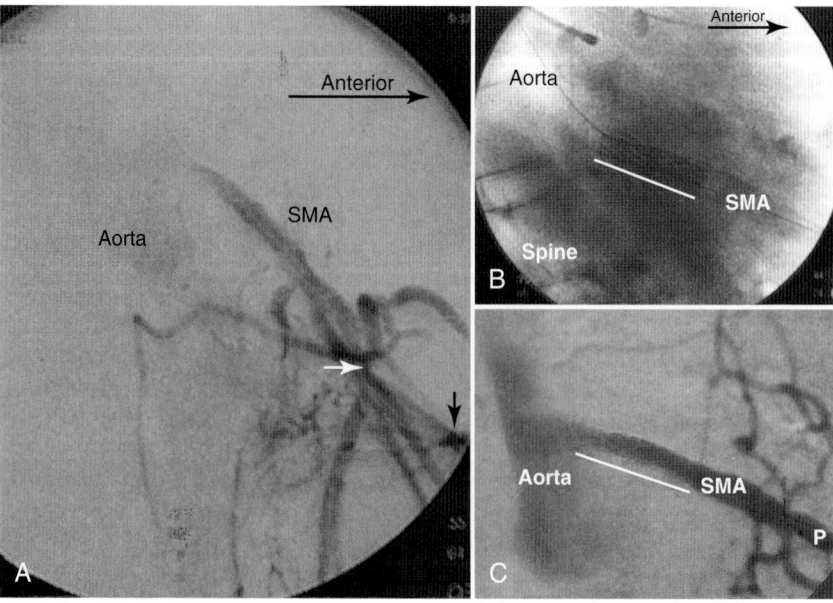

Figure 149-17 Retrograde open mesenteric stenting. **A,** Intraoperative arteriogram during retrograde superior mesenteric artery (SMA) injection. Note the proximity of the sheath's point of entry (*black arrow*) and the sheath's tip (*white arrow*) to the proximal SMA occlusion. There is no reflux of contrast material into the aorta. **B,** Intraoperative lateral fluoroscopic image of two stents (underscored by a *white line*) deployed in the SMA origin with the 0.018-inch wire still in place. Note the lumbar vertebral bodies to the left. **C,** Completion retrograde arteriogram with free reflux of contrast material into the aorta and no residual angiographic stenosis. P, approximate location of SMA patch angioplasty. *(From Wyers MC, Powell RJ, Nolan BW, Cronenwett JL. Retrograde mesenteric stenting during laparotomy for acute occlusive mesenteric ischemia. J Vasc Surg. 2007;45:269-275.)*

group suffered only 17% in-hospital mortality, compared with 80% among five patients treated with conventional mesenteric bypass. Recurrent stenosis after ROMS, as with all forms of mesenteric stenting,[59,94] happens frequently and relatively early, so we recommend duplex surveillance for the first month and every 3 months thereafter. Most patients with recurrent stenosis can be re-treated with a percutaneous approach as outpatients. Many of these patients remain poor operative candidates and have limited life expectancies because of co-morbidities.[100] In this situation, even repeated SMA dilatations are a viable, safe option. For patients who make a good recovery and are nutritionally sound, a more durable operative bypass may be considered.[93] ROMS during emergent laparotomy for AMI is a promising technique and an attractive alternative to emergent surgical bypass. This method needs to be tested by others to determine its true value in comparison to traditional methods.

OTHER CONSIDERATIONS

Second-Look Surgery

Even after reperfusion and careful assessment, bowel viability cannot be determined with certainty at the time of initial exploration. The frequency of bowel resection is routinely higher during second-look surgery (53%) compared with the initial exploration and revascularization procedure (31%).[11] The decision to perform this second-look surgery is made at the time of initial operation. This plan is essentially inviolate, regardless of the clinical status of the patient. Typically, at the conclusion of the initial procedure, the surgeon leaves transected ends of the intestine stapled shut without reanastomosis. Likewise, the abdominal fascia can be left open if bowel edema is significant, in anticipation of a return to the operating room within the next 48 hours. Certainly, if the patient's clinical condition deteriorates at any point, reoperation is

immediate. This strategy allows the preservation of as much bowel as possible, resecting only areas of bowel that are clearly nonviable at each procedure. The patient is returned to the operating room 12 to 48 hours later, and the abdomen is re-explored. By this time, the viability of the bowel has usually declared itself, but occasionally a third look is required. This mandatory return protects the patient from ongoing bowel necrosis before irreversible physiologic changes develop and before perforation that would risk further sepsis, abscess, or graft infection. Mesenteric blood flow is reassessed, and the bowel anastomoses are performed if the condition of the bowel is satisfactory.

Intraoperative Vasodilators

Splanchnic vasospasm may persist for variable periods of time, causing continued bowel ischemia after a successful revascularization.[12,101] Low flow after ischemia can also result from relative hypovolemia, myocardial depression, and sepsis. To improve local vasospasm in the mesenteric arcades, papaverine can be administered selectively in the SMA. Alternatively, intravenous glucagon administration increases cardiac output and flow to all layers of the small and large intestine and liver while inhibiting gastrointestinal motility and secretory function. This has been shown to improve survival in an animal model[102,103] but has not been tested extensively in humans. Glucagon administration should be coupled with additional volume resuscitation to avoid vasodilatation-mediated hypotension.

Duplex Follow-up

Duplex ultrasound seems to be the most reasonable, cost-effective way to obtain objective data for clinical decision making after various forms of mesenteric revascularization. Robust reports of Doppler ultrasound follow-up after mesenteric bypass have been lacking, however. In a recent article by Liem and coworkers, duplex-derived flow velocities in mesenteric artery bypass grafts were characterized for the first time.[104] Postprandial scans were performed in a longitudinal follow-up of 43 mesenteric grafts, for a total of 167 duplex examinations. Midgraft flows were higher in smaller diameter grafts (6 mm) and saphenous vein grafts compared with larger diameter grafts (7 mm) but were not affected by graft orientation or inflow source. Two grafts failed during the follow-up interval, but unfortunately, no duplex scan characteristics were found to predict graft thrombosis.

Restenosis is common and happens early after mesenteric stenting,[59,94] including ROMS patients. Therefore, frequent duplex surveillance is required to judge the need for re-intervention. Although the published data on Doppler ultrasound of native (unstented) mesenteric arteries are very good,[105-107] the literature that focuses on stented mesenteric vessels is meager. Our experience at Dartmouth with mesenteric duplex following interventional visceral artery therapy is promising but still empirical, based on an anticipated high rate of restenosis. We have not identified an absolute velocity threshold that indicates the need for prompt re-intervention. However, the traditional velocity criteria for native vessels seem to provide reasonably accurate information to guide clinical decision making.

SELECTED KEY REFERENCES

Aschoff AJ, Stuber G, Becker BW, Hoffmann, MH, Schmitz BL, Schelig H, Jaeckle T. Evaluation of acute mesenteric ischemia: accuracy of biphasic mesenteric multi-detector CT angiography. *Abdom Imaging.* 2009;34:345-357.
Good example of CTA technique.

Kassahun WT, Schulz T, Richter O, Hauss J. Unchanged high mortality rates from acute occlusive intestinal ischemia: six year review. *Langenbecks Arch Surg.* 2008;393:163-171.
Good review article.

Kazmers A. Operative management of acute mesenteric ischemia. *Ann Vasc Surg.* 1998;12:187-197.
Excellent illustrations of operative technique.

Kirkpatrick ID, Kroeker MA, Greenberg HM. Biphasic CT with mesenteric CT angiography in the evaluation of acute mesenteric ischemia: initial experience. *Radiology.* 2003;229:91-98.
Establishes CTA as the best diagnostic imaging choice.

Kougias P, Lau D, El Sayed HF, Zhou W, Huynh TT, Lin PH. Determinants of mortality and treatment outcome following surgical interventions for acute mesenteric ischemia. *J Vasc Surg.* 2007;46:467-474.
Good look at factors that influence patient survival.

Oldenburg WA, Lau LL, Rodenberg TJ, Edmonds HJ, Burger CD. Acute mesenteric ischemia: a clinical review. *Arch Intern Med.* 2004;164:1054-1062.
Good review article.

Park WM, Gloviczki P, Cherry KJ Jr, Hallett JW Jr, Bower TC, Panneton JM, Schleck C, Ilstrup D, Harmsen WS, Noel AA. Contemporary management of acute mesenteric ischemia: factors associated with survival. *J Vasc Surg.* 2002;35:445-452.
Good contemporary series and discussion.

Wyers MC, Powell RJ, Nolan BW, Cronenwett JL. Retrograde mesenteric stenting during laparotomy for acute occlusive mesenteric ischemia. *J Vasc Surg.* 2007;45:269-275.
Description of new technique for revascularization of the SMA.

REFERENCES

The reference list can be found on the companion Expert Consult Web site at *www.expertconsult.com.*

CHAPTER 150

Mesenteric Vascular Disease: Venous Thrombosis

Stefan Acosta and Martin Björck

Splanchnic venous thrombosis can occur within the portal, superior and inferior mesenteric, and splenic veins. Mesenteric venous thrombosis (MVT) is defined as thrombosis within the superior mesenteric vein with or without extension to the portal or splenic vein. Recovery following resection of infarcted intestine secondary to mesenteric vessel occlusion was first reported by Elliot in 1895.[1] MVT was recognized as an entity distinct from mesenteric arterial occlusion by Warren and Eberhard in 1935.[2]

EPIDEMIOLOGY

MVT is most commonly encountered in middle-aged and elderly patients, with an equal gender distribution.[3,4] In a population-based study with an average autopsy rate of 87%, MVT was found to be present in 63 of 402 patients (16%) with acute mesenteric ischemia (Fig. 150-1).[5,6] Additionally, the overall incidence of MVT with transmural intestinal infarction was estimated to be 1.8 per 100,000 person-years in Malmö, Sweden, between 1970 and 1982, and the cause-specific mortality ratio was 0.9 per 1000 autopsies.[5] The overall incidence of MVT increased to 2.7 per 100,000 person-years in the same city between 2000 and 2006.[4] An important factor contributing to a decrease in the incidence estimate was the declining autopsy rate, from 87% to 10%, between the two periods. In contrast, factors increasing the incidence estimate over time were the growing proportion of elderly in the population and the greater diagnostic activity and quality. Patients with MVT were diagnosed at autopsy, at operation, or with computed tomography (CT) in 12% (6 of 51), 19% (10 of 51), and 69% (35 of 51) of cases, respectively,[4] during the latter period.

PATHOGENESIS

Etiology

Primary MVT is defined as spontaneous, idiopathic thrombosis of the mesenteric veins not associated with any other disease or etiologic factor. Patients with any condition known to predispose to MVT (Box 150-1) are considered to have secondary MVT.[7] Approximately 90% of MVTs are secondary,[8] due to direct injury, local venous congestion or stasis, or hypercoagulable states. Inherited thrombophilia[9-12] has been reported in 42% (13 to 31)[3] to 55% (16 of 29)[4] of patients with MVT. Primary cytomegalovirus infection has also been associated with MVT.[13] However, neither liver cirrhosis nor abdominal cancer was a risk factor in a population-based case-control study based on autopsies.[5] Synchronous venous thromboembolism in the systemic circulation occurs frequently in patients with MVT, especially pulmonary embolism.[5]

Risk Factors

Several conditions are associated with MVT (see Box 150-1), and these can be divided into three main categories: direct injury, local venous congestion or stasis, and thrombophilia. Factor V Leiden mutation (activated protein C resistance) was present in 45% of the patients with MVT in Malmö, Sweden,[4] which was considerably higher than the known prevalence rate of 7% in the background population.[14] Although factor V Leiden mutation is a genetic defect, peripheral venous thrombotic manifestations are frequently delayed until adulthood, even in homozygotes.[14,15] Obesity is also a risk factor,[5]

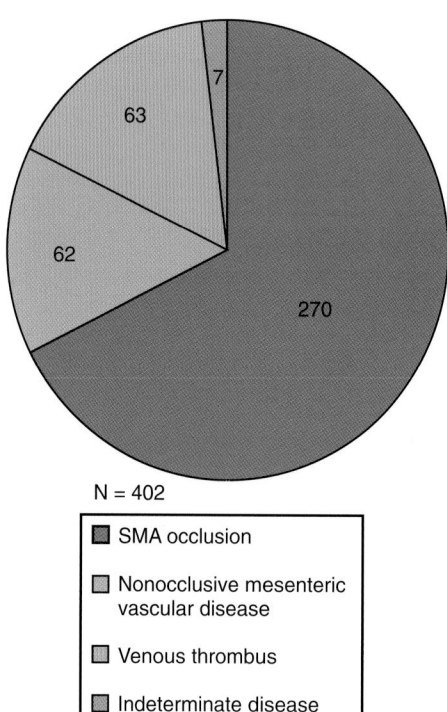

N = 402

- ■ SMA occlusion
- ▨ Nonocclusive mesenteric vascular disease
- ▤ Venous thrombus
- ▦ Indeterminate disease

Figure 150-1 Acute mesenteric ischemia: distribution of etiologies in 402 patients in Malmö, Sweden, between 1970 and 1982.[4,5] SMA, superior mesenteric artery.

Box 150-1 Conditions Associated with Mesenteric Venous Thrombosis

DIRECT INJURY
- Abdominal trauma (blunt and penetrating)
- Postsurgical (particularly postsplenectomy)
- Intra-abdominal inflammatory states (pancreatitis, inflammatory bowel)
- Peritonitis and abdominal abscess

LOCAL VENOUS CONGESTION OR STASIS
- Portal hypertension; cirrhosis of the liver
- Congestive heart failure
- Hypersplenism
- Obesity
- Increased abdominal pressure; abdominal compartment syndrome

THROMBOPHILIA
- Protein C and protein S deficiency
- Antithrombin III deficiency
- Activated protein C resistance (factor V Leiden gene mutation)
- Presence of 20210 A allele of prothrombin gene
- Methylenetetrahydrofolate reductase mutations
- Neoplasms (particularly pancreatic and colonic)
- Oral contraceptive use
- Polycythemia vera
- Heparin-induced thrombocytopenia
- Lupus anticoagulant-antiphospholipid syndrome
- Cytomegalovirus infection
- Extramesenteric venous thromboembolism

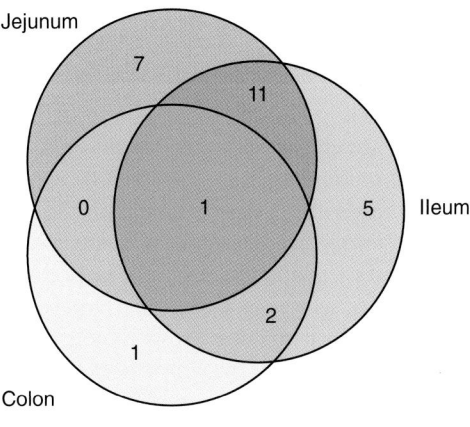

Figure 150-2 Venn diagram showing the extent of intestinal infarction in 27 patients with mesenteric venous thrombosis and transmural intestinal infarction.

and splenectomy is a risk factor for the development of thrombus propagation to the portomesenteric venous system.[16]

NATURAL HISTORY

It is difficult to pinpoint the natural history of MVT. The disease is uncommon, patients often have diffuse symptoms, and the condition is not always detected, even with contemporary diagnostic routines. Thus, we have no absolute knowledge of the total number of patients with symptomatic and asymptomatic disease. However, in a population-based study with a high autopsy rate (87%) covering the years 1970 to 1982, it was found that 35 of 31,015 patients (0.1%) examined post mortem had MVT.[5] The majority of patients with MVT at autopsy (27 of 35, or 77%) had a transmural intestinal infarction, judged to be the cause of death. The patients diagnosed at explorative laparotomy all had transmural intestinal infarction and required bowel resection for survival. Portal venous thrombosis (PVT) was studied in the same cohort, and there were some interesting differences: PVT was 10 times more common than MVT at autopsy, patients with PVT more often had asymptomatic disease, and PVT was seldom considered the cause of death.[17] A recent study suggested that superior MVT, in contrast to isolated PVT, is associated with symptoms in the overwhelmingly majority of

cases and is diagnosed mainly by imaging.[18] From these data, we conclude that MVT is very often symptomatic and often results in bowel gangrene, although we do not know exactly how often.

PATHOLOGY AND MANIFESTATIONS

The degree of intestinal ischemia that develops depends on the extent of venous thrombosis within the splanchnic venous circulation and whether there is occlusion and collateral flow. Patients with isolated PVT without distal propagation to the superior mesenteric vein are asymptomatic in the majority of cases and almost never experience intestinal infarction.[17,18]

At operation, MVT is characterized by a limited segment of intestinal ischemia, with edema, swelling, and reddish discoloration of the affected small bowel and its adjacent mesentery and a palpable pulsatile flow in the superior mesenteric artery (SMA) and its branches.[19] In contrast, intestinal ischemia due to arterial occlusive or nonocclusive disease is often characterized by extensive ischemia that includes the jejunum, ileum, and colon,[20] with patchy cyanosis, reddish black discoloration, and no palpable pulsations. MVT can be confirmed during surgery if an infarcted bowel segment is removed. Division of a small part of the adjacent mesentery, without previous vessel ligation, reveals thrombosis within the veins, whereas a pulsatile hemorrhage arises from the arteries. The extent of intestinal infarction is often limited to the jejunum or the ileum (Fig. 150-2).[5]

DIAGNOSIS

Patients with symptoms of less than 4 weeks' duration are classified as having acute MVT. Those with symptoms lasting longer than 4 weeks but without bowel infarction, or those with clinically insignificant MVT diagnosed incidentally on abdominal imaging, are classified as having chronic MVT. The majority of patients—71% and 74% in two large clinical series[4,7]—have acute MVT.

Recognition by History and Physical Examination

Acute and particularly chronic MVT is a difficult diagnosis among patients presenting with acute or subacute abdominal pain. Awareness of the disease, a careful risk factor evaluation, and positive findings at physical examination should lead the clinician to the diagnosis. The onset of acute MVT is often insidious, and diffuse abdominal pain may be present for days or weeks. Diarrhea, nausea and vomiting, lower gastrointestinal bleeding, and constipation are common complaints.[7,8] Typically, a middle-aged patient with a personal history or a family history of deep venous thrombosis presents with abdominal pain of a few days' duration, abdominal distention, and signs of intestinal obstruction, as well as a clearly raised C-reactive protein level. The patient may have localized peritonitis. With progression to transmural intestinal infarction, peristalsis ceases, and signs of generalized peritonitis occur.

Laboratory Testing

There are no accurate plasma biomarkers for diagnosing intestinal ischemia. D-dimer has been reported to be a sensitive but not a specific marker of acute thromboembolic occlusion of the SMA.[26] From a theoretical point of view, we have reason to believe that a normal D-dimer level may be useful to exclude MVT as well. This view is supported by experience from a small series of patients.[4]

Further, because inherited thrombophilic factors are common in MVT, it is recommended that all patients with MVT should be screened for the following inherited disorders: factor V Leiden mutation, prothrombin gene mutation, protein C deficiency, protein S deficiency, and antithrombin deficiency. Simultaneously, the patient should be checked for acquired disorders such as lupus anticoagulant and cardiolipin antibodies.

Noninvasive and Invasive Testing

Multidetector computed tomography (MDCT) of the abdomen, with intravenous contrast injection and imaging in the portal venous phase, is the most important and sensitive diagnostic tool.[21,22] The protocol for acute CT of the abdomen varies with the clinical history provided by the referring physician who requests the examination. However, MVT is seldom suspected by the clinician before ordering CT; in fact, the diagnosis is often first made by the radiologist.[23] In one series, MVT or intestinal ischemia was suspected prior to CT in only one patient with congenital portal vein occlusion out of 20 with verified MVT.[23]

The vascular and intestinal findings of MVT on MDCT (Figs. 150-3 to 150-5) are summarized in Table 150-1.[23] MDCT often demonstrates extensive thrombosis of the portomesenteric system, with extension of thrombosis to at least the extrahepatic portal vein and the splenic vein. Intestinal findings are less common and more subtle. Hence, the radiologist should always examine the mesenteric vessels in cases

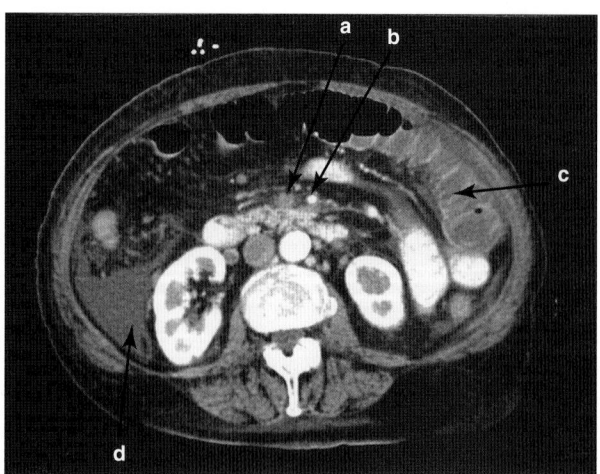

Figure 150-3 MDCT of the abdomen in the portal venous phase, with multiplanar reconstruction in the axial projection, shows thrombosis of the superior mesenteric vein (a), an open superior mesenteric artery (b), dilated and edematous small bowel loops (c), and ascites (d).

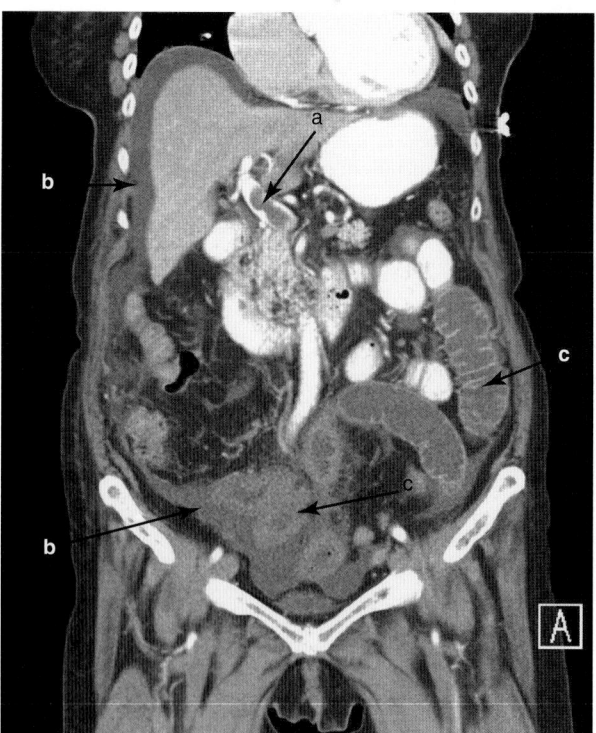

Figure 150-4 MDCT with multiplanar reconstruction in the coronal view shows thrombosis in the extrahepatic portion of the portal vein (a), ascites (b), and dilated and edematous small bowel loops (c).

of an acute or unclear abdomen. MVT can be diagnosed using routine MDCT techniques not optimized for MVT. However, a more dedicated CT protocol for the follow-up of patients with MVT, to assess both thrombotic status within the portomesenteric venous circulation and intestinal ischemia, is warranted (Table 150-2).[23] This protocol can also be useful in MVT patients in whom the discontinuation of oral vitamin K antagonist (VKA) treatment is being considered or when

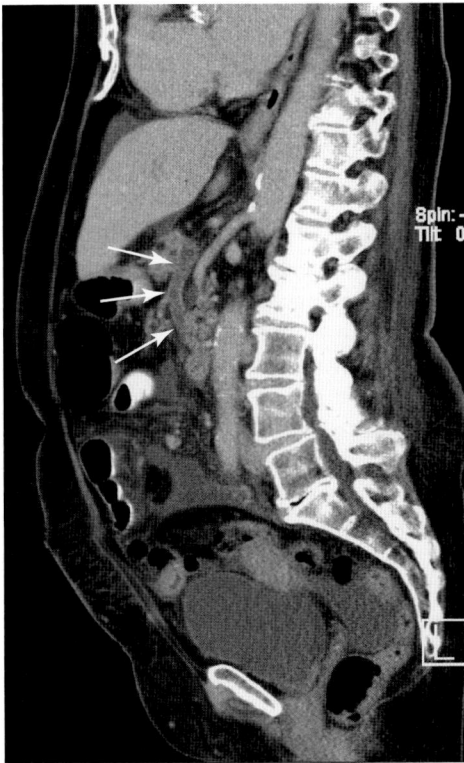

Figure 150-5 MDCT with multiplanar reconstruction in the sagittal view shows thrombosis in the superior mesenteric vein (*arrows*).

Table 150-2 Computed Tomographic Protocol for Mesenteric Venous Thrombosis

Criteria	Protocol
Scanner	Siemens
Kilovolts	120
Effective milliamperes	225
Rotation time	0.5 sec
Detector collimation	0.75 mm
Slice thickness	0.75 mm
Feed/rotation	12.0 mm
Kernel	B30f medium smooth
Increment	0.75 mm × 0.5 mm (3D)
	5 mm × 5 mm (filming)
Image order	Craniocaudal
Oral contrast	1000 mL water
Intravenous contrast	120 mL Omnipaque 400
Injection rate	3-5 mL/sec
Scan delay	Arterial: 25-30 sec
	Venous: 30 sec later (55-60 sec) or
	ROI in upper abdominal aorta
	100 HU + 15 sec
3D technique	MPR and MIP

Note: Dual-phase imaging allows the evaluation of both arterial and venous patency as well as definition of the pattern of bowel wall enhancement.
HU, Hounsfield unit; MIP, maximum intensity projection; MPR, multiplanar reconstruction; ROI, region of interest; 3D, three-dimensional.
Modified from Elliot K Fishman, MD, and www.ctisus.com.

Table 150-1 Findings with Multidetector Computed Tomographic Venography of the Abdomen in 20 Patients with Mesenteric Venous Thrombosis

Finding	Frequency (%)
Vascular	
Mesenteric venous thrombosis	20 (100)
Central* mesenteric venous thrombosis	20 (100)
Peripheral mesenteric venous thrombosis	6 (30)
Portal venous thrombosis	17 (85)
Extrahepatic portal venous thrombosis	17 (85)
Intrahepatic portal venous thrombosis	9 (45)
Splenic venous thrombosis	15 (75)
Venous collaterals	12 (80)
Intestinal	
Mesenteric edema	10 (50)
Small bowel wall edema	5 (25)
Local small bowel dilatation†	4 (20)
Gas in portomesenteric venous system	0 (0)
Ascites	8 (40)

*The first 5 cm of the proximal superior mesenteric vein is defined as central.
†Greater than 4 cm in diameter.

patients on anticoagulation treatment are suffering from abdominal pain or experiencing a general deterioration in their condition.

Explorative laparoscopy or laparotomy will continue to be a necessary diagnostic tool for some patients, especially those presenting with unclear peritonitis, even after CT. In experienced hands, laparoscopy can be the preferred method to assess intestinal viability.[24,25] Major obstacles for full visualization and macroscopic evaluation of the small intestines are extensive paralysis and prior adhesions.

TREATMENT AND RESULTS

Medical treatment is instituted as soon as the diagnosis has been established. The patient should be kept fasting and receive total parenteral nutrition through a central venous line. Initial anticoagulation with heparin is the treatment of choice in patients without peritonitis. Systemic thrombolysis in MVT has not been evaluated systematically, and at present, there is only one report in which a patient with extensive MVT was successfully treated with recombinant tissue plasminogen activator (rt-PA; total dose of 100 mg for 48 hours).[27] After initial anticoagulation, continued treatment with low-molecular-weight heparin (LMWH) or VKA is advocated. Uncertainties about bowel viability are assessed through laparotomy or laparoscopy; it is safer to perform a laparotomy to check for bowel viability in patients with signs of peritonitis and rebound tenderness. Bowel resection should be performed in cases of severe ischemic or frank necrotic intestinal segments.

Endovascular treatment in combination with heparin infusion, with or without bowel resection, is an additional treatment tool. The role of different endovascular techniques, such as aspiration and mechanical thrombectomy, stenting, and local thrombolysis, seems promising in selected patients. Local thrombolysis, through catheters placed endovascularly, has been successful in some cases, even after bowel surgery.[28,29] However, patients with recent cerebral infarction (within 6 weeks), history of cerebral hemorrhage, malignant tumor, arteriovenous malformation in the brain, severe diabetic retinopathy, gastrointestinal hemorrhage, or esophageal varices should not undergo thrombolysis. Older age correlates with an increased bleeding risk and is a relative contraindication to thrombolysis.

Thus, for the majority of patients with MVT without peritonitis, initial treatment with heparin alone is sufficient; a minority of patients with peritonitis may require laparotomy and bowel resection. In cases in which there is extensive thrombosis within the portomesenteric venous system, progression of thrombosis despite heparin treatment, or continued pain despite anticoagulation, adjunctive endovascular management may be appropriate for a more rapid clearance of extensive thrombotic clots and a prompt restoration of flow.

Medical Treatment

Full anticoagulation with a continuous infusion of unfractionated heparin is used in nonoperated as well as in operated cases to obtain an activated partial thromboplastin time of 50 to 70 seconds monitored at 4-hour intervals. If necessary, protamine can promptly reverse the anticoagulation effect. Patients should initially be closely observed, with repeated abdominal evaluations and body temperature readings and daily C-reactive protein and leukocyte measurements. In the absence of recovery or in the case of slight clinical deterioration, repeat CT with intravenous contrast can show alterations, such as extension of venous thrombosis, and the severity of ischemic bowel lesions, providing help in the decision-making process.[30]

When gastrointestinal function has normalized, LMWH or oral VKA is advocated. The anti-inflammatory effects of heparin and LMWH may be advantageous in the early follow-up period.[31] Lifelong treatment with VKA is recommended owing to the high recurrence rate of MVT—36% in one report.[7] Long-term treatment with LMWH is reserved for patients with liver dysfunction or other conditions in which VKA treatment is contraindicated. Most patients can be treated conservatively if they are diagnosed in a timely manner.[8] A recent series showed that MDCT in the portal venous phase was diagnostic in all 20 investigated patients, and conservative management was possible in 19 (95%).[23]

In-hospital mortality among identified and actively treated patients has decreased toward 20%, probably due to earlier detection with CT.[3,8] The decreasing mortality rates in contemporary series can also be explained by differences in the case mix: in older series, most patients required laparotomy, whereas with modern CT, many less severe cases are identified. Anticoagulation with or without bowel resection in patients with acute MVT has also improved survival in comparison with observation alone.[7] The overall 30-day survival in a contemporary series was 80% (41 of 51), and the estimated 5-year survival for the 51 patients was 70%.[4]

Gastrointestinal bleeding,[7] late small bowel perforation, and intestinal stricture[8] have been described as specific gastrointestinal complications. The thrombotic status within the splanchnic venous system after VKA treatment has not been evaluated systematically with repeated CT scans, but it seems that most thrombosis shows either no change or regression after a short period (3 months) of VKA treatment.[23]

Endovascular Treatment

A number of endovascular procedures for the treatment of MVT have been developed in recent years, including percutaneous transjugular intrahepatic portosystemic shunting (TIPS) with mechanical aspiration thrombectomy and direct thrombolysis,[32] percutaneous transhepatic mechanical thrombectomy,[28] percutaneous transhepatic thrombolysis,[33] thrombolysis via the SMA,[34] and thrombolysis via an operatively placed mesenteric vein catheter.[29] Rapid thrombus removal or dissolution can be achieved through these techniques, especially after TIPS and stent placement to create a low-pressure runoff.[35] Mechanical thrombectomy is performed using a variety of thrombectomy devices and is most effective in cases of acute rather than chronic thrombus. Local direct thrombolysis into the portomesenteric circulation through the transjugular or transhepatic route is useful for clearing residual clots and restoring venous flow. Indirect thrombolytic therapy via the SMA may be less effective and more time-consuming, may require longer infusion times and higher doses of thrombolytic agent, and may be associated with an increased bleeding risk. There is some experience with both rt-PA and urokinase as thrombolytic agents.[34] Balloon angioplasty is an alternative technique of clot fragmentation in cases of refractory thrombus and fixed venous stenosis. Aspiration thrombectomy is performed with a stiff, large-diameter (at least 8 Fr), angled catheter connected to a Luer-Lok syringe to create a vacuum effect.[32]

Endovascular techniques have been successful in terms of survival, patency of the portomesenteric veins, low complication rates, and avoidance of bowel resection in selected patients. However, in a larger series of 17 patients with MVT treated with local thrombolysis, 2 had complete lysis, 11 had partial lysis, and 3 had no lysis of the superior MVT.[34] Local thrombolysis was associated with significant bleeding complications in 60% of patients, including intra-abdominal bleeding, bleeding from the access site, perihepatic hematoma, nosebleed, and hematuria.[34] In another report, re-intervention for the extension of one stent had to be performed in a patient undergoing TIPS due to occlusion of the primary stent before clot fragmentation.[32] Accumulation of blood from the portal vein in the right pleural space, causing right-sided hemothorax, has been reported during percutaneous transhepatic thrombectomy and thrombolysis,[36] as have deaths due to gastrointestinal hemorrhage and sepsis.[34,36]

Patients should be anticoagulated with heparin following endovascular treatment, and the bowel should be rested. VKA replaces heparin when gastrointestinal function is normalized. Patency of the portal system after TIPS can be evaluated by follow-up Doppler ultrasound at 1 and 3 months, and then again at 6 months to check the portal system and shunt function.[32] Thrombotic status should be evaluated by repeat CT scan after 6 months in all patients to guide further anticoagulation treatment.

Surgical Treatment

The indications for surgery are peritonitis, severe gastrointestinal bleeding, late small bowel perforation, and intestinal stricture; the last is often associated with chronic diarrhea. When a clear clinical deterioration or peritonitis develops in a patient with MVT, laparotomy is indicated. Bowel resection should be performed in cases of frank transmural intestinal necrosis, uncertain bowel viability, or severe ischemic bowel lesions (Fig. 150-6). However, signs of peritonitis are not always associated with transmural intestinal infarction, and some patients with rebound tenderness can still be treated

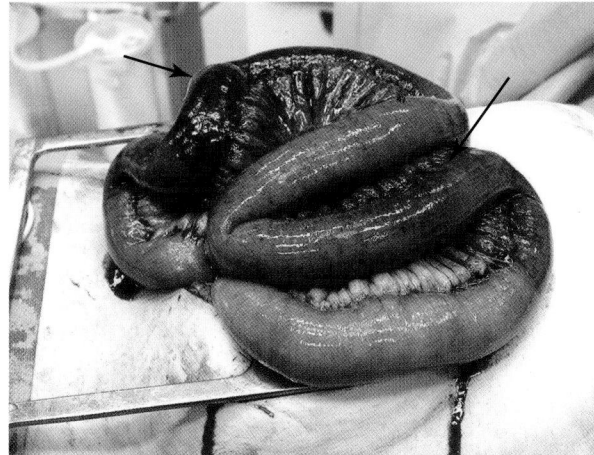

Figure 150-6 Resected bowel. A 47-year-old man with a history of deep venous thrombosis (DVT) and pulmonary embolism treated with a vena cava filter and vitamin K antagonist presented with a 3-day history of lower abdominal pain and obstipation. He had discontinued vitamin K antagonist treatment 4 days previously. At admission, plasma D-dimer was 9.6 mg/L (reference value, <0.2 mg/L), and plasma lactate was 1.0 mmol/L (reference value, 0.5 to 2.2 mmol/L). He developed signs of generalized peritonitis with rebound tenderness in the abdomen 12 hours after admission. Laparoscopy showed signs of small bowel ischemia in the proximal ileum due to mesenteric venous thrombosis. At laparotomy, 1.2 m of the small bowel was ischemic. It was decided to remove the two most reddish, discolored, and severely ischemic segments (*arrows*) by resecting a total length of 0.4 m, followed by one small bowel anastomosis. Note the edema of the affected small bowel loops and their adjacent mesentery. Treatment with a DVT dose of low-molecular-weight heparin was started at the end of surgery. Second-look laparotomy was performed after 30 hours. After the removal of 800 mL of red-colored peritoneal fluid, a reassessment of bowel viability showed that 0.5 m of the small bowel and its adjacent mesentery above the anastomosis was edematous. However, this intestinal segment showed normal turgor and color, and the anastomosis was intact. Recovery thereafter was uneventful, and the patient was prescribed lifelong treatment with vitamin K antagonist. Histopathology of the resected bowel did not show fully developed transmural infarction but did show infarcted mucosa and venous thrombosis.

conservatively.[8] Primary bowel anastomosis after resection is recommended. This is a straightforward treatment in the typical patient in whom a short segment of the small bowel is affected. In the less common situation in which a longer segment of the intestines is threatened, an alternative is to staple off the infarcted intestine and delay reconstruction until a second-look laparotomy, when the viability of the remaining small intestine can be evaluated. At the second look, areas of intestinal ischemia may show recovered viability, or there may be a clearer demarcation of infarcted segments. The purpose of the second-look laparotomy is to reduce unnecessary bowel resections at the primary exploration and detect insufficient bowel anastomoses.

Initially after surgery, a heparin infusion is administered. The patient should be on bowel rest and receiving total parenteral nutrition for a few days. All patients should then receive anticoagulation with either LMWH or VKA. Lifelong treatment should be considered for most patients owing to the high recurrence rate and the often fatal outcome of recurrence. The value of a postoperative CT scan to evaluate the extension of thrombosis and the frequency of thrombus recanalization is unclear. However, a repeat CT scan after 6 months of anticoagulation therapy may be helpful in determining the duration of treatment if lifelong treatment is not being considered.

Morbidity rates in cases managed with and without surgery are similar,[8] although it must be recognized that these are different groups of patients, and no randomized studies exist. The short-term[3] and 2-year[8] survival rates are also comparable between groups undergoing surgery and medical treatment. The survival rate after bowel resection is around 80%.[3,7] The most common complications following surgery are pneumonia, wound infection, renal failure, sepsis, and gastrointestinal bleeding.[7,8] Fortunately, the occurrence of short-bowel syndrome after bowel resection for MVT is rare.[2,7] In a recent series, none of the 12 patients who underwent bowel resection developed short-bowel syndrome.[4] The median length of the resected intestinal segment in that series was 0.6 m (range, 0.1 to 2.2 m). The relatively high frequency (23%) of short-bowel syndrome in patients with acute MVT in an older study might be attributable to unnecessarily extensive bowel resections or suboptimal pharmacologic therapy.[7] Among patients with MVT, bowel resection should always be conservative.

SELECTED KEY REFERENCES

Acosta S, Alhadad A, Svensson P, Ekberg O. Epidemiology, risk and prognostic factors in mesenteric venous thrombosis. *Br J Surg.* 2008;95:1245-1251.
Most recent large review with updates. It highlights the importance of MDCT with portal phase contrast enhancement and for screening and diagnosing inherited thrombophilic disorders.

Acosta S, Ögren M, Sternby N-H, Bergqvist D, Björck M. Mesenteric venous thrombosis with transmural intestinal infarction: a population-based study. *J Vasc Surg.* 2005;41:59-63.
Strong epidemiologic work based on a high autopsy rate of 87%.

Brunaud L, Antunes L, Collinet-Adler S, Marchal F, Ayav A, Bresler L, Boissel P. Acute mesenteric venous thrombosis: case for nonoperative management. *J Vasc Surg.* 2001;34:673-679.

Modern review strengthening the role of conservative management.

Morasch M, Ebaugh J, Chiou A, Matsumara J, Pearce W, Yao J. Mesenteric venous thrombosis: a changing clinical entity. *J Vasc Surg.* 2001;34:680-684.
Modern review of the fast evolution of CT techniques.

Rhee Ry, Gloviczki P, Mendonca CT, Petterson TM, Serry RD, Sarr MG, Johnson CM, Bower TC, Hallett JW Jr, Cherry KJ Jr. Mesenteric venous thrombosis: still a lethal disease in the 1990s. *J Vasc Surg.* 1994;20:688-697.
Large review.

REFERENCES

The reference list can be found on the companion Expert Consult Web site at *www.expertconsult.com.*

Trauma and Acute Limb Ischemia

Section **19**

Fred A. Weaver

CHAPTER 151

Vascular Trauma: Epidemiology and Natural History

Raul Coimbra and David B. Hoyt

Vascular trauma results from penetrating, blunt, or iatrogenic injuries. This chapter focuses on the epidemiology and natural history of vascular injuries. It emphasizes the evolution of the management of vascular injuries, initially based on military experience and subsequently applied to civilian trauma, and describes the clinical presentations of various forms of arterial injuries.

EPIDEMIOLOGY

Approximately 2.6 million people are hospitalized annually in the United States as a result of accidental injury. Each year, 35 million to 40 million emergency department visits are made for the evaluation and treatment of traumatic injuries.[1] Most patients are between 25 and 44 years of age, and 20% are between 15 and 24 years. People younger than 45 years sustain almost 80% of all injuries and account for 75% of the total lifetime costs of injury.

Young males are at highest risk, owing to their propensity to engage in high-risk activities. According to data from the National Center for Injury and Prevention, 56.6% of all trauma-related deaths in 1997 occurred in the 15- to 49-year age group, predominantly in males. Overall, males have a seven times higher risk of dying following injury than do females.[2]

In addition to morbidity and mortality data, another important variable related to the societal cost of injury is years of productive life lost (YPLL). This reflects the potential productivity lost owing to premature death. Injury-related deaths result in higher YPLL compared with cancer and cardiovascular deaths. For each traumatic death there are, on average, 36 YPLL, compared with 16 for cancer and 12 for cardiovascular diseases.[3]

The leading causes of injury include motor vehicle crashes, falls, wounds from firearms, wounds from cutting or piercing instruments, and burns. Fatalities after injury are mainly due to motor vehicle accidents (32%), gunshot wounds (22%), and falls (9%).[4] The three leading causes of traumatic death for persons younger than 35 years are the same in all groups: motor vehicle accidents, homicide, and suicide.[3] Alcohol ingestion and the use of other drugs, such as marijuana and cocaine, have also been implicated in increased trauma-related fatalities.[5]

Peripheral vascular injuries account for 80% of all cases of vascular trauma, and the great majority of patients are young males. Most of the injuries involve the lower extremities. Most injuries are caused by high-velocity weapons (70% to 80%), followed by stab wounds (10% to 15%) and blunt trauma (5% to 10%). The incidence of vascular trauma in the military is comparable to that in the civilian population and varies from 0.2% to 4% of injured patients.[6-12] Table 151-1 depicts the incidence of vascular trauma in survivors during military conflicts and in large comprehensive civilian series in distinct geographic areas.

Most civilian penetrating vascular injuries occur in the extremities, and the incidence of extremity vascular injuries in the military is even higher. Frykberg analyzed a large series of civilian survivors of trauma from 1960 to 1989 and reported that the incidence of extremity vascular trauma was 51%, compared with 93.7% in the military setting.[16] Explanations for these differences include the torso protective gear worn by soldiers and the high-velocity weapons used in military conflicts, which tend to cause immediate death when major vessels of the torso are injured. Extremity vascular injuries occur more commonly than major torso vessel injuries because torso protective gear does not protect the extremities. Also,

Table 151-1 Incidence of Vascular Injuries in Military Conflicts and Civilian Practice

	Total Number of Vascular Injuries	Number of Extremity Vascular Injuries	Extremity Vascular Injuries (%)	Penetrating Mechanism (%)
World War I[13]	443	Unknown	–	Unknown
World War II[6]	2471	2409	97.5	Almost all
Korean War[14]	304	286	94.1	Almost all
Vietnam War[8]	1000	910	91.0	98.9
Georgia[15]	Unknown	99	–	All
Houston, TX[10]	5760	2131	37.0	93.0
North Carolina[9]	978	632	65.0	63.0
Australia[12]	175	79	45.0	11.4
San Diego, CA[12]	664	263	40.0	67

the total number of injuries to the major vessels in the chest, abdomen, and pelvis that occur in military conflicts may be underestimated or underreported. In general, most vascular injuries in the military setting are caused by a penetrating mechanism. In the civilian setting, although a penetrating mechanism predominates,[16] the relative incidence of blunt injuries increases (see Table 151-1).

NATURAL HISTORY

The natural history of untreated vascular injuries varies with the extent and type of injury. Occult vascular injuries are usually composed of intimal flaps, segmental narrowing, and hemodynamically insignificant arteriovenous fistulae or pseudoaneurysms. There is growing evidence that most of these injuries heal spontaneously or stabilize without further compromising the distal circulation and perfusion.[17-19] These findings have been confirmed by independent studies in animals[20,21] and by two human studies.[22,23] Potential complications of untreated peripheral vascular trauma include hemorrhage, thrombosis, pseudoaneurysm, arteriovenous fistula, and compartment syndrome.

BIOMECHANICS OF INJURY

Classically, injury mechanisms are divided into penetrating or blunt. Following blunt trauma, tissue injury is produced by local compression or rapid deceleration. In penetrating trauma, the injury is produced by crushing and separation of tissues along the path of the penetrating object. Understanding the biomechanics of specific injuries is important in guiding the initial evaluation, because the natural history of arterial injuries is related to injury type and location, hemodynamic consequences, and mechanism of injury.

Injury severity is proportional to the amount of kinetic energy (KE) transferred to the tissues, which is a function of the mass (M) and velocity (V): $KE = M \times V^2/2$. This is valid for both blunt and penetrating mechanisms. Changes in velocity alter the kinetic energy transfer more significantly than do changes in mass. This is critical when evaluating high- and low-velocity gunshot wounds and their corresponding injury potential.

Another important concept in understanding the biomechanics of vascular injury is that of cavitation. Cavitation is a phenomenon that occurs as tissue recoils from the point of impact by a moving object away from that object. After blunt trauma, the resulting transient tissue cavity may be caused by rapid acceleration or deceleration. Extreme strain occurs at points of anatomic fixation during the formation of these temporary cavities. Forces can be produced both along the longitudinal axis (tensile or compression strain) and across the transverse axis (shear strain). These types of forces cause deformity, tearing, and tissue failure or fracture. Following penetrating trauma, temporary cavitation is caused by the transfer of kinetic energy from the projectile to adjacent tissue, which is followed by the formation of a permanent cavity caused by tissue displacement. This mechanism explains why vessels can be injured even without being in contact with projectiles or bone fragments.[24]

CLINICAL PRESENTATION

The clinical presentation of an arterial injury varies, based on the anatomic location and the type of injury. In general, clinical evidence of an arterial injury is manifested in one of four ways: external bleeding, end-organ or extremity ischemia, pulsatile hematoma, or internal bleeding accompanied by signs of shock.

Neck

The presentation of vascular injuries in the neck is straightforward. Direct bleeding, a large hematoma, or any compromise of the airway indicates significant vascular injury. Injury to the carotid might be accompanied by altered mental status, suggesting early neurologic compromise. In the absence of clear signs of vascular injury, a workup that includes computed tomographic angiography (CTA) or plain-film angiography can confirm the diagnosis of vascular injury. In the event of obvious bleeding or airway compromise, direct transfer to the operating room is indicated.

Thorax

Most major penetrating vascular injuries in the chest are identified intraoperatively after a chest tube is placed to treat a hemothorax. Depending on the amount of blood loss, signs of shock may be present, leading to operative exploration and identification. After blunt trauma, the great majority of arterial injuries in the chest are tamponaded by the mediastinal structures and adventitial containment. Suggestive signs on plain chest films (e.g., apical cap, extrapleural hematoma, tracheal deviation, widened mediastinum, blurred aortopulmonary window) suggest a vascular injury.

Abdomen

In the abdomen, the type of clinical presentation depends on the presence of retroperitoneal tamponade. Patients with an intact retroperitoneum may be hypotensive or hemodynamically stable on presentation; this group has the greatest chance of survival. When the retroperitoneal tamponade is lost, signs of shock and acute hypovolemia are present. Usually these injuries are identified during surgical exploration for a penetrating abdominal injury. Blunt injuries to major abdominal vessels are rare. Major injuries to large vessels in the mesentery (e.g., superior mesenteric artery) usually cause significant hemoperitoneum and shock.

Extremity

Knowledge of the clinical presentation and natural history of vascular trauma is of utmost importance when dealing with the extremities. External bleeding is a rare presentation and is associated mostly with high-velocity gunshot wounds in the presence of massive destruction of soft tissues and, consequently, loss of tissue tamponade. Prehospital information on vital signs, as well as the amount and characteristics of blood lost at the scene (e.g., pulsatile, bright red), is helpful during the resuscitation phase. Most patients are hypotensive without external blood loss, although external bleeding may resume during fluid resuscitation owing to expansion of the intravascular compartment and subsequent increases in arterial blood pressure. The most common presentation of extremity arterial injury is acute ischemia. This occurs most commonly after stab wounds, low-velocity gunshot wounds, and blunt trauma associated with fractures and dislocations.

Classically, signs and symptoms of arterial injury are divided into hard and soft categories. Hard signs include absence of distal pulses, active external arterial hemorrhage, signs of ischemia, pulsatile hematoma, and bruit or thrill. The presence of a pseudoaneurysm or arteriovenous fistula should be suspected following a penetrating injury to the extremity in the presence of a pulsatile hematoma accompanied by a bruit or a thrill. The clinical signs of ischemia are rest pain, paresthesias, paralysis, paleness, and poikilothermy, associated with decreased or absent distal pulses. Soft signs include diminished distal pulses, injury in the proximity of a major vessel, neurologic deficit, and hypotension or shock. A detailed and complete physical examination, including inspection, palpation, and auscultation, is usually sufficient to identify the acute signs of ischemia.

Detection of an extremity arterial injury depends on the thoroughness of the workup. Injury severity depends on the mechanism, type, and location of the arterial injury and the duration of ischemia, if present. In the absence of clinical findings, there is still debate about whether an angiogram should be obtained in patients with penetrating extremity injuries when the wound tract is near major vessels. However, any patient with a significant mechanism of injury presenting with soft clinical signs should undergo an objective evaluation of the distal circulation. The most practical way of doing so in the trauma resuscitation area is to measure the ankle-brachial index (ABI). An ABI less than 1.0 in either the ankle (dorsalis pedis, posterior tibial artery) or wrist (radial, ulnar artery) suggests a proximal arterial injury and should prompt further diagnostic investigation. The ABI is also useful in monitoring the status of extremity distal circulation over time in patients with other life-threatening injuries that require operative intervention (craniotomy, thoracotomy, laparotomy) before the extremity arterial injury is addressed or in patients who are too unstable to undergo operative exploration of an extremity arterial injury. For a more detailed discussion of the diagnosis of extremity arterial injuries, refer to Chapter 155: Vascular Trauma: Extremity.

Injury Type

The most common arterial injuries are partial lacerations and complete transections. In general, complete transections lead to retraction and thrombosis of the proximal and distal ends

Table 151-2 Types of Arterial Injuries and Possible Clinical Presentations

Type of Injury	Clinical Presentation
Partial laceration	Decreased pulse, hematoma, hemorrhage
Transection	Absent distal pulses, ischemia
Contusion	Initial exam may be normal; may progress to thrombosis
Pseudoaneurysm	Initial exam may be normal; bruit or thrill, decreased pulses
Arteriovenous fistula	Same as pseudoaneurysm
External compression	Decreased pulses; normal pulses when fracture aligned

of the vessel, with subsequent ischemia. In contrast, partial lacerations cause persistent bleeding or pseudoaneurysm formation. Partial lacerations as well as contusions may be accompanied by intimal flaps, which may progress to thrombosis. Small arterial contusions with limited intimal flaps may not cause distal hemodynamic compromise and may be undiagnosed. These are sometimes classified as "occult or minimal arterial injuries" when seen on angiography. Although these injuries carry a small risk of thrombosis, several studies have documented spontaneous healing.[17-23] Concomitant arterial and venous injuries may lead to the formation of an arteriovenous fistula. The correlation between injury type and clinical presentation is shown in Table 151-2.

EPIDEMIOLOGY AND NATURAL HISTORY OF SPECIFIC ARTERIAL INJURIES

Neck

Carotid Artery

Blunt carotid artery disruption accounts for about 3% to 10% of all carotid injuries. The most commonly injured structures in the neck are the blood vessels. The incidence of major vascular trauma following a penetrating neck injury is 20%.[25] The incidence of neck arterial injuries following blunt trauma is extremely low, although there has been an increase in reported blunt carotid injuries owing to aggressive screening.[26,27] Blunt carotid artery disruption accounts for about 3% to 10% of all carotid injuries.[28-30]

More than 90% of blunt injuries involve the internal carotid artery, often distally, rather than the common carotid artery. Bilateral injury has been reported in 20% to 50% of cases. The overall incidence of carotid artery injury in blunt trauma has been variously reported as 0.08% to 0.33%, and as many as half of affected patients show no signs of cervical trauma or neurologic deficit at presentation. The low incidence, anatomic site, and variable presentation have made the determination of optimal diagnostic and management strategies difficult.[29-41]

Four mechanisms of injury are recognized: (1) cervical hyperextension-rotation (most common), (2) direct blow to the neck, (3) intraoral trauma, and (4) basilar skull fracture.

Injury can result in dissection, thrombosis, pseudoaneurysm, carotid-cavernous sinus fistula, or complete arterial disruption.[28] In one series, 85 blunt carotid injuries in 67 patients were reported during an 11-year period.[26] The most common mechanism of injury was motor vehicle crash (82%), followed by motorcycle crash (7%) and assault (6%).

The mortality rate of blunt carotid injury varies from 20% to 40%, and permanent neurologic impairment occurs in 25% to 80% of survivors.[26,27,30,42] Outcomes are dependent on several factors, but the size and location of the arterial injury are key factors.

Vertebral Artery

The identification of vertebral artery injuries has increased in recent years, probably owing to the liberal use of screening tests (CTA or neck angiography) following both penetrating and blunt injuries. The incidence of vertebral artery injury caused by a penetrating mechanism varies from 1% to 7.5%.[43] This variation is related to the indications for angiography, and some of these injuries may not need surgical intervention. The incidence of blunt vertebral artery injury is low. These injuries are commonly associated with cervical vertebral fractures.[44,45]

Thorax

Aorta

Blunt aortic injury occurs following abrupt deceleration. This causes shear forces at the aorta's points of anatomic fixation, leading to transmural injuries. Most injuries are located distal to the takeoff of the left subclavian artery (65%), although other segments of the thoracic aorta, such as the arch (10%), the descending aorta (12%), or multiple sites (13%), may be injured.[46] Frontal and side-impact motor vehicle collisions are the most frequent mechanism.

Penetrating injuries to the ascending aorta are commonly caused by stab wounds, whereas gunshot wounds are the usual mechanism of injury in the descending portion of the thoracic aorta.

Subclavian and Axillary Arteries

Because the subclavian and axillary arteries are protected by overlying bone and muscle, injuries to these vessels are relatively uncommon. The incidence varies from 0.9% to 3%, depending on the mechanism of injury (stab or gunshot wound). Blunt trauma is rare.[47,48] Because of the close proximity to a variety of structures, subclavian or axillary trauma is usually associated with major musculoskeletal fractures and brachial plexus and venous injuries. These injuries occur following high-speed frontal motor vehicle crashes, with significant deceleration causing fracture of the clavicle or first and second ribs. An associated injury of particular importance is a fracture-dislocation of the posterior portion of the first rib. The mortality of these injuries is high, and most patients do not reach the hospital alive.[49]

Abdomen

In contrast to military data, major abdominal vascular injuries are common in civilian practice. These injuries account for approximately 30% of all vascular injuries. Most injuries (90% to 95%) are caused by a penetrating mechanism.[50]

Earlier reviews of vascular injuries reported a very low incidence of penetrating abdominal vascular injuries. DeBakey and Simeone reported 2471 arterial injuries during World War II, which included only 49 abdominal arterial injuries (2%).[6] Similarly, Rich and coworkers, in a study of 1000 arterial injuries from the Vietnam War, reported only 29 abdominal arterial injuries (2.9%).[8] However, in civilian penetrating injuries, the incidence of abdominal vascular trauma is significantly higher. Approximately 10% of patients undergoing surgical exploration following a stab wound to the abdomen and 20% to 30% of those undergoing surgical exploration following a gunshot wound to the abdomen sustain a major vascular injury.[51]

The incidence of vascular injuries in patients with blunt abdominal trauma undergoing exploratory laparotomy is 3%.[52] Blunt abdominal trauma may cause vascular injury by one of three mechanisms: (1) rapid deceleration, as in high-speed traffic accidents or falls from heights, which may cause damage to abdominal vessels by avulsion or intimal tear and subsequent thrombosis; (2) direct anteroposterior crushing, as in seat-belted car passengers or direct blows to the anterior abdomen; and (3) direct laceration of a major vessel by a bone fragment, as in severe pelvic fractures.

Abdominal arterial and venous injuries occur with the same incidence. In a review of 302 abdominal vascular injuries, the incidence of arterial injuries was 49% and that of venous injuries was 51%. The most commonly injured abdominal vessel was the inferior vena cava (IVC), accounting for 25% of injuries, followed by the aorta (21%), the iliac arteries (20%), the iliac veins (17%), the superior mesenteric vein (11%), and the superior mesenteric artery (10%). Overall, patients with penetrating trauma had an average of 1.6 vascular injuries.[50]

Hospital mortality rates vary from 30% to 80% for abdominal aortic injuries and from 30% to 65% for IVC injuries. Many patients do not reach the hospital alive, dying at the scene or during transport.[53-58] Death is usually due to exsanguination, despite aggressive resuscitation and early operation.[54,59,60] The location of abdominal vascular injuries also determines survivability. Ease of surgical access for control directly correlates with increased survivability.[53]

Aorta

Blunt injury to the abdominal aorta is extremely rare, diagnosed in 0.04% of all blunt trauma admissions or 0.07% of patients with an Injury Severity Score greater than 15. Motor vehicle injuries account for about half of all reported cases, and direct blows to the abdomen, falls, and explosions account for the rest.[53,61-63] Fractures of the thoracolumbar spine and seat-belt injuries are associated with an increased risk of abdominal aortic injuries.[64]

Penetrating injuries are by far the most common cause of abdominal aortic injuries. In a review of 1218 patients with abdominal gunshot wounds from our center, there were 33 abdominal aortic injuries (2.7%). In 529 stab wounds to the abdomen, the aorta was injured in 8 (1.5%).[65] In another review of 302 abdominal vascular injuries, the aorta was involved in 63 cases (21%) and was the second most commonly injured vessel after the IVC.[50]

The infrarenal aorta is injured in 50% of cases, the supraceliac aorta in 25%, and the aorta between the celiac trunk and the renal arteries in 25%.[53,65]

Visceral Vessels

Traumatic injuries to the portal vein and superior mesenteric vein are uncommon; few surgeons have significant experience with their treatment, and mortality remains high.[66-71] The technical difficulty in isolating the injured vessel and the frequent occurrence of associated abdominal injuries with massive bleeding are the most common causes of death. Previous publications have reported mortality rates ranging from 50% to 70%.[67-73]

The mechanism of trauma differs among studies, and it has a marked impact on mortality. Stone and colleagues, in a series of 83 patients with injuries to the portal vein and superior mesenteric vein during a 23-year period, reported that 93% of the injuries were due to penetrating trauma.[67] The mortality rate according to the mechanism of injury was 39% in gunshot wounds, 64% in shotgun wounds, 11% in stab wounds, and 67% in blunt trauma. Coimbra and associates, analyzing 18 patients with traumatic injury to the portal venous system, reported a mortality rate of 78% in gunshot wounds, 67% in stab wounds, and 66.7% in blunt trauma.[70] In other series with only portal vein injuries, the mortality rate ranged from 25% to 57% in gunshot wounds, 0% to 33% in stab wounds, and 35% to 75% in blunt trauma.[69,72-75]

Renal Artery

Renovascular injuries account for about 16% of all abdominal vascular injuries. The incidence of renal artery injuries is less than 1% of all blunt trauma admissions. The left renal artery is 1.3 to 1.6 times more likely to be injured than the right renal artery. It has been suggested that the right renal artery is protected from deceleration injuries because of its course underneath the IVC. Rapid deceleration accidents may cause intimal tears and subsequent arterial thrombosis at a later stage. In about 50% of cases of blunt renal artery injury, there is thrombosis or an intimal flap. Avulsion of the artery occurs in 12% of cases. In 9% to 14% of renovascular injuries, the renal artery is involved bilaterally.[76-81]

Inferior Vena Cava

The IVC is the most commonly injured abdominal vessel and accounts for about 25% of abdominal vascular injuries.[50] Blunt trauma is responsible for about 10% of IVC injuries,

and it usually involves the retrohepatic part of the vein. In about 18% of patients with penetrating IVC injuries, there is an associated aortic injury.[53,56,82,83]

Iliac Vessels

Early experience from World War II, the Korean War, and the Vietnam War reported a low incidence of iliac vascular injuries, ranging from 1.7% to 2.6% of all arterial injuries.[6,8,14] More recent studies from urban trauma centers have reported that iliac injuries represent about 10% of all abdominal vascular injuries, or about 2% of all vascular injuries.[50,84]

Iliac vein injuries account for about 10% of all abdominal vascular injuries. About 10% of 1310 patients undergoing laparotomy for gunshot wounds and 2% of 638 patients undergoing laparotomy for stab wounds were found to have iliac vascular injuries. About 26% of patients with iliac vascular injuries have combined arterial and venous injuries.[85]

Penetrating injuries usually involve the common iliac vessels, whereas blunt trauma usually affects branches of the internal iliac artery. Injury to the common or external iliac artery due to blunt trauma is uncommon. Direct laceration of the iliac vessels from a pelvic fracture or stretching of the iliac artery over the pelvic wall, resulting in an intimal tear and subsequent thrombosis, is the usual mechanism of injury following blunt trauma.

Extremity

The overall incidence of arterial injury following penetrating injury to the extremity (upper or lower) is approximately 10%, in contrast to 1% following blunt trauma.[11,86,87] The brachial, femoral, and popliteal arteries are the most frequently injured vessels in both civilian and military series of penetrating trauma.[6,8,10,87,88]

Most femoral artery injuries are the result of a penetrating mechanism, usually a gunshot wound.[89] In contrast, a blunt mechanism accounts for 20% to 75% of popliteal artery injuries, although in some series, a penetrating mechanism predominates. These injuries account for 19% of all extremity arterial injuries. Recently, Frykberg compiled 1209 cases of civilian popliteal artery injury and reported that 56% were secondary to penetrating injury, with a 10.5% amputation rate, compared with an amputation rate of 27.5% following blunt trauma.[90] Recent published series have demonstrated a significant decrease in the amputation rate, which reflects a significant improvement in the management of these serious injuries.

The incidence of vascular injuries below the popliteal fossa is difficult to determine because most of these injuries, when isolated, cause no vascular compromise. One study analyzing 755 patients sustaining gunshot wounds below the knee reported 136 injuries below the popliteal fossa identified on angiography—an incidence of 18%.[91]

The association between arterial injuries and orthopedic lesions (fractures and dislocations) is well known. Table 151-3 summarizes the most common orthopedic injuries and their respective arterial injuries.

Table 151-3 Orthopedic Injuries Commonly Associated with Vascular Trauma

Orthopedic Injury	Arterial Injury
Supracondylar fracture of the humerus	Brachial artery
Clavicular, first rib fracture	Subclavian artery
Shoulder dislocation	Axillary artery
Elbow dislocation	Brachial artery
Distal femur fracture	Superficial femoral, popliteal artery
Posterior knee dislocation	Popliteal artery
Proximal tibia fracture	Popliteal artery, distal vessels

SELECTED KEY REFERENCES

Dennis JW, Frykberg ER, Veldenz HC, Huffman S, Menawat SS. Validation of nonoperative management of occult vascular injuries and accuracy of physical examination alone in penetrating extremity trauma: 5- to 10-year follow-up. *J Trauma*. 1998;44:243-253.
Proposes that physical examination alone and nonoperative management of clinically occult arterial injuries of the extremities are safe and effective and should be considered the standard of care.

Fabian TC, Patton JH Jr, Croce MA, Minard G, Kudsk KA, Pritchard FE. Blunt carotid injury: importance of early diagnosis and anticoagulant therapy. *Ann Surg*. 1996;223:513.
Evaluates the incidence, associated injury pattern, diagnostic factors, risk of adverse outcome, and efficacy of anticoagulant therapy in the setting of blunt carotid injury. The authors conclude that blunt carotid injury is more common than appreciated, that treatment with heparin is efficacious and reduces neurologic morbidity and

mortality, and that screening for blunt carotid injury should be liberal, leading to earlier diagnosis and improved outcome.

Frykberg ER, Dennis JW, Bishop K, Laneve L, Alexander RH. The reliability of physical examination in the evaluation of penetrating extremity trauma from vascular injury: results at one year. *J Trauma*. 1991;31:502-511.
Prospective study determining that physical examination alone is safe and accurate for the evaluation of vascular injury of the extremities. This study supports the concept that the incidence of significant vascular injury is negligible following clinically occult penetrating extremity trauma.

Jurkovich GJ, Hoyt DB, Moore FA, Ney AL, Morris JA Jr, Scalea TM, Pachter HL, Davis JW. Portal triad injuries. *J Trauma*. 1995;39:426-434.
Large multicenter study characterizing the incidence, management, and outcome of portal triad injuries. The authors conclude that intraoperative exsanguination is the primary cause of death, and hemorrhage control should be the first priority.

Wall MJ, Hirshberg A, LeMaire SA, Holcomb J, Mattox K. Thoracic aortic and thoracic vascular injuries. *Surg Clin North Am*. 2001;81:1375-1394.
Well-written review of the mechanism of injury, natural history, and diagnosis of, and surgical approach to, major thoracic vascular injuries.

REFERENCES

The reference list can be found on the companion Expert Consult Web site at *www.expertconsult.com*.

CHAPTER 152

Vascular Trauma: Head and Neck

Zachary M. Arthurs and Benjamin W. Starnes

Cervical vascular injuries are notoriously difficult to evaluate and manage owing to very complex anatomy confined to a relatively narrow anatomic space. The initial evaluation of these injuries is often obscured by associated injuries in the head, chest, or abdomen. In addition, signs of cerebral ischemia, cranial nerve deficits, or cervical nerve compression may not be present on initial evaluation. The appropriate evaluation and management of this injury pattern have been controversial and continue to evolve. Advances in noninvasive imaging (primarily computed tomography) have revolutionized the evaluation of stable patients with cervical vascular injuries, aerodigestive injuries, and associated fractures. Endovascular surgery has added another facet to the care of these trauma patients. Injuries to the distal internal carotid, proximal common carotid, subclavian, and vertebral arteries are now amenable to endovascular adjuncts to arrest hemorrhage, exclude dissections or pseudoaneurysms, or assist with open repair. This chapter addresses the presentation, evaluation, and treatment of cervical vascular injuries.

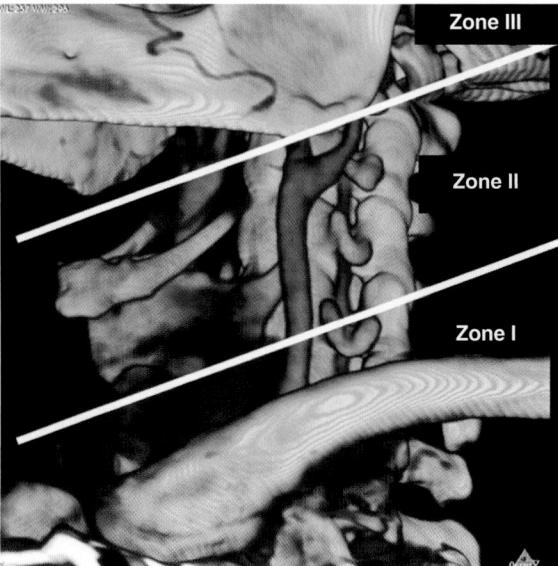

Figure 152-1 Anatomic zones of the neck for penetrating neck injuries.

CAROTID ARTERY

Penetrating Injury

Following penetrating cervical trauma, cervical blood vessels are the most commonly injured structures in the neck, accounting for a 7% to 27% stroke rate and a 7% to 50% mortality rate.[1] Eighty percent of deaths in this population are stroke related.

Clinical Presentation

The neck has classically been divided into three zones that dictate the diagnostic evaluation and treatment (Fig. 152-1):
- *Zone I:* Below the cricoid cartilage—proximal control obtained in the chest.
- *Zone II:* Between the cricoid cartilage and the angle of the mandible—proximal and distal control obtained in the neck.
- *Zone III:* Above the angle of the mandible—distal control difficult to obtain.[2]

Zone II is the most commonly injured (47%), followed by zone III (19%) and zone I (18%). It is not uncommon for an injury to traverse two zones of the neck.[3] In addition to location, the physical examination triages patients based on hard signs (mandating exploration) and soft signs (observation or

further diagnostic evaluation) of vascular injury. Hard signs include shock, refractory hypotension, pulsatile bleeding, bruit, enlarging hematoma, and loss of pulse with stable or evolving neurologic deficit. Soft signs include history of bleeding at the scene of injury, stable hematoma, nerve injury, proximity of the injury track, and unequal upper extremity blood pressure measurements. Ninety-seven percent of patients with hard signs have a vascular injury, as opposed to only 3% of those with soft signs.[3]

Based on mechanism of injury, gunshot wounds are more likely to cause a large neck hematoma and vascular injury (27%) than are stab wounds (15%).[3] Shotgun wounds, blast injuries, and transcervical (crossing the midline) gunshot wounds have a higher rate of vascular injury and should be approached with a high index of suspicion. Associated injuries to the tracheobronchial tree, esophagus, and spinal cord are present in 1% to 7% of patients.[3] In addition to hard signs of a vascular injury, patients may present with hard signs of a tracheobronchial injury (respiratory distress or air bubbling from the wound), mandating operative exploration. Soft signs of a cervical neck injury include painful swallowing, subcutaneous emphysema, hematemesis, and signs of nerve injury (cranial nerves IX, X, XI, and XII) or brachial plexus injury (axillary, musculocutaneous, radial, median, and ulnar nerves). A focused and detailed clinical evaluation reliably identifies

2318

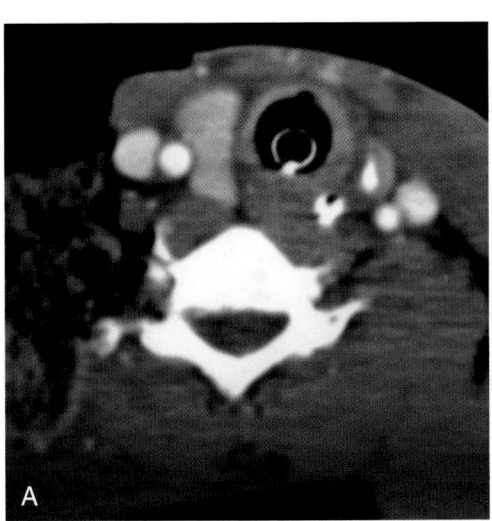
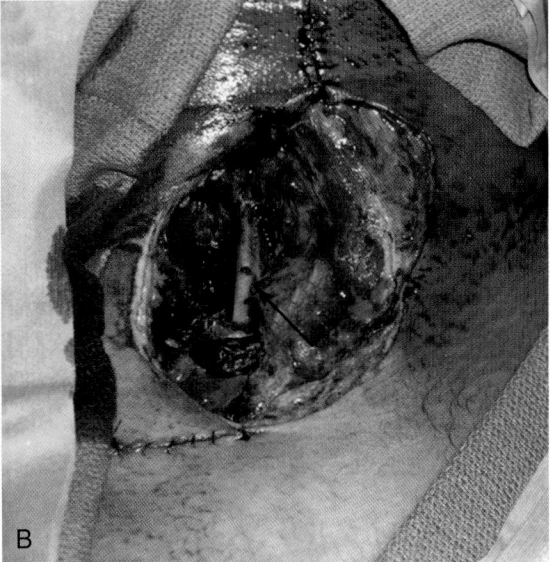

Figure 152-2 This patient sustained a high-velocity gunshot wound to zone I of the neck. On initial evaluation, he did not have hard signs of a vascular injury. **A,** CTA demonstrates no injury to the internal jugular vein or common carotid artery. In addition, there is no injury to the aerodigestive tract. **B,** The patient's wound was débrided in the operative suite; the *arrow* marks the cords of the brachial plexus.

patients with vascular injuries that require treatment. A negative physical examination with observation has a negative predictive value of 90% to 100% for vascular injuries.[4]

Special consideration should be given to patients who present with coma, dense hemispheric stroke, or documented carotid thrombosis. The treatment of this specific injury pattern has come full circle—from revascularization in the 1950s to routine ligation in the 1970s and back to revascularization as the current mainstay of treatment. In the 1970s authors reported only a few patients with dense hemispheric strokes who developed hemorrhagic strokes after revascularization, leading to the recommendation of internal carotid artery ligation distal to the thrombus.[5-7] Follow-up studies demonstrated that the extent of anoxic brain injury (not hemorrhagic conversion of the injury) and the development of reperfusion injury, cerebral edema, and resultant uncal herniation accounted for worsening neurologic status and death.[8,9] However, to date, there is no preoperative marker other than time (>24 hours from the time of injury) that predicts which patients are unlikely to benefit from revascularization. Early revascularization has consistently demonstrated improvement or stabilization of neurologic symptoms in patients with dense hemispheric strokes (100%), even in those who present obtunded (50%).[1,10]

Diagnostic Evaluation

Patients with hard signs of a vascular injury should proceed to the operative suite. All patients should have plain radiographs of the neck and chest to determine the track of the injury and to diagnose occult hemothorax or pneumothorax. There have been several advances in the treatment of penetrating neck injuries, and there are now sufficient data to support selective exploration in hemodynamically stable patients who have no hard signs of a vascular or tracheobronchial injury. Exploration of cervical injuries based on platysma muscle penetration carries an unacceptably high negative exploration rate of 50% to 90%.[11]

Computed tomography is the modern workhorse for trauma evaluation and should be the initial diagnostic step in patients with penetrating neck injuries but no hard signs of vascular or aerodigestive injury. Contrasted axial imaging with reformatting software allows an exact determination of the injury track, vascular injuries, proximity to the esophagus or trachea, spinal fractures and cord involvement, and extension to the head or chest (Fig. 152-2). In the setting of penetrating cervical injuries, computed tomographic angiography (CTA) has a 90% sensitivity and 100% specificity for vascular injuries that require treatment.[12,13] CTA may be limited in the setting of missile fragments (especially shotgun injuries) or bone fragments obscuring the cervical vasculature; arteriography should be used for these patients as a confirmatory study. Ultrasonography has been used for penetrating neck trauma, but its utility is limited to zone II neck injuries.[14] In addition, subcutaneous air, fragments, and hematomas make ultrasound less reliable.

Medical Treatment

Occult injuries (intimal flaps, dissections, pseudoaneurysms) identified during the evaluation for penetrating cervical injury should be managed the same as those caused by blunt trauma (see "Blunt Cerebrovascular Injury"). Isolated intimal flaps are rare in penetrating trauma, and dissections occur in only 2% of cases. Pseudoaneurysms are the most common occult injury identified. Large pseudoaneurysms should be considered for early intervention, whereas small pseudoaneurysms should be treated with antithrombotic therapy and early follow-up imaging. The natural history of these lesions is not known; however, patients should be closely monitored for the development of embolic symptoms.

Endovascular Treatment

An endoluminal approach to neck injuries may avoid the morbidity of a median sternotomy, high thoracic incision, or difficult dissection at the base of the skull. Another benefit is that endoluminal therapy can be performed with the patient under local anesthesia, allowing direct assessment of the patient's neurologic status. For zones I and III injuries, endovascular exclusion of a pseudoaneurysm, partial transection, or arteriovenous fistula remains a viable option, depending on the location of the injury and the patient's clinical status. Self-expanding covered stents can be safely delivered to these locations with limited morbidity.[15-18] Zone II injuries should be treated by operative repair.

Surgical Treatment

Proximal and Distal Control in the Neck.
Obtaining control of the injury in each zone presents unique challenges. For all patients, the proximal thighs (potential vein conduit) and chest (potential proximal control) should be prepared and included in the operative field. Zone I injuries that present with hard signs may be approached through a cervical incision, but obtaining proximal control requires a median sternotomy or high anterolateral thoracotomy. If the patient is in shock, endovascular attempts at proximal control should not delay the performance of a median sternotomy. Depending on the patient's hemodynamic status and the injury location, proximal control of the great vessels may be performed from a femoral approach in the operative suite with balloon occlusion (a large 33-mm compliant balloon catheter). Alternatively, if the proximal vessel can be visualized from a cervical approach but not secured with a vascular clamp, a compliant balloon or Fogarty catheter can be passed retrograde for temporary proximal control. Once the vessel is properly exposed, the balloon can be replaced with a vascular clamp.

An overt injury in zone II can be readily approached through a cervical incision, and repair performed under direct visualization. The most common vessel injured by penetrating mechanisms is the internal jugular vein, followed by the common carotid artery. The operative feasibility, ability to examine the aerodigestive tract, and relatively low risk of exploration in this region favor open exploration over endovascular techniques in emergent situations.

Hemorrhage from a zone III injury can be devastating, and an immediate operative exploration through a cervical incision can be used initially to control inflow and assess the injury pattern. Even after subluxation of the mandible and division of the posterior belly of the digastric muscle, the distal extent of the injury may not be visualized. If the vessel is transected, with an inadequate length for clamp application, distal control can be obtained by placing a Fogarty balloon (No. 3 or 4) within the vessel lumen. If the vessel is lacerated, a sheath can be placed in the common carotid artery, and a Fogarty catheter can be passed antegrade through the injury to control backbleeding. Once the Fogarty is inflated, an arteriogram can be performed through the sidearm of the sheath to delineate the injury with respect to the skull base and further guide operative exposure. Once the hemorrhage is arrested, the surgeon must decide whether to proceed with operative repair, embolization of the carotid artery, endoluminal stenting, or temporary shunting or to return the patient to the intensive care unit for resuscitation, imaging of the brain, and delayed repair. If a damage-control approach is used, the patient should have serial imaging to evaluate evolving cerebral edema, and cerebral perfusion pressures should guide further resuscitative maneuvers.

Surgical Repair of Cervical Vessels.
Once the injury has been delineated and controlled, the surgeon must decide whether to ligate, repair, or temporarily shunt the vessel. The internal jugular vein and external carotid artery can be ligated with limited morbidity. Ligation of the internal carotid artery results in a 45% mortality rate and should be reserved only for injuries at the base of the skull that are not amenable to reconstruction.[1] Clean-based lacerations caused by stab wounds can be repaired primarily; however, gunshot wounds, fragmentation wounds, and shotgun injuries typically require reconstruction of the common carotid or internal carotid artery. Shunts should be used in patients who are already at risk for cerebral hypoperfusion secondary to shock and to injuries of the internal carotid artery. If the distal clamp can be placed below the carotid bulb, the internal carotid artery will receive adequate backbleeding through the external carotid artery. Heparin should be given before the clamps are placed.

The great saphenous vein is a good size match with the internal carotid artery and when used as an interposition graft has demonstrated excellent patency and limited risk of infection. The external carotid artery can also be transposed to the internal carotid artery for injuries to the proximal internal carotid. In addition, the superficial femoral artery can be used in the common or internal carotid artery, but it requires an additional reconstruction in the lower extremity with polytetrafluoroethylene (PTFE).[19] A PTFE graft is typically a better size match than the great saphenous vein in the common carotid artery, and in this location, there is no difference in patency rates between the two conduits. In the setting of associated aerodigestive injuries, autogenous conduits should be used, the esophageal repair should be drained away from the vascular repair, and a muscle pedicle (cervical strap muscle, omohyoid muscle, digastric muscle, or sternal head of the sternocleidomastoid) should be placed between the two repairs.

After repair of the vascular injury, all patients must be monitored for signs of cerebral edema and intracranial hypertension. If a clinical neurologic examination cannot be performed, direct intracerebral pressure monitoring or serial head imaging should be obtained.

Blunt Cerebrovascular Injury

The overall incidence of blunt cerebrovascular injury (BCVI) has been universally reported as less than 1% of all admissions for blunt trauma, but this relatively small population of patients has stroke rates ranging from 25% to 58% and mortality rates of 31% to 59%.[20-22] The incidence of BCVI is 0.19% to 0.67% for unscreened populations and 0.6% to 1.07% for screened populations.[20]

Clinical Presentation

The recognition and treatment of BCVI have evolved dramatically over the past 2 decades. As imaging technology has improved with respect to both image quality and acquisition times, it has become a fundamental diagnostic tool in blunt trauma evaluation. Paralleling advances in noninvasive imaging, a heightened awareness of BCVI has emerged. Through aggressive screening, these injuries are increasingly recognized before devastating neurologic ischemia results.

Mechanism of Injury.
Three basic mechanisms of injury are encountered: (1) extreme hyperextension and rotation, (2) direct blow to the vessel, and (3) vessel laceration by adjacent bone fractures.[23] The most common mechanism of blunt carotid injury is hyperextension of the carotid vessels over the lateral articular processes of C1-C3 at the base of the skull, which is typically a result of high-speed automobile crashes. There are also scattered case reports of BCVIs resulting from chiropractic manipulation[24] and rapid head turning with exercise.[25] A direct blow to the artery typically occurs in the setting of a misplaced seat belt across the neck during a motor vehicle crash or in the setting of hanging. This injury pattern typically occurs in the proximal internal carotid artery as opposed to the distal aspect. Basilar skull fractures involving the petrous or sphenoid portions of the carotid canal can injure the vessel at this location.

Common mechanisms of injury associated with BCVI include motor vehicle crash (41% to 70%), direct cervical blow (10% to 20%), automobile versus pedestrian (12% to 18%), fall from height (5% to 15%), and hanging events (5%).[20,22] The most common associated injuries at the time of diagnosis include closed head injuries (50% to 65%), facial fractures (60%), cervical spine fractures (50%), and thoracic injuries (40% to 51%).[20,22]

Signs and Symptoms.
Case reports as early as 1967 described BCVI with recognized symptoms of cerebral ischemia, and all patients were symptomatic at the time of diagnosis.[26] Carotid injuries typically present with a contralateral sensory or motor deficit, decreased mental status, or neurologic deficits not explained by closed head injury. A carotid-cavernous fistula may present with orbital pain, proptosis, hyperemia, cerebral swelling, or seizure. Depending on whether the vessel is occluded or whether the resultant injury is a nidus for embolic events, the symptoms may be variable.

Patients typically have coexisting traumatic brain injuries that may mask signs and symptoms of BCVI.

Patients may present to the trauma center with obvious signs of BCVI; however, many patients are initially asymptomatic and develop symptoms after a latent period. Several authors have reported the development of symptoms from 1 hour to several weeks after injury.[27-30] Evaluating an unscreened trauma population, Berne and coworkers found a median time to diagnosis of 12.5 hours for survivors of BCVI and 19.5 hours for nonsurvivors, suggesting a sufficient window of opportunity for diagnosis and treatment.[22] Neither admission Glasgow Coma Scale (GCS) score nor baseline neurologic examination correlates with the subsequent development of symptoms attributed to BCVI.

Screening.
Although there is no consensus on the ideal screening protocol for BCVI, several authors have found an association with signs, symptoms, and risk factors identified on admission. The first and most comprehensive screening protocol was initiated at the Denver Health Medical Center (Table 152-1).[20,31] With this screening protocol, the authors reported an overall BCVI incidence of 0.86%. Exactly 4.8% of all trauma patients were screened based on defined risk criteria, and 18% of screened patients were found to have an injury. Fifty-two percent of these screened patients were asymptomatic. Neurologic morbidity was 16%, and BCVI-associated mortality was 15%.[20] Using the Memphis criteria (see Table 152-1), the incidence of BCVI was 1.03%, 3.5% of all blunt trauma patients were screened, and 29% of screened patients were found to have an injury.[32] Both screening regimens mandate four-vessel cerebral angiography if the patient meets at least one of the screening criteria.

Several authors have evaluated a more restricted screening protocol in an effort to reduce the cost of screening and limit the number of negative examinations. A cervical seat-belt sign has been evaluated in several prospective studies but was not found to be predictive of BCVI.[20,33] Biffl and colleagues performed a multivariate analysis on a prospectively screened population and found four clinical findings predictive of BCVI (listed in Table 152-1).[34] Patients with one finding had a 41% risk of BCVI; two findings, 56% to 74%; three findings, 80% to 88%; and all four, 93%; however, 20% of patients with BCVI did not have any of the findings. The bulk of the available literature supports an appropriate screening protocol, and all major trauma centers should have predetermined screening criteria for BCVI.

Diagnostic Evaluation

Duplex Ultrasound.
Duplex scanning has been evaluated in multiple trauma centers for diagnosing BCVI. In the evaluation of carotid artery stenosis, duplex ultrasound is limited for identifying lesions causing less than 60% stenosis; likewise, duplex often cannot identify small intimal tears or nonocclusive dissections. It may be difficult to obtain adequate visualization of the internal carotid artery at the base of the skull, where the majority of these injuries occur. The

Table 152-1 Screening Criteria for Blunt Cerebrovascular Injury

Denver Criteria*	Memphis Criteria†	Biffl's Modified Criteria‡ (Odds Ratio)
Signs and Symptoms	**Signs and Symptoms**	**Signs and Symptoms**
Arterial hemorrhage or expanding hematoma Cervical bruit Neurologic exam inconsistent with head CT findings Stroke on follow-up head CT Focal neurologic deficit	Neurologic exam not explained by brain imaging Horner's syndrome Neck soft tissue injury (seat-belt sign, hanging, or hematoma)	GCS < 6 (1.98)
Risk Factors	**Risk Factors**	**Risk Factors**
Le Fort II or III fracture pattern Basilar skull fracture with involvement of carotid canal Diffuse axonal injury with GCS < 6 Cervical spine fracture Near-hanging with anoxic brain injury	Le Fort II or III fracture pattern Basilar skull fracture with involvement of carotid canal Cervical spine fracture	Le fort II or III fracture pattern (3.7) Petrous fracture (2.64) Diffuse axonal injury (3.09)

*Adapted from Biffl WL, Moore EE, Ryu RK, et al. The unrecognized epidemic of blunt carotid arterial injuries: early diagnosis improves neurologic outcome. *Ann Surg.* 1998;228(4):462-470.
†Adapted from Miller PR, Fabian TC, Croce MA, et al. Prospective screening for blunt cerebrovascular injuries: analysis of diagnostic modalities and outcomes. *Ann Surg.* 2002;236(3):386-393; discussion 393-395.
‡Adapted from Biffl WL, Moore EE, Offner PJ, et al. Optimizing screening for blunt cerebrovascular injuries. *Am J Surg.* 1999;178:517-522.
CT, computed tomography; GCS, Glasgow Coma Scale score.

sensitivity of duplex ultrasound for detecting BCVI ranges from 38% to 86%[29,35]; therefore, it should not be used as a screening modality.

Digital Subtraction Angiography.

Selective digital subtraction angiography (DSA) is the diagnostic "gold standard" for screening patients with suspected BCVI. The Denver group proposed an angiographic grading system that has become the standard for reporting BCVI (Table 152-2).[36] Most important, the grading scale has prognostic value for patients' risk of subsequent stroke.

DSA has several limitations that make it a difficult diagnostic tool. First and foremost, it is an invasive procedure with technical limitations and a complication profile that includes a risk of stroke (<1%).[20] Performing screening DSA on all patients at risk for BCVI may impose too great a burden on the angiography suite—both economically and in terms of workload; some institutions cannot support this type of demand.

Table 152-2 Blunt Cerebrovascular Injury Grading Scale

Grade	Angiographic Findings	Stroke Risk (%)	Mortality (%)
I	Luminal irregularity or dissection; intramural hematoma with <25% luminal narrowing	3	11
II	Dissection or intramural hematoma with ≥25% luminal narrowing	11	11
III	Pseudoaneurysm	33	11
IV	Vessel occlusion	44	22
V	Vessel transection	100	100

Adapted from Biffl WL, Moore EE, Offner PJ, et al. Blunt carotid arterial injuries: implications of a new grading scale. *J Trauma.* 1999;47:845-853.

Computed Tomographic Angiography.

Helical CTA offers several potential advantages over conventional DSA. It is a noninvasive study that can be obtained in less than 5 minutes and, as opposed to cerebral angiography, CTA obtains three-dimensional images of the vessel wall (Fig. 152-3). In addition, the workup of blunt trauma patients inevitably involves computed tomography (CT) of the head,

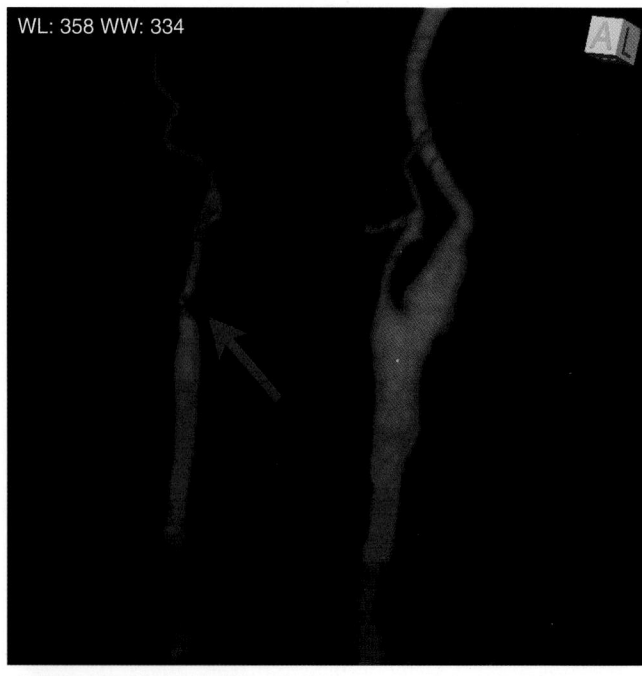

WL: 358 WW: 334

Figure 152-3 Three-dimensional CTA reconstruction with bone subtraction demonstrates occlusion of the right internal carotid artery. This patient presented with a zone II neck hematoma and a seat-belt mark across the right neck after an automobile crash. The *arrow* marks the occlusion at the origin of the internal carotid artery.

chest, abdomen, or all of these. CTA of the carotid-vertebral circulation can easily be obtained during this examination, sacrificing little in terms of time (60 seconds per scan), contrast burden (approximately 100 mL), or radiation exposure.

The ability to use CTA for screening depends on the quality of the scanner at the host institution. Utilizing early-generation single-slice and four-slice CT scanners, two prospective comparative studies (performed by the Denver and Memphis groups) found that CTA had a sensitivity of 47% to 68% and a specificity of 67% to 99% when compared with DSA.[32,37] CTA missed 55% of grade I, 14% of grade II, and 13% of grade III injuries.[37] CTA technology rapidly improved over the ensuing years, such that the number of detectors progressively increased and postimaging processing became readily available. Bub and associates prospectively compared multidetector CTA (four- and eight-slice scanners) to DSA and found a sensitivity of 83% to 92% and a specificity of 88% to 98% with CTA from three different radiologists.[38] The interobserver reliability was also higher for CTA than for DSA.

In 2005, Biffl and colleagues reported their experience using 16-slice CTA for the diagnosis of BCVI, and unlike the prior study by the Denver group, DSA was not used as the gold standard.[39] Over an 11-month period, 331 patients were screened, and 5.4% were diagnosed with BCVI. In this study, negative CTA scans were followed with clinical observation, and no patients developed neurologic symptoms consistent with a delayed presentation of missed BCVI. All positive examinations were confirmed with DSA. Of the 18 injuries identified by CTA, 17 were correctly graded; one patient was upstaged to grade III on DSA owing to a small pseudoaneurysm not identified on CTA (false-positive rate, 1.2%).[39]

In 2006, a prospective comparative study validated 16-slice CTA as a primary screening modality for BCVI.[40] In this series, CTA was performed in addition to DSA in 162 consecutive patients; 20 carotid and 26 vertebral injuries were diagnosed. This resulted in an incidence of 1.25% and a screening yield of 28%, which is comparable to historic controls. CTA and DSA were 100% concordant for blunt carotid injuries, resulting in a sensitivity of 100% and a specificity of 100%.[40] This is the only study comparing conventional 16-slice CTA directly to DSA and demonstrating equivalence. Based on these findings, 16-slice CTA should be considered the primary screening modality for BCVI.

Magnetic Resonance Angiography. Magnetic resonance angiography (MRA) is an attractive noninvasive modality because of the image resolution obtained in this anatomic region, the infinite number of projections of the vessel, and the ability to assess the intracranial architecture for signs of stroke.[41,42] Limitations include availability and the time required for image acquisition. This modality is impractical in a trauma patient with multiple competing injuries. In comparative studies of DSA versus MRA, MRA performed poorly, with sensitivities of 50% to 95%.[32,43] The latest report is from 2002, and improved technology may change the role of MRA in BCVI.

Medical Treatment

The mainstay of treatment for BCVI is antithrombotic therapy; however, there are no randomized controlled trials to support this recommendation. Fabian and coworkers reported the first prospective observational study demonstrating improved neurologic outcome associated with the early use of antithrombotic therapy.[21] Their analysis revealed the benefit of heparin therapy for decreasing the rate of neurologic deterioration after the development of symptoms and for decreasing the rate of new neurologic events. Heparin therapy was associated with a dramatic reduction in neurologic morbidity (29%) compared with no treatment (73%). Biffl and colleagues confirmed that patients benefit from early anticoagulation, documenting the greatest benefit among those who were asymptomatic at the time heparinization.[20] In the asymptomatic group, only one patient developed subsequent stroke. Analyzing the symptomatic cohort, 93% of patients had improvement in their neurologic deficits with anticoagulation, compared with only 67% without anticoagulation. Based on these two studies, anticoagulation became the first-line treatment for BCVI.

Complications associated with anticoagulation occur in 25% to 54% of the trauma population.[20] Most concerning is intracranial hemorrhage, but more common are gastrointestinal bleeding, retroperitoneal hemorrhage, blunt solid organ injury with hemorrhage, and rebleeding from surgical wounds. Eachempati and associates noted that few patients were able to receive heparin therapy at the time of the BCVI diagnosis (14%), and they found a complication rate of 16% among those who received heparin therapy.[44]

Because of the complication profile of full anticoagulation therapy, several authors have focused on antiplatelet therapy as an alternative. A prospective comparison of antiplatelet therapy versus anticoagulation for BCVI does not exist. One study by Biffl and colleagues reported that anticoagulation (heparin with transition to warfarin) was superior to antiplatelet therapy (aspirin or clopidogrel), with stroke rates of 1% versus 9%.[20] Several follow-up studies have failed to confirm this result. Miller and coworkers found that resultant stroke rates after BCVI treated with heparin and with antiplatelet therapy were similar (5% and 3%, respectively).[45] Follow-up studies demonstrated no difference in stroke rates for patients treated with heparin (5% to 8%) compared with those treated with antiplatelet therapy (3% to 7%).[32,31,46]

Either heparin or antiplatelet therapy can be used with similar results. If the patient has no contraindications to anticoagulation, a prudent protocol would be heparin therapy (goal, activated partial thromboplastin time of 50 to 60 seconds) and transition to warfarin (goal, international normalized ratio of 2.0) for 3 months. Antiplatelet therapy should be used for the same period.

All patients treated medically should undergo serial 16-slice CTA or DSA at 1-week and 3-month follow-up. At 3 months one can expect 72% of grade I injuries to be completely healed.[47] Grade II injuries are fairly evenly distributed: 33% are improved, 33% are stable, and 33% progress to pseudoaneurysms.[47] Grade III injuries tend to either remain unchanged (50%) or enlarge (40%). Grade IV injuries do not improve and probably do not warrant follow-up imaging after discharge.[47]

Follow-up imaging of BCVI treated with antithrombotic therapy is imperative. Pseudoaneurysms are unlikely to resolve with medical management,[48] and 33% of acute nonocclusive dissections treated with anticoagulation develop pseudoaneurysms on follow-up arteriography.[21] These lesions have a very low risk of rupture, but they tend to be the source of chronic embolic events or thrombosis.[49,50]

Endovascular Treatment

Endovascular therapy has been reserved primarily for evolving dissections that are surgically inaccessible, pseudoaneurysms that persist after antithrombotic treatment, or patients with worsening neurologic symptoms. When a patient develops a symptomatic injury, a pseudoaneurysm, or a chronic dissection, endoluminal treatment with either a bare-metal or a covered stent is an alternative to open repair.[51,52] Balloon-expandable and self-expanding stents have been used in this location, and in all cases, apposition of the dissection to the wall was achieved, with no neurologic events reported.[52,53]

Because of the potential for embolic stroke, pseudoaneurysms that fail to resolve with antithrombotic therapy, enlarge, or result in ischemic complications should be excluded from the cerebral circulation. Based on the location of these lesions in the distal internal carotid artery, endovascular therapy offers several advantages over open repair. Self-expanding covered stents can be safely delivered to these locations with limited morbidity.[15-18]

Initial reports from Parodi and coworkers relied on balloon-expandable bare Palmaz stents (Cordis, Johnson and Johnson, Miami Lakes, FL) to cover the orifice of the pseudoaneurysm.[54] Covering the orifice typically promotes thrombosis of the pseudoaneurysm, but if the sac fails to thrombose, one option is to coil-embolize the sac through the interstices of the bare stent.[55] In these series, the mean follow-up was 3.5 years without neurologic sequelae, but thrombosis, embolic potential, and restenosis are concerns after the endovascular placement of devices in the carotid artery.[56] Although thromboembolic complications are most common immediately after stent placement, patients require lifelong follow-up for unforeseen complications such as stent fracture.[57] Post-stent therapy is variable; based on an extrapolation of data from carotid artery stenting for atherosclerotic disease, a regimen of dual antiplatelet therapy (aspirin and clopidogrel) appears adequate to prevent stent thrombosis and embolic ischemic events.[58] If antiplatelet therapy is discontinued, stent thrombosis and resultant stroke are inherent risks.[16]

Cothren and colleagues reported their 3- to 6-month follow-up analysis of post-traumatic carotid pseudoaneurysms treated with carotid stents.[59] Patients with a persistent pseudoaneurysm 7 to 10 days after injury were considered candidates for stent therapy. Twenty-three patients were treated with carotid Wallstents (Boston Scientific, Natick, MA), and

three of those patients (13%) experienced ischemic complications (two periprocedural and one attributed to medication noncompliance).[59] Edwards and associates placed 22 carotid stents for BCVI: 18 patients had pseudoaneurysms, and 4 patients were treated for extensive dissections.[47] They experienced no periprocedural complications. Twelve patients were treated with postprocedural antiplatelet therapy, and 8 received anticoagulation. With a mean angiographic follow-up of 7 months, there were no occlusions (100% patency). Follow-up is imperative in this patient cohort, and additional prospective studies with long-term follow-up are needed to determine the risks and efficacy of carotid stents for BCVI. Compliance with medications and follow-up surveillance should be considered when planning appropriate therapy for trauma patients.

Surgical Treatment

The indications for surgical intervention parallel those for endovascular intervention.[21,60] Patients with evolving dissections, pseudoaneurysms that persist or enlarge after antithrombotic treatment, or worsening neurologic symptoms should undergo repair. Whether an open or an endovascular repair is performed should be based on the patient's associated injuries, the location of the BCVI, and the patient's ability to comply with an antiplatelet regimen and long-term follow-up.

Schievink and coworkers addressed blunt carotid pseudoaneurysms with operative repair in 22 patients.[61] To exclude the lesions, 5 patients required carotid ligation, 13 underwent resection with reconstruction, and 4 required cervical–to–intracranial carotid bypass. In their series, 2 patients experienced ischemic stroke, and the most common complications were cranial nerve neurapraxia secondary to high surgical exposure. This series illustrates the difficulty of treating these lesions at the base of the skull and the resultant morbidity.

If the injury is located at the base of the skull, the only option for treatment may be endovascular exclusion. When the lesion is located in the proximal internal carotid or common carotid artery, the vessel should be approached via an anterior exposure. The vessel may be repaired primarily or, more commonly, with patch angioplasty using either the great saphenous vein or a prosthetic graft.

■ VERTEBRAL ARTERY

Vertebral artery injuries (VAIs) are rare, with an incidence of 0.20% to 0.77% among all trauma admissions.[20,21] The first portion of the vertebral artery (V1) is readily accessible; however, the second (V2, within the bony foramen of the cervical canal), third (V3, as the vessel exits the bony foramen and enters the base of the skull), and fourth (V4, the intracranial segment to the basilar artery) portions can be extremely difficult to control.

Clinical Presentation

Penetrating injuries are most commonly due to gunshot or stab wounds.[62] Life-threatening hemorrhage is rare from an isolated VAI (mortality, 4%); however, penetrating injuries frequently involve the common carotid artery, subclavian artery, internal jugular vein, and subclavian vein, which may be life threatening. Patients are typically asymptomatic or complain of associated neurologic injury secondary to either compression from hematoma or direct injury.[62]

The most common mechanism of blunt VAI is fracture of the transverse foramen through which the vessel courses (C2-C6).[63] The vertebral vessels are relatively fixed throughout the vertebral canal, making the V2 segment susceptible to hyperextension and stretch injuries. Because of the rich collateral circulation in the neck, unilateral VAI is asymptomatic in 80% of cases. With regard to dissection, patients may complain of subtle neck pain or posterior headache. Vertebrobasilar ischemia may present with protean symptoms, including dizziness, vertigo, nausea, tinnitus, dysarthria, dysphagia, ataxia, visual deficits, or hoarseness. The degree of ischemia is determined by the extent of distal propagation into the basilar or posterior inferior cerebellar arteries. Patients with bilateral VAI may present with more severe symptoms: coma, fixed pupils, and loss of respiratory drive. Approximately 25% of patients have bilateral blunt VAIs, and 33% have an associated blunt carotid injury.[64]

Diagnostic Evaluation

VAI typically presents with penetrating neck injury. If the patient presents with refractory shock, hard signs of a vascular injury, or hard signs of a tracheal injury (continuous air bubbling from the wound), the injury should be diagnosed in the operating room, and management is straightforward. Plain films in the emergency department are useful for determining the track of the missile and any foreign bodies within the wound. Hemodynamically stable patients with normal GCS scores who do not have hard signs of a vascular injury should undergo 16-slice CTA of the neck. The head and chest should be included in the evaluation to identify associated injuries and the track of the missile or knife. This mechanism of injury should also prompt a high suspicion for aerodigestive injuries, which may require additional evaluation (bronchoscopy, rigid esophagoscopy, upper gastrointestinal swallow studies).

Blunt VAIs were originally diagnosed using DSA, and the same grading criteria were applied to the vertebral artery as to the carotid artery (see Table 152-2). In contrast to blunt carotid injuries, the grade of a blunt VAI does not correlate with an increasing risk of stroke. The stroke risk of blunt VAIs is 20%, irrespective of grade.[64] The same controversy regarding screening and imaging for blunt carotid trauma surrounds the evaluation of blunt VAIs. The same screening criteria are also applied (see Table 152-1); however, cervical spine fracture is the only factor independently associated with blunt VAI (odds ratio, 14.5).[34]

All imaging modalities are less accurate at diagnosing blunt VAIs than carotid injuries. Duplex evaluation of the vertebral vessels is extremely limited; however, the use of color flow allows one to assess vessel patency. MRA has the previously stated limitations in the setting of trauma. For the evaluation of blunt VAI, CTA has a sensitivity and specificity of 40% to 60% and 90% to 97%, respectively.[38] If there is a high index of suspicion based on cervical fracture, a confirmatory study should be obtained. MRA is an acceptable option when available; however, if concern persists, DSA should be performed.

Medical Treatment

Medical management has no role in penetrating injuries, but it does have a role in blunt injuries identified during the diagnostic evaluation. The posterior circulation stroke rate attributed to blunt VAI is 24%, with an associated mortality of 8%.[64] Symptomatic patients should be treated with heparin and monitored for hemorrhagic conversion with serial neurologic examinations. Heparin therapy was first evaluated in asymptomatic patients and was found to reduce neurologic events in the posterior circulation, from 20% to 35% with no anticoagulation to 0% to 14% with heparin therapy.[45,64] In patients who could not tolerate anticoagulation, the efficacy of aspirin treatment was similar to that of heparin. Follow-up studies have increasingly used aspirin to avoid the bleeding complications associated with heparin therapy. Miller and coworkers treated 43 patients with VAIs; 32 received aspirin or clopidogrel, and only 8 patients received heparin therapy.[45] None of the patients developed stroke. Symptomatic patients or those without contraindications to anticoagulation should be treated with 3 to 6 months of anticoagulation with radiographic follow-up. Asymptomatic patients should be treated with either 3 to 6 months of anticoagulation or dual antiplatelet therapy; there are insufficient data to recommend any one treatment at this time.

Endovascular Treatment

Endovascular treatment of the vertebral artery is used for hemorrhage not controlled by surgery, backbleeding from the V3 segment, pseudoaneurysm, or symptomatic patients who cannot tolerate anticoagulation (Fig. 152-4). The endovascular technique of crossing the vertebral artery confluence at the basilar artery is technically challenging, but both proximal and distal ends of the transected or lacerated vessel should be treated with embolization when possible. If the vessel is intact, the injury may be crossed from an antegrade approach, allowing embolization of both outflow and inflow (trapdoor technique). In nearly half of VAIs evaluated with endovascular techniques, the vessel was thrombosed and required no treatment at all.[65] Preservation of the vertebral artery may be a concern when other extracranial blood supply has been compromised. In these complex cases, endovascular stenting of the vertebral artery has been performed as a salvage procedure.[45] There are no data to support routine stenting for blunt VAI.

Surgical Treatment

Operative management is reserved for patients with active bleeding from the vertebral artery at the time of neck

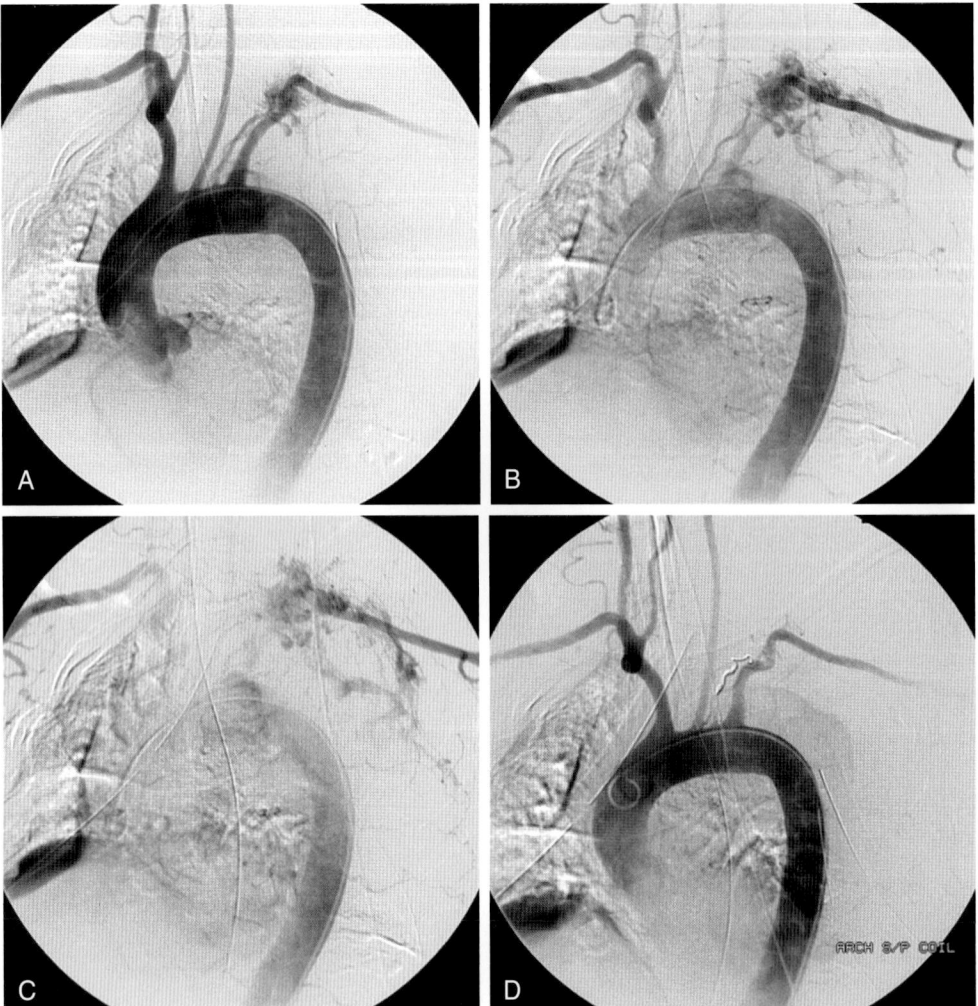

Figure 152-4 Penetrating vertebral artery injury secondary to a stab wound at the base of the left neck. Aortic arch angiography demonstrates initial contrast extravasation from the left vertebral artery originating directly from the aorta and no flow into the distal vertebral artery (**A**), contrast within the soft tissues of the neck (**B** and **C**), and successful embolization of the vertebral artery (**D**).

exploration. In a review of the largest series of penetrating VAIs, 50% of patients who underwent open exploration required postoperative endoluminal embolization to arrest bleeding or control arteriovenous fistulae.[65] Controlling the vertebral artery can be challenging for even the most experienced trauma or vascular surgeon. Unilateral surgical ligation results in a stroke rate of 3% to 5%.[66]

The approach is the same as that described previously for the exploration of the carotid artery. Once the sternocleidomastoid muscle (SCM) has been retracted laterally, the V1 segment can be visualized by transecting the SCM from the sternum and clavicle. Next, the scalene fat pad is divided vertically, and care is taken to identify and protect the phrenic nerve coursing from lateral to medial across the anterior scalene muscle. Division of the anterior scalene muscle from the first rib allows visualization of the first portion of the subclavian artery and the origin of the vertebral artery, thyrocervical trunk, and internal mammary artery. On the right side, the recurrent laryngeal nerve should be protected, and care should be taken on the left

side to avoid injury to the thoracic duct. Partial manubrium and clavicle resection can be performed to gain exposure in this location.

The V2 segment is more challenging to control, and most surgeons should simply ligate the proximal V1 segment because repair of the vertebral artery is futile and exposure of the V2 segment is fraught with venous bleeding. Exposure of V2 involves retracting the SCM laterally, dividing the omohyoid muscle, and retracting the carotid sheath medially. Identification of the cervical spinal bodies and the associated prevertebral fascia is mandatory. The sympathetic chain ganglia should be protected as they course through this region. Longitudinal opening of the anterior longitudinal ligament and paraspinous muscles allows identification of the transverse processes of the spinal bodies. Removal of the anterior aspect of the transverse processes using a hand-held rongeur allows exposure of the vertebral artery. Posterior to the vessel lie the cervical nerve roots. Hemorrhage in this location should be controlled with proximal ligation of V1. Bone wax can be packed into the bony canal, and postoperative embolization of the distal vertebral artery can be performed if needed.

Most vascular and trauma surgeons are unfamiliar with the V3 segment at the base of the skull. Rather than undergoing a timely dissection, the patient may be better served by proximal ligation of the V1 segment; packing the wound with bone wax or gauze or by balloon occlusion; and proceeding to endoluminal embolization. To expose the V3 segment for ligation, the incision is extended posteriorly behind the ear onto the mastoid process.[67] The SCM is retracted medially and may be divided from the skull base. During this step, the spinal accessory nerve should be identified and preserved. The transverse process of C1 is identified anterior and below the mastoid process. The muscle attachments to C1 and C2 are cleared with a periosteal elevator, and after resecting the lateral process of C1, the vertebral artery is exposed.

■ SUBCLAVIAN ARTERY

Injuries to the thoracic outlet are often lethal. Prehospital mortality is 50% to 80%, and of those patients who survive transport, 15% die during treatment.[68]

Clinical Presentation

Blunt injuries to the subclavian vessels are extremely rare, but when they occur, patients typically have associated clavicular fractures, mediastinal injuries, and pulmonary contusions. Penetrating injuries account for the majority of trauma to the subclavian vessels; in one U.S. trauma center, gunshot wounds accounted for 74% and stab wounds for 26% of injuries.[69] These patients often present to the emergency department in cardiac arrest, and consideration of resuscitative thoracotomy must be based on time from injury and signs of life. Those patients who survive transport may present with hard signs of vascular injury as described earlier, mandating immediate operative exploration. All other patients with soft signs of vascular injury should undergo further diagnostic evaluation. A normal radial pulse does not reliably exclude an upper extremity vascular injury. Concomitant cervical and thoracic injuries are common, occurring in 70% of patients.

The upper extremities rarely suffer from ischemia, owing to intense collateral circulation; however, long-term morbidity may be secondary to brachial plexus injuries. Brachial plexus injuries can be caused by penetrating injuries that directly transect nerve roots, blunt injuries that result in shear or traction forces, and operative exposure, which can result in iatrogenic injury. Blunt injury to the brachial plexus typically occurs secondary to stretch injuries to the upper extremity or to bone fractures.

Diagnostic Evaluation

In an unstable patient, there are few options other than immediate exploration. However, owing to the fibrous attachments surrounding the subclavian vessels, injuries frequently result in a contained extrapleural hematoma that may extend into the supraclavicular fossa. If time allows, CTA can be invaluable for identifying the location of injury and evaluating the mediastinum. Hemodynamically stable patients with an asymmetric pulse or neurologic deficits should undergo evaluation with CTA of the chest, neck, and upper extremity. Injury to the axillary vessels can range from intimal disruption, pseudoaneurysm, dissection, or even thrombosis. In addition, axial imaging can evaluate the mediastinum, cervical vasculature, and associated bone fractures.

Medical Treatment

Intimal disruptions and dissections that are not flow limiting should be treated with clinical observation. Anticoagulation or antiplatelet therapy can be added at the discretion of the surgeon. If the patient develops embolic symptoms, antithrombotic therapy should be instituted, with arteriography of the injury.

Endovascular Treatment

Endovascular treatment in this area can obviate the need for extensive dissection at the base of the neck. Covered stent-grafts have increasingly been used in this location, with several authors reporting immediate technical success in treating pseudoaneurysm, laceration, arteriovenous fistula, and even complete transection (Fig. 152-5).[70,71] Approximately 42% to 50% of patients are candidates for endovascular treatment.

These injuries can be approached from a transfemoral, transbrachial, or combined technique. Acute thrombosis in patients with malperfusion symptoms can be treated through a retrograde brachial approach, and after flow is restored, a covered stent can be used to treat the injury. Most transected vessels can be crossed with a hydrophilic wire. Undoubtedly, endovascular techniques reduce the morbidity of operative exposure and potential nerve injury in a blood-stained field. There are relatively few contraindications to this approach. The patient must be hemodynamically stable. Some consider a large supraclavicular hematoma with brachial plexus compression a relative contraindication; however, the injury can be treated with a covered stent followed by hematoma evacuation in a controlled field.

Mobility and compression between the first rib and clavicle raise concern about long-term patency in the young trauma population; it is imperative to follow these patients for late sequelae. In addition, endovascular repair does not preclude stent explantation with formal open repair; ideally, this approach can reduce the potential for iatrogenic nerve injury in the acute setting. In one of the largest reported series, three early stent thromboses were encountered in 56 patients.[70] All three were opened with a secondary intervention, and no patient experienced upper extremity ischemia.[70] Endovascular therapy in the thoracic outlet offers rapid, less invasive treatment and has the added benefit of avoiding injury to the brachial plexus, which has long-term implications for a functional recovery.

Section **19** Trauma and Acute Limb Ischemia

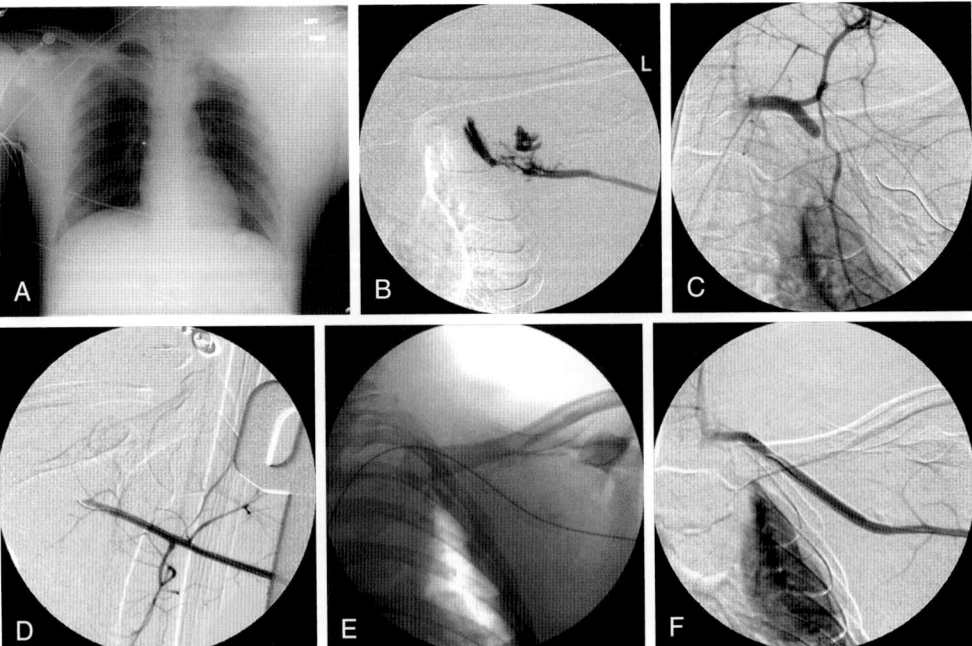

Figure 152-5 Blunt subclavian artery transection. The patient presented with a large stable hematoma in the supraclavicular fossa and extending into the axilla after a high-speed motorcycle crash. **A,** Chest radiograph demonstrates soft tissue density over the left clavicle. **B,** From the left brachial approach, there is extravasation at the level of the junction of the subclavian and axillary arteries. **C,** From the right groin, a left subclavian artery selective angiogram was performed. **D,** A curved glide wire was used to cross the transection. **E,** Once the transection was crossed, the brachial wire was snared within the hematoma, obtaining femoral-brachial wire access. The transection was treated with a covered stent. **F,** Completion angiogram demonstrates complete exclusion of the transected segment and no residual extravasation.

Surgical Treatment

Injuries to the thoracic outlet can be difficult to expose in an acute setting; it is important to prepare and include the neck, chest, and groins in the surgical field. Proximal control requires either a median sternotomy for the innominate and right subclavian arteries or a high left anterolateral thoracotomy with potential clavicular resection for the left subclavian artery. Rather than directly exploring the hematoma, the surgeon can place a remote occlusion balloon either from the groin or retrograde from the brachial artery. The surgeon can then perform an arteriogram, and with proximal control, the operative tempo changes from emergent to semi-urgent. The surgeon can undertake endovascular treatment or proceed with a meticulous dissection at the base of the neck and avoid either a sternotomy or a thoracic incision.

If the patient is in extremis, subclavian artery ligation rarely results in upper extremity ischemia. When repairing the vessel, the injury typically requires an interposition graft. PTFE works well in this location and has excellent patency.[72,73] If the field is grossly contaminated, saphenous vein, internal jugular vein, or superficial femoral artery have all been used in this location. It is important to note that nearly 50% of penetrating subclavian artery injuries have an associated subclavian vein injury.[72]

CERVICAL VENOUS INJURY

Venous injuries to the neck and thoracic outlet are invariably due to penetrating injuries. Blunt venous injuries are extremely rare and should be considered with sternal and clavicular fractures. Injuries to the internal jugular vein occur in 20% of cases of penetrating neck trauma, and subclavian vein injuries occur in 50% of penetrating subclavian injuries.[73,74]

Clinical Presentation

When patients present in extremis, the venous injury is typically identified in the operative suite. Isolated venous injuries present with hard or soft signs of a vascular injury, but patients are rarely hypotensive.[75]

Diagnostic Evaluation

The diagnostic evaluation should parallel the evaluation described earlier for each arterial anatomic region. If the patient undergoes CTA for suspicion of a vascular injury, delayed acquisition (30 seconds to 3 minutes) can provide improved imaging of the venous anatomy once the contrast material has cleared the associated arterial anatomy.

Endovascular Treatment

Endovascular stents have been used in the central venous system for subclavian and superior vena cava chronic thromboses. The efficacy of covered stents for venous trauma has been noted only in case reports, with good technical results.[76,77] This technology will increasingly be used for isolated venous injuries in hemodynamically stable patients.

Surgical Treatment

The surgical approach to each vein is identical to the arterial exposure described earlier. If the patient has hard signs of a vascular injury and is in extremis, the neck and subclavian veins can be ligated with limited morbidity. If the internal jugular vein is ligated, the patient should be monitored for cerebral edema; however, this is a rare occurrence, even with bilateral internal jugular vein ligation. Internal jugular vein reconstructions (using either spiral vein grafts or externally re-enforced PTFE) in the setting of bilateral neck dissections have an 18-month patency of 64%; elevated stump pressures (>30 mm Hg) may improve patency.[78] When the subclavian vein is ligated, the upper extremity should be elevated and placed in compression; transient edema typically resolves over the course of 7 to 10 days, and long-term venous stasis is rare.[74] Simple lacerations of the vein can be repaired with lateral venorrhaphy if less than 50% of the wall is involved.[74] All repairs are at risk for eventual thrombosis; mechanical and chemical thromboprophylaxis should be considered. Extensive vein repairs (end-to-end, venous interposition, or spiral panel grafts) typically do not have a role in penetrating neck injuries (as opposed to lower extremity injuries) when time is critical.

SELECTED KEY REFERENCES

Biffl WL, Moore EE, Ryu RK, Offner PJ, Novak Z, Coldwell DM, Franciose RJ, Burch JM. The unrecognized epidemic of blunt carotid arterial injuries: early diagnosis improves neurologic outcome. *Ann Surg.* 1998;228:462-470.
Large retrospective registry review comparing an unscreened population with a screened population for blunt carotid injury. This study increased the awareness of blunt carotid injury and noted a trend toward improvement in neurologic outcome if the injury was treated with heparin.

Cothren CC, Moore EE, Biffl WL, Ciesla DJ, Ray CE Jr, Johnson JL, Moore JB, Burch JM. Anticoagulation is the gold standard therapy for blunt carotid injuries to reduce stroke rate. *Arch Surg.* 2004;139: 540-545; discussion 545-546.
Prospective, nonrandomized, noncontrolled observational study that demonstrated reduced neurologic events in patients with BCVI treated with systemic heparin, low-molecular-weight heparin, or antiplatelet agents.

Demetriades D, Theodorou D, Cornwell E, Berne TV, Asensio J, Belzberg H, Velmahos G, Weaver F, Yellin A. Evaluation of penetrating injuries of the neck: prospective study of 223 patients. *World J Surg.* 1997;21:41-47; discussion 47-48.
Prospective evaluation of penetrating neck injuries that validated physical examination for detecting arterial injuries requiring treatment.

Eastman AL, Chason DP, Perez CL, McAnulty AL, Minei JP. Computed tomographic angiography for the diagnosis of blunt cervical vascular injury: is it ready for primetime? *J Trauma.* 2006;60:925-929; discussion 929.
Prospective comparative study that demonstrated equivalence between 16-slice CTA and DSA for screening BCVIs.

Fabian TC, Patton JH Jr, Croce MA, Minard G, Kudsk, KA, Pritchard FE. Blunt carotid injury. Importance of early diagnosis and anticoagulant therapy. *Ann Surg.* 1996;223:513-522; discussion 522-525.
Large retrospective registry review that compared patients with blunt carotid injury who were treated with and without heparin. Heparin therapy resulted in improved neurologic function and improved survival.

REFERENCES

The reference list can be found on the companion Expert Consult Web site at *www.expertconsult.com.*

Section **19** Trauma and Acute Limb Ischemia

CHAPTER 153

Vascular Trauma: Thoracic

William T. Brinkman and Joseph E. Bavaria

Based in part on a chapter in the previous edition by Matthew J. Wall, Jr., MD; Joseph Huh, MD; and Kenneth L. Mattox, MD.

Injury to the great vessels of the thorax—the aorta and its brachiocephalic branches—can occur following blunt and penetrating trauma. When confronted with injuries to these vessels, the surgeon's goal is twofold: prevention of acute hemorrhage, and prevention of delayed hemorrhage due to post-traumatic aneurysm or pseudoaneurysm rupture.

Greater than 90% of injuries to the great vessels of the thorax are caused by penetrating trauma.[1] Gunshots, stab wounds, shrapnel, and even iatrogenic misadventures are frequently reported causes.

The innominate artery, pulmonary veins, venae cavae, and thoracic aorta (most common) are susceptible to blunt injury. Aortic blunt injuries usually involve the proximal descending aorta, but injuries to other segments such as the ascending aorta or transverse arch (10% to 14%), mid–distal descending aorta (12%), and even multiple sites (13% to 18%) have been reported.[2,3]

■ DIAGNOSTIC STUDIES

Chest Radiograph

A supine anteroposterior chest radiograph should be obtained routinely in trauma patients. All emergency room physicians, radiologists, and surgeons should have experience in interpreting supine portable chest radiographs, because many patients are clinically unstable or have suspected spinal injuries, making "upright" posteroanterior chest radiographs unsafe. Assessment of a supine chest radiograph can rapidly rule out significant pathology such as pneumothorax, hemothorax, and fractures. If possible, an upright chest radiograph should be obtained. A normal upright chest radiograph has a negative predictive value of approximately 95% to 98%.[4]

When presented with penetrating injuries, marking the entrance and exit sites with radiopaque markers is useful. Radiographic findings suggestive of penetrating great vessel injury include a large hemothorax; foreign bodies or their trajectory close to the great vessels; a confusing trajectory, which may indicate a migrating endovascular course; or a "missing" missile, suggesting embolization.[5]

Radiographic findings suggestive of blunt injury to the thoracic aorta include fractures of the sternum, scapula, clavicle, first rib, or multiple left-sided ribs. Indirect mediastinal clues include obliteration of the aortic knob, depression of the left mainstem bronchus, loss of the paravertebral pleural stripe, an apical pleural cap, deviation of a nasogastric tube,

and lateral displacement of the trachea at the T4 level.[4] Pathologic widening of the mediastinum, defined as greater than 8 cm at the level of the aortic knob or a mediastinum width–to–chest width ratio exceeding 25%, has a reported sensitivity of 81% to 100% and a specificity of 60%. However, determination of the presence of mediastinal widening has significant interreader variability, even among experienced radiologists. The radiologist's overall impression of the mediastinum, rather than any one measurement, is a more sensitive predictor of traumatic aortic injury.[6]

Computed Tomography

Contrast-enhanced computed tomography (CT) using multislice detector technology has now replaced angiography as the screening modality for traumatic aortic injury.[7] In the past decade there has been a dramatic change in the diagnosis of and screening for traumatic thoracic vascular injury. Traditional "step and shoot" CT scanners were not deemed acceptable screening tools owing to slow acquisition, motion artifact, and poor spatial resolution.[8] However, with the arrival of multidetector CT (MDCT), concerns about image acquisition time and spatial resolution have been minimized. An MDCT study from the base of the skull through the symphysis pubis can be performed in less than 1 minute.

At many trauma centers, all blunt multitrauma patients receive MDCT. Using bolus tracking with a threshold of 90 Hounsfield units set in the proximal ascending aorta, a 16- by 0.75-mm scan or a 16- by 1.5-mm scan (in large patients) of the entire chest is performed. The data can then be reconstructed at 3- or 5-mm intervals. Thin-section reconstructions can also be performed, allowing for multiplanar reformatting, maximum intensity projection analysis, and volumetric and endovascular reformatting.[9]

The protocol for multisystem evaluation usually includes nonionic contrast at 3 to 4 mL/sec, for a total volume of 90 to 125 mL. Collimation of 3.2 mm with a pitch of 1.25 is used to reconstruct images at 1.6-mm intervals. Multiplanar reformulations are then used to evaluate vascular structures, including the aorta. Using this protocol at the Ryder Trauma Center over a 4-year period, 48 cases of traumatic aortic injury were identified. All 48 cases were diagnosed using direct signs of injury. Direct signs include active extravasation of contrast material, pseudoaneurysm formation, intimal flaps, and filling defects. Indirect signs of aortic injury include periaortic hematoma and mediastinal hematoma.[10] Direct

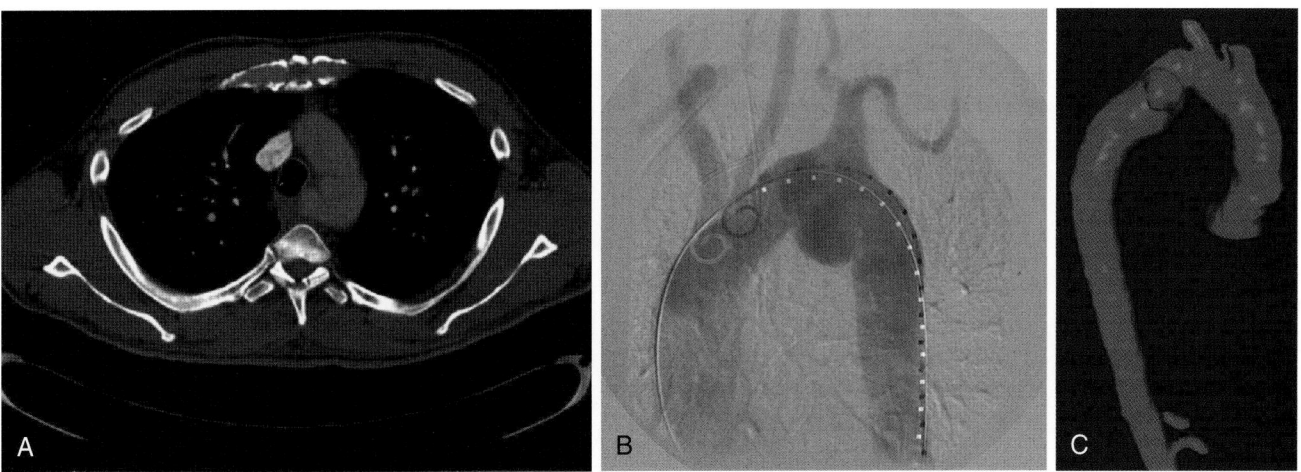

Figure 153-1 Blunt isthmic aortic injury as visualized by MDCT (**A**), intraoperative angiography (**B**), and three-dimensional CT reconstruction (**C**). Angulation of the aortic isthmus necessitates a more proximal landing zone at the left common carotid orifice.

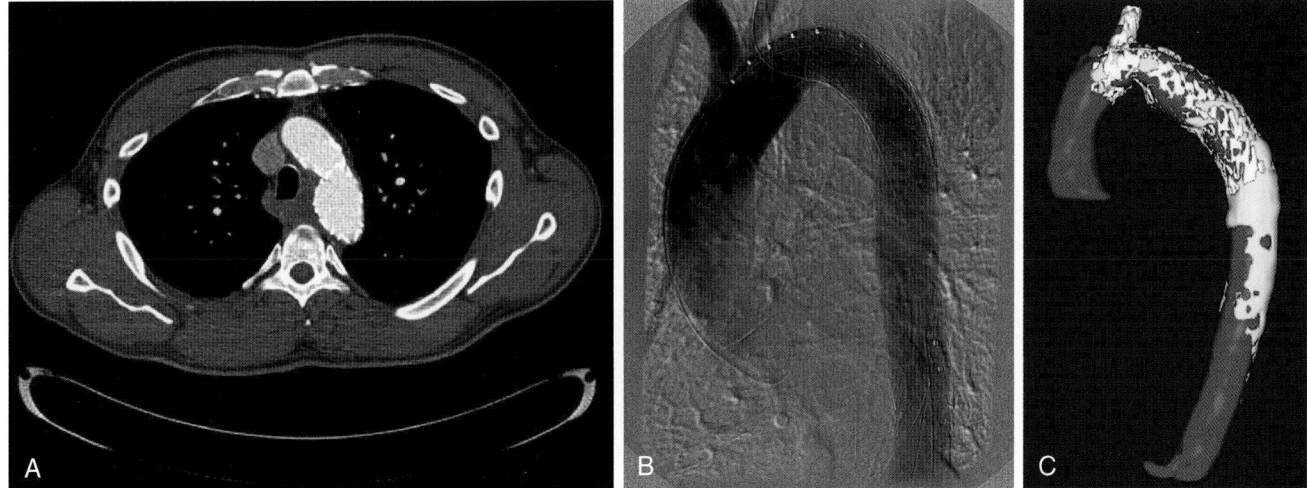

Figure 153-2 Blunt isthmic aortic injury seen in Figure 153-1 after thoracic endovascular repair as visualized by MDCT (**A**), intraoperative angiography (**B**), and three-dimensional CT reconstruction (**C**). Additional stent placement in the left common carotid artery was performed to ensure left carotid patency owing to the short proximal landing zone. Note the wire in the left common carotid artery in the angiographic image (**B**).

signs of aortic injuries are more accurate diagnostically than indirect signs.[11] Traditionally, periaortic hematomas without direct signs on CT were considered suspicious for aortic injury. Aortography was then recommended as a standard of care.[12,13] Since the development of MDCT, the presence of periaortic hematomas in the absence of a direct sign of aortic injury does not necessarily require aortography. However, this depends on the confidence of the radiologist and the quality of the scanner and the study.[14] There have been reports of positive aortograms with no direct signs of aortic injury, but all these cases were performed on older-generation helical scanners, not MDCT scanners.[12,13]

The traditional "gold standard" for the diagnosis of traumatic aortic injury, with a sensitivity and specificity approaching 100%, is aortography. However, multiple studies using single-slice helical CT for the diagnosis of traumatic aortic injury have shown sensitivities and specificities equal to those of aortography.[15,16] MDCT's ability to accurately diagnose aortic injury as well as injuries elsewhere in the body makes it the more useful diagnostic tool in trauma patients. In addition, MDCT has proved to be cost-effective and is available 24 hours a day, 7 days a week. In addition, MDCT can be used for stent-graft sizing if an endovascular approach is planned for repair (Figs. 153-1 and 153-2).

Transesophageal Echocardiography

Transesophageal echocardiography (TEE) is a useful tool for the evaluation of traumatic aortic injury. Multiple authors have demonstrated TEE's ability to visualize cardiac and vascular structures, making it a useful decision-making tool in cases of chest trauma. In addition, TEE can be applied quickly at the bedside or in the emergency room while resuscitation is ongoing. Some authors promote TEE as a first-line test in the initial evaluation of trauma patients with high-velocity deceleration injuries, regardless of the mediastinal width on the chest radiograph.

The accuracy of TEE in the published literature is varied. There are no prospective randomized trials of TEE in trauma patients. However, in a meta-analysis of studies of TEE in the setting of traumatic aortic injury, the sensitivity and specificity of TEE were approximately 97%. In a direct comparison with aortography, TEE's sensitivity and specificity were slightly lower (93% versus 95%). The findings of these studies were adversely affected by small enrollment numbers.[17-19] The main findings of this meta-analysis were that (1) overall, TEE has a high diagnostic performance for the detection of traumatic aortic injury; and (2) in general application, there are no differences in the diagnostic performance of TEE and aortography.

In fact, TEE performed better in patients with small aortic injuries that did not require surgery. These small aortic lesions can be missed by aortography because they do not cause any change in aortic shape.[20] These small lesions require careful diagnosis and follow-up because of their unpredictable behavior. Three trials followed patients with minor nonsurgical aortic injuries. In these studies, TEE results were consistently positive, whereas in 10 of 12 patients, aortography or CT results were negative. It is unclear whether the use of MDCT would have increased the sensitivity for nonsurgical aortic injuries. In these studies, TEE was used to follow the progressive healing of nonsurgical aortic lesions. The clinical application of these data is debatable because of the small sample size, inconsistent follow-up, and unknown sensitivity of TEE for small nonsurgical aortic injuries. However, TEE seems promising for the diagnosis and follow-up of these lesions. Additional studies to determine the incidence of nonsurgical traumatic aortic injuries, their long-term prognosis, and the role of TEE in their management are necessary.[17,19-21]

Unfortunately, TEE requires specific training and expertise and may not be as readily available as CT or angiography. This can lead to significant time delays in a patient population in which rapid decisions are critical. TEE may also be difficult to use in patients with neck injuries or when cervical spine "clearance" is pending. In addition, TEE does not visualize the ascending aorta or aortic branches well, owing to acoustic shadowing from the trachea and bronchi.[22,23]

Aortography

Angiography of the aorta has been and remains the gold standard for significant blunt aortic injury, although some question its use with the advent of MDCT and TEE. There is a small incidence of false-positive angiograms from known anatomic abnormalities such as ductus diverticulum and aberrant brachiocephalic arteries. However, physicians interpreting angiograms should be familiar with these variants.[24-26]

Magnetic Resonance Angiography

Long examination times and limited access have hindered the application of magnetic resonance imaging (MRI) to acute aortic pathology. However, with the development of fast MRI techniques (requiring only a few minutes), it can now be used even in critically ill patients. The use of MRI to detect traumatic aortic rupture in comparison with angiography and CT (not MDCT) was reported in a series of 24 patients. The diagnostic accuracy was 100% for MRI, 84% for angiography (two false-negatives), and 69% for CT (two false-negatives and three false-positives).[27] MRI is most useful for detecting the hemorrhagic component of a traumatic lesion. An aortic tear limited to the anterior or posterior wall can be visualized and followed if nonoperative management is chosen. Determination of the extent of aortic hematoma may be of prognostic significance. MRI is currently not commonly used to evaluate acute injury to the thoracic great vessels. However, when an aortic injury is being followed nonoperatively, MRI can be an excellent tool. This is especially true if there is a contraindication to computed tomographic angiography (CTA), such as renal insufficiency.[28]

The following sections discuss specific thoracic aortic and other arterial and venous injuries.

◼ BLUNT AORTIC INJURY

Incidence

The exact incidence of blunt aortic disruption is not known, but it is estimated to be responsible for approximately 8000 deaths each year in the United States.[29] Autopsy series of blunt trauma patients have reported aortic rupture rates from 12% to 23%. Aortic injury is the second most common cause of death in blunt trauma patients, after brain injury.[30] Vesalius in 1557 was the first to describe a patient's death from a ruptured aorta after being thrown from a horse.[31] In large part, however, traumatic blunt aortic injury (BAI) is a condition of modern society. The first successful repair accomplished by Klassen was reported by Passaro and Pace in 1957.[32] Before this report, prominent medical journals advised physicians to avoid surgery for traumatic aortic aneurysms.[33] Parmley and coworkers from the Armed Forces Institute of Pathology first emphasized the lethality of blunt traumatic aortic disruption in 1958 with a combined autopsy and clinical study.[34] The death rate at the accident scene was 85%. Of the patients who arrived at the hospital alive, most died from aortic rupture within a few days.

Pathology

The degree of BAI, first described by Parmley and coworkers,[34] is a continuum from subintimal hemorrhage to total aortic disruption. They classified the lesions into six groups: (1) intimal hemorrhage, (2) intimal hemorrhage with laceration, (3) medial laceration, (4) complete laceration of the aorta, (5) false aneurysm formation, and (6) periaortic hemorrhage. Patients who arrive at the hospital alive have generally sustained incomplete, noncircumferential lesions to the media and intima. The tunica adventitia and mediastinal pleura then prevent free rupture. Remarkably, there are examples in the literature of patients with complete aortic transections who have survived long enough to allow intervention.[35]

Any part of the aorta, from the aortic root to the iliac bifurcation, can be involved with BAI; however, it tends to be confined to a few specific locations. The "classic" site of BAI is in the descending aorta at the isthmus. BAI may also occur in the ascending aorta proximal to the origin of the brachiocephalic, aortic arch, and distal descending or abdominal aorta. Most patients suffer a single injury, but there are examples of multiple BAIs in a single patient.[36] Autopsy series have found that 36% to 54% of BAIs occur at the aortic isthmus, 8% to 27% at the ascending aorta, 8% to 18% at the arch, and 11% to 21% at the distal descending aorta.[3,34,37,38] However, most surgical series demonstrate a much higher percentage of aortic isthmic injuries—80% to 100%—with only 3% to 10% in the ascending aorta, arch, or distal descending aorta. This discrepancy suggests that the peri-isthmic aortic adventitia may be more durable than other segments of the aorta, allowing containment of the rupture. This assertion is contradicted by tensile tests conducted by Lundevall on aortic wall samples.[39]

Pathogenesis

Several different mechanical forces act in the pathogenesis of BAI. The relative importance of these forces remains a subject of debate (Fig. 153-3).

Stretching

The earliest proposed mechanism of BAI was "stretching" of the aortic wall. This was supported by tensile test data demonstrating the inherent weakness of the isthmus, as well as the relative immobility of the fixed distal descending aorta relative to the ascending aorta and arch. The isthmus lies at the junction of these two segments. Arguing against this hypothesis are data showing that the aortic wall is capable of sustaining

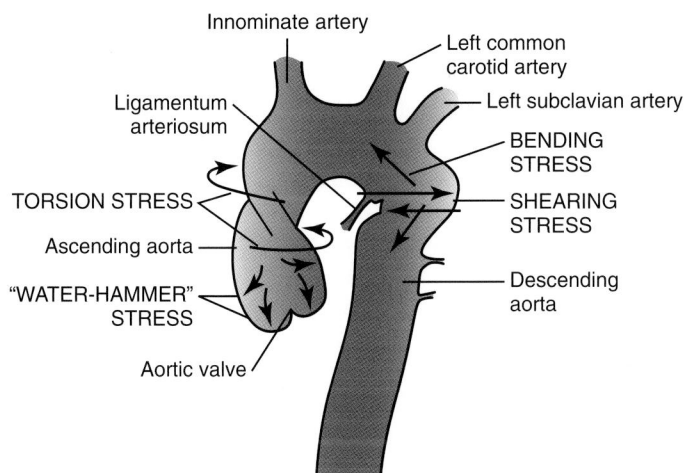

Figure 153-3 Demonstration of the putative forces acting through the aorta during blunt traumatic injury. *(Redrawn from Symbas P. Cardiothoracic Traumas. London: WB Saunders; 1989.)*

strains up to 80% before rupturing. Therefore, the area stretched must be very localized to reach the required strain within the thoracic cage (see Fig. 153-3).[40,41]

Sudden Blood Pressure Elevation

Others have proposed a sudden rise in blood pressure as the cause of BAI. A number of investigators have dismissed this, rationalizing that an isotropic cylinder under pressure ruptures longitudinally rather than transversely. Transverse tears (as seen with BAI) occur only if the transverse strength is more than twice the longitudinal strength.[35] Tensile data from Mohan and Melvin on aortic wall samples demonstrated that the transverse-to-longitudinal strength was almost the required 2:1 ratio. In addition, their test samples consistently failed in a transverse manner.[40] However, these bench tensile data have little clinical relevance. Zehnder in 1956 (as cited in the Kirklin and Barrett-Boyes text) calculated that an intravascular pressure of 2500 mm Hg is necessary to produce rupture of the aorta.[42]

Osseous Pinch

The novel hypothesis reported by Crass and colleagues is that aortic rupture is due to entrapment of the aorta between the anterior thoracic bony structures and the vertebral column.[43] A similar mechanism was reported by Symbas, who proposed that the aorta was forced onto and stretched over the spine in high-impact injuries.[44]

Water-Hammer Effect

When the flow of a noncompressible fluid is suddenly obstructed, a high-pressure reflected wave is generated. If, during a vehicle impact, the aorta is suddenly occluded at the diaphragm, a reflected wave would be generated. The pulse pressure generated by this reflected wave would be greatest at the aortic arch owing to the curvature reflection and further intensification. This phenomenon has been studied in simple analytical models only.[45] Symbas concluded that torsion stress and stress from the water-hammer effect are most likely responsible for injuries to the ascending aorta, and bending and shearing stresses effect the aortic isthmus.[41]

Multivariate Hypotheses

The most likely explanation is that multiple forces, including shear, torsion, and stretch, combined with hydrostatic forces, cause BAIs.[35]

Clinical Presentation

Blunt aortic disruption is caused primarily by motor vehicle accidents and falls. Motor vehicle crashes account for approximately 80% of BAIs. Head-on collisions are the most common mechanism, but side and rear impacts can also cause BAI. Patients with BAI tend to be young (mean age, 39 years). In a review of automobile crashes in the 1990s from the United Kingdom, patients with blunt aortic rupture had a 9% survival rate at the scene and an overall mortality of 98%. Scenarios were variable, but most common was impact from the side. Interestingly, 81% of the people who died were using seat belts, air bags, or both at the time of the crash.[46] Substance abuse is common and is a factor in more than 40% of the motor vehicle crashes resulting in aortic disruption. Seat-belt use decreases risk by a factor of 4. Ejection from a vehicle doubles the risk of aortic disruption.[47,48] For drivers and front-seat passengers, steering wheel deformity is an independent predictor of serious thoracic injury.[49] Even the deployment of air bags in automobile crashes has been associated with BAI—in some instances, at speeds as low as 10 miles per hour. Falls that result in aortic injury are generally from a height of 3 m or greater.

Table 153-1 lists the frequency of injuries associated with BAI, based on data compiled from the 1970s to the late 1990s. The American Association for the Surgery of Trauma compiled prospective data on 274 cases of BAI from 50 trauma centers throughout the United States and Canada. It reported that 50% of patients with BAI have associated brain injury. Other series have reported that the occurrence of associated brain injuries is as low as 30%.[50] Associated chest injuries, pelvic or long-bone fractures, and severe abdominal injuries are also frequently reported.

Diagnosis

All patients with thoracic trauma should have a chest radiograph. Surgeon-performed subxiphoid pericardial ultrasound to evaluate for pericardial fluid should also be routinely performed during the initial trauma evaluation. If there is suspicion of a vascular thoracic injury based on the mechanism of injury, physical examination, or any diagnostic finding, the next test is MDCT of the chest with contrast enhancement. Many times, CT of the chest is combined with head and abdominal CT. It is best to minimize the patient's time in the radiology suite during the diagnostic evaluation in the emergency department.

Management

Timing of Operation

Once the diagnosis of a blunt or penetrating aortic injury is made, immediate repair is recommended. This practice began with the landmark paper from Parmley and coworkers, discussed earlier.[34] Most important was their observation that of the 38 patients who made it to the hospital alive, 23 died of rupture within 7 days of admission. In their conclusions, they stated that to save lives, early diagnosis and immediate surgical intervention are required. However, in the 1990s Pate and associates pointed out that the observations by Parmley's group had been made in the "pre-surgical era" and that the injury pattern had changed since then.[51] Rupture at the aortic isthmus was reported in only 45% of Parmley's cases, whereas the percentage in recent surgical series is generally over 80%.[52-54] These findings seemed to indicate a change in cause. Motor vehicle crash is now the most common mechanism for BAI. Moreover, injuries at the aortic isthmus seem to be more stable than injuries at other locations of the thoracic aorta.[7]

Surgical management in patients with BAI is challenging, and operative mortality rates may be as high as 30%. Multiple associated severe injuries are common and are most likely the cause of this excess morbidity and mortality. Because of this reality, immediate operative repair may not be possible. The Western Association of Trauma multicenter study group identified age and preexisting cardiac disease as major contributing factors in operative mortality. That group concluded that patients may benefit from a longer preoperative workup or nonoperative management, noting that there was no difference in outcome between stable patients who had operations immediately and those whose surgery was delayed longer than 24 hours.[55]

Patients who may benefit from initial medical management and delayed surgical repair include those with (1) cardiac risk factors, such as segmental wall motion abnormality on echocardiography, ongoing angina, prior coronary artery bypass graft, and need for inotropic support; (2) head injury, such as abnormal CT (hemorrhage or edema); (3) pulmonary injury, such as pulmonary contusion on imaging combined with any one of the following: Pao_2/Fio_2 less than 300 mm Hg, positive end-expiratory pressure requirement of 7.5 cm H_2O to maintain adequate oxygenation, or inability to tolerate single-lung ventilation; (4) coagulopathy, including extensive nonsurgical bleeding, international normalized ratio greater than 1.5, or laboratory evidence of consumption, such as increased fibrin-split products or platelets less than 100,000; and (5) severe

Table 153-1 Injuries Associated with Blunt Aortic Injury

Injury	Number of Patients (N = 274) (%)
Closed head injury	140* (51)
Multiple rib fractures	123 (46)
Flail chest	34 (12)
Pulmonary contusion	103 (38)
Myocardial contusion	10 (4)
Diaphragm rupture	20 (7)
Splenic injury	39 (14)
Liver injury	61 (22)
Small bowel injury	19 (7)
Other abdominal injury	38 (14)
Spinal cord injury	10 (4)
Pelvic injury	84 (31)
Femoral injury	67 (24)
Tibial injury	60 (22)
Upper extremity injury	54 (20)
Maxillofacial injury	36 (13)
Cervical spine injury	12 (4)
Thoracic spine injury	11 (4)
Lumbar spine injury	10 (4)
None	0 (0)

*Thirty-four patients (24%) had intracranial hemorrhage.
From Fabian T, Richardson J, Croce M. Prospective study of blunt aortic injury: Multicenter Trial of the American Association for the Surgery of Trauma. *J Trauma*. 1997;42:374-380.

abdominal solid organ injury and pelvic fractures, when the use of heparin may need to be temporarily avoided.[55,56]

It is generally recognized that patients admitted with blunt traumatic aortic injuries fall into two distinct categories: stable and unstable. The hemodynamically unstable group has been associated with an all-cause mortality exceeding 90%. In the hemodynamically stable group, there is generally time for a workup and staging of any intervention; mortality in this group is as low as 25%.[57] Fabian and colleagues demonstrated that an aggressive antihypertensive regimen can significantly reduce the rate of rupture in BAIs.[58-60] They recommend maintenance of systolic blood pressure below 100 mm Hg or mean arterial pressure less than 80 mm Hg and control of the heart rate (<100 beats/min) using an intravenous beta blocker such as esmolol or labetalol. A vasodilator can be added if a satisfactory blood pressure is not achieved with beta blockade alone.[58-60] As has been well described, the combination of a beta blocker and a vasodilator reduces aortic wall shearing force by lowering the ventricular ejection dynamic (dP/dt).

Factors that may cause the abandonment of a delayed or nonoperative strategy for BAI include a rapid increase in the size of a mediastinal hematoma or pleural effusion, anuria persisting for more than 6 hours, limb ischemia, or the free leak of contrast medium within the thorax. Transient hypotension in association with these factors is an ominous sign and indicates impending rupture.[61]

Surgical Repair

Technique. Standard vascular principles of proximal and distal control facilitate a precise hemostatic repair. Clamp sites are selected, and the patient is heparinized. For BAI of the aortic isthmus, a fourth interspace left thoracotomy is usually selected, and the proximal clamp is placed between the left common carotid artery and the left subclavian artery. A separate clamp site is obtained for the left subclavian artery. Frequently, generous lymphatics can be seen overlying the subclavian artery. These should be ligated before division. Careful attention is paid to the location of the phrenic and vagus nerves, which can be difficult to ascertain in the midst of a large hematoma. Sharp division of the ligamentum arteriosum, followed by blunt dissection between the proximal right pulmonary artery and the lesser curve of the aortic arch proximal to the left subclavian artery, can facilitate proximal clamp site exposure. Knowledge of esophageal and bronchial anatomy is paramount to avoid injuries. The distal clamp is placed as proximal as possible to maximize spinal cord blood flow.

In general, some form of distal aortic perfusion is used during the repair of injuries to the descending thoracic aorta. For example, the most expeditious technique with blunt injury of the aortic isthmus is the use of left atrial (via the left inferior pulmonary vein)–to–distal descending aortic bypass (Fig. 153-4). In the rare event that a proximal clamp site is untenable, the patient is placed on full cardiopulmonary bypass through the groin (right atrium–to–left femoral artery bypass). This technique allows for maximal control of perfu-

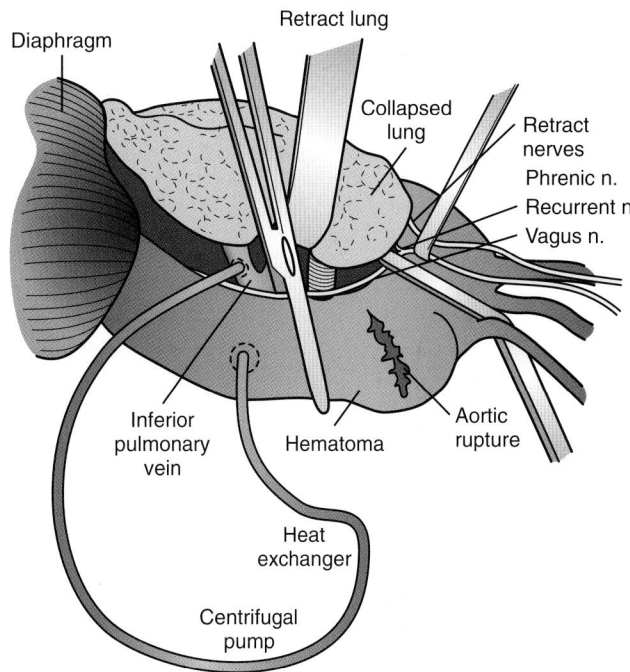

Figure 153-4 Intraoperative setup for distal aortic perfusion using left atrial–to–descending aortic bypass.

sion and oxygenation and the ability to perform circulatory arrest. If circulatory arrest is necessary, careful venting of the left ventricle is critical during cooling and rewarming (venting via the left atrium is usually adequate, but occasionally the ventricle is vented directly via the left ventricular apex). TEE is useful in general, but it is especially important to rule out concomitant cardiac contusion or valvular insufficiency, which can complicate perfusion strategies.

Before the initiation of partial bypass, an intravenous cocktail of agents to decrease cardiac dysrhythmias and decrease spinal cord injury is given (MgSO$_4$ 1 g, lidocaine 200 mg, and Solu-Medrol 250 mg). Following de-airing, partial bypass is initiated, maintaining proximal mean aortic pressure about 10 mm Hg higher than distal aortic pressure (70 to 80 mm Hg proximal/50 to 60 mm Hg distal) and cooling to 32°C. Generally, flows of 2 to 3 L/min are adequate. If perfusion in the circuit is satisfactory, the proximal and distal clamps are placed. The periaortic hematoma can then be entered in a controlled manner. Devitalized aortic tissue is débrided, and primary repair versus interposition graft is contemplated. A 3-0 or 4-0 Prolene suture with an SH needle facilitates a quick anastomosis with generous bites. Re-enforcement of the anastomosis with polytetrafluoroethylene felt and the judicious use of Bioglue is recommended. It is important to preserve the aortic adventitia and incorporate it into the anastomosis. Remember that the periaortic tissues are the aortic surgeon's "friend."

If a significant portion of the descending aorta requires replacement, two or three sets of intercostals (usually in the T6 to L1 region) are reimplanted. This can be done with a separate side graft or with a Carrel patch technique. Fortunately, this is rarely necessary in the setting of BAI. Once

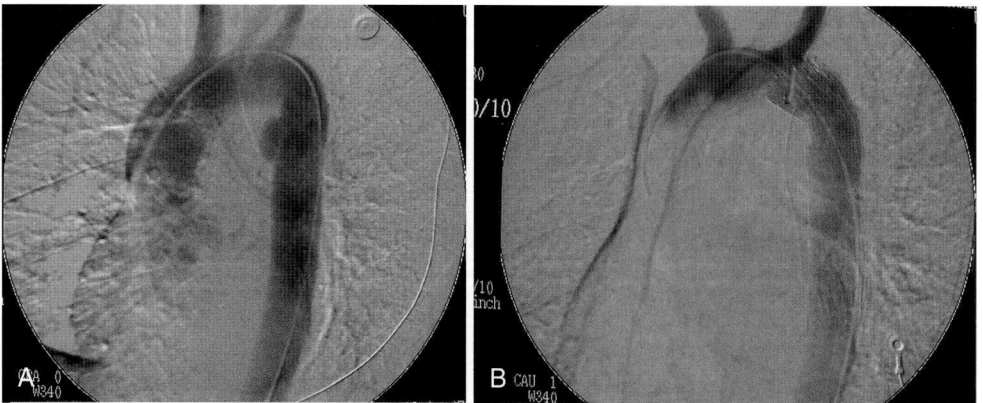

Figure 153-5 Traumatic aortic transection before (**A**) and after (**B**) endovascular stent-graft repair. The stent's proximal margin is distal to the left subclavian artery.

clamps are removed, rewarming is commenced. In general, warming is stopped at a core temperature of 37° C. This usually results in patients arriving in the intensive care unit at 35.5° C to 36° C. Gentle rewarming is then restarted.

Other than the execution of a technically sound vascular repair, spinal cord protection and distal end-organ protection are the predominant concerns during operative repair of a blunt injury to the aortic isthmus or descending thoracic aorta (Fig. 153-5). Spinal cord injury can occur either during operative repair or in the postoperative period. Interruption of blood flow with aortic cross-clamping is thought to be the causative event. Hypertension proximal to the aortic cross-clamp will occur if no measures are taken to unload the left ventricle. This hypertension can result in the production of increased spinal fluid and may decrease spinal cord perfusion.[62] Delayed paraplegia can manifest up to 21 days following repair. This delayed response is believed to be from intraoperative hypotension followed by reperfusion injury to the cord. The duration of cross-clamping is related to the duration of ischemia.[62]

Location of the aortic cross-clamp is an important factor in preserving spinal cord perfusion. Commonly, the proximal aortic clamp site in an open aortic transection repair is between the left common carotid artery and the left subclavian artery. With application of a clamp proximal to the left subclavian, important collaterals to the spinal cord (e.g., the internal mammary artery) are occluded. Active augmentation of distal perfusion can minimize spinal cord ischemia while a beveled anastomosis incorporating the left subclavian artery is fashioned.

Spinal Cord Protection. The optimal method of spinal cord protection during repair is a source of continued debate in the surgical literature. Traditionally a "clamp and sew" approach has been used. However, it has become clear that cross-clamp times greater than 30 minutes are associated with paraplegia rates of 15% to 30%.[63]

In general, spinal cord perfusion is dependent on radicular arteries, which arise from the posterior intercostal and lumbar arteries. Collateral blood supply to the cord is supplemented from the left subclavian artery and internal iliac arteries.

Because the blood supply to the spinal cord is somewhat variable and the risk of paraplegia is difficult to predict in any given patient, a spinal protective strategy is important in all patients. In the lower thorax and upper abdomen, the anterior spinal artery is less well developed. This increases the reliance on adjacent intercostal and lumbar arteries. In 25% of patients, the artery of Adamkiewicz (which can arise anywhere from T8 to L4) is essential for lower thoracic spinal cord perfusion owing to discontinuity of the anterior spinal artery.[64,65]

Important causative factors of postoperative paraplegia are the duration of cross-clamping, the level and length of aorta excluded by the cross-clamp, the perfusion pressure of the aorta distal to the cross-clamp, increased cerebrospinal fluid pressure, total-body and spinal cord temperature, systemic arterial hypotension, and the number of intercostal arteries ligated during surgery. Of note, patients with traumatic aortic injury do not have a well-developed collateral circulation to the spinal cord, in contrast to patients with coarctation and chronic aneurysmal disease of the aorta.[51]

Multiple adjuncts have been used to reduce the incidence of paraplegia following the repair of descending thoracic and thoracoabdominal pathology. The great variety of techniques is a testament to the complex pathophysiology involved. Generalized and local hypothermia,[66,67] steroids,[68] naloxone hydrochloride,[69] barbiturates,[70] papaverine hydrochloride,[71] reattachment of intercostal arteries,[72] and cerebrospinal fluid drainage[73] have all been used for this purpose. Neurologic outcomes are also undoubtedly influenced by the extent of aortic injury, cross-clamping times, and concomitant medical issues such as renal insufficiency, systemic hypertension, and diabetes.[74]

Spinal cord ischemia is the result of the interaction of several factors: cord perfusion, oxygenation, metabolic rate, reperfusion injury, and microcirculation patency. Svensson and Loop in 1988 proposed a model of ischemic time versus deficit risk to assess various techniques.[75] Techniques that decrease spinal cord injury shift the curve to the right; conversely, a left shift is harmful (Fig. 153-6). For example, the effects of active systemic cooling, cerebrospinal fluid drainage, and intrathecal papaverine infusion cause progressive shifts to the right.[71]

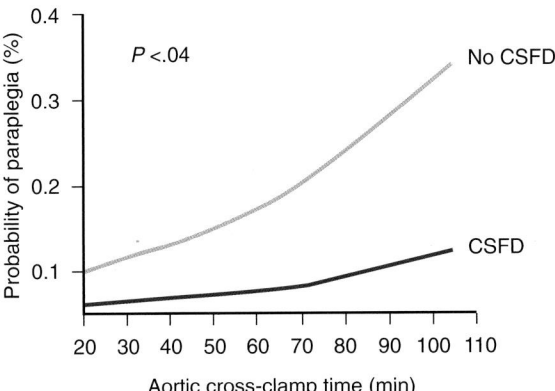

Figure 153-6 Logistic regression curves show a reduction in the risk of paraplegia or paraparesis associated with cerebrospinal fluid drainage (CSFD). *(From Coselli J, LeMaire S, Koksoy C, et al. Cerebrospinal fluid drainage reduced paraplegia after thoracoabdominal aortic aneurysm repair: results of a randomized clinical trial.* J Vasc Surg. *2002;35:631-639.)*

The passive augmentation of distal circulation to decrease postoperative paraplegia was first reported by Gott in 1972.[76] Subsequently, Molina and coworkers published experimental data indicating that the passive flow provided by the Gott shunt was inadequate to consistently prevent paraplegia.[77] The length of the tube and its inner diameter were constraints to adequate flow. To address these limits imposed by the laws of fluid dynamics, Oliver and colleagues used heparin-bonded tubing between the left atrium and the femoral artery and a centrifugal pump to actively augment distal perfusion. In their first nine cases, there were no instances of paraplegia.[78] Currently, surgeons are debating the relative merits of left atrium–femoral artery bypass (LA-FA, or left heart bypass) versus femoral artery–femoral vein (FA-FV) partial cardiopulmonary bypass techniques for the prevention of postoperative paraplegia.

Left Atrium–Femoral Artery Bypass. The believed advantages of LA-FA bypass are left ventricular unloading, distal perfusion, and minimal or no heparinization required in LA-FA circuits. Unloading of the left heart can be especially important in the setting of a concomitant myocardial contusion. If 1 L/min flow and a distal aortic pressure of 50 mm Hg are maintained, systemic heparin is not required in most LA-FA circuits. However, there have been reports of posterior cerebral infarctions associated with nonheparinized LA-FA circuits when the cross-clamping times exceeded 30 minutes.[79] Because of this, most surgeons use 10,000 units of heparin if clamp times are expected to exceed 30 minutes.[80] The two main disadvantages of LA-FA bypass are occasional injury to the left atrial appendage or pulmonary veins and occasional inadequate pump flows.

Femoral Artery–Femoral Vein Bypass. FA-FV bypass involves partial cardiopulmonary bypass using a pump and oxygenator with full heparinization. FA-FV bypass minimizes the occurrence of hypoxia, which can be critical in the setting of one-lung ventilation, pulmonary contusion, and pulmonary insufficiency. In addition, FA-FV bypass provides excellent distal perfusion while decreasing preload to the heart. The main disadvantage of FA-FV bypass is the need for full heparinization. A retrospective analysis by Weisman and colleagues in 2006 showed a higher paraplegia rate in patients repaired with LA-FA bypass versus FA-FV bypass.[80] This difference, though not significant, occurred even with decreased cross-clamping times in the LA-FA group. Full heparinization should be used cautiously in multitrauma patients, and it has been associated with increased mortality in some series.[81]

Thoracic Endovascular Stent-Graft Repair

Even with recent advances in surgical and anesthetic techniques, the open repair of traumatic aortic injuries is still associated with significant morbidity and mortality. Because of this, the use of thoracic endovascular aortic repair (TEVAR) of BAI is currently being investigated.[82] Endovascular stent-grafts have been used for the definitive treatment of infrarenal aortic aneurysms since 1991, with excellent results. Stimulated by this success, endovascular technology is now being applied to diseases of the thoracic aorta.[83-89]

Indications. The most useful application of endovascular technology appears to be for patients with severe nonaortic blunt injuries who would otherwise be denied surgical repair of the aortic injury. However, TEVAR in this group of severely injured patients may not significantly improve overall survival, with these patients eventually dying from their nonaortic traumatic injuries. More evidence and long-term follow-up are needed before definitive conclusions can be made.

Technique. The current generation of thoracic stent-grafts was designed for aneurysmal disease processes. Because the aorta is usually of normal size in an acute transection, thoracic stent-grafts are occasionally too large for endovascular repair. With aortas less than 24 mm in diameter, current devices that have received Food and Drug Administration approval are inadequate. In these situations, extension cuffs from abdominal aneurysm supplies and peripheral vascular stents have been used. Caution is required when considering the off-label use of such products in aortic trauma patients.[90]

In emergent and urgent cases, the anatomy of the vertebral, carotid, and vertebrobasilar system usually is not known. Coverage of the left subclavian artery is frequently required in the acute situation and is generally well tolerated. Mild ischemic symptoms may be noted post repair. In these patients a left subclavian–to–left common carotid bypass can be performed in a later procedure.[86] Arm ischemia following repair of acute aortic transections is relatively rare and generally well tolerated. The main issue, however, is the chance of increased ischemic damage to the posterior cerebral circulation with vertebral artery occlusion.

Section **19** Trauma and Acute Limb Ischemia

Outcome

Surgical Repair

Multiple studies have reported the safety of delayed surgical repair of BAI in multitrauma patients by first addressing the life-threatening injury or adopting a nonoperative strategy. Maggisano and colleagues reported a 90% survival rate following delayed aortic repair in 44 patients with severe concomitant injuries or sepsis.[56] Holmes and coworkers, in a subgroup analysis of 30 patients with delayed management, found 15 patients managed nonoperatively.[57] (Delayed management was defined as not performing operative repair within 24 hours of injury.) Three patients exhibited progression of their aortic injuries within 5 days of the event, and two died. Of the 15 patients managed with a delayed operation, three deaths occurred (one rupture and two intraoperative arrests). The 15 patients managed without an operation were followed for a mean of 2.5 years. Ten patients survived without the need for further surgery; five had complete resolution, and five were left with radiographically stable pseudoaneurysms. The five deaths in the nonoperated patients were all due to head trauma. The authors concluded that selected patients with multiple severe injuries or high-risk premorbid conditions can undergo delayed aortic repair or nonoperative management. They did, however, mandate serial radiographic examinations during the first week of hospitalization.

The results of various spinal cord protection strategies during open repair are mixed. The benefits of "active" distal perfusion during aortic cross-clamping in reducing spinal cord injury have been supported by multiple surgical series.[91-93] Forbes and associates, in a review of 30 patients who underwent repair of descending aortic transections, reported no neurologic deficits in the 21 patients who had distal perfusion while 4 of the 9 patients who underwent clamp and sew had new neurologic deficits.[92] Read and colleagues subsequently reported a retrospective series of 16 consecutive patients with descending aortic disruptions repaired with left heart bypass and a centrifugal pump.[93] They demonstrated an 88% operative survival and no cases of paraplegia. Fabian and coworkers reported prospective data on 207 cases of stable BAI undergoing repair.[30] Twelve of the 73 patients treated with a clamp-and-sew procedure developed paraplegia, whereas only 6 of the 134 patients treated with left heart bypass had postoperative paraplegia ($P < .004$). The authors concluded that distal aortic perfusion significantly lowers paraplegia rates compared to a clamp-and-sew approach (Fig. 153-7).

Von Oppell and colleagues, in a meta-analysis of spinal cord protection during aortic surgery in the absence of collateral circulation, noted that the risk of paraplegia increased progressively as the cross-clamp time lengthened if simple aortic cross-clamping was used.[81] They noted a cutoff time of 30 minutes of cross-clamping, after which the rate of paraplegia began to increase markedly if no method of distal perfusion was used. The rates of paraplegia in their meta-analysis were 19% with simple cross-clamp application, 8.2% if passive distal perfusion was used, and 2.3% if active augmentation of distal aortic perfusion was used ($P < .00001$ versus simple cross-clamp application or passive shunts). However, mortal-

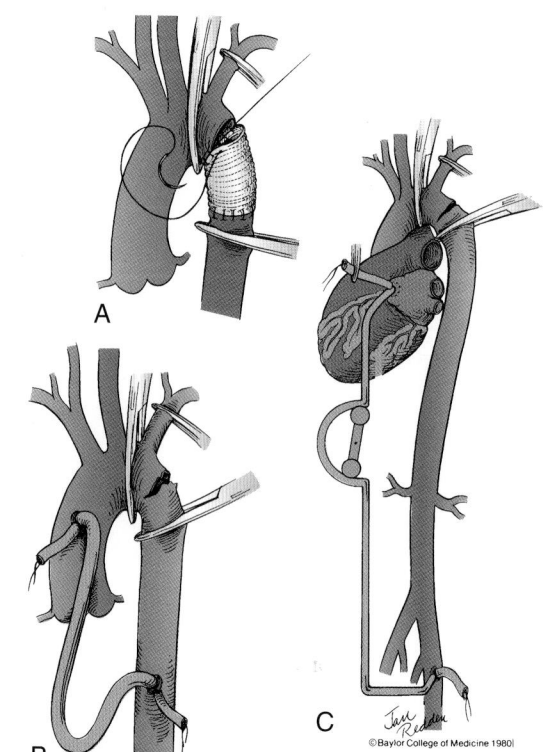

Figure 153-7 Various techniques for spinal cord protection during open repair of the descending thoracic aorta. **A,** Clamp and sew. **B,** Passive distal aortic perfusion. **C,** Active distal aortic perfusion.

ity was higher in multitrauma patients who were perfused distally with methods requiring full systemic heparinization (18.2%) compared with methods not requiring full heparinization (11.9%; $P < .01$).

Most individual series have failed to demonstrate a clear benefit of active distal perfusion due to poor statistical power.[52] Some authors still advocate the clamp-and-sew technique. Sweeney and associates reported a series of 71 patients undergoing repair of traumatic aortic injuries with an average cross-clamping time of 24 minutes, overall mortality of 12%, and a paraplegia rate of 1.5%.[94] It appears that in experienced hands, good results can be obtained with a simple clamp-and-sew technique. In actual surgical practice, it is impossible to predict whether a repair can be performed in less than 30 minutes. Of note, in a prospective analysis of North American repairs of BAI reported by Fabian and coworkers in 1997, only 33% were performed in less than 30 minutes.[30]

Endovascular Stent-Graft Repair

The early and midterm results of TEVAR for BAI are promising. However, these repairs must be followed with serial imaging, unlike traditional open repairs. Long-term follow-up data are needed to better define the role of TEVAR in acute aortic transections. It seems apparent that even if the long-term success is not equivalent to that of open repair, the ability to convert an emergent or urgent intervention to a later elective repair is beneficial to multitrauma patients.

Multiple series with limited patient numbers and limited follow-up indicate that TEVAR is a viable alternative to open repair for traumatic aortic injuries. In fact, perioperative mortality and paraplegia rates appear to compare favorably with those of traditional open repair, despite increased intercostal artery occlusion and more frequent coverage of the left subclavian artery with TEVAR. The reason for this is unclear, but it may be due to the fact that mean arterial pressures can be run higher after stent repair than after open repair.

Leurs and colleagues, in an analysis of the EuroSTAR database, reported on 50 patients treated for traumatic aortic transections; they cited an operative mortality of 6% and a paraplegia rate of 6%.[95] Reed and coworkers recently reviewed their experience with traumatic transections over a 5-year period from 2000 to 2005.[96] A total of 51 patients presented with the diagnosis of traumatic transection. Twenty-seven patients (52%) died before intervention. Of the remaining 24 patients, 9 patients underwent emergent conventional open repair. Thirteen patients underwent delayed TEVAR, with a mean interval from diagnosis to treatment of 6 days. Technical success with complete exclusion of the transection was achieved in all 13 patients. Thirty-day mortality was 23% (n = 3). Tehrani and coworkers reported on 30 patients with traumatic aortic transection and severe concomitant nonaortic injuries treated with TEVAR.[97] Technical success was 100%, with angiographic evidence of complete exclusion of the disruption. There were two perioperative deaths and no incidence of paraplegia. With a mean follow-up of 11.6 months, there was no evidence of endoleak, stent migration, or late pseudoaneurysm formation. Other smaller series have demonstrated similar findings, with a mean follow-up of up to 21 months.[86,98-100] Perioperative mortality rates ranged from 0% to 11%, with no incidence of paraplegia. All endovascular stent-graft deployment was performed using no heparin or low-dose heparin. Stroke was rare, with one series reporting one patient suffering a cerebrovascular accident.[86,89,98]

CHRONIC TRAUMATIC AORTIC ANEURYSM

Chronic traumatic aortic aneurysms are rarely found in the clinical setting, and natural history data are incomplete. Management guidelines are not well delineated in the literature. Most believe that if such lesions are detected more than 2 years after the initial trauma, they can be followed for the onset of symptoms or radiologic changes. Thus, once the acute period is over, their management is similar to that of a true thoracic aneurysm.[101-103] Rarely, chronic post-traumatic aneurysms have been reported to form fistulae to the pulmonary artery[104] and bronchus.[105,106] Symptomatic compression of mediastinal and hilar structures has also been reported.[107]

Open repair of chronic traumatic aneurysms has a mortality rate of 5% to 18% and a morbidity rate of 11% to 50%. More recently, endovascular repair of chronic aortic injuries has been performed using covered stents. Short-term mortality and morbidity are improved with aortic stenting versus open repair, but improvements in long-term outcomes remain to be seen.[108] Midterm data on the endovascular management

of descending aortic aneurysms are promising. Significant reductions in operative mortality have been seen with endovascular approaches to thoracic aneurysms. In addition, reintervention rates and paraplegia rates are similar in open and endovascular cohorts.[109]

NONISTHMIC AORTIC AND ARTERIAL LACERATION

Ascending Aorta and Transverse Arch

Rupture of the ascending and transverse aorta is uncommon, but the exact incidence is unknown owing to the lethality of these injuries. A widened mediastinum and cardiac tamponade are frequently associated with ascending aortic ruptures. Repair of ascending aortic injuries requires full heparinization via a median sternotomy and frequently the institution of cardiopulmonary bypass (Fig. 153-8). Management of the aortic tear may be primary or with interposition graft. Special attention should be paid to the status of the aortic valve. Injuries to the aortic arch may require hypothermic circulatory arrest and associated antegrade and retrograde cerebral perfusion techniques. Survival depends primarily on the severity of associated injuries.[110,111]

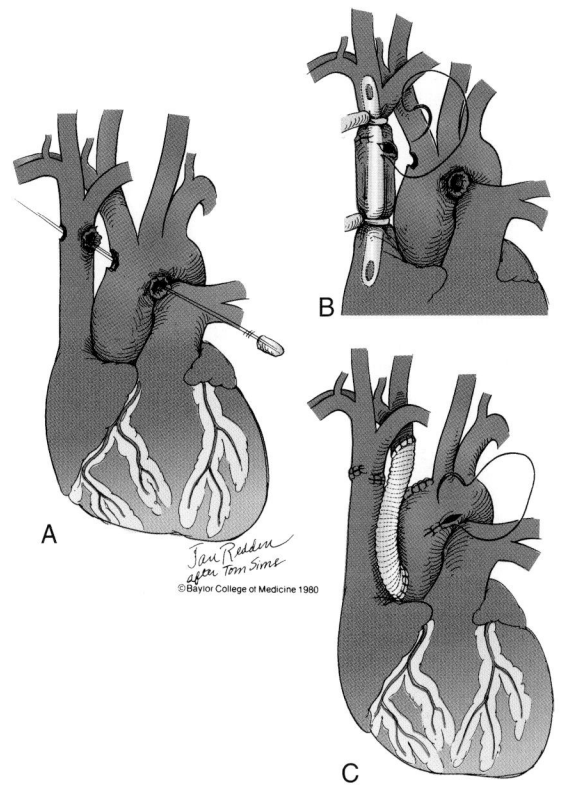

Figure 153-8 Penetrating injury to the superior vena cava and ascending aorta. Before repair, full heparinization should be achieved, and cardiopulmonary bypass should be considered. **A,** Injury to the superior vena cava, innominate artery, and ascending aorta. **B,** Repair of the superior vena cava. **C,** Repair of the innominate artery and ascending aorta. *(From Baylor College of Medicine, 1980.)*

Innominate Artery

Innominate artery injuries can generally be repaired via a median sternotomy with a right cervical extension when necessary. Blunt injury typically involves the base of the innominate artery. This is most expeditiously repaired with a bypass to the distal innominate artery from the ascending aorta, followed by oversewing of the innominate base (Fig. 153-9). Division of the innominate vein is occasionally required for exposure. Shunts or cardiopulmonary bypass should not be needed. Avoidance of the injured area until completion of the bypass leads to a technically easier repair.[112]

Left Common Carotid Artery

The surgical approach to injuries of the proximal left carotid artery mirrors that of the innominate artery—a sternotomy with a left cervical extension if needed. With injuries of the left carotid origin, bypass graft repair is generally preferred over end-to-end reanastomosis.[5] The management of a carotid injury in the setting of neurologic disturbances is controversial. Generally, if the patient is evaluated soon after injury, revascularization is recommended because hypotension (rather than ischemic infarct) is the most likely cause of morbidity.[113] In young trauma patients the use of shunts is gener-

ally not necessary, except when profound hypotension is present or when concomitant clamping of the innominate or right carotid artery is necessary.[114] Chapter 152 (Vascular Trauma: Head and Neck) contains additional information on carotid injuries.

Recently, traumatic carotid lesions have been managed with endovascular techniques such as the implantation of balloons or porous or covered stents; embolic materials such as coils or glue have also been used. An endovascular approach is especially useful for extensive lesions with involvement near the skull base, where obtaining proximal and distal vascular control may result in increased morbidity.[115] The goal of endovascular therapy is the elimination of a fistula, aneurysm, or stenosis while preserving native flow patterns to the brain. There have been multiple reports on the successful management of traumatic carotid injuries with endovascular techniques.[115-119] Specifically, the use of covered and porous stents has revolutionized the treatment of extracranial carotid lesions. The use of stents introduces new considerations, however, such as the probability of late in-stent thrombosis. The administration of postprocedural medications such as aspirin and clopidogrel can minimize the incidence of these complications.[120]

Subclavian Vessels

Injuries to the subclavian vessels are usually caused by penetrating wounds. Subclavian vascular injuries require preoperative imaging (generally CTA) for appropriate incision planning. Injuries to the right subclavian are best addressed via a median sternotomy with a right cervical extension. Proximal control of left-sided subclavian injuries can be obtained via a left anterior thoracotomy. A separate supraclavicular incision can be used for distal control. These two incisions can be connected with a sternotomy to facilitate exposure (the "book" thoracotomy; Fig. 153-10). This incision should be used sparingly because of reports of postoperative "causalgia" neurologic symptoms.[121,122] In addition, the second or third portion of the subclavian artery can usually be exposed without the need for clavicular resection or sternotomy. When necessary, a clavicular resection can be performed without a sternotomy. After completion of the repair, the clavicular fragment can be resecured.[123]

Endovascular approaches to innominate, intrathoracic carotid, and subclavian arterial injuries have been described.[115,124-127] The long-term results of this approach are not known, but it can be an attractive option in a multitrauma patient who is not a good candidate for traditional open repair. Additional information on subclavian injuries can be found in Chapter 152 (Vascular Trauma: Head and Neck).

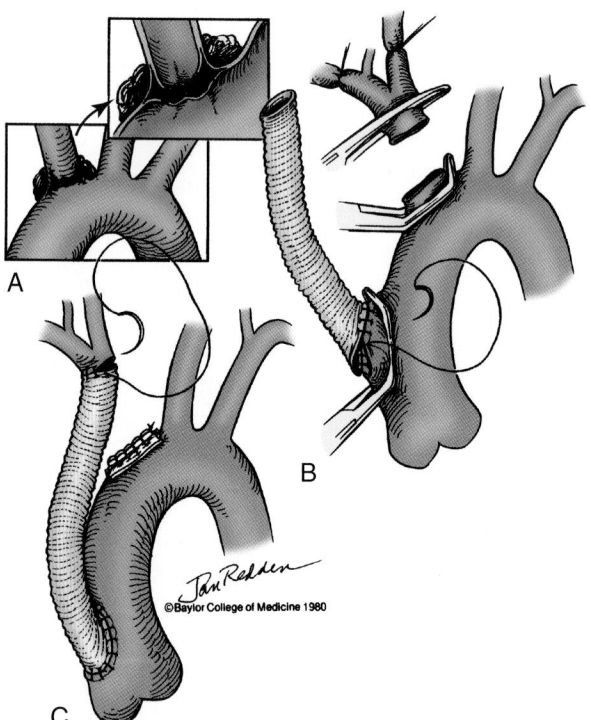

Figure 153-9 Bypass principle used to repair blunt injury to the proximal innominate artery–aortic arch. **A,** Blunt injury to the innominate artery. **B,** Vascular control of the injury and creation of a proximal ascending aorta–innominate bypass anastomosis. **C,** Completed ascending aorta–innominate bypass with oversewing of the innominate artery stump. *(From Baylor College of Medicine, 1980.)*

■ PULMONARY VASCULAR INJURY

Pulmonary vascular injuries are rare in blunt trauma. In a series of 585 fatal traffic accidents, the thoracic aorta was involved in 46 patients and the pulmonary veins in 5 patients.[128,129] Sudden deceleration may cause tears at the

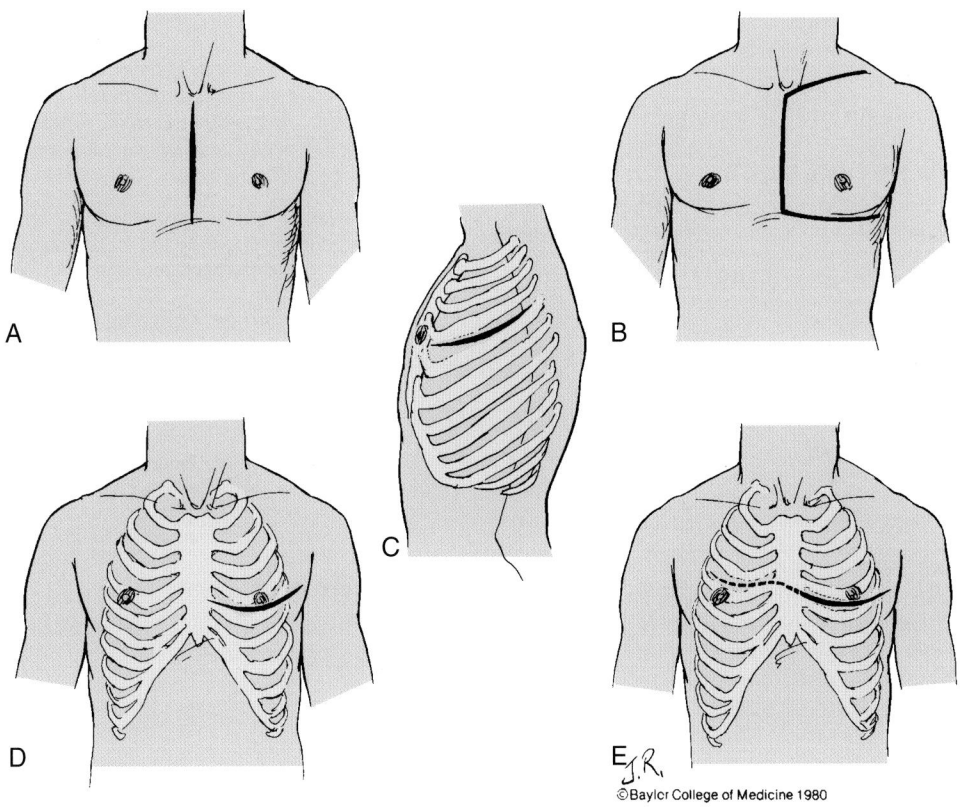

Figure 153-10 Incisions for thoracic trauma. **A,** Median sternotomy. **B,** "Book" thoracotomy (more commonly, the sternal connection is not needed). **C,** Posterolateral thoracotomy. **D,** Anterolateral thoracotomy (the "utility" incision for patients in extremis). **E,** Extension of the anterolateral thoracotomy to the opposite chest as a "clamshell" incision. *(From Baylor College of Medicine, 1980.)*

points of anatomic fixation, such as the junction of the pulmonary veins and the left atrium.

Massive hemothorax on presentation or continued chest tube output greater than 200 mL/hr should prompt consideration of thoracotomy. Because the pulmonary circulation is a low-pressure system, patients with significant injuries can maintain transient hemodynamic stability. When filled with blood, the pleural space may generate modest positive pressure, impeding further bleeding and acting as a blood reservoir. In this situation, the abrupt institution of closed-suction drainage of the pleural space may induce a rapid loss of intravascular volume. Therefore, in the setting of a large hemothorax, physicians must be prepared for a rapid thoracotomy if hemodynamic instability ensues following chest tube placement with substantial output. Following thoracotomy, pulmonary venous bleeding can usually be controlled by digital pressure and hilar clamping if needed. Careful attention to the entrainment of air in the left atrium must be maintained at all times when dealing with lacerations of the pulmonary veins.

Injuries to the pulmonary veins may be accompanied by cardiac, pulmonary arterial, and bronchial injuries.[128,130-133] Some of these injuries may remain undiagnosed during the initial treatment period, resulting in arteriovenous fistulae and pseudoaneurysms, necessitating later repair.[134-137]

VENA CAVA INJURY

Blunt injury to the inferior vena cava (IVC) or superior vena cava (SVC) is rare but can be lethal. Mortality rates up to 50% have been reported. Rapid deceleration and a mobile heart can cause lacerations of both the SVC and IVC. The injuries resulting from blunt trauma tend to occur at pericardial reflections, where the cavae are fixed and vulnerable to sheer forces (e.g., the diaphragm).[138-140] Associated retrohepatic IVC and hepatic vein injuries are not uncommon. Another proposed mechanism of caval injuries is downward deceleration of the liver, resulting in IVC laceration.[141] Other have proposed the Valsalva effect and sudden abdominal compression as a cause of caval rupture.[138] Penetrating injuries to the cavae are more common, but their location is not predictable.

Diagnostic evaluation of caval injuries should follow the Advanced Trauma Life Support (ATLS) protocol, with a chest radiograph followed by surgeon-performed subxiphoid echocardiography in the trauma resuscitation unit. CT can identify pericardial fluid, but the test of choice is ultrasound, either transthoracic or transesophageal.[142]

Repair of these injuries is usually straightforward and can be done without cardiopulmonary bypass. However, with extensive injuries to the SVC, IVC, or retrohepatic vena cava, atrial-caval shunts and cardiopulmonary bypass with femoral venous drainage may be necessary.[143] Stenosis must be avoided when repairing the cavae. Native or bovine pericardial patch angioplasty should be used liberally to prevent difficult problems such as SVC syndrome or IVC occlusion or stenosis.

SELECTED KEY REFERENCES

Appoo JJ, Moser WG, Fairman RM, Cornelius KF, Pochettino A, Woo EY, Kurichi JE, Carpenter JP, Bavaria JE. Thoracic aortic stent grafting: improving results with newer generation investigational devices. *J Thorac Cardiovasc Surg.* 2006;131:1087-1094.
Early TEVAR results from a single busy aortic center.

Fabian T, Richardson J, Croce M. Prospective study of blunt aortic injury: Multicenter Trial of the American Association for the Surgery of Trauma. *J Trauma.* 1997;42:374-380.
Prospective multicenter trial of BAI with important clinical management implications—specifically, the use of active distal aortic perfusion during repair.

Mattox K, Feliciano D, Beal A. Five thousand seven hundred and sixty cardiovascular injuries in 4459 patients; epidemiologic evolution 1958-1988. *Ann Surg.* 1989;209:698-705.
This extensive civilian series presents epidemiologic profiles that are distinctly different from military reports and serves as a guide for current trauma center and health planners.

Mirvis S. Thoracic vascular injury. *Radiol Clin North Am.* 2006;44: 181-197.
CTA is the screening study of choice for aortic injury; it has replaced thoracic angiography almost completely for screening patients with chest trauma. Angiography remains a potential problem solver for uncertain CT results and for planning and guiding endovascular aortic stent-graft placement.

Nagy K, Fabian T, Rodman G, Fulda G, Rodriguez A, Mirvis S. Guidelines for the diagnosis and management of blunt aortic injury: an EAST Practice Management Guidelines Work Group. *J Trauma.* 2000;48:1128-1143.
Consensus guidelines for the management of BAI.

Symbas P. *Cardiothoracic Traumas.* London: WB Saunders; 1989.
Excellent overview of cardiothoracic trauma by an excellent clinician and investigator.

Von Oppell U, Dunne T, DeGroot M, Zilla P. Traumatic aortic rupture: twenty-year meta analysis of mortality and risk of paraplegia. *Ann Thorac Surg.* 1994;58:585-593.
Important meta-analysis of various management techniques in BAI.

REFERENCES

The reference list can be found on the companion Expert Consult Web site at *www.expertconsult.com.*

CHAPTER 154

Vascular Trauma: Abdominal

Demetrios Demetriades and Kenji Inaba

Abdominal vascular injuries are the most common cause of death after penetrating abdominal trauma. The surgical exposure and associated intra-abdominal injuries may challenge the skills and judgment of even the most experienced surgeons. Rapid transportation to a trauma center, early recognition of the injuries, early surgical intervention, excellent knowledge of the anatomy, and good surgical judgment are critical for the patient's survival.

▮ SURGICAL ANATOMY

For vascular trauma purposes, the abdomen is conventionally divided into three anatomic areas (Fig. 154-1):

- *Zone 1*, which includes the midline retroperitoneum extending from the aortic hiatus to the sacral promontory. This zone is subdivided into the supramesocolic and inframesocolic areas. The supramesocolic area contains the suprarenal aorta and its major branches (celiac axis, superior mesenteric artery [SMA], and renal arteries), the supramesocolic inferior vena cava (IVC) with its major branches, and the superior mesenteric vein (SMV). The inframesocolic area contains the infrarenal aorta and IVC.
- *Zone 2* (left and right), which includes the kidneys, paracolic gutter, and renal vessels.
- *Zone 3*, which includes the pelvic retroperitoneum and contains the iliac vessels.

Some authors include a fourth zone in the perihepatic area that contains the hepatic artery, portal vein, retrohepatic IVC, and hepatic veins.

▮ MECHANISM OF INJURY

Penetrating trauma is responsible for most abdominal vascular injuries and accounts for about 90% of cases in urban trauma centers.[1] Low-velocity missiles cause direct injury to the vessel. High-velocity missiles and blasts can also cause vascular trauma by means of the shock wave and transient cavitation. Some of these injuries may manifest as early or late thrombosis or hemorrhage.

In patients who undergo exploratory laparotomy for injury, the incidence of vascular trauma is 14.3% for gunshot injuries,[2] 10% for stab wounds,[3] and 3% for blunt injuries.[4]

Blunt abdominal trauma may cause vascular injuries by one of three mechanisms:

1. Rapid deceleration, as occurs in high-speed vehicular accidents or falls from heights: this mechanism may cause

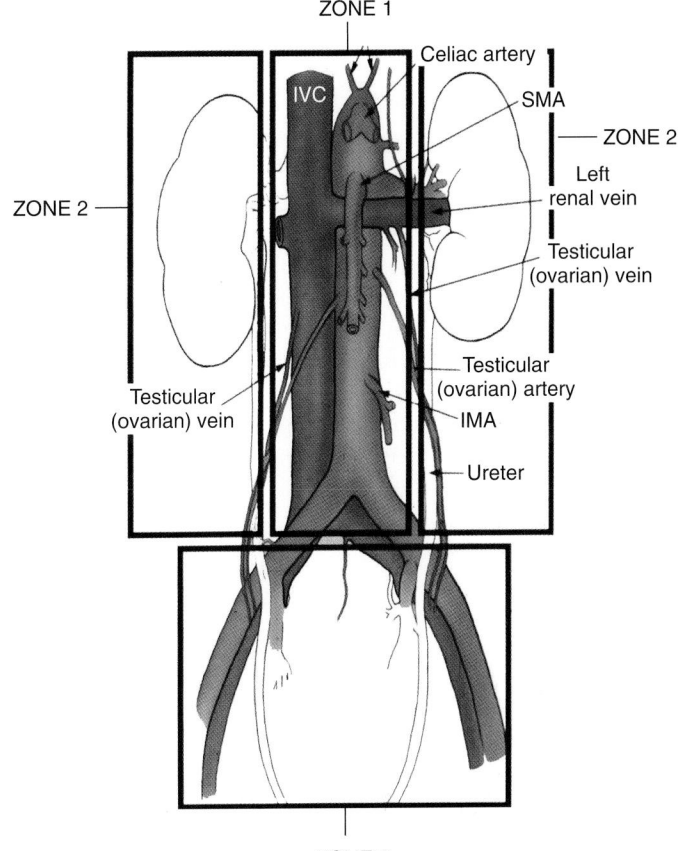

Figure 154-1 Retroperitoneal vascular zones. Zone 1 includes the midline vessels from the aortic hiatus to the sacral promontory; zone 2 includes the paracolic gutter and the kidneys; and zone 3 includes the pelvic retroperitoneum. IMA, inferior mesenteric artery; IVC, inferior vena cava; SMA, superior mesenteric artery.

damage to abdominal vessels by avulsion or intimal tear and subsequent thrombosis.

2. Direct anteroposterior crushing, as occurs in car passengers wearing seat belts or from direct blows to the anterior abdomen.

3. Direct laceration of a major vessel by a bone fragment, as occurs in severe pelvic fractures.

Abdominal arterial and venous injuries occur with the same incidence. In a review of 302 abdominal vascular injuries from our center, the incidence of arterial injuries was 49% and that of venous injuries was 51%.[1] The most commonly injured abdominal vessel was the IVC (accounting for 25% of injuries), followed by the aorta (21%), iliac arteries (20%), iliac veins (17%), SMV (11%), and SMA (10%). Overall, patients with penetrating trauma had an average of 1.6 vascular injuries.[1]

CLINICAL PRESENTATION

Many patients with major abdominal vascular injuries die at the scene and never reach medical care. Of the patients who are transported to hospitals, about 14% lose vital signs during transportation or in the emergency department.[1] The clinical presentation depends on the injured vessel, the size and type of the injury, the presence of associated injuries, and time elapsed since the injury.

Penetrating injuries to the abdomen associated with hypotension and abdominal distention are highly suggestive of vascular injury. Asymmetric femoral pulses may indicate iliac artery injury. Many patients may be normotensive on admission only to decompensate a few minutes later. Some patients present in a hemodynamically stable condition because of thrombosis of the vessel or effective containment of the bleeding in the retroperitoneum. In most cases the diagnosis is made intraoperatively. Vascular injuries due to blunt trauma are often missed on initial examination or even during the initial hospitalization, unless they are associated with significant bleeding or early ischemic changes.

DIAGNOSTIC EVALUATION

In most patients with penetrating abdominal vascular injuries no investigations are needed because of the patient's critical condition and the obvious need for immediate laparotomy. Radiographic evaluation of the torso should be reserved only for gunshot wounds, if the patient is hemodynamically stable. The location of any bullets or missile fragments may be useful in planning the operation (Fig. 154-2) or in diagnosing other extra-abdominal injuries. About 30% of victims with gunshot injuries to the abdomen have multiple gunshot wounds,[2] and an abdominal radiograph may provide useful information. Finally, early radiographic diagnosis of gunshot wounds to the spine or other bones may be useful in prescribing antibiotic prophylaxis. In blunt trauma, radiographic diagnosis of complex pelvic fractures may increase the suspicion of iliac vascular injuries.

Computed tomography (CT) has little or no role in suspected vascular injuries resulting from penetrating trauma during the acute stage. However, it may play a useful role in blunt trauma by identifying large hematomas, false aneurysms, or vessel occlusions (Fig. 154-3). In selected cases with penetrating trauma, elective CT after the intravenous administration of a contrast agent may identify false aneurysms or arteriovenous fistulae (Figs. 154-4 and 154-5). Angiography has no role in suspected vascular injuries resulting from penetrating trauma during the acute stage. However, it has an important role in the evaluation of suspected late complications such as false aneurysms or arteriovenous fistulae. It remains a valuable tool in the evaluation of patients with blunt

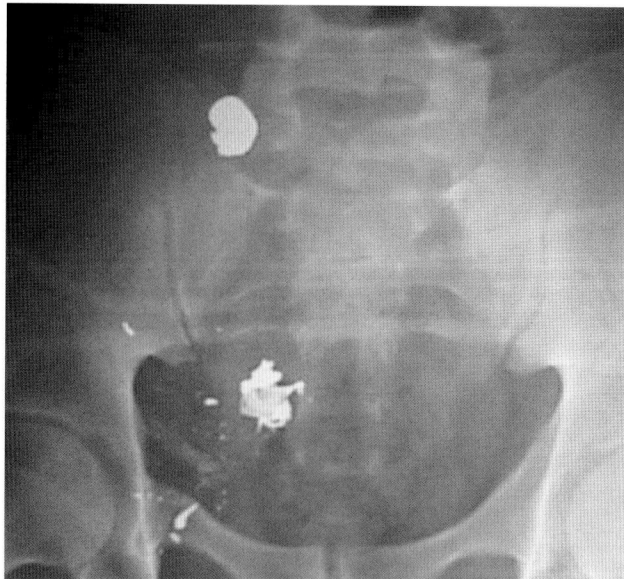

Figure 154-2 The pelvic location of the missile on the abdominal radiograph, combined with hypotension, is highly suggestive of an iliac vascular injury.

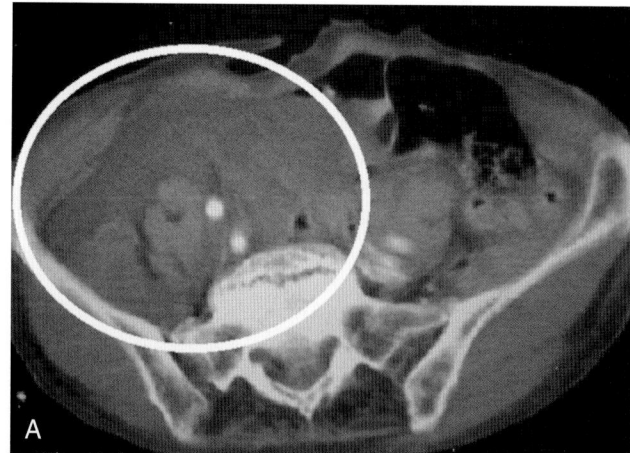

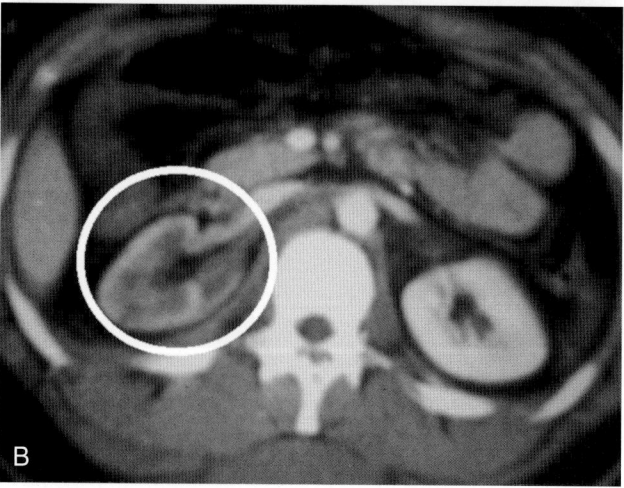

Figure 154-3 A, CT of a traffic accident victim shows a large pelvic hematoma (*circle*) due to injury of the right common iliac artery. **B,** CT scan with intravenous contrast material in a patient who fell from a significant height shows poor contrast uptake in the right kidney due to occlusion of the renal artery (*circle*).

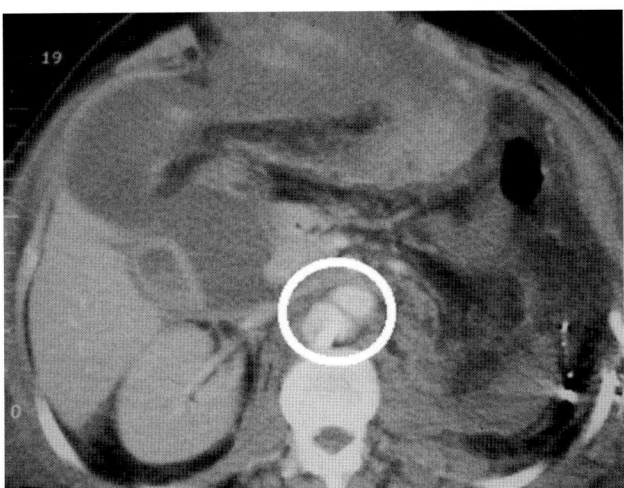

Figure 154-4 Postoperative CT scan of a patient with a gunshot wound shows an abdominal aortic false aneurysm (*circle*).

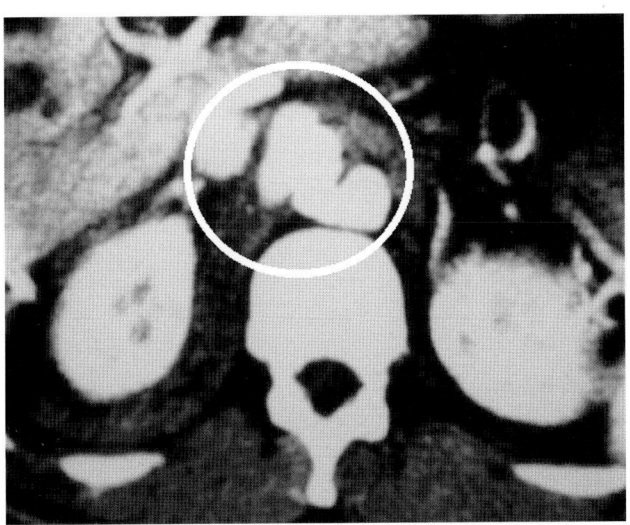

Figure 154-5 Postoperative CT scan of a patient with a gunshot wound shows an aortocaval fistula (*circle*).

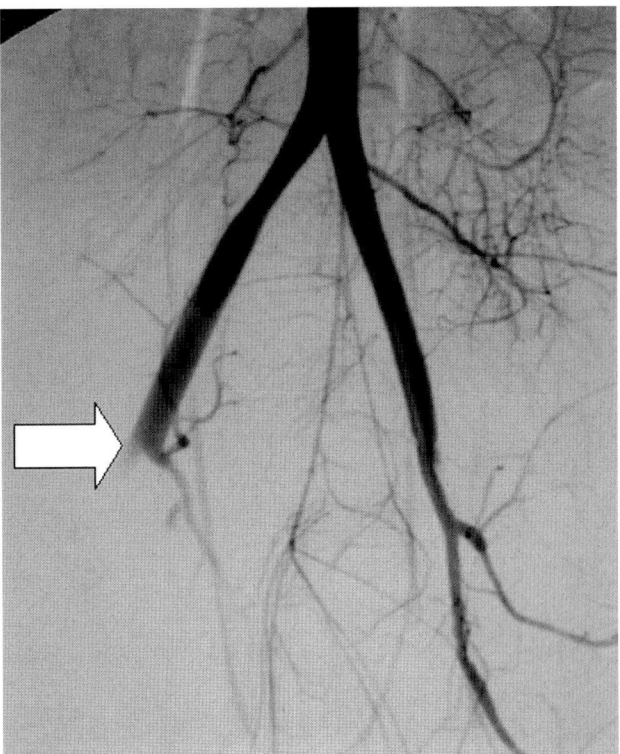

Figure 154-6 A 5-year-old child presented with a severe pelvic fracture and absent right femoral pulse. Angiography shows a complete occlusion of the right common iliac artery (*arrow*).

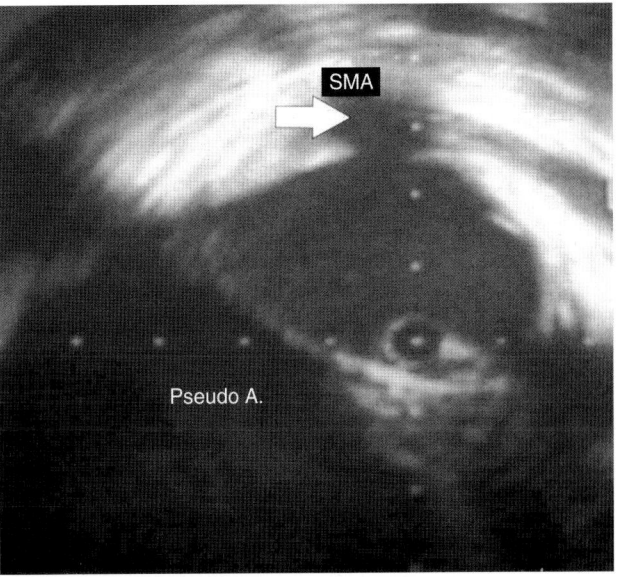

Figure 154-7 Intravascular ultrasound shows a false aortic aneurysm (Pseudo A.) at the level of the superior mesenteric artery (SMA; *arrow*) after a gunshot wound to the aorta.

trauma, especially those with pelvic fractures who are suspected of having vascular injuries (Fig. 154-6).

Other investigations such as intravascular ultrasonography may be useful in selected cases involving late abdominal vascular complications. In these cases, ultrasound may more accurately define the anatomy of a vascular lesion (Fig. 154-7).

■ TREATMENT

Prehospital Treatment

The most important factor for the survival of salvageable patients with vascular injuries is rapid transportation to a trauma center followed by immediate surgical control of the bleeding. Prehospital advanced life support (ALS) has no place in penetrating trauma, especially in an urban environment. A policy of "scoop and run" is currently the recommended approach. The role of prehospital intravenous fluid administration is controversial, with some studies showing improved survival with fluid restriction and others showing no effect on survival.[5,6] Experimental work on abdominal aortic injuries has shown that in the presence of uncontrolled bleeding, aggressive fluid resuscitation increases mortality and the rate and volume of hemorrhage.[7,8] However, avoiding all fluid resuscitation in near-fatal hemorrhage may result in cardiac arrest before bleeding is controlled.[9] It seems that some degree of controlled hypotension is beneficial and prevents massive exsanguination while avoiding the risk of cardiac arrest due to massive blood loss and severe hypotension.[7,10] In many trauma systems the prehospital intravenous resuscitation protocol recommends the insertion of intravenous lines and crystalloid resuscitation in the ambulance on the way to the hospital.

Emergency Department Treatment

The presence of hypotension or tachycardia (>120 beats/min) or a gunshot wound to the torso is a criterion for trauma team activation in most trauma systems. The type and duration of evaluation and resuscitation in the emergency department depend on the clinical condition of the patient. Endotracheal intubation and a resuscitative thoracotomy should be performed in the emergency department when patients are admitted in cardiac arrest or when cardiac arrest is imminent. A left anterolateral thoracotomy is performed, the thoracic aorta is cross-clamped, and the heart is massaged as necessary. If cardiac activity returns, the operation is completed in the operating room. The survival rate after emergency department resuscitative thoracotomy for abdominal vascular injuries is about 2%.[1] We occasionally combine the emergency department thoracotomy with a laparotomy to control bleeding by direct compression, but the results are poor.

In patients with suspected vascular injuries and in no need of resuscitative thoracotomy, time should not be wasted on fluid resuscitation or diagnostic investigations, with the exception of plain radiographs. Large-bore intravenous catheters should be placed in the upper extremities or the central veins of the thoracic inlet in case the victim has an injury to the IVC or the iliac veins. The concept of controlled hypotension should be borne in mind, and aggressive fluid resuscitation should not be attempted in the emergency department. Except for patients in cardiac arrest or at risk for imminent cardiac arrest, endotracheal intubation should be avoided in the emergency department because rapid-sequence induction is often associated with cardiovascular decompensation.

Surgical Treatment

General Principles

All possible steps should be taken to diminish hypothermia and its detrimental effects. The operating room should be warm, the infused fluids should be prewarmed to 40°C to 42°C, and the patient's extremities should be covered with a warming blanket. Rapid-infusion devices should be ready, and the blood bank should be notified. The patient's entire torso, from the neck to the knees, should be prepared and draped in case thoracotomy or saphenous vein harvesting is necessary. The surgical team should be ready, and the skin preparation should be performed before induction of anesthesia because the latter is often associated with rapid hemodynamic decompensation in these patients.

Some surgeons have advocated a preliminary left thoracotomy and aortic cross-clamping to prevent cardiovascular collapse after anesthesia and laparotomy.[11,12] The effectiveness of this procedure has been challenged by other authors.[13] We believe that this approach should be considered only for patients in cardiac arrest or at risk for imminent cardiac arrest. A thoracotomy is an additional traumatic insult that may aggravate hypothermia and coagulopathy and has little effect on the control of bleeding from major venous injuries. We advocate an immediate laparotomy, temporary control of bleeding by direct compression, and aortic cross-clamping, if necessary, at the diaphragm. In our experience, this is almost always possible, even in obese patients. To facilitate aortic exposure, division of the left crux of the diaphragm may be necessary. In cases in which a retroperitoneal hematoma extends high toward the aortic hiatus, infradiaphragmatic exposure of the aorta is difficult, and a left thoracotomy may be necessary for aortic control.

The abdomen should be entered through a long midline incision. The operative findings depend on the nature and site of the vascular injury and the presence of other associated injuries. In penetrating trauma, the usual findings include various degrees of intraperitoneal bleeding, a retroperitoneal hematoma, or a combination of the two. In blunt trauma, the most likely finding is a retroperitoneal hematoma, which may or may not be expanding or pulsatile. In some patients with intimal tear and thrombosis, the hematoma may be unremarkable, and the only findings may be dark bowel or an absent or diminished femoral pulse. Some injuries may be missed only to manifest at a later stage with thrombosis, false aneurysm, or arteriovenous fistula.

Retroperitoneal Hematoma

The management of retroperitoneal hematomas depends on the mechanism of injury. As a general rule, almost all hematomas due to penetrating trauma should be explored, irrespective of size. Underneath a small hematoma there is often a vascular or hollow viscus perforation. The only exception to this recommendation is a stable and nonexpanding retrohepatic hematoma. Surgical exploration of the retrohepatic vena cava or the hepatic veins is difficult and potentially dangerous.

Retroperitoneal hematomas due to blunt trauma rarely require exploration because of the very low incidence of underlying vascular or hollow viscus injuries requiring surgical repair. In patients with zone 2 hematomas due to renal trauma, surgical exploration may result in the unnecessary loss of the kidney. Similarly, exploration of a zone 3 hematoma due to pelvic fractures may cause severe bleeding that may be uncontrollable. Exploration of retroperitoneal hematomas should be limited to patients with expanding, pulsatile, or leaking hematomas. In addition, zone 3 pelvic hematomas associated with an absent ipsilateral femoral pulse should be explored because of the potential for an iliac artery injury. Paraduodenal hematomas also need exploration to exclude an underlying duodenal injury. Finally, hematomas at the root of the mesentery in the presence of ischemic bowel may harbor an injury to the SMA and should be explored. Exploration of these hematomas is technically difficult and potentially dangerous and should not be performed in the absence of ischemic bowel. Unexplored hematomas should be evaluated postoperatively by means of color-flow Doppler studies (which may be difficult because of bowel gas), CT angiography, or angiography.

In the presence of severe active bleeding, the immediate priority is to control the bleeding by direct compression. Once this critical task is achieved, the next step is to identify the bleeding vessel and obtain proximal and distal control. If control is difficult or the patient is severely hypotensive, the abdominal aorta can be compressed digitally or with an aortic compressor at the aortic hiatus. After dissection of the peritoneum over the aorta and, if necessary, division of the left crux of the diaphragm (at the 2 o'clock position to avoid bleeding), the aorta can be cross-clamped.

The exploration of the area of bleeding or hematoma should proceed systematically. Each anatomic zone requires a different technical maneuver. Zone 1 supramesocolic bleeding or hematomas are the most difficult to approach because of the dense concentration of major vessels (aorta, celiac artery, SMA, renal vessels, IVC), the difficult exposure of many of these vessels, and the difficult proximal control of the infradiaphragmatic aorta. For some injuries, the only safe way to achieve proximal aortic control is through a left thoracotomy. The supramesocolic aorta, along with the origins of its major branches, is best exposed by mobilization and medial rotation of the viscera in the left upper abdomen. The first step of this approach is to divide the peritoneal reflection lateral to the left colon, the splenic flexure of the colon, and the spleen. The fundus of the stomach, spleen, tail of the pancreas, colon, and left kidney are then rotated to the right. This maneuver provides exposure of the aorta, origin of the celiac axis, SMA, and left renal vessels (Fig. 154-8). Some surgeons prefer not to include the left kidney in the medial rotation.[14] However, for injuries involving the posterior wall of the aorta, inclusion of the left kidney in the visceral rotation improves the exposure. In suspected supramesocolic IVC injuries, zone 1 should be explored through a medial rotation of the right colon and hepatic flexure and Kocher mobilization of the duodenum and head of the pancreas (Fig. 154-9). The inframesocolic zone 1 area can be approached by retracting the transverse colon cephalad and displacing the small bowel to the right. The peritoneum over the aorta and IVC is then incised, and the vessels are exposed. An alternative approach is medial rotation of the right or left colon.

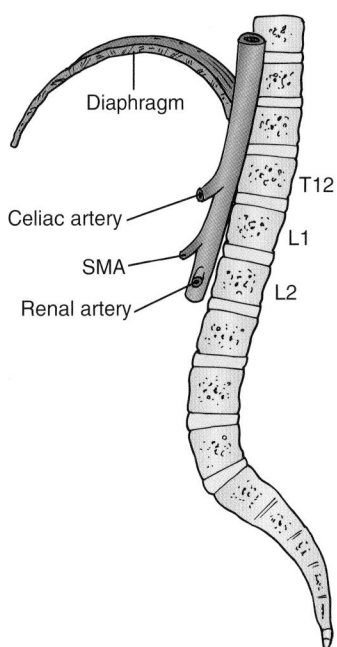

Figure 154-8 Medial left visceral rotation provides good exposure of the supramesocolic aorta and the origin of the celiac axis, superior mesenteric artery (SMA), and left renal vessels.

Zone 2 bleeding or hematomas are explored by mobilization and medial rotation of the right colon, duodenum, and head of the pancreas on the right side, or the left colon on the left side. The source of bleeding in zone 2 is the renal vessels or the kidneys.

Zone 3 vessels are explored by dissection of the paracolic peritoneum and medial rotation of the right or left colon. In some cases, direct dissection of the peritoneum over the vessels provides the necessary exposure.

The reconstruction of major vessels with synthetic grafts in the presence of intestinal spillage poses significant risks for graft infection. Copious irrigation before graft placement, use of polytetrafluoroethylene (PTFE) grafts when possible, and omental wrapping or soft tissue coverage reduce the risk of infection.

Damage-Control Procedures

Many patients with major abdominal vascular injuries require massive blood transfusions, are hypotensive, and become severely hypothermic, acidotic, and coagulopathic intraoperatively. Persistent attempts to reconstruct or repair all abdominal injuries are ill advised and result in increased mortality. These patients may benefit from early damage control and definitive reconstruction at a later stage when their general condition improves. Earlier reports recommended that damage-control procedures be considered in patients in extremis who had exhausted their physiologic reserves and were in danger of irreversible shock and death. The criteria included coagulopathy, hypothermia less than 35°C, base deficit greater than 15 mEq/L (15 mmol/L), and severe bowel edema. However, these criteria are now considered very late manifes-

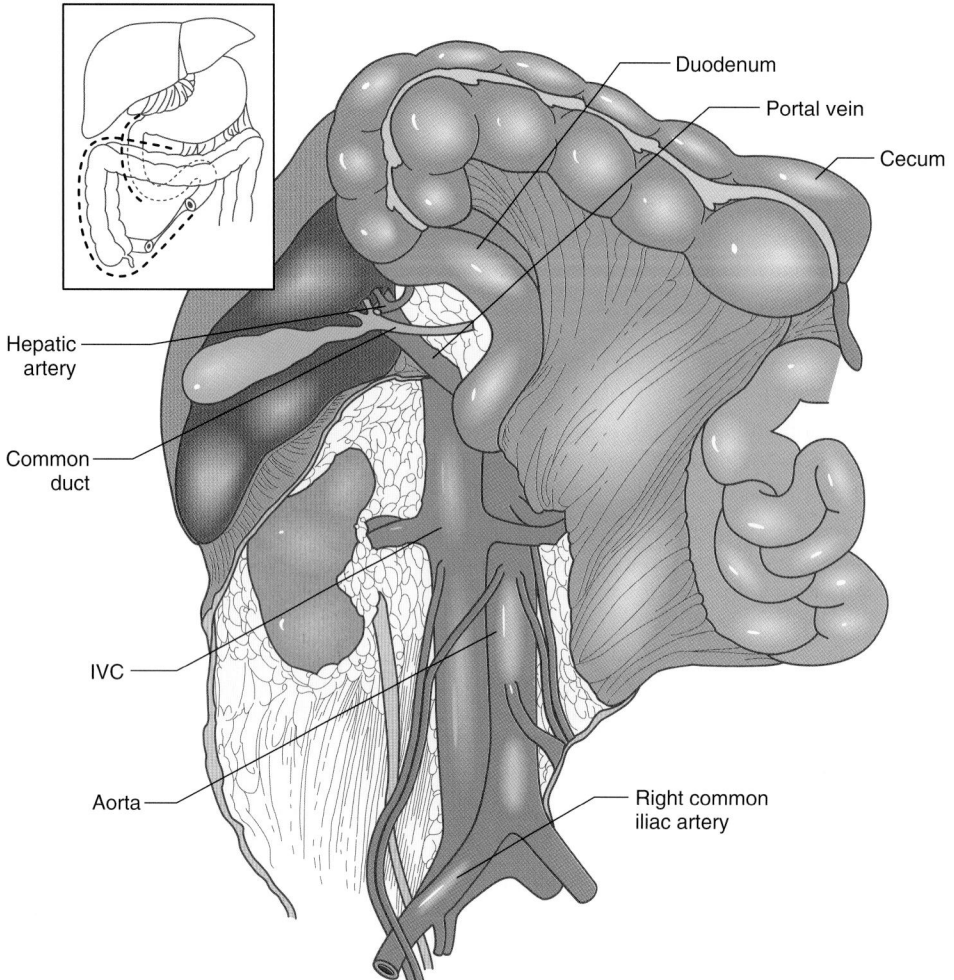

Figure 154-9 Medial rotation of the right colon and hepatic flexure and Kocher mobilization of the duodenum and pancreas provide excellent exposure of the inferior vena cava (IVC) and the origins of the renal veins. *(From Buckman RF, Pathak AS, Badelino MM, Bradley KM. Injuries of the inferior vena cava. Surg Clin North Am. 2001;81:1431-1447.)*

tations, at which point damage control might be ineffective. Damage control should not be a procedure of last resort but should be considered at a much earlier stage, before the patient becomes severely hypotensive and coagulopathic. This concept is even more important in patients with major co-morbidities, such as older age or chronic medical problems, and in suboptimal environments, such as small community hospitals or combat zones.

With the damage-control approach, all complex venous injuries are ligated, arterial injuries may be shunted, and any diffuse retroperitoneal or parenchymal bleeding is controlled by tight gauze packing. Temporary intraluminal shunts can be constructed from sterile intravenous or nasogastric tubing. The shunt is secured with proximal and distal ligatures (Fig. 154-10). The abdomen is then closed temporarily with a prosthetic material or vacuum dressing techniques (Fig. 154-11), and the patient is transferred to the intensive care unit (ICU) for further resuscitation. The abdomen should never be closed primarily because of the very high incidence of abdominal compartment syndrome (ACS). Some patients may benefit from early angiointervention before admission to the

ICU. The patient is returned to the operating room after resuscitation and stabilization for definitive vascular repair and abdominal wall closure.

Abdominal Compartment Syndrome

The normal intra-abdominal pressure (IAP) in the resting supine position is near zero. Elevation of the IAP above 25 to 30 cm H_2O can cause severe organ dysfunction and result in ACS. ACS is characterized by a tense abdomen, tachycardia with or without hypotension, respiratory dysfunction with high peak inspiratory pressures in mechanically ventilated patients, and oliguria. However, significant organ dysfunction may begin long before classic ACS manifests.

All patients with severe abdominal trauma, especially vascular trauma, are at risk of developing ACS. Major risk factors include massive blood transfusions, prolonged hypotension, hypothermia, aortic cross-clamping, damage-control procedures, and tight closure of the abdominal wall. After severe trauma, the abdomen should never be closed under tension. Similarly, after damage-control procedures, the abdominal

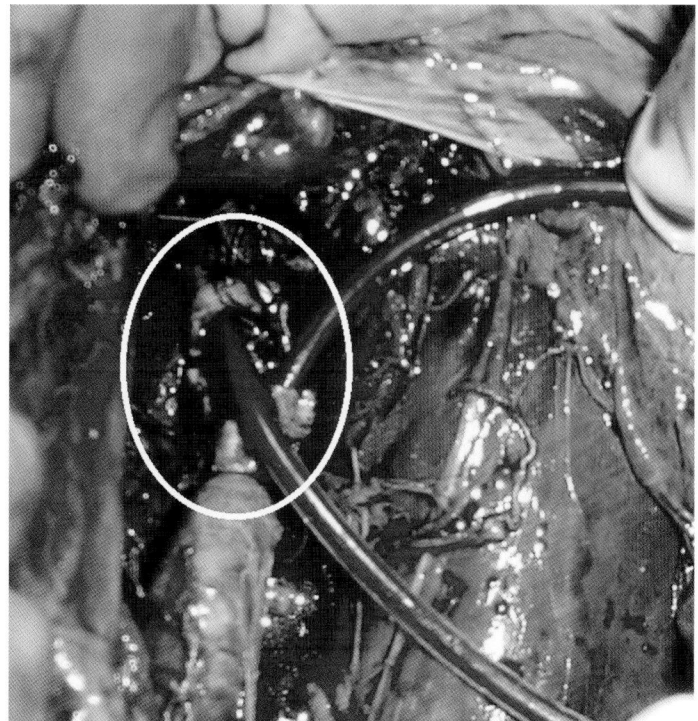

Figure 154-10 Temporary arterial shunt for damage control in a hemodynamically unstable patient with a gunshot wound and complete transection of the iliac artery (*circle*).

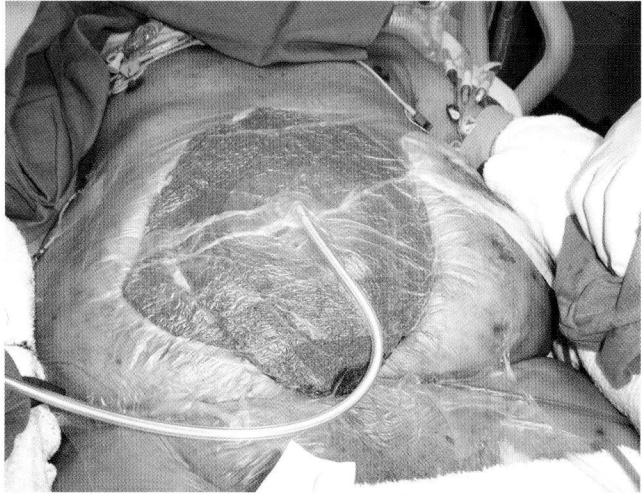

Figure 154-11 Temporary closure of the abdomen using vacuum dressing techniques. After damage-control procedures, the abdomen should never be closed primarily because of the risk of abdominal compartment syndrome.

wall should not be closed because postoperative bowel edema results in ACS in most patients.

The diagnosis of ACS is based on clinical examination and IAP measurements. All high-risk patients and those with a tense abdomen on palpation should be monitored closely with serial IAP measurements. The IAP can be measured reliably through the bladder catheter. In general, pressures higher than 30 cm H_2O are considered strong indicators for surgical decompression of the abdomen. The abdomen can be opened

in the operating room or even in the ICU if necessary. Temporary abdominal wall closure can be achieved with the use of a prosthetic material or vacuum dressing techniques (see Fig 154-11). When the bowel edema improves, usually within 2 to 3 days, the patient is returned to the operating room for definitive abdominal wall closure. The technical details of temporary or permanent wall closure are beyond the scope of this chapter.

■ SPECIFIC VASCULAR INJURIES

Abdominal Aorta Injuries

Anatomy

The aorta descends into the retroperitoneum between the two crura of the diaphragm at the T12-L1 level and bifurcates into the common iliac arteries at the L4-L5 level, which roughly corresponds to the level of the umbilicus. The first branches of the abdominal aorta are the phrenic arteries that originate from its anterolateral surface. Immediately below is the celiac trunk that originates from the anterior surface of the aorta, and 1 to 2 cm below is the SMA; the renal arteries are next, at 1 to 1.5 cm below the origin of the SMA; and finally, the inferior mesenteric artery (IMA) is 2 to 5 cm above the bifurcation of the aorta.

Mechanism of Injury

Blunt injury to the abdominal aorta is extremely rare, diagnosed in 0.04% of all blunt trauma admissions.[15] Fractures of the thoracolumbar spine and seat-belt injuries are associated with an increased risk of abdominal aortic injuries.[15,16] Intimal dissection and thrombosis are the most common lesions in patients reaching the hospital alive (Fig. 154-12). False aneurysms occur less frequently. Patients with free ruptures die at the scene and rarely receive medical care.[16,17]

Penetrating injuries are by far the most common cause of abdominal aortic injuries. In a review of 1218 patients with abdominal gunshot injuries from our center, there were 33 abdominal aortic injuries (2.7%). In 529 knife wounds to the abdomen, the aorta was injured in 8 (1.5%).[18] The infrarenal aorta is injured in 50% of patients, the supraceliac aorta in 25%, and the aorta between the celiac trunk and the renal arteries in 25% of patients.[19]

Clinical Presentation

The clinical presentation depends on the mechanism of injury (blunt or penetrating), the type of aortic injury, the presence of free intraperitoneal bleeding or retroperitoneal hematoma, associated injuries, and time elapsed since the injury. In blunt trauma, two thirds of patients have acute symptoms of bleeding or visceral or lower extremity ischemia. The diagnosis is made during the initial hospitalization by means of CT or angiography or at laparotomy. In one third of cases the diagnosis is made many months or even years after the injury.[15-17]

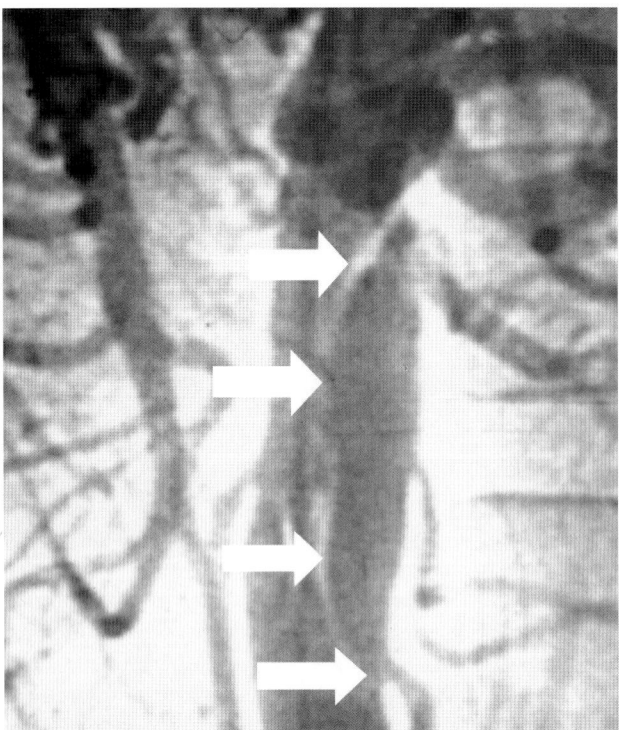

Figure 154-12 Angiography shows a dissecting aneurysm of the abdominal aorta (*arrows*) after a motor vehicle accident. Management with an endovascular stent was successful.

The clinical presentation of penetrating aortic injuries is usually dramatic. Many victims die at the scene and never receive medical care. Of those who are treated, about 28% have an unrecordable blood pressure, and about 21% require an emergency resuscitative thoracotomy.[18] In about 18% of cases the bleeding is temporarily contained in the retroperitoneum, and the patients are normotensive on admission.[19] On rare occasion the injury is missed at operation only to manifest at a later stage as a false aneurysm or arteriovenous fistula (see Figs. 154-4 and 154-5).

Endovascular Treatment

Endovascular management has a definitive role in selected cases of infrarenal aortic injury. Patients with limited infrarenal aortic dissection, false aneurysms, or aortocaval fistulae have been treated successfully with angiographically placed stents (see Fig. 154-12).[20,21]

Surgical Treatment

The surgical exposure of the vascular structures in zone 1 is achieved by medial visceral rotation, as described under the heading "Retroperitoneal Hematoma" (see Fig. 154-8). For high supramesocolic injuries, a left thoracotomy may be necessary for cross-clamping of the aorta. About 93% of patients with penetrating trauma have other associated intra-abdominal injuries, the most common being injuries to the small bowel (45% of cases), the colon (30%), and the liver (28%).[18] Before any definitive management that requires a prosthetic graft, all enteric spillage should be controlled, and the peritoneum should be washed out. Lateral aortorrhaphy is possible in most cases. More complex repairs with prosthetic grafts may be necessary.[22] Many authors do not consider the presence of enteric spillage a contraindication for the use of prosthetic material.[22]

Mortality

The prognosis of abdominal aortic injuries after blunt trauma is significantly better than that of injuries due to penetrating trauma. The reported overall mortality in blunt trauma is 27%.[16] The mortality after penetrating trauma in two large series with 146 patients was 67%.[18,22] In another series of 57 patients with gunshot wounds, the mortality rate was 85%.[23] Suprarenal aortic injuries have a significantly worse outcome than infrarenal injuries.[19] The mortality in patients undergoing emergency center resuscitative thoracotomy is almost 100%.[18,19] The prognosis of penetrating abdominal aortic injuries is significantly better than that of injuries to the thoracic aorta, most likely owing to the retroperitoneal containment of bleeding in abdominal injuries. In a comparison of 67 abdominal aortic injuries with 26 thoracic aortic injuries, the mortality rates were 76% and 92%, respectively.[18]

Celiac Artery Injuries

Anatomy

The celiac artery originates from the anterior wall of the abdominal aorta, immediately below the aortic hiatus, at the level of T12-L1 (see Fig. 154-8). The main trunk is 1 to 1.5 cm long, and at the upper border of the pancreas it has three branches (the tripod of Haller): the common hepatic artery, the left gastric artery, and the splenic artery. Because of the extensive fibrous, ganglionic, and lymphatic tissues that surround the trunk, surgical dissection may be tedious.

Mechanism of Injury

Injuries to the celiac artery are rare and almost always due to penetrating trauma. In a review of 302 abdominal vascular injuries, the celiac artery was involved in 10 cases (3.3%).[1]

Surgical Treatment

The surgical exposure can be achieved either by direct dissection over the upper abdominal aorta through the lesser sac or by medial rotation of the upper abdominal viscera, as described previously. The rotation does not need to include the left kidney. The celiac artery can be ligated without ischemic sequelae to the stomach, liver, or spleen because of the rich collateral circulation of these organs. The left gastric and splenic arteries may also be ligated with impunity. Ligation of the common hepatic artery is usually well tolerated because of adequate supply from the portal vein and the gastroduodenal artery.

Mortality

The reported mortality rate of celiac axis injuries ranges from 38% to 75%.[24] However, among the 50 collectively reported cases of celiac axis injuries, most patients had other vascular injuries that contributed to the high mortality.

Superior Mesenteric Artery Injuries

Anatomy

The SMA originates from the anterior surface of the aorta, immediately below the celiac artery, behind the pancreas at the L1 level (see Fig. 154-8). It then proceeds over the uncinate process of the pancreas and the third part of the duodenum and enters the root of the mesentery. The SMA has the following branches: inferior pancreaticoduodenal artery, middle colic artery, arterial arcade with 12 to 18 intestinal branches, right colic artery, and ileocolic artery. SMA injuries are divided into the four zones:

- *Zone 1*, between the aortic origin and the inferior pancreaticoduodenal artery
- *Zone 2*, between the inferior pancreaticoduodenal artery and the middle colic artery
- *Zone 3*, distal to the middle colic artery
- *Zone 4*, the segmental intestinal branches

As a general rule, ligation of the SMA in zones 1 and 2 results in severe ischemia of the small bowel and right colon. Ligation of zones 3 and 4 may result in localized ischemia of the small bowel that requires segmental resection.

Another anatomic classification of SMA injuries uses only two zones: the short retropancreatic segment and the segment below the body of the pancreas, where it courses over the uncinate process of the pancreas and the third part of the duodenum.[25]

Mechanism of Injury

The SMA is second to the renovascular system as the most commonly injured abdominal vessel after blunt trauma. Blunt trauma is responsible for between 10% and 20% of all SMA injuries[26,27] and can cause thrombosis of the artery by a direct blow, crushing of the abdomen, or seat-belt injuries. Deceleration injuries may cause avulsion of the vessel from its origin in the aorta or intimal tear and subsequent thrombosis. Penetrating injuries are the most common mechanism of injury. Because of the anatomic location of the artery, multiple significant associated injuries are common.[25]

Clinical Presentation

The clinical presentation depends on the mechanism of injury, nature of the vascular injury, presence of associated intra-abdominal injuries, and time elapsed since injury. Isolated thrombosis of the SMA due to blunt trauma may be missed during the initial evaluation, only to manifest at a later stage with bowel necrosis. Most patients with penetrating trauma present in severe shock. Patients with contained hematomas may be normotensive or mildly hypotensive on admission.

Surgical Treatment

The operative findings may include various degrees of hemoperitoneum, hematoma around the SMA, ischemic bowel, or any combination of these (Fig. 154-13A).

After temporary control of the bleeding by direct compression and, if necessary, cross-clamping of the aorta, the SMA should be explored.

Exposure. Exposure of the retropancreatic SMA can be achieved by medial rotation of the left colon, gastric fundus, spleen, and tail of the pancreas, as described earlier. The kidney does not need to be rotated unless injury to the posterior wall of the aorta is suspected. In cases of severe bleeding when immediate exposure is critical, stapled division of the neck of the pancreas may provide fast and direct exposure of the SMA and the portal vein. Exposure of the infrapancreatic SMA can be achieved by cephalad retraction of the inferior border of the pancreas and direct dissection, or it can be achieved through the root of the small bowel mesentery by incising and dissecting the tissues to the left of the ligament of Treitz. An extensive Kocher maneuver may be required to

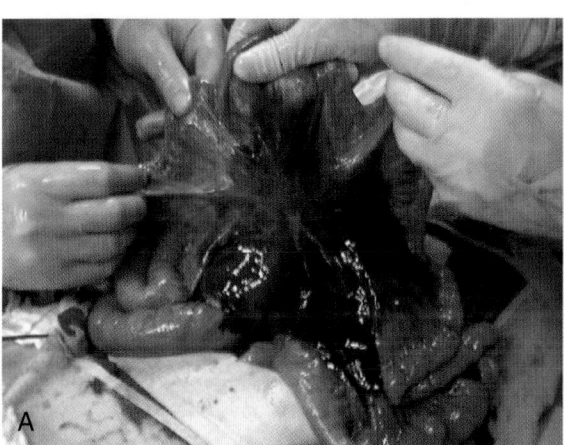
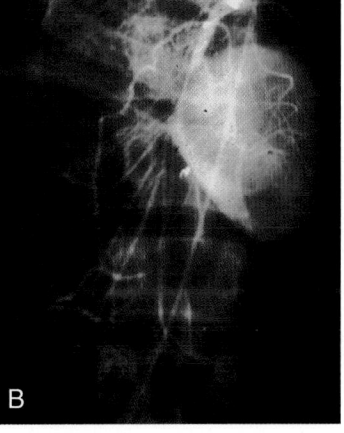

Figure 154-13 A, Traffic accident victim with a large hematoma at the base of the mesentery found at laparotomy. This is suggestive of a superior mesenteric artery (SMA) injury and needs to be evaluated by angiography, preferably postoperatively. **B,** Postoperative angiography shows a large SMA false aneurysm.

expose this segment of the SMA. More distal sections of the SMA can be approached directly.

Exploration of a hematoma at the root of the mesentery is always a difficult and potentially dangerous task, even in the hands of experienced surgeons. In penetrating trauma or blunt trauma with ischemic bowel, all hematomas around the SMA should be explored. However, it is our practice and recommendation not to explore stable hematomas after blunt trauma in the absence of bowel ischemia. In these patients, the SMA is evaluated postoperatively by means of angiography, CT angiography, or color-flow Doppler imaging (Fig. 154-13B).

Operative Management. Sharp partial transections of the SMA, such as those inflicted by knife wounds, can be managed with lateral arteriorrhaphy using 6-0 vascular sutures. This approach is possible in about 40% of cases.[28] Because mobilization of the SMA is restricted by the surrounding dense neuroganglionic tissue and its multiple branches, an end-to-end anastomosis is rarely possible.

Depending on the site of SMA injury, the condition of the patient, and the color of the bowel, these injuries can be managed by ligation or an interposition graft. Ligation of the SMA below the middle colic artery is usually associated with a moderate risk of bowel ischemia. Ligation of the proximal SMA results in ischemic necrosis involving the small bowel and the right colon. The first 10 to 20 cm of the jejunum may survive via collaterals from the superior pancreaticoduodenal artery. Ligation of the SMA proximal to the origin of the inferior pancreaticoduodenal artery may preserve critical collateral circulation to the proximal jejunum and is preferable to a more distal ligation. Ligation of the proximal SMA should be performed only in the presence of necrotic bowel. Ligation should be avoided in all other circumstances because of the catastrophic consequences of the short bowel syndrome. In patients in critical condition with severe hypothermia, acidosis, and coagulopathy, a damage-control procedure with a temporary endoluminal shunt should be considered.[29]

Definitive reconstruction is performed at a later stage after resuscitation and correction of the patient's physiologic parameters. The reconstruction can be performed with a saphenous vein or PTFE graft between the distal stump of the SMA and the anterior surface of the aorta. In the presence of an associated pancreatic injury, the vascular anastomosis should be performed away from the pancreas, and every effort should be made to protect it from pancreatic enzymes by use of omentum and surrounding soft tissues.

Postoperative Considerations. Postoperatively, the patient should be monitored closely for any signs of bowel ischemia. The threshold for second-look laparotomy within the first 24 hours of operation should be low. Failure to improve postoperatively and the persistence of metabolic acidosis despite adequate fluid resuscitation should prompt the surgeon to re-explore the abdomen to rule out bowel ischemia. Some authors practice mandatory second-look laparotomy. Damage-control techniques allow inspection of the bowel through the transparent material used for temporary closure of the abdomen.

Mortality

The mortality directly related to SMA injuries is difficult to assess because most patients have multiple severe injuries, including other major vascular injuries. The reported mortality varies from 33% to 68%.[26-28,30]

Renovascular Injuries
Anatomy

The renal arteries originate from the aorta at the L2 level (see Fig. 154-8). The right renal artery emerges at a slightly higher level and is longer than the left and courses under the IVC. About 30% of the population has more than one renal artery, often an accessory one to the lower pole of the kidney. The renal veins lie in front of the renal arteries (Fig. 154-14). The left renal vein is significantly longer than the right and courses in front of the aorta. It has collateral branches from the left gonadal vein inferiorly, the left adrenal vein superiorly, and a lumbar vein posteriorly.

Mechanism of Injury

Renal artery injuries account for about 0.05% of all blunt trauma admissions.[31] The left renal artery is 1.3 to 1.6 times more likely to be injured than the right renal artery.[31,32] It has been suggested that the right renal artery is protected from deceleration injuries because of its course underneath the IVC (see Fig. 154-14).[33] Rapid deceleration accidents may cause intimal tears and subsequent arterial thrombosis at a later stage. In about 50% of cases with blunt renal artery injury, there is thrombosis or an intimal flap (Fig. 154-15; see also Fig. 154-3B). Avulsion of the artery occurs in 12% of cases.[34] In 9% to 14% of renovascular injuries the renal artery is involved bilaterally.[32,34]

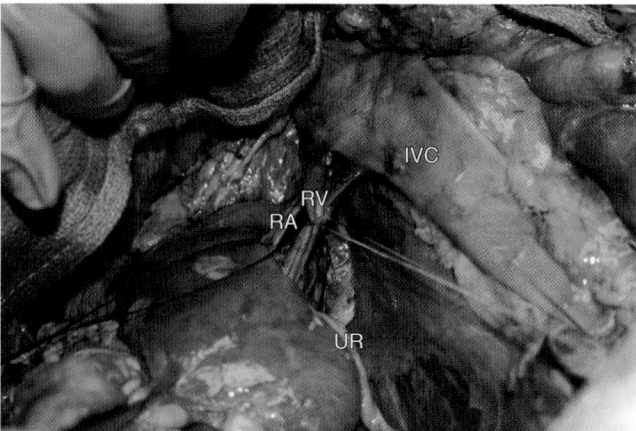

Figure 154-14 Anatomy of the hilum of the right kidney. Note the position of the renal artery (RA; black ligature) behind the renal vein (RV; white ligature) and inferior vena cava (IVC). UR, ureter.

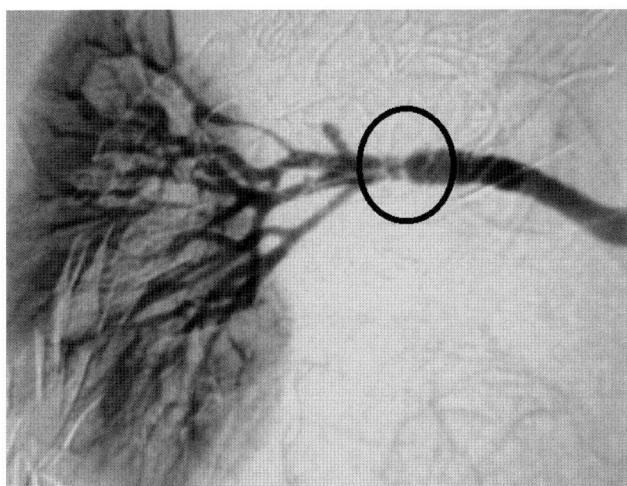

Figure 154-15 Angiography shows an intimal tear of the right renal artery (*circle*) due to a fall from a height. Management with an endovascular stent was successful.

Clinical Presentation

The diagnosis of renovascular injury after penetrating trauma is almost always made intraoperatively. However, in blunt trauma, the diagnosis is usually made during routine CT evaluation of the abdomen (Fig. 154-16; see also Fig. 154-3B). The clinical presentation is subtle and nondiagnostic, and the diagnosis is often delayed. In earlier reports, when CT evaluation of the abdomen was not as common, up to 50% of patients did not receive timely treatment because of delayed diagnosis.[34] Abdominal contrast-enhanced CT is highly sensitive in diagnosing renovascular trauma and should be the first-line investigation (see Fig. 154-3B).[35] In addition, CT provides useful information about associated injuries. Angiography is usually required for confirmation of the CT findings. Intravenous pyelography has a limited role, and many patients with renovascular injuries have normal studies.

Endovascular Treatment

Endovascular treatment may play an important role in selected cases of blunt renovascular trauma, and it should be consid-

ered the first-line therapeutic option in patients in stable condition with intimal tears, acute occlusions, false aneurysms, and arteriovenous fistulae (see Fig. 154-16). The experience with this technique is still limited, and the follow-up is short. However, it is very promising and most likely will increase the number of patients undergoing revascularization.[36-38]

Surgical Treatment

The management of renovascular injuries depends on the mechanism of injury, time of diagnosis, ischemia time, general condition of the patient, and presence of a contralateral normal kidney. In penetrating injuries, the diagnosis is almost always made early during the exploratory laparotomy, and depending on the extent of the injury and the condition of the victim, reconstruction of the vessels or nephrectomy is performed.

Revascularization. As a general rule, all zone 2 hematomas resulting from penetrating trauma should be explored. The only exception may be a stable perinephric hematoma away from the hilum.[39] However, in blunt trauma, the management of renal artery injuries is complicated by the often delayed diagnosis and prolonged ischemia of the kidney. Renal function is severely affected after 3 hours of total ischemia and 6 hours of partial ischemia, although with collateral circulation from the renal capsule or surrounding soft tissues, kidney function may be preserved despite prolonged ischemia.[35]

In stable patients diagnosed with renovascular trauma within 4 to 6 hours of injury, the general recommendation is revascularization.[35,40] However, revascularization is rarely performed, even in patients with no other injuries. In a study based on the National Trauma Data Bank, which is maintained by the Committee on Trauma of the American College of Surgeons, only 9% of the 517 patients with renal artery injury due to blunt trauma underwent revascularization. Of the remaining cases, 73% had no kidney exploration, and 18% underwent immediate nephrectomy. In the group of 87 patients with isolated renal artery injuries, 8% underwent revascularization, 8% had early nephrectomy, and 84% were

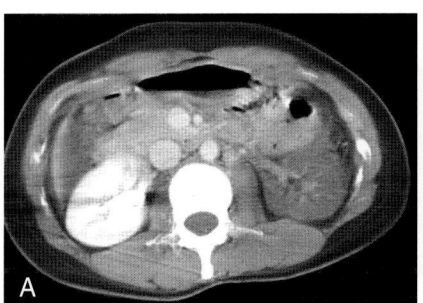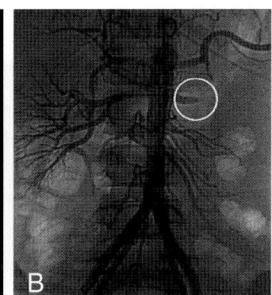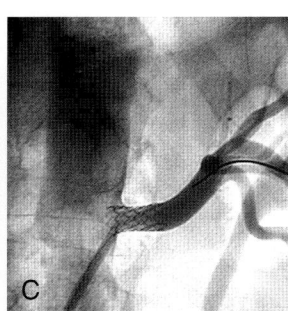

Figure 154-16 A, CT shows a nonfunctioning left kidney after a traffic injury. **B,** Angiography shows complete thrombosis of the renal artery (*circle*). **C,** Revascularization with an angiographically placed endovascular stent.

observed. Multiple-regression analysis adjusting for age, injury severity score, and severe associated injuries showed that patients treated with revascularization had a significantly longer ICU and hospital stay than observed patients.[31] In patients with bilateral injuries or injury to a solitary kidney, some authors recommend revascularization up to 20 hours after trauma.[40] Most surgeons avoid revascularization in patients diagnosed more than 6 hours after trauma, unless the injury involves both kidneys or a solitary kidney. The results after revascularization are generally disappointing, and successful surgical revascularization has been reported mainly by surgeons with extensive experience in renovascular surgery. The cumulative success rate of revascularization is 28%.[32] Even after successful revascularization, subsequent hypertension develops in 12% to 57% of patients, and most require elective nephrectomy.[32,40,41] The overall poor long-term results have led some authors to suggest that revascularization should be considered only in patients with bilateral renal artery occlusion or those with injury to a solitary kidney.[32,40]

Nonoperative management is certainly an acceptable option, especially in patients with delayed diagnosis, those with other major extra-abdominal injuries or significant hemodynamic instability, and those with a contralateral normally functioning kidney. Thirty-two percent to 40% of patients managed nonoperatively develop renovascular hypertension.[32,34,40] In most patients the hypertension develops within 1 year of the injury, with a mean of about 3 months.[32] We recommend revascularization only in renovascular injuries diagnosed intraoperatively, provided that the patient's condition is fairly stable, or in the rare case of bilateral injuries or injury to a solitary kidney. For the remainder, we advocate observation and long-term monitoring for hypertension.

Surgical Reconstruction. Surgical reconstruction of a renal artery injury can be achieved by simple arteriorrhaphy, vein patch, resection and anastomosis, and interposition grafting. For complex, time-consuming arterial reconstructions, the kidney should be perfused intermittently with iced heparinized lactated Ringer's solution or University of Wisconsin solution. Postrevascularization administration of mannitol may improve the parenchymal blood flow and alleviate the reperfusion injury.

Venous Injuries. Renal vein injuries can be managed by lateral venorrhaphy if feasible. Extensive injuries should be managed by ligation. Complex reconstruction, especially in a hemodynamically unstable patient, should be avoided. Ligation of the left renal vein near the IVC is well tolerated because of satisfactory venous drainage through the left gonadal vein, left adrenal vein, and lumbar veins. Ligation of the right renal vein should always be followed by nephrectomy.

Mortality

The true mortality rate of renovascular injuries is difficult to estimate because in most cases there are other major injuries.

The reported mortality rate varies from 0% to 57%.[35] The mortality in renovascular injuries due to blunt trauma is low because of the occlusive nature of most arterial injuries.[31]

Inferior Mesenteric Artery Injuries

Anatomy

The IMA originates from the anterior surface of the aorta 3 to 4 cm above the aortic bifurcation. It provides blood supply to the left colon, sigmoid, and upper part of the rectum. It communicates with the SMA through the marginal artery of Drummond.

Mechanism of Injury

Injuries of the IMA are rare, almost always due to penetrating trauma, and account for 1% of all abdominal vascular injuries.[1]

Surgical Treatment

The diagnosis of IMA injury is made intraoperatively. Ligation is well tolerated, and no cases of colorectal ischemia have been reported in trauma cases.

Iliac Vascular Injuries

Anatomy

The abdominal aorta bifurcates into the two common iliac arteries at the L4-L5 level. The common iliac arteries divide into the external and internal iliac arteries over the sacroiliac joint. The ureter crosses over the bifurcation of the common iliac artery.

The common iliac veins join at the L5 level, below the level of the aortic bifurcation and underneath the right common iliac artery, to form the IVC (Fig. 154-17).

Mechanism of Injury

Penetrating trauma is by far the most common cause of iliac vascular injuries. About 10% of patients who undergo laparotomy for gunshot wounds and 2% of patients with laparotomies due to stab wounds have iliac vascular injuries.[42] Injury to the common or external iliac artery due to blunt trauma is not common, although there are many case reports. Direct laceration of the iliac vessels from a pelvic fracture or stretching of the iliac artery over the pelvic wall, resulting in intimal tear and subsequent thrombosis, is the usual mechanism of injury after blunt trauma (see Fig. 154-6).[43] About 26% of patients with iliac vascular injuries have combined arterial and venous injuries.[42] Penetrating injuries usually involve the common iliac vessels, whereas blunt trauma usually affects branches of the internal iliac artery.

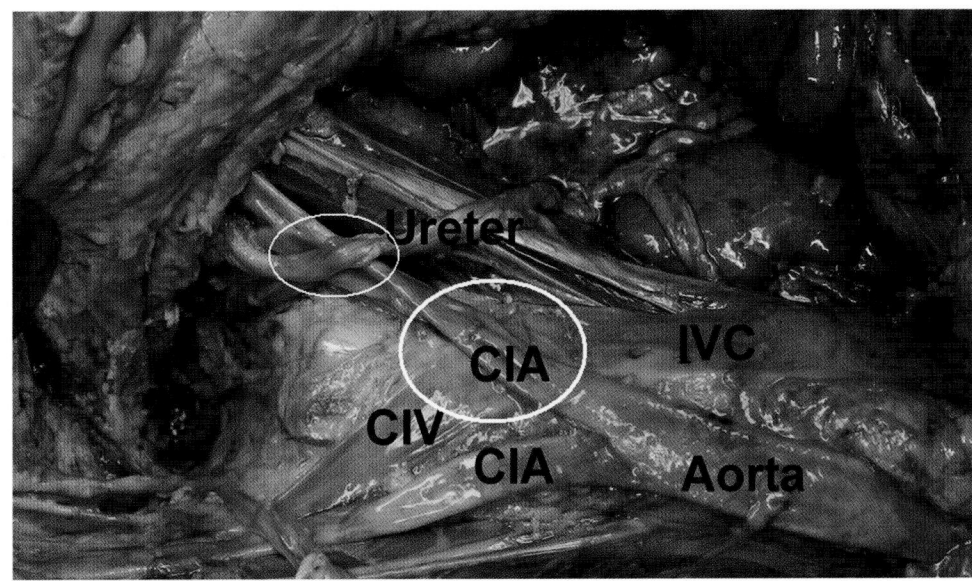

Figure 154-17 Anatomy of the iliac vessels. Note the confluence of the two common iliac veins (CIV) behind the proximal right common iliac artery (CIA; *large circle*). Also note the position of the ureter over the bifurcation of the common iliac artery (*small circle*). IVC, inferior vena cava.

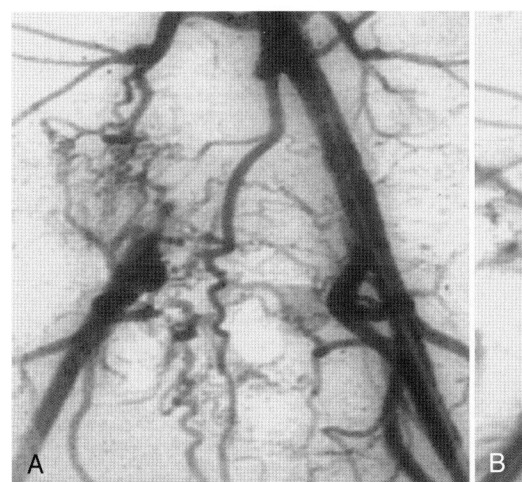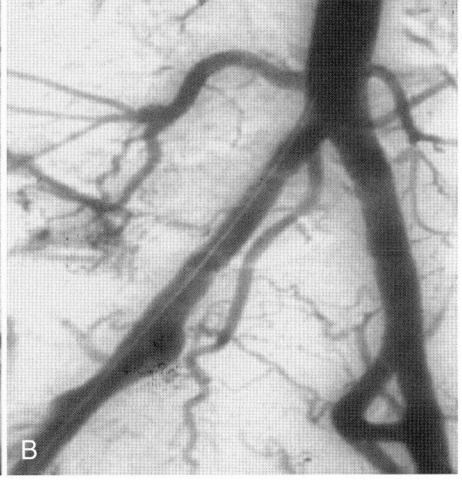

Figure 154-18 A, Right common iliac artery thrombosis in a 16-year-old patient diagnosed many months after a motor vehicle accident. **B,** Management with an endovascular stent was successful.

Clinical Presentation

The presence of a penetrating injury in the lower abdomen associated with severe hypotension and abdominal distention is highly suggestive of iliac vascular injuries. An absent or diminished femoral pulse in a young patient with penetrating abdominal trauma or pelvic fracture is diagnostic of an injury to the common or external iliac artery. In rare cases of blunt trauma, thrombosis of the iliac artery may not be diagnosed early during the initial hospitalization because of the subtle clinical symptoms. In other patients with blunt trauma, the diagnosis is made during the routine abdominal CT evaluation.

Endovascular Treatment

Endovascular techniques may play an important role in selected cases of iliac artery injury, especially after blunt trauma. Patients with false aneurysms, arteriovenous fistulae, or major intimal tears with or without thrombosis may benefit from angiographically placed endovascular stents (Fig. 154-18).[44,45] Because of its safety and low complication rate, this should be the first-line therapeutic option in elective cases in patients with subacute or chronic traumatic lesions of the common or external iliac arteries.

Surgical Treatment

Exposure. The operative findings may include free intraperitoneal bleeding, a zone 3 pelvic hematoma, or a combination of the two (Fig. 154-19). Zone 3 hematomas due to blunt trauma should be explored only if there is associated intraperitoneal leak, if they are expanding rapidly, or if there is an absent or diminished femoral pulse. In penetrating trauma, all hematomas should be explored. Any active bleeding is initially exposed by direct dissection of the overlying peritoneum, although medial rotation of the right or left colon may provide

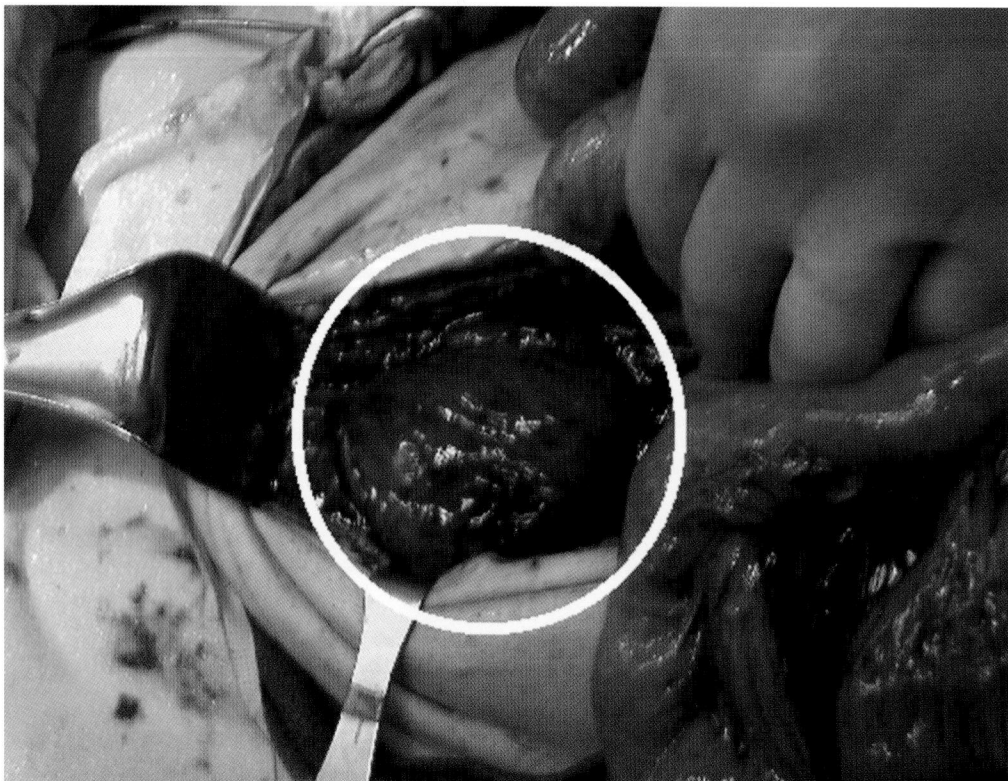

Figure 154-19 Large hematoma in the pelvis (*circle*) after a gunshot wound. This is highly suggestive of an iliac vascular injury, and proximal control should be obtained as soon as possible.

better exposure. The ureter, which crosses over the bifurcation of the common iliac artery, should be identified and protected during the dissection. In addition, care should be taken to avoid iatrogenic injury to the iliac veins that lie directly under the arteries. Isolation and control of the internal iliac artery are essential in arterial injuries because bleeding may persist despite proximal and distal control. If exposure of the distal iliac vessels is difficult, especially in males with a narrow pelvis, extension of the midline incision by adding a transverse lower abdominal incision or longitudinal incision over the groin and dividing the inguinal ligament may be necessary.[42]

Arterial Injuries. Small arterial injuries can be repaired with 4-0 or 5-0 vascular sutures, with care taken to avoid significant stenosis of the vessel. If necessary, a venous or PTFE patch can be used to avoid stenosis. In most gunshot injuries and in all patients with blunt trauma, reconstruction by an end-to-end anastomosis or with a prosthetic graft (size 6 or 8) is usually necessary. Local heparin solution should be administered to prevent thrombosis during the repair. A balloon-tipped catheter should always be passed proximally and distally to remove any clots. Complex arterial reconstructions with an extra-anatomic bypass or with a mobilized internal iliac artery have little or no role in the acute management of trauma. Extra-anatomic bypass should be considered only in late cases with severe purulent peritonitis or infected grafts. There is evidence that the presence of enteric contamination

is not a contraindication for synthetic graft use.[46] However, many vascular surgeons still recommend that in the presence of significant enteric contamination, an extra-anatomic bypass be considered. If prosthetic material is used, it is important that any enteric spillage be controlled and that the peritoneal cavity be meticulously cleaned before prosthetic graft repair.

Ligation of the common or external iliac arteries should never be performed, even in patients in critical condition. Ligation is poorly tolerated by most patients, it is associated with a high incidence of limb loss, and subsequent attempts to revascularize the leg may cause severe reperfusion injury and organ failure or death. In patients in critical condition who need damage control, the continuity of the injured artery can be established with a temporary intraluminal shunt (see Fig. 154-10); definitive reconstruction of the vessel is performed at a later stage when the patient's condition has stabilized.

Venous Injuries. Iliac venous injuries can be technically more challenging than arterial injuries because of the difficult exposure caused by the anatomic arrangement behind the arteries. This problem is even more difficult on the right side because of the location of the right common iliac artery and the confluence of the two common iliac veins behind the right common iliac artery. Despite these difficulties, the recommendation to transect the iliac artery to access the underlying vein[47] is extreme and should rarely be considered. In most cases, careful mobilization and retraction of the artery provides satisfactory exposure of the vein. Ligation and division of the internal iliac artery may be helpful in providing a better exposure. Repair of the iliac veins by means of lateral venorrhaphy should be considered only if it can be performed without producing major stenosis. Ligation is generally preferable to a repair that produces severe stenosis because of the risk of thrombosis and pulmonary embolism.[42] There is no experience with vena caval filters in cases with narrowed iliac veins. Complex reconstruction with spiral grafts or prosthetic materials, especially in a critically ill patient, is not recommended. Ligation is usually well tolerated, although many patients develop transient leg edema. On rare occasion, ligation results in massive edema of the leg and compartment syndrome that requires fasciotomy. The management of iliac venous injuries in the presence of associated iliac artery injuries is even more controversial. We do not recommend complex venous reconstruction because patients with combined arterial and venous injuries are invariably in extremely critical condition, and any procedures that prolong the operation or increase blood loss should be avoided. However, many authors recommend venous reconstruction with patch venoplasty or PTFE grafts, although there is no evidence of improved outcome with this approach.

Compartment Syndrome. Many patients with iliac vascular injuries develop extremity compartment syndrome. In this case, fasciotomy should be performed without delay, often before arterial reconstruction. The role of prophylactic fasciotomy, however, is controversial and has been challenged by many authors. Prophylactic fasciotomy is a major procedure that is often associated with increased bleeding due to coagulopathy and increased venous pressures if an iliac vein ligation is performed.[48,49] If fasciotomy is not performed, the patient should be monitored closely with frequent clinical examinations and compartment pressure measurements. Fasciotomy should be performed at the first signs of compartment syndrome.[42] Perioperative administration of mannitol may play a beneficial role in reducing the effects of reperfusion injury and inhibiting the development of compartment syndrome and the need for fasciotomy.[49,50]

Mortality

The reported overall mortality varies from 30% to 50% in arterial injuries and 25% to 40% in venous injuries. In isolated iliac vascular injuries, the mortality is about 20% for arterial injuries and about 10% for venous injuries.[42]

Inferior Vena Cava Injuries
Anatomy

The IVC is formed by the confluence of the two common iliac veins in front of the L5 vertebra and underneath the right common iliac artery. It ascends over the spine to the right of the aorta; at the level of the renal veins it deviates farther to the right, courses behind the liver, crosses the diaphragm,

and, after a short course of 2 to 3 cm in the chest, drains into the right atrium of the heart. In its course the IVC receives four or five pairs of lumbar veins, the right gonadal vein, the renal veins, the right adrenal vein, the hepatic veins, and the phrenic veins. All lumbar veins are below the renal veins, and except for the right adrenal vein, there are no other venous branches between the renal veins and hepatic veins. Besides the three major hepatic veins, there are six to eight accessory veins inferiorly. Some of the accessory veins are large and may bleed profusely in the case of injury or iatrogenic avulsion.

Mechanism of Injury

The IVC is the most commonly injured abdominal vessel and accounts for about 25% of abdominal vascular injuries.[1] Blunt trauma is responsible for about 10% of IVC injuries, and it usually involves the retrohepatic part of the vein.[51] In about 18% of patients with penetrating IVC injuries, there is an associated aortic injury.[52]

Clinical Presentation

More than half the patients with IVC injuries who reach the hospital alive are hypotensive, and about 18% require emergency thoracotomy.[52,53] Many patients with contained hematomas may be hemodynamically stable on admission. The diagnosis is almost always made intraoperatively.

Surgical Exposure

Many injuries to the IVC, especially those involving the infrarenal IVC, present with stable hematomas. As a rule, all hematomas due to penetrating trauma should be explored. An exception to this approach is stable retrohepatic hematomas. Exploration of these hematomas is extremely difficult and may lead to uncontrollable hemorrhage and death. The infrarenal and juxtarenal IVC are best exposed by mobilization and medial rotation of the right colon, the hepatic flexure of the colon, and the duodenum (see Fig. 154-9). Exposure of the retrohepatic IVC is technically challenging and usually requires extensive mobilization of the liver by dividing its ligaments and extending the incision to include a right subcostal incision, right thoracotomy, or sternotomy. In our experience, a subcostal incision provides excellent exposure and is preferred. A median sternotomy is performed if an atriocaval shunt is anticipated. These additional incisions should be considered only if perihepatic packing is not effective in controlling the hemorrhage. In cases in which packing is not effective and the additional incisions are not sufficient for adequate visualization and repair of the IVC or hepatic veins, other more radical maneuvers may be considered. Such maneuvers include hepatic vascular isolation, an atriocaval shunt, or division of the liver.

Hepatic Vascular Isolation. Hepatic vascular isolation involves cross-clamping the infradiaphragmatic aorta, suprahepatic IVC, infrahepatic IVC above the renal veins, and portal triad. Failure to clamp the aorta as a first step may result in severe hypotension and possible cardiac arrest, owing to the reduced venous return after occlusion of the IVC. The suprarenal IVC can be cross-clamped in the space between the superior surface of the liver and the diaphragm. If a thoracotomy is performed, the IVC is controlled in the pericardium.[53] Despite the hepatic isolation there is still backbleeding.

Atriocaval Shunt. The atriocaval shunt requires placing a tube through a purse-string suture in the appendage of the right atrium and directing it into the IVC, distal to the caval injury. Tourniquets should be applied around the intrapericardial IVC and the suprarenal IVC.[54] A large-bore thoracostomy tube or a large endotracheal tube with clamp occlusion of the proximal end and one or two holes created to correspond to the endoatrial part of the tube can be used as shunts. If an endotracheal tube is used, the inflated balloon can replace a tourniquet around the suprarenal IVC (Fig. 154-20). This is preferable to dissection around the IVC for tourniquet placement. Although numerous reports have highlighted the extremely poor results with atriocaval shunts, a few patients have survived when the shunt was used early. This approach obviously entails a major escalation of the operation, but in appropriate cases, it should be used early in the operation.

Division of the Liver. Some authors have recommended dividing the liver along the gallbladder-IVC plane to provide

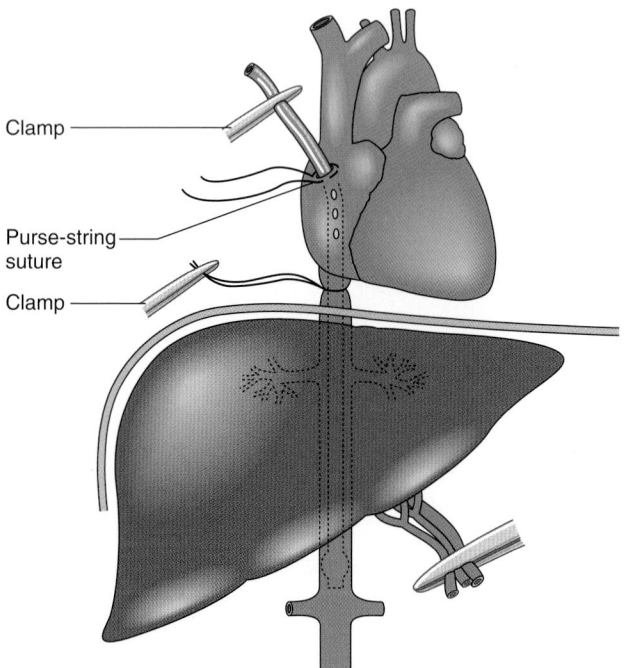

Figure 154-20 Atriocaval shunt for severe retrohepatic inferior vena cava (IVC) injuries. An endotracheal tube is placed through a purse-string suture in the right atrial appendage, and the cuff is inflated above the renal veins. A tourniquet is applied in the intrapericardiac IVC. Note the extra holes in the endoatrial part of the tube. This technique should be considered when liver packing does not control hemorrhage.

direct exposure to the IVC. This approach increases bleeding, especially in an already coagulopathic patient, and should be avoided except when the liver is severely injured and the IVC can be exposed with a brief dissection.

Surgical Options

In most patients the IVC can be repaired by lateral venorrhaphy with 3-0 or 4-0 vascular suture material. Most posterior caval wounds can be exposed and repaired by rotating the IVC. In some patients with anterior and posterior caval injuries, the posterior wound can be exposed and repaired from within the vein by extending the anterior wound. Ligation of the vein should be considered in hemodynamically unstable patients with severe infrarenal injuries or when repair produces major stenosis. Ligation of the suprarenal IVC is not an acceptable option because it results in renal failure. In these cases, reconstruction of the vein with a patch or a ringed prosthetic graft can be attempted, but it is rarely successful because of the patient's poor hemodynamic status.

Postoperatively, patients with IVC ligation should have their lower extremities wrapped with firm elastic bandages and elevated. Most of them develop temporary edema that subsides within a few weeks. However, some patients develop extremity compartment syndrome and require fasciotomy.

In patients with severe IVC stenosis after lateral venorrhaphy, there is a risk of thrombosis and pulmonary embolism. If this cannot be avoided, a caval filter or clips should be deployed above the site of stenosis.

Mortality

About half the patients with IVC injuries die before reaching medical care, and among those who arrive at the hospital with signs of life, the mortality ranges between 20% and 57%.[51] In a study of 136 cases with IVC injuries, Kuene and associates reported an overall mortality of 52%.[51] In patients reaching the operating room alive, the mortality was 35%. The mortality was significantly higher in suprarenal injuries.

Portal Vein System Injuries

Anatomy

The portal vein is 6 to 10 cm long and is formed by the confluence of the SMV and the splenic vein behind the neck of the pancreas, to the right of L2, and to the left of the IVC. It passes behind the first part of the duodenum and enters the hepatoduodenal ligament. In the hepatoduodenal ligament it courses between and behind the common bile duct to the right and the hepatic artery to the left. In the hilum of the liver it splits into right and left branches. The portal vein has no valves and provides about 80% of the hepatic blood flow. The SMV trunk crosses over the third part of the duodenum and the uncinate process of the pancreas. It then passes behind the neck of the pancreas, where it joins the slightly smaller splenic vein to form the portal vein. The splenic vein courses along the superior border of the pancreas and drains the inferior mesenteric vein, just before the confluence with the SMV.

Mechanism of Injury

Injury to the portal vein trunk is relatively rare and is found in about 1% of patients undergoing laparotomy for trauma.[55] More than 90% of portal vein injuries are due to penetrating trauma. Because of its close proximity to other major vessels, the incidence of associated vascular injuries is high, ranging from 70% to 90% of cases.[56]

Clinical Presentation

Most patients with penetrating injuries to the portal venous system present with signs of hemorrhagic shock and require emergency laparotomy. In blunt trauma, the injury usually involves the SMV and is due to a direct blow to the abdomen or deceleration forces. These mechanisms often result in thrombosis of the vessels and occasionally avulsion and bleeding. In cases with thrombosis, the diagnosis is delayed and is often made on abdominal CT evaluation.

Surgical Treatment

The operative findings usually include a combination of local hematoma and various degrees of hemorrhage. Exposure of the retropancreatic portal vein and its major branches can be achieved by mobilization and medial rotation of the right colon and hepatic flexure of the colon and extensive Kocher mobilization of the duodenum. However, this approach often does not provide satisfactory exposure, especially in patients with associated injuries to the SMA. In these cases, stapled division of the neck of the pancreas provides excellent exposure and should be considered early (Fig. 154-21). The suprapancreatic portal vein can be exposed by a combination of mobilization and medial rotation of the right colon and hepatic flexure and a Kocher maneuver.

The portal vein and SMV should be repaired if this can be achieved with lateral venorrhaphy. Complex reconstructive procedures, such as interposition grafts, are rarely feasible or advisable because of the patient's poor condition. About 80% of patients have other vascular injuries that contribute to blood loss and coagulopathy. Complex reconstruction should be undertaken only in patients with associated hepatic artery injury that cannot be repaired. Ligation of both the portal vein and the hepatic artery is not compatible with life. In these cases, reconstruction of the portal vein with a saphenous vein graft should be considered.[56]

Ligation of the portal vein with a patent hepatic artery is compatible with life, and the survival ranges from 55% to 85%.[57,58] After ligation of the portal vein or SMV the bowel becomes massively edematous, and patients can develop patchy bowel wall necrosis. The abdomen should never be closed primarily because, without exception, all patients develop ACS. Temporary abdominal wall closure with pros-

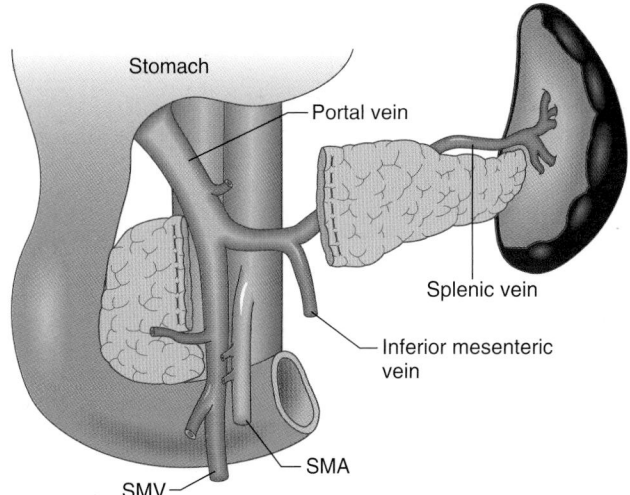

Figure 154-21 Stapled division of the neck of the pancreas provides good exposure of the retropancreatic portal vein and the superior mesenteric vessels. SMA, superior mesenteric artery; SMV, superior mesenteric vein.

thetic material should be performed. Second-look laparotomy should be performed in 48 to 72 hours to remove any abdominal packs and check the viability of the bowel.

Postoperatively, massive fluid replacement is required because of sequestration in the splanchnic bed. Over the next few days there is significant improvement of bowel edema owing to enlargement of the collateral circulation, and abdominal wall closure may be possible. Experience with the long-term effects of portal ligation is limited, but there is evidence that most survivors do not develop portal hypertension.[55,57,58]

Mortality

The mortality in portal vein injuries is high and ranges between 50% and 72%.[1,57,58] Most patients have other major injuries, making it difficult to assess the mortality directly related to isolated portal vein injuries.

ADVANCES IN THE MANAGEMENT OF ABDOMINAL VASCULAR INJURIES

There have been some significant advances in the management of abdominal vascular injuries in the past decade. Introduction of the policy of "scoop and run" and early surgical control of bleeding have now become the standard of care and have improved survival in patients with vascular injuries. The concept of damage control has gained popularity and acceptance, and as a result, many patients with vascular injuries have been saved. The recognition of ACS and the use of temporary abdominal wall closure are also important steps in improving outcomes. Endovascular technology has revolutionized the management of selected patients with specific vascular occlusions, arteriovenous fistulae, and false aneurysms. Finally, research into powerful new hemostatic agents is promising, and these agents may have a major impact on the management of abdominal vascular injuries.

SELECTED KEY REFERENCES

Bickell WH, Wall MJ, Pepe PE, Martin RR, Ginger VF, Allen MK, Mattox KL. Immediate versus delayed fluid resuscitation for hypotensive patients with penetrating torso trauma. *N Engl J Med.* 1994; 331:1105-1109.

Dutton RP, Mackenzie CF, Scalea TM. Hypotensive resuscitation during active hemorrhage: impact on in-hospital mortality. *J Trauma.* 2002;52:1141-1146.

Leppaniemi A, Solter R, Burris D, Pikoulis E, Waasdorp C, Ratigan J, Hufnagel H, Malcolm D. Fluid resuscitation in a model of uncontrolled hemorrhage: too much too early, or too little too late? *J Surg Res.* 1996;63:413-418.
This three-study series (two human, one animal) demonstrates the impact of controlled resuscitation in traumatic hemorrhagic shock. The first study by Bickell and associates in hypotensive patients who sustained penetrating torso injuries demonstrated improved outcomes, including survival, with delayed fluid resuscitation. The second study randomized penetrating and blunt trauma patients in hemorrhagic shock to resuscitation targeted at conventional (>100 mm Hg) versus low (70 mm Hg) systolic blood pressure, with no difference in mortality. In the penetrating aortic injury model of uncontrolled hemorrhage used in the animal study, the response to varied fluid infusion rates raises the possibility that a more moderate resuscitation strategy may be the key to maximizing survival.

Buckman RF, Pathak AS, Badelino MM, Bradley KM. Injuries of the inferior vena cava. *Surg Clin North Am.* 2001;81:1431-1447.

Buckman RF, Pathak AS, Badelino MM, Bradley KM. Portal vein injuries. *Surg Clin North Am.* 2001;81:1449-1462.
These reviews summarize the anatomy, clinical presentation, diagnostic workup, and management options for injuries to the IVC and portal vein.

Demetriades D, Murray JA, Asensio JA. Iliac vessel injuries. In: Rich N, Mattox KL, Hirshberg A, eds. *Vascular Trauma.* Philadelphia: WB Saunders; 2004:339-351.
This comprehensive overview of vascular trauma provides in-depth reference material covering all aspects of iliac vascular trauma.

Demetriades D, Theodorou D, Murray J, Asensio JA, Cornwell EE 3rd, Velmahos G, Belzberg H, Berne TV. Mortality and prognostic factors in penetrating injuries of the aorta. *J Trauma.* 1996;40: 761-763.
This major epidemiologic review of penetrating aortic injuries summarizes the epidemiology and outcomes after penetrating aortic trauma and highlights the differences between injuries to the thoracic and abdominal segments.

Lee JT, White RA. Endovascular management of blunt traumatic renal artery dissection. *J Endovasc Ther.* 2002;9:354-358.
This article describes the clinical diagnosis and endovascular approach to the treatment of blunt renal artery injuries.

Sangthong B, Demetriades D, Martin M, Salim A, Brown C, Inaba K, Rhee P, Chan L. Management and hospital outcomes of blunt renal artery injuries: analysis of 517 patients from the National Trauma Data Bank. *J Am Coll Surg.* 2006;203:612-617.
This study describes the epidemiology and outcomes after blunt renal artery injuries, including the impact of both operative and nonoperative management strategies.

Voellinger DC, Saddakni S, Melton SM, Wirthlin DJ, Jordan WD, Whitley D. Endovascular repair of a traumatic infrarenal aortic dissection: a case report and review. *Vasc Surg.* 2001;35:385-389.
This case demonstrates the challenges in the clinical diagnosis of blunt abdominal vascular injury and highlights contemporary endovascular management techniques.

REFERENCES

The reference list can be found on the companion Expert Consult Web site at *www.expertconsult.com.*

CHAPTER 155

Vascular Trauma: Extremity

Kaushal R. Patel and Vincent L. Rowe

Approximately 90% of all peripheral arterial injuries occur in an extremity. In civilian studies the majority of arterial injuries are in the upper extremity, whereas in the military experience lower extremity injuries are more common.[1] During World War II, extremity arterial injuries were routinely ligated. For popliteal artery injuries, the amputation rate was 73%.[2] The poor results of arterial ligation prompted Hughes to perform formal repair of peripheral arterial injuries during the Korean War.[1,3] Rich and associates reported further refinements of arterial repair during the Vietnam War, decreasing the amputation rate for popliteal artery injuries to 32%.[4] Continuing refinements in arterial surgery over the ensuing decades have reduced limb loss in most civilian series to less than 10% to 15%[5-7]; however, long-term disability, predominantly from associated skeletal and nerve injuries, is a persistent problem for 20% to 50% of patients.[8]

MECHANISM OF INJURY

The initial and ultimate outcomes of vascular injury depend in large part on the wounding agent or mechanism of injury. Determining the mechanism of injury—whether blunt trauma, high-velocity penetrating trauma, or low-velocity penetrating trauma—is of the utmost importance if the surgeon is to use the available diagnostic and treatment options appropriately. Peripheral vascular injuries in an urban environment most often result from penetrating trauma from knives or bullets. In a series of penetrating injuries, arterial injuries were caused by gunshot wounds in 64%, knife wounds in 24%, and shotgun blasts in 12%.[9]

Traditionally, high-velocity firearm injuries occurred in the battlefield, but with increasing frequency they are the causative agent in civilian vascular trauma as well. In addition to the vascular injury, extensive associated musculoskeletal injury is common. Vascular injuries in this setting result from the dissipation of energy into the surrounding tissues, fragmentation of the projectile or of bone, and the blast effect.[10] Experimental studies have demonstrated a positive correlation between muzzle velocity and the microscopic extent and "length" of damage to the vessel wall.[11] In many ways, these wounds mimic lower velocity shotgun injuries in their devastating combination of penetrating and blunt tissue injury.[12]

Motor vehicle accidents and falls are the most common causes of blunt injury and are becoming more frequent with the increasing mobility of modern society.[11,13] The morbidity of blunt vascular injuries can be magnified by associated fractures, dislocations, and crush injuries to muscles and nerves.

DIAGNOSTIC EVALUATION

Physical Findings

Extremity arterial injuries have varied clinical presentations. A minority of patients present with obvious clinical evidence, or hard signs, of an arterial disruption, such as pulsatile external bleeding, an enlarging hematoma, absent distal pulses, or an ischemic limb (Box 155-1). For patients with overt signs of arterial injury, immediate surgical exploration in the operating room, without further diagnostic testing, is preferred. When arteriography is required, an intraoperative arteriogram is usually sufficient to identify the location and extent of injury and guide the surgical repair.

A large majority of arterial injuries are clinically occult and pose a diagnostic challenge. The diagnostic approach has changed substantially since the Korean War. Initially, the severity of soft tissue destruction typical of military wounds prompted the recommendation that all penetrating extremity wounds near a neurovascular bundle be explored routinely. When applied to civilian injuries, this practice detected normal intact vessels in a large percentage of cases, up to 84% in one series.[14] These patients had thus undergone expensive, nontherapeutic operations that occasionally resulted in additional morbidity.

Box 155-1 Signs of Traumatic Vascular Injury

HARD SIGNS
- Observed pulsatile bleeding
- Arterial thrill by manual palpation
- Bruit auscultated over or near an area of arterial injury
- Absent distal pulse
- Visible expanding hematoma

SOFT SIGNS
- Significant hemorrhage by history
- Neurologic abnormality
- Diminished pulse compared with contralateral extremity
- Proximity of bony injury or penetrating wound

Doppler Indices and Selective Arteriography

With the availability of arteriography in most trauma centers, this diagnostic modality supplanted wound exploration for penetrating extremity trauma. As was the case with wound exploration, mandatory or routine screening arteriography for proximity wounds, in the absence of other suspicious clinical findings, resulted in a large proportion of normal arteriograms (90%), at significant cost. In addition, arteriograms were found to be less than perfect, having a low but real incidence of false-negative and false-positive findings. Because of its invasive nature and the potential nephrotoxicity of contrast media, arteriography also occasionally results in serious complications, thus increasing patient morbidity and further increasing the cost of care.

Several studies have documented that selective rather than routine arteriography is appropriate and safe for patients who may have an occult extremity arterial injury.[15-18] In one study of 373 patients with a unilateral penetrating injury to an upper or lower extremity, arteriography was obtained. In the 216 patients with one or more abnormal physical findings, an arterial injury was identified by arteriography in 65 (30%), whereas in the absence of physical findings (157 patients), only minor injuries were identified in 17 (11%). Only a pulse deficit, neurologic deficit, or shotgun injury correlated with arteriographic evidence of a major arterial injury ($P < .05$).

A follow-up study investigated the ability of Doppler indices to detect occult arterial injuries in a consecutive cohort of 514 patients with unilateral, isolated penetrating extremity injuries.[19] Arteriography was limited to patients with a pulse deficit, neurologic deficit, shotgun injury, or one or more soft signs or a Doppler ankle-brachial index (ABI) of less than 1. All patients with arteriographic evidence of a major arterial injury had either a pulse deficit or an ABI below 1.

The selective use of angiography to evaluate patients with penetrating extremity trauma was recently confirmed by Conrad and associates, who retrospectively reviewed 538 patients.[16] Similar to previous studies, angiography was limited to patients presenting with an abnormal pulse examination or Doppler indices less than 1. Patients with a normal physical examination and Doppler indices of 1 or greater were discharged home without further workup. Of the 300 asymptomatic patients discharged home, 51% were available for an average follow-up of 9.8 months. There were no missed injuries or late complications identified in that group.

For blunt extremity trauma, the indications for arteriography parallel what has been established for penetrating injuries. A prospective study analyzed the results of arteriography in 53 patients with unilateral blunt lower extremity trauma.[20] Thirty-one patients had physical findings suggestive of an arterial injury, and an arterial injury was demonstrated in 15. A pulse deficit or decreased capillary refill correlated significantly with arteriographic evidence of injury ($P < .05$). Of the 15 arterial injuries, 12 were found in patients who had one or both of these findings, and 4 of those injuries required repair. In the remaining 22 patients with neither a pulse deficit nor

decreased capillary refill, three minor injuries were found, none of which required repair.

Another series of blunt injuries focused on 115 patients with knee dislocations.[21] Popliteal artery injury was demonstrated arteriographically in 27 of 115 patients (23%). An abnormal pedal pulse identified popliteal artery injuries with a sensitivity of 85% and a specificity of 93%. All injuries that required intervention were associated with a diminished pulse. Dennis and colleagues reported an identical experience in 37 patients with knee dislocations.[22] In all patients who required popliteal repair, pedal pulses were absent. More recently, Abou-Sayed and Berger confirmed the sensitivity of physical examination in 52 patients with blunt popliteal artery injuries.[15] Twenty-three patients with normal pulse examinations did not undergo angiography and required no vascular interventions. Angiography was performed in 13 patients with normal pulse examinations (at the discretion of the attending surgeon), and no clinically significant lesions that required intervention were identified. Again, the assertion that the clinical examination can define a subset of high-risk patients who need arteriography and possibly surgical repair was validated.

Similar evidence of the reliability of the clinical examination combined with noninvasive pressure measurements has been provided by Lynch and Johansen.[23] In a series of 100 patients with blunt or penetrating limb trauma, all patients had ABI measurements and arteriography. Arterial injuries that required intervention were discovered in 14 cases, and an ABI less than 0.90 predicted the injury with 87% sensitivity and 97% specificity. Because two of the arteriograms were falsely positive, the sensitivity and specificity of ABIs less than 0.90 were even higher—95% and 97%, respectively—when clinical outcome was the standard.

Based on these published reports, the consensus is that for penetrating or blunt extremity trauma, arteriography is indicated only for patients with either an abnormal extremity pulse examination or a Doppler index less than 1.00. Careful physical examination and pressure measurements appropriately select the vast majority of patients (>95%) who have significant arterial injury and require arteriography. With these principles in mind, the diagnostic algorithm shown in Figure 155-1 was constructed.[24]

Color-Flow Duplex Ultrasonography

Because of continued improvements in noninvasive vascular imaging, color-flow duplex (CFD) ultrasonography has been suggested as a substitute for or complement to arteriography.[25] CFD has several obvious advantages. It is noninvasive and painless. It is portable and can easily be brought to the patient's bedside or the emergency room or operating room. Repeat and follow-up examinations are easily performed without morbidity and are relatively inexpensive.

Bynoe and colleagues reported a sensitivity of 95%, specificity of 99%, and accuracy of 98% when CFD was used to evaluate blunt and penetrating injuries of the neck or extremities,[26] and Fry and coworkers documented 100% sensitivity

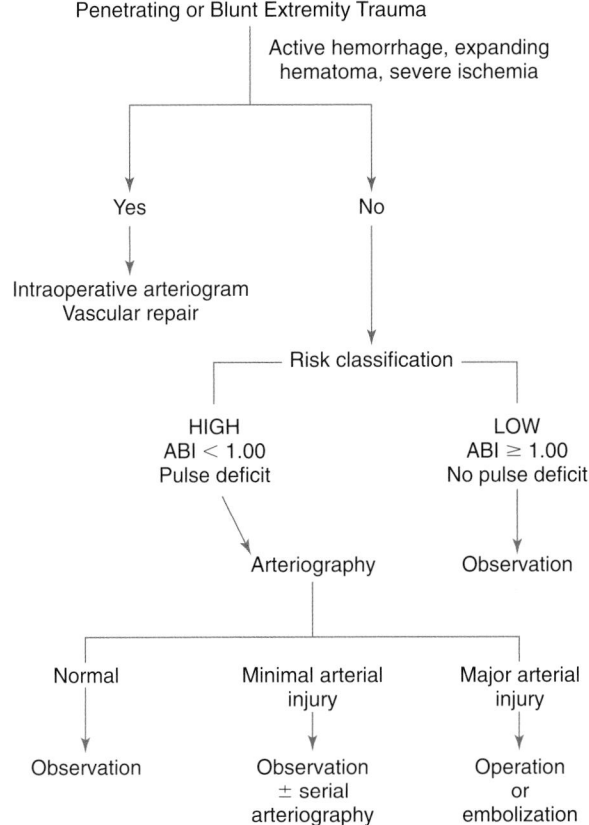

Figure 155-1 Diagnostic algorithm for extremity arterial trauma. ABI, ankle-brachial index. *(From Hood DB, Yellin AE, Weaver FA. Vascular trauma. In: Dean R, ed.* Current Vascular Surgical Diagnosis and Treatment. *Norwalk, CT: Appleton & Lange; 1995:405.)*

and 97.3% specificity in a similar series.[27] In these two studies, however, a comparison arteriogram was available for only a minority of patients. Bergstein and associates reported on 67 patients who had 75 penetrating extremity injuries, all of whom underwent both CFD and arteriography.[28] Using arteriography as the "gold standard," CFD had two false-negative results and one false-positive result (sensitivity 50%, specificity 99%). Gagne and coworkers published a series of 37 patients with proximity injuries in 43 extremities.[29] Arteriography identified three injuries to the deep femoral, superficial femoral, and posterior tibial arteries that were not identified by CFD; however, CFD detected a superficial femoral artery intimal flap that arteriography missed.

Despite some uncertainty about CFD's ability to detect all arterial injuries, these reports suggest that nearly all major injuries that require therapeutic intervention can be identified.[25] Ordog and colleagues estimated a multimillion-dollar saving if CFD and outpatient follow-up, rather than arteriography and inpatient observation, were used to exclude extremity arterial injuries.[30]

Our own experience with CFD in the evaluation of extremity trauma has produced an important caveat: CFD is highly operator dependent and, to be used effectively, requires an institutional investment in experienced vascular technologists

and interpreting physicians.[31] This expense could be lessened over the long term if the current effort to train surgeons in the use of diagnostic ultrasound for intracavitary trauma were extended to include extremity vessels.

Magnetic Resonance Angiography

Magnetic resonance angiography (MRA) has increased in popularity for the diagnosis of vascular disorders; however, its application to trauma patients is not widely accepted. Compared with other modalities, MRA has the advantage of imaging multiple anatomic areas simultaneously and being noninvasive, preventing the need for contrast agents. Unfortunately, MRA is not easily accessible in the majority of hospitals, and the presence of metallic orthopedic instrumentation limits its widespread use for trauma patients.[32]

Computed Tomographic Angiography

With advances in technology, computed tomographic angiography (CTA) is challenging the need for digital angiography in the evaluation of trauma patients with suspected vascular injuries. Current scanners with multiplanar and three-dimensional reformatting capabilities allow the rapid acquisition of high-resolution images. Compared with digital angiography for trauma patients, CTA has the distinct advantage of being readily available and providing simultaneous imaging of surrounding body structures and adjacent anatomic locations in a single examination.

Soto and colleagues performed one of the early comparisons of CTA and digital angiography for the evaluation of suspected vascular injuries in extremity trauma patients.[33] In this study, all extremity trauma patients referred for digital angiography underwent CTA. Two independent observers documented sensitivity and specificity levels greater than 90% for the diagnosis of vascular injuries, with an interobserver agreement of 0.9 (kappa statistics). More recently, trauma centers are reporting the benefits of CTA not only for the diagnosis of extremity vascular injuries but also for surgical planning.[34-36] However, if an endovascular treatment option is contemplated, the deleterious effects of sequential intravenous contrast boluses must be considered.

■ TREATMENT OF ARTERIAL INJURIES

Nonoperative Management

The management of minimal, nonocclusive, clinically asymptomatic arterial injuries detected by arteriography remains controversial (Fig. 155-2).[37] Some surgeons continue to insist that all detected arterial injuries should be repaired, whereas we[38] and others[22,39] have proposed using a nonoperative approach when the following clinical and radiologic criteria are present: low-velocity injury, minimal (<5 mm) arterial wall disruption for intimal defects and pseudoaneurysms, adherent or downstream protrusion of intimal flaps, intact distal circulation, and no active hemorrhage. When this approach is

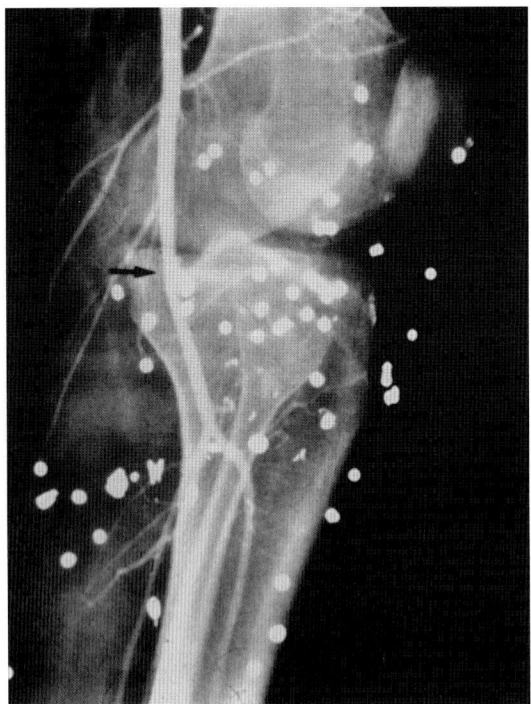

Figure 155-2 Popliteal artery shotgun injury with a small false aneurysm (*arrow*) that was managed nonoperatively.

selected, follow-up vascular imaging is advisable to document healing or stabilization. Knudson's group suggested that CFD may be used instead of arteriography for serial follow-up.[40]

In a study by Stain and coworkers, 24 nonocclusive, minimal arterial injuries were managed nonoperatively and subsequently studied arteriographically at 1 to 12 weeks after injury.[38] Resolution, improvement, or stabilization of the injury occurred in 21 injuries (87%). Progression was noted in three, and only one required repair. There were no cases of acute thrombosis or distal embolization. A similar experience in a group of patients with minimal arterial injuries identified on diagnostic arteriography was reported by Frykberg.[39] Resolution or stability of detected injuries occurred in 89% of cases during 27 months of follow-up. Frykberg's follow-up has now been extended to 10 years, with comparable excellent results, further confirming the wisdom of this approach.[22]

Endovascular Management

During the last decade there has been an increasing interest in the use of endovascular interventions in the management of traumatic vascular injuries. Once used strictly for diagnosis, with the advent of new endovascular devices, angiography has quickly assumed a role in the treatment of many vascular injuries. Applications range from vascular reconstruction with stents to control of bleeding vessels with coil embolization. In some instances, endovascular interventions may be used as a bridge to definitive open treatment once patients have recovered from other injuries. In a retrospective review of 12,732 arterial injures from the National Trauma Data Bank

between 1994 and 2003, the number of endovascular procedures performed annually increased 27-fold, from 4 in 1997 to 107 in 2003.[41]

Transcatheter Embolization

Transcatheter embolization with hemostatic agents or coils can be used to manage selected arterial injuries such as low-flow arteriovenous fistulae, false aneurysms, and active bleeding from noncritical arteries, particularly in remote anatomic sites. Coils are particularly useful for occluding bleeding vessels and arteriovenous fistulae (Fig. 155-3). Coils are made from stainless steel and have wool or Dacron tufts. Introduced via a 5 or 7 Fr catheter, they can be extruded at the vessel site that requires occlusion. Once deployed, the coils expand and lodge at the site of extrusion. The Dacron or wool tuft promotes thrombosis of the vessel. If flow persists 5 minutes after deployment, a second coil is introduced. For arteriovenous fistulae, the coil embolus is used to occlude the arterial side of the fistula, preferably by isolating the fistula site with proximal and distal coils. The diameter of the coil must be approximately the same as the diameter of the artery to be embolized; otherwise, it may dislodge and embolize peripherally or centrally.

McNeese and colleagues reported on 11 patients with post-traumatic arteriovenous fistulae, arterial false aneurysms, or uncontrolled bleeding from noncritical vessels who were treated by embolization.[42] Eight patients were treated by wire coil embolization or gelatin clot emboli, and one was treated

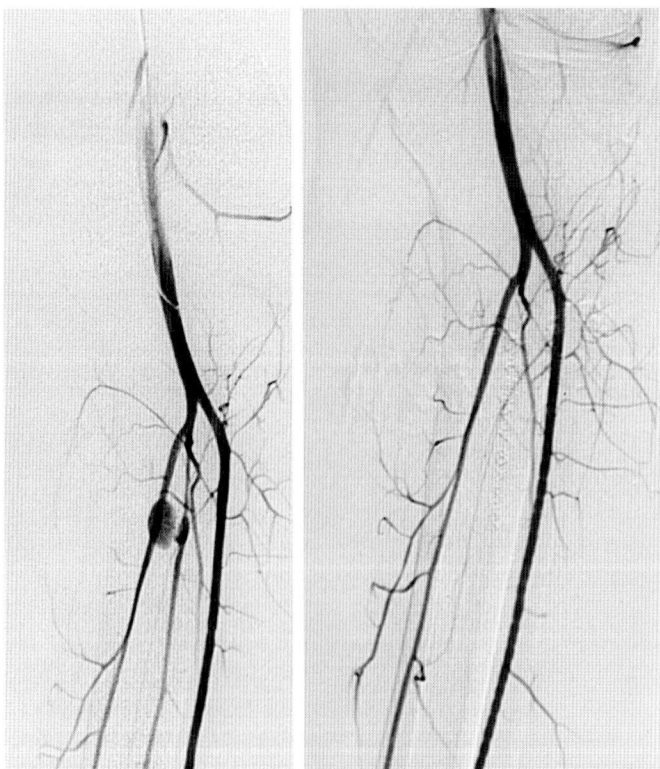

Figure 155-3 Large peroneal artery false aneurysm (*left*) that was successfully treated by coil embolization (*right*).

with selective injection of barium-impregnated silicone-like (Silastic) beads sized to the vessel lumen. The latter technique was found to be useful in treating arteriovenous fistulae fed by multiple small arteries. Four of six fistulae were permanently obliterated. No ischemia distal to an obliterated vessel occurred, and no major complications directly related to the embolization were reported.

Endografts

Another endovascular approach to extremity injuries uses endograft technology. By combining a fixation device such as a stent with a graft, endoluminal repair of false aneurysms or large arteriovenous fistulae is possible. Marin and coworkers reported the successful treatment of seven vascular injuries by endografts.[43] Since this early study, numerous small series and anecdotal reports have documented the successful management of traumatic arterial injuries with endografts.[44-47] Compiled results from multiple institutions in the National Trauma Data Bank demonstrate a statistically significant survival advantage for those undergoing endovascular repair of all traumatic vascular injuries, even after controlling for the number of associated injuries.[4] Patients with thoracic aortic injuries seem to benefit most from endovascular covered stent placement, with a 3% mortality for that procedure, compared with 19% for open surgical repair.[4] The potential disadvantages of endovascular interventions relate to the endografts used. Ongoing surveillance for graft migration, endoleak development, or in-stent stenosis is needed long term. Considering the relatively young age of most trauma patients, the long-term durability of endografts is also an issue.

In centers with sufficient experience and personnel to perform the procedure expediently, endovascular treatment of arterial lesions should be considered, especially in high-risk patients with multiple concomitant injuries. As hospital infrastructure for endovascular intervention improves (e.g., the development of more angiography-capable operating rooms) and surgeons become more adept in endovascular treatment modalities, the expeditious diagnosis and management of traumatic arterial injuries can be expected in the future.

Operative Management

General Principles

Once the decision is made for operative intervention, the patient should be transported to the operating room in an expeditious manner. Preoperative antibiotics with strong gram-positive coverage should be instituted before making the skin incision. In patients with known bony injuries, microbial coverage for gram-negative organisms is prudent. Anticipating the need for an intraoperative angiogram or bony manipulations, a fluoroscope-compatible operating room table should be used. The entire injured extremity should be prepared and draped to ensure adequate proximal control and offer multiple options for revascularization. In addition, an uninjured extremity should be included in the operative field

in the event an autogenous vein graft is required. In most cases, harvesting vein from the injured limb should be avoided owing to associated venous injuries and a potential worsening of postoperative swelling.

The initial goal in operative intervention is obtaining proximal control, especially in the case of hemorrhaging wounds. In most instances, extremity incisions are placed longitudinally, directly over the injured vessel, and extended proximally or distally as necessary. Proximal and distal arterial control is obtained before exposure of the injury. When proximal control of the traumatized vessel is problematic, as in some axillary and subclavian injuries, endoluminal balloon occlusion of the proximal artery via catheters placed under fluoroscopic guidance from a remote arterial site can provide temporary control. Occasionally, a proximally placed pneumatic tourniquet may help minimize operative blood loss.

Once control is established, a careful evaluation of the extent of arterial injury, as well as venous and nervous tissue damage, should be carried out. Débridement of all macroscopically injured or contused tissue is key to a successful outcome. In both blunt and penetrating traumatic injuries, the level of intimal damage can extend far beyond the obvious area of injury. Fogarty catheters should be passed gently, both proximal and distal to the arterial injury, to remove any intraluminal thrombus. It is extremely important not to overinflate the balloon, lest the endothelial lining be damaged and arterial spasm or thrombosis result. Both proximal and distal arterial lumina are flushed with heparinized saline solution. Systemic heparinization, particularly for popliteal artery injuries, is a helpful adjunct to prevent thrombosis or thrombus propagation when systemic anticoagulation is not contraindicated.[5,16]

Intraluminal Shunts

Temporary intraluminal shunting may be of value for some injuries when the limb is severely ischemic and revascularization will be delayed because of fracture fixation, complex soft tissue injury, or associated life-threatening injuries.[48-50] This technique allows early restoration of limb perfusion, which lessens the likelihood of ischemic damage and distal thrombosis. Débridement, fasciotomy, fracture fixation, neurorrhaphy, or vein repair can then be performed in a deliberate and unhurried fashion, before arterial reconstruction.

This adjunct has been extensively evaluated in the military setting, where revascularization often needs to be delayed. Rasmussen and colleagues reported on the military's experience over 1 year during Operation Iraqi Freedom.[51] Shunt patency varied, based on location: 86% at a proximal location (above the elbow or knee), and 12% at a distal location (below the elbow or knee). Most shunts were in place for less than 2 hours, but patency was noted in proximally placed shunts for up to 18 hours without the use of systemic heparin. Early limb viability was seen in 92% of shunted limbs. Several investigators have documented shunt patency for longer than 3 hours without systemic heparinization.[52-55] A recent report from Belfast demonstrated that the routine use of intraluminal arterial and venous shunting reduced the need for fasciotomy and the rate of amputation.[56]

There are many important technical considerations when placing intraluminal shunts. Chambers and associates, reporting on the military's experience with shunting, identified several technical factors that contribute to shunt occlusion.[57] Early occlusion was noted in several limbs in which major venous outflow had not been established before shunt placement. Although most civilian wounds do not have the same soft tissue and collateral venous injury seen in military wounds, simple venous ligation may contribute to shunt occlusion. If simple repair cannot be performed in an expedient manner, venous shunting should also be considered until definitive treatment is possible. The development of unrecognized and untreated compartment syndrome after arterial shunting for ischemic injuries increases the likelihood of shunt occlusion. Prophylactic fasciotomies or frequent compartment monitoring should be considered if prolonged ischemia precedes shunt placement. Shunt angulation or looping can increase flow resistance and contribute to thrombosis; this can easily be avoided by splinting the affected limb in a position that ensures that the shunt lies in a straight line. Finally, ensuring adequate intraluminal shunt length can prevent dislodgement and recurrent bleeding. However, deep shunt placement should be avoided because it can occlude side branches and runoff vessels, as noted in one patient in Chambers and colleagues' study.

Arterial Repair

Once the decision to perform definitive repair is made, the type of repair is dictated by the extent of arterial damage. Repair of injured vessels can be accomplished by lateral suture patch angioplasty, end-to-end anastomosis, interposition graft, or, when adjacent soft tissue injury is extensive, bypass graft. Extra-anatomic bypass grafts are useful in patients with extensive soft tissue injury or sepsis. Stain and coworkers reported on three axillofemoral, four femorofemoral, one obturator, and one extra-anatomic femoropopliteal graft performed in nine patients who had extensive soft tissue injuries.[58] In seven patients (78%), functional extremities were salvaged.

Autogenous vein grafts were first used successfully to repair arterial injuries during the Korean War.[3] The later development of prosthetic graft material—expanded polytetrafluoroethylene (ePTFE)—made possible the routine use of prosthetic conduits as a substitute for autogenous grafts. Surgical experience suggests that ePTFE is more resistant to infection than other prosthetic grafts and has acceptable patency rates when used in the above-knee position.[59,60]

In a 5-year experience with PTFE, Feliciano and associates reported the results of 236 grafts placed after traumatic injury.[61] Graft infection did not occur in the absence of adjacent osteomyelitis or exposed graft in large soft tissue defects. In a retrospective civilian series of 188 patients with lower extremity vascular trauma, Martin and coworkers reported equivalent patencies when ePTFE and vein grafts were used

to repair the iliac, femoral, and superficial femoral arteries.[62] There were no infections of ePTFE or vein grafts. A significant difference in immediate patency was apparent, however, when the distal arterial anastomosis was at or below the popliteal artery: failure was more common in patients with ePTFE grafts. Blunt trauma was associated with a higher graft failure rate (35%) than penetrating trauma (1.2%), and graft failure always resulted in amputation. Similarly, in a series of 550 patients with lower extremity traumatic arterial injuries, Hafez and associates identified the following significant independent risk factors for amputation after arterial repair: occluded bypass graft, combined above- and below-knee injury, a tense compartment, arterial transection, and associated compound fracture.[63]

We believe that the greater saphenous vein harvested from the uninjured extremity provides the most durable arterial repair. Dorweiler and colleagues recently documented an 81% patency rate at a mean follow-up of 59 months in patients with vein grafts used to repair extremity arterial injuries.[64] ePTFE grafts are used only when autogenous vein is inadequate or unavailable, when the patient is unstable and expeditious repair of the arterial injury is mandatory, or when a large size discrepancy between a vein graft and the native artery would result.

Monofilament 5-0 or 6-0 sutures are suitable for most peripheral vascular repairs, and all completed repairs should be tension free and covered by viable soft tissue. With major soft tissue injury, it may be prudent to enlist the assistance of a plastic or orthopedic reconstructive surgeon to rotate a muscle flap adequate for soft tissue coverage. We consider intraoperative completion arteriography or duplex scanning mandatory to document the technical perfection of the vascular reconstruction, visualize arterial runoff, and detect persistent missed distal thrombi. Intra-arterial vasodilators such as papaverine or tolazoline may be helpful, particularly in pediatric patients, to reverse severe spasm in the distal arterial tree or the repaired arterial segment.

Reperfusion Injury

The period immediately following limb reperfusion is an important determinant of ultimate outcome after injury. During reperfusion, toxic oxygen-derived free radicals are generated and overwhelm inherent protective enzyme-scavenging systems such as superoxide dismutase, glutathione peroxidase, and catalase, producing cell injury and death. A more detailed description of the biochemical events can be found in Chapter 6 (Ischemia-Reperfusion).

Viewed clinically, these effects are manifested by the accelerated muscle edema and necrosis seen in compartmental hypertension. Experimentally, superoxide dismutase, catalase, mannitol, and allopurinol can interrupt this pathogenetic cascade at various levels and protect against reperfusion injury; decreased muscle necrosis and edema are observed in animals pretreated with these agents.[65]

Wright and colleagues documented similar benefits in animals pretreated with heparin before reperfusion of an ischemic limb.[66] In addition to the experimental evidence that heparin has a mitigating effect on reperfusion injury, its beneficial effects include prevention of thrombosis of distal outflow vessels and collaterals. In fact, a retrospective review of 150 patients with lower extremity arterial injuries documented that the incidence of limb loss was significantly higher in patients who developed compartment syndrome (41% versus 7%) or did not receive perioperative anticoagulation (15% versus 3%).[67] For all these reasons, the surgeon must be aware of the deleterious effects of reperfusion injury, and systemic mannitol or heparin infusion should be considered before an ischemic limb is reperfused. The clinical manifestation of reperfusion injury—compartmental hypertension—must be sought assiduously and treated aggressively.[68]

Compartment Syndrome

Compartment syndrome is a frequent manifestation of reperfusion injury following a traumatic extremity injury. The potential for compartment syndrome depends on the specific vessel injured, the time from injury to arterial repair, and the presence of associated venous, orthopedic, and soft tissue injuries. The incidence of compartment syndrome and the need for fasciotomy following extremity trauma are increased with occlusive injuries to the popliteal artery, when the time from injury to repair extends beyond 6 hours, and when one or more associated injuries are present. For a more complete discussion, the reader is referred to Chapter 159 (Compartment Syndrome).

Specific Arterial Injuries

Axillary Artery

Anatomy and Mechanism of Injury. The axillary artery is the continuation of the subclavian artery as it passes from the lateral border of the first rib and extends to the lateral border of the teres major muscle. Injury to the axillary artery is more common than injury to the subclavian artery (which is protected by the overlying bone and muscle) and is most commonly due to penetrating trauma.[69,70] Anterior shoulder dislocation or fracture of the humeral neck can also result in axillary artery injury. Because of the close proximity of a variety of structures, subclavian-axillary trauma is usually associated with major musculoskeletal fractures and brachial plexus and venous injuries.[69-71] Surgical exposure can pose a significant challenge, especially in the presence of active hemorrhage. Subclavian arterial injuries are discussed further in Chapter 152 (Vascular Trauma: Head and Neck).

Diagnosis. Critical ischemia of the upper extremity is uncommon following axillary artery injuries owing to the rich collateral circulation around the shoulder. In one report, only 20% of patients had decreased or absent pulses.[72] Therefore, a high index of suspicion, careful pulse examination, measurement of Doppler arterial pressure indices, and liberal use of arteriography are mandatory for the reliable diagnosis of these injuries.

Endovascular Treatment. In selected patients, endovascular therapy has a high technical success rate for blunt and penetrating subclavian-axillary arterial injuries.[47,71,73] Ideal candidates include patients who are hemodynamically stable or are diagnosed with traumatic arteriovenous fistulae and false aneurysms. The use of endovascular stent-grafts should be considered for arterial lesions near the origins of the vertebral or right common carotid artery. Xenos and associates reviewed 23 patients who underwent intervention for traumatic subclavian-axillary artery injuries.[47] Only 12 patients had lesions suitable for endovascular repair, and of those, only 7 underwent treatment with a covered stent, owing to surgeon preference. Compared with open repair, endovascularly treated patients had significantly shorter operative times and less blood loss ($P < .05$) while attaining similar patency rates.

Surgical Treatment. The axillary artery is surgically approached through a horizontal infraclavicular incision, but proximal supraclavicular subclavian control may be necessary for arterial injuries at the thoracic outlet. Resection of the middle third of the clavicle is rarely necessary, but it is an alternative approach for certain injuries at the axillary-subclavian junction. Multiple chest incisions to achieve proper proximal control and adequate exposure for the vascular reconstruction may also be necessary.

Brachial, Radial, and Ulnar Arteries

Mechanism of Injury. Brachial artery injuries are usually due to penetrating trauma and are frequently iatrogenic, caused by endovascular access. Blunt brachial artery injuries are most often associated with supracondylar fractures of the humerus. The location of the brachial artery injury has implications with regard to associated clinical findings; injuries below the origin of the profunda brachii may not show signs of ischemia owing to the robust collateral networks present.

Surgical Treatment. Single-vessel injury in the forearm need not be repaired but may be ligated or embolized. Repair is mandatory when one of the vessels, either the radial or ulnar artery, was previously traumatized or ligated or when the palmar arch is incomplete. Incomplete superficial palmar arches are estimated to occur in 3.6% to 21.5% of patients.[74,75] When both radial and ulnar arteries are injured, the ulnar artery should be repaired preferentially because it is the dominant vessel.

External Iliac Artery

For proximal control of the external iliac artery, a retroperitoneal approach is ideal. The surgeon extends the femoral incision through the inguinal ligament or makes a separate incision parallel to the lateral border of the rectus sheath and 2 cm above the inguinal ligament (Fig. 155-4). The rectus

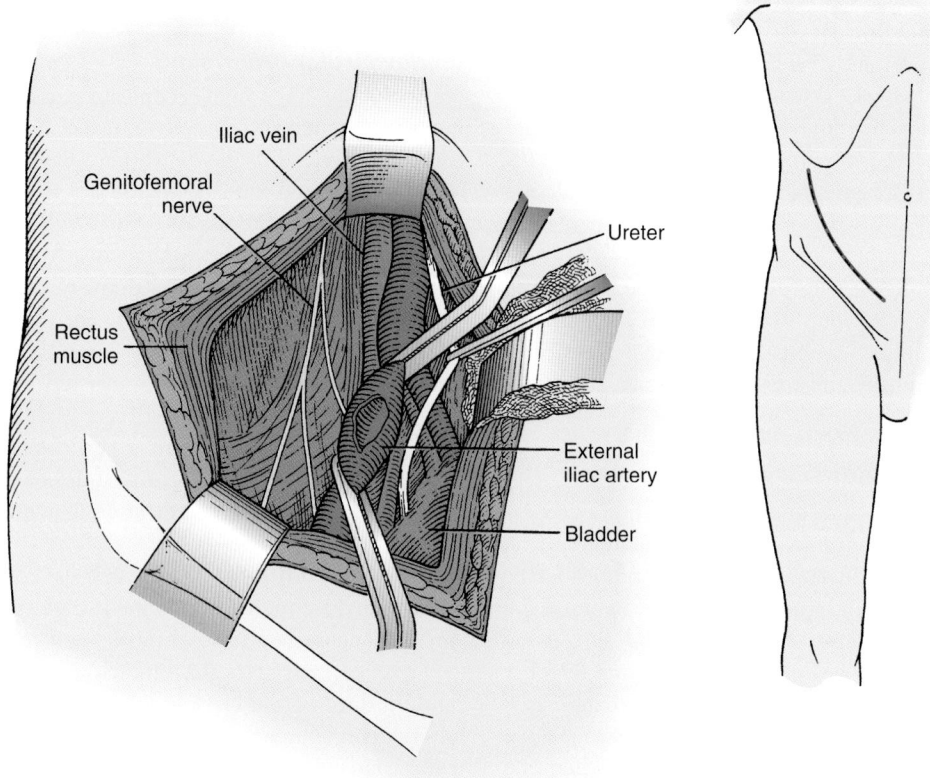

Figure 155-4 Retroperitoneal exposure for proximal control of the iliac and proximal common femoral arteries. *(From Yellin AE, Weaver FA. Vascular system. In: Donovan AJ, ed. Trauma Surgery. St. Louis: Mosby-Year Book; 1994.)*

muscle is retracted medially, the transversalis fascia is incised, and the retroperitoneal space is entered. The peritoneum and its contents are reflected medially to provide exposure of the distal aorta and the iliac vessels.

Iliac artery injuries are one of the most lethal arterial injuries sustained by trauma patients (see Chapter 154: Vascular Trauma: Abdominal). Mortality rates range from 24% to 40% and can exceed 50% when combined with an aortic or iliac venous injury.[76,77] In a recent series from our institution analyzing iliac vessel injuries, Asensio and colleagues reported a 51% overall survival, which diminished to 38% when concomitant iliac venous injuries were present.[78]

Femoral Arteries

Exposure of the common femoral, proximal deep femoral, and proximal superficial femoral arteries is accomplished through a longitudinal thigh incision over the femoral triangle. The common femoral artery lies within the femoral sheath; the common femoral vein lies medial to it, and the femoral nerve is lateral. Careful dissection is required to avoid iatrogenic injury to the deep femoral artery.

Blunt and penetrating injuries to the superficial femoral artery are very common and are repaired with the techniques described earlier under "Operative Management." Injuries to

the proximal deep femoral artery should always be repaired in hemodynamically stable patients because of this artery's contribution to the collateral supply of the lower extremity.[79]

Popliteal Artery

Mechanism of Injury. Popliteal artery injuries are among the most challenging of all extremity vascular injuries. The outcome of a penetrating popliteal artery injury depends predominantly on the mechanism of injury. The amputation rate for shotgun wounds approaches 20% because of the associated soft tissue injury and septic sequelae. In contrast, for single-missile injuries and stab wounds associated with minimal musculoskeletal injury, amputation rates approach zero. The popliteal vein, infrapopliteal arteries, and tibial nerve are frequently involved in penetrating popliteal injuries (20% to 38% of cases).

Surgical Treatment. A popliteal artery injury above the knee joint is best repaired through a medial thigh incision; a similar below-knee injury requires a leg incision. An isolated penetrating injury directly behind the knee can be approached from behind (Fig. 155-5). When this approach is used, the contralateral lesser saphenous vein can be harvested if an autogenous graft is required.

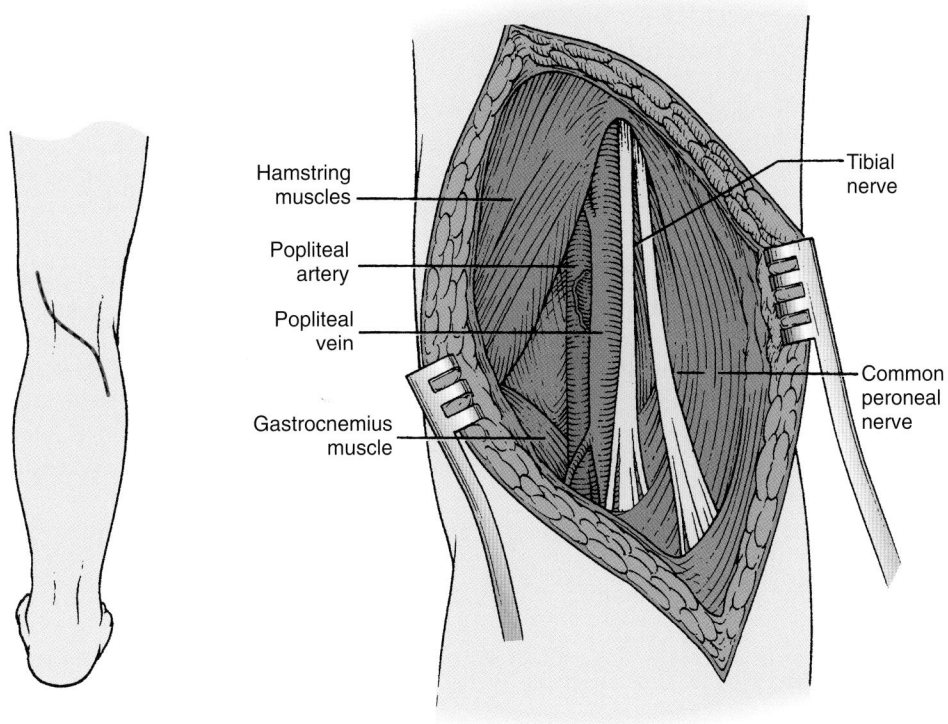

Figure 155-5 Posterior approach for a penetrating popliteal injury behind the knee. *(From Yellin AE, Weaver FA. Vascular system. In: Donovan AJ, ed. Trauma Surgery. St. Louis: Mosby-Year Book; 1994.)*

During the past decade there has been a dramatic reduction in the rate of amputation after civilian popliteal artery injuries. Amputation rates at our institution have decreased from 23% to 6% for blunt injuries and from 21% to 0% for penetrating trauma.[6,7] In a series of 100 blunt popliteal artery injuries reported from our institution, popliteal artery thrombosis or transection occurred in 97% of cases; concomitant popliteal vein injury was present in 29%.[6] Repair of the artery was accomplished by end-to-end anastomosis in 49%, vein interposition in 43%, intimal repair and vein patch in 2%, and thrombectomy in 1%. Ten amputations were required because of failure of the arterial repair, and five were necessitated by invasive limb sepsis or massive soft tissue injury. Prior to 1980, 12 amputations were necessary; after 1980, only three limbs were amputated. Factors that positively influenced limb salvage included systemic (heparin) anticoagulation, arterial repair accomplished either laterally or end to end, and palpable pedal pulses within the first 24 hours. Conversely, severe soft tissue injury, deep soft tissue infection, and preoperative ischemia were negative predictors of limb salvage (Table 155-1). Attention to the possibility of compartment syndrome, along with rapid treatment by complete dermatomy or fasciotomy if present, is crucial for these patients.[68]

In a more recent series, Melton and associates reported a similar experience. In 102 patients with penetrating or blunt popliteal injuries, systemic heparin or local thrombolytic therapy significantly reduced the amputation rate, whereas all severely traumatized limbs (characterized by a Mangled Extremity Severity Score [MESS][80] greater than 8)

Table 155-1 Amputation Rates in Association with Perioperative Risk Factors in Blunt Popliteal Artery Trauma (N = 100)

Risk Factor	Present (%)	Absent (%)	P Value*
Severe soft tissue injury	13/31 (42)	2/69 (3)	<.0001
Deep soft tissue infection	9/17 (53)	6/83 (7)	<.0001
Preoperative ischemia	15/64 (23)	0/36 (0)	<.001
Preoperative delay >6 hr	10/40 (25)	5/24 (21)	NS
Preoperative delay >12 hr	2/14 (14)	13/50 (26)	NS
Systemic anticoagulation	6/71 (8)	9/29 (31)	<.01
Primary arterial repair	3/49 (6)	12/51 (24)	<.05
Palpable pedal pulse within 24 hr	4/55 (7)	11/45 (24)	<.05
Trifurcation arterial injury	6/29 (21)	9/71 (13)	NS
Popliteal vein injury	6/29 (21)	9/71 (13)	NS
Ligation of venous injury	2/6 (33)	4/23 (17)	NS
Fasciotomy (operative or delayed)	11/61 (18)	4/39 (10)	NS
Delayed fasciotomy	1/4 (25)	14/96 (15)	NS
Preoperative compartment syndrome	2/17 (12)	13/83 (16)	NS

*Two-tailed Fisher exact test.
NS, not statistically significant.
Modified from Wagner WH, Caulkins E, Weaver FA, et al. Blunt popliteal artery trauma: 100 consecutive cases. *J Vasc Surg.* 1988;7:736.

required amputation.[5] Likewise, Dar and colleagues retrospectively reviewed 272 patients with traumatic popliteal injuries, 95% of which were secondary to penetrating trauma.[81] In their series, the amputation rate was 5.5%. Significant variables associated with amputation included concomitant bone fracture and delay in vascular repair greater than 12 hours. The early evaluation of popliteal artery injuries from our institution concurred with the finding by Dar and colleagues that lower total ischemia time improves outcome. Of note, in our analysis, MESS was not predictive of amputation.

Tibial Arteries

Isolated occlusive injury to one infrapopliteal artery rarely results in limb ischemia and does not, as a rule, require therapeutic intervention. A single actively bleeding traumatized vessel or arterial pseudoaneurysm can be treated by simple ligation or angiographic embolization; however, when the tibioperoneal trunk or two infrapopliteal arteries are injured, repair is required.[82] Associated nerve, bone, and soft tissue injuries are the essential determinants of limb salvage. In a study by Whitman and colleagues, no amputations occurred in limbs with less than two of these associated injuries; however, for limbs with all three associated injuries, the amputation rate was 54%.[83]

■ SPECIAL CONSIDERATIONS
Pediatric Extremity Arterial Injuries

Management principles for noniatrogenic arterial injuries in children parallel those for adult trauma, and recent studies suggest that the judicious use of arteriography and arterial repair in pediatric vascular injury provides results equivalent to those achieved in adults.[14,18,60,84-87] Considerations unique to the management of pediatric injuries include the severity of arterial spasm, the unknown long-term consequences of autogenous grafts placed in children, and the long-term effects of diminished blood flow on limb length. The intense arterial spasm associated with pediatric vascular injuries can compromise any arterial repair. Pharmacologic agents that may impede the vasoactive response include papaverine (injected topically or into the adventitia) and nitrates. Warm saline applied topically may also be helpful.[86] Diagnostic arteriography can exacerbate vasospasm and limb ischemia. Consequently, when diagnostic studies are indicated, a noninvasive alternative such as CFD should be considered. In a viable, neurologically intact limb with an occlusive injury, the arterial repair can be deferred; in a very young child, this may be preferable.[88] If repair is not performed, careful follow-up of limb growth is necessary, and arterial repair is indicated if a limb-length discrepancy develops. Harris and Hordines reported long-term outcomes in 9 of 19 pediatric patients who underwent revascularization for traumatic vascular injuries.[86] With a mean follow-up of 35 months, 7 patients (78%) were able to resume normal physical activities. The 2 patients unable to regain full function had combined orthopedic, soft tissue, and vascular trauma. No limb-length discrepancy or aneurysmal changes within the vein grafts were found.

Extremity Venous Injuries

The most commonly injured major veins of the extremities are the superficial femoral vein (42%), followed by the popliteal vein (23%) and the common femoral vein (14%).[89] When the venous injury is localized and end-to-end or lateral venorrhaphy is possible, repair should be performed unless the patient is hemodynamically unstable. When more extensive venous injuries exist, an interposition, panel, or spiral graft can be configured for repair. However, the indications for and benefits of such complex repairs remain controversial.[41,90]

Meyer and coworkers studied 36 patients with traumatic venous injuries who underwent venous repair.[89] Repairs were studied venographically 7 days after operation. Fourteen (39%) of the venous repairs had thrombosed. Moreover, when an interposition vein graft was used, the thrombosis rate rose to 59%. Limb salvage was 100% successful and was not affected by failure of the venous repair. Timberlake and Kerstein reported a similar outcome, with transient edema in 36% and long-term permanent edema in only 2% of patients with venous injuries.[91] The finding of edema was not related to whether the vein was repaired or ligated. Kuralay and colleagues evaluated the outcome of venous repairs using postoperative duplex scanning to assess not only patency but also blood flow velocity.[92] In 130 patients suffering military and civilian trauma, repair of vein injuries were most successful in the proximal venous segments, which correlated with the highest postoperative flow rates. Repaired common femoral, superficial femoral, and popliteal veins had patency rates of 100%, 100%, and 86%, respectively, at 1 year and 89%, 78%, and 60%, respectively, at 6 years. Earlier studies from Baylor Medical Center with ePTFE as conduits in venous injury repair showed near universal stenosis or occlusion on follow-up venography. However, repaired patients had less bleeding from distal blast defects and fasciotomy sites.[61] This experience and others suggest that repair of major venous injuries in a stable patient is a reasonable undertaking; however, when venous repair would be complex or the patient is hemodynamically unstable, simple ligation is appropriate. When venous ligation is necessary, postoperative edema can be controlled by elevation of the extremity and elastic wrapping. For patients undergoing venous repair, patency should be monitored with a hand-held Doppler or duplex scan.

When venous injury occurs with an ischemic arterial injury, the vein should be repaired before the arterial repair is initiated. This sequence provides improved hemostasis in the operative field and venous drainage of the leg during the arterial reconstruction. In patients with significant limb ischemia times, approximately 200 mL of distal venous blood should be removed before restoring in-line flow to help minimize the reperfusion insult.[57]

Orthopedic, Soft Tissue, and Nerve Injuries

The surgical treatment of combined vascular and orthopedic injuries is one of the most difficult problems in the management of trauma patients.[93] The incidence of combined vascular injury and skeletal fractures is reportedly 0.3% to 6.4%.[94-97] Although combined injuries are uncommon, the duration of ischemia is critical to the outcome. Therefore, we believe that the arterial repair should be performed first to restore circulation to the limb before orthopedic stabilization is addressed. Sometimes, however, massive musculoskeletal trauma renders a limb so unstable that external fixation must be accomplished before the vascular procedure. Selective use of intraluminal shunts and rapid installation of an external fixator can minimize limb ischemia in this setting, thus allowing an unhurried orthopedic and vascular repair.[48,49,98] When the vascular repair is performed before orthopedic fixation, the surgeon must inspect the vascular reconstruction before final wound closure and before the patient leaves the operating room. Patency of the repair must be documented by palpable pulses, arteriography, or CFD.

In patients with major soft tissue injuries, débridement of all clearly nonviable tissue is mandatory. Frequent and early returns to the operating room, as often as every 24 to 48 hours, may be required. In these patients, unexplained fever and leukocytosis are assumed to be due to deep tissue infection until proved otherwise. Re-exploration of the wound and débridement of necrotic tissue or hematoma are essential for minimizing septic sequelae. Ultimate wound coverage by delayed primary closure, rotational flaps, or free tissue transfer when the soft tissue bed is clean minimizes the risk of invasive sepsis.

Nerve injuries occur in about 50% of upper extremity and 25% of lower extremity vascular injuries. The nerve injury usually determines the long-term functional status of the injured extremity.[99] If a major nerve has been cleanly transected by a sharp object, primary repair can be performed at the time of vascular repair; however, for most penetrating and all blunt nerve injuries, immediate repair is rarely possible or indicated. Rather, both ends of the injured nerve should be tagged with nonabsorbable suture at the initial operation. This facilitates identification of the nerve at the time of eventual nerve repair or grafting.

Vascular repairs are now performed with such a high rate of success that they exert little influence on ultimate extremity function. Rather, the associated orthopedic, nerve, and soft tissue injuries are the critical factors that determine long-term limb function. A number of scores or indices have been proposed in an attempt to predict early limb salvage and to limit protracted reconstructive efforts aimed at restoring limb function. The MESS incorporates the associated soft tissue injury based on mechanism of injury, level of arterial ischemia, patient age, and level of hemodynamic shock. Durham and colleagues retrospectively evaluated four different systems (Mangled Extremity Syndrome Index, MESS, Predictive Salvage Index, and Limb Salvage Index) used to predict limb salvage and functional outcome.[100] None of the indices could predict functional outcome. Other studies have also failed to predict functional limb salvage reliably.[5,101]

Primary Amputation versus Reconstruction

One of the more difficult decisions in the trauma setting is whether to undertake the reconstruction of a severely injured extremity as opposed to a primary amputation. As previously discussed, injury severity indices routinely fail to accurately predict individual limb functional outcomes. The involvement of a multidisciplinary team comprising a trauma surgeon, plastic or reconstructive surgeon, and orthopedic surgeon is very helpful. From the vascular injury standpoint, much has been made of the "magical" 6-hour maximum for the toleration of ischemia. This period stems from data provided by Miller and Welch in a canine model of hind limb occlusion.[102] Extremity salvage rates dramatically decrease as ischemia time increases: 90% for less than 6 hours of ischemia, 50% for 12 to 18 hours of ischemia, and 20% for ischemia in excess of 24 hours. Although these times are useful as a guide, strict reliance on them to determine the need for primary amputation is not followed at our institution. In the majority of situations, vascular reconstruction can be accomplished. Unfortunately, revascularization does not reincarnate an insensate limb to a functional one. Therefore, the decision to proceed with primary amputation should not be based solely on the vascular injury. Currently, for limbs with massive orthopedic, soft tissue, and nerve injuries, primary amputation rather than complex reconstruction should be considered, because permanent and total functional limb disability, ultimately requiring amputation, is common.[83,93,103] Primary amputation should also be considered in hemodynamically unstable patients in whom a complex vascular repair might jeopardize survival. Finally, in cases in which rigor is present, any attempt at limb salvage should be aborted.

Intra-arterial Drug Injection

An often-neglected, frequently misdiagnosed and mistreated arterial injury is that caused by the inadvertent intra-arterial injection of medications not intended for intra-arterial use or the accidental injection of illegal street drugs into an artery rather than a vein.

Clinical Presentation

The most common site of intra-arterial drug injection (IADI) is the brachial artery. Iatrogenic IADI is usually associated with the injection of barbiturates during the induction of anesthesia. Self-injected, illegal, nonsterile street drugs are often complicated by the presence of a variety of insoluble additives. Whether an IADI is iatrogenic or self-administered, an accurate history may be difficult to obtain. If possible, a site of injection should be located and noted.

IADI is followed immediately by severe, unremitting pain, often accompanied by edema, numbness, discoloration, cyanosis, or mottling of the skin. This reaction occurs as the concentrated drug flows into the smaller distal arteries, resulting in an intense inflammatory response with endothelial injury and thrombosis. If the injection is in the upper extremity, the hand is typically held in a clawlike position. Sensory loss is usually present. The entire wrist and hand might be involved, but changes are most severe in the distal digits. Depending on the anatomy of the palmar arch and digital circulation, one or more fingers might be spared. The fingers are usually cool, and the fingertips are deeply cyanotic. Motor function is diminished. Pulses at the wrist are usually present and might be accentuated owing to the outflow obstruction. Distal pulses are usually absent, even by Doppler.

Diagnosis

The diagnosis can usually be made clinically based on the history and clinical findings. CFD should be used to identify the remaining patent arteries. Although angiography provides a vivid picture of the pathology and may even demonstrate the venous microcirculatory damage, it is rarely helpful in guiding therapy and could promote further thrombosis. Therefore, we do not use angiography in our diagnostic or therapeutic regimen unless we suspect thrombosis of a major artery.

Treatment

Our therapeutic regimen is based on the premise that once the intravascular damage occurs and arterial thrombosis is present, revascularization is not a realistic option. Our goal is to preserve all collateral circulation and prevent further propagation of clot. If inflammation, edema, stasis, and thrombosis can be minimized, functional recovery usually follows. This regimen has now been used in more than 50 patients with IADI.[104,105]

Therapy consists of the following:

- Heparin sodium 10,000 units intravenously, followed by a continuous drip to keep the partial thromboplastin time at one and a half to two times control to prevent further clotting.
- Dexamethasone 4 mg intravenously every 6 hours to reduce inflammation and stabilize cellular membranes.
- Dextran 40 intravenously at 20 mL/hour to prevent platelet aggregation and thrombosis.
- Appropriate pain control, including opiates as needed.
- Elevation of the extremity to reduce edema.
- Aggressive physical therapy to minimize contractures.

This regimen is continued until the condition resolves or is fully stabilized, which occurs in 72 hours to 1 week. Débridement of ischemic tissue is deferred until it is clear what is viable and what is not. Long-term physical therapy is frequently necessary to restore function.

Various other treatment regimens have been reported, including the use of nerve blocks, local and systemic vasodilators, and thrombolytic agents. Experience with these modalities is confined to small groups of patients.[106] It is possible that thrombolytic therapy may be effective in selected cases, but its role remains to be defined.

Complications

Complications of IADI may include soft tissue infection (abscess, cellulitis), mycotic aneurysm, and arterial thrombosis and ischemia.

Soft Tissue Infection. Soft tissue cellulitis or localized abscesses are common sequelae of illegal drug use. Increasingly, drug-resistant gram-positive organisms are the culprits. *Staphylococcus aureus* is a common pathogen; however, oral flora such as streptococcal species and anaerobic species such as *Peptostreptococcus* and *Bacteroides* are often present. Appropriate parenteral antibiotic therapy combined with incision, drainage, and débridement are the hallmarks of therapy.

Mycotic Aneurysm. When the soft tissue infection is in the vicinity of a major blood vessel, and particularly when there is a painful, tender pulsatile mass, a mycotic aneurysm must be suspected. However, less than half of these aneurysms are pulsatile. Therefore, before any attempt at drainage, CFD must be performed to rule out the presence of a mycotic aneurysm. Management of a mycotic aneurysm requires careful consideration of the options: ligation, with possible acute ischemia, versus repair, possibly followed by secondary infection and hemorrhage. Treatment is further complicated by the fact that autologous vein conduits might not be readily available in drug abusers. Brachial mycotic aneurysms can invariably be ligated without ischemic consequences. Similar outcomes are expected following ligation of the deep femoral or superficial femoral arteries, and less than 50% of patients with common femoral artery ligation develop ischemia. Therefore, in the presence of severe local soft tissue destruction, ligation followed by careful observation for evidence of ischemia is a prudent choice. Doppler flow and pressures can be used as a guide. If distal flow is present, limb ischemia is uncommon. This algorithm has been used successfully by others.[107] Delayed in-line revascularization in clean tissue is an option for the rare patient with subsequent persistent claudication. If there is acute ischemia, revascularization may be necessary. A conduit, preferably autogenous, should be placed in a clean tissue plane and anastomosed to healthy artery proximally and distally, thereby restoring flow. Numerous extra-anatomic routes have been used. All vascular anastomoses should be covered by healthy muscle, which might require rotation of a local muscle flap.

Arterial Thrombosis and Ischemia. Downstream arterial thrombosis following IADI can have catastrophic consequences owing to obliteration of the small-vessel collateral circulation by the injected agent. The primary problem is not one of spasm but of almost immediate endothelial damage to the arterial and venous microcirculations, leading to intimal necrosis, thromboxane release, platelet aggregation, norepinephrine release, vasoconstriction, and thrombosis.[105] The initial occlusive injury is likely to involve the small venules that accompany the arterioles. The resultant venous outflow obstruction leads to increased interstitial edema, secondary arterial insufficiency, thrombosis, tissue hypoxia, neurologic deficit, and soft tissue necrosis.

SELECTED KEY REFERENCES

Chambers LW, Green DJ, Sample K, Gillingham BL, Rhee P, Brown C, Narine N, Uecker JM, Bohman HR. Tactical surgical intervention with temporary shunting of peripheral vascular trauma sustained during Operation Iraqi Freedom: one unit's experience. *J Trauma.* 2006;61:824.
Clinical outcomes and technical aspects of temporary shunt placement in vascular injuries.

Dennis JW, Frykberg ER, Veldenz HC, Huffman S, Menawat SS. Validation of nonoperative management of occult vascular injuries and accuracy of physical examination alone in penetrating extremity trauma: 5- to 10-year follow up. *J Trauma.* 1998;44:243.
Outcomes of nonoperative treatment of clinically occult vascular injuries with short-term and long-term follow-up.

Durham RM, Mistry BM, Mazuski JE, Shapiro M, Jacobs D. Outcome and utility of scoring systems in the management of the mangled extremity. *Am J Surg.* 1996;172:569.
Retrospective review of four systems for predicting limb salvage and functional outcome.

Schwartz MR, Weaver FA, Bauer M, Siegel A, Yellin AE. Refining the indications for arteriography in penetrating extremity trauma: a prospective analysis. *J Vasc Surg.* 1993;17:116.
Validates the role of selective angiography in patients with suspected vascular injuries and describes predictive risk factors.

Smith C, Green RM. Pediatric vascular injuries. *Surgery.* 1981;90:20.
Technical and management considerations in pediatric vascular injuries.

Weaver FA, Yellin AE, Bauer M, Oberg J, Ghalambor N, Emmanuel RP, Applebaum RM, Pentecost MJ, Shorr RM. Is arterial proximity a valid indication for arteriography in penetrating extremity trauma? A prospective analysis. *Arch Surg.* 1990;125:1256.
Confirms the safety of clinical examination and selective arteriography in the management of suspected extremity vascular injuries.

REFERENCES

The reference list can be found on the companion Expert Consult Web site at *www.expertconsult.com.*

CHAPTER 156

Vascular Trauma: Military*

Todd E. Rasmussen and Charles J. Fox

Vascular injury in the military has special significance. Combat-related injuries to major vessels present unique technical challenges and result in hemorrhage that is responsible for 80% of potentially preventable deaths on the battlefield.[1] The most lethal vascular injuries are those to the torso, which includes the chest and abdomen. Torso injury is reportedly the cause of half of potentially survivable hemorrhagic deaths, followed by extremity vascular injury, which is responsible for one third.[1] The front lines of a battleground are chaotic, located in harsh environments, and vary widely, depending on the goal and scope of military operations. Surgical care may be rendered in tents or buildings of opportunity that lack suitable light and ventilation or in more established and well-equipped forward surgical hospitals. These austere conditions, combined with the technical demands associated with the treatment of vascular injury, necessitate the early and deliberate preparation of military medics and surgeons at all levels of care to ensure the successful management of vascular trauma.[2]

■ HISTORIC ADVANCES THROUGH MILITARY CONFLICT

Contributions from the armed conflicts of the 20th century have defined the standards for vessel ligation or repair of arterial and venous injuries in resource-limited situations. Since the Vietnam War there has been considerable modernization of the battlefield environment, which has translated into a measurable survival advantage.[2,3] Forward surgical capability, expeditious evacuation, and new and effective resuscitation strategies have provided the foundation for innovation and progress. Lessons learned during current U.S. military operations continue to advance the practice of vascular trauma surgery, and these techniques are directly translated to surgical practices in trauma centers around the world.

World War II

A classic paper by DeBakey and Simeone illustrated the challenges of vessel repair during wartime, revealing only 81 repairs of 2471 arterial injuries during World War II.[4] Saphenous bypass grafts were impractical at the time, and all but three injuries were repaired by lateral suture. Amputation followed vessel ligation in nearly half of extremity vascular injuries during this era. Therefore, during World War II, evacuation delays, practical difficulties, and poor physiologic conditions led to the conclusion that vessel ligation, though not the "procedure of choice, is one of necessity."[4]

Korean War

In 1952, during the Korean War, arterial repair of vascular injury was introduced by Frank Spencer and a team of U.S. Marine Corps medics; it originally consisted of a cadaveric femoral artery used as an interposition graft conduit in the injured extremity.[5] A surgical research team based at Walter Reed Army Hospital and led by Captain John Howard was established to study these reported successes and other challenges associated with vascular injury in an effort to optimize management strategies.[6] Several more comprehensive reports on successful arterial repair performed during the Korean War followed, including classic papers from Colonel Carl Hughes, which gained the attention of the Office of the Army Surgeon General.[6-8] Hughes demonstrated an impressive reduction in the amputation rate among 269 repairs—from 49% in World War II to 13% during the Korean War. Despite the introduction of rotary wing casualty evacuation (CASEVAC) during the Korean War, significant time delays and resuscitation requirements remained the primary Achilles heel of successful vascular injury management.[6]

Vietnam War

Forward surgical capabilities and advances in CASEVAC continued to reduce ischemic time and commonly led to successful arterial reconstructions during the Vietnam War. The management of complex injuries, such as those involving the popliteal artery and vein or those associated with severe open contaminated fractures, became the focus of attention during this period.[9-12] Under the guidance of Major Norman Rich, the Vietnam Vascular Registry provided details of the treatment of more than 1000 wartime vascular injuries and confirmed and extended the experience of Hughes and others in the Korean War. The Vietnam Vascular Registry now serves as a reference standard for the application of vascular surgery during the modern conflicts of the 21st century.[13]

*The views expressed in this chapter are those of the authors and do not reflect the official policy of the Department of Defense, the United States Army or Air Force, or other departments of the United States government.

Global War on Terror

For decades, the vascular injury experience of past wars was thought to be unapproachable with regard to the duration of conflict and the number of injuries. However, now in its seventh year and with more than 35,000 combat-related injuries, the global war on terror (GWOT) has proved to be a formidable and sustained military campaign. During this conflict, modern advances have allowed for a concerted effort to reduce deaths from potentially survivable vascular injuries and improve the quality of functional extremity salvage (i.e., saving life *and* limb).[1]

At the beginning of the GWOT, the Department of Defense implemented a testing, training, and fielding program for battlefield tourniquets.[14-16] The effectiveness of early tourniquet application observed in Iraq and Afghanistan has led to doctrinal changes that have produced a surge of patients with vascular injuries who, in the past, would not have reached a field hospital alive (Fig. 156-1).[17,18] Although current military endeavors regarding the appropriateness of tourniquet use began with trepidation, the forward deployment of surgical capabilities has limited tourniquet duration, thus increasing the effectiveness of tourniquets and reducing the rate of associated complications. Additionally, the development of the Joint Theater Trauma System has improved surgical care and reduced mortality by implementing clinical practice guidelines and performing outcomes research emerging from the Joint Theater Trauma Registry. The GWOT Vascular Initiative is a comprehensive registry designed to study patterns of vessel injury and methods of vascular repair and to provide more complete long-term analysis of patient outcomes.

Other modern advances include the routine use of personal protective gear (body armor), the deployment of level II facili-

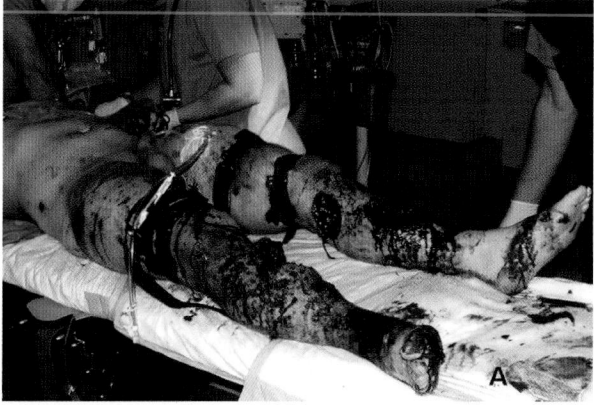

Figure 156-1 Patient with severe injuries to both lower extremities with two tourniquets on each leg. In such cases, the presence or absence of a vascular injury may not be determined until the tourniquets are released at the appropriate time and the patient is warmed and resuscitated. Note that the patient is in the operating room and that all the tourniquets remain in place while the anesthesia team tends to resuscitation needs. In this case, the tourniquets were released slowly in sequence, allowing the anesthesia team to treat any untoward effects of reperfusion. The patient is positioned on the table so that fluoroscopy can be performed during the operation to assess for fracture or so that arteriography can be performed.

ties at more forward locations, and the selective application of surgical adjuncts (e.g., temporary vascular shunts, fasciotomies).[19-24] Progress in the management of complex soft tissue wounds associated with vascular injury, such as closed negative-pressure wound therapy (NPWT), has been impressive; also impressive is the increased complexity of in-theater repair, which now includes tibia-level reconstruction for select patterns of injury.[25] Last, the extension of endovascular technologies to diagnose and treat certain types of vascular, pelvic, and solid organ war-related injuries has been reported.[26,27] In the aggregate, modern-day endeavors rooted in the wartime efforts and academic accomplishments of the past make the topic of wartime vascular injury not just relevant but enthralling.

■ EPIDEMIOLOGY

Rates of Wartime Vascular Injury

In the Vietnam War, vascular injuries accounted for 2% to 3% of battle-related injuries.[11] Published reports from the GWOT and Operation Iraqi Freedom (OIF) demonstrate that the contemporary rate of vascular injury is considerably higher, at 4% to 6% of battle-related injuries.[19-24] Additionally, early data from the GWOT Vascular Initiative suggest that the rate of vascular injury may be as high as 10% among those injured in combat. The increased incidence of vascular injury may have several explanations, including an increased awareness of and attention to recording such injuries. Undoubtedly, the effectiveness of tourniquets and modern body armor and the strategic forward placement of surgical capabilities also allow the treatment of vascular injuries that would have been fatal in past wars. Regardless of the reason, the distinct increase in the rate of vascular injuries during modern war underscores the importance of training and the maintenance of competency within the military surgical ranks.

Demographics

Not surprisingly, the overwhelming majority of combat troops sustaining wartime vascular injuries are young (mean age, 23 years) and male (95%).[19-24] Most commonly, this group of patients has no preexisting cardiovascular disease or morbidity. However, depending on the location of the military surgical facility and the concept of operations of the wartime setting, military surgeons may be faced with vascular injuries in patients at both ends of the age spectrum.[25,28] The availability of surgical care to segments of the local civilian population at U.S. theater hospitals during the GWOT has provided an uncommon experience in the management of wartime vascular injuries in pediatric and elderly patients. Peck and coworkers documented this experience in patients with extremity vascular injuries who were as young as 5 years and as old as 65 years.[25] Reconstruction of vascular injuries is unique in children, given the technical challenges related to the repair of small vessels that are not yet fully developed. Additionally, depending on age and stage of development, pediatric patients have a propensity for collateralization and better potential tolerance of axial vessel ligation compared with adults. This fact makes observation or even ligation of certain extremity vascular injuries a more prudent course of action than attempting a highly complex vascular intervention or reconstruction in certain pediatric patients.

Anatomic Patterns

Contemporary patterns of wartime injury are similar to historical reports, with extremity vascular injuries being most common (Fig. 156-2).[19-24] An in-theater report by Clouse and colleagues on nearly 350 vascular injuries among both U.S. forces and the local population showed that extremity injuries were most common, and the rate of extremity injury was higher among U.S. forces (81%) than among civilians (70%).[20] In addition, there was a proportionate lower incidence in truncal vascular injuries among U.S. forces (4%) compared with the local population (13%; see Fig. 156-2). These figures suggest the effectiveness of modern body armor available to those in combat.

Lower extremity vascular injuries occur at approximately two times the rate of upper extremity injuries, reflecting the relative length of axial vessels and the exposed position of the lower extremity away from the protection of the torso. The anatomic distribution of arterial and venous injuries is roughly the same, although there is a slightly higher percentage of venous injuries in the neck and a lower percentage of upper extremity venous injuries (Tables 156-1 and 156-2).[19,20] In the lower extremity, the superficial femoral artery is most commonly injured (33% to 37%), followed by the popliteal and tibial arteries (25% each). Injuries to the proximal common femoral artery and profunda femoris are less common because of their proximity to the protective structures of the torso and their lethality when they do occur. In a detailed analysis of penetrating femoropopliteal injuries during modern warfare, Woodward and colleagues showed that nearly 50% of lower extremity vascular injuries had a combined arterial and venous component.[22] Arterial injury in the neck constitutes roughly 15% of all arterial trauma and is equally distributed among the common, external, and internal carotid arteries and the vertebral artery, whereas all venous injuries in the neck are to the jugular vein (see Tables 156-1 and 156-2).[20]

Because nearly all vascular injuries in wartime are caused by blast or high-velocity weaponry, approximately one third of those with vascular injuries have associated orthopedic

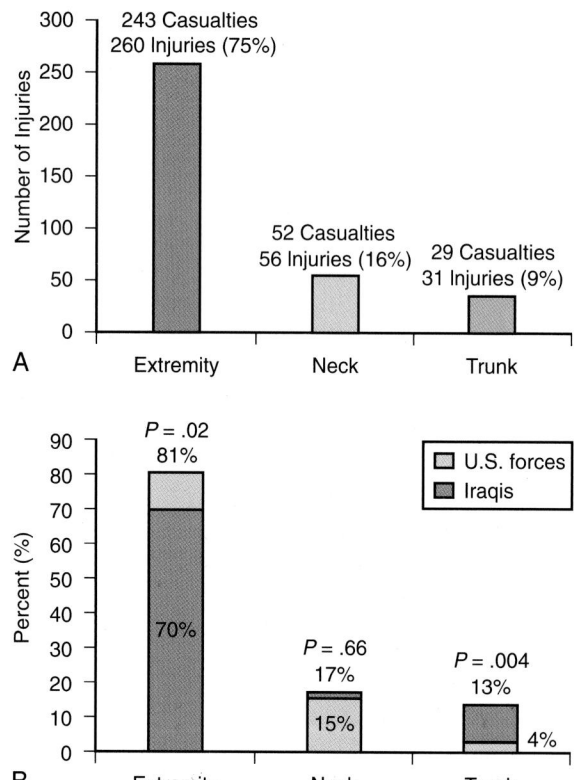

Figure 156-2 Distribution of vascular injuries at the 332nd Expeditionary Medical Group, Air Force theater hospital at Balad Air Base, Iraq, from September 1, 2004, through August 31, 2006. **A,** Distribution of vascular injuries by anatomic location (N = 347). **B,** Anatomic distribution of vascular injuries among U.S. forces and among the local population (N = 347). There are significant differences between these two groups in terms of the proportion of patients with extremity and trunk injuries, suggesting the efficacy of military body armor.

Table 156-1 Location of Arterial Injuries in Military Trauma*

Artery	Number	%
Neck	42	14.0
Common carotid	13	4.3
Internal carotid	11	3.7
External carotid	9	3.0
Vertebral	9	3.0
Upper Extremity	76	25.3
Subclavian-axillary	11	3.7
Brachial	42	14.0
Forearm	23	7.6
Chest	7	2.3
Supra-aortic trunk	4	1.3
Thoracic aorta	3	1.0
Abdomen	18	6.0
Abdominal aorta	5	1.7
Renovisceral	4	1.3
Common iliac	4	1.3
Internal iliac	2	0.7
External iliac	3	1.0
Lower Extremity	158	52.5
Common femoral	9	3.0
Profunda femoris	12	4.0
Superficial femoral	53	17.6
Popliteal	40	13.3
Tibial	44	14.6
Total	**301**	**100.0**

*Location of arterial injury by anatomic location and injured vessel in 301 arterial injuries over 24 months.
Data from Clouse WD, Rasmussen TE, Peck MA. In-theater management of vascular injury: 2 years of the Balad Vascular Registry. *J Am Coll Surg.* 2007;204:625-632.

Table 156-2 Location of Venous Injuries in Military Trauma*

Vein	Number	%
Neck	24	22.4
Internal jugular	24	22.4
Upper Extremity	9	8.4
Subclavian-axillary	9	8.4
Chest	3	2.8
Brachiocephalic	2	1.9
IVC	1	0.9
Abdomen	9	8.4
IVC	4	3.7
Common iliac	2	1.9
External iliac	3	2.8
Lower Extremity	62	58.0
Common femoral	5	4.7
Profunda femoris	4	3.7
Superficial femoral	28	26.2
Popliteal	25	23.4
Total	107	100.0

*Location of venous injury by anatomic location and injured vessel in 107 venous injuries over 24 months.
IVC, inferior vena cava.
Data from Clouse WD, Rasmussen TE, Peck MA. In-theater management of vascular injury: 2 years of the Balad Vascular Registry. *J Am Coll Surg.* 2007;204:625-632.

injuries, and up to 20% have partial- or full-thickness burns[21]; the same percentage has an additional head or torso injury. All these associated injuries impact the decision making related to the triage and ultimate treatment of vascular injury.

Mechanism of Injury

Penetrating mechanisms of injury are by far the most common, with explosive devices and gunshot wounds responsible for nearly all vascular injuries in wartime.[4,6,11,19-21] In OIF, improvised explosive devices were the cause of vascular injury in 55% of patients, and gunshot wounds accounted for 39% of injuries.[19-21] Although the cause of vascular injury is often difficult to ascertain, and definitions of types of explosive devices may vary slightly, the proportion of gunshot wounds (25% to 45%) versus explosive devices (55% to 75%) responsible for vascular injuries has remained roughly the same in every conflict since World War II. In contrast to slight variations in the cause of vascular injury, which may vary depending on the operational setting (e.g., traditional versus asymmetric), the anatomic distribution is largely constant, with extremity injuries always most prevalent.[19-21]

LEVELS OF CARE

The organization of surgical care in the theater of war requires the distribution of surgical capabilities to facilities and locations referred to as *levels of care* (Fig. 156-3).[24,29] Each level of care (previously referred to as *echelons*) functions uniquely in the management of wartime vascular injury, attempting to prevent hemorrhage and optimize functional outcome. There are five levels of care, ranging from level I (combat medic) to level V (facilities within the United States).[29] The highest level of care in the area of responsibility (AOR), which encompasses the theaters of Iraq and Afghanistan, is level III surgical capability. Levels of care are part of an organizational pattern and may change according to the type of battlefield, events on the ground, and the distribution of surgical expertise. The evacuation of injured troops through the various levels of care has specific terminology to allow uniform communication, tracking, and study of this step in the care of the wounded. The in-theater movement of casualties from the site of injury or from a level I location to a level II or III facility is referred to as casualty evacuation (CASEVAC). In-theater movement between levels II and III facilities is termed medical evacuation, or MEDEVAC; evacuation out of theater is designated air evacuation, or AIREVAC (Fig. 156-4).

Level I

Level I care is provided by the tactical combat casualty medic, who performs lifesaving measures and initiates movement of the wounded to treatment facilities such as Army Battalion Aid Stations or Marine Corps Shock Trauma Platoons. Level I care includes establishment of an airway; hemorrhage control, with or without application of a field dressing or tourniquet; and intravenous access. Because bleeding is the leading cause of potentially preventable death on the battlefield, the availability and use of certain tools to stop hemorrhage have become standardized among level I medics.[14-16] The distribution of the Special Operations Forces Tactical Tourniquet (SOFTT) or the Combat Applications Tourniquet System (CATS) for hemorrhage control is one such change. Although improvised tourniquet devices have been used for hundreds of years, the more formal discussion of their safety and efficacy and the purchase of commercial devices have occurred since the experience with vascular injury in the Vietnam War.

SOFTT and CATS are designed to be placed with one hand and are carried by nearly all combat forces in Iraq and Afghanistan. Despite the potential harmful effects of inappropriate or prolonged application of tourniquets, experience with the use of tourniquets for hemorrhage control has been favorable.[20-22,24] In rare cases, tourniquets have been applied unnecessarily or inappropriately; examples include application on extremities with isolated venous injuries or on extremities without injuries to major axial vessels. However, in these cases, the tourniquets were evaluated at level II or III facilities and removed in less than an hour, with few adverse effects.[24] Preliminary data from the GWOT Vascular Initiative show that tourniquet use is documented in approximately one third of extremity vascular injuries.

In addition to the use of tourniquets, there has been a proliferation of commercially available topical hemostatic agents that can be applied by medics at the scene of the injury to assist with hemorrhage control. The two most common are

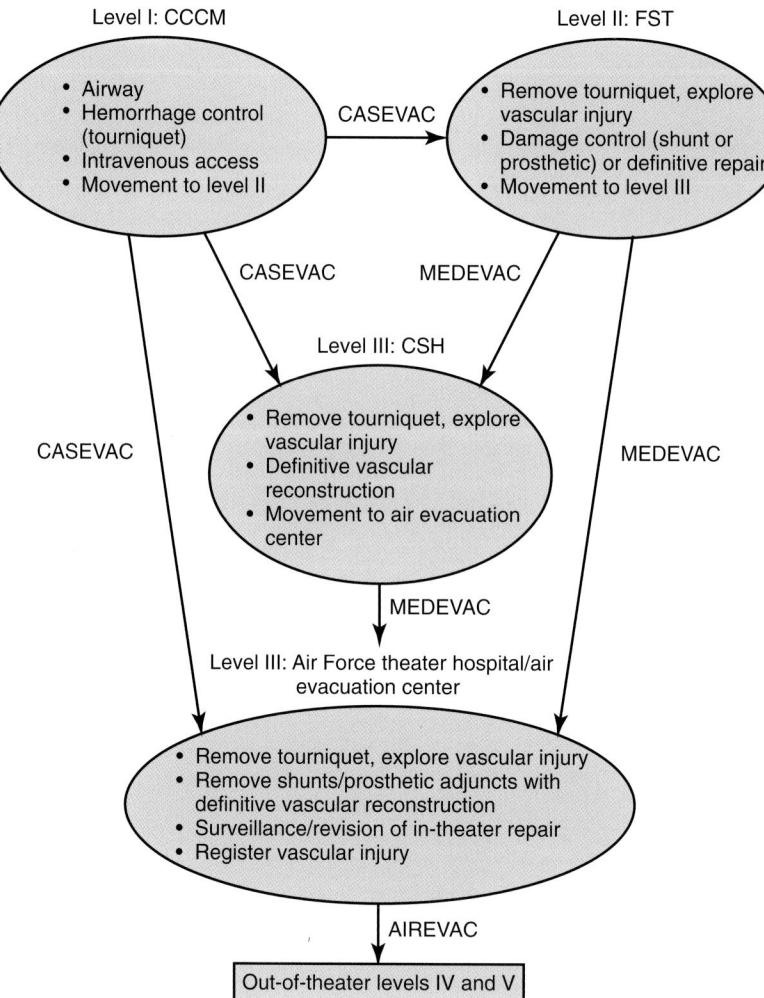

Figure 156-3 Evacuation scheme for injured troops through all five levels of care. Levels I, II, and III are in the theater of war. Level IV care is provided at Landstuhl Regional Medical Center in Germany. Level V represents tertiary military medical centers in the United States. CASEVAC, casualty evacuation; CCCM, combat casualty care medic; CSH, combat support hospital; FST, forward surgical team; MEDEVAC, medical evacuation; AIREVAC, air evacuation.

HemCon (HemCon Medical Technologies Inc., Portland, OR) and QuickClot (Z-Medica Corp., Wallingford, CT).[30-32] HemCon is a chitosan dressing that adheres strongly to soft tissues, sealing the wound site and concentrating red blood cells and clotting factors, including platelets. The active ingredient in QuickClot is zeolite granules, which avidly absorb water, concentrating red blood cells and clotting factors at the bleeding site in a significant exothermic reaction. In-theater experience with these agents is generally favorable, although each has potential complications and can make definitive vascular reconstruction more difficult.

Currently, the potential downside of using hemostatic adjuncts, topical agents, or tourniquets is accepted, knowing that the use of these tools will prevent death from hemorrhage in a percentage of wounded soldiers with select patterns of vascular injury.

Level II

In past military conflicts, capabilities at level II facilities were not well defined; however, in the decades since the Vietnam War, advances in the forward deployment of surgical resources have been formalized to provide a damage-control capacity within minutes of injury. The GWOT represents the first prolonged military conflict in which this strategy and its impact on vascular injury have been tested. Each military service has a different level II unit with similar surgical capabilities. The Army deploys a level II medical treatment facility, a forward surgical team, or a combination of both. The Air Force deploys an expeditionary medical support unit, a mobile field surgical team, or a combination thereof. The Navy provides casualty receiving and treatment ships, and the Marine Corp has a forward resuscitative surgery system.[28,33]

The full impact of level II capability on vascular outcomes is unknown, although preliminary experience is favorable. In a report of the Marine Corps' forward resuscitative surgical system, Chambers and coworkers demonstrated that wounded were received at their level II facility within 30 minutes of injury.[33] By comparison, during the Vietnam War, 85% of those with missile wounds underwent initial operation within 90 minutes of injury (at a level III facility, by today's definitions).[34] Woodward and colleagues reported that over a 32-month period, 58 of 142 casualties (38%) with penetrating femoropopliteal injuries were seen at a level II facility before being evacuated to the Air Force theater hospital at Balad Air Base, a level III facility.[22] This more forward level II capacity allows the earlier removal of tourniquets and more immediate identification and exploration of vascular injuries. This trans-

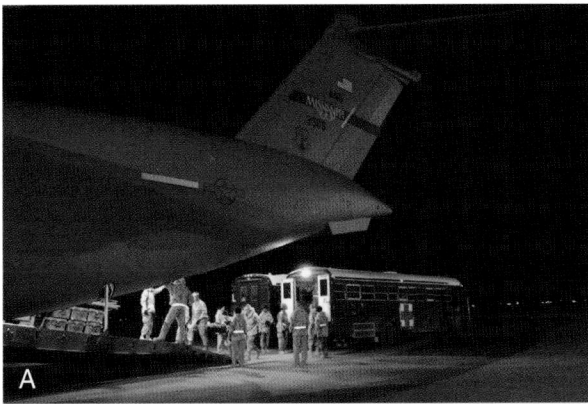
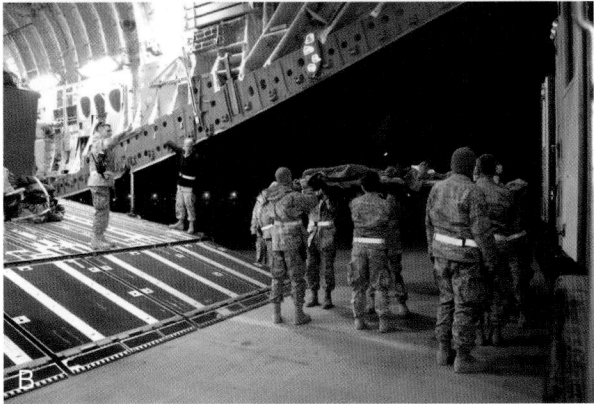

Figure 156-4 A and **B,** Loading of an AIREVAC flight aboard the Air Force's C-17 Globemaster.

lates to earlier thrombectomy, application of heparin to the injured vessel, vascular reconstruction, placement of temporary shunts, and fasciotomy, all noted priorities in emergency wartime surgery.[20-24,29,33]

In contrast to the reported experience from the Vietnam Vascular Registry, a significant percentage of extremity vascular injuries are now managed with temporary vascular shunts to restore axial flow to the extremity.[20-24,33] Currently, during periods of high casualties, temporary vascular shunts are most commonly placed as damage-control adjuncts at level II facilities as part of the triad of thrombectomy, restoration of flow, and fasciotomy.[20,23,33]

Data from the Balad Vascular Registry indicate that temporary vascular shunts have been used in 33% to 50% of extremity vascular injuries and that shunts placed in proximal injuries (e.g., femoropopliteal, axillosubclavian) are most effective. Patency of shunts in proximal vessels is greater than 90% when these injuries are re-explored at level III facilities following MEDEVAC.[23] The patency rates of vascular shunts in wartime are achieved without the use of systemic heparinization, which reflects the preliminary large animal data from Dawson and colleagues.[35] At level III facilities, the vascular injuries are re-explored, the shunts are removed, and definitive vascular reconstruction is performed. Anecdotal cases of successful arterial and venous shunting are not uncommon in injuries of the femoral vessels. Data from our group show that despite the poor patency of shunts placed in more distal vascular injuries (e.g., forearm, tibia), the early limb salvage rate

in such cases is not compromised.[23] Use of temporary vascular shunts in more distal vessels should be the exception and should be considered only when the procedure is technically straightforward, with exposed vessels and a good size match. In the case of most distal vascular injuries, ligation without shunting represents an important component of damage control. The extremity should then be assessed for perfusion with continuous wave Doppler. In most instances, the collateral circulation around such distal vascular injuries is sufficient to keep the extremity viable until a more complete evaluation can be performed. In these cases, the utility of continuous wave Doppler to demonstrate the presence or absence of even a weak arterial signal cannot be overemphasized.

Although there is appropriate concern regarding the use of shunts for long periods over extended evacuation distances, under the current system, patients treated at level II facilities arrive at level III facilities within 2 hours of injury (and often within 30 to 60 minutes).[23,33] In a review of in-theater evacuation patterns, the average time from loading on a helicopter to arrival at a level III facility was 46 minutes.[24] Rapid movement of patients with vascular shunts and effective communication between surgeons at both levels of care can increase the likelihood of shunt usefulness and minimize complications such as shunt thrombosis or dislodgment. Currently, the use of temporary vascular shunts is encouraged in select patterns of proximal vascular injuries (including venous injuries) as part of the triad of early thrombectomy, restoration of flow, and fasciotomy.

Level III

Level III facilities in Iraq and Afghanistan include the Army's combat support hospitals and the Air Force's theater hospitals.[24,29] Level III care is the highest level of care in both theaters. In light of the evacuation time to the level IV facility in Germany (8 to 12 hours), much of the operating historically performed at level IV facilities has now been pushed forward to level III locations in theater. This is especially true for vascular injuries, and the goal has been to place trained peripheral vascular surgeons at level III facilities. As part of this model, nearly all vascular injuries are definitively repaired prior to AIREVAC out of Iraq and Afghanistan, including the removal of all temporary shunts and the repair of extremity vascular injuries with autologous vein.[24]

Level III facilities are equipped with vascular instrument sets, continuous wave Doppler, intraoperative fluoroscopy, blood banks, and intensive care units. In addition, there are accessories such as prosthetic graft material for aortic and great vessel repair, embolectomy catheters, thrombolytic agents, and permanent as well as removable vena cava filters. Recent reports from our group described the forward deployment of endovascular capabilities to a level III facility to provide the rare but often critical intervention offered by endovascular techniques.[26] Examples include coil embolization of hemorrhage from pelvic fractures or select solid organ injuries, placement of covered stents in certain arterial injury patterns, and placement of temporary vena cava filters in patients unable to receive chemoprophylaxis because of associated solid-organ or intracranial injuries.[26] Removable filters are especially useful in the setting of concomitant pelvic or long-bone fractures, which place patients who are unable to receive heparin at high risk for pulmonary embolus during extended AIREVAC.

Level IV

One level IV facility in Germany currently receives all injured troops evacuated by air from the AOR. At this fixed U.S. hospital facility, patients with vascular injuries are further stabilized and frequently undergo additional washout and débridement of soft tissue wounds. In this context, coverage of any vascular anastomosis is carefully considered before AIREVAC to level V facilities in the United States. Additionally, vascular reconstruction is checked for patency using continuous wave Doppler, duplex ultrasound, computed tomographic angiography (CTA), and even angiography in select cases. If soft tissue coverage is lacking or there are concerns about graft disruption or thrombosis, patients may undergo additional procedures to ensure coverage (e.g., advancement or pedicle flaps) or remain at this level IV facility for an extended period. Although there have been no reports of vascular reconstruction thrombosis or blowout during transport from the level IV facility in Germany to level V facilities in the United States, there have been anecdotal cases of early anastomotic disruption with hemorrhage soon after arrival at a level V facility. The untoward complications of graft thrombosis or blowout due to wound contamination or compromised soft tissue coverage are rare but should be recognized as serious and especially relevant in this scenario, given the rapid evacuation of those with vascular injuries out of the theater of war. The average time from point of injury in the AOR to arrival at a level V facility in the United States has been a fairly constant 4 to 5 days.[19]

Level V

Several level V facilities exist in various regions of the United States. Reports from Walter Reed have documented the role of these tertiary facilities in the management of wartime vascular injuries.[19,27,36] In addition to the completion of soft tissue wound management associated with vascular injury, surveillance of vascular repairs is paramount. In the rare cases when a hemodynamically significant defect in a vascular reconstruction is detected, operative or endovascular intervention can be performed to obtain assisted primary patency. Level V facilities are also responsible for detecting, diagnosing, and treating vascular injuries that may have been missed at previous levels of care or that present in a delayed fashion (e.g., traumatic pseudoaneurysm). Whether these injuries are actually missed or represent the delayed presentation of an evolving injury is debatable, but it is generally accepted that 5% of wartime vascular injuries present or are detected in a belated fashion.[19,27,36]

The Walter Reed group has demonstrated the utility of several diagnostic modalities in the surveillance of vascular injuries, including duplex ultrasonography, CTA, and arteriography.[19,27,36] The first reports on the utility of endovascular modalities to diagnose and treat wartime vascular injuries came from this group and were largely responsible for the advancement of endovascular capabilities to in-theater level III facilities, closer to the point of injury.[19,26,27] Level V facilities are also responsible for removing vena cava filters inserted at level III facilities, once the patient is able to ambulate or receive chemoprophylaxis or anticoagulation. Finally, patient education related to vascular injury should occur at level V facilities. This includes discussing with the patient and the family the natural history of vascular reconstruction and the need for appropriate lifelong surveillance. In some cases, long-term antiplatelet therapy or anticoagulation may be indicated, although data with regard to this topic are lacking.

CLINICAL PRESENTATION

The presentation of vascular injury can be divided into two familiar categories: patients presenting with hard signs of vascular injury and those presenting with soft signs. Approximately half of wartime vascular injuries manifest hard signs, including hemorrhage from a penetrating wound or bleeding into a closed space as evidenced by an expanding hematoma, most commonly in an extremity or the neck. About 30% of extremity vascular injuries present with an associated fracture or dislocation. Extremity ischemia is another hard sign of vascular injury commonly encountered. Careful physical examination, including use of a stethoscope, may detect the hard sign of a palpable thrill or audible bruit associated with a traumatic arteriovenous fistula. Frequently, these injuries are associated with hemorrhagic shock, with reports of significant blood loss at the scene of the injury or during evacuation. Hemorrhage from a torso vascular injury may present as hemoperitoneum or hemothorax discovered at the time of chest tube placement, thoracotomy, or laparotomy. Alternatively, in patients who are hemodynamically stable and able to undergo contrast computed tomography, vascular injury may be diagnosed by the presence of blood in the abdomen or chest or an abnormality of a large vessel (e.g., pseudoaneurysm, extravasation).

DIAGNOSTIC EVALUATION

Patients with hard or obvious signs of vascular injury are generally taken to the operating room for exploration, and there is often no time to perform a more detailed diagnostic evaluation. Therefore, the diagnostic evaluation pertains mostly to patients with soft signs of vascular injury or penetrating wounds or fragments proximal to a major axial vessel. In this context, the surgeon is attempting to determine whether an occult major vascular injury is present. In addition to a thorough physical examination looking for signs of vascular injury, the three most useful modalities in diagnosing combat-related vascular injuries are continuous wave Doppler, contrast-enhanced CTA, and standard angiography.

Clinical Findings

The clinical evaluation of wartime vascular injury is often complicated by the capacity of young individuals to vasoconstrict or "clamp down" the peripheral circulation to support the central circulation. This phenomenon is especially evident in the setting of slight degrees of hypotension and hypothermia, the latter of which is worsened during rotary wing evacuation. The vascular examination therefore relies heavily on the presence or absence of Doppler signals in an injured extremity and is, by necessity, a dynamic measurement repeated several times over the first hour of the patient's resuscitation. What may initially appear to be an ischemic limb in a patient with a systolic blood pressure of 90 mm Hg and a core temperature of 96°F (35°C) often improves with resuscitation and warming. Continuous wave Doppler in this setting is quick and useful to confirm perfusion to an extremity on initial presentation. Calculation of a more sensitive injured extremity index (IEI) can be performed if perfusion is still a concern after the patient has been warmed and resuscitated.

Liberal use of continuous wave Doppler either alone or to calculate the IEI allows for the selective application of angiography in cases in which soft signs of vascular injury are present. This approach avoids the overuse of arteriography, which is important in the setting of multiple casualties and limited angiographic capabilities or operating room space. If available, contrast-enhanced CTA is another useful tool to evaluate patients with soft signs of vascular injury; it is particularly germane to the evaluation of the vessels of the supra-aortic trunk and neck. Regardless of location, it is important to note that soft signs of vascular injury allow the surgeon time to evaluate injuries to other body regions and then return to the area of concern to repeat diagnostic testing as needed, perhaps when the patient is improved physiologically.

Another challenging scenario unique to wartime relates to significant penetrating wounds at multiple levels of the same extremity without hard signs of vascular injury. A common example is a patient with significant wounds in proximity to the femoral, popliteal, and tibial vessels of the same leg. In these instances, arteriography is especially useful to detect the injury and determine the specific level or levels affected.[2]

Doppler Indices

Lavenson, Rich, and Strandness were among the first to describe the utility of continuous wave Doppler in wartime, and its efficacy has been sustained in the modern combat environment.[20,21,24,40] Often, determining the initial presence and quality of an arterial signal (monophasic versus biphasic) beyond the zone of injury is all that is required early in patient assessment (secondary survey). More detailed information about extremity perfusion can be gleaned by calculating the IEI, which is an extension of the more familiar ankle-brachial index used to assess age-related vascular disease. To calculate

the IEI, the distal occlusion pressure of the arterial Doppler signal in the injured extremity—arm or leg—is divided by the arterial occlusion pressure of the uninjured extremity. If the IEI is greater than 0.9, the likelihood of significant arterial injury is 5% or less in most series.

Computed Tomographic Angiography

Contrast-enhanced CTA is useful to evaluate the vessels of the supra-aortic trunk and neck. Cox and associates demonstrated the utility of CTA in evaluating such vascular injuries in soldiers returning from combat at a level V facility.[36] Because CTA is available at most if not all level II and III facilities in theater, it should be used to determine which patients with penetrating wounds to the chest or neck require exploration. Although we have not used CTA to evaluate extremity vascular injuries, given the advances in imaging speed and quality, one can foresee that this technique will become increasingly useful in the evaluation of all combat vascular injuries. The advantages of CTA over standard arteriography are its speed and noninvasiveness, as well as the important fact that CTA does not occupy an operating room, which may be in short supply during times of high casualties.

Arteriography

The use of standard arteriography in the acute setting of war was initially advocated by Starnes and coworkers in the early phases of OIF.[2] Their report on extremity vascular injury emphasized the usefulness of arteriography in the evaluation of an extremity with penetrating wounds at multiple levels. Although arteriography is useful in select clinical scenarios, its overuse for diagnostic purposes in the combat setting should be discouraged. Extremity arteriography in young patients who are even slightly hypotensive or hypothermic may result in an apparent abnormality that leads to confusion or even unnecessary exploration in some cases. Arteriography of the distal extremity vessels (e.g., forearm, tibia) can be especially tricky to interpret in the combat setting, and we often rely on the Doppler examination and the appearance of the leg or foot rather than angiography. Because most combat vascular injuries can be diagnosed by physical examination, continuous wave Doppler, and CTA, arteriography should be reserved for unusual situations, such as when CTA is not available or in the case of multiple levels of penetrating wounds to the same extremity.[2] We have also found arteriography to be useful to exclude vascular injury in the setting of orthopedic injuries that have a propensity to cause vascular trauma, such as posterior knee dislocation, supracondylar femur fracture, displaced tibial plateau fracture, and humerus fracture. However, because patients with these types of injuries will be evacuated before the original surgeon can act, we have a lower threshold for evaluating these injuries with arteriography before patient transport.

In a 2004 report from Walter Reed, we examined the use of catheter-based techniques in the evaluation of soldiers returning to a level V facility.[19] In our experience, nearly two thirds (63%) underwent angiography less than a week after injury, and half were found to have some type of occult vascular injury. A more recent report from our group found that half of soldiers with an occult injury identified by arteriography underwent further intervention or repair.[27] In many respects, our level V experience has established the relevance of endovascular techniques to wartime injury management, providing momentum to extend that capability into the theater of war closer to the site of wounding.[26]

■ TRIAGE

Hemorrhage Control: Initial Triage

The four categories used to triage patients in a wartime setting are immediate, delayed, expectant, and minimal.[29] These terms should be kept in mind when considering vascular trauma, although most if not all vascular injuries are considered to be in the immediate or delayed category. *Immediate* implies that instant or urgent action is required, such as placement of a tourniquet, a vascular clamp, or manual pressure to stop hemorrhage. The *delayed* category implies that there is no active bleeding and the injury can be addressed by ligation or reconstruction within a matter of minutes or hours. Like patient triage, the process of prioritizing vascular injury is dynamic, requiring reassessment or re-triage once bleeding is controlled, and is dependent on multiple factors.

Hemorrhage from a vascular injury, regardless of body region, falls into the immediate category until the bleeding is controlled. Once this has been achieved, attention should be turned to patient resuscitation (i.e., damage-control resuscitation) and the evaluation of other life-threatening injuries in the abdomen, thorax, or cranium. In this context, we consider severe physiologic derangement (i.e., shock) that results from blood loss a life-threatening condition that should be at least partially treated with warming, resuscitation, and correction of physiologic parameters *before* embarking on extremity vascular reconstruction.

If tourniquets are in place, we recommend a well-timed and careful approach to their release, keeping in mind that this may result in additional blood loss, acidosis, hyperkalemia, and hypotension. Tourniquets should be released only at a calculated time during the patient's resuscitation, and only after communication with the anesthesia team, which may need to volume-load the patient and have medications such as bicarbonate ready for administration. For example, one should consider leaving an extremity tourniquet in place if a patient requires a laparotomy, thoracotomy, or neck exploration for bleeding (Fig. 156-5). In many circumstances, tourniquets should remain in place until the treatment of life-threatening intracranial injuries has been accomplished. Regardless of the scenario, a stepwise approach directed by the primary surgeon can avoid a situation in which a tourniquet is released haphazardly, resulting in physiologic insult to the patient. These triage steps are not necessary for every tourniquet, but they are important to consider in the wartime setting, where patients often have multiple injuries in more than one body location.

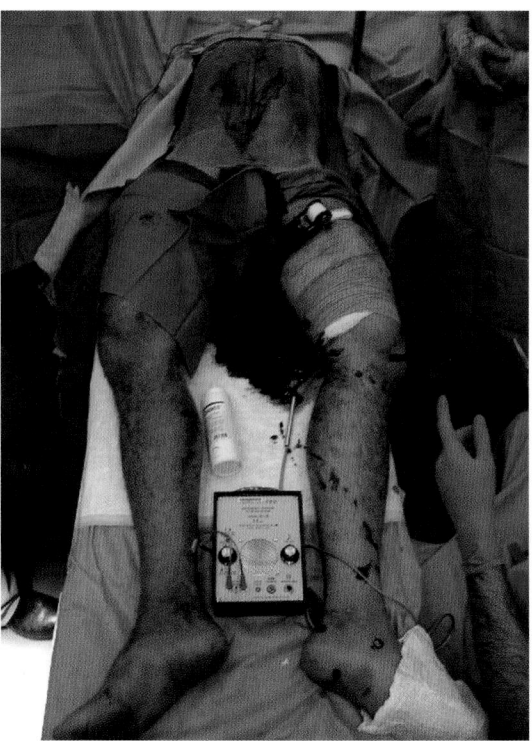

Figure 156-5 Patient in vascular injury triage category II (see Box 156-1). He has a left femoral artery injury as well as life-threatening intra-abdominal hemorrhage from a solid-organ injury. In this case, the tourniquet device was a load strap applied by those on the scene; it was left in place while the intra-abdominal hemorrhage was stopped and resuscitation initiated. Following lifesaving laparotomy, the extremity injury was addressed after slow release of the tourniquet, allowing the anesthesia team to treat any untoward effects of reperfusion. Premature release of this tourniquet in a patient with hemorrhagic shock and severe physiologic derangements from intra-abdominal hemorrhage may have led to additional physiologic insult from reperfusion (e.g., hyperkalemia, hypotension, bleeding), resulting in the patient's death.

Post-Hemorrhage Control: Re-triage

After hemorrhage control, extremity vascular injury can be re-triaged into one of four categories to assist with prioritization during combat surgical operations (Box 156-1). These categories represent guidelines, and the treatment of individual patients within each category varies, depending on resuscitation status, available technical expertise, blood bank resources, and casualty numbers.

Category I: Isolated Vascular Injury

If the injury is isolated (i.e., no other body regions are injured) and the patient has been resuscitated, vascular repair should be undertaken, including repair of venous injury and even complex procedures such as tibia-level reconstructions for limb salvage. In this category, limb salvage takes priority, and lengthier vascular reconstructions with anticipated blood loss may be attempted that would otherwise not be considered. In the case of an isolated extremity vascular injury, a two-team approach may be useful when vein harvest is required; otherwise, one surgical team typically manages this category.

Box 156-1 Triage Categories and Management Guidelines for Wartime Extremity Vascular Injuries

CATEGORY I: ISOLATED VASCULAR INJURY

- One surgical team required
- Vascular injury, restoration of flow, reconstruction, and limb salvage take priority
- Extremity tourniquet may be removed in the operating room in coordination with the anesthesia team
- Venous injury should be repaired
- Complex or lengthy reconstructions acceptable

CATEGORY II: VASCULAR INJURY IN CONJUNCTION WITH OTHER NON–LIFE-THREATENING INJURIES

- Two-team approach preferable to treat vascular and other injury
- Vascular injury, restoration of flow, reconstruction, and limb salvage take priority
- Extremity tourniquet may be removed in the operating room in coordination with the anesthesia team
- Venous injury should be repaired
- Complex or lengthy reconstructions acceptable

CATEGORY III: MULTIPLE VASCULAR INJURIES

- Two-team approach preferable to treat multiple vascular injuries
- Vascular injury, restoration of flow, reconstruction, and limb salvage take priority
- Extremity tourniquet may be removed in the operating room in coordination with the anesthesia team
- Diminished role for venous injury repair
- Diminished role for complex or lengthy reconstructions

CATEGORY IV: VASCULAR INJURY IN CONJUNCTION WITH LIFE-THREATENING INJURIES

- Two-team approach optional after life-threatening injury is stabilized
- Life-threatening torso, neck, or head injury takes priority
- Extremity tourniquets should remain in place until the life-threatening injury* is stabilized
- Diminished role for venous injury repair
- Diminished role for complex or lengthy reconstructions

*Includes severe physiologic derangement from shock (e.g., severe acidosis, anemia, coagulopathy, hypothermia, electrolyte disorder).

Category II: Vascular Injury in Conjunction with Other Non–Life-Threatening Injuries

If other non–life-threatening injuries are present in conjunction with a vascular injury and the patient is physiologically well, vascular repair should occur before or in conjunction with treatment of the other injuries. This scenario includes associated abdominal or thoracic injuries that do not involve hemorrhage, dislocated fractures, and other soft tissue injuries. In this setting, we recommend judicious tourniquet release in the operating room, exploration of the vascular injury, and quick restoration of perfusion to the extremity. In the case of concomitant torso, neck, or face injuries, we commonly work on the extremity vascular injury while another surgical team operates on these areas (a two-team approach).

In the case of concomitant orthopedic injuries, we recommend exploration of the vascular injury, thrombectomy, placement of a temporary vascular shunt, and performance of a fasciotomy prior to or simultaneous with orthopedic fixation. Removal of the shunt and definitive vascular repair follow orthopedic fixation. This stepwise strategy applies to proximal extremity injuries (e.g., humerus, femur, knee) more so than distal injuries (e.g., forearm, tibia).

Category III: Multiple Vascular Injuries

Though unusual in the civilian setting, combat wounds may result in vascular injury to more than one limb or at more than one level in a given extremity. In this challenging situation, priority should be given to the reconstruction of proximal vessels first, with the lower extremity taking priority over the upper extremity owing to the collateral circulation of the arm and its relatively small size. The goal is to achieve perfusion of the largest area of muscle first. In this category, a temporary vascular shunt can be effective in restoring flow through one injury zone while another vascular injury is repaired. Alternatively, a two-team approach is preferable to shorten operative time. In a patient with more than one extremity vascular injury, the role of venous repair and complex distal reconstruction is diminished, given the operative time required to manage both extremities.

Category IV: Vascular Injury in Conjunction with Life-Threatening Injuries, Including Severe Shock

In this category, once hemorrhage control is achieved at the vascular injury site, attention should be turned to life-threatening injuries in the abdomen, thorax, or cranium. In addition, damage-control resuscitation should have already been initiated. In cases of extremity vascular injury, tourniquets should be left in place and definitive repair delayed until other more pressing injuries have been addressed. Examples include laparotomy for splenic injury, thoracotomy for bleeding lung injury, or craniotomy for intracranial hematoma (see Fig. 156-5). If a tourniquet is not in place or not available, other options include ligation of the injured extremity vessel or placement of a temporary vascular shunt. Definitive vascular repair should be considered only after the life-threatening injury has been managed, depending on the patient's physiologic status. In this scenario, vascular repair should not include lengthy, complex reconstructions, and the role of venous injury repair is diminished.

■ MANAGEMENT

Resuscitation and Surgical Planning

As noted, military vascular trauma usually involves the extremities and is often part of an injury complex in patients with exsanguinating hemorrhage presenting to a field hospital. Optimal management requires proper planning and recognition of the essential priorities to prevent immediate hemorrhagic death. Blast-associated injury, the most common vascular wounding pattern, involves fractures, thermal injury, and embedded fragments over a majority of the body surface. Following immediate airway control, attention is directed at controlling hemorrhage and obtaining vascular access. External bleeding is often hidden by warming blankets or military gear because wounded casualties usually arrive in full body armor and may have field tourniquets applied to one or more limbs. Direct pressure is the most effective way to control hemorrhage, although a volume-depleted patient may not always manifest active arterial bleeding at the time of admission.

Prehospital tourniquets should be inspected and may be left in place as the primary and secondary surveys of the patient take place. Readjustment or replacement of these tourniquets is often best accomplished in the operating room as resuscitation restores adequate peripheral perfusion. For active arterial bleeding, the narrow prehospital tourniquets are commonly exchanged for the much wider EMT pneumatic type (Delfi Medical, Vancouver, Canada), and the wound is explored in the operating room.[37]

Intravenous access may be hindered by shock, but immediate intraosseous access to the tibia or sternum is easily and rapidly achieved in adults. Initial laboratory studies depict the degree of physiologic distress, which is used to guide resuscitation and early operative planning. Damage-control resuscitation, a strategy of liberal blood product administration, minimal crystalloid use, and selective use of recombinant factor VIIa, should begin early in the emergency room and continue intraoperatively.[38] The goal is to achieve hemostasis, restore normal physiology, and potentially complete a vascular reconstruction on arrival in the intensive care unit. Blood products should be transfused within minutes of arrival, with an emergency release of 4 units of type O packed red blood cells and 2 units of thawed AB plasma sent on demand from the blood bank. Blood products are best transfused through a Belmont rapid-infuser system (Belmont Instrument Corporation, Billerica, MA) in the admitting area.

Unstable patients with truncal injuries or those with more than one mangled extremity are considered in extremis and should trigger a massive transfusion protocol. This involves a standardized release and transfusion of packed red blood cells, thawed plasma, cryoprecipitate, and platelets. Unusual in civilian practice, fresh whole blood, obtained from a pre-screened donor pool, has been used in every major U.S. military conflict since World War I. The use of fresh whole blood is safe and can be very effective in remote locations where the supply is limited or in patients who require massive transfusions.[39]

Recognizing the need for vascular reconstruction early during a trauma admission is crucial for success; indecision and a progressive ischemic burden can result in ultimate graft failure and subsequent limb loss. Radiographs provide reliable clues to the existence of extremity vascular injuries and are

therefore an important part of the assessment. For instance, supracondylar femur and tibial plateau fractures are frequently associated with injuries to the popliteal artery. Deformed extremities are straightened, and the onset of additional hemorrhage is controlled with direct pressure, gauze packing, hemostatic dressings, or additional tourniquets.

Alternatively, in stable patients without active bleeding, prehospital tourniquets may be carefully loosened by the surgeon to determine the degree of vascular injury, if any. A Doppler assessment is advisable to confirm the presence or absence of arterial signals and therefore perfusion. Additionally, the more sensitive IEI can be measured if Doppler signals are reduced or there is a particularly high index of suspicion for injury. A patient assessment done in concert with an orthopedic surgeon can facilitate discussion of the appropriate operative sequence and the techniques of external fixation that can best aid in the anticipated vascular exposure. Important information to relay to the entire surgical team includes ideal patient positioning, the plan for vein harvesting in a contralateral extremity, and the desire for a C-arm unit or arteriography. Special instruments located in "peel packs" can ease the apprehension of not having the right instruments when they are needed quickly.

Operating Room Considerations

A dedicated two-team approach is recommended for the management of categories II, III, and IV military vascular injuries (see Box 156-1). For extremity injuries, this practice reduces ischemic time: while the primary team is preoccupied with thoracotomy or laparotomy for the treatment of other soft tissue wounds (see "Triage"), the second team can be applying external fixation, performing fasciotomies, beginning peripheral vascular exposure, or harvesting vein from a noninjured or amputated extremity. The patient should always be positioned to enable unimpeded access to another body cavity or limb in the event of unexpected deterioration or the need for additional vein harvesting.

Hemorrhage is often initially controlled by digital occlusion using an assistant's hand prepped directly into the bleeding wound bed with povidone-iodine (Betadine) spray. This is followed by a careful dissection proximal and distal to the site of injury. Balloon catheters can also be used to tamponade hemorrhage when a tourniquet or manual pressure is not effective, but blind insertion of surgical instruments can be unproductive or harmful and is discouraged. Tourniquets are left in place until the anesthesia team has had sufficient time to resuscitate the patient and prepare for the anticipated reperfusion phenomena (e.g., bleeding, acidosis, hyperkalemia) upon tourniquet release. Proximal femoral injuries are best managed by division of the inguinal ligament or a retroperitoneal approach to control the external iliac artery. For proximal axillosubclavian wounds, sternotomy or left anterior thoracotomy and clamping of the subclavian artery eliminate the error of uncontrolled dissection through an expanding hematoma of the chest.

Surgical Treatment

Methods of Repair

Although used fairly infrequently for wartime vascular injuries, primary end-to-end repair is preferred when lateral sutures are not sufficient to repair the vessel. Advantages of primary end-to-end repair include a single anastomosis and use of autologous tissue. Dividing nearby branches, even if patent, may afford the surgeon some length in noncalcified vessels, but this method should be both expedient and tensionless. Complete débridement of any disrupted tissue is an essential step, and sacrifices made to avoid an interposition conduit should be passionately resisted. Because most combat vascular injuries result in too much vessel damage to allow a safe, tension-free primary end-to-end anastomosis, interposition graft placement using reversed saphenous vein is most common. Clouse and colleagues demonstrated that autogenous vein graft was used in more than half of the 301 arterial injuries from the Balad Vascular Registry, and primary repair was accomplished in only 18% of cases[20] (Table 156-3). The complexity and additional operative time required for a vein harvest and interposition graft or bypass make these cases more taxing and technically involved, so the operative plan and estimated time should be communicated to the entire surgical team.[6,42]

Ballistic trauma can transmit kinetic energy and result in intimal injury well beyond the transected arterial segment. Therefore, a vigilant débridement is performed, focusing on the quality of the luminal surface, the strength of the vessel, and the arterial inflow relative to the patient's hemodynamic state. Fogarty thromboembolectomy catheters should be used liberally proximally and distally before arterial repair because the use of prehospital tourniquets and the lack of anticoagulation in the setting of trauma may result in thrombus accumulation. Failure to recognize and clear such thrombus with Fogarty catheters is a likely cause of early graft failure in the wartime setting.

In military trauma, the lack of adequate lighting, fine surgical instruments, monofilament sutures, and loupe magnification may adversely affect the careful tissue handling that is

Table 156-3 Methods of Arterial Repair

Location	Primary	AVG/P	Prosthetic	Ligation	Endovascular	Nonoperative
Neck						
CCA	2	10		1		
ICA	4	3		3	1	
ECA				7	2	
Vertebral	4			2		3
Upper Extremity						
SC/A	5	4		2		
Brachial	6	35	1			
Forearm	4	8		11		
Chest						
SAT	1	1	1	1		
TA	3					
Abdomen						
Aorta	3	1			1	
Renovisceral	3			1		
CIA	2	1	1			
IIA				1	1	
EIA		1	1		1	
Lower Extremity						
CFA	4	4	1			
PFA	2			9	1	
SFA	8	42	3			
Popliteal	2	38				
Tibial	3	22		19		
Total	**56** (18.6%)	**170** (56.5%)	**8** (2.7%)	**57** (18.9%)	**7** (2.3%)	**3** (1.0%)

*Method of repair in 301 arterial injuries by anatomic location.
AVG/P, autogenous vein graft or patch angioplasty; CCA, common carotid artery; CFA, common femoral artery; CIA, common iliac artery; ECA, external carotid artery; EIA, external iliac artery; ICA, internal carotid artery; IIA, internal iliac artery; PFA, profunda femoris artery; SAT, supra-aortic trunk; SC/A, subclavian-axillary; SFA; superficial femoral artery; TA, thoracic aorta.
Data from Clouse WD, Rasmussen TE, Peck MA. In-theater management of vascular injury: 2 years of the Balad Vascular Registry. *J Am Coll Surg.* 2007;204:625-632.

Section **19** Trauma and Acute Limb Ischemia

crucial to a successful vascular operation. Given these expected obstacles, a four-quadrant, heel-to-toe anastomosis that is well spatulated is the easiest method to teach and perform in difficult situations. Small Heifitz clips or bulldog clamps can also minimize the chance of a clamp injury. Special precautions are worthwhile and should include habitual flushing of the graft and native artery with heparinized saline to dislodge fibrin strands and platelet debris. This form of regional heparinization is especially important because most patients with combat vascular injuries cannot receive systemic anticoagulation because of other injuries.

The saphenous vein is the preferred conduit for interposition grafts used to restore flow in military vascular injuries (see Table 156-3). This practice is based on the poor historical results obtained with prosthetic materials used in contaminated war wounds, an experience that has been confirmed in recent wartime reports.[43] A number of authors have suggested that prosthetic conduits yield satisfactory results; however, in our experience, prosthetic grafts should be reserved for use in larger vessels such as the supra-aortic trunk, aorta, and iliac arteries. The inferior long-term patency of prosthetic materials and the potential for infection or poor incorporation in war wounds have restricted their widespread use in combat-related extremity wounds.[44-46] There have even been anecdotal cases in which a patent prosthetic conduit in the extremity was removed electively or preemptively in favor of a saphenous vein conduit to facilitate incorporation and reduce infection risk.[20,24]

Temporary Vascular Shunts

The use of temporary vascular shunts in the management of vascular injuries was described as early as 1959 by the French in the Algerian War (1959-1961), with scattered reports and smaller series appearing in the literature since that time. Only recently has this technique been described in a sustained military conflict and its usefulness in certain injury patterns confirmed on a large scale.[23,33,52] In select injury patterns, shunts can serve as a bridge to delayed reconstruction, maintaining extremity perfusion during patient transport, orthopedic reduction and fixation, or harvesting of vein conduit.[23,52-55] The value of temporary shunting should be weighed against the consequences of vessel ligation or clamping, with a prolongation of ischemia, during these same maneuvers. During the periods of highest casualties during OIF, we noted that 33% to 50% of patients with extremity vascular injuries treated at level II facilities had temporary vascular shunts placed as damage-control measures before MEDEVAC to our level III location.[20,22] As noted earlier, experience with shunts during the GWOT has demonstrated their particular effectiveness in more proximal vascular injuries, both arterial and venous.[23,33] Specifically, temporary vascular shunts placed in proximal vessels (e.g., subclavian-brachial, femoropopliteal) have very high (90%) patency rates during patient evacuation, treatment of other injuries, and vein harvest, with few complications. Shunts have also proved effective to restore flow and maintain perfusion at the site of one vascular injury while a second vascular injury is repaired. When applied appropriately as part of the triad of early thrombectomy, restoration of flow, and fasciotomies, shunts reduce ischemic time to peripheral muscle and nerve and may assist in efforts to improve not just statistical limb salvage but also quality or functional limb salvage. Currently, small-diameter shunts such as the Sundt, Argyle, or Javid, which are designed for elective carotid artery surgery, are most commonly used in the battlefield. The maximum internal diameter of these shunts is 1.7 to 2.5 mm, and efforts are under way to explore the effectiveness of larger diameter (4 to 5 mm) trauma-specific shunts with regard to extremity ischemia and reperfusion in the setting of injury.

Associated Soft Tissue Injuries

Military munitions produce large cavitary wounds, with numerous disruptions of the skin and loss of underlying muscle. As a result, it may be difficult to achieve suitable graft coverage. When confronted with this situation, a longer vein graft tunneled completely around the zone of injury is often preferable to a shorter, poorly covered vein interposition conduit.[21] Appropriately applied external fixation should take this issue into consideration, and the options must be discussed before fasciotomy and external fixation incisions are made. Devitalized tissue is excised and irrigated under low pressure, with careful evaluation of the viability of muscle tissue. A lengthy débridement at the outset is not always necessary, and many of these wounds look much better in a few days, after subsequent washouts and the use of closed NPWT.[47] Peck and coworkers demonstrated the effectiveness of a strict wound management strategy in the setting of extremity vascular injury using the VAC device (KCI Inc., San Antonio, TX).[25] In this report on 134 extremity vascular injuries with extensive soft tissue wounds, more than half the wounds were successfully closed in a delayed primary fashion using a strategy that involved repeat operative washouts, NPWT, and initiation of closure. In this report, one third of all soft tissue wounds were able to be covered with split-thickness skin grafts as a form of secondary closure.[25]

Limb Salvage versus Early Amputation

The decision to amputate versus salvage an extremity should consider the patient's physiologic condition, severity of associated injuries, location, and, most important, definitive orthopedic care and physical rehabilitation that will be necessary (see Box 156-1, categories III and IV). The Mangled Extremity Severity Score may be useful when factoring in the patient's age, limb ischemia, shock, and degree of tissue injury.[41] No one situation or scoring system can replace the surgical judgment of an experienced team.

Upper Extremity Vascular Injury

Upper extremity vascular injuries on the battlefield should not be underestimated and often require significant blood transfusions and special technical considerations. Clouse and colleagues reported the particular challenges associated with wartime vascular injuries in the upper extremity, demonstrating that the early amputation rate was nearly two times that of the lower extremity.[48] In their report, the amputation rate associated with upper extremity vascular injury was nearly 10%, which likely reflects the severity of injuries in which limb salvage is pursued. Owing to the deployment of forward surgical teams close to the site of injury and the liberal use of tourniquets, surgeons in combat are now presented with complex upper extremity injuries for which limb salvage might not have been an option in past wars. Significant soft tissue defects, orthopedic injuries, and wound expansion in response to injury highlight the importance of the careful tunneling of vein grafts in the upper extremity, which, given its relatively small size, can be challenging. In the report from Clouse's group, almost 15% of vascular reconstructions in the arm failed because of poor tissue coverage, infection, or early thrombosis.[48] Although this is still a low rate of early failure, it is three times that in the lower extremity.

Extremity Venous Repair

There has been sustained interest in the repair of venous injuries to improve functional limb salvage and avoid the morbidity from venous hypertension or chronic edema in both the upper and lower extremities.[49,50] In a contemporary wartime report from Quan and associates, the thrombosis rate following extremity venous repair was only 16%.[51] Although ligation remained the most common method of managing venous injury (64% of injuries were ligated), this report demonstrated the short-term and midterm success rates of venous repair and found that the rate of pulmonary embolus following venous repair was no higher than that following ligation.[51] The results of this landmark study laid to rest the hypothetical concerns about such complications and support venous repair in extremity injuries when circumstances allow (see Box 156-1, categories I and II). The authors emphasized that venous repair is particularly important in anatomic watershed areas responsible for significant venous outflow, such as the iliofemoral, popliteal, and internal jugular venous segments. With combined injuries, arterial repair usually precedes venous repair to minimize the ischemic burden, unless repair of the vein would require very little effort. As an alternative, we have placed temporary vascular shunts in the venous injury to maintain venous drainage of the extremity while arterial repair is accomplished.[20,23]

Endovascular Treatment

The established effectiveness of endovascular therapies in the treatment of specific patterns of acute injury has led the military to incorporate the capacity to perform endovascular techniques on the modern battlefield.[26,56-62] These concepts, originally promoted in urban trauma centers, have continued to evolve and have proved useful in the early management of isolated wartime injuries.[19,26,58] Specifically, coil embolization

of certain pelvic fractures and solid organ injuries is useful, and covered stents to treat central aortic and proximal great vessel injuries are effective if not preferable. Our group recently reported on 150 catheter-based procedures performed at a level III facility in Iraq, demonstrating the utility of endovascular capability in wartime.[26] Based on this experience, endovascular therapies can be divided into three categories: embolization, covered stent placement, and miscellaneous techniques, including snare removal of missile emboli. More than 60% of diagnostic angiographic procedures demonstrated a positive finding (i.e., vascular injury), and 70% of these patients underwent either open or endovascular repair. Advances in endovascular capability have followed the imaging improvements achieved with portable C-arm units capable of performing digital subtraction angiography. The logistics of maintaining a robust inventory in a field hospital continues to limit the ability to carry out many of these interventions in combat. Equipment shortages are not uncommon, and surgical expectations have to be adjusted to comply with the mission of a mobile hospital unit. Despite logistical and skill set challenges, the potential for endovascular treatment to improve the care of those acutely injured in war should not be minimized.[26]

◾ POSTOPERATIVE CARE

Early postoperative care in patients with wartime vascular injuries is focused on patient warming, resuscitation, and frequent surveillance of the vascular repair. In the case of extremity vascular reconstruction, such surveillance takes the form of frequent pulse or Doppler checks using the continuous wave Doppler machine. The presence of palpable pulses and normalization of the IEI (>0.9) may be delayed until appropriate resuscitation has occurred. Patients should remain in the intensive care unit for at least 24 hours while resuscitation and vascular surveillance are performed. In addition to monitoring perfusion, careful assessment for the development of compartment syndrome is essential, although we advocate four-compartment fasciotomies in all patients who have undergone reconstruction of lower extremity vascular injuries. Routine fasciotomies are especially important, given that patients are transferred out of the care of the original surgeon to providers who are unfamiliar with the postoperative examination. Although the degree of reperfusion and edema may appear limited in the operating room, many patients who sustain wartime vascular injuries require ongoing resuscitation, which can cause such benign-appearing extremities to develop compartment syndrome in the ensuing hours or days. The importance of soft tissue wound management following vascular injury has already been discussed, and one wartime strategy of using repeat operative washouts and the VAC device for NPWT was recently detailed by Peck and colleagues[25] and Leininger and associates.[47]

Although there is a paucity of clinical data to guide the use of antiplatelet or anticoagulation therapy following wartime vascular injury, our practice is to use some form of such therapy in patients who have no contraindications related to other injuries (e.g., closed head injury, solid organ injury). Specifically, patients who are awake and able to tolerate oral intake are given an aspirin early in the postoperative period and also receive low-molecular-weight heparin as prophylaxis for deep venous thrombosis. If the patient is unable to take aspirin orally, we administer an aspirin suppository or occasionally forgo aspirin and simply use a prophylactic dose of low-molecular-weight heparin administered subcutaneously. Full anticoagulation using low-molecular-weight heparin (1 mg/kg subcutaneously twice daily) or intravenous unfractionated heparin is reserved for rare cases of severely compromised outflow after prolonged ischemic times or after early failure of an arterial reconstruction that requires revision. If associated injuries preclude the use of anticoagulation, these therapies are withheld. The same guidelines are used for venous repair, although we have a lower threshold for the use of full-dose anticoagulation with low-molecular-weight or unfractionated heparin if possible. The other important adjunct following extremity venous repair is application of an intermittent pneumatic compression device distal to the repair. Pneumatic compression devices use mechanical force to intermittently augment venous flow through the venous repair, reducing the likelihood of stasis and thrombosis.

■ EVACUATION

Evacuation within the theater and out of the AOR was outlined previously (see Fig. 156-3).[24] Currently, patients who have sustained major vascular injuries are evacuated by air out of the theater by a critical care air transport team.[63] This team, comprising a critical care physician, flight nurse, and medical and respiratory technician, constitutes a mobile intensive care unit capable of providing full intensive care en route to a level IV or V facility aboard the Air Force's C-17 Globemaster (see Fig. 156-4). Although rapid evacuation is a priority, a patient who is recovering from a major vascular injury should not be rushed through the AIREVAC system, given the often complicated nature of the postoperative course. Specifically, a patient with a vascular reconstruction that is particularly tenuous or that has failed early in the postoperative period, requiring revision, is better served by remaining under the care of the original surgeon for a period of days rather than being placed in the MEDEVAC system. In these cases, more aggressive use of heparin may be indicated, and the surgeon is immediately available should operative intervention be required (e.g., early graft failure, postoperative bleeding). As of the end of 2007, critical care air transport teams had completed nearly 10,000 missions to evacuate the most critically injured U.S. troops out of Afghanistan and Iraq.

SELECTED KEY REFERENCES

Clouse WD, Rasmussen TE, Peck MA. In-theater management of vascular injury: 2 years of the Balad Vascular Registry. *J Am Coll Surg.* 2007;204:625-632.
Two-year report on the management of 347 consecutive wartime vascular injuries from the 332nd Expeditionary Medical Group, Air Force theater hospital, Balad Air Base, Iraq.

Fox CJ, Gillespie DL, Cox ED, Mehta SG, Kragh JF Jr, Salinas J, Holcomb JB. The effectiveness of a damage control resuscitation strategy for vascular injury in a combat support hospital: results of a case control study. *J Trauma.* 2008;64(2 Suppl):S99-S106.
Case-control study of the effectiveness of a novel, component-based damage-control resuscitation strategy used during the management of wartime vascular injuries.

Holcomb JB, McMullin NR, Pearse L, Caruso J, Wade CE, Oetjen-Gerdes L, Champion HR, Lawnick M, Farr W, Rodriguez S, Butler FK. Causes of death in US Special Operations Forces in the global war on terrorism 2001-2004. *Ann Surg.* 2007;245:986-991.
First autopsy-based study of cause of death on the modern battlefield. It found that 32% of potentially survivable deaths were due to compressible hemorrhage or hemorrhage amenable to tourniquet placement.

Kragh JF Jr, Walters TJ, Baer DG, Fox CJ, Wade CE, Salinas J, Holcomb JB. Practical use of emergency tourniquets to stop bleeding in major limb trauma. *J Trauma.* 2008;64(2 Suppl):S38-S49.
Modern report on 428 tourniquets applied to 309 injured extremities, demonstrating low-risk morbidity and a positive risk-benefit ratio on the modern battlefield.

Quan RW, Gillespie DL, Stuart BS, Chang AS, Wittaker DR, Fox CJ. The effect of vein repair on the risk of venous thromboembolic events: a review of more than 100 traumatic military venous injuries. *J Vasc Surg.* 2008;47:571-577.
First contemporary follow-up report on venous injury management, demonstrating good midterm patency of venous repairs and low rates of thromboembolic events.

Rasmussen TE, Clouse WD, Jenkins DH, Peck MA, Eliason JL, Smith DL. Echelons of care and the management of wartime vascular injury: a report from the 332nd EMDG/Air Force Theater Hospital Balad Air Base Iraq. *Perspect Vasc Surg Endovasc Ther.* 2006;18:91-99.
Contemporary review of vascular injury management strategies employed at the five levels of combat casualty care.

Rasmussen TE, Clouse WD, Jenkins DH, Peck MA, Eliason JL, Smith DL. The use of temporary vascular shunts as a damage control adjunct in the management of wartime vascular injury. *J Trauma.* 2006;61:8-12.
First significant wartime series demonstrating the utility of temporary vascular shunts as an adjunct in the management of extremity vascular injuries.

Rasmussen TE, Clouse WD, Peck MA, Bowser AN, Eliason JL, Cox MW, Woodward EB, Jones WT, Jenkins DH. Development and implementation of endovascular capabilities in wartime. *J Trauma.* 2008;64:1169-1176.
First report on the utility of endovascular capabilities and a trauma-specific endovascular inventory to manage acute wartime injuries at a level III field hospital.

Starnes BW, Beekley AC, Sebesta JA, Andersen CA, Rush RM Jr. Extremity vascular injuries on the battlefield: tips for surgeons deploying to war. *J Trauma.* 2006;60:432-442.
Early report from the invasion phase of Operation Iraqi Freedom detailing the practical aspects of vascular injury management in an austere environment.

REFERENCES

The reference list can be found on the companion Expert Consult Web site at *www.expertconsult.com.*

CHAPTER 157

Acute Ischemia: Evaluation and Decision Making

Jonothan J. Earnshaw

Acute ischemia of the limb represents one of the toughest challenges encountered by vascular specialists. The diagnosis and initial assessment are largely clinical, and diagnostic errors can result in a high price to the patient—amputation or even death. Amputation and death rates remain high despite intervention, which is in contrast to major advances in the treatment of many other vascular diseases. Acute ischemia is often an end-of-life condition that presents in a patient with multiple medical co-morbidities. Therefore, careful clinical assessment of the individual is as important as assessment of the limb. Unlike many other vascular conditions, there is no one definitive treatment; a variety of modalities are available, including anticoagulation, operative intervention, thrombolysis, and mechanical thrombectomy. Selection of the most appropriate intervention or combination of interventions can be critical to the eventual outcome.

■ ETIOLOGY AND PATHOLOGY

Acute ischemia is the result of a sudden deterioration in the arterial supply to the limb. Excluding trauma and iatrogenic causes, there are two main reasons for acute ischemia to occur: arterial embolism and thrombosis. The distinction between thrombosis and embolism is important in terms of diagnosis and prognosis, but it may not be crucial when deciding on the form of treatment.

Embolism

Embolism (from the Greek *embolos*, or "plug") is the result of material passing through the arterial tree and obstructing a peripheral artery. Usually the source of the embolus is the heart, and the material is mural thrombus that has accumulated and detached. The other main cause is atherosclerotic debris from a diseased proximal artery, often the thoracic aorta, in individuals with a heavy burden of atherosclerotic disease.

Once the embolus detaches, it passes easily through large arteries and lodges peripherally, usually at an arterial bifurcation, where vessels naturally narrow. Emboli can occlude any artery, but in the legs, the common femoral and popliteal arteries are commonly obstructed. Only large emboli, so-called saddle emboli, occlude the normal aortic bifurcation.

Embolic ischemia is usually catastrophic because it often occurs in otherwise normal arteries, without any established collaterals. Typically, the patient presents with an acute white

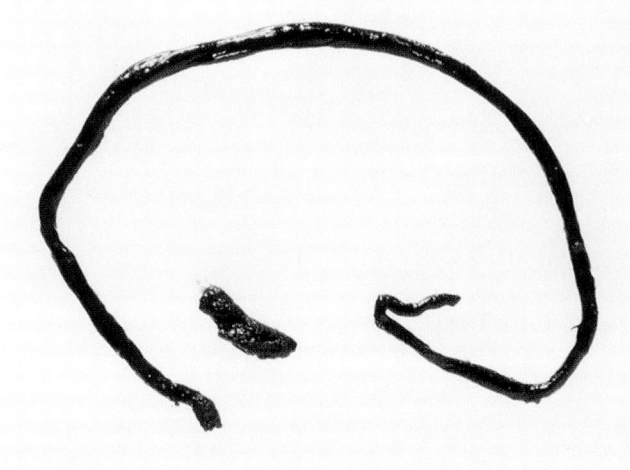

Figure 157-1 Embolus with secondary thrombus removed at embolectomy.

leg, including a complete neurosensory deficit. Embolic occlusion is also progressive; the ischemia worsens as secondary thrombus forms both proximal and distal to the occlusion. The secondary thrombus is the plum-colored clot removed at embolectomy (Fig. 157-1). It is particularly important that this secondary thrombus be removed because it may be responsible for obstruction in smaller distal vessels. If the presentation is delayed, the secondary thrombus adheres to the arterial wall, making it particularly resistant to removal with an embolectomy catheter and less easily lysed by thrombolytics.

Cardiac Embolism

Atrial and Ventricular. Embolism may occur in patients with otherwise normal arteries, with the embolic material usually arising from the heart. Embolic material from the heart usually consists of platelet-rich thrombus. Often it is organized, giving it the characteristic white surface on removal at embolectomy. The most common cause is atrial fibrillation; thrombus forms in the left atrial appendage as a result of stasis due to incoordinate contractions of the atrium and ventricle.

Mural thrombus, as a result of acute myocardial injury due to infarction, is a particularly dangerous cause of embolism; the patient has not only an ischemic extremity but also a high-

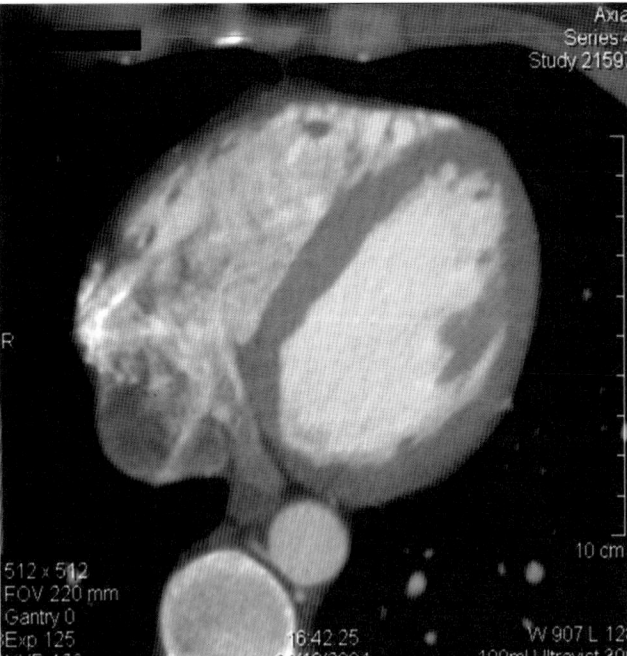

Figure 157-2 Computed tomogram of the heart showing mural thrombus that caused brachial embolus (same patient as in Fig. 157-9).

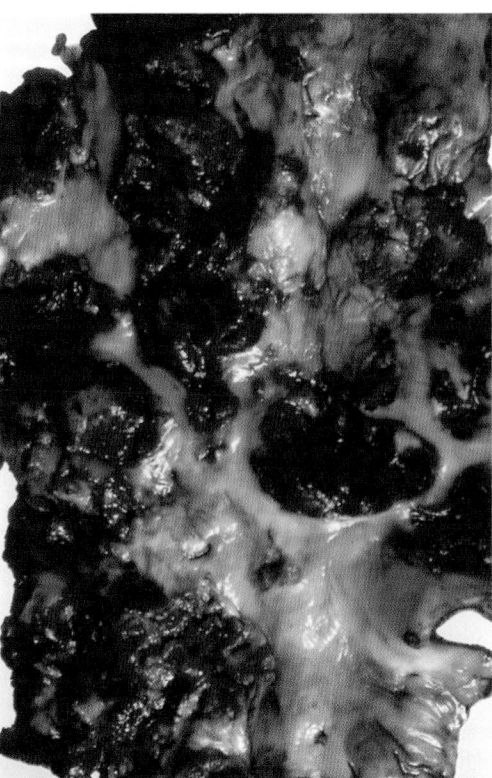

Figure 157-3 Ulcerated aortic atheroma at autopsy.

risk medical condition (Fig. 157-2). Left ventricular aneurysm is also a high-risk cause of embolism because these patients have a low cardiac output as a result of the previous infarcts that caused the aneurysm.

In the past, cardiac valve disease was the main cause of arterial embolism, but the active management of these patients and advances in cardiac surgery have virtually eliminated this as a cause.[1-3] Instead, many patients now have artificial heart valves, and those with metal valves are usually anticoagulated. Embolism is rare in patients with porcine replacement heart valves.

Paradoxical. Paradoxical embolism occurs when a clot from the venous system, usually a deep venous thrombosis, travels through a patent foramen ovale into the arterial system. The clinical clue is acute arterial ischemia in a patient with known deep venous thrombosis.[4]

Endocarditis. Bacterial endocarditis is an infrequent diagnosis since the introduction of widespread echocardiography and antibiotics. However, certain patient groups are at risk, including intravenous drug users, patients with indwelling arterial or venous lines, and those who are immunocompromised.

Cardiac Tumor. Atrial myxoma is a benign tumor of the left atrium that may fragment as it enlarges. Surgeons are advised that if there is anything atypical about the material removed at embolectomy, or if the patient is young with no obvious reason for embolic disease, the specimen should be sent for histology.[5]

Noncardiac Embolism

Atheroembolism. Along with foreign bodies and material introduced during vascular intervention (which is increasingly common), another source of embolism is the native arteries themselves. Particularly in patients with extensive atherosclerotic disease in major arteries such as the aortic arch or the descending thoracic aorta, fragments of plaque or adherent thrombus may detach and cause symptoms that mimic cardiac embolism (Fig. 157-3). The embolic material may be variable and may consist entirely of platelet-rich thrombus, similar to embolism. More sinister are fragments of atheromatous plaque, which may contain cholesterol elements, that detach (Fig. 157-4); these are more difficult to remove at embolectomy and may irreversibly occlude small distal vessels (see Chapter 160: Atheromatous Embolization).

Aortic Mural Thrombi. Occasionally, patients with hypercoagulable conditions develop an aortic mural thrombus in the absence of aortic pathology, which then embolizes to a limb. This should be suspected in a patient without atherosclerotic vascular disease and in whom the cardiac evaluation is negative. Although the acutely ischemic limb may need urgent treatment, the underlying aortic pathology can often be treated simply by anticoagulation, with resolution of the thrombus.[8]

Thrombosis

Thrombosis results from blood clotting within an artery, which can be caused by progressive atherosclerotic obstruction, hypercoagulability, or aortic or arterial dissection.

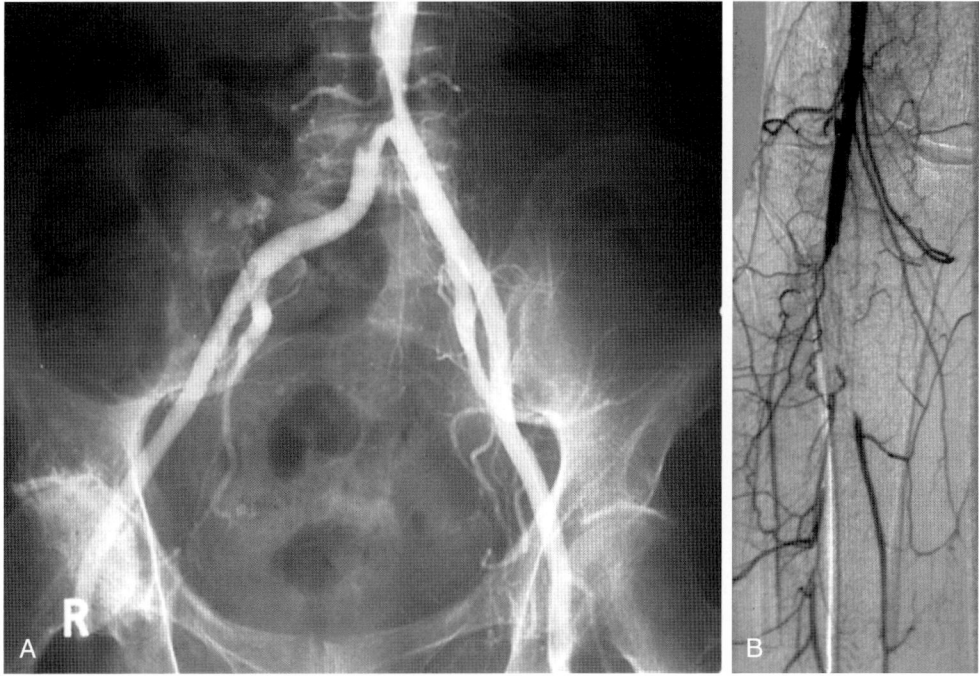

Figure 157-4 Angiogram showing aortic plaque (**A**) causing distal popliteal thromboembolism (**B**).

Atherosclerotic Obstruction

Thrombotic occlusion is most commonly the result of progressive atherosclerotic narrowing in peripheral arteries of the leg. Once a stenosis becomes critical, platelet thrombus develops on the stenotic lesion, leading to an acute arterial occlusion. The clinical manifestations are seldom as dramatic as those of embolization because the progressive process of atherosclerotic narrowing results in the development of robust collateral circulation. Patients with atherosclerosis deteriorate in a stepwise fashion as thrombosis supervenes on an arterial stenosis. The resulting symptoms of ischemia (usually the acute onset of claudication) improve as collateral vessels expand. Critical ischemia is the end result when this process occurs at multiple levels. Acute stroke or myocardial infarction is the result of atherosclerotic plaque disruption[6] (this plaque can be examined at carotid endarterectomy or autopsy). In the extremities, it is not known whether plaque disruption is a cause of acute-on-chronic arterial thrombosis, because the offending plaque is rarely available for examination. It is possible, however, that the process of plaque disruption is the etiology in certain cases.

In patients with extensive atherosclerotic peripheral vascular disease, a reduction in cardiac output may produce acute limb ischemia by a global reduction in limb arterial perfusion. For example, if a patient with severe claudication develops complicated diverticulitis, the onset of shock may cause low cardiac output and result in acute critical limb ischemia in the absence of thrombosis. It is important to recognize this phenomenon because it is the underlying disease, not the leg, that needs urgent treatment.

Hypercoagulable States

In situ vessel thrombosis can also occur in the absence of atherosclerotic disease in states of hypercoagulability, low arterial flow, or hyperviscosity. These hypercoagulable states are associated predominantly with venous thrombosis, but thrombocythemia in particular can cause arterial occlusion, usually in small vessels. Malignant disease is also linked mainly to venous thrombosis, but several authors have observed an association with acute arterial ischemia.[7] It may be worth screening patients with acute leg ischemia for an underlying malignancy. Because the vessel thrombosis is often a marker of advanced malignancy, the outcome in these patients is poor.

Vascular surgeons occasionally encounter heparin-induced thrombocytopenia, in which a patient on heparin develops progressive vessel thrombosis with a falling platelet count. Other hypercoagulable conditions that may cause arterial thrombosis and result in acute limb ischemia are discussed in Chapter 37 (Hypercoagulable States).

Aortic or Arterial Dissection

Another condition that requires a high index of suspicion for diagnosis is aortic dissection, which may involve the aortic bifurcation and give the appearance of iliac artery thrombosis.[9] These patients typically have back pain and may be hypotensive. Another clinical clue is renal failure if the dissection involves the renal arteries. Isolated arterial dissections of vessels supplying the lower extremity are uncommon but can occur from traumatic or fibrodysplastic causes.

Bypass Graft Occlusion

Another significant cause of acute limb ischemia is the occlusion of an existing patent bypass graft. Clearly, the rate depends on how many bypass grafts exist in a community.[10,11] In areas that are well endowed with vascular services, patients frequently present emergently with graft thrombosis. In the United Kingdom, a national survey in 1996 reported that graft or angioplasty occlusion was responsible for 15% of acute limb ischemia.[12] The diagnosis is usually easy, and the cause is more likely to be thrombosis than embolism. Assessment and treatment are similar to that for native vessel ischemia, but decisions about treatment can be much more difficult because of the variety of options available (see Chapter 109: Infrainguinal Disease: Surgical Treatment).

■ CLINICAL PRESENTATION

The symptoms caused by vascular occlusion depend on the size of the artery occluded and whether collaterals have developed beforehand. Sudden occlusion of a proximal artery without existing collaterals leads to an acute white leg, whereas occlusion of the superficial femoral artery in the presence of well-established collaterals may be entirely asymptomatic. This is borne out by the number of individuals who are found to have occult femoropopliteal occlusive disease on population screening. Acute ischemia affects sensory nerves first; therefore, loss of sensation is one of the earliest signs of acute leg ischemia. Motor nerves are affected next, causing muscle weakness; then skin and finally muscles are affected by the reduction in arterial perfusion. This is why muscle tenderness is one of the end-stage signs of acute leg ischemia. Once ischemia is established, the skin's initial pallor becomes dusky blue as capillary venodilatation occurs. At this stage, pressure over the discolored skin leaves it white because the vessels are still empty (Fig. 157-5). The terminal stage of skin ischemia is caused by extravasation of blood owing to capillary disruption; digital pressure over the discolored skin produces no blush. At this stage, the skin is nonviable, and revascularization of necrotic tissue risks compartment syndrome and renal failure without salvaging the extremity (Fig. 157-6).

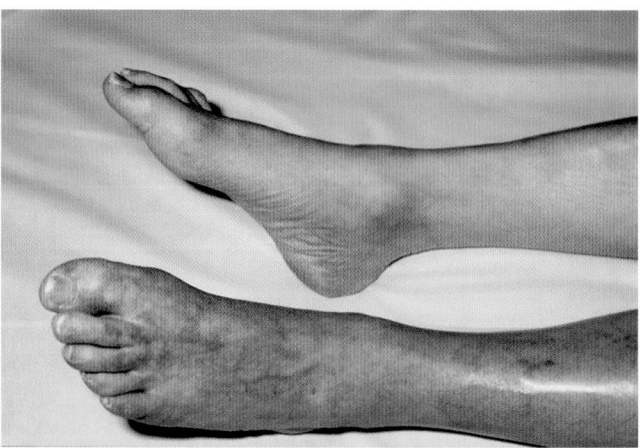

Figure 157-6 Acute ischemia class III—irreversible.

Historical series of patients with acute leg ischemia reveal a preponderance of embolic occlusion, usually secondary to valvular heart disease; however, this cause has essentially been eradicated owing to modern cardiovascular surgical expertise.[1-3] The usual cause of cardiac emboli is atrial fibrillation as a result of ischemic heart disease, possibly mediated by conduction abnormalities. This means that the affected population tends to be much older than it was 50 years ago, and patients often have established atherosclerotic disease of the arteries. This can produce the confusing picture of a patient with an embolus as well as peripheral vascular disease. Another effect is the gradual increase in the incidence of acute ischemia as the population ages.[13,14]

■ CLINICAL ASSESSMENT

The initial assessment of acute critical ischemia involves an evaluation of both the limb and the patient as a whole.

History

The severity of the initial symptoms depends on the severity of ischemia and can range from incapacitating pain to the sudden onset of mild claudication. Obviously, the more severe the ischemia, the faster the patient seeks medical attention. Severe acute ischemia is usually obvious, with extreme pain and loss of sensation and power in the limb. Less severe ischemia can be difficult to diagnose and may be confused with musculoskeletal pain, sciatica, and other causes of limb discomfort. The duration of symptoms is the most important part of the history; in patients with severe ischemia, irreversible muscle necrosis occurs within 6 to 8 hours if the condition is untreated. Patients with an acute white leg require urgent intervention. The symptoms of sensory loss and muscle pain are also evidence of critical ischemia.

The history should include an attempt to define the cause of the ischemia. Historically, patients with emboli had valvu-

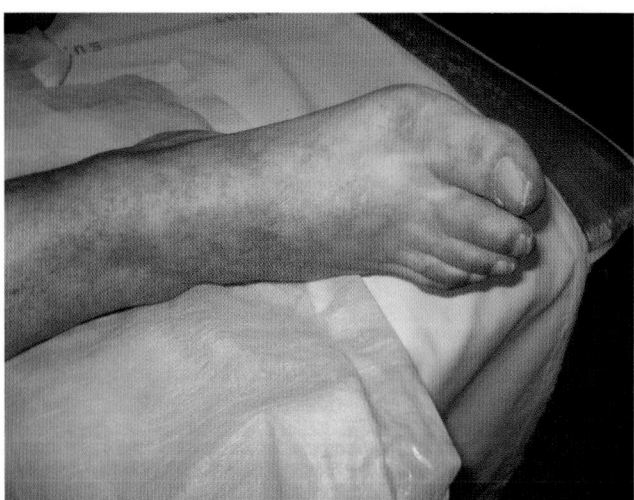

Figure 157-5 Acute ischemia class IIb—immediately threatened.

lar heart disease but no evidence of peripheral vascular disease or other atherosclerotic conditions; however, the presence of atherosclerosis no longer rules out embolism. Patients with acute-on-chronic thrombosis often give a history of prior intermittent claudication in the ipsilateral or contralateral leg. A full medical history is important because it may reveal other associated diseases such as diabetes mellitus. Risk factors for atherosclerotic disease should be sought, including smoking, hypertension, high cholesterol, and family history.

Physical Findings

Examination of the leg is used to define the severity of the ischemia and is therefore fundamental. The well-known rule of P's—pain, pallor, paresis, pulse deficit, paresthesia, and poikilothermy—remains a good guide to both symptoms and signs. The color of the skin reflects its vascular supply. Marble-white skin is associated with acute total ischemia. Slow capillary refill is a sign that at least a small degree of distal flow is present and runoff vessels are probably patent. Sensation may be lost completely and the foot may be numb, but more often there is loss of fine touch and proprioception, which should be tested specifically. Muscle tenderness, particularly in the calf, is a sign of advanced ischemia. Acute ischemia is associated with the loss of peripheral pulses, which also helps define the level of the occlusion. Palpable normal pulses in the contralateral leg points toward embolism as the cause.

A full vascular examination reveals the level of the occlusion by the loss of arterial pulsation. A strong pulse can, however, mask an occlusion at that level because of the water-hammer effect. Other possible sources of embolization may become apparent, such as aortic or popliteal aneurysm or cardiac abnormalities such as atrial fibrillation. Patients with acute leg ischemia are often elderly with multiple co-morbidities, and a full physical examination should be undertaken because the final outcome may depend as much on associated conditions as on the severity of the leg ischemia.

Hand-held Doppler examination is also a basic part of the examination. Pedal arterial signals may be absent or reduced. The presence of normal biphasic signals excludes the diagnosis. Soft monophasic signals are associated with patent distal vessels but proximal arterial occlusion. Absent Doppler signals in the ankle arteries is a poor prognostic sign. The arteries may be patent but with little flow, or they may be occluded with thrombus. In severe ischemia, ankle Doppler pressures are impossible to measure, partly due to the lack of signal but also due to muscle tenderness. In less severe ischemia, an ankle pressure of 30 to 50 mm Hg can be expected, and an ankle-brachial index of about 0.3 is diagnostic of subcritical acute ischemia. Doppler can also be used to examine the extremity veins. In particular, lack of a venous signal in the popliteal fossa suggests popliteal venous occlusion, which is a particularly poor prognostic sign in a patient with acute arterial ischemia.

CLASSIFICATION OF ACUTE LIMB ISCHEMIA

Acute limb ischemia used to be classified according to cause—thrombosis or embolism—because this had implications for treatment and prognosis. Patients with thrombosis tended to be younger but had a higher risk of major amputation. Patients with emboli tended to be older and had a higher risk of dying after treatment.[15,16] It has become clear that this is not a useful classification because there is no way of proving definitively whether an occlusion is thrombus or embolus. A more valuable method of classification is based on the severity of the arterial ischemia, which is helpful in determining the urgency of intervention and has implications for outcome.[17,18]

The Society for Vascular Surgery and the International Society for Cardiovascular Surgery have published definitions of acute leg ischemia that are valuable for treatment and prognosis (Table 157-1).[19,20] These standards were modified in 2007 by a larger group—the Trans-Atlantic Inter-Society Consensus—which defined acute ischemia as any sudden decrease in limb perfusion causing a potential threat to limb viability.[21] The categories of ischemia are based on clinical findings and Doppler measurements, which can be performed at the bedside and are immediately available. In patients with class I ischemia (viable) or acute-onset claudication, intervention, particularly with thrombolysis, may be risky, and there is an argument for conservative treatment consisting of exercise and best medical therapy. In class III or irreversible ischemia, there is no indication to improve the blood supply,

Section 19 Trauma and Acute Limb Ischemia

Table 157-1 Classification of Acute Limb Ischemia

| Category | Description/Prognosis | Findings | | Doppler Signals | |
		Sensory Loss	Muscle Weakness	Arterial	Venous
I. Viable	Not immediately threatened	None	None	Audible	Audible
II. Threatened					
a. Marginally	Salvageable if promptly treated	Minimal (toes) or none	None	Inaudible	Audible
b. Immediately	Salvageable with immediate revascularization	More than toes, associated with rest pain	Mild, moderate	Inaudible	Audible
III. Irreversible	Major tissue loss or permanent nerve damage inevitable	Profound, anesthetic	Profound, paralysis (rigor)	Inaudible	Inaudible

From Rutherford RB, Baker JD, Ernst C, et al. Recommended standards for reports dealing with lower extremity ischemia: revised version. *J Vasc Surg.* 1997;26:517-538.

which may risk rhabdomyolysis, so the decision is between major amputation and conservative treatment.

Patients with class II ischemia require intervention, and the distinction between IIa (marginally threatened) and IIb (immediately threatened) is crucial. Any delay in treating the latter risks irreversible muscle necrosis, whereas in patients with IIa ischemia, there is time for investigation and semi-elective intervention. Class II ischemia encompasses the majority of patients with acute leg ischemia, and it may be helpful to think of class IIa as acute subcritical ischemia and class IIb as acute critical ischemia.[18] The three findings that best differentiate IIa from IIb ischemia are pain at rest, sensory loss, and muscle weakness.[21]

DIAGNOSIS

Following clinical assessment and classification, the anatomic location of the arterial occlusion can be diagnosed with a high degree of reliability.

Aortic Occlusion

The diagnosis of an aortic occlusion is usually obvious. Paralysis of the legs is often the presenting feature; patients are unwell, with mottled skin discoloration that often extends above the inguinal ligament onto the lower abdomen and no palpable extremity pulses. This is a particularly high-risk condition, and urgent treatment is indicated.[22] The kidneys are especially at risk, particularly if the aortic occlusion is due to an aortic dissection. The dissection or occlusion may already involve the renal arteries, in which case the patient presents in established renal failure. Successful revascularization restores the blood supply to a large muscle mass, but the effects of ischemia-reperfusion may cause further renal damage.

Iliac Occlusion

The findings are similar to those for aortic occlusion, but unilateral. The femoral pulse is lost on the affected side, and mottling usually extends to the inguinal level. Aortic dissection should be excluded if there is time for investigation or if symptoms are suggestive.

Femoropopliteal Occlusion

Femoropopliteal occlusion is the most common situation in those with acute leg ischemia. The severity of the ischemia depends on whether the profunda femoris remains patent. The symptoms are more severe if the profunda is involved. Although the femoral pulse may be strongly palpable (owing to the water-hammer effect), the artery may be occluded.

Popliteal and Infrapopliteal Occlusion

In popliteal and infrapopliteal occlusion, the calf muscles are ischemic with a palpable femoral pulse. In young patients, rare

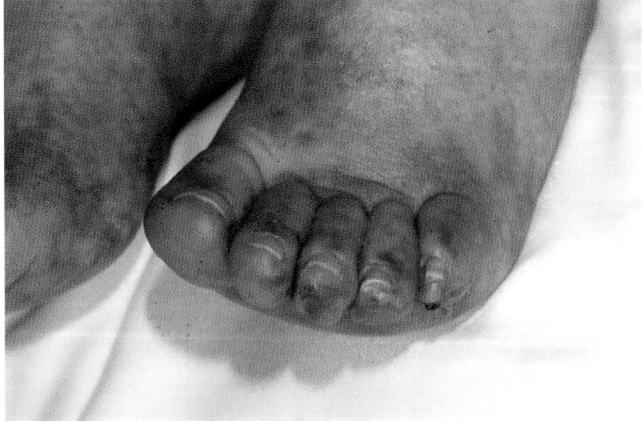

Figure 157-7 Distal ischemia due to occlusion of small vessels (acute blue toe syndrome).

diagnoses include popliteal thrombosis due to muscular entrapment or cystic adventitial disease. The most sinister cause is popliteal aneurysm thrombosis or embolization. This diagnosis should be suspected if a generous popliteal pulse is palpable in either leg or there is a nonpulsatile mass in the popliteal fossa of the affected leg. The outcome of this condition is particularly poor, despite aggressive treatment.[23] Chronic embolization of thrombus from within the aneurysm gradually occludes the distal vessels and arterial outflow; the aneurysm then thromboses, leaving no distal arterial targets for revascularization. Tibial embolism is an infrequent diagnosis, because most emboli that produce symptoms are large and obstruct proximal arteries (Fig. 157-7). Very distal emboli can be challenging to treat because the embolectomy catheter is least valuable in small distal vessels. Some authors recommend approaching tibial emboli from below via pedal arteries.[24]

INVESTIGATION

Investigation may be valuable in confirming the clinical diagnosis and planning the appropriate treatment for patients with acute ischemia. However, when the ischemia is critical, there may be no time for investigation if direct operative intervention is required. It is possible to employ on-table angiography to assist in decision making in the operating room. Time permitting, a number of methods can be used to definitively determine the site and nature of the arterial occlusion.

Transfemoral Arteriography

Arteriography has been the mainstay of investigation for acute leg ischemia, provided at least one femoral pulse is palpable. Brachial puncture can be used in the absence of femoral pulses, but patients with aortic occlusion often require hyper-acute treatment, leaving little time for investigation. The angiogram can document the level of occlusion and sometimes its nature. Thrombotic occlusion is likely if there are established collateral arteries and evidence of arterial atherosclerosis. Sometimes emboli can be seen in several vessels,

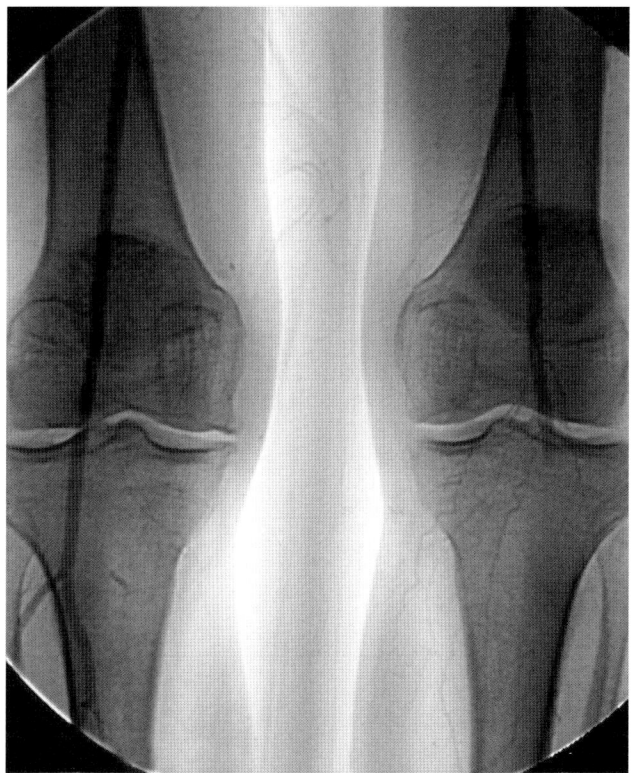

Figure 157-8 Angiogram showing popliteal embolus. Note the meniscal-type cutoff, with no existing collaterals.

establishing the diagnosis (Fig. 157-8). The best reason to perform angiography is when an endovascular solution to the arterial occlusion is likely, because thrombolysis, percutaneous thrombectomy, angioplasty, or stenting can be done at the same sitting. Arteriography may not visualize all the distal vessels in the acute situation because the lack of collaterals and associated spasm limit visualization. It may still be worth exploring distal vessels surgically when contemplating a distal bypass in this situation, although an alternative would be to consider intra-arterial thrombolytic therapy (see Chapter 158: Acute Ischemia: Treatment).

Ultrasound

Imaging with duplex ultrasonography is the mainstay of investigation for chronic arterial ischemia. It may not be available in all hospitals, but it can be employed in cases of acute ischemia to define the level of the arterial occlusion and the patency of other vessels. Many vascular specialists are becoming expert in duplex imaging, and portable ultrasound machines are getting smaller, so they may be available for bedside use by trained clinicians.

Computed Tomographic Angiography

New-generation computed tomography (CT) scanners acquire images at very high speed and are available in most emergency suites. Intravenous contrast injection with current CT technology provides images that are similar in quality to

intra-arterial arteriography. The images sometimes require manipulation to produce the best results, but this is an acquired skill of many young vascular specialists. These images are particularly good for aortoiliac occlusions. Because of its immediate and widespread availability, computed tomographic angiography is the investigation of choice for acute ischemia.

Magnetic Resonance Angiography

Magnetic resonance angiography with gadolinium enhancement is less useful than either CT or ultrasound in the context of acute limb ischemia. It is often unavailable at off hours, takes time for images to be acquired, and is generally inconvenient for sick patients.

Echocardiography

Debate continues about the role of echocardiography. In practical terms, the investigation seldom alters management because most patients are anticoagulated for life after successful treatment for acute ischemia. Some surgeons, however, regard the investigation as a vital part of management. There are certainly some conditions that require echocardiography to make a diagnosis, such as valvular disease (including vegetations), septal defect, and cardiac tumor. Problems associated with the routine application of echocardiography include the variability in results between transthoracic and transesophageal techniques and among different technicians, the inability to visualize the left atrial appendage, the fact that failure to visualize the source of an embolus does not rule out its existence, and the test's lack of influence on overall management.[25] A pragmatic view would be that echocardiography is indicated in young patients, those in whom a cardiac diagnosis is suspected, and those in whom the results might affect decisions about long-term anticoagulation.[26]

■ INITIAL MANAGEMENT

Once the diagnosis of acute ischemia has been established and its severity classified, a number of immediate interventions are possible. These are discussed briefly here and elaborated on in greater detail in Chapter 158 (Acute Ischemia: Treatment).

Anticoagulation

The threat to the limb escalates with secondary thrombosis of underperfused distal vessels, particularly in patients with emboli. Therefore, immediate anticoagulation with intravenous calcium heparin can stabilize the condition of the leg and prevent deterioration. Whereas low-molecular-weight heparin is a valuable therapy for many conditions, the potential for immediate reversal with protamine makes calcium heparin the drug of choice in this situation. An initial bolus of 5000 U is appropriate for most patients, followed by an intravenous infusion commencing at 1000 U/hr. If urgent operation is not undertaken, the infusion should be monitored using the activated partial thromboplastin time, aiming for a ratio of 2 to 3. It is vital not to assume that anticoagulation is being accomplished while heparin is being administered; there is a wide variation in response to the drug, and careful monitoring by protocol is needed.

Ancillary Supportive Measures

Other first-aid measures that are beneficial in patients with leg ischemia include the use of oxygen delivered by facemask. This has been shown to improve skin perfusion, even in the ischemic limb.[27] Patients with acute ischemia are often dehydrated, and an intravenous infusion of fluid is necessary, together with catheter monitoring of urine output. Many radiologic maneuvers involve the use of contrast agents that can damage the kidneys, and adequate renal perfusion is important. As part of the diagnostic workup, a full blood screen for blood urea nitrogen and a full blood count are indicated. In patients with recurrent thrombosis, a full thrombophilia screen should be performed at this stage, if indicated, because therapeutic anticoagulation renders these investigations inaccurate.[28,29] These tests are indicated in patients with a strong family history of arterial and venous thrombosis or those with recurrent disease.[30,31] Patients are often in severe pain, and adequate analgesia is important. Intramuscular opiates are contraindicated in a patient who may receive thrombolysis, and patient-controlled intravenous analgesia is a good alternative.

■ TREATMENT

Options

Once the initial assessment is complete, a decision should be made about the intervention required and its timing. The following options are available: anticoagulation alone, operative intervention, and endovascular intervention via mechanical thrombectomy or thrombolysis.

Anticoagulation

Heparin anticoagulation has no direct thrombolytic effect; it is employed to stabilize clot formation and prevent further secondary thrombosis. Use of anticoagulation alone as a treatment implies that the limb is likely to remain viable or that other therapeutic options are limited, perhaps by age or comorbidity. Before anticoagulants were available, treatment of acute leg ischemia was largely expectant, and historical series documented high morbidity and mortality rates, despite amputation. Heparin and then warfarin made an immediate impact after their introduction.[32,33] Anticoagulation for stable class I ischemia, followed several weeks later by intervention (usually endovascular) if collaterals do not become established, is safe and effective. Anticoagulation has been shown to improve results after embolectomy.[34] In class III irreversible ischemia, anticoagulation allows stabilization of the

patient while his or her medical condition is improved, pending major amputation at a later date. Otherwise, anticoagulation may be a component of treatment but does not constitute definitive treatment for acute leg ischemia.

Operative Intervention

After Fogarty and coworkers described the embolectomy catheter for the remote removal of clot via a groin incision in 1963, surgery became the main treatment for acute leg ischemia.[35] Before this, surgeons had used a variety of ingenious methods to remove clots, often with little success. The new embolectomy procedure could be performed with the patient under local anesthesia, through a relatively small incision, and in combination with anticoagulation; it marked an immediate improvement in outcome. Over the years, the pattern of disease has changed, and emboli now occur in patients with ischemic heart disease, often in association with peripheral vascular disease. Thus, the embolectomy procedure has become more complicated, and the results are inferior in patients who may have an acute thrombosis.[36,37] Increasingly, surgical bypass techniques are required in this situation and in the expanding category of acute arterial thrombosis as Western populations live longer. A modern vascular surgeon should be able to offer a full range of bypass procedures to patients with acute leg ischemia, which may include on-table diagnostic angiography and even therapeutic intraoperative thrombolysis. This development has implications for the delivery of treatment. Acute leg ischemia should no longer be managed by occasional operators because specialized vascular procedures are often required to achieve optimal outcomes.[38]

Endovascular Intervention

The last 20 years have witnessed an incredible change in the delivery of vascular services from open surgery toward less invasive endovascular interventions. Two nonsurgical options are available for the removal of obstructing thrombus: mechanical thrombectomy and thrombolysis.

Mechanical Thrombectomy. Mechanical thrombectomy uses homemade (aspiration embolectomy) or commercially available custom-built devices. The procedure is performed in the angiography suite, and in expert hands, it can yield good results in selected patients, particularly those with bypass graft occlusions. If unsuccessful, it can be followed promptly by surgical intervention or thrombolysis.

Thrombolysis. Percutaneous thrombolysis is now an established intervention for all forms of acute arterial occlusion. All current thrombolytic agents are plasminogen activators that accelerate plasmin production with the degradation of fibrin (see Chapter 35: Thrombolytic Agents). A potential advantage of thrombolysis is that unlike surgical embolectomy, which simply removes thrombus from the large arteries, thrombolysis lyses clot in both large and small arteries as

Box 157-1 Contraindications to Local Thrombolysis for Acute Limb Ischemia

ABSOLUTE
- Recent stroke or neurosurgery within 2 months
- Major surgery (including bypass grafts) within 2 weeks
- Patients at significant risk of bleeding or with a bleeding tendency (e.g., recent gastrointestinal bleed)

RELATIVE
- Any surgery within 1 month
- Uncontrolled hypertension
- Hepatic failure
- Bacterial endocarditis
- Pregnancy
- Limb ischemia including neurologic deficit
- Occluded retroperitoneal Dacron graft

well as arteriolar and capillary beds. Box 157-1 lists the contraindications to thrombolysis.

Selection

The choice of intervention depends on the available expertise and the severity of the leg ischemia.

Acute Critical Ischemia

Patients with acute critical (class IIb) ischemia need urgent intervention. In institutions where vascular and endovascular services are limited, the choice may be restricted to surgical intervention. Where expertise is limited, consideration should be given to transferring the patient to an institution with a full range of vascular and endovascular services; this clinical setting has been shown to improve outcomes.[38]

If endovascular treatment is offered for acute critical ischemia, there should be no delay. Percutaneous thrombectomy is a valuable option where expertise exists. Low-dose intra-arterial thrombolysis is contraindicated because it usually takes 12 to 24 hours to be effective. Accelerated thrombolysis may be an option in experienced units, using either high-dose bolus infusion techniques[39] or pulse spray thrombolysis.[40] However, with these few exceptions, most patients with acute class IIb critical limb ischemia are best treated in the operating room. This can usually be rapidly arranged, and a full range of interventions are available, from embolectomy through reconstruction to on-table angioplasty or thrombolysis.

Acute Subcritical Ischemia

The treatment of patients with stable (class IIa) acute ischemia should be individualized, given the greater number of options and the greater time available for deliberation. These decisions are often best made by multidisciplinary teams reflecting local expertise. Obvious emboli may be treated most appropriately by embolectomy. With this exception, the primary option for class IIa ischemia is intra-arterial thrombolysis with or without adjunctive mechanical thrombectomy. There has been much debate about the advantages and disadvantages of thrombolysis versus a surgical approach, and a number of large randomized trials have compared the two modalities.[41] Premier vascular units are familiar with both surgery and thrombolysis and can make treatment decisions on an individual basis.[42] For instance, many patients with acute leg ischemia are in poor general health and at high risk for complications following operative intervention, particularly if general anesthesia is required. If a good surgical option exists, it is probably best that this be undertaken in a fit patient. Thrombolysis is particularly indicated when the surgical options are poor and the runoff vessels in the leg appear occluded. A meta-analysis of the available trials suggested that thrombolysis was best for short-duration ischemia and bypass graft occlusions.[43]

In Gloucestershire a clinical pathway has been used for the past decade that requires urgent embolectomy or thrombectomy in a patient with the acute onset of ischemia (<24 hours), an obvious embolic source, class IIb ischemia, and normal pulses in the contralateral leg. All other patients with class IIb acute critical ischemia require consultation with a specialist vascular surgeon on admission. The remainder with subcritical (class IIa) ischemia are anticoagulated overnight and treated by a vascular specialist in the morning.[44]

PROGNOSIS

The medical state of a patient who presents with acute leg ischemia is a good prognostic index of survival.[45] In particular, patients with acute myocardial infarction or poor cardiac output have a high mortality rate.[46,47] Outcome can also be predicted from pretreatment POSSUM (Physiological and Operative Severity Score for the Enumeration of Mortality and Morbidity) physiology scores.[48] Despite active intervention, the outcome after treatment for acute limb ischemia is often poor. In some patients, limb ischemia is a manifestation of the end of life. Such agonal thrombosis may be recognized in the very elderly with multiple co-morbidities, particularly in hospitalized patients,[49] and is an indication for palliative care rather than active intervention.[50]

UPPER LIMB ISCHEMIA

There are a number of significant differences between acute ischemia of the arm and leg. Patients with acute arm ischemia tend to be, on average, about 4 years older than those with acute leg ischemia (mean age, 74); arm ischemia is seldom limb threatening, and treatment decisions are less urgent.[51,52] The main reason for treating arm ischemia is to prevent late complications such as arm claudication and pain.[53] Most arm ischemia is due to cardiac embolism (Fig. 157-9); atherosclerosis is rare in upper limb arteries.

Patients often present with a cold feeling and numbness rather than pain in the arm. The diagnosis is clinical and can be confirmed by duplex imaging. The arm often improves

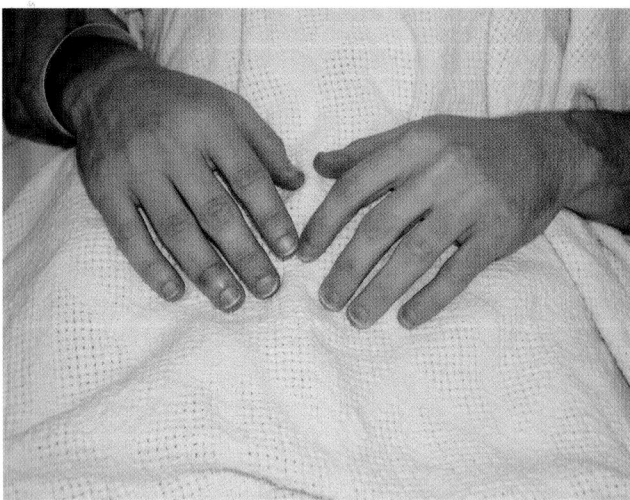

Figure 157-9 Acute arm ischemia due to brachial embolus of cardiac origin (same patient as in Fig. 157-2).

after initial anticoagulation, and decisions about whether to perform embolectomy can be difficult. Up to 50% of patients have late symptoms of arm pain if untreated; consequently, there should be a low threshold to undertake embolectomy under local anesthesia if there is doubt about limb viability.[53] A small number of patients present with class IIb critical ischemia and should undergo urgent surgical intervention.[52] Failed surgery in this situation risks ischemic contracture (Fig. 157-10) or even arm amputation on occasion. The threat to the arm is generally low, but up to 20% of patients with acute arm ischemia do not survive the acute event, usually owing to cardiac complications.[54] Like acute leg ischemia, there is a high attrition rate after successful treatment; only 60% of patients survived 3 to 5 years in one typical series.[54]

Rare causes of arm emboli include thoracic outlet syndrome and proximal subclavian artery aneurysm. The increasing use of arteriovenous fistulae for dialysis also causes a number of complications, including thrombosis and aneurysm formation.

SELECTED KEY REFERENCES

Blaisdell FW, Steele M, Allen RE. Management of acute lower extremity arterial ischaemia due to embolism and thrombosis. *Surgery.* 1978; 84:822-834.
These authors were the first to suggest that the severity of acute ischemia should influence its management.

Campbell WB, Ridler BM, Szymanska TH. Current management of acute leg ischaemia: results of an audit by the Vascular Surgical Society of Great Britain and Ireland. *Br J Surg.* 1998;85:1498-1503.
Large-scale audit of practice in the United Kingdom and Ireland.

Campbell WB, Ridler BM, Szymanska TH. Two year follow-up after acute thromboembolic limb ischaemia: the importance of anticoagulation. *Eur J Vasc Endovasc Surg.* 2000;19:169-173.
Follow-up to the national audit defined the importance of anticoagulation after treatment for acute limb ischemia.

Davies B, Braithwaite BD, Birch PA, Poskitt KR, Heather BP, Earnshaw JJ. Acute leg ischaemia in Gloucestershire. *Br J Surg.* 1997;84: 504-508.
Thorough investigation of acute ischemia over 1 year in a defined area.

Kuukasjarvi P, Salenius JP. Perioperative outcome of acute lower limb ischaemia on the basis of the national vascular registry. The Finnvasc Study Group. *Eur J Vasc Surg.* 1994;8:578-583.
Longitudinal analysis of outcomes.

Ljungman C, Holmberg L, Bergqvist D, Bergstrom R, Adami HO. Amputation risk and survival after embolectomy for acute arterial ischaemia. Time trends in a defined Swedish population. *Eur J Vasc Endovasc Surg.* 1996;11:176-182.
Careful longitudinal survey over 20 years.

Norgren L, Hiatt WR, Dormandy JA, Nehler MR, Harris KA, Fowkes FG, TASC II Working Group. Inter-Society Consensus for the Management of Peripheral Arterial Disease (TASC II). *J Vasc Surg.* 2007;45(suppl):S5-S67.
Comprehensive and detailed manual with definitions of and recommended treatments for all types of vascular disease, including acute ischemia.

Ouriel K, Veith FJ, Sasahara AA, for the Thrombolysis or Peripheral Arterial Surgery (TOPAS) Investigators. A comparison of recombinant urokinase with vascular surgery as initial treatment for acute arterial occlusion of the legs. *N Engl J Med.* 1998;338:1105-1111.
Large randomized trial that defined the role of thrombolysis.

Palfreyman SJ, Booth A, Michaels JA. A systematic review of intra-arterial thrombolytic therapy for acute leg ischaemia. *Eur J Vasc Endovasc Surg.* 2000;19:143-157.
Scientific overview of the role of thrombolysis.

Whitman B, Foy C, Earnshaw JJ, on behalf of the Thrombolysis Study Group. National Audit of Thrombolysis of Acute Leg Ischemia (NATALI): clinical factors associated with early outcome. *J Vasc Surg.* 2004;39:1018-1025.
Largest database concerning patients treated with intra-arterial thrombolysis.

REFERENCES

The reference list can be found on the companion Expert Consult Web site at *www.expertconsult.com*.

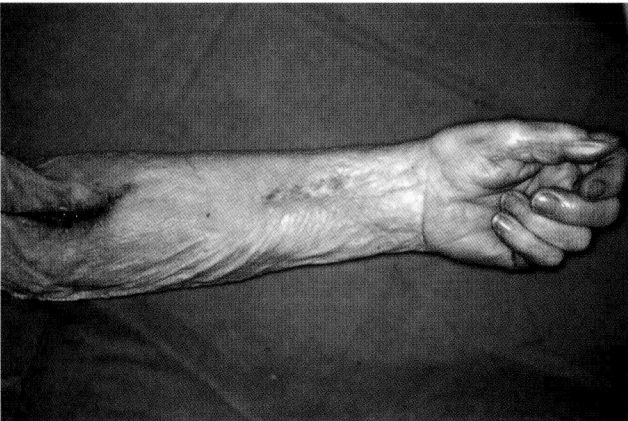

Figure 157-10 Failed embolectomy with wound dehiscence resulting in ischemic contracture.

CHAPTER 158

Acute Ischemia: Treatment

Karthikeshwar Kasirajan

Acute limb ischemia (ALI) threatens the viability of the extremity and the patient's survival because of systemic acid-base, electrolyte, and other abnormalities. Moreover, successful reperfusion may result in the release of highly toxic free radicals, further compromising these critically ill patients.

Chapter 157 (Acute Ischemia: Evaluation and Decision Making) covers in detail the evaluation of an acutely ischemic limb. This chapter focuses on the therapeutic approaches.

◼ TREATMENT SELECTION

Treatment for ALI depends largely on the degree of limb ischemia present clinically. Rutherford developed a classification of ALI that is helpful in determining the appropriate therapeutic intervention (Table 158-1).[1] The classification is as follows:

- *Class I:* Viable, nonthreatened extremity, no neurologic deficit, audible Doppler signal.
- *Class II:* Threatened extremity, manifested by neurologic deficit and sluggish or absent Doppler signals in the affected limb. Class II has been divided into IIa, which is characterized by mild sensory deficits, and IIb, which is associated with both motor and sensory deficits.
- *Class III:* Irreversible ischemic nerve and soft tissue injury.

Class I ALI may require only medical therapy, such as anticoagulation. Revascularization, if contemplated, can be performed electively and can consist of either thrombolytic or open surgical intervention. Treatment selection depends on the duration of ALI, the location and cause of the occlusion, the presence of underlying atherosclerotic occlusive disease, and the patient's overall medical condition.

Class II ALI requires a flexible approach to intervention. All patients with class II ALI require revascularization to preserve the functional integrity of the extremity. For patients with class IIa ischemia, immediate revascularization is not necessary. Consequently, either endovascular or surgical options can be considered. When planning therapy for a patient with class IIa ALI, the duration of symptoms is of prime importance. Percutaneous endovascular options are more effective in patients with ischemia of less than 2 weeks' duration, whereas ischemic symptoms of greater than 2 weeks' duration are better served by surgical revascularization.[2] For a duration of symptoms of less than 14 days, prospective studies comparing thrombolytic and surgical intervention favor the initial use of thrombolytic therapy, with surgical intervention reserved for those limbs that do not respond to lytic therapy. Because the ischemic insult in class IIa ALI is mild, whatever therapy is selected can be instituted on an urgent rather than emergent basis.

More severe ALI (class IIb), manifested by both sensory and motor deficits, requires urgent attention. Because time is a factor, surgical revascularization has been preferred; however, recent advances in catheter-based thrombolytic delivery and percutaneous mechanical thrombectomy devices have shortened the time to reperfusion. Consequently, these techniques are increasingly being used as first-line therapy in patients with class IIb ALI.

Class III ALI is manifested by a profound neurologic deficit (insensate, paretic limb), muscle rigidity, and the absence of Doppler signals in the affected vascular bed. Whether these findings are irreversible is a matter of clinical judgment, but when rigor is present, revascularization is futile and may in fact be harmful owing to the development of significant myoglobinuria.

Table 158-1 Clinical Categories of Acute Limb Iischemia

Category	Sensory Change	Motor Change	Doppler Signals	
			Arterial	Venous
Class I: Viable	None	None	Audible	Audible
Class II: Threatened	Rest pain	Moderate	Inaudible	Audible
Class III: Irreversible	Anesthesia	Paralysis	Inaudible	Inaudible

From Rutherford RB, Baker DJ, Ernst C, et al. Recommended standards for reports dealing with lower extremity ischemia: revised version. *J Vasc Surg.* 1997;26:517-538.

◼ ANTICOAGULATION ALONE

In 1978, Blaisdell and coworkers introduced the concept of early heparinization to prevent proximal and distal propagation of thrombus, in combination with delayed intervention.[3] Today, early heparinization is still one of the mainstays in the treatment of ALI. For unclear reasons, immediate full-dose heparinization can result in symptomatic improvement in some patients, either from the anticoagulation effects of heparin or from volume expansion Most importantly, immediate and adequate anticoagulation prevents proximal and distal thrombus propagation and preserves the microcirculation.

ENDOVASCULAR TREATMENT

The search for less invasive revascularization strategies is ongoing, seeking to lessen procedure-related morbidity without compromising the satisfactory rate of limb salvage that has been achieved with contemporary surgical procedures. Catheter-directed thrombolysis (CDT) and, more recently, percutaneous mechanical thrombectomy (PMT) have potential in this regard. Both techniques can clear the occluding thrombus from a peripheral artery in a minimally invasive fashion, restoring blood flow to the extremity and allowing the identification of any underlying lesion responsible for the occlusive event. The culprit lesion can then be addressed in a directed fashion with endovascular procedures such as angioplasty and stenting.

Catheter-Directed Thrombolysis

The introduction of CDT has challenged 3 decades of dominance by Fogarty catheter thrombectomy. Thrombolytic agents are widely used to dissolve the occluding arterial or venous thrombus, reconstitute blood flow, and improve the status of the tissue bed supplied by the involved vascular segment.

All thrombolytic agents in clinical use today are actually plasminogen activators. As such, they do not directly degrade fibrinogen. Rather, they are trypsin-like serine proteases with a highly specific activity directed at the cleavage of a single peptide bond in the plasminogen zymogen, converting it to plasmin. Plasmin is the active molecule that cleaves fibrin polymer to cause the dissolution of thrombus. Peripheral thrombolytic therapy is administered through a catheter-directed approach to achieve regional thrombus dissolution with minimal systemic fibrinolysis. However, a moderate systemic proteolytic state often results from the use of thrombolytic agents, limiting their use to patients with no contraindications (Box 158-1).[4-6]

The concurrent use of a therapeutic dose of heparin increases the risk of hemorrhagic complications. Nevertheless, a fixed dose of heparin in the range of 500 units/hr or less is routinely used to prevent pericatheter thrombosis; this may also increase the likelihood of successful thrombolysis. A complete discussion of the available pharmacologic lytic agents and their actions is provided in Chapter 35 (Thrombolytic Agents).

Technique

Most physicians prefer a contralateral approach when dealing with ALI. Ipsilateral femoral access carries a higher risk of hemorrhagic complications and increases the risk of wound infection if an open vascular procedure becomes necessary following thrombolysis. I routinely use a micropuncture needle to minimize the risk of femoral hematoma; some authors recommend routine ultrasound-guided femoral artery puncture.

Box 158-1 Contraindications to Pharmacologic Thrombolytic Agents

ABSOLUTE CONTRAINDICATIONS
- Active bleeding disorder
- Gastrointestinal bleeding within 10 days
- Cerebrovascular event within 6 months
- Intracranial or spinal surgery within 3 months
- Head injury within 3 months

RELATIVE CONTRAINDICATIONS
- Major surgery or trauma within 10 days
- Hypertension (systolic >180 mm Hg or diastolic >110 mm Hg)
- Cardiopulmonary resuscitation within 10 days
- Puncture of noncompresssible vessel
- Intracranial tumor
- Pregnancy
- Diabetic hemorrhagic retinopathy
- Recent eye surgery
- Hepatic failure
- Bacterial endocarditis

Once access is obtained, a short 6 Fr sheath is introduced. After the initial abdominal aortogram, the target vessel or location is imaged. It is important to perform a complete evaluation of the runoff vessels before attempting to cross the occlusion. This assists in the recognition of embolic events and also provides a target vessel for outflow in the event of failed thrombolytic therapy. I routinely use a vertebral catheter (Cook Inc., Bloomington, IN) with an angled glide wire and liberal roadmapping techniques to cross the occlusion. Multiple oblique angiographic views to visualize the proximal stump of a thrombosed bypass graft may be required for access.

Occasionally, if a graft cannot be crossed, ultrasound-guided direct puncture may be helpful. This is also used in patients with thrombosed axillofemoral grafts, with two separate counterpunctures and sheaths directed toward each other. Patients with prior aortobifemoral bypass grafts present a unique challenge in that it is often very difficult to get up and over these grafts. The thrombosed limb is usually best approached by an ultrasound-guided puncture of the ipsilateral proximal superficial femoral artery. Occasionally, I approach the thrombosed limb of an aortobifemoral graft by placing an up-and-over Simmons I catheter and then infusing the lytic agent via a Katzen wire placed through the Simmons catheter into the occlusion.

Once the occlusion has been crossed, a distal angiogram is performed to confirm the catheter's location in the true lumen distal to the occluded graft or native vessel. If using urokinase (ImaRx, ImaRx Therapeutics Inc., Tucson, AZ), an initial bolus dose of 240,000 units is given and then a drip at 60,000 units/hr. If using recombinant tissue plasminogen activator (rt-PA; Alteplase, Genentech, South San Francisco, CA), a 1-mg bolus and then a drip at 0.5 mg/hr are used. Heparin is administered through the proximal 6 Fr sheath at 500 units/

hr to prevent perisheath thrombosis. I do not routinely place contralateral sheaths during the infusion. The most common infusion catheter is the Unifuse (Arrow International, Inc., Reading, PA), with the choice of catheter length depending on the length of the occlusion. When patients return for recheck angiograms, I routinely perform the angiogram via the infusion catheter.

Results

Thrombolysis with agents such as urokinase, rt-PA, streptokinase (Streptase, Astra Pharmaceutical, Eatontown, NJ), and reteplase (Retevase, Centocor, Malvern, PA) has been investigated in uncontrolled trials as a therapeutic alternative to operation for acute peripheral arterial occlusion. In the 1990s, three multicenter randomized trials were published comparing thrombolysis with operation for arterial occlusion (Table 158-2).[7-9]

The first trial, the Rochester study, randomly assigned 114 patients with acute limb-threatening ischemia to thrombolysis with urokinase (57 patients) or to immediate operation (57 patients).[7] At 1 year, the amputation-free survival rates were 75% and 52%, respectively, a statistically significant difference. A closer analysis revealed this finding to be the result of a higher mortality rate in the operative group caused by perioperative cardiopulmonary complications. It appeared that taking patients with severe limb ischemia directly to operation without the opportunity for preparation resulted in a high frequency of complications that culminated in death.

The second large multicenter evaluation was the Surgery versus Thrombolysis for Ischemia of the Lower Extremity (STILE) trial.[8] In this study, 393 patients were randomly assigned to surgery or to thrombolysis with either rt-PA or urokinase. Clinical outcomes for the rt-PA and urokinase groups were similar, so the data were combined for an overall comparison of thrombolysis and surgery. Post hoc stratification of patients into two subgroups on the basis of duration of symptoms before enrollment (greater or less than 14 days) showed that among patients with symptoms of longer duration, the surgical group had lower amputation rates than the thrombolysis group at 6 months (3% versus 12%). In contrast, among patients with symptoms of shorter duration, patients assigned to thrombolysis had lower amputation rates than did surgical patients (11% versus 30%).

The third multicenter trial to evaluate thrombolytic therapy was the Thrombolysis or Peripheral Arterial Surgery (TOPAS) trial.[9] Recombinant urokinase (r-UK) (4000 IU/min for 4 hours, followed by 2000 IU/min) was compared to primary operation in 544 patients with lower extremity native artery or bypass graft occlusions of 14 days' duration or less. There was no significant difference in amputation-free survival rates or mortality rates at the time of discharge from the hospital. Likewise, the amputation-free survival rates 6 months after randomization were not significantly different: 71.8% in the r-UK group and 74.8% in the operative group. At the end of 6 months, 31.5% of the patients in the r-UK group had avoided amputation or death without the need for anything more than a percutaneous procedure. By contrast, the vast majority of the patients randomized to primary operation underwent open surgery (94.2%), a rate that was not unexpected owing to the design of the trial. The median length of hospitalization was 10 days in both treatment groups. Among the patients assigned to thrombolysis, those with occlusions in bypass grafts had better clinical outcomes, better rates of clot dissolution, and lower rates of major hemorrhagic complications than did those with native artery occlusions.

Complications

Hemorrhagic complications are the primary cause of morbidity following CDT. In the TOPAS trial, major hemorrhagic complications occurred in 32 patients (12.5%) in the r-UK group, compared with 14 patients (5.5%) in the surgery group.[9] Patient age, duration of infusion, and activated partial thromboplastin time at baseline were unrelated to the risk of bleeding. Intracranial hemorrhage occurred in four patients in the r-UK group (1.6%), one of whom died. There were no instances of intracranial hemorrhage in the surgery group. The risk of bleeding was significantly greater when therapeutic heparin was used. In 102 patients who received therapeutic heparin, bleeding occurred in 19 patients (19%). By contrast, in the 150 patients in whom therapeutic heparin was not used, bleeding occurred in only 13 patients (9%).

Although not widely reported, distal embolization during CDT is not uncommon. Symptoms may worsen, or patients may lose a distal Doppler signal during the initial phase of lytic infusion. This is often easily managed by a transient (2 to 3 hours) increase in the dose of thrombolytic agent. More significant distal embolization that does not resolve in a few hours requires immediate re-imaging, with the occasional need to reposition the catheter to a more distal location.

Table 158-2 Outcome of Patients Treated with Initial Thrombolytic Therapy or Primary Operation for Acute Limb Ischemia						
			Thrombolytic Therapy		**Primary Operation**	
Series	**Number of Patients**	**Period (months)**	**Amputation (%)**	**Death (%)**	**Amputation (%)**	**Death (%)**
Rochester[7]	114	12	18	16	18	42
STILE[8]	393	6	12	6.5	11	8.5
TOPAS-II[9]	544	12	15	20	13.1	17

STILE, Surgery versus Thrombolysis for Ischemia of the Lower Extremity; TOPAS, Thrombolysis or Peripheral Arterial Surgery.

Table 158-3 Mechanical Thrombectomy Devices for Acute Limb Ischemia

Catheter	Sheath Size (Fr)	Guide Wire	Working Length (cm)	Mechanism	Thrombus Extraction
Hydrodynamic Devices					
AngioJet Xpeedior	6	0.035	110	Venturi effect	Yes
Hydrolyser	6, 7	0.025	65, 100	Venturi effect	Yes
Oasis	6	0.018	65, 100	Venturi effect	Yes
Rotational Devices					
Amplatz	6, 8	0.018*	55, 90	Microfragmentation	No
Helix	7	0.018*	75, 120	Microfragmentation	No
Arrow-Trerotola	5	0.025	65	Microfragmentation	No
Castañeda brush	6	0.035	65	Microfragmentation	No
Cragg brush	6	Incompatible	65	Microfragmentation	No
Other Mechanical Adjuncts					
Trellis	8	0.035	80, 120	Fragmentation/mixing	Yes
EKOS	6	0.035	106, 135	Ultrasound/infusion	No
OmniWave	7	0.035	100	Ultrasound/cavitation	No

*Device cannot be activated with guide wire in place.

Percutaneous Mechanical Thrombectomy

PMT devices can be classified as hydrodynamic, rotational, and other mechanical adjuncts to CDT (Table 158-3).

Hydrodynamic Devices

Three percutaneously delivered devices can remove thrombus from the peripheral arteries using a stream of fluid and hydrodynamic forces to extract the thrombotic material from the lumen.[10-13] These devices are the AngioJet Xpeedior (Possis Medical, Minneapolis, MN), the Hydrolyser (Cordis, Warren, NJ), and the Oasis catheter (Boston Scientific, Natick, MA). They differ in their method of fluid delivery; the AngioJet uses a dedicated fluid delivery machine to achieve rapid flow rates, and the other two devices employ a standard angiographic injector. At present, the AngioJet is the only PMT device that has been approved by the Food and Drug Administration for use in the peripheral arterial circulation.

Of the mechanical thrombectomy devices available, the AngioJet has the greatest clinical history.[2,11,12] Its thrombectomy system consists of three major components: the catheter, the pump set, and the drive unit (Fig. 158-1). The Oasis and Hydrolyser systems use the same principle, but without a dedicated pump drive. The pump set and drive unit are responsible for producing a controlled, high-velocity saline jet (350 to 450 km/hr) that is redirected at the tip of a dual-lumen catheter back into the effluent lumen of the catheter. The inflow lumen is a low-profile stainless steel tube that forms a transverse loop at the distal end of the catheter and has multiple 25- to 50-μm-diameter orifices directed retrograde toward the inflow lumen. Saline solution from the pump drive unit is driven at 50 to 60 mL/min at 8000 to 10,000 pounds per square inch, resulting in a high-velocity jet at the catheter tip. The velocity of the saline jets produces

an area of extremely low pressure (Venturi effect) that is exposed to the intra-arterial lumen only at the catheter tip. Thrombus surrounding the catheter tip is fragmented (99.8% is <100 μm)[14] and rapidly evacuated through the effluent lumen in an isovolumic manner (fluid instilled equals fluid and blood removed). Because thrombus removal is achieved not by the actual mechanical force of the saline but by an indirectly created negative pressure zone (–760 mm Hg), luminal endothelial damage is kept to a minimum.

Rotational Devices

A variety of "brushes," rotating wires, and mechanical thrombectomy devices that simply fragment thrombus without actually aspirating the fragments have been designed to establish arterial recanalization. This class of devices includes the Amplatz thrombectomy device (Clot Buster; Microvena Corporation, White Bear Lake, MN), Arrow-Trerotola PTD (Arrow International Inc., Reading, PA), and Castañeda and Cragg brushes (Micro Therapeutics Inc., Aliso Viego, CA).[15-17] Although these devices have gained a foothold in the treatment of dialysis access graft occlusion, clinicians have been reluctant to use them in the periphery for fear of injuring the vessel wall. Another potential limitation of this class of device involves the risk of distal embolization of macroparticles of thrombus.

Amplatz. The Amplatz device is designed to create a vortex that draws the thrombus to an area surrounding the catheter tip, where it is macerated into microfragments. The catheter tip design and the impeller are shown in Figure 158-2. The impeller is housed within a 1-cm-long metal cage located at the distal tip of the catheter. The metal cage at the tip protects the vessel from direct contact with the rotating impeller blades. Thrombus that is sucked into the catheter tip exits via

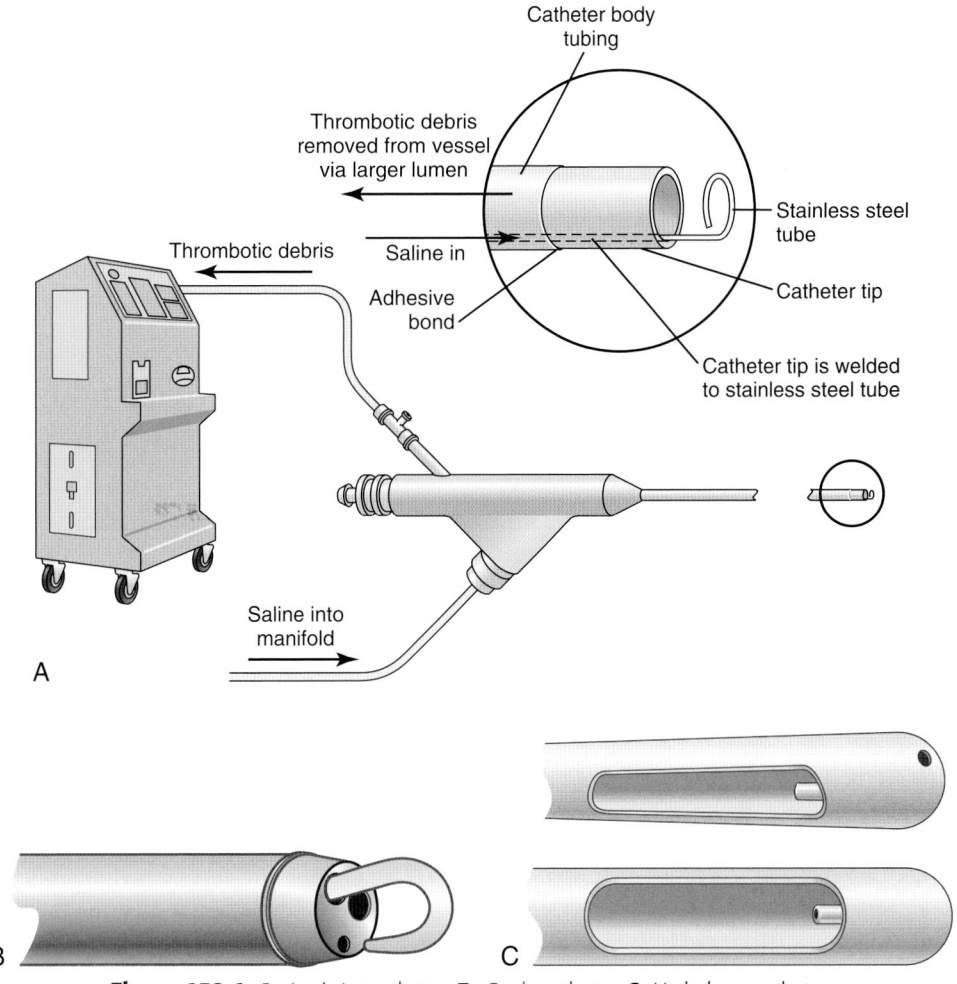

Figure 158-1 A, AngioJet catheter. **B,** Oasis catheter. **C,** Hydrolyser catheter.

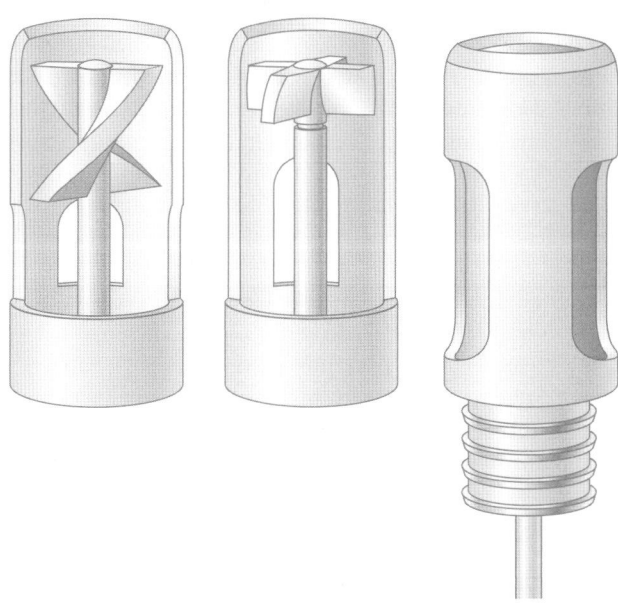

Figure 158-2 Amplatz thrombectomy device.

the three side holes. Thrombus exiting the side ports is subject to recirculation and refragmentation. The impeller is attached to a flexible coil driveshaft within the catheter that spins at 100,000 revolutions per minute (rpm) when activated.[17] Compressed air or nitrogen is used to power the driveshaft, controlled by a foot pedal. The presence of a proximal side port in the catheter allows the infusion of a cooling solution to the impeller; it can also be used to infuse a variety of other solutions, such as thrombolytic agents or contrast material. The device is available in 6 or 8 Fr version in lengths of 55 or 90 cm. Although the device can be passed over a 0.018-inch wire, it cannot be activated with the guide wire in place. A guiding catheter can be used to direct the tip of the catheter, helping to overcome its poor steerability, and to aspirate thrombus. Preclinical evaluation of the new Helix impeller design demonstrated a 24% increase in thrombus resolution; it is available as a 7 Fr catheter in lengths of 75 and 120 cm.

Arrow-Trerotola. The catheter tip of the Arrow-Trerotola nonaspirating device consists of a 9-mm-diameter self-expanding nitinol basket attached to a wire driveshaft (Fig. 158-3). The wire driveshaft is attached to a hand-held disposable rotator drive unit that spins at 3000 rpm. Thrombus is

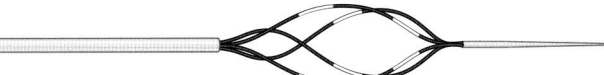

Figure 158-3 Arrow-Trerotola thrombectomy device.

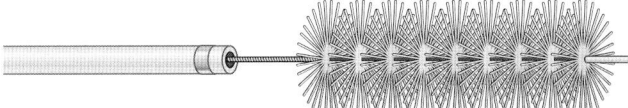

Figure 158-4 Castañeda/Cragg thrombectomy brush.

rapidly fragmented and stripped off the graft wall by the spinning motion of the basket, which maintains wall contact. The thrombus fragments are usually less than 1 mm but can occasionally be as large as 3 mm.[16] The device is available as a 5 Fr catheter with a 65-cm usable length. It is recommended only for graft thrombectomy. A newer over-the-wire (maximal wire size 0.025 inch) design is available. Although the device itself is nonaspirating, thrombus can be aspirated through the outer sheath as long as flow has not been restored.

Castañeda and Cragg Brushes. Both of these devices were developed as adjuncts to pharmacologic thrombolytic therapy, to decrease the dose and duration of thrombolytic agents. A rapidly rotating brush is located at the tip of the catheter (Fig. 158-4). The brush fragments the thrombus while dispersing the thrombolytic agent. The Castañeda brush is 6 mm in diameter, 10 mm long, and made of many short strands of polyamide material. It is available as a 6 Fr coaxial system and can be passed over a 0.035-inch guide wire. The working length of the catheter is 65 cm, and it is attached to a hand-held motor unit that spins the brush at 3000 rpm. The Cragg brush is made of soft nylon material (the bristles are 0.003 inch in diameter) and is similar to the Castañeda brush except that it is not an over-the-wire system.

Other Mechanical Adjuncts

These devices are intended to be used in conjunction with lytic agents. Mechanical mixing (Trellis) or ultrasound (EKOS, OmniSonics) energy is used to accelerate the speed to lysis. The resultant decrease in the dose and duration of lytic agents has the potential to minimize the bleeding risk associated with standard CDT and speed the time to reperfusion. These are relatively new devices with few published clinical data.

Trellis Catheter. The Trellis drug dispersion and thrombectomy catheter (Bacchus, Santa Clara, CA) is an 8 Fr coaxial system that can be passed over a 0.035-inch guide wire. The proximal portion of the device, which remains outside the patient, has five separate entry ports (Fig. 158-5). Two of these ports are used to inflate the compliant balloons located at each end of the infusion and dispersion segment. The balloons can be inflated to a maximal diameter of 14 mm. When inflated, the balloons are designed to isolate the treatment

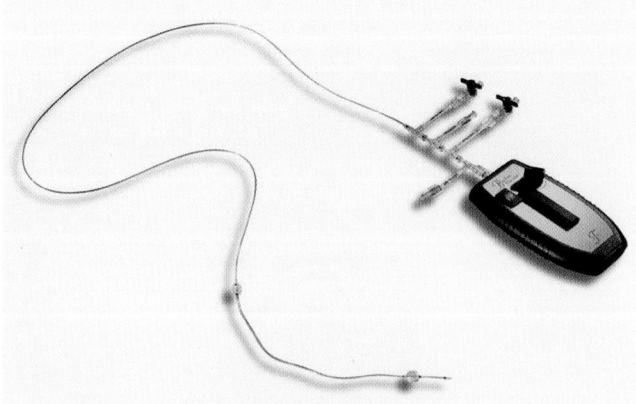

Figure 158-5 Trellis device.

zone and maintain the thrombolytic agent locally at the infused concentration. The balloons also help prevent downstream or upstream release of embolic debris. After balloon isolation of the treatment zone, the thrombolytic agent is infused through a separate proximal infusion port. A fourth, separate guide wire flush port facilitates the performance of distal runoffs while the device is in place or can be used for the distal infusion of thrombolytic agents. The proximal-end hole accommodates the guide wire or the dispersion wire through the central lumen.

Once the device is in place, the distal balloon is first inflated with a 3 : 1 concentration of angiographic dye. The thrombolytic agent is then introduced through the infusion port, followed by inflation of the proximal balloon with the contrast agent. The guide wire is then exchanged for the dispersion wire within the central lumen of the catheter. The dispersion wire is a sheathed, shape-set nitinol cable. Once it is placed, the sinusoidal shape-set region of the dispersion wire resides between the two balloons, within the isolated treatment zone. The proximal end of the dispersion wire is connected to a hand-held oscillation drive unit, which has three knobs: the on-off switch, the rate-control knob, and the translation bar. The device is first placed in the "on" mode. Then the oscillation of the dispersion wire is gradually increased to achieve optimal wire movement in the selected conduit, which is fluoroscopically confirmed. The translation bar is used to move the wire back and forth every 2 minutes to optimize mechanical dispersion of the thrombolytic agent simultaneous with mechanical thrombus fragmentation. After 10 minutes the proximal balloon is deflated, an 8 Fr sheath is passed to the level of the distal balloon, and the liquefied thrombus is aspirated as the sheath is gradually withdrawn to the proximal site of the treatment zone. At this point the distal balloon is deflated, and a completion angiogram may be performed through the 8 Fr sheath (Fig. 158-6). Although this device was initially developed for both ALI and deep venous thrombosis, the recent focus has been the treatment of acute deep venous thrombosis.[18-20]

EKOS Endowave System. The EKOS device (EKOS Corporation, Bothell, WA) uses the principle of ultrasound

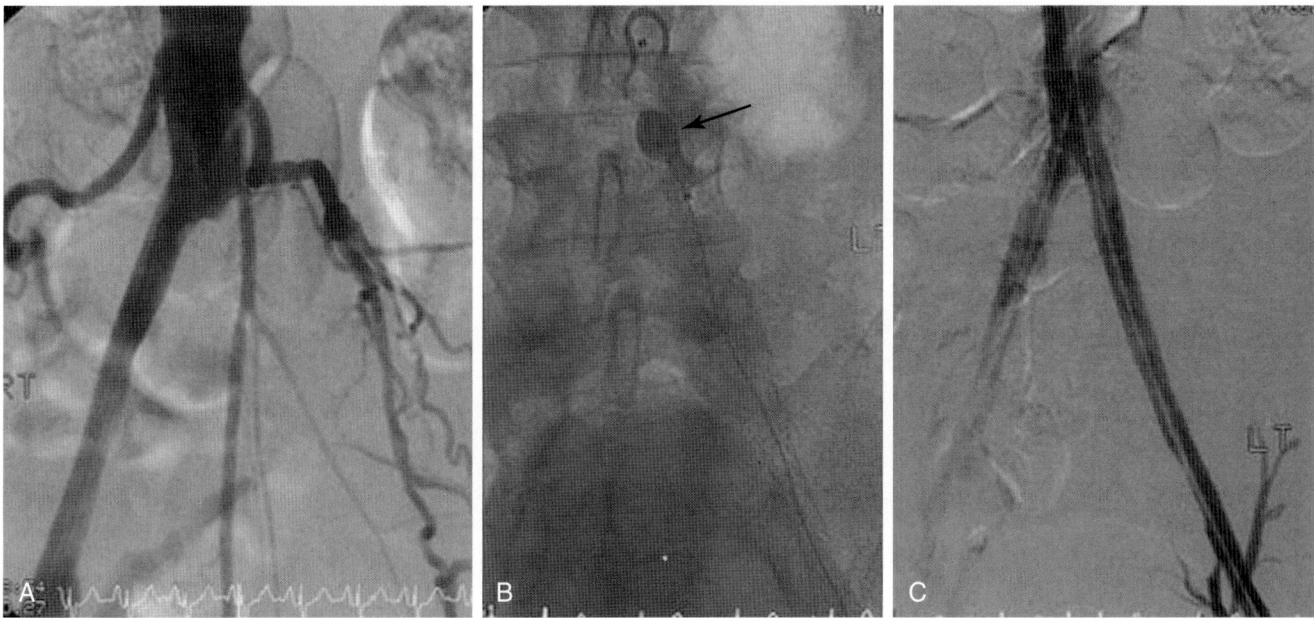

Figure 158-6 A, Acute left iliac occlusion. **B,** Trellis balloon (*arrow*) seen inflated at the site of the proximal extent of the thrombus. **C,** Complete thrombus resolution with 15 minutes of Trellis thrombectomy.

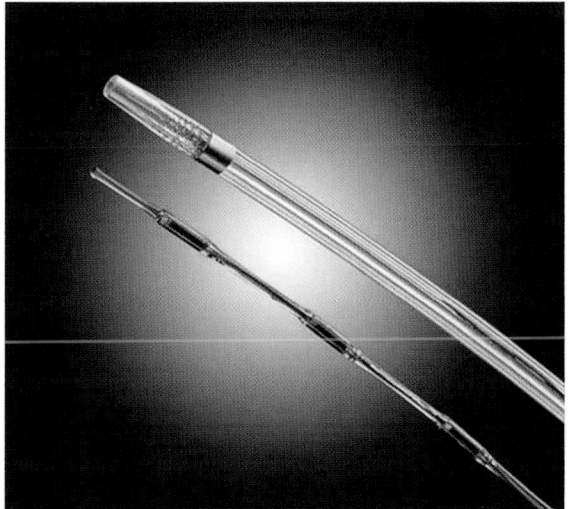

Figure 158-7 EKOS infusion catheter and the ultrasound core wire.

to facilitate clot penetration by the lytic agent, thereby accelerating thrombolysis. The device consists of a 5.2 Fr multilumen drug delivery catheter and a coaxial ultrasound core wire. The active treatment zone of the catheter is available in lengths from 6 to 50 cm; catheter selection is based on the length of the occlusion (Fig. 158-7).

Once the thrombus has been crossed with a standard 0.035-inch guide wire, the drug delivery catheter is placed over the guide wire. The guide wire is then exchanged for the ultrasound core wire, which contains a series of transducer elements (2.2 MHz, 0.45 W) spaced about 1 cm apart. In addition to the guide wire (ultrasound core) lumen, the back end of the catheter has two other ports—one for infusion of

the lytic agent, and the other for infusion of normal saline as a coolant. The ultrasound energy is delivered via the core wire simultaneous with the infusion of lytic agent and coolant. The endowave system control unit monitors the temperature and alters the ultrasound power to prevent overheating. Theoretically, maximal ultrasound power is reached with complete thrombus dissolution, as the free flow of blood and coolant prevents the thermocouples from overheating. The control unit displays a continuous graph of the power generated, which may help determine when the patient needs to have a recheck angiogram (Fig. 158-8).

In preclinical studies, thrombus exposed to ultrasound absorbed 48% more t-PA in 1 hour, 84% more in 2 hours, and 89% more in 4 hours than thrombus not exposed to ultrasound.[21] This phenomenon is thought to be secondary to thrombus deformation by the ultrasound waves, thereby exposing a greater surface area to the infused lytic agent.

Microbubble Technology. The OmniWave endovascular system (OmniSonics Medical Technologies Inc., Wilmington, MA) is a catheter-based device that uses transverse ultrasound technology to remove thrombus and enhance the dispersion of lytic agents in patients with ALI. The mechanical vibration of the wave guide produces microbubbles that cause cavitation, resulting in thrombus breakdown (Figs. 158-9 and 158-10). Additionally, the constant motion of the wave guide causes microstreaming that brings fresh thrombus in contact with the active element. The working length of the catheter is 100 cm, and the active treatment zone is 10 cm. Its 7 Fr sheath is compatible with the ability to treat vessels from 5 to 12 mm. Early clinical experience appears promising, although no published clinical data are available.

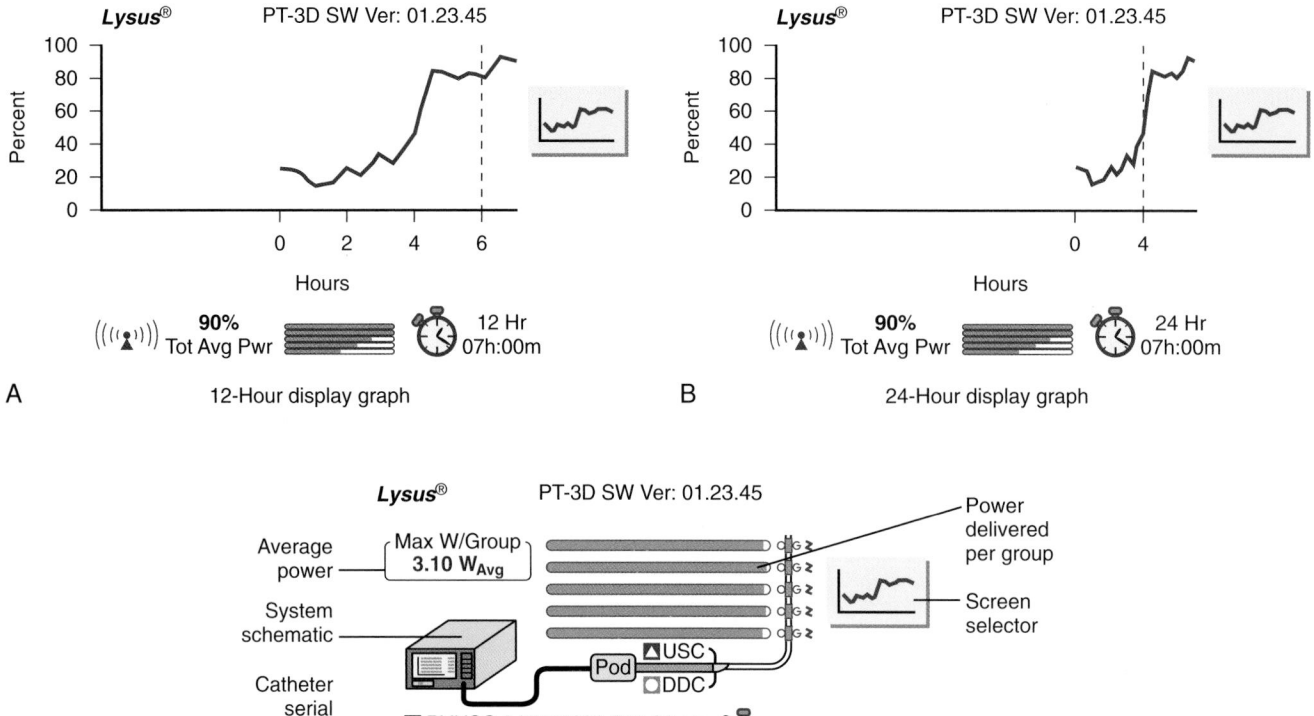

Figure 158-8 A–C, EKOS device demonstrates the power log that indirectly defines the extent of thrombus resolution.

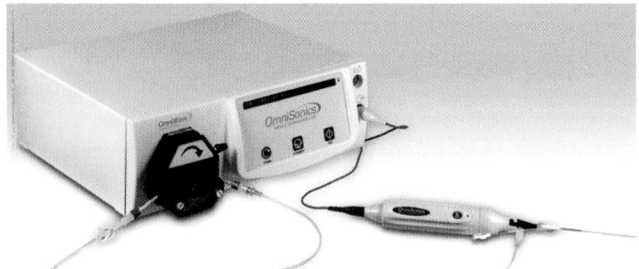

Figure 158-9 OmniWave endovascular system.

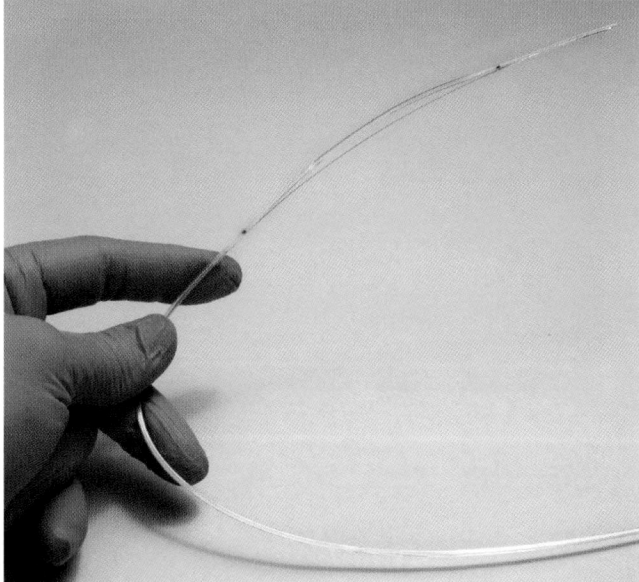

Figure 158-10 Endowave catheter with the active working element.

Results

The ability of percutaneous devices to rapidly restore arterial perfusion is an attractive addition to pharmacologic thrombolysis alone. In patients with significant ischemia that precludes the obligatory delay associated with pharmacologic thrombolysis, percutaneous thrombectomy devices may rapidly clear a channel through the occluded segment. Partial reperfusion of the extremity may provide enough improvement to allow complete removal of thrombus with thrombolytic infusions thereafter. Initial thrombus debulking may also significantly reduce the dose and duration of thrombolytic agents, thereby decreasing the risk of hemorrhagic complications associated with pharmacologic thrombolysis.[2,10,11,13] Finally, the devices may be employed as sole therapy in patients with contraindications to thrombolytic administration, such as those who have recently undergone major surgical procedures.

It appears unlikely that mechanical thrombectomy devices will completely eliminate the need for pharmacologic thrombolysis or open surgery.[10,11,15,17,22] In all but one clinical report,[12] a significant number of patients required adjunctive thrombolytic therapy for complete thrombus removal. The advantage of mechanical devices, however, lies in the ability to rapidly debulk the thrombus (Fig. 158-11), significantly

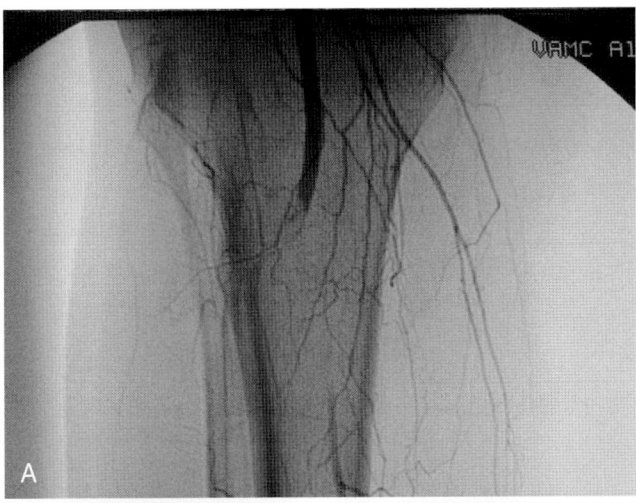

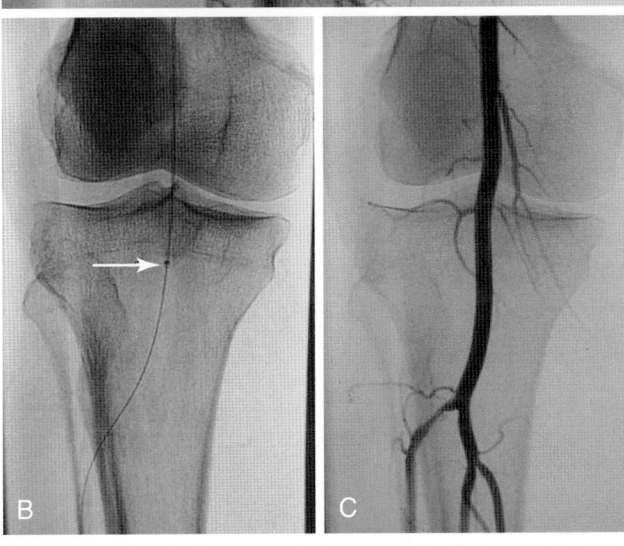

Figure 158-11 A, Acute popliteal artery embolization. **B,** AngioJet catheter (*arrow*) used to aspirate the embolic debris. **C,** Complete thrombus resolution following AngioJet thrombectomy.

reducing the duration of ischemia and increasing the exposure of the residual thrombus and distal vessels to pharmacologic thrombolytic agents. The reduced dose and time needed to achieve complete thrombolysis may result in considerable cost savings and fewer bleeding complications.[9]

In patients with contraindications to pharmacologic thrombolysis and at high risk for open surgery, mechanical thrombectomy may represent the best therapeutic option. Braithwaite and coworkers managed 15 patients with ALI due to infirmity or surgical or thrombolytic contraindications with anticoagulation alone, resulting in dismal 30-day limb salvage and mortality rates of 33% and 60%, respectively.[22]

My colleagues and I compared patients with ALI treated with the AngioJet catheter and historic controls treated with standard open surgical techniques.[23] The 65 patients in the AngioJet group received stand-alone treatment (n = 21) or subsequent adjunctive pharmacologic thrombolysis (n = 44). They were compared with 79 patients who underwent open surgical revascularization. No difference was noted in the 1-month amputation rate (11% versus 14%; $P = .57$); however, a reduction in the rate of early mortality was observed in the AngioJet group (7.7% versus 22%; $P = .037$). A lower event rate for local ($P = .002$) and systemic ($P < .001$) complications was observed for the AngioJet treatment group.

The EKOS endowave system has also been studied. In a series of 25 patients presenting with ALI, total clot removal was achieved in 22 (88%) after 16.9 hours (range, 5 to 24) using a mean dosage of 17 mg (range, 5 to 25) rt-PA. In 8 cases, total clot removal of the main lesion was achieved after 6 hours with 6 mg of rt-PA.[4] A prospective randomized study is currently under way comparing the EKOS system to standard CDT to evaluate the time to complete lysis (Fig. 158-12). Other clinical trials using a variety of PMT and adjunctive devices for ALI are shown in Table 158-4.[10,11,16,17,25-30]

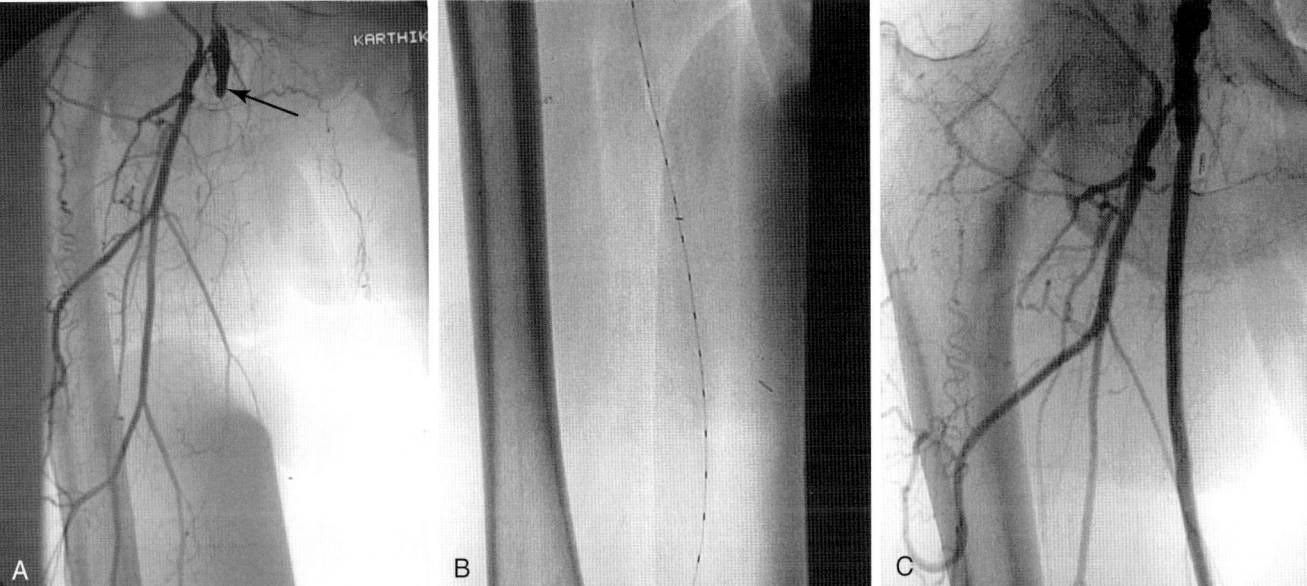

Figure 158-12 A, Patient with a right femoropopliteal artery graft occlusion (*arrow*). **B,** EKOS ultrasound catheter placed in the femoropopliteal graft. **C,** After 8 hours of lytic infusion, complete thrombus resolution is noted.

Table 158-4 Review of Mechanical Thrombectomy Devices Used for Peripheral Arterial Occlusion

Series	Year	Device	Number of Patients	Conduit	Duration	Results			
						Device Success	Adjunctive Procedure	Primary Patency	Complications
Höpfner et al.[25]	1999	Oasis	51	Native 44 (86%) Graft 7 (14%)	All acute	6 (11.8%)	PTA 20, SA 3, PAT 15, lysis 5	64% at 1 mo 54% at 6 mo	Hemorrhage 8% Emboli 4.8% Acute occlusion 37% Amputation 17.7% Mortality 8%
Müller-Hülsbeck et al.[26]	2000	AngioJet	115	Native 99 (86%) Graft 16 (14%)	All acute	71%	PTA 68, lysis 20, PAT 11	68% at 6 mo 60% at 2 yr 58% at 3 yr	Embolization 9.8% Dissection 8% Perforation 3.6% Amputation 1.8% Mortality 7%
Kasirajan and Ouriel[27]	2000	AngioJet	83	Native 52 (63%) Graft 31 (37%)	Acute 62 Chronic 21	Complete 51 (61%) Partial 19 (23%)	Lysis 50, PTA 47	90% at 3 mo 78% at 6 mo	Hemorrhage 10.5% Emboli 2.3% Dissection 3.5% Perforation 2.3% Amputation 11.6% Mortality 9.3%
Silva et al.[11]	1998	AngioJet	22	Native 13 (59%) Graft 9 (41%)	All acute	21 (95%)	PTA 21	NA	Hemorrhage 10% Embolism 9% Dissection 5% Occlusion 18% Amputation 5% Mortality 14%
Wagner et al.[10]	1997	AngioJet	50	Native 39 (78%) Graft 11 (22%)	All acute	26 (52%)	Lysis 15, PTA 34, PAT 9	69% at 1 yr	Hemorrhage 6% Emboli 6% Dissection 6% Perforation 4% Amputation 8% Mortality 0
Reekers et al.[28]	1996	Hydrolyser	28	Native 11 (39%) Graft 17 (61%)	Acute 23 Chronic 5	23 (82%)	Lysis 11, PTA 20, PAT 2	50% at 1 mo	Embolization 18% Hemorrhage 0 Acute occlusion 10.7% Amputation 11% Mortality 0
Henry et al.[29]	1998	Hydrolyser	41	Native 28 (68%) Graft 8 (20%) Other 5 (12%)	All acute	34 (83%)	Lysis 10, PTA 29, PAT 17	73% at 1 mo	Acute occlusion 12% Emboli 2.4% Amputation 0 Mortality 0
Rilinger et al.[16]	1997	Amplatz	40	All native	All acute	30 (75%)	Lysis, PTA, or SA 9	NA	Hemorrhage 2.5% Device failure 7.5% Emboli 0 Amputation 5% Mortality 0
Tadavarthy et al.[17]	1994	Amplatz	14	Native 2 (14%) Graft 10 (71%) Other 2 (14%)	Acute 9 Chronic 5	10 (71%)	Lysis 4, PTA or SA 11	43% at 6 mo	Hemorrhage 14.3% Emboli 14% Device failure 7% Amputation 0 Mortality 0
Görich et al.[30]	1998	Amplatz	18	All native	All acute	14 (78%)	PAT 9, lysis 12	NA	Hemorrhage 6% Device failure 6% Amputation 6%

NA, not applicable; PAT, percutaneous aspiration thrombectomy; PTA, percutaneous transluminal angioplasty; SA, Simpson atherectomy.

Complications

With these devices, there is always the possibility of inducing distal embolization as the device is passed through the thrombus. This problem is being addressed by the development of a distal occlusion balloon called the "guard-dog" to be used in association with the AngioJet catheter (Fig. 158-13). The efficacy of the device is limited by the diameter of the cylindrical "core" of thrombus that can be extracted with each pass of the catheter—a property dependent on the size of the device. This limitation, however, must be balanced by the convenience of placing the device through a relatively small-bore sheath, as well as the increased safety associated with the use of a smaller device in the tibial vessels. Another limitation of current devices is the amount of potential red blood cell damage. Hemolysis with hemoglobinemia and hemoglobinuria can occur, especially with repeated passes of the device.

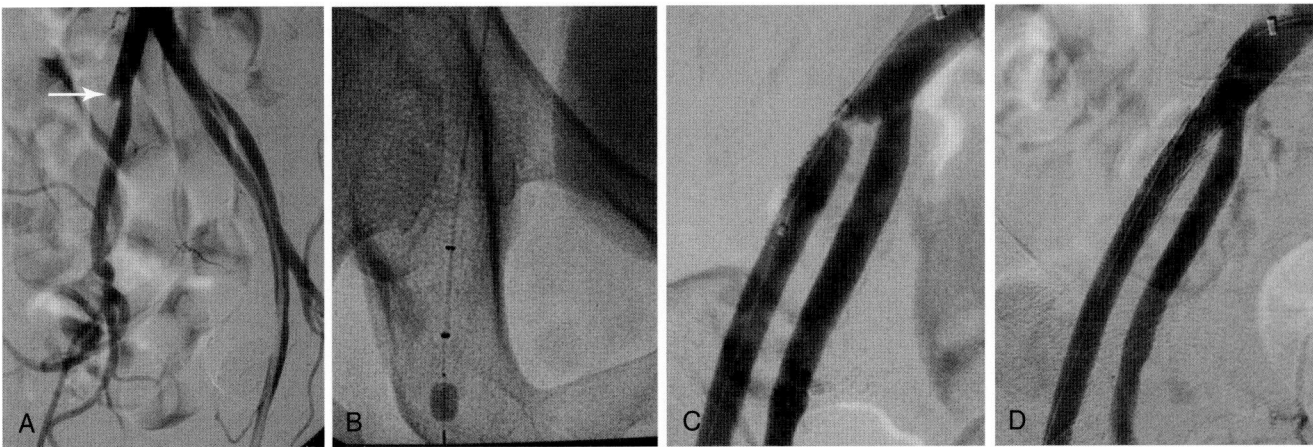

Figure 158-13 A, Acute occlusion of the right external iliac artery (*arrow*). **B,** "Guard-dog" occlusion to prevent distal embolization, with proximal AngioJet thrombectomy. **C,** Complete thrombus resolution after AngioJet thrombectomy, with underlying stenosis. **D,** Treatment of stenosis with angioplasty and stenting.

Last, fluid overload can develop if one does not carefully monitor the amount of intravascular irrigation instilled. Despite these theoretical limitations, fluid overload and hemolysis have not proved to be problems in preliminary clinical trials.[10-13]

In vitro studies comparing endothelial denudation with the AngioJet and the Fogarty thrombectomy catheter have demonstrated significantly greater mean endothelial loss in vessels treated with the Fogarty balloon catheter (58.0% versus 88.0%).[14] Particulate embolization was uncommon, and 99.83% of particles were smaller than 100 μm.[14] Hemolysis equivalent to that resulting from lysis of 75 mL of blood was seen after a standard pump run, but no elevation in blood urea nitrogen or creatinine was noted.[14]

SURGICAL REVASCULARIZATION

Balloon catheter thrombectomy, first introduced by Fogarty and coworkers,[31] became the cornerstone of therapy in the 1960s and 1970s.[27] Interestingly, this marked the beginning of catheter-based endovascular options that introduced the concept of *remote* rather than *direct* open surgical intervention for the management of occlusive vascular disease.

Techniques

Techniques for salvage of an ischemic limb include (1) balloon catheter thrombectomy or embolectomy (Fig. 158-14), (2) bypass procedures to direct blood flow beyond the occlusion, (3) endarterectomy with or without patch angioplasty, and (4) intraoperative isolated limb thrombolysis. Additional technical details of these procedures can be found in Chapter 83 (Technique: Open Surgical).

Balloon Catheter Thrombectomy or Embolectomy

These techniques are commonly used when dealing with an embolic event or graft thrombosis. In situ native vessel throm-

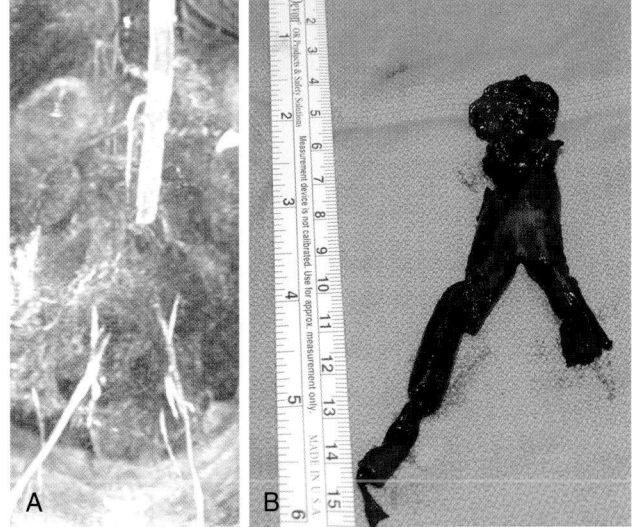

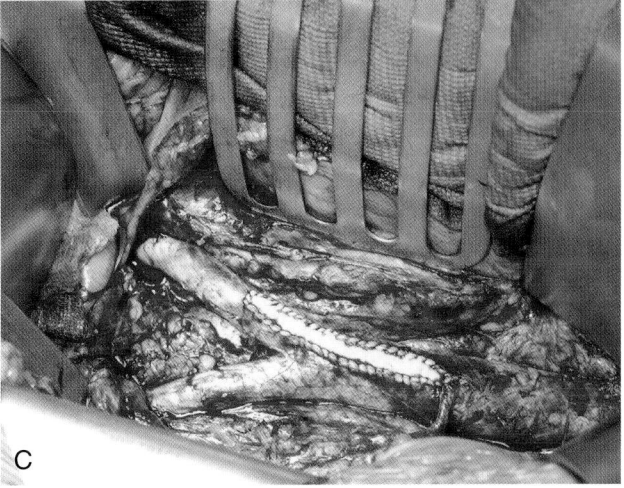

Figure 158-14 A, Acute embolic occlusion of the aortic bifurcation. **B,** Embolectomy, with occlusive material removed by a direct open surgical approach. **C,** Patch closure after embolectomy.

bosis superimposed on chronic occlusive disease is best treated surgically with a bypass graft. The technique involves exposure of the vessel (usually the common femoral artery) followed by proximal and distal control with vessel loops. Depending on the size of the vessel and associated atherosclerotic disease, a transverse or longitudinal arteriotomy is performed. Balloon embolectomy catheters are then passed proximally and distally until no visible thrombus is removed or a good pulse or backflow is established. Completion angiograms are helpful in evaluating the completeness of thrombus removal. Clinical examination alone may miss a culprit lesion that may result in early rethrombosis.

Bypass Procedures

Bypass procedures are more commonly performed in patients with known peripheral arterial disease or after failed open balloon thrombectomy. Proximal and distal targets can be evaluated by an on-table angiogram; however, if the clinical scenario permits, a preoperative angiogram from a contralateral femoral approach provides the best guide to open intervention. The ideal bypass conduit is an ipsilateral single-segment saphenous vein of adequate caliber (>3 mm). Otherwise, the contralateral saphenous vein, arm veins, or lesser saphenous vein should be used if below-knee revascularization is required. For above-knee revascularization, synthetic grafts can be used.

Endarterectomy

Endarterectomy is uncommonly used for limbs with ALI, but when it is, it is most often performed for in situ occlusion of the common femoral artery. After the diagnostic angiogram confirms occlusion of the common femoral artery, the target vessel is usually approached by a longitudinal groin incision. The common femoral, deep femoral, and proximal superficial femoral arteries should be adequately exposed and controlled. Atherosclerotic plaque often extends into the superficial femoral and profunda femoris orifices. Distal endpoints that extend into the superficial femoral artery or profunda femoris may require tacking sutures. Some type of patch material, either autogenous or synthetic, is required in most cases to prevent narrowing of the common femoral artery.

Intraoperative Isolated Limb Thrombolysis

This technique is seldom used, primarily because of the risk of bleeding at the operative site. The technique and lytic dose are variable, with the most common being a bolus infusion of urokinase (250,000 units in 10 mL of normal saline) or 1 mg of rt-PA injected through a cannula into the distal vessel via the arteriotomy. Some authors close the arteriotomy and then use a needle to infuse the lytic agent into the distal target.

In my opinion, this is a desperate measure in a patient with few remaining options. In general, the infusion of lytic agents proximal to the thrombus burden fails because the lytic agent bypasses the thrombus via patent collaterals. This is why wire

Table 158-5 Amputation, Mortality, and Long-term Limb Salvage for Open Surgery for Acute Limb Ischemia

Series	Year	Number of Patients	Results		
			Amputation (%)	Mortality (%)	Limb Salvage
Campbell et al.[4]	1998	474	16	22	NR
Nypaver et al.[5]	1998	71	7	10	62% at 1 yr
Pemberton et al.[6]	1999	107	12	25	75% at 2 yr

NR, not reported.

and catheter traversal of the occluding thrombus is necessary for CDT to be effective. Measures such as a proximal tourniquet followed by cannulation of the artery and vein for lytic infusion via an extracorporeal pump have also been described, but with limited success.

Results

Although improvements in open surgical technique have diminished the rate of limb loss associated with ALI, the mortality rate remains unacceptably high (Table 158-5).[2] In fact, patient survival has not changed dramatically since the report of Blaisdell and colleagues more than 30 years ago. The discordance of limb salvage and patient survival is explained by the specific factors controlling the two events. Mortality occurs as a result of medical co-morbidities and the fragile baseline medical state of patients presenting with ALI, whereas limb loss is related to an unsuccessful revascularization procedure. As such, the rate of amputation has diminished over the decades, presumably because of improvements in surgical technique. Unfortunately, the ability to rapidly restore arterial flow to the extremity with an operative procedure represents a significant insult to medically compromised individuals—one that all too frequently culminates in the patient's death.

■ SPECIAL CONSIDERATIONS

Myoglobinuria

Myoglobinuria is not uncommon after the treatment of ALI. It is rarely a significant problem except in patients with pre-existing renal failure, when associated with the use of greater than 150 mL of ionic contrast agent, or when combined with hemoglobinuria. Hemoglobinuria is not uncommon after the use of certain PMT devices, especially with run times greater than 5 minutes. Patients with any of these risk factors are monitored for myoglobinuria, and a urine output of greater than 100 mL/hour is maintained. Alkalization of the urine is achieved by adding sodium bicarbonate to intravenous fluids. Acute renal failure due to myoglobinuria may require temporary dialysis until the kidney function improves.

Fasciotomy

Compartment syndrome is most commonly seen in patients who have undergone open surgical revascularization or in those treated with PMT devices, owing to the speed of revascularization (see Chapter 159: Compartment Syndrome). Fasciotomy for compartment syndrome is less frequently required in patients undergoing CDT owing to the more gradual resolution of ALI. In addition, fasciotomies in patients receiving CDT is associated with significant bleeding. Any patient with early motor changes (Rutherford class IIb or III) should have fasciotomy after open surgical revascularization or successful PMT. It has been my practice to perform anterolateral and posterior release (a medial and lateral incision). Any patient not receiving a fasciotomy should be monitored on an hourly basis for any signs of compartment syndrome. It is also important to remember that a decrease in distal pulses and footdrop are late signs, and irreversible muscle and nerve damage may already have resulted at this stage. Any disparity in calf tension or tenderness compared with the normal contralateral leg requires an urgent fasciotomy. Compartment pressures can also be measured to confirm an elevation of pressure.

SELECTED KEY REFERENCES

Kasirajan K, Gray B, Beavers FP, Clair DG, Greenberg R, Mascha E, Ouriel K. Rheolytic thrombectomy in the management of acute and subacute limb threatening ischemia. *J Vasc Interv Radiol.* 2001;12: 413-421.
Explores use of the AngioJet in managing patients with ALI.

Ouriel K, Veith FJ, Sasahara AA, for the Thrombolysis or Peripheral Arterial Surgery (TOPAS) investigators. A comparison of recombinant urokinase with vascular surgery as initial treatment for acute arterial occlusion of the legs. *N Engl J Med.* 1998;338:1105-1111.
Largest randomized controlled study of CDT versus open surgery. A dosing study was done before randomization to avoid any dose-dependent bias.

Rutherford RB, Baker DJ, Ernst C, Johnston KW, Porter JM, Ahn S, Jones DN. Recommended standards for reports dealing with lower extremity ischemia: revised version. *J Vasc Surg.* 1997;26:517-538.
Establishes guidelines for reporting on limb ischemia to facilitate a more universal practice pattern.

The STILE Trial: Results of a prospective randomized trial evaluating surgery versus thrombolysis for ischemia of the lower extremity. *Ann Surg.* 1994;220:251-266.
One of the first large, randomized trials comparing open surgery to CDT. Failure of CDT was thought to be primarily due to the duration of ischemia, and many patients were treated for chronic limb ischemia (6 months' duration) with this technique. Currently, most physicians limit the use of CDT for symptoms of less than 2 weeks' duration. Additionally, the dose of t-PA used in the STILE study is rarely administered with a cautious approach to systemic anticoagulation.

Wissgott C, Richter A, Kamusella P, Steinkamp HJ. Treatment of critical limb ischemia using ultrasound-enhanced thrombolysis (PARES Trial): final results. *J Endovasc Ther.* 2007;14:438-443.
Large study that evaluates a new and promising tool to help decrease the dose and duration of thrombolytic therapy in the hope of lowering the risk of hemorrhagic complications.

REFERENCES

The reference list can be found on the companion Expert Consult Web site at *www.expertconsult.com.*

Section 19 Trauma and Acute Limb Ischemia

CHAPTER 159

Compartment Syndrome

J. Gregory Modrall

Compartment syndrome is a recognized complication of several conditions treated by vascular surgeons. Failure to arrive at a timely diagnosis of compartment syndrome increases the risk of short- and long-term morbidity, including limb loss or permanent disability. Conversely, prompt recognition and appropriate management of compartment syndrome can optimize the chances of a full recovery. This chapter address the pathogenesis, diagnosis, and treatment of compartment syndrome of the lower leg and other less common sites. Abdominal compartment syndrome is discussed in Chapter 154 (Vascular Trauma: Abdominal).

PATHOGENESIS

The unifying feature that defines all compartment syndromes, regardless of cause or anatomic location, is an increase in intracompartmental pressure (ICP) that impairs tissue perfusion.

Local Hemodynamics

The adverse consequence of elevated ICP on tissue perfusion can be understood by applying Poiseuille's law

$$F = \frac{\pi r^4 \Delta P}{8 \eta L}$$

to capillary blood blow within a muscle compartment. In this equation, F represents capillary blood flow, ΔP is the pressure gradient from the precapillary arteriole to the postcapillary venule, and r is proportional to the radius of the capillary to the fourth power. The viscosity of blood (η) and length of capillary (L) remain unchanged. Increasing ICP alters two variables in this equation: ΔP and R. As ICP rises, pressure is transmitted to the postcapillary venules, increasing the venous pressure and decreasing the arterial-venous pressure gradient (ΔP). Furthermore, increased ICP may collapse capillaries, decrease their radius, and increase the resistance to flow.[1,2]

Compartment Pressures

Critical Closing Pressure

Matsen suggested that there is a "critical closing pressure" above which capillaries collapse from transmural pressure and blood flow is arrested.[2] The pressure at which capillary blood flow ceases has been debated over the decades. Using wick catheters inserted into the anterolateral compartment of dogs, Hargens and colleagues demonstrated that baseline capillary

hydrostatic pressure in normotensive dogs was 25 ± 3 mm Hg, while hydrostatic pressure in postcapillary venules was 16 ± 4.4 mm Hg.[1] They proposed that capillary perfusion pressure would drop precipitously if ICP exceeded 30 mm Hg. Using vital microscopy to observe the response of isolated rat cremasteric muscle to increased external pressure, Hartsock and coworkers found that a pressure gradient between ICP and mean arterial pressure (MAP) of 25.5 ± 14 mm Hg arrested capillary blood flow.[3] Interestingly, they saw no significant collapse of arterioles, capillaries, or venules. Another study saw no significant collapse of arterioles with increased ICP but a modest reduction ($\leq 25\%$) in the diameter of venules.[4] Together, these studies disproved the "critical closing theory" proposed by Matsen and suggested instead that the arterial-venous pressure gradient is the critical determinant of capillary blood flow.[2-4] This conclusion has direct implications for determining the threshold ICP that defines compartment syndrome.

Absolute ICP Threshold

Defining the threshold ICP that produces tissue injury and cell death is an important step in determining the pressure at which fasciotomy is advisable. Hargens and colleagues found that an absolute ICP of 30 mm Hg for 8 hours universally produced muscle necrosis in normotensive dogs, whereas pressures less than 30 mm Hg produced no muscle necrosis.[5] Interestingly, tissues differ in their susceptibility to increased ICP. Early signs of endoneurial injury were observed at pressures of 30 mm Hg for 8 hours.[6,7] Tissues' different susceptibility to injury may explain those cases in which a delayed fasciotomy fails to restore full neurologic function despite viable muscle in the compartment.

Dynamic ICP Threshold

Defining compartment syndrome based on an absolute pressure threshold is appealing in its simplicity but ignores the role of arterial blood pressure in compartment blood flow. Changes in arterial pressure affect the arterial-venous pressure gradient, altering compartment blood flow. Thus, some authors have proposed defining compartment syndrome using a pressure threshold relative to MAP or diastolic pressure. Heppenstall and associates found that uninjured muscle in dogs developed evidence of tissue ischemia on ^{31}P magnetic resonance spectroscopy when the difference between MAP and ICP (MAP – ICP) dropped below 30 mm Hg.[8] Injured muscle showed greater sensitivity to ischemia, and tissue ischemia became evident when the difference between MAP and ICP was less than 40 mm Hg. In a small series of patients, Heppenstall and associates found that a dynamic pressure threshold (MAP – ICP) less than 40 mm Hg prevented unnecessary fasciotomy in a number of patients with absolute ICPs exceeding 30 mm Hg.[8] Using the diastolic blood pressure as their reference point in a dog study, Heckman and coworkers found a dramatic increase in tissue injury and necrosis when the difference between the diastolic blood pressure and the ICP was less than 10 mm Hg.[9] Comparing ICP criteria, McQueen and Court-Brown found that an absolute ICP threshold of 30 mm Hg would have resulted in fasciotomy in 43% of patients, whereas a dynamic ICP threshold of 30 mm Hg less than diastolic pressure resulted in only three fasciotomies.[10] These studies provide compelling data suggesting that a dynamic ICP threshold relative to MAP or diastolic pressure is a more appropriate criterion for selecting patients for fasciotomy.

■ CLINICAL ETIOLOGIES

Vascular Causes

ICP is elevated by conditions that either increase compartment volume or produce external compression on the compartment. The most common vascular causes of compartment syndrome are ischemia-reperfusion (I/R) injury associated with acute ischemia, arterial and venous traumatic injuries, phlegmasia cerulea dolens, and hemorrhage within a compartment.

Ischemia-Reperfusion

Compartment syndrome may complicate up to 21% of cases of acute ischemia.[11,12] The I/R phenomenon, described in detail in Chapter 6 (Ischemia-Reperfusion), is believed to play a central role in the pathogenesis of compartment syndrome due to acute ischemia. I/R increases compartment volume by causing muscle tissue injury that results in tissue and interstitial edema. With increasing duration and extent of ischemia, increased microvascular permeability permits the efflux of plasma proteins and progressive interstitial edema.[13] With reperfusion, oxygen radical generation causes lipid peroxidation of cell membranes, further augmenting microvascular permeability and exacerbating interstitial edema.[13] In a series of 194 fasciotomies performed for acute arterial occlusion, Papalambros and colleagues identified several risk factors for compartment syndrome after acute arterial ischemia, including prolonged ischemia time (>6 hours), young age, insufficient arterial collaterals, acute time course for arterial occlusion, hypotension, and poor backbleeding from the distal arterial tree at embolectomy.[11]

Trauma

Both arterial and venous trauma may produce compartment syndrome. Occlusive arterial injuries result in distal ischemia that initiates the I/R phenomenon, whereas venous injuries

may compromise venous outflow. The impact of compromised venous outflow is discussed below. The incidence of fasciotomy for trauma varies from 11.3% for blunt trauma to 28% for penetrating vascular trauma.[12,14] The need for fasciotomy also varies according to the type of vascular injury. In one series, fasciotomy was performed for 29.5% of isolated arterial injuries, 15.2% of isolated venous injuries, and 31.6% of combined arterial and venous injuries. Injuries to the popliteal artery have a notoriously higher risk of requiring fasciotomy (61% incidence) compared with injuries above the knee (19% incidence).[14]

Venous Outflow Obstruction

Conditions that dramatically impede venous outflow may predispose a limb to compartment syndrome. Examples include phlegmasia cerulea dolens and harvesting of the deep veins of the thigh. Uncomplicated deep venous thrombosis (DVT) often increases ICP, depending on the extent of DVT, but compartment syndrome is rare in the absence of phlegmasia cerulea dolens.[15] The extensive DVT of phlegmasia impairs venous outflow and produces profound tissue swelling. With increased venous hypertension, the arterial-venous pressure gradient is altered and capillary blood flow is impaired. With reduced capillary blood flow, muscle cell injury ensues, exacerbating tissue edema. This cycle continues until eventually the postcapillary venules thrombose and venous gangrene develops.

Iatrogenic interruption of venous outflow, such as when harvesting the superficial femoral vein for use as a conduit for arterial reconstruction, is associated with the development of compartment syndrome in 17.8% of limbs.[16] Risk factors for compartment syndrome after superficial femoral vein harvest are a low preoperative ankle-brachial index and concurrent harvest of the ipsilateral great saphenous vein.[16]

Hemorrhage

Hemorrhage may be the source of a rapid increase in compartment pressure. Thigh compartment syndrome has been described as the presenting symptom for rupture of a popliteal artery aneurysm[17] or postoperative hemorrhage after joint replacement surgery in an anticoagulated patient.[18]

Nonvascular Causes

Fracture

Fractures of the tibia or forearm are the most common orthopedic causes of acute compartment syndrome. These fractures injure the surrounding muscles and cause bleeding within the compartment, elevating ICP. The incidence of compartment syndrome with fracture ranges from 1% to 29%.[10,19-21] The anterior compartment of the leg and the flexor compartment of the forearm are most prone to this phenomenon. Comminuted fractures are more likely to result in compartment syndrome, owing to the greater energy absorbed in such injuries.[20]

Crush Injury

Crush injuries are another form of trauma that may cause compartment syndrome. Prolonged immobility due to intoxication, pinning of a victim beneath heavy equipment at industrial sites or large structures during earthquakes, and blunt trauma from assault are potential causes of crush injuries.[22,23] In such cases, compartment syndrome results from direct compartment pressure with underlying muscle ischemia. Rhabdomyolysis frequently complicates crush injuries and carries a 4% to 33% risk of acute renal failure.[24]

Iatrogenic

Iatrogenic causes of compartment syndrome include extravasation of large volumes of fluid within a muscle compartment, extravasation of caustic medications such as contrast agents, inadvertent arterial injections, and hemorrhage related to arterial or venous punctures in coagulopathic or anticoagulated patients.[25-27] Additional mechanisms include the compression injuries associated with prolonged intraoperative immobilization, as occurs in the dorsal lithotomy position, and cast immobilization for fractures.[28,29]

Secondary Compartment Syndrome

Rarely, compartment syndrome develops in the upper or lower extremities of a trauma patient with no overt evidence of extremity trauma. This phenomenon has been termed *secondary compartment syndrome*, and it is believed to result from diffuse microvascular permeability resulting from a trauma-induced systemic inflammatory response syndrome in concert with massive fluid resuscitation.[30] It is a local manifestation of a systemic illness that may rarely necessitate compartment decompression.

■ CLINICAL EVALUATION

The diagnosis of acute compartment syndrome begins with a high index of suspicion.

History and Examination

Symptoms of compartment syndrome include pain that is disproportionate to the magnitude of the injury and paresthesia in the distal extremity.[31] The pain is typically not relieved by immobilization or reduction of fractures and responds poorly to analgesic medications. Paresthesia represents an early symptom of ischemia of the nerves traversing the muscle compartment in question.

On examination, the most common findings are a tense, swollen compartment with pain elicited by passive movement of the muscles in that compartment. A careful neurologic examination should document sensory and motor function distal to the compartment, focusing on the nerves that traverse the compartment at risk. For example, a compartment syndrome affecting the anterior compartment of the lower leg

may be accompanied by dysfunction of the deep peroneal nerve, causing numbness at the first dorsal web space of the foot or inability to extend the great toe. Loss of two-point discrimination is a sensitive indicator of developing compartment syndrome.[32]

Clinical examination, including a pulse examination, should also exclude ongoing ischemia because this must be addressed expeditiously. The sensitivity of examination findings for compartment syndrome is dubious, however. In a meta-analysis of compartment syndromes related to tibial fractures, Ulmer found that clinical findings had low sensitivity (13% to 19%) for diagnosing compartment syndrome, and the negative predictive value was high (97% to 98%).[33] Ulmer concluded that although the presence of positive findings on clinical examination may not secure the diagnosis, the absence of such findings is helpful in excluding the diagnosis of compartment syndrome.

Laboratory finding such as elevated creatinine phosphokinase may indicate muscle ischemia or injury, but they are generally not helpful for diagnosing compartment syndrome.

Compartment Pressure Measurement

Measurements of ICP are not required to ascertain the diagnosis of compartment syndrome in most cases. Pressure measurement should be reserved for equivocal cases, unconscious patients, and pediatric patients in whom compartment syndrome is suspected. When the diagnosis is apparent from the history or examination, measuring ICP is superfluous and risks delaying definitive therapy.

Technique

Measuring ICP requires an instrument for measuring compartment pressures and a working knowledge of the muscle compartments of the limb. ICP has been measured using a host of techniques and instruments, including simple manometers, wick catheters, slit catheters, side-ported needles, and fiberoptic transducers.

There are two components in each system: (1) a needle to access the compartment and (2) a pressure measurement system. The most commonly used ICP measuring systems are the arterial line manometer, hand-held Stryker system, and Whiteside manometer. The arterial line manometer is ideal for use in the intensive care unit and operating room, where pressure transducers and monitors are readily available. In the emergency room, the hand-held Stryker system is particularly convenient. In environments where neither of these approaches is feasible, the Whiteside manometer technique offers a simple, inexpensive alternative (Fig. 159-1).[34]

The most comprehensive comparison of the accuracy of the various ICP measurement devices was performed by Boody and Wongworawat using a graduated cylinder to generate a known pressure.[34] They found that side-port needles and slit catheters were more accurate than straight

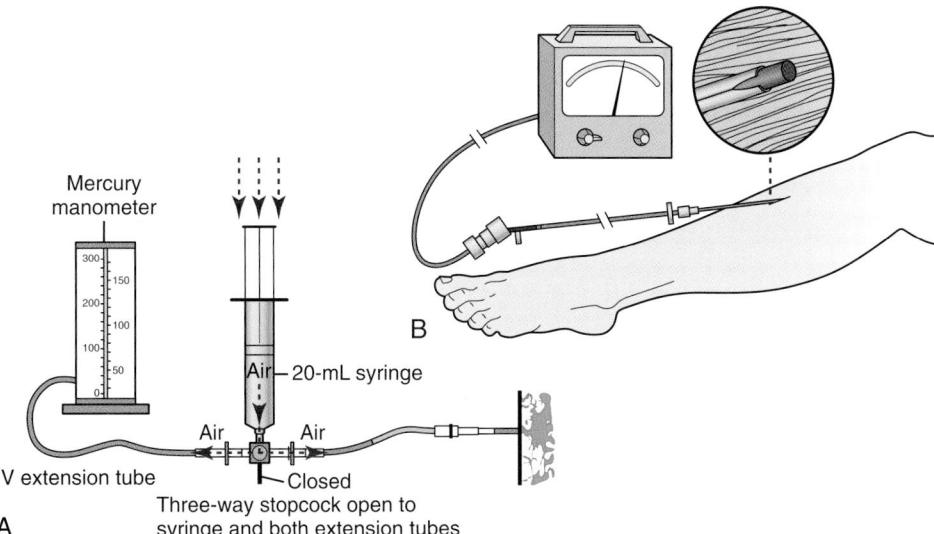

Figure 159-1 Whiteside technique for measuring intracompartmental pressure. **A,** Essential equipment includes a sterile 18-gauge (1.25-inch) needle, sterile intravenous (IV) extension tubing, three-way stopcock, second section of IV extension tubing, and blood pressure manometer, which are connected sequentially. A 20-mL syringe filled 15 mL of air is connected to the stopcock. The syringe is inserted into a bag of sterile saline, and saline is aspirated until it fills approximately half the first length of IV extension tubing. **B,** The stopcock is turned off, and the needle is inserted into the muscle compartment using aseptic technique. The stopcock is turned so that both sections of the extension tubing are open to the syringe. Air is gently injected until the saline meniscus in the tube begins to move. The pressure at which this occurs represents the compartment pressure.

needles, which tended to overestimate pressure. The arterial line manometer and hand-held Stryker device were more accurate than the Whitesides manometer. For this reason, I favor an arterial line manometer or hand-held Stryker device.

The choice of compartments for pressure measurement should be guided by the clinical examination. The most symptomatic or turgid compartment should be interrogated first, remembering that the anterior compartment of the lower leg and flexor compartment of the forearm are most prone to compartment syndrome. Ultimately, it is advisable to obtain compartment pressures from all compartments at risk. If necessary, multiple readings should be obtained. ICP, MAP, and diastolic pressure should be recorded for the medical record. The pressure criteria that define compartment syndrome are discussed later under "Criteria for Fasciotomy." A normal compartment pressure is 10 to 12 mm Hg or less.

Alternative Objective Techniques

Near-infrared spectroscopy has been proposed as a noninvasive means of continuously monitoring tissue oxygen saturation in critically ill patients. Its proponents have suggested that it may have utility in determining when tissue oxygen saturation declines owing to increased ICP. A pilot study with nine patients confirmed that tissue oxygenation was lower in limbs with confirmed compartment syndrome compared with the uninjured extremity.[35] Laser Doppler flowmetry is another tool that can detect decreased flow to a muscle compartment.[36] Data supporting the clinical use of these techniques are not currently available.

Unusual Presentations

Compartment syndrome can affect any myofascial compartment. Although less common than in the lower leg, compartment syndromes have been described in the upper extremity, hand, thigh, foot, and buttock. For any of these compartment syndromes, pain and swelling remain the hallmarks. In some cases, passive motion may exacerbate the pain. The presence of neurologic symptoms is highly variable and is not required to secure the diagnosis.

Hand compartment syndromes are usually associated with crush injuries or fractures of the carpal bones. Compartment syndrome can affect any of the 10 compartments of the hand. The classic symptoms are pain and local paralysis at the intrinsic muscles.[37] Forearm compartment syndromes are typically associated with direct blows, crush injuries, or distal radius fractures.[38] Pain, swelling, and neurologic symptoms are the classic indicators of increased ICP in the forearm.

Thigh compartment syndrome is usually caused by blunt trauma from motor vehicle accidents or contusion,[39] although bleeding complications in the thigh and exercise-induced injuries have been implicated.[17,18,40] I/R injury rarely results in a compartment syndrome of the thigh. The anterior thigh compartment is most commonly involved and universally presents with pain on passive motion. Paresthesia and paralysis may also be present.[39]

Gluteal compartment syndrome has been associated with hypogastric artery ligation or embolization during aortic aneurysm repair, hip arthroplasty, and prolonged compression during operative procedures.[41-44] Gluteal compartment syndrome has been cited as a cause of rhabdomyolysis, renal failure, and sciatic nerve palsy.[41]

ADJUNCTIVE MEASURES

Prevention of Compartment Syndrome

A variety of adjuncts have been proposed to mitigate muscle swelling and prevent the development of compartment syndrome.

Pharmacologic

The most common approach has been pharmacologic therapy to blunt the I/R phenomenon. These pharmacologic interventions are aimed primarily at modulating oxygen radical formation during reperfusion of an ischemic limb to minimize I/R injury. Mannitol, allopurinol, superoxide dismutase, deferoxamine, and thromboxane A_2 have shown promise in reducing oxygen radical formation and lowering compartment pressures in animal models.[45-48] Their use in humans is limited to anecdotal reports of benefit.[49,50]

Clinical Protocol

In cases of impending compartment syndrome, Mars and Hadley proposed a protocol of "first aid to hypoxic cells."[51] Their protocol includes (1) maintaining normal blood pressure, because hypotension reduces perfusion pressure; (2) removing any constricting bandages; (3) maintaining the limb at heart level (with no elevation) to avoid reducing the arterial-venous pressure gradient; and (4) administering supplemental oxygen to optimize oxygen saturation. This protocol represents a simple, rational approach to minimizing the risk of compartment syndrome based on its pathophysiology.

Prevention of Systemic Sequelae

Myonecrosis is a recognized complication of compartment syndrome. With myonecrosis, large quantities of intracellular potassium, phosphate, myoglobin, and creatine phosphokinase are liberated. Treatments designed to prevent systemic sequelae of compartment syndrome are aimed at preventing further complications related to the electrolyte disturbances or myoglobinuria that results from extensive myonecrosis.

Hyperkalemia with cardiac arrest has been described among patients with significant myonecrosis, especially those with crush injuries.[52] Treatment of hyperkalemia with oral binding resins, loop diuretics, or insulin and glucose may be inadequate, especially with concurrent acidosis or acute renal failure. Daily hemodialysis or continuous hemofiltration may be required to control hyperkalemia.[53]

Myoglobinuria exerts its nephrotoxic effects by inducing renal vasoconstriction, tubular cast formation, and direct heme protein–induced cytotoxicity.[54] The management of myoglobinuria includes aggressive crystalloid infusion, forced diuresis with mannitol, and alkalinization of the urine with bicarbonate. The rationale for crystalloid and bicarbonate infusion is based on the observation that heme proteins have minimal nephrotoxicity in the absence of hypovolemia and aciduria.[54] Clinical data affirm that early resuscitation with crystalloid diminishes the risk of progression to acute renal failure.[54-56] The data supporting mannitol and bicarbonate are more circumstantial. In a review of 217 patients with acute renal failure due to myoglobinuria, Brown and colleagues found no difference in the incidence of acute renal failure, need for dialysis, or mortality between patients receiving mannitol and bicarbonate and those receiving crystalloid infusion alone.[57] Nonetheless, most authorities continue to advocate the use of mannitol and bicarbonate based on their theoretical benefit in minimizing tubular deposition of heme proteins and cytotoxicity.[54,58-60]

Myoglobin is poorly cleared by conventional dialysis membranes owing to its relatively large molecular weight (17,000 Da), so hemodialysis is not useful in preventing renal injury due to myoglobinuria.[61] Renal replacement therapy should be reserved for standard indications, including the management of severe hyperkalemia.

FASCIOTOMY

Performing an adequate fasciotomy is critical to complete decompression of a compartment syndrome. Conversely, poor technique may lead to incomplete decompression, with a risk of permanent disability or limb loss. The technical details and relevant anatomy for fasciotomy are outlined in this section. Lower and upper extremity fasciotomies are considered separately, beginning with the more common anatomic sites.

Criteria for Fasciotomy

The decision to proceed to fasciotomy may be reached on clinical grounds or based on ICP measurements.

Clinical Criteria

Clinical criteria for fasciotomy include a swollen, tense compartment; pain with passive motion of the muscle groups traversing that compartment; and neurologic findings referable to the compartment. Not all these criteria are required to proceed to fasciotomy. The presence of a turgid compartment with either of the other two criteria (pain with passive motion and neurologic changes) is sufficient to warrant fasciotomy. Any neurologic finding referable to a tense compartment is an absolute indication for expeditious fasciotomy because nerve injury is ongoing. The presence of a tense compartment alone places the limb in an equivocal category for which fasciotomy or continued serial examination is an option. Patients who are obtunded or require other operations are poor candidates for serial examination, making fasciotomy the best option. An important consideration is the likely evolution of muscle swelling over the next several hours. In an equivocal case in which additional muscle swelling is inevitable, a "prophylactic" fasciotomy may be prudent. If serial examination is pursued, it must be done by an experienced surgeon. In equivocal cases, ICP measurement may assist in decision making.

ICP Measurements

The threshold ICP for the diagnosis of compartment syndrome remains controversial, but the data favor the use of a dynamic ICP threshold related to MAP or diastolic pressure.[8-10] Fasciotomy is warranted if the difference between the ICP and MAP falls to less than 40 mm Hg or the difference between ICP and diastolic pressure is less than 10 mm Hg.

Lower Extremity Technique

Lower Leg

The lower leg is the most common site for compartment syndrome. The lower leg is subdivided into four anatomic compartments: anterior, lateral, superficial posterior, and deep posterior. Single- and double-incision techniques have been described for decompression of the four compartments.[62-64]

Single-Incision Technique. The single-incision technique (Fig. 159-2) involves a lateral incision over the fibula from the fibular neck to 3 to 4 cm above the lateral malleolus.[64] A subcutaneous flap is developed in an anterior direction to access the anterior and lateral compartments. Longitudinal fascial incisions are used to decompress these compartments. A posterior subcutaneous flap is developed to access the superficial posterior compartment for a longitudinal fascial incision. The interval between the lateral and superficial posterior compartments is exposed. The flexor hallucis longus muscle is identified and dissected off the fibula in a subperiosteal plane. The fascial attachment of the posterior tibial muscle to the fibula is incised to open the deep posterior compartment. Most surgeons no longer perform a fibulectomy. The primary advantage of the single-incision approach is the ability to decompress all four compartments through one incision, but it is a relatively tedious approach to fasciotomy, with the potential to injure the peroneal artery and nerve. Most vascular surgeons now favor the double-incision technique.

Double-Incision Technique. The double-incision technique (Fig. 159-3) for lower leg fasciotomy involves a lateral incision over the intermuscular septum between the anterior and lateral compartments, through which these compartments are opened longitudinally. A second incision is placed

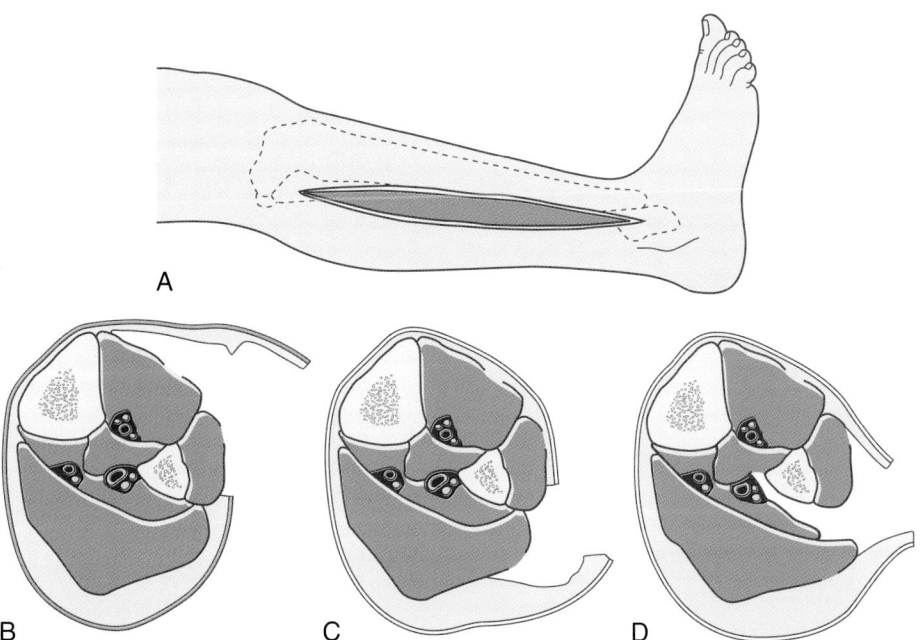

Figure 159-2 Single-incision fasciotomy of the lower leg. **A,** Lateral skin incision from the fibular neck to 3 to 4 cm proximal to the lateral malleolus. **B,** The skin is undermined anteriorly, and a fasciotomy of the anterior and lateral compartments is performed. **C,** The skin is undermined posteriorly, and a fasciotomy of the superficial posterior compartment is performed. **D,** An interval between the superficial posterior and lateral compartments is developed. The flexor hallucis longus muscle is dissected subperiosteally off the fibula and retracted posteromedially. The fascial attachment of the posterior tibial muscle to the fibula is incised to decompress the muscle. *(From Davey JR, Rorabeck CH, Fowler PJ. The tibialis posterior muscle compartment: an unrecognized cause of exertional compartment syndrome. Am J Sports Med. 1984;12:391-397.)*

on the medial aspect of the leg immediately posterior to the tibia for decompression of the two posterior compartments. The advantage of the two-incision technique is its relative simplicity, allowing rapid decompression of the four compartments of the lower leg.

The length of the skin incisions required to ensure complete decompression of the compartments is an important variable. Jensen and Sandermann found that 12% of subcutaneous fasciotomies using minimal incisions resulted in

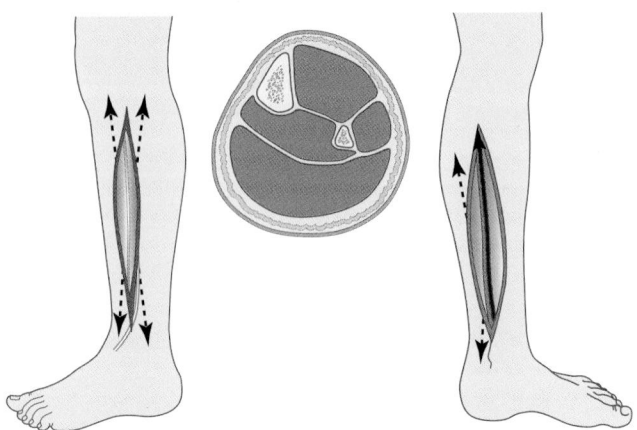

Figure 159-3 Double-incision (anterolateral and medial) fasciotomy of the lower leg. A longitudinal incision lateral to the tibia and overlying the intermuscular septum is used to visualize the anterior and lateral compartments. Parallel fascial incisions are used to decompress these compartments. A medial incision immediately posterior to the tibia is used to access both posterior compartments. The soleus muscle must be detached from the tibia to decompress the deep posterior compartment. *(From Janzing H, Broos P, Rommens P. Compartment syndrome as a complication of skin traction in children with femoral fractures. J Trauma. 1996;41:156.)*

incomplete decompression requiring reoperation to extend the skin incision.[31] They hypothesized that the skin itself could prevent adequate decompression of the compartment syndrome. This observation was shared by Cohen and coworkers, who noted that an 8-cm skin incision decreased the mean ICP in the anterior compartment of the lower leg from 48 to 25 mm Hg, but full decompression of all compartments of the lower leg required incisions 12 to 20 cm long.[65] Some authors have advocated using limited incisions when the muscle swelling is expected to be minimal, reserving extensive open incisions for cases of dramatic muscle swelling.[66] Unfortunately, it is often difficult to predict the extent of postoperative swelling.

Thigh

The thigh contains three compartments: anterior, posterior, and medial. In most cases a single lateral incision can be used to decompress the posterior and medial compartments (Fig. 159-4); the anterior compartment rarely requires decompression.[67] An incision is placed along the lateral thigh, beginning just distal to the intertrochanteric line and extending distally to the lateral epicondyle. The iliotibial band is exposed and incised longitudinally along the length of the skin incision to decompress the anterior compartment. The vastus lateralis is reflected medially to expose the lateral intermuscular septum. The intermuscular septum is incised over the length of the skin incision to release the posterior compartment. The medial compartment pressure should be measured. Decompression of the medial compartment is rarely necessary, but a separate incision over the adductor muscle group can be used to decompress this compartment.

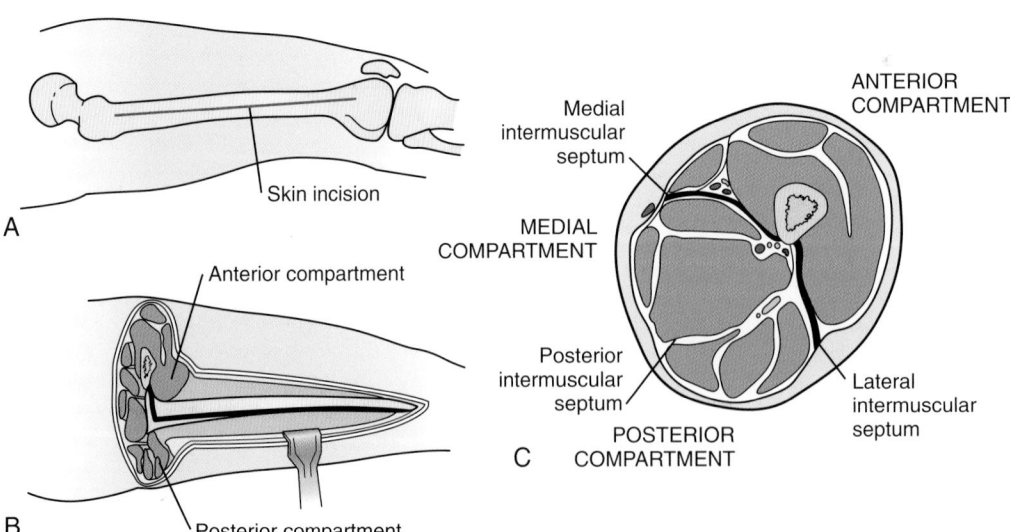

Figure 159-4 Fasciotomy of the thigh. **A,** The incision extends from the intertrochanteric line to the lateral epicondyle. **B,** The anterior compartment is opened by incising the fascia lata. The vastus lateralis is retracted medially to expose the lateral intermuscular septum, which is incised to decompress the posterior compartment. **C,** Thigh compartments and appropriate incision. *(A and B, redrawn from Tarlow SD, Achterman CA, Hayhurst J, et al. Acute compartment syndrome in the thigh complicating fracture of the femur: a report of three cases. J Bone Joint Surg Am. 1986;68:1439.)*

Foot and Buttock

Compartment syndromes of the foot and buttocks are rare, but vascular surgeons should be familiar with the approaches to decompressing these sites. The compartments of the foot are the medial, central, lateral, and interosseous. A variety of approaches have been described, although two dorsal incisions are most commonly employed for decompression of the foot.[68,69] In the gluteal compartment there are three compartments—gluteus maximus, gluteus medius, and gluteus minimus—and all three must be decompressed by fasciotomy to fully decompress a gluteal compartment syndrome. Decompression is accomplished through a posterior incision, although there is no consensus on the optimal orientation of that incision.[70,71]

Upper Extremity Technique

Forearm

The forearm is the most frequent site of compartment syndrome in the upper extremity. Within the forearm there are three compartments: the superficial and deep (volar) flexor compartments and the extensor (dorsal) compartment. The volar compartments more commonly develop increased ICP than the dorsal compartment. The volar, or Henry, approach (Fig. 159-5) uses a single incision to decompress both the superficial and deep flexor compartments.[32,72] A curvilinear incision begins proximal to the antecubital fossa, medial to the biceps tendon; it crosses the antecubital crease and extends to the radial side of the forearm, where is extends distally along the medial border of the brachioradialis muscle. From the distal forearm the incision extends across the carpal tunnel along the thenar crease. The fascia overlying the superficial flexor compartment is incised along the entire length of the skin incision. The radial nerve and brachioradialis muscle are retracted to the radial side of the forearm, and the flexor carpi radialis and radial artery are retracted to the ulnar side. The fascia overlying each of the muscles of the deep flexor

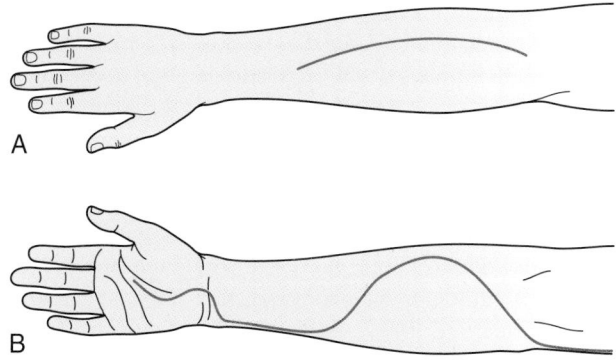

Figure 159-5 Fasciotomy of the volar forearm for severe Volkmann's contracture. **A,** Extensive opening of the fascia of the dorsum of the forearm for dorsal compartment syndromes. **B,** Incision used for anterior forearm compartment syndromes. The skin and underlying fascia are released completely throughout.

compartment is incised to complete the volar fasciotomy. If the dorsal ICP is elevated, a long incision from the lateral epicondyle to the wrist is used to perform a fasciotomy between the extensor carpi radialis brevis and the extensor digitorum communis.[32]

Hand

The hand is a rare location for compartment syndrome. The hand has 10 compartments—hypothenar, thenar, and adductor pollicis compartments; four dorsal interosseous compartments; and three volar interosseous compartments—which complicates decision making. Fasciotomies for the hand should be tailored to symptoms.[25] All patients should have a carpal tunnel release, and most require one or two dorsal interosseous fasciotomies. Many patients also require thenar or hypothenar fasciotomy. All hand fasciotomies should be performed through longitudinal dorsal hand incisions.

■ FASCIOTOMY WOUND MANAGEMENT

Fasciotomy may solve the problem of increased ICP, but it creates wounds that may be the source of considerable short- and long-term morbidity.[73,74] The goal of early wound care after fasciotomy is preventing further muscle injury or necrosis until muscle swelling subsides sufficiently to permit closure. When muscle viability is questionable, periodic saline dressings permit caregivers the opportunity to inspect and débride the wound at regular intervals. Vacuum-assisted closure (VAC) therapy is an alternative means of wound coverage, although the wound should be inspected at frequent intervals early after fasciotomy. Once tissue viability is ensured and wound swelling has subsided, the priority shifts to wound closure.

Fasciotomy wounds can be closed through a variety of approaches. The options include delayed primary closure, closure by secondary intention, gradual dermal apposition, split-thickness skin grafting, and myocutaneous flap coverage. Each of these approaches has a role, depending on the clinical circumstances. Delayed primary closure offers the simplicity of direct closure but should be reserved for cases in which muscle swelling is minimal or nonexistent. Wiger and colleagues found that 7 of 12 fasciotomy wounds had increased ICP (>30 mm Hg) with attempted delayed primary closure on postoperative days 3 or 4, so early closure should be undertaken with caution and ICP monitoring.[75]

Closure by secondary intention should be reserved for patients who are either medically or nutritionally ill suited for any other option, because this approach is the least expeditious in achieving wound closure. The addition of VAC therapy accelerates the process of closure by secondary intention and has been employed with success for fasciotomy wounds.[76-78]

To accelerate closure further, various forms of gradual dermal apposition have been advocated, including the Sure-Close suturing system, Marburger Skin Approximation

System, Wisebands device, progressive closure with Silastic vessel loops, or cutaneous sutures placed at surgery.[79-83] Anecdotal reports have documented success with each approach, although the Marburger system has been associated with dermal necrosis in some cases.[80]

Finally, several authors have proposed closing fasciotomy wounds using split-thickness skin grafts.[11,31,73,84] Early closure may decrease the rate of wound complications associated with closure by secondary intention and truncate the length of hospital stay.[11,73] Myocutaneous flaps are generally reserved for coverage of neurovascular structures or exposed bone in a limb that remains functional. My preferred approach is to use gradual dermal apposition with the shoelace technique or cutaneous sutures. When this approach is contraindicated, VAC therapy is a reasonable option to accelerate closure by secondary intention. I often use both approaches in combination to accelerate dermal apposition.

OUTCOMES

Outcomes of fasciotomy are determined largely by the patient's functional status at hospital discharge. Neurologic deficits or amputation in the early postoperative period are harbingers of long-term disability. Even in the subset of patients discharged without amputation or neurologic deficits, a fasciotomy predisposes the limb to future problems. Fitzgerald and colleagues noted at late follow-up that 77% of fasciotomy sites were associated with impaired sensation at the margins of the wound, 7% had tethered tendons, and 13% had recurrent ulcerations.[85] A small subset (7.5%) of patients requires late amputation (between 30 days and 1 year), usually due to a neurologically devastated limb or ischemia.[86,87] At a mean follow-up of 37 months, Bermudez and colleagues found that a significant proportion of patients (47%) had clinical evidence of chronic venous insufficiency after lower leg fasciotomy, despite a mean age of only 37 years.[88] In that study, air plethysmography documented a lower mean calf ejection fraction and residual volume fraction compared with control patients. These findings suggest that fasciotomy compromises calf muscle pump function, predisposing the limb to the development of chronic venous insufficiency.

COMPLICATIONS
Early Complications

Systemic complications of compartment syndrome are related primarily to myonecrosis and may include hyperkalemia, hypocalcemia, elevated liver enzymes, disseminated intravascular coagulation, and myoglobinuria.[58,89] Renal failure is a rare complication after compartment syndrome except after fasciotomy for crush injury, in which renal failure may complicate up to 44% of cases.[24] The mortality rate for patients undergoing fasciotomy ranges from 11% to 15% and is directly related to the underlying cause of the compartment syndrome.[31,86,90]

Local complications are frequent in limbs with compartment syndrome. Major amputations are required in 5% to 21% of limbs.[31,86,90] Neurologic deficits occur in 7% to 36% of limbs.[86,90,91] Wound complications are common (4% to 38%)[73,74,90] and are more frequent if fasciotomy is delayed more than 6 hours (37%, versus 25% for fasciotomy performed within 6 hours).[74,92]

Sequelae of Missed Compartment Syndrome

A delayed or missed compartment syndrome has devastating consequences for the patient and the limb, increasing the risk of neurologic deficit, amputation, and renal failure. Sheridan and Matsen found that the overall complication rate increased dramatically if fasciotomy was delayed more than 12 hours (54%) compared with early fasciotomy (4.5%).[84] Nearly half the patients with delayed fasciotomies required amputation, and 92% had significant neuropathy. Not surprisingly, delay of fasciotomy for more than 36 hours almost invariably results in amputation. After 3 to 4 days, decompression of compartment syndrome is not indicated because the rate of infection and muscle necrosis is prohibitively high.

The classic late consequence of a missed compartment syndrome or incomplete decompression is Volkmann's contracture. In this state, the ischemic muscle and nerve tissues are replaced by fibrosis, leaving the compartment firm, contracted, and largely nonfunctional.[93] Adjacent joints become stiff and immobile. Treatment consists of contracture and joint capsule release.[94] Orthopedic consultation for immediate and long-term management is advisable.

CHRONIC COMPARTMENT SYNDROME

Chronic exertional compartment syndrome is a syndrome of exercise-induced pain and tightness that usually affects the muscles of the lower leg, especially the anterior compartment.[95,96] The syndrome is believed to result from increased ICP and resulting muscle ischemia.[97]

The typical patient is a young (20 to 30 years), athletic runner.[95] Recently, the syndrome has also been described in nonathletes.[98] The syndrome is characterized by pain that begins 20 to 30 minutes after the onset of exercise and abates with 15 to 30 minutes of rest. Paresthesia often occurs in the distribution of peripheral nerves traversing the compartment. Symptoms are bilateral in 82% of cases. Physical examination often shows tenderness of the affected muscle compartment.

The differential diagnosis includes fascial hernia, medial tibial syndrome (for anterior compartment symptoms), and claudication due to popliteal entrapment syndrome (for calf symptoms). Although magnetic resonance imaging and other tests may rule out other causes of leg pain, measurement of ICP is required to secure the diagnosis. Pedowitz and colleagues established pressure criteria for the diagnosis: (1) resting ICP greater than 15 mm Hg, (2) ICP greater than 30 mm Hg 1 to 2 minutes after the completion of exercise, or (3) ICP greater than 20 mm Hg 5 minutes after the completion of exercise.[99] One or more of these criteria is sufficient for the diagnosis when the characteristic symptoms are reproducible with exercise.

Treatment for chronic exertional compartment syndrome is either avoidance of the precipitating exercise or surgical decompression of the affected compartment. Avoidance is poorly accepted by athletic patients, so fasciotomy is typically the treatment of choice.

In his review of the treatment of 796 patients with chronic exertional compartment syndrome, Turnipseed suggested that open fasciotomy produced a lower wound complication rate (5.5%) and recurrence rate (2%) compared with subcutaneous fasciotomy (13% and 17%, respectively).[96] Turnipseed currently advises fasciectomy as the treatment of choice in most cases of chronic compartment syndrome.

SELECTED KEY REFERENCES

Boody AR, Wongworawat MD. Accuracy in the measurement of compartment pressures: a comparison of three commonly used devices. *J Bone Joint Surg Am*. 2005;87:2415-2422.
This article compares various methods of measuring compartment pressures to a known standard.

McQueen MM, Court-Brown CM. Compartment monitoring in tibial fractures. The pressure threshold for decompression. *J Bone Joint Surg Br*. 1996;78:99-104.
This paper compares the number of fasciotomies that would be performed using two different thresholds: an absolute ICP versus a dynamic pressure threshold based on diastolic blood pressure.

Sheridan GW, Matsen FA III. Fasciotomy in the treatment of the acute compartment syndrome. *J Bone Joint Surg Am*. 1976;58:112-115.
This often quoted article reports the difference in outcome for early versus delayed fasciotomies.

Turnipseed WD. Clinical review of patients treated for atypical claudication: a 28-year experience. *J Vasc Surg*. 2008;40:79-85.
This article reviews the management and outcome of a large series of patients with chronic exertional compartment syndrome.

REFERENCES

The reference list can be found on the companion Expert Consult Web site at *www.expertconsult.com*.

CHAPTER 160

Atheromatous Embolization

Jeffrey W. Olin and John R. Bartholomew

Atheromatous embolization is a poorly recognized and under-diagnosed multisystem disorder that is associated with high mortality from cardiovascular and other causes.[1] There are myriad clinical manifestations occurring across all specialties, making the differential diagnosis broad and the diagnosis difficult. In addition, atheromatous embolization is a confusing entity because it is known by many different names (cholesterol embolization, cholesterol crystal embolization, blue toe syndrome, purple toe syndrome, atheroembolism, and pseudovasculitis). Once atheroembolism has occurred, therapy involves three major strategies: treat the end-organ that is the recipient of the embolization, prevent further embolization from occurring, and prevent future cardiovascular morbidity and mortality. Therefore, it is critical for clinicians to have a high index of suspicion and to recognize the clinical manifestations of this syndrome.

INCIDENCE

The incidence of atheromatous embolization varies, based on population characteristics, diagnostic criteria, and study design. Among unselected autopsy series, the incidence of atheromatous embolization ranges from 0.18% to 2.4%.[2,3] However, autopsy studies performed in selected patients with atherosclerosis and those who have undergone aortic manipulation report a greater prevalence of atheromatous embolization, ranging from 12% to 77%.[4-6] In autopsy studies of patients with known advanced atherosclerosis who had recently undergone an arteriogram or a cardiac or vascular surgical procedure, the incidence is also high.[7] Blauth and coworkers identified atheroemboli in 22% of their post–cardiac surgery autopsy cases,[7] whereas Ramirez and colleagues reported a 27% incidence in patients who had undergone arteriography prior to death.[8] In general, retrospective autopsy studies may overestimate the frequency of the disease because of the detection of subclinical cases as well as the selection bias inherent in obtaining information after necropsy. In contrast, clinically significant atheroembolic disease may be missed in clinical studies because of short follow-up. The prevalence of atheroembolic disease in clinical studies has been estimated to be between 1% and 4%.[9-13]

PATHOGENESIS

The first description of atheromatous embolization was published more than a century ago by the German pathologist Panum.[14] However, Flory is credited with accurately describing the syndrome in 1945.[15] Among 267 consecutive autopsies, he observed 9 instances of cholesterol crystal embolism: none in 63 cases in which aortic plaque ulceration was absent, 2 instances in 147 cases (1.4%) with moderate aortic plaque erosion, and 7 instances in 57 cases (12.8%) with severe aortic plaque ulceration. Since that seminal paper, it has become clear that the risk of atheromatous embolization is directly related to the severity of aortic atherosclerosis (Fig. 160-1).

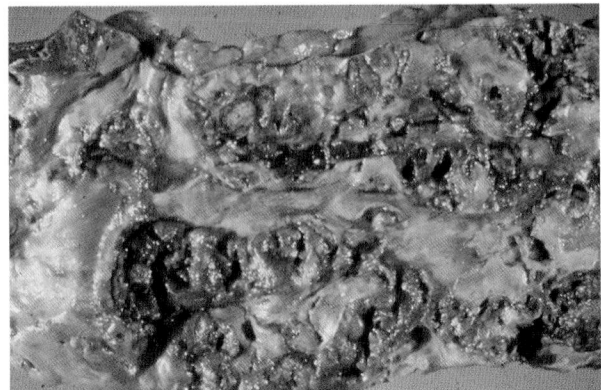

Figure 160-1 Gross autopsy specimen from a patient with a severely diseased aorta and atheroembolization syndrome.

Atherosclerotic plaque consists of a fibrous cap under which there are macrophages, necrotic debris, and cholesterol crystals. The most vulnerable plaque, or the plaque at the highest risk of rupture, is that with a thin fibrous cap surrounding a large, lipid-rich core.[16] Atheromatous embolization is a process in which emboli from proximal lesions produce ischemia in distal arterial beds. Emboli may consist of thrombus, platelet-fibrin material, or cholesterol crystals either individually or in combination. Macroemboli may arise from thrombus originating in aortic or peripheral aneurysms or atheromatous ulcers or from the dislodgement of atheromatous plaques. Microemboli are platelet-fibrin emboli or cholesterol crystals.[17]

Cholesterol crystals are white and rhomboid or rectangular. They can also be elongated, biconvex, and needle shaped and range in size from 250 μm to less than 10 μm in diameter (Fig. 160-2).[10] In paraffin-fixed sections the cholesterol crystals are dissolved, leaving needle-like clefts (Fig. 160-3). Frozen or wet formalin-fixed sections reveal doubly refractile cholesterol crystals, and with Schultz histochemical stain, these crystals stain blue-green.[18]

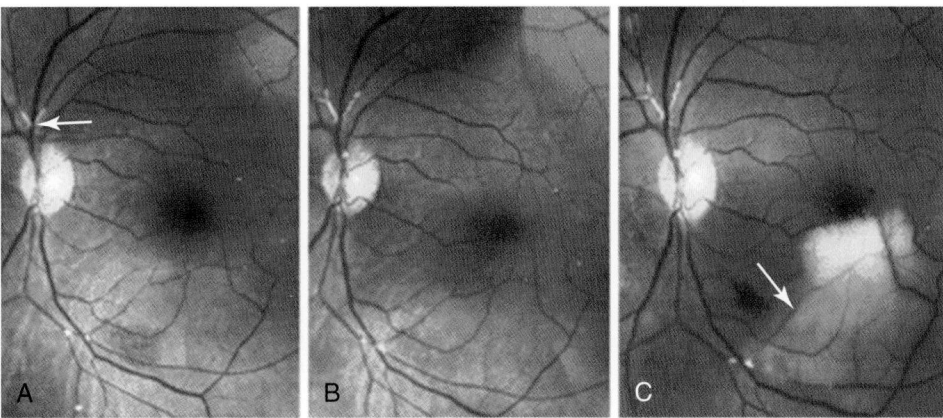

Figure 160-2 A 59-year-old man underwent stenting of the left internal carotid artery. **A,** Two months later, examination of the left eye shows multiple tiny, refractile retinal arteriolar cholesterol emboli and a saddle embolus superior to the optic nerve (*arrow*). **B,** Two months later, repeat examination shows an increase in the number of cholesterol emboli. **C,** Four weeks later, the patient experienced a sudden, painless loss of the left superior visual field. Examination reveals whitening in the inferior macular region (*arrow*), a finding consistent with an occlusion at the second major bifurcation of the inferior temporal branch of the retinal artery. *(From Colucciello M. Images in clinical medicine. Retinal arteriolar cholesterol emboli.* N Engl J Med. *2008;358:826.)*

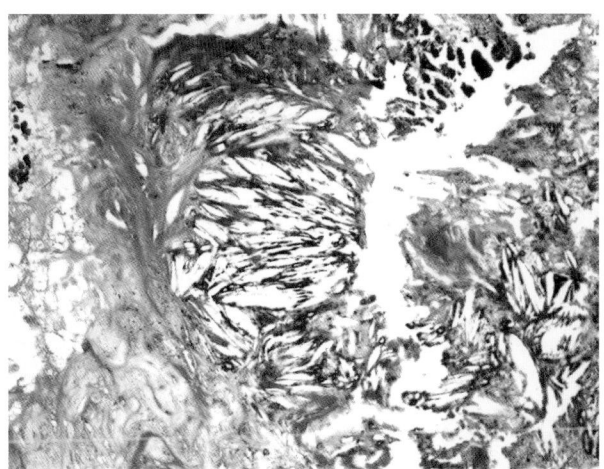

Figure 160-3 Typical appearance of cholesterol clefts in a specimen from a carotid artery plaque. The convex-shaped crystals dissolve during the fixation process, leaving the "ghosts" seen in the histopathology (H&E; ×200).

Because they are lightweight and hydrophobic, cholesterol crystals pass quickly through blood vessels until they are stopped by arterial bifurcations or the narrowing of the vessel lumen or when they reach the end of the arterial circulation.[10] Cholesterol emboli tend to be diffuse and lodge in arteries 100 to 200 μm,[12] although small crystals have been observed in capillaries in the end-arterial circulation.

Cholesterol crystals that lodge in the arterioles immediately incite an inflammatory response characterized by varying degrees of polymorphonuclear and eosinophilic infiltration.[10,15,19,20] By 2 to 4 weeks, a more chronic inflammatory infiltrate is seen. Cholesterol crystals become embedded in multinucleated giant cells and smooth muscle cells.[19] Endothelial proliferation and fibrous tissue can be found surround-

ing the crystals, ultimately leading to luminal obliteration.[19,20] At 1 to 2 months, crystals may become extruded out of the vessel lumen and buried in the adventitia, or they may remain in the lumen embedded within organized thrombus that may recanalize.[19] The crystals are resistant to breakdown by macrophages and have been shown to persist in tissue for up to 9 months.[21,22] Arterial lumina are eventually occluded by the accumulation of cells and fibrous material. These pathologic changes result in tissue effects distal to the cholesterol crystal emboli; ischemia and, rarely, infarction can occur, depending on the extent of organ involvement. This type of foreign body reaction is the reason it may take weeks to months for serum creatinine levels to rise in patients with atheroembolic renal disease and illustrates why renal function usually does not recover.[21,23,24]

RISK FACTORS AND SIMPLE PREVENTIVE STRATEGIES

The most important risk factor for atheromatous embolization is established atherosclerosis. In 1945, Flory was the first person to hypothesize such a relationship between cholesterol crystal embolism and a diseased, atherosclerotic aorta.[15] More recently, Blauth and associates reported on 46 patient autopsies in which severe atherosclerosis of the ascending aorta was accompanied by evidence of atheroemboli in other vascular beds.[7] In their study, significant risk factors for atheromatous embolization included peripheral arterial disease, hypertension, older age, and coronary artery disease.[7]

Several precipitating factors have been implicated in the occurrence of plaque instability and consequent atheromatous embolization, including trauma, vascular surgery,[25,26] angiographic and endovascular procedures,[1,21,24,27] anticoagulation,[9,28,29] and thrombolysis.[30-33] Although spontaneous atheromatous embolization was once the most common presentation, endovascular revascularization techniques are now the most frequent underlying cause of atheromatous embolization syndrome.[23,24,34-36] In 354 subjects followed for an average of 2 years, Scolari and associates found that the atheroembolic disease was spontaneous in only 23.5% of cases.[24]

Coronary Interventions

Manipulation of the aorta with catheters or guide wires can cause mechanical trauma and dislodgement of atheromatous material from the arterial wall.[37] One study evaluating the retrieval of atherothrombotic material during the placement of coronary catheters found that 0.5% of 7621 patients had macroscopically visible atherothrombotic debris.[38] None of these patients, however, had clinically apparent atheroembolic disease. In a review of 4587 cardiac catheterizations, Drost and coworkers found 7 cases of clinical atheromatous embolization (0.002%).[39] Colt and colleagues found 8 cases after 3733 procedures (0.002%) involving heart catheterization, percutaneous transluminal angioplasty, and intra-aortic balloon pump insertion.[40] Coronary angiography with angioplasty and stenting is considered the most common arteriographic procedure inciting atheromatous embolization.[12,24] Saklayen and colleagues, in a prospective analysis of 267 patients undergoing coronary angiography, found the incidence of cholesterol embolism to be less than 2%.[41] Similar statistics were found in a more recent prospective analysis by Fukumoto and coworkers, who reported clinically apparent cholesterol embolism (livedo pattern on the feet, blue toe syndrome, digital gangrene, or renal failure) in 1.4% of 1786 patients undergoing left heart catheterization.[42]

Although it is impossible to predict the risk of atheromatous embolization in a given patient, the presence of severe peripheral arterial disease, aortic aneurysm, protruding mobile atheroma by transesophageal echocardiography (TEE),[43] or aortic plaque greater than 4 mm thick[44] increases the risk of distal embolization and should therefore influence the vascular approach.[41,45-47] Use of long guide wire (260 cm) exchanges is recommended, and backbleeding from guiding catheters (once the wire is removed) allows the removal of debris. Advancement and removal of catheters should occur over a guide wire to straighten the catheter and minimize contact with the aortic wall.[48] Brachial and radial access may minimize embolization from the abdominal aorta but not from the ascending aorta or arch. However, a prospective study of 1579 patients undergoing coronary angioplasty found no significant differences between the brachial and femoral approaches.[49] In another study involving 3733 procedures, there were no cases of atheromatous embolization after cardiac catheterization when the brachial artery was used.[40]

Aortography

Catheter manipulation of the aorta is frequently performed during the diagnosis and evaluation of patients with vascular disease prior to revascularization, and as with coronary angiography, the risk of atheromatous embolization is a serious concern. Ramirez and associates, in a retrospective study of 71 autopsies, reported a 27% incidence of atheromatous embolization in patients who had arteriography before death, compared with a 4.3% incidence of spontaneous cholesterol emboli in an age- and disease-matched control group that did not undergo arteriography.[8] The rigidity of the catheter used, as well as the force of the contrast injection, appears to contribute to the risk of embolization. Although some advocate the use of softer, more flexible catheters to avoid such a complication,[8,50] the most important risk factor remains the severity of atherosclerotic disease in the aorta. It should be understood, however, that the studies reporting a significant incidence of atheromatous embolization after angiography were conducted nearly 25 years ago. With the advent of better, smaller, and more flexible catheters, guide wires, and balloons, as well as superior operator technique and the use of the "no-touch" technique,[51] the incidence of atheromatous embolization following angiography is much less than it was 3 decades ago.

Endovascular Therapy

Endovascular therapy for patients with peripheral vascular disease has become a widely used alternative to surgical revascularization. Clinically important atheromatous embolization appears to be a relatively infrequent, but not absent, complication of endovascular therapy. In a retrospective analysis of 493 patients who underwent a total of 565 aortoiliac stent placements, Lin and coworkers found the incidence of atheroembolism to be 1.6%.[52] This figure is comparable to the findings of previous clinical studies, in which the incidence ranged between 1.3% and 3.6%.[53,54] In a study using duplex ultrasound at the time of renal artery stenting, microembolic signals were detected in the renal parenchyma in every case.[1,55] In addition, when embolic protection devices are used in carotid stent procedures[56] or renal artery stent procedures,[57-63] visible atherosclerotic debris occurs frequently. Several studies have shown that distal protection devices used at the time of renal artery stenting are associated with less deterioration in renal function compared with stenting without the use of these devices.[57,61,62] In a small prospective randomized trial, Cooper and associates demonstrated that during renal artery stenting, the combination of distal embolic protection and the glycoprotein IIb/IIIa inhibitor abciximab resulted in an improvement in renal function compared with the use of either one alone.[62]

The presence of a shaggy aorta and diffuse, soft, ulcerative plaque on TEE clearly identifies a high-risk population.[44] Hence, heightened awareness; proper patient selection; use of the most advanced catheters, guide wires, and balloons; use of embolic protection devices; and greater operator expertise may have a favorable impact on the incidence of atheromatous embolization during endovascular interventions. In some cases, endovascular procedures using covered stent-grafts may be effective (see under "Treatment").

Vascular Surgery

The effect of atheromatous embolization after major vascular surgery was first recognized by Thurlbeck and Castleman in 1957.[64] In their series, atheromatous embolization was present at autopsy in more than 75% of patients who died after aortic aneurysm surgery. Atheromatous embolization was the cause of death or significantly contributed to mortality in nearly half the patients in this series. Subsequently, numerous studies have confirmed the importance of vascular surgery as a precipitator of atheromatous embolization. Vascular surgery procedures may disrupt plaque when the vessel is manipulated, cross-clamped, or incised during surgery. Other vascular surgery procedures known to precipitate atheromatous embolization include aortoiliac and aortofemoral bypass, carotid endarterectomy, and renal artery revascularization.[12]

Cardiac Surgery

Atheromatous embolization is a recognized complication of cardiac surgery and has profound medical and economic consequences. Doty and associates, in a retrospective analysis of 18,402 patients who underwent cardiac surgery, found evidence of atheromatous embolization in 0.2% of patients at autopsy.[26] The clinical presentation of atheromatous embolization in this study was broad and included five distinct organ systems: heart, central nervous system, gastrointestinal (GI) tract, kidneys, and lower extremities. In 21% of the cases, death was directly attributable to atheromatous embolization. Kolh and colleagues documented a significant increase in intensive care unit stay, overall hospital stay, and total hospital cost in patients with documented atheromatous embolization after cardiac surgery.[65] TEE can identify significant aortic plaque preoperatively, with a sensitivity and specificity in excess of 90%.[66] Multidetector computed tomographic angiography (CTA) may also be a valuable imaging tool for evaluating the aorta and iliac arteries.[67] Alteration of the cannulation site and avoidance of aortic manipulation for coronary artery bypass based on such findings may reduce the incidence of atheromatous embolization.

It is clear that the most effective strategy for the management of atheroemboli in vascular surgery is prevention. In high-risk surgical patients, noninvasive procedures such as magnetic resonance imaging, TEE, or CTA are excellent techniques to screen for the presence of aortic atherosclerosis preoperatively. When shaggy aortas are visualized, alternative surgical procedures should be considered to minimize aortic manipulation. Appropriate surgical techniques to prevent atheroemboli during operation are now well recognized and documented.[68]

Anticoagulation

An increased risk of atheromatous embolization with anticoagulation, and clinical improvement when anticoagulation was removed, has been noted in case reports for more than a quarter of a century.[9,12,28] One hypothesis is that anticoagulation may prevent thrombus formation over unstable atherosclerotic plaque, thus allowing exposed cholesterol crystals to embolize. Another hypothesis is that these agents may initiate the disruption of a complex plaque by causing intraplaque hemorrhage.[69-73] Based on these small case series and case reports, some investigators have recommended that warfarin be discontinued, when feasible, in patients who have had an episode of atheromatous embolization for which no other cause can be identified.

The data, however, are not entirely clear in terms of assessing anticoagulation safety in patients with large amounts of aortic plaque. The assumption that anticoagulation precipitates cholesterol emboli syndrome was not confirmed by the Stroke Prevention in Atrial Fibrillation (SPAF-3) trial, in which patients with documented aortic plaque identified by TEE and assigned to adjusted-dose warfarin therapy had a low annual rate of atheromatous embolization (0.7% per patient-year; 95% confidence interval, 0.1% to 5.3%).[74] Furthermore, atheromatous embolization was not seen in patients with documented aortic arch plaque greater than 1 mm thick who were treated with warfarin in a French study.[44] More recently, Fukumoto and coworkers, in a prospective evaluation of 25 patients with cholesterol emboli syndrome after cardiac catheterization, failed to show any significant association between the use of anticoagulants and cholesterol embolism.[42] In addition, anticoagulation has been advocated for patients with crescendo transient ischemic attacks (TIAs), a syndrome caused by atheromatous embolization to the eye or brain. Therefore, whether anticoagulation is associated with a higher incidence of atheroemboli remains controversial, but current literature suggests that it is safe to continue anticoagulation therapy in patients with a compelling reason to do so, such as atrial fibrillation or venous thromboembolism.

Thrombolysis

Atheromatous embolization has also been associated with thrombolytic therapy in case reports and small series,[30,31,33] but again, this is controversial. Thrombolytic agents act by converting plasminogen to plasmin, and plasmin directly degrades fibrin. Theoretically, any therapy that causes the thrombus to undergo lysis may leave atherosclerotic plaque uncovered, thus placing the patient at risk for embolization. In one small prospective study, however, no relationship between thrombolytic therapy and cholesterol emboli syndrome was found.[75]

EPIDEMIOLOGY

Atheromatous embolization usually affects elderly persons who have multiple risk factors for atherosclerosis, but it may occur in younger individuals with advanced atherosclerosis.[2] In a recent prospective study to identify risk factors for cholesterol embolism in patients undergoing cardiac catheterization, Fukumoto and coworkers confirmed that cholesterol emboli syndrome occurs more frequently in patients with generalized atherosclerosis such as multivessel coronary disease and cerebrovascular disease.[42] In addition, the authors found a significant relationship between C-reactive protein and cholesterol embolism (odds ratio 4.6 [P = .01] using multivariate analysis), indicating an important possible association between systemic inflammation and cholesterol emboli syndrome.

The increased frequency of this disease in males may be explained by the difference in the prevalence of atherosclerosis between the genders.[76] In addition, atheroemboli occur almost exclusively in patients older than 50 years.[76] A race predilection has also been reported, with atheroemboli less likely to occur in blacks than whites (32 : 1 ratio).[76,77] However, because blacks appear to have an increased prevalence of atherosclerosis, it has been suggested that this may actually represent a failure to recognize the classic features of this syndrome because of skin pigmentation and the propensity of black patients to develop renal failure secondary to poorly controlled blood pressure.

■ CLINICAL MANIFESTATIOS

Patients almost always have symptomatic atherosclerosis manifested clinically by angina, myocardial infarction, TIA, stroke, renal artery disease, mesenteric ischemia, or peripheral arterial disease and claudication.[78] Atheromatous embolization can present with myriad symptoms (Box 160-1).[17,79] In

---

Box 160-1 Clinical Manifestations of Atheromatous Embolization

SKIN
- Purple or blue toes
- Gangrenous digits
- Livedo reticularis
- Nodules

RENAL
- Uncontrolled hypertension
- Renal failure

NEUROLOGIC
- Transient ischemic attack
- Amaurosis fugax
- Stroke
- Hollenhorst plaque

CARDIAC
- Myocardial infarction or ishemia

GASTROINTESTINAL
- Abdominal pain
- Gastrointestinal bleeding
- Ischemic bowel
- Acute pancreatitis

CONSTITUTIONAL SYMPTOMS
- Fever
- Weight loss
- Malaise
- Anorexia

From Bartholomew JR, Olin JW. Atheromatous embolization. In: Young JR, Olin JW, Bartholomew JR, eds. *Peripheral Vascular Diseases.* 2nd ed. St. Louis: C.V. Mosby; 1996.

---

general, the organs involved by cholesterol embolism depend on the location of the embolic source. Atheroemboli from the ascending aorta and proximal aortic arch usually manifest with central nervous system or retinal pathology, whereas cholesterol crystal emboli originating from the descending thoracic or abdominal aorta affect the visceral organs and extremities. In general, bilateral lower extremity atheroemboli signify a source proximal to the aortic bifurcation, whereas unilateral emboli may originate either proximally or in any artery distal to the aortic bifurcation. Patients with macroemboli arising from one or more large atheromatous plaques may present with a catastrophic event such as an acutely ischemic limb or renal or mesenteric infarction.[34] Conversely, patients with microemboli may have milder localized signs or a clinical picture that suggests a systemic illness. There may be a delay of up to 8 weeks between the inciting event and clinical findings (especially for renal failure).[17]

Cutaneous Manifestations

Skin manifestations are among the most common clinical manifestations of atheromatous embolization, and the most common cutaneous features are livedo reticularis and blue toes.[80,81] The appearance of cutaneous signs can be delayed, with 50% of patients in one series showing skin signs of atheromatous embolization more than 30 days after their procedure or other inciting event.[80]

Livedo Reticularis

Livedo reticularis is a blue-red mottling or discoloration of the skin that occurs in a netlike pattern, most commonly seen on the buttocks, thighs, or legs (Fig. 160-4). A detailed skin examination performed with the patient in both the supine and the upright postures is necessary because livedo reticularis

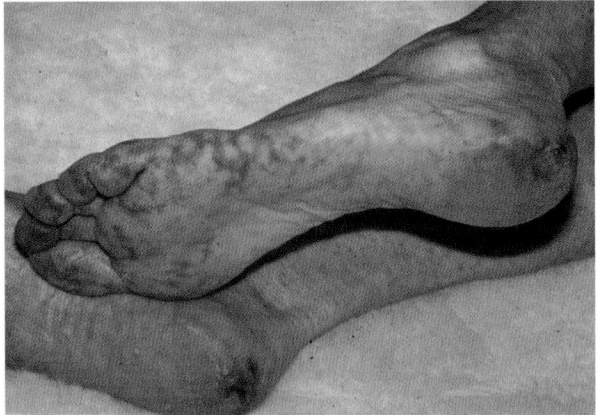

Figure 160-4 Classic livedo reticularis on the lateral portion of the left foot and on both heels. Note the blue (cyanotic) second and fourth toes. The involvement of both heels indicates that the lesion is above the aortic bifurcation. *(From Bartholomew JR, Olin JW. Atheromatous embolization. In: Young JR, Olin JW, Bartholomew JR, eds. Peripheral Vascular Diseases. 2nd ed. St Louis: C.V. Mosby; 1996.)*

is more readily demonstrable with the patient upright.[82] Livedo reticularis is most likely caused by the obstruction of small arteries, capillaries, or venules in the deep dermis.[12,24] When the skin is biopsied in patients with atheromatous embolization, cholesterol crystals may be seen in the dermal blood vessels. Livedo reticularis is not pathognomonic of atheroemboli, however; it has an extensive differential diagnosis, including but not limited to other causes of intravascular obstruction (e.g., antiphospholipid antibody syndrome, cryoglobulinemia, endocarditis, left atrial myxoma), vasculitis, and drug reactions (e.g., quinidine, quinine, amantidine, catecholamines).[83] There are also physiologic (cutis marmorata) and idiopathic (livedoid vasculitis) forms of livedo reticularis.[83] Livedo can occur in healthy young women and appears to be related to abnormal sensitivity of the dermal blood vessels to cold. The livedo reticularis pattern usually disappears on rewarming. Such patients should be reassured that there is no serious circulatory abnormality present.

Blue Toe Syndrome

Classically, blue toe syndrome presents as the sudden appearance of a cool, cyanotic, and painful toe in the presence of palpable distal pulses (Fig. 160-5A).[69,70,72,80] Discoloration may also be seen on the sole of the foot. The discoloration may be patchy, and comparison of both feet shows that the distribution is not symmetric. These lesions may progress to ulcer-

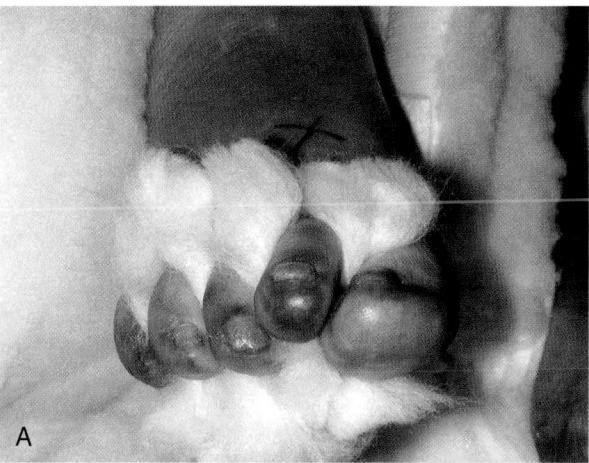
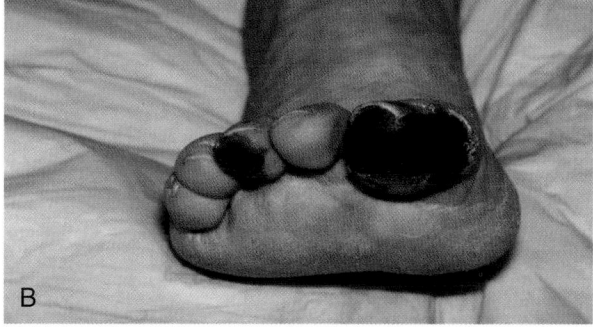

Figure 160-5 A, Typical appearance of the blue or purple toes that may occur with atheromatous embolization. **B,** More severe cases may progress to gangrene.

ation, necrosis, and frank gangrene (Fig. 160-5B).[12] Accessory lesions may be present on the lateral and posterior aspects of the heels, which later develop into linear fissures with skin-edge gangrene and a dark, necrotic base.

Other Skin Manifestations

Other skin manifestations include splinter hemorrhages, petechiae, purpura, ulcers,[84] and raised nodules that result from subepidermal inflammation surrounding the cholesterol crystals.[12,80] These nodules are painful, appear violaceous, have a necrotic center, and may mimic a necrotizing vasculitis such as polyarteritis nodosa or leukocytoclastic vasculitis. Ulceration of the penis and scrotum has also been described.[85]

Renal Involvement

The kidneys are a prime target for atheromatous embolization owing to the enormous amount of blood that flows through them, as well as the close proximity of the proximal renal arteries to the abdominal aorta, where atheromatous plaque is common.[23,24]

Incidence

Mayo and Swartz, in a review of 402 nephrology consultation charts, found that at least 4% of all inpatients examined had clinically detectable atheromatous embolization, representing approximately 5% to 10% of the acute renal failure patients encountered.[11] In 2000, Scolari and colleagues estimated that they encountered at least one case of atheroembolic renal disease each month.[12] Since that report, these investigators have accumulated 354 subjects who have been followed for an average of 2 years.[24] Most investigators believe that this condition is significantly underdiagnosed.[23,24]

Pathology

Pathologically, the classic lesion of atheroembolic renal disease is the occlusion of medium-sized arterioles (150 to 200 μm in diameter) and glomerular capillaries with cholesterol emboli.[12] In addition to the ischemic obstructive mechanical phenomenon produced at the onset, this pathologic condition produces an inflammatory reaction within the arterioles. The initial stages, occurring several days to weeks after the inciting event, are characterized by an inflammatory infiltration consisting of polymorphonuclear leukocytes, macrophages, and multinucleated giant cells. The cellular infiltrate leads to thickening and fibrosis of the arterioles, and later stages are characterized by glomerular sclerosis, tubular atrophy, and interstitial fibrosis.[17,23,86] A kidney biopsy specimen from a single patient may reveal different stages of histologic evolution as dislodged atheromatous debris is showered into the circulation at different times.[86] Furthermore, the involvement tends to be patchy, so a renal biopsy may not always show the classic pathologic lesions of this disease.[86]

Clinical Features

The net effect of this pathogenic process, when combined with varying amounts of atheromatous embolization, results in three somewhat different clinical presentations.[12,23,24] Marked renal impairment with an acute onset is the easiest form of atheroembolic renal disease to recognize. It has the closest temporal relationship to the inciting event and is generally considered the consequence of massive embolization. The subacute form of atheroembolic renal disease, the most frequently observed, is more insidious in onset, occurring a few weeks after the inciting event. Renal impairment may worsen over weeks to months owing to a foreign body reaction or the cyclic occurrence of cholesterol crystal embolic showers. This form of atheroembolism is more difficult to diagnose because patients usually come to medical attention with advanced renal failure and few clues that can identify the exact onset of renal impairment. Chronic stable renal impairment is the third form of atheroembolic renal disease and is generally asymptomatic. Clinical features tend to be similar to those of ischemic nephropathy and nephrosclerosis. The role of atheromatous embolization in this setting is somewhat unclear, and many patients are misdiagnosed because a renal biopsy is not performed or, if it is performed, atheromatous embolization is missed owing to the patchy distribution of the emboli.

Atheroembolic renal disease is often associated with poorly controlled hypertension.[17,71,72,87] When large segments of small arterioles are occluded, ischemic atrophy of substantial portions of the kidney occurs. As glomerular filtration declines, the renin-angiotensin-aldosterone system is activated, causing hypertension.[17] Severe, accelerated, labile, and malignant hypertension have all been reported, and atheroembolic renal disease should be strongly considered in patients who present with resistant hypertension.[87,88]

Prognosis

The renal outcome for patients with atheroembolic renal disease is variable. In early reports, the renal outcome was uniformly dismal, with progression over weeks or months to end-stage renal failure.[70,71] Over the past decade, however, spontaneous recovery of renal function in patients with atheroembolic renal disease has been reported in the literature, even after variable periods of dialysis support.[9,27,89,90] The improvement in renal function may be related to the reversal of inflammation, resolution of acute tubular necrosis in ischemic areas, and hypertrophy of surviving nephrons.[12,91] Despite these promising case reports, most patients with atheroembolic renal disease continue to have advanced chronic renal insufficiency or progress to end-stage renal disease requiring dialysis. In the large study by Scolari and associates, of the 354 subjects followed for an average of 2 years, 116 patients (32.7%) required dialysis therapy.[24] Eighty-three patients remained on maintenance dialysis therapy, and 33 were able to discontinue dialysis. Five patients restarted dialysis within 2 to 6 months of stopping therapy. Cumulative

renal survival probability was reduced by the presence of heart failure ($P < .001$), baseline chronic kidney disease categories ($P < .001$), age older than 70 years ($P < .039$), iatrogenic atheromatous embolization ($P < .001$), acute or subacute onset ($P < .001$), and leg ($P < .007$) or GI ($P < .001$) involvement. Statin treatment was associated with protective effects when already in place at the time of diagnosis and when initiated after diagnosis ($P < .001$). Multivariate analysis showed that the same factors plus diabetes were associated with a significantly increased risk of end-stage renal disease.

Gastrointestinal Involvement

Although this site is frequently overlooked, atheromatous embolization commonly occurs in the GI tract.

Incidence

The preferential involvement of the GI tract is probably a result of its rich vascular supply. Sites of GI involvement include the colon (up to 42% of cases), the small bowel (33%), and the stomach (12%).[4,92-94] Other areas of the digestive system that may be affected are the pancreas, liver, and gallbladder.[92,93,95,96] The pancreas and liver are frequent sites of atheromatous embolization, as indicated by autopsy reports; however, clinically overt pancreatitis and hepatitis are exceedingly rare presentations of atheromatous embolization.[96] In contrast, atheromatous embolization to the gallbladder, though even rarer, tends to be clinically significant, with a presentation ranging from chronic acalculous cholecystitis to acute gangrenous cholecystitis.[93]

Clinical Features

The most common manifestations of GI tract involvement are abdominal pain, diarrhea, and blood loss.[92] Abdominal pain may be caused by bowel ischemia, with or without infarction, or by fibrous stricture and bowel obstruction as a consequence of tissue repair after repeated showers of atheromatous embolization.[12] The pathogenesis of diarrhea may be related to multiple mechanisms, including mucosal inflammation, accumulation of luminal blood, and malabsorption.[92] GI bleeding is caused by superficial mucosal ulceration, erosions, and microinfarcts.[94]

The diagnosis of atheromatous embolization is rarely made by endoscopy alone. A variety of nonspecific lesions can be detected, including congestive or erythematous mucosa, erosions, ulcerations, necrosis, inflammatory polyps, and strictures.[2,9,94,96] Mucosal punch biopsies from the stomach, duodenum, or colon may be helpful in making the diagnosis, occasionally demonstrating the typical appearance of cholesterol crystals.[94]

Prognosis

The prognosis of patients with GI involvement tends to be poor, and the overall death rate is high. Patients with GI involvement commonly have multisystem atheromatous embolization syndrome. In a retrospective review of 10 patients with histologically proved cholesterol crystal emboli diagnosed by endoscopic GI biopsy, 5 patients died of atherosclerotic complications within 3 months after diagnosis (multisystem failure in 3, stroke in 1, and ruptured abdominal aortic aneurysm in 1). All these patients also had cutaneous manifestations and end-stage renal disease.[94]

Central Nervous System and Eye Involvement

Atheromatous embolization commonly occurs in the brain and eye and causes significant morbidity and mortality.[2]

Retinal

The culprit atherosclerotic plaques are located in the ascending aorta, aortic arch, carotid arteries, or vertebral arteries.[97,98] Patients may develop visual disturbances such as amaurosis fugax or variable degrees of blindness caused by central or branch retinal artery occlusion.[10] Retinal atheromatous embolization is evident as yellow, highly refractile plaques (Hollenhorst plaques) at arterial bifurcations on ophthalmoscopic examination (see Fig. 160-2).[10,99] In a study conducted from 2000 to 2005, 130 patients were analyzed with either Hollenhorst plaques or branch retinal artery occlusions.[100] There was a low rate of significant extracranial carotid artery disease among these patients (<30% in 68%, 30% to 60% in 22%, and >60% in 8%). Only 6 patients underwent carotid endarterectomy or stenting. With a medium follow-up of 22 months, no stroke or TIA occurred, and overall survival was 94% in this group of patients. Another group found that among the 3654 survivors of the Blue Mountain Eye Study, the cumulative incidence of retinal emboli was only 2.9%.[101] The authors believed that this was an underestimation of the true incidence, however, owing to the transient nature of emboli and differential loss to follow-up. The same authors assessed the relationship between retinal emboli and mortality in elderly patients.[102] Of the 8384 patients with retinal photographs available, 2506 (30%) died over a 10- to 12-year period. The cumulative mortality was higher in subjects with emboli than without (all causes, 56% versus 30%; stroke-related mortality, 12% versus 4%; cardiovascular mortality, 30% versus 16%).

Cerebral

Cerebral cholesterol embolism may manifest as TIA, stroke, confusional state, headache, dizziness, or organic brain syndrome.[9,97,103] In a retrospective review of 29 patients with autopsy-proven brain cholesterol emboli, encephalopathy was the predominant finding on neurologic examination.[104] This is most likely due to the diffuse and bihemispheric nature of atheromatous embolization. Involvement of the spinal cord artery, which can lead to lower extremity paralysis, has been rarely reported.[105] A case history comprising a procedure involving the ascending thoracic aorta, acute renal failure, and encephalopathy in an elderly patient should raise the suspicion of cholesterol emboli to the brain. Radiologic studies can be helpful by showing multiple small ischemic lesions or border-zone infarcts.

Other Areas

Atheromatous embolization can occur in virtually any organ. Cardiac manifestations include angina pectoris and myocardial infarction. The usual source in these circumstances is the aortic root or proximal coronary artery.[106] Pulmonary involvement has rarely been reported in the context of cholesterol embolism.[107,108] Hemoptysis and dyspnea are the most common respiratory symptoms described. The pathogenesis of pulmonary involvement may be related to direct deposition of atheroemboli in the lungs[109] or de novo production of pulmonary lesions as a result of systemic inflammation associated with cholesterol embolism.[110] Atheromatous emboli have also been demonstrated in the spleen, bone marrow,[111] muscle, prostate, thyroid, and adrenal glands in autopsy studies.[2,69-71] Nonspecific findings such as fever, weight loss, headache, and myalgia have been reported and may suggest a multisystem illness (see Box 160-1).[9,27,112]

DIAGNOSIS

The diagnosis of atheromatous embolization syndrome remains a significant challenge for physicians. The symptoms and signs are nonspecific and diverse, which explains why this disease is sometimes referred to as the "great masquerader."[13,112] For this reason, a high index of suspicion and a thorough understanding of the various clinical manifestations are needed to make the correct diagnosis antemortem. The diagnosis can often be made on clinical grounds alone, without histologic evaluation, in a patient who has a precipitating event, acute or subacute renal failure, difficult-to-control hypertension, and evidence of peripheral embolization.[9]

In the absence of obvious clinical clues, definitive diagnosis may require a biopsy. The highest yield for histologic confirmation is in the skin in patients exhibiting livedo reticularis or in an affected organ, such as an amputated extremity in a patient presenting with gangrenous toes, the kidney in a patient with new-onset renal failure, or the GI tract in a patient with abdominal pain and GI bleeding. However, in one older series, random biopsies of the gastrocnemius and quadriceps muscles were helpful in making the diagnosis.[113] It is rarely necessary to pursue a blind biopsy to make a diagnosis of atheromatous embolization.

Laboratory Tests

No specific laboratory tests are diagnostic of atheromatous embolization. Eosinophilia can be found in up to 80% of cases and is probably related to the generation of complement C5, which has chemotactic properties for eosinophils.[114] The eosinophilia, however, tends to be transient and short-lived.[2,22]

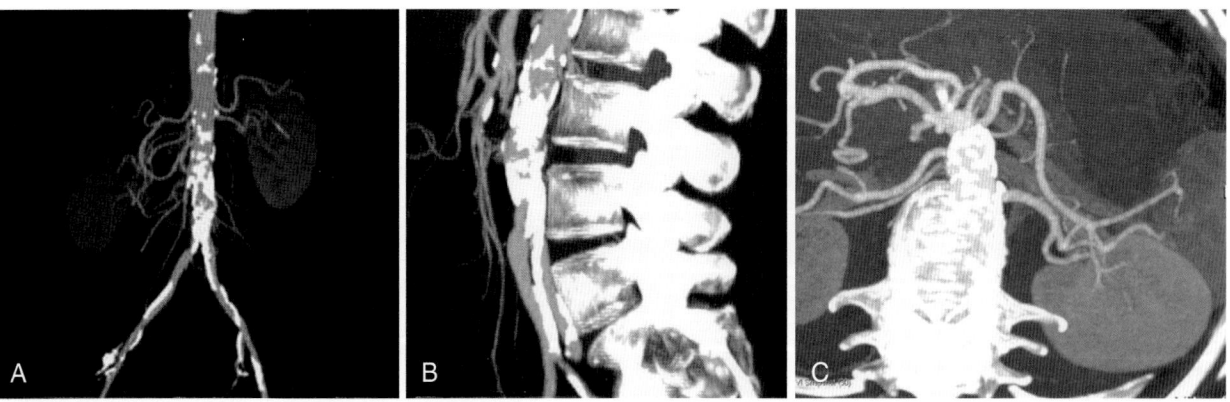

Figure 160-6 Reformatted anteroposterior (**A**), lateral (**B**), and axial (**C**) views from 64-slice multidetector CTA demonstrate marked calcified atherosclerotic disease in the abdominal aorta.

Laboratory markers of inflammation, including C-reactive protein, fibrinogen, and erythrocyte sedimentation rate, are elevated in many patients.[70] Other reported laboratory findings include leukocytosis, anemia, thrombocytopenia, and decreased complement levels.[69,70,115] Laboratory data may also reflect specific organ involvement. Elevations in serum levels of amylase, hepatic transaminases, blood urea nitrogen and creatinine, and creatinine phosphokinase may be seen with involvement of the pancreas, liver, kidney, and muscle, respectively. Mild proteinuria, microhematuria, and hyaline or granular casts are the most common urinary findings in patients with confirmed cholesterol embolism.[70,116] Nephrotic-range proteinuria and eosinophiluria have been reported less commonly.[21,116,117]

Imaging Modalities

Invasive vascular procedures requiring aortic instrumentation should be avoided as a diagnostic modality owing to the risk of producing recurrent atheroembolism. Noninvasive imaging studies such as multidetector CTA, magnetic resonance angiography, and TEE can assist in confirming the diagnosis if a markedly irregular and shaggy aorta is demonstrated (Fig. 160-6). These imaging modalities only show that the patient has significant underlying atherosclerosis; they cannot determine whether the patient has embolized from these atherosclerotic lesions.

■ DIFFERENTIAL DIAGNOSIS

Diseases that should be considered in the differential diagnosis include, but are not limited to, contrast nephropathy, acute tubular necrosis (ATN) from ischemic injury, necrotizing vasculitis, leukocytoclastic vasculitis, thrombotic thrombocytopenic purpura, antiphospholipid antibody syndrome, and multiple myeloma. Thromboembolism from the heart or aneurysms and other cardiac sources of emboli, such as atrial myxoma, nonbacterial thrombotic endocarditis, and infective endocarditis, should always be excluded.[118]

No laboratory test uniformly helps in the diagnosis of atheroembolic disease. The peripheral blood eosinophilia,

hypocomplementemia, elevated sedimentation rate, and increased level of C-reactive protein seen in these patients are nonspecific findings that can also occur in patients with systemic or renal vasculitis.[112,119] Atheroembolic disease should be distinguished from vasculitis on the basis of other clinical findings and histology. The urine sediment in patients with atheroembolic renal disease is usually benign or shows only microhematuria. Rarely, eosinophiluria may be present.[120] By contrast, the urine sediment in patients with ATN often demonstrates pigmented (dirty-brown) casts and renal tubular cells. Atheroembolic renal disease can be further differentiated from ATN or contrast nephropathy based on the time frame of renal impairment. In contrast nephropathy and ATN, the renal failure occurs within 48 to 72 hours after the inciting event, whereas in patients with atherombolic renal disease, the rise in creatinine is often delayed for 7 to 10 days.[17,23,24,79] In addition, full recovery of renal function is the rule for contrast nephropathy and ATN if the underlying precipitating factor is corrected, whereas it is the exception in atheroembolic renal disease.[12,17] There are, however, examples of late recovery of renal function in patients with atheroemboli.[121] ATN is further characterized by normal blood pressure levels, as opposed to the severe and refractory hypertension present in many patients with atheroembolic renal disease. Other disorders mentioned earlier that can mimic atheromatous embolization owing to their multisystem involvement should be excluded through appropriate diagnostic studies.

■ TREATMENT

There have been no randomized controlled trials of any therapeutic intervention for patients with atheromatous embolization, and no agent has been strongly correlated with favorable outcomes in case series. Clearly, as noted earlier, the most important aspect of therapy is prevention. Once atheromatous embolization has occurred, therapy is mostly supportive. Avoiding other inciting events such as aortic manipulation, good control of hypertension and heart failure, dialysis support, and adequate nutrition are the mainstays of treatment.[9,72] Symptomatic care of the end-organ where the emboli are located and risk factor modification to prevent myocardial infarction, stroke, and progression of atherosclerotic disease are also important treatment goals.[79,122]

Medical Therapy

Pathologic descriptions of cholesterol embolism highlight the severe inflammatory reaction that contributes to vascular obstruction. Although the inflammatory process caused by atheromatous embolization may suggest a role for anti-inflammatory agents,[22] the use of corticosteroids has had conflicting results. Dahlberg and associates report a rapid and dramatic improvement in the manifestations of peripheral embolization in two patients given prednisone (60 mg/day) or methylprednisolone (80 mg/day) for 5 days.[73] More recent case reports describe improvement in renal function in patients with suspected atheromatous embolization given corticosteroid therapy.[123-127] Corticosteroid administration is also helpful in relieving symptoms related to mesenteric ischemia, such as abdominal pain and food intolerance, and for ischemic leg pain.[9] In contrast, in a series of 67 patients, 18 of whom were treated with corticosteroids, no survival benefit could be attributed directly to this therapy.[9] Finally, in a large retrospective series, Falanga and colleagues found that corticosteroid use was associated with 100% mortality.[80] Based on the available literature, corticosteroid use cannot be recommended on a routine basis for this patient population.

Statins are reportedly beneficial in the treatment of livedo reticularis caused by atheromatous embolization,[128] as well as in the treatment of renal[129] and lower limb cholesterol emboli syndrome.[130] Furthermore, in a retrospective analysis of 519 patients with severe thoracic aortic plaque visualized on TEE, multivariate analysis showed that statin use was independently protective against recurrent embolic events ($P = .0001$).[131] The mechanism of the beneficial effects of statin therapy is most likely related to the plaque-stabilizing activity of these drugs.

Iloprost, a prostacyclin analogue, is a potent vasodilator and antiplatelet agent. In a report of four cases of atheromatous embolization, intravenous iloprost improved both ischemia of the distal extremities and renal failure.[132] Another report suggested that prostaglandin E_1 was helpful in improving renal failure and blue toe syndrome in a single patient.[133] Anecdotally, the prostaglandin analogues appear to be beneficial in the healing of ischemic ulcerations associated with atheroemboli. It is not known whether this class of drug is effective in patients with atheroembolic renal failure.

Low-density lipoprotein (LDL) apheresis, with or without the addition of steroids, is effective in improving skin manifestations.[134,135] Hasegawa and Sugiyana showed that combining corticosteroids and LDL apheresis improved atheroembolism related to blue toe syndrome.[134] The mechanism is unknown; however, it is postulated to improve blood viscosity by removing high- molecular-weight substances, decreasing total and oxidized LDL, improving endothelial function, and reducing circulating inflammatory cytokines and chemokines.[134,135]

Other forms of therapy that have been advocated include antiplatelet agents such as aspirin[69,70,136] and dipyridamole, low-molecular-weight dextran, intra-arterial papaverine, pentoxifylline,[137] and platelet infusions to help stabilize the source of atheroemboli.[30] Unfortunately, no controlled trials have shown that any of these therapies are beneficial.

All patients should receive aggressive risk factor modification with an antiplatelet agent (aspirin, clopidogrel, or both), a statin, and an angiotensin-converting enzyme inhibitor, all of which can improve mortality in patients with underlying atherosclerotic disease.[79,138-143]

Surgical Therapy

Surgical therapy for atheroembolic disease includes, first and foremost, elimination of the embolic source and, secondarily, arterial reconstruction of any hemodynamically significant proximal occlusive disease to encourage healing through improved end-arterial bed perfusion. Two prospective series reported favorable outcomes with vascular resection of atherosclerotic segments of large arteries identified as the source of previous cholesterol crystal embolism.[144,145] However, when the suprarenal aorta was involved, greater mortality rates were observed, likely related to the risk for visceral and renal ischemia or atheroemboli.[144] Thus, according to some investigators, surgical elimination of the presumed source of atheromatous embolization should be reserved for patients with lower limb ischemia and an infrarenal source of embolization.[12]

Given the frequent instability of these lesions, surgical treatment has been perceived as safer than endovascular approaches because the surgeon can clamp the artery proximal and distal to the lesion before manipulating the diseased vessel in an attempt to decrease the risk of recurrent embolization.[146] Lin and coworkers, in a retrospective study, found that recurrent atheroembolism and amputation rates in surgically treated patients were 0% and 20%, respectively; this was in sharp contrast to the outcomes of patients treated with endovascular therapy, whose recurrent atheroembolism and amputation rates were 33% and 66%, respectively.[52] Thromboendarterectomy or resection and graft replacement have been the surgical approaches most commonly used.[147] In patients who are too weak for major surgical intervention, ligation of the external iliac arteries or common femoral arteries followed by an extra-anatomic bypass (e.g., axillobifemoral bypass) has been advocated.[147,148] Ligation prevents further embolization from reaching the legs, although embolization to the kidneys and intestines may still occur.

Endovascular Therapy

There are several reports of intra-arterial treatment of embolizing lesions, including thrombolytic administration,[149,150] percutaneous atherectomy,[151,152] balloon angioplasty,[149,150] and stent implantation.[153,154] Intra-arterial thrombolytic administration in isolation is controversial. By destroying the platelet-fibrin thrombus that covers the atheromatous, ulcerated plaques, fibrinolysis may allow the liberation of the cholesterol crystals into the arterial circulation, with consequent microembolization. There are no data on whether the adjunctive use of tissue plasminogen activator augments clot extraction in combination with endovascular interventions.

In percutaneous transluminal angioplasty, the intima is cracked and remolded; thus, theoretically, the chance of distal embolization may be increased. However, anecdotal reports of this approach have shown symptomatic improvement in leg pain, re-establishment of peripheral pulses, and no evidence of recurrent embolization. Stent placement in conjunction with angioplasty may provide a protective scaffold to help secure these lesions. However, a potential risk of recurrent atheroembolism may exist owing to either plaque dislodgement or extrusion of atheromatous material through stent interstices at the time of stent placement.

The possibility of distal embolization caused by stent placement was highlighted in a recent study by Ohki and associates that demonstrated a significant risk of distal embolization secondary to intra-arterial stent placement in an ex vivo carotid endarterectomy model.[155] Lin and coworkers found that operative procedures, either bypass or endarterectomy, appeared to provide a superior result over intraluminal stent placement.[52] This was evidenced by no recurrent atheroembolism in the surgical patients, whereas 66% of patients treated with iliac stents developed recurrent atheroembolism. In contrast, Matchett and colleagues, in a retrospective report of 15 patients treated with stent placement for blue toe syndrome, found no procedure-related embolization and only one recurrent embolization in follow-up.[153] Renshaw and coworkers reported successful angioplasty with stenting in eight patients with unilateral blue toe syndrome.[156] Symptoms resolved in all patients over the ensuing month, and there were no recurrences with a mean follow-up of 18.5 months.

The short-term results in studies of percutaneous atherectomy, in which the plaque is shaved off the wall of the vessel and removed through a collection device, are similar to those of percutaneous transluminal angioplasty or surgery.[151,152]

The availability of covered stent-grafts has raised the question of their potential utility in the management of patients with distal atheroembolic lesions. Covered stents offer the advantage of completely excluding the diseased segment, preventing the escape of thrombus or plaque debris. Kumins and colleagues reported on the successful use of the Wallgraft endoprosthesis in two patients with distal microembolism from common iliac artery pathology.[157]

Carroccio and associates recently reported on endovascular stent-graft repair of abdominal aortic aneurysms in 16 patients presenting with atheromatous embolization syndrome.[158] The 30-day mortality was 0%, and the aneurysm was successfully excluded in 88% of patients. Resolution of foot ischemia and prevention of further atheromatous embolization occurred in 89% of the patients still alive at 1 year. Six patients died during a mean follow-up of 26 months, illustrating the high mortality in this patient population.

Because of the limited studies available regarding the role of endovascular therapy for atheromatous embolization, its clinical efficacy is difficult to compare with operative treatment. Undoubtedly, further clinical evaluation is warranted to further validate endovascular therapy in the treatment of atheroembolism.

Pain Control

Pain control is a critical aspect of the management of peripheral cholesterol embolism. The degree of pain associated with lower extremity ischemic and necrotic lesions secondary to cholesterol embolism is generally severe and disproportionate to the extent of tissue involvement. Sympathectomy has received attention as a surgical method for the palliation of atheroembolic lesions. Lee and associates demonstrated that adjunctive sympathectomy resulted in improved healing of distal digital ischemic ulcers.[159] Sympathectomy is easily performed during aortic procedures, or it can be achieved postoperatively through lumbar sympathetic block or laparoscopic techniques.

More recently, Ghilardi and coworkers reported on two cases of inferior limb ischemia secondary to cholesterol embolism treated with the temporary surgical implantation of spinal cord stimulation devices.[160] Spinal cord stimulation provided rapid and effective pain control in the reported cases as well as improvement in peripheral microcirculation, manifested by the rapid resolution of necrotic lesions within 4 to 6 weeks. In addition to being an adjunct to the direct surgical treatment of the offending arterial segment, these procedures may be useful to control the pain of severe atheroembolic lower extremity lesions in patients who are not candidates for direct reconstruction of the embolic source or when correction of the embolic source does not improve distal perfusion.

◼ OUTCOME

In general, the prognosis of patients with atheroembolic disease is poor, most likely related to the severe and diffuse atherosclerosis in this patient population. The course varies, however, depending on the clinical presentation. Patients with symptoms limited to an extremity tend to have a better prognosis than those with disseminated cholesterol crystal embolization, particularly when there is evidence of visceral and renal involvement. The reported 1-year mortality in four different reports varied from 64% to 81%.[21,70,72,73] Causes of death were multifactorial and included cardiac, central nervous system, and GI ischemia.

◼ SPECIAL CONSIDERATIONS
Atheroembolism Arising from the Thoracic Aorta

The importance of the thoracic aorta as a source of cerebral and peripheral vascular emboli has been ascertained only recently.

Epidemiology

Tunick and coworkers, in a retrospective study comparing 122 patients with a history of stroke, TIA, or peripheral emboli with 122 age- and sex-matched controls, found protruding atheromas to be an independent risk factor for embolic symptoms.[161] Plaques located proximal to the ostium of the left subclavian artery were found in 60% of patients 60 years of age or older with ischemic stroke; plaques greater than 4 mm thick had the strongest association.[162] Similar results were found in an autopsy study in which ulcerated plaques in the ascending aorta and aortic arch, which included both atheromatous material and thrombus, were significantly more prevalent in those who had suffered cerebral embolic events.[163]

A separate issue—the role of aortic plaque as a predictor of subsequent stroke and other embolic events—has been evaluated in prospective studies.[164,165] Three studies, in which patients who had sustained recent strokes were followed prospectively, showed an association between aortic arch atherosclerosis and cerebral or peripheral embolic events.[166-168] Tunick and colleagues found a 33% annual event rate of vascular events in patients who had protruding plaques greater than 5 mm thick in the thoracic aorta, compared with 7% in matched control subjects.[167] In a similar study, Mitusch and associates found a significantly higher rate of vascular events in patients with complex plaques (>5 mm thick or with mobile components) on echocardiographic examination compared with those having only moderate atherosclerosis (13.7% versus 4.1% per 100 person-years, respectively).[168] Davila-Roman and colleagues, in a prospective, long-term follow-up study of 1957 patients undergoing cardiac surgery, found atherosclerosis of the ascending aorta to be an independent predictor of long-term neurologic events and mortality.[166] Based on these echocardiographic and pathologic studies, the overall vascular risk arising from advanced atherosclerosis of the thoracic aorta may be as high as that from established sources of embolism, including nonvalvular atrial fibrillation, left atrial thrombi, or severe stenosis of the internal carotid artery origin.[162]

Risk Profile

The vascular risk attributable to complex atherosclerosis of the thoracic aorta appears to be correlated mainly with plaque thickness and the morphologic parameters associated with plaques. TEE of the ascending aorta and aortic arch has been used to identify plaque size and morphology as risk factors for embolic events (Fig. 160-7). A review from the French Study of Aortic Plaques in Stroke Group included 331 patients with an initial ischemic stroke who were followed for 2 to 4 years.[44] Patients were divided into groups based on aortic plaque thickness: greater than 4 mm, 1 to 3.9 mm, and less than 1 mm. At follow-up, the patients with plaque thickness greater than 4 mm had a significantly greater incidence of recurrent stroke and vascular events (Table 160-1). Analysis of a 788–person-year follow-up to determine the effect of plaque morphology on the risk of ischemic disease demonstrated that

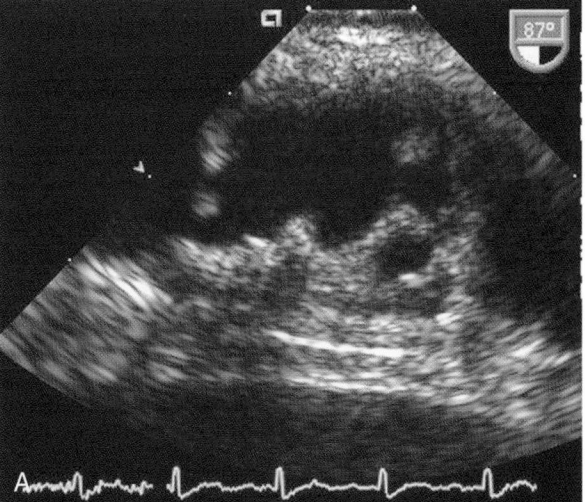
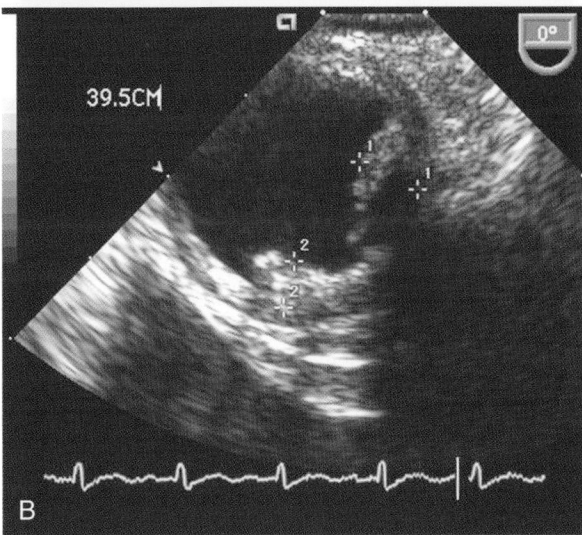

Figure 160-7 Transesophageal echocardiogram demonstrates mobile (seen on real-time imaging), protruding aortic atheromas located in the aortic arch (**A**) and descending thoracic aorta (**B**). This patient had multiple strokes due to atheromatous embolization from the ascending aorta and aortic arch.

the only plaque morphology that increased the risk of ischemic events was the absence of plaque calcification.[162] Ulceration and hypoechoic plaques had no predictive value in evaluating vascular events. Overall, it was determined that aortic plaques greater than 4 mm thick increase the risk of vascular events, and this risk is further increased by the lack of plaque calcification. These authors hypothesized that noncalcified plaques are probably lipid-laden plaques with thin, fibrous caps, which are unstable and prone to ulceration, rupture, and thrombosis.[169] Pedunculated, mobile plaques have also been associated with an increased risk of recurrent embolization.[161,170,171]

Treatment

In addition to being valuable markers of severe, widespread atherosclerosis,[162,163] complex thoracic aortic plaques identify

Table 160-1 Incidence of Vascular Events Relative to Plaque Thickness in the Aortic Arch Proximal to the Ostium of the Left Subclavian Artery

Plaque Thickness (mm)	Recurrent Brain Infarction			Any Vascular Event*		
	Person-Years of Follow-up	Number of Events	Incidence per 100 Person-Years of Follow-up	Person-Years of Follow-up	Number of Events	Incidence per 100 Person-Years of Follow-up
<1	359.3	10	2.8	354.0	21	5.9
1-3.9	312.6	11	3.5	308.2	28	9.1
≥4	92.4	11	11.9	88.4	23	26.0

*Includes brain infarction, myocardial infarction, peripheral embolism, and death from vascular causes.
From The French Study of Aortic Plaques in Stroke Group. Atherosclerotic disease of the aortic arch as a risk factor for recurrent ischemic stroke. *N Engl J Med.* 1996;334:1216-1221.

individuals at high risk for cardiovascular events—approximately 26 per 100 person-years in one study.[44] There are no clear guidelines on the most appropriate therapy for these patients. Data concerning the efficacy of anticoagulation in patients with complex thoracic aortic plaques are conflicting. Ferrari and coworkers used TEE in a prospective cohort to compare antiplatelet therapy with anticoagulation therapy and found that patients treated with antiplatelet agents had more combined vascular events and a higher mortality rate than patients treated with oral anticoagulants.[172] Similar results were reported by Dressler and colleagues, who found that patients with mobile aortic atheromas not receiving warfarin had a higher incidence of vascular events than those receiving warfarin treatment (27% of the former had strokes, versus 0% of the latter).[171] Conversely, a recent retrospective study showed that warfarin had no significant effect on the risk of vascular events.[131] Based on the evidence to date, it seems reasonable to follow the recommendation of the 2001 Sixth American College of Chest Physicians Consensus Conference on Antithrombotic Therapy, which is to prescribe warfarin therapy in patients with mobile aortic atheromas or aortic plaques greater than 4 mm as measured by TEE who have had an embolic event.[173] It should be recognized that this recommendation is not based on randomized controlled trials.

Lipid-lowering therapy, primarily with a statin, is warranted in all patients with symptomatic atherosclerotic vascular disease.[143] In a retrospective analysis of patients with complex aortic arch plaques, statin therapy independently and significantly reduced the risk of embolic events.[167]

Finally, surgical treatment of thoracic aorta atherosclerosis may be considered. Surgical therapy cannot be recommended routinely for asymptomatic patients because the risks of such a complex procedure outweigh the benefits.[174] However, performing aortic arch endarterectomy or aortic resection along with a planned cardiac procedure if severe atheromatous disease is discovered has been addressed. Stern and coworkers reported a large increase in intraoperative stroke and mortality when surgery was performed to limit the risk of stroke after cardiopulmonary bypass.[175] At this time, in the absence of randomized controlled trials, surgical indications for aortic endarterectomy should be restricted to highly selected patients with a low operative risk who have had multiple documented embolic events despite optimal medical treatment.[169]

SELECTED KEY REFERENCES

Belenfant X, Meyrier A, Jacquot C. Supportive treatment improves survival in multivisceral cholesterol crystal embolism. *Am J Kidney Dis.* 1999;33:840-850.
A standardized treatment program for patients with disseminated cholesterol embolization to address the leading causes of death: recurrent embolization, cardiovascular events, renal failure, and nutrition.

Falanga V, Fine MJ, Kapoor WN. The cutaneous manifestations of cholesterol crystal embolization. *Arch Dermatol.* 1986;122:1194-1198.
Detailed review of the skin findings in patients with atheromatous embolization.

The French Study of Aortic Plaques in Stroke Group. Atherosclerotic disease of the aortic arch as a risk factor for recurrent ischemic stroke. *N Engl J Med.* 1996;334:1216-1221.
Using TEE, the authors demonstrated that the thicker the plaque in the aorta, the greater the likelihood of recurrent brain infarction and cardiovascular events.

Kronzon I, Tunick PA. Aortic atherosclerotic disease and stroke. *Circulation.* 2006;114:63-75.
Comprehensive review by two experienced clinicians of the role of aortic atherosclerosis in recurrent stroke and cardiovascular events.

Mittal BV, Alexander MP, Rennke HG, Singh AK. Atheroembolic renal disease: a silent masquerader. *Kidney Int.* 2008;73:126-130.
Comprehensive review of atheroembolic renal disease.

Scolari F, Ravani P, Gaggi R, Santostefano M, Rollino C, Stabellini N, Colla L, Viola BF, Maiorca P, Venturelli C, Bonardelli S, Faggiano P, Barrett BJ. The challenge of diagnosing atheroembolic renal disease: clinical features and prognostic factors. *Circulation.* 2007; 116:298-304.
Large series with a detailed discussion of the clinical manifestations and outcomes of patients with atheroembolic renal disease.

Tunick PA, Nayar AC, Goodkin GM, Mirchandani S, Francescone S, Rosenzweig BP, Freedberg RS, Katz ES, Applebaum RM, Kronzon I; NYU Atheroma Group. Effect of treatment on the incidence of stroke and other emboli in 519 patients with severe thoracic aortic plaque. *Am J Cardiol.* 2002;90:1320-1325.
Retrospective study of 519 patients with severe aortic plaque on TEE demonstrating that statins are protective against recurrent atheroembolic events, whereas antiplatelet agents and warfarin are not.

REFERENCES

The reference list can be found on the companion Expert Consult Web site at *www.expertconsult.com.*

CHAPTER 161

Complex Regional Pain Syndrome

Ali F. AbuRahma

Complex regional pain syndrome (CRPS), previously called post-traumatic pain syndrome (PTPS), causalgia, or reflex sympathetic dystrophy (RSD), is one of the most poorly understood and frequently misdiagnosed entities encountered in clinical practice. This painful condition can develop after damage to peripheral nerves in a variety of settings. In susceptible patients, the initiating event may be relatively insignificant or even obscure.

ETIOLOGY AND INCIDENCE

The exact incidence of CRPS is unknown, but it has been estimated to occur in at least 1% to 12% of patients with peripheral nerve injury.[1] Three causes of CRPS have been identified: traumatic, nontraumatic, and idiopathic.

Traumatic

Traumatic causes include fracture, dislocation, sprain, crush injury, burn, and iatrogenic injury. Most cases of CRPS are post-traumatic. CRPS has been reported in 0.2% to 11% of patients with Colles fracture[2] and in 12% to 20% of patients with hemiplegia.[3] The incidence of CRPS type II (as defined later) has varied from as low as 1.5% in the Vietnam War to 8% in the Persian Gulf War[4] to as high as 32% in the Civil War.[5] CRPS has also been reported in patients with spinal cord and brain injuries, with an incidence of 5% to 12%.[4,6]

Recently, Hassantash and colleagues reported the results of a meta-analysis of the literature on causalgia.[7] The 110 articles contained a total of 1528 cases of causalgia. High-velocity missiles caused at least 77% of the injuries. The median nerve, alone or in combination with other nerves (56%), and the sciatic nerve (60%) were most commonly involved. In 92% of cases the nerve injury was incomplete.

Nontraumatic

Nontraumatic causes include prolonged bed rest, neoplasm, metabolic bone disease, deep venous thrombosis, myocardial infarction, and stroke. The incidence of CRPS in patients with myocardial ischemia is between 5% and 20%.[4] Chronic painful conditions of the upper extremity subsequent to myocardial infarction have been grouped into a category designated *shoulder-hand syndrome*. These conditions have been reported in 15% of patients,[1] but this percentage has been reduced significantly because of much more rapid postinfarct mobilization.[8]

Idiopathic

In idiopathic CRPS, no cause can be identified.

CLASSIFICATION AND TERMINOLOGY

Box 161-1 lists more than 40 terms that describe CRPS. The most common include *causalgia*, both minor and major (*causalgia* is derived from the Greek *causos*, meaning "heat," and *algos*, meaning "pain"—that is, a burning pain)[9]; *minor* and *major traumatic dystrophy*, describing the intensity of the syndrome when it develops after an injury that does not damage a peripheral nerve; *shoulder-hand syndrome*, or RSD involving the entire upper extremity; and *Sudeck's atrophy*, a post-traumatic reflex dystrophy with bone involvement demonstrable on radiographs.

To resolve the confusion surrounding the various terms used to describe this syndrome, Stanton-Hicks and associates convened a consensus committee of the International Association for the Study of Pain to discuss the nomenclature of causalgia and RSD.[10] As a result, the term *complex regional pain syndrome* was developed to replace the terms *causalgia* and *reflex sympathetic dystrophy*. CRPS includes a spectrum of conditions with somewhat similar clinical manifestations that often are grouped together for the sake of clinical utility.[11] Hallmarks of this syndrome include dysfunction and pain of a duration or severity out of proportion to what might be expected from the initiating event. The new classification scheme is based on a descriptive method that should allow future modifications to reflect new scientific findings.[10-12]

Summary of Key Features

Three components characterize CRPS:

1. *Complex.* This term denotes the dynamic and varied nature of the clinical presentation in a single person over time and among persons with seemingly similar disorders. It also reflects the autonomic, cutaneous, motor, inflammatory, and dystrophic changes that distinguish this syndrome from other forms of neuropathic pain.
2. *Regional.* This term describes the wide distribution of clinical symptoms and findings beyond the area of the original lesion. This is considered a key characteristic of the syn-

Box 161-1 Terms Used to Describe Complex Regional Pain Syndrome

- Acute atrophy of bones
- Algodystrophy
- Algoneurodystrophy
- Causalgia
- Causalgia-like states
- Chronic segmental arterial spasm
- Chronic traumatic edema
- Disuse phenomenon
- Homans' minor causalgia
- Major causalgia
- Mimocausalgia
- Minor causalgia
- Mitchell's causalgia
- Painful osteoporosis
- Peripheral trophoneurosis
- Post-traumatic dystrophy
- Post-traumatic fibrosis
- Post-traumatic neurovascular pain syndrome
- Post-traumatic osteoporosis
- Post-traumatic pain syndrome
- Post-traumatic painful osteoporosis
- Post-traumatic spreading neuralgia
- Post-traumatic sympathalgia
- Post-traumatic sympathetic dysfunction
- Post-traumatic sympathetic dystrophy
- Post-traumatic vasomotor disorder
- Reflex dystrophy
- Reflex dystrophy of the extremities
- Reflex nervous dystrophy
- Reflex neurovascular dystrophy
- Reflex sympathetic dystrophy
- Shoulder-hand syndrome
- Steinbrocker's shoulder-hand syndrome
- Sudeck's atrophy
- Sudeck's osteodystrophy
- Sudeck's syndrome
- Sympathalgia
- Sympathetic neurovascular dystrophy
- Traumatic angiospasm
- Traumatic edema
- Traumatic neuralgia
- Traumatic vasospasm

drome. The distal part of a limb is usually affected, but occasionally CRPS occurs in other parts of the body (e.g., the face or torso) and may spread to other body parts.

3. *Pain.* The hallmark of CRPS is pain that is out of proportion to the initiating event. The designation refers to spontaneous burning pain and thermally or mechanically induced allodynia (i.e., pain from stimuli that are not normally painful).

Syndrome Types

Two types of CRPS have been recognized. Type I corresponds to the former term *RSD*, and type II corresponds to

the former term *causalgia*. The definitions of CRPS types I and II contain criteria that exclude (1) pain and other findings that are physiologically, anatomically, and temporally appropriate to some form of injury, and (2) myofascial pain syndrome. The terms *sympathetically maintained pain* (SMP) and *sympathetically independent pain* (SIP) are used to describe types of pain that can be associated with a variety of pain disorders, including CRPS types I and II.

Diagnostic Criteria

The diagnostic criteria for CRPS type I, as adapted from Stanton-Hicks and coworkers[12] and Merskey and Bogduk,[13] are as follows:

- History of an inciting noxious event.
- Spontaneous pain, hyperalgesia, or allodynia beyond the territory of a single peripheral nerve and disproportionate to the initiating event.
- Edema, skin blood-flow abnormality, or abnormal sudomotor activity in the region of the pain that has developed since the initiating event.
- Absence of other conditions that would account for the degree of dysfunction and pain.

The diagnostic criteria for CRPS type II are as follows:

- History of a nerve injury.
- Spontaneous allodynia or pain is not necessarily limited to the region of the injured nerve.
- Edema, temperature and skin blood-flow changes, abnormal sudomotor activity, or motor dysfunction in the region of the pain that has developed since the original nerve injury.
- Absence of other conditions that would account for the degree of dysfunction and pain.

■ PATHOGENESIS
Theories and Components

Many theories have been proposed to explain CRPS, but none has been universally accepted. Most were developed to explain the causalgia associated with nerve injury (CRPS type II).

Artificial Synapses. The most popular theory is that of "artificial synapses" occurring at the site of a nerve injury, as first proposed by Doupe and colleagues.[14] According to this theory, a "short circuit" occurs at the point of partial nerve interruption or demyelinization, which allows efferent sympathetic impulses to be relayed back along afferent somatic fibers. Such an artificial synapse has been demonstrated experimentally in crushed nerves,[14] and the interruption of sympathetic efferent impulses may explain the warm, red, dry extremity seen initially in cases of major causalgia.

One piece of evidence weighing against this theory is the demonstration that nerve blockade with local anesthetic beyond the site of the nerve injury (and presumably beyond this artificial synapse) sometimes brings relief.[15,16]

Vicious Circle of Reflexes. In the late 1930s, Livingston proposed that causalgia consists of a vicious circle of reflexes with three components: (1) chronic irritation of a peripheral sensory nerve with increasingly frequent afferent impulses, (2) abnormal heightened activity in the "internuncial pool" in the anterior horn of the spinal cord, and (3) increased efferent sympathetic activity.[17] Livingston's theory explains a number of characteristics of CRPS type I that cannot be accounted for by the artificial synapse theory. In particular, it explains the high incidence of sympathetic overactivity observed in these patients and the modifying effect of emotional or sensory stimuli, all of which could act by heightening the background activity in this internuncial pool. It follows that anything that breaks this vicious circle—be it interruption of sympathetic efferents by spinal anesthesia or interruption of somatic nerve conduction—should relieve pain.

Gate Control Theory. Modern neurophysiology has led to the "gate control" theory of pain mediation.[18] In the substantia gelatinosa of the dorsal horns of the spinal cord, the synapses between the peripheral nerves and those that relay impulses up the long tracts to the brain are modulated by sympathetic input. In simplified terms, it is as if a gate exists at this point of relay and transmission, and the gate controls the relationship between the number or frequency of incoming peripheral impulses and the number or frequency of outgoing pulses reaching the brain. High-frequency stimulation of the latter pathways in awake patients is perceived as burning pain. Thus, when the gate is open—an effect of increased sympathetic activity—sensations of touch or pressure, for example, which would normally result in relaying of lower frequency impulses to the brain, might instead be perceived as burning pain because of the higher frequency of the impulses passing through the open gate. This theory offers an explanation for causalgia and the role of sympathetic tone, associated peripheral sympathetic activity, and relief by sympathectomy, which closes the gate.

Exaggerated Local Inflammatory Response. Several authorities have suggested that CRPS can be secondary to an exaggerated local inflammatory response to injury, resulting in disruption of the autoregulation of blood flow and giving rise to the classic phases of CRPS.[8] Likewise, some of the clinical features of early-stage CRPS can be explained by an inflammatory response.[8] This theory is supported by the fact that corticosteroids are often successful in treating patients with acute CRPS.[19] In one study, venous blood samples from affected extremities showed increased levels of the cytokines interleukin-6 and tumor necrosis factor-α as evidence of local inflammation.[20] In addition, serum concentrations of calcitonin gene-related peptide were elevated in CRPS patients as a marker of neurogenic inflammation.[20] It has also been suggested that localized neurogenic inflammation may be involved in the production of vasodilatation, acute edema, and increased sweating.

Other Theories

Recent studies have reviewed the mechanisms underlying the plasticity of dorsal root ganglia and dorsal horn neurons that leads to central pain from a peripheral nerve injury. Evidence points to molecular changes in the nociceptive terminals, ectopic firing of afferent pain fibers at the level of the dorsal root ganglia, and physiologic changes in the N-methyl-D-aspartate receptor that cause chronic nociceptive pain. Central sensitization is the physiologic manifestation of several severe peripherally induced pain states.[21] Other authorities have questioned whether genetic factors are involved in the pathophysiology of patients with CRPS.[8,22]

Sympathetically Maintained Pain and Sympathetically Independent Pain

SMP and SIP are not separate disorders but types of pain that can characterize a variety of pain syndromes, including CRPS types I and II. The role of the sympathetic nervous system in the pain associated with CRPS is unclear. Because of the poor understanding of pathophysiologic mechanisms, it was decided that words with mechanistic connotations, such as those involving the sympathetic nervous system, would not be included in the new nomenclature for CRPS.

Recently, the term *SMP* has been used to describe the pain maintained by sympathetic efferent innervation, circulating catecholamines, or neurochemical action and relieved by pharmacologic blockade or local anesthetic blockade of the sympathetic ganglia serving the painful area.[23,24] *SIP* refers to pain states not sustained by the sympathetic nervous system. SMP may vary over time, and a patient may have a pain syndrome in which part of the pain is sympathetically maintained and another part is sympathetically independent (i.e., a patient can have both SIP and SMP at the same time, or a patient may have SMP at one time and SIP at another).[11]

■ CLINICAL PRESENTATION

CRPS type I can occur in any age group, with a female-male ratio of 2:1. Although type I has been reported in children,[25,26] it is not as disabling as in adults.

Clinical Stages

Drucker and colleagues divided the natural history of PTPS into three clinical stages[27]:

Stage 1, acute (0 to 3 months). Stage 1 is characterized by warmth, erythema, burning, edema, hyperalgesia, hyperhidrosis, and, after a few months, patchy osteoporosis. At this stage, a good result can be expected with Bier blockade or chemical sympathectomy, and relief often lasts longer than the normal duration of a blockade. Spontaneous resolution may occur, and the clinical course is reversible.

Stage 2, dystrophic (3 to 6 months). Stage 2 is characterized by coolness, mottling of the skin, cyanosis, brawny edema, dry and brittle nails, continuous pain, and diffuse osteoporosis. Symptoms are present for a fixed interval, and spontaneous resolution is rare. There is a good response to sympathetic blockade. A bone scan is positive, and changes in bone structure are seen on plain films.

Stage 3, atrophic (>6 to 12 months). Pain extends beyond the area of injury, and florid trophic changes occur, including atrophy of the skin and its appendages and fixed joint contractures. Radiographs show severe demineralization and ankylosis.

Although these stages oversimplify the condition, they provide a framework for the diagnosis, treatment, and prognosis of CRPS. For example, among patients who are in stage 1 or 2, prompt treatment may produce permanent pain relief, and sympathectomy may not be required by those with stage 1 disease. For patients in stage 3, the likelihood of a poor result is greater, and even sympathectomy may not provide lasting relief.

Symptoms and Signs

The clinical criteria for the diagnosis of CRPS, as outlined by Stanton-Hicks and colleagues, are summarized in Figure 161-1 and Box 161-2.[10,12]

Pain. Pain is a necessary symptom for the diagnosis of CRPS. This pain is located in the affected extremity and is disproportionate to what would be expected from the initial event. It may be spontaneous or evoked and is usually reported as burning or diffuse pain. The pain may also be described as throbbing or aching, intermittent or continuous, and exacerbated by physical or emotional stress. The pain is not consistent with the distribution of a peripheral nerve, even if the initial injury involved such a nerve. This important feature distinguishes CRPS from pain of other causes and from more specific neuropathic pain disorders. The patient often adopts a protective posture to guard the affected extremity.

Sensory Changes. Sensory changes of CRPS are usually reported at some stage and include allodynia and hyperesthesia in the region of the pain. Allodynia may occur in response to thermal stimulation (cold or warm), deep pressure, light touch, or joint movement.

Sympathetic Dysfunction. Sympathetic dysfunction in CRPS is reported as a sudomotor or vasomotor instability in the affected extremity compared with the unaffected extremity. This dysfunction may vary in severity at different times.

Box 161-2 Diagnostic Criteria for Complex Regional Pain Syndrome

CLINICAL SYMPTOMS AND SIGNS
- Burning pain
- Hyperpathia or allodynia
- Temperature or color changes
- Edema
- Hair or nail growth changes

LABORATORY RESULTS
- Thermometry or thermography
- Bone radiography
- Three-phase bone scan
- Quantitative sweat test
- Response to sympathetic block

INTERPRETATION
If total number of positive findings is:
- >6: Reflex sympathetic dystrophy probable
- 3-5: Reflex sympathetic dystrophy possible
- <3: Reflex sympathetic dystrophy unlikely

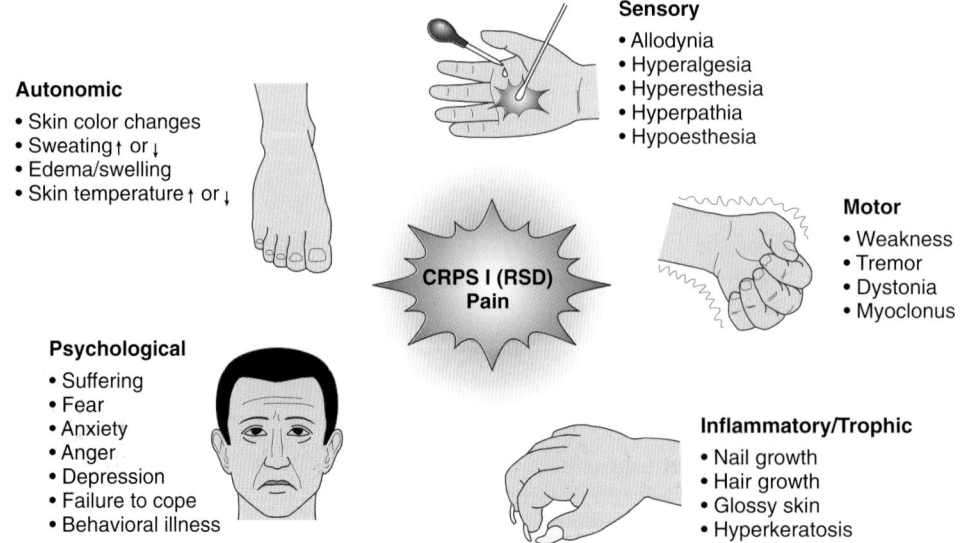

Figure 161-1 Clinical features of complex regional pain syndrome (CRPS) type I (reflex sympathetic dystrophy [RSD]).

The patient may report that the extremity is warm and red or cold and blue, purple, or mottled. Veldman and associates reported that 92% of patients had altered skin temperature.[28] Sweating, particularly of the palms or soles, may be reported as increased, decreased, or unchanged. Normal sympathetic function may be present at certain times. Swelling can occur at any stage of the syndrome and is typically peripheral; it may be intermittent or permanent and may be exacerbated by the dependent position of the extremity. There can also be pitting or brawny edema.

Trophic Changes. Trophic changes of the skin may occur later in the course of the syndrome. The nails may be atrophic or hypertrophic. Hair growth and texture may be decreased or increased, and the skin may become atrophic. Motor dysfunction includes dystonia, tremor, and loss of strength of the affected muscle groups. Joint swelling and stiffness may also be reported, particularly of the digits.

Advanced Diagnostic Criteria

Advanced diagnostic criteria have been published to facilitate the clinical diagnosis of CRPS.[29] In addition to continuing pain that is disproportionate to the inciting event, the patient must report at least one symptom in each of the following four categories:
1. *Sensory:* hyperesthesia
2. *Sudomotor, edema:* sweating changes, edema, or sweating asymmetry
3. *Vasomotor:* skin color changes, temperature asymmetry, or skin color asymmetry
4. *Motor, trophic:* decreased range of motion, motor dysfunction (weakness, tremor, dystonia), or trophic changes (hair, nail, skin)

The patient must display at least one sign in two or more of the following categories:
1. *Sensory:* evidence of allodynia (to light touch) or hyperalgesia (to pinprick)
2. *Sudomotor, edema:* evidence of sweating changes, edema, or sweating asymmetry
3. *Vasomotor:* evidence of skin color changes, temperature asymmetry, or skin color asymmetry
4. *Motor, trophic:* evidence of decreased range of motion, motor dysfunction (weakness, tremor, dystonia), or trophic changes (hair, nail, skin)

Comprehensive Adjunctive Clinical Tests

With the foregoing features in mind, the clinical evaluation can be enhanced by focusing on particular aspects or using adjunctive tests.

Sensory Examination. Sensory impairment can be positive (allodynia, mechanical and thermal hyperalgesia) or negative (hyperesthesia, hypalgesia). These sensory impairments can be localized (glovelike) or generalized. Quantitative sensory testing to confirm the clinical findings of sensory

abnormalities can be applied; however, this is not specific for patients with CRPS.[30]

Sudomotor Sympathetic Examination. Resting heat output can be estimated by skin impedance,[31] by quinizarin or cobalt blue testing,[32] or as part of the quantitative sudomotor axon reflex test,[33] which measures resting sweat output by hygrometry and changes evoked by iontophoresis of acetylcholine into the skin.[34] These tests are useful diagnostic tools, but they are difficult to conduct and are generally not recommended for the routine diagnosis of CRPS.[30,35]

Vasomotor Examination. Simultaneous temperature measurements of both the affected and unaffected extremities are taken at corresponding anatomic sites. The temperature of the digit pads, palms, soles, forearms, and calves can be measured with noncontact thermometry or thermography. Serial measurements should be taken, because peripheral temperatures vary widely under normal circumstances. Skin perfusion can be evaluated visually or by pulse oximetry.

Edema. Edema is judged clinically by comparing one extremity to the other. Most volume displacement methods are too cumbersome.

Trophic Changes. The skin, hair, and nails of the two sides are compared.

Motor Dysfunction. The presence of dystonia, tremor, and changes in strength can be measured clinically. Objective measurements should be taken (e.g., apposition and opposition pinch strength, grip, weight bearing on the lower extremity).

Psychological Testing. Psychological testing has not been validated in CRPS. The psychiatrist generally uses familiar instruments as part of the initial assessment and follow-up.

Neurophysiologic Testing. The diagnosis of CRPS type II requires a peripheral nerve lesion, and CRPS may develop following a central nervous system lesion (brain tumor or brain infarct). It is therefore important to confirm or exclude peripheral nerve and central nervous system lesions. Nerve conduction studies may show discrete abnormalities secondary to edema or peripheral vasoconstriction.[30] Distinct abnormalities exceeding 20% of normal values should be observed and may indicate a peripheral nerve lesion, which can be noted in patients with carpal tunnel syndrome or CRPS type II. Somatosensory evoked potentials after ulnar-median or tibial nerve stimulation testing are usually normal in patients with CRPS type I; however, these tests can be abnormal in patients with CRPS type II. Electromyograms are usually not performed in patients with CRPS because they are painful and may exaggerate the pain of CRPS. Overall, these tests can be useful in the diagnosis of CRPS types I and II and to confirm peripheral nerve or central nerve system lesions; however, the findings are not specific.

Inflammatory Assessment. Neuroinflammatory media-tors such as substance P, bradykinin, and calcitonin gene-related peptide are usually increased in patients with CRPS; however, other systemic inflammatory markers, such as C-reactive protein, erythrocyte sedimentation rate, and leukocyte count, are not elevated.[36]

DIAGNOSTIC EVALUATION
Radiographic Findings

The primary radiographic manifestations in patients with CRPS are diffuse osteoporosis with severe patchy deminer-alization, especially of the periarticular regions, and subperios-teal bone resorption.[30,37] However, these changes are late and nonspecific.

Three-Phase Bone Scans. Bone scans have been used for the diagnosis of CRPS for 3 decades.[38,39] Accelerated blood flow in the diseased limb combined with increased, diffuse activity during the blood-pool phase and increased periarticu-lar uptake in the delayed static phase is considered pathogno-monic for CRPS (Fig. 161-2). A meta-analysis of 19 articles on the use of three-phase bone scans in patients with CRPS revealed a poor sensitivity of 50%. Therefore, many believe that bone scans are not accurate enough for the diagnosis of CRPS.[30]

Magnetic Resonance Imaging. Magnetic resonance imaging (MRI) may reveal characteristic findings during the course of the disease.[30] Skin thickening and changes in bone

signal intensity in carpal and metacarpal bones, along with effusions in adjacent joints, may be related to the acute and early stages of CRPS. However, several studies have sug-gested that the consequences of surgery or trauma may mimic CRPS type I–like MRI findings; therefore, MRI is usually not used as a screening method, but it may be helpful in excluding other disease entities.

Diagnostic Sympathetic Blockade

The validity of a clinical diagnosis of CRPS can be greatly strengthened by a positive response to sympathetic blockade. If there is no relief from pain for the duration of the complete sympathetic blockade, the diagnosis of CRPS is less likely. A documented increase in skin temperature of 1°C to 3°C confirms the success of sympathetic blockade. Patients should be encouraged to quantify the degree of pain relief experi-enced (e.g., 100% relief, 50% relief). The degree of pain relief a patient experiences with such a blockade is an excellent predictor of how much relief can be expected from surgical sympathectomy.[40] Caution should be exercised, however, because sympathectomy can provide some degree of nonspe-cific relief of almost any pain, including ischemic pain.[40,41] CRPS pain is usually dramatically relieved by sympathetic blockade (almost always 75% to 100% relief), whereas relief of pain from other causes is usually only mild to moderate (25% to 50% at most).

Sympathetic blockade can be achieved by the intravenous delivery of an alpha-blocking agent (e.g., phentolamine), intravenous regional blockade with bretylium, Bier blockade, differential spinal blockade, epidural blockade, and local anes-thetic blockade of the paravertebral lumbar sympathetic chain. Many consider paravertebral lumbar blockade using lidocaine or bupivacaine most effective because it blocks both sensory and motor nerves.[40]

Differential Diagnosis

Causalgia-like pain can occur if a nerve is caught in a suture, entrapped by scar, or compressed by surrounding structures. Nerve entrapment must be considered when causalgia appears immediately after an operation, but because a nerve can be irritated or injured by any compressing or pinching mecha-nism, there may be a causalgia component to the pain associ-ated with any nerve compression. This consideration is important because relieving the compression may only par-tially relieve the pain, and the causalgia component may persist. If peripheral nerve entrapment is the cause, there is often a "trigger point" where focal application of pressure causes sharp pain. The pain can be relieved by the infiltration of a small amount of local anesthetic at that point.

Patients who present with cutaneous signs and symptoms characteristic of Drucker's stage 2 are sometimes thought to have Raynaud's syndrome; however, with Raynaud's, the patient's symptoms should be intermittent, related principally to cold exposure, and relieved by warmth. Further, hyperes-thesia is rare in Raynaud's syndrome, and its characteristic pain is not severe or burning.

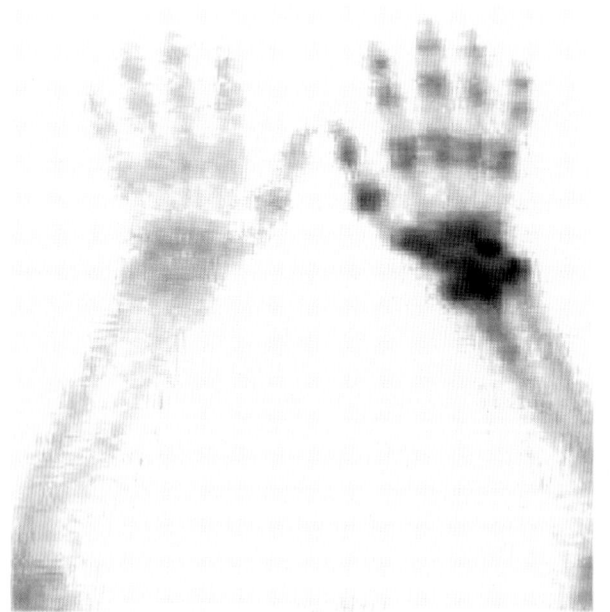

Figure 161-2 Three-phase bone scan in complex regional pain syndrome of the left hand. *(From Schurmann M, Gradl G, Rommel O. Early diagnosis in post-traumatic complex regional pain syndrome. Orthopedics. 2007;30:450-456.)*

The pain of peripheral neuritis is often burning and associated with hyperesthesia and vasomotor phenomena. However, the clinical syndrome associated with peripheral neuritis is more anatomically diffuse and gradual in onset, and the patient has no history of trauma or another discrete precipitating event. Other conditions must be kept in mind, including inflammatory or infectious disorders, such as rheumatic arthritis, and unilateral vascular occlusive disease.

◼ NONSURGICAL TREATMENT

In the past, when there was no effective treatment, CRPS frequently resulted in chronic invalidism, emotional deterioration, and drug addiction. Thus, the proper treatment of CRPS is based on prevention and early recognition. For patients known to be susceptible to CRPS, such as those who have hemiplegia or myocardial infarction, early mobilization of an injured extremity is critical. When early sympathetic dystrophic changes occur, pain relief and active use of the hand, arm, or leg are indicated. Passive motion by physical therapists should be avoided because it may increase the pain and edema. Opiate analgesics, when needed, should be used conservatively. Splinting the hand in a functional position may help.

Few evidence-based treatment modalities for CRPS are available. In fact, the few literature reviews of outcome studies provide discouragingly inconsistent information about the various pharmacologic and other therapies for CRPS.[42,43] Treatment of CRPS usually requires a multidisciplinary approach, including a neurologist, anesthesiologist, vascular surgeon, orthopedic specialist, psychologist, and physical therapist.

Physical Therapy

Physical therapy should be considered not only essential but also the first line of treatment for patients with CRPS. Intensive physical therapy should be initiated, including full range-of-motion exercises and whirlpool exercises. Aggressive therapy should be avoided, however, because patients with CRPS have an exaggerated response to painful and nonpainful stimuli,[44] and any pain may exaggerate the syndrome. The primary objective of physical therapy is goal-oriented functional restoration, which includes (1) mobilization, swelling control, and isometric strengthening; (2) desensitization of the affected region; (3) stress loading, isotonic strengthening, range of motion, postural normalization, and aerobic conditioning; and (4) vocational rehabilitation.[12] Physical therapy should be combined with pharmacologic therapy.

Mirror Visual Feedback. Mirror visual feedback has been used in the early stages of CRPS type I. The effect of this therapy is based on findings that visual input from a moving, unaffected limb re-establishes the pain-free relationship between sensory feedback and motor execution of the affected limb. McCabe and coworkers reported good results in patients with early stages of CRPS type I.[45]

Transcutaneous Electrical Nerve Stimulation. Transcutaneous electrical nerve stimulation (TENS) has been used to treat CRPS.[44,46,47] Results have been mixed, but because TENS is easily administered and safe, it may be tried before more aggressive treatment is attempted. In the hands of an experienced practitioner, the success or failure of TENS will be apparent by the third to fifth treatment.[48]

Acupuncture and Electroacupuncture. Chan and Chow reported on the use of acupuncture in more than 20 patients with CRPS after hand injuries.[49] Acupuncture needles were inserted in the affected limb and connected to a stimulator; a monophasic electrical pulse was passed for 20 to 30 minutes, and this was repeated 5 to 10 times. A total of 14 patients experienced marked permanent improvement, and 4 had some improvement.

Pharmacologic Therapy

Pharmacologic therapy, particularly as it applies to stage 1 or early stage 2 disease, can be combined with intermittent sympathetic blockades and physical therapy. Drug therapy may require nonspecific analgesics, but these should be superimposed, only when necessary, on a "background" of medication designed to attenuate the symptoms by direct effect. Of these, phenytoin, amitriptyline, carbamazepine, and baclofen can be effective, and they are usually used in that order owing to increasing side effects. Benson recommends the tricyclic antidepressant amitriptyline hydrochloride (Elavil) in doses of 50 to 75 mg nightly or divided during the day (150 mg maximum).[50] Benson also recommends a phenothiazine such as fluphenazine hydrochloride (Prolixin), which potentiates opiate analgesic effects, possesses an analgesic property of its own, and depresses the response to peripheral stimuli. The recommended dosage is 1 mg three times daily, but doses as large as 10 mg/day can be used.

A summary of pharmacologic therapies for CRPS follows.

Opioids. Opioids inhibit central nociceptive neurons through interaction with μ-receptors. There are no long-term studies of oral opioids in the treatment of neuropathic pain, including CRPS; however, the expert opinion of pain clinicians is that opioids should be part of a comprehensive pain regimen protocol. Opioids should be tried early in the course of CRPS, not as a "last resort."

Tricyclic Antidepressants. Tricyclic antidepressants are some of the best-studied drugs in the treatment of neuropathic pain, and they have shown an analgesic effect. They inhibit the reuptake of monoaminergic transmitters. There is solid evidence that the reuptake and noradrenaline blocker amitriptyline and the selective noradrenaline blocker desipramine produce pain relief in several neuropathies.

GABA-Agonists. GABA-agonists such as gabapentin (Neurontin) have also been used in the treatment of CRPS. The action of gabapentin probably includes the inhibition of calcium channels.

α-Adrenergic Blocking Agents. The use of α-adrenergic blockers is based primarily on the fact that patients with CRPS have altered blood flow as a result of increased local secretion of norepinephrine and vascular endothelial hypersensitivity. Inhibition of the receptors leading to vascular dilatation and increased blood flow may be helpful. Pain relief following intravenous phentolamine administration has been suggested as a diagnostic tool as well as a prognostic guide for favorable response to sympathetic blockade.[44,51] Its 15-minute plasma half-life precludes its use as a therapeutic modality. Other medications include phenoxybenzamine and prazosin.[44,52]

Oral β-Blocking Agents. Propranolol, which antagonizes serotonin, has been partially successful.[44]

Oral Calcium Channel Blocking Agents. These agents produce smooth muscle relaxation of the arteriole walls, leading to increased blood flow. Treatment with either nifedipine or the alpha-sympathetic blocker phenoxybenzamine was assessed in 59 patients with early and chronic CRPS, and cure rates of 92% and 40% were achieved in early and late CRPS, respectively.[53]

Bisphosphonate Therapy. This therapy is based on the concept that pain results from osteopenia as part of CRPS. Adami and colleagues reported that this therapy was beneficial in patients with CRPS.[54]

Antiarrhythmic Agents. The efficacy of bretylium and mexiletine has been studied in patients with CRPS, with mixed results.[55] These medications suppress the spontaneous discharge of injured neurons and depress C fiber–mediated reflexes at the level of the spinal cord.

Nonsteroidal Anti-inflammatory Drugs. These drugs inhibit the enzyme cyclooxygenase, which leads to decreased production of the prostaglandins and thromboxanes that increase nociceptor sensitivity to painful stimuli and promote vascular constriction. There are no published trials of their use in patients with CRPS.

Steroid Therapy. These are potent anti-inflammatory agents that decrease tissue edema, which decreases pain and improves joint motion. Prednisone, prednisolone, and methylprednisolone are commonly used.[44,56] A course of steroids should be tried when the response to physical therapy or TENS is poor. Kozin and collaborators reported a fair to excellent response to steroids in 63 of 67 CRPS patients.[39] The usual starting dose of prednisone is 60 mg/day. The dose is tapered every 3 days by 5 mg, so the total course of therapy lasts about 5 weeks.

Sympathetic Blockade

Because many patients experience at least a temporary response to nonoperative treatment in the early stages of CRPS, a common error in management is to carry conservative therapy too far, persisting with such treatments too long and shifting repeatedly from one to another. This subjects patients to wasted time and expense and prolonged suffering, and it may also compromise their chances of obtaining complete and lasting relief by surgical sympathectomy. Thus, if the measures described earlier are not effective in relieving the patient's symptoms promptly, or if the symptoms are exacerbated over the course of several days, the physician should proceed directly to sympathetic blockade, which is both diagnostic and therapeutic.

An initial sympathetic blockade is appropriate early in stage 1 to confirm the diagnosis and test the procedure's therapeutic potential. The rapid pain relief gained from a sympathetic blockade can be extremely helpful psychologically. Also, the condition may be reversible at this stage, and complete remission can sometimes be achieved, particularly in patients who experience long-lasting relief from serial sympathetic blockade, thus allowing aggressive physical therapy. When relief is short-lived, however, repeated blockade is counterproductive and expensive.

Sympathetic blockade of the affected extremity has been used as an alternative therapy for patients with CRPS, but proof of its effectiveness is scanty.[8,42,57] Several uncontrolled studies have reported on the effect of sympathetic blockade in patients with CRPS. About 85% of patients reported positive results, but fewer patients (60%) reported long-term relief.[6] Other authorities have questioned the role of the sympathetic system in the pathogenesis of CRPS and, therefore, its role in treatment.[58,59] A Cochrane review of local anesthetic sympathetic blockade for CRPS concluded that the published evidence is too scarce to support the use of sympathetic blockade as the "gold standard" treatment for CRPS.[60]

Chemical sympathectomy (injections of alcohol and phenol) have been used instead of surgical sympathectomy, but a significant incidence of incomplete or transient blockade is associated with this approach.[1] Radiofrequency ablation has been proposed as a more precise method of achieving percutaneous sympathetic denervation.[61]

Lumbar Sympathetic Blockade Technique

The point of the needle must be placed precisely adjacent to the sympathetic chain. Landmarks for this blockade are L1, situated at the level of the junction of the 12th rib and erector spinae muscles, and L4-L5, at the level of a line drawn between the posterior iliac crests. Preferably, the patient should lie in the lateral position. Complete sympathetic blockade may be obtained with a single injection of 15 mL of bupivacaine (Marcaine) at the level of L2. Better results may be obtained using two or even three needles, with one point inserted at L2 and the others at L3 and L4 (Fig. 161-3).

Upper Extremity Sympathetic Blockade Technique

See Chapter 121: Thoracic Sympathectomy.

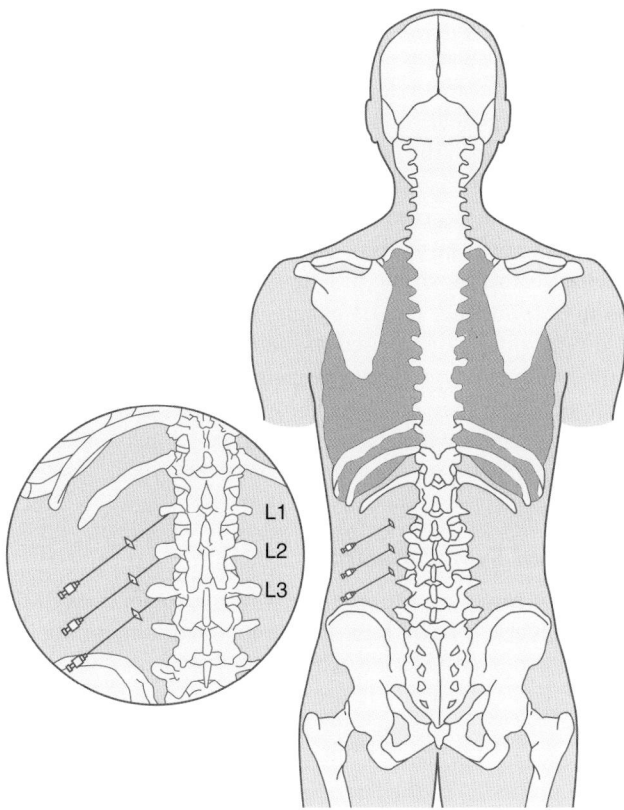

Figure 161-3 Lumbar sympathetic blockade (three-needle technique).

Epidural and Intrathecal Drug Therapy

Continuous epidural anesthesia or an intrathecal narcotic pump allows low-dose narcotics or local anesthetics to be administered, which may result in fewer systemic side effects than intravenous application. Local narcotic use can elevate the pain cycle, whereas the anesthetic agent provides a relatively selective sympathetic blockade. Successful outcomes with placement of an indwelling morphine pump[62] or the administration of continuous epidural anesthesia in conjunction with continuous passive motion[63] have been reported. Owing to the risk and cost of this modality, its use has been limited. Continuous epidural anesthesia also requires hospitalization and carries the risk of urinary retention, hypertension, and skin breakdown. Intrathecal morphine pumps are usually expensive and require refilling of the narcotic reservoir. One double-blinded controlled trial reported that epidural clonidine is beneficial in CRPS patients. Intrathecal baclofen therapy has been suggested for CRPS patients who are refractory to conventional modalities.[64]

Neuromodulation

Neuromodulation modalities include peripheral nerve, spinal cord, and thalamic stimulation. Implantable devices such as spinal cord stimulators are increasingly used in patients with intractable CRPS for symptomatic pain relief. In a prospective randomized controlled study, patients with CRPS who received spinal cord stimulation with physical therapy obtained greater pain relief and improvement in health-related quality of life than those who received physical therapy alone.[65] Spinal cord stimulation also produced analgesia in patients with CRPS who had undergone previous sympathectomy, which suggests that spinal cord stimulation can provide analgesia without inhibiting sympathetic function in CRPS patients.[65] The mechanism of action is somewhat diverse and likely involves neurochemical changes at both spinal and supraspinal targets, although it inhibits sympathetic outflow.

Taylor reported on a systematic review and meta-analysis of the use of spinal cord stimulation in CRPS.[66] The results supported the use of spinal cord stimulation in patients with refractory neuropathic back and leg pain and failed back surgery syndrome (grade B evidence), CRPS type I (grade A evidence), and CRPS type II (grade D evidence). Taylor noted that spinal cord stimulation not only reduces pain but also improves quality of life, reduces analgesic consumption, allows some patients to return to work, is associated with minimal significant adverse events, and may result in significant cost savings over time.

Psychotherapy

Recently, the International Association for the Study of Pain consensus report recommended that patients with CRPS seek psychotherapy, including psychometric testing, if their pain persists beyond 2 months.[11] This includes the treatment of anxiety, depression, and personality disorders. Counseling, behavioral modification, relaxation therapy, biofeedback, group therapy, and self-hypnosis should be considered in these patients.

Summary of Treatment Guidelines

Following are the generally accepted guidelines for the treatment of patients with CRPS type I:

Stage 1. Physical therapy with or without TENS is usually useful. A local nerve or sympathetic blockade may be necessary for patients who experience severe pain and are unable to undergo physical therapy. If these measures fail, a course of steroid therapy should be given.

Stage 2. Physical therapy, TENS, and steroid therapy should be combined. Sympathetic blockade and surgical sympathectomy should be considered if these measures fail.

Stage 3. Steroid therapy or sympathetic blockade and surgical sympathectomy should be considered but may be unsuccessful. Neuromodulation (spinal cord stimulation) may be used. Manipulation of joint contractures under general anesthesia, antidepressants, and vocational guidance may be used.

In Cooney's treatment protocol,[67] the first step is to differentiate sympathetic pain from somatic pain (see Box 161-2). The RSD score can be helpful. When the pain is somatic, treatment options include isolated nerve blockade, continuous nerve blockade, TENS (external), direct electrical nerve stimulation (internal), and nerve ablation. If the pain is sympathetic in origin, treatment should include protection of the limb (with a garment or splint) combined with active use, sympathetic blockade (single or continuous), and sympathectomy.

■ SYMPATHECTOMY

Once CRPS has been temporarily relieved by sympathetic blockade, the question arises whether to try to achieve this degree of relief more permanently by sympathectomy.

Indications

The decision to perform a sympathectomy depends on the clinical stage of the disease, the severity of symptoms, and the degree and duration of relief obtained by sympathetic blockade. This applies to both upper and lower extremity CRPS. For example, if a patient with pain of recent onset experiences pain relief from sympathetic blockade that lasts well beyond the known duration of the anesthetic agent used, it is advisable to continue with nonoperative measures. A patients whose condition has persisted for several months, whose pain is disabling, and who experiences nearly total relief from sympathetic blockade, but only for the typical duration of the anesthetic, may be considered a candidate for immediate surgical sympathectomy. A patient with symptoms of long duration (many months to years) and associated trophic changes, whose symptoms are less "classic" and less severe, and who receives only mild to moderate relief from sympathetic blockade should be advised that the long-term results are likely to be disappointing. These examples correspond to Drucker's three stages; this is deliberate because sympathectomy is, for the most part, best applied in stage 2—before progression to stage 3 and after stage 1—in patients who are unresponsive to nonoperative therapy.

For CRPS of the upper extremity, surgical cervical or dorsal sympathectomy (lower stellate ganglion and T2 and T3) is indicated, whether through the open or the thoracoscopic approach (see Chapter 121: Thoracic Sympathectomy). For patients with CRPS of the lower extremity, lumbar sympathectomy is usually indicated. If surgical sympathectomy is limited to patients who obtain excellent relief from sympathetic blockade with local anesthetic, nearly 90% of patients experience long-term relief.[40,68]

Upper Extremity Sympathectomy

See Chapter 121 (Thoracic Sympathectomy) for a description of the open or thoracoscopic technique.

Lumbar Sympathectomy

Anatomic Considerations

Sympathetic outflow to the lower extremities originates in spinal cord segments T10 to L3. Preganglionic fibers from these segments form extensive synaptic connections in para-

vertebral ganglia from L1 to S3 for innervation of the entire lower extremity and pelvic region. Sympathetic innervation of the foot and lower leg is conveyed primarily through the L2 and L3 ganglia; the proximal leg region is innervated primarily through the L1 to L4 ganglia. Overall, three lumbar ganglia are most commonly found, with fusion of the L1 and L2 ganglia most commonly accounting for the reduced number. Crossover fibers occur in 15% of patients, with most leaving via the fourth and fifth lumbar ganglia. For most clinical indications, L2 and L3 ganglionectomy is sufficient, but also removing L4 is advised to reduce the possibility of collateral reinnervation. Extensive ganglionectomy is usually not warranted and may result in ejaculatory disturbances in preclimacteric men when bilateral high ganglionectomies (i.e., including L1) are performed.

Chemical Sympathectomy

The high response rate achieved with percutaneous sympathetic blockade with local anesthetics led to attempts to achieve extended blockade with phenol or alcohol injections via the same approach. To accomplish this, the tips of three needles are placed against the bodies of the L2, L3, and L4 vertebrae (see Fig. 161-3). Their positions must be confirmed radiographically. In the lateral view, the needle points should barely reach the anterior border of the vertebral bodies. In the anteroposterior view, the points should lie over them. After proper needle positioning has been ascertained, 3 mL of 6.5% to 7% phenol dissolved in water, or 3 mL of absolute alcohol, is injected through each needle.

Experience with phenol lumbar sympathectomy is limited in the United States but is increasing. Long-term results have not been reported. The clinical impressions are that this approach produces a less complete and less durable effect than surgical sympathectomy; in addition, painful side effects occasionally mar its use. In view of the current low risk, durability, and precision of surgical sympathectomy, percutaneous techniques require improvement before they can be accepted as an alternative to surgery to produce lasting sympathetic denervation. Chemical sympathectomy must not be taken lightly, because phenol or alcohol injections can cause significant inflammation and scarring, making subsequent surgical sympathectomy, if needed, difficult or unsafe.

Open Technique

The open technique for lumbar sympathectomy is illustrated in Figure 161-4. It begins with proper positioning of the patient so that the interval between the costal margin and the iliac crest is "opened." The surgeon can accomplish this objective by raising the flank region approximately 30 degrees.

An oblique incision is begun at the lateral edge of the rectus muscle, extending toward the middle of the space between the ribs and the iliac crest and ending at the anterior axillary line. The musculofascial layers of the external and internal oblique as well as the transversalis muscles are split in the direction of their fibers. The lateral plane between the

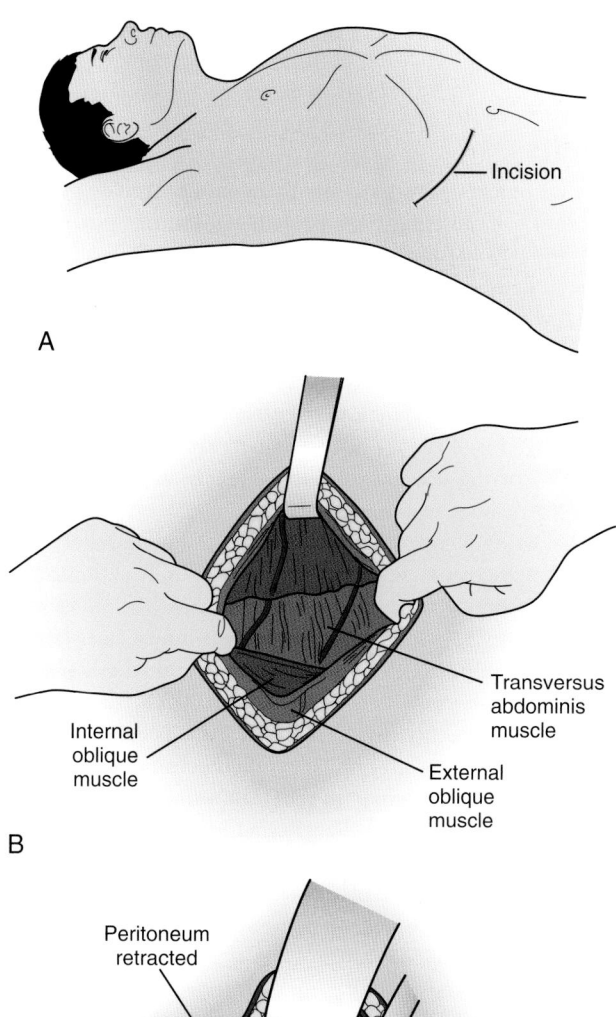

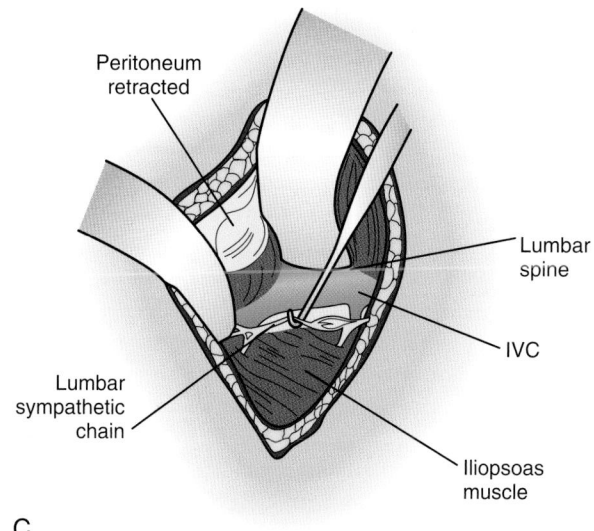

Figure 161-4 Open technique for lumbar sympathectomy. **A,** Incision site. **B,** The external oblique, internal oblique, and transversus abdominis muscles have been split and retracted. **C,** The retracted peritoneum and position of the lumbar sympathetic chain. IVC, inferior vena cava.

transversalis fascia and the peritoneum is easily developed by blunt finger dissection directed toward the vertebral column. Continued separation of the peritoneum is gently performed in medial, caudad, and cephalad directions to maximize retroperitoneal exposure. Dissection should stay anterior to the psoas muscle. The ureter and gonadal vessels are left attached to overlying peritoneum and are lifted off the psoas muscle as

the dissection proceeds medially. The lumbar sympathetic chain is located medial to the psoas muscle and lies over the transverse processes of the lumbar spine. The lumbar chain should not be confused with the genitofemoral nerve, which lies more laterally over the medial third of the psoas muscle itself. On the left, the lumbar ganglia lie adjacent and lateral to the abdominal aorta; on the right, the chain lies just beneath the edge of the inferior vena cava.

Tactile identification of the lumbar chain by plucking discloses a characteristic "snap" as a result of tethering of the nodular chain by rami communicantes. Other vertical, band-like structures in this region (genitofemoral nerve, paravertebral lymph nodes, ureter) do not recoil as briskly. Once identified, the midportion of the sympathetic chain is dissected free of surrounding tissues and retracted with a right-angle clamp or a nerve hook to draw it up under tension from the surrounding tissue. The ganglia are mobilized by division of the tethering rami with prior metal clip application. The surgeon facilitates orientation and ganglion numbering by identifying the sacral promontory and an adjacent lumbar vein that usually crosses the sympathetic chain in front of or behind the third lumbar ganglion. Once the chain, with at least two lumbar ganglia, is removed, hemostasis is secured, and the incision is closed in layers.

This anterolateral approach of Flowthow is most popular because the incision is well tolerated, dissection remains retroperitoneal, and exposure is adequate.[69] The anterior transperitoneal approach of Adson is applicable only for sympathectomy combined with an abdominal aortic or other intraperitoneal procedure.[70] The right lumbar chain is dissected along the right lateral aspect of the inferior vena cava. Exposure of the left lumbar chain is accomplished by medial reflection of the left colon along the white line of Toldt.

Laparoscopic Technique

The technique of laparoscopic lumbar sympathectomy has been described by several authorities[71-73] (Figs. 161-5 and 161-6). A 12- to 15-mm incision is made midway between the iliac crest and the costal margin at the anterior axillary line. This is carried down through the external and internal oblique muscles, which are separated along their respective fibers to reach the retroperitoneal space. Using blunt dissection, the areolar fatty tissue is dissected while the peritoneal sac is gently pushed forward, which creates a safe space for insertion of the distention balloon system into the retroperitoneum. The balloon is inflated under direct vision via a 30-degree scope introduced into the balloon trocar. A Hasson trocar is introduced into the space created and secured with two sutures to the fascia to avoid gas leakage. The space created is insufflated with carbon dioxide to a pressure of 10 to 12 mm Hg. Two or three additional 5-mm ports are inserted under direct vision into the retroperitoneal space along a line 2 to 3 cm posterior to the first trocar, at the mid and posterior axillary lines.

Decompression of the peritoneal cavity can also be accomplished using a Veres needle, which equalizes pressures. The

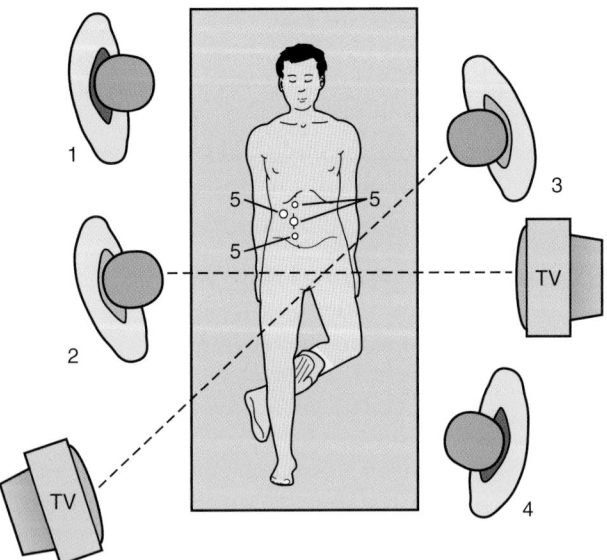

Figure 161-5 Diagram showing the positions of the camera operator (1), surgeon (2), assistant (3), scrub nurse (4), and port placements (5) for laparoscopic lumbar sympathectomy.

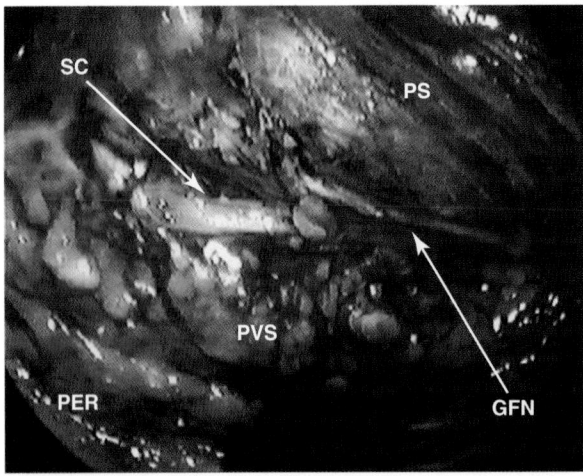

Figure 161-6 Retroperitoneoscopic view of the operative field. GFN, genitofemoral nerve; PER, peritoneum; PS, psoas muscle; PVS, prevertebral space; SC, sympathetic chain. *(From Beglaibter N, Berlatzky Y, Zamir O, et al. Retroperitoneoscopic lumbar sympathectomy. J Vasc Surg. 2002;35:815-817.)*

surgeon and assistant should stand in front of the patient so they can clearly identify the peritoneal sac, which is pushed backward and medially, and the psoas muscle, which is in front and upward. The gonadal vessels and ureters should be clearly identified. The genitofemoral nerve is visualized descending obliquely along the psoas muscle. Two instruments are used for dissection, traction, clipping, and cutting, and a third instrument is sometimes used for retraction of the psoas muscle and for suction, if needed. The sympathetic chain is identified along the inner margin of the psoas muscle, and small communicating rami and blood vessels are divided with cautery, clips, and endoscissors. The sympathetic chain is then transected between clips at the level of L2 and L4. The retroperitoneal space is deflated, the trocars are removed,

the fascia at the large port site is sutured, and the skin incisions are closed.[71-73]

Results

The first reports of surgical sympathectomy (stellate ganglionectomy) for causalgia were probably those of Spurling[74] in 1930 and Kwan[75] in 1935. In Thompson's 1979 series, 82 patients with causalgia (upper and lower extremity) were treated with sympathectomy, and 93% had excellent or good pain relief.[18] Olcott and associates reported 91% good to excellent results in 35 patients (17 upper extremity and 18 lower extremity).[76] Some form of postsympathectomy neuralgia occurred in 4 (23%) of the upper extremity cases and in 12 (67%) of the lower extremity cases. In all instances, the neuralgia resolved spontaneously.

Mockus and coworkers reported 97% pain relief in 31 patients, which was sustained in 94%.[68] In 9 patients with upper extremity causalgia, 12 dorsal sympathectomies were performed; in 22 patients with lower extremity causalgia, 23 lumbar sympathectomies were performed. In the 9 patients who had dorsal sympathectomies, all 9 (100%) had early pain relief, and 8 patients (89%) had late pain relief. Of the 22 patients who underwent lumbar sympathectomies, 21 patients (95%) had early and late pain relief. In a similar, more recent series of 28 patients, my colleagues and I reported 95% long-term success in patients who had experienced an excellent response to sympathetic blockade.[40]

An interesting subgroup of patients was identified in two of the aforementioned reports.[40,68] In the first series,[68] patients with causalgia persisting after disk surgery enjoyed pain relief following sympathectomy equal to that in other patients.

Bandyk and associates reported sympathectomy results in 73 patients with CRPS type I (46 were video-assisted thoracoscopic lumbar sympathectomies).[77] At 3 months after sympathectomy, 90% of patients experienced a more than 50% reduction in pain, with pain severity scores decreasing from a mean of 8.7 before surgery to 3.4 after surgery. Overall, patient satisfaction was 77% and was not significantly influenced by patient age, CRPS duration, or extremity involvement (84% lumbar, 72% cervicodorsal).

Similarly, Singh and associates reported the results of sympathectomy in 42 patients with CRPS type II of the upper extremity.[78] Thoracoscopic dorsal sympathectomy was successful in 32 patients, and 10 had successful open sympathectomy.

Hassantash and colleagues reviewed 110 articles containing 1528 cases of causalgia.[7] Response to sympathetic blockades was noted in 88%, and 94% of patients undergoing sympathectomy were cured. However, in a recent Cochrane systematic review of the literature, Cepeda and associates analyzed patients who obtained at least 50% pain relief shortly after sympathetic blockade (30 minutes to 2 hours) and those with pain relief at 48 hours or longer after blockade.[60] They concluded that it was not possible to determine the effect of sympathetic blockade on long-term pain relief because the studies evaluated different outcomes.

Complications

Complications may include injury to the genitofemoral nerve, ureter, lumbar veins, aorta, and inferior vena cava. The most common complication is postsympathectomy neuralgia, which occurs in up to 50% of patients from 5 to 20 days after sympathectomy.[40,68,79] The cause is still speculative. The pain is characterized as an annoying "ache" in the anterolateral thigh region that is worse at night and is unaffected by activity or level of cutaneous stimulation. The discomfort responds to moderate analgesics and spontaneously remits within 8 to 12 weeks after onset.

Retrograde ejaculation can occur in 25% to 50% of male patients undergoing bilateral L1 sympathetic ganglionectomy.[80] This complication rarely occurs after unilateral ganglionectomy, especially when the surgeon takes care to preserve the first lumbar ganglion. Although potency should not be affected, many experienced surgeons insist that such derangements in sexual function do occur in men. Careful preoperative questioning about sexual function is important to evaluate any changes reported after lumbar sympathectomy.

Systemic arterial steal syndromes resulting from lumbar sympathectomy have been reported but are largely unsubstantiated by careful analysis. Nonetheless, paradoxical gangrene of the contralateral extremity has been reported, but this was due to intrinsic arterial occlusion of the affected leg rather than selective hypoperfusion at the aortoiliac level.[81] Similarly, mesenteric arterial insufficiency with bowel infarction has been attributed to intrinsic mesenteric occlusive disease rather than to aortoiliac steal.

Although sympathectomy was once associated with significant morbidity and even death when performed on elderly patients with advanced arteriosclerosis, current techniques carry negligible risk and produce few permanent adverse sequelae in the typically younger patients.

◼ OVERALL RESULTS OF TREATMENT

Most studies indicate that patients with early diagnosis and treatment (within 6 to 12 months) have an overall good outcome.[82-84] Most authorities also agree that spontaneous resolution can occur if CRPS is diagnosed and managed early.[83,85]

Failure to promptly recognize and treat CRPS type I results in irreversible changes, including wasting of skin and muscles, fixed joint contractures,[46] and severe demineralization of bone. It is generally believed that initiating treatment in the early stage carries a better prognosis. Patients who are diagnosed later are more refractory to treatment.[82,83,86] In patients with CRPS, restricted movement of the knee joint is very common.[82] Patella baja (an abnormally low position of the patella) and changes in the mechanics of the tibiofemoral joint may occur, leading to chronic degeneration.[86]

In Katz and Hungerford's series of 36 patients undergoing sympathetic blockade for CRPS affecting the knee, 10 patients treated within 1 year from the onset of symptoms did significantly better than those with symptoms of more than a year's duration before sympathetic blockade was initiated.[82]

SELECTED KEY REFERENCES

AbuRahma AF, Robinson PA, Powell M, Bastug D, Boland JP. Sympathectomy for reflex sympathetic dystrophy: factors affecting outcome. *Ann Vasc Surg.* 1994;8:372-379.
Analysis of the various factors affecting the outcome of patients with RSD, with an emphasis on the response to epidural sympathetic block and sympathectomy.

Bandyk DF, Johnson BL, Kirkpatrick AF, Novotney ML, Back MR, Schmacht DC. Surgical sympathectomy for reflex sympathetic dystrophy syndromes. *J Vasc Surg.* 2002;35:269-277.
Modern study of the results of surgical sympathectomy for RSD syndromes, a significant number of which were thoracoscopic- or laparoscopic-assisted sympathectomies.

Beglaibter N, Berlatzky Y, Zamir O, Spira RM, Freund HR. Retroperitoneoscopic lumbar sympathectomy. *J Vasc Surg.* 2002;35:815-817.
Nice illustration of the retroperitoneoscopic technique, which has been advocated for lumbar sympathectomy.

Bryant PR, Kim CT, Millan R. The rehabilitation of causalgia (complex regional pain syndrome—type II). *Phys Med Rehabil Clin N Am.* 2002;13:137-157.
Study highlighting the causes, definitions, and clinical features of this syndrome, with an emphasis on rehabilitation.

Dowd GSE, Hussein R, Khanduja V, Ordman AJ. Complex regional pain syndrome with special emphasis on the knee. *J Bone Joint Surg Br.* 2007;89:285-290.
Modern, up-do-date review article on the cause, pathophysiology, clinical manifestation, and treatment of CRPS.

Drucker WR, Hubay CA, Holden WD, Bukovnic JA. Pathogenesis of posttraumatic sympathetic dystrophy. *Am J Surg.* 1959;97:454-465.
Classic paper that divides CRPS into three stages, which is critical for the diagnosis and management of patients with this syndrome (causalgia).

Hassantash SA, Afrakhteh M, Maier RV. Causalgia: a meta-analysis of the literature. *Arch Surg.* 2003;138:1226-1231.
Meta-analysis of 110 articles containing a total of 1528 cases of causalgia, highlighting the various causative factors, clinical manifestations, and response to sympathetic block and sympathectomy.

Schurmann M, Gradl G, Rommel O. Early diagnosis in post-traumatic complex regional pain syndrome. *Orthopedics.* 2007;30:450-456.
Study highlighting the early diagnosis of post-traumatic CRPS, which is critical for proper management and the prevention of complications.

Stanton-Hicks M, Baron R, Boas R, Gordh T, Harden N, Hendler N, Koltzenburg M, Raj P, Wilder R. Complex regional pain syndromes: guidelines for therapy. *Clin J Pain.* 1998;14:155-166.
Landmark paper highlighting the guidelines for therapy after the consensus conference that analyzed the concepts and terminology of CRPS.

Wasner G, Schattschneider J, Binder A, Baron R. Complex regional pain syndrome—diagnostic, mechanisms, CNS involvement and therapy. *Spinal Cord.* 2003;41:61-75.
Review article highlighting the cause, pathogenesis, diagnosis, and management of patients with CRPS.

REFERENCES

The reference list can be found on the companion Expert Consult Web site at *www.expertconsult.com.*

AAA, abdominal aortic aneurysm
ABFB, aortobifemoral bypass
ABI, ankle-brachial index
ACA, anterior cerebral artery
ACE, angiotensin-converting enzyme
ACT, activated clotting time
ADA, American Diabetes Association
ADP, adenosine diphosphate
AEF, aortoenteric fistula
AF, atrial fibrillation
AFB, aortofemoral bypass
AGE, advanced glycosylation end product
AHA, American Heart Association
AHRQ, Agency for Healthcare Research and Quality
AI, aortoiliac
AIDS, acquired immunodeficiency syndrome
AKA, above-knee amputation
AMP, adenosine monophosphate
APC, activated protein C
APG, air plethysmography
aPTT, activated partial thromboplastin time
ARB, angiotensin receptor blocker
ARDS, acute respiratory distress syndrome
ARF, acute renal failure
ASA, acetylsalicylic acid
ATN, acute tubular necrosis
ATP, adenosine triphosphate
AVF, arteriovenous fistula
AVG, arteriovenous graft
AVM, arteriovenous malformation
AVP, ambulatory venous pressure

bFGF, basic fibroblast growth factor
BKA, below-knee amputation
BSA, body surface area
BUN, blood urea nitrogen

CABG, coronary artery bypass grafting
CAD, coronary artery disease
cAMP, cyclic adenosine monophosphate
CAS, carotid artery stenting
CAVH, continuous arteriovenous hemofiltration
CAVHDF, continuous arteriovenous hemodiafiltration
CCA, common carotid artery

CCB, calcium channel blocker
CDC, Centers for Disease Control and Prevention
CEA, carotid endarterectomy
CEAP, clinical, etiologic, anatomic, pathologic [staging system]
CFA, common femoral artery
CFV, common femoral vein
cGMP, cyclic guanosine monophosphate
CI, confidence interval
CIA, common iliac artery
CK-MB, MB isozyme of creatine kinase
CLI, critical limb ischemia
CMS, Centers for Medicare and Medicaid Services
CNS, central nervous system
CO, carbon monoxide
CO$_2$, carbon dioxide
COPD, chronic obstructive pulmonary disease
COX, cyclooxygenase
CRI, chronic renal insufficiency
CRP, C-reactive protein
CRPS, complex regional pain syndrome
CSF, cerebrospinal fluid
CT, computed tomography
CTA, computed tomographic angiography
CTD, connective tissue disease
CTV, computed tomographic venography
CVI, chronic venous insufficiency
CVP, central venous pressure
CVVH, continuous venovenous hemofiltration
CVVHDF, continuous venovenous hemodiafiltration

2D, two-dimensional
3D, three-dimensional
DBI, digital-brachial index
DBP, diastolic blood pressure
DDAVP, desmopressin
DES, drug-eluting stent
DFU, diabetic foot ulcer
DIC, disseminated intravascular coagulation
DM, diabetes mellitus
DNA, deoxyribonucleic acid
2,3-DPG, 2,3-diphosphoglycerate
DRIL, distal revascularization–interval ligation
DSA, digital subtraction angiography
DSE, dobutamine stress echocardiography
DTAA, descending thoracic aortic aneurysm

DUS, duplex ultrasound
DVT, deep venous thrombosis

EC, endothelial cell
ECA, external carotid artery
ECG, electrocardiogram
EC-IC, extracranial-intracranial [bypass]
ECM, extracellular matrix
ED, erectile dysfunction
EDS, Ehlers-Danlos syndrome
EDV, end-diastolic velocity
EEG, electroencephalography
EF, ejection fraction
EIA, external iliac artery
ELAM-1, endothelial leukocyte adhesion molecule-1
ELISA, enzyme-linked immunosorbent assay
ELT, euglobulin lysis time
EMG, electromyography
eNOS, endothelial nitric oxide synthase
ePTFE, expanded polytetrafluoroethylene
ESR, erythrocyte sedimentation rate
ESRD, end-stage renal disease
EVAR, endovascular aneurysm repair

FDA, Food and Drug Administration
FDP, fibrin/fibrinogen degradation product
FEV$_1$, forced expiratory volume in 1 second
FFP, fresh frozen plasma
FGF, fibroblast growth factor
FMD, fibromuscular dysplasia
FRC, functional residual capacity
FVC, forced vital capacity

GA, general anesthesia
GFR, glomerular filtration rate
GI, gastrointestinal
GMP, guanosine monophosphate
G6PD, glucose-6-phosphate dehydrogenase
GP-IIb/IIIa, glycoprotein IIb/IIIa
GSM, gray-scale median
GSV, great saphenous vein
GSW, gunshot wound
GTP, guanosine triphosphate
GUI, graphic-user interface
GW, guide wire

HD, hemodialysis
HDL, high-density lipoprotein
HIPPA, Health Insurance Portability and Accountability Act
HIT, heparin-induced thrombocytopenia
HIV, human immunodeficiency virus
HLA, human leukocyte antigen
HMG-CoA, 3-hydroxy-3-methylglutaryl coenzyme A

HR, hazard ratio
HRQoL, health-related quality of life
hsCRP, high-sensitivity C-reactive protein
5-HT, serotonin
HTN, hypertension

ICA, internal carotid artery
ICAM-1, intercellular adhesion molecule-1
ICAVL, Intersocietal Commission for the Accreditation of Vascular Laboratories
ICH, intracerebral hemorrhage
ICU, intensive care unit
IDL, intermediate-density lipoprotein
IEL, internal elastic lamina
IFN, interferon
IFU, instructions for use
IGF, insulin-like growth factor
IH, intimal hyperplasia
IL-6, interleukin-6
IMA, inferior mesenteric artery
iNOS, inducible nitric oxide synthase
IOM, Institute of Medicine
IPC, intermittent pneumatic compression
IPG, impedance plethysmography
IPPB, intermittent positive pressure breathing
I/R, ischemia-reperfusion
IVC, inferior vena cava
IVUS, intravascular ultrasound

JAK-2, Janus kinase-2
JNK, jun N-terminal kinase

K/DOQI, Kidney Disease Outcomes Quality Initiative
KM, Kaplan-Meier

LAO, left anterior oblique
LDL, low-density lipoprotein
LMWH, low-molecular-weight heparin
LOS, length of stay
Lp(a), lipoprotein (a)
LS, lumbosacral
LV, left ventricular
LVEDP, left ventricular end diastolic pressure
LVEDV, left ventricular end diastolic volume
LVH, left ventricular hypertrophy

MAP, mean arterial pressure
MCA, middle cerebral artery
MI, myocardial infarction
MIP, maximum intensity projection
MMP, matrix metalloproteinase
MOF, multiple organ failure

MRA, magnetic resonance angiography
MR, magnetic resonance
MRI, magnetic resonance imaging
MRSA, methicillin-resistant *Staphylococcus aureus*
MRV, magnetic resonance venography
MTHFR, 5,10-methylenetetrahydrofolate reductase

NAC, *N*-acetylcysteine
NAD⁺, oxidized nicotinamide dinucleotide
NADH, reduced nicotinamide adenine dinucleotide
NADPH, reduced nicotinamide adenine dinucleotide phosphate
NAIS, neo-aortoiliac system
Nd:YAG, neodymium:yttrium-aluminum-garnet
NF-κB, nuclear factor κB
NIH, National Institutes of Health
NIS, National Inpatient Sample
NOS, nitric oxide synthase
NPV, negative predictive value
NSAID, nonsteroidal anti-inflammatory drug
NSQIP, National Surgical Quality Improvement Program

OR, odds ratio
OTW, over-the-wire

PA, pulmonary artery
PAD, peripheral arterial disease
PAI, proximalization of arterial inflow
PAI-1, plasminogen activator inhibitor-1
PAOD, peripheral arterial occlusive disease
PBI, penile-brachial index
PBRCs, packed red blood cells
PCA, posterior cerebral artery
PCI, percutaneous coronary intervention
PCNA, proliferating cell nuclear antigen
PCWP, pulmonary artery wedge pressure
PD, peritoneal dialysis
PDE, phosphodiesterase
PDGF, platelet-derived growth factor
PE, pulmonary embolism
PECAM-1, platelet–endothelial cell adhesion molecule-1
PEEP, positive end-expiratory pressure
PEG, polyethylene glycol
PET, positron emission tomography
PF4, platelet factor 4
PFA, profunda femoris artery
PFT, pulmonary function test/testing
PGE₂, prostaglandin E₂
PGI₂, prostaglandin I₂
PKC, protein kinase C
PMN, polymorphonuclear neutrophil
PPG, photoplethysmography
PPV, positive predictive value
PRBCs, packed red blood cells

PSA, pseudoaneurysm
psi, pounds per square inch
PSV, peak systolic velocity
PT, prothrombin time
PTA, percutaneous transluminal angioplasty
PTFE, polytetrafluoroethylene
PTT, partial thromboplastin time
PVI, peripheral vascular intervention
PVR, pulse volume recording

QALY, quality-adjusted life year
QoL, quality of life

RAAA, ruptured abdominal aortic aneurysm
RAGE, receptor for advanced glycosylation end products
RAO, right anterior oblique
RAS, renal artery stenosis
RBC, red blood cell
RCT, randomized controlled trial
Re, Reynolds number
RFA, radiofrequency ablation
RGD, Arg-Gly-Asp
RI, resistive index
RIND, reversible ischemic neurologic deficit
RP, retroperitoneal
RR, relative risk
RS, Raynaud's syndrome
rt-PA, recombinant tissue plasminogen activator
RUDI, revision using distal inflow

SBP, systolic blood pressure
SD, standard deviation
SE, standard error
SEPS, subfascial endoscopic perforator surgery
SF-36, Short Form (36) Health Survey
SFA, superficial femoral artery
SFJ, saphenofemoral junction
SK, streptokinase
SLE, systemic lupus erythematosus
SMA, superior mesenteric artery
SMC, smooth muscle cell
SOD, superoxide dismutase
SPECT, single-proton emission computed tomography
SPJ, saphenopopliteal junction
SSV, small saphenous vein
STEMI, ST-segment myocardial infarction
SVC, superior vena cava
SVS, Society for Vascular Surgery

TAA, thoracic aortic aneurysm
TAAA, thoracoabdominal aortic aneurysm
TAAD, thoracic aortic aneurysm and dissection
TAO, thromboangiitis obliterans

TASC, Trans-Atlantic Inter-Society Consensus for the
   Management of Peripheral Arterial Disease
TCD, transcranial Doppler
TEE, transesophageal echocardiography
TEVAR, thoracic endovascular aortic repair
TF, tissue factor
TGF-β, transforming growth factor-β
TIMP-1, tissue inhibitor of matrix metalloproteinase-1
TIPS, transjugular intrahepatic portosystemic shunting
TLR, target lesion revascularization
TMA, transmetatarsal amputation
TNF-α, tumor necrosis factor-α
TOS, thoracic outlet syndrome
t-PA, tissue plasminogen activator
TT, thrombin time
TTE, transthoracic echocardiography
TXA$_2$, thromboxane A$_2$

UFH, unfractionated heparin
UK, urokinase
u-PA, urinary plasminogen activator (urokinase)
USPSTF, U.S. Preventive Services Task Force

VATS, video-assisted thoracoscopic surgery
VCAM-1, vascular cell adhesion molecule-1
VEGF, vascular endothelial growth factor
VFI, venous filling index
VLDL, very-low-density lipoprotein
VSMC, vascular smooth muscle cell
VSS, Venous Severity Score
VTE, venous thromboembolism
vWF, von Willebrand factor

WBC, white blood cell
WIQ, Walking Impairment Questionnaire

Index

Note: Page numbers followed by the letter f refer to figures; those followed by t refer to tables; and those followed by b refer to boxed material.